Disinfection, Sterilization,
and Preservation

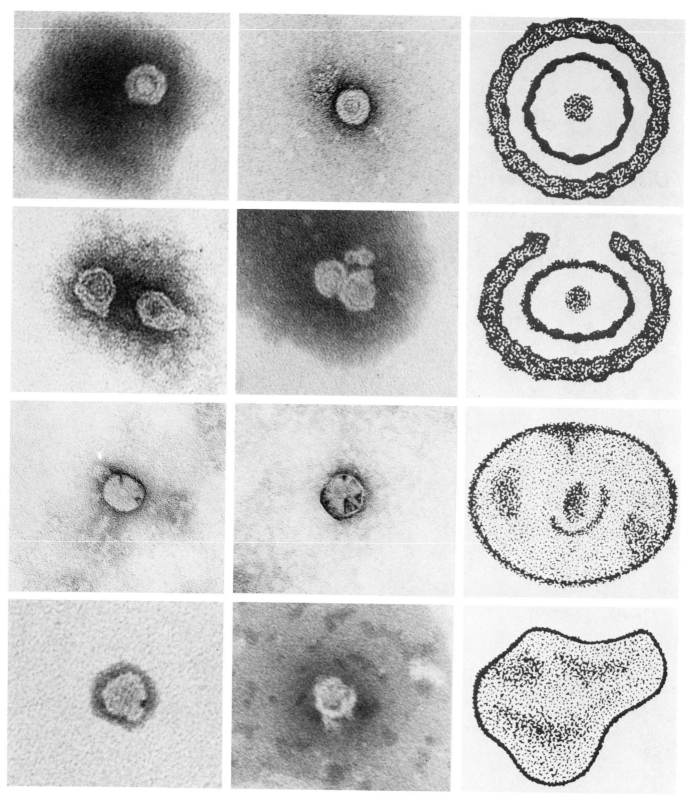

Morphological alteration and disintegration of hepatitis B virus particles (HBV) after exposure to different reagents (Thraenhart et al., (1987)). The left and middle column show electron photomicrographs (Prof. Dermietzel, Regensburg, Germany) of representative HBV of the three alteration phases, schematically drawn in the right column. Alteration increased from intact HBV (upper line; alteration phase 0), alteration of the envelope (2nd line; alteration phase 1), alteration of all structures, which are, however, still visible (3rd line; alteration phase 2) to structureless HBV (4th line; alteration phase 3). HBV was exposed to double distilled water for 15 minutes (upper line), 2% (v/v) formaldehyde reacted with HBV for 15 minutes (left column, 2nd line) and for 60 minutes (left column, 3rd and 4th line). HBV was exposed to 5% succinicdialdehyde for 2 minutes (middle column, 2nd and 3rd line) and for 15 minutes (middle column, 4th line).

Disinfection, Sterilization, and Preservation

Fourth Edition

SEYMOUR S. BLOCK, Ph.D.

Professor Emeritus of Bioengineering
Department of Chemical Engineering
University of Florida
Gainesville, Florida

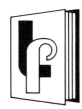

Lea & Febiger   Philadelphia • London

Williams & Wilkins
Rose Tree Corporate Center, Building II
1400 North Providence Road, Suite 5025
Media, PA 19063-2043 USA

Library of Congress Cataloging-in-Publication Data

Disinfection, sterilization, and preservation / [edited by] Seymour S. Block.—4th ed.
  p. cm.
  Includes bibliographical references and index.
  ISBN 0-8121-1364-0
  1. Disinfection and disinfectants. 2. Antiseptics.
3. Sterilization. I. Block, Seymour Stanton, 1918-
RA761.L33 1991
  614.4′8—dc20   90-22653
                                                                                   CIP

PRINTED IN THE UNITED STATES OF AMERICA

Print number: 5

Dedication

This volume is dedicated to many devoted investigators: pioneers of the past, workers of the present who have contributed these chapters, those listed in the references, and many more whose names remain unmentioned but who have contributed to achieving our common goal of a world free of the deleterious effects of microorganisms.

Preface

In the span of man's development the field of disinfection is quite new. Only 100 years have elapsed since the time of Lister, Pasteur, and Koch, which is just a moment when compared to our knowledge of such fields as metal working and agriculture. Progress in our technology has been great in this short time, but we are still faced with new problems and the need to improve old techniques. When different laboratories running the official standard use-dilution carrier test for evaluating disinfectants get widely different results, something is wrong and needs to be corrected. When we think we have discovered all the common infectious bacteria in our part of the world and suddenly over 100 Legionnaires at a convention in Philadelphia come down with an illness that kills 28 of them, and comes from a common organism in water all around us, we have more work to do. When by employing proper sanitation with disinfectants, we are able to curb age-old diseases like cholera, but thousands of people in South America and Asia still contract this disease, something must be done. When several common disinfectants of different chemical structures contain live bacteria which infect patients, then we have more investigation ahead. We also have to find disinfectants that work better in the presence of proteins that can reduce antimicrobial activity by as much as 50 times. We need disinfectants that will penetrate and kill microorganisms that produce biofilms and slimes that protect the organisms from disinfectants.

Since its appearance 23 years ago, this book has attempted to assist investigators in coping with the problems that face us. According to the reviewers of the last edition, a sampling of which follows, it has filled an important niche:

Journal of the Canadian Dental Association: "It will remain a classic work in this area."

ASM (American Society for Microbiology) News: "This third edition represents the single most comprehensive book available on the subject. It is a must for all who are involved in any activity requiring knowledge and use of sterilization, disinfection, and preservation principles and techniques."

Laboratory Practice: "It is a rare opportunity to have all major aspects of an important field of technology in a single book. The authors of various sections are acknowledged experts and many are responsible for major advances in the subjects contained within the book."

Society for Industrial Microbiology: "It is an ambitious goal to attempt to compile a broad spectrum basic primer on the scope indicated by the title, but the editor and contributing authors have succeeded admirably."

Cosmetics and Toiletries: "The third edition is a masterful accomplishment. My sincere congratulations to Dr. Block

and his 58 authors for completing a most difficult task. Their efforts will be more than appreciated by microbiologists worldwide."

If we are to include all aspects of this important technology in a single book, as the reviewer stated, some important new subjects should be treated in this edition. Of the 65 chapters grouped in 10 sections of this edition, 17 chapters appear for the first time. Among these are chapters on veterinary medicine, viral hepatitis, AIDS, sporicidal agents, infection control, kinetics of disinfection, aseptic packaging of foods, building-related illness, and disinfection design of medical instruments. Others are sanitation in food manufacturing, microbial corrosion of metals, germ-free technology, polymeric antimicrobials, organotin compounds, ozone, copper and zinc compounds, and food and water-infecting microorganisms.

This edition is not only enlarged but entirely revised. For example, with the increasing problem of viral infections, the chapter on viral transmission and control has been greatly expanded. With the national attention drawn to the problem of medical wastes following ocean dumping and contamination of eastern beaches, the chapter on the treatment and sanitary disposal of medical wastes has also been revised. Up-to-date data have been provided on important, changing areas, such as the government regulation of antimicrobial pesticides and the business and marketing of antimicrobial agents. The very valuable section on testing methods has also been updated. This edition touches on all important aspects of antimicrobial agents and practices. It ranges from the prevention of mold and bacterial damage to paintings, statuary and other works of art, to the microbial-initiated corrosion of pipelines that carry petroleum from offshore oil wells in the ocean; from the disinfection of catheters that explore the deepest recesses of the human body to the disinfection of swimming pools.

In this edition, we are fortunate to have retained most of the distinguished authorities who contributed to the last edition as well as enlisting a number of others including experts in Sweden, Japan, Britain, France, Germany, South Africa, Austria and both northern and southern Ireland. That seems only right and proper since science has no national boundaries, and neither do microorganisms.

It may come as a surprise but the company that is publishing this book was founded almost 100 years before Pasteur and Lister did their great work. It is now 25 years since I began my association with Lea & Febiger to edit this book, and it has always been a most cordial

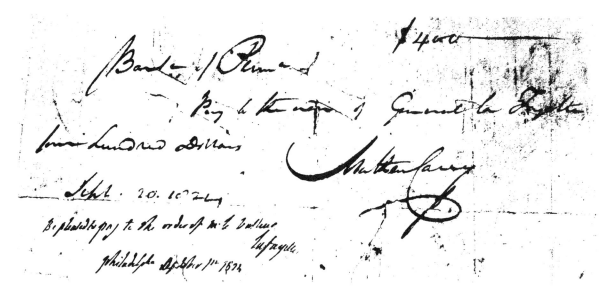

association. Five years before that, browsing in a small bookshop and, being especially interested in Benjamin Franklin, I bought an old book dated 1785, which contained articles by Franklin and others. The book, entitled *The American Museum*, was a Reader's Digest of those days and was dedicated to General George Washington, who had not yet been elected President. When I first visited Lea & Febiger in their offices in Philadelphia, just two blocks from Independence Hall where the Declaration of Independence and the Constitution were signed, I stopped in the lobby to look at the portrait of the founder of the company, Mathew Carey. To my amazement, he was the fellow who had published my old book.

Mathew Carey was a young Irish reformer who got into trouble with the British and made his way to France to avoid arrest. In Paris he worked for Benjamin Franklin on his private printing press, which had been used during the Revolutionary War to turn out American propaganda. When Carey left Paris he went to Philadelphia and started his own publishing business with $400 he borrowed from General Lafayette. *The American Museum* was one of his first publishing ventures. An annual edition was published for several years and was said to be Washington's favorite reading matter. Carey published various sorts of books, including a biography of George Washington written by an itinerant preacher, Parson Weems, who sold books for Carey. Weems was an inventor; his most famous invention was his story of young Washington chopping down the cherry tree.

Like Franklin, Carey was active in community affairs. When the great yellow fever epidemic struck Philadelphia in 1793, everyone who was able to leave the city did so. Carey, however, remained to care for the sick and dying. He wrote and published pamphlets opposing sweatshop working conditions of women in factories. He donated funds to charities and helped start the Franklin Institute for Science in Philadelphia. When Lafayette came back to visit America in 1824, Carey paid him back the $400 he had borrowed. That $400 check is owned by Lea & Febiger and is reproduced here.

Carey also published books by early American authors—James Fenimore Cooper, Washington Irving, and Edgar Allen Poe. His family firm later started the *Encyclopedia Americana*, and eventually became a publisher of medical books with classics like Gray's *Anatomy* and Sir William Osler's seven volume *Modern Medicine*. In 1985, I attended the company's 200th anniversary celebration. Having bought and read his first book and having become acquainted with his life, I felt like a representative of the founder himself.

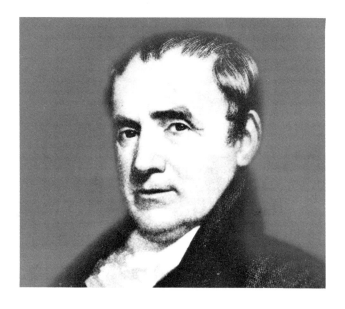

Gainesville, Florida   Seymour S. Block, Ph.D.

Contributors

W. E. Barkley, Ph.D.

Director of Laboratory Safety
Howard Hughes Medical Institute
Bethesda, Maryland

C. M. Beck-Sague, M.D.

Medical Epidemiologist
Epidemiology Branch
Hospital Infections Program
Centers for Disease Control
Atlanta, Georgia

Charles B. Beiter, B.S.

Senior Project Chemist
Atochem North America Inc.
Branchburg Technical Center
Somerville, New Jersey

Robert Berube, Ph.D.

Microbiology Specialist
Health Care Microbiology/Sterilization Services
3M Center
St. Paul, Minnesota

Seymour S. Block, Ph.D.

Professor Emeritus of Bioengineering
Department of Chemical Engineering
University of Florida
Gainesville, Florida

Walter W. Bond, M.S.

Research Microbiologist
Hospital Infections Program
Centers for Disease Control
Atlanta, Georgia

Mary K. Bruch

Vice President
MicroBioTest, Inc.
Chantilly, Virginia

F. F. Busta, Ph.D.

Professor and Head of Department
Department of Food Science and Nutrition
University of Minnesota
St. Paul, Minnesota

Arturo E. Castillo, B.S.

Federal Regulatory Consultants, Inc.
Arlington, VA

John H. S. Chen, D.V.M., M.V.Sc.

Principal Virologist
Hazard Evaluation Division
Office of Pesticide Programs
Environmental Protection Agency
Washington, D.C.

A. Cremieux

Professor of Microbiology and Hygiene
Faculty of Pharmacy
University of Marsailles
Marsailles, France

Graham W. Denton, C.Biol., M.I.Biol.

Product Information Manager
Medical Affairs Department
ICI Pharmaceuticals
Macclesfield, Cheshire, England

George R. Dychdala, M.S.

Manager, Technical Information
Ecolab Research Center
Blue Bell, Pennsylvania

Reza A. Fassihi, B.Pharm., Ph.D., H.P.A.

Chairman and Head, Department of Pharmacy
Medical School
University of the Witwatersrand
Johannesburg, South Africa

Martin F. Favero, Ph.D.

Hospital Infections Program
Centers for Disease Control
Atlanta, Georgia

J. Fleurette

Professor of Bacteriology-Virology
Faculty of Medicine Alexis Carrel
Biologiste des Hospitaux–Hopital Edouard Herriot
Lyon, France

Peggy M. Foegeding, Ph.D.

Associate Professor
Department of Food Science
North Carolina State University
Raleigh, North Carolina

Kathleen A. Franke

Public Health Advisor
Center for Devices and Radiological Health
Food and Drug Administration
Rockville, Maryland

Glen R. Gale, Ph.D.

Research Career Scientist
Department of Veterans Affairs Medical Center and
    Professor of Pharmacology
Medical University of South Carolina
Charleston, South Carolina

Melvin H. Gitlitz, Ph.D.

Senior Staff Chemist
Branchburg Technical Center
Atochem North America Inc.
Somerville, New Jersey

Sean P. Gorman, Ph.D.
Lecturer
School of Pharmacy
The Queens University of Belfast
Belfast, Northern Ireland

Waldemar Gottardi, Ph.D.
Associate Professor in Technical Hygiene
Institute of Hygiene
University of Innsbruck
Innsbruck, Austria

Dieter H. M. Gröschel, M.D.
Professor of Pathology and Internal Medicine
University of Virginia School of Medicine
Charlottesville, Virginia

Inge Gurevich, R.N., M.A.
Coordinator, Infection Control Department
Winthrop University Hospital
Mineola, New York
Assistant Clinical Professor
School of Nursing
Adelphi University
Garden City, New York

Richard G. Holcomb, Ph.D.
Medical Device Consultant
Minneapolis, Minnesota

C. George Hollis
Vice President, Research and Development
Buckman Laboratories International, Inc.
Memphis, Tennessee

Christon J. Hurst, Ph.D.
Microbiologist
U.S. Environmental Protection Agency
Cincinnati, Ohio

William R. Jarvis
Chief, Epidemiology Branch
Hospital Infection Program
Centers for Disease Control
Atlanta, Georgia

Larry J. Joslyn, B.S.
President, Joslyn Sterilizer Corporation
Macedon, New York

Harry B. Kostenbauder, Ph.D.
Associate Dean for Research
College of Pharmacy
University of Kentucky
Lexington, Kentucky

William S. LaGrange
Extension Food Scientist
Iowa State University
Ames, Iowa

Elaine Larson, R.N., Ph.D., F.A.A.N., C.I.C.
Nutting Professor in Clinical Nursing
The Johns Hopkins University School of Nursing
Baltimore, Maryland

Timothy J. Leahy, Ph.D.
Consulting Scientist
Millipore Corporation
Bedford, Massachusetts

Stanley E. Leland, Jr., Ph.D.
Professor of Parasitology
Department of Laboratory Medicine
College of Veterinary Medicine
Associate Director
Agricultural Experiment Station
Kansas State University
Manhattan, Kansas

Richard V. Levy
Manager, Microbiology and Process Applications
Millipore Corporation
Bedford, Massachusetts

John A. Lopes, Ph.D., C.L.D.
Director of Technology
Microcide, Inc.
Troy, Michigan

Raymond J. Lukens, Ph.D.
CEO, R.J. Lukens & Associates
Agricultural & Microbiological Consultants
Modesto, California

Milton Manowitz, Ph.D.
Consultant
Givaudan Corporation
Clifton, New Jersey

Anthony J. Marisca, B.A., M.B.A.
Senior Consultant
Kline and Company
Fairfield, New Jersey

Oscar W. May, B.S.
Development Manager
Buckman Laboratories International, Inc.
Memphis, Tennessee

Jack E. McCracken, Ph.D.
Staff Scientist
Center for Devices and Radiological Health
Food and Drug Administration
Rockville, Maryland

Robert W. McKinney, Ph.D.
Director, Division of Safety
National Institutes of Health
Bethesda, Maryland

John J. Merianos, Ph.D.
Associate Director Research and Development
Sutton Laboratories
Chatham, New Jersey

Chris H. Miller, Ph.D.
Professor and Chairman
Department of Oral Microbiology
Indiana University School of Dentistry
Indianapolis, Indiana

Harry E. Morton, Sc.D.

Emeritus Professor of Bacteriology
Department of Pathology and Laboratory Medicine
University of Pennsylvania
Former Chief of Microbiology
William Pepper Laboratory
Hospital of the University of Pennsylvania
Philadelphia, Pennsylvania

Robert F. Morrissey, Ph.D.

Director, Sterilization Sciences Group
Johnson & Johnson Corporation
New Brunswick, New Jersey

Deirdre M. O'Connor, A.B. Chem.

Director of Product Development
Lehn & Fink Products Group
Sterling Drug Inc.
Montvale, New Jersey

Nobuhiko Ohnishi, Ph.D.

Assistant Professor
Department of Microbiology
School of Medicine
Tokai University
Kanagawa, Japan

Robert A. Oppermann, Ph.D.

Montville, New Jersey

Beverly J. Ott, C.G.C.

Endoscopy Services Coordinator
Division of Gastroenterology
Department of Internal Medicine
Mayo Clinic
Rochester, Minnesota

Gordon S. Oxborrow, M.P.H.

3M Company
St. Paul, Minnesota

Charles John Palenik

Associate Professor of Oral Microbiology
Indiana University School of Dentistry
Indianapolis, Indiana

Anthony N. Parisi, Ph.D.

Director of Laboratories
Baxter Healthcare Corporation
Pharmaseal Division
Valencia, California

I. G. Pflug, Ph.D.

Professor of Food Sciences and Nutrition
University of Minnesota
St. Paul, Minnesota

G. Briggs Phillips, Ph.D.

Petra, Inc.
St. Michaels, Maryland

Daniel L. Prince, Ph.D.

President
Gibraltar Biological Laboratories, Inc.
Fairfield, New Jersey

Herbert N. Prince

Scientific Director
Gibraltar Biological Laboratories, Inc.
Fairfield, New Jersey
Associate Professor
School of Graduate Medical Education–St. Michael's
    Medical Center
Seton Hall University
Newark, New Jersey

Richard N. Prince, Ph.D.

Director, Quality Assurance
Gibraltar Biological Laboratories
Fairfield, New Jersey

Timothy L. Pruett, M.D.

Assistant Professor of Surgery and Internal Medicine
University of Virginia Medical Center
Charlottesville, Virginia

P. J. Quinn, M.V.B., Ph.D., M.R.C.V.S.

Professor of Veterinary Microbiology and Parasitology
Department of Veterinary Microbiology and Parasitology
Faculty of Veterinary Medicine
University College Dublin
Dublin, Ireland

H. W. Rossmoore, Ph.D.

Professor of Biological Sciences
Wayne State University
Detroit, Michigan

Jeffrey Rubin, M.D.

County Public Health Director
Bradford, Union, and Levy Counties
Starke, Florida

Joseph R. Rubino, M.A.

Group Leader, Microbiology
Lehn & Fink Products Group
Sterling Drug Inc.
Montvale, New Jersey

A. D. Russell, D.Sc., Ph.D., F.R.C. Pathl., F.R.Pharm.S.

Reader in Pharmaceutical Microbiology
Welsh School of Pharmacy
University of Wales College of Cardiff
Cardiff, Wales

Shogo Sasaki, M.D.

Professor, Department of Microbiology
Dean, School of Medicine
Tokai University
Kanagawa, Japan

I. L. Schechmeister, Ph.D.

Emeritus Professor of Microbiology
Microbiology Department
Southern Illinois University
Carbondale, Illinois

Eileen M. Scott, Ph.D.

Senior Lecturer
School of Pharmacy
The Queens University of Belfast
Belfast, Northern Ireland

Fred Sharpell, M.S.
Manager, Biotechnology
Givaudan Corporation
Clifton, New Jersey

Jose R. Sifontes
Former Professor and Chief of Chemical
Engineering Department
Universidad de Carabobo, Venezuela
Department of Agricultural Engineering
University of Florida
Gainesville, Florida

Gerald J. Silverman, Ph.D.
Chief, Microbiology Section
U.S. Army Natick Research Development and Engineering
Center
Natick, Massachusetts

Otis J. Sproul, D.Sc.
Dean, College of Engineering and Physical Sciences
University of New Hampshire
Durham, New Hampshire

Olaf Thraenhart, D.M.V.
Lecturer in Medical Virology
Acting Director, Institute for Medical Virology and
Immunology
University of Essen
Director, WHO Collaborating Centre for Reference and
Research on Neurological Zoonoses
Essen, Germany

Bernard von Bockelmann, Ph.D.
AB Tetra Pak
Lund, Sweden

Ernest M. Walker, Jr., M.D., Ph.D.
Professor of Pathology
University of Arkansas for Medical Sciences
Assistant Chief, Laboratory Service
John L. McClellen Memorial Veterans Hospital
Little Rock, Arkansas

Homer W. Walker
Professor Emeritus
Department of Food Science and Human Nutrition
Iowa State University
Ames, Iowa

A. G. Wedum, M.D., Ph.D.*
Consultant, Frederick Cancer Research Facility
Frederick, Maryland

G. B. Wickramanayake, Ph.D., P.E.
Senior Consulting Engineer
Environ Corporation
Princeton, New Jersey

Charles C. Yeager
Owner, Registration Consulting Associates
Auburn, California

William E. Young
Director, Sterility Assurance
I.V. Systems Division
Baxter Healthcare Corporation
Round Lake, Illinois

*Deceased

Contents

Disinfectants and Antiseptics. B. By Type of Microorganisms

Part IV   Chemical and Physical Sterilization

Part V   Medical and Health-Related Applications

Part IX Methods of Testing

PART I

Introduction

HISTORICAL REVIEW

Seymour S. Block

Although the scientific application of disinfectants, sterilants, and preservatives is limited to, at most, the past 150 years, empiric practices that were more or less effective go back to ancient times. The Bible is filled with injunctions on cleanliness: strict dietary rules, regulations regarding lepers, care regarding wastes. These matters were almost an obsession. For example, the biblical requirement that campsites be moved daily was an obvious attempt to avoid contagion arising from human wastes. Soldiers returning from battle were required to disinfect their equipment and clothing with heat. "Everything that may abide fire" had to be put into the fire; the rest had to be immersed in boiling water (Numbers 31:21–24). Aristotle understood the need to avoid disease and instructed Alexander the Great to require his armies to boil their drinking water and bury the dung. Alexander was also aware of the need for preservatives, for he is reported to have ordered timber for bridge-building to be covered with olive oil as a precaution against decay. This process was followed by the Roman emperors for all wooden construction that was exposed to severe moisture conditions. Interestingly enough, much of the empiric knowledge of the Jews and early Greeks on the transmission of disease was lost in the later Greek and the Roman period, and the Hippocratic treatises contain no reference to contagion as it is viewed today (Bulloch, 1960).

The first disinfectant to be reported was sulfur in the form of sulfur dioxide, and the reporter was the Greek poet Homer. In *The Odyssey* XXII, Odysseus, returning home after a long absence, killed his wife's suitors and, having disposed of their bodies, turned to his old nurse and said "bring me some disinfectant sulfur, and make me a fire so that I can fumigate the house" (Rieu, 1952). This was about 800 BC. Sulfur, burned to sulfur dioxide, was used in this way during the great plagues of the Middle Ages, and sulfur dioxide is still used as a disinfectant and preservative for dried fruit, fruit juices, and wine.

EARLY WORK

Preservation of food by heating, drying, smoking, salting, sugaring, fermenting, acidifying, and impregnating with spices and aromatics has been practiced in one form or another by most primitive peoples, ancient and modern. They did not know why they did it, except that it worked. Some scientific progress was made during the Middle Ages. The Hindu physician, Susruta, writing about 500 A.D., instructed surgeons to clean and fumigate the operating room with disinfecting vapors before and after all operations. The Swiss physician Paracelsus (1493–1541), called the Luther of Medicine, reformed the pharmacopeia and introduced compositions of mercury, lead, arsenic, copper, iron, and sulfur. It remained for Nicolas Appert in France in 1810 to develop our modern method for sterilizing food with heat and preserving it in closed containers, referred to today as canning. The more modern investigators recognized a relationship between decomposition, as in the case of putrefaction and fermentation, and contagious disease long before microorganisms were demonstrated to be the causative agents. One of the earliest of these "moderns" was Girolamo Fracastoro (1478–1553), a classmate of Copernicus at the University of Padua in Italy (Fig. 1–1). Fracastoro wrote three books on contagion in which he proposed that infection was caused by the passage from one person to another of minute bodies capable of self-multiplication. He differentiated contagion from the "corruption" (putrefaction) that occurs in milk or meat. He recognized three different sources of contagion: by contact alone, by fomites (a word he first used), and at a distance (through the air). He described many diseases and classified them according to the three categories. He referred to the seeds or germs of disease and included the spread of infection that appears among fruits, as from apple to apple and grape to grape, as well as contagion in man and cattle in his broad considerations. Unfortunately, as in so many other cases, his work was forgotten, and the knowledge had to be rediscovered much later (Bulloch, 1960; Wright, 1930). Fracastoro's one claim to

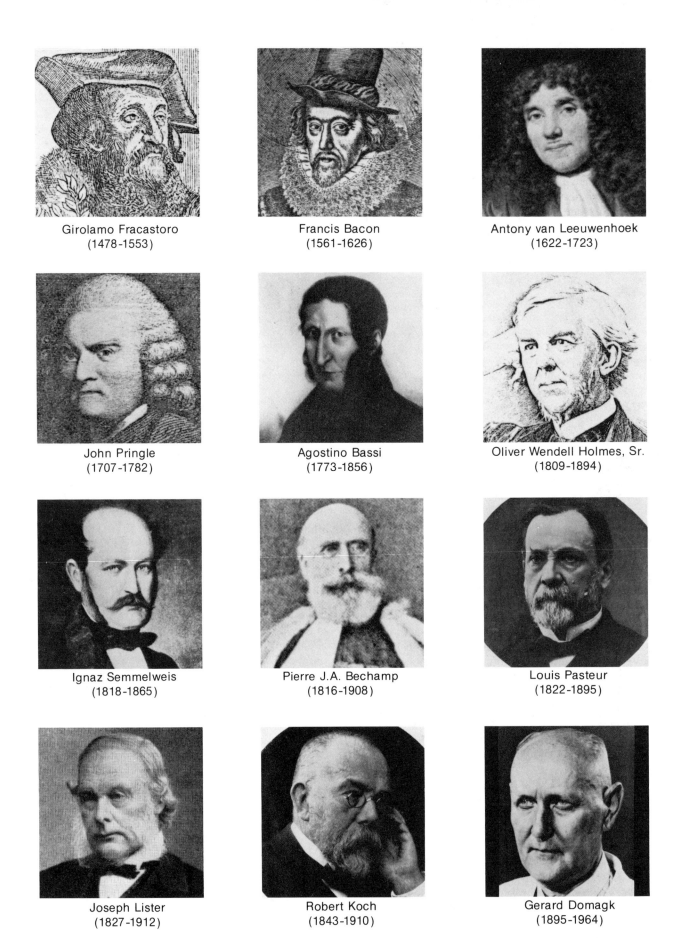

Girolamo Fracastoro
(1478-1553)

Francis Bacon
(1561-1626)

Antony van Leeuwenhoek
(1622-1723)

John Pringle
(1707-1782)

Agostino Bassi
(1773-1856)

Oliver Wendell Holmes, Sr.
(1809-1894)

Ignaz Semmelweis
(1818-1865)

Pierre J.A. Bechamp
(1816-1908)

Louis Pasteur
(1822-1895)

Joseph Lister
(1827-1912)

Robert Koch
(1843-1910)

Gerard Domagk
(1895-1964)

Fig. 1–1. Pioneers in disinfection.

fame rests on a poem he wrote in which his hero, Syphilus, named after a character in Greek mythology, was punished with a dread and odious disease. Thus syphilis got its name.

Nevertheless, practical measures to fight contagion were begun early. During the Great Plagues, the clothes of victims were destroyed by burning them in a fire. The bodies themselves were skewered on poles at least 10 feet in length to avoid contact with the bearers and carried outside the city for disposal. Supposedly, this practice led to the expression, "I wouldn't touch him with a 10-foot pole." Physicians who attended patients suffering from plague were careful to protect themselves with a unique costume that included gloves, mask, hat, and long coat (Fig. 1–2). The mask resembled a chicken's head, no doubt to confuse the evil spirits, and the large beak contained perfumes to counteract the foul odor of the sickroom that was associated with the contagion. Fortuitously, the perfumes contained volatile oils that in some cases may have had disinfectant properties (Fig. 1–2).

Venice was far ahead of all other cities in its control of sanitation, and in 1438 it created its Magistry of Health, which fumigated ships' cargoes. Infectious diseases were observed to spread along trade routes, which made these cargoes suspect. Incidentally, the mail routes coincided with the trade routes, making mail also suspect. From the fifteenth to the early twentieth century, mail was fumigated or perfumed to cleanse and disinfect it. Meyer, in his unusual book on disinfected mail (1962), notes that a letter dated 1485 still exists that apparently was treated with vinegar to disinfect it.

In 1663, the famous scientist Robert Boyle had the foresight to observe that fermentation and disease were somehow related, and he predicted that discovery of the cause of fermentation would lead to the knowledge of the cause of disease. Thus, Boyle prophesied the great discoveries of Pasteur, still two centuries away.

The great scholar of the English renaissance, Sir Francis Bacon, in his *Natural History*, 1625, stated, "It is excellent to inquire into the means of preventing [that] which makes [up] a great part of physic [medicine] and surgery," whereupon he stated, "Removing that which caused putrefaction, does prevent and avoid putrefaction." Having related gangrene to putrefaction, he then listed 10 methods or substances for preventing putrefaction. These included astringency, sulfuric acid (oil of vitriol), salting, souring, sugaring, and excluding air (Fig. 1–3). It is interesting to note that as late as 1867, 242 years later, medical opinion had regressed rather than progressed. In the journal *Lancet*, a paper appeared that expressed the prevailing thought on this subject. Savory, a physician, acknowledged that chemicals known as antiseptics were effective in arresting the decomposition of dead organic matter but questioned whether they could successfully be used for living tissues that develop similar symptoms, as evidenced by appearance and odor. The

work of Lister, which was published in *Lancet* 1 month later, was to provide his answer: they could be.

If someone were to ask when did the first person knowingly use chemicals to kill microorganisms, the answer would be the year 1676. And who was that person? A Dutch cloth merchant and amateur microscope maker named Anton van Leeuwenhoek. As the first human being to see microorganisms (Fig. 1–4), he first examined the effect of pepper on the "little animals," He wrote: "When there was much of the water of the pounded pepper . . . the said animals soon died." A fellow of insatiable curiosity, Leeuwenhoek examined microscopically the scurf of film from his teeth and saw a great number of very small objects moving with a swift motion, like eels. This was the first observation ever of bacteria. Then, he said, "I took a little wine-vinegar and mixed it with the water in which the scurf was dissolved, whereupon the animals died presently (Fig. 1–5)." Leeuwenhoek gave the first description of a pathogenic protozoan, *Giardia lamblia*, when he had the curiosity to examine his stools during a bout of diarrhea. This is an organism that has created a lot of disinfection interest lately. An Englishman, Edmund King, in 1693 followed up the work of Leeuwenhoek by testing a number of substances on the "animalcules," as Leeuwenhoek referred to the little creatures. These included sulfuric acid, sodium tartarate, salt, sugar, wine, blood, and ink. He observed their effect on the rate of kill, the mobility, and the shape of the organisms. All the materials appeared to kill, but with salt the animalcules recovered when fresh water was applied.

Although these investigators did not consider the practical potential of their experiments, the little animals of Leeuwenhoek suggested to others a germ theory of disease. This included in America a most unlikely individual, the Puritan minister and prosecutor of the Salem witch trials, Cotton Mather. Mather had studied medicine before switching to the ministry and continued his interest by reading scientific papers from England. In 1720, he was the first person in America to initiate the vaccination for smallpox, after reading about Lady Mary Wortly Montagu's report on that subject. This described the Chinese method that used the actual smallpox virus from scabs and pus of infected persons; Mather's experiment took place some 80 years before Jenner developed his safe cowpox vaccination. Although some smallpox deaths resulted from this method, the number of deaths was much smaller than when the infection occurred naturally.

An English physician, John Pringle, who has earned the title of father of military medicine, made significant discoveries. He noted the relationship of human waste to a variety of human fevers and developed a method of sanitary trench disposal of wastes, far removed from the barracks. His observations of the relationship of putrefaction to disease, which he credited to the writing of Sir Francis Bacon, led him to do experiments in which

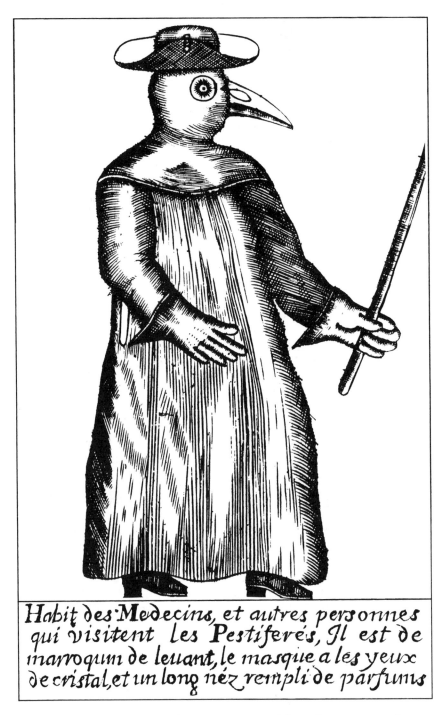

Habit des Medecins, et autres personnes qui visitent les Pestiferés, Il est de marroquin de leuant, le masque a les yeux de cristal, et un long néz rempli de parfums

Fig. 1–2. Plague physician's protective clothing, seventeenth century. Courtesy of the Wellcome Trustees, from Maurice, *Traité de la peste*, Geneva, 1721.

Century IV.

The Tenth is, by *Time, and the Work and Procedure of the Spirits themselves*; which cannot keep their Station; Especially if they be left to themselves; And there be not Agitation or Locall Motion. As we see in Corn not stirred; And Mens Bodies not exercised.

338

All *Moulds* are Inceptions of *Putrefaction*; As the *Moulds* of *Pyes*, and *Flesh*; the *Moulds* of *Orenges*, and *Limmons*; which *Moulds* afterwards turn into Wormes, or more odious *Putrefactions*: And therefore (commonly) prove to be of ill Odour. And if the Body be Liquid, and not apt to putrifie totally, it will cast up a *Mother* in the Top; As the *Mothers* of *Distilled Waters*.

339

Mosse is a Kinde of *Mould*, of the Earth and Trees. But it may be better sorted as a *Rudiment* of *Germination*; To which we referre it.

340

It is an *Enquirie* of Excellent use, to Enquire of the *Meanes of Preventing or Staying of Putrefaction*; For therein consisteth the *Meanes of Conservation of Bodies*; For *Bodies* have two Kindes of *Dissolutions*; The one by *Consumption*, and *Desiccation*; The other by *Putrefaction*. But as for the *Putrefactions* of the *Bodies of Men*, and *Living Creatures* (as in Agues, Wormes, Consumptions of the Lungs, Impostumes, and Vlcers both Inwards and outwards) they are a great *Part of Physicke*, and *Surgery*. And therefore we will reserve the *Enquiry* of them to the proper Place, where we shall handle *Medicinal Experiments of all Sorts*. Of the rest we will now Enter into an Enqniry: wherin much light may be taken, from that which hath been said, of the *Meanes* to *Enduce* or *Accelerate Putrefaction*: For the Removing that, which caused *Putrefaction*, doth Prevent and Avoid *Putrefaction*.

Experiments in Consort, touching Prohibiting and Preventing Putrefaction.

The First *Meanes* of *Prohibiting* or *Checking Putrefaction, is Cold*: For so we see that Meat and Drink will last longer, Unputrified, or Unsowred, in Winter, than in Summer: And we see that Flowers, and Fruits; put in Conservatories of Snow, keep fresh. And this worketh by the *Detention* of the *Spirits*, and *Constipation* of the *Tangible Parts*.

341

The Second is *Astriction*: For *Astriction* prohibiteth *Dissolution*: As we see (generally) in *Medicines*, whereof such as are *Astringents* doe inhibit *Putrefaction*: And by the same reason of *Astringency*, some small Quantity of Oile of Vitrioll, will keep Fresh Water long from *Putrifying*. And this *Astriction* is in a Substance that hath a *Virtuall Cold*; And it worketh (partly) by the same Meanes that Cold doth.

342

The Third is, the Excluding of the *Aire*; And again, the *Exposing to the Aire*: For these Contraries, (as it commeth often to passe,) work the same Effect, according to the Nature of the Subject-Matter. So we see, that *Beere*, or *Wine*, in Bottles close stopped, last long; That the *Garners under Ground* keepe Corne longer than those above Ground; And that *Fruit closed in Wax* keepeth fresh: And likewise *Bodies* put in *Honey*, and *Flower*, keep more fresh: And *Liquors*, *Drinks*, and *Juyces*, with a little *Oyle* cast on the Top, keep fresh. Contrariwise, we see that *Cloth* and *Apparell*, not *Aired*, doe breed Moaths, and Mould; and the Diversitie is, that in *Bodies*

343

H 2　　　　　　　　　　　　　　　　　　　　　　　that

Fig. 1–3.　Page from Francis Bacon's book, *A Natural History*.

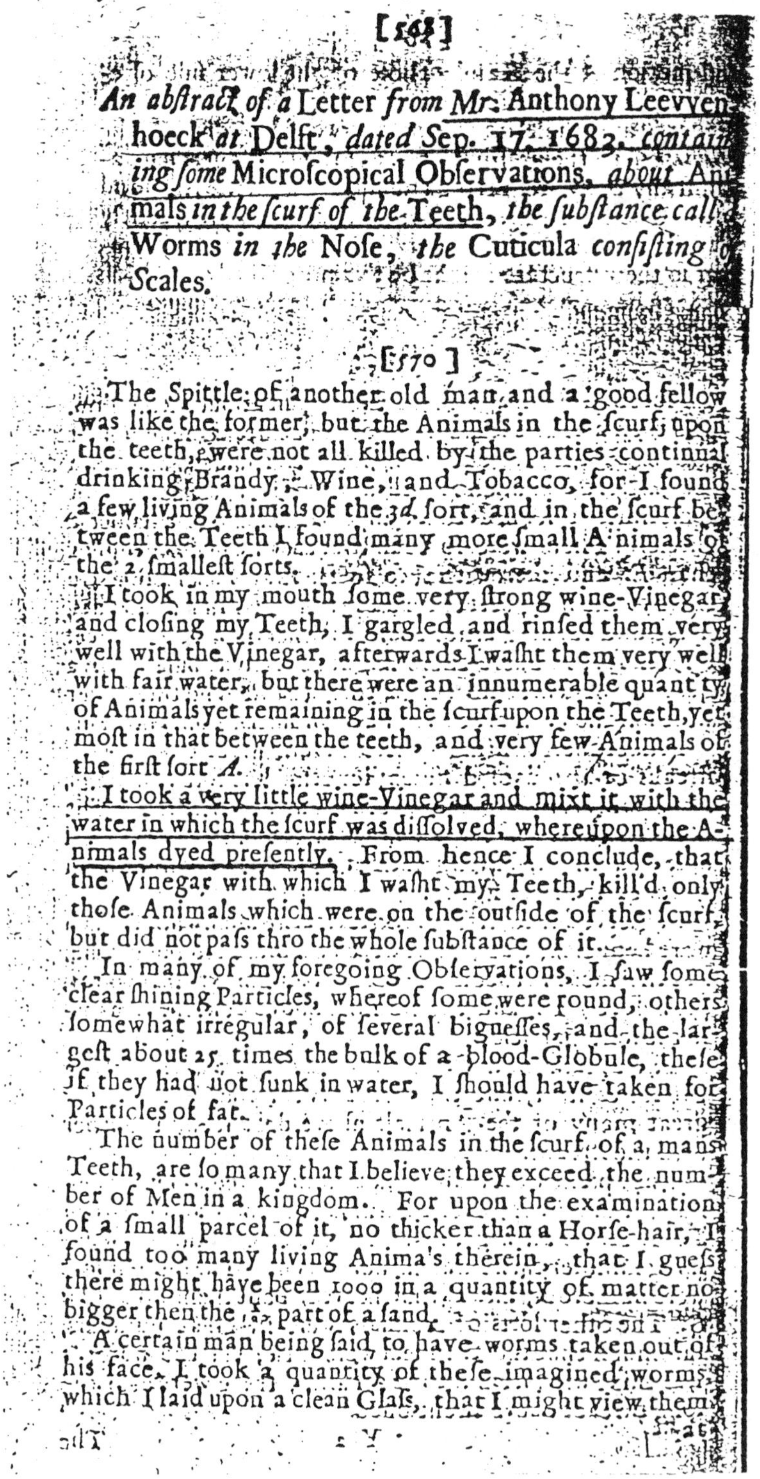

[568]

An abstract of a Letter *from* Mr. Anthony Leevven-
hoeck *at* Delft, *dated* Sep. 17. 1683. *containing some* Microscopical Observations, *about Animals in the scurf of the* Teeth, *the substance call'd*
Worms *in the* Nose, *the* Cuticula *consisting of
Scales.*

[570]

The Spittle of another old man and a good fellow
was like the former; but the Animals in the scurf upon
the teeth, were not all killed by the parties continual
drinking Brandy, Wine, and Tobacco, for I found
a few living Animals of the 3d. sort, and in the scurf between the Teeth I found many more small Animals of
the 2 smallest sorts.

I took in my mouth some very strong wine-Vinegar,
and closing my Teeth, I gargled and rinsed them very
well with the Vinegar, afterwards I washt them very well
with fair water, but there were an innumerable quantity
of Animals yet remaining in the scurf upon the Teeth, yet
most in that between the teeth, and very few Animals of
the first sort A.

I took a very little wine-Vinegar and mixt it with the
water in which the scurf was dissolved, whereupon the A-
nimals dyed presently. From hence I conclude, that
the Vinegar with which I washt my Teeth, kill'd only
those Animals which were on the outside of the scurf,
but did not pass thro the whole substance of it.

In many of my foregoing Observations, I saw some
clear shining Particles, whereof some were round, others
somewhat irregular, of several bignesses, and the largest about 25 times the bulk of a blood-Globule, these
if they had not sunk in water, I should have taken for
Particles of fat.

The number of these Animals in the scurf of a mans
Teeth, are so many that I believe they exceed the number of Men in a kingdom. For upon the examination
of a small parcel of it, no thicker than a Horse-hair, I
found too many living Anima's therein, that I guess
there might have been 1000 in a quantity of matter no
bigger then the 1/1000 part of a sand.

A certain man being said, to have worms taken out of
his face, I took a quantity of these imagined worms,
which I laid upon a clean Glass, that I might view them

Fig. 1–4. Page from 1684 paper by van Leeuwenhoek describing how he killed bacteria with vinegar.

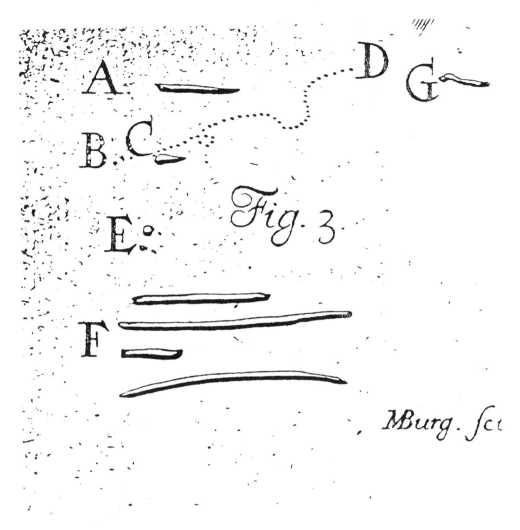

Fig. 1–5. Bacteria, scraped off the teeth, as sketched by van Leeuwenhoek in 1684, and killed by immersion in vinegar.

a fresh egg was more readily putrefied when infected with a drop from an already spoiled egg:

> Lord Bacon, as well as some of the Chemists, have hinted at a putrid Fermentation, analogous to what is found in Vegetables, and this having so near a Connexion with Contagion, I made the following Experiment. . . . In the Yolk of an Egg, already putrid, a small Thread was dipped, and a small Bit of this was cut off and put into a Phial, with Half of the Yolk of a new laid Egg diluted with Water. The other Half, with as much Water, was put into another Phial, and both being corked, were set by the Fire to putrefy. The Result was, that the Thread infected the fresh Yolk; for the Putrefaction was sooner perceived in the Phial that contained it, than the other.

Pringle published three papers in 1750 in which he compared the resistance to putrefaction offered by substances that he was the first to call "antiseptics." He used ordinary sea salt as his standard of comparison and made a table of salt coefficients (Fig. 1–6), much the same as the phenol coefficient of Rideal and Walker 150 years

later. Among his most active antiseptics were acids and alkalies, but camphor with a coefficient of about 300 he found to be the best.

In 1757 James Lind wrote a paper on hygiene at sea for the British navy. It calls for disinfection, filtration of water through sand or charcoal, cleanliness and ventilation of the sick berth, and special clothes for surgeons. In 1768 he wrote another paper on diseases in hot climates in which he advised people to live on high ground and avoid stagnant water to escape the "effluvia" that were believed to cause fevers.

It is interesting to examine the official pharmacopeia of the U.S. Navy in 1778, during the American Revolution, which contained 100 medicants. The first in the list was "acidulated water," termed a universal antiseptic potion made of wine or cider vinegar, cream of tartar, and water. Vinegar, first mentioned by the Roman, Celsus, as a purifying wash for abdominal wounds, was an ingredient of many of the formulations; interestingly

A Table *of the comparative Powers of Salts in refifting Putrefaction.*

Sea-Salt	1
Sal Gemmæ	1+
Tartar vitriolated	2
Spiritus Mindereri	2
Tartarus folubilis	2
Sal diureticus.	2+
Crude *Sal Ammoniac.*	3
Saline Mixture	3
Nitre	4+
Salt of Hartfhorn	4+
Salt of Wormwood	4+
Borax	12+
Salt of Amber	20+
Alum	30+

Fig. 1–6. Pringle's table of salt coefficients (1750).

enough, dilute acetic acid has recently been employed for the topical treatment of wounds infected with *Pseudomonas aeruginosa*. Mercury was also present in a number of the formulations, including ointments and pills, as well as in a solution of mercuric chloride.

PLANT DISEASE

The cause of contagious disease and the means of its prevention and treatment with chemicals were to be discovered in the case of plants prior to disease in humans. Pier Antonio Micheli, a botanist of Florence, Italy, published his work with higher plants and fungi in 1729, in which he examined different fungi (*Mucor*, *Botrytis*, and *Aspergillus*) microscopically and identified their "seeds." He scattered the spores on leaves and the cut surfaces of fruits and showed that the "seeds" produced crops of their own kind. His work was one of the great hammer blows against the theory of spontaneous generation, long before it succumbed. A French experimenter, Tillet, in 1755 produced proof that the disease known as bunt of wheat is contagious, although he did not recognize its origin. He showed that the black dust from diseased plants produced the disease on bunt-free plants. Further, a century before Semmelweis and Lister were to make their monumental demonstrations that chemical disinfectants would prevent disease, Tillet treated bunt-infected wheat seeds with a saltpeter solution and lime and found that these chemicals partially prevented the disease.

The man who deserves the laurel wreath for having first recorded adequate experimental proof as well as for having interpreted the role of a microorganism in the causation of disease is Isaac-Benedict Prevost of Montauban, France. He also used chemical disinfectants and showed in field tests that they were effective in preventing infection. In 1807 Prevost published "Mémoire sur la cause immédiate de la carie ou charbon des blés, et de plusiers autres maladies des plantes, et sur les préservatifs de la carie." In it, he showed that the immediate cause of bunt is a fungus of the genus *Uredos* or a nearly related genus. He found that copper salts—used in 1761 by Schulthess and in 1783 by Tessier (McCallan, 1967)—as well as distilled water in which metallic copper had been left, and various other substances would prevent germination of spores of the bunt fungus. He further distinguished between inhibitory and lethal effects, and experimented on the concentrations of the toxic agent and the time and temperature as related to toxic effects. In field tests, he obtained excellent control of the disease by steeping seed wheat in copper sulfate solution and made detailed recommendations for practical, large-scale seed treatment. Prevost was ahead of his time, for the autogenetic theory of disease, which viewed diseases as arising from the plant because of abnormalities in the plant juices, was prevalent, and the authorities of the time rejected Prevost's brilliant work. His expressed disbelief in spontaneous generation, which was still accepted, did his own thesis no good. It was unfortunate that Prevost's experiments remained unrecognized, for in 1845 and 1846, the potato blight in Ireland, which might have been prevented with copper treatments, caused the starvation of hundreds of thousands of people (Keitt, 1959).

The empirically minded gardeners by this time were beginning to obtain practical results with sulfur, which had been known and used as a disinfectant in antiquity. Forsyth recorded its use on fruit trees as early as 1802. Robertson, in 1824, used a preparation of sulfur and soap in water on peach mildew, which he correctly recognized to be caused by a fungus. The powdery mildew disease spread rapidly through Europe's vineyards in the 1850s,

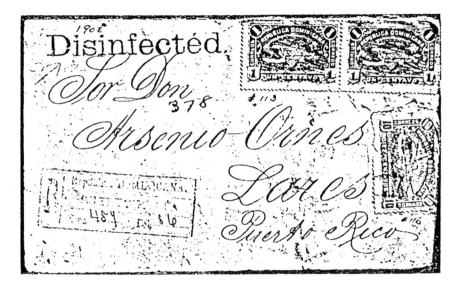

Fig. 1–7. From 1500 to the present century, mail was sometimes fumigated to prevent outbreaks of contagious diseases. From Meyer's book *Disinfected Mail* (1962).

but gardeners had a weapon in sulfur. Edward Tucker, in England in 1845, examined it microscopically and satisfied himself that he was dealing with a fungus, whereupon he applied an aqueous suspension of sulfur and slaked lime to the leaves. This controlled the disease in his glasshouses, whereas it continued to develop in the next garden. Grison, a French gardener, in 1851 obtained control of mildew disease with a diluted preparation made from sulfur and freshly slaked lime boiled in water. This treatment received a favorable comment from an investigating commission and it became the "eau Grison," a precursor of our present-day lime-sulfur fungicide. When the renowned plant pathologist De Bary published on the cause of powdery mildew in 1853, the battle against the autogeneticists had been already won (Keitt, 1959).

TOWARD MODERN TIMES

The eighteenth century ushered in the age of chemistry and with it the discovery of chlorine in 1774 by the Swedish chemist Scheele, followed by the discovery of hypochlorites by the French chemist Bertholet in 1789. These chemicals possessed the dramatic property of counteracting noxious odors, and the demonstration that they could prevent putrefaction further confirmed the mistaken belief that putrefaction and unpleasant odors were the causative factors of contagious diseases. Labarraque (1825), in France, reported the use of calcium hypochlorite in the general sanitation of morgues, sewers, privies, stables, hospital wards, ships, and prisons, where the atmosphere was "loaded with the effluvia of animal or vegetable matter," as indicated by the horrible stench. More important, he reported that Parisian surgeons obtained great success in cases of carbuncle, hospital gangrene, ulcers, and burns, where the wounds were covered with dressings of an aqueous 1 to 8 solution

of hypochlorite. In England, Alcock in 1827 recommended the use of chlorine for the purification of drinking water. He also reported these favorable French surgeons' results, but in 1832 the British Board of Health, while acknowledging that chlorine and hypochlorites could nullify stenches, vehemently disavowed both their usefulness as disinfectants and their medical value. They gave reports that chlorine gas was ineffectual in reducing the spread of infectious fever and smallpox when used in the wards of hospitals. They disassociated odors from contagious disease and even suggested statistical evidence that putrid, intolerable odors were indicative of "the healthiest of all our functions" (a reference, no doubt, to the bowel function).

In this same paper, experiments by a Mr. Faraday were reported in which the cowpox inoculum was destroyed by a 1:50 dilution of chlorine gas and could no longer produce a reaction when used to vaccinate persons. Could this have been the famous scientist Michael Faraday? Faraday was working with chlorine at this time in his experiments to liquefy it, but I have found no biographic evidence linking him with this demonstration of the killing of a virus with a chemical disinfectant. It is likely that he supplied the chlorine used in this work, and it is possible that he was the Faraday who conducted the experiments.

In his 1827 paper on the disinfectant powers of hypochlorite, Alcock relates an interesting account of a Frenchman named Bourcier, which I would be remiss if I did not report: Bourcier, it seems,

"was a married man and lived very happily with his wife, but lately had been much annoyed by the visits of a Greek . . . who was very constantly in the shop with his (B's) wife! . . . This was a source of many quarrels between Bourcier and his spouse. About the end of June, 1823, Bourcier was attacked with symptoms of acute inflammation of the stomach . . . The disease proved fatal . . . On the very day of her husband's death . . . and on the day of his interment, Bourcier's widow was seen at balls with her Greek lover . . . This led the neighbors to suspect that some unfair means had been used to get rid of him (Bourcier)."

An investigation followed. On August 1, the body of Bourcier, who had died a month before, was exhumed. The temperature was 17 or 18°C that day. The body was carried to a large and well aired place, but the odor became intolerable; "The corpse had become swollen in a very manifest degree since it was taken out of the ground." The attendants began their work by sprinkling the subject with a solution of sodium hypochlorite "which produced a marvelous effect . . . the infected odor was instantaneously destroyed, and it became possible to begin the operation."

Alcock now intrigues us with "the reader may like to know the sequel." He tells us that arsenic was found in the intestines. The Greek was sought but had escaped. The widow was brought to trial and though the presumptive evidence was strong, there was no proof she had administered the arsenic; therefore she was acquitted. Bourcier aside, the hypochlorites were yet to make their mark in disinfection history.

Robert Collins in 1829, in an attempt to check an epidemic of puerperal fever, and Eisenmann in 1837 recommended the use of chlorine solutions for this disease. And again in 1843, Lefevre recommended chlorine water to prevent its spread. Credit, however, goes to Oliver Wendell Holmes in Boston and Ignaz Semmelweis in Vienna for illuminating the cause of the disease and its prevention.

Holmes, father of the famous Supreme Court justice and a physician who was better known for his poetry, was in 1843 the first person to elucidate the infectious nature of puerperal (childbed) fever and its transmission by doctors and nurses. Childbed fever had reached epidemic proportions, leading to death in a large percentage of cases, but Holmes, by checking the English registry statistics, had found that formerly it had been a rare disease with a fatality of only three in a thousand cases. By obtaining data from many physicians, he concluded that it was carried from patient to patient by doctors and nurses on their hands and clothing. The patients of one physician who had reported washing his hands with calcium hypochlorite solution between visits had been unusually free of the disease. Four years later Semmelweis, a physician in Vienna, not knowing of Holmes' work, independently discovered the same relationship. His work was classic, covering his detailed statistical results in a large hospital and published in 1861 in his famous book *Aetiologie*. Semmelweis noted that when medical students came directly from the autopsy room and examined patients in the maternity ward, the rate of infection was greater than when they were not present. He noted the odor of the autopsy room when they were present and, suspecting decomposing organic matter, insisted that they wash their hands with chloride of lime on leaving the autopsy room and before examining obstetric patients. The decrease in the death rate was spec-

tacular, yet the personal relationship between Semmelweis and the director of the hospital, as well as with other physicians, was such that despite his dramatic results, he created a storm of opposition.

The work of these two men was historic but unfortunately in their time it was overlooked. The first reason was the nature of their publication. Holmes published first in a minor journal and didn't publish again on this subject for 12 years. Semmelweis didn't publish for 14 years and when he did it was in such a manner that his message was obscured. Further, the work was rejected by many physicians because they did not want to acknowledge responsibility for the death of their patients. Holmes coldly responded to these physicians, "The pestilence-carrier of the lying-in chamber must look to God for pardon for man will never forgive him." Semmelweis, a tragic figure who went insane because of his rejection, painfully cried out in response to all the unnecessary deaths: "Murder must cease!"

Two important players had come on the scene but their work, in other areas, was not known to Holmes or Semmelweis. These were Agostino Bassi and Theodore Schwann, who made their significant contributions consecutively in 1835 and 1836 in Italy, and in 1836 in Germany, respectively. Bassi, making careful observations with a microscope, demonstrated that a disease of silkworms was contagious and was caused by a fungus. This was the first clear demonstration of the microbial origin of disease in animal life. Further, he developed a theory of contagion originating from living parasites in infected wounds, in gangrene, cholera, syphilis, plague, typhus, etc. He suggested the use as germicides, mentioning alcohol, acids, alkalies, chlorine, and sulfur. For diseases such as cholera he advocated immediate isolation of the patient and disinfection of the clothes and excreta. His work, however, received little attention outside of Italy. The most amazing thing about Bassi is that he was by training neither physician nor scientist, but a lawyer.

Schwann, the co-discoverer of the yeast cell, showed by experiment that fermentation and putrefaction were of microbial origin. He also disproved spontaneous generation: with sterile flasks and media he demonstrated that it was microorganisms in the air that produced putrefaction or fermentation of substances. Alcohol was produced when yeast was added to a sugar solution. When sterile media were exposed to the air they decomposed, but if the air was sterilized by heat no decomposition occurred. Schwann reasoned that the air contained living germs that produced the putrefaction because arsenic and mercuric chloride, which were known to kill living things, also prevented putrefaction. These were the same kind of experiments Pasteur was to perform a quarter-century later. Schwann was the originator but Pasteur got the recognition. That is not to belittle Pasteur, for his many achievements earned him his place in history.

Another French chemist, Antoine Bechamp, in a series of experiments from 1854 to 1858, studied the hydrolysis of a sucrose solution. When the sucrose was hydrolyzed he noted mold growing in the solution. When he boiled the solution or added mercuric chloride or creosote to it, it did not hydrolyze. Bechamp concluded that the mold, coming from the air, caused the hydrolysis and that only those chemicals considered to be antiseptic prevented it. He thus further clarified the role of antiseptic chemicals.

Louis Pasteur's achievements in chemistry, bacteriology, and medicine demonstrate his genius and his intense devotion to his work. His careful experiments helped create the science of microbiology, and his example inspired other scientists in microbiology's rapid development in the conquest of microbial diseases and the preservation of food and beverages. Pasteur had to battle ignorance and prejudice in convincing physicians that invisible microorganisms cause disease. When he advised surgeons to put their instruments through a flame before using them, they could not understand why they should do so, and he had to explain (Vallery-Radot, 1923): If the instrument "were examined under a microscope, it would be seen that its surface presents grooves where dusts are harbored. Fire entirely destroys those organic dusts; in my laboratory, where I am surrounded by dust of all kinds, I never make use of an instrument without previously putting it through a flame." He encouraged hospital personnel to heat-sterilize bandages that were put on open wounds. He saved the lucrative French wine industry, whose wines were being rejected because of off-flavors resulting from bacterial fermentations, by prescribing a process of heating the wine briefly at 50 to 60°C, a procedure we know today as "pasteurization," which is used for milk and other products.

Pasteur's experiments had the fortunate effect of enlisting the attention of Lister, who knew nothing of Schwann's experiments or of Bechamp's. Lister represented the prepared mind Pasteur spoke of when he made his famous observation, "Chance favors only the prepared mind." Lister had published on the subject of inflammation of wounds and he wondered why in compound fractures, where the skin was broken, the wound became inflamed and infected, often resulting in death of the patient, whereas in equally severe but simple fractures, where the skin was not broken, there was no infection and the patient usually recovered. Pasteur had supplied the answer: the putrefaction of the wound resulted from the microbes in the air. Lister looked for an antiseptic that would kill these organisms. Connecting putrefaction with inflammation, he chose phenol because he had heard about the remarkable results produced by carbolic acid (phenol) for the town of Carlisle in preventing the odor of the sewage used to irrigate pastures. Phenol, in this treatment, also caused the destruction of the entozoa, the protozoan parasites that infested the cattle that grazed on these pastures.

If ignorance is bliss, Lister was indeed a happy man. He was blissfully unaware of the French surgeons and their use of hypochlorite as an antiseptic. He was un-

aware that phenol, known since 1834, had been used by Kuchenmeister in Germany in 1860 as a dressing for wounds and by Lemaire successfully in France in 1860 as a wound antiseptic. He did not know of the published report in England by Lund in 1862 on the use of carbolic acid in wounds, nor of the 750-page book by Lemaire describing his work in surgery and theory of infection, which was in print in 1863, before Lister began his work. Further, Lister was later to admit that his basic hypothesis that the air was the source of infection was faulty and that the major source of the infective microorganisms was the surgeon's dirty hands and instruments. In addition, he could not know of and hence be discouraged by the results 14 years later of Robert Koch, who showed, however erroneously, that phenol was worthless as a germicide, when tested by Koch's method using anthrax spores. Neither was he hindered by the fact that undiluted phenol, as he used it, irritated and inflamed the patient's wound.

In spite of, or perhaps because of the fact that he was oblivious to these matters, Lister proceeded full force, despite early failures and over considerable resistance by other surgeons, to institute this system of antiseptic surgery that would save multitudes of lives every year. He succeeded because he had great confidence that his method would work, and he pursued it doggedly despite the initial failures and opposition. It worked because phenol was indeed a germicide that killed vegetative bacteria, if not spores, and by the way Lister literally poured it on all parts of the wound, the walls, and the floor; it literally floated away the spores if it did not kill them. Phenol used full-strength was toxic to the tissue, but it was less harmful than the infection, and in his later surgery Lister found that phenol diluted 1:20 and even 1:40 was still effective. His method succeeded because it worked; the wounds healed and the patients got well. Furthermore, it succeeded because he was a dedicated spokesman for it, in written and oral reports. In 1867 in one of his first reports, Lister commented that prior to his antiseptic surgery his wards were among the unhealthiest in the Glasgow hospital, but since he adopted his antiseptic treatment the wards changed character "so that during the last nine months not a single instance of pyaemia, hospital gangrene, or erysipelas has occurred in them." He left no doubt that the cause of this change was his system of antiseptic surgery. His conviction persuaded others to try it, and they also reported dramatic success. For example, in the General Hospital in Berlin, his method reduced the infection rate from 90 to 15%. Lister received many honors. He was knighted and even had a mouthwash named after him.

Another giant on the scene in the development of microbiology and medicine was Robert Koch. He ushered in the era of modern bacteriology with sterile technique, pure cultures and solid media. Using the achromatic microscope, invented by Lister's father, Koch demonstrated conclusively that bacteria did indeed invade the tissues and produce disease. In the area of disinfection, he wrote in 1881 a comprehensive research paper titled simply "On Disinfection." Forty-eight pages in length, it examined the ability of over 70 chemicals at different concentrations, in aqueous, oil, or alcoholic solutions, and at different temperatures to kill anthrax spores. Among the most active he found chlorine, bromine, and iodine, mercuric chloride, potassium permanganate, and osmic acid. Of somewhat lesser activity were hydrochloric acid, ferric chloride, arsenic, calcium hypochlorite, ammonium sulfide, formic acid, chloropicrin, quinine, and oil of turpentine. Phenol had to be greater than 3% to kill the spores.

Kronig and Paul, in their classic research published in 1897, laid the foundation of modern, scientific knowledge of chemical disinfection. They noted that bacteria are not all killed at the same time, but at a rate that depends upon the concentration of the chemical and the temperature. They observed that disinfectants can be compared accurately only when tested under controlled conditions. The number of bacteria must be constant and must be brought into contact with the disinfectant without the interference of other organic matter such as the nutritive medium. The action of the disinfectant must be arrested promptly after a stated period and the bacteria transferred to the most favorable medium at optimal temperature. The result of tests is determined by accurate count of survivors in plate cultures.

These principles were put into practice in 1903 by Rideal and Walker in their famous phenol coefficient method of testing disinfectants. They rigidly standardized all conditions of the test and employed specific bacteria in a prescribed broth medium. Further, they employed phenol as a basis for comparison. In 1908, Chick and Martin modified the method when they introduced organic matter in the disinfectant solution to make it conform to the more rigorous conditions frequently encountered in use. These methods received other modifications in the years to follow, but they served to lay the groundwork for disinfectant testing procedures.

CHEMICAL DISINFECTANTS

Chlorine and hypochlorites continued to find their areas of application. They were used for treatment of sewage and for deodorization and disinfection of hospital wards as early as 1854. Traube in 1894 established the disinfecting properties of hypochlorites in water treatment, where chlorine found its greatest use. In 1915 Dakin introduced a solution of 0.5% sodium hypochlorite with alkali, which was used for disinfection of open wounds in World War I. Hypochlorite solutions are major household disinfectants today and are also used in treating swimming pools. Organic chloramines, which are a stabilized form of chlorine, were introduced by Dakin with chloramine-T. Chlorine dioxide, which is employed by paper mills for destroying bacterial slimes, was tested in 1947 and put into a stabilized formulation in 1955.

Iodine was used in medicine for the treatment of goiter in 1816, but the first reference to its use in wounds was in 1839 by Davies. The tincture of iodine, a 5% solution of iodine in diluted alcohol, was admitted to the U.S. Pharmacopeia in 1830. It was used with success in the U.S. Civil War in 1862 to treat battle wounds. Its use against the anthrax bacillus and a whole host of pathogenic microorganisms soon followed. It was tested as an antiseptic by Davaine in 1873 and 1875, and in 1905 Senn declared it to be the safest and most potent of all known antiseptics. As the tincture, it gained wide acceptance as an effective skin antiseptic despite its staining properties, odor, and toxicity. Organic iodine compounds have come into use as a means of eliminating these properties. The major ones are iodoform, which was used as a dusting powder earlier in this century, and the iodophors, which are complexes of iodine with water-soluble polymers. Iodophors are presently popular because they have good wetting properties, emulsify fat deposits, and penetrate organic soil to deliver the germicide.

Knowledge of mercury and its uses goes back to early civilizations in China, India, and Egypt. Mercury shares with sulfur the longest history of continued use of a disinfectant. Knowledge of the medical uses of mercury was introduced into Europe through Arab physicians and was first mentioned in European literature in 1140 by Matthaeus Platearius. It was used in the treatment of syphilis when that disease first reached epidemic proportions in Italy in 1429. The outstanding results of Koch with the bichloride popularized the use of that germicide. Its toxicity, however, led to the search for other mercurials, which in the early part of the twentieth century produced such organic mercurials as Metaphen, Merthiolate, and Mercurochrome, and the phenylmercury and ethylmercury salts, which demonstrated higher antimicrobial activity. Mercurials also found extensive use in agriculture as plant and seed protectants and in industry as preservatives and antimicrobial agents.

Alcohol (ethanol) is another antiseptic with a long history of use. Wine was used liberally throughout history, both externally and internally, to heal all sorts of ailments. Unfortunately the concentration of alcohol in wine is so low that it has relatively no value as an antiseptic. Distilled spirits, which became available in Europe in the sixteenth and seventeenth centuries, provided a higher concentration of alcohol, but the value of ethanol as an antiseptic was not appreciated until it was demonstrated in tests by Reinicke in 1894 and by Epstein in 1897.

Harrington and Walker in 1903 showed that a 60 to 70% solution was the most effective, but that no concentration would kill bacterial spores. Isopropyl alcohol was also shown to have activity like that of ethyl alcohol.

Phenol or carbolic acid, like chlorine, found use first as a deodorant to prevent the foul odors of sewage and garbage and then to prevent wound infections, which were considered a form of putrefaction. Although phenol was discovered in 1834, it was some years later before it was used to treat wounds. Lemaire first used it in wounds in 1860, although creosote, which contains a mixture of different phenols, nitrogen bases, and aromatic hydrocarbons, had been employed earlier for this purpose. Savory, in 1867, reported on the treatment of pyemia, stating, "Among the most useful of these are . . . solutions of carbolic acid, chlorine, chlorinated soda . . . or iodine."

The interest in phenol resulting from Joseph Lister's work led to a search for other phenols with greater antimicrobial activity. Coal tar creosote, which contained, among other things, a mixture of alkyl phenols, was emulsified with soap and was patented in 1877. A version of that emulsion with a mixture of cresols was marketed and sold under the name Lysol, a name still used today, although the ingredients may have changed. In 1906 Bechhold and Ehrlich published on beta naphthol and polyhalogentated phenols. In 1921 the alkylresorcinols with the popular hexylresorcinol appeared. The xylenols and alkylchlorophenols appeared in 1933. The chlorophenols, such as pentachlorophenol, gained wide acceptance as wood and industrial preservatives, and alkylparahydroxybenzoates became popular as preservatives for cosmetics, drugs, and foods. Arylphenols, including the bisphenols, added more potent weapons to the phenol arsenal. Early work by Bechhold and Ehrlich in 1906 and by Gump in 1941 showed the high antibacterial activity of the halogenated bisphenols, which found a large market in antiseptic soaps (Cade, 1944).

The chemical structure of hydrogen peroxide was reported by Thenard in 1818, and its ability to do away with foul odors was discovered by an English physician, B.W. Richardson, in 1858, who subscribed to the then-popular idea connecting odor and infection and therefore proposed its use as a disinfectant. It was put on the market under the name Sanitas. The 3% solution became popular and was found in almost every medicine chest in the 1920s through 1950s. Unfortunately, in living tissues it was shown to be quickly destroyed by the catalase in the tissue. At present, more concentrated solutions are proving useful in producing sterile cartons for non-refrigerated milk and fruit juices (Chapter 48).

The quaternary ammonium compounds represent an important group of disinfectants in wide use today. Although knowledge of their antimicrobial activity was reported in 1916, it was not until 1935, when Gerard Domagk reported the much greater activity of the long-chain derivatives, that they came into commercial use. Domagk was awarded the Nobel prize (which Hitler didn't let him accept) in 1939, but it wasn't for the quaternaries but for the discovery of the antibacterial activity of the sulfonamide drugs. In the latter case he had made a lucky mistake. Having been a student of the famous Paul Ehrlich, he pursued the antimicrobial activity of textile dyes as Erhlich had done. The red dye Prontisil, which he found to have remarkable activity in killing microorganisms in the body when used as a chemotherapeutant, actually functioned because it decomposed

in the body to produce sulfanilamide, which was not a dye but a white, crystaline compound.

A paper by Kinnaman in 1905 gives us a resume and bibliography of the work of several investigators on disinfectant action of chemicals thought to be of value at that time. These included bichloride of mercury, phenol, ethanol, hydrogen peroxide, iodine, iodoform, formaldehyde, lysol, benzoic acid, salicylic acid, potassium permanganate, and turpentine, among others.

The twentieth century, with its great advances in chemistry, particularly in organic chemistry, has brought us many new disinfectants, and our chemical disinfectants serve us in many different ways. They protect our food from destructive microorganisms while it is growing, when it is processed, and when it is shipped and stored. They preserve many of our products, like wood and tents, from rotting and deterioration. They protect electronic equipment from electrical leakage due to moisture from mold growth, and prevent jet fuel from clogging engines with slime from bacterial growth. But most important, they protect our bodies from those tiny invaders that threaten us in the air we breathe, in the water we drink, in the food we eat, and even in the things we touch. Before there were disinfectants, few people survived surgery, and even a simple cut often proved fatal. It is well documented in history that during war more soldiers commonly died from disease and infection than from direct battle injuries, and it was not until World War II, when disinfectants were in common use, that these statistics were reversed.

HEAT AND FILTRATION

In biblical and medieval times, heat was employed in the form of fire to destroy clothes and corpses of diseased persons. Spallanzani, in his experiment disproving spontaneous generation published in 1776, noted that the microorganisms that were thought by other investigators to have appeared spontaneously in a medium could be killed by heat, but that some organisms were more resistant than others, and to kill these resistant ones, the liquids had to be boiled for 1 hour. In 1718, Joblot sterilized a hay infusion by boiling it for 15 minutes and then sealing the container. Appert, in 1810, applied this procedure for preserving food.

In 1831, William Henry undertook the problem of destroying infectious matter of the plague on Egyptian cotton brought into England. He considered using chlorine, but abandoned it because of possible damage to the cotton and spinning machinery. Based on the knowledge that plague ceases when the weather becomes hot, he thought heat below the temperature of boiling water might solve the problem. Since Jenner had already developed his vaccination for smallpox using cowpox, Henry employed cowpox as the infectious agent, heating it and then injecting it into children in the usual way for vaccination. His experiments showed that the vaccine was inactivated at 140°F after 3 hours but was still active at 120°F. Henry's work was ignored for almost 50 years, but in 1878, Lister recommended the heating of glassware at 150°F for 2 hours to produce sterilization, and in 1881, Koch published on the relative values of hot air and steam as sterilizing agents. John Tyndall had discovered the benefit of discontinuous heating (Tyndallization) and Pasteur discovered the sterilizing effectiveness of superheated steam. Modern autoclaves modeled after the principle of Papin's "digestor or engine for softening bones" of 1681 were made for laboratory use under the name of Chamberland's autoclave about 1884 by the Parisian engineering firm of Wiesnegg (Bulloch, 1960).

Filtration as a means of water purification had been practiced since early times, but it was not until the nineteenth century that science entered the picture. Schröder and von Dusch filtered air sterilely through cotton wool in 1854, and in 1884, the ceramic, Pasteur-Chamberland bacterial filter for fluids arrived, followed by the Berkefeld candle in 1891.

Tyndall's careful experiments in 1876 and 1877 clearly demonstrated the effectiveness of filtration in producing sterility and simultaneously dealt a final death blow to the persistent belief in spontaneous generation. By demonstrating that dust and microorganisms suspended in air could be seen easily by the naked eye by passing a ray of light through a dark room (the Tyndall cone), he showed that air that was rendered free of visible particles would not infect sterile solutions that were left open to this air, but that were readily infected by air containing particulate matter.

RADIATION

The antimicrobial effects of light on microorganisms were investigated by Downes and Blunt in 1877, who demonstrated the sterilization of a bacterial culture after 9 hours' exposure to sunlight. In 1893, Ward observed from his experiments with different colored lights that "the very dim blue light . . . is far more bactericidal than the much brighter orange light." However, it was not until 1928 that Gates noted the bactericidal action of different wavelengths of ultraviolet light and remarkably indicated the relationship between the germicidal wavelength and that absorbed by DNA. The antimicrobial activity of x-rays was described by Rieder in 1898, shortly after their discovery by Roentgen in 1895, when he showed that they were toxic to the common pathogens. The inhibitory action of radioactive substances was demonstrated by Strebel in 1900 when he subjected *Serratia marcescens* to radium (McCullough, 1945).

PRESERVATION

In the preservation field, empirical results were reduced to practice earlier than in the case of disease-preventive treatments for plants, animals, and man. Wood preservation may be taken as a specific example. In America in 1716, the Province of South Carolina granted its first wood-preserving patent to Dr. William Crook for a preservative containing "the Oyle or Spirit

of Tarr" and advocated it for the protection of ship planking against decay and shipworm. Mercuric chloride was used for preserving wood as early as 1705 by Homberg and was patented in England by John Kyan in 1832. Copper sulfate was recommended by Boissieu and Bordenare in 1767 and patented in 1837 by Margary in England. Zinc chloride was recommended for use in wood in 1815 by Thomas Wade and was patented by William Burnett in England in 1838. Coal-tar creosote, which has been regarded as the standard wood preservative, was patented in 1838 by John Bethell in England; his treatment involved the injection of the creosote into the wood under pressure. This process has been used with slight modification up to the present time, thus demonstrating the early establishment of the wood-preserving industry (Hunt and Garratt, 1953).

This chapter has given the reader a glimpse of some of the highlights in the early developments of disinfection, sterilization, and preservation. More detailed accounts will be found in the references, and more recent history will be found in the individual treatments of the specialized chapters in this volume.

REFERENCES

Alcock, Thomas. 1827. An essay on the use of chloreuts of oxide of sodium and zinc, as powerful disinfecting agents. Lancet, *11*, 643–648.

Appert, N. 1810. The art of preserving all kinds of animal and vegetable substances for several years. Translated from the French. New York. D. Longworth, 1812. New York, C.S. Van Winkle.

Bacon, Francis. 1635. Sylva Sylvarum or a Natural History. 2nd Edition. London, John Haviland and William Lee. Century IV, p. 75.

Bassi, Agostino. 1836. On the Mark Disease (Del Mal Del Signo). Translated from the Italian by P.J. Yarrow. The American Phytopathological Society. 1958. Baltimore, Monumental Printing.

Béchamp, M.A. 1855. Note on the influence that pure water and certain salt solutions exert on cane sugar. Comptes Rendues, *40*, 436–438.

Béchamp, M.A. 1858. The effect that pure water or saturated solutions of different salts exercise in the cold on cane sugar. Comptes Rendues, *46*, 44–47. See also Annales de Chimie et de Physique, 3rd Series, *54*, 28–42.

Bechhold, H., and Ehrlich, P. 1906. Relation between chemical constitution and disinfecting action. Z. Physiol. Chem., *47*, 173–199.

Board of Health Report. 1832. Alleged disinfecting properties of chlorine. Lancet, *1*, 594–600.

Bulloch, W. 1960. *The History of Bacteriology.* London, Oxford, 1938. Reprinted 1960.

Cade, A.R. 1944. Halogenated dihydroxydiphenylmethanes as disinfectants. Soap Sanit. Chem., *20*, 111–115.

Chick, H., and Martin, C.J. 1908. The principles involved in the standardization of disinfectants and the influence of organic matter upon germicidal value. J. Hyg., *8*, 654–697.

Dakin, H.D. 1915. The antiseptic action of hypochlorites. Br. Med. J., *2*, 809–810.

Davaine, C. 1873. *Dictionnaire Encyclopedique des Science Med.* p. 335.

Davaine, C. 1875. On the discovery of bacteria. Bull. Acad. Med., *4*, 581–584.

Domagk, G. 1935. A new class of disinfecting agents. Dtsch. Med. Wochenschr., *61*, 829–832.

Downes, A., and Blunt, T.P. 1877. Researches on the effect of light upon bacteria and other organisms. Proc. R. Soc., *26*, 488–500.

Epstein, F. 1897. On the question of alcohol disinfection. Z. Hyg. Infektionskr., *24*, 1–21.

Fracastoro, G. 1546. *Contagion, Contagious Diseases and Their Treatment.* Translated from the Latin by Wilmer C. Wright. 1930. New York, Putnam.

Gates, F.L. 1928. Nuclear derivatives and the lethal action of ultraviolet light. Science, *68*, 479–480.

Gump, W.S. 1941. Dihydroxyhexachlorodiphenylmethane and method of producing same. U.S. Patent No. 2,250,408.

Harrington, C., and Walker, H. 1903. The germicidal action of alcohol. Boston Med. Surg. J., *148*, 548–552.

Henry, W. 1832. Experiments on the disinfecting powers of increased temperatures. Lancet, *2*, 92–93.

Holmes, O.W. 1843. The contagiousness of puerperal fever. N. Engl. Quart. J. Med. Surg., *1*(4), 503–530.

Holmes, O.W. 1855. *Puerperal Fever, as a Private Pestilance.* Boston, Ticknor and Fields.

Hunt, G.M., and Garratt, G.A. 1953. *Wood Preservation.* New York, McGraw-Hill.

Joblot, L. 1718. *Descriptions and Use of Several New Microscopes.* Paris.

Keitt, G.W. 1959. History of plant pathology. In *Plant Pathology.* Volume 1. Edited by J.G. Horsfall and A.E. Dimond. New York, Academic Press, pp. 62–91.

King, E. 1693. Several observations and experiments on the animalcula in pepper water, etc. Philos. Trans. Roy. Soc. London, *17*(203), 861–865.

Kinnaman, G.C. 1905. The antimicrobic action of iodin. JAMA, *45*, 600–607.

Koch, R. 1881. On disinfection. Mittheilungen aus dem Kaiserlichen Gesunheitsamte, *1*, 234–282.

Kronig, B., and Paul, T.L. 1897. The chemical foundations of the study of disinfection and of the action of poisons. Z. Hyg. Infekt. Ionskr., *25*, 1–112. For English translation (condensed), see Brock, T. 1965. *Milestones in Microbiology.* Englewood Cliffs, NJ, Prentice-Hall, pp. 163–176.

Kuchenmeister, G.F.H. 1860. On disinfecting action in general, carbolic acid and its therapeutic application in particular. Deutsche Klinik, *12*, 123.

Labarraque, A.-G. 1825. *The Use of Sodium and Calcium Hypochlorites.* Paris, Huzard.

van Leeuwenhoek, A. 1684. An abstract of a letter from Mr. Anthony Leeuwenhoek at Delft dated Sept. 17, 1683 about some microscopical observations about animals in the scurf of the teeth. Phil. Trans. R. Soc. London, *14*, 568–574.

Lefevre, G. 1843. Observations on some of the popular remedies of German practitioners. Lancet, *1*, 143–148.

Lemaire, F.-J. 1860. Saponified coal tar, an effective disinfectant in stopping fermentations, its applications in hygiene, in therapy, and general background. Paris, Germer-Bailliere.

Lind, J. 1757. Essay on the most effectual means of preserving the health of seamen in the Royal Navy. London.

Lind, J. 1768. An essay on the diseases incidental to Europeans in hot climates. London.

Lister, J. 1867. On a new method of treating compound fracture, abscess, etc., with observations on the conditions of suppuration. Lancet, *1*, 326–329; 352–359; 387; 389; 507–509. *2*, 95–96.

Lister, J. 1867. On the antiseptic principle in the practice of surgery. Lancet, *2*, 353–356; 668–669.

McCallan, S.E.A. 1967. History of fungicides. In *Fungicides.* Edited by D.C. Torgeson. New York, Academic Press, p. 4.

McCullough, E.C. 1945. *Disinfection and Sterilization.* Philadelphia, Lea & Febiger, Chapter 4.

Meyer, K.F. 1962. *Disinfected Mail.* Holton, KS, The Gossip Printery.

Papin, D. 1681. A new digester or engine for softening bones. London.

Pringle, J. 1750. Some experiments on substances resisting putrefaction. R. Soc. Phil. Trans., *46*, 480–488.

Pringle, J. 1750. II. A continuation of the experiments on substances resisting putrefaction. R. Soc. Phil. Trans., *46*, 525–534.

Pringle, J. 1750. V. Further experiments on substances resisting putrefaction; with experiments upon the means of hastening and promoting it. R. Soc. Phil. Trans., *46*, 550–558.

Reinicke, E.A. 1894. Bacteriological investigations on the disinfection of the hands. Zentralbl. Gynakol., *18*, 1189–1199.

Reddish, G.F. 1957. *Antiseptics, Disinfectants, Fungicides, and Chemical and Physical Sterilization.* Historical Review. Philadelphia, Lea & Febiger, pp. 15–22.

Richardson, B.W. 1891. On peroxide of hydrogen, or ozone water, as a remedy. Lancet, *1*, 707–709, 760–763. See also Trans. Med. Soc., London, *2*, 51 (1862).

Rideal, S., and Walker, J.T.A. 1903. The standardization of disinfectants. J. R. Sanit. Inst., *24*, 424–441.

Rieu, E.V. 1952. Homer, *The Odyssey.* London, Methuen, p. 324.

Savory, W.S. 1867. On pyemia. Lancet, *1*, 139–142.

Schroder, H., and von Dusch, T. 1854. On filtration of the air in relation to putrefaction and fermentation. Ann. Chem. Pharm., *89*, 232–243.

Semmelweis, I.P. 1861. The etiology, conception and prophylaxis of childbed-fever. Pest, Vienna, and Leipzig, Hartleben.

Senn, N. 1905. Iodine in surgery with special reference to its use as an antiseptic. Surg. Gynecol. Obstet., *1*(1), 1–10.

Spallanzani, L. 1776. Observations and experience about the animalcules of the infusion. In writings on the natural animals and vegetables of the Abbey Spallanzani, Modena, *1*, 3–221.

Tyndall, J. 1877. The optical deportment of the atmosphere in relation to the phenomena of putrefaction and infection. Phil. Trans. R. Soc. London, *166*, 27–74.

Tyndall, J. 1881. Essays on the floating matter in the air and in relation to putrefaction and infection. London.

Vallery Radot, Rene. 1923. *Pasteur.* New York, Doubleday, p. 240.

Ward, H.M. 1893. Further experiments on the action of light on *Bacillus anthracis.* Proc. R. Soc., *53*, 23–45.

CHAPTER 2

DEFINITION OF TERMS

Seymour S. Block

Words are meant to convey meaning, but we cannot be sure that any word will convey the same meaning to every person. People have different backgrounds and outlooks and derive different meanings from the same word. Further, language is, in a sense, a living organism, and words change their meaning with time. Thus we have some trouble reading Shakespeare and even more with Chaucer. It is said that if something looks like a duck, quacks like a duck, and waddles like a duck, it is a duck. This is not necessarily so. Most people think they know what the term "whiskey" means, but they could be wrong, for it is a word with a legal as well as a popular meaning. Legally, whiskey is a malted beverage made from small grains distilled in a certain way, containing a certain amount of ethyl alcohol, and aged in new, charred-oak barrels. A product having the same color, odor, taste, and chemical composition might not satisfy the legal definition.

Definitions are man-made; they do not come to us from on high. They attempt to make boundaries around terms but these boundaries are often vague and indistinct. Yet we must work with them as best we can. Death is not exact. When is a person dead? When he is no longer breathing? When he is brain dead? When all the cells in his body are dead? When is a product sterile? When all life in it has been killed or when it has been heated at x temperature for y minutes or when its microbial population is reduced by z D values? It is what we say it is according to the way we construct our definition.

Definitions by lexicographers and lawyers serve the useful purpose of giving all persons the opportunity of common understanding of what they mean when they use a word. When manufacturers label a product as an antiseptic or disinfectant, it is imperative that their product does what these terms say it should do. Under the original Food and Drugs Act, a judicial decision states, "Language used in the label is to be given the meaning ordinarily conveyed by it to those to whom it was addressed." This is difficult to do where meanings are vague. Dictionaries and legal definitions clarify the meanings and give them greater stability. Words such as "antiseptic," "disinfectant," and "sanitizer" are excellent examples of words that had loosely accepted meanings until they were more strictly defined. Austin M. Patterson, a lexicographer of scientific terms, made a thorough study of many of these words in 1932, which served to crystallize their meanings. Many of the definitions that follow are of his preparation. Some of the others are from Reddish (1957) and various dictionaries, with comments by myself.

Disinfectant

A disinfectant is an agent that frees from infection, usually a chemical agent but sometimes may be a physical one, such as x rays or ultraviolet light, that destroys disease or other harmful microorganisms but may not kill bacterial spores. It refers to substances applied to inanimate objects.

The legal definition (Reddish, 1957) is similar but more detailed: An agent that frees from infection; usually a chemical agent that destroys disease germs or other harmful microorganisms or inactivates viruses. The term is most commonly used to designate chemicals that kill the growing forms, but not necessarily the resistant spore forms of bacteria, except when the intended use is specifically against an organism forming spores or a virus, in which case the spores, too, must be killed or the virus inactivated. Proper use of a disinfectant is contingent upon the purpose for which it is employed or the type of infectious agent that there is reason to suspect may be present.

Comments. The word "disinfect" first appeared in the seventeenth century when certain "effluvia" or mysterious emanations were thought to cause disease and could be destroyed by chemical substances such as burning sulfur. Because disease was associated with foul odors, disinfectants were expected to destroy or mask the odors to get rid of the infection. Patterson (1932) studied 143 definitions of *disinfectant* used from 1854 to 1930. Of these, 25, mostly of earlier date, made no mention of microorganisms. Of the rest, 95 defined disinfectants as germ destroyers. The word still carries with it much of its original connotation, namely, the cleaning of sickrooms, clothing, bedding, lavatories, stables, etc. The use of "disinfectant" for antimicrobial chemicals used on the body, as in the case of "skin disinfectant," is frowned upon. The OTC Antimicrobial I Drug Review Panel (1974) states that disinfection properly refers to the use of such chemicals on inanimate objects and not on the human body. A hard distinction insofar as governmental regulation is concerned is that disinfectants or antimicrobial chemicals labeled for use on inanimate objects are considered economic poisons under the Federal Environmental Pesticide Control Act (7 U.S.C. 136), whereas agents such as antiseptics labeled for use on human or animal tissue are regulated as drugs under the Federal Food, Drug and Cosmetic Act. Whereas disinfectants are commonly associated with chemicals, the official definition of *disinfection* by the American Public Health Association (1950), U.S. Public Health Service, and British Ministry of Health includes physical agents as well: *Disinfection*—killing of pathogenic agents by chemical or physical means directly applied.

It is now about 60 years since Patterson made his study of the existing definitions of the word disinfectant. I have attempted to update Patterson's study by examining and analyzing the definitions given by 15 modern dictionaries: eight medical, two chemical, two legal, and three general. The results are given in Table 2–1. It will be noted that there are five elements in the definition of disinfection that have been given in the discussion above. These are that a disinfectant (1) removes infection, (2) kills, not just inhibits, microorganisms in the vegetative stage, (3) does not necessarily kill spores, (4) is ordinarily a chemical but can be a physical agent, and (5) is used only on inanimate objects, not on the human or animal body. It is important to make these distinctions if we are to distinguish the term disinfectant from other terms that follow, such as antiseptic, sporicide, and bacteriostat.

It will be noted from Table 2–1 that only one of the dictionaries, *Taber's Medical Dictionary*, contained all five elements of the definition. *Taber's* also was the only dictionary that specifically stated that a disinfectant could be chemical or physical. Others merely used the words "an agent" and were given credit in our table for either chemical or physical. All of the dictionaries perpetuated the oldest aspect of the definition, namely, freeing from infectious disease. *Black's Law Dictionary* defines disinfected as "Made free from injurious or contagious disease. Immunization." Injurious disease might be noninfectious diseases like arthritis or diabetes, and how immunization is equivalent to disinfection, only the writers of that dictionary can explain. *Taber's Medical Dictionary* states that a disinfectant prevents infection by killing bacteria. No mention of fungi, viruses, or protozoans. Some dictionaries use terminology such as "a disinfectant destroys, eliminates, neutralizes, or inhibits

growth or activity of harmful microorganisms, or renders them inert." If it just inhibits or renders inert it would not be considered a disinfectant but a bacteriostatic, fungistatic, or other agent. The *Random House Dictionary* refers to a disinfectant as any chemical agent that destroys harmful organisms. That definition would include insecticides that kill malaria mosquitos, because they are harmful organisms. *Steadman's* includes the elimination of toxins or vectors as well as pathogenic microorganisms. Vectors might also include the malaria mosquitos.

Three dictionaries, *Steadman's*, *International*, and *Hawley's*, define "complete" and "incomplete disinfection." They state complete disinfection kills both vegetative organisms and spores, whereas incomplete disinfection kills only the vegetative form. These terms relate to "levels of disinfection" proposed by Spaulding (Lawrence and Block, 1968) for rating disinfectants used for medical instruments. He designated three levels of disinfection action: high-level which kill all microorganisms (sporicides); low-level, which kill only vegetative cells and some viruses; and intermediate-level, which kill vegetative cells, most viruses, and some spores. This system has been accepted by the Centers for Disease Control (Garner and Favero, 1985) in their guideline for "Cleaning, Disinfecting, and Sterilizing Patient Care Equipment." It is important, however, to use the term sterilization or sporicidal where all forms are killed and not to use disinfection or complete disinfection. The APIC (Association for Practitioners in Infection Control) proposed levels, which include sterilization, high-level disinfectant, and low-level disinfectant (Rutala, 1990), would therefore be preferred. Another definition, given by Random House, for disinfection is "to cleanse (clothing, wounds, etc.) to destroy harmful microorganisms." *Black's Medical* tells us that disinfection is the "process of rendering harmless any persons, articles, rooms, and the like which are liable to communicate disease." In today's understanding of the term we do not disinfect people or wounds. We treat them with antiseptics. The idea of cleaning goes hand-in-hand with disinfection, and the distinction may be confused. The legal dictionary, *Words and Phrases*, tells of a court case in which a company that disinfected a railroad for carrying food left it dirty and was sued. The judge explained that disinfection did not mean that all dirt had to be removed, as long as it did not contain living microorganisms capable of doing harm; thus the case was lost. Whereas the word disinfectant was originally and still is used primarily with regard to pathogenic microorganisms in a medical setting, the more general use would cover a range of nonmedical organisms and applications such as a toilet bowl disinfectant, water cooling-tower disinfectant, or drilling-mud disinfectant. It can be concluded from this analysis that dictionary definitions in this area can not be counted on for strict, modern meanings. They can be used as a beginning, but one would be better advised to consult professionals actively working in the field for more accurate, complete interpretation of the terms.

Table 2–1. *A Comparison of 15 Dictionaries on 5 Elements of the Definition of Disinfection*

Criteria	Dorland's Medical 27th, 1988 W.B. Saunders	Gould's Medical 3rd, 1972 McGraw-Hill	Webster's Medical 1986 Merriam-Webster	Steadman's Medical 25th, 1990 Williams & Wilkins
1. Removes infection	+	+	+	+
2. Kills microorganisms	−	−	+	+
3. May not kill spores	−	−	+	−
4. May be chemical or physical	−	+	+	−
5. Used only on inanimate objects	+	+	−	−

Criteria	Taber's Medical 16th, 1989 F.A. Davis	Mosby's Medical 3rd, 1990 C.V. Mosby	Black's Medical 35th, 1987 Barnes & Noble	International Medical & Biology 1986 Wiley
1. Removes infection	+	+	+	+
2. Kills microorganisms	+	+	+	+
3. May not kill spores	+	−	+	−
4. May be chemical or physical	+	−	−	−
5. Used only on inanimate objects	+	−	−	+

Criteria	Condensed Chemical 1961 Rheinhold	Hawley's Condensed Chemical 1987 Van Nostrand-Rheinhold	American Heritage General 1973 Houghton Mifflin	Random House General 1968 Random House
1. Removes infection	+	+	+	+
2. Kills microorganisms	+	+	−	+
3. May not kill spores	+	+	−	−
4. May be chemical or physical	−	−	+	−
5. Used only on inanimate objects	+	+	+	−

Criteria	Oxford English General 2nd, 1989 Oxford	Black's Law 1954 West	Words & Phrases Law 1954 West
1. Removes infection	+	+	+
2. Kills microorganisms	+	−	+
3. May not kill spores	−	−	−
4. May be chemical or physical	−	−	−
5. Used only on inanimate objects	−	−	−

+ Includes this element of the definition
− Doesn't include this element of the definition

A chemical may have different antimicrobial designations depending on its application. For example, Fraser (1987) mentions a number of designations for peracetic acid: "It should be noted the terms used for disinfectants vary between industries, e.g., 'sanitizers' in food and brewing industries, 'terminal disinfectants' in dairies, 'biocides' in municipal water purification, 'ovicides' in agricultural waste stabilization, 'sterilants' in medicinal and pharmaceutical applications." Of course, peracetic acid may be bacteriostatic under certain conditions with short contact time, bactericidal with longer time, and sporicidal or biocidal with even longer time. Each is a proper designation for the conditions of use. On the other hand, some industries may employ terminology peculiar to that industry with no regard to properly accepted definitions. It would be desirable to have definitions accepted internationally but they are not; therefore there may be different interpretations of the terms as they are used in different countries.

Antiseptic

An antiseptic is a substance that prevents or arrests the growth or action of microorganisms either by inhibiting their activity or by destroying them. The term is used especially for preparations applied topically to living tissue.

The legal definition (Federal Food, Drug and Cosmetic Act, 1938) states: The representation of a drug in its labeling as an *antiseptic* shall be considered to be a representation that it is a germicide, except in the case of a drug purporting to be, or represented as, an *antiseptic* for inhibitory use as a wet dressing, ointment, dusting powder, or other such use as involves prolonged contact with the body. For a more complete definition and discussion of the use of the term antiseptic, refer to Chapter 58.

Comments. The word "antiseptic," derived from the Greek "against putrefaction," was used by Pringle in 1750 (see Chapter 1) to record the ability of substances to prevent the spoilage of organic matter such as egg and meat. After Lister's research in the use of antimicrobial agents in surgery, the term acquired a second meaning, that of a substance used to destroy pathogenic microorganisms. There was some difference of opinion in regard to the second meaning—whether an antiseptic merely inhibited the growth of microorganisms, killed them, or both. Patterson examined 165 definitions of *antiseptic* used between 1819 and 1930, of which 20 make no mention of bacteria; 27 state that they arrest but do not destroy, 12 that they destroy, 10 that they inhibit growth but do not indicate how, 66 that they do one or the other, and 30 that antiseptics act to neutralize toxins, etc. A similar survey in 1921 shows that 37 of 53 citations described an antiseptic as inhibiting microorganisms without necessarily killing them, whereas only 6 held that they functioned by killing. The mode of action of course may depend upon such criteria as concentration used, time of contact, temperature, pH, nature of the organism, organic matter present, etc., and such conditions have been included in more restrictive definitions of many of these terms. For example, formerly under the Federal Food and Drug Act of 1938, mouthwashes, douches, and gargles that are allowed to remain in contact with the tissue for short periods were permitted to be labeled as antiseptics only if they destroy organisms in the dilutions recommended for use. Currently, the FDA (1974) specifies clinical verification of infection prevention.

Germicide

A germicide is an agent that destroys microorganisms, especially pathogenic organisms.

Comment. The word "germ" is a popular one and has been used to form the convenient term *germicide*, which finds extensive use in the technical as well as the popular literature. As commonly used, the term is associated with the death of all disease-producing microorganisms but, like the word disinfectant, to which it is similar, it does not necessarily include the capability of destroying bacterial spores. Since germicide is a popular term it is often misused to include sporicides, as in the phrase "high level germicides," which includes sporicides like ethylene oxide. It should be stated that usage eventually determines meaning and if a word is generally used in a certain way, its meaning will change to conform to its common use, regardless of authority's efforts to the contrary. This seems to be occurring with the term germicide. It applies to use on both living tissue and inanimate objects. It refers to chemical agents, but the adjective "germicidal" may refer to physical agents, as for example, *germicidal* lamps.

Bactericide

A bactericide is an agent that kills bacteria.

Comment. This term is applied to chemical agents that kill all bacteria, both pathogenic and nonpathogenic, but not necessarily bacterial spores. It is used for both living tissue and inanimate objects. It differs from *germicide* in that is does not include fungi, viruses, and other microorganisms that are not bacteria, although it may kill them but does not claim to do so.

Fungicide

A fungicide is an agent that kills fungi.

Comment. This term is associated with chemicals and includes substances applied to both living tissue and inanimate objects. Unlike the definition of *bactericide*, no mention is made to exclude spores; therefore, the assumption should be made that fungus spores are also killed.

Virucide

A virucide is an agent that destroys or inactivates viruses, especially a chemical substance used on living tissue.

Comment. The word virucide is a misnomer because the ending "cide" means kill and the virus, by itself, is not a living entity. Thus we do not say a virus is killed, but that a virus is inactivated. The spelling "viricide" is sometimes used but is not preferred.

Sporicide

A sporicide is an agent that destroys microbial spores, especially a chemical substance that kills bacterial spores. The term is commonly used in reference to substances applied to inanimate objects. Because spores are more resistant than vegetative cells, a *sporicide* might be a sterilizing agent, killing such resistant forms as amoebic cysts.

Biocide

A biocide is a substance that kills all living organisms, pathogenic and nonpathogenic.

Comment. Because a *biocide* kills spores as well as vegetative cells, it is presumably a sterilizing agent. The definition includes all species of living organisms, micro and macro, but the term is commonly used with reference to microorganisms.

Bacteriostat

A bacteriostat is an agent, usually chemical, that prevents the growth of bacteria but that does not necessarily kill them or their spores. Similarly, a *fungistat* and a *biostat* refer to the prevention of growth of fungi and of all living organisms, respectively. Sometimes the only difference as to whether a chemical is bacteriostatic or bactericidal depends on the conditions of application, such as time, temperature, or pH.

Fungitoxic

An agent is termed *fungitoxic* that inhibits but does not necessarily kill fungi. It is equivalent to the term *fungistatic*.

Antibiotic

An antibiotic is an organic chemical substance produced by microorganisms that has the capacity in dilute solutions to destroy or inhibit the growth of bacteria and other microorganisms, used most often at low concentrations in the treatment of infectious diseases of man, animals, and plants.

Sterilization

Sterilization is the act or process, physical or chemical, that destroys or eliminates all forms of life, especially microorganisms.

Comment. Because of the misuse of this term, the council on Pharmacy and Chemistry of the American Medical Association (1936) officially went on record stating that sterilization was intended to convey an absolute meaning, not a relative one. A substance cannot be partially sterile. Nevertheless, the word is still used in the partial sense, as noted by Lawrence (1968), for mechanically filtered solutions called "sterile" although, while being free of bacteria and fungi and their spores, they may contain active viruses that are not removed by the filter.

Because it cannot be known with certainty whether all microorganisms of all types have been killed because we may not even be aware of the existence of some species or have media suitable for culturing all organisms, and furthermore, because we can never prove the achievement of a negative absolute (species once claimed to be extinct occasionally turn up), it becomes more practical, as pointed out by Bruch and Bruch (1971), to employ a process definition of sterilization. By this definition, sterilization is the process by which living organisms are removed or killed to the extent that they are no longer detectable in standard culture media in which they previously have been found to proliferate. According to this definition, both the process used to achieve sterility and the methods for testing for it are equally important.

Microorganisms of the same species vary in their resistance to chemical and physical agents, and if even one of a billion organisms survives, there is the possibility of rapid multiplication and contamination of the material. Although, as stated, the term sterile implies an absolute, in practice it becomes a matter of probability whether sterility has been achieved. Different operations require different degrees of certainty of sterility, as measured by the percent reduction or number of logarithmic reductions (D values) in initial count brought about by the treatment.

Criteria of Sterilization

Thermal Death Time. The time required to kill all spores at a specified temperature.

D Value, D₁₀ Value, or Decimal Reduction Time (DRT). This value is defined as the time required to inactivate 90% of the cells present or to reduce the microbial population to one-tenth its number, that is, a one-logarithm reduction.

F Value. The F value is the time in minutes required to kill all the spores in suspension when at a temperature of 121° C or 250° F.

Z Value. The Z value is a measure of the way the D value changes with temperature for a particular organism. It may be considered the slope of the logarithm of the thermal death time against temperature. Mathematically, it is defined:

$$Z = \frac{T_2 - T_1}{\log\left(\dfrac{D_2}{D_1}\right)},$$

where T is in °F.

Q₁₀ Value. Like the Z value, the Q_{10} value is also a measure of inactivation rate with temperature. It is defined as the ratio of inactivation rate constants at two temperatures 10° C apart.

Sanitizer

A sanitizer is an agent that reduces the number of bacterial contaminants to safe levels as judged by public health requirements. It is commonly used with substances that are applied to inanimate objects.

Comment. This term is associated with the cleaning of eating and drinking utensils and dairy equipment and is restricted to cleaning operations, as in the case of a *detergent sanitizer*, which combines both cleaning and antibacterial properties. According to the official sanitizer test (See Chapter 60), a sanitizer is a chemical that kills 99.999% of the specific test bacteria in 30 seconds under the conditions of the test.

Prophylactic

A prophylactic agent is one that contributes to the prevention of infection and disease.

Comment. This word is wide in scope. It is used for rubber condoms and antiseptic lotions and may even refer to fresh air and a nutritious diet when these serve to ward off disease.

Preservation

Preservation is the process by which chemical or physical agents prevent biologic deterioration of materials.

Biologic Indicator

A biologic indicator (BI) is a preparation of microorganisms, usually bacterial spores, that is carried either directly by some of the items to be sterilized or by adventitious carriers such as filter paper, threads, and porcelain cylinders, and that serves as a challenge to the efficiency of a given sterilization process or cycle.

Soaps and Skin Preparations

Several additional terms to receive formal definition (OTC Antimicrobial I Drug Review Panel, 1974) relate to antimicrobial substances for application to the skin:

Antimicrobial Soap: A soap containing an active ingredient with in-vitro and in-vivo activity against skin microorganisms.

Health-Care Personnel Handwash: A safe, nonirritating preparation designed for frequent use that reduces the number of transient microorganisms on intact skin to an initial baseline level after adequate washing, rinsing, and drying. If the preparation contains an antimicrobial agent, it should be broad spectrum, fast acting, and, if possible, persistent.

Patient Preoperative Skin Preparation: A safe, fast-acting, broad-spectrum antimicrobial-containing preparation that significantly reduces the number of microorganisms on intact skin.

Skin Antiseptic: A safe, nonirritating, antimicrobial-containing preparation that prevents overt skin infection. Claims stating or implying an effect against microorganisms must be supported by controlled human studies that demonstrate prevention of infection.

Skin Wound Cleanser: A safe, nonirritating liquid preparation (or product to be used with water) that assists in the removal of foreign material from small superficial wounds and does not delay wound healing.

Skin Wound Protectant: A safe, nonirritating preparation applied to small cleansed wounds that provides a protective (physical and/or chemical) barrier and neither delays healing nor favors the growth of microorganisms.

Surgical Hand Scrub: A safe, nonirritating, antimicrobial-containing preparation that significantly reduces the number of microorganisms on the intact skin. A surgical hand scrub should be broad spectrum, fast acting, and persistent.

Some Other Words

Algicide: A substance that kills algae; unicellular chlorophyll-containing plants.

Antimicrobial Agent: Any agent that kills or suppresses the growth of microorganisms.

Asepsis: Prevention from contamination with microorganisms. Includes sterile conditions in tissues, on materials, and in rooms, as obtained by exclusion, removing, or killing organisms.

Bioburden: The excess microbiologic load, that is, the number of contaminating organisms in the product prior to sterilization. For example, it will be more difficult to sterilize a product heavily loaded with spores than one lightly loaded.

Biodeterioration: The deterioration of valuable materials due to biological activity. The vectors are usually microbiological but may be insects, rodents, or higher animals or plants. Deterioration may be due to the breakdown of the material, biodegeneration, as in decay of timber, or it may be due to aesthetic depreciation, as in staining of works of art.

Chemisterilant: A chemical used to kill all microorganisms, including spores.

Chemitherapeutant: A chemical used inside the body that kills or suppresses microorganisms to control disease, as for example, quinine taken for malaria control or sulfadrugs for various microbial diseases.

Contamination: The introduction of microorganisms into tissues or sterile materials.

Decontamination: Disinfection or sterilization of infected articles to make them suitable for use.

Degerming Agent: A disinfecting agent.

Disinfestation: Extermination or destruction of insects, rodents, or other animal forms that transmit disease, which may be on a person, his belongings, his clothing, or his surroundings.

Fumigation: Exposure of an area or object to disinfecting fumes.

Inactivation: Removal of the activity of microorganisms by killing or inhibiting reproduction or enzyme activity. When referring to an antimicrobial agent, inactivation means neutralizing its activity by any means.

Ovicide: A substance that kills the eggs of very small infectious animals, such as the eggs of tapeworms.

Pasteurization: A process developed by Louis Pasteur of heating milk, wine, or other liquids to around 60°C for about 30 minutes to significantly reduce or kill the number of pathogenic and spoilage organisms.

Pathogen: Any disease-producing microorganism. In current circumstances in which drugs, radiation, or AIDS may cause immunosuppression, the distinction between pathogens and nonpathogens may no longer be significant.

Planktonic: Describes growth of microbiological organisms dispersed in solution, as in the case of free-swimming plankton.

Prions: Little-understood virus-like infectious agents that cause serious diseases of man and animals. Prions are thought to differ from viruses by containing neither DNA or RNA, only protein. They are extremely resistant to inactivation by heat and disinfecting agents.

Sessile: Describes growth of microorganisms growing attached to a body, not freely dispersed in planktonic growth.

Tyndallization: A process of heat treatment for killing microorganisms by which the treated material is heated to less than sterilization temperatures then allowed to cool and stand to incubate any spores that would germinate. This process is successively repeated for several days to destroy all vegetative forms and germinated spores.

Viroids: Virus-like infectious agents that produce diseases in higher plants. They differ from true viruses in that they are believed to contain no protein, only low-molecular-weight ribonucleic acid.

Origin of Terms

It might be of interest to examine the origin of a few of the terms we use now that we have considered their meanings. One will find that the terms follow closely the history of disinfection, which is presented in Chapter 1. Some are as old as the English language; others are quite recent. The word disinfectant was first recorded in writing in 1598, with the meaning "to cure, to heale," but in 1658 it was used in the more modern sense, to remove infection: "They use to make great fires, where there is household stuffe of men that died of the Pestilence to dis-infect them." (See the *Oxford English Dictionary*, OED, 1989, for references to quotations in this section.) In those days it was believed that contagious diseases arose from effluvia, a flowing-out of invisible particles from the diseased person or corpse, or from miasmas, which were noxious disease-bearing exhalations from putrefying organic matter emanating from damp, unhealthful places like malarial swamps. Miasmas were referred to in medical writing as early as 1665. The word *disease*, coming from the French, meaning absence of ease, or discomfort, appeared in English about 1330 and was used by Chaucer in 1386. Chaucer was aware of the spread of infection by such means as coughing, for in 1386 he wrote, "Hoold cloos thy mouth . . . Thy cursed breeth infecte wole us alle." (Hold closed your mouth . . . your cursed breath will infect us all.) The word *antiseptic* is credited to John Pringle, whose experiments in 1750 are described in Chapter 1. He was familiar with the word *septic,* first recorded in 1605, which means putrefying. As a physician, he had written "The miasma or septic ferment being received into the blood," and when he found chemicals that prevented putrefaction, the word *antiseptic* was generated.

Although Leeuwenhoek first saw bacteria in 1676, the term was not recorded in use until 1847 to 1849. Leeuwenhoek just referred to "the little animals" or, in English, *animalcules,* a term first recorded in 1599 to refer to any small animal and in 1677 to mean those seen only under the microscope. It should be recognized that the terms discussed in this section may have been in oral use much earlier, but the written record gives the only dates that can be depended upon. After bacteria, we find Tyndall using the adjective *bactericidal* in 1878; *bactericide* follows in 1884, the year that the word *bacteriology* appeared: "Permanganate of potash is not a bactericide of great activity," but by 1894 we see that "A solution of formaldehyde appears to be a very powerful bactericide."

The familiar word *microbe* did not arise by spontaneous generation, despite the strong belief by many respectable scientists in that mechanism of origin of microorganisms. It was the invention of the French surgeon, Charles Sédillot, an admirer of Pasteur and one of the first French physicians to apply Lister's antiseptic method. He wanted a word that would include bacteria and all the other tiny organisms that could be seen only with the microscope. The philologists criticized the word because its Greek root suggested an animal with a short life rather than an infinitesimally small animal. But with terminology for the tiny creatures in an uncertain state, with terms like *bacteridites* being used, Pasteur adopted the term and it was accepted worldwide. It was in 1878 that Sédillot presented his paper with the new word. By 1880 we had *microorganism*, by 1885 *microbiologist* and *microbiocide* in *Science* and *The British Medical Journal*, respectively, and the field of *microbiology* in 1888 in *Popular Science Monthly.* The adjective *microbiocidal* didn't arrive until 1897.

The word *fungus* goes back much further, because mushrooms and other fungi didn't require a microscope to be seen. Fungus, spelled *fungous*, first appeared in the English language in 1420 and was used as a human infection in 1674 to 1677. The word *fungicide*, however, didn't show up until 1889, when it appeared in *The Voice*, a New York City newspaper. It is probable that earlier use in technical publications was not uncovered by the OED researchers. As in the case of *bactericidal*, the adjective *germicidal*, in a medical journal, preceded in 1880 the noun *germicide*, in 1881, in the London *Times*. The word *germ*, in relation to a smallpox infection, was printed in 1803. *Germifuge* is listed in one medical dictionary as an obsolete term for disinfectant, but I could find no reference to its actual use.

In reading an article on disinfection written in the early 1800s I was surprised to see the word *virus* used in connection with a disease. This was many years before bacteria were known to cause disease, and viruses could not even have been seen with the microscope. On looking into the matter I discovered that virus was the Latin word for poison and was used, as such, as early as 1599. Its use eventually became more restricted to a substance related to contagious disease, as in the 1728 description, "a corrosive or contagious pus." In 1880 Pasteur stated, "The virus is a microscopic parasite which may be multiplied by cultivation outside the body of an animal." The adjective *virucidal* was first noted in 1925, and to our surprise the OED does not contain the word *virucide*. The term *biocide*, to mean destruction of tissues of the human, was first recorded in 1947, and in 1963 Rachel Carson used biocide in her book *Silent Spring* to mean "genocide." In 1968, at a biodeterioration symposium, it was finally used in the way we define it, as referring principally to microorganisms, being a sterilizing agent. *Sterilization*, as in "Sterilization by heat or organic liquids," was written in 1874, but the word *sterile* did not appear until 1877; in 1891 the steam *sterilizer* was mentioned in print. *Antibiotic* did not come into use until after penicillin, appearing in *Lancet* in 1944. The term *sanitizer* appeared first in the *Journal of Milk and Food Technology* in 1950. The second mention of *sanitizer* listed by the OED was in 1968 and referred to the first edition of this book, where Chapter 4 gave methods for testing sanitizers and bacteriostatic substances. Thus, this book not only records the history of disinfection but itself has become part of that history.

REFERENCES

American Medical Association, 1936. Report of the Council on Pharmacy and Chemistry. Use of the terms "sterile," "sterilize," and "sterilization." JAMA, 107, 38.

American Public Health Association, 1950. *The Control of Communicable Diseases in Man.* 7th Edition. p.11.

Bruch, C.W., and Bruch, M.K. 1971. Sterilization. In *Husa's Pharmaceutical Dispensing,* Edited by E.W. Martin. Easton, Pa., Mack Publishing Co., pp. 592–623.

Dorland's Illustrated Medical Dictionary, 24th Edition. 1969. Philadelphia, W.B. Saunders Co.

Federal Food, Drug, and Cosmetic Act. 1938. Chapter II. Sec. 201, par. (0).

Fraser, J.A.L. 1987. Novel applications of peracetic acid in industrial disinfection. Specialty Chemicals, 7(3), 178, 180, 182, 184, 186.

Garner, J.S. and Favero, M.S. 1986. Guideline for handwashing and hospital environmental control, 1985. Am. J. Infect. Control, *14*, 110–126.

Lawrence, C.A. 1968. In *Disinfection, Sterilization, and Preservation*. 1st Edition. Edited by C.A. Lawrence and S.S. Block. Philadelphia, Lea & Febiger, pp. 10–11.

OTC Antimicrobial I Drug Review Panel. 1974. Food and Drug Administration. OTC topic antimicrobial products and drug and cosmetic products. Fed. Register, *39*, (179), 33114.

Oxford English Dictionary. 2nd Edition. 1989. Oxford, Clarendon Press.

Patterson, A.M. 1932. Meaning of antiseptic, disinfectant, and related words. Am. J. Public Health, *22*, 465–472.

Reddish, G.F. 1957. *Antiseptics, Disinfectants, Fungicides and Chemical and Physical Sterilization*. 2nd Edition. Philadelphia, Lea & Febiger, pp. 23–29.

Richards, J.W. 1968. Introduction to industrial sterilization. London, Academic Press, pp. 67–75.

Rutala, W. 1990. APIC Guideline for selection and use of disinfectants, APIC, 1990. Am. J. Infect. Control, *58*, 99–117.

Spaulding, E.H. 1968. Chemical disinfection of medical and surgical materials. In *Disinfection, Sterilization, and Preservation*. Edited by C.A. Lawrence, and S.S. Block, Philadelphia, Lea & Febiger, pp. 517–531.

PART II

Fundamental Principles
of Activity

CHAPTER 3

PRINCIPLES OF ANTIMICROBIAL ACTIVITY

A.D. Russell

Antimicrobial agents may be of several different types, either physical or chemical or, sometimes, a combination of the two. Table 3–1 depicts the various processes that are available. Several physical processes such as moist heat, dry heat, and ionizing radiations generally can be relied upon to kill all types of microorganisms, including bacterial spores, and thus will achieve sterilization. Temperatures well below 100°C may be of value in pasteurization or in the preparation of certain bacterial vaccines when the aim is to inactivate all the cells without affecting their antigenic identity. Ultraviolet (UV) radiation can kill spores but is considered a surface sterilizer only, and it thus effects disinfection rather than sterilization. Hydrostatic pressure is a method that uses the high pressures exerted by liquids on bacterial spores and other microorganisms. Some organisms, the so-called slow-growing viruses, are highly resistant to physical and chemical processes (Russell, 1990a).

Of the chemical agents, some are used as disinfectants and others as antiseptics, whereas some find uses as preservatives for pharmaceuticals, cosmetics, or foods. Borick (1968) introduced the term "chemosterilizer" to denote a substance that possesses sporicidal activity. It is true, of course, that many chemical agents act as sporicides, for example, glutaraldehyde (pentanedial), formaldehyde (methanal), hypochlorites, and ethylene oxide. Their activity against bacterial spores is often slow, however, and is influenced by many factors (Russell, 1982a,b) such as the condition of the spores (present in liquid suspension or dried onto test objects), the concentration and pH of the agent, and the presence of organic matter. With ethylene oxide, an additional consideration is the relative humidity of the environment or, perhaps more accurately, the microenvironmental water content. The general term "biocide" is used to denote a chemical that possesses antiseptic, disinfectant, or preservative activity.

Chemotherapeutic agents are those that are used orally or systemically for the treatment of microbial infections of man and animals. The most important agents are antibiotics together with synthetic compounds, such as those listed in Table 3–1, which may be used for their antibacterial, antifungal, or antiviral properties.

Methods of potentiating the activity of an agent are obviously important. The activity of most compounds increases with an increase in temperature (Russell, 1982a, 1989; Russell and Hugo, 1987), and in the United Kingdom, a process of heating with a bactericide was until recently employed for many years as one method of sterilizing certain parenteral and eye preparations. Ultrasonic radiation has been shown to increase the sporicidal activity of glutaraldehyde (Boucher, 1979) and of hydrogen peroxide (Ahmed and Russell, 1975). Attention has also focused on the process of thermoradiation, which is the simultaneous use of ionizing radiation and high temperatures. In the field of chemotherapy, β-lactamase-producing bacteria have posed a considerable problem, and consequently, the development of β-lactamase inhibitors such as clavulanic acid is an important advance (Cole, 1980; Fisher and Knowles, 1980; Reading and Cole, 1986).

The response of microorganisms to adverse agents depends on the type of organism, the agent itself, and the intensity (e.g., concentration of a chemical, temperature of exposure, radiation dose) and duration of exposure of the cells. In bacterio- or fungistasis, reversible inhibition of growth and multiplication can be achieved by restoring the organism to favorable conditions. Organisms injured but not killed by a particular process may be able to repair the damage inflicted on them, and such damaged cells may pose a problem, e.g., in the design of sterilization and disinfection processes, in their detection and enumeration, and as a health hazard in processed foods. The subject is considered in greater detail by Andrew and Russell (1984). In particular, the contributions by Gould (1984), Gilbert (1984), Moseley (1984), and Waites and Bayliss (1984) are worthy of further attention. It may also be necessary to use an appropriate antagonist or neutralizing agent (inactivator, inactivating agent, neutralizer, antidote) to distinguish between a lethal effect

Table 3–1. *Types of Antimicrobial Processes*

Type of Process	Agent	Application	Comments
Physical	Dry heat (160°C or higher)	Sterilization	Less effective than moist heat
	Moist heat (121°C or higher)	Sterilization	Use of autoclave
	Moist heat (below 100°C)	Disinfection	Inactivation of bacterial cells (56°C) in vaccine production
	Cold/freezing	Preservation	See text
	Ionizing radiation	Sterilization	
	Ultraviolet radiation	Disinfection	Considered a surface sterilizer only
	Hydrostatic pressure	Disinfection(?)	Activity dependent on concentration and temperature
Chemical (vapor phase)	Ethylene oxide Propylene oxide Formaldehyde β-propiolactone	Disinfection	Ethylene oxide also used as sterilizing agent Possible carcinogenic activity of β-propiolactone
Chemical (low selectivity)	Acids and esters, alcohols, aldehydes and aldehyde-releasing agents, halogens (including chlorine-releasing agents), metals, phenols and cresols, quaternary ammonium compounds, biguanides	Disinfection or preservation	Glutaraldehyde (pentanedial): has been considered a "chemosterilizer" Quaternary ammonium compounds: also used as antiseptics Chlorhexidine salts are important antiseptics, disinfectants, and preservatives
Chemical (moderate selectivity)	Antibiotics (bacitracin and polymyxins)	Topical chemotherapy	Injectable polymyxins also available (nephrotoxic)
	Dyes (acridines, triphenyl methane)	Antisepsis	
	Metal chelate complexes	Antisepsis	
	Organic arsenic compounds	Chemotherapy	
	Organic mercury compounds	Preservation or antisepsis	Important pharmaceutical preservatives
	Silver compounds	Application to wounds	Effective against *Pseudomonas aeruginosa*
Chemical (high selectivity)	Synthetic antibacterial agents (*p*-aminosalicylic acid, isonicotinic acid hydrazine, sulfonamides, trimethoprim, metronidazole, 4-quinolone derivatives)	Chemotherapy	
	Synthetic antifungal agents (imidazole derivatives)	Chemotherapy	
	Synthetic antiviral agents (amantadine, idoxuridine, cytarabine, acyclovir, zidovudine (azidothymidine, AZT))	Chemotherapy	
	Antibacterial antibiotics (aminoglycoside-aminocyclitol, chloramphenicol, β-lactams, β-lactamase inhibitors, lincomycins, macrolides, rifamycins, tetracyclines)	Chemotherapy	Widely used in treating various types of bacterial infections.
	Antifungal antibiotics (griseofulvin, amphotericin, nystatin, imidazoles)	Chemotherapy	Comparatively few agents available
Other	Bacterial vaccines and toxoids Viral vaccines Rickettsial vaccines	Prophylaxis	
	Antisera	Therapy	
	Antiviral protein (interferon)	Chemotherapy	Possible highly significant role in near future
Combined processes	Heat + chemical	Sterilization	Method until recently used in U.K. to sterilize certain injections and eyedrops
	Irradiation + chemical	Sterilization	
	Thermoradiation	Sterilization	Use of lowered radiation dose in combination with substerilizing temperature
	Heat + hydrostatic pressure	Sterilization(?)	
	Chemical + ultrasonics	Sterilization(?)	

and mere inhibition in cells exposed to disinfectants, antiseptics, preservatives, or antibiotics. The theoretic principles in using neutralizing agents have been fully discussed by Russell et al. (1979) and a more practical orientation presented by Russell (1981). Table 3–2 summarizes the uses of neutralizing agents and comments on any particular problems, such as the unwanted toxicity some such agents have for some types of microorganisms. Moreover, in some instances (e.g., mercury and -SH compounds, sulfonamides, and p-aminobenzoic acid), the chemical nature of the neutralizing agent may provide a clue to the mechanism of action of the inhibitor.

SELECTIVE TOXICITY

Selective activity is defined as injury to one kind of living organism without harming another that is intimately associated with it (Albert, 1979). The principle of selective toxicity is used in agriculture, pharmacology, and diagnostic microbiology, but its most dramatic application is the systemic chemotherapy of infectious disease.

Selective action against microorganisms is based on differences in the cell physiology of the parasite and the mammalian host. Despite the general similarity of nutritional requirements, enzyme composition, and nucleic acid structure among all forms of life, there are many differences between microbes and man, especially in the processes of cell synthesis. Energy-yielding processes do not offer the same possibilities for selective toxicity. Chemicals that inhibit a particular step in a metabolic pathway that is vital to the parasite, but that does not occur or is not accessible in the cells of the host, exhibit selective toxicity. The treatment of bacterial infections is more successful than that of viral disease because viruses depend on many enzymes of the host cell for their replication.

The requirement for selective toxicity increases from disinfectants, which are used only on inanimate surfaces, through skin disinfectants and wound antiseptics, to systemic chemotherapeutic agents. A high degree of selective toxicity may be associated with a narrow antimicrobial spectrum and with the emergence of drug-resistant organisms.

CELLULAR TARGETS OF ANTIMICROBIAL ACTION

It is not easy to elucidate the exact mechanism of action of a chemical agent or physical process. The reason for this is that more than one cell constituent may be affected, and consequently the problem is to distinguish

Table 3–2. *Agents That Neutralize Antimicrobial Compounds**

Inhibitor (Antimicrobial Compound)	Neutralizing Agent	Comment
Aldehydes	Dilution to subinhibitory level; glycine better	Sodium sulfite not recommended (may itself be toxic)
Phenolics	Dilution to subinhibitory level	Tween 80 is possible alternative
Organic acids and their esters	Dilution to subinhibitory level	Tween 80 is possible alternative
Acridines	Nucleic acid or nucleotide	Satisfactory?
Hydrogen peroxide	Catalase	Rapid effect
Mercury compounds	-SH compounds	Possible toxicity of sodium thioglycollate
Alcohols	Dilution to subinhibitory level	
Quaternary ammonium compounds, biguanides	Letheen broth (or agar); Lecithin + Lubrol W	
Tego compounds	Tween 80	
EDTA and related chelating agents	Dilution	Mg^{++} useful
Hypochlorites, iodine	Sodium thiosulfate	Staphylococci may be sensitive to thiosulfate
Streptomycin	Nutrient broth—sodium chloride	See Kogut and Carrier (1980)
Chloramphenicol	Chloramphenicol acetyltransferase	
Tetracyclines	Mg^{++}?	
β-Lactam antibiotics	Appropriate β-lactamase	"Broad-spectrum" β-lactamases available
Trimethoprim	Thymidine	Thymine much less active
Sulfonamides	p-Aminobenzoic acid	

*Membrane filtration may be alternative method.

Data from Russell, A.D., Ahonkai, I., and Rogers, D.T. 1979. Microbiological applications of the inactivation of antibiotics and other antimicrobial agents. J. Appl. Bacteriol., 46, 207–245; Russell, A.D. 1981. Neutralization procedures in the evaluation of bactericidal activity. In *Disinfectants. Their Use and Evaluation of Effectiveness.* Edited by C.H. Collins, M.C. Allwood, S.F. Bloomfield, and A. Fox. Society for Applied Bacteriology Technical Series No. 16. New York, Academic Press, pp. 45–59; Russell, A.D., Furr, J.R., and Rogers, D.T. 1984. Laboratory uses of antibiotic-inactivating enzymes. J. Antimicrob. Chemother., 14, 567–570.

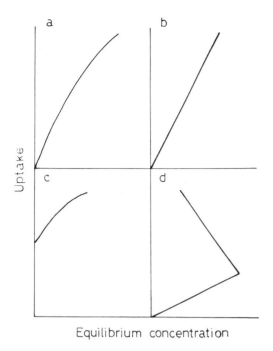

Fig. 3–1. Examples of adsorption isotherms: *a*, L-pattern; *b*, C-pattern; *c*, H-pattern; and *d*, Z-pattern.

The determination of the binding or uptake (Fig. 3–1) of an antimicrobial agent by microbial cells or their components is a necessary part of any attempt to elucidate its mechanism of action. The basic principles are (1) the addition of the drug to the potential binding materials; (2) the separation of bound from unbound drug, and (3) the assay of the free and/or bound drug. When an unlabeled compound is used, it is usually necessary to use thick suspensions of binding material to detect the amount bound. Sensitivity can be increased by the use of a radioactive drug, and the higher the specific activity, the greater the sensitivity. Initial studies are usually carried out with whole cells, but investigations of the interaction of certain compounds with cellular fractions have also been rewarding, e.g., (1) the interaction of acridines, triphenylmethane dyes, and mitomycins with DNA, and (2) the binding of aminoglycoside antibiotics to bacterial ribosomes (or 30S or 50S subribosomal units). More recently, the detection of penicillin-binding proteins (PBPs; see later section) in *Escherichia coli* and other bacteria and the interaction of various β-lactam antibiotics with these PBPs has furthered understanding of the morphologic changes induced in bacteria by these antibiotics (Spratt, 1980).

Cell envelope mutants, with defects in the lipopolysaccharide core and especially the protein components of the outer membrane of gram-negative bacteria (including *Neisseria gonorrhoeae*) have yielded useful information about the reasons for bacterial resistance (Nikaido and Nakae, 1979; Hancock, 1984; Nikaido and Vaara, 1985; Russell and Chopra, 1990). These studies, coupled with those involving changes in target sites, e.g., alteration in PBPs or ribosomes and enzymes, provide additional knowledge about the overall mechanism of an action of an agent.

the primary effect from the secondary effects, which may, however, contribute to cell death. In general, the most useful information is obtained by studying the effects of low concentrations of a drug, or the effects of a low radiation dose or short exposure time at a particular temperature, on the organism being tested. For example, when heated at temperatures of 50° to 60°C, *Staphylococcus aureus* leaks amino acids, K$^+$, and 260-nm-absorbing material, whereas at much higher temperatures (100°C), protein coagulation is a complicating issue (Allwood and Russell, 1970). Similarly, low concentrations of chlorhexidine induce leakage of intracellular materials; at high (bactericidal) concentrations, however, leakage is reduced as a result of intracellular precipitation (Hugo and Longworth, 1966; Longworth, 1971; Hugo, 1982).

Information as to the cellular target can be obtained in various ways, which can be summarized as follows (Russell et al., 1973). Drug treatment of cells under conditions of growth (e.g., in broth) or nongrowth (use of washed suspensions) indicates whether the test substance inhibits some biosynthetic process, in which case nongrowing cells will be unaffected. Further preliminary experiments can then be carried out to determine whether the agent inhibits synthesis of the cell wall, protein, ribonucleic acid (RNA), or deoxyribonucleic acid (DNA). Other useful experiments include studies on the possible lytic potency of the test drug and on the leakage of low-molecular-weight materials; in the latter context, proton flux across the cytoplasmic membrane should now be an indisputable experimental technique (Harold et al., 1974; Hugo, 1976a and b, 1982; Russell and Hugo, 1988) and is considered in a later section.

EFFECTS OF PHYSICAL AGENTS ON MICROORGANISMS

The most important physical agents are those described in Table 3–1. Ionizing radiation is a process in which electrons are stripped from the atoms of the material through which the radiation passes, whereas UV radiation possesses insufficient energy to eject an electron, and instead causes excitation of the atoms. UV is not, therefore, an ionizing radiation. Both types of radiation damage DNA, although again, the nature of the damage is different.

Thermal processes involve heating in the presence (e.g., autoclaving) or absence (dry heat) of moisture. Bacterial spores are much more resistant to both processes than are vegetative bacteria, and the possible reasons for this are considered later in this section. At the other extreme, cold (especially freezing and freeze-drying) can have deleterious effects on microorganisms.

Hydrostatic pressure is believed to induce germination of spores and then to kill the germinated cell.

Ionizing Radiation

Types of ionizing radiation are x-rays, γ-rays, high-speed electrons (β-rays), protons and α-rays (positively charged helium atoms). In practice, β-rays and especially γ-rays (usually produced from a ^{60}Co source) are used; α-particles are charged and heavy and have little penetrating power.

Bacterial spores are generally more resistant than nonsporulating bacteria to ionizing radiations. The most resistant organism found to date, however, is the gram-positive coccus *Deinococcus (Micrococcus) radiodurans*, which possesses an efficient repair process for both ionizing and ultraviolet radiations (Bridges, 1976; Moseley and Williams, 1977; Moseley, 1984, 1988).

Ionizing radiation is believed to exert its effect by bringing about single-strand or double-strand breakages in DNA, the latter being more lethal (Pollard, 1969; Pollard and Davis, 1970; Goldblith, 1971; Davies, 1976).

Several reasons have been given for the comparatively high resistance of bacterial spores. These include the presence of radioprotective substances in the spore coat (an explanation that is now discounted), the water content of the spore, the possible differences in the DNA of spores and nonsporing cells, and the ability of damaged cells to repair damage (Tallentire, 1970). Single-strand scission in spores has been shown to be repaired during postirradiation germination (Terano et al., 1969), but this rejoining is not inhibited by chloramphenicol, an inhibitor of protein synthesis during outgrowth (Terano et al., 1971). According to Durban et al. (1974), a highly radiation-resistant strain of *Clostridium botulinum* can rejoin single-strand breaks in DNA under nonphysiologic conditions at 0°C and in the absence of germination. Such repair of single-strand breaks within these dormant, ungerminated spores may result from DNA ligase activity. Irradiation injury is manifest as an inability of spores to outgrow or as an increased sensitivity to environmental stresses at the outgrowth stages. Irradiated spores are capable of initiating germination and swelling (Russell, 1982 and 1984; Gould, 1984).

Ultraviolet Radiation

Ultraviolet (UV) radiation has a wavelength range between about 328 and 210 nm, with maximal bactericidal activity near the wavelength (260 nm) of peak absorption of DNA. This point is important when one considers that DNA is the target of the action of UV radiation (Moseley, 1988).

Bacterial spores are generally more resistant to UV light than are vegetative cells, although, as with ionizing radiation, *Deinococcus radiodurans* is the most resistant organism. The possible reasons for this are discussed in the following.

When nonsporing bacteria are exposed to UV light, thymine dimers are formed between adjacent thymine molecules in the same strand of DNA (Fig. 3–2). Other dimers may also be formed, such as a uracil-thymine heterodimer. The induction of dimers is sufficient to explain the lethal nature of UV radiation. Some bacteria, however, are capable of repairing this damage, and this property is most highly developed in *Deinococcus radiodurans* (Howard-Flanders, 1973; Bridges, 1976; Witkin, 1976). In *E. coli*, most of the inducible genes that code for DNA repair proteins are members of either (1) the SOS network, a term used to describe the physiologic changes after UV radiation (or other DNA-damaging treatment), and controlled by RecA and LexA proteins; or (2) the adaptive response network, controlled by the Ada protein (Walker, 1985; Moseley, 1988). LexA is a *repressor* of every SOS gene so far identified. Exposure of cells to UV light or to a treatment interfering with DNA replication generates an inducing signal that is responsible for activating RecA molecules.

Repair mechanisms existing in *E. coli* are (1) photoreactivation; (2) excision repair; (3) postreplication recombination repair; and (4) error-prone repair (see Moseley, 1984, 1988).

In the frozen state, strains of various types of nonsporing bacteria are usually supersensitive to UV light (Ashwood-Smith and Bridges, 1967). An exception is *Deinococcus radiodurans*. Photoreactivating light is ineffective following irradiation at −79°C. When bacterial spores are exposed to UV light, thymine-containing photoproducts accumulate that are different from the cyclobutane-type thymine dimers found in vegetative cells (Fig. 3–2) (Donnellan and Setlow, 1965). The spore photoproduct, 5-thyminyl-5,6-dihydrothymine (TDHT) (Fig. 3–3) (Varghese, 1970) is identical to that found in frozen, UV-irradiated nonsporing bacteria, described previously, and cannot be removed by photoreactivation.

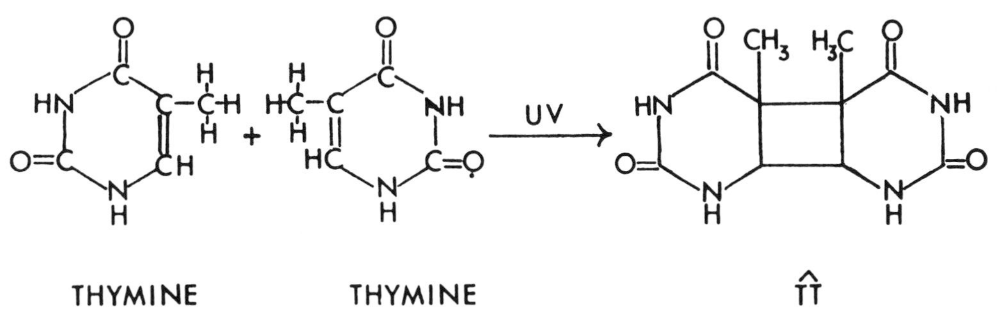

Fig. 3–2.   Formation of thymine dimers (T̂T) in the DNA of irradiated nonsporulating bacteria.

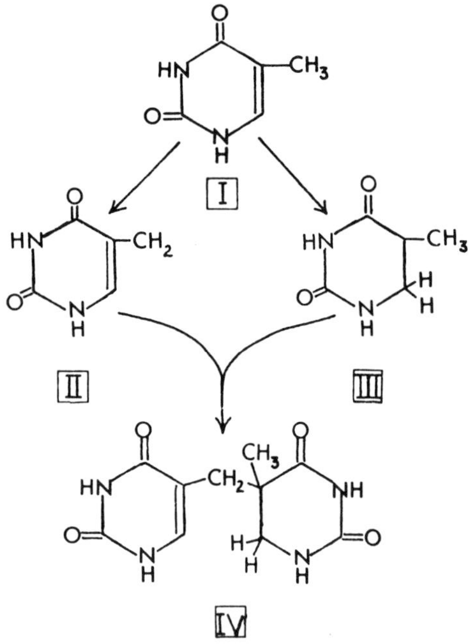

Fig. 3–3. Postulated formation of thymine photoproducts in the DNA of ultraviolet-irradiated bacterial spores. I, Thymine; II, thyminyl radical; III, thymyl radical; IV, 5-thyminyl-5,6-dihydrothymine (TDHT).

Bacterial spores themselves do not seem capable of removing TDHT. Nevertheless, it has been found that UV-sensitive mutants of UV-resistant spores form the same spore photoproduct (TDHT) and to the same extent for a given radiation dose as the parent (resistant) spores. It may thus be inferred that resistance to UV radiation is linked to the ability to remove TDHT (Munakata and Rupert, 1972). Elimination of TDHT has been shown to occur early during germination or during further development towards the vegetative cell (Munakata and Rupert, 1974).

Moist Heat

Surprisingly, the precise manner in which bacteria and their spores are killed on exposure to water or steam at high temperatures remains to be elucidated. When suspensions of nonsporing bacteria are heated, several changes occur in the cells (Allwood and Russell, 1970; Tomlins and Ordal, 1976; Welker, 1976; Hurst, 1984). These include leakage of low-molecular-weight material, RNA and DNA breakdown, protein coagulation, and alterations in the appearance of the cell itself. In *S. aureus*, Mg^{2+} is lost from wall teichoic acid and a mutant lacking teichoic acid is more sensitive than the parent. In *E. coli*, structural damage occurs to the outer membrane, and the cells become more sensitive to selective agents. Ribosomes from heat-injured cells of *Salmonella typhimurium* or *Staphylococcus aureus* have a sedimentation coefficient of 47S, with no 30S particles. Ribosomal RNA (rRNA) from heat-injured cells of *S. typhimurium* suffers complete degradation of the 23S species. Single- and double-strand breaks in DNA have been reported in

Escherichia coli cells held at 52°C, similar to those induced by ionizing radiation. The possibility of the same repair processes being involved in the recovery from both types of damage has been considered (Tomlins and Ordal, 1976).

DNA repair-deficient mutants of *E. coli* are more heat sensitive than the wild type. Cell revival appears to be related to repair of DNA breaks and is inhibited by inhibitors of DNA synthesis. Furthermore, mild heating causes an increase in mutation frequency.

During heating at 50°C, *E. coli* can synthesize a small number of proteins, the "heat-shock" proteins, which may demonstrate the cells' capacity to express new information that might be needed to repair the multitarget damage induced by moist heat (Pellon and Sinskey, 1984).

When bacterial spores are lethally heated, intracellular constituents are released and there is a progressive loss of dipicolinic acid (DPA) and calcium, the rate of release being temperature dependent (Rode and Foster, 1960). It would appear that viability loss precedes DPA leakage (Warth, 1980), and consequently, leakage cannot be considered a primary effect.

DPA might have a role to play, however, in the resistance of bacterial spores to inactivation by moist heat. Thus, it has been shown that higher growth temperatures enhance the thermal resistance of spores, and that the ratio of total cation content to DPA content increases with increasing growth temperature (Lechowich and Ordal, 1962). Murrell and Warth (1965) found that the heat resistance of spores was related directly to their Ca content and inversely to their Mg content. In species with more than a 700-fold range in heat resistance, there was only a small range in DPA content. Thus, DPA does not appear to be directly involved in the heat-resistant mechanism, although it might contribute by reducing or preventing thermally induced denaturation of proteins (Mishiro and Ochi, 1966). DPA is located in the spore core (Leanz and Gilvarg, 1973), as is almost all the spore calcium, magnesium, and manganese (Stewart et al., 1980).

The role of DPA in heat resistance, however, still remains the subject of conjecture. DPA-less mutants have been described, a mutant of *Bacillus cereus* T being heat-sensitive, while the mutant of *B. subtilis* strain 168 is as thermoresistant as the wild-type strain (Zytkovicz and Halvorson, 1972). Balassa et al. (1979) have observed a direct relationship between DPA content and resistance in a mutant of *B. subtilis* that produces heat-sensitive spores.

The water content of the spore is likely to be a controlling factor in its sensitivity to moist heat. Lewis et al. (1960) proposed that the water content of the protoplast is reduced by a mechanical contraction of the cortex about the protoplast (the "contractile cortex" theory). In an alternative "expanded cortex" theory, an osmoregulatory hypothesis predicts that germinating spores heated in high concentrations of the nonpenetrating solute, sucrose, regain their heat resistance because of the decrease in water content of the cell. This theory also assumes a low water content of the spore core (see also Algie, 1983) brought about initially during the sporulation process by osmotic dehydration by the mother cell, which is then maintained in the mature spore by electronegative peptidoglycan and positively charged counterions in the cortex (Gould and Dring, 1975; Lewis, 1975; Gould, 1983, 1984, 1985).

Warth (1978, 1985) has proposed an alternative theory for the high heat resistance of spores. This envisages an anisotropic cortex, in which layers parallel to the surface are in tension, so the swelling pressure is confined to a radial, as opposed to uniform, direction.

Maintenance of the integrity of the cortex, by whatever means, is essential for the heat resistance of spores because removal of exosporium (if present) and of coats has no effect on heat resistance, whereas additional removal of cortex produces heat-sensitive protoplasts.

The thermoresistance of spores depends on three factors affecting the protoplast (Gerhardt, 1988): (1) dehydration; (2) mineralization, heat resistance decreasing if spores are demineralized and regained if remineralized; and (3) thermal adaptation, because spores of a given species are most resistant when grown at maximum temperatures. Of these three factors, however, dehydration predominates.

Dry Heat

Heat in the absence of moisture is a much less efficient process than moist heat, and thus, much higher temperatures for longer periods of time must be used in practice.

Destruction of microorganisms by dry heat has been considered primarily an oxidation process (Sykes, 1965). If this were true, one would expect bacterial spores heated in oxygen to be more sensitive to dry heat than when heated in the presence of other gases. The results of Pheil et al. (1967), who obtained D values (minutes) of 1.40, 1.46, 1.47, 1.63, and 1.96 for *Bacillus subtilis* spores heated in carbon dioxide, air, oxygen, helium, and nitrogen, respectively, indicate that this hypothesis is not necessarily true. Consequently, although oxidation may play an important part in the destruction of microorganisms, other possibilities must also be considered.

An effect on DNA is one such possibility (Russell, 1982b). Sublethal temperatures have been shown to induce mutants in *B. subtilis* spores (Zamenhof, 1960) as a result of depurination (Northrop and Slepecky, 1967), and Molin (1977) claims that the dry-heat sensitivity of spores could result from the genetically determined differences in the water content, or in the water-retaining capacity, of the spores. The water content of spores is, in fact, an important factor in determining their inactivation by dry heat. Rowe and Silverman (1970) have postulated that only a relatively small amount of water is needed to protect the heat-sensitive site in spores, and that dry-heat resistance depends mainly on the location of water, rather than the amount, in the spore, together with the nature of its association with other molecules.

Inactivation by Cold

Growth of microorganisms slows down and eventually stops if they are exposed to reduced temperatures. Some microorganisms can grow at temperatures approaching 0°C; these are termed "psychrophilic" and may be important as food-spoilage organisms (Russell and Fuller, 1979). Environmental factors such as nutrient status, pH, and water activity can alter the minimum growth temperature (Ingram and Mackey, 1976). Differences between mesophiles and psychrophiles at near-zero temperatures might be related to differences in membrane composition (Hagen, 1971).

Cold shock refers to a process in which organisms are suddenly chilled without freezing, and cell death has been shown to occur with gram-positive and gram-negative bacteria, but not with yeasts (MacLeod and Calcott, 1976; Rose, 1976). Several factors influence the response of cells, notably, the age of culture, because exponential-phase (but not stationary-phase) cultures are susceptible to cold shock. Likewise, the composition of the medium is an important factor, and various divalent cations protect the cells against chilling. Low-molecular-weight materials are released from chilled cells as a consequence of an increase in the permeability of the bacterial cell membrane, which in turn occurs because of a phase transition in membrane lipids (Rose, 1976).

A modification of this treatment is cold osmotic shock, in which bacteria are suspended in a hypertonic sucrose solution containing EDTA and are then resuspended in ice-cold magnesium chloride solution. This treatment does not cause death of the cells but does induce the release of periplasmic enzymes, including β-lactamases, from gram-negative bacteria. The procedure, with appropriate modifications, has also been used in preparing outer membranes of some gram-negative organisms.

Another aspect of inactivation by low temperatures must be mentioned, namely, freezing and thawing. Membrane damage occurs, as evidenced by the leakage of intracellular materials and the increased penetrability into cells of certain compounds that are normally excluded. Damage to the outer membrane of the cell envelope has also been shown, because frozen and thawed cells of *Escherichia coli* become sensitive to lysozyme. Comprehensive accounts of freezing and thawing and of the repair of damage are provided by MacLeod and Calcott (1976) and Mackey (1984).

Hydrostatic Pressure

Hydrostatic pressure, in the present context, refers to the effects of high pressure on microorganisms. Some organisms can exist at the bottom of deep oceans, where they are subjected to high hydrostatic pressure (Dring, 1976). Bacterial spores are more resistant to hydrostatic pressure than are nonsporulating bacteria or germinated spores. Within a certain pressure range, which may vary with different types of spores, the number of survivors decreases as the pressure increases. Above this pressure range, increasing pressure has a *reduced* effect (Sale et al., 1970; Gould, 1973; Wills, 1974). The sporicidal effect is related to temperature, both during and after treatment, i.e., the combined effect of temperature and hydrostatic pressure can be further potentiated if an additional heat treatment is given after pressurization. Thus, a proportion of spores has been heat sensitized by the pressure (Sale et al., 1970; Gould, 1973).

These facts are relevant to an understanding of the mechanism of action of hydrostatic pressure (Gould, 1984). When spores are pressurized, they are induced to germinate, and the germinated cells are then inactivated (Clouston and Wills, 1969, 1970; Murrell and Wills, 1977). Pressurized spores release DPA, calcium, and hexosamine-containing material and become phase bright (Sale et al., 1970). Mercuric chloride, a germination inhibitor, also inhibits the germination induced by hydrostatic pressure (Gould and Sale, 1970).

EFFECTS OF CHEMICAL AGENTS ON MICROORGANISMS

Cellular Uptake of Antimicrobial Agents

It was stated earlier that uptake of an antimicrobial agent by a cell represents an early manifestation in the effect of that agent. If the uptake of the drug (usually expressed as μg taken up per mg dry weight of cells) is plotted against the equilibrium concentration, a whole range of different curves may be obtained (Giles et al., 1960, 1974; Gilbert et al., 1978; Hugo, 1982), some of which are described in Figure 3–1. An S-shaped pattern indicates a monofunctional drug molecule that gives rise to a vertical packing pattern on the cell. The Langmuirian (L-shaped) pattern (Fig. 3–1a) denotes a situation in which, as sites of uptake on the cells are filled by drug molecules, additional molecules have increasing difficulty in finding vacant sites. The C (constant-partition) pattern, depicted in Figure 3–1b, occurs when the solute molecules penetrate more readily into the adsorbate than into the solvent. The H (high-affinity) pattern demonstrates that the drug molecule has a high affinity for the cells (Fig. 3–1c). These four types have been well documented over the past 20 years (see Hugo, 1982). A comparatively recent finding has been the Z-uptake curve (Gilbert et al., 1978) (Fig. 3–1d); this has been taken to suggest that above certain critical applied concentrations, the agents in question (2-phenoxyethanol and phenoxypropanol) induce structural changes in the membrane, so a considerable increase in the surface area available for uptake would ensue.

Mechanism of Action

An immense amount of time and effort has been spent studying the effects of chemical agents on microorganisms, yet the precise mechanism of action of many inhibitory compounds remains unclear (Table 3–3). The penicillins may be cited as a case in point. Several years ago, benzylpenicillin was shown to induce the accumulation of cell wall precursors, uridine nucleotides (Park

nucleotides) (Park and Strominger, 1957). Subsequently, it was demonstrated that the antibiotic irreversibly inhibited a late, crosslinking (transpeptidation) stage in cell wall peptidoglycan synthesis (Tipper and Strominger, 1965). The development of newer penicillins, and the introduction of cephalosporins and cephamycins (7-α-methoxycephalosporins) with differing effects on bacteria, reawakened interest in the mechanism of action of the β-lactam group of antibiotics, and these drugs are considered in the following section.

In addition to understanding how particular substances achieve their lethal or inhibitory antimicrobial effect, two other questions must be considered: Why are some agents toxic to bacteria and not to fungi, or vice versa? How does resistance to antimicrobial compounds arise? The first question is considered in this section, whereas the second question is discussed in the following section.

Inhibitors of Bacterial Cell Wall Synthesis

The basic unit of the bacterial cell wall is composed of peptidoglycan (murein, mucopeptide), which confers mechanical rigidity on the cell and protects the delicate, underlying cytoplasmic membrane. In gram-positive bacteria, the wall consists of a thick layer of peptidoglycan interspersed with teichoic acid or another such acidic polymer. A typical gram-negative rod has a much thinner peptidoglycan layer closest to the cytoplasmic membrane; external to the peptidoglycan is the periplasmic space (in which may be found any β-lactamase enzyme); the outermost region is termed the outer membrane. This complex outer part contains lipoprotein (covalently linked to the peptidoglycan layer), lipopolysaccharide, and phospholipids.

Substantial changes in peptidoglycan crosslinking and in the extent to which *S. aureus* teichoic acid is substituted with D-alanyl ester occur in *S. aureus* grown under different growth conditions (Archibald, 1988). Changes in outer membrane components of gram-negative bacteria can also take place thereby modifying responses in disease and to biocides (Brown and Williams, 1985; Costerton et al., 1987).

In brief, the stages of cell wall synthesis can be envisaged as follows. Uridine diphosphate (UDP)-N-acetylmuramic acid (MurNAc) is formed from N-acetylglucosamine (GlcNAc), uridine triphosphate and phosphoenol pyruvate. D-alanine (D-ala) is obtained from L-alanine (L-ala) by means of the enzyme L-alanine racemase, and two molecules of D-ala combine, under the influence of D-ala synthetase, to give the peptide D-ala—D-ala. Three amino acids, namely, L-ala, D-glutamic acid (D-glu), and L-lysis (L-lys) (or *meso*-diaminopimelic acid [DAP] in some organisms) are added sequentially to the carboxyl group of UDP-MurNAc, followed by the dipeptide D-ala—D-ala. Each step is catalyzed by a specific enzyme and requires ATP.

UDP-MurNAc ——————→ UDP-MurNAc
|————— 4 ATP-requiring —————|————————|
steps   pentapeptide

Table 3–3. *Cellular Targets of Antimicrobial Action*

Target	Agents	Effect
Cell wall	Penicillins, cephalosporins, D-cycloserine (oxamycin), phosphonomycin, vancomycin	Inhibition of cell wall synthesis (see text and Table 3–4)
	Lysozyme	Attacks peptidoglycan (β,1–4 links)
	Aldehydes	Interaction with -NH$_2$ groups
	Lysostaphin	Peptidase liberates *N*-terminal glycine and alanine
	Anionic surfactants	High concentrations: lysis
Outer membrane	EDTA (and similar chelating agents)	Chelates cations, induces release of up to 50% of lipopolysaccharide of outer membrane
	Lactoferrin, transferrin	Iron-binding proteins with effects similar to EDTA
	Polycations, e.g., polylysine	Displace cations
	Polymyxins	Displace cations
Cytoplasmic membrane	Moist heat, polymyxins, phenols, quaternary ammonium compounds, biguanides, parabens, novobiocin, ionophorous antibiotics, hexachlorophene	Leakage of low-molecular-weight material; proton flux (for more specific information, see Table 3–6)
	Polyenic antibiotics (antifungal only)	Bind to sterols in fungal membrane
Protein synthesis	Aminoglycoside antibiotics, tetracyclines, lincomycins, macrolides, chloramphenicol, fucidin	Affect protein synthesis in different ways (see Table 3–7)
Nucleic acids	Acridines, mitomycins, actinomycins, dyes, nalidixic acid, novobiocin, rifamycins, alkylating agents, ionizing and ultraviolet radiations	Possible binding of agents to nucleic acids extensively studied (see text and Table 3–8)
Folate synthesis or utilization	Sulfonamides, trimethoprim	Potentiation of action by use of combination in vitro
Enzymes or proteins	Metal ions	-SH groups of enzymes, which may be membrane associated
	Alkylating agents, oxidizing agents	May also combine with DNA or RNA

In the next stage, UDP-MurNAc-pentapeptide reacts with membrane-bound undecaprenyl phosphate (C$_{55}$-prenyl phosphate), and uridine monophosphate (UMP) is lost. Another molecule of GlcNAc, via UDP-GlcNAc with the loss of UDP, now reacts to give a β, 1-4 disaccharide link between GlcNAc and MurNAc. These additions thus may be depicted as follows:

UDP-MurNAc⟶MurNAc-P-P-lipid⟶
pentapeptide · pentapeptide

GlcNAc-MurNAc-P-P-lipid
pentapeptide

In *Staphylococcus aureus*, five molecules of glycine are added to the ϵ-amino group of lysine. This requires glycyl-tRNA, but is independent of the ribosomes.

The next stage involves linear polymerization, i.e., the formation of a polymer containing alternating GlcNAc and MurNAc-decapeptide residues (in *Staphylococcus aureus*) or alternating GlcNAc and MurNAc-pentaptide residues (in *Escherichia coli*). The linkage to the membrane lipid is severed, leading to the release of C$_{55}$-prenyl pyrophosphate, which, under the influence of an enzyme (pyrophosphatase) is converted to C$_{55}$-prenyl phosphate and reutilized in the cycle just described. The linear polymer forms by attachment to an acceptor group, a growing point in the cell wall structure.

$$\left[\begin{array}{c} \text{GlcNAc-MurNAc} \\ | \\ \text{decapeptide} \end{array} \right]_n$$

in *Staphylococcus aureus*

or

$$\left[\begin{array}{c} \text{GlcNAc-MurNAc} \\ | \\ \text{pentapeptide} \end{array} \right]_n$$

in *Escherichia coli*

The final stage is a transpeptidation stage (Fig. 3–4), in which crosslinking occurs between the linear polymers, the peptidoglycan structure thereby being considerably strengthened. The terminal D-ala molecules are removed, e.g., by a specific carboxypeptidase in *E. coli* (Reynolds, 1985).

An important early discovery was that penicillin induced the intracellular accumulation of uridine diphosphate nucleotides (Park and StromGinger, 1957), significant in that these were precursors in peptidoglycan synthesis, and that penicillin interrupted this synthesis at some specific point.

Other antibiotics have also been shown to inhibit peptidoglycan synthesis (Table 3–4). D-cycloserine, an ana-

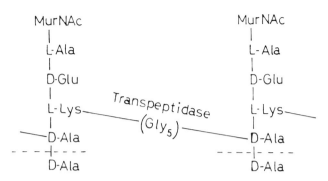

Fig. 3–4. Crosslinking: the penicillin-sensitive reaction in *Staphylococcus aureus.*

log of D-alanine (Fig. 3–5), is a competitive inhibitor of both the racemase and synthetase enzymes. Vancomycin is believed to inhibit cell wall synthesis by binding to the D-ala—D-ala group on the peptide chain of a membrane-bound intermediate.

Bacitracin induces the intracellular accumulation of uridine nucleotides, and has been shown to inhibit the enzymic conversion of C_{55}-isoprenyl pyrophosphate to C_{55}-isoprenyl phosphate (Storm and Toscano, 1979).

These antibiotics thus act at an earlier stage in cell wall synthesis than the β-lactam group. It has been proven conclusively that members of the latter group

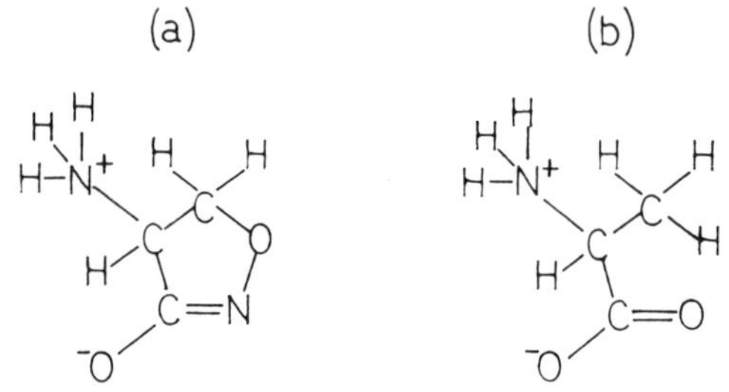

Fig. 3–5. Structural similarity between D-cycloserine *(a)* and D-alanine *(b)*.

inhibit the transpeptidation reaction (Tipper and Strominger, 1965; Tipper, 1979). The only bacterial enzymes that are specifically inhibited by β-lactam antibiotics are the transpeptidase and D-ala carboxypeptidase (see Frère et al., 1980), although inhibition of the latter is not lethal (Blumberg and Strominger, 1971). The combination between the transpeptidase and antibiotic is covalent and irreversible. Penicillins and cephalosporins are analogs of the donor substrate, acyl-D-alanyl-D-alanine (Tipper and Strominger, 1965; Virudachalam and Rao, 1977).

There are, however, multiple targets with differential sensitivity to different β-lactam antibiotics (Tipper, 1979). These have been reviewed by Spratt (1980, 1983). Multiple penicillin-sensitive enzymes (PSEs) have been detected and studied as penicillin-binding proteins (PBPs) on sodium dodecyl sulfate polyacrylamide gels. In *Escherichia coli*, three (numbers 1B, 2, and 3) of the seven PBPs (with molecular masses of 40,000 to 91,000) in the cytoplasmic membrane have been identified as killing targets for penicillins and cephalosporins. The β-lactam antibiotics can induce different types of morphologic variants in *E. coli* and other gram-negative bacteria.

In *Staphylococcus aureus* four PBPs have been found. PBP 4 is considered to be responsible for the high degree of crosslinking, and PBPs 1, 2, and 3 are believed to be the primary targets for β-lactam action.

Lederberg (1956) was the first to demonstrate that, in the presence of an osmotic stabilizer, benzylpenicillin induced spheroplasts in gram-negative organisms (for a detailed account of spheroplasts and protoplasts, see McQuillen, 1960). It has since been noted, however, that different members of the β-lactam group induce different types of morphologic variants in *E. coli* and other gram-negative bacteria. Cephaloridine and cefoxitin, which bind to PBP 1B (Table 3–5) induce lysis (or spheroplasts in a hypertonic medium), whereas mecillinam (a 6-β-amidinopenicillin binding to PBP 2), irrespective of concentration, induces osmotically stable round forms. Benzylpenicillin and other antibiotics, such as ampicillin, cephalexin, and cefotaxime, bind most strongly to PBP

Table 3–4. *Inhibitors of Bacterial Cell Wall Synthesis*

Stage	Inhibitor	Comment
L-alanine racemase	D-cycloserine (oxamycin)	Competitive inhibition.
D-alanine synthetase	D-cycloserine	Note similarity in structure of D-alanine and D-cycloserine (Fig. 3–5)
Binds to D-ala—D-ala group on peptide chain of membrane-bound intermediate	Vancomycin, teicoplanin	Inhibit transfer of linear glycan acceptor in wall to MurNAc-pentapeptide—GlcNAc on its lipid carrier
Release of undecaprenyl pyrophosphate from linkage with *N*-acetylmuramic acid	Bacitracin	Bacitracin forms complex with the C_{55}-prenyl pyrophosphate, preventing hydrolysis to C_{55}-prenyl phosphate
Transpeptidase	Penicillins, cephalosporins	Irreversible binding } see also
Carboxypeptidase	Penicillins, cephalosporins	Not lethal } Table 3–5
Hydrolases (autolysins)	Chloramphenicol (CMP)	CMP prevents lysis of penicillin-treated bacteria (reason for antagonism between CMP and penicillin?)

Table 3–5. *Penicillin-binding Proteins: Properties and Inhibition*

PBP number	Physiologic Role	Examples of a β-Lactam as Inhibitor
1B	Cell elongation	Cephaloridine, cefoxitin
2	Cell shape	Mecillinam, imipenem
3	Cell division	Benzylpenicillin, ampicillin, cephalexin, cefotaxime

3, and these induce long forms at low to moderate concentrations (if affinity is 3>1B>2, filaments without bulges are induced; if 3>2>1B, filaments with bulges); lysis occurs at higher drug concentrations.

This increasingly complex picture is further complicated by the role of peptidoglycan hydrolases (autolysins), enzymes that do not react directly with the penicillin molecule. The studies of Tomasz and colleagues (reviewed by Tomasz, 1979, 1980, 1983) indicate that lysis and loss of viability are not always synonymous. Autolysin-defective mutants of various gram-positive and gram-negative bacteria (Rogers and Forsberg, 1971; Tomasz, 1979, 1980) are resistant to penicillin-induced lysis. Thus, it appears that the activity of the hydrolases is triggered in penicillin-treated bacteria and that the hydrolases (Tomasz, 1980) are involved in autolytic cell wall degradation.

All the inhibitors described here are inactive against fungi, in which the structure and synthesis of the cell wall differ considerably from the bacterial situation.

Other Agents Acting on the Cell Wall or Outer Membrane

Whereas β-lactam antibiotics, D-cycloserine, and vancomycin are active only against growing cells, other substances are known that are active against growing or nongrowing cells.

The enzyme lysozyme (EC 3.2.1.17) induces lysis of some gram-positive organisms such as *Bacillus megaterium*, *Micrococcus lysodeikticus* and *Sarcina lutea* (McQuillen, 1960). *Staphylococcus aureus*, fungi, and typical gram-negative bacteria are resistant to its action, which is effected by hydrolysis of the β, 1-4 links between GlcNAc and MurNAc in cell wall peptidoglycan. Cell lysis ensues, but this can be prevented if the treatment is carried out in the presence of an appropriate concentration of an osmotic stabilizer, such as sucrose, so protoplasts are formed. With gram-negative bacteria such as *Escherichia coli*, lysozyme does not penetrate the outer membrane of plasmolysed cells, but does so when the outer membrane is destabilized with ethylenediamine-tetraacetic acid (EDTA) (Witholt et al., 1976).

EDTA itself has proved to be a useful agent in studies involving antibacterial agents (Russell, 1971; Leive, 1974; Wilkinson, 1975; Russell and Gould, 1988; Russell and Chopra, 1990). It is not a powerful bactericide in its own right; indeed, it generally has no effect on gram-positive bacteria and some effect on some types of gram-negative bacteria, but causes significant lysis of *Pseu-*

domonas aeruginosa. Its usefulness resides in the fact that it can potentiate the activity against gram-negative bacteria of chemically unrelated antibacterial compounds and, in so doing, has provided an insight into one of the reasons for the resistance of these organisms. EDTA is a chelating agent that combines with cations associated with the outer membrane of gram-negative bacteria. At the same time, large amounts of outer-membrane lipopolysaccharide are released. EDTA has no apparent effect on gram-positive bacteria and does not increase their sensitivity to antibacterial agents (Russell, 1971; Russell and Furr, 1977). EDTA has no apparent effect on yeast and molds, except on yeast protoplasts suspended in stabilizing medium containing glucose (Russell, 1971).

Polymyxin, a polycationic amphipathic antibiotic, disorganizes the outer membrane of gram-negative bacteria (Chopra, 1988a, b) thereby promoting its own entry to its ultimate target, the inner membrane. Other polycationic agents such as polylysine (lys_{20}) and salmine sensitize smooth stains of *E. coli* and *Salmonella typhimurium* to hydrophobic antibiotics (Vaara and Vaara, 1983a, b; Nikaido and Vaara, 1985). The permeability increase, however, is slower than that occurring with polymyxin.

Two iron-binding proteins, lactoferrin and transferrin, lose antibacterial activity if blocked with iron, implying that bacteriostasis results from an iron-deficient environment. They also damage the outer membrane of gram-negative bacteria, although transferrin is a less powerful chelator (Ellison et al., 1988).

These "permeabilizing agents" are of considerable use in studying the mechanisms of impermeability of gram-negative bacteria to antibiotics and biocides.

The mechanism of action of glutaraldehyde (pentanedial) has yet to be fully elucidated. Studies in my laboratory and elsewhere (reviewed by Russell and Hopwood, 1976; Gorman et al., 1980) have demonstrated that this dialdehyde has the following effects on bacteria: (1) crosslinking of the peptidoglycan in gram-positive bacteria such that reduced lysis occurs with lysozyme (*Bacillus subtilis*) or lysostaphin (*Staphylococcus aureus*); (2) interaction with protein in the cell walls of gram-negative bacteria so that lysis by sodium lauryl sulfate or EDTA-lysozyme is reduced; (3) reaction with spore cortex constituents, this being assisted by the action of inorganic cations; and (4) increased resistance to lysis of protoplasts and spheroplasts.

The reaction of glutaraldehyde with nucleic acids follows pseudo-first-order kinetics at high temperatures, but even at the higher temperatures, there is little evidence for the formation of intermolecular crosslinks (Hopwood, 1975). Glutaraldehyde inhibits synthesis of protein, RNA, and DNA in *E. coli*, but this is believed to arise from an inhibition of precursor uptake as a consequence of aldehyde-protein interaction in the outer structures of the cell (Gorman et al., 1980). Glutaraldehyde thus affects the bacterial cell wall and probably the fungal wall also (Gorman et al., 1980).

Low concentrations of phenol, formaldehyde, hypochlorite, and mercuric chloride have been reported to induce lysis of *E. coli* (reviewed by Hugo, 1982). The effects of these agents at low and high concentrations perhaps should be reconsidered.

Lysostaphin is an extracellular lytic enzyme, produced from a staphylococcus, that lyses viable or heat-killed cells of other *Staphylococcus aureus* strains (Schindler and Schuhardt, 1964). The rate of cell lysis of cells or walls depends on temperature, pH, lysostaphin concentration, and ionic strength of the test medium. Lysostaphin attacks the peptidoglycan in the staphylococcus cell wall, resulting in the formation of spheroplasts when the cells are treated in hypertonic medium (Watanakunakorn et al., 1969). The lytic principle is a peptidase that liberates *N*-terminal glycine and alanine from the cell wall; lysostaphin also contains a (nonlytic) hexosaminidase that is specific for the glucosaminyl-muramic acid bond of the carbohydrate backbone (Zygmunt and Tavormina, 1972). Other bacteria, as well as fungi, are resistant to the action of lysostaphin.

Lysostaphin is an important in vitro agent because it is used to lyse staphylococci prior to examining DNA plasmid profiles.

Membrane-Active Antimicrobial Agents

A range of diverse chemical agents has been shown to attack the cytoplasmic membrane. Some of these affect both fungi and bacteria, whereas others (e.g., polyenic antibiotics) have a selective action against yeast and fungi; the reasons for this are discussed in the following.

Several substances are known to disrupt the cytoplasmic membrane. These agents cause the leakage of intracellular materials, although other effects have also been reported (Lambert, 1978). Thus, phenol has been found to cause cell lysis; chlorhexidine in low concentrations induces leakage, but at much higher drug concentrations, leakage is reduced as a consequence of the interaction of chlorhexidine with cytoplasmic protein and nucleic acid (Hugo and Longworth, 1966; Longworth, 1971). Chlorhexidine at bacteriostatic concentrations has also been found to inhibit membrane-bound adenosine triphosphatase (ATPase) (Harold et al., 1969), and cetyltrimethylammonium bromide, the proton-motive force (Hugo, 1978; see the following). Modern thinking, however, is inconsistent with the concept that membrane-bound ATPase is the primary target of chlorhexidine action (Chopra et al., 1987). Chlorhexidine (Longworth, 1971) and quaternary ammonium compounds (Gilby and Few, 1960) will lyse bacterial protoplasts and spheroplasts. The polymyxins also impair the integrity

of the cytoplasmic membrane of gram-negative bacteria (Newton, 1956), gram-positive bacteria generally being resistant. Recent interest in the polymyxins has been centered on their interaction with the components of the outer membrane of gram-negative organisms as a means towards a better understanding of sensitivity and resistance (Brown, 1975).

Both polymyxin B and polymyxin B nonapeptide affect the inner membrane of *Escherichia coli* inducing leakage of K^+ and other intracellular constituents, but only the former agent is bactericidal. A possible reason is that it, but not the nonapeptide, promotes leakage of cytoplasmic proteins (Dixon and Chopra, 1986).

Polyenic antibiotics, such as nystatin and amphotericin, are antifungal and not antibacterial; the reason for this is that the fungal membrane contains sterol, with which a polyene combines (Lampen et al., 1962; Gottlieb and Shaw, 1970). Interestingly, *Acholeplasma laidlawii* cells can be grown with or without sterol and are or are not, respectively, sensitive to polyene antibiotics (De Kruijff et al., 1974). Resistance to polyenes in *Candida* species has been found to be associated with changes in the ergosterol content of the cells (Athar and Winner, 1971).

Both polyenes and antifungal synthetic imidazole derivates act on the fungal cytoplasmic membrane (Gale, 1986; Kerridge, 1986). The polyenes affect the structural integrity of the membrane, as do the imidazoles at fungicidal concentrations; at fungistatic concentrations, however, the antimycotic imidazoles inhibit synthesis of membrane constituents.

Over the last 20 years, knowledge about the cytoplasmic membrane, oxidative phosphorylation, and active transport has increased dramatically (Kaback, 1986; Booth, 1988). Mitchell's chemosmotic theory (Mitchell, 1966, 1972) couples electron transport (oxidative chain) to ATP synthesis. The flow of electrons through the carrier system drives protons across the bacterial (or other cellular) membrane. As a result, a transmembrane electrochemical proton gradient is created, with the interior of the cell alkaline and negative. The proton-motive force also may be generated by the hydrolysis of ATP by ATPase (Hinkle and McCarty, 1978).

Proton-motive force consists of two components, a difference in H^+ concentration and a difference in electrical potential. Mitchell derived an equation to show that:

$$\Delta p = \Delta \psi - z\Delta pH$$

in which Δp is the proton-motive force, $\Delta \psi$ the membrane potential (measured in mV), ΔpH the transmembrane pH, and z (approximately 60 at 25°C) a factor converting pH into mV. Cetyltrimethylammonium bromide, at its bacteriostatic concentration, discharges the pH component of Δp in *Staphylococcus aureus* (Hugo, 1978).

It has been known for many years that several agents can uncouple oxidative phosphorylation. These uncoupling agents inhibit ATP synthesis in a different manner from ATPase inhibitors (Hammond, 1979). Uncoupling agents such as 2,4-dinitrophenol (DNP), tetrachlorsalicylanilide (TCS), and carbonylcyanide-*m*-chlorophenyl-hydrazone (CCCP) are lipid soluble; they dissolve in biologic membranes, dissociating oxidation from phosphorylation, effectively short-circuiting the proton-motive force, and thus causing a rapid backflow of protons into the cell and the collapse of Δp. TCS has been found to discharge $\Delta\psi$ in *Streptococcus faecalis* (Harold and Papineau, 1972; see also Hamilton, 1975; Hugo 1976a and b, 1982).

Hammond (1979) has divided the true inhibitors of Mg^{++}-ATPase into two groups: (1) those acting on both the soluble and membrane-bound ATPase; and (2) those inhibiting only the membrane-bound enzyme. Enzymes coupling the diffusion of protons back through the membrane to ATP synthesis are globular bodies protruding from the surface of the membrane. The protruding knob (F_1), a soluble protein made up of five types of subunit, is attached to the membrane through another set of proteins (F_0) embedded in the membrane. F_1 is readily removed, F_0 only when the membrane is destroyed (Hinkle and McCarty, 1978). Examples of agents acting at the F_0 site include N_1N^1-dicyclohexylcarbodiimide (DCCD) and the antifungal compound oligomycin (although they appear to act in different ways). The best-known example of an agent acting at the F_1 site is chlorhexidine, which directly inhibits membrane-bound and solubilized Mg^{++}-ATPase (Harold et al., 1969). As pointed out earlier, however, this is not considered to be the primary effect of the biguanide (Chopra et al., 1987).

Hexachlorophene inhibits the membrane-bound electron transport chain in *Bacillus megaterium*; menadione (an artificial electron carrier) reverses this inhibition (Frederick et al., 1974).

Other ion conductors of importance are: (1) K^+-conducting ionophores, notably the antibiotic valinomycin (the prototype of this group) and the chemically unrelated nonactin; they form lipid-soluble complexes with metal ions that are transported across the membrane and will also uncouple oxidative phosphorylation (Harold et al., 1974); and (2) cation-antiport ionophores, e.g., nigericin and monensin; these catalyze electroneutral exchange of alkali metals of H^+. Nigericin exchanges K^+ for H^+, whereas monensin exchanges Na^+ for H^+. Because no charge is translocated, the membrane potential is not affected, and oxidative phosphorylation consequently is not uncoupled (Harold et al., 1974).

Detailed studies have been made on the interaction of a polymeric biguanide, polyhexamethylene biguanide (PHMB). This binds to the negatively charged *Escherichia coli* cell surface, impairs the outer membrane and interacts with inner membrane phospholipids (Ikeda et al., 1983, 1984). K^+ loss occurs, and eventually there is a complete loss of membrane function with precipitation of intracellular constituents (Broxton et al., 1984; Woodcock, 1988).

Mercury compounds are well known as being able to combine with the -SH groups of enzymes (Hugo, 1982). Of course, this could occur with membrane-associated enzymes or with enzymes and proteins found in the cytoplasm. A summary of the effects of membrane-active agents is given in Table 3–6.

Inhibitors of Protein Synthesis

Protein synthesis arises from polypeptide chains formed by amino acids linked together by peptide (-CO-NH-) bonds. Synthesis occurs at the ribosomes (the "protein workshops" of the cell), made up of rRNA and protein. Each bacterial (70S) ribosome is assembled from two subunits: the smaller (30S) particle contains 16S RNA and approximately 20 proteins, and the larger (50S) particle contains 5S and 23S RNA and approximately 34 proteins (Nomura, 1973). Mammalian cells have 80S ribosomes, but mitochondrial ribosomes resemble those of bacteria. The order of attachment of amino acids to the growing peptide chain is coded by the base sequence of an mRNA molecule, each codon containing three bases (Tai and Davis, 1985).

In brief, protein synthesis (Fig. 3–6) can be considered to consist of the stages described in the following. The first event (and subsequent events, as described) in the chain elongation process involve the operation of certain factors known as *extension* (or elongation) factors. One such factor catalyzes the hydrolysis of guanosine triphosphate (GTP) in the attachment process (Stage 1), while another frees guanosine diphosphate (GDP) from a complex with the first factor. *Initiation* factors aid in the formation of an initiation complex involving mRNA, ribosomes, and *N*-formylmethionine (fMet)-tRNA and GTP, e.g., IF-2 directs the binding of fMet-tRNA to the 50S ribosomal subunit and IF-3 that of mRNA to the 30S subunit. The various stages can then be considered as follows:

1. Initiation. An initiation complex is formed between mRNA, the 30S ribosome, fMet-tRNA, and GTP.
2. Attachment of amino acid complex to the acceptor (A) (aminoacyl-tRNA) site, with the peptidyl-tRNA binding to the donor (P) site.
3. Peptide bond formation. This results from the action of peptidyl transferase located in the 50S ribosomal subunit, whereby the peptidyl moiety carried by peptidyl-tRNA on the P site is transferred to the aminoacyl-tRNA at the A site. Thus, peptidyl-tRNA increased by the new amino acid is bound at the A site.
4. Translocation. The peptidyl-tRNA is translocated to the P site, the tRNA originally occupying this site having been released. As a result of translocation, the mRNA is also moved and the next codon exposed at the A site, which is then able to accept the new incoming aminoacyl-tRNA.
5. Termination. The overall process is repeated until one of the three termination codons (UAA, UAG, UGA) is reached. The ester linkage between the polypeptide and tRNA is hydrolyzed by peptidyl transferase, with polypeptide release.

Several structurally unrelated drugs have been shown to inhibit bacterial protein synthesis (Pestka, 1971, 1977).

Table 3–6. *Membrane-Active Antimicrobial Agents*

Antibacterial Agent(s)	Effect on Cell	Mechanism of Action
Phenol	Leakage; possible cell lysis; protein denaturation	Generalized membrane damage
Quaternary ammonium compounds	Leakage; protoplast lysis; interaction with membrane phospholipid; discharge of pH component of Δp in protonmotive force	Generalized membrane damage
Chlorhexidine	Leakage at low concentrations, interactions of high concentrations with cytoplasmic constituents; protoplast and spheroplast lysis (both also concentration dependent); high concentrations inhibit membrane-bound ATPase	Concentration-dependent effect: low concentrations affect membrane integrity; higher ones congeal protoplasm
Hexachlorophene	Leakage, protoplast lysis (maximum at concentrations > bactericidal level); inhibits respiration	Membrane-bound electron transport chain
Phenoxyethanol	Leakage; low concentrations stimulate total oxygen uptake and uncouple oxidative phosphorylation; H^+ translocation and K^+ permeability are independent actions	Proton-conducting uncoupler
Fentichlor	Collapse of proton potential; relationship between bactericidal action and leakage; no leakage at bacteriostatic concentration	Uncoupler
Tetrachlorsalicylanilide	Inhibition of energy-dependent (not -independent) transport of phosphate and amino acids into *S. aureus*; increase of oxygen uptake in presence of glucose; increased permeability to Cl^-	Uncoupler
Sorbic acid	Transport inhibition (conflicting results reported); inhibition of pH across cytoplasmic membrane	Transport inhibitor (effect on pmf); possibly another unidentified mechanism
Parabens	Leakage of intracellular constituents; transport inhibition; selective inhibition of ΔpH across membrane	Concentration-dependent effect; low concentrations inhibit transport; higher ones affect membrane integrity
Valinomycin, nonactin	Formation of lipid-soluble, positively charged complex with K^+ and diffusion of complex across membrane; inhibition of active transport of sugars and amino acids	K^+-conducting ionophores
Nigericin, monensin	Catalysis of electroneutral exchange of alkali metals (K^+: nigericin; Na^+: monensin) for H^+; no translocation of charge, membrane potential thus unaltered	Cation-antiport ionophores
Polymyxins	Leakage of intracellular constituents, gross cytologic changes, interaction with components of outer membrane also	Disruption of inner membrane
Polyenic antibiotics	Antifungal, not antibacterial; interaction with sterols in fungal membrane	Sterol-binding agents
Antifungal imidazoles	Low concentrations inhibiting ergosterol synthesis (fungistatic); high concentrations inducing gross membrane damage (fungicidal)	Direct membrane damage (fungicidal concentrations)

These may be subdivided into three groups, described as follows (see also Table 3–7).

Inhibitors of 30S Subunit Functions. The aminoglycoside antibiotics act here (Pestka, 1977; Wallace et al., 1979; Gale et al., 1981; Greenwood, 1983; Davis et al., 1986). The primary target appears to be initiation (Table 3–7), as fMet-tRNA is released from the initiation complex, and this is followed by ribosomal breakdown. The subunits are released, but reassemble to form 70S particles, which recycle on to mRNA to form a blocked initiation complex (Garvin et al., 1973).

This is not, however, the only effect of streptomycin and other members of this group. At chemotherapeutic concentrations, they act to fix the initiation complex, whereas at subinhibitory doses, they stimulate misreading (miscoding). The latter occurs with ribosomes already engaged in chain elongation, so that there is a less drastic distortion of the ribosome, which continues its protein synthesis but with impaired accuracy. See Franklin and Snow (1981) for a comprehensive account. Furthermore, streptomycin has been shown to affect the permeability of the cytoplasmic membrane of *Escherichia coli* (Anand and Davis, 1960). An essential step in the bactericidal action of streptomycin and other aminoglycosides appears to be the creation of membrane channels as a consequence of protein misreading (Davis et al., 1986).

The mechanism of action of streptomycin has been re-examined by Kogut and Carrier (1980), whose hypothesis correlates an irreversible inhibition of growth and the inability of drug-affected ribosomes to recover, i.e., to

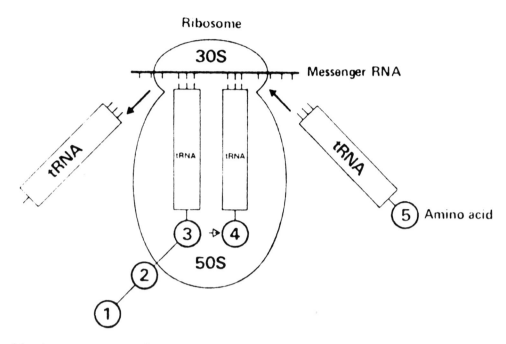

Fig. 3–6. Role of the ribosome in protein synthesis.

carry out correct translation of mRNA. Inhibition of growth and of protein synthesis are complete at approximately one molecule of streptomycin per ribosome.

Neomycin and kanamycin have effects similar to those of streptomycin but induce more extensive miscoding (Pestka, 1977).

The tetracyclines at low concentrations inhibit protein synthesis by preventing the binding of aminoacyl-tRNA to the ribosome acceptor site. Higher concentrations inhibit initiation and peptide bond synthesis (Pestka, 1977).

Inhibitors of 50S Subunit Functions. The chemical structure of puromycin indicates that it is an analog of the 3'-O-aminoacyladenosine portion of aminoacyl-tRNA, and it reacts with peptidyl-tRNA in the P site to form peptidyl puromycin (reviewed by Harris and Pestka, 1977, and Pestka, 1977). This contains a newly formed peptide bond. If peptidyl-tRNA is in the acceptor (A) site, it must be translocated to the P site before reaction with puromycin can occur.

Chloramphenicol acts by inhibiting peptide bond formation (transpeptidation). It has been shown to inhibit substrate binding to the acceptor (A) but not to the donor (P) site (Pongs, 1979).

Lincomycin is another antibiotic that inhibits peptide bond synthesis by prokaryotic ribosomes. It prevents formation of peptidyl puromycin, and it inhibits the peptidyl transferase reaction by interfering with the binding of aminoacyl-tRNA to the A site (Chang, 1979).

The macrolides bind to a common site on 50S ribosomal subunits. This is likely to be that site near the donor peptidyl-tRNA site. Another effect of erythromycin is considered briefly in the following section.

Table 3–7. *Inhibitors of Bacterial Protein Synthesis*

Inhibition	Inhibitor	Comments
Initiation	Streptomycin and other amino-glycoside antibiotics	Misreading also may occur: see text
Recognition	Puromycin	Puromycin is analog of terminal aminoacyl adenosine of tRNA; premature release of nascent polypeptide chain
Binding of aminoacyl-tRNA to 30S ribosomal subunit	Tetracyclines	Inhibit protein synthesis on 80S ribosomes, also (but no energy-dependent active transport system as with 70S ribosomes)
Peptidyl transferase	Chloramphenicol Lincomycin	Selective for 70S ribosomes; bind to 50S subunit
Translocase	Erythromycin*	Inhibits release of tRNA from P site*
	Fusidic acid* (Fucidin)	Forms 1:1 complex with extension factor associated with GDP on ribosome

*See text also.

Inhibitors of Translocation. Fucidin (fusidic acid) has been shown to inhibit the translocation process. It inhibits the enzymic activity of EF-G and increases the stability of the ternary complex (EF-G·GDP·ribosome) by forming highly stable 1:1 complexes, EF-G·GDP·ribosome·fusidic acid (Brot, 1977). According to Cundliffe (1979), the sequestering of EF-G and GDP on ribosomes results in inhibition of the ribosomal binding of aminoacyl-tRNA and means that Fucidin should not be regarded as an inhibitor of translocation.

Erythromycin does not prevent the migration of peptidyl-tRNA from the A site, but it has been found to inhibit the release of tRNA from the P site and is thus an inhibitor of the translocation process, since the incoming peptidyl-tRNA is prevented from occupying its proper position on the P site. This type of effect may occur, however, only at high concentrations of the antibiotic (Pestka, 1977). Chang (1979) has stated that it interferes primarily with the translocation of peptidyl-tRNA from the A site, following transpeptidation to the P site.

Agents Acting on Nucleic Acids

Antimicrobial agents acting on nucleic acids (DNA and/or RNA) can do so by different mechanisms (Table 3–8).

Mitomycin C is a potent bactericide and also exhibits antitumor activity. In susceptible bacteria, it inhibits DNA synthesis, giving rise to filament formation in gram-negative organisms. Covalent linking occurs between mitomycin D and the DNA of bacteria cells in such a manner that crosslinks are formed between complementary DNA strands. There is a correlation between the C-G (cytosine-guanine) content of DNA and the degree of crosslinking (Goldberg and Friedman, 1971), and although the crosslinking affects only about 1 base pair in 1000, this is sufficient to block transcription by RNA polymerase (Franklin and Snow, 1981).

Actinomycin D has antibacterial and cytostatic activity and acts by inhibiting RNA synthesis in susceptible bacteria. It binds strongly to helical double-stranded DNA, but not to RNA, and inhibits the DNA-dependent RNA polymerase (Leive, 1974). DNA polymerase is much less sensitive.

Nalidixic acid is active mainly against gram-negative organisms, and in growing cultures, treated cells become greatly elongated, but are not osmotically fragile. It has been found to inhibit DNA synthesis at a drug concentration corresponding to the minimum bactericidal level. Nalidixic acid does not inhibit DNA polymerase I or polynucleotide ligase. Its main effect is on DNA gyrase (Crumplin et al., 1980). New 4-quinolone drugs have been synthesized, many of which are more effective and with a broader antibacterial spectrum than nalidixic acid. They inhibit the A subunit of the essential DNA gyrase; gyrA mutant strains carry an alteration in the structural gene for the A subunit and are thus resistant (Smith, 1985).

Rifampicin (rifampin), the most important member of the rifamycin group of antibiotics, is inactive against DNA polymerase and RNA polymerase from animal cells. It is, however, specifically active towards bacterial RNA polymerase (Wehrli and Staehelin, 1970). This enzyme is responsible for transcription, whereby, based on a DNA template, it transfers the information from DNA into relatively small RNA molecules.

Novobiocin, an antibiotic with a fairly broad spectrum of activity, has several different effects on microorganisms (Morris and Russell, 1971). It induces filamentation in gram-negative rods and chaining in streptococci, prevents or reduces penicillin-induced spheroplast formation, causes a nonspecific inhibition of cell wall synthesis, produces a magnesium deficiency (considered an unlikely explanation for the mechanism of action of the antibiotic) (Morris and Russell, 1971), induces leakage of intracellular constituents, and inhibits DNA synthesis (Smith and Davis, 1967), with a lesser effect on synthesis of RNA and protein. Staudenbauer (1975) has shown that the primary action of novobiocin in *Escherichia coli* is a specific inhibition of semiconservative DNA replication. Novobiocin inhibits DNA gyrase (Staudenbauer, 1975), an enzyme that introduces negative superhelical turns into covalently closed, circular, double-stranded DNA molecules (Ryan, 1979).

The supercoiling of *E. coli* gyrase (topoisomerase II) β-subunits is the primary target site for the action of

Table 3–8. *Antimicrobial Compounds and Nucleic Acids*

Effect	Antimicrobial Compound	Comments
Covalent linking to DNA	Mitomycin C	Interaction between antibiotic and DNA guanine
Binds to helical double-stranded DNA	Actinomycin D	Less affinity for denatured or single-stranded DNA; does not bind to RNA. Prevents transcription of RNA
Inhibition of bacterial RNA polymerase	Rifampicin	
Inhibition of function of DNA gyrase	4-Quinolones	Multiple other effects noted
Specific inhibition of semiconservative DNA replication	Novobiocin	DNA gyrase affected (see text)
Intercalation to DNA	Acridines	DNA synthesis inhibited. Binding to other macromolecules observed
Alkylation	Ethylene oxide	Alkylation of phosphated guanine responsible for antibacterial effect?
Alkylation	Formaldehyde	Alkylation responsible for antibacterial action?

novobiocin (Smith, 1985). 4-Quinolones and novobiocin, acting at different sites on the enzyme, produce synergism when used in combination.

The antibacterial activity of the acridines increases with the degree of ionization (Albert, 1979). Ionization is, in fact, the most important factor governing their activity, but it must be cationic in nature. Acridine derivatives that are ionized to form anions or zwitterions are only poorly antibacterial by comparison. A considerable amount of research has been done on the mechanism of their antibacterial action (Foster and Russell, 1971). They induce filamentous forms in gram-negative bacteria, inhibit DNA synthesis, and combine strongly to DNA, although binding to other sites, such as RNA, cell envelopes, and ribosomes, has also been reported. Binding to DNA has been studied extensively (Neidle, 1979). The classic studies of Lerman (1961) resulted in the hypothesis that the planar drug molecules become intercalated (sandwiched) between adjacent base pairs. Thus, with proflavine, the compound is bound through the two primary amino groups, which are held in ionic linkage by two phosphoric acid residues of the Crick-Watson spiral, with the flat skeleton of the acridine ring resting on (and held by Van der Waals forces to) the purine and pyrimidine molecules. Binding to DNA occurs by two distinct mechanisms (Peacocke and Skerrett, 1956; Waring, 1965). The first shows a first-order reaction, with one molecule of proflavine binding to every four to five nucleotides, the second a slower, higher order of reaction with one molecule per nucleotide.

Although of little clinical importance, the acridines are useful laboratory tools because of their role in "curing" plasmids.

Alkylation is defined as the conversion:

$$\text{H-X} \longrightarrow \text{R-X}$$

where R is an alkyl group (Price, 1958). Biologic activity of alkylating agents is indicated by reaction with nucleophilic groups (Stacey et al., 1958).

Epoxides, of which ethylene oxide is one example, are known to interact with amino acids and proteins (Phillips, 1952; Ross, 1958). Ethylene oxide causes hydroxyethylation of amino acids (Starbuck and Busch, 1963) with the phosphate group of nucleic acids to form a triester (Alexander and Stacey, 1958) and with guanine to give 7-(2′-hydroxyethyl)guanine (Brooks and Lawley, 1964). Alkylation of phosphated guanine in nonsporing bacteria has been proposed as the primary reason for the lethal effect of ethylene oxide (Michael and Stumbo, 1970) (see Russell, 1976 and 1982a, for a more detailed discussion).

The general antimicrobial activity of ethylene oxide (CH_2CH_2O) and related substances parallels their activity as alkylating agents (Phillips, 1952). Thus, cyclopropane ($CH_2CH_2CH_2$), which is not an alkylating agent, has no antimicrobial action, whereas ethylene sulfide (CH_2CH_2S) has equal activity, and ethylene imine (CH_2CH_2NH) has greater activity.

Formaldehyde is another agent that has been suggested to act by its alkylating effect. Binding of formal-

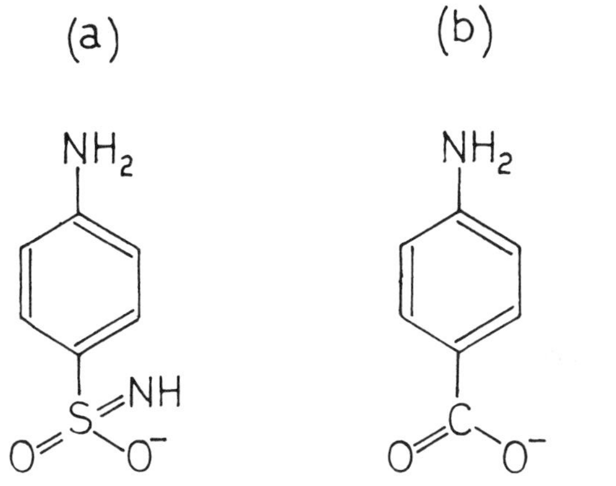

Fig. 3–7. Structural similarity between sulfanilamide (a) and p-aminobenzoic acid (4-aminobenzoic acid) (b).

dehyde to RNA is reversible up to a point (Staehelin, 1958). Grossman et al. (1961) demonstrated the interaction of formaldehyde with T2 bacteriophage DNA. Interaction with protein has also been described (Russell and Hopwood, 1976; Gorman et al., 1980).

Inhibitors of Tetrahydrofolate Synthesis

Most bacteria synthesize dihydrofolic acid (DHFA) from its components, namely, p-aminobenzoic acid (PAB; 4-aminobenzoic acid), pteridine, and glutamic acid. Others require it as a growth factor, and man, lacking this synthetic capacity, obtains it preformed in his diet. This, taken in conjunction with the fact that bacteria that synthesize dihydrofolate are impermeable to exogenous folates, demonstrates a potentially valuable area of selective chemotherapy (Smith, 1979; Wise and Reeves, 1979).

It was shown several years ago that PAB would reverse the antibacterial activity of sulfanilamide (Woods, 1940). This was a competitive antagonism, with 1 molecule of PAB antagonizing the inhibitory action of 300 sulfanilamide molecules. This suggested that the antibacterial action of the sulfonamides was based on their structural resemblance to PAB (Fig. 3–7). It is now known (Brown, 1962) that the sulfonamides competitively inhibit the enzyme dihydropteroate synthetase, which is responsible for the condensation of a pteridine derivative with PAB.

DHFA as such plays no important part in bacterial metabolism. It is reduced, however, to tetrahydrofolic acid (THFA), which is involved in the production of purines, thymine constituents of nucleic acid, etc. (Hitchings, 1973). The enzyme responsible for the reduction of DHFA to THFA is dihydrofolate reductase, which is competitively inhibited by trimethoprim. The dihydrofolate reductase in human cells is much less sensitive to this inhibition (Burchall and Hitchings, 1965; Hitchings and Burchall, 1965).

A large family of drugs has been derived from sulfanilamide by substitution of hydrogen in the sulfonamide (SO_2NH_2) group. They are all PAB analogs, as the substituents do not interfere with the structural resemblance, but they differ in solubility and other pharmacologic properties. The amino group directly attached to the ring cannot be altered or displaced without loss of activity. Other PAB analogs are known. p-Aminosalicylic acid (PAS) is used in combination with more potent drugs for tuberculosis treatment. The dihydrofolate synthetase of *Mycobacterium tuberculosis* utilizes the inhibitor, but the product is not acceptable to the next enzyme in the reaction sequence. Thus, the pteridine moiety of folic acid is also immobilized.

Combinations of a sulfonamide, sulfamethoxazole, and trimethoprim are synergistic in vitro because they inhibit sequential stages in the biosynthesis of THFA. Unfortunately, the situation in vivo is less clearcut, because it might be difficult to achieve the optimal ratios of the two drugs at the site of infection. In fact there is a tendency now to use trimethoprim alone as a chemotherapeutic agent (see Smith, 1979, for an alternative viewpoint).

Certain R-factors have been shown to confer resistance to trimethoprim (Amyes and Smith, 1978). These appear to code for the presence of an additional target enzyme, dihydrofolate reductase, that is much less susceptible to trimethoprim than the host enzyme. Another less common type of resistance involving thymineless mutants has also been described; these lack thymidylate synthetase and, if they are supplied with a source of thymine, are highly resistant to trimethoprim (Amyes and Smith, 1975).

Chelating Agents

The effects of EDTA in chelating Mg^{++} and Ca^{++} in the outer membrane of gram-negative bacteria have already been described, as have the effects of polycations, lactoferrin, and transferrin. The tetracyclines can also chelate metals, especially Ca^{++}, and although this is an important consideration in their in vivo chemotherapeutic use, it has not been claimed to be responsible for their mechanisms of antibacterial action. It must be added that divalent cations can reduce the activity of other antibiotics, notably members of the aminoglycoside group, but this may be the result of competition for binding sites on or in the bacterial cell.

Streptomycin and gentamicin, which are polycationic aminoglycosides, are known to interact with divalent cation-binding sites on the lipopolysaccharide (LPS) of *Pseudomonas aeruginosa*, thereby increasing outer membrane permeability (Hancock, 1984).

Although antimony, arsenic, mercury, and silver are the only metals that are active as free ions, many others confer bactericidal activity on organic chelating agents, or ligands. These organic compounds show little or no activity alone, indicating that they do not act by depriving the organisms of essential trace metals; nor do they act as simple carriers of metal into the cell, because the metals alone are nontoxic. The mechanisms of chelation and associated antimicrobial activity will be described by reference to studies on 8-hydroxyquinoline, or oxine. Of the eight isomers, only the one in which the hydroxyl anion and the ring nitrogen atom are correctly positioned

Oxine anion · · · · Unsaturated (1:1) complex · · · · Saturated (2:1) complex

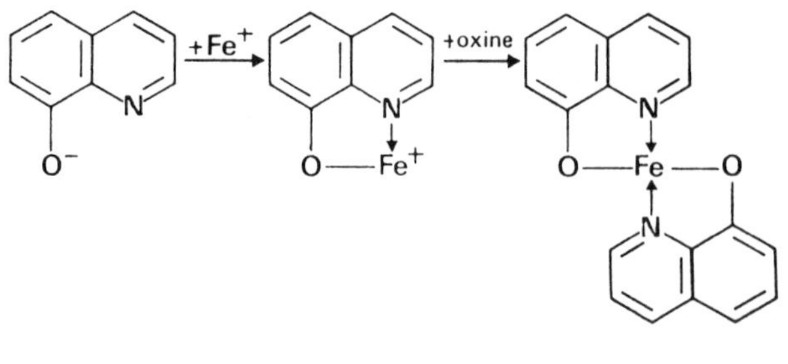

Fig. 3–8. Complexes formed between oxine and a divalent metal.

for chelation is bactericidal. Methylation of the hydroxy group abolishes activity. The metal is held in a clawlike linkage that is partly ionic and partly covalent. The complexes that may be formed between oxine and a divalent metal are illustrated in Figure 3–8.

Oxine is bactericidal to gram-positive cocci at a concentration of M/100,000 in nutrient broth, but is inactive in distilled water unless an equivalent amount of divalent or trivalent iron or divalent copper is added (Albert et al., 1953). The activity in broth is caused by metal impurities. The necessity for extracellular reaction between metal and ligand indicates that activity depends on the saturated or unsaturated complexes. The saturated complexes of oxine are unlikely to be active, but would give the best chance of entering the cell. Provided that excess oxine, which abolishes activity, is not present, they could be expected to break down within, giving rise to the reactive unsaturated complexes.

Iron and copper are the only metals that are active with oxine. Cobalt and nickel, which have greater affinity for oxine than the divalent forms of iron and copper, act as antagonists. Reversal by nickel is competitive, but cobalt is effective in trace amounts. It is known to break chain oxidation reactions involving ascorbic acid, which are catalyzed by iron or copper, and may prevent oxidative destruction of lipoic acid (Albert, 1979).

Derivatives of 1,10-phenanthroline combine with a greater variety of metals, including copper, manganese, nickel, and ruthenium, to give both saturated and unsaturated complexes active against gram-positive or gram-negative bacteria (Butler et al., 1969; Dwyer et al., 1969) or pathogenic fungi (Cade et al., 1970). Two nitrogen atoms are involved in the chelate bond, and the antimicrobial spectrum depends on the metal. The saturated complexes are active because they carry a positive charge on the whole molecule, but their bactericidal action is relatively slow.

Many other antimicrobial agents are capable of chelation. It may have nothing to do with their activity, but could be responsible for beneficial or undesired side effects. Tetracyclines chelate iron and calcium; consequences of this may be suppression of absorption from the intestine, failure to cure bovine mastitis, accumulation in bones and teeth, or deprivation of calcium that is needed for some body functions. Combination with metals enhances the antimicrobial activity of bacitracin (zinc), isonicotinic acid hydrazide, and p-aminosalicylic acid (Weinberg, 1961).

Sporicidal and Sporistatic Chemicals

Comparatively few chemicals are sporicidal, and many powerful bactericidal agents, such as phenols and quaternary ammonium compounds, have little effect on the viability of bacterial spores. Nevertheless, such agents will be inhibitory at certain stages in the overall life cycle, and consequently, there are three general areas in which a lethal or inhibitory effect may prevail. These are (1) during the various stages of sporulation; (2) on the mature spore itself; and (3) during germination and/or outgrowth.

Sporulation is a complex process, and the development of a mature spore from a vegetative cell is characterized by seven distinct stages (Young and Mandelstam, 1979). Penicillin and other antibiotics inhibit the septation stage (Stage II), although it has also been shown (Lawrence et al., 1971) that there are two distinct phases of penicillin binding, the second occurring during Stage IV (cortex formation). Nonantibiotic agents can be lethal if added before a certain stage of spore development. For example, resistance to octanol and butanol occurs at Stage V (synthesis of the spore coats) and to phenol at Stage VI (spore maturation, increase in refractility) (Balassa et al., 1979).

The following agents have been found to kill mature spores: glutaraldehyde, formaldehyde, hypochlorites, iodine, hydrogen peroxide, and ethylene oxide. The reasons for this effect, however, are poorly understood. Glutaraldehyde is believed by Gorman et al. (1980) to interact with protein, enzymes, and loosely crosslinked peptidoglycan in the cortex. This action may be assisted by the action of inorganic cations. As a rather loose explanation, penetration of the disinfectants into the spore has been invoked as the underlying factor in their action (Sykes, 1970; see also Russell, 1982b, 1983).

Several studies show clearly that chemicals that are not sporicidal, as well as those that are, might be inhibitory during the germination and/or outgrowth processes. Certain agents such as phenols and cresols inhibit germination, whereas others (e.g., quaternary ammonium compounds) inhibit outgrowth. Further examples are provided in Table 3–9. Interesting though these findings undoubtedly are, no significant studies have been carried out to indicate what changes occur in the spores during germination and outgrowth that will correlate with an altered sensitivity to disinfectant-type agents at certain times. The situation with specific antibiotic inhibitors of macromolecular syntheses is somewhat different, because it is known that these biosynthetic processes occur during outgrowth. Thus, in this order, actinomycin D inhibits mRNA synthesis, chloramphenicol and tetracycline inhibit protein synthesis, and mitomycin C inhibits DNA synthesis. In *Bacillus cereus*, the cells are relatively stable to penicillin (an inhibitor of cell wall synthesis) during the early phase of postgerminative development, but become highly sensitive to this antibiotic during the later phase of elongation and first division (Vinter, 1971). The effects of various agents on bacterial spores are considered by Russell (1983 and 1990b) and Russell et al. (1989).

MICROBIAL RESISTANCE TO CHEMICAL AGENTS

A review of the principles of antimicrobial activity would be incomplete if the complex problem of microbial resistance (Table 3–10) were not considered. In this section, the mechanisms of resistance only to antimicrobial chemicals are considered, because possible mechanisms of resistance of bacteria (especially spores) to thermal and radiation processs have been described earlier. The general nature of resistance has been well considered by Bryan (1979).

"Sensitivity" and "resistance" are relative terms. Microorganisms are said to be resistant when they are not killed by a concentration of a chemotherapeutic drug

Table 3–9. *Inhibitors of Germination or Outgrowth of Bacterial Spores**

Stage	Inhibitor(s)	Comment
Germination	Phenols, cresols, esters of p-hydroxybenzoic acid	Reversible
	Mercury compounds	Reversible? Thioglycollate might be toxic
	Alcohols	Reversible
	Glutaraldehyde, formaldehyde	
Outgrowth	Quaternary ammonium compounds	Retention by spores?
	Chlorine disinfectants	High concentrations prevent germination also
	Ethylene oxide	
	Actinomycin D	Inhibits RNA synthesis
	Chloramphenicol	Inhibits protein synthesis
	Mitomycin C	Inhibits DNA synthesis

*See Russell, 1982b, 1983 and 1990b.

Table 3–10. *Mechanisms of Resistance to Antimicrobial Agents*

Mechanism of Resistance	Example	Comment
Enzymatic inactivation	Chloramphenicol	Acetyltransferase found in *Staphylococcus aureus* (inducible) and R+ *Escherichia coli* (constitutive)
	Aminoglycoside-amino-cyclitol antibiotics*	Phosphotransferase, acetyltransferase or adenylase enzymes, usually coded for by R-factors
	β-Lactam antibiotics	β-Lactamases: different types of enzymes. Various penicillins and (especially) cephalosporins may be resistant (see Table 3–11)
	Mercury compounds	Vaporization: usually associated with R+ bacteria
Permeability barrier (outer membrane, gram-negative bacteria)	β-Lactam antibiotics	Gram-negative rods; likely in gonococci also
	Tetracyclines	Note R+ bacteria (see text)
	Biguanides	*Providencia stuartii* may be highly resistant
	Quaternary ammonium compounds	*Pseudomonas aeruginosa* highly resistant
	Polymyxins	*Proteus* and *Serratia* highly resistant
	Triphenylmethane dyes	
	Hydrophobic molecules	
Permeability barrier (spore coat and/or cortex)	Ethylene oxide	Spore coat is barrier?
	Hydrogen peroxide	Coats are barrier in *Clostridium bifermentans* (not in *Bacillus cereus*)
	Octanol	Barrier is cortex?
	Chlorine disinfectants	Coats are barrier
Tolerance	β-Lactam antibiotics	Found in autolysin-defective pneumococci and certain other bacteria
Efflux mechanism	Mercury compounds	
	Tetracyclines	Found in some MRSA† strains
	Quaternary ammonium compounds, acridines, ethidium bromide	
Decreased affinity of target enzyme	β-Lactam antibiotics	Altered penicillin-sensitive enzymes (PSEs) in resistant strains of gonococci
	Trimethoprim	Altered dihydrofolate reductase
	Sulfonamides	Altered dihydropteroic synthetase
Alteration in binding site	Streptomycin	Altered 30S ribosomal subunits
	Erythromycin	Altered 50S ribosomal subunits

*Drug modification, rather than drug inactivation, is a better term when applied to this group of antibiotics.
†MRSA, methicillin-resistant *Staphylococcus aureus* strains.

normally attainable in vivo (e.g., serum concentration) or of a disinfectant at a concentration used in practice, when they are not killed by a concentration of drug that kills the majority of cells in a culture, or when a strain is not killed by an agent that kills similar strains at a specified concentration.

In the simplest possible terms, resistance may be natural, i.e., characteristic of particular species or strains, or acquired (arising by mutation in sensitive cell populations or by transfer of resistance). Transferable resistance, which is considered more fully in the following section, occurs usually between mating cells of gram-negative bacilli during the process of conjugation. The possibility that mutations conferring drug resistance are induced by exposure of bacteria to the drug is unlikely

to be important in the majority of cases, because the replica-plating technique of Lederberg and Lederberg (1952) allowed *indirect* selection of mutant clones and their development into large, uniformly resistant populations.

Selection by exposure to an antimicrobial agent is the most important factor in the emergence and spread of drug-resistant bacteria in hospitals. Without this selection procedure it is likely that rare resistant mutants would not normally survive and naturally resistant strains such as β-lactamase-producing staphylococci and multiresistant enteric bacilli would constitute only a small proportion of the organisms isolated in hospitals.

As early as 1911, Ehrlich postulated that resistance to drugs would be a problem. This prediction has been amply confirmed, and resistance to many important chemotherapeutic and biocides has been observed.

This section examines the mechanisms of resistance of nonsporing bacteria to antibiotics and biocides and the possible relationship and significance between the two groups. The role of plasmids is considered, as are the mechanisms whereby inhibitors enter bacterial cells (bacterial spores are dealt with in another chapter).

Transferable Drug Resistance

Genetic material can be transferred from one bacterial cell to another in three ways: (1) by transduction, in which a transducing phage might "pick up" a stretch of DNA containing a drug-resistant determinant and transfer this to another cell; (2) by transformation, in which DNA extracted from the cells of one strain may be absorbed by a second strain ("competent" cells) in which heritable changes occur; or (3) by conjugation, in which cell-to-cell contact is necessary. This process will be considered in the following.

In the late 1950s, during a dysentery outbreak in Japan, a *Shigella* strain was observed to be resistant to four chemically different chemotherapeutic agents. It was unlikely that this strain arose by spontaneous mutation during the outbreak. Other multiresistant strains of gram-negative bacteria were also isolated, and researchers suggested that blocks of resistance genes were being transferred among bacteria of the same or different species.

In conjugation, cell-to-cell contact occurs via a cytoplasmic bridge (pilus) between mating bacteria. Male bacteria (donors) possess sex factors that promote conjugation to female bacteria (recipients). In the context of resistance, conjugation between donors and recipients is promoted by a resistance transfer factor (RTF), to which may be attached one or more fragments of resistance determinants that confer drug resistance. The RTF and resistance determinant(s) together comprise the resistance (R-) factor or resistance (R-) plasmid. A plasmid is a small, extrachromosomal element composed of double-stranded DNA that replicates independently within host cells. It remains extrachromosomal and is thus distinguishable from another type of extrachromosomal element, an episome, which undergoes reversible integration into the chromosome. Excellent accounts of plasmids and of their role in resistance are provided by Novick (1980), Levy (1982), and Hardy (1986). Moreover, plasmids can be transferred from cell to cell by transduction.

A transposable element (transposon, designated Tn) is a DNA segment that can insert into several sites on a genome (Cohen, 1976; Levy, 1982). Transposons are structurally defined and genetically discrete units and are capable of moving from plasmid to plasmid or from plasmid to chromosome. Several drug-resistance determinants are located on these transposable elements. Plasmid RP1, for example, codes for resistance to carbenicillin, tetracycline, and kanamycin; acquisition of the mercury transposon Tn 501 produces a new plasmid pUB

1351, which now combines the properties of RP1 and that coded for by Tn501.

Transferable (infective) drug resistance is thus important in the spread of bacterial resistance (Richmond et al., 1980). Plasmids have also been associated with bacterial resistance to biocides, and antibiotic and biocide resistance have been proposed to be linked.

The role of plasmids in bacterial resistance to biocides has not been studied extensively. There are examples where acquisition of a plasmid can alter surface properties (Curtis and Richmond, 1974; Hesslewood and Smith, 1974). The RP1 plasmid appears to be responsible for cell envelope changes and can additionally specify resistance to the antibiotics carbenicillin, tetracycline, and neomycin/kanamycin, but not to Hg^{2+} or organomercury. $RP1^+$ strains of *Escherichia coli* and *Pseudomonas aeruginosa* show the same order of sensitivity to quaternary ammonium compounds, chlorhexidine, phenolics, and organomercurials as the isogenic plasmidless strains (Ahonkhai and Russell, 1979). The closely related RP4 plasmid has been found to increase the sensitivity of *E. coli*, *Proteus mirabilis*, and *Serratia marcescens* to the bactericidal action of chlorhexidine, whereas other plasmids decreased sensitivity (Michel-Briand et al., 1986). Acquisition of transposon (Tn)501 specifying Hg^{2+} resistance in *E. coli* does not alter biocide response (Ahonkhai et al., 1984). Introduction of the F-like plasmid R124 into an OmpC mutant of *E. coli* confers greater sensitivity to quaternary ammonium compounds (Rossouw and Rowbury, 1984). In *P. aeruginosa*, the RP1 plasmid has been claimed to confer resistance to hexachlorophane (hexachlorophene; Sutton and Jacoby, 1978), but not to other biocides. Plasmid-mediated resistance to formaldehyde in *S. marcescens* has been described (Kaulfers et al., 1987; Heinzel, 1988), with a significant increase in uptake of the aldehyde by the-resistant strain as compared to the sensitive, plasmid-free, strain and transfer of resistance to an *E. coli* recipient. Col V plasmids confer F-like transfer properties on enterobacteria and permit them to synthesize the colicin V toxin as well as an outer membrane protein VmpA. Col^+ strains are more hydrophobic than Col^- strains and show an increasing sensitivity to acid and to hydrophobic agents; when attached to glass beads, however, the Col^+ strains are more resistant to chlorine than are unattached bacteria (Hicks and Rowbury, 1986).

Plasmid-mediated resistance to some cationic bactericides has been described with some strains of *Staphylococcus aureus* (see "Efflux mechanisms," later in this chapter). Generally, however, no strong evidence indicates that plasmids are involved to any great extent in the resistance of gram-negative bacteria to biocides. Resistance that occurs is usually intrinsic and not transferable (Russell, 1985; van Cuyck-Gandre et al., 1985; Russell et al., 1986; Hammond et al., 1987).

The biochemical mechanisms of chromosomal and plasmid-mediated resistance to antibiotics and other agents are discussed in the following. Resistance to an antimicrobial agent can arise in several ways (Bryan, 1984; Jacoby, 1985; Table 3–10). Bacteria may produce inactivating enzymes, exclude the drug, show tolerance, present changes in the target enzyme or other target site, or remove the drug or biocide by an efflux mechanism.

Inactivation of Antimicrobial Agents

Bacterial enzymes are often responsible for the inactivation of antibiotics. Some organisms produce an enzyme (chloramphenicol acetyltransferase) that inactivates chloramphenicol (Shaw, 1971, 1984; Mitsuhashi et al., 1977; Davies and Smith, 1978). In gram-negative plasmid-bearing strains, the enzyme is constitutive, whereas in *S. aureus*, it is inducible.

Aminoglycoside-inactivating enzymes are frequently described, although perhaps the term "aminoglycoside-modifying enzymes" should be used because, unlike with chloramphenicol (discussed previously) and β-lactam antibiotics (to be discussed), not all the antibiotic is inactivated, and one cannot isolate modified antibiotic from the culture medium. Thus, complete detoxification of the molecule of aminoglycoside does not occur. The drug-modifying enzymes coded for by R⁻ plasmids appear to be located in the periplasmic space (Davies and Smith, 1978; Shannon and Phillips, 1983; Phillips and Shannon, 1984).

Probably the most widely studied drug-inactivating enzymes are the β-lactamases (Hamilton-Miller and Smith, 1979; Medeiros, 1984). Soon after the introduction of benzylpenicillin into clinical use, it became clear that β-lactamase-producing staphylococci would pose a problem to its efficacy. The development of β-lactamase-resistant penicillins and cephalosporins was thus significant. More recently, considerable numbers of resistant strains of gram-negative bacteria have been isolated, and many of these have been shown to produce β-lactamases. Some of these enzymes (Table 3–11) are of the penicillinase type (with predominant activity against penicillins), and others are of the cephalosporinase type (with predominant activity against cephalosporins); the remainder have a broad spectrum of activity and are coded by R-plasmids. Several different types of β-lactamases are known (Table 3–11), and considerable information is now available about their substrate profiles (the relative rates at which β-lactams are hydrolyzed), inhibition by cloxacillin and *p*-chloromercuribenzoate, inducibility, and role in bacterial resistance (Sykes and Matthew, 1976; Richmond, 1978; Sykes, 1982; Nayler, 1987; Dürckheimer et al., 1988). O'Callaghan (1980) has considered structure-activity relationships in the β-lactam antibiotics with β-lactamase resistance.

Inactivation of metallic compounds is also known. Some bacteria, notably R⁺ strains, are capable of producing enzymes that can vaporize inorganic (and possibly organic) mercury salts to mercury. This example of resistance has been well discussed by Chopra (1982, 1987). Because of its toxicity, mercuric chloride is no longer widely used as a disinfectant. Organomercury compounds such as thiomersal, phenylmercuric nitrate (PMN), and acetate (PMA), however, may still be used as preservatives. Mercury resistance is plasmid borne, not chromosomal (Foster, 1983; Silver and Misra, 1988), and may be transferred from donor to recipient cells by conjugation or transduction. Such plasmids are of two types, "narrow-spectrum" and "broad-spectrum." Plasmids have also been described that encode increased sensitivity to Hg^{2+}. Several resistance determinants that are located on DNA segments can transpose from one bacterial replicon to another. Plasmid-determined resistance to silver (Ag^+) and to other cations as well as to some anions has also been demonstrated.

Permeability Barriers

Significant differences exist in the outer layers of gram-positive and gram-negative bacteria. The cell walls of staphylococci, for example, are composed predominantly of peptidoglycan and teichoic acids and protect the delicate, underlying lipoprotein cytoplasmic membrane. No specific receptor molecules or permeases exist to assist biocide or antibiotic penetration, and the exclusion limit of the cell wall of *Bacillus megaterium* has been calculated as being at least 30,000 daltons (Lambert, 1983; Hammond et al., 1984). Thus, most antibacterial agents readily enter nonsporing, nonmycobacterial, gram-positive bacteria, and such organisms are generally more sensitive than gram-negative bacteria.

In gram-negative bacteria, the outer layers are more complex and diverse. Gram-negative organisms possess two membranes, an outer and an inner (cytoplasmic) membrane. The inner membrane again consists of lipoprotein, and between the two membranes is the periplasmic space incorporating the peptidoglycan, which is smaller and less extensively crosslinked than in staphylococci.

The outer membrane of gram-negative bacteria is composed of lipopolysaccharide, protein, and lipid. It plays an important role in acting as a barrier to the entry of diverse chemical agents (Costerton et al., 1974; Costerton, 1977; Witholt et al., 1976; Nikaido, 1976; Nikaido and Nakae, 1979; El-Falaha et al., 1983; Nikaido and Vaara, 1985).

The presence of lipid in the cell envelope of gram-negative organisms has long been claimed to be related to the fact that they are more highly resistant than are gram-positive bacteria to antibacterial agents. Chaplin (1952) developed strains of *Serratia marcescens* that were highly resistant to quaternary ammonium compounds and, on the basis of electrophoretic studies, observed that the most resistant strains had a greater amount of cell-surface lipid, which was associated with insusceptibility. Lipid is normally present only in small amounts in the cell wall of staphylococci. If this is increased (by growing the cells in the presence of glycerol), however, the organisms become more resistant to penicillins (Hugo and Stretton, 1966) and to certain phenols (Hugo and Franklin, 1968). The lipid content of cell walls of mycobacteria is believed to be associated with their

Table 3–11. *β-Lactamases of Gram-Negative Bacteria*

Class*	Gene Location†	Constitutive (Con) or Inducible (Ind)	Substrate Preference
I	C	Mostly Ind	Cephalosporins
II	C	Con	Penicillins
III	P	Con	Penicillins + cephalosporins
IV	C	Con	Penicillins Cephalosporins
V	P	Con	Penicillins + cephalosporins

*Class III enzymes are inhibited by cloxacillin. Class V enzymes are not inhibited by cloxacillin, which may act as a substrate for these Class V β-lactamases.

†C, chromosome; P, plasmid-mediated.

frequently above-average resistance to disinfectants (Croshaw, 1971; Russell and Chopra, 1989).

Tamaki et al. (1971) studied the sensitivities to various antibiotics of novobiocin-supersensitive strains of *Escherichia coli* that had defects in their outer-membrane lipopolysaccharide. The lipopolysaccharide of these mutants contained significantly different levels of heptose, phosphate, glucose and galactose, and the cells were sensitive to some antibiotics (e.g., novobiocin, actinomycin D), but not to others (such as benzylpenicillin). Lipopolysaccharide-defective mutants of *Pseudomonas aeruginosa* strain PAO show increased susceptibility to sodium deoxycholate, quaternary ammonium compounds, and some antibiotics (Kropinski et al., 1978). A considerable amount of outer membrane lipopolysaccharide is released when gram-negative cells are exposed to EDTA (Leive, 1974). The organisms are not usually killed by such treatment (although *P. aeruginosa* is more sensitive to EDTA than other bacteria), but are rendered more sensitive to a variety of chemically unrelated disinfectants and antibiotics (Russell, 1971; Brown, 1975; Wilkinson, 1975; Haque and Russell, 1976). These studies all suggest that the lipopolysaccharide component of the outer membrane plays an important role in conferring resistance to antibacterial agents. EDTA may additionally damage the inner membrane, however, because actinomycin D does not penetrate the sucrose-lysozyme spheroplasts of *P. aeruginosa* unless the cells are also treated with EDTA (Cheng et al., 1973). Nonetheless, EDTA-induced damage is more severe to the outer than to the inner membrane (Matsushita et al., 1978).

Studies by Nikaido and his colleagues (Ames et al., 1974; Nikaido and Nakae, 1979; Nikaido and Vaara, 1985) have demonstrated that alterations in the structure of the outer membrane lipopolysaccharide also affect the composition of outer membrane proteins. Deep rough mutants, which are defective in the inner region of the core, are sensitive to a variety of dyes and detergents. Nevertheless, Ames et al. (1974) concluded that the increased permeability of the deep rough mutants could be either a direct consequence of defective (or decreased) lipopolysaccharide or of a lowered level of outer membrane proteins. Subsequent investigations by Nakae (1976) demonstrated that the reconstitution of the outer membrane of vesicles permeable to small hydrophilic molecules (such as sugars) requires the presence of three species of proteins in *Salmonella typhimurium*, but only one kind of protein in *E. coli*, in addition to phospholipids and lipopolysaccharide. These major proteins are responsible for producing nonspecific water channels (pores) through the outer membrane; these are termed "porins" by Nakae (1976; see also Benz, 1988). This theme has been explored further by Nikaido (1976), who found, as described earlier, that deep rough mutants of *S. typhimurium* were much more sensitive than the wild-type strains to certain antibiotics and dyes (mostly hydrophobic, molecular weights generally above 1200), but not to others (mainly hydrophilic, molecular weights usually less than 650). From this, it has been proposed that most small hydrophilic substances (e.g., benzylpenicillin, ampicillin) penetrate the outer membrane by means of the porins. Evidence for this has been obtained by the reduced diffusion of cephaloridine in porin-deficient mutants of *Salmonella* (Nikaido et al., 1977). Nikaido and Nakae (1979) have suggested that the increased permeability of deep rough mutants results from extensive changes in the organization of the outer membrane as a consequence of lipopolysaccharide defects. Reorganization of phospholipid in the outer membrane could allow the penetration of hydrophobic molecules by dissolution and diffusion in the lipid.

Permeability barriers to the entry of antibacterial agents thus exist in the outer membrane of gram-negative bacteria. The composition of the outer membrane (and hence the cellular response to chemical agents) can be varied by changing the growth conditions, and especially by limiting the amount of a specific component; thus, magnesium-limited cells of *P. aeruginosa* are more resistant to EDTA and polymyxin (Brown, 1975). In this organism, the exclusion limit of the porins has been claimed to be much higher (around 6000) than in other gram-negative bacteria (Nikaido and Nakae, 1979), leading to the concept that either *P. aeruginosa* possesses fewer porins or that many of them are nonfunctional. An exclusion limit of about 300 has also been proposed, however (Caulcott et al., 1984).

The surface of smooth gram-negative bacteria is hydrophilic in nature; deep rough (heptoseless) mutants, on the other hand, tend to be much more hydrophobic. In wild-type strains, the intact lipopolysaccharide molecules prevent ready access of hydrophobic biocides or antibiotics to the cell interior, probably by shielding phospholipids, many of which are not in the classic membrane structure. In deep rough strains, which lack the O-specific side chain and most of the core polysaccharide, as well as in EDTA-treated cells, phospholipid patches appear at the cell surface. The sensitivity of wild-type and outer membrane mutants of *Escherichia coli* and *Salmonella typhimurium* to a range of biocides has recently been studied. The parabens (esters of *para*(4)-hydroxybenzoic acid) are most useful in this context because they have a range of hydrophobicities. Antibacterial activity increases against smooth strains as the homologous series is ascended and even more against deep rough strains (Russell and Furr, 1986a, b; Russell et al., 1985, 1987). Similar findings have been made with the phenolics phenol, cresol, and chlorocresol (Russell and Furr, 1986a, b; Russell et al., 1987; Russell and Gould, 1988).

In addition to the hydrophilic and hydrophobic pathways considered previously, a third pathway has been proposed for cationic bactericides. Biguanides and quaternary ammonium compounds (QACs) both interact with phospholipids and LPS, and it has been suggested that these biocides, as well as polymyxins, damage the outer membrane, thereby promoting their own uptake (Hancock, 1984). There are, however, significant differences in the response of gram-negative bacteria to these agents. The QACs are considerably less active against wild-type than deep rough strains, whereas chlorhexidine has the same order of activity against wild-type and envelope mutants of *E. coli*, although deep rough strains of *S. typhimurium* are more sensitive than the parent (Russell, 1986; Russell and Furr, 1986b).

A particularly resistant gram-negative organism is *Providencia stuartii* (Stickler et al., 1983, 1987; Hawkey, 1984; Stickler and Chawla, 1987). Together with other gram-negative bacteria such as *Pseudomonas aeruginosa* and *Proteus mirabilis* isolated from urinary tract infections in patients in a paraplegic unit these organisms showed resistance to cationic bactericides and to several antibiotics. This has led to the suggestion that the widespread use of chlorhexidine might be responsible for selecting antibiotic-resistant strains, but all attempts to demonstrate any plasmid-linked association of antibiotic and chlorhexidine resistance have been unsuccessful. Resistance appears to be associated with the outer rather than the inner membrane (Ismaeel et al., 1986, 1987; Russell and Gould, 1988), although the exact mechanism has yet to be elucidated.

MRSA strains may be a considerable problem in the context of hospital infections (Shanson, 1987), but no evidence indicates that exclusion is a major factor in their resistance.

Role of the Glycocalyx: Bacterial Biofilms

The interaction of bacteria is initially reversible and eventually irreversible. The process of irreversible adhesion is initiated by the binding of bacteria to the surface by means of exopolysaccharide glycocalyx polymers (Brown and Williams, 1985; Costerton et al., 1987). Sister cells produced as a result of cell division are bound within the glycocalyx matrix. The development of adherent microcolonies leads eventually to the production of a continuous biofilm on the colonized surface. Although mucoexopolysaccharide production is sometimes associated with antibiotic-supersensitive cells, e.g. of *Pseudomonas aeruginosa* (Slack and Nichols, 1982), bacteria within biofilms tend to be much more resistant to antibiotics and biocides than cells in batch-type culture (Marrie and Costerton, 1981; Costerton et al., 1987). There are two possible reasons: (1) physiologic changes in the cells; and (2) penetration barriers presented by the exopolysaccharide matrix. Subculture of cells in vitro results in loss of the glycocalyx and reimposition of biocide sensitivity.

Tolerance

The term "tolerance" has been used in the context of bacteria that are able to resist the irreversible effects (lysis) of penicillin. *Streptococcus pneumoniae* cells (pneumococci) have demonstrable autolysin (peptidoglycan hydrolase) activity, whereas tolerant pneumococci do not. Penicillin-tolerant strains of other organisms (*Escherichia coli*, staphylococci) have also been described; autolysin-defective mutants of staphylococci have been isolated from clinical specimens (Sabath, 1980). For an excellent review on tolerance, consult Tomasz (1980).

Altered Target Sites

The binding of antibiotics to specific enzymes or sites, such as penicillin-binding proteins and ribosomal binding, has been mentioned previously. Changes in these enzymes or sites thus would be expected to result in an altered susceptibility.

Spratt (1978) has described a mutant of *E. coli* that is resistant to mecillinam at 30°C or below because it produces an altered PBP 2 (see Table 3–5), which has a decreased affinity for this antibiotic. Giles and Reynolds (1979) have isolated cloxacillin-resistant mutants of *Bacillus megaterium* in which increasing resistance to cloxacillin is related to an increase in the ratio of PBP 3 to PBP 1. Reynolds and Fuller (1986) have demonstrated that a methicillin-resistant strain of *Staphylococcus aureus* possessed a PBP 3 with a decreased affinity for β-lactam antibiotics and contained an additional PBP (PBP 2).

The site of action of streptomycin has been shown to be the 30S ribosomal subunit. The S12 ribosomal protein determines whether or not the ribosome binds this antibiotic, and alterations in S12, although it itself does not bind streptomycin, alter the availability of streptomycin attachment sites (Wallace et al., 1979). Likewise, alteration in the 50S ribosomal subunit is believed to be associated with resistance to erythromycin (Pestka, 1977).

Low concentrations of novobiocin inhibit purified DNA gyrase from novobiocin-sensitive *E. coli* strains, whereas a similarly purified enzyme from a resistant strain is not inhibited by high concentrations of the antibiotic (Ryan, 1979).

Alterations in target enzymes (dihydropteroate synthetase and dihydrofolate reductase) have been found to be reasons for increased bacterial resistance to sulfonamides and trimethoprim, respectively (Smith, 1979).

Efflux Mechanisms

An interesting research mechanism is one involving efflux of antibiotics or biocides. This has been known for many years as one mechanism conferring resistance to tetracyclines (Chopra, 1988a, b, c) and has also been claimed to occur with methicillin-resistant *Staphylococcus aureus* (MRSA) strains and various antibacterial agents. For example, resistance to ethidium bromide, originally considered to arise by a diminished uptake to resistant cells, is now known to be caused by an efflux system whereby it is extruded from the cell interior (Jones and Midgeley, 1985). A similar mechanism is believed to operate in these strains with acridines and quaternary ammonium compounds (QACs). Further studies along these lines with MRSA and other strains might well show that this mechanism is more widespread than is currently believed.

Possible Linked Antibiotic-biocide Resistance

There has been a tendency to consider antibiotic resistance and biocide resistance as separate events. Some have claimed, however, that not only can antibiotic and biocide resistances be linked and plasmid-mediated, but also biocides are responsible for the selection of antibiotic-resistant strains. As already stated, Stickler and his colleagues (Stickler et al., 1983, 1987; Stickler and Chawla, 1987) found that about 15% of gram-negative strains (*Pseudomonas aeruginosa*, *Proteus mirabilis* and *Providencia stuartii*) isolated from urinary tract infections in a paraplegic unit showed resistance to cationic bactericides (QACs, chlorhexidine) and to at least five antibiotics (see Russell, 1985, Russell et al., 1986, and Russell and Gould, 1988, for further details). This led to the suggestion that the widespread use of these biocides was responsible for selecting antibiotic-resistant strains, although all attempts to demonstrate any plasmid-linked association of antibiotic and chlorhexidine resistance have failed.

Multiple-antibiotic-resistant bacteria have been isolated from drinking water (Armstrong et al., 1981, 1982). Disinfection and purification of water may augment the occurrence of antibiotic-resistant bacteria, and chlorination may select or induce such changes (Murray et al., 1984).

Disinfectants have been shown to induce changes in the antibiotic sensitivity and phage typing pattern in *Staphylococcus aureus* (Sivaji et al., 1986). The persistence and spread of a determinant conferring acridine, ethidium bromide, and QAC resistances ($Ac^REb^RQa^R$) in MRSA strains have been claimed to result from the extensive use of acriflavin and QACs as antiseptics and disinfectants (Gillespie et al., 1986; Lyon and Skurray, 1987). The level of resistance to QACs of these MRSA strains is low, however; MIC values are considerably below in-use concentrations, and further, acridines are now used only infrequently.

Obviously, the genetic basis of linked antibiotic-biocide resistance is one of potential clinical and public health significance, and it is hoped that further progress will be made toward a better understanding of the problem.

REFERENCES

Ahmed, F.I.K., and Russell, C. 1975. Synergism between ultrasonic waves and hydrogen peroxide in the killing of micro-organisms. J. Appl. Bacteriol., 39, 31–40.

Ahonkhai, I., and Russell, A.D. 1979. Response of RP1+ and RP1- strains of *Escherichia coli* to antibacterial agents and transfer of resistance to *Pseudomonas aeruginosa*. Curr. Microbiol., 3, 89–94.

Ahonkhai, I., Pugh, W.J., and Russell, A.D. 1984. Sensitivity to antimicrobial agents of some mercury-sensitive and -resistant strains of gram-negative bacteria. Curr. Microbiol., 11, 183–185.

Albert, A. 1979. Selectivity in the service of man. In *Selective Toxicity*. 5th Edition. London, Methuen and Co.

Albert, A., Gibson, M.I., and Rubbo, S.D. 1953. The influence of chemical constitution on antibacterial activity. Part VI. The bactericidal action of 8-hydroxyquinoline (oxine). Br. J. Exp. Pathol., 34, 119–130.

Alexander, P., and Stacey, K.A. 1958. Comparison of the changes produced by ionizing radiations and by the alkylating agents: evidence for a similar mechanism at the molecular level. Ann. N.Y. Acad. Sci., 68, 1225–1237.

Algie, J.E. 1983. The heat resistance of bacterial spores and its relationship to the contraction of the forespore protoplasm during sporulation. Curr. Microbiol., 9, 173–175.

Allwood, M.C., and Russell, A.D. 1970. Mechanisms of thermal injury in nonsporing bacteria. Adv. Appl. Microbiol., 12, 89–119.

Ames, G., Spudich, E., and Nikaido, H. 1974. Protein composition of the outer membrane of *Salmonella typhimurium*: effect of lipopolysaccharide mutations. J. Bacteriol., 117, 406–416.

Amyes, S.G.B., and Smith, J.T. 1975. Thymineless mutants and their resistance to trimethoprim. J. Antimicrob. Chemother., 1, 85–89.

Amyes, S.G.B., and Smith, J.T. 1978. R-factor mediated dihydrofolate reductases which confer trimethoprim resistance. J. Gen. Microbiol., 107, 263–271.

Anand, N., and Davis, B.D. 1960. Effect of streptomycin on *Escherichia coli*. Nature, 185, 22–23.

Andrew, M.H.E., and Russell, A.D. (Eds.) 1984. *The Revival of Injured Microbes*. Society for Applied Bacteriology Symposium Series No. 12. London, Academic Press.

Archibald, A.R. 1988. Bacterial cell wall structure and the ionic environment. FEMS Symp. No. 44, 159–173.

Armstrong, J.L., Calomaris, J.J., and Seidler, P.J. 1982. Selection of antibiotic-resistant standard plate count bacteria during water treatment. Appl. Environ. Microbiol., 44, 308–316.

Armstrong, J.L., Shigend, D.S., Calomaris, J.J., and Seidler, P.J. 1981. Antibiotic-resistant bacteria in drinking water. Appl. Environ. Microbiol., 42, 277–283.

Ashwood-Smith, M.J., and Bridges, B.A. 1967. On the sensitivity of frozen micro-organisms to ultraviolet radiation. Proc. R. Soc. London., B, 168, 194–202.

Athar, M.A., and Winner, H.I. 1971. The development of resistance by *Candida* species to polyene antibiotics *in vitro*. J. Med. Microbiol., 4, 505–517.

Balassa, G., et al. 1979. A *Bacillus subtilis* mutant requiring dipicolinic acid for the development of heat-resistant spores. J. Gen. Microbiol., 110, 365–379.

Benz, R. 1988. Structure and function of porins from gram-negative bacteria. Annu. Rev. Microbiol., 42, 359–393.

Blumberg, P.M., and Strominger, J.L. 1971. Inactivation of D-alanine carboxypeptidase by penicillins and cephalosporins is not lethal in *Bacillus subtilis*. Proc. Natl. Acad. Sci., U.S.A., 68, 2814–2817.

Booth, I.R. 1988. Control of proton permeability: its implications for energy translation and pH homeostasis. FEMS Symp. No 44, 1–12.

Borick, P.M. 1968. Chemical sterilizers (Chemosterilizers). Adv. Appl. Microbiol., *10*, 291–312.

Boucher, R.M.G. 1979. Ultrasonics. A tool to improve biocidal efficacy of sterilants or disinfectants in hospital and dental practice. Can. J. Pharm. Sci., *14*, 1–12.

Bridges, B.A. 1976. Survival of bacteria following exposure to ultraviolet and ionizing radiations. In *The Survival of Vegetative Microbes*. Edited by T.R.G. Gray and J.R. Postgate. Symposium 26, Society for General Microbiology. Cambridge, Cambridge University Press, pp. 183–208.

Brooks, P., and Lawley, P.D. 1964. Alkylating agents. Br. Med. Bull., *20*, 91–95.

Brot, N. 1977. Translocation. In *Molecular Methods of Protein Biosynthesis*. Edited by H. Weissback and S. Pestka. New York, Academic Press, pp. 375–411.

Brown, G.M. 1962. The biosynthesis of folic acid. Inhibition by sulfonamides. J. Biol. Chem., *237*, 536–540.

Brown, M.R.W. 1975. The role of the cell envelope in resistance. In *Resistance of Pseudomonas aeruginosa*. Edited by M.R.W. Brown, London, John Wiley & Sons, pp. 71–107.

Brown, M.R.W., and Williams, P. 1985. The influence of environment on envelope properties affecting survival of bacteria in infection. Annu. Rev. Microbiol., *39*, 527–556.

Broxton, P., Woodcock, P.M., Heatley, D., and Gilbert, P. 1984. Interaction of some polyhexamethylene biguanides and membrane phospholipids in *Escherichia coli*. J. Appl. Bacteriol., *57*, 115–124.

Bryan, L.E. 1979. Resistance to antimicrobial agents: the general nature of the problem and the basis of resistance. In *Pseudomonas aeruginosa: Clinical Manifestations of Infections and Current Therapy*. Edited by R.G. Doggett. New York, Academic Press, pp. 219–270.

Bryan, L.E. 1984. *Antimicrobial Drug Resistance*. London, Academic Press.

Burchall, J.J., and Hitchings, G.H. 1965. Inhibitor binding analysis of dehydrofolate reductases from various species. Mol. Pharmacol., *1*, 126–136.

Butler, H.M., Hurse, A., Thursky, E., and Shulman, A. 1969. Bactericidal action of selected phenanthroline chelates and related compounds. Aust. J. Exp. Biol. Med. Sci., *47*, 541–552.

Cade, G., et al. 1970. The treatment of dermatological infections with a manganese phenanthroline chelate. A controlled clinical trial. Med. J. Aust., *2*, 304–309.

Caulcott, C.A., Brown, M.R.W., and Gonda, I. 1984. Evidence for small pores in the outer membrane of *Pseudomonas aeruginosa*. FEMS Microbiol. Lett., *21*, 119–123.

Chang, F.N. 1979. Lincomycin. In *Antibiotics V. Part 1: Mechanism of Action of Antibacterial Agents*. Edited by F.E. Hahn. Berlin, Springer-Verlag, pp. 127–134.

Chaplin, C.E. 1952. Bacterial resistance to quaternary ammonium disinfectants. J. Bacteriol., *63*, 453–458.

Cheng, K.-J., Costerton, J.W., Singh, A.P., and Ingram, J.M. 1973. Susceptibility of whole cells and spheroplasts of *Pseudomonas aeruginosa* to actinomycin D. Antimicrob. Agents Chemother., *3*, 399–406.

Chopra, I.C. 1982. Microbial resistance: plasmids. In *Principles and Practice of Disinfection, Preservation and Sterilization*. Edited by A.D. Russell, W.B. Hugo, and G.A.J. Ayliffe. Oxford, Blackwell Scientific Publications, pp. 199–206.

Chopra, I. 1987. Microbial resistance to veterinary disinfectants and antiseptics. In *Disinfection in Veterinary and Farm Animal Practice*. Edited by A.H. Linton, W.B. Hugo, and A.D. Russell, Oxford, Blackwell Scientific Publications, pp. 43–65.

Chopra, I. 1988a. Molecular mechanisms involved in the transport of antibiotics into bacteria. Parasitology, *96*, S25–S44.

Chopra, I. 1988b. Mechanisms of resistance to antibiotics and other chemotherapeutic agents. J. Appl. Bacteriol. Symp. Suppl., 149S–166S.

Chopra, I. 1988c. Efflux of antibacterial agents from bacteria. FEMS Symp. No. 44, 146–158.

Chopra, I., Johnson, S.C., and Bennett, P.M. 1987. Inhibition of *Providencia stuartii* cell envelope enzymes by chlorhexidine. J. Antimicrob. Chemother., *19*, 743–751.

Clouston, J.G., and Wills, P.A. 1969. Initiation of germination and inactivation of *Bacillus pumilus* spores by hydrostatic pressure. J. Bacteriol., *97*, 684–690.

Clouston, J.G., and Wills, P.A. 1970. Kinetics of initiation of germination of *Bacillus pumilus* spores by hydrostatic pressure. J. Bacteriol., *103*, 140–143.

Cohen, S.N. 1976. Transposable genetic elements and plasmid evolution. Nature, *263*, 731–738.

Cole, M. 1980. 'β-lactams' as β-lactamase inhibitors. Phil. Trans. R. Soc. London., *B289*, 207–223.

Costerton, J.W. 1977. Cell envelope as a barrier to antibiotics. In *Microbiology 1977*. Edited by D. Schlessinger. American Society for Microbiology, Washington, D.C., pp. 151–157.

Costerton, J.W., Ingram, J.M., and Cheng, K.-J. 1974. Structure and function of the cell envelope of Gram-negative bacteria. Bacteriol. Rev., *38*, 87–110.

Costerton, J.W., et al. 1987. Bacterial biofilms in nature and disease. Annu. Rev. Microbiol., *41*, 435–464.

Croshaw, B. 1971. The destruction of mycobacteria. In *Inhibition and Destruction of the Microbial Cell*. Edited by W.B. Hugo. New York, Academic Press, pp. 419–449.

Crumplin, G.C., Midgley, J.M., and Smith, J.T. 1980. Mechanism of action of nalidixic acid and its congeners. In *Topics in Antibiotic Chemistry*. Edited by P.G. Sammes. Volume 3. Chichester, England, Ellis Horwood Ltd., pp. 9–38.

Cundliffe, E. 1979. Thiostrepton and related antibiotics. In *Antibiotics V. Part 1: Mechanism of Action of Antibacterial Agents*. Edited by F.E. Hahn. Berlin, Springer-Verlag, pp. 329–343.

Curtis, N.A.C., and Richmond, M.H. 1974. Effect of R-factor mediated genes on some surface properties of *Escherichia coli*. Antimicrob. Agents Chemother., *6*, 666–671.

Davies, J., and Smith, D.I. 1978. Plasmid-determined resistance to antimicrobial agents. Annu. Rev. Microbiol., *32*, 469–518.

Davies, R. 1976. The inactivation of vegetative bacterial cells by ionizing radiation. In *Inhibition and Inactivation of Vegetative Microbes*. Edited by F.A. Skinner and W.B. Hugo. Society for Applied Bacteriology Symposium Series No. 5. New York, Academic Press, pp. 239–255.

Davis, B.D., Chen, L., and Tai, P.C. 1986. Misread protein creates membrane channels: an essential step in the bactericidal action of aminoglycosides. Proc. Natl. Acad. Sci. U.S.A., *83*, 6164–6168.

De Kruijff, B., et al. 1974. Polyene antibiotic-sterol interactions in membranes of *Acholeplasma laidlawii* cells and lecithin liposomes. I. Specificity of the membrane permeability changes induced by the polyene antibiotics. Biochim. Biophys. Acta, *339*, 30–43.

Dixon, R.A., and Chopra, I. 1986. Polymyxin B and polymyxin B nonapeptide after membrane permeability in *Escherichia coli*. Antimicrob. Chemother., *18*, 557–563.

Donnellan, J.E., and Setlow, R.B. 1965. Thymine photoproducts but not thymine dimers found in ultraviolet-irradiated bacterial spores. Science, *149*, 308–310.

Dring, G.J. 1976. Some aspects of the effects of hydrostatic pressure on microorganisms. In *Inhibition and Inactivation of Vegetative Microbes*. Edited by F.A. Skinner and W.B. Hugo. Society for Applied Bacteriology Symposium Series No. 5. New York, Academic Press, pp. 257–277.

Durban, E., Grecz, N., and Farkas, J. 1974. Direct enzymatic repair of deoxyribonucleic acid single strand breaks in dormant spores. J. Bacteriol., *118*, 129–138.

Dürckheimer, W., Adam, F., Fischer, G., and Kirrstetter, R. 1988. Recent developments in the field of cephem antibiotics. Adv. Drug Res., *17*, 62–234.

Dwyer, F.P., et al. 1969. The biological actions of 1,10-phenanthroline and 2,2′-bipyridine hydrochlorides, quaternary salts and metal chelates and related compounds. I. Bacteriostatic action on selected Gram-positive, Gram-negative and acid-fast bacteria. Aust. J. Exp. Biol. Med. Sci., *47*, 203–218.

Ehrlich, P. 1911. *Theorie und Praxis der Chemotherapie*. Leipzig, Klinkhardt.

El-Falaha, B.M.A., Russell, A.D., and Furr, J.R. 1983. Sensitivities of wild-type and envelope-defective strains of *Escherichia coli* and *Pseudomonas aeruginosa* to antibacterial agents. Microbios, *38*, 99–105.

Ellison, R.T., Giehl, T.J., and LaForce, F.M. 1988. Damage of the outer membrane of enteric gram-negative bacteria by lactoferrin and transferrin. Infect. Immun., *56*, 2774–2781.

Fisher, J.F., and Knowles, J.R. 1980. The inactivation of β-lactamase by mechanism-based reagents. In *Enzyme Inhibitors as Drugs*. Edited by M. Sandler. London, Macmillan Press, pp. 209–218.

Foster, J.H.S., and Russell, A.D. 1971. Antibacterial dyes and nitrofurans. In *Inhibition and Destruction of the Microbial Cell*. Edited by W.B. Hugo. New York, Academic Press, pp. 185–208.

Foster, T.J. 1983. Plasmid-determined resistance to antimicrobial drugs and toxic metal ions in bacteria. Microbiol. Rev. *47*, 361–409.

Franklin, T., and Snow, G.A. 1981. *Biochemistry of Antimicrobial Action*. 3rd Edition. London, Chapman and Hall.

Frederick, J.J., Corner, T.R., and Gehardt, P. 1974. Antimicrobial actions of hexachlorophene: inhibition of respiration in *Bacillus megaterium*. Antimicrob. Agents Chemother., *6*, 712–721.

Frère, J.M., et al. 1980. Mode of action of β-lactam antibiotics at the molecular level. In *Enzyme Inhibitors as Drugs*. Edited by M. Sandler. London, Macmillan Press, pp. 183–207.

Gale, E.F. 1986. Nature and development of phenotypic resistance to amphotericin B in *Candida albicens*. Adv. Microb. Physiol., *27*, 277–320.

Gale, E.F., et al. 1981. *Molecular Basis of Antibiotic Action*. 2nd Edition. London, John Wiley.

Garvin, R.T., Rosset, R., and Gorini, L. 1973. Ribosomal assembly influenced by growth in the presence of streptomycin. Proc. Natl. Acad. Sci. U.S.A., *70*, 2762–2766.

Gerhardt, P. 1988. The refractory homeostasis of bacterial spores. FEMS Symp. No. 44, 41–49.

Gilbert, P. 1984. The revival of microorganisms sublethally injured by chemical inhibitors. In *The Revival of Injured Microbes*. Edited by M.H.E. Andrew and A.D. Russell. Society for Applied Bacteriology Symposium Series No. 12. London, Academic Press, pp. 175–197.

Gilbert, P., Beveridge, E.G., and Sissons, I. 1978. The uptake of some membrane-active drugs by bacteria and yeast: possible microbiological examples of 'Z'-curve adsorption. J. Coll. Interface Sci., *64*, 377–379.

Gilby, A.R., and Few, A.V. 1960. Lysis of protoplasts of *Micrococcus lysodeikticus* by ionic detergents. J. Gen. Microbiol., *23*, 27–33.

Giles, A.F., and Reynolds. P.E. 1979. *Bacillus megaterium* resistance to cloxacillin accompanied by a compensatory change in penicillin binding proteins. Nature, *280*, 167–168.

Giles, C.H., Smith, D., and Huitson, A. 1974. A general treatment and classification of the solute adsorption isotherm. I. Theoretical. J. Coll. Interface Sci., *47*, 755.

Giles, C.H., MacEwan, T.H., Nakhara, S.N., and Smith, D. 1960. Studies in adsorption. XI. A system of classification of solution adsorption isotherms and its use in the diagnosis of adsorption mechanisms and in measurement of specific surface areas of solids. J. Chem. Soc., 3973–3993.

Gillespie, M.T., May, J.W., and Skurray, R.A. 1986. Plasmid-encoded resistance to acriflavin and quaternary ammonium compounds in methicillin-resistant *Staphylococcus aureus*. FEMS Microbiol. Lett., *34*, 47–51.

Goldberg, I.J., and Friedman, P.A. 1971. Antibiotics and nucleic acids. Annu. Rev. Biochem., *40*, 775—810.

Goldblith, S.A. 1971. The inhibition and destruction of the microbial cell by radiations. In *Inhibition and Destruction of the Microbial Cell*. Edited by W.B. Hugo. New York, Academic Press, pp. 285–305.

Gorman, S.P., Scott, E.M., and Russell, A.D. 1980. Antimicrobial activity, uses and mechanisms of action of glutaraldehyde. J. Appl. Bacteriol., *48*, 161–190.

Gottlieb, D., and Shaw, P.D. 1970. Mechanism of action of antifungal antibiotics. Annu. Rev. Phytopathol., *8*, 371–402.

Gould, G.W. 1973. Inactivation of spores in food by combined heat and hydrostatic pressure. Acta Aliment., *2*, 377–383.

Gould, G.W. 1983. Mechanisms of resistance and dormancy. In *The Bacterial Spore*. Edited by A. Hurst and G.W. Gould. Volume 2. London, Academic Press, pp. 173–209.

Gould, G.W. 1984. Injury and repair mechanisms in bacterial spores. In *The Revival of Injured Microbes*. Edited by M.H.E. Andrew and A.D. Russell. Society for Applied Bacteriology Symposium Series No. 12. London, Academic Press, pp. 199–220.

Gould, G.W. 1985. Modification of resistance and dormancy. In *Fundamental and Applied Aspects of Bacterial Spores*. Edited by G.J. Dring, D.J. Ellar, and G.W. Gould. London, Academic Press, pp. 371–382.

Gould, G.W., and Dring, G.J. 1975. Role of an expanded cortex in resistance of bacterial endospores. In *Spores VI*. Edited by P. Gerhardt, R.N. Costilow, and H.L. Sadoff. American Society for Microbiology, Washington D.C., pp. 541–546.

Gould, G.W., and Sale, A.J.H. 1970. Initiation of germination of bacterial spores by hydrostatic pressure. J. Gen. Microbiol., *60*, 335–346.

Greenwood, D. 1983. *Antimicrobial Chemotherapy*. London, Baillière Tindall.

Grossman, L., Levine, S.S., and Allison, W.S. 1961. The reaction of formaldehyde with nucleotides and T2 bacteriophage DNA. J. Mol. Biol., *3*, 47–60.

Hagen, P.-O. 1971. The effect of low temperatures on microorganisms: conditions under which cold becomes lethal. In *Inhibition and Destruction of the Microbial Cell*. Edited by W.B. Hugo. New York, Academic Press, pp. 39–76.

Hamilton, W.A. 1975. Energy coupling in microbial transport. Adv. Microb. Physiol., *12*, 1–53.

Hamilton-Miller, J.J.T., and Smith, J.T. 1979. *Beta-Lactamases*. London, Academic Press.

Hammond, S.A., Morgan, J.R., and Russell, A.D. 1987. Comparative susceptibility of hospital isolates of gram-negative bacteria to antiseptics and disinfectants. J. Hosp. Infect., *9*, 255–264.

Hammond, S.M. 1979. Inhibitors of enzymes of microbial membranes: agents affecting Mg^{2+}-activated adenosine triphosphatase. In *Progress in Medicinal Chemistry*. Edited by G.P. Ellis and G.B. West. Volume 16. Amsterdam, Elsevier/North-Holland Biomedical Press, pp. 223–256.

Hammond, S.M., Lambert, P.A., and Rycroft, A.N. 1984. *The Bacterial Cell Surface*. London, Croom Helm.

Hancock, R.E.W. 1984. Alterations in outer membrane permeability. Annu. Rev. Microbiol., *38*, 237–264.

Haque, H., and Russell, A.D. 1976. Cell envelopes of Gram-negative bacteria: composition, response to chelating agents and susceptibility of whole cells to antibacterial agents. J. Appl. Bacteriol., *40*, 89–99.

Hardy, K. 1986. *Bacterial Plasmids*. 2nd Edition. Walton-on-Thames, Surrey, Nelson & Sons.

Harold, F.M., and Papineau, D. 1972. Cation transport and electrogenesis in *Streptococcus faecalis*. I. The membrane potential. J. Memb. Biol., *8*, 27–44.

Harold, F.M., Altendorf, K.H., and Hirata, H. 1974. Probing membrane transport mechanisms with ionophores. Ann. N.Y. Acad. Sci., *235*, 149–160.

Harold, F.M., Baarda, J.R., Baron, C., and Abrams, A. 1969. Dio 9 and chlorhexidine: inhibitors of membrane bound ATPase and of cation transport in *Streptococcus faecalis*. Biochim. Biophys. Acta, *183*, 129–136.

Harris, R.J., and Pestka, S. 1977. Peptide bond formation. In *Molecular Mechanisms of Protein Biosynthesis*. Edited by H. Weissbach and S. Pestka. New York, Academic Press, pp. 413–442.

Hawkey, P.M. 1984. *Providencia stuartii*: a review of multiply antibiotic-resistant bacteria. J. Antimicrob. Chemother., *13*, 209–226.

Heinzel, M. 1988. The phenomena of resistance to disinfectants and preservatives. In *Industrial Biocides*. Edited by K.R. Payne. Society of Chemical Industry. Chichester, John Wiley & Sons, pp. 52–67.

Hesslewood, S.R., and Smith, J.T. 1974. Envelope alterations produced by R factors in *Proteus mirabilis*. J. Gen. Microbiol., *85*, 146–152.

Hicks, S.J., and Rowbury, R.J. 1986. Virulence plasmid-associated adhesion of *Escherichia coli* and its significance for chlorine resistance. J. Appl. Bacteriol., *61*, 209–218.

Hinkle. P.C., and McCarty, R.E. 1978. How cells make ATP. Sci. Am., *238*, 104–123.

Hitchings, G.H. 1973. The biochemical basis for the antimicrobial activity of Septrin. In *Trimethoprim/Sulphamethoxazole in Bacterial Infections*. Edited by L.S. Bernstein and A.J. Salter. London, Churchill Livingstone, pp. 7–16.

Hitchings, G.H., and Burchall, J.J. 1965. Inhibition of folate biosynthesis and function as a basis for chemotherapy. Adv. Enzymol., *27*, 417–468.

Hopwood, D. 1975. Reactions of glutaraldehyde with nucleic acids. Histochem. J., *7*, 267–276.

Howard-Flanders. P. 1973. DNA repair and recombination. Br. Med. Bull., *29*, 226–235.

Hugo, W.B. 1976a. Survival of microbes exposed to chemical stress. In *The Survival of Vegetative Microbes*. Edited by T.R.G. Gray and J.R. Postgate. Symposium 26, Society for General Microbiology. Cambridge, Cambridge University Press, pp. 383–413.

Hugo, W.B. 1976b. The inactivation of vegetative bacteria by chemicals. In *Inhibition and Inactivation of Vegetative Microbes*. Edited by F.A. Skinner and W.B. Hugo. Society for Applied Bacteriology Symposium Series No. 5. New York, Academic Press, pp. 1–11.

Hugo, W.B. 1978. Membrane-active antimicrobial drugs: a reappraisal of their mode of action in the light of the chemiosmotic theory. Int. J. Pharm., *1*, 127–131.

Hugo, W.B. 1982. Mechanism of action of antibacterial agents. In *Principles and Practice of Disinfection, Preservation and Sterilization*. Edited by A.D. Russell, W.B. Hugo, and G.A.J. Ayliffe. Oxford, Blackwell Scientific Publications, pp. 158–185.

Hugo, W.B., and Franklin, I. 1968. Cellular lipid and the antistaphylococcal activity of phenols. J. Gen. Microbiol., *52*, 365–373.

Hugo, W.B., and Longworth, A.R. 1966. The effect of chlorhexidine on the electrophoretic mobility, cytoplasmic constituents, dehydrogenase activity and cell walls of *Escherichia coli* and *Staphylococcus aureus*. J. Pharm. Pharmacol., *18*, 569–578.

Hugo, W.B, and Stretton, R.J. 1966. The role of cellular lipid in the resistance of Gram-positive bacteria to penicillins. J. Gen. Microbiol., *42*, 133–138.

Hurst, A. 1984. Revival of vegetative bacteria after sublethal heating. In *The Revival of Injured Microbes*. Edited by M.H.E. Andrew and A.D. Russell. Society for Applied Bacteriology Symposium Series No. 12. London, Academic Press, pp. 77–104.

Ikeda, T., Tazuke, S., and Watanabe, M. 1983. Interaction of biologically active molecules with phospholipid membranes. I. Fluorescence depolarization studies on the effect of polymeric biocide bearing biguanide groups in the main chain. Biochim. Biophys. Acta, *735*, 380–386.

Ideda, T., Ledwith, A., Bamford, C.H, and Hann, R.A. 1984. Interaction of polymeric biguanide biocide with phospholipid membranes. Biochim. Biophys. Acta, *769*, 57–66.

Ingram, M., and Mackey, B.M. 1976. Inactivation by cold. In *Inhibition and Inactivation of Vegetative Microbes*. Edited by F.A. Skinner and W.B. Hugo. Society for Applied Bacteriology Symposium Series No. 5. New York, Academic Press, pp. 111–151.

Ismaeel, N., Furr, J.R., and Russell, A.D. 1986. Resistance of *Providencia stuartii* to chlorhexidine: A consideration of the role of the inner membrane. J. Appl. Bacteriol., *60*, 361–367.

Ismaeel, N., Furr, J.R., and Russell, A.D. 1987. Inhibitory and lethal effects of chlorhexidine and a polymeric biguanide on some strains of *Providencia stuartii*. Lett. Appl. Microbiol., *5*, 23–26.

Jacoby, G.A. 1985. Genetics and epidemiology of resistance. In *The Scientific Basis of Antimicrobial Chemotherapy*. Edited by D. Greenwood and F. O'Grady. Symposium 38, Society for General Microbiology. Cambridge, Cambridge University Press, pp. 185–218.

Jones, I.G. and Midgley, M. 1985. Expression of a plasmid borne ethidium resistance determinant from *Staphylococcus* in *Escherichia coli*: evidence for an efflux system. FEMS Microbiol. Lett., *28*, 355–358.

Kaback, H.R. 1986. Active transport in *Escherichia coli*: passage to permease. Annu. Rev. Biophys. Biophys. Chem., *15*, 279–319.

Kaulfers, P.-M., Karch, H., and Laufs, R. 1987. Plasmid-mediated formaldehyde resistance in *Serratia marcescens* and *Escherichia coli*: alterations in the cell surface. Zentralbl. Bakteriol. Mikrobiol. Hyg. [A], *266*, 239–248.

Kerridge, D. 1986. Mode of action of clinically important antifungal drugs. Adv. Microb. Physiol., 27, 1–72.

Kogut, M., and Carrier, M.J. 1980. A new look at the antibiotic action of streptomycin: the unitary hypothesis revisited. FEMS Microbiol. Lett., 9, 245–253.

Kropinski, A.M.B., Chan, L., and Milazzo, F.H. 1978. Susceptibility of lipopolysaccharide-defective mutants of *Pseudomonas aeruginosa* strain PAO to dyes, detergents and antibiotics. Antimicrob. Agents Chemother., 13, 494–499.

Lambert, P.A. 1978. Membrane-active antimicrobial agents. In *Progress in Medicinal Chemistry*. Edited by G.P. Ellis and G.B. West. Volume 15. Amsterdam, Elsevier/North-Holland Biomedical Press, pp. 87–124.

Lambert, P.A., 1983. The bacterial surface and drug resistance. In *Role of the Envelope in the Survival of Bacteria in Infection*. Edited by C.F. Easmon, J. Jeljaszewicz, M.R.W. Brown, and P.A. Lambert. London, Academic Press, pp. 1–19.

Lampen, J.O., Arnow, P.M., Borowska, Z., and Laskin, A.I. 1962. Location and role of sterols in nystatin-binding sites. J. Bacteriol., 84, 1152–1160.

Lawrence, P.J., Rogolsy, M., and Hanh, V.T. 1971. Binding of radioactive benzylpenicillin to sporulating *Bacillus* cultures: chemistry and fluctuation in specific binding capacity. J. Bacteriol., 108, 662–667.

Leanz, G.R., and Gilvarg, C. 1973. Dipicolinic acid location in intact spores of *Bacillus megaterium*. J. Bacteriol., 114, 455–456.

Lechowich, R.V., and Ordal, Z.J. 1962. Influence of the sporulation temperature on the heat resistance and composition of bacterial spores. Can. J. Microbiol., 8, 287–295.

Lederberg, J. 1956. Bacterial protoplasts induced by penicillin. Proc. Natl. Acad. Sci. U.S.A., 42, 574–577.

Lederberg, J., and Lederberg, E.M. 1952. Replica plating and indirect selection of bacterial mutants. J. Bacteriol., 63, 399–406.

Leive, L. 1974. The barrier function of the Gram-negative envelope. Ann. N.Y. Acad. Sci., 235, 109–129.

Lerman, L. 1961. Structural considerations in the interactions of DNA with acridines. J. Mol. Biol., 3, 18–30.

Levy, S.B. 1982. Microbial resistance to antibiotics: an evolving and persistent problem. Lancet, 2, 83–88.

Lewis, J.C. 1975. Ca²⁺-peptidoglycan interactions. In *Spores VI*. Edited by P. Gerhardt, P.N. Costilow, and H.L. Sadoff. American Society for Microbiology, Washington D.C., pp. 547–549.

Lewis, J.C., Snell, N.S., and Burr, H.K. 1960. Water permeability of bacterial spores and the concept of a contractile cortex. Science, 132, 544–545.

Longworth, A.R. 1971. Chlorhexidine. In *Inhibition and Destruction of the Microbial Cell*. Edited by W.B. Hugo. New York, Academic Press, pp. 95–106.

Lyon, B.R., and Skurray, R.A. 1987. Antimicrobial resistance of *Staphylococcus aureus*: genetic basis. Microbiol. Rev., 51, 88–134.

Mackey, B.M. 1984. Lethal and sublethal effects of refrigeration, freezing and freeze-drying on micro-organisms. In *The Revival of Injured Microbes*. Edited by M.H.E. Andrew and A.D. Russell. Society for Applied Bacteriology Symposium Series No. 12. London, Academic Press, pp. 45–75.

Macleod, R.A., and Calcott, P.H. 1976. Cold shock and freezing damage to microbes. In *The Survival of Vegetative Microbes*. Edited by T.R.G. Gray and J.R. Postgate. Symposium 26, Society for General Microbiology. Cambridge, Cambridge University Press, pp. 81–109.

Marrie, T.J., and Costerton, J.W. 1981. Prolonged survival of *Serratia marcescens* in chlorhexidine. Appl. Environ. Microbiol., 42, 1093–1102.

Matsushita, K., Adachi, O., Shinegawa, E., and Ameyama, M. 1978. Isolation and characterization of outer and inner membranes from *Pseudomonas aeruginosa* and effect of EDTA on the membranes. J. Biochem., 83, 171–181.

McQuillen, K. 1960. Bacterial protoplasts. In *The Bacteria*. Edited by I.C. Gunsalus and R.Y. Stanier. Volume 1. New York, Academic Press, pp. 249–359.

Medeiros, A.A. 1984. β-lactamases. Br. Med. Bull., 40, 18–27.

Michael, G.T., and Stumbo, C.R. 1970. Ethylene oxide sterilization of *Salmonella senftenberg* and *Escherichia coli*: death kinetics and mode of action. J. Food Sci., 35, 631–634.

Michel-Briand, Y., Laporte, J.M., Bassignot, A., and Plesiat, P. 1986. Antibiotic resistance plasmids and bactericidal effect of chlorhexidine on Enterobacteriaceae. Lett. Appl. Microbiol., 3, 65–68.

Mishiro, Y., and Ochi, M. 1966. Effect of dipicolinate on the heat denaturation of proteins. Nature, 211, 1190.

Mitchell, P. 1966. Chemiosmotic coupling in oxidative and photosynthetic phosphorylation. Biol. Rev., 41, 445–502.

Mitchell, P. 1972. Chemiosmotic coupling in energy transduction: a logical development of biochemical knowledge. Bioenergetics, 3, 5–24.

Mitsuhashi, M., Yamagishi, S., Sawai, T., and Kawabe, H. 1977. Biochemical mechanism of plasmid-mediated resistance. In *R-factor Drug Resistance Plasmid*. Edited by S. Mitsuhashi. Baltimore, University Park Press, pp. 195–251.

Molin, G. 1977. Inherent genetic differences in dry heat resistance of some *Bacillus* spores. In *Spore Research 1976*. Edited by A.N. Barker et al. New York, Academic Press, pp. 487–500.

Morris, A., and Russell, A.D. 1971. The mode of action of novobiocin. In *Progress in Medicinal Chemistry*. Edited by G.P. Ellis and G.B. West. Volume 8. London, Butterworths, pp. 39–59.

Moseley, B.E.B. 1984. Radiation damage and its repair in non-sporulating bacteria. In *The Revival of Injured Microbes*. Edited by M.H.E. Andrew and A.D. Russell. Society for Applied Bacteriology Symposium Series No. 12. London, Academic Press, pp. 147–174.

Moseley, B.E.B. 1988. The microbial response to DNA damage. FEMS Symp. No. 44, 194–205.

Moseley, B.E.B., and Williams, E. 1977. Repair of damaged DNA in bacteria. Adv. Microb. Physiol., 16, 99–156.

Munakata, N., and Rupert, C.S. 1972. Genetically controlled removal of "spore photoproduct" from deoxyribonucleic acid of ultraviolet-irradiated *Bacillus subtilis* spores. J. Bacteriol., 111, 192–198.

Munakata, N., and Rupert, C.S. 1974. Dark repair of DNA containing "spore photoproduct" in *Bacillus subtilis*. Mol. Gen. Genet., 130, 239–250.

Murray, G.E., Tobin, R.S., Jenkins, B., and Kushner, D.J. 1984. Effect of chlorination on antibiotic resistance profiles of sewage-related bacteria. Appl. Environ. Microbiol., 48, 73–77.

Murrell, W.G., and Warth, A.D. 1965. Composition and heat resistance of bacterial spores. In *Spores III*. Edited by L.L. Campbell and H.O. Halvorson. Ann Arbor, American Society for Microbiology, pp. 1–24.

Murrell, W.G., and Wills, P.A. 1977. Initiation of *Bacillus* spore germination by hydrostatic pressure: effect of temperature. J. Bacteriol., 129, 1272–1280.

Nakae, T. 1976. Identification of the outer membrane protein of *E. coli* that produces transmembrane channels in reconstituted vesicle membranes. Biochem. Biophys. Res. Commun., 71, 877–884.

Nayler, J.H.C. 1987. Resistance to β-lactams in gram-negative bacteria: relative contributions of β-lactamase and permeability limitations. J. Antimicrob. Chemother., 19, 713–732.

Neidle, S. 1979. The molecular basis for the action of some DNA-binding drugs. In *Progress in Medicinal Chemistry*. Edited by G.P. Ellis and G.B. West. Volume 16. Amsterdam, Elsevier/North-Holland Biomedical Press, pp. 151–221.

Newton, B.A. 1956. The properties and mode of action of the polymyxins. Bacteriol. Rev., 20, 14–27.

Nikaido, H. 1976. Outer membrane of *Salmonella typhimurium*: transmembrane diffusion of some hydrophobic substances. Biochim. Biophys. Acta, 433, 118–132.

Nikaido, H., and Nakae, T. 1979. The outer membrane of Gram-negative bacteria. Adv. Microb. Physiol., 20, 163–250.

Nikaido, H., and Vaara, T. 1985. Molecular basis of bacterial outer membrane permeability. Microbiol. Rev., 49, 1–32.

Nikaido, H., Song, S.A., Shaltiel, L., and Nurminen, M. 1977. Outer membrane of salmonella. XIV. Reduced transmembrane diffusion rates in porin-deficient mutants. Biochem. Biophys. Res. Commun., 76, 324–330.

Northrop, J., and Slepecky, R.A. 1967. Sporulation mutations induced by heat in *Bacillus subtilis*. Science, 155, 838–839.

Novick, R.P. 1980. Plasmids. Sci. Am., 243, 76–90.

O'Callaghan, C.H. 1980. Structure-activity relations and β-lactamase resistance. Phil. Trans. R. Soc. Lond., B289, 197–205.

Park, J.T., and Strominger, J.L. 1957. Mode of action of penicillin. Biochemical basis for the mechanism of action of penicillin and for its selective toxicity. Science, 125, 99–101.

Peacocke, A.R., and Skerrett, J.N.H. 1956. The interaction of aminoacridines with nucleic acids. Trans. Faraday Soc., 52, 261–279.

Pellon, J.R., and Sinskey, A.J. 1984. Heat-induced damage to the bacterial chromosome and repair. In *The Revival of Injured Microbes*. Edited by M.H.E. Andrew and A.D. Russell. Society for Applied Bacteriology Symposium Series No. 12. London, Academic Press, pp. 105–125.

Pestka, S. 1971. Inhibitors of ribosome functions. Annu. Rev. Microbiol., 25, 487–562.

Pestka, S. 1977. Inhibitors of protein synthesis. In *Molecular Mechanisms of Protein Biosynthesis*. Edited by H. Weissbach and S. Pestka. New York, Academic Press, pp. 467–553.

Pheil, C.G., Pflug, I.J., Nicholas, R.C, and Augustin, J.L. 1967. Effect of various gas atmospheres on the destruction of microorganisms by dry heat. Appl. Microbiol., 15, 120–124.

Phillips, C.R. 1952. Relative resistance of bacterial spores and vegetative bacteria to disinfectants. Bacteriol. Rev., 16, 135–138.

Phillips, I., and Shannon, K.P. 1984. Aminoglycoside resistance. Br. Med. Bull., 40, 28–35.

Pollard, E.C. 1969. The biological action of ionizing radiation. Am. Sci., 57, 206–236.

Pollard, E.C., and Davis, S.A. 1970. The action of ionizing radiation on transcription (and translation) in several strains of *Escherichia coli*. Radiat. Res., 41, 375–399.

Pongs, O. 1979. Chloramphenicol. In *Antibiotics V*. Part 1: *Mechanism of Action of Antibacterial Agents.* Edited by F.E. Hahn. Berlin, Springer-Verlag, pp. 26–42.

Price, C.C. 1958. Fundamental mechanisms of alkylation. Ann. N.Y. Acad. Sci., *68*, 663–668.

Reading, C., and Cole, M. 1986. Structure-activity relationships among β-lactamase inhibitors. J. Enz. Inhib., *1*, 83–104.

Reynolds, P.E. 1985. Inhibition of bacterial cell wall synthesis. In *The Scientific Basis of Antimicrobial Chemotherapy.* Edited by D. Greenwood and F. O'Grady. Symposium 38, Society for General Microbiology. Cambridge, Cambridge University Press, pp. 13–40.

Reynolds, P.E., and Fuller, C. 1986. Methicillin-resistant strains of Staphylococcus aureus: presence of identical additional penicillin-binding protein in all strains examined. FEMS Microbiol. Lett., *33*, 251–254.

Richmond, M.H. 1978. Factors influencing the antibacterial action of β-lactam antibiotics. J. Antimicrob. Chemother., *4*(Suppl. B), 1–14.

Richmond, M.H., et al. 1980. The genetic basis of the spread of β-lactamase synthesis among plasmid-carrying bacteria. Phil. Trans. R. Soc. Lond., *B289*, 349–359.

Rode, L.J., and Foster, J.W. 1960. Action of surfactants on bacterial spores. J. Bacteriol., *79*, 1772–1778.

Rogers, H.J., and Forsberg, C.W. 1971. Role of autolysins in the killing of bacteria by some bactericidal antibiotics. J. Bacteriol., *108*, 1235–1243.

Rose, A.H. 1976. Osmotic stress and microbial survival. In *The Survival of Vegetative Microbes.* Edited by T.R.G. Gray and J.R. Postgate. Symposium 26, Society for General Microbiology. Cambridge, Cambridge University Press, pp. 135–182.

Ross, W.J.C. 1958. *In vitro* reactions of biological alkylating agents. Ann. N.Y. Acad. Sci., *68*, 669–681.

Rossouw, F.T., and Rowbury, R.J. 1984. Effects of the resistance plasmid R124 on the level of the OmpF outer membrane protein and on the response of *Escherichia coli* to environmental agents. J. Appl. Bacteriol., *56*, 63–79.

Rowe, J.A., and Silverman, G.J. 1970. The absorption-desorption of water by bacterial spores and its relation to dry heat resistance. Dev. Ind. Microbiol., *11*, 311–326.

Russell, A.D. 1971. Ethylenediamine tetraacetic acid. In *Inhibition and Destruction of the Microbial Cell.* Edited by W.B. Hugo. New York, Academic Press, pp. 209–225.

Russell, A.D. 1976. Inactivation of non-sporing bacteria by gases. In *Inhibition and Inactivation of Vegetative Microbes.* Edited by F.A. Skinner and W.B. Hugo. Society for Applied Bacteriology Symposium Series No. 5. New York, Academic Press, pp. 61–88.

Russell, A.D. 1981. Neutralization procedures in the evaluation of bactericidal activity. In *Disinfectants. Their Use and Evaluation of Effectiveness.* Edited by C.H. Collins. M.C. Allwood, S.F. Bloomfield, and A. Fox. Society for Applied Bacteriology Technical Series No. 16. New York, Academic Press, pp. 45–59.

Russell, A.D. 1982a. Factors influencing the activity of antimicrobial agents. In *Principles and Practice of Disinfection, Preservation and Sterilization.* Edited by A.D. Russell, W.B. Hugo, and G.A.J. Ayliffe. Oxford, Blackwell Scientific Publications, pp. 107–133.

Russell, A.D. 1982b. *The Destruction of Bacterial Spores.* London, Academic Press.

Russell, A.D. 1983. Mechanisms of action of chemical sporicidal and sporistatic agents. Int. J. Pharm., *16*, 127–140.

Russell, A.D. 1985. The role of plasmids in bacterial resistance to antiseptics, disinfectants and preservatives. J. Hosp. Infect., *6*, 9–19.

Russell, A.D. 1986. Chlorhexidine: antibacterial action and bacterial resistance. Infection, *14*, 212–215.

Russell, A.D. 1990a. The effects of chemical and physical agents on microbes: disinfection and sterilization. In *Topley and Wilson's Principles of Bacteriology, Virology and Immunity.* Edited by H.M. Dick and A.H. Linton. 8th Edition. Volume 1. London, Edward Arnold.

Russell, A.D. 1990b. Bacterial spores and chemical sporicidal agents. Clin. Microbiol. Rev., *3*, 99–119.

Russell, A.D. and Chopra, I. 1990. *Understanding Antibacterial Action and Resistance.* Chichester, Ellis Horwood.

Russell, A.D., and Fuller, R. (Eds.) 1979. *Cold-Tolerant Organisms in Spoilage and the Environment.* Society for Applied Bacteriology Technical Series No. 13. London, Academic Press.

Russell, A.D., and Furr, J.R. 1977. The antibacterial activity of a new chloroxylenol preparation containing ethylenediamine tetraacetic acid. J. Appl. Bacteriol., *43*, 253–260.

Russell, A.D., and Furr, J.R. 1986a. The effects of antiseptics, disinfectants and preservatives on smooth, rough and deep rough stains of *Salmonella typhimurium.* Int. J. Pharm., *34*, 115–123.

Russell, A.D., and Furr, J.R. 1986b. Susceptibility of porin and lipopolysaccharide-deficient stains of *Escherichia coli* to some antiseptics and disinfectants. J. Hosp. Infect., *8*, 47–56.

Russell, A.D., and Furr, J.R. 1987. Comparative sensitivity of smooth, rough and deep rough stains of *Escherichia coli* to chlorhexidine, quaternary ammonium compounds and dibromopropamidine isethionete. Int. J. Pharm., *36*, 191–197.

Russell, A.D., and Gould, G.W. 1988. Resistance of Enterobacteriaceae to preservatives and disinfectants. J. Appl. Bacteriol., Symp. Suppl., 167S–195S.

Russell, A.D., and Hopwood, D. 1976. Biological uses and importance of glutaraldehyde. In *Progress in Medicinal Chemistry.* Edited by G.P. Ellis and G.B. West. Volume 13. Amsterdam, Elsevier/North-Holland Publishing Co., pp. 271–301.

Russell, A.D., and Hugo, W.B. 1987. Chemical disinfectants. In *Disinfection in Veterinary and Farm Animal Practice.* Edited by A.H. Linton, W.B. Hugo, and A.D. Russell. Oxford, Blackwell Scientific Publications, pp. 12–42.

Russell, A.D., and Hugo, W.B. 1988. Perturbation of homeostatic mechanisms in bacteria by pharmaceuticals. FEMS Symp. No. 44, 206–219.

Russell, A.D., Ahonkhai, I., and Rogers, D.T. 1979. Microbiological applications of the inactivation of antibiotics and other antimicrobial agents. J. Appl. Bacteriol., *46*, 207–245.

Russell, A.D., Dancer, B.N., and Power, E.M.G. 1990. Effects of chemical agents on bacterial sporulation, germination and outgrowth. Society for Applied Bacteriology Technical Series. Oxford, Blackwell Scientific Publications.

Russell, A.D., Furr, J.R., and Pugh, W.J. 1985. Susceptibility of porin- and lipopolysaccharide-deficient mutants of *Escherichia coli* to a homologous series of esters of p-hydroxybenzoic acid. Int. J. Pharm., *27*, 163–173.

Russell, A.D., Furr, J.R., and Pugh, W.J. 1987. Sequential loss of outer membrane lipopolysaccharide and sensitivity of *Escherichia coli* to antibacterial agents. Int. J. Pharm., *35*, 225–232.

Russell, A.D., Furr, J.R., and Rogers, D.T. 1984. Laboratory uses of antibiotic-inactivating enzymes. J. Antimicrob. Chemother., *14*, 567–570.

Russell, A.D., Hammond, S.A., and Morgan, J.R. 1986. Bacterial resistance to antiseptics and disinfectants. J. Hosp. Infect., *7*, 213–225.

Russell, A.D., Morris, A. and Allwood, M.C. 1973. Methods for assessing damage to bacteria induced by chemical and physical agents. In *Methods in Microbiology.* Edited by D.W. Ribbons and J.R. Norris. Volume 8. New York, Academic Press, pp. 95–182.

Ryan, M.J. 1979. Novobiocin and coumermycin A₁. In *Antibiotics V. Part 1: Mechanism of Action of Antibacterial Agents.* Edited by F.E. Hahn. Berlin, Springer-Verlag, pp. 214–234.

Sabath, L.D. 1980. Achievements and problems from the vew of a physician. Phil. Trans. R. Soc. Lond., *B289*, 251–256.

Sale, A.J.H., Gould, G.W., and Hamilton, W.A. 1970. Inactivation of bacterial spores by hydrostatic pressure. J. Gen. Microbiol., *60*, 323–334.

Schindler, C.A., and Schuhardt, V.T. 1964. Lysostaphin: a new bacteriolytic agent for the staphylococcus. Proc. Natl. Acad. Sci. U.S.A., *51*, 414–421.

Shannon, K.P., and Phillips, I. 1983. Detection of aminoglycoside-modifying strains of bacteria. In *Antibiotics: Assessment of Antimicrobial Activity and Resistance.* Edited by A.D. Russell and L.B. Quesnel. Society for Applied Bacteriology Technical Series No. 18. London, Academic Press, pp. 183–198.

Shaw, W.V. 1971. Comparative enzymology of chloramphenicol resistance. Ann. N.Y. Acad. Sci., *182*, 234–242.

Shaw, V.W. 1984. Bacterial resistance to chloramphenicol. Br. Med. Bull., *40*, 36–41.

Shanson, D.C. 1987. Staphylococcal infections in hospitals. Br. J. Hosp. Med., *35*, 312–320.

Silver, S., and Misra, T.K. 1988. Plasmid-mediated heavy metal resistance. Annu. Rev. Microbiol., *42*, 717–743.

Sivaji, Y., Mandal, A., and Agaswal, D.S. 1986. Disinfectant-induced changes in the antibiotic sensitivity and phage typing pattern in *Staphylococcus aureus.* J. Hosp. Infect., *7*, 236–243.

Slack, M.P.E., and Nichols, W.W. 1982. Antibiotic penetration through capsules and exopolysaccharides. J. Antimicrob. Chemother., *10*, 368–372.

Smith, D.H., and Davis, B.D. 1967. Mode of action of novobiocin in *Escherichia coli.* J. Bacteriol., *93*, 71–79.

Smith, J.T. 1979. Some biochemical mechanisms of antibiotics acting together on bacterial folate metabolism. In *Antibiotic Interactions.* Edited by J.D. Williams. New York, Academic Press, pp. 87–98.

Smith, J.T. 1985. The 4-quinolone antibacterials. In *The Scientific Basis of Antimicrobial Chemotherapy.* Edited by D. Greenwood and F. O'Grady. Symposium 38, Society for General Microbiology. Cambridge, Cambridge University Press, pp. 69–94.

Spratt, B.G. 1978. *Escherichia coli* resistance to β-lactam antibiotics through a decrease in the affinity of a target for lethality. Nature, *274*, 713–715.

Spratt, B.G. 1980. Biochemical and genetical approaches to the mechanism of action of penicillin. Phil. Trans. R. Soc. Lond., *B289*, 273–283.

Spratt, B.G. 1983. Penicillin-binding proteins and the future of β-lactam antibiotics. J. Gen. Microbiol., *127*, 1247–1260.

Stacey, K.A., Cobb, M., Cousens, S.F., and Alexander, A. 1958. The reactions of the "radiomimetic" alkylating agents with macromolecules *in vitro.* Ann. N.Y. Acad. Sci., *68*, 682–701.

Staehelin, M. 1958. Reactions of tobacco mosaic virus nucleic acid with formaldehyde. Biochim. Biophys. Acta, *29*, 410–417.

Starbuck, W.C., and Busch, H. 1963. Hydroxyethylation of amino acids in plasma albumin with ethylene oxide. Biochim. Biophys. Acta, *78*, 594–605.

Staudenbauer, W.L. 1975. Novobiocin—a specific inhibitor of semiconservative DNA replication in permeabilized *Escherichia coli* cells. J. Mol. Biol., *96*, 201–205.

Stewart, M., et al. 1980. Distribution of calcium and other elements in cryosectioned *Bacillus cereus* T spores determined by high resolution scanning electron probe X-ray microanalysis. J. Bacteriol., *143*, 481–491.

Stickler, D.J., and Chawla, J.C. 1987. The role of antiseptics in the management of patients with long-term indwelling bladder catheters. J. Hosp. Infect., *10*, 219–228.

Stickler, D.J., Clayton, C.L., and Chawla, J.C. 1987. The resistance of urinary trace pathogens to chlorhexidine bladder washouts. J. Hosp. Infect., *10*, 28–39.

Stickler, D.J., Thomas, B., Clayton, C.L., and Chawla, J.C. 1983. Studies on the genetic basis of chlorhexidine resistance. Br. J. Clin. Pract., Symp. Suppl. 25, 23–28.

Storm, D.R., and Toscano, W.A., Jr. 1979. Bacitracin. In *Antibiotics V. Part 1: Mechanism of Action of Antibacterial Agents.* Edited by F.E. Hahn. Berlin, Springer-Verlag, pp. 1–17.

Sutton, L.A., and Jacoby, G.A. 1978. Plasmid-determined resistance to hexachlorophene in *Pseudomonas aeruginosa*. Antimicrob. Agents Chemother., *13*, 634–636.

Sykes, G. 1965. *Disinfection and Sterilization.* 2nd Edition. London, F. & N. Spon.

Sykes, G. 1970. The sporicidal properties of chemical disinfectants. J. Appl. Bacteriol., *33*, 147–156.

Sykes, R.B. 1982. The classification and terminology of enzymes that hydrolyze β-lactam antibiotics. J. Infect. Dis., *145*, 762–765.

Sykes, R.B., and Matthew, M. 1976. The β-lactamases of Gram-negative bacteria and their role in resistance to β-lactam antibiotics. J. Antibiot. Chemother., *2*, 115–157.

Tai, P.C., and Davis, B.D. 1985. The actions of antibiotics on the ribosome. In *The Scientific Basis of Antimicrobial Chemotherapy.* Edited by D. Greenwood and F. O'Grady. Symposium 38, Society for General Microbiology. Cambridge, Cambridge University Press, pp. 44–68.

Tallentire, A. 1970. Radiation resistance of spores. J. Appl. Bacteriol., *33*, 141–146.

Tamaki, S., Sato, T., and Matsuhishi, M. 1971. Role of lipopolysaccharides in antibiotic resistance and bacteriophage absorption of *Escherichia coli* K12. J. Bacteriol., *105*, 968–975.

Terano, H., Tanooka, H., and Kadota, H. 1969. Germination-induced repair of single-strand breaks of DNA in irradiated *Bacillus subtilis* spores. Biochem. Biophys. Res. Commun., *37*, 66–71.

Terano, H., Tanooka, H., and Kadota, H. 1971. Repair of radiation damage to deoxyribonucleic acid in germinating spores of *Bacillus subtilis.* J. Bacteriol., *106*, 925–930.

Tipper, D.J. 1979. Mode of action of β-lactam antibiotics. Rev. Infect. Dis., *1*, 39–53.

Tipper, D.J., and Strominger, J.L. 1965. Mechanism of action of penicillins: a proposal based on their structural similarity to acyl-D-alanyl-D-alanine. Proc. Natl. Acad. Sci. U.S.A., *54*, 1133–1141.

Tomasz, A. 1979. The mechanism of the irreversible antimicrobial effects of penicillins: how the β-lactam antibiotics kill and lyse bacteria. Annu. Rev. Microbiol., *38*, 113–137.

Tomasz, A. 1980. On the mechanism of the irreversible antimicrobial effects of β-lactams. Phil. Trans. R. Soc. Lond., *B289*, 303–308.

Tomasz, A. 1983. Mode of action of β-lactam antibiotics—a microbiologist's view. In *Antibiotics Containing the β-Lactam Structure.* Edited by A.L. Demain and N.A. Solomon. Handbook of Experimental Pharmacology. Volume 67. Berlin, Springer-Verlag, pp. 15–47.

Tomlins, R.I., and Ordal, Z.J. 1976. Thermal injury and inactivation in vegetative bacteria. In *Inhibition and Inactivation of Vegetative Microbes.* Edited by F.A. Skinner and W.B. Hugo. Society for Applied Bacteriology Symposium Series No. 5. New York, Academic Press, pp. 153–190.

Vaara, M., and Vaara, T. 1983a. Polycations sensitize enteric bacteria to antibiotics. Antimicrob. Agents Chemother., *24*, 107–113.

Vaara, M., and Vaara, T. 1983b. Polycations as outer membrane-disorganizing agents. Antimicrob. Agents Chemother., *24*, 114–122.

Van Cuyck Gandre, H., Moulin, G., and Cenatiempo, Y. 1985. Étude de la résistance plasmidique aux antiseptiques. Pathol. Biol., *33*, 623–627.

Varghese, A.J. 1970. 5-thyminyl-5,6-dihydrothymine from DNA irradiated with ultraviolet light. Biochem. Biophys. Res. Commun., *38*, 484–490.

Vinter, V. 1970. Germination and outgrowth: effect of inhibitors. J. Appl. Bacteriol., *33*, 50–59.

Virudachalam, R., and Rao, V.S.R. 1977. Theoretical studies on β-lactam antibiotics. Int. J. Pept. Protein Res., *10*, 51–59.

Waites, W.M., and Bayliss, C.E. 1984. Damage to bacterial spores by combined treatments and possible revival and repair processes. In *The Revival of Injured Microbes.* Edited by M.H.E. Andrew and A.D. Russell. Society for Applied Bacteriology Symposium No. 12. London, Academic Press, pp. 221–240.

Walker, G.C. 1985. Inducible DNA repair systems. Annu. Rev. Biochem., *54*, 425–457.

Wallace, B.J., Tai, P.-C., and Davis, B.D. 1979. Streptomycin and related antibiotics. In *Antibiotics V. Part 1: Mechanism of Action of Antibacterial Agents.* Edited by F.E. Hahn. Berlin, Springer-Verlag, pp. 272–303.

Waring, M.J. 1965. The effects of antimicrobial agents on ribonucleic acid polymerase. Mol. Pharmacol., *1*, 1–13.

Warth, A.D. 1978. Molecular structure of the bacterial spore. Adv. Microb. Physiol., *17*, 1–45.

Warth, A.D. 1980. Heat stability of *Bacillus cereus* enzymes within spores and in extracts. J. Bacteriol., *143*, 27–34.

Warth, A.D. 1985. Mechanisms of heat resistance. In *Fundamental and Applied Aspects of Bacterial Spores.* Edited by G.J. Dring, D.J. Ellar, and G.W. Gould. London, Academic Press, pp. 209–225.

Watanakunakorn, C., Goldberg, L.M., Carleton, J., and Hamburger, M. 1969. Staphylococcal spheroplasts and L-colonies. III. Induction by lysostaphin. J. Infect. Dis., *119*, 67–74.

Wehrli, W., and Staehelin, M. 1970. Actions of the rifamycins. Bacteriol. Rev., *35*, 290–309.

Weinberg, E.D. 1961. Known and suspected role of metal coordination in actions of antimicrobial drugs. Fed. Proc., *20(Suppl. 10)*, 132–135.

Welker, N.E. 1976. Microbial endurance and resistance to heat stress. In *The Survival of Vegetative Microbes.* Edited by T.R.G. Gray and J.R. Postgate. Symposium 26, Society for General Microbiology. Cambridge, Cambridge University Press, pp. 241–277.

Wilkinson, S.G. 1975. Sensitivity to ethylenediamine tetracetic acid. In *Resistance of Pseudomonas aeruginosa.* Edited by M.R.W. Brown. London, John Wiley & Sons, pp. 145–188.

Wills, P.A. 1974. Effects of hydrostatic pressure and ionizing radiation on bacterial spores. Atomic Energy Aust., *17*, 2–10.

Wise, R., and Reeves, D.S. (Eds.) 1979. Advances in therapy with antibacterial folate inhibitors. J. Antimicrob. Chemother., *5 (Suppl. B.)*.

Witholt, B., Van Heerikhuizen, H., and De Leij, L. 1976. How does lysozyme penetrate through the bacterial outer membrane? Biochim. Biophys. Acta, *443*, 534–544.

Witkin, E.M. 1976. Ultraviolet mutagenesis and inducible DNA repair in *Escherichia coli.* Bacteriol. Rev., *40*, 869–907.

Woodcock, P.M. 1988. Biguanides as industrial biocides. In *Industrial Biocides.* Edited by K.R. Payne. Society of Chemical Industry. Chichester, John Wiley & Sons, pp. 19–36.

Woods, D.D. 1940. The relation of p-aminobenzoic acid to the mechanism of action of sulphanilamide. Br. J. Exp. Pathol., *21*, 74–90.

Young, M., and Mandelstam, J. 1979. Early stages during bacterial endospores formation. Adv. Microb. Physiol., *20*, 103–162.

Zamenhof, S. 1960. Effect of heating dry bacteria and spores on their phenotype and genotype. Proc. Natl. Acad. Sci. U.S.A., *46*, 101–105.

Zygmunt, W.A., and Tavormina, P.A. 1972. Lysostaphin: model for a specific enzymatic approach to infectious disease. In *Progress in Drug Research.* Edited by E. Jucker. Volume 16. Basel, Birkhäuser Verlag, pp. 310–333.

Zytkovicz, T.H., and Halvorson, H.O. 1972. Some characteristics of dipicolinic acid-less mutant spores of *Bacillus cereus, Bacillus megaterium* and *Bacillus subtilis.* In *Spores V.* Edited by H.O. Halvorson, R. Hanson, and L.L. Campbell. Washington, D.C., American Society for Microbiology, pp. 49–52.

CHAPTER 4

PHYSICAL FACTORS INFLUENCING THE ACTIVITY OF ANTIMICROBIAL AGENTS

Harry B. Kostenbauder

Discussion of the influence of physical factors in this chapter is directed primarily toward a consideration of the effect of environment upon the antimicrobial activity of chemical agents. Extremes of environmental factors such as temperature, radiation, or pH often provide an efficient means of controlling or combating microorganisms. More subtle changes in environment, which in themselves might have only a minor influence on microbial growth, can be significant factors in the control of microorganisms by virtue of their influence on the antimicrobial activity of a chemical agent.

In the development that follows, it is assumed that a finite minimum concentration of a biologically active chemical species in the continuous aqueous phase in contact with a microorganism elicits a desired antimicrobial effect. This assumption is not restricted by the nature or definition of the response. Using fundamental physical chemical principles, it is then possible to predict with reasonable accuracy the total quantity of antimicrobial agent that might be required to achieve the desired antimicrobial effect in systems considerably more complex than simple aqueous solutions.

The intensity of antimicrobial activity of a chemical agent can often be correlated with the rate at which the antimicrobial agent gains access to the biophase or the site at which it acts. The driving force that determines this rate of transport of the toxic substance to the site of action is the difference in chemical potential or partial molal free energy of the agent at the site at which it acts and in the external aqueous phase in contact with the microorganism. If the chemical potential of the antimicrobial agent at the site of action can be considered to be small relative to the chemical potential of the agent in the aqueous phase, then the driving force is the chemical potential of the agent in the aqueous phase.

Ferguson (1939) first considered the relationship between toxicity of a substance and the tendency of the toxic substance to transfer from a surrounding external aqueous phase to the biophase or site of action. He used principles of chemical equilibrium to illustrate that, for substances for which biologic response might be related to the equilibrium concentration of toxic substance in the biophase, biologic response could be correlated not with the stoichiometric concentration in the aqueous phase but with the chemical potential of the substance. The chemical potential or partial molal free energy is commonly expressed as a function of thermodynamic activity.*

In its original application, the Ferguson postulate was restricted to processes considered to be directly related to the level of accumulation of nonspecific chemical agents in the biophase at equilibrium. Allawala and Riegelman (1953d) extended the Ferguson concepts to nonequilibrium processes such as dynamics of disinfection by utilizing the term "availability," a term describing the rate of transport of a toxic substance to the site at which it acts. Allawala and Riegelman demonstrated that, for potentially rate-determining steps such as permeation of a membrane, adsorption on a surface, diffusion, or transfer across an interface, the driving force that determines the rate of transport can be related to the thermodynamic activity of the toxic agent in the surrounding aqueous phase.

Unfortunately, because the original application of the Ferguson postulate was to permit comparison of the relative toxicity of a series of chemical agents, and was thus concerned with compounds that were nonspecific in biologic activity, it is sometimes implied that the physical chemical principles on which the concept is based are also restricted in application to nonspecific agents. The use of these principles to correlate the availability and toxicity of a single chemical agent under different con-

---

*The thermodynamic activity of a solute may be defined as the ratio of the escaping tendency of the solute in solution to the escaping tendency of the solute in some standard state. The pure solute is often taken as the standard state.

ditions of application is equally valid for agents that are either specific or nonspecific in action. Availability determines the access of an agent to its site of action, and certainly an agent that does not gain access to its site of action cannot exhibit the expected biologic activity.

EFFECT OF SOLVENTS

The use of solvents other than water as the continuous external phase or the addition of cosolvents to an aqueous phase can influence antimicrobial activity by virtue of the inherent toxicity of the solvent or cosolvent or through the effect of solvent or cosolvent on the thermodynamic activity of an antimicrobial agent. The observed effect of various solvents on the antimicrobial activity of a germicide therefore is a summation of these sometimes opposing factors.

Toxicity of Solvent

The use of ethyl alcohol as a solvent in concentrations that are highly toxic to microorganisms might represent an example of enhancement of effectiveness of an antimicrobial agent by action of the solvent. Propylene glycol at 10% concentration inhibits many microorganisms (Barr and Tice, 1957a; Selenka, 1963) and, in combination with antimicrobial agents, may produce an enhanced activity (Neipp, 1957), provided there is little or no interaction between the antimicrobial agent and the glycol. It has been suggested that considerable antimicrobial activity can be contributed to a formulation by selecting as solvents, emulsifiers, chelators, and antioxidants food-grade chemicals that are hostile to microorganisms (Kabara, 1981).

Solvents such as glycerin and sorbitol appear to have little influence on microbial growth unless they are used in concentrations of the order of 20 to 50% (Barr and Tice, 1957b), and the inhibition observed at these relatively high concentrations have been attributed to an osmotic effect. No increase in germicidal activity was noted when 10% glycerin was used as a solvent for the same agents that showed increased activity in 10% propylene glycol (Neipp, 1957).

Thermodynamic Activity of Antimicrobial Agent

If the standard state is taken as that of pure solute, then all saturated solutions of an antimicrobial agent will have unit thermodynamic activity, regardless of the solvent used and the actual concentration of antimicrobial agent required to produce saturation. Thus, methylparaben would have the same thermodynamic activity in a saturated aqueous solution containing 0.25 g/100 ml methylparaben and in a saturated solution in a solvent of 10% polyethylene glycol—90% water containing 0.55 g/100 ml methylparaben. A useful approximation for predicting activity of sparingly soluble nonelectrolytes in different solvents is that solutions of the same fractional saturation with respect to a specific antimicrobial agent exhibit similar thermodynamic activity.

Cooper (1945, 1947, 1948; Cooper and Goddard, 1957)

has extensively investigated the effect of solvents on germicides. In general, nontoxic solvents such as glycerin invariably decrease the antimicrobial activity of a fixed concentration of any agent that has greater affinity for the glycerin-containing solvent than for pure water. The germicidal activity of phenol is diminished by glycerin, but the activity of less water-soluble phenols such as thymol, chlorophenol, and hexylresorcinol is depressed by glycerin to a much greater degree than is that of phenol (Cooper, 1948). Solvents such as dilute aqueous acetone or alcohol have some toxicity and generally enhance the germicidal activity of relatively water-soluble antimicrobial agents; however, germicides of low water solubility may show greater affinity for the acetone- or alcohol-containing solvent, and their thermodynamic activity may be diminished considerably. Thus, 12.5% aqueous acetone increases significantly the germicidal activity of phenol, increases the germicidal activity of *p*-cresol to a small extent, and fails to increase the germicidal activity of thymol (Cooper, 1945).

The presence of nonaqueous solvents such as carbon tetrachloride will diminish the germicidal activity of the more lipophilic antimicrobial agents, sometimes reversing the order of activity observed for a series of compounds in an aqueous medium (Endres and Rohr, 1942).

EFFECT OF pH

Extremes of acidity or alkalinity can effectively limit growth of microorganisms, pH 4.5 to 9 being a limiting range for many organisms. Moreover, the activity of antimicrobial agents that occur as different species within the pH range compatible with microbial growth may be profoundly influenced by relatively small changes in the pH of the medium.

For many weak acids, the antimicrobial activity is primarily or solely attributed to the undissociated molecule (Albert, 1985). The equilibrium between undissociated acid and the less active anion is a function of pH:

$$HA \rightleftharpoons H^+ + A^- \qquad K_a = (H^+)(A^-)/(HA) \qquad (1)$$

$$\text{Fraction of Weak Acid Undissociated} = \frac{(HA)}{(HA) + (A^-)}$$

$$= \frac{1}{1 + K_a/(H^+)} = \frac{(H^+)}{(H^+) + K_a} \qquad (2)$$

The concentration of undissociated acid is therefore given by:

$$(HA) = (\text{Total Weak Acid})(H^+)/[(H^+) + K_a] \qquad (3)$$

If μ is the required concentration of the biologically active undissociated weak acid in the aqueous phase, then the total concentration of the weak acid required in the system at any pH can be readily calculated.

$$(\text{Total Weak Acid}) = \mu[(H^+) + K_a](H^+) \qquad (4)$$

Table 4–1. *Fraction of Weak Acids Undissociated At Various pH Values*

Salicylic Acid pKa 3.0		Benzoic Acid pKa 4.2		Hypochlorous Acid pKa 7.5	
pH	Undissoc.	pH	Undissoc.	pH	Undissoc.
	(%)		(%)		(%)
1	98.4	2	99.4	5	99.7
2	90.4	3	94.3	6	96.9
3	48.5	4	62.5	7	75.7
4	8.6	5	13.7	8	23.8
5	0.9	6	1.6	9	3.9

Table 4–1 illustrates the fraction of total weak acid undissociated at various pH values for several common weak acids for which antimicrobial activity has been attributed primarily to the concentration of undissociated acid (Rahn and Conn, 1944; Marks and Strandskov, 1950). Reference to Table 4–1 indicates that the total benzoate required to preserve a solution at pH 6 might be expected to be approximately 60 times that required at pH 3. Such information can readily eliminate from consideration agents that might be inefficient for a specific system.

Should the anion be the effective species, the expression used is that giving the concentration of anion as a function of pH.

$$(A^-) = (\text{Total Weak Acid}) \, K_a/[K_a + (H^+)] \qquad (5)$$

For weak bases such as the acridines, the biologic activity has been correlated with the concentration of cationic species (Albert, 1985), and analogous equations can be developed to show concentration of active species as a function of pH.

EFFECT OF ELECTROLYTES

The ionic environment may affect the growth of microorganisms through direct effects such as specific ionic effects or osmotic effects, or salts may indirectly affect microorganisms by altering the thermodynamic activity of antimicrobial agents in the system. It is often impossible to isolate the several factors unless one effect is of overwhelming importance.

Effect of Salt on Microorganisms

Brown (1964) concluded that the effect of ionic environment on bacteria can be attributed largely to specific ionic effects, whereas osmotic factors are of lesser importance. Although sodium and chloride ions are among those exhibiting the lowest order of toxicity for microorganisms, even 0.5% sodium chloride can inhibit growth of some microorganisms (Naylor, 1965).

Effect of Salts on Activity of Antimicrobial Agents

The addition of an electrolyte such as sodium chloride to an aqueous solution of an antimicrobial agent such as phenol has a "salting-out" effect on the phenol. The af-

finity of the solvent for the phenol is reduced, and there is an increase in fractional saturation or thermodynamic activity. The increased escaping tendency of phenol on the addition of sodium chloride can be demonstrated by the increase in the oil/water partition coefficient of the phenol on the addition of sodium chloride (Reichel, 1909a). The greatly increased rate of disinfection by phenol in the presence of 10 and 20% sodium chloride (Reichel, 1909b) is largely attributed to the increased thermodynamic activity of the phenol.

The addition of much lower concentrations of sodium chloride has been shown to enhance the antimicrobial activity of organic acids (Oka, 1960) and hexylresorcinol (Beckett et al., 1959a and b). Although there was an increased uptake of germicide by the cells, the relative importance of the increased thermodynamic activity and specific ionic effects in these systems was less obvious.

Salts found in hard water may influence the activity of antimicrobial agents either through an effect on the growth of an organism or by interfering with the mechanism of action of the agent (Bennett, 1962). Special consideration is required for those antimicrobial agents that form either active or inactive chelates with metal ions (Weinberg, 1957). Moreover, chelating agents such as ethylene-diaminetetraacetate increase the activity of cationic antimicrobial agents such as polymyxin B, benzalkonium, and chlorhexidine, presumably by removing calcium or magnesium ions from microbial cell membranes and altering cell permeability (Brown and Richards, 1965).

Other salt effects may be encountered if, for example, added electrolyte forms an insoluble salt or an inactive complex with the antimicrobial agent. In the presence of excess chloride ion, phenylmercuric ion might be precipitated as the relatively insoluble chloride, and in the presence of iodide ion, iodine would exist largely in the form of the inactive species, I_3^-.

$$PhHg^+ + Cl^- \longrightarrow PhHgCl \downarrow \qquad (6)$$

$$I_2 + I^- \rightleftharpoons I_3^- \qquad (7)$$

COMPLEX FORMATION AND ADSORPTION

Complexing or binding of an antimicrobial agent present in solution at a concentration less than that corresponding to saturation must result in decreased thermodynamic activity and therefore a decrease in the availability of the agent. Correlation of antimicrobial activity and thermodynamic activity in such systems has been adequately documented (Allawala and Riegelman, 1953b; Pisano and Kostenbauder, 1959; Anton, 1960).*

---

*In these studies, antimicrobial activity has been correlated with the concentration of free or unbound antimicrobial agent. In dilute solution, however, the assumption of direct proportionality between thermodynamic activity and concentration of free agent is acceptable.

Complexes Between Antimicrobial Agent and Small Molecules or Ions

If A represents unbound antimicrobial agent in the aqueous phase and B is some component, that complexes reversibly with A, for the simplest case of a 1:1 interaction, the equilibrium might be represented as:

$$A + B \rightleftharpoons AB \quad K = (AB)/(A)(B) \tag{8}$$

If the constant K is unknown, it may be readily obtained by experimentally determining concentration of free A as a function of concentration of B.

If A_τ and B_τ represent total A and total B, respectively, then $(A) = (A_\tau) - (AB)$, $(B) = (B_\tau) - (AB)$, and substituting these equalities in equation 8 gives:

$$K = [(A_\tau) - (A)]/(A) [(B_\tau) - (AB)] \text{ or}$$
$$(A_\tau) - (A) = K(A)[(B_\tau) - (AB)] \tag{9}$$

If $(B_\tau) \gg (AB)$, then $[(B_\tau) - (AB)] \approx (B_\tau)$, and equation 9 can be simplified to:*

$$(A_\tau) - (A) = K(A) (B_\tau)$$
$$\text{or} \tag{10}$$
$$(A_\tau)/(A) = 1 + K(B_\tau)$$

For conditions under which equation 10 is valid, a plot of $(A_\tau)/(A)$ versus B_τ will be linear. From such a plot one can readily determine the ratio, R, of total to free agent at any concentration of B.

$$[(A_\tau)/(A)]_{B_\tau} = R \tag{14}$$

If μ is the required concentration of A in absence of B, then for any concentration of B (or B_τ) for which R is

---

*The conditions for which this simplification is valid (Garrett, 1966) can be illustrated as follows:

$$\text{Since } (B) = \frac{(B)}{(B) + (AB)} \cdot (B_\tau)$$
$$= \frac{B_\tau}{1 + K(A)} \tag{11}$$
$$= \frac{1/K (B_\tau)}{1/K + (A)}$$

equation 9 can be rewritten as:

$$(A_\tau) - (A) = K(A)(B) = (A)(B_\tau)/[1/K + (A)] \tag{12}$$

If $1/K \gg (A)$, then

$$[(A_\tau) - (A)]/(A) = K(B_\tau) \text{ or } (A_\tau)/(A) = 1 + K(B_\tau) \tag{13}$$

---

known, the total antimicrobial agent required is given by:*

$$(A_\tau) = R \cdot \mu \tag{15}$$

Binding to Macromolecules

If, instead of one binding site B, there are n equivalent and independent sites per mole of macromolecule M, then the amount of agent bound is $n(AB)$, and equation 9 becomes:

$$(A_\tau) - (A) = nK(A)[(M_\tau) - (AB)] \tag{18}$$

Equation 18 can be written as:

$$[(A_\tau) - (A)]/(A) = nKM$$
$$\text{or} \tag{19}$$
$$(A_\tau)/(A) = 1 + nKM$$

provided $1/K \gg (A)$ or $nM \gg [(A_\tau) - (A)]$, so that the fractional saturation of sites is small.† The linearity of a plot of $(A_\tau)/(A)$ versus M_τ, and therefore the validity of the simplifications introduced, has been demonstrated for many practical systems involving binding of antimicrobial agents to macromolecules (Patel and Kostenbauder, 1958; Miyawaki et al., 1959; Bahal and Kostenbauder, 1964). Figure 4–1 illustrates data for binding of chlorobutanol by polyvinylpyrrolidone plotted according to equation 19.

Adsorption to Solids

Suspended solids in contact with a solution of an antimicrobial agent may modify the activity of the agent. Quaternary ammonium compounds such as cetylpyridinium chloride and benzalkonium chloride are adsorbed by solids such as talc and kaolin, and the binding can be treated as Langmuir-type adsorption (Batuyios and Brecht, 1957). Adsorption isotherms have also been determined for the binding of quaternary ammonium com-

---

*If a plot of $(A_\tau)/(A)$ should be nonlinear, the model can be tested by rearranging equation 12 to:

$$\frac{(B_\tau)}{(A_\tau) - (A)} = \frac{1/K + (A)}{(A)} = \frac{1/K}{(A)} + 1 \tag{16}$$

and a plot of $(B_\tau)/[(A_\tau) - (A)]$ versus $1/(A)$ will be linear. The expression for calculation of total antimicrobial agent required is then

$$(A_\tau) = u\left[\frac{K}{1 + K\mu} + 1\right] \tag{17}$$

where μ has the same significance as in equation 15.

†This represents a limiting case of the classical Klotz (1953) treatment of protein binding. Where the simplification is not valid equation 18 may be written in the form:

$$\frac{(M_\tau)}{(A_\tau) - (A)} = \frac{1/K}{n(A)} + \frac{1}{n} \tag{20}$$

and a plot of $(M_\tau)/[(A_\tau) - (A)]$ versus $1/(A)$ will be linear. The total antimicrobial agent required can be calculated from:

$$(A_\tau) = \mu\left[\frac{nKM_\tau}{1 + K\mu} + 1\right] \tag{21}$$

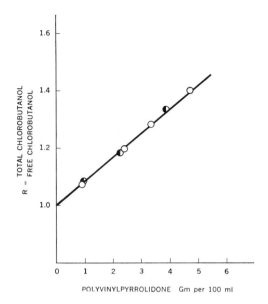

Fig. 4–1. Binding of chlorobutanol by polyvinylpyrrolidone in aqueous solution at 30°C. Data plotted according to equation 19 in the text. Total chlorobutanol in solution: ●, 2.87×10^{-2} M; ○, 5.77×10^{-2} M. From Bahal, C.K., and Kostenbauder, H.B. 1964. Interaction of preservatives with macromolecules. V. Binding of chlorobutanol, benzyl alcohol, and phenylethyl alcohol by nonionic agents. J. Pharm. Sci., 53, 1027–1029.

pounds to cellulosic fibers (Sexsmith and White, 1959a). Horn et al. (1971) found that adsorption of preservatives such as 8-hydroxyquinoline, phenylmercuric nitrate, quaternary ammonium compounds, benzoic acid, *o*-chlorobenzoic acid, dehydroacetic acid, and methylparaben from aqueous solution by 15 common pharmaceutical powders was sufficient to anticipate diminished preservative effectiveness. Because antimicrobial activity is dependent upon the preservative concentration in the aqueous phase after adsorption equilibrium is established (Bean and Dempsey, 1967), it should be possible to use data for adsorption by solids in accordance with methods outlined previously for adjusting preservative concentrations to compensate for binding of antimicrobial agents to macromolecules in solution.

EFFECTS OF SURFACTANTS

Surface Tension

A decrease in surface tension per se appears to be of relatively minor significance in combating microorganisms. Correlations of decrease in surface tension with increasing antimicrobial activity can be obtained in solutions of anionic and cationic surfactants, but the decrease in surface tension in such solutions simply indicates an increase in the concentration of the toxic anionic or cationic surfactant ion. Nonionic surface-active agents are relatively nontoxic to microorganisms and, at concentrations below the critical micelle concentration, show either no effect or only slight enhancement of the activity of most antimicrobial agents. In many practical

applications, however, such as disinfection of porous surfaces, the addition of a surfactant to a solution of a germicide may be an important factor in bringing the solution into contact with the organism.

Micellar Solubilization

Alexander and Trim (1946) clearly illustrated the effect of surfactant on the uptake of hexylresorcinol by the *Ascaris* worm. At surfactant concentrations below the critical micelle concentration (CMC), there is an increase in the rate of uptake of hexylresorcinol. Above the CMC of the surfactant, however, the hexylresorcinol is preferentially associated with the surfactant micelles, and the decreased thermodynamic activity results in a greatly decreased rate of absorption of the phenol by the worm. The influence of micelle-forming surface-active agents on antimicrobial agents can usually be satisfactorily interpreted according to this model. Below the CMC, either ionic or nonionic surfactants may show slight enhancement of the rate of uptake of an antimicrobial agent and increased antimicrobial activity; when surfactant concentrations are in excess of the CMC, however, antimicrobial agents that have affinity for the surfactant micelle may show greatly diminished activity (Alexander and Johnson, 1950; Bean and Berry, 1951; Allawala and Riegelman, 1953b; Aoki et al., 1956; Pisano and Kostenbauder, 1959). Agents that have no affinity for surfactant micelles are not influenced or are slightly more effective in presence of surfactant (Bliss and Warth, 1950). Enhancement of the action of the antibiotic polymyxin B on *Pseudomonas aeruginosa* by small concentrations of polysorbate 80 is one of the more impressive examples of synergism between surfactants and antimicrobial agents (Brown and Winsley, 1971).

Allawala and Riegelman (1953b) used a partition method to determine free and bound iodine in the presence of a nonionic, micellar surface-active agent and clearly demonstrated that the rate of kill in the iodine-surfactant solution was strictly a function of the concentration of free or unbound iodine (Fig. 4–2).

Patel and Kostenbauder (1958) used nylon membrane equilibrium dialysis to determine free and bound methylparaben and propylparaben in the presence of the nonionic surfactant polysorbate 80. They demonstrated that the interaction of the antimicrobial agent with the micellar surfactant can be treated as a Langmuir-type adsorption, and in useful preservative concentration ranges, the interaction is adequately described by the simplified binding equation, equation 10. At a concentration of 5% surfactant, 78% of the total methylparaben and 95.5% of the total propylparaben was bound to the surfactant. According to equation 15, to obtain adequate antimicrobial activity under these conditions would require the use of methylparaben in a concentration 4.5 times that required in absence of the surfactant, and propylparaben would be used in a concentration 22 times that required in absence of surfactant.

Microbiologic studies of the paraben-polysorbate system (Pisano and Kostenbauder, 1959) confirmed that the

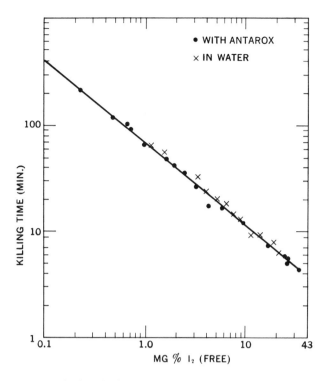

Fig. 4–2. A log-log plot showing that 99% killing time (*Bacillus cereus* [*metiens*]) is a function of the concentration of free iodine both in the presence and in the absence of added surface-active agent. From Allawala, N.A., and Riegelman, S. 1953. The properties of iodine in solutions of surface-active agents. J. Am. Pharm. Assoc., Sci. Ed., *42*, 396–401.

antimicrobial activity is a function of the concentration of unbound preservative (Fig. 4–3) and that equation 15 permits a prediction of the increased concentration of preservative from a knowledge of the required paraben concentration in absence of surfactant and the ratio, R, of total to free paraben at the surfactant concentration of interest. Figure 4–4 illustrates agreement between predicted and experimental inhibitory concentration.

The high degree of interaction with nonionic surfactants and the accompanying decrease in activity is not limited to phenolic preservatives, but has been demonstrated for organic acids, aromatic alcohols, chlorobutanol, and quaternary ammonium compounds. Representative binding data are presented in Figure 4–5 for several common preservatives, and the extremely high degree of interaction of quaternary ammonium compounds with the nonionic polysorbate is indicated by Table 4–2.

Self-Micellization

Not only are the antimicrobial quaternary ammonium compounds adsorbed to other surfactant micelles, but because they undergo self-micellization, the concentration and activity of the antimicrobial long-chain cation also passes through a maximum in the vicinity of the

critical micelle concentration. This maximum can be shown to occur (Sexsmith and White, 1959b) for any micellar equilibrium of the form:

$$aQ^+ + bX^- \rightleftharpoons Q_a^+ X_b^- \text{ where a} > b \geq 2 \qquad (22)$$

The binding of quaternary ion to nonionic macromolecules also passes through a maximum (Sexsmith and White, 1959b; DeLuca and Kostenbauder, 1960) as illustrated in Figure 4–6. Furthermore, the adsorption of quaternary ion can be suppressed by any factor that might cause the critical micelle concentration to be shifted to lower values and thus cause a decrease in the maximum in individual quaternary ion concentration.

It is recognized that increasing the chain length of a quaternary ammonium ion from, for example, C_{12} to C_{16-18} increases the antimicrobial activity, but a further increase in chain length of C_{20} may result in a decrease in antimicrobial activity (Cella et al., 1952). The increase

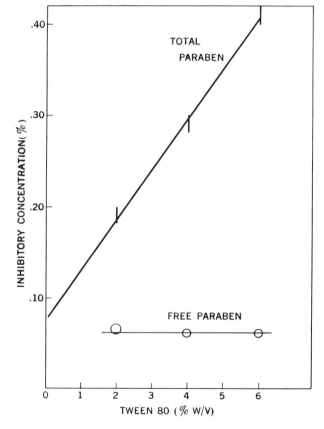

Fig. 4–3. A comparison of the total methylparaben concentration and the free methylparaben concentration required to inhibit growth of *Aerobacter aerogenes* in the presence of polysorbate 80. From Pisano, F.D., and Kostenbauder, H.B. 1959. Interaction of preservatives with macromolecules. II. Correlation of binding data with required preservative concentrations of p-hydroxybenzoates in the presence of Tween-80. J. Am. Pharm. Assoc., Sci. Ed., *48*, 310–314.

Table 4–2. *Influence of Nonionic Surfactant on Concentrations of Cationic Agent Required to Inhibit* Aerobacter aerogenes

| Nonionic | Inhibitory Concentration | |
	Cetylpyridinium Cl	Benzalkonium Cl
0	1–100,000 to 1–250,000	No growth at 1–100,000
0.5% Polysorbate 80	1–2,500 to 1–5,000	—
2.0% Polysorbate 80*	1–250 to 1–500	—
3.0% Polysorbate 80†	1–100 to 1–250	1–500 to 1–1000

*Commercial sample
†Treated with ion exchange resin before use
From DeLuca, P.P., and Kostenbauder, H.B. 1960. Interaction of preservatives with macromolecules. IV. Binding of quaternary ammonium compounds by nonionic agents. J. Am. Pharm. Assoc., Sci. Ed., *49*, 430–437.

in chain length causes the quaternary ion to have a greater tendency to adsorb to macromolecules or microorganisms. The increased chain length also increases the tendency for self-micellization, however, and, if micellization occurs at a sufficiently low concentration, the maximum concentration of the nonmicellar quaternary ion may be insufficient to produce the desired response. This model is illustrated in Figure 4–7.

Several workers have correlated antimicrobial activity of quaternary ammonium compounds with fractional micellar concentration, using either bulk phase (Ecanow and Siegel, 1963) or surface concentrations (Weiner et al., 1965). The critical micelle concentration does not provide a standard state of uniform chemical potential for the quaternary ion, however, as illustrated by equation 22, the chemical potential of the quaternary ion at the critical micelle concentration is a function of the concentration of anion present.

DISTRIBUTION BETWEEN IMMISCIBLE LIQUID PHASES

The distribution of antimicrobial agents between aqueous and nonaqueous phases is an important factor in both the preservation and the efficacy of emulsion systems encountered as foods, pharmaceuticals, and cosmetics and in numerous industrial applications.

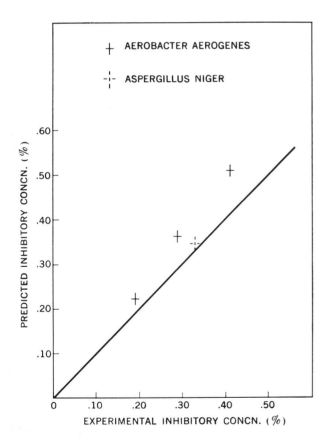

Fig. 4–4. A comparison of experimental inhibitory concentrations of methylparaben in various concentrations of polysorbate 80 with predicted inhibitory concentrations calculated according to equation 15 in the text. From Pisano, F.D., and Kostenbauder, H.B. 1959. Interaction of preservatives with macromolecules. II. Correlation of binding data with required preservative concentrations of p-hydroxybenzoates in the presence of Tween-80. J. Am. Pharm. Assoc., Sci. Ed., *48*, 310–314.

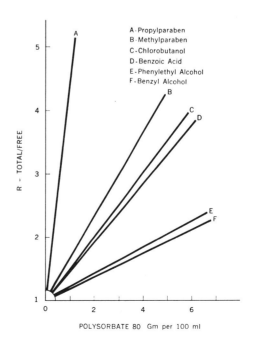

Fig. 4–5. Binding of representative preservatives by a nonionic surface-active agent, polysorbate 80, in aqueous solution at 30°C.

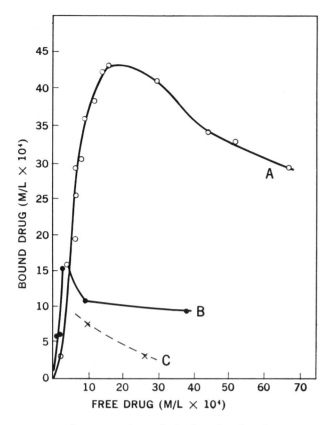

Fig. 4–6. Adsorption isotherms for binding of cetylpyridinium chloride and cetyldimethylbenzylammonium chloride in 0.2% polysorbate 80 at 30°C. These curves illustrate the degree of binding occurring at concentrations of the quaternary ammonium compounds both above and below their normal critical micelle concentrations. A, Cetylpyridinium chloride; B, benzalkonium chloride (CDBAC); C, cetylpyridinium chloride, 0.05 M sodium chloride. Curve C illustrates the influence of electrolyte on the degree of interaction. From DeLuca, P.P., and Kostenbauder, H.B. 1960. Interaction of quaternary ammonium compounds by nonionic agents. J. Am. Pharm. Assoc., Sci. Ed., 49, 430–437.

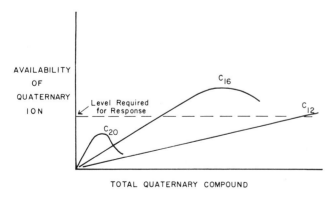

Fig. 4–7. Model illustrating the effect of self-micellization on the availability of quaternary ammonium cation.

Simple Partition

In the case of a simple distribution of an antimicrobial agent between an oil and water, the equilibrium is expressed by the distribution coefficient or partition coefficient. In the following equations, (A_{H_2O}) and (A_{oil}) represent the concentration of antimicrobial agent in the water and oil phases, respectively. D is the partition coefficient, and (A_T) is the concentration of antimicrobial agent based on the total volume, V, of the emulsion system.

$$A_{H_2O} \rightleftharpoons A_{oil} \qquad D = (A_{oil})/A_{H_2O} \qquad (23)$$

$$(A_{oil}) = D (A_{H_2O}) \qquad (24)$$

$$A_T = \frac{\text{Total Agent}}{\text{Volume of System}}$$

$$= \frac{(A_{H_2O}) V_{H_2O} + (A_{oil}) V_{oil}}{V_{H_2O} + V_{oil}} \qquad (25)$$

Substituting equation 24 into equation 25:

$$(A_T) = \frac{(A_{H_2O}) V_{H_2O} + (A_{H_2O}) D V_{oil}}{V_{H_2O} + V_{oil}}$$

$$= (A_{H_2O}) \left[\frac{V_{H_2O} + D V_{oil}}{V_{H_2O} + V_{oil}} \right] \qquad (26)$$

If μ represents the concentration of antimicrobial agent required in the aqueous phase, then the total concentration of antimicrobial agent required for the system is:

$$(A_T) = \mu \left[\frac{V_{H_2O} + D V_{oil}}{V_{H_2O} + V_{oil}} \right] \qquad (27)$$

Dimerization of Antimicrobial Agent in the Oil Phase

The simple distribution law is not always sufficient to describe the system. For example, carboxylic acids such as benzoic acid exist in polar solvents as monomers, but in nonpolar solvents as dimers. If A_2 represents the dimer and K'' represents the dimerization constant, the distribution of such a compound between water and a hydrocarbon solvent might be represented as follows:

$$A_{H_2O} \rightleftharpoons A_{oil} \qquad D = (A_{oil})/(A_{H_2O}) \qquad (28)$$

$$2A_{oil} \rightleftharpoons A_{2oil} \qquad K'' = (A_{2oil})/(A_{oil})^2 \qquad (29)$$

From equation 28 to equation 29:

$$(A_{2oil}) = K''(A_{oil})^2 = K''[D (A_{H_2O})]^2 \qquad (30)$$

Letting (A_T) represent the concentration of antimicrobial agent based on the total volume of the emulsion system:

$$(A_T) = \frac{\text{Total Agent}}{\text{Volume of System}}$$

$$= \frac{(A_{H_2O})\, V_{H_2O} + [(A_{oil}) + 2\,(A_{2oil})]\, V_{oil}}{V_{H_2O} + V_{oil}} \quad (31)$$

$$(A_T) = \frac{(A_{H_2O})\, V_{H_2O} + [(A_{H_2O})\, D + 2\, K''\, D_2\, (A_{H_2O})^2]V_{oil}}{V_{H_2O} + V_{oil}} \quad (32)$$

If μ is the required concentration of antimicrobial agent in the aqueous phase, one can substitute this term for (A_{H_2O}) in equation 32 and obtain:

$$(A_T) = \mu\left[\frac{V_{H_2O} + [D + 2\, K''\, D^2\, \mu]V_{oil}}{V_{H_2O} + V_{oil}}\right] \quad (33)$$

INTERFACIAL PHENOMENA

Bean et al. (1962) demonstrated that greater antimicrobial activity is observed when mineral oil is dispersed in an aqueous phenol solution than without the oil. Investigation of this system indicated that both microorganisms and phenol were in higher concentration at the interface than in the bulk aqueous phase, and the increased activity of the dispersion was attributed to this interfacial adsorption. Although data have not yet been obtained for more complex dispersions, such as systems containing emulsion stabilizers, it appears that the interfacial factor may be more significant than has previously been recognized.

Solid-liquid interfaces may also increase the efficiency of antimicrobial agents. Aalto et al. (1953) observed that solutions containing excess solid butylparaben could be effective inhibitors of microbial growth, although the saturated supernatant alone was ineffective. On the assumption that this result might be attributed to increased capacity of the system containing excess solid paraben, a saturated solution was prepared in an aqueous solution containing sufficient polysorbate 80 to just dissolve the excess paraben. Although the thermodynamic activity and the capacity were identical in both systems, the aqueous dispersion of solid paraben prevented growth, whereas the paraben-saturated surfactant solution failed to prevent growth. Upon addition of excess paraben to the surfactant solution, inhibition could also be obtained in this system (Kostenbauder and Bahal, 1960).

CAPACITY

In the preceding discussions in this chapter, maintenance of an adequate level of antimicrobial activity for whatever time interval was required has been assumed, without consideration of possible depletion of the anti-microbial agent. Depletion in fact may occur through processes such as consumption of an agent in interaction with microorganisms, loss from the system via volatilization, chemical decomposition, or even metabolism of the antimicrobial agent by the microorganism. In the in vivo application of antibiotics or chemotherapeutic agents in humans or animals, the concentration of drug in the body may be depleted through excretion of intact drug or metabolism to inactive derivatives. Many of these processes result in a first-order rate of depletion.

First-order elimination data are routinely used to determine the initial dose of a drug required if the desired blood level of drug is to be maintained above a minimum effective concentration for a specified time. Garrett (1966) pointed out that a similar approach might be used to determine initial preservative concentrations when antimicrobial activity is to be maintained during storage of a product for perhaps several years. Preservatives are generally relatively stable compounds, but typical examples of depletion during storage are chemical decomposition such as hydrolysis of chlorobutanol (Nair and Lach, 1959), loss of preservative by diffusion through or adsorption by rubber closures or plastic containers, or possible microbial decomposition of preservatives such as the hydrolysis of methylparaben by *Cladosporium resinae* (Sokolski et al., 1962).

If the rate of depletion of the antimicrobial agent is known, it is possible to calculate the initial concentration of agent necessary to ensure adequate activity after any specified time. For example, if the rate of disappearance is first order, the concentration of agent present at any time t is given by:

$$(A) = (A_0)e^{-kt} \quad (34)$$

where (A_0) is the initial concentration at zero time, and k is the first-order rate constant in appropriate units. For simplicity in treating the data, it is desirable that the rate constant be known for the disappearance of the antimicrobial agent from the total system under study, be it a test tube, a packaged emulsion, or a living animal. If it is desired to have a minimum concentration μ of antimicrobial agent after some time interval t, the initial concentration of antimicrobial agent required (A_0) can be obtained from a transformation of equation 34:

$$(A_0) = \mu e^{kt} \quad (35)$$

Although correlation between thermodynamic activity and antimicrobial response has been emphasized throughout this chapter, for sparingly soluble chemicals, a further consideration is required. A saturated aqueous solution of iodine or of hexachlorophene would have maximum thermodynamic activity, yet neither of these solutions would be of practical value as a germicide because of rapid depletion of the minute quantity of agent that can be dissolved in water. The performance of an antimicrobial solution is therefore dependent on both an "intensity" factor, the thermodynamic activity, and a "capacity" factor (Allawala and Riegelman, 1953b). A saturated solution of iodine or hexachlorophene in an aqueous surfactant solution is an effective germicide because the thermodynamic activity is maximum and the solubilized agent provides a reservoir of agent so the activity can be maintained. For surfactant solutions that contain iodine or hexachlorophene at concentrations less than saturation, and when capacity is adequate, the relative antimicrobial activity of such solutions can be predicted with the aid of equation 14.

PREDICTION OF ACTIVITY OF ANTIMICROBIAL AGENTS IN COMPLEX SYSTEMS

It is evident that not all factors influencing antimicrobial activity can be treated quantitatively. When some of the important factors can be quantified, however, it is possible to make a reasonable estimate of the feasibility or economy of employing a specific agent. Although such methods cannot replace microbiologic evaluation under actual conditions of use, they often can reduce labor and provide more effective use of testing facilities.

Several important factors have been considered individually, but they can be combined as required to treat more complex systems (Kostenbauder, 1962; Garrett, 1966). For example, to preserve a vegetable oil emulsion with a weak acid preservative for which the undissociated acid is the effective species, that partitions between vegetable oil and water, that binds to surfactant present as an emulsion stabilizer, and that disappears from the system at a first-order rate, the required concentration of preservative can be predicted from a combination of equations 4, 15, 27, and 35. If the required concentration of undissociated acid in the aqueous phase is μ, then the total preservative concentration (A_T) required in the system is:

$$(A_T) = \mu \left[\frac{[K_a/(H^+) + R]V_{H_2O} + D\, V_{oil}}{V_{H_2O} + V_{oil}} \right] e^{kt} \quad (36)$$

Correlations of mathematically predicted preservative availability with antimicrobial activity have been demonstrated for complex systems such as emulsions (Kazmi and Mitchell, 1978).

COMBINATION OF ANTIMICROBIAL AGENTS

A number of applications of combinations of antimicrobial agents can be readily justified from both theoretic and practical considerations. Where contamination may involve a variety of microorganisms that have different susceptibilities to a single antimicrobial agent, a combination of antimicrobial agents may be desirable to provide a broad spectrum of activity. A further indication might arise when the applicable concentration of a single agent is limited for reasons of solubility or toxicity. For example, if a saturated solution of a single preservative does not provide sufficient capacity, the required capacity might be achieved by the inclusion of several chem-

ically similar agents. Within a series of compounds, such as phenols, the solubilities will be independent, but the antimicrobial activity might be expected to be additive. The use of a combination of three sparingly soluble sulfonamides in therapeutics, prior to the introduction of the modern, more soluble sulfonamides, was based on this principle.

On theoretic grounds (Marcus et al., 1965), it would also be expected that if a relatively insoluble antimicrobial agent is to be used in a formulation in a concentration in excess of its solubility (a suspension, for example), greater activity would be expected if the excess solid consisted of two or three different chemical species than if only a single agent were used. Because the rate of uptake of total agent by the microorganism would be a function of the summation of the individual thermodynamic activities, greater response would be expected for the combination. This statement assumes that the antimicrobial activity of the agents is additive, an assumption not unwarranted for a series of agents such as phenols.

The desirability of using combinations of antimicrobial agents in solution to combat a single type of microorganism, except where combinations have been shown to delay emergence of resistant strains, has been a subject of considerable controversy. Garrett (1958) critically reviewed the criteria used in attempts to demonstrate superior performance of combinations of agents and suggested kinetic models as a foundation for the terminology and design of studies of combined antimicrobial action. It has been emphasized that in assessment of activity of combinations, it is not fractional kills but the first-order rates of kill of organisms in the maximum growth phase that are additive. Garrett has used postulates of (1) *additivity*, to describe two agents that act independently and produce a combined response that is additive with respect to responses of the individual agents, and (2) *equivalence*, to describe two agents that act in the same manner, with the same dose-response curve, except for a difference in the weight of a unit dose. The introduction of the equivalence term prevents such anomalies as classification of two doses of the same agent as synergistic or antagonistic because of a nonlinear dose-response curve. It has been pointed out that many claims for synergistic activity are, in fact, the expected additive response (Garrett, 1958, 1966). Growth rate studies show that some combinations of preservative agents produce effects that are more than additive, however (Richards and McBride, 1971; Hugbo, 1977). For example, phenylethyl alcohol enhancement of activity of several other preservatives has been attributed to an effect on the cell envelope such that higher concentrations of another bactericide may enter the cell than would enter in the absence of phenylethyl alcohol (Richards and McBride, 1973).

Maccacaro (1961), in a notable review, has collected and compared the varied methods applied to evaluate combinations of antimicrobial agents.

TEMPERATURE DEPENDENCY OF ANTIMICROBIAL ACTIVITY

The temperature dependency of the antimicrobial activity of a chemical agent represents a complex situation. The observed effects of temperature change include terms for the temperature dependency of the growth rate and the temperature dependency of thermal death rate, as well as the temperature dependency of the antimicrobial properties of the chemical agent. A number of investigators have attempted to study the relationship between temperature and time for disinfection in a manner that would provide some insight into the nature of the temperature dependency and the mechanism of the disinfection process (Tilley, 1942; Jordan and Jacobs, 1945; Kondo, 1957).

The temperature dependency of the rate of a simple chemical reaction can usually be illustrated by an expression of the form (Alberty, 1987):

$$\log k = \frac{-E_a}{2.303 \, R} \cdot \frac{1}{T} + \text{constant} \qquad (37)$$

where k is the rate constant, R is the gas constant, T is absolute temperature, and E_a is the activation energy. A plot of the logarithm of the rate constant against the reciprocal of the absolute temperature produces a straight line with a slope proportional to the activation energy, E_a. The larger the value of the activation energy, the more sensitive is the rate of the reaction to change in temperature. For many chemical reactions, the activation energy is of the order of 12 to 50 kilocalories (kcal) per mole. For other reactions such as protein denaturation, the activation energy may be of the order of 100 kcal. Application of equation 37 indicates that, in the vicinity of room temperature, a reaction having an activation energy of 12 kcal would exhibit a 10° temperature coefficient (Rate$_{T+10°}$/Rate$_T$) of approximately 2, whereas a reaction having an activation energy of 50 kcal would have a 10° temperature coefficient of approximately 14.*

For limited ranges of temperature, it has been shown that the temperature dependency of rate of microbial growth and death might be described by an expression analogous to that applied to simple chemical reactions, k representing the apparent first-order rate constant for growth or death. For microorganisms under conditions favorable to growth, an increase in temperature may increase growth rate with an apparent activation energy of about 10 kcal (Johnson and Lewin, 1946a; Senez, 1962). At higher temperatures, where organisms are subject to rapid destruction by heat, the death rate may show an apparent activation energy of the order of 100 kcal (Johnson and Lewin, 1946b).

Because the temperature coefficient of disinfection

*It should be noted that the 10° temperature coefficient is not a constant, but is dependent upon the temperature range under consideration. Whereas a reaction with an activation energy of 100 kcal would exhibit approximately a 250-fold change in rate for a 10° change in temperature in the vicinity of room temperature, the same reaction would show only a 33-fold change in rate for a 10° change in temperature in the vicinity of 100°C.

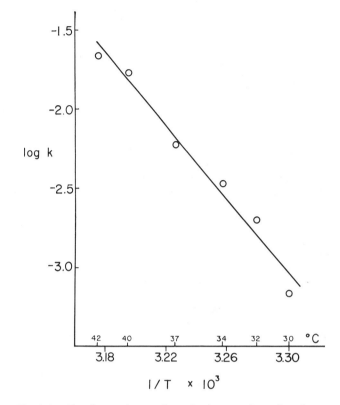

Fig. 4–8. Plot showing linear relationship between logarithm of rate constant for disinfection of *E. coli* by phenol and reciprocal of absolute temperature. From Kondo, W. 1957. Studies on the mechanism of resistance of bacteria. VII. The measure of thermodynamical quantities in the disinfection of phenol against *E. coli*. Bull. Tokyo Med. Dent. Univ., *4*, 81–98.

may be a complex summation of the effect of temperature change on rate of growth, rate of thermal death, and rate of chemical disinfection, this factor is difficult to analyze. For narrow concentration ranges of phenol (0.035 to 0.1 M), and narrow temperature limits (30° to 42°C), Kondo (1957) observed a linear relationship for a plot of logarithm of first-order rate constant for disinfection against reciprocal of absolute temperature, with an apparent overall activation energy of approximately 52 kcal (Fig. 4–8). Such linearity can be expected only over relatively narrow concentration and temperature ranges where the rate of disinfection greatly exceeds both rate of growth and rate of thermal destruction of the microorganisms (Table 4–3).

Although difficult to apply quantitatively, information such as apparent activation energy for disinfection can be useful in a qualitative way in practical applications. For example, if one wished to use a disinfectant at a temperature considerably above room temperature, greater efficiency might be achieved by selecting an agent with a large energy of activation. The rate of disinfection with such an agent would be expected to be highly temperature dependent, and the agent would be

Table 4–3. *Temperature Dependence of Rate of Kill of Microorganisms by Phenol, Benzyl Alcohol, and Benzalkonium Chloride in Aqueous Medium*

| Organism | Phenol (pH 6.1) | | Benzyl Alcohol (pH 7.1) | | Benzalkonium Cl (pH 6.1) | |
	E_a kcal/mol	Q_{10}	E_a kcal/mol	Q_{10}	E_a kcal/mol	Q_{10}
A. niger	10.7	2.0–1.8	15.5	2.4–2.3	32.0	6.1–5.5
C. albicans	14.1	2.5–2.2	35.9	7.7–6.7	18.3	3.2–2.7
E. coli	22.2	4.1–3.5	18.7	3.3–2.9	20.5	3.7–3.2
P. aeruginosa	17.2	3.0–2.7	20.1	3.6–3.0	18.2	3.2–2.7
S. aureus	21.7	4.0–3.5	19.4	4.3–3.4	22.1	4.1–3.2

E_a, Activation energy; Q_{10}, Death rate increase with 10° rise in temperature. Data from Karabit, M.S., Juneskans, O.T., and Lundgren, P. 1985. Studies on the evaluation of preservative efficacy. I. The determination of antimicrobial characteristics of phenol. Acta Pharm. Suec., *22*, 281–290; Karabit, M.S., Juneskans, O.T., and Lundgren, P. 1986. Studies on the evaluation of preservative efficacy. II. The determination of antimicrobial characteristics of benzylalcohol. J. Clin. Hosp. Pharm., *11*, 281–289; Karabit, M.S., Juneskans, O.T., and Lundgren, P. 1988. Studies on the evaluation of preservative efficacy. III. The determination of antimicrobial characteristics of benzalkonium chloride. Int. J. Pharm., *46*, 141–147.

expected to become considerably more effective as temperature increased. For use at temperatures considerably below room temperature one might select an agent having a relatively low activation energy, and therefore, an agent relatively independent of change in temperature. The large E_a and Q_{10} values shown in Table 4–3 for the antimicrobial action of benzalkonium chloride against *Aspergillus niger* indicate that benzalkonium chloride becomes less effective against this organism as temperature is decreased. One is therefore not surprised that 0.014% benzalkonium chloride may be fungicidal against *A. niger* at 20° but not at 3° (Karabit, et al., 1988). It is also obvious from Table 4–3, however, that the temperature dependency of antimicrobial activity appears to show organism specificity. Much more data on these effects are needed before any broad conclusions may be drawn with respect to practical application against a wide spectrum of organisms.

REFERENCES

Aalto, T.R., Firman, M.C., and Rigler, N.E. 1953. p-Hydroxybenzoic acid esters as preservatives. I. Uses, antibacterial and antifungal studies, properties and determination. J. Am. Pharm. Assoc., Sci. Ed., *42*, 449–457.

Albert, A. 1985. *Selective Toxicity.* 7th Edition. New York, John Wiley & Sons, pp. 420–423.

Alberty, R.A. 1987. *Physical Chemistry.* 7th Edition. New York, John Wiley & Sons, p. 693.

Alexander, A.E., and Johnson, P. 1950. *Colloid Science.* London. Oxford University Press, p. 696.

Alexander, A.E., and Trim, A.R. 1946. Biological activity of phenolic compounds: The effect of surface-active substances upon the penetration of hexylresorcinol into Ascaris lumbricoides var. suis. Proc. R. Soc. Lond. (B), *133*, 220–234.

Allawala, N.A., and Riegelman, S. 1953a. The release of antimicrobial agents from solutions of surface-active agents. J. Am. Pharm. Assoc., Sci. Ed., *42*, 267–275.

Allawala, N.A., and Riegelman, S. 1953b. The properties of iodine in solutions of surface-active agents. J. Am. Pharm. Assoc., Sci. Ed., *42*, 396–401.

Anton, A.H. 1960. The relation between the binding of sulfonamides to albumin and their antibacterial efficacy. J. Pharmacol. Exp. Ther., *129*, 282–290.

Aoki, M., Kamata, A. Yoshioka, I., and Matsuzaki, T. 1956. Application of surface-active agents to pharmaceutical preparations. I. Effect of Tween-20 upon the antifungal activities of p-hydroxybenzoic acid esters in solubilized preparations. J. Pharm. Soc. Jap., *76*, 939–943.

Bahal, C.K., and Kostenbauder, H.B. 1964. Interaction of preservatives with macromolecules. V. Binding of chlorobutanol, benzyl alcohol, and phenylethyl alcohol by nonionic agents. J. Pharm Sci., *53*, 1027–1029.

Barr, M., and Tice, L.F. 1957a. A study of the inhibitory concentrations of glycerin-sorbitol and propylene glycol-sorbitol and propylene glycol combinations on growth of microorganisms. J. Am. Pharm. Assoc., Sci. Ed., *46*, 217–218.

Barr, M., and Tice, L.F. 1957b. A study of the inhibitory concentrations of various sugars and polyols on the growth of microorganisms. J. Am. Pharm. Assoc., Sci. Ed., *46*, 219–221.

Batuyilos, N.H., and Brecht, E.A. 1957. An investigation of the incompatibilities of quaternary ammonium germicides in compressed troches. I. The adsorption of cetylpyridinium chloride and benzalkonium chloride by talc and kaolin. J. Am. Pharm. Assoc., Sci. Ed., *46*, 524–531.

Bean, H.S., and Berry, H. 1951. The bactericidal activity of phenols in aqueous solutions of soap. II. The bactericidal activity of benzylchlorophenol in aqueous solutions of potassium laurate. J. Pharm. Pharmacol., *3*, 639–655.

Bean, H.S., and Dempsey, G. 1967. The bactericidal activity of phenol in a solid-liquid dispersion. J. Pharm. Pharmacol., *19* (Suppl.), 197s–202s.

Bean, H.S., Richards, J.P., and Thomas, J. 1962. The bactericidal activity against *Escherichia coli* of phenol in oil-water dispersions. Boll. Chim. Farm., *101*, 339–346.

Beckett, A.H., Patki, S.J., and Robinson, A.E. 1959a. The interaction of phenolic compounds with bacteria. II. The effects of various substances on the interaction of hexylresorcinol with *Escherichia coli*. J. Pharm. Pharmacol., *11*, 367–373.

Beckett, A.H., Patki, S.J., and Robinson, A.E. 1959b. The interaction of phenolic compounds with bacteria. III. Evaluation of the antibacterial activity of hexylresorcinol against *Escherichia coli*. J. Pharm. Pharmacol., *11*, 421–426.

Bennett, E.O. 1962. Factors involved in the preservation of metal-cutting emulsions. Dev. Ind. Microbiol., *3*, 273–285.

Bliss, E.A., and Warth, P. 1950. The effect of surface-active agents on antibiotics: An informal report. Ann. N.Y. Acad. Sci., *53*, 38–41.

Brown, A.D. 1964. Aspects of bacterial response to the ionic environment. Bacteriol. Rev., *28*, 296–329.

Brown, M.R.W., and Richards, R.M.E. 1965. Effect of ethylenediamine tetraacetate on the resistance of Pseudomonas aeruginosa to antibacterial agents. Nature, *207*, 1391.

Brown, M.R.W., and Winsley, B.E. 1971. Synergism between polymyxin and polysorbate 80 against Pseudomonas aeruginosa. J. Gen. Microbiol., *68*, 367–373.

Cella, J.A., et al. 1952. The relation of structure and critical concentration to the bactericidal activity of quaternary ammonium salts. J. Am. Chem. Soc., *74*, 2061–2062.

Cooper, E.A. 1945. The influence of organic solvents on the bactericidal action of the phenols. J. Soc. Chem. Ind. (Lond.), *64*, 51–53.

Cooper, E.A. 1947. The influence of organic solvents on the bactericidal action of the phenols. Part II. J. Soc. Chem. Ind. (Lond.), *66*, 48–50.

Cooper, E.A. 1948. The influence of ethylene glycol and glycerol on the germicidal power of aliphatic and aromatic compounds. J. Soc. Chem. Ind., *67*, 69–70.

Cooper, E.A., and Goddard, A.E. 1967. Influence of solvents on the bacteriostatic and bactericidal action of organic acids. J. Appl. Chem., *7*, 613–619.

DeLuca, P.P., and Kostenbauder, H.B. 1960. Interaction of preservatives with macromolecules. IV. Binding of quaternary ammonium compounds by nonionic agents. J. Am. Pharm. Assoc., Sci. Ed., *49*, 430–437.

Ecanow, B., and Siegel, F.P. 1963. Ferguson principle and the critical micelle concentration. J. Pharm. Sci., *52*, 812–813.

Endres, G., and Rohr, R. 1942. Bactericidal action. I. The disinfecting power of alcohols in nonaqueous solvents. Annalen, *552*, 167–175.

Ferguson, J. 1939. The use of chemical potentials as indices of toxicity. Proc. R. Soc. Lond. (B), *127*, 387–404.

Garrett, E.R. 1958. Classification and evaluation of combined antibiotic activity. Antibiot. Chemother., 8, 8–20.

Garrett, E.R. 1966. A basic model for the evaluation and prediction of preservative action. J. Pharm. Pharmacol., 18, 589–601.

Horn, N.R., McCarthy, T.J., and Price, C.H. 1971. Interaction between preservatives and suspension systems. Am. Perfum. Cosmet., 86, 7, 37–40.

Hugbo, P.G. 1977. Additivity and synergism *in vitro* as displayed by mixtures of some commonly employed antibacterial preservatives. Cosmet. Toil., 92, 52–56.

Johnson, F.H., and Lewin, I. 1946a. The growth rate of *E. coli* in relation to temperature, quinine and coenzyme. J. Cell. Comp. Physiol., 28, 47–75.

Johnson, F.H., and Lewin, I. 1946b. The influence of pressure, temperature and quinine on the rates of growth and disinfection of *E. coli* in the logarithmic growth phase. J. Cell. Comp. Physiol., 28, 77–97.

Jordan, R.C., and Jacobs, S.E. 1945. Studies in the dynamics of disinfection. III. The reaction between phenol and *Bacterium coli:* The effect of temperature and concentration: with detailed analysis of the reaction velocity. J. Hyg., 44, 210–220.

Kabara, J.J. 1981. The medium is the preservative. Cosmet. Toil., 96, 63–67.

Karabit, M.S., Juneskans, O.T., and Lundgren, P. 1985. Studies on the evaluation of preservative efficacy. I. The determination of antimicrobial characteristics of phenol. Acta Pharm. Suec., 22, 281–290.

Karabit, M.S., Juneskans, O.T., and Lundgren, P. 1986. Studies on the evaluation of preservative efficacy. II. The determination of antimicrobial characteristics of benzylalcohol. J. Clin. Hosp. Pharm., 11, 281–289.

Karabit, M.S., Juneskans, O.T., and Lundgren, P. 1988. Studies on the evaluation of preservative efficacy. III. The determination of antimicrobial characteristics of benzalkonium chloride. Int. J. Pharm., 46, 141–147.

Kazmi, S.J.A., and Mitchell, A.G. 1978. Preservation of solubilized and emulsified systems. I: Correlation of mathematically predicted preservative availability with antimicrobial activity. J. Pharm. Sci., 67, 1260.

Klotz, I.M. 1953. *The Proteins.* Volume I, Part B. Edited by H. Neurath and K. Bailey. New York, Academic Press, p. 763.

Kondo, W. 1957. Studies on the mechanism of resistance of bacteria. VII. The measure of thermodynamical quantities in the disinfection of phenol against *E. coli*. Bull. Tokyo Med. Dent. Univ., 4, 81–98.

Kostenbauder, H.B. 1962. Physical chemical aspects of preservative selection for pharmaceutical and cosmetic emulsions. Dev. Ind. Microbiol., 3, 286–295.

Kostenbauder, H.B., and Bahal, S.M. 1960. Unpublished results.

Maccacaro, G.A. 1961. The assessment of interaction between antibacterial drugs. Prog. Ind. Microbiol., 3, 173–210.

Marcus, A.D., Dempski, R.E., Higuchi, T., and DeMarco, J.D. 1965. Mutual independence of release rates of steroids from a topical vehicle. Implications for potentially optimal formulations. J. Pharm. Sci., 54, 495–496.

Marks, H.C., and Strandskov, F.B. 1950. Halogens and their mode of action. Ann. N.Y. Acad. Sci., 53, 163–171.

Miyawaki, G.M., Patel, N.K., and Kostenbauder, H.B. 1959. Interaction of preservatives with macromolecules. III. Parahydroxybenzoic acid esters in the presence of some hydrophilic polymers. J. Am. Pharm. Assoc., Sci. Ed., 48, 315–318.

Nair, A.D., and Lach, J.L. 1959. The kinetics of degradation of chlorobutanol. J. Am. Pharm. Assoc., Sci. Ed., 48, 390–395.

Naylor, P.G.D. 1965. Inhibition of growth of *Aerobacter aerogenes* by sodium chloride. Nature, 205, 420–421.

Neipp, L. 1957. The effect of propylene glycol and other alcohols on the action of antibacterial substances. Schweiz. Z. Allgem. Pathol. Bakteriol., 20, 150–160.

Oka, S. 1960. Transfer of antiseptics to microbes and their toxic effect. II. Relation between adsorption of acid antiseptics on yeast cells and their toxic effect. Bull. Agric. Chem. Soc. Jap., 24, 338–343.

Patel, N.K., and Kostenbauder, H.B. 1958. Interaction of preservatives with macromolecules. I. Binding of parahydroxybenzoic acid esters by polyoxyethylene-20 sorbitan monooleate (Tween-80). J. Am. Pharm. Assoc., Sci. Ed., 47, 289–293.

Pisano, F.D., and Kostenbauder, H.B. 1959. Interaction of preservatives with macromolecules. II. Correlation of binding data with required preservative concentrations of *p*-hydroxybenzoates in the presence of Tween-80. J. Am. Pharm. Assoc., Sci. Ed., 48, 310–314.

Rahn, O., and Conn, J.E. 1944. Effect of increase in acidity on antiseptic efficiency. Ind. Eng. Chem., 36, 185–187.

Reichel, H. 1909a. The theory of disinfection. The disinfecting action of phenols. I. Biochem. Z., 22, 149–176.

Reichel, H. 1909b. The theory of disinfection. The disinfecting action of phenols. III. Biochem. Z., 2, 201–231.

Richards, R.M.E., and McBride, R.J. 1971. Phenylethanol enhancement of preservatives used in ophthalmic preparations. J. Pharm. Pharmacol., 23 (Suppl.), 141s–146s.

Richards, R.M.E., and McBride, R.J. 1973. Effect of phenylethanol on *Pseudomonas aeruginosa*. J. Pharm. Pharmacol., 25, 841–842.

Selenka, F. 1963. Activity of propylene glycol on bacteria: Influence on growth rate in a liquid medium. Arch. Hyg. Bakteriol., 147, 189–200.

Senez, J.C. 1962. Some considerations of the energetics of bacterial growth. Bacteriol. Rev., 26, 95–107.

Sexsmith, F.H., and White, H.J., Jr. 1959a. The absorption of cationic surfactants by cellulosic materials. I. The uptake of cation and anion by a variety of substrates. J. Colloid. Sci., 14, 598–618.

Sexsmith, F.H., and White, H.J, Jr. 1959b. The absorption of cationic surfactants by cellulosic materials. III. A theoretical model for the absorption process and a discussion of maxima in adsorption isotherms for surfactants. J. Colloid. Sci., 14, 630–639.

Sokolski, W.T., Chidester, C.G., and Honeywell, G.E. 1962. The hydrolysis of methyl p-hydroxybenzoate by *Cladosporium resinae*. Dev. Ind. Microbiol., 3, 179–187.

Tilley, F.W. 1942. An experimental study of the influence of temperature on the bactericidal activities of alcohols, and phenols. J. Bacteriol., 43, 521–525.

Weinberg, E.D. 1957. The mutual effects of antimicrobial compounds and metallic cations. Bacteriol. Rev., 1, 46–68.

Weiner, N.D., Hart, F., and Zografi, G. 1965. Application of the Ferguson principle to the antimicrobial activity of the quaternary ammonium salts. J. Pharm. Pharmacol., 17, 350–355.

CHAPTER 5

KINETICS OF THE INACTIVATION
OF MICROORGANISMS

G.B. Wickramanayake and Otis J. Sproul

Microbial inactivation is a kinetic process wherein the viability of organisms exposed to an inactivation agent varies as a function of time. Inactivation kinetics depends on the type of organism, type and concentration of biocide, and, for some disinfectants, environmental conditions such as temperature and pH. Additional attributes, such as the complexity of cell physiology and differences in inactivation mechanisms, make the analysis and interpretation of inactivation kinetics even more complex. An understanding of microbial inactivation kinetics is important in determining the efficacy of various biocides and the rate and extent of inactivation under different exposure conditions, however. If the inactivation data are generated experimentally for a limited set of environmental conditions, mathematic or statistical approaches can then be used to develop formulas to predict the inactivation data for a universe that includes the given conditions. As far as the practical applications in disinfection and sterilization processes are concerned, such kinetic-based models can play an important role in predicting the extent of inactivation of microorganisms under a variety of environmental conditions.

The purpose of this chapter is to describe previously established kinetic-based approaches for disinfection or sterilization processes that can be adapted to treat water, wastewater, infectious wastes, bioprocessing wastes, equipment (surfaces), and food. The commonly used procedures in the inactivation data analysis and comparison of biocidal efficiencies are presented with some mechanistic and empiric disinfection models. Also discussed are the effects of environmental factors on the rate and extent of inactivation.

ANALYSIS OF CELL INACTIVATION DATA

Survival curves, which are semilog plots of the ratio of the concentration of surviving organisms to the initial number versus time, are commonly used to present in-

activation data and to interpret the inactivation kinetics of microorganisms. Typical curves, as shown in Figure 5–1, may be linear, but are frequently nonlinear. Nonlinear curves have sigmoidal, concave upward, or concave downward configurations. A number of concepts, based on theoretic and mechanistic approaches, have been developed to explain the various curve configurations.

Assuming the resistance of different individuals of apparently similar microorganisms to be different, Lee and Gilbert (1918) presented a vitalistic concept to explain the sigmoidal or upward concaving survival curves. They suggested that organisms possessing an average degree of resistance would be found in the majority, whereas those possessing a maximum or minimum degree of resistance would be found in the minority. Consequently, the survival times were expected to be normally distributed, but according to Cerf (1977), no experimental evidence was available to verify this concept. Withell (1942), however, demonstrated that the logarithm of survival time for some organisms was normally distributed. This indicates that the microorganisms resisting in a minimum degree are present in the greatest number, in contrast to the vitalistic concept of Lee and Gilbert (1918). In a comprehensive analysis of disinfection kinetics, Koch (1966) presented several theoretic and practical drawbacks of this vitalistic concept and indicated the need for further experimental evidence to substantiate the concept. Following experiments on the inactivation of enteroviruses with ozone, Roy et al. (1982) doubted that the heterogeneity of the viral population could explain the curved nature of survival curves.

The shoulder associated with many microorganism survival curves (curve 1 in Fig. 5–1) has been analyzed in different ways. The expressions developed from the multitarget (Morris, 1970) and multihit (Oliver and Shepstone, 1964) phenomena were able to generate survival curves that were concave upward. The multitarget ap-

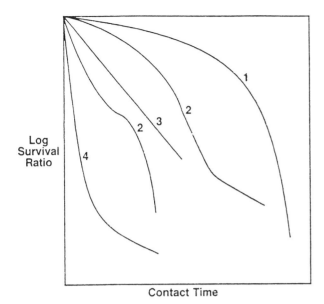

Fig. 5–1. Typical configuration for survival curves. 1, Concave upward; 2, sigmoidal; 3, linear (exponential kinetics); and 4, concave downward.

proach assumed that the microorganisms possess several vital sites, each of which must be hit once before inactivation. The multihit concept is based on the assumption of only one sensitive target that requires several hits for inactivation. These approaches did not prove to be satisfactory in fitting data for some studies (Taylor and Johnson, 1974), but they were successful in fitting data for other studies (Severin et al., 1983).

In another approach, Berg et al. (1964) considered that the virus devitalization by iodine was first order and that the nonlinearity was caused by the multihit effect necessary to inactivate the organisms that remained as clumps. Moreover, they deduced that a typical lagging curve (curve 1 in Fig. 5–1) occurs if all the virions form clumps of about equal numbers of infectious particles. In contrast, Young and Sharp (1977) demonstrated that survival curves for the chlorine inactivation of single virion preparations of poliovirus type 1 (Mahoney) at low pH also resemble typical lagging curves. Floyd et al. (1979), using the same organism and disinfectant at pH 6, reported a similar curve configuration that was concave upward. Wickramanayake et al. (1984) demonstrated that the inactivation of a suspension of clump-free protozoan cysts with ozone produced typical lagging curves. Similar observations have been made by Rubin et al. (1983) and Chen et al. (1985) in the inactivation of protozoan cysts by chlorine and chlorine dioxide, respectively. Thus, existence of an initial lag in microbial inactivation may not be attributed to simple aggregation of particles.

In a study on inactivation of *Naegleria gruberi* cysts with iodine, Wei and Chang (1975) showed that the inactivation rate of a single-cell suspension followed first-order kinetics. They also ascribed the shoulder of survival curves (curve 1 in Fig. 5–1) to aggregation of cysts. Sub-

sequently, a multi-Poisson distribution model was developed to explain their cyst inactivation kinetics assuming that the destruction of each individual of the clump was first order. Two other assumptions were also made in the derivation of the model. First, the rate of inactivation of clumped organisms is directly proportional to the concentration of clumps of a specific size. Second, the destruction of a clump is sequential with only one individual inactivated at a time. Although no experimental evidence substantiated the last two assumptions, the multi-Poisson distribution model appeared successful in fitting their data.

Prokop and Humphrey (1970) were able to explain different configurations of survival curves using a deterministic approach. The development of such models is based on the assumption that the reaction is chemical in nature and thus obeys the law of mass action, and the organism undergoes an intermediate sensitive stage during the inactivation. Some of these models were subsequently modified and verified by Haas (1980) for the inactivation of viruses by chlorine and Roy et al. (1982) by ozone. Lack of understanding of the inactivation mechanism has hampered the use of the models developed by Prokop and Humphrey (1970), however.

It is evident from the preceding discussion that none of these hypotheses can be considered entirely correct because they have not been subjected to adequate independent verifications. A common kinetic theory has difficulty in its universal application because different microorganisms behave differently under similar experimental conditions, and the same microorganism may behave differently under various experimental conditions. The kinetics based on empiric or mechanistic approaches can be used with confidence, however, for engineering applications such as designing full-scale treatment units or predicting the extent of inactivation under different hydraulic and mixing conditions. For example, using the multitarget and series-event kinetic parameters generated from batch data, Severin et al. (1983) successfully predicted the response of microorganisms to ultraviolet (UV) inactivation in flow-through reactors.

Depending on the type of organism and waste characteristics, the kinetics of the inactivation of relevant subcellular components such as DNA and RNA may also need to be established experimentally if the inactivation of those components is deemed necessary. Inactivation kinetics can be established for different viability end points as needed. For example, kinetic data can be established for the inactivation of the organism as well as denaturation of the genetic materials in it if such treatments are deemed necessary based on the risk associated with the release of the specific organism. Such applications may be required in the treatment of infectious wastes and bioprocessing facility wastes that contain genetically engineered organisms. Similar to the microorganisms, inactivation kinetics can be established for genetic elements ex vivo. Once the kinetics are established, the extent of inactivation of biological agents can then be predicted for a variety of conditions such as different biocide concentration, pH value, and temperature.

COMPARISON OF INACTIVATION EFFICIENCY

Selection of an appropriate disinfection and/or sterilization process is determined by a number of criteria:

1. Effectiveness of the biocide to inactivate microorganisms and, if necessary, the subcellular components.
2. Applicability of the method to different media (e.g., air, wastewater, sludge, surfaces).
3. The effect of "chemical demand."
4. Detoxification requirements and lack of toxic by-product formation.
5. Hazard associated with the biocide and treatment process.
6. Ease of handling and application.
7. Capital and operating costs.

The effectiveness of different decontaminants is generally evaluated by comparing the decontaminant concentration-exposure time (C·t) data for the inactivation of the organisms to a given level (e.g., 99% inactivation). For a successful comparison, data should be generated at identical experimental conditions. For example, inactivation data need to be generated using the same suspension of organisms in a given medium (water or wastewater). Environmental conditions such as pH and temperature should also be the same. Experiments need to be conducted using appropriate reactors (e.g., batch versus continuous flow) for which data will be applied.

The C·t (concentration-time) data can also be used to compare the relative resistance of different microorganisms to a given inactivation agent. This information is necessary when the waste stream contains several different microorganisms and subcellular components. In this case, inactivation data need to be obtained for each of the biologic agents of concern under identical environmental conditions.

A convenient way to evaluate C·t data is to compare the times required to inactivate 99% (2-log) of the organisms when exposed to a certain concentration (e.g., 1 ppm) of each of the biocides. A unique concentration for all the inactivation agents does not seem to be feasible, however, because of the significant variations in the effectiveness of decontaminant and resistance of microorganisms. For example, when *Escherichia coli* was exposed to 0.07 mg/L of ozone at pH 7.2 and 1°C in a batch reactor, the time required to achieve 99% inactivation was only about 5 seconds (Katzenelson et al., 1974). In contrast, Berman and Hoff (1984) reported that time required to inactivate simian rotavirus (SA11) by 10 mg/L of preformed chloramine at pH 8 and 5°C was over 6 hours. As a result of these wide variations, the concentration (C) and contact time (t) product for 99% inactivation were compared by several groups for a range of decontaminant concentrations (Safe Drinking Water

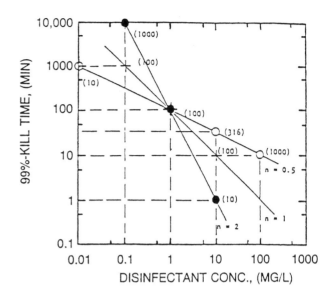

Fig. 5–2. Effect of n value on C·t values at different disinfectant concentrations (C·t values given in parentheses). From Hoff, J.C. 1986. *Inactivation of Microbial Agents by Chemical Disinfectants.* EPA–600/2–86–067. Cincinnati, Water Engineering Research Laboratory, United States Environmental Protection Agency.

Committee, 1980; Hoff and Geldreich, 1981; Wickramanayake et al., 1984; Leahy, 1985; and Hoff, 1986).

The "C·t" concept appears to be based on an empiric relationship reported by Watson (1908) in the following form:

$$C^n \cdot t = k \qquad (1)$$

where C = concentration of decontaminant
 n = coefficient of dilution
 t = exposure time required to obtain a given level of inactivation (e.g., 99%)
 k = empirical parameter that varies with the decontaminant, microorganism, and extent of inactivation for a specific environmental condition.

When n = 1, the C·t product is constant for a given range of values. When n >1, C is the dominant factor that determines the extent of inactivation and the C·t value decreases with increasing C. When n <1, the dominant factor is contact time and the C·t value increases with increasing C. The effects of various n values on C·t are presented in Figure 5–2.

A set of n values for different chemicals and microorganisms is given in Table 5–1. Reported n values ranges from 0.34 to 4.76. Data also indicate that, in some cases, n falls reasonably close to 1. Under these conditions, C·t values can be used to compare the efficiencies of different biocides to inactivate the same organism or resistance of different microorganisms to a given biocide. Some C·t data to compare the resistance of different

Table 5–1. *Coefficient of Dilution (n) For Free Chlorine, Chlorine Dioxide, and Ozone*

Disinfectant	Organism	pH	Temp. (°C)	Range Disinfectant Concentration (mg/L)	n	Reference
Free chlorine	N. gruberi	5.0	25	0.49–2.68	0.96	Rubin et al. (1983)
		7.0	25	0.78–3.44	1.19	
		9.0	25	11.6–72.6	0.93	
Free chlorine	G. muris	7.0	5	0.41–2.73	0.34	Leahy (1985)
		7.0	5	11.1–78.5	1.52	
		7.0	5	186–244	4.76	
Free chlorine	G. muris	5.0	25	4.9–13.0	1.35	Leahy (1985)
		7.0	25	2.87–7.12	1.59	
		9.0	25	15.5–84.1	0.90	
Chlorine dioxide	Poliovirus type 1	7.0	5	0.4–1.0	1.05	Brigano (1979)
		7.0	25	0.4–0.8	1.02	
Chlorine dioxide	E. coli	6.5	5	0.25–0.75	1.08	Bernarde et al. (1967)
		6.5	10	0.25	1.18	
		6.5	20	0.25	1.08	
Chlorine dioxide	G. muris	7.0	5	1.20	1.20	Leahy (1985)
Chlorine dioxide	G. muris	5.0	25	1.22	1.22	Leahy (1985)
		7.0	25	1.30	1.30	
		9.0	25	1.37	1.37	
Chlorine dioxide	N. gruberi	5.0	25	0.53–1.2	1.09	Chen et al. (1985)
		7.0	25	0.41–1.3	0.93	
		9.0	25	0.48–1.1	0.94	
Ozone	N. gruberi	5–9	25	0.21–1.05	1.0	Wickramanayake et al. (1984)
		7	5–30		1.1	
Ozone	G. muris	5–9	25	0.02–0.19	1.2	
		7	5–25	0.03–0.7	1.1	

From Hoff, J.C. 1986. *Inactivation of Microbial Agents by Chemical Disinfectants.* EPA–600/2–86–067. Cincinnati, Water Engineering Research Laboratory, United States Environmental Protection Agency.

Table 5–2. *Concentration-Time (C·t) Data for 99% Inactivation of Cysts with Ozone*

Temperature (°C)	pH	Naegleria gruberi			Giardia muris		
		C mg/L	t min	C·t mg-min / L	C mg/L	t min	C·t mg-min / L
25	5	0.3–1.2	4.4–1.1	1.33	0.04–0.1	5.0–2.0	0.201
25	6	0.3–1.1	5.2–1.4	1.55	—	—	—
25	7	0.3–1.2	4.3–1.1	1.29	0.03–0.15	9–1.8	0.27
25	8	0.25–0.8	5.4–1.7	1.36	—	—	—
25	9	0.35–1.1	6.1–1.9	2.12	0.015–0.01	7.5–1.1	0.112
5	7	0.55–2.0	7.8–2.1	4.23	0.15–0.7	12.9–2.8	1.94
15	7	0.3–0.9	6.8–2.3	2.04	0.05–0.3	7.5–1.3	0.375
30	7	0.3–1.0	4–1.2	1.21	—	—	—

C, Ozone concentration; t, time for 99% kill; C·t, values for average of 3 or more experiments; n, values for *N. gruberi* and *G. muris* are 1.0–1.1 and 1.0–1.2, respectively.

From Wickramanayake, G.B. 1984. *Kinetics and Mechanism of Ozone Activation of Protozoan Cysts.* Ph.D. dissertation. Columbus, Department of Civil Engineering, The Ohio State University.

organisms are given in Table 5–2. Reported inactivation data are for protozoan cysts *Naegleria gruberi* and *Giardia muris* exposed to aqueous ozone in batch reactors under different pH and temperatures. The coefficient of dilution (n) for each organism was approximately 1. Comparison of C·t values for both organisms at pH 7 and 25°C indicates that *N. gruberi* is about 5 times more resistant than *G. muris*. The higher the C·t value, the more resistant the organism. C·t values can also be used to compare the pH and temperature effects. For example, with an increase in temperature from 5 to 15°C at pH 7, the resistance of *G. muris* to inactivation by ozone was decreased about 5 times. In the case of *N. gruberi*, the decrease of resistance for similar conditions was only by a factor of 2.

The C·t values also can be used to compare the efficiency of different inactivation agents for the same organism. Table 5–3 contains data with which the efficacy of ozone, chlorine dioxide, chlorine, and chloramines against a number of microorganisms can be compared. In this case, the lower the C·t value, the higher is the efficacy of the decontaminants. Consequently, ozone, with C·t values ranging from 0.006 to 2.0 mg-min/L, appears to be most effective among the four chemical decontaminants. Chlorine dioxide and free chlorine are more or less comparable to each other in disinfection efficiency. Chloramines are the least effective, with C·t values ranging from 95 to 6476 mg-min/L.

The C·t data for the inactivation of microorganisms also can be presented as log-log plots of time versus concentration. A graph developed by Baumann and Ludwig (1962) to compare the resistance of different organisms to inactivation by free available chlorine is given in Figure 5–3. The inactivation lines for the most sensitive organisms fall closer to the origin of X-Y axes, and the lines for resistant organisms fall further away from the origin. For example, *Escherichia coli* at pH 7 is the most sensitive and *Bacillus anthracis* at pH 8.0 is the most resistant to chlorine inactivation at 20 to 29°C (Fig. 5–3).

Hoff (1986) completed a thorough literature study on disinfection data available for chlorine, chloramine, chlorine dioxide, and ozone. One of the objectives of this study was to evaluate the applicability of the C·t concept in developing disinfection requirements for these chemical agents. His conclusions appear to be pertinent to the scope of this chapter:

The C·t values provide a basis for comparing the effectiveness of different disinfectants for inactivation of specific microorganisms and for comparing the relative resistance of different microorganisms to specific disinfectants. In some cases, the C·t values derived from exposure to different concentrations of the same disinfectant under specific pH and temperature conditions show little variation while in other cases a wide range of C·t values is seen. Almost always it is difficult to discern the reasons when widely different values are found either when considering the results of only one investigation or when considering results from several different investigations. These factors make it difficult to pinpoint disinfection requirements precisely. The use of C·t values to evaluate disinfection practice or establish disinfection criteria for use in the field must be done with considerable caution and incorporation of appropriate safety factors into the C·t values is necessary. Some major problems in applying the results of C·t values in developing disinfection requirements are: (a) the failure of disinfection data to follow the exponential rates described by the empirical C·t equation; (b) differences in disinfection resistance between different isolates of the same species and between different species within groups (bacteria, viruses, cysts); (c) "state of the microorganism" effects such as aggregation, prior growth conditions and protective effects that cannot be factored into the values; (d) influence of experimental conditions (reactor configuration, mixing intensity, disinfectant concentration variations, etc.) on inactivation rates; (e) problems relating to relevance of laboratory data to field conditions.

Information presented so far has focused on microbial inactivation by chemical agents. An approach similar to the C·t concept can be applied to evaluate the inactivation data for physical agents such as UV radiation and heat. In the case of UV radiation, the intensity of the UV source falling on the treatment medium is given as power per unit area (e.g., milliwatts per square centimeter, mW/cm²). The dose is given by the product of intensity and time (mW-sec/cm²) which is similar to the

Table 5–3. *Summary of Concentration-Time (C·t) Value Ranges (mg-min/L) for 99% Inactivation of Various Microorganisms by Chemical Disinfectants at 5°C*

| Microorganism | Disinfectant | | | |
	Free Chlorine pH 6 to 7	Preformed Chloramine pH 8 to 9	Chlorine Dioxide pH 6 to 7	Ozone pH 6 to 7
E. coli	0.034–0.05	95–180	0.4–0.75	0.02
Poliovirus type 1	1.1–2.5	768–3740	0.2–6.7	0.1–0.2
Rotavirus	0.01–0.05	3806–6476	0.2–2.1	0.006–0.06
Phage f₂	0.08–0.18	—	—	—
G. lamblia cysts	47–150	—	—	0.5–0.6
G. muris cysts	30–630	—	7.2–18.5	1.8–2.0

From Hoff, J.C. 1986. *Inactivation of Microbial Agents by Chemical Disinfectants.* EPA–600/2–86–067. Cincinnati, Water Engineering Research Laboratory, United States Environmental Protection Agency.

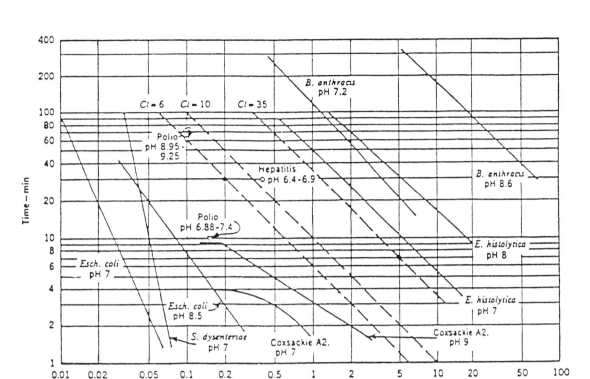

Fig. 5–3. Inactivation of bacteria and viruses by free available chlorine at 20 to 90°C. From Baumann, E.R., and Ludwig, D.D. 1962. Free available chlorine residuals for small nonpublic water supplies. J. Am. Water Works Assoc., *54*, 1379–1388.

C·t product in the chemical inactivation. In the case of heat, a temperature-time product (θ·t) can be used in place of the C·t product.

The C·t values generated from laboratory or pilot scale experiments can be used for the design of full scale treatment units for rDNA process wastes. Extrapolation of C·t values should be done with considerable caution, however, and should be limited to the reported ranges of chemical concentrations, environmental conditions, and reactor type(s).

EFFECTS OF ENVIRONMENTAL CONDITIONS

The environmental factors that affect the rate and extent of the inactivation of microorganisms include temperature, pH, chemical demand exerted on the inactivation agent, and accessibility of the biocide to the targeted organisms. These issues are discussed briefly in this section.

Temperature

The trend of the effects of temperature changes on chemical reactions and inactivation kinetics appears to be similar. The efficacy of chemical inactivation increases with increasing temperature. The ratio of times required to achieve the same level of inactivation of an organism with the same chemical agent and concentration as the temperature increased by 10°C is referred to as the Q_{10} value. If n is close to 1, Q_{10} is the ratio of C·t values as

the temperature is decreased by the corresponding 10°C. The Q_{10} values estimated for free chlorine, chlorine dioxide, chloramines, and ozone for inactivation of different microorganisms are given in Table 5–4. Q_{10} ranged from 1 to 5, with most of the values falling between 1.5 and 2.5. According to some empirical rules, chemical reaction rates increase by a factor of 2 to 3 for each 10°C rise in temperature (Weber, 1972). Clarke and Chang (1959) and Hoff (1986) identified the similarities between changes in chemical reaction and inactivation rates.

In addition to the inactivation rates, temperature changes can affect the chemical disinfectants in different ways. A decrease in temperature results in increased solubility of inactivation agents such as chlorine and ozone gas. Ozone decomposition is accelerated with rising temperature. All these issues related to temperature need to be considered in determining efficacy and stability of a biocide in rDNA process waste treatment.

pH

The pH of the medium during the decontamination process is important, especially with certain chemicals. For example, the distribution of free chlorine species, which have different disinfection efficiencies, is governed by the solution pH. At pH 3 and above, with chlorine concentration less than 1000 mg/L, elemental chlorine is completely hydrolyzed to hypochlorous acid. Hypochlorous acid dissociates to form hydrogen and hypo-

Table 5–4. *Effects of 10°C Changes in Temperature (Q_{10}) on Microorganism Inactivation Rates*

Disinfectant	Organisms	Temp. (°C)	pH	Q_{10}	Reference
Free chlorine	E. coli	5–25	7	1.65	Fair et al. (1948)
			8.5	1.42	
			9.8	2.13	
			10.7	2.5	
	E. histolytica cysts	—	—	2.1	
Chloramines	E. coli	5–25	7.0	2.09	Fair et al. (1948)
			8.5	2.28	
			9.5	3.35	
	Poliovirus type 2	5–15	9.0	1.5	Scarpino et al. (1979)
		15–25	9.0	4.0	(99% inactivation)
	Poliovirus type 1	5–15	9.0	2.0	Scarpino et al. (1979)
		15–25	9.0	1.9	(90% inactivation)
	Poliovirus type 1	5–15	4.5	2.5	
Chlorine dioxide	Poliovirus type 1	5–15	7	2.26	Scarpino et al. (1979)
		15–25	7	1.99	(monodispersed virus)
		5–15	7	4.12	Cronier et al. (1978)
		15–25	7	1.34	
Ozone	Poliovirus type 1	10–20		1.5	Roy et al. (1981)
	N. gruberi	5–15	7	2.07	Wickramanayake et al. (1984)
		15–25	7	1.58	
	G. muris	5–15	7	5.17	Wickramanayake et al. (1984)
		15–25	7	1.39	

From Hoff, J.C. *Inactivation of Microbial Agents by Chemical Disinfectants.* EPA–600/2–86–067. Cincinnati, Water Engineering Research Laboratory, United States Environmental Protection Agency.

chlorite ions above pH 4. Hypochlorous acid is completely dissociated above pH 10 when chlorine concentration is less than 5000 mg/L. As with chlorine, the speciation of other halogens such as bromine and iodine also depend on pH, which, as a result, affects the disinfection efficiencies.

Chloramines, which are less effective disinfectants than chlorine in equivalent doses, are considered potential alternatives in drinking water disinfection because (1) they provide longer lasting residuals, and (2) they are less of a health hazard. Distribution of the three inorganic chloramine species (monochloramine, dichloramine, and trichloramine) is a function of the solution pH and the chlorine-ammonia ratio. Increasing pH and ammonia concentration favors the formation of monochloramine, which is a less effective disinfectant than dichloramine.

In addition to chemical speciation, pH affects the stability of chemicals or resistance of microorganisms by changing its biochemical properties. The stability of aqueous ozone can be improved by decreasing the pH. Olivieri et al. (1975) reported that the reason for the effectiveness of the hypobromite ion as a virucide may be that the high pHs of the solutions make the f_2 phage more sensitive to the ion. Chen et al. (1984) speculated that decreased microbial resistance to chlorine dioxide at higher pH observed by Bernarde et al. (1967) and Scarpino et al. (1979) could have been caused by the changes in microorganisms at increased pH in the environment.

Chemical Disinfectant Demand

Most of the chemical inactivation agents are oxidative compounds. Therefore, the chemical biocides can be consumed by reduced inorganic and organic compounds present in the medium to be treated. A classic example for initial chemical reactions is the "chlorine demand" exerted in the presence of organic nitrogen and ammonia. The chemical demand, in this case the chlorine demand, is defined as the difference between the amount of chemical applied and the quantity of chemical available after a specified contact period. The effects of ammonia-nitrogen on chlorine demand are presented in Figure 5–4. In the presence of 1 mol of nitrogen, it is necessary to apply almost 2.5 mol of chlorine to obtain 1 mol of free chlorine.

In chemical inactivation of microorganisms, the most important issue is not the amount of chemical applied, but the residuals in the medium after demand has been exerted. In the case of waste treatment, a significant chemical demand can be introduced by organic matter in the medium. Consequently, adequate residuals should be maintained to ensure the extent of desired microbial inactivation.

Chemical Accessibility to Targeted Organisms

Most of the microorganisms that need to be inactivated by disinfection or sterilization processes may not be found in free suspension as discrete particles. For example, in sludges, bioprocessing wastes, and infectious

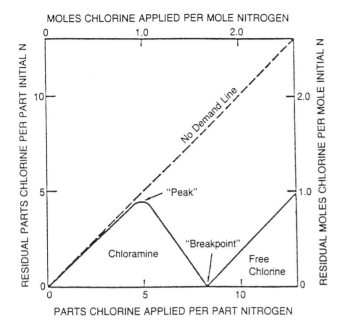

MOLES CHLORINE APPLIED PER MOLE NITROGEN

Fig. 5–4. Diagrammatic representation of completed breakpoint reaction. From Safe Drinking Water Committee. 1980. The disinfection of drinking water. In *Drinking Water and Health*. Volume 2. Washington, D.C., National Academy Press, pp 5–138.

chlorine dioxide inactivation decreased by factors of 1.5 and 5.9, respectively. The smaller value for chloramine may be attributed to the extended contact times provided with this inactivation agent. In the case of chlorine dioxide, where a rapid decontamination is expected, the efficiency has dropped significantly (about 6 times). Similarly, Hejkal et al. (1979) observed during the inactivation of fecal associated poliovirus that the occluded viruses required a fourfold combined residual chlorine level, as compared to free or secondarily adsorbed viruses, to achieve the same degree of inactivation. Therefore, the effects of the association of organisms or subcellular components with suspended matter need to be thoroughly studied in developing disinfection/sterilization data and designing waste-treatment unit processes.

EFFECTS OF REACTOR CONFIGURATION

The reactors used in environmental engineering waste-treatment processes are categorized on the basis of mixing and hydraulic characteristics. The types of reactors that are likely to be used in the treatment of wastewater include:

1. Completely mixed batch (CMB) reactor.
2. Completely mixed flow-through (CMF) reactor that is also known as continuous stirred-tank reactor (CSTR).
3. Plug flow (PF) reactor.

Data for the inactivation of microorganisms by physical and chemical agents have been developed for these types of reactors. Extrapolation of inactivation data generated for a given type of reactor from bench or pilot scale to full scale is permitted if the same type of reactor is used in a full-scale system and the hydraulic characteristics are maintained. Data generated from the use of different reactors should not be compared unless the appropriate changes are made for kinetic and hydraulic differences. For example, C·t data generated for a CMF reactor should not be compared directly with that of a CMB reactor. The scope of this chapter does not permit an extensive discussion on CMB, CMF, and PF reactors. Detailed descriptions of reactor configuration, theory and design are given in Weber (1972), Municipal Wastewaters Disinfection Manual (U.S. EPA, 1986), and Wastewater Disinfection Manual (WPCF, 1986).

wastes, they may be found either as clumps or attached to other cellular debris. Consequently, the accessibility of the inactivation agent to microorganisms may be hampered to different degrees, depending on their physical stage.

Research conducted with the organisms associated with suspended particles indicate that biocidal activity has been significantly reduced when compared to those found freely in suspension (Hejkal et al., 1979; Boardman and Sproul, 1977; Boyce et al., 1981; Berman and Hoff, 1984). In addition, Berman et al. (1988) reported that coliforms associated with larger particles were more difficult to inactivate by chlorine than those adsorbed to smaller particles.

Some data generated with the inactivation of simian rotavirus, when present as virus particles and associated with cell debris, are given in Table 5–5. Comparison of C·t values indicates that the efficacy of chloramine and

Table 5–5. *Reduced Inactivation Efficiency in Cell Associated Viruses: Data for 99% Inactivation of Simian Rotavirus*

				Range				
Test	Chemical	Temp. (°C)	pH	Disinfectant Concentration (mg/L)	Time (min)	Concentration-Time (C·t)	Mean C·t	Exp. No.
a	Chloramine	5	8	9.98–10.00	366–402	3806–4261	4034[a]	2
b	Chloramine	5	8	9.78–10.28	570–636	5472–6476	6124[b]	3
a	Chlorine dioxide	5	6	0.49–0.99	0.20–0.56	0.19–0.30	0.22[a]	4
b	Chlorine dioxide	5	6	0.45–1.0	1.15–4.75	1.03–2.14	1.3[b]	6

Tests: [a]virus only; [b]virus-cell debris complex.

From Berman, D., and Hoff, J.C. 1984. Inactivation of simian rotavirus SA 11 by chlorine, chlorine dioxide and monochloramine. Appl. Environ. Microbiol., *48*, 317–323.

MATHEMATICAL MODELING

Inactivation data can be generated by bench or pilot scale tests only for a few points in a broad range of environmental conditions. In data analysis, simple methods such as the C·t concept can be applied to a limited number of cases for which the data are available. Mathematical models are preferable in representing inactivation kinetics because they can estimate inactivation data for the entire subset within a given range. Generally, the mathematical models are developed from empirical or mechanistic approaches to fit the laboratory data. Development of mathematical models, however, can be extremely complex because inactivation kinetics depend on a large number of defined and undefined variables. In spite of these difficulties, models have been developed to predict the inactivation of microorganisms with a reasonable accuracy (Hom, 1972; Majumdar et al., 1973; Roy et al., 1981; Severin et al., 1983; Haas and Karra, 1984; Wickramanayake and Sproul, 1988). The purpose of this section is to discuss briefly some of the models developed to interpret the kinetics of microbial inactivation processes.

Much of the data analysis and model development in disinfection is based on empirical approaches. Chick (1908), who conducted a study on the laws of disinfection, pointed out that inactivation of bacterium *Bacillus paratyphosus* is strictly analogous to a chemical reaction in which individual bacterium can be made to resemble a molecule. The inactivation of bacterial spores by different chemical disinfectants was observed to be first order and expressed in the form of Chick's Law where the rate of inactivation is given by:

$$-\frac{dN}{dt} = KN. \tag{2}$$

In this equation, N is the concentration of microorganisms at time t, and K is the first order inactivation rate constant. Subsequent studies with different organisms, however, showed that the inactivation kinetics frequently deviated from Chick's Law.

Watson (1908) analyzed the laboratory data generated by Chick (1908) to establish Watson's Law which is given in equation 1. Watson's Law was later used to compare the disinfection efficiency in the form of C·t product.

Hom (1972) derived a mathematical model assuming the disinfectant (chlorine) concentration and the contact time are the major controllable variables. The hypothesis derived by Hom is that the combined effects of time-concentration relationships of the effect of chlorine on bacteria could be expressed as:

$$\frac{dN}{dt} = -kNt^mC^n \tag{3}$$

where, K is the inactivation rate constant, m is m-order reaction rate constant, and n is the coefficient of dilution. Assuming equation 1 holds, equation 3 was resolved to:

$$\log \frac{N}{N_o} = \frac{-Kk't^m}{m} \tag{4}$$

in which N_o is the initial concentration of microorganisms, K is the first-order reaction rate constant, and k' is the Watson's Law constant. Hom (1972) reported that equation 4 can be used to describe the inactivation of coliform bacteria in wastewater. One of the limitations in this model is that m, which was defined as a constant, decreases significantly with increasing chlorine dosage. However, Polprasert and Rajput (1984) were later able to fit their coliform inactivation data into a similar model that also incorporates the effects of algae concentration in waste stabilization pond effluents.

Majumdar et al. (1973) developed a kinetic model based on the inactivation of poliovirus by ozonation in a completely mixed batch reactor. The rate equation for inactivation of poliovirus in water and wastewater was presented as:

$$\frac{dN}{dt} = -k_1N^nC^m \tag{5}$$

Further analyses of data indicated that the survival ratio (N/N_o) can be correlated in the form of:

$$Ct = a\left(\frac{N}{N_o}\right)^b \tag{6}$$

where, a and b are constant for a given range of experiment conditions. Majumdar et al. (1973) also concluded that the inactivation data obtained from batch studies can be successfully used for continuous flow-through reactors.

Roy et al. (1981) developed a model based on equations 1 and 5 for enterovirus inactivation by ozone. The test data were generated at three different temperatures (5 to 20°C) where experiments were conducted in a continuous flow-through reactor. Analyses of test data resulted in the following simplified model:

$$\frac{dN}{dt} = -kCN^{0.69} \tag{7}$$

Roy et al. (1981) also reported that the overall inactivation rate constant and the absolute temperature can be correlated by the classical Arrhenius equation.

$$k = Ae^{-E/RT} \tag{8}$$

Subsequent studies by Chen et al. (1985) and Wickramanayake et al. (1988) also showed that the above relationship held for the inactivation of protozoan cysts by chlorine dioxide and ozone, respectively.

Gard (1957) developed the following equation to express the declining rate of microbial inactivation with contact time (even when the disinfectant concentration held steady):

$$-\frac{dS'}{dt} = \frac{kCS}{1 + k'Ct} \tag{9}$$

where, S is the survival ratio. This expression, however, gives a maximum rate of disinfection at zero contact time that is not necessarily true for some organisms and disinfectants. Consequently, the model was modified by Collins and Selleck (1975) as follows:

$$-\frac{dS}{dt} = \frac{nC}{b} S^{(n+1)/n} \tag{10}$$

where, b is an empirical constant. A simplified version of this model by Selleck et al. (1978) and White (1972) in the following form:

$$\ell n(N/N_o) = -n \, \ell n(1+bCt) \tag{11}$$

was used by Haas and Karra (1984b) who concluded that the use of this empiric model for description and analysis of coliform decay kinetics in wastewater (including other systems containing chlorine demand) is justifiable as an approximation to rational kinetic behavior.

Haas (1980) developed a mechanistic model to represent lag-survival curves observed for batch reactors. The process was assumed to be analogous to a chemical reaction in the following form:

$$D + S <= = = => DS \xrightarrow{k_f'} \text{inactive microbe}$$

Here, D, S, and DS are disinfectant molecules, organism, and disinfectant-organism complex, respectively; and k values are the reaction kinetic coefficients. The model, which has the form of the classic Monod model, was reported to be successful in fitting data for the chlorine inactivation of single poliovirus particles. Roy et al. (1982) used a similar mechanistic concept to derive a formulation for the inactivation kinetics in a completely mixed flow-through reactor. The model is reported to fit well with the data generated for ozone inactivation of a group of viruses. In another study by Wickramanayake (1984), a mechanistic model based on the chemical diffusion theory was developed to predict the rate and extent of the inactivation of protozoan cysts. The model was successful in estimating cyst inactivation by chlorine, chlorine dioxide, and ozone.

Haas and Karra (1984a) reviewed the kinetics of microbial inactivation by chlorine in demand-free systems. They performed a critical analysis of the available data on microbial inactivation by free and combined chlorine using the Monod model (described previously), Hom's model (equation 3) and the Chick-Watson model, in the following form:

$$\ell n(N/N_o) = -kC^n t. \tag{12}$$

Based on the free and combined chlorine inactivation data for bacteria, viruses, protozoan cysts, and fungi, Haas and Karra (1984a) concluded that the Chick-Watson model produces an adequate fit and, in general, no substantial improvement in the fit to experimental data is obtained by the other two models.

Wickramanayake and Sproul (1988) derived an empirical formulation to define microbial inactivation ki-

netics using a modified Chick-Watson equation that can be written as:

$$\log \frac{N}{N_o} = K_o C^n (t - t_o) \tag{13}$$

where K_o is the overall inactivation rate constant and t_o is the lag time. The model derivation by Wickramanayake and Sproul (1988) was based on data for protozoan cyst inactivation with ozone. The empirical formulation was then used to predict the inactivation rate constant variation with temperature and ozone level (Fig. 5–5) and the survival ratio at different ozone concentrations and contact time (Fig. 5–6).

In addition to mechanistic approaches, statistical methods are also used to derive empirical disinfection models. For example, regression analysis of coliform response on the logarithm of the disinfectant dose is typical for dose-response models for water and wastewater disinfection (Finch et al., 1988). For the inactivation of *Escherichia coli* by ozone, the following dose response model was proposed:

$$\log(N/N_o) = a + bC + ct \tag{14}$$

where, C and t are independent variables, and a, b, and c are the model parameters. Although the variance analyses revealed a lack of fit, Finch et al. (1988) found that for practical applications, an adequate dose-response model for 0 to 99.99% reduction of *E. coli* could be developed using the logarithm of utilized ozone as the dose function.

Clark et al. (1989) compiled and analyzed the chlorine inactivation data for *Giardia lamblia* to develop concentration-time (C·t) values for the treatment of drinking water. The regression model developed for 99.99% inactivation of *Giardia* cysts was:

$$t = RC^a pH^b temp^c \tag{15}$$

where, pH is the water pH, temp is the temperature (°C), and a, b, c are the constants.

In the development of empiric models, sequential linear regression, nonlinear least square regression, or maximum likelihood estimation is commonly used. Haas (1988) compared these three statistical methods and reported that the maximum likelihood estimation procedure produced estimates of inactivation parameters of lesser bias and variance than the other two procedures.

The disinfection models discussed so far have been developed for the chemical inactivation agents. Similar kinetic models have been generated for physical treatment processes such as irradiation and heat, however. One of the approximations used in ultraviolet (UV) disinfection (WPCF, 1986; Haas and Sakellaropoulos, 1979) is:

$$N = N_o exp(-kIt) \tag{16}$$

where, I is the intensity of the germicidal UV energy, generally expressed as $\mu W/cm^2$.

In a pilot-scale study to demonstrate the application

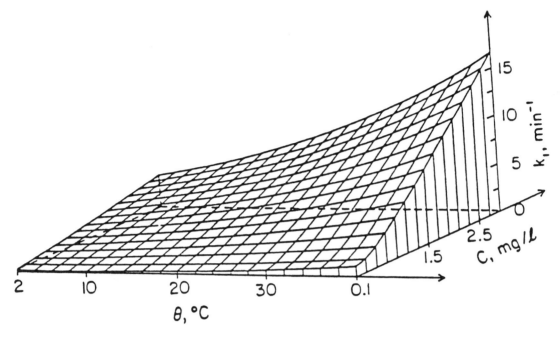

Fig. 5–5. Variation of the inactivation rate constant with temperature and ozone concentration. From Wickramanayake, G.B., and Sproul, O.J. 1988. Ozone concentration and temperature effects on disinfection kinetics. Ozone Sci. Eng., *10*, 123–135.

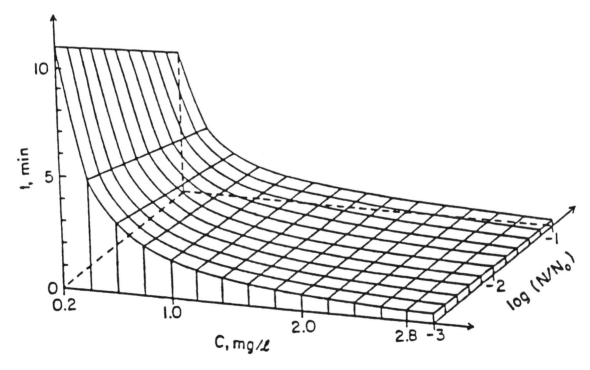

Fig. 5–6. Survival curves for 1 through 3 logs of inactivation of *Naegleria gruberi* cysts with ozone at pH 7 and 25°C. From Wickramanayake, G.B., and Sproul, O.J. 1988. Ozone concentration and temperature effects on disinfection kinetics. Ozone Sci. Eng., *10*, 123–135.

of UV disinfection to secondary wastewater effluent, Scheible et al. (1986) empirically evaluated the performance of UV units by a series of multiple linear regression analyses. The dependent variable in all cases was the log-survival ratio, whereas the independent variables included suspended solids concentration, turbidity, wastewater flow rate, and UV absorbance coefficients. The inactivation rate of coliform related well to the calculated intensity of the UV reactor. The study also demonstrated that coliforms, which are occluded by suspended particles, are not affected by UV light intensity.

Qualls and Johnson (1985) developed a model to predict bacterial survival in flow-through systems that takes into account the complex intensity patterns, nonideal flow patterns, and nonlinear curves of log survival versus UV dose. The general form of the model is:

$$N_s = \sum_{i=1}^{m} N_{oi} f(I_j t_i) \qquad (17)$$

where, N_s is the number of organisms surviving irradiation, N_{oi} is the initial number of organisms in ith fraction, and $f(I_j t_i)$ is a function described by the experimental dose survival curve. Qualls and Johnson (1985) reported that the model corresponded well with the measured survival in a ultraviolet pilot plant study.

Severin et al. (1983, 1984a,b) analyzed the kinetics of the inactivation of E. coli, Candida parapsilosis, and bacterial virus f_2 by UV irradiation and chemical disinfection. They developed a "series-event kinetic model" where the inactivation of single organisms was viewed as undergoing a series of damaging reactions or events. The damage is considered to occur in integer steps, and the rate at which an organism passes from one event to the next is first order with respect to chemical concentration. Then, a threshold exposure, n, or the lethal number of reactions for a single organism was postulated. For closed-batch reactors, the fraction survival is given by the model:

$$\frac{N}{N_o} = e^{-kCt} \sum_{i=0}^{n-1} \frac{(kCt)^i}{i!} \qquad (18)$$

where C is the disinfection concentration (mg/L) or UV light intensity ($\mu W/cm^2$).

Severin et al. (1983) tested the multitarget and series-event kinetic models for their ability to scale between batch results and flow-through reactor results. Using the respective best-fit kinetic parameters for each model from batch data, the response of the organisms in the flow-through reactor could be predicted by using either of the two models. Severin et al. (1983) concluded that ". . . since two different models can be used to describe the data, the simple agreement between experimental data and model predictions does not necessarily prove that either model is mechanistically correct. . ." The importance of mathematic models in disinfection/sterilization kinetics, however, lies in their ability to predict the viability of microorganisms under a variety of environ-

mental conditions and for scale-up of laboratory data to design large-scale treatment units.

REFERENCES

Baumann, E.R., and Ludwig, D.D. 1962. Free available chlorine residuals for small nonpublic water supplies. J. Am. Water Works Assoc., 54, 1379–1388.

Bernarde, M.A., Snow, W.B., and Oliveri, V.P. 1967. Chlorine dioxide disinfection temperature effects. J. Appl. Bacteriol., 30, 159–167.

Berg, G., Chang, S.L., and Harris, E.K. 1964. Devitalization of microorganisms by iodine. 1. Dynamics of the devitalization of enteroviruses by elemental iodine. Virology, 22, 469–481.

Berman, D., and Hoff, J.C. 1984. Inactivation of simian rotavirus SA 11 by chlorine, chlorine dioxide and monochloramine. Appl. Environ. Microbiol., 48, 317–323.

Berman, D., Rice, E.W., and Hoff, J.C. 1988. Inactivation of particle-associated coliforms by chlorine and monochloramines. Appl. Environ. Microbiol., 54, 507–512.

Boardman, G.D., and Sproul, O.J. 1977. Protection of viruses during disinfection by adsorption to particulate matter. J. Water Pollut. Control Fed., 49, 1857–1862.

Boyce, D.S., Sproul, O.J., and Buck, C.E. 1981. The effect of bentonite clay on ozone disinfection of bacteria and viruses in water. Water Res., 15, 759–767.

Brigano, F.A.O. 1979. The Effects of Particulates on the Inactivation by Chlorination Dioxide of Enteroviruses in Water. Ph.D. thesis, Cincinnati Department of Civil and Environmental Engineering, University of Cincinnati, 1979.

Cerf, O. 1977. A review: Tailing of survival curves of bacterial spores. J. Appl. Bacteriol., 43, 1.

Chen, Y.S.R., Sproul, O.J., and Rubin, A.J. 1985. Inactivation of Naegleria gruberi cysts by chlorine dioxide. Water Res., 19, 783–789.

Chick, H. 1908. An investigation of the laws of disinfection. J. Hyg., 8, 90–156.

Clark, R.M., Read, E.J., and Hoff, J.C. 1989. Analysis of inactivation of Giardia lamblia by chlorine. J. Environ. Eng., 115, 80–90.

Clarke, N.A., and Chang, S.L. 1959. Enteric viruses in water. J. Am. Water Works Assoc., 51, 1299–1317.

Collins, H.F., and Selleck, R.E. 1971. Process Kinetics of Wastewater Chlorination. Report No. 72–5. Richmond, CA, Sanitary Engineering Research Laboratory, University of California.

Cronier, S., Scarpino, P.V., and Zink, M.L. 1978. Chlorine dioxide destruction of viruses and bacteria in water. In Water Chlorination Environmental Impact and Health Effects. Volume 2. Edited by R.L. Jolly, et al. Ann Arbor, MI, Ann Arbor Science, pp. 651–658.

Fair, G.M., et al. 1948. The behavior of chlorine as a water disinfectant. J. Am. Water Works Assoc., 10, 1051–1061.

Finch, G.R., Smith, D.W., and Stiles, M.E. 1988. Dose-response of Escherichia coli in ozone demand-free phosphate buffer. Water Res., 22, 1563–1570.

Floyd, R., Sharp, D.G., and Johnson, J.D. 1979. Inactivation by chlorine of single poliovirus particles in water. Environ. Sci. Technol., 13, 438.

Gard, S. 1957. Chemical inactivation of viruses. In Nature of Viruses. CIBA Found. Symp., 123–146.

Haas, C.N. 1980. A mechanistic kinetic model for chlorine disinfection. Environ. Sci. Technol., 14, 339.

Haas, C.N. 1988. Maximum likelihood analysis of disinfection kinetics. Water Res., 22, 669–677.

Haas, C.N., and Karra, S.B. 1984a. Kinetics of microbial inactivation by chlorine-I. Review of results in demand-free systems. Water Res., 18, 1443–1449.

Haas, C.N., and Karra, S.B. 1984b. Kinetics of microbial inactivation by chlorine-II. Kinetics in the presence of chlorine demand. Water Res., 22, 669–677.

Haas, C.N., and Sakellaropoulos, G.G. 1979. Rational analysis of ultraviolet disinfection reactors. In Proceedings of the National Conference on Environmental Engineering, American Society of Civil Engineering, pp. 540–547.

Hejkal, T.W., Wellings, F.M., LaRock, P.A., and Lewis, A.L. 1979. Survival of poliovirus within organic solids during chlorination. Appl. Environ. Microbiol., 38, 114–118.

Hoff, J.C. 1986. Inactivation of Microbial Agents by Chemical Disinfectants. EPA-600/2–86–067. Cincinnati, Water Engineering Research Laboratory, United States Environmental Protection Agency.

Hoff, J.C. and Geldreich, E.F. 1981. Comparison of the biocidal efficiency of alternative disinfectants. J. Am. Water Works Assoc., 73, 40–44.

Hom, L.W. 1972. Kinetics of chlorine disinfection in an ecosystem. J. Environ. Eng. Div., Am. Soc. of Civil Eng., 98(SA1), 183–194.

Katzenelson, E., Kett, B., and Shuval, H.I. 1974. Inactivation kinetics of virus and bacteria in water by use of ozone. J. Am. Water Works Assoc., 66, 730–733.

Koch, A.L. 1966. The logarithm in biology, II. Distribution simulating the log-normal. J. Theor. Biol., *23*, 251.

Lee, R.E., and Gilbert, C.A. 1918. Application of the mass law to the process of disinfection being a contribution to the mechanistic theory as opposed to the vitalistic theory. J. Phys. Chem., *22*, 348.

Leahy, J.G. 1985. Inactivation of *Giardia muris* cysts by chlorine and chlorine dioxide. M.S. thesis, Columbus, Ohio State University, Department of Civil Engineering.

Majumdar, S.B., Ceckler, W.H., and Sproul, O.J. 1973. Inactivation of poliovirus in water by ozonation. J. Water Pollut. Control Fed., *45*, 2433.

Morris, J.C. 1970. Disinfectant chemistry and biocidal activities. In *Proceedings of the National Specialty Conference on Disinfection*. American Society of Civil Engineering, New York.

Oliver, M.A., and Shepstone, B.J. 1964. Some practical considerations in determining the parameters for multi-target and multi-hit survival curves. Phys. Med. Biol., *9*, 167.

Olivieri, V.P., et al. 1975. The comparative action of chlorine, bromine, and iodine on f_2 bacterial virus. In *Disinfection: Water and Wastewater*. Edited by J.D. Johnson. Ann Arbor, MI, Ann Arbor Science, pp. 145–162.

Polprasert, C., and Rajput, V.S. 1984. Study on the chlorine disinfection of stabilization pond effluent. Water Res., *18*, 513–518.

Prokop, A., and Humphrey, A.E. 1970. Kinetics of disinfection. In *Disinfection*. Edited by M.A. Bernarde. New York, Marcel Dekker, pp. 61–83.

Qualls, R.G. and Johnson, J.D. 1985. Modeling and efficiency of ultraviolet disinfection systems. Water Res., *19*, 1039–1046.

Roy, D., Chian, E.S.K., and Engelbrecht, R.S. 1981. Kinetics of enteroviral inactivation by ozone. J. Env. Eng. Div. ASCE. *107*, 887–901.

Roy, D., Chian, E.S.K., and Engelbrecht, R.S. 1982. Mathematical model for enterovirus inactivation by ozone. Water Res., *16*, 667.

Rubin, A.J., Engle, R.P., and Sproul, O.J. 1983. Disinfection of amoebic cysts in water with free chlorine. J. Water Pollut. Control Fed., *55*, 1174–1182.

Safe Drinking Water Committee. 1980. The disinfection of drinking water. In *Drinking Water and Health*, Volume 2. Washington, D.C., National Academy Press, pp. 5–138.

Scarpino, P.V., Brigano, F.A.O., Cronier, S., and Zink, M. 1979. *Effect of particulates on disinfection of enteroviruses in water by chlorine dioxide*. EPA–600/2–79–054. United States Environmental Protection Agency.

Scheible, O.K., Casey, M.C., and Forndran, A. 1986. *Ultraviolet Disinfection of Wastewaters from Secondary Effluent and Combined Sewer Overflows*. EPA–600/2-86/005. Cincinnati, United States Environmental Protection Agency.

Selleck, R.E., et al. 1978. Kinetics of bacterial deactivation with chlorine. J. Environ. Eng. Div., Am. Soc. Civil Eng., *104*, 1197–1212.

Severin, B.F., Suidan, M.T., and Engelbrecht, R.S. 1983. Kinetic modeling of U.V. disinfection of water. Water Res., *17*, 1669–1678.

Severin, B.F., Suidan, M.T., and Engelbrecht, R.S. 1984a. Series-event kinetic model for chemical disinfection. J. Environ. Eng., *110*, 430–439.

Severin, B.F., Suidan, M.T., and Engelbrecht, R.S. 1984b. Mixing effects in U.V. disinfection. J. Water Pollut. Control Fed., *56*, 881–888.

Taylor, D.G., and Johnson, J.D. 1974. Kinetics of viral inactivation by bromine. In *Chemistry of Water Supply, Treatment, and Distribution*. Edited by A.J. Rubin. Ann Arbor, MI, Ann Arbor Science.

United States Environmental Protection Agency. 1986. *Design Manual: Municipal Wastewater Disinfection*. EPA–625/1–86/021. Cincinnati, Water Engineering Research Laboratory, United States Environmental Protection Agency.

Watson, H.E. 1908. A note in the variation of the rate of disinfection with change in the concentration of the disinfectant. J. Hyg., *8*, 536–592.

Weber, W. 1972. *Physiochemical Processes for Water Quality Control*. New York, Wiley-Interscience.

Wei, J.H., and Chang, S.L. 1975. A Multipoisson Distribution Model for Treating Disinfection Data. In *Disinfection: Water and Wastewater*. Edited by J.D. Johnson. Ann Arbor, MI, Ann Arbor Science, pp. 11–48.

White, G.C. 1972. *Handbook of Chlorination*. New York, Van Nostrand Reinhold.

Wickramanayake, G.B. 1984. Kinetics and Mechanism of Ozone Inactivation of Protozoan Cysts. Ph.D. dissertation. Columbus, Department of Civil Engineering, The Ohio State University.

Wickramanayake, G.B., and Sproul, O.J. 1988. Ozone concentration and temperature effects on disinfection kinetics. Ozone: Sci. Eng., *10*, 123–135.

Wickramanayake, G.B., Rubin, A.J., and Sproul, O.J. 1984. Inactivation of *Naegleria* and *Giardia* cysts in water by ozonation. J. Water Pollut. Control Fed., *56*, 983–988.

Wickramanayake, G.B., Rubin, A.J., and Sproul, O.J. 1985. Effects of ozone and storage temperature on *Giardia* cysts. J. Am. Water Works Assoc., *77*, 74–77.

Withell, E.R. 1942. The significance of the variation in shape of time-survivor curves. J. Hyg., *42*, 124.

WPCF (Water Pollution Control Federation). 1986. *Wastewater Disinfection: Manual of Practice FD-10: Facilities Development*. Alexandria, VA, WPCF.

Young, D.C., and Sharp, D.G. 1979. Poliovirus aggregates and their survival in water. Appl. Environ. Microbiol., *33*, 168.

CHAPTER 6

PRINCIPLES OF THE THERMAL DESTRUCTION OF MICROORGANISMS

I.J. Pflug and R.G. Holcomb

In the study of the heat destruction of microorganisms, we are dealing with destruction of life at the single cell level. Today we relate heat stress and microbial death. Undoubtedly, in the future, study of the death of single cells will be based upon exact knowledge of the effect of heat on vital cell molecules through a precise path leading from the lethal heat energy to the ultimate cessation of organized cell metabolism, or death of the cell.

Schmidt (1954) states, "The only single practical criterion of the death of microorganisms is the failure to reproduce when, as far as is known, suitable conditions for reproduction are provided. This means that any organism which fails to show evidence of growth when placed under what are considered, in the light of our present knowledge of bacterial nutrition and growth requirements, adequate growth conditions is considered as dead." As is well pointed out by Schmidt, death is defined as the loss of the cell's ability to reproduce. In the destruction of cells and spores of microorganisms by heat, the end objective is to destroy the life processes. We are not satisfied, however, simply to discuss rates of death or factors that influence conditions for death. We believe that it is important to try to understand more about the basic mechanisms that cause or result in death, so we will be better able to predict destruction rates for conditions that we have not been able to duplicate in the laboratory.

In this discussion of the death of microorganisms, the lethal agent is heat or, more precisely, a molecular energy state capable of producing changes in the cell that prevent the cell from reproducing either by direct effects on the reproductive mechanism or by disrupting cellular metabolic systems that provide energy and chemical intermediates for reproduction. In discussing the death of microorganisms brought about by high levels of heat energy, most of our attention is directed toward bacterial spores, which are the microbial systems most able to tolerate high molecular energy levels.

Research dealing with the heat destruction of microorganisms can be divided into two areas: (1) studies carried out at the molecular level directed toward understanding what takes place inside the cell or spore from a physiologic and genetic standpoint; and (2) studies of the heat destruction of populations of microorganisms of different species subjected to heat stress under different conditions. For an up-to-date review of the present knowledge at the molecular level inside of microbial cells and spores, the reader is directed to *Spores VII* (Gerhardt and Murrell, 1978), *The Destruction of Bacterial Spores* (Russell, 1982), and *Fundamental and Applied Aspects of Bacterial Spores* (Dring et al., 1985). In this presentation, we concentrate on the cell or spore as an entity and try to relate how an external heat treatment affects the ability of the cell or spore to germinate, grow, and reproduce.

The material is divided into three sections: (1) discussion of theories and models of microbial death; (2) factors affecting the heat destruction of microorganisms; and (3) the art of gathering and analyzing microbial heat-destruction data. Although we can treat this topic in parts, we cannot completely separate all subjects; therefore, the reader will find reference to survivor curves, z values, and other important subjects appearing in all sections of this presentation.

THEORIES AND MODELS OF MICROBIAL DEATH

Both theoretic and practical reasons exist for quantifying the effect of a lethal stress on a microbial population. The end result of a testing program should be broadly meaningful. In developing microbial destruction data, we start with a suspension of microorganisms, an inoculum. The inoculum can be either heterogeneous or homogeneous. A heterogeneous microbial culture is typical of a sample of the large universe of microbial contamination that occurs in or on real material. Homogeneous is the term for a pure culture of microorganisms in which all the organisms have identical physical and biochemical properties. The usefulness of the results of a testing program in which a heterogeneous inoculum is used is different from that of a homogeneous inoculum. The utility of the results of a study using heterogeneous inocula is limited, whereas the utility of the results of a study using homogeneous inocula may be almost unlimited.

A heterogeneous inoculum is what is readily available in the real world. For example, a field sample of raw product normally contains a heterogeneous microbial population. There will be heterogeneity in species of microorganisms as well as variation in resistance within each species present. Variability among organisms in the test inoculum precludes our relating the lethal stress with the rate of destruction of a specific microorganism. All we can do is develop data regarding the gross change in the numbers of viable organisms with stress. Evaluation of the heat-destruction characteristics of this heterogeneous population will probably result in a curvilinear semilogarithmic survivor curve that indicates the presence of large numbers of low-resistance organisms, plus small numbers of organisms with high resistance. Interpretation of the results is limited to the test condition and cannot be meaningfully extrapolated beyond the last data point.

When we evaluate a homogeneous spore suspension (a pure culture that has been grown so ideally all spores have identical characteristics), we obtain destruction rate data for the specific microorganism as a function of the lethal stress. A homogeneous inoculum, subjected to varied levels of lethal stress and treated identically, should produce data that can be treated analytically to yield rate of kill data. We can use these data in mechanism of death studies and with models to be used in sterilization process design.

Heat-destruction models are idealistic in their requirements; therefore, for the microorganisms to fit the model, the test program must meet all the requirements of the model: (1) the inoculum must be homogeneous; (2) the lethal stress must have a uniform effect regardless of heating time; (3) the recovery medium must act in an equal optimal manner on both heated and unheated spores; and (4) there must be no environmental factors in the testing program that will tend to cause deviation from the ideal reaction of the spores to the test stress.

Meeting all these criteria in a biologic system in which the microorganisms themselves are able to sense and respond to levels of chemicals, water, and other factors in the environment that may be below the threshold of measurement even with today's sophisticated instrumentation, should indicate to the potential researcher the magnitude of the environmental control problem. Because all these possible obstacles to obtaining accurate results exist, Cerf (1977) and others have pointed out that a tailing effect and other peculiarities that result from survivor-curve experiments may be artifacts unless special care is taken and additional testing carried out to prove that these conditions are real.

The design of the testing program and the controls that need to be used to ensure repeatability of technique and consistency of media and other supplies are the most important parts of determining the heat resistance of a microbial population.

Semilogarithmic Graph as a Tool for Examining Experimental Microbial Survivor Data

In experiments to evaluate the effect of heat stress on a microbial population, all conditions except the heating time are usually held as constant as possible. If we subject aliquots of a suspension of microorganisms to heat for several different time periods and then enumerate the survivors using the plate count technique, the resulting data will be the number of colony-forming units (cfu) for each heating time. In addition, we usually determine the number of organisms in the unheated control. In most heat-destruction experiments designed to yield survivor curves, the initial microbial populations are of the order of 10^6 to 10^7 organisms per unit, with the final number of survivors as low as 10 or 100 per unit. To communicate these results visually, a survivor curve graph is prepared, in which the number of survivors is shown as a function of the length of heating time at temperature T. A survivor curve graph in which both the numbers of survivors and time are plotted on an arithmetic scale is shown in Figure 6–1. A change in the number of organisms from 10^6 to 10^2 cannot be presented meaningfully on an arithmetic scale. In Figure 6–2, a survivor graph is shown in which the numbers of survivors has been plotted on a logarithmic scale as a function of time on an arithmetic scale. This is an appropriate way to treat microbial survivor data because in sterilization studies we are interested in the rate of destruction of microorganisms as we approach zero survivors.

The semilogarithmic graph is one of the most important tools we use when studying the heat destruction of microorganisms. Perhaps, because of its wide use, it was inevitable that confusion should arise regarding its use and meaning. Because of its importance, we will try to separate and clarify the use and meaning of this important tool. We recommend that results of a microbial destruction test be plotted on a semilogarithmic graph so we can visually examine the data; subsequently, we may correlate the data using the semilogarithmic model. These two procedures are separate; plotting data on the semilogarithmic graph is a general first step and should always be done, whereas correlating the data using the semilogarithmic model is a second step and should only be carried out if it seems appropriate.

When the logarithm of the number of survivors is plotted as a function of heating time (referred to as a semilogarithmic survivor curve), usually part or all of the survivor curve is a straight line, or the survivor curve can be represented by two straight lines. Not all experimentally obtained semilogarithmic survivor curves are

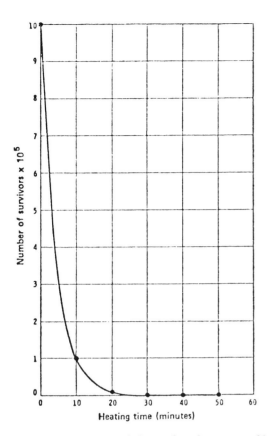

Fig. 6–1. A survivor curve with the number of survivors and heating time both plotted on an arithmetic scale.

single straight lines, however, nor can they be described by two straight lines. The literature has many examples in which the semilogarithmic survivor curves for heat or other lethal stress are parabolic or in some cases even sigmoid in shape.

The shape of the semilogarithmic survivor curve varies depending on the organism and the test system. Four common types of survivor curve shapes are shown in Figure 6–3. The shape of the semilogarithmic curve for a specific culture of microorganisms in a specific test system at a particular temperature is reproducible so long as the test system is not altered. When a homogeneous culture of microorganisms is subjected to assumed identical environmental stress conditions and widely varying results are obtained, this variation is often attributed to the microorganisms; however, fluctuations in the environment are probably responsible for the variation. The microbial cell is extremely sensitive and responds predictably to changes in environmental conditions to integrate the effect of chemical and physical changes acting over time. Meaningful results cannot be obtained where fluctuations in the environment produce responses in the microorganisms comparable to the responses produced and measured by the experiment itself. It is vital that all environmental variables be controlled.

The shape of the semilogarithmic survivor curve for a specific spore crop may change with the test temperature

or a change in the test system, and when another similar spore crop is produced by a different spore production method. The semilogarithmic survivor curves for both wet- and dry-heat destruction of pure cultures of microorganisms are similar in their response to the three points just mentioned; however, there appears to be no relationship between the shape of the semilogarithmic survivor curve of a homogeneous culture of microorganisms subjected on the one hand to wet-heat and on the other hand to dry-heat conditions. All four shapes of survivor curves shown in Figure 6–3 have been obtained in both wet- and dry-heat studies.

The survivor curves for aliquots of a mixed natural flora, for example, found in soil or as a food or drug product contaminant, usually are similar in shape to the curve shown in Figure 6–4. A natural flora almost always contains varying numbers of organisms and heat-resistance levels within and among species. Ignoring species, these natural cultures usually have a large population of low-resistance organisms and a relatively small population of high-resistance organisms.

Rahn's Heat-Destruction Model

Rahn (1945b) suggested that microbial destruction was due to the inactivation of a single critical molecule in the

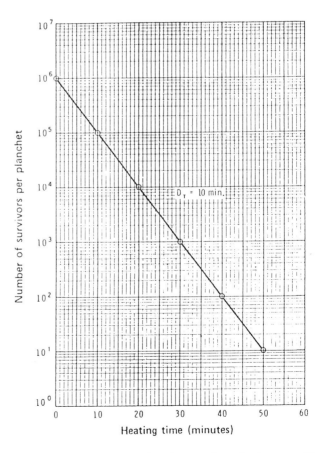

Fig. 6–2. A survivor curve plotted on semilogarithmic paper with the number of survivors plotted on the logarithmic scale.

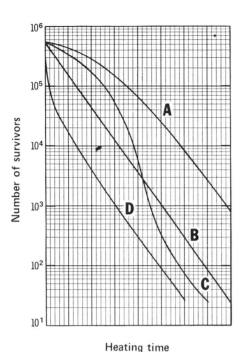

Fig. 6–3. An exponential survivor curve (B) and three commonly observed nonexponential survivor curves (A, C, and D). From Moats, W.A. 1971. Kinetics of thermal death of bacteria. J. Bacteriol., *105,* 165–171.

cell, and, therefore, could be assumed to follow first-order kinetics:

$$\frac{dN(t)}{dt} = -kN(t) \qquad (1)$$

where $N(t)$ is the number of microorganisms, k is the reaction rate constant, and t is time.

Integrating this differential equation and letting N_0 equal the initial number of microorganisms, we find:

$$N(t) = N_0 e^{-kt} \qquad (2)$$

If we replace t with U, which is conventionally used as the symbol for equivalent time at heating medium temperature, and change from base e to base 10 logarithms and convert from a temperature coefficient k to a unit D $\left(k = \dfrac{2.3026}{D}\right)$, our equation becomes:

$$\log N(U) = -\frac{U}{D} + \log N_0 \qquad (3)$$

If we plot the logarithm of the numbers of surviving organisms as a function of heating time U, the result will be a straight line with the slope equal to $(-1/D)$. The D value will also be the time required for the population N to change by a factor of 10, or for the survivor curve

to traverse one log cycle. This is usually referred to as "Rahn's logarithmic order of death." If the viable number of organisms in aliquots of a homogeneous suspension of microorganisms subjected to identical heat stress conditions is reduced according to this model, the resulting survivor curve will be a straight line through the point N_0, with the D value being a measure of the slope of this survivor curve. The D-value is a function of temperatures so it should be indicated as D_T.

We estimate that approximately one-third of the experimentally determined semilogarithmic survivor curves for homogeneous cultures of microorganisms subjected to what are thought to be identical heat stress conditions will fit Rahn's logarithmic order of death model (B in Fig. 6–3). Curves A and D of Figure 6–3 probably constitute another third of the experimentally determined survivor curves. During the initial heating time period, these survivor curves have a higher or lower death rate than the major straight-line portion. For the data that form a straight line on the semilogarithmic graph, the use of the D_T value as a measure of the destruction characteristics of the microbiologic population is most appropriate. For approximately two-thirds of the data where one sees either a reduction in the death rate during the initial period (curve A) or an increase in the death rate (curve D) during the initial period, a meaningful D_T value can be calculated for the straight-line portion of the survivor curve, but this value is not applicable to the initial period. Suggested treatment of this type of experimental data is covered in the last section of this chapter.

Additional Microbial Heat-Destruction Models

Moats (1971) developed a model for the death of bacteria on the basis of the assumption that a bacterium has many critical sites and several of these sites must be

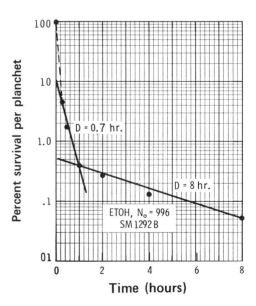

Fig. 6–4. An example of a semilogarithmic survivor curve for a sample of mixed natural flora (substrate is soil suspended in ethanol).

inactivated before death occurs. The inactivation of the individual sites was assumed to take place at random, and the inactivation of each site followed first-order kinetics. This model produces survivor curves of shapes A, B, C, and D (Fig. 6–3), depending on the magnitude of the parameters. Parameters can be estimated from experimental data.

Prokop and Humphrey (1972) describe a model based upon cytologic changes in bacterial spores during heating. They assume that, following heat treatment, a spore is in one of three sequentially occupied states: heat shocked, heat sensitive, and nonviable. A sequential first-order model is assumed, with sequential reaction rates k_1 and k_2.

Several models for microbial destruction have been developed by Brannen (1968b). He describes a multihit model based on chemical reaction kinetics in which nonlogarithmic survival is inherent in the organism. Brannen (1968a) discusses a similar model that can be used to obtain all four types of survivor curves shown in Figure 6–3. Brannen (1970) investigated, via models, the consequences of the assumption that genetic homogeneity and DNA chemical homogeneity of a microbial population are not equivalent.

Frederickson (1966) describes probabilistic microbial death models that are similar to the models mentioned previously and applies the results to an idealized fermentation process. He observes that, in such models, the extinction time of the "last" organism is a random variable and the modeled survival curve shows sudden, unpredictable drops as the population size gets smaller.

In studies in which the semilogarithmic survivor curve was concave downward, Alderton and Snell (1970) used a model in the form $(\log N_0/N)^a = kt + c$ to analyze their data.

Schalkowsky and Wiederkehr (1968) developed a model in which they assumed that the incremental death time of heated microorganisms is directly proportional to prior exposure time and concluded that the log of the survival time is normally distributed. They derive the normal distribution for survival times by assuming that prior exposure time does not produce a cumulative effect on the destruction process. Analyses of experimental data show an early normal distribution followed by a log normal distribution of survival times. The authors indicate that these observations are consistent with the idea that environmental effects are dominant in early stages, and time-cumulative effects are stronger later in the heating process.

Shull et al. (1963) consider a thermal death model for spores that obeys first-order kinetics and has a first-order dormant spore activation component. They describe how this model may explain the initial lag period often observed in semilogarithmic survivor curves.

Temperature Coefficient Models

In some heat sterilization processes, the lethal effect must be integrated over a range of temperatures; in others, it must be possible to determine an equivalent process at another temperature. Both these situations require the use of a temperature coefficient model.

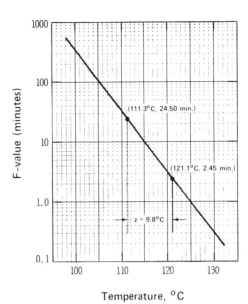

Fig. 6–5. Thermal death time curve for *Clostridium botulinum* spores. Data from Townsend, C.T., Esty, J.R., and Baselt, F.C. 1938. Heat resistance studies on spores of putrefactive anaerobes in relation to determination of safe processes for canned foods. Food Res., 3, 323–346.

The temperature coefficient of a process is the change in the rate of the process with a change in temperature. The Q_{10} value is widely used by the scientific community as a measure of the temperature coefficient of chemical and biologic reactions. Q_{10} is defined as the change in the reaction rate constant, k, for a change in temperature of 10°C. In equation form:

$$Q_{10} = \frac{K_{(T + 10°C)}}{K_T} \qquad (4)$$

The Q_{10} value of many chemical and biologic reactions is 2; however, Q_{10} values for the heat destruction of bacteria are larger, ranging from 2.2 to 4.6 for dry heat and from 6.8 to 100 for wet heat.

Bigelow (1921) observed that, if the logarithm of the destruction time was plotted against temperature on an arithmetic scale, the result over the range of temperatures studied was a straight line. This method of plotting thermal resistance and thermal death time data must be judged as empiric. The simplicity of this type of analysis and the ready adaptation of the analysis to analytic manipulation has encouraged its use.

The temperature coefficient model of Bigelow (1921) is shown graphically in Figure 6–5. The equation of this model is

$$\log F_T^Z = \frac{1}{z} (T_B - T) + \log F_{T_B}^Z \qquad (5)$$

where T_B is the base temperature, $F_{T_B}^Z$ is specified, and

T is the new temperature corresponding to F_T^z. The z value is a measure of the slope of the thermal death time curve (log F vs. temperature) and is the number of degrees necessary to change F by a factor of 10. It is also the number of degrees of temperature change necessary to change the D value by a factor of 10. The z value is related to Q_{10} by the equation

$$z°C = \frac{10}{\log Q_{10}} \tag{6}$$

The graphic presentation of the Bigelow temperature coefficient model is commonly called a thermal resistance curve if the logarithms of the D values are plotted against the temperature. It is referred to as a thermal death time curve if the logarithms of the F values are plotted against temperature.

The Bigelow model is empiric. The lack of a theory as to why thermal destruction data should respond and form straight lines when plotted in this manner caused researchers to look for a theory that could be used to reinforce this method of analysis or to develop another method that had a sound theoretic basis.

The Arrhenius analysis is a method for handling established kinetic data of either zero, first, or second order. In making an Arrhenius analysis, the logarithm of k is plotted against the reciprocal of the absolute temperature. The Arrhenius equation is:

$$k = A \exp\left(-\frac{E^*}{RT}\right) \tag{7}$$

where
k = the specific reaction rate constant (time^{-1})
A = a constant, the frequency factor (time^{-1})
$\exp$ = exponential function of the Napierian base e
E^* = activation energy
R = gas constant
T = absolute temperature

This equation can be used to find activation energy, because the slope of the curve resulting when ln k is plotted against 1/T is the constant $\frac{E^*}{R}$. Integration between the limits $k = k_1$, at $T = T_1$ and $k = k_2$ at $T = T_2$ using base 10 logarithms and constant E^*, will give:

$$\log \frac{k_2}{k_1} = \frac{E^*}{2.303R} \left(\frac{T_2 - T_1}{T_1 T_2}\right) \tag{8}$$

which can be used to determine the activation energy of the reaction from two values of D or k. The z value can be related to the energy of activation using the equation:

$$E^* = 2.303 \, RT^2/z \tag{9}$$

where E^* is the activation energy, R is the gas constant, and T is the absolute temperature.

In present-day chemical kinetics, the fundamental equation of Eyring (1935) and Glasstone et al. (1941) is used instead of the generally empiric Arrhenius relationship. This relationship,

$$k = \frac{RT}{Nh} \exp\left(\frac{\Delta S_a}{R}\right) \exp\left(\frac{-\Delta H_a}{RT}\right) \tag{10}$$

in which N is Avogadro's number, h is Planck's constant, and ΔS_a is the entropy of activation change, is sophisticated and requires a large quantity of reaction rate data before meaningful results are obtained. The ΔH_a, the enthalpy of activation, of the Eyring equation is essentially equal to the experimental energy of activation of the Arrhenius equation. In general, the same type of graph, ln k vs. 1/T, is used in the Eyring analysis as is used in the Arrhenius analysis.

Although the experimental data in the literature for developing thermal destruction curves normally do not extend over more than 30°C (54°F), the general agreement that most thermal destruction curves are straight lines cannot be dismissed lightly. It is impossible to find in the literature a consistent trend for thermal resistance curves to be either concave upward or downward; this fact suggests that no strong basic trend exists.

It is generally recognized that in the biologic system we are working with chemicals and chemical inactivation rates; however, the reaction laws are different for these chemical inactivations in an organized metabolic system than in pure chemical solutions. The Arrhenius plot may be open to some question because of the reciprocal of the absolute temperature type plot, which would seem to have little relationship to living microbial systems where, at 0 to 55°C (32 to 131°F), the system will actually reproduce itself and, instead of chemical destruction, there will be chemical reactions constructing new biologic units. When thermal destruction data for heat-resistant bacterial cells are plotted on a thermal resistance or Arrhenius graph against temperature or the reciprocal of absolute temperature to give a straight line, this data area is remote in regard to temperature from the area in which cell growth takes place. It is doubtful that these curves can be extrapolated into the temperature area in which growth occurs. In the range of temperatures in which microbial growth takes place, the basic time necessary for the organism to die from a heat effect is probably infinite; therefore, the thermal resistance or Arrhenius curve would be expected to become asymptotic to the temperature line of optimum growth.

These two methods of plotting data for temperature coefficient determination, thermal resistance or thermal death time method and the Arrhenius method should produce curves with different shapes. If a thermal resistance data plot is a straight line, an Arrhenius plot will be a curve. If the activation energy is constant over a wide temperature range, then the Arrhenius plot will be a straight line, and the corresponding thermal resistance plot will be a curve where the z value of a thermal destruction plot will change so T^2/z (absolute temperature) is a constant value.

Ball (1958), in discussing the work of Amaha and Sakaguchi (1957), transforms the Arrhenius equation into a form that is generally identical to the equation of the thermal destruction curve. The Arrhenius equation, however, is in terms of an absolute zero temperature base, whereas the thermal destruction curve is in terms of a convenient base, usually 250°F.

Experimental results do not conclusively support either the thermal resistance or Arrhenius plot methods. For example, Esselen and Pflug (1956) investigated the thermal destruction of *Clostridium sporogenes* (PA 3679) in vegetables in the temperature range 121.1 to 143.3°C (250 to 290°F) and found that all seven vegetables gave curves concave upward with a smaller z value in the 121.5 to 132.2°C (250 to 270°F) range, z = 8.8°C (15.9°F), than in the 132.2 to 143.3°C (270 to 290°F) range, z = 12.2°C (22.0°F). Licciardello and Nickerson (1963), on the other hand, found that the thermal resistance curve for *C. sporogenes* in phosphate buffer was concave downward; between 90 and 105°C (194 and 221°F) the z value was 12°C (21.6°F) and between 105 and 120°C (221 and 248°F) the z value was 9°C (16.2°F). Wang et al. (1964) correlate data for *Bacillus stearothermophilus* using both an Arrhenius and thermal resistance plot and conclude that a thermal resistance curve is a poor way to correlate data. In their report, however, points between 127.2 and 143.8°C (261 and 291°F) where the flow system was used appear to form a straight line on the thermal resistance curve; these points appear to have a different slope from the capillary tube data.

In these three studies, we have one set of data that is concave upward on a thermal resistance plot suggesting that an Arrhenius plot would give a straight line, a second set of data that is concave downward on a thermal resistance plot that would show more curvature on an Arrhenius plot, and a third set of data that is reported to fit the Arrhenius plot but that apparently will give a straight-line fit on a thermal resistance plot when the data are limited to the same apparatus system.

The debate regarding which method, the Arrhenius or Bigelow temperature coefficient model, is most correct from a scientific standpoint is inconclusive; however, from a practical standpoint for use in the design and evaluation of sterilization processes, the choice is the temperature coefficient model of Bigelow on the basis of simplicity. Sophisticated methods exist today for the design and evaluation of heat sterilization processes, all based on the Bigelow model. Details of these methods are found in Ball (1923, 1928), Ball and Olson (1957), Stumbo (1973), and Pflug (1990).

FACTORS AFFECTING THE WET-HEAT DESTRUCTION OF MICROORGANISMS

Wet-heat sterilization represents a single unique water content condition. Liquid water must be present, or sufficient water must be available to produce 100% relative humidity at the sterilization temperature. Heating under less than saturated water conditions must be considered dry heat.

It is difficult to appraise the factors affecting thermal resistance from any survey of the literature. The many variables introduced by the type of organism studied, the techniques used, and the unrecognized involvement of the many factors make a sound interpretation of previously reported data difficult. We believe that a detailed critical analytic review of past work that evaluates the conclusions reached by individual workers in the light of the techniques used, and at the same time attempts to sort out in usable form only that work that is not invalidated or rendered questionable by techniques or procedures later shown to be faulty, is a necessary foundation to the most productive future development of this field of study. Under present limitations, however, we must follow the accepted procedure of citing the results and conclusions as given in the literature in an attempt to portray to some degree the effect of the various factors that may influence the thermal resistance of microorganisms.

There may be three general types of factors affecting thermal resistance:

1. Inherent resistance.
2. Environmental influences active during the growth and formation of cells or spores.
3. Environmental influences active during the time of heating of the cells or spores.

Inherent resistance is illustrated by the finding that, in the same medium and under the same growth conditions, different strains of the same species or same general type of organism may produce cell or spore suspensions having widely different degrees of resistance. This is shown for obligate thermophilic flat sour types (Bigelow and Esty, 1920), *Clostridium botulinum* (Esty and Meyer, 1922; Esty, 1923; Dickson et al., 1925). A similar type of behavior has been shown for vegetative cells of bacteria (Beamer and Tanner, 1939a) and yeasts (Beamer and Tanner, 1939b).

Environmental influences active during the formation of cells or spores are illustrated by the effects of age, incubation temperature, and composition of the nutrient medium considered in relation to any one particular organism.

Environmental influences active during the heating of the suspension comprise all those variables such as pH, ionic strength, carbohydrate, protein, and fat content of the substrate, colloidal systems such as starch or soil, salt, and many other soluble organic or inorganic compounds that might be present.

When several cultures are compared on one arbitrarily selected medium, what may appear to be inherent differences in resistance may be the effects of environmental conditions. If the same cultures are studied in relation to some selected environmental variable, and the relative resistances of two organisms appearing in one suspending medium such as phosphate buffer are either accentuated or minimized by suspending in another substrate, all comparisons and evaluations become difficult and elusive, as do the previously attempted distinctions.

Age

Esty and Meyer (1922) found young moist spores to be more resistant than old moist spores. Magoon (1926b) reported complex interrelationships between length of storage, storage temperature, and humidity upon the resistance of spores of *Bacillus mycoides*. The total range of time of survival within which differences were regarded as significant was 3 to 7 minutes at 100°C. Sommer (1930) found the maximum resistance of spores of *Clostridium botulinum* to develop in 4 to 8 days. Curran (1934) found that aging up to 1 year slightly increased resistance. Williams (1936), however, could find no correlation between age and resistance of spores of several different species of spore-forming organisms.

There appears to be no possibility of reaching any general conclusion with regard to the effect of aging upon the resistance of bacterial spores based upon the data available in the literature. Furthermore, it may be questioned whether many of the data reported were adequate to measure the effect of age, even though age was defined as one of the variable factors.

Growth Phase

It has been generally observed that vegetative microbial cells show differing degrees of susceptibility to adverse influences at various stages of the growth cycle (Sherman and Albus, 1923; Sherman and Cameron, 1934). Robertson (1928) and Stark and Stark (1929) found young cells to be more susceptible to heat destruction than older and more mature cells. Anderson and Meanwell (1936) found increased resistance of thermoduric streptococci to heat destruction during the early logarithmic phase, whereas Ellicker and Frazier (1938), working with *Escherichia coli*, found greater heat resistance during the initial stationary phase, with decreasing resistance when reproduction began and a minimum resistance during the period of most rapid reproduction. Evidence is sufficient in these and other publications to demonstrate that destruction-rate studies of nonspore-forming organisms must take into consideration the factors of growth phase and age.

Growth Temperature

The effect of growth temperature has been studied extensively. Weil (1899) found the resistance of spores of *Bacillus anthracis* to increase with growth temperature. Sames (1900) studied the resistance of spores of thermophilic members of the *Bacillus* group and found that spores produced at higher temperatures are more resistant than spores produced at lower temperatures. Williams (1929), Curran (1934), and Sobernheim and Mündel (1936) have also found resistance of spores to increase with incubation temperature. Theophilus and Hammer (1938) found that the spores of cultures from evaporated

milk showed maximum resistance at the optimum growth temperature. Several subcultures at a given temperature were necessary before the maximum effect of temperature became apparent. Lamanna (1942) presented a general relationship between maximum growth temperature and spore resistance of various members of the *Bacillus* group; however, only organisms of comparatively low resistance, not over 45 minutes at 100°C, are included. Sugiyama (1951) reported that spores of *Clostridium botulinum* produced at higher temperatures have higher resistance than those produced at lower temperatures. Williams and Robertson (1954) found that increasing the temperatures of sporulation increased the resistance of spores of ten strains of aerobic-thermophilic bacilli. El-Bisi and Ordal (1956b) found the resistance of spores of a strain of *Bacillus coagulans (thermoacidurans)* to be greater with increased sporulation temperature. Schmidt and Nank (1958) found that spores of *B. subtilis* 5230 grown at 37°C had greater heat resistance than spores grown at 30°C; however, spores grown at 45°C were not more resistant than those grown at 37°C. Lechowich and Ordal (1962) reported that the heat resistance of spores of *B. subtilis* grown at 45°C was greater than at 30°C, and that the heat resistance of spores of *B. coagulans* grown at 30°, 45°, and 52°C increased with increasing spore crop growth temperature.

Nutrient Conditions

Williams (1929) has reviewed the earlier literature and conducted extensive studies of the effect of nutrient conditions and other factors on the resistance of spores of a strain of *Bacillus subtilis*. Many of the nutrient conditions tested either increased or decreased the resistance compared to one standard nutrient condition. Different brands of peptone may result in differing resistance, although resistance appeared to be independent of concentration with any one peptone. Various digest media resulted in spores of low resistance, except casein digest, which enhanced resistance. Spores of high resistance were found in all media prepared from vegetable extracts and also in isoelectric gelatin. The addition of either phosphate or magnesium to the standard peptone medium increased resistance. The addition of available carbohydrates, organic acids, or amino acids in some cases increased resistance. The increases in resistance obtained with varying nutrient conditions were reflected only in the specially produced spores; transfer to a standard medium restored the original resistance. Curran (1935) found that spores produced and aged on soil or oats were more resistant than those from artificial media, whereas Görtzen (1937) found no significant difference in the resistance of spores of anaerobic organisms taken directly from soil and those from cultures, except for one organism, *Clostridium sphenoides*. Sobernheim and Mündel (1938) found that the time required to sterilize soil containing spores was six to eight times longer than for a similar number of spores cultured from the spores in the soil. Gillespy (1947), working with thermophilic anaerobes, found an appreciable increase in resistance of the spores when soil was included in the medium. Sugiyama (1951), using *C. botulinum*, found the resistance of the spores to be influenced by the composition of the culture medium. Reduction of iron or calcium concentration decreased resistance. The inclusion of fatty acids, notably the long-chain unsaturated fatty acids, tended to increase resistance. Extraction of the medium with chloroform or petroleum ether reduced the resistance of the spores produced on the extracted medium. El-Bisi and Ordal (1956a) observed a decrease in resistance of spores of *Bacillus coagulans* with the presence of high phosphate concentration (1% KH_2PO_4) in the sporulation medium. Amaha and Ordal (1957) found that an increase in the phosphate concentration of the medium reduced thermal resistance of spores of *B. coagulans*, whereas the addition of calcium and manganese caused an increase and the addition of magnesium produced no effect. Nank and Schmidt (1958) reported that the addition of 1 ppm manganese to nutrient agar significantly increased the thermal resistance of spores of two strains of *Bacillus stearothermophilus* by 20 to 90% in either M/15 phosphate buffer or cream-style corn. Schmidt and Nank (1958) found that the addition of 1 ppm of manganese to nutrient agar did not increase the resistance of spores of *B. subtilis* 5230 in M/15 phosphate buffer, nor did the addition of 75 ppm of calcium to the nutrient agar containing manganese.

pH

In general, the greatest thermal resistance is in a fairly broad pH zone centering on the neutral point, pH 7. Although variations exist among individual organisms, resistance is at a maximum in the pH range 6.0 to 8.0. This zone is broader or narrower depending upon the species, the particular suspension, the suspending medium (buffer or food substrate), the techniques used, and the subculture conditions (Bigelow and Esty, 1920; Esty and Meyer, 1922; Williams, 1929; Lang, 1935; Nichols, 1940; Gillespy, 1948; Townsend et al., 1954; and many others). Sognefest et al. (1948) studied the resistance of spores of *Clostridium botulinum* and PA 3679 heated and incubated in pureed food products adjusted to various pH levels packed in thermal death-time cans and concluded that, in the pH range 4.5 to 9, the lower the pH the lower the heat required to prevent spoilage. Between pH 6 and 9, the change in resistance was comparatively minor, whereas in the region of pH 5.5 and below, thermal resistance fell off sharply. In this case, resistance is measured by both destruction and the ability of any surviving spores to germinate in the product at that particular pH. Somewhat different results may be found after heating spores in the acid pH range, followed by subculturing survivors into a neutral medium. The effects of pH on thermal resistance and spore germination in food products are complex, because pH changes not only may directly affect the organism, but also, by altering the degree of dissociation of many substances in solution in the product or by producing a shift in the oxidation-reduction potential, may indirectly affect either survival

or the ability of surviving organisms to develop. Generally, spore suspensions heated in food products at or below pH 6.0 and then subcultured in a more neutral medium have longer indicated survival times (Sognefest et al., 1948; Reed et al., 1951; Reynolds et al., 1952). Anellis et al. (1954) reported that the resistance of strains of *Salmonella* in liquid eggs was a continuous function of pH between 6.1 and 8.5, with maximum resistance at pH 6.1.

Aref and Cruess (1934) found yeasts to be slightly more resistant at pH 3.8 to 4.0 than at a more neutral pH, whereas Beamer and Tanner (1939b) found all but one of the yeasts tested to have greater resistance at pH 6.8 than at pH 3.8. Gillespy (1936–1937) reported the ascospores of *Byssochlamys fulva* to have a maximum resistance at pH 5.0, with resistance greater at 3.0 than at 7.0. Among other studies on the effect of pH upon the thermal resistance of nonspore-forming organisms are those of Levine and Fellers (1940) and Skillinglaw and Levine (1943). Further references to the extensive literature on this subject may be found in most of the papers cited.

Carbohydrates

High concentrations of soluble carbohydrates generally result in an increase in heat resistance of yeasts (Peterson et al., 1927; Wallace and Tanner, 1931; Corry, 1976a and b); nonspore-forming bacteria (Fay, 1934; Baumgartner and Wallace, 1934; Baumgartner, 1938; Corry, 1974, 1976b); and bacterial spores (Weiss, 1921; Rahn, 1928; Von Angerer and Küster, 1939; Braun et al., 1941; Anderson et al., 1949; Sugiyama, 1951). Amaha and Sakaguchi (1954), however, found no effect with the addition of 10 to 50% sucrose, glucose, or glycerol to phosphate buffer on the survival time at 240°F of spores of PA 3679. The increase in resistance has been attributed to partial dehydration of the protoplasm. Fay (1934), Von Angerer and Küster (1939), and Sugiyama (1951) have observed decreases in turbidity or increases in light transmission for cells or spores suspended in carbohydrate solutions. Rahn (1945a) and Sugiyama (1951) do not believe the theory of dehydration is sufficient to fit all the facts, because protection is not proportional to molarity. Gould and Dring (1975) and Gould (1977) postulate that suspending bacterial spores in high-concentration solutes (e.g., sucrose) dehydrates the central core osmotically, thus increasing heat resistance. The magnitude of the effect is great, in some cases resulting in increases of resistance of 200 to 300%.

The marked and general effect of soluble carbohydrates in increasing the thermal resistance of almost all organisms tested offers a point of approach to the study of the mechanisms of thermal destruction that should be exploited more fully by further investigation.

Salt

Weiss (1921) found that 3% salt decreased the resistance of *Clostridium botulinum* spores. Esty and Meyer (1922), however, found an increase in resistance with 1 to 2% salt and a decrease in resistance above 8%. Viljoen (1926), working with spores of thermophilic flat sour organisms, found resistance in a pea liquor, prepared by processing peas with distilled water, to be increased by the addition of salt. Increasing the amount of salt up to 3% increased the heat resistance. The addition of 0.25% salt to water decreased the resistance of the same organisms. It is apparent that the protective effect of salt in this case is related to some constituent of the pea liquor. In view of the striking results reported by Viljoen, it is surprising that further work along these lines has not been conducted.

Headlee (1931) found that 2.5% salt increased the resistance of spores of *Clostridium welchii*, whereas 10% led to a definite decrease. Yesair and Cameron (1942) found that 3.5% salt in phosphate buffer decreased the resistance of spores of *C. botulinum* at temperatures below 230°F, but there was no appreciable effect at 230 to 235°F. Anderson et al. (1949) added 1%, 2%, 4%, and 8% salt to tomato juice and found that increasing salt concentrations decreased the destruction time of spores of *Bacillus coagulans*. Sugiyama (1951) obtained an increase in resistance on the addition of 0.15 M (0.8%) salt to phosphate buffer. Apparently, the effect of sodium chloride, and perhaps of other salts, varies depending upon the suspending medium and the particular test organism used.

Jaynes, Pflug, and Harmon (1961a) and Jaynes et al. (1961) studied the effect of pH and brine concentration on gas production and thermal resistance of PA 3679 in a processed cheese spread and found that when the pH was reduced from 7.0 to 6.0, the lag time for gas production increased; gas production was completely inhibited at pH 5.6 and below. As the brine concentration increased, the lag time for gas production increased, and there was a decrease in the rate, total amount, and duration of gas production. Gas production was completely inhibited at a brine concentration of 7.6% or more; in general, relatively small levels of heat prevented gas production, whereas a large amount of heat was required to kill the spores.

Roberts et al. (1966) found that the heat-destruction rates of spores of PA 3679 were the same in water and in 3 and 6% NaCl solutions. However, spores heated in water or 3% NaCl to give 0.1% survival were more sensitive to inhibition by NaCl in the recovery medium; the percent recovery of survivors decreased as the salt concentration in the recovery medium increased from 0 to 6%. Roberts and Ingram (1966) reported that both *Bacillus* and *Clostridium* spores surviving heat treatments were inhibited to various degrees by concentrations of NaCl, KNO_3, and $NaNO_2$ in the recovery medium. In general, for a given level of heat treatment, the degree of inhibition increased with increasing concentration of the chemical in the recovery medium. More severe heat treatments made the spores more sensitive to inhibition, and in general, a lower level of heat was required to produce an effect with two *Bacillus* than with three *Clos-*

tridia species. The inhibitory effect of $NaNO_2$ was increased approximately tenfold when the pH was reduced from 7.0 to 6.0.

The use of sodium nitrite, in conjunction with sodium chloride, water activity, pH, Eh, product composition, microbial contamination, and packaging and storage conditions, plays a major role in retarding *Clostridium botulinum* growth and toxin production in cured meat products (Silliker, 1959; Riemann, 1963; Pivnick et al., 1970; Wolf and Wasserman, 1972; Baird-Parker and Baillie, 1974). During the 1970s, the addition of nitrite to cured meat products caused controversy because of reports that nitrite served as a precursor to carcinogenic nitrosamines (Magee and Barnes, 1967; Sebranek and Cassens, 1973). Cured meat products contain both nitrite (up to 200 μg/g meat) (Binkerd and Kolari, 1975) and amines, thus producing a potential for nitrosamine formation, given the right conditions. Fazio et al. (1973) and Havery et al. (1976), among others, have found nitrosamines present in cooked bacon; Kushnir et al. (1975) reported finding nitrosoproline in uncooked bacon.

Recent research has focused on finding a way to eliminate or reduce the nitrite concentration in cured meat products and at the same time to maintain botulinal safety. Ivey et al. (1978) evaluated low nitrite (0 and 40 μg/g) and potassium sorbate (0.13 and 0.26%) concentrations in bacon inoculated with 1100 spores per gram. The results indicated that potassium sorbate reduced the number of toxic swollen packages. Several investigators (Tompkin et al., 1974; Wada et al., 1975; Tanaka et al., 1977) have reported that the protective effect of sorbate is effective only at a pH below 6.0 to 6.5. Other researchers (Robach et al., 1978; Ivey and Robach, 1978; Sofos et al., 1979a) reported that low-nitrite (20 to 156 μg/g) sorbate (0.1 and 0.2%) combinations greatly extend the botulinal safety of cured meats over that of nitrite or sorbate alone. A comprehensive review of this problem is presented by Sofos et al. (1979b).

Antibiotics

The study of the effects of antibiotics was stimulated by the report of Andersen and Michener (1950) of the successful use of subtilin and mild heat to preserve a variety of foods. Subsequent investigations by a number of workers failed to confirm these results. The main conclusion reached was that the effect was not lethal but rather sporostatic; the antibiotic apparently acted to inhibit the outgrowth of the germinated spores. In many cases, the effect appeared to be of a transient nature. The effect of antibiotics and related substances on the heat destruction of microorganisms has been reviewed by Hirsch (1953), Lewis et al. (1954), Campbell and O'Brien (1955), and Schmidt (1957).

In recent years, nisin and tylosin have been studied extensively as potential additives to permit a reduction in the heat processes of a variety of foods. The early investigative work on nisin was summarized by Hawley (1957); since then, several workers have reported evidence that nisin added to various food products may permit a reduction in the thermal processes; the thermal process would still remain above a minimum botulinum process in the case of nonacid foods (Campbell and Sniff, 1959; Denny et al., 1961a and b; Wheaton and Hays, 1964; Heinemann et al., 1964; Gibbs and Hurst, 1964; Segmiller et al., 1965).

Tylosin, an antibiotic of more recent origin, has been studied for its effect on spore-forming organisms in thermal processed foods by Denny et al. (1961a and b), Greenberg and Silliker (1962, 1964), Malin and Greenberg (1964), Poole and Malin (1964), Wheaton and Hays (1964), and Segmiller et al. (1965).

Although most of the reports indicate favorable effects with both nisin and tylosin in reducing the thermal process requirement necessary to prevent spoilage, either with the normal flora or in the presence of added spores of representative spoilage organisms, the results may be influenced by the nature and pH of the product, the level of spore contamination present, the level of survivors following the heat process, the nature of the contaminating organism, and the stability of the antibiotics both to the thermal process and during storage (Gibbs and Hurst, 1964; Segmiller et al., 1965).

Denny et al. (1961a and b) demonstrated that tylosin had no effect on spore destruction rates, suggesting that the favorable effect found when tylosin was added to a food product was due to inhibition. Greenberg and Silliker (1962) showed that tylosin did not prevent the germination of spores of PA 3679, but rather it prevented the outgrowth and vegetative multiplication of the germinated spores. Unpublished work by Schmidt demonstrated that the rate of germination of spores of *Bacillus subtilis* 5230 in a glucose L-alanine germination system was the same with or without tylosin. Gould (1964) also demonstrated that the effect of nisin on a variety of *Bacillus* spores was to prevent outgrowth rather than to prevent germination.

It is possible that both nisin and tylosin may have a significant role in the future in reducing the thermal process requirements of a number of food products; however, much additional study will be required to determine the optimal dose level and level of heat processing for normal or higher-than-normal contamination levels of naturally occurring flora. The reality of the effectiveness of these antibiotics perhaps can only be tested by a large-scale pack of at least 100,000 cans containing the antibiotic and processed at such a level that the controls would show significant spoilage.

The use of nisin as an additive to canned foods is permitted in many countries of the world including Australia, Bahrain, Italy, Singapore, Spain, the United Arab Emirates, and the United Kingdom (H.M.S.O., 1959; Hurst, 1983). The Joint Food and Agriculture Organization/World Health Organization Expert Committee on Food Additives accepted nisin as a food additive with an unconditional average daily intake of 0 to 33,000 units/kg body weight (40 units = 1 μg of pure nisin) (Hurst, 1983). Nisin at a maximum of 250 ppm (Federal Register, 1988), was recently approved by the Food and Drug Administration of the United States for use in pasteurized process cheese spreads and pasteurized process cheese to inhibit the growth of *Clostridium botulinum*. Nisin has been found to have no effect on animals in studies of subchronic or chronic toxicity, reproduction, or sensitization, and no indication exists that it produces cross-resistance in microorganisms to therapeutic antibiotics (Federal Register, 1988). Although neither nisin nor tylosin are currently permitted in the United States for use as adjuncts to thermal processing, the approval of nisin in pasteurized process cheeses may allow for expanded use of the compound in the future.

There may be many substances of comparatively simple chemical structure that may either increase or decrease the thermal destruction rates of microorganisms. Almost any inorganic or organic chemical compound might be included in this class, and its presence in a food substrate may be primarily responsible for the particular thermal destruction rate if the rate is determined using a product incubation technique, because a chemical may either directly affect the lethal action of the heat treatment or indirectly affect the outgrowth potential of surviving organisms. Continued investigation of the effects of chemicals of known nature added to the simple and complex substrates upon the thermal destruction rates of microorganisms may contribute considerably to both the theoretic and practical aspects of heat sterilization.

Pressure

ZoBell and Johnson (1949) studied the effect of pressures of 300 to 600 atmospheres on the growth and viability of microorganisms at 20°, 30°, and 40°C. They found that at 20 to 30°C, although all cultures developed well at normal pressure, most of the species failed to develop at 400 or 500 atmospheres and none at 600 atmospheres. Surprisingly, some of the species that did not develop at 20 or 30°C at 600 atmospheres did grow at 600 atmospheres when the temperature was increased to 40°C. The reciprocal effect of pressure and temperature is explained by analyzing the effect of these factors on the large molecules of the biologic systems. The volume changes in the large protein type of molecules upon activation are great; "at higher temperatures the critical enzyme undergoes a reversible denaturation that proceeds with an even larger volume increase of reaction." High pressures that oppose volume increases tend to retard denaturation. ZoBell and Johnson (1949) concluded, "The influence of pressure on pure cultures in all cases depended upon the temperature."

Chemical State of Spores

Alderton and co-workers (1963, 1964, 1969a and b, 1970) have demonstrated, using *Bacillus megaterium* and *B. stearothermophilus* spores, that heat-destruction characteristics of bacterial spores can be altered significantly by chemical treatment. They have observed that if spores are placed in, for example, a tryptone-glucose-starch medium adjusted to pH 1.1 using 3N HCl at 20°C overnight, they lose heat resistance and are in the "sensitive" state. If the same spores are now placed in a 0.02 M calcium acetate solution adjusted to pH 9.7 with aqueous $Ca(OH)_2$ at 20°C overnight, the spores bind cations and are in the "heat-resistant" state. The reaction is reversible; heat resistance is decreased by stripping to the hydrogen form and increased by loading with metal cations. The rates of cation uptake suggest two binding sites: the initial rapid uptake rate exerts only a small effect on heat resistance, with the later slow uptake producing a large increase in heat resistance. These investigators observed that when unequalized spores with low initial heat resistance were heated in calcium buffers, survivor curves that were concave upward resulted, compared to straight-line survivor curves for the fully equalized cells and concave-downward curves when equalized spores were placed in a low-pH buffer. These results indicate that the heat resistance of spores can change during the heating period if there are chemical changes in spores. Alderton and Snell (1963) determined the changes in the survivor curves of Bacillus megaterium that occur as a function of several different chemical treatments. The D values of "resistant" spores may be as much as ten times as large as the D values for "sensitive" spores.

The empiric methods used for growing and storing spores probably unknowingly produce spores that are in the "resistant" state chemically. The effect of this parameter should be evaluated especially if spores of maximum heat resistance are desirable. The chemical state of the solutions in which the spores are stored and heated is important in that: (1) differences in the chemical state of substrates in which spores are suspended during heating may be responsible for the differences in resistance in the different solutions; and (2) when the chemical state of the suspension in which the spores are heated is different from the chemical state of the solution in which spores are stored, it may be impossible to determine accurately the effect of the heat treatment because of a simultaneous change in the chemical state of the spores.

The work of Alderton and co-workers has demonstrated the effect of the chemical state on the heat resistance of bacterial spores. Consideration of the chemical state should now be a requisite part of any study of heat resistance. The chemical state during spore crop growth, storage, or testing can affect heat resistance; uncontrolled, it will contribute at a minimum to the overall experimental variation and may produce grossly erroneous results.

Effect of Variation in Physical Environmental Conditions

Under certain conditions when spores (dried on paper carriers and placed in nonhermetic envelopes) were heated in saturated steam, spore destruction rates were greater than when the spores were in a liquid substrate at the time of heating. The nature and sequence of operations appear to be critical, as is, perhaps, the species of microorganism.

Anderson (1959) tested the heat resistance of spores of Bacillus subtilis strain 5230 using a thermoresistometer: (1) when the suspension was dried in cups; (2) when there was visible moisture in the cups; and (3) when a paper disk was used in the cup with the spore suspension deposited directly on the paper disk (free moisture was present). He reported that his data "show no significant difference (at the 95% confidence level) between dry and moist spore suspensions."

Chapman and Pflug (1973) describe an "enclosure effect" on heat resistance. They found that when Bacillus stearothermophilus spores were dried on filter paper disks and placed in nonhermetic paper or foil envelopes, which in turn were heated in saturated steam, survival times were shorter than when no envelope was used. In subsequent studies (Pflug and Smith, 1977; Smith et al., 1982), these observations were verified in that spores suspended directly in trypticase soy broth (TSB) survived longer heat treatments than spores dried on filter paper disks, with the disks placed in TSB after heating. The shortest survival times were for spores dried on filter paper disks, placed in nonhermetic glassine paper envelopes and heated in saturated steam. In observations by Chapman and Pflug (1973), the two factors that appeared to play a role in reducing times of B. stearothermophilus spores heated in saturated steam were: (1) drying spores on filter paper; and (2) enclosing spores dried on filter paper in a nonhermetic envelope. The results of Anderson (1959) do not appear to contradict those of Chapman and Pflug (1973), because Anderson did not dry his spores on filter paper, nor did he enclose the spore disks in envelopes.

In 1991 there is general recognition that if the $D_{121.1C}$ of B. stearothermophilus spores heated in water or buffer is 5 min., aliquots of the same spore suspension deposited on paper strips that are in glassine paper envelopes when heated will have a $D_{121.1C}$ value in the vicinity of 2 minutes.

FACTORS AFFECTING THE DRY-HEAT DESTRUCTION OF MICROORGANISMS

Dry heat has been used throughout the world for sterilizing glassware and hospital supplies that could not be sterilized in saturated steam. It is amazing that with this wide usage, so little is known about its overall effectiveness. Bruch (1966) notes that the United States Pharmacopeia specifies that containers for pharmaceutical products be held at 170°C for 2 hours for dry-heat sterilization; in contrast, the British Pharmacopeia states that 150°C for 1 hour is satisfactory for the vessels and containers to be used in parenteral injections. Lastly, the State Pharmacopeia of the Union of Soviet Socialist Republics indicates that heating in a drying cabinet for 1 hour at 160 to 170°C is adequate for containers to be used to hold various pharmaceutical preparations. These variations in dry-heat recommendations undoubtedly reflect the fact that dry heat is not so easily defined as wet heat. Wet-heat sterilization is a relatively easily defined condition in that the relative humidity (RH) is 1.00 or 100%, depending on whether it is expressed as a ratio or a percentage.

If the relative humidity is 100%, then some water is present in the liquid state. Dry heat is the sterilization condition in which water is not present in the liquid state. Therefore, in dry-heat sterilization, the relative humidity of the system will be less than 100%; it can be any value between 0 and 100%. Because the destruction rate of dry microbial cells is a function of their water content, which in turn is determined by the relative humidity of the atmosphere surrounding the cells, the destruction rate will vary with the relative humidity of the system. Therefore, in dry-heat sterilization, the relative humidity conditions must be specified in addition to temperature to establish the relative sterilization effect.

Relative humidity is used because the response of biologic materials more nearly parallels vapor pressure than water content, and vapor pressure of the gas atmosphere surrounding dry microbial cells is more easily measured and controlled than the water content inside the microbial cell. The term relative humidity in gaseous systems corresponds to water activity in liquid systems. The water vapor pressure in the gas surrounding the spore can be measured by psychrometric methods. It can be reported in several ways, but relative humidity is the most widely used.

At equilibrium, the relative humidity of the atmosphere surrounding the microbial cell is theoretically equal to the water availability inside the cell, which is called water activity (A_w*).

The concept of water activity of solutions adopted by Scott (1957) has been extended in some cases to microbial cells and spores. Because it is possible to confuse terms, the following are suggested to clarify the description of water in dry microbial systems. *Relative humidity* is a real, physical unit that is the ratio of two measured quantities: the actual water vapor pressure in a system and the saturated water vapor pressure at the same temperature. It is used with gaseous systems, for example, to describe the water condition in the atmosphere surrounding bacterial cells or spores. *Water activity*, A_w, is a term used to describe the relative water availability inside a microbial cell or spore. It is a theoretic term that cannot be directly measured. If the water in a cell or spore is in equilibrium with the surrounding atmosphere, the water activity of the spore is theoretically equal to the external relative humidity.

In discussing and reporting on dry-heat test data, it is suggested that if, in a microbial destruction rate test, the relative humidity is measured and controlled, the results should be reported as a function of relative humidity, not water activity. Whenever a relative humidity value is reported, the temperature at which it was measured should be included, for example, 0.2% RH (110°C).

*A_w = a_w value throughout this chapter.

Dry-Heat Destruction of the Natural Microorganisms Associated With Soil or Soil Particles

When an object is in contact with people and ambient air, it will accumulate a microflora that in general can be divided into two groups: (1) naked or unprotected microbial cells from human or other animal origin, individual or clumps of naked cells that are a residue from food or other organic media that remain on the object to be sterilized; and (2) spores associated with particles of dirt or dust that fall upon the object to be sterilized, either from the air or from the activity of persons or apparatus working near the object to be sterilized. These spores will have originated in the soil and will have been transported to the object by air or human carrier. In general, naked microbial cells are easily killed by a dry-heat sterilization treatment; however, some of the microflora associated with the soil particles are difficult to kill.

It often seems that we know the least about those things close by. Only in recent years have we been learning about the microflora associated with soil particles. The decision by the National Aeronautics and Space Administration (NASA) to use dry heat for the terminal sterilization cycle of the Viking Lander stimulated a large research effort regarding the dry-heat resistance of microbial spores. The results of the findings to date regarding the dry-heat destruction characteristics of the microflora associated with soil particles suggest that:

1. The normal microflora of soil is widely variable; the semilogarithmic survivor curve for microorganisms in soil is nonlinear. A typical survivor curve for microorganisms in soil is shown in Figure 6–6.
2. There are some soil organisms that are highly resistant to dry heat. One such organism, *Bacillus xerothermodurans*, was isolated by Bond et al. (1973) and found to have a $D_{125°C}$ value of 139 hours.
3. Moderately resistant organisms such as *Bacillus subtilis* can be very resistant to dry heat when encapsulated in particles.
4. The best estimate today is that, in soil, 1 spore in 10^3 and 10^5 is very resistant to dry heat.
5. The fallout dirt or dust in a facility is part of the area dirt that has become airborne and is carried into the plant by air or on clothing or equipment that moves into the facility.
6. The role of the ambient relative humidity on the rate of destruction of spores in soil heated in open systems has been studied, but the results are not conclusive. It is possible that the bound water in the soil particles overshadows the effect of the ambient humidity level on the spore destruction rate.

The normal microflora of soil varies widely and includes both vegetative cells and spores. The survivor curve in Figure 6–6 at 125°C is for 0.1-g samples of Minnesota soil. As is evident in Figure 6–6, this Minnesota soil contains a large fraction of spores very resistant to dry heat, and not only are there large numbers of

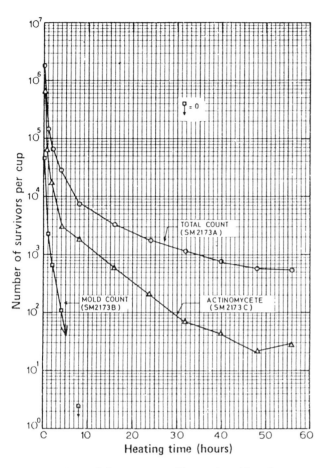

Fig. 6–6. Survival characteristics of bacterial, mold, and actinomycete spores associated with dry Minnesota soil, heated at 125°C, 0.1 g soil per TDT cup. From Smith, G., and Pflug, I.J. 1972. Dry heat destruction rates of microorganisms on surfaces. In *Progress Report No. 8. Environmental Microbiology as Related to Planetary Quarantine.* NASA NGL 24–005–160, University of Minnesota.

bacterial spores resistant to dry heat, but also there are large numbers of actinomycetes relatively resistant to dry heat.

Koesterer (1965a and b) reports on studies of the survival of organisms in 0.1 g of a sample of dry soil. Survivor curves for temperatures in the range of 120 to 160°C are shown in Figure 6–7. There is surprising similarity between the 125°C dry-heat survivor curves for Koesterer FG soil from upstate New York and the Minnesota soil, even though the Minnesota soil has a larger resistant population.

At the present time, no survivor curve model exists for microorganisms in soil. Therefore, the D value cannot be used because it is a parameter of the straight-line semilogarithmic survivor curve. The semilogarithmic survivor curve for microorganisms in soil has been described as being biphasic; in general, soil contains a large low-resistance population and a small high-resistance population of microorganisms. However, neither the low- nor the high-resistance population is homogeneous.

Soil contains some organisms resistant to dry heat. If

the surviving organisms of dry-heat tests are cultured in the laboratory, spore crops with high dry-heat resistance can be produced. Koesterer (1965a), Bond et al. (1971), and Campbell (1974) have all cultured resistant organisms from soil. The resistance of these "hardy organisms" is variable; $D_{125°C}$ values range from 5 to 139 hours.

When some of the surviving organisms of dry-heat tests are cultured in the laboratory, the resulting spore crops have resistance levels of the order of *Bacillus subtilis* var. *niger.* Doyle and Ernst (1967) and Mullican and Hoffman (1968) have shown that when spores are encapsulated in crystals, the dry-heat resistance can be increased more than tenfold. In many soil particles, crystals with large waters of hydration may cause organisms normally of low dry-heat resistance to become superresistant spores.

In soil, the possible variation in numbers and species of microflora and the physical conditions of their location are almost unlimited; the spores can be of a range of species all produced under widely varying unknown conditions, and the soil particles can vary in size and composition. The spores can be located at any point on or within the soil particles. It seems probable that, through soil wetting and drying cycles, spores can be completely encapsulated in soil particles, which in itself could increase dry-heat resistance by a factor of 10.

Studies carried out by Puleo and co-workers (1975) suggest that the relative number of resistant spores is small. They estimated that 1 spore in between 10^3 and 10^5 will survive a dry-heat treatment of about 30 hours at 110°C.

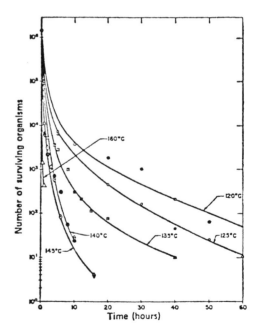

Fig. 6–7. Survivor curves for the indigenous mesophilic population in 0.1-g samples of dry FG soil to dry heat in the temperature range 120 to 160°C. From Koesterer, M.G. 1965. *Studies for Sterilization of Space Probe Components.* NASA Contract No. NASW–879. Rochester, NY, Wilmot Castle Co.

When objects are manufactured under ambient air conditions, with adequate opportunity for soil particles to be deposited on the units to be sterilized, then the sterilization cycle will have to be based on the resistance of the spores in or on the soil particles. If manufacturing is carried out under closely controlled conditions such as in a Class-100 clean room, it is possible that the number of soil particles per object will be reduced to the point at which they are not the critical design criterion. The naked microorganisms from the people working with the objects or grown in the product will become the critical microbial load, and the sterilization cycle will be based on the resistance of these naked organisms, rather than the organisms associated with soil particles. Weather can have a major effect on dry-heat sterilization requirements. Humid conditions reduce, and dry conditions increase, soil particle movement. High wind velocities and dry soil and air conditions will increase the number and size of soil particles that move into production areas, which will obviously increase the number of soil particles and accompanying microbial load on objects to be sterilized.

Dry-Heat Destruction of Laboratory-Grown Spores

From 1963 to 1973, NASA supported a great deal of research in the dry-heat area. A large part of this work involved model systems. Spores of *Bacillus subtilis* var. *niger* were used extensively. The results of these studies led to certain general conclusions regarding the dry-heat destruction of homogeneous cultures of spores: (1) the semilogarithmic survivor curves in general are straight lines if we exclude the N_0 point from the analysis; (2) the destruction rate of the spores starting at time zero is greater than the steady-state destruction rate and increases with a decrease in spore water content.

The mode of action of dry heat has three primary and three secondary variables. The primary variables are temperature, water content, and time; the secondary variables are open and closed systems, physical and chemical properties of the microorganism and adjacent

support, and the gas atmosphere. The secondary variables all play an important role in determining the microbial water content during heating and will be discussed as part of that section.

Effect of Temperature

Temperature, which is the measure of the heat energy level, is the most important variable in the dry-heat destruction of microorganisms; its action is a function of time. Thermal destruction curves for *Bacillus subtilis* var. *niger* spores in five different systems (data of Angelotti et al., 1968a) are shown in Figure 6–8. Dry-heat resistance values for several species of microorganisms are shown in Table 6–1.

The z value of the Bigelow (1921) model is one measure of the change in destruction rate with temperature. Reported z values for dry-heat destruction of microbial spores range from about 15 to 30°C (27 to 54°F) with Q_{10} values of 4.6 to 2.2. In the temperature range of 105 to 135°C, the average z value is about 21°C; Q_{10} is 3.0. A z value of 21°C was adopted by NASA (1969). The z values for microbial spores subjected to wet heat are in the range of 5 to 12°C, with Q_{10} values of 100 to 6.8. This major difference in z or Q_{10} value is the basis for the assumption that the mechanism of dry-heat destruction is different from the mechanism of wet-heat destruction.

Effect of Microbial Water Content

The role of water in the heat inactivation of intracellular molecules has long been a subject for speculation among microbiologists. Recently, evidence has been provided that water has a direct influence on microbial resistance to destruction by dry heat.

The effect of water on the dry-heat destruction rate of spores was first reported by Murrell and Scott (1957). This initial report has been supported by additional studies by Murrell and Scott (1966) and Angelotti et al. (1968a). In addition to these studies dealing directly with water and dry-heat destruction, a large number of studies in recent years have reported dry-heat destruction rates

Table 6–1. *Dry-Heat Resistance Values*

Organism	$D^*_{120°C(248°F)/min}$	z °C	z °F	Testing Conditions	Source
Bacillus subtilis (5230)	195–295	18.3	33	Hermetic cup-TDT-can system using He, N₂, O₂, CO₂, and air	Pheil et al. (1967)
Clostridium sporogenes (PA 3679)	115–195	21.7–22.8	39–41	Hermetic cup-TDT-can system using He, CO₂, and air	
B. subtilis (niger)	38–55	27.2	49	Filter paper strips in 150 × 16 mm screw-cap tubes in aluminum block	Bruch et al. (1963)
B. stearothermophilus (FS 1518)	19	24.4	44		
B. subtilis (niger)	36–240	23.3	42	Added to or trapped in solids	Bruch et al. (1963)
B. subtilis (5230)	154	23.3	42	Superheated steam in thermo-resistometer (300 to 350°F)	Pflug (1960)

*D is the symbol used to describe the slope of the straight-line semilogarithmic survivor curve. D is the equivalent time required to reduce the microbial population by 90% or, on semilogarithmic paper, the time required for the curve to traverse one log cycle. The temperature at which the D value was measured is shown as a subscript.

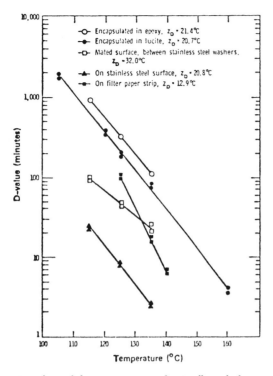

Fig. 6–8. Thermal destruction curves for *Bacillus subtilis* var. *niger* spores. From Angelotti, R., et al. 1968. Influence of spore moisture content on the dry heat resistance of *Bacillus subtilis* var. *niger*. Appl. Microbiol., *16*, 735–745.

Table 6–2. *Moisture Content of Six Bacterial Species of Spores Equilibrated to Various Relative Humidities*

Relative Humidity	Range of Water Content (% dry weight)
0.1	4.8–8.2
0.2	5.5–10.2
0.4	7.3–12.4
0.6	9.5–16.0
0.8	12.1–25.5
0.9	38.5–57.0

From Marshall, B.J., Murrell, W.G., and Scott, W.J. 1963. The effect of water activity, solutes, and temperature on the viability and heat resistance of freeze-dried bacterial spores. J. Gen. Microbiol., *31*, 451–460.

is between 5.5 and 12.4% of the dry weight of the spores, depending on the species (see Table 6–2).

Figure 6–9 shows a curve of D value vs. spore water content; the data are from Angelotti et al. (1968a). The zero value is for an open system; it is added here along with the dotted line to indicate the probable D value when spore water content approaches zero.

Brannen and Garst (1972) determined D values at 105°C for relative humidities from 3×10^{-4} to 2×10^{-3}. They found that when log D was plotted against log relative humidity (RH) between an RH of 1×10^{-3} and 1×10^{-2}, the data points formed a straight line. Jacobson and Pflug (1972) studied the dry-heat destruction rates

for specific conditions (Pflug, 1960; Jacobs et al., 1965; Pheil et al., 1967; Paik et al., 1967; Green et al., 1967; Fox and Pflug, 1968; Silverman, 1968; Hoffman et al., 1968; Bruch and Smith, 1968; Bond et al., 1970).

At this time, it appears that the dry-heat destruction rate of microbial spores is a function of the quantity of water in the cell at the time of heating, which will be constant only under certain conditions. In most conditions, the moisture content of the cell can change so that initial cell water content, the physical and chemical properties of the cell and adjacent support, and the water vapor pressure of the surrounding gas atmosphere may act as variables and cause confusion in the analysis of research results.

The movement of water to or from microorganisms on surfaces will be determined by the water vapor pressure in the atmosphere surrounding the cell (Pflug, 1970). By increasing the humidity in air passing over microbial spores from near zero to 0.20, Silverman (1968) was able to consistently increase the D value by a factor of 100, and his data suggest that the maximum was not reached.

In the temperature range of 100 to 135°C, spores of an intermediate moisture content (equilibrated at relative humidities between 0.1 and 0.6) are more resistant to the effects of heat (larger D values) than spores of either greater or lesser moisture content. According to Marshall et al. (1963), who measured the moisture content of spores of six bacterial species equilibrated to various water levels at 25°C, the critical moisture content

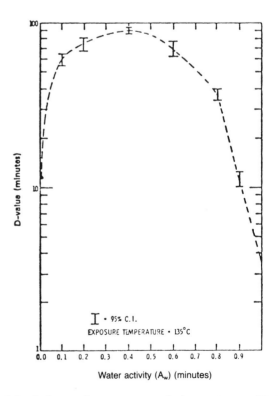

Fig. 6–9. Influence of water activity on dry heat resistance of *Bacillus subtilis* var. *niger* spores encapsulated in Lucite. From Angelotti, R., et al. 1968. Influence of spore moisture content on the dry heat resistance of *Bacillus subtilis* var. *niger*. Appl. Microbiol., *16*, 735–745.

of spores of *Bacillus subtilis* var. *niger* at 90°, 110°, and 125°C at atmospheric water contents from about 5 to 13,000 ppm, *volume per volume* (at 110°C, this is a RH range from 7×10^{-6} to 7×10^{-3}). They found that, in the range studied, the D values decreased continuously as the RH calculated at test temperature decreased. When log D was plotted as a function of log RH at each test temperature, the data points formed straight lines. The lines for data at 90°, 110°, and 125°C were parallel. A decrease in the RH from 1×10^{-2} to 1×10^{-6} resulted in a 90% reduction in the D value. The z value was about 20°C and appeared to be constant over the temperature and RH ranges studied.

It is generally agreed that at heating temperatures from 90 to 125°C, the maximum D value occurs at an RH between 0.2 and 0.5, and the z value is about 21°C in this area and is in the range of 8 to 10°C when RH is 1.00 (wet heat). On the basis of the data reported, it appears that in the temperature range from 90 to 125°C, the z value does not change as the RH decreases below about 0.35.

Control of Spore Water Content During Heating

The terms "open system" and "closed system" were suggested by Pflug (1968) to indicate the relative control of the heating environment on spore water loss or gain. In general, in an open system, the spore water content is determined by the environmental atmosphere surrounding the spore, whereas in a closed system, the spore water content is a function of conditions inside an enclosure and is not influenced by the heating environment.

Closed System. In the closed system (shown diagrammatically in Fig. 6–10), water movement and water availability to the cells are restricted. The quantity of water that is available, or that can be transferred to or from the cell, is limited by the quantity of water initially present in the enclosure.

There are two important parameters regarding cells in a closed system: initial water content and enclosure volume. The water concentration in the cell during heating will be determined by the relative humidity of the atmosphere in the enclosure at the time of sealing the enclosure and by the total volume of the enclosure. Changing either the quantity of water initially in the

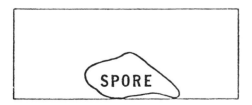

Fig. 6–10. Diagrammatic concept of a microorganism in a closed system. From Pflug, I.J. 1968 Some observations regarding factors important to dry heat sterilization. In *Sterilization Techniques for Instruments and Materials as Applied to Space Research.* Edited by P.N.A. Sneath. Paris, Muray-Print, pp. 57–58. (COSPAR Techn. Man. No. 4.)

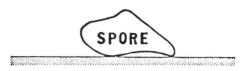

Fig. 6–11. Diagrammatic concept of a microorganism in an open system. From Pflug, I.J. 1968. Some observations regarding factors important to dry heat sterilization. In *Sterilization Techniques for Materials and Instruments as Applied to Space Research.* Edited by P.N.A. Sneath. Paris. Muray-Print, pp. 57–58. (COSPAR Techn. Man. No. 4.)

enclosed volume or the enclosed volume itself alters the relative humidity and, in turn, the water content in the spore during the heating cycle.

Open System. In the open system (shown diagrammatically in Fig. 6–11), microbial cells are heated, during which time water can be lost or gained by the cells almost without limit. In an infinite time, the cells will be in equilibrium with the water condition of the environment. This definition places no restrictions on the rate of water transfer; the cells may lose or gain water either rapidly or slowly, depending on the nature of the spore and the physical system.

Encapsulation of Spores in Crystals and Solids

Doyle and Ernst (1967) and Mullican and Hoffman (1968) both produced crystals in which spores of *Bacillus subtilis* var. *niger* were encapsulated. Doyle and Ernst reported a ninefold increase in the dry-heat resistance of spores encapsulated in calcium carbonate crystals compared to the nonencapsulated controls. Mullican and Hoffman found that spores were 5 to 24 times more resistant in glycine crystals and 6 times more resistant in sodium chloride crystals than the nonencapsulated spore controls. Encapsulating the spores increased the wet-heat resistance 900 times. It was not possible to sterilize the crystals containing spores with ethylene oxide. The spores inside crystals were in a "closed system" compared to the spore controls, which were in an "open system." The vapor tightness of the crystals is verified by the fact that ethylene oxide did not sterilize even after 48 hours.

The "wet-heat" results suggest that wet-heat conditions existed on the outside of the crystal, but that inside the crystal (closed system), dry-heat conditions existed. The results of the encapsulation-in-crystal studies are similar to the results of Angelotti et al. (1968a and b) where the survival times were longer when spores were encapsulated in Lucite. The high dry-heat resistance of encapsulated spores is probably due to the presence of the optimum amount of water in the spores to give near-maximum dry-heat resistance.

Bruch et al. (1963) reported D values for spores of *Bacillus subtilis* deposited on paper strips, sand, and glass tubes. The D values were lowest when spores were deposited on the paper strips and highest when spores were deposited on sand. They also studied the effect of the material in which the spores were entrapped. Table

Table 6–3. *Thermal Death Times and D Values (in hours) at 120°C (248°F) for Spores of* Bacillus Subtilis *var.* Niger *Entrapped in Several Solids*

Compounds	Time to Sterilize (hr)	D Values* (hr)
Solid rocket propellant	24	2.5
Asbestos patching cement	20	2.1
Plaster of Paris	12	1.7
Glue-base marble patching plaster	30	4.0
Dental materials:		
Inlay investment A	4.5	0.6
Inlay investment B	30	3.2
Inlay die material	30	3.6
Bridge model material	15	1.6

*The D values were calculated from levels of spore contamination found by assay of the solid materials. The weight of samples for a given solid was held constant and was in the range of 0.5 g for all materials. Samples solidified around thermocouples showed that all solids reached temperature in 10 minutes.

From Bruch, C.W., Koesterer, M.G., and Bruch, M.K. 1963. Dry-heat sterilization: Its development and application to components of exobiological space probes. Dev. Ind. Microbiol., *4,* 334–342.

6–3 includes data from Bruch et al. (1963) for *B. subtilis* var. niger entrapped in several solids. (For reference, the resistance of the suspension of *B. subtilis* var. niger on a paper strip was 0.91 hours.) It would be of considerable value to know whether these heat-resistance values correlate with water activity of the particular material or the water activity of the microarea in which the spores may be contacting the carrier. Are these differences a reflection of the hygroscopic characteristics of these carriers, and as such, do they act as protectors of spore death in the manner that Greaves (1960) has described as a protective colloid and buffer system to maintain a minimum moisture level in freeze-dried spores?

Gas Atmosphere

Pheil et al. (1967) evaluated the effect of the gas atmosphere surrounding dry spores of *Bacillus subtilis* strain 5230 and *Clostridium sporogenes* strain PA 3679 over the temperature range 121.1 to 160°C (250 to 320°F). In all cases they found that the effect of the different dry gases was small; *B. subtilis* showed slightly more resistance in the inert gases nitrogen and helium than in oxygen, air, and carbon dioxide. The PA 3679 exhibited highest resistance in helium, least resistance in air, with carbon dioxide generally between the two but nearer the resistance in helium. The z value was 18.3°C (33°F) for *B. subtilis* in the five gases tested, 21.7°C (39°F) for PA 3679 in helium and carbon dioxide, and 22.8°C (41°F) in air. Bruch (1966) included data from Koesterer (1962) in which microorganisms showed the greatest heat resistance in an air atmosphere, with decreasing resistance in a helium atmosphere and in a vacuum. The reported relative D value effect of air and helium is approximately 2 to 1, whereas Pheil et al. (1967) found a relative air-to-helium D value effect of 5 to 6. These differences may be related to the type of experi-

mental system; Pheil et al. (1967) used a closed system, while Koesterer (1962) used an open system.

Simko et al. (1971) determined the dry-heat resistance of spores of *Bacillus subtilis* var. *niger* on mated surfaces in an air, nitrogen, and helium atmosphere. They found no difference in the resistance of the spores to the two dry gases, nitrogen and helium. The spores had a significantly greater resistance in air. Because ambient air was used, its higher water content was probably responsible for the higher spore resistance in air.

Davis et al. (1963) found that the survival of dry spores at 60°C and high vacuum was consistently lower than that of dry spores held at atmospheric pressure for the same length of time, whereas at 25°C there was little difference between atmospheric pressure and a high vacuum. At a temperature of 88°C, growth (upon subculturing) was considerably less than at 60°C and at 100°C; in general, there was no growth (upon subculturing) after 4 to 5 days at high vacuum. The relative vapor pressures of water at these temperatures are: 25°C, 23.756 mm Hg; 60°C, 149.38 mm Hg; 88°C, 487.1 mm Hg; 100°C, 760 mm Hg. Comparison of the vapor pressure values, a measure of the rate of dehydration when measured against a hard vacuum, points out that the drying rate is more than six times faster at 60°C than at 25°C, more than three times faster at 88°C than at 60°C, and 50% faster at 100°C than at 88°C. Destruction rates seem to approximately parallel drying rates. These data appear to parallel data of Marshall et al. (1963) and Murrell and Scott (1957), who have reported that spore viability decreases when spores are exposed to a near zero water activity or, in other words, subjected to a severe drying stress.

Bruch et al. (1963) observed, when discussing their data and those of Davis et al. (1963), that "Clearly, the presence or lack of gaseous environment surrounding microbial spores during dry heat sterilization influences the rate of spore destruction. The composition and stability of the gaseous atmosphere also may be important and may be the factor responsible for the high dry heat resistance of spore samples on sand and soil samples."

When microbial spores are heated in a superheated steam atmosphere, they are subject to dry-heat conditions; at equilibrium, no liquid water is present, and the relative humidity is less than 1.00. It is perhaps confusing but true that we can have a 100% water vapor atmosphere and still have a relative humidity below 100% and dry-heat conditions. In a 100% superheated steam atmosphere, the relative humidity is determined by the pressure and temperature of the system. The saturated vapor pressure is determined by the temperature of the system. The vapor pressure will be the actual pressure of the system. Reducing the pressure while holding temperature constant will reduce the relative humidity.

Heat Destruction of Microorganisms in Lipids

Interest in the heat resistance of microorganisms in various lipids has existed for more than 65 years. Bartlett and Kline (1913) demonstrated that the longest survival time for *Bacillus subtilis* at 100°C in glycerin was 75 minutes; in oil, 50 minutes; and in water, 3 minutes. They further demonstrated that, at 112°C, the longest survival times were 15 minutes, 10 minutes, and less than 5 minutes, respectively. Similar patterns of enhanced heat resistance in lipids have been reported for other *Bacillus* species (Molin and Snygg, 1967; Zakula, 1969).

The influence of lipids on the heat-resistance characteristics of nonspore-forming organisms has also been investigated. An enhanced effect has been reported for pneumococci, *Pseudomonas*, *Micrococcus*, *Streptococcus*, yeast, and other microorganisms (Gay et al., 1931; Hansen and Reimann, 1963; Yesair et al., 1946; Zuccaro et al., 1951; Jensen, 1954; Thuillot et al., 1968; Zaleski et al., 1971; Senhaji and Loncin, 1977). From these reports, it can be concluded that microorganisms, either vegetative cells or spores, present in lipids are capable of resisting heating conditions that would be lethal in an aqueous system.

Possible mechanisms have been proposed to account for the protective effect of oil. It has been suggested that oil requires more time to reach the desired temperature. Consequently, spores in oil were exposed for a shorter period of time to high temperatures (Dickson et al., 1925). Another mechanism proposed was the localized absence of moisture around the spore (Mudd and Mudd, 1924; Yesair et al., 1946).

If enhancement of heat resistance is indeed due to the localized absence of moisture around the spore, then the spore, when heated, could be considered to be subjected to dry-heat conditions. Spores have longer survival times under dry- than under wet-heat conditions (Murrell and Scott, 1966; Alderton and Snell, 1969b; Harnulv and Snygg, 1972) and, as has been already shown here, microorganisms are more heat resistant in lipids than in aqueous systems.

Little direct experimental attention has been given to the similarity between heating microorganisms in lipids and heating microorganisms under dry-heat conditions, though several authors have alluded to a possible connection (Dickson et al., 1925; Hansen and Reimann, 1963). One study directly addresses this issue. Yesair et al. (1944) studied dried micrococci in moist fat under wet-heat conditions and in dried fat under dry-heat conditions at 100°C. The killing times were 15 to 20 minutes and 135 to 150 minutes, respectively. When dry micrococci were exposed to dry air at 110°C, the killing time was 135 to 150 minutes. Thus, these authors concluded that micrococci, when in dried fat, essentially were being subjected to the equivalent of dry-heat conditions. Later, Yesair et al. (1946) reported the same findings for dried streptococci. Dickson et al. (1925) came to similar conclusions when heating spores of *Clostridium botulinum* in oil, although, based on the studies they conducted, their conclusion would be better termed a conjecture.

If heating microorganisms in oil is equivalent to subjecting them to dry-heat conditions, as has been suggested, the addition of some water to the system should influence how closely the environment in oil approximates a dry-heat situation. A number of reports in the literature treat the effect of adding small amounts of water on the heat-survival characteristics of microorganisms in oil. Several are presented in Table 6–4. Molin and Snygg (1967) reported on the effect of adding 0, 1, 3, and 30 μl water per ml of soy oil on the percentage of *Bacillus cereus* spores surviving 15 minutes exposure at 121°C. The results were 25.0%, 0.06%, 0.04%, and 0.01% survivors, respectively. Thuillot et al. (1968) heated *Staphylococcus aureus* in dry peanut oil and calculated a $D_{250°F}$ value of 9 minutes and a z value of 38°F. When they added 3 parts water per 1000 parts of oil, they experimentally arrived at a $D_{150°F}$ value of 15 minutes and a z value of 14°F. Zaleski and co-workers in 1971 reported heating *S. aureus* in dried soy oil with the following amounts of water added per liter of oil: 0, 1.0, 2.0, and 3.0 ml. The z values obtained were 23°, 15°, 14°, and 13°C, and in nutrient broth, 6.5°C. Thus, the addition of water resulted in a reduction of the protective effect seen in oil.

Lang and Dean (1934) reported the opposite finding, namely, that the protective effect of fat was best demonstrated with the addition of some water. This has been interpreted by some as contradicting the postulated relationship between the lack of water in lipids and the protective effect of lipids. For example, Molin and Snygg (1967) reported a decreased resistance of bacteria upon the addition of water (see Table 6–4). By applying the finding of Murrell and Scott of maximum dry-heat resistance at A_w values of 0.2 to 0.4, however, the data of Lang and Dean can be reconsidered. Assuming that their "dry" fat had an A_w approaching 0.00, then, upon the addition of water to the lipid, an A_w in the range of 0.2 to 0.4 could be achieved and maximum protection demonstrated. Thus, their findings can be considered as not contradicting those of Molin and Snygg.

When dealing with systems containing lipids and water, a logical question could be raised as to the location of bacteria in such a system. Mudd and Mudd (1924) made observations germane to this point studying various enterobacteria and members of the genus *Bacillus*. They reported a concentration of bacteria at the interface of the oil-water mixture with an infrequent and apparently passive entry into the oil phase, whereas they found numerous situations in which bacteria entered the aqueous phase. We would conclude that under conditions akin to those used by Mudd and Mudd, bacteria tend to concentrate in the aqueous phase.

Two reports (Senhaji, 1977; Senhaji et al., 1976) have examined the effect of added water on the survival of *Bacillus subtilis* spores in soy oil by a unique method. They investigated the effect of agitating a 2.5% water-in-oil mixture so that the A_w approached 1.00 throughout the entire course of heating. In this study, they found a striking reduction in spore resistance with agitation, whereas without agitation, spore resistance was shown

Table 6–4. *Summary of Key Reports in Literature on Heat Resistance of Bacteria in Lipids*

Organism	Test Conditions		Findings or Results		Reference
B. subtilis			*Longest Survival Time (min)*		Bartlett and Kline (1913)
	Water Bath at 100°C		In glycerin. 75		
			In oil 50		
	In Autoclave ~112°C		In water. 3		
			In oil 15		
			In glycerin. 10		
			In water. . . . . <5		
C. botulinum	Thermal death times at 121°C for 3 strains:				Dickson et al. (1925)
	oil/broth mixture 23, 23, 15 min				
	broth alone 4, 5, 3 min				
Streptococcus	*Condition of Bacteria*	*Temp °C*	*Kill Time (min)*		Yesair et al. (1944)
	moist, in broth	55	Moist Heat	30–45	
	dried, in broth	55		30–45	
	dried, in moist fat	100		15–20	
	dried	110	Dry Heat	135–150	
	dried in dry fat	100		135–150	

	Water Activity (A_w)	*0.0*	*0.2–0.4*	*1.00*	Murrell and Scott (1966)
B. stearothermophilus	D Value	15.8	501	25.1	
B. megaterium	at 110°C	39.8	316	0.12	
C. botulinum B		0.5	1259	0.5	

B. cereus	$D_{121°C}$ in soy oil = 34 min			Molin and Snygg (1967)
	Percent Water Added to Oil	*Percent Survival at 15 min*		
	0	25.0		
	1	0.06		
	3	0.04		
	30	0.01		

B. subtilis	*Conditions*	$D_{95°C}$ *(min)*		Senhaji (1977)
	pure soy oil	167		Senhaji et al. (1976)
	oil + 2.5% water	137		
	oil + 2.5% water agitated during heating	7		
	buffer	4.8		

B. subtilis	*Conditions*	$D_{95°C}$ *(min)*	$D_{105°C}$ *(min)*	Senhaji and Loncin
	pure soy oil		71	(1975, 1977)
	33% oil in buffer, 2 phases	142	38	
	same, but shaken to make "emulsion"	53	0.9	
	1–2 drops oil on top of 1 ml buffer	10	1.0	
	buffer	12	0.6	
		7.3		

S. aureus	Heated in peanut oil			Thuillot et al. (1968)
	Dry oil	$D_{250°F}$ = 9 min z = 38°F		
	Dry oil + 0.3% water	$D_{150°F}$ = 15 min z = 14°F		

S. aureus	Heated in soy oil	*z Value °C*	Zaleski et al. (1971)
	Dried oil	23	
	Dried oil + 0.1% H_2O	15	
	Dried oil + 0.2% H_2O	14	
	Dried oil + 0.3% H_2O	13	
	Nutrient broth	6.5	

to be like that occurring in the total absence of water. Their findings are summarized in Table 6–4. By using numeric simulation of oil-water mixtures, these authors reported additional confirmation of the proposal that the heat resistance of spores in oil occurs as a result of a reduction of the water activity during heating. These findings suggest that when the A_w of oil is maintained close to 1.0, the resistance characteristics of bacterial spores in oil approximate those of spores in an aqueous system.

In another series of studies, Senhaji and Loncin (1975, 1977) examined the survival characteristics of *Bacillus subtilis* spores inoculated in soy oil in four oil-water systems: (1) soy oil; (2) 33% v/v oil and buffer in a two-phase system; (3) 33% v/v oil and buffer handshaken to create an "emulsion"; and (4) 1 to 2 drops of oil layered on top of 1 ml of buffer. For comparison, spores were also inoculated into buffer. Their results are presented in Table 6–4. Although some question exists as to the clean level of the spore preparations used and the stability of the oil-in-water emulsion generated by handshaking, their findings definitely contribute to our understanding of the survival of spores in oil-water mixtures. The results can be summarized as follows: survival of spores in the two-phase system appeared to resemble that of spores in a single oil phase, whereas spore survival in the 33% oil-in-buffer "emulsion" and in the 1 to 2 drops of oil on top of 1 ml of buffer did not seem to differ from that in phosphate buffer at any of three temperatures used. Similar patterns were found for the vegetative bacterium *Pseudomonas fluorescens*.

Discussion of Dry-Heat Destruction of Microorganisms

Lea et al. (1950) demonstrated the critical nature of relative humidity or water activity on certain chemical reactions associated with dry living cells, mainly those involving proteins in work directed toward preservation of cells by freeze-drying. These authors found reaction rates expressed as Q_{10} (in the range 20 to 30°C) to range from 4.8 to 8.5. They found that the low reaction rates are associated with low water contents, increasing reaction rates with increasing water contents. The temperature coefficients that these authors found for the rate of loss of amino groups in dry human blood plasma containing added glucose and citrate are not materially different from those being found for dry-heat-destruction of microorganisms. This work suggests that the z value of the thermal destruction curve will decrease with increased moisture.

Greaves (1960) suggested that the beneficial effect of glucose in the drying medium for the preservation of freeze-dried cultures was due to its buffering effect on the residual moisture content. If the organisms were dried too far, they were killed during the drying operation; on the other hand, if they were not dried far enough, they survived poorly on storage. Greaves (1962) concluded that the most important factor in determining the percentage of survival both immediately and after

drying and for long-term storage was the medium in which the organisms are suspended for drying. In reviewing this area, he noted that Fry and Greaves (1951) suggested the use of a serum, which they felt acted as a protective colloid and as a support medium to give a final dried cake, and that the glucose in this serum exerted its effect by acting as a buffer on the residual moisture content, preventing the organisms from becoming too dry.

Greaves (1960) concluded that a drying medium for bacteria should contain: (1) a protective colloid, for example, 5% dextran containing no glucose; (2) a buffer to control the residual moisture content to around 1%, e.g., 5 to 10% sucrose or 5 to 10% sodium glutamate; (3) a neutralizer of carbonyl groups, e.g., broth or 1% sodium glutamate.

ART OF GATHERING AND ANALYZING MICROBIAL HEAT-DESTRUCTION DATA

Scientists and engineers working in the physical sciences or engineering have few problems with measurement, whereas those of us gathering microbial heat-destruction data have many problems with measurements and standards; we will discuss the source of some of these problems.

The concept of using standards in the physical sciences, including the chemical area, and the use of physical measurements in everyday life cannot be extended to the biologic world. The biologic world is different, it is an entity unto itself. There is no standard man or woman, monkey, or microorganism. Each biologic entity is unique and different from all others. There are no standard bacterial spores. We describe a biologic population using the statistical measures of the critical parameters. For example, in the sterilization area we determine the mean D_T value and its variation. Each spore is unique, each spore crop is different from all previous spore crops. Therefore, if a new *Bacillus stearothermophilus* spore crop is grown in our laboratory, we must test this spore crop to determine its characteristics. We cannot use the D_T value for an old spore crop or go into the literature and get a D_T value for John Doe's *B. stearothermophilus* and have these D_T values be meaningful for our new spore crop.

Working with a biologic system places a number of constraints on us that we must accept and meet if our experiments are to produce meaningful results. As mentioned previously we must keep in mind that each biologic organism or product is a unique entity.

Because we do not have standard microorganisms, including bacterial spores, we must test to a point where we essentially make each spore crop a standard. We accomplish this by carrying out survivor curve tests at several temperatures (at least three), by repeating each survivor curve test at least a second time on a different day from the first test, and evaluating all the data statistically (each test must be complete in that it has an N_0

test plus four to five heating times where the change in the initial population N_0 is at least three log cycles).

In heat-destruction studies we have a second biologic variable, the recovery or growth medium (Schmidt 1955a). Agar is a biologic product, hence it is variable on a lot-to-lot basis. Most recovery media contain other biologic products in addition to agar. It has been amply demonstrated by Pflug et al. (1981) and Pflug (1989) that commercial dehydrated media have a lot-to-lot variability that will produce a significant lot-to-lot variability in the D_T value. The simplest way of eliminating the media effect is to obtain enough of a single lot of medium at the beginning to last for the whole project. The performance of each lot of medium should be validated.

We need to be aware of and have an understanding of sampling science because it may tell us when variation in results are due to microbial variability and when due to environmental variability. If I have a vial of bacterial spores and I test these in system A today and again in an identical manner in system A tomorrow, I should get the same results within the tolerance limits of experimental variation. If the results of today's experiment are different from the results of tomorrow's experiment, I should not blame the spores because ample data indicate that spores are relatively stable and will not change from today to tomorrow. Therefore, what has happened is that an environmental variable has produced this variation, and we must find and eliminate the cause of the variation before we have a meaningful test result.

Design of Thermal Destruction Tests

The objective of the thermal destruction test and the procedure for accomplishing that objective should be carefully studied as part of the design on the overall experiment to ensure that the results satisfy the objective. Most testing procedures are of the multiple replicate type; the specific procedure usually depends on the objectives of the experiment and the type of apparatus available.

Three to five replicate units should be tested at each time-temperature condition; the number of multiple replicate units (n) should be constant throughout the experiment. In general, the precision of the result is a function of n; however, when we increase n by a factor of four, we only increase our precision by a factor of two. The physical effort varies directly with the number of replicates. In end-point fraction-replicate-unit-negative (FN) tests, the time intervals should be selected so all the multiple replicate units are positive at the shortest time period and all are negative at the longest time period, with intermediate times showing both positive and negative results.

Heating times can be spaced uniformly, or the interval may increase logarithmically with increasing time (Townsend et al., 1956). It is doubtful whether a strong case can be made for either logarithmic or uniform increments; therefore, factors such as convenience and personal preference must govern this judgment.

Thermal resistance experiments with the exception of

preliminary runs should be conducted at a minimum of four temperatures and preferably at five. Thermal resistance temperature coefficient data obtained at three temperatures are valid, but these z values usually do not have the degree of accuracy of z values determined at four or five temperatures.

In general, biologic systems are well known for their variability; however, the behavior of microbial cells and spores in heat-destruction experiments appears to be an exception to this general association. Microbial spores are probably some of the most accurate heat and nutrient transducers available to man today. If equal numbers of a uniform suspension of microbial spores are subjected to successively longer increments of heating, and these spores are treated identically in all respects other than heating time, the results will be increasing numbers of negative tubes with increasing heating times. Variation in this pattern indicates variation in testing technique. Organisms that die at the times when they are supposed to survive in fact have received a lethal dose of heat, and organisms that survive at heating times when the researcher thinks they should have died did not receive a lethal dose of heat. It is doubtful that man can produce as accurate a transducer as these living organisms, and it is perhaps the alert and prudent investigator who realizes and makes use of the unique attributes of this biologic system to monitor and improve his experimental technique.

Measuring Wet-Heat-Destruction Rates of Microorganisms

The food microbiologist has been actively engaged in measuring the heat-destruction rates of microorganisms for about 100 years; during this time, a number of methods have been developed for obtaining data leading to heat-destruction rates of microorganisms. Each investigator has developed his own novel and unique method for measuring heat destruction; however, many of the methods are similar in part, and it now appears desirable to look at heat-destruction measurement from an overall vantage point and describe these measurements in terms of the principles of the several major procedures.

Study of the thermal destruction of microorganisms is directed toward analysis of the destruction pattern and the final destruction end point. Two general types of techniques for studying the effect of heat have evolved: (1) successive sampling and plating of a suspension of microorganisms during heat treatment; (2) evaluation of a number of small replicate samples subjected to several time-temperature conditions on a growth/no growth basis.

The "successive sampling method" can be thought of as a beaker of substrate and inoculum heated in a controlled temperature water bath in which, at successive time intervals, an aliquot is removed, usually using a pipette, and appropriate dilutions are made and plated. The result is a destruction rate curve relating numbers of survivors with heat treatment. Although this method is simple in concept, it is usually quite involved in practice because:

1. Substrate and inoculum should be brought to testing temperature in a known reproducible time.
2. When heat-sensitive organisms are studied, times are short, requiring precise time and temperature control.
3. Evaluation of the thermal resistance of spores above 100°C requires a pressure system with the accompanying pressure sealing and sampling problem.

A precise successive sampling type study provides valuable data on the effect of heat on the microbial population; however, it is usually limited in regard to the minimum number of organisms that can be evaluated.

The "multiple replicate unit system," using the growth/no growth method, involves the evaluation of individual replicate samples; a minimum testing program at one temperature would consist of 5 replicate units at each of 5 to 10 successive time intervals for a total of 25 to 50 units per temperature condition.

The multiple replicate unit system relies on a large number of tests to arrive at a precise statistical answer. The precision of the method is improved by increasing the number of replicates and decreasing the time interval. The advantages of the multiple replicate unit methods are that the thermal destruction characteristics of the organism are measured in the fractional survival range, and incubation times and conditions are relatively nonrestricted. When studies must be made above 100°C, some of the multiple replicate unit systems are still simple, thereby neatly bypassing inoculation and sampling under pressure.

When using the multiple replicate system to obtain a survivor curve by direction enumeration, at least three, but usually no more than five, units are subjected to the same heat-stress environment (heating time). For each survivor curve that is to be developed, the number of surviving organisms is determined at five to seven heating times. Heating times are chosen so survivor curve data are developed from the initial concentration of microorganisms of the sample to perhaps as few as ten surviving organisms per sample.

A number of laboratory methods have been developed for both the successive sampling method and the multiple replicate unit system. In general, high-quality thermal resistance data can be produced by all of the methods; however, each method usually excels in certain aspects and at the same time has certain limitations. An attempt will be made to note the points of excellence and the limitations of each method.

Successive Sampling Systems

Several individual methods for determining thermal destruction rates can be grouped together and categorized as mixing methods, whereby some type of system is used to bring a small volume of inoculum into a larger quantity of substrate, i.e., at the heating medium temperature, and then to remove samples in a sort of dynamic system so that heating and cooling lags are minimized. All the successive sampling systems are similar, but at the same time they differ slightly in certain aspects. The objective of all systems is the same—to determine the effect of a holding time at a specific temperature on the microbial population.

Heating in a Flask. In this method, probably the most reliable results have been obtained through the use of a Woulfe bottle with three necks, as described by Levine et al. (1927). These bottles are obtainable in sizes from 250 ml to several liters. For use in thermal-destruction studies, a small mechanical stirrer is introduced through one neck and a thermometer through a second, and the third neck serves as an entry for introduction of the inoculum and withdrawal of the samples. All holes should be closed with stoppers or cotton plugs to prevent contamination during the test. Townsend et al. (1956) also describe a procedure for successive sampling using a flask.

Atmospheric Mixing Method. Kaufmann and Andrews (1954) described an apparatus for the study of milk pasteurization in which the heating unit was a large water bath provided with an electric heater and temperature control. The test chamber is placed in a 4-L beaker that is supplied with continuously flowing liquid from the water bath. To minimize temperature change during mixing, only 1 ml of inoculum is used for 200 ml of presterilized milk. After inoculation, samples are removed from the test chamber by means of a 5-ml syringe and immediately transferred to a test tube in an ice-water bath. The samples are plated and results expressed as a survivor curve.

Tank Method. Williams et al. (1937) developed a metal container system for succession sampling at temperatures above 100°C. The advantages of this method are that bacteria can be studied in a food suspension under conditions thought to parallel those that exist in the food container. A disadvantage of the system is the specialized equipment required.

Nitrogen Pressure Mixing Method. In this method, nitrogen gas under pressure is used to force a controlled amount of hot liquid medium and spore suspension into a mixing chamber (Wang et al., 1964). In the mixing chamber, temperature equilibration is accomplished in 0.6 ms; after temperature has been obtained, it is maintained for the designed holding time by having the mixture flow through a constant-temperature reactor pipe. The holding time is controlled by changing either the flow rate through the reactor pipe or the length of reactor pipe. At the end of the treatment, the suspension is cooled by instantaneous expansion of the test fluid from reactor pressure to atmospheric pressure in a flash chamber provided with a cold water condenser. The sample is collected and plated to determine the viable count. The results are expressed as a survivor curve.

Multiple Replicate Unit Testing Systems

The multiple glass tube, multiple capillary tube, multiple metal tube, multiple can, multiple cup, and thermoresistometer methods differ basically in the geometry and size of the inoculum-containing unit and the heating equipment required. The several types of multiple replicate units are compared in Table 6–5, and the heating equipment required is compared in Table 6–6. The details of each system are described below.

Glass Tube Method (Sealed, Cotton-Plugged, and Screw-Capped). The heating of a suspension of microorganisms in sealed Pyrex glass tubes has been widely used since the method was first described by Bigelow and Esty (1920) and revised by Esty and Williams (1924).

Microbial suspensions of a near-water consistency are the most convenient to use with the tubes since a thin solution can be pipetted into and poured out of the tubes for subculture. The normal inoculum for 9-mm OD (7-mm ID) tubes is 2 ml. Solid or viscous products may be introduced into the tubes with a modified grease gun (Stumbo et al., 1945); these materials are difficult to subculture and are usually incubated in the tubes for fraction-negative analysis.

After the tubes have been subjected to the heat treatment, the contents are normally subcultured in a growth medium. The tubes are scratched approximately half an inch from the end and, after flaming to sterilize the outside, are broken; the contents are poured into the subculture medium tubes.

A method developed by Schmidt (1950) eliminated the sealing through a miniature retort modification that made possible the use of cotton-plugged tubes.

Screw-capped Pyrex glass test tubes can be used in the same manner as the special 9-mm tubes just described. The screw-capped tubes are more easily used in substrate incubation tests, especially where a viscous food product must be evaluated. A liquid substrate in cotton-plugged or screw-capped tubes can also be plated for direct enumeration of surviving organisms. The heating-lag correction of screw-capped glass tubes is large; probably the screw-capped tubes should be used only in a miniature retort.

Kooiman and Geers (1975) developed a screw-capped glass tube technique that allows accurate heating at temperatures above 100°C. In this method, the tubes containing the test substrate are preheated in an oil bath, and a 0.1-ml sample of spores is added to each preheated tube of substrate, through a neoprene septum, with a 100-μl Hamilton syringe. After heating, the tubes are cooled in an ice bath. This method eliminates the need to correct for heating and cooling lags and can be used for both fraction-negative and plate count analyses. A disadvantage is that when a viscous substrate is evaluated, it is essential to shake the tubes to mix the spore suspension.

Capillary Tube Methods. Capillary tube methods, described by Stern and Procter (1954) and Wilder and Nordan (1957), can be considered a modification of the glass tube method just described. In this method, the tube is reduced to capillary size so that heating takes place rapidly and, by using a sterile heating and cooling bath, the heated capillary tube can be subcultured by breaking the tube and depositing the broken tube directly into the subculture tube.

Table 6–5. *Widely Used Types of Inoculum-Substrate Containers Used in Multiple Replicate Unit Testing Methods*

Unit	Volume of Inoculum Plus Substrate (ml)	Type of Heating Apparatus Required	Suitability of Method for Substrate Incubation or Subculture	Heating-Lag Correction $z = 10°C$ or $18°F$, minutes
Glass tube, sealed	2	Water bath to 90°C; above 90°C, oil bath, miniature autoclave or retort	Subculture or substrate incubation	0.9–1.2 in steam
Glass tube (cotton-plugged or screw-capped)	2–5	Water bath to 90°C; above 90°C, oil bath, miniature autoclave or retort	Subculture or substrate incubation	2.0 minute for 5 ml water in 18 × 150 mm test tubes
Metal tube Al., 150 × 3 mm	1	Water bath to 90°C; above 90°C, oil bath, miniature autoclave or retort	Subculture only	0.2 for 1 ml water
Capillary tube, glass	0.01	Special heating oil bath, cooling bath, and transfer mechanism	Subculture only	
TDT Can*	13–16	Water bath to 90°C; above 90°C, oil bath, miniature autoclave or retort	Substrate incubation	0.6–2.0 in steam
Cup	0.01–0.02	Miniature autoclave	Subculture only	Negligible
Cup-can system	0.01–0.02	Water bath to 90°C; above 90°C, oil bath, miniature autoclave or retort	Subculture only	
Cup-thermoresistometer	0.01–0.02	Thermoresistometer	Subculture only	Negligible

*Thermal Death Time Cans 208 × 006 (63.5 mm diameter × 9.52 mm deep).

Table 6–6. *Heating Equipment Used in Multiple Replicate Unit Testing Methods*

Heating Equipment	Type of Multiple Unit that Can Be Accommodated	Capacity of Replicate Units	Degree of Complexity of Operation	Utilities Required	Relative Cost
Water bath	Glass tubes: sealed, cotton-plugged, screw-capped; Metal tubes TDT cans	Limited only by physical size of apparatus	Simple	Low-pressure steam or 115V AC	Low
Oil bath	Glass tubes, sealed Metal tubes TDT cans	Limited only by physical size of apparatus	Simple	115V AC	Low
Miniature steam autoclave or retort BIER* vessel	Glass tubes: sealed, screw-capped; Metal tubes TDT cans Cups Cups in cans	Limited only by physical size of apparatus	Simple	80 psig steam	Moderate
Thermoresistometer	Cups	5 or 6 cups, depending on design	Complex	80 psig steam 115V AC	Expensive

*The Association for the Advancement of Medical Instrumentation (AAMI), Arlington, VA 22209, developed standards for laboratory equipment to evaluate biologic indicators used to validate and monitor sterilization processes using the steam autoclave. The equipment was designated as a BIER/steam vessel (Biological Indicator–Evaluation Resistometer for saturated steam); this terminology is now often used to mean a small (miniature) saturated/steam autoclave or retort where the test temperature can be accurately controlled.

The capillary tubes are 0.8 mm ID, 1.5 mm OD, and 3 inches long. The column of bacterial suspension is approximately half an inch long after the tubes are sealed in a gas flame. A 0.01-ml bacterial suspension is placed into each sterile capillary tube using a precision syringe; Wilder and Nordan (1957) developed a capillary tube evacuation and filling system to generally improve this method.

The advantages of the capillary tube method are that shorter times with correspondingly higher temperatures can be used; the subculturing operation is simplified. Disadvantages are that special heating and cooling equipment is required, filling and sealing the tubes are probably more laborious than with standard tubes, and the volume of bacterial suspension is small.

Metal Tube Method. The metal tube method used by Odlaug and Pflug (1977) and by Mayou and Jezeski (1977) is a cross between the capillary tube and the 7- or 15-mm OD glass tube methods. The column of substrate in the metal tube is about 150 mm long and 3 mm in diameter with a volume of about 1 ml. The metal surrounding this column of substrate has a high heat conductivity, which results in a low lag-correction factor. The tubes, which are reusable, are internally threaded at both ends and are closed with a plastic cap screw and O-ring. The advantages of the metal tube system are: (1) closing and opening are simple; (2) shorter heating times with correspondingly higher temperatures can be used; and (3) no special heating equipment is required. Metal tubes used with a precision-type miniature retort system give good results with heating times as short as 0.5 minutes.

Can Method. Special metal cans 2.5 inches in diameter by 0.375 inches high or, in sanitary can terminology, 208 × 006, were designed by the American Can Company (Townsend et al., 1938) for thermal resistance studies using nutrient media or food product. These special cans make possible the study of the effect of heat on microorganisms in foods consisting of solid pieces of food product in brine or syrup, or foods of heavy consistency that either cannot be readily introduced into thermal death time tubes or where it is desirable to incubate the organisms in the same food product in which they are heated.

The multiple can method is ideally suited for use with gas-producing bacteria where growth of the test microorganisms can be evaluated by the swelling of the can. The approximate maximum capacity of the 208 × 006 cans is 20 g. The amount of material per can varies, but generally it is in the range of 13 to 16 ml. It is important that a system be used that will ensure that the microbial inoculum is uniform on a can-to-can basis and is uniformly distributed throughout the cans. Before use, the cans and lids should be thoroughly cleaned. The cans should be sealed in a vacuum of at least 15 inches of mercury.

Advantages of the can method: it is possible to study thermal destruction in viscous and particulate food products, to have direct incubation of the heated organisms in the food substrate, the operation is mechanized in that the cans can be rapidly closed on conventional mechanical closing equipment, and relatively high temperatures and short times can be used because of the geometry of the can and the fact that it is a metal object. Disadvantages of the can method are that a relatively large amount of substrate is required, and the substrate cannot be easily subcultured, thereby increasing the labor required if non-gas-forming organisms are evaluated.

The cans may be heated in a water bath if temperatures are below 100°C, or in miniature steam retorts (BIER/steam vessels) or oil baths for temperatures above 100°C. The miniature steam retorts are the ideal heating units and make possible minimum times and maximum temperatures.

Metal Cup Method. Metal cups with straight sides and flat bottoms 0.433 inches OD and 0.333 inches high were developed as inoculum-substrate containers in the cup-thermoresistometer thermal resistance testing system. They have since been used extensively in two other systems—directly in miniature retorts for thermal resistance studies at or above 100°C and in thermal resistance cans for oil-bath heating at lower temperatures.

Pflug and Augustin (1962) developed a procedure whereby small metal cups containing a bacterial inoculum are heated directly in miniature retorts before being subcultured in tubes of growth media. An inoculum consisting of 0.01 ml of spore suspension is pipetted into the thermal resistometer cups; conventionally, the suspension is dried in a vacuum oven and the replicate cups are placed in a small carrier tray in a special holder that is then placed in the miniature retort. In this manner, the cups and the spore suspension in the cups are directly heated by the steam. After the desired heating period, the pressure in the miniature retort is released and the cups are allowed to cool, after which they are aseptically transferred to sterile petri plates, carried to the plating room, and then subcultured into tubes of growth medium. The surviving spores can also be plated; the heated cup is placed in a tube or flask containing dilution buffer and exposed to ultrasonic energy (NASA, 1968) to remove the spores from the cup. The diluent is plated using standard microbiologic procedures. The advantages of this method are that the cups are relatively inexpensive and can be easily prepared in quantity, heating times can be short, and high temperatures, compared to the 9-mm OD glass tube method, can be used. Disadvantages of this method are that a small, highly concentrated inoculum is required, a miniature retort system with precise temperature control is required, and the bacterial inoculum cannot be suspended at a high dilution level in a food product.

Pheil and Pflug (1964) adapted a technique they developed for dry-heat testing for use in wet-heat thermal resistance testing below 100°C. They used the metal cups described previously but loaded them into modified thermal resistance cans (208×006). Ten cups are placed in each can with about 2 ml of distilled water on filter paper in the bottom of the can; the cans are sealed. The 208×006 cans were modified by punching a recess in the bottom to accommodate the 0.333-inch high cups. After sealing, the cans are heated in an oil bath. Following heating and cooling, the cans are aseptically opened and the cup subcultured into suitable growth media or the inoculum plated.

Advantages of the cup-can system are that cups are easier and less expensive to prepare than tubes, and the ten cups in the same can receive an identical treatment. The chief disadvantage is that the inoculum is in a concentrated condition.

Cup-Thermoresistometer Method. The cup-thermoresistometer method (Stumbo, 1948b; Pflug and Esselen, 1953; Pflug, 1960) is a combination of two unique devices—the small metal inoculum-substrate container and a mechanical apparatus designed specifically to move the small metal cup into and out of a steam atmosphere. The thermoresistometer is described more fully later in this chapter.

In the cup-thermoresistometer system, the cups, described previously, are heated in steam under controlled time and temperature conditions. The rapid operation and high-pressure design make possible thermal resistance testing under wet-heat conditions at temperatures up to 150°C, for times as short as 0.02 minute. The advantages of the thermoresistometer and the metal cup system are that heating-lag corrections are negligible, studies can be made at high temperatures and short times that are impossible with other multiple-unit testing systems, and the output rate at high temperatures and short times is high. The only true disadvantage is the low output with longer times and lower temperatures.

Heating Equipment for Multiple-Unit Replicate Testing System. Because all thermal resistance data are keyed to a temperature, the control of the temperature must be continuous and the measurement of the temperature accurate. The measurement and control of temperature are sciences unto themselves; however, the scientist interested in thermal destruction not only must become acquainted with temperature measurement and control but also must master them to the degree that he can use the methods and equipment accurately.

Water Bath. The water bath is the ideal heating unit for temperatures to 90°C. Water baths come in all sizes, can be heated by electricity or low-pressure steam, are operated as still water baths or are equipped with stirring devices to agitate the water.

The temperature cycle of any water bath used for thermal resistance testing should be determined before testing is started; if the temperature cycle exceeds ±0.15°C, the equipment should be modified to bring it within these limits.

Lag-correction factors for tubes or cans heated in the water bath should be determined under the same conditions as those used for the test.

Oil Bath. The oil bath is used for thermal destruction testing over the range of temperatures of 90 to 120°C. The upper temperature limit is usually imposed by the heating lag, the lower limit by the more convenient use of a water bath when the temperature permits.

The heating-lag correction is much larger for oil than for water or steam. The lag correction must be determined for the product and container under actual oil bath heating conditions.

Miniature Retort (BIER/Steam Vessel). The miniature retort (Pilcher, 1947; Schmidt et al., 1955) is, as its name implies, a small-sized retort with a fast come-up to temperature capability. Miniature retorts are usually operated from a large ballast tank where the steam temperature is accurately controlled; the miniature retort is connected to the ballast tank using large piping and quick-action type valves.

A miniature retort system should include at least two units but probably no more than four. The miniature retorts can be constructed directly above the ballast or reservoir tank or adjacent to it, or they may be constructed adjacent to a large retort where the retort serves as the ballast tank.

Thermoresistometer. The thermoresistometer is the coined name first applied to an apparatus designed by Stumbo (1948b) for studying the thermal resistance of spores at temperatures generally in the 120 to 140°C range, where the heating times are so short that other methods cannot be used because of the heating and cooling lags. The apparatus consists of a system for moving five or six small cups into a steam chamber maintained at a controlled temperature, followed by subculturing of the cups into tubes of appropriate media. An apparatus similar in function was developed by Pflug and Esselen (1953) that was operable at temperatures as high as 150°C. Pflug (1960) designed a special type of thermoresistometer that was usable for both wet- and dry-heat resistance studies. Read (1963) described a thermoresistometer type apparatus that can be used for heat-resistance studies in the temperature range of 45 to 100°C.

The advantage of the thermoresistometer is its ability to expose samples of microorganisms in metal cups to high temperatures for controlled short time periods. When time periods are short, the production rate of thermal resistance data using the thermoresistometer is high. Disadvantages of the system are that it is a specialized piece of apparatus, it is expensive, and it requires considerable maintenance to keep it operating efficiently. For intermediate temperatures, the thermoresistometer is not efficient, because only one replicate set of samples can be evaluated at any one time, and the number of replicates is limited by the design of the apparatus.

Measuring the Dry-Heat Destruction Rate of Microorganisms

In studies of the dry-heat destruction rate of microorganisms, both the temperature and the water in the spore at the time of heating must be known and controlled if the test results are to be meaningful. Many adequate temperature control systems are in use today; the problem area in temperature control is in ensuring that the temperature that the controller senses and the sample temperature are the same or, if they are not the same, that the relationship between them is known.

When multiple replicate units are used in dry-heat testing, the rate of heating of the several units at their different locations must be evaluated. Changes in the design of a system after initial evaluation will require a re-evaluation. It is a good practice in dry-heat testing to have one planchet or cup fitted with a thermocouple so

that a continuous record can be made of the temperature of this unit during each test.

Where air is used as the heat transfer medium, its low heat capacity, as well as its low heat transfer rate, must be taken into account in the design of the experimental system.

The system for controlling the water content of the spores must be designed to have the same amount of water in the spores in all tests or, if the effect of water concentration is to be evaluated, provision must be made for varying the quantity of water in the spores. The relative humidity of the gas surrounding the spore during heating determines the amount of water in the spore. It would be desirable to know the quantity of water in the spores and support; however, this is usually not possible because of the small mass. Therefore, spore water content is indirectly measured and controlled by measuring and controlling the relative humidity of the gas surrounding the spores.

Dry-heat resistance studies can be carried out in either an open or a closed system. Open and closed systems (Pflug, 1968), as has already been pointed out, represent extremes in water movement to or from the spores during heating. Spores in a closed system are inside a container of finite size that has a gas-impermeable wall. In contrast, spores in an open system are usually located on surfaces, so when they are subjected to a dry-heat process, they are in intimate and continuous contact with the surrounding atmosphere of the oven or room. The relative location of the microbial cell, in either a closed or an open system, is important because of the effect of the physical system on water vapor transfer to and from the cell.

In the typical open system in which naked microorganisms are on surfaces, the three following important parameters affect the spore destruction rate: (1) the initial water content of the cell; (2) the relative humidity or water vapor pressure of the gas surrounding the cell during heating; and (3) the mass transfer rate of water to or from the cell. The quantity of water in the spores at the start of heating can be controlled by equilibrating the system at a controlled relative humidity for 48 to 72 hours immediately before the start of the tests. During heating, the ambient relative humidity controls the final equilibrium spore water content. Theoretically, the movement of water to or from the cell would be determined by analysis, because this is a typical diffusion problem. At present, however, it is not always possible to make this analysis because of the nonavailability of rates of diffusion data of water vapor to and in microorganisms. Practically, the effect of the mass transfer rate will be controlled indirectly by having the same constant physical conditions (especially gas velocities across the spores) for all tests.

The rate of water gain and loss from naked spores on surfaces is rapid. Exposing spores to a high- or low-humidity environment between the equilibration and heating parts of a test program for even a few minutes will change the water content of the spores.

In a closed system, the water initially present in the enclosure is the water in the spores plus the water in the gas in the enclosure, and adsorbed on the walls of the enclosure. (All materials adsorb water, and this variable must be included if it is a significant contributor of water.) During heating, the relative humidity in the enclosure is determined by the quantity of water present when the closed system is established, the enclosure volume, and the test temperature.

In the open type of experimental system, spores are deposited on metal planchets, on plastic or glass strips, or in cups. Following deposition, they are equilibrated for approximately 24 hours under controlled temperature and humidity conditions, after which time they are subjected to a dry-heat treatment in a system located inside a controlled environmental (relative humidity and temperature) room, or heating can itself be carried out in a closed environmental chamber where the relative humidity is controlled.

A closed system can be used—a screw-cap test tube, a sealed thermal death time tube, thermal death time can, or heat block or any other hermetic container. To control the relative humidity during heating, the water content of the closed system is controlled by assembling the units in a controlled environmental chamber plus, in some cases, the addition of measured quantities of water to the enclosure prior to sealing.

Open Type of Test System

Planchet-Oven System. Depositing spores on stainless steel planchets and then heating the planchets in a specially equipped oven is a practical way of studying dry-heat destruction of microorganisms on surfaces. Bond et al. (1970) modified an oven so that holders with planchets could be dropped into the oven from the top. Drummond and Pflug (1970) inserted planchets through small holes cut in the door of the oven. Smith et al. (1971) inserted racks of planchets into a controlled environment oven through special openings 6 inches in diameter that could be easily opened or tightly sealed. A requisite of the planchet-oven system is that the humidity as well as the temperature in the oven must be known and controlled. This can be accomplished by placing the oven in a controlled environmental clean room (Bond et al., 1970) or by using an environmental chamber where temperature and humidity are both controlled (Smith et al., 1971).

Planchet-Hotplate System. Depositing spores on planchets and then heating the planchets on a hotplate is a method of duplicating the dry-heat effect on metal surfaces and has been used by Hoffman et al. (1968) and Drummond (1972).

The planchet-boat-hotplate system has been used extensively at the University of Minnesota to gather dry-heat destruction data for spores deposited on stainless steel surfaces. The hotplates were 10 inches wide, 10 inches long, and 2 inches thick. The top was milled flat. Four 150-watt cartridge heaters were inserted into holes

drilled into the side of the plate. A cartridge-type unit containing a thermistor (the sensor for the temperature controller) and a copper-constantan thermocouple (to monitor the block temperature) was located in a fifth hole drilled in the center of one edge of the block.

Spores were deposited on and (after heating) recovered from 0.5- ×0.5-inch planchets cut from 0.015-inch stainless steel shim stock; burrs from the cutting were carefully removed.

Copper plates, 2.5 inches long, 0.75 inches wide, and 0.179 inches deep with a slot 0.5 inches wide and 0.054 inches deep milled the length of the plate, were used as planchet holders to facilitate moving the thin planchets onto and off of the hotplate. These copper plates were called boats and held up to five planchets. Copper boats 2.5 inches long, 0.75 inches wide, and 0.384 inches deep with five holes each 0.375 inches in diameter by 0.3 inches deep machined into the length of the boat were made to hold thermal death time cups so that the dry-heat destruction of microorganisms associated with soil particles could be studied.

The temperature of the hotplate was controlled and monitored. There was approximately a 2°C temperature drop as heat flowed from the hotplate to the planchets. The hotplate temperature was adjusted to 2°C above the test temperature so the planchets were at the desired test temperature.

The hotplates were located in a room or chamber where temperature and humidity were controlled.

Dry-Heat Thermoresistometer. Pflug (1960) developed a device that used hot gas to heat four or five replicate samples. The gas flowed into the small heating chamber through a manifold; flow was continuous through the chamber. This system is usable for heat-resistance studies using superheated steam or hot dry gases. The long heating times of dry cells tend to make thermal destruction evaluation using this device a laborious task unless temperatures in the range of 150 to 180°C are being studied. The apparatus described by Pflug (1960) and devices similar to it appear to be practical ways for evaluating the heat destruction of microorganisms in superheated steam.

Flow Apparatus. Fox and Pflug (1968) developed a flow oven that could be used to expose spores dried in small metal cups to flowing hot gases. Silverman (1968) also developed a special apparatus in which spores deposited on planchets could be heated in flowing hot gases. With a flow apparatus and a gas humidity control system such as that described by Garst and Lindell (1970), microbial spores can be exposed to an almost limitless range of test conditions.

Closed Type of Test System

Glass Tube Systems. Murrell and Scott (1957, 1966) and Marshall et al. (1963) used sealed glass tube systems in their tests. Angelotti et al. (1968a) also used sealed glass tubes that were heated in an oil bath. The technique is identical to that used in wet-heat testing, except that the sample in the tube is dry.

Bruch et al. (1963) used aluminum blocks with a centrally located heating element, a thermoswitch, a thermometer or thermocouple well and six ports to hold 150-× 16-mm screw-cap test tubes. The thermometer and tube ports were covered with a lid. They reported that 1 to 2 minutes were required for samples on paper strips or glass to reach block temperature.

Cup-Can Systems. Pflug and Augustin (1962) developed the cup-thermal death time can technique, in which the small cups were placed inside a thermal death time can, and the can was sealed and then heated in saturated steam in a miniature retort. They found that the lag correction factor was surprisingly small and that it was possible to obtain 30 or more replicate samples as easily as 5 replicates were obtained using the thermoresistometer. Later, Pheil et al. (1967) found that, through the use of a plastic isolation chamber, it was possible to control the type of gas inside the can so they could study the effect of the gas atmosphere on thermal resistance.

Campbell (1969) describes a system in which stainless steel cups 0.312 inches in diameter by 0.375 inches deep inoculated with spores were loaded and sealed into 206×300 metal cans. Approximately 120 cups can be placed in each can. The sealing operation was carried out in a controlled environmental chamber. The atmosphere in the chamber was the atmosphere that surrounded the cups when the cans were sealed. The water content of the atmosphere in this area was controllable, so that the effect of a range of atmosphere water contents could be evaluated.

Heat Block System. Moore et al. (1969) used heat blocks for closed-system experiments. A heat block consisted of cylindrical top and bottom units made of stainless steel, sealed with a Teflon gasket and held together with cap screws. The top unit had a cavity 1.185 inches in diameter by 0.5 inches deep machined into the inside surface. The assembled heat blocks were 2.75 inches in diameter and 1.00 inch high. Spores to be heated in the heat block system were either deposited on a stainless steel disk or placed in thermal death time cups. Each heat block held five thermal death time cups. To give the desired relative humidity at the test temperature, the amount of water in the sealed block was controlled either by assembling and sealing the block in a controlled environmental chamber or by adding a calculated amount of water to the block at the time of sealing. The blocks were heated in either an oil bath or a fluidized bed sand bath.

Evaluating and Correcting for Heating and Cooling Lags Incurred in Thermal Resistance Testing

Ideally, thermal resistance testing should be done where the corrections for heating and cooling lags are zero. This is not possible for the majority of thermal resistance testing devices; therefore, corrections must be made for the lag in heating and the lag in cooling. Continuing with this reasoning, it becomes evident that the larger the mass and thermal capacity of the object being heated in the thermal resistance test, the larger will be the heating and cooling lags with correspondingly larger corrections.

Pflug and Esselen (1955) note that, when the sample under study fails to reach approximately 0.1°F below the exposure temperature, the data obtained are not truly representative of the thermal resistance at that temperature and should be discarded. Therefore, the time required for the sample to reach approximately 0.1°F below the heating medium temperature should be calculated at the same time that the heating- and cooling-lag corrections are evaluated; the time required for the sample to reach approximately 0.1°F below heating medium temperature should be the minimum heating time used in a thermal resistance testing program.

In carrying out tests to evaluate the heating and cooling lags, it is necessary to measure temperatures during heating and cooling of the thermal resistance test unit. Problems in the measurement of the heating rate of thermal resistance devices and in the determination of lag-correction factors are discussed by Sognefest and Benjamin (1944), Townsend et al. (1956), Ball and Olson (1957), Jaynes et al. (1961), Pflug (1960), and Augustin (1964). An extensive review of the heating and cooling lag problem, of the calculation of lag-correction factors, and of some lag-correction factor data has been prepared by Pflug (1988).

Data logging devices available today from many instrument manufacturers not only measure temperatures as a function of time, but also calculate the equivalent time for any specified temperature and z value. These instruments are useful in determining the lag-correction factors and are used routinely in some laboratories to determine the equivalent time received by the microorganism in the test system.

ANALYSIS OF HEAT-DESTRUCTION DATA

In the study of the heat destruction of microorganisms, the researcher is constantly confronted by the desire and need to measure and at the same time by the inability to measure. Direct enumeration of colonies formed by surviving organisms has many advantages, one of which is high statistical precision (Meynell and Meynell, 1965), but is not usable for product incubation and when the total number of survivors per replicate unit is less than about 100. End-point and FN (fraction-negative) or quantal methods are applicable to lower levels of survival, but are limited to the maximum population that can be measured. The sensitive nature of microorganisms to environmental conditions in general precludes combining data obtained from different experimental systems, for example, survivor curve and FN or end point.

Most of the practical uses of microbial heat destruction data require that the data be in semilogarithmic survivor curve form; if the semilogarithmic survivor curve is other than a straight line, direct use of the data is difficult. Data use limitations have encouraged researchers (1) to attempt to describe the patterns formed by the survivor data on the semilogarithmic graph by a single straight line, regardless of its true shape; and (2) to gather FN type data and then use an end-point method of analysis where D_T-values are calculated directly without facing the "shape of the survivor curve" problem.

In the discussion of the theory of death of microorganisms by heat, we observed that not all researchers obtain straight-line survivor curves. In fact, the variations in the shape of survivor curves are so great that one of the objectives of a thermal destruction test should be to determine the actual shape of the survivor curve, the other objective being the measurement of the rate of destruction of the organism. There is a separate and distinct survivor curve for each heating temperature; also, each substrate tested probably produces its own distinct survivor curve even though similar spores are used.

Once measurements are made, the experimenter must choose an appropriate and adequate method of analysis to use the data he has gathered and interpret them meaningfully. In the following paragraphs, we discuss the analysis of information collected from observations on microorganisms subjected to heat stress. The discussion falls into two categories: (1) treatment of counts made by direct enumeration of colonies formed by surviving organisms; and (2) treatment of data where there is only a dichotomous response by the organisms: growth or no growth.

The proper circumstances under which a researcher will choose to use either of the two broad types of analysis will become clear as the topics are developed.

Survivor Curve by Direct Enumeration

The most straightforward method of establishing a survivor curve is to heat representative aliquots of the suspension of microorganisms for different lengths of time and then estimate the number of survivors by plating aliquots of the heated suspension and, after incubation, counting colonies. The semilogarithmic survivor curve is generated when the logarithm of the numbers of surviving organisms is plotted as a function of heating time. Prior to the heat treatment, a known number of organisms are deposited in or on identical carrier units. These may be glass tubes, metal cups, metal disks, glass plates, or paper strips. Groups of the carrier units are subjected to the same heat stress environment for different lengths of time. The longest heating times are shorter than the shortest heating time for fraction-negative (FN) or quantal analysis. Heating times must be corrected for heating and cooling lags; therefore, the heating and cooling rate of the suspension in the test system is critical.

Following heating, appropriate dilutions are made in the recovery system, and aliquots are plated according to a standard microbiologic technique. An estimated number of survivors at each heating time is calculated, using the dilution factor and the appropriate plate counts. The experimental design regarding the number of replicate units heated, the number of serial dilutions made, and the number of replicate plates poured is critical if

total labor is to be minimal for the required data reliability.

Survivor curve determinations involve considerable technical difficulties in establishing the true shape of the curve. Any measurement of resistance in terms of survivors always involves two phases: (1) the actual or true survival of the organism following exposure to the lethal agent; and (2) the ability of the surviving organism to germinate, if a spore, and to reproduce and grow through a sufficient number of generations to be recognized as a colony of survivors under the subculture conditions used. Factors in the determination of the resistance of bacterial spores with reference to spore germination and its inhibition have been reviewed (Schmidt, 1955b). An altered reaction of the survivors, either favorable or unfavorable, to the recovery value of a given subculture medium may occur during the course of a given heat treatment, and this effect will be reflected in the survivor curve. If particulate matter is present in the suspending menstruum, difficulties in counting colonies may occur. Finally, in many cases, the important information to be determined is the resistance in a product based on the ability of the survivors to develop in the product. It is almost impossible to develop survivor curves where a food product must be used as the medium for the enumeration of survivors.

Researchers have observed that when the logarithm of the estimated number of surviving organisms is plotted against heating times on semilogarithmic paper, the survivor curve is often well described by a single straight line. This relationship is given the name of the logarithmic order of death model, which is described mathematically in the following paragraphs.

Let N_0 be the initial population of organisms, t the heating time, N the number of surviving organisms after time t, and D a parameter that depends on the temperature used for heating and other heat stress conditions. The semilog equation for the model is:

$$N(t) = N_0 10^{-\frac{t}{D}} \tag{11}$$

The parameter D is the time necessary for the microbial population to be reduced by 90%. This 90% reduction is equivalent to the straight line given by equation 11 crossing one log cycle on the semilog plot. Equivalent forms for equation 11 are:

$$\log N(t) = \log N_0 - t/D \tag{12}$$

$$N(t) = N_0 e^{-kt} \tag{13}$$

where $k = 2.3026/D$.

Equation 12 shows clearly the linear relationship between log N(t) and the heating time t. The representation in equation 13 becomes a useful form for mathematic manipulations. Once points are plotted from experimentally produced survivor data on semilog paper and the decision is made to represent the data by a straight line, the question arises as to how to fit the best straight line to the data. We are concerned here with an estimation problem; we seek to estimate a theoretic straight line from our sample values. We give here the least-squares method as an estimation procedure. The least-squares method makes the following assumptions: (1) the true model describing the relationship between the logarithm of the number of surviving organisms and heating time is a linear one; (2) the deviation in the log number of survivors from the straight line is a random variable with expected value zero; (3) the expected deviation is the same for all heating times; and (4) the deviations for different heating times are uncorrelated. Thus, the model we are postulating is the following:

$$y = \alpha + \beta t + \epsilon \qquad (14)$$

where, $y = \log N(t)$, the logarithm of the number of survivors at time t, t = heating time, α = the y-intercept at t = 0, β = slope of the line, ϵ = deviation component, a random variable with mean zero, constant variance equal to some value σ^2, and which is uncorrelated for different heating times.

If k observations have been made at various heating times $(t_1, t_2, \ldots t_k)$, not all necessarily distinct, we can derive estimates of α and β, which will be denoted $\hat{\alpha}$ and $\hat{\beta}$. This will be done by choosing α and β so as to minimize the following sum of squared deviations:

$$S = \sum_{i=1}^{k} \epsilon_i^2 = \sum_{i=1}^{k}[y_i - (\alpha + \beta t_i)]^2 \qquad (15)$$

By taking the partial derivatives $\dfrac{\partial S}{\partial \alpha}$ and $\dfrac{\partial S}{\partial \beta}$, we get two equations that, when set equal to zero and solved simultaneously for α and β, give:

$$\hat{\beta} = \frac{\sum_{i=1}^{k}(t_i - \bar{t}) y_i}{\sum_{i=1}^{k}(t_i - \bar{t})^2} \qquad (16)$$

$$\hat{\alpha} = \bar{y} - \hat{\beta}\bar{t} \qquad (17)$$

where

$$\bar{t} = \sum_{i=1}^{k} t_i/k, \quad \bar{y} = \sum_{i=1}^{k} y_i/k$$

An unbiased estimate of the variance σ^2 of the random variable ϵ is given by

$$\hat{\sigma}^2 = \frac{\sum_{i=1}^{k}(y_i - \hat{\alpha} - \hat{\beta}t_i)^2}{k-2} \qquad (18)$$

Similarly, estimates of the standard errors of $\hat{\alpha}$ and $\hat{\beta}$ can be given using the result for $\hat{\sigma}^2$:

$$S\hat{E}(\hat{\alpha}) = \left[\frac{\sum_{i=1}^{k} t_i^2}{k \sum_{i=1}^{k}(t_i - \bar{t})^2}\right]^{0.5} \hat{\sigma} \qquad (19)$$

$$S\hat{E}(\hat{\beta}) = \frac{\hat{\sigma}}{\left[\sum_{i=1}^{k}(t_i - \bar{t})^2\right]^{0.5}} \qquad (20)$$

Equations 15 to 20 are defining equations and can be expanded and put into a simpler form for computation.

Because there are estimates and α and β and standard errors of those estimates, we can form confidence intervals for the two parameters. The 95% confidence intervals based on our experimental data would be:

$$\hat{\alpha} \pm t_{.975}(k-2)\, S\hat{E}(\hat{\alpha}) \qquad (21)$$

$$\hat{\beta} \pm t_{.975}(k-2)\, S\hat{E}(\hat{\beta}) \qquad (22)$$

where $t_{.975}(k-2)$ is the 0.975 percentage point of the Student's t distribution with (k-2) degrees of freedom.

These confidence intervals for the intercept and slope parameters have the following interpretation in our survivor model: If the experiment is carried out in exactly the same way (using the same heating times, recovery techniques) for a large number of times, then we would expect the confidence intervals calculated from each set of data to cover the true values of α and β about 95% of the time.

Figure 6–12 illustrates an example of experimental data plotted on semilogarithmic paper with a straight line fitted by the least-squares procedure just described.

Draper and Smith (1966) treat the least-squares problem in greater detail. They discuss the implications of the assumptions we made on our fitted line as well as answers to the questions about the quality of fit of the line and fitting the best line.

One empiric method used in the laboratory to examine whether a single straight line describes well the observed data over the whole heating time interval is to look at $\hat{\alpha}$, the y-intercept of the fitted line, and $\log N_0$, the total number of organisms on each carrier unit at time zero. If a single straight line is a good fit to the data, then $\hat{\alpha}$ should estimate $\log N_0$. We define the ratio of $\hat{\alpha}$ to $\log N_0$ as the *intercept ratio* (IR).

$$IR = \frac{\hat{\alpha}}{\log N_0}$$

For values of $\hat{\alpha}$ close to $\log N_0$, the ratio will be nearly equal to unity. Stumbo (1973) gives examples of circum-

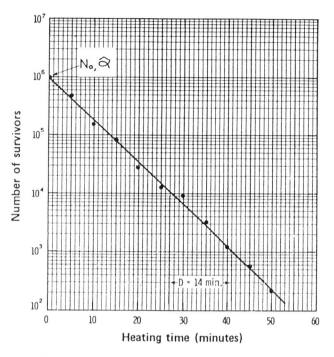

Fig. 6–12. Least-squares line fitted to semilogarithmic survivor data.

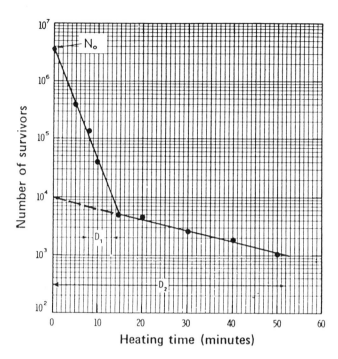

Fig. 6–14. Two least-squares lines fitted to a semilogarithmic survivor curve.

stances in which there are deviations from the straight line fit and provides possible explanations. Figure 6–13 shows an example of a survivor curve for which the IR value is not equal to 1 because of the deviation from linearity in the first portion of the heating interval.

In cases such as that seen in Figure 6–13, it is sometimes appropriate to leave out the data point for the initial

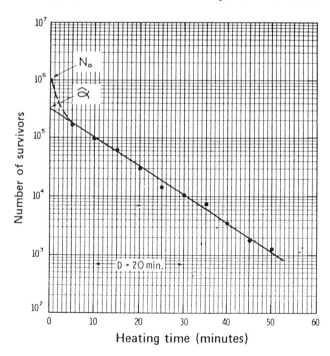

Fig. 6–13. Least-squares line fitted to semilogarithmic survivor data with the data point $(0, N_0)$ omitted.

number N_0 and fit the straight line to the remaining data points. It is justified when the initial nonlinear portion can be shown to be a reproducible phenomenon. The linear model given in equation 14 is redefined for only those heating times strictly greater than zero.

The parameter D defined in equation 11 is often the object of interest. The value D is a destruction rate index dependent on the type of organisms heated, temperature, relative humidity, and other heat stress parameters. An estimate of D, call it $\hat{D}$, can be obtained by comparing equations 11 and 14.

We see that $\hat{\beta}$ is an estimate of $\left(-\dfrac{1}{D}\right)$. From this we can get an estimate of D.

$$\hat{D} = -\frac{1}{\hat{\beta}} \qquad (23)$$

The estimate in equation 23 is called the quasi-least-squares estimator of D, in the terminology of Sundararaj (1971) and McHugh and Sundararaj (1972). The D just defined is not a true least-squares estimator of D, since the minimization of the sum of squares in equation 15 was with respect to $\beta = \left(-\dfrac{1}{D}\right)$ and not D. McHugh and Sundararaj (1972) describe various methods for estimating D, including quasi-least-squares and the weighted and unweighted least-squares methods, and the method of maximum likelihood.

An approximate 95% confidence interval for D can be

obtained from equation 23. If $\hat{\beta}_1 = \hat{\beta} - t_{.975}$ (k-2) $S\hat{E}$ $(\hat{\beta})$ and $\hat{\beta}_2 = \hat{\beta} + t_{.975}$ (k-2) $S\hat{E}$ $(\hat{\beta})$, the 95% C.I. for D is:

$$\left(-\frac{1}{\hat{\beta}_1}, -\frac{1}{\hat{\beta}_2}\right) \qquad (24)$$

It may be that, after plotting a survivor curve, the asumption of a single straight line is clearly not warranted. Such is the case in the example presented in Figure 6–14. The data may be well described, however, by fitting two straight lines simultaneously to two separate subintervals during the heating period, as indicated in Figure 6–14. There is little practical experience with such multiple regression fitting procedures with heat survivor data. The possibility remains here for future work to give a usable statistical tool for this kind of survivor data. It is important that the decision to fit two or three straight lines to survivor curve data be made on the basis of sufficient information. There is clearly a danger involved in assuming and fitting any model on the basis of two few data points. If, however, there is reproducible evidence to indicate that the model is well described by multiple lines, then an analysis scheme can be developed accordingly.

The straight lines fitted to survivor data and the corresponding D-value estimates can be usable tools in examining heat sterilization effects. The D value as an index to the behavior of organisms under heat stress environments has seen wide use. The D value itself is a tool that must be used with prudence to prevent misuse. To the previous discussion must be added a few additional notes. A single D value estimated from a least-square fitted line will not summarize well data that are essentially curvilinear. It is a parameter taken from a straight line and will more or less be an accurate index depending upon the viability of the straight line hypothesis. A survivor curve that is broken up into straight line segments for various portions of the heating interval may give rise to separate D-value estimates for each segment. The D-value concept is a usable tool here only if this multiple line model is an accurate, reproducible description of reality.

The applicability of the D-value index should also be restricted to those ranges of experimental times actually observed. There is a chance for potentially misleading results to occur when one extrapolates the model into areas where no observations were made. The straight lines fitted to the log number of surviving organisms are experimentally verified for only those time intervals in which observations took place.

A further discussion about the appropriateness of a D-value analysis and some of its limitations can be found in Pflug and Holcomb (1980).

Conclusions. The use that is to be made of thermal destruction survivor data is an important consideration in the type of data required and the amenability of the data to mathematic treatment. If data are to be used for a 99.00 or 99.90% reduction in number of organisms or

as a calibration curve for survival or biologic indicator tests, then it is necessary that an accurate survivor curve be available in the area of use. If, on the other hand, the thermal resistance data are ultimately to be used where N_0 is in the range of 10^4 and the probability of survival is 10^{-3} or 10^{-8}, then the direction or D value is critical, and FN or quantal-type of analysis coupled with knowledge of the survivor curve shape will give maximum information.

Survivor Curves From Fraction-Negative or Quantal Data

Fraction-negative (FN) data (quantal data) are experimental results in the form of a dichotomous response: the unit tested is either positive (showing growth) or negative (showing no growth).

In the design of sterilization processes, the objective is for all units to be free from microbial growth; therefore, it is logical to evaluate the efficiency of sterilization processes at conditions in which sterilization takes place. However, the heating of a single test unit containing a microbial inoculum to the point at which it is sterile tells the researcher little regarding the heat destruction characteristics of the microbial inoculum. As the science of sterilization microbiology progressed, researchers found that heating replicate inoculated units at a range of heating times in which, at the short heating times, all the units were positive, while at the long heating times, they were all negative, provided more information on the resistance of the microbial inoculum. When the number of replicate units tested was increased along with the number of heating times, still more information could be obtained from an experiment. Typical data are shown in Table 6–7. As the experimental procedures were improved, the methods of analysis of the data were refined. In recent years, the statistical characteristics of this quantal response region, or region between where all units show growth and all units are negative, have been explored. Understanding the relationship of heating time and the number of the fraction-multiple-replicate units negative in the quantal area is important in heat-resistance studies where complete sterility is desired or in evaluating the performance characteristics of biologic indicator units where several biologic indicators are placed in a load and where a single positive unit indicates a process failure.

In this discussion of the development of microbial survivor curves using data gathered in the quantal area, we: (1) discuss the historically important end-point methods that led to quantal analysis; (2) give a probability basis for quantal analysis; (3) describe the analysis of quantal data using the Spearman-Karber method; (4) discuss the design of experiments to gather data in the quantal range; and (5) discuss some problems in gathering and analyzing quantal data.

End-Point Method of Analysis

Bigelow and Esty (1920) describe a method of evaluating the thermal destruction of microorganisms that

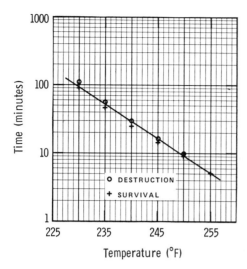

Fig. 6–15. Thermal death time curve for spores of PA 3679 in beef and gravy in thermal death time cans. From Pflug, I.J., and Schmidt, C.F. 1968. Thermal destruction of microorganisms. In *Disinfection, Sterilization and Preservation.* 1st Edition. Edited by C.A. Lawrence and S.S. Block. Philadelphia, Lea & Febiger.

they termed the "thermal death point in relation to time." Bigelow (1921) shortened the name to "thermal death time." In this method, the positive or negative results of multiple replicate unit tests as a function of time were indicated on a log time versus temperature graph by a plus sign when any of the replicate units were positive and a zero when all units at a given time were negative. The thermal death time was assumed to be between the longest heating time when a positive unit was obtained and the shortest heating time when all units were negative. Initially a single unit was tested at each time-temperature condition. Esty and Williams (1924) called attention to the fact that a "skip" (survival of organisms at a time beyond that at which sterility is indicated) often occurred when single tubes were used and suggested that if several units were tested at each time-temperature condition, this source of error or uncertainty could be eliminated. The present-day basis for end-point analysis was developed by Townsend et al. (1938), who used multiple times and replicated units for determining thermal death times.

End-point data treated as recommended by Townsend et al. (1938) to develop a thermal death time curve are shown in Figure 6–15. The data were obtained using a 10,000-spore inoculum of PA 3679 in beef and gravy using thermal death time cans and product incubation. This curve is almost ideal, because the straight line can be drawn above every survival point and below or through every destruction point, $F_0 = 9.5$ minutes, $z = 20°F$. Many curves will not fit the data quite as closely as this, although they may do so as the number of replicate units heated at each time interval is increased. The end-point method of analysis does not consider either the effect of the initial number of organisms or the number of replicate units in the test system. The end-point

methods were brought into the practical realm by using large initial numbers of organisms with small numbers (5 to 20) of replicate units to study commercial conditions where N_0 is relatively small but larger numbers of units are produced.

Analysis of Quantal Data Using MPN (Most-Probable-Number) Technique

Data in which a fraction of the replicate units are negative can be analyzed statistically using the MPN technique to yield the probable number of survivors at the respective heating time. Thermal destruction data developed specifically for MPN analysis are shown in Table 6–7, in which there are five test times when fraction-negative (FN) data were obtained.

Methods of evaluation of thermal destruction data have evolved relatively slowly; the most sophisticated methods are of relatively recent origin. The first step in the development of the MPN technique was an improvement of the then-used end-point analysis methods. Stumbo (1948a) proposed that each positive tube in a multiple replicate unit thermal destruction testing program where quantal data existed be considered to contain one viable organism. Subsequently, Stumbo et al. (1950) suggested that the MPN equation of Halvorson and Ziegler (1933) be used to evaluate more accurately the number of survivors when quantal data were obtained using a multiple replicate testing program.

The Halvorson and Ziegler (1933) equation,

$$N_U = \ln (n/r) = 2.303 \log_{10} (n/r) \qquad (25)$$

where n = number of units heated and r = number of units sterile, is the foundation of MPN analysis. It is the probability of the "no survivors term" of the Poisson equation.

The number of organisms in thermal destruction testing will be based on the number of organisms per replicate unit. N_0 is taken as the inital population per multiple replicate unit; N_U is the population per multiple replicate unit after a heat treatment of time U. (When we developed equation 11 we used t as the symbol for heating time. We have now switched to the symbol U— the equivalent or net heating time—the time corrected for any log in heating or cooling.) This standardization will in effect simplify the use of the equation $D_T = U/(\log N_0 - \log N_U)$; N_U is found using equation 25 (given previously) and $N_U = (n - r)/n$ when the Stumbo (1948a) method is used (which is quite accurate when the number of positive replicates is small).

Table 6–8 shows the relative survivors N_U as a function of the number of positive replicate units on the basis of 5, 10, and 20 replicate units. Figure 6–16 is a modified piece of multicycle semilogarithmic paper in which the percentage lines have been drawn so, if the initial number of organisms and approximate D_T value are known, the curve can be plotted on the paper and both the approximate level of survivors and the approximate num-

Table 6–7. *Thermal Destruction Rate Data for* Clostridium botulinum *Type B Spores Suspended in M/15 Sorensen's Phosphate Buffer (pH 7.0) and Heated at 110.0°C*

U Corrected Time (min)	n Number of Replicate Units Heated	n–r Number Showing Growth	r Number Sterile
3.90	6	6	0
5.90	6	6	0
7.90	6	4	2
9.90	6	3	3
11.90	6	1	5
13.90	6	0	6

$N_0 = 4.2 \times 10^7$ organisms per unit

ber of positive multiple replicate units can be determined directly from the graph.

The final result of an FN test is a time value U and the number of survivors N_U. These data can be used in either of two ways: (1) If large numbers of multiple replicates are evaluated, the values of U and N_U can be plotted as a survivor curve; and (2) using the equation $D_T = U/(\log N_0 - \log N_U)$, the D_T value can be calculated.

If we assume as an example the use of 100 replicates per time interval, it is possible to develop a survivor curve over the approximate 2½ log cycles between fractions negative of $\frac{1}{100}$ to $\frac{99}{100}$. It seems probable that when 20 or more replicate units are used per time interval, the experimenter could well develop a survivor curve over the area where his FN determinations are valid. Whenever the objective of the experiment is simply to develop general thermal resistance data, however, there

is a tendency to reduce the number of replicate units to 5 or 10, in which case there are usually not enough data to indicate the direction of the survivor curve.

The calculation of D values from MPN data is based on the assumption that the survivor curve is a straight line between N_0 and N_U. It has been mentioned previously that FN-MPN data can be used to establish a survivor curve. If the survivor curve established by MPN data is not coincident with the line connecting N_0 and N_U, then the D values calculated for various values of U and N_U using the methods of Stumbo (1948a) or Stumbo et al. (1950) will vary depending on the value of N_U, as discussed by Pflug and Esselen (1954).

The method of analysis of FN data using the MPN approach has been the subject of much work and discussion. There is general agreement that N_U can be estimated by the method of Stumbo (1948a) and that the Stumbo et al. (1950) use of the Halvorson and Ziegler (1933) equation gives a more precise estimate. It seems

Table 6–8. *Most Probable Number of Survivors**

n = 5	r n = 10	n = 20	$\frac{n}{r}$	$\log_{10}\frac{n}{r}$	N	$\log_{10} N$
			1			
		1	20.000	1.30103	2.9961	0.4766
	1	2	10.000	1.00000	2.3029	0.3623
		3	6.667	0.82391	1.8974	0.2782
1	2	4	5.000	0.69897	1.6097	0.2068
		5	4.000	0.60206	1.3865	0.1419
	3	6	3.333	0.52288	1.2041	0.0807
		7	2.857	0.45593	1.0500	0.0212
2	4	8	2.500	0.39794	0.9164	−0.0379
		9	2.222	0.34678	0.7986	−0.0977
	5	10	2.000	0.30103	0.6932	−0.1591
		11	1.818	0.25963	0.5957	−0.2250
3	6	12	1.667	0.22185	0.5109	−0.2918
		13	1.538	0.18709	0.4308	−0.3657
	7	14	1.429	0.15491	0.3567	−0.4477
		15	1.333	0.12494	0.2877	−0.5411
4	8	16	1.250	0.09691	0.2232	−0.6513
		17	1.176	0.07058	0.1625	−0.7892
	9	18	1.111	0.04575	0.1054	−0.9772
		19	1.053	0.02228	0.0513	−1.290
5	10	20	1.000	0.00000	—	

*Calculated using equation 25 (see text).

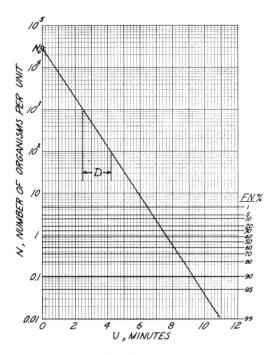

Fig. 6–16. A convenient chart for use in planning multiple replicate unit type of thermal destruction tests.

that problems of analysis usually stem from data problems; for example, the data are either skewed, inconsistent, or inadequate. From an overall analysis standpoint, it appears today that the methods of analysis are more precise than the experimental techniques. So long as this is the case, simplicity in understanding and use is the important factor in selecting a method for use. Perhaps we should note that the character of the data and the ultimate use of the data are really the determining factors; if we are limited to only one or two FN values, we have no choice but to use the method of Stumbo et al. (1950) to calculate individual D values and average these D values. Again, the method recommended for treating the data will depend on the ultimate use of the data. If the data are to be subjected to statistical treatment where heating media, subculture media, or other phases of the experiment are to be evaluated, then a method should be used that will allow the researcher to calculate a confidence interval for the D_T values.

Analysis of Quantal Data Using a Probability Model Combined with the Spearman-Karber Estimator, Identified as the Spearman-Karber Method

Equations 11 to 13 provided a vehicle for looking at survivor data gathered when a given number of organisms N_0 are subjected to a lethal heat agent for various times. If the N_0 organisms are heated for a long enough period, then it is clear by equation 11 that at some point the number of surviving organisms will be less than one. The equations treat the number of organisms as a continuous number, when in reality the number of organisms takes on integer values. We shall treat data gath-

ered in these extended heating periods by introducing the concept of the probability of sterility. (Note: in describing the Spearman-Karber method we will use "t" instead of "U" as the symbol for the corrected heating time and μ as the expected time until sterility; the estimated value is $\hat{\mu}$. The estimated value $\hat{\mu}$ is sometimes identified as the U_{SK} value.)

We will assume that equations 11 to 13 describe the mean or expected number of organisms recovered after any heating time t. Experimental variability would cause some deviation about these values even if the mechanism of death was exactly as described by these relationships. For any heating time t, it will be assumed that the surviving organisms follow a Poisson distribution, with the mean given by any of the equivalent forms of equation 11. If N(t), the mean number of surviving organisms, follows a Poisson distribution, at any time t, the probability of no organisms being present is given by the first term in the Poisson model:

$$P(t) = e^{-N(t)} \tag{26}$$

Substituting for the mean value N(t) from equation 13, we have:

$$P(t) = \exp\left[-N_0 \exp\left(-kt\right)\right] \tag{27}$$

The use of the Poisson model in the assay of organisms recovered from water or milk sampling has been discussed by Halvorson and Ziegler (1933) and by Cochran (1950). The justification for use of the Poisson model for estimating the probability of sterility for the logarithmic model has been investigated by Lewis (1956).

Equation 27 gives the probability of sterility (no growth) after a heating time t, given an N_0 and k_T value (or an equivalent D_T value). The shape of the curve described by equation 27 is given in Figure 6–17 for $N_0 = 10^6$ organisms and $k_T = 2.3026$ ($D_T = 1$ minute).

The function P(t) just defined in equation 27 is a cumulative distribution function in the probability sense, because it gives the probability of sterility at any time up to and including the time t. The probability density function associated with P(t) is defined as the derivative of P(t) with respect to t.

$$p(t) = \frac{dP(t)}{dt} \tag{28}$$

$$p(t) = N_0 k \exp\left(-kt\right) \exp\left[-N_0 \exp\left(-kt\right)\right]$$
$$\tag{29}$$

The function p(t) associated with the curve in Figure 6–17 is shown in Figure 6–18.

If we have the probability density function p(t), we

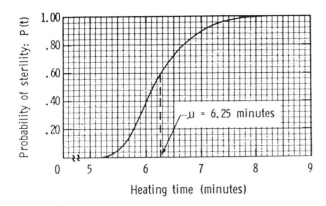

Fig. 6–17. The probability of sterility versus heating time ($N_0 = 10^6$ organisms, $D_T = 1$ minute).

can calculate the expected time μ until sterility. The result is given in equations 30 and 31:

$$\mu = \int_0^\infty t\, p(t)\, dt \tag{30}$$

$$\mu = \frac{\gamma + \ln N_0}{k} \tag{31}$$

where $\gamma = .57722$, Euler's constant.

The heating time μ is the time we expect to observe before a sample of N_0 organisms with a given k value becomes sterile. Because the function $p(t)$ is not symmetric, the mean and median t values for the function are not the same. As given in Figures 6–17 and 6–18, the mean for the given curve is $\mu = 6.25$, corresponding to the point where the probability of sterility is $P(6.25) = 0.57$.

The median is given by the point $t = 6.16$ where $P(6.16) = 0.50$ for the data.

Other Properties of p(t)

If t has a probability density function given by $p(t)$, then the mean value of t is given by equation 31. The

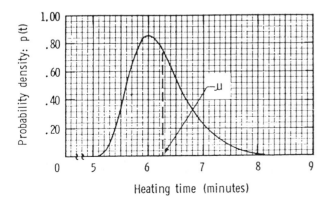

Fig. 6–18. The probability density function for the cumulative distribution in Figure 6–17.

variance of t is an indication of the spread of the curve $p(t)$ on the t-scale and is given in equations 32 and 33:

$$var\ (t) = \int_0^\infty (t - \mu)^2\, p(t)\, dt \tag{32}$$

$$var\ (t) = (\beta - \gamma^2)/k^2 \tag{33}$$

where $\gamma = .57722$, Euler's constant.

$$\beta = \int_0^\infty (\ln y)^2\, e^{-y}\, dy = 1.978$$

The variance of t for $N_0 = 10^6$ organisms and $k = 2.3026$ (Fig. 6–18) is approximately:

$$var\ (t) = 1.645/k^2 = 0.310$$

The mode or maximum value of $p(t)$ is found by solving equation 34 for t:

$$\frac{dp(t)}{dt} = 0 \tag{34}$$

When we solve equation 34 for t we find that the maximum value of $p(t)$ results when:

$$t_{mode} = \ln N_0/k \tag{35}$$

$$Max\ p(t) = p(\ln N_0/k) = k/e \tag{36}$$

For the data in Figure 6–18: $t_{mode} = 6.00$, $p(t_{mode}) = 0.847$

It can also be shown that changing the N_0 by a factor A to AN_0 translates the curve on the t axis by a factor ln A/k, where the sign of ln A determines whether the shift is to the right or left.

In conclusion, we can say that the mean or placement of the curve $p(t)$ on the t axis depends on both N_0 and k, but that the variance or spread of the curve depends only on k. This information can be useful in the design of quantal assays where prior estimates of the k or the D value are available.

Sampling Procedure

In the direct enumeration experiment, we heat N_0 organisms for a period of time t and then count the number of survivors recovered and plated on culture medium. The heating times in the quantal assay experiment will be longer, and we will record only growth or no growth of survivors in the recovery medium. If we subject n replicate carriers, each with N_0 organisms, to heat for a time t, and r of the carriers show no survivors after recovery, then we have an estimate of $P(t)$ for the time t.

$$P(t) = \frac{r}{n} \tag{37}$$

The data used in our analysis of quantal experiments will consist of these estimates $\hat{P}(t_i)$ for heating times (t_1, t_2, . . . t_k) and an estimate of N_0, the number of organisms at time zero.

Generally, the N_0 will have greater precision than the other estimates calculated from the data in the experiments and for this reason will be assumed to be a known constant and not a random variable in the analysis.

Spearman-Karber Estimation

The use of the Spearman-Karber (S-K) estimator has been discussed by many authors, including Armitage and Allen (1950), Lewis (1956), Finney (1964), and Church and Cobb (1975). Application of the S-K procedure in analyzing serial dilution assays, a problem similar to the one discussed here, is treated in a paper by Johnson and Brown (1961). An extensive investigation of the properties of the S-K estimation procedure in bioassay has been reported by Brown (1959).

We are using the S-K procedure to estimate the mean time until sterility μ, defined in equation 31, from a set of experimental data gathered in the quantal region. The quantal region in microbial heat destruction tests are those data sets where the probability of sterility is significantly different from either 0 or 1, for example, between the values of $P(t) = 0.01$ and $P(t) = 0.99$. The estimate of μ, called $\hat{\mu}$, is useful in comparing sets of quantal data. The k or D value can be estimated using equation 31 if we have an estimate of μ and a value for N_0.

When r_i is the number of sterile replicates out of n_i heated to a time t_i, then the S-K estimate of μ is given by:

$$\hat{\mu} = \sum_{i=1}^{k-1} \left(\frac{t_{i+1} + t_i}{2} \right) \left(\frac{r_{i+1}}{n_{i+1}} - \frac{r_i}{n_i} \right) \qquad (38)$$

If successive times differ by a constant d and the same number of replicates n is heated at all times, we can write equation 38 as:

$$\hat{\mu} = t_k - \frac{d}{2} - \frac{d}{n} \sum_{i=1}^{k-1} r_i \qquad (39)$$

The reasoning behind the S-K value given in equations 38 and 39 may not be clear. Actually, the S-K value is nothing more than the quantal version of an arithmetic mean. The heating interval (t_1, t_2, . . . t_k) should be chosen to cover completely the quantal region. The first time t_1 should show zero sterile replicates or $r_1 = 0$. The last time interval t_k should have all sterile replicates or $r_k = n_k$. If a set of experimental data has been gathered, the first t_1 should be chosen so that no times less than t_1 have replicates that are sterile. Similarly, the time t_k should be chosen so that no replicates at times larger than t_k show growth.

It can be seen from equation 38 that a sequence of all

positive replicates at times less than t_1 will add nothing to the estimate of μ. Likewise, a sequence of all sterile replicates at times larger than t_k contribute nothing to the estimation of μ.

Properties of $\hat{\mu}$

The S-K value $\hat{\mu}$ is actually a biased estimate of μ, with the bias depending on the t_1 chosen and the spacing of the heating times. The t_1 determines, for equal spacing d, the placing of the observation mesh on the quantal region and thus affects the determination of $\hat{\mu}$. The bias is independent, however, of the number of replicates n_i used at each heating time. Brown (1959) discusses this bias component, and Johnson and Brown (1961) give some numeric results. They conclude that, if t_1 is chosen randomly, d is reasonably small, and the observations span the quantal region well ($P(t_1) \leq 0.01$ and $P(t_k) \geq 0.99$), then the bias component is negligible and the expected value of $\hat{\mu}$ given a particular t_1 is μ, to a good approximation.

The variance of $\hat{\mu}$ can also be shown to be conditional on the t_1 chosen. The expression for the variance of $\hat{\mu}$ given the equal spacing and number of replicates in equation 39 can be written as:

$$V(\hat{\mu}|t_1) = \frac{d^2}{n} \sum_{i=1}^{k-1} P(t_i) \left[1 - P(t_i) \right] \qquad (40)$$

The estimated variance for the $\hat{\mu}$ defined in equation 39 is given by:

$$\hat{V}(\hat{\mu}|t_1) = \frac{d^2}{n^2 (n-1)} \sum_{i=1}^{k-1} r_i (n - r_i) \qquad (41)$$

When t_1 is randomly chosen and the heating times cover the quantal region well, then the estimate for $\hat{V}(\hat{\mu}|t_1)$ may be taken as a good estimate for the unconditional variance $V(\hat{\mu})$. If d, in addition, is small compared to the length of the quantal region, the following approximation for $V(\hat{\mu})$ is given by Johnson and Brown (1961):

$$\hat{V}(\hat{\mu}) \doteq \frac{d \ln 2}{n} \qquad (42)$$

The approximate 95% confidence interval for μ is given by:

$$\hat{\mu} \pm 2\sqrt{\hat{V}(\hat{\mu})} \qquad (43)$$

Estimation of D from $\hat{\mu}$

Solving equation 31 for k, we get the following expression:

$$k = \frac{.57722 + \ln N_0}{\mu} \qquad (44)$$

and since $k = 2.3026/D$, we have:

$$D_T = \frac{2.3026\ \mu}{.57722 + \ln N_0} \qquad (45)$$

To get an estimate for D when N_0 is known, we put in the S-K value for μ, giving:

$$\hat{D}_T = \frac{2.3026\ \hat{\mu}}{.57722 + \ln N_0} \qquad (46)$$

or

$$\hat{D}_T = \frac{\hat{\mu}}{.2507 + \log N_0} \qquad (47)$$

The 95% confidence interval for D_T can be estimated by putting in equation 47 the lower and upper 95% confidence points for μ.

Sample Calculations

Some sample calculations for the data in Table 6–9 will be made using the Spearman-Karber estimate procedure.

Using equation 39:

$$\hat{\mu} = 13.90 - \left(\frac{2}{2}\right) - \frac{2}{6}(0 + 2 + 3 + 5)$$
$$= 9.57\ \text{min.}$$

Using equation 41:

$$\hat{V}(\hat{\mu}) = \frac{(2)^2}{(6)^2(5)}\,[(0)\,(6) + (2)\,(4)$$
$$+ (3)\,(3) + (5)\,(1)] = 0.49$$

The 95% confidence interval for μ:

Lower: $9.57 - 2\sqrt{.49} = 8.17$ minutes

Upper: $9.57 + 2\sqrt{.49} = 10.97$ minutes

Using equation 47:

$$\hat{D}_T = \frac{9.57}{.2507 + \log(4.2 \times 10^7)} = 1.22\ \text{min.}$$

The 95% confidence interval for D_T:

Lower: $\dfrac{8.17}{.2507 + \log(4.2 \times 10^7)} = 1.04\ \text{min.}$

Upper: $\dfrac{10.97}{.2507 + \log(4.2 \times 10^7)} = 1.39\ \text{min.}$

Designing the Experiment

In applying the procedures just described, the first heating time must be chosen to result in all replicate tubes being positive for growth. Similarly, the last heating time should produce all sterile replicate tubes. Range-finding experiments may be necessary to discover the quantal region so that an experiment can be designed to satisfy these restrictions. It is recommended as a minimum that three heating times be represented in the quantal data between the times showing all growth and the times with complete sterility.

It can be seen from the variance formula for $\hat{\mu}$ that a better estimate of μ and hence D_T can be obtained in two ways: increasing the number of heating times sampled in the quantal region, thus decreasing d, and increasing the number of replicate tubes of each heating time. The implication of equation 42 is that doubling the number of heating times (halving the size of d) would have the same effect on the variance estimate of $\hat{\mu}$ and the confidence interval for μ as doubling the number of replicate units at each heating time. Decreasing the size of d also decreases the bias in estimating μ. There is a practical lower limit, however, on the size of d, which may depend on equipment and human factors.

The parameter (N_0), the initial number of organisms, has been considered a known constant throughout the preceding calculations. In a given situation, the exact value of N_0 may never be known with exact certainty.

Table 6–9. *Microbial Heat Destruction Data (From Table 6–7) Analyzed for Use in Spearman-Karber Estimation Procedure*

Corrected Heating Time t, minutes		Number of Replicate Units Heated, n	Number Showing Growth n-r	Number Sterile r
3.90		6	6	0
5.90		6	6	0
7.90	↑	6	4	2
9.90	Quantal region	6	3	3
11.90	↓	6	1	5
13.90		6	0	6

$N_0 = 4.2 \times 10^7$ organisms per unit; $d = 2$ minutes; $n = 6$

t_1 longest heating time where none of the units are negative (at all shorter heating times, all units are positive) = 5.90 minutes

t_k first heating time where all units are negative (at all longer heating times, all units are negative) = 13.90 minutes

Using a value of N_0 that is higher or lower than the true value may lead to some error in the estimation of D_T. It can be shown, for example, that assuming N_0 to be 10^6 organisms when the true value is 0.5×10^6 can lead to a 5% underestimate in the calculation of D_T. It becomes important, therefore, to accurately determine N_0 to improve the estimation of the D_T value in an experimental setting.

It has also been tacitly assumed in the discussion up to this point that the D_T value, though unknown, is constant across an experimental series. Variation in the estimated D_T values may occur owing to slight changes in the resistance of the test organisms or to minor fluctuations in the delivered sterilization cycle. It is not possible to tell from the data of a single quantal experiment whether or not there is time-to-time variation in the underlying D_T value. Comparisons must be made between replicated quantal experiments to discover whether additional sources of variability are present in these estimation procedures.

USE OF SURVIVOR CURVE DATA FOR THE DESIGN OF HEAT STERILIZATION PROCESSES

When the results of the heat-resistance tests are available either in the form of a D_T value or a semilogarithmic survivor curve, then we can proceed to establish the F_T or sterilization value of the processes. One approach to process design is to use the equation $F_T = nD_T$, where n is the number of logs of destruction that we are seeking. As an example, let us assume that we wish to obtain an F_T sterilizing value for a clean drug product in bottles in which there are no more than 100 resistant organisms per bottle and where the most resistant organism has a $D_{121.1°C}$ value not exceeding 1.0 minute. If we want the poststerilization probability of a contaminated bottle not to exceed 10^{-6}, we must design for a reduction of eight logs. Using the equation $F_T = nD_T$, we calculate:

$$F_{121.1°C} = 8(1.0 \text{ minute}) = 8.0 \text{ minutes}$$

A second approach to sterilization process design that is possible in some situations is to develop a survivor curve in which the reduction in the numbers of organisms from the beginning to the end of the survivor curve approximates the reduction that will occur in practice under worse case conditions. In the drug example, we anticipate at most an eight-log reduction. Therefore, if we can develop a survivor curve starting where $N_0 = 10^9$ per unit and extending through $N_U = 10$ per unit, we can determine directly from this survivor curve graph the F_T value or sterilization time. The values calculated previously are usually just the starting point for the design of commercial sterilization processes, because neither the resistance levels of the natural microflora nor the numbers of organisms of each different resistance level are known. The usual practice is to evaluate the

resistance of the most resistant organism that we think will be in the product. Because spore crops of this most resistant organism have to be produced in a laboratory, there is the question of the relative resistance of laboratory-grown spores compared to the spores in nature. The general procedure that we follow today is to assume that spores in nature are at least as resistant as the spores grown in the laboratory. As we proceed to make more accurate sterilization process design, will have to know more about the relative resistance of organisms in nature versus those grown in the laboratory.

Somewhere in the design of sterilization processes, an allowance must be made for unknown factors and errors. The sterilization process design, F_T, is a convenient place to include provision for the process unknown. Therefore, the final design value will be a judgment based on the laboratory survivor data and process reliability experience.

DETERMINING THE TEMPERATURE COEFFICIENT OF MICROBIAL DESTRUCTION

In some heat-sterilization processes, the lethal effect must be interpreted over a range of temperatures; in others it must be possible to determine an equivalent process at another temperature. Both these situations require the use of a temperature coefficient model. The different temperature coefficient models have been discussed in the introductory section of this chapter. Although several models are available, only that of Bigelow (1921) has been set into an overall system where it is readily usable in sterilization process design and evaluation. The key value in the Bigelow model is the z value, which is used along with the general method and the method of Ball (1923, 1928), Ball and Olson (1957), and Stumbo (1973) for heat process calculations where the lethal effect must be integrated over a range of temperatures and for calculating equivalent sterilizing values at other temperatures.

The Bigelow model only provides the temperature coefficient. End-point data in the form of F_T or D_T values can be plotted on a log scale against temperature on an arithmetic scale, and the resulting temperature coefficient graph can be analyzed for the z value. The z value is the number of degrees of temperature change required for the F or D value to change by a factor of 10. The temperature coefficient (z) can also be calculated when D or F value data are available at two different temperatures (T_1, T_2) using the following equations:

$$z = \frac{T_2 - T_1}{\log D_1 - \log D_2} \quad (48)$$

$$z = \frac{T_2 - T_1}{\log F_1 - \log F_2} \quad (49)$$

The authors gratefully acknowledge the assistance of Geraldine Smith in the revision of this chapter.

REFERENCES

Alderton, G., and Snell, N. 1963. Base exchange and heat resistance in bacterial spores. Biochem. Biophys. Res. Commun., 10, 139–143.

Alderton, G., and Snell, N. 1969a. Bacterial spores: chemical sensitization to heat. Science, 163, 1212–1213.

Alderton, G., and Snell, N. 1969b. Chemical states of bacterial spores: dry heat resistance. Appl. Microbiol., 17, 745–749.

Alderton, G., and Snell, N. 1970. Chemical states of bacterial spores: dry heat resistance and its kinetics at intermediate water activity. Appl. Microbiol., 19, 565–572.

Alderton, G., Thompson, P.T., and Snell, N. 1964. Heat adaptation and ion exchange in Bacillus megaterium spores. Science, 143, 141–143.

Amaha, M., and Ordal, Z.J. 1957. Effect of divalent cations in the sporulation medium on the thermal death rate of Bacillus coagulans var. thermoacidurans. J. Bacteriol., 74, 596.

Amaha, M., and Sakaguchi, K. 1954. Effects of carbohydrates, proteins and bacterial cells in the heating media on the heat resistance of Clostridium sporogenes. J. Bacteriol., 68, 338–345.

Amaha, M., and Sakaguchi, K. 1957. The mode and kinetics of death of the bacterial spores by moist heat. J. Gen. Appl. Microbiol., 3, 163–193.

Andersen, A.A., and Michener, H.D. 1950. Preservation of foods with antibiotics. I. The complementary action of subtilin and mild heat. Food Technol., 4, 188–189.

Anderson, E.B., and Meanwell, L.J. 1936. Studies in bacteriology of low temperature pasteurization. Part II. The heat resistance of a thermoduric streptococcus grown at different temperatures. J. Dairy Res., 7, 182–191.

Anderson, E.E., Esselen, W.B., and Fellers, C.R. 1949. Effect of acids, salts, sugars, and other food ingredients on thermal resistance of Bacillus thermoacidurans. Food Res., 14, 499–510.

Anderson, T.E. 1959. Some Factors Affecting the Thermal Resistance Values of Bacterial Spores as Determined with a Thermoresistometer. M.S. Thesis, Michigan State University.

Anellis, A., Lubas J., and Rayman, M.M. 1954. Heat resistance in liquid eggs of some strains of the genus Salmonella. Food Res., 19, 377–395.

Angelotti, R., et al. 1968a. Influence of spore moisture content on the dry heat resistance of Bacillus subtilis var. niger. Appl. Microbiol., 16, 735–745.

Angelotti, R., et al. 1968b. Protective mechanisms affecting dry heat sterilization. In Sterilization Techniques for Instruments and Materials as Applied to Space Research Edited by P.N.A. Sneath. Paris, Muray-Print, pp. 59–74. (CO-SPAR Tech. Man. No. 4.)

Aref, H., and Cruess, W.V. 1934. An investigation of thermal death point of Saccharomyces ellipsoideus. J. Bacteriol., 27, 443–452.

Armitage, P., and Allen, I. 1950. Methods of estimating LD50 in quantal response data. J. Hyg., 48, 298–322.

Augustin, J.A.L. 1964. Recovery Patterns of Putrefactive Anaerobe No. 3679 in Various Subculture Media Following Moist and Dry Heat Treatment. Ph.D. Thesis, Michigan State University.

Baird-Parker, A.C., and Baillie, M.A.H. 1974. The inhibition of Clostridium botulinum by nitrite and sodium chloride. In Proceedings of the International Symposium on Nitrite in Meat Products. Edited by B. Krol and B.J. Tinbergen. Wageningen, The Netherlands.

Ball, C.O. 1923. Thermal process time for canned food. Bull. Natl. Res. Council, 7, Part 1, No. 37, 76 pp.

Ball, C.O. 1928. Mathematical solution of problems on thermal processing of canned foods. Univ. Calif. Publ. Public Health, 1, 230 pp.

Ball, C.O. 1958. Discussion of a paper by Mikio Amaha and Kinichiro Sakaguchi titled: "The mode and kinetics of death of the bacterial spores by moist heat." J. Gen. Appl. Microbiol., 4, 312–316.

Ball, C.O., and Olson, F.C.W. 1957. Sterilization in Food Technology. New York, McGraw-Hill.

Bartlett, C.J., and Kline, F. 1913. Resistance of microorganisms suspended in glycerine or oil to the sterilizing action of heat. Science, 38, 372 (N.S.).

Baumgartner, J.G. 1938. Heat sterilized reducing sugars and their effect on the thermal resistance of bacteria. J. Bacteriol., 36, 369–382.

Baumgartner, J.G., and Wallace, M.D. 1934. The destruction of microorganisms in the presence of sugars. Part I. The role of sucrose in the commercial processing of canned fruits. J. Soc. Chem. Ind., 53, 294–297T.

Beamer, P.R., and Tanner, F.W. 1939a. Resistance of non-sporeforming bacteria to heat. Zentralbl. Bakteriol. Parasitenk., II, 100, 81–98.

Beamer, P.R., and Tanner, F.W. 1939b. Heat resistance studies on selected yeasts. Zentralbl. Bakteriol. Parasitenk., II, 100, 202–211.

Bigelow, W.D. 1921. The logarithmic nature of thermal death time curves. J. Infect. Dis., 29, 528–536.

Bigelow, W.D., and Esty, J.R. 1920. Thermal death point in relation to time of typical thermophilic organisms. J. Infect. Dis., 24, 602.

Binkerd, E.F., and Kolari, O.E. 1975. The history and use of nitrate and nitrite in the curing of meat. Food Cosmet. Toxicol., 13, 655–661.

Bond, W.W., Favero, M.S., and Korber, M.R. 1973. Bacillus Sp. ATCC 27380: A spore with extreme resistance to dry heat. Appl. Microbiol., 26, 614–616.

Bond, W.W., Favero, M.S., Petersen, N.J., and Marshall, J.H. 1970. Dry heat inactivation kinetics of naturally occurring spore populations. Appl. Microbiol., 20, 573–578.

Bond, W.W., Favero, M.S., Petersen, N.J., and Marshall, J.H. 1971. Relative frequency distribution of D125c values for spore isolates from the Mariner-Mars 1969 spacecraft. Appl. Microbiol., 21, 832–836.

Brannen, J.P. 1968a. A rational model for thermal sterilization of microorganisms. Math. Biosci., 2, 165–170.

Brannen, J.P. 1968b. On logarithmic extrapolation of microbial survivor curves for planetary quarantine requirements. Space Life Sci., 1, 150–152.

Brannen, J.P. 1970. On the role of DNA in wet heat sterilization of microorganisms. J. Theor. Biol., 27, 425–432.

Brannen, J.P., and Garst, D.M. 1972. Dry heat inactivation of Bacillus subtilis var. niger spores as a function of relative humidity. Appl. Microbiol., 23, 1125–1130.

Braun, O.F., Hays, G.L., and Benjamin, H.A. 1941. Use of dry sugar in sweetening foods canned in syrup. Part II. Bacteriological aspects. Decrease in lethal value of sterilization process results from use of dry sugar in packing sweet potatoes. Food Ind., 13, 64–65.

Brown, B. 1959. Some properties of the Spearman estimator in bioassay. Techn. Rept. No. 6, Contract Nonr2582(00), Task NR 042–200.

Bruch, C.W. 1966. Dry-heat sterilization for planetary-impacting spacecraft. Proc. Natl. Conf. Spacecraft Sterilization Technol. NASA SP-108.

Bruch, C.W., Koesterer, M.G., and Bruch, M.K. 1963. Dry-heat sterilization: Its development and application to components of exobiological space probes. Dev. Ind. Microbiol., 4, 334–342.

Bruch, M.K., and Smith, F.W. 1968. Dry heat resistance of spores of Bacillus subtilis var. niger on Kapton and Teflon film at high temperatures. Appl. Microbiol., 16, 1841–1846.

Campbell, J.E. 1969. Ecology and thermal inactivation of microbes in and on interplanetary space vehicle components. In 18th Quarterly Report of Progress. NASA Research Project R-R-36-015-001.

Campbell, J.E. 1974. Ecology and thermal inactivation of microbes in and on interplanetary space vehicle components. In 37th Quarterly Report of Progress. NASA Order No. W-13411.

Campbell, L.L., Jr., and O'Brien, R.T. 1955. Antibiotics in food preservation. Food Technol., 9, 461.

Campbell, L.L., and Sniff, E.E. 1959. Effect of subtilin and nisin on spores of Bacillus coagulans. J. Bacteriol., 77, 766–770.

Cerf, O. 1977. Tailing of survivor curves of bacterial spores. J. Appl. Bacteriol., 42, 1–19.

Chapman, P.A., and Pflug, I.J. 1973. Effect of the biological indicator envelope on the heat destruction rate of Bacillus stearothermophilus spores. Bacteriol. Proc., 73, E144.

Chick, H. 1908. An investigation of the laws of disinfection. J. Hyg., 8, 92–158.

Church, J.D., and Cobb, E.B. 1975. An improved Spearman-type estimator for the exponential parameter. Biometrics, 31, 913–920.

Cochran, W.G. 1950. Estimation of bacterial densities by means of the 'the most probable number.' Biometrics, 6, 105–116.

Corry, J.E.L. 1974. The effect of sugars and polyols on the heat resistance of salmonellae. J. Appl. Bacteriol., 37, 31–43.

Corry, J.E.L. 1976a. The effect of sugars and polyols on the heat resistance and morphology of osmophilic yeasts. J. Appl. Bacteriol., 40, 269–276.

Corry, J.E.L. 1976b. Sugar and polyol permeability of Salmonella and osmophilic yeast cell membranes measured by turbidimetry, and its relationship to heat resistance. J. Appl. Bacteriol., 40, 277–284.

Curran, H.R. 1934. The influence of some environmental factors upon thermal resistance of bacterial spores. J. Bacteriol., 27, 26.

Curran, H.R. 1935. The influence of some environmental factors upon the thermal resistance of bacterial spores. J. Infect. Dis., 56, 196–202.

Davis, N.S., Silverman, G.J., and Keller, W.H. 1963. Combined effects of ultra high vacuum and temperature on the viability of some spores and soil organisms. Appl. Microbiol., 11, 202–211.

Denny, C.B., Reed, J.M., and Bohrer, C.W. 1961a. Effect of tylosin and heat on spoilage bacteria in canned corn and canned mushrooms. Food Technol., 15, 338–340.

Denny, C.B., Shaope, L.E., and Bohoer, C.W. 1961b. Effect of tylosin and nisin on canned food spoilage bacteria. Appl. Microbiol., 9, 108–110.

Dickson, E.C., Burke, G.S., Beck, D., and Johnston, J. 1925. Studies on thermal death time of spores of Clostridium botulinum. J. Infect. Dis., 36, 472–483.

Doyle, J.E., and Ernst, R.R. 1967. Resistance of Bacillus subtilis var. niger spores occluded in water-insoluble crystals to three sterilization agents. Appl. Microbiol., 15, 726–730.

Draper, N.R., and Smith, H. 1966. Applied Regression Analysis. New York, John Wiley & Sons.

Dring, G.J., Ellar, D.J., and Gould, G.W. (Eds.). 1985. Fundamental and Applied Aspects of Bacterial Spores. London, Academic Press.

Drummond, D.W. 1972. Effects of humidity, location, surface finish, and separator thickness on the dry heat destruction of Bacillus subtilis var. niger spores located between mated surfaces. Ph.D. thesis, Division of Environmental Health, University of Minnesota.

Drummond, D.W., and Pflug, I.J. 1970. Dry heat destruction of Bacillus subtilis spores on surfaces: effect of humidity in an open system. Appl. Microbiol., 20, 805–809.

El-Bisi, H.M., and Ordal, Z.J. 1956a. The effect of certain sporulation conditions on the thermal death rate of Bacillus coagulans var. thermoacidurans. J. Bacteriol., 71, 1–9.

El-Bisi, H.M., and Ordal, Z.J. 1956b. The effect of sporulation temperature on the thermal resistance of Bacillus coagulans var. thermoacidurans, J. Bacteriol., 71, 10–16.

Ellicker, P.R., and Frazier, W.C. 1938. Influence of time and temperature of incubation on heat resistance of Escherichia coli. J. Bacteriol., 36, 83–98.

Esselen, W.B., and Pflug, I.J. 1956. Thermal resistance of putrefactive anaerobe No. 3679 spores in vegetables in the temperature range of 250–290°F. Food Technol., *10*, 557–560.

Esty, J.R. 1923. The heat resistance of *B. botulinus* spores. Am. J. Public Health, *13*, 108–113.

Esty, J.R., and Meyer, K.F. 1922. The heat resistance of the spores of *B. botulinus* and allied anaerobes. XI. J. Infect. Dis., *31*, 650–663.

Esty, J.R., and Williams, C.C. 1924. Heat resistance of bacterial spores. J. Infect. Dis., *34*, 518–528.

Eyring, H. 1935. The activated complex and the absolute rate of chemical reactions. Chem. Rev., *17*, 65–77.

Fay, A.C. 1934. The effect of hypertonic sugar solution on the thermal resistance of bacteria. J. Agric. Res., *48*, 453–468.

Fazio, T., White, R.H., Dusold, L.R., and Howard, J.W. 1973. Nitrosopyrrolidine in cooked bacon. J. Assoc. Off. Anal. Chem., *56*, 919–921.

Federal Register. 1988. Nisin preparation: affirmation of GRAS status as a direct human food ingredient. *53*, 11247.

Finney, D.J. 1964. *Statistical Method in Biological Assay.* 2nd Edition. London, Charles Griffin.

Fox, K., and Pflug, I.J. 1968. Effect of temperature and gas velocity on the dry-heat destruction rate of bacterial spores. Appl. Microbiol., *16*, 343–348.

Frederickson, A.G. 1966. Stochastic models for sterilization. Biotechnol. Bioeng., *8*, 167–182.

Fry, R.M., and Greaves, R.I.N. 1951. The survival of bacteria during and after drying. J. Hyg., *49*, 220.

Garst, D.M., and Lindell, K.F. 1970. *A Precisely Controlled, Low Range Humidity System.* NASA Contract No. W-12853, Report SC-RR-70-775. Albuquerque, NM, Sandia Laboratories.

Gay, F.P., Atkins, K.N., and Holden, M. 1931. The resistance of dehydrated pneumococci to chemicals and heat. J. Bacteriol., *22*, 295–307.

Gerhardt, P., and Murrell, W.G. 1978. Basis and mechanism of spore resistance: a brief preview. In *Spores VII.* Edited by G. Chambliss and J.C. Vary. Washington, D.C., American Society for Microbiology.

Gibbs, B.M., and Hurst, A. 1964. Limitations of nisin as a preservative in non-dairy food. In *Proceedings 4th International Symposium on Food Microbiology.* Göteburg, SIK, pp. 151–165.

Gillespy, T.G. 1936–1937. Studies on the mould *Byssochlamys fulva.* Progress report. Annu. Rep. Fruit Veg. Presvn. Stn. Campden, 68–75.

Gillespy, T.G. 1947. The heat resistance of the spores of thermophilic bacteria. II. Thermophilic anaerobes. Annu. Rep. Fruit Veg. Presvn. Stn. Campden, 40–54.

Gillespy, T.G. 1948. The heat resistance of spores of thermophilic bacteria. III. Thermophilic anaerobes (con't). Ann. Rep. Fruit Veg. Presvn. Stn. Campden, 34–43.

Glasstone, S., Laidler, K.J., and Eyring, H. 1941. *The Theory of Rate Processes.* New York, McGraw-Hill Book Co.

Görtzen, S. 1937. Untersuchungen über die Widerstandsfähigkeit nativer anaerober Erdsporen gegen siedehitze. Zentralbl. Bakteriol. Parasitenk., 1 Orig, *138*, 227–241.

Gould, G.W. 1964. Effect of food preservatives on the growth of bacteria from spores. In *Proceedings 4th International Symposium on Food Microbiology.* Göteburg, SIK, pp. 17–35.

Gould, G.W. 1977. Recent advances in the understanding of resistance and dormancy in bacterial spores. J. Appl. Bacteriol., *42*, 297–309.

Gould, G.W., and Dring, G.J. 1975. Heat resistance of bacterial endospores and concept of an expanded osmoregulatory cortex. Nature, *258*, 402–405.

Greaves, R.I.N. 1960. Some factors which influence the stability of freeze-dried cultures. In *Recent Researches in Freezing and Drying.* Edited by A.S. Parkes and A.V. Smith. Oxford, Blackwell, pp. 203–215.

Greaves, R.I.N. 1962. Recent advances in freeze-drying. J. Pharm. Pharmacol., *14*, 621–640.

Green, R.H., Olson, R.L., Gustan, E.A., and Pilgrim, A.J. 1967. Microbial survival in propellants before and after rocket firings. Dev. Ind. Microbiol., *8*, 227–234.

Greenberg, R.A., and Silliker, J.H. 1962. The action of tylosin on spore-forming bacteria. J. Food Sci., *27*, 64–68.

Greenberg, R.A., and Silliker, J.H. 1964. Spoilage patterns in *Clostridium botulinum* inoculated canned foods treated with tylosin. In *Proceedings 4th International Symposium on Food Microbiology.* Göteburg, SIK, pp. 97–103.

Halvorson, H.O., and Ziegler, N.R. 1933. Application of statistics in bacteriology, I. A means of determining bacterial population by the dilution method. J. Bacteriol., *25*, 101–121.

Hansen, N.H., and Reimann, H. 1963. Factors affecting the heat resistance of nonsporing organisms. J. Appl. Bacteriol., *26*, 314–333.

Harnulv, B.G., and Snygg, B.G. 1972. Heat resistance of *Bacillus subtilis* spores at various water activities. J. Appl. Bacteriol., *35*, 615–624.

Havery, D.C., et al. 1976. Survey of food products for volatile N-nitrosamines. J. Assoc. Off. Anal. Chem., *59*, 540–546.

Hawley, H.B. 1957. Nisin in food technology. Food Mfg., *32*, 370–373, 430-434.

Headlee, M.R. 1931. Thermal death point. III. Spores of *Clostridium welchii.* J. Infect. Dis., *48*, 328–329.

Heinemann, R., Stumbo, C.R., and Scuolock, A. 1964. Use of nisin in preparing beverage-quality sterile chocolate-flavored milk. J. Dairy Sci., *47*, 8–12.

Hirsch, A. 1953. Antibiotics in food preservation. Proc. Soc. Appl. Bacteriol., *16*, 100–106.

H.M.S.O. 1959. Food Standards Committee Report on Preservatives in Foods. H.M.S.O., London.

Hoffman, R.K., Gambill, V.M., and Buchanan, L.M. 1968. Effect of cell moisture on the thermal inactivation rate of bacterial spores. Appl. Microbiol., *16*, 1240–1244.

Hurst, A. 1983. Nisin and other inhibitory substances from lactic acid bacteria. In *Antimicrobials in Foods.* Edited by A.L. Branen and P.M. Davidson. New York, Marcel Dekker Inc.

Ivey, F.J., and Robach, M.C. 1978. Effect of potassium sorbate and sodium nitrite on *Clostridium botulinum* growth and toxin production in canned comminuted pork. J. Food Sci., *43*, 1782–1785.

Ivey, F.J., Shaver, K.J., Christiansen, L.N., and Tompkin, R.B. 1978. Effect of potassium sorbate on toxinogenesis of *Clostridium botulinum* in bacon. J. Food Prot., *41*, 621–625.

Jacobs, R.A., Nicholas, R.C., and Pflug, I.J. 1965. Heat resistance of *Bacillus subtilis* spores in atmospheres of different water content. Mich. Agric. Exp. Stat. Q. Bull., *48*, 238.

Jacobson, R.L., and Pflug, I.J. 1972. Dry heat destruction of bacterial spores A. Study of destruction rates at low levels of water at 90, 110 and 125°C. In *Progress Report No. 9. Environmental Microbiology as Related to Planetary Quarantine.* NASA NGL 24-005-160. University of Minnesota, Minneapolis, MN, pp. 19–31.

Jaynes, J.A., Pflug, I.J., and Harmon, L.G. 1961a. Effect of pH and brine concentration on gas production by a putrefactive anaerobe (PA 3679) in a processed cheese spread. J. Dairy Sci., *44*, 1265–1271.

Jaynes, J.A., Pflug, I.J., and Harmon, L.G. 1961b. Some factors affecting the heating and cooling lags of processed cheese in thermal death time cans. J. Dairy Sci., *44*, 2171–2175.

Jaynes, J.A., Pflug, I.J., Harmon, L.G., and Costilow, R.N. 1961c. Effect of pH and brine concentration on the thermal resistance of PA 3679 in a processed cheese spread. J. Dairy Sci., *44*, 1997–2003.

Jensen, L.B. 1954. *Microbiology of Meat.* 3rd Edition. Champaign, IL, Gerrard Press, pp. 273–274.

Johnson, E., and Brown, B. 1961. The Spearman estimator for serial dilution assays. Biometrics, *17*, 79–88.

Kaufmann, O.W., and Andrews, R.H. 1954. The destruction rate of psychrophilic bacteria in skim milk. J. Dairy Sci., *37*, 317–327.

Koesterer, M.G. 1962. *Sterilization of Space Probe Components.* Final Report of Contract NASr-31, NASA, Washington, D.C.

Koesterer, M.G. 1965a. *Studies for Sterilization of Space Probe Components.* NASA Contract No. NASW-879. Rochester, Wilmot Castle Co.

Koesterer, M.G. 1965b. Thermal death studies on microbial spores and some considerations for the sterilization of spacecraft components. Dev. Ind. Microbiol., *6*, 268–276.

Kooiman, W.J., and Geers, J.M. 1975. Simple and accurate technique for the determination of heat resistance of bacterial spores. J. Appl. Bacteriol., *38*, 185–189.

Kushnir, J., et al. 1975. Isolation and identification of nitrosoproline in uncooked bacon. J. Food Sci., *40*, 427–428.

Lamanna, C. 1942. Relation of maximum growth temperature to resistance to heat. J. Bacteriol., *44*, 29–35.

Lang, O.W. 1935. Thermal processes for canned marine products. Univ. Calif. Publ. Health, *2*, 1–175.

Lang, O.W., and Dean, S.J. 1934. Heat resistance of *Clostridium botulinum* in canned sea foods. J. Infect. Dis., *55*, 39–59.

Lea, C.H., Hannan, R.S., and Greaves, R.I.N. 1950. The reaction between proteins and reducing sugars in the 'dry' state. Biochem. J., *47*, 626–629.

Lechowich, R.V., and Ordal, Z.J. 1962. The influence of the sporulation temperature on the heat resistance and chemical composition of bacterial spores. Can. J. Microbiol., *8*, 287–295.

Levine, A.S., and Fellers, C.R. 1940. Action of acetic acid on food spoilage microorganisms. J. Bacteriol., *39*, 499–514.

Levine, M., Buchanan, J.H., and Lease, G. 1927. Effect of concentration and temperature on germicidal efficiency of sodium hydroxide. Iowa State Coll. J. Sci., *1*, 379.

Lewis, J.C. 1956. The estimation of decimal reduction times. Appl Microbiol., *4*, 211.

Lewis, J.C., Michener, H.D., Stumbo, C.R., and Titus, D.S. 1954. Additives accelerating death of spores by moist heat. J. Agric. Food Chem., *2*, 298.

Licciardello, J.J., and Nickerson, J.T.R. 1963. Some observations on bacterial thermal death time curves. Appl. Microbiol., *11*, 476–481.

McHugh, R.B., and Sundararaj, N. 1972. Decimal reduction time estimation in thermal microbial sterilization. In *Progress Report No. 9. Environmental Microbiology as Related to Planetary Quarantine.* NASA Grant NGL 24-005-160, University of Minnesota. Minneapolis, MN.

Madsen, T., and Nyman, M. 1907. Zur Theorie der Desinfection. Z. Hyg. Infectionsk., *57*, 388–404.

Magee, P.N., and Barnes, J.M. 1967. Carcinogenic nitroso compounds. Adv. Cancer Res., *10*, 163–246.

Magoon, C.A. 1926b. Studies on bacterial spores. II. Thermal resistance as affected by age and environment. J. Bacteriol., *11*, 253–283.

Malin, B., and Greenberg, R.A. 1964. The effect of tylosin on spoilage patterns of inoculated and non-inoculated cream style corn. Proceedings 4th International Symposium on Food Microbiology. Göteburg, Sweden, SIK, pp. 87–95.

Marshall, B.J., Murrell, W.G., and Scott, W.J. 1963. The effect of water activity, solutes, and temperature on the viability and heat resistance of freeze-dried bacterial spores. J. Gen. Microbiol., *31*, 451–460.

Mayou, J.L., and Jezeski, J.J. 1977. Effect of sporulation media on the heat resistance of *Bacillus stearothermophilus* spores. J. Food Prot., *40*, 232–233.

Meynell, G.G., and Meynell, E. 1965. *Theory and Practice in Experimental Bacteriology.* Cambridge, Cambridge University Press.

Moats, W.A. 1971. Kinetics of thermal death of bacteria. J. Bacteriol., *105*, 165–171.

Molin, N., and Snygg, B.G. 1967. Effect of lipid materials on heat resistance of bacterial spores. Appl. Microbiol., *15*, 1422–1426.

Moore, B., Pflug, I.J., and Haugen, J. 1969. Dry heat destruction rates of *B. subtilis* var. *niger* in a closed system. In *Progress Report No. 3. Environmental Microbiology as Related to Planetary Quarantine.* NASA Grant NGL 24-005-160, University of Minnesota. Minneapolis, MN.

Mudd, S., and Mudd, E.H. 1924. The penetration of bacteria through capillary spaces. IV. A kinetic mechanism in interfaces. J. Exp. Med., *40*, 633–645.

Mullican, C.L., and Hoffman, R.K. 1968. Dry heat or gaseous chemical resistance of *Bacillus subtilis* var. *niger* spores included within water-soluble crystals. Appl. Microbiol., *16*, 1110–1113.

Murrell, W.G., and Scott, W.J. 1957. Heat resistance of bacterial spores at various water activities. Nature, *179*, 41.

Murrell, W.G., and Scott, W.J. 1966. The heat resistance of bacterial spores at various water activities. J. Gen. Microbiol., *43*, 411–425.

Nank, W.K., and Schmidt, C.F. 1958. The effect of the addition of manganese to a nutrient agar sporulation medium upon the resistance of thermophilic flat sour spore crops. Bacteriol. Proc., p. 42.

NASA. 1968. *NASA Standard Procedures for the Microbiological Examination of Space Hardware.* National Aeronautics and Space Administration Document No. NHB5340.1A. October, 1968 edition. Washington, D.C., Government Printing Office.

NASA. 1969. *Planetary Quarantine Provisions for Unmanned Planetary Missions.* National Aeronautics and Space Administration Document No. NHB 8020.12. April 1969 edition. Washington, D.C., Government Printing Office.

Nichols, A.A. 1940. The effect of variations in the fat percentage and in the reaction (pH) of milk media on the heat resistance of certain milk bacteria. J. Dairy Sci., *11*, 274–291.

Odlaug, T.E., and Pflug, I.J. 1977. Thermal destruction of *Clostridium botulinum* spores suspended in tomato juice in aluminum thermal death time tubes. Appl. Environ. Microbiol., *34*, 23–29.

Paik, W.W., Michael., S.C., Smith, C.D., and Stern, J. 1967. Dry heat resistance of bacterial spores (Bacillus globigii) on selected spacecraft surface material. In *Space Programs Summary 37–46,* Vol. IV. Pasadena, California, Jet Propulsion Laboratory, pp. 43–48.

Peterson, E., Levine, M., and Buchanan, J. 1927. A study of the preparation of syrups. Iowa State Coll. J. Sci., *2*, 31–41.

Pflug, I.J. 1960. Thermal resistance of microorganisms to dry heat: design of apparatus, operational problems and preliminary results. Food Technol., *14*, 483–487.

Pflug, I.J. 1968. Some observations regarding factors important to dry heat sterilization. In *Sterilization Techniques for Instruments and Materials as Applied to Space Research.* Edited by P.N.A. Sneath. (COSPAR Techn. Man. No. 4.) Muray-Print, Paris.

Pflug, I.J. 1970. Dry heat destruction rates for microorganisms on open surfaces, in mated surface areas and encapsulated in solids of spacecraft hardware. In *Life Sciences and Space Research,* VII. Amsterdam, North-Holland Publishing.

Pflug, I.J. 1988. Collecting wet-heat microbial-destruction data using a miniature retort system: operation, temperature calibration, lag correction factors, and minimum heating times. In *Selected Papers on the Microbiology and Engineering of Sterilization Processes.* Edited by I.J. Pflug. Environmental Sterilization Laboratory, University of Minnesota, Minneapolis, MN.

Pflug, I.J. 1989. Biologically validating the sterilization process delivered to particles in a heat-hold-cool system. In *Proceedings of the First International Congress on Aseptic Processing Technologies.* Department of Food Science and Nutrition, Purdue University, Lafayette, Indiana.

Pflug, I.J. 1990. *Microbiology and Engineering of Sterilization Processes,* 7th Ed. Environmental Sterilization Laboratory, University of Minnesota, Minneapolis.

Pflug, I.J., and Augustin, J.A.L. 1962. Dry heat destruction of microorganisms. Progress report on Project 830, Food Science Department, Michigan State University.

Pflug, I.J., and Esselen, W.B. 1953. Development and application of apparatus for study of thermal resistance of bacterial spores and thiamine at temperatures above 250°F. Food Technol., *7*, 237.

Pflug, I.J., and Esselen, W.B. 1954. Observations on the thermal resistance of putrefactive anaerobe No. 3679 spores in the temperature range of 250°–300°F. Food Res., *19*, 92.

Pflug, I.J., and Esselen, W.B. 1955. Heat transfer into open metal thermoresistometer cups. Food Res., *20*, 237–246.

Pflug, I.J., and Holcomb, R.G. 1980. The use of bacterial spores as sterilization process monitoring devices: a discussion of what they can do and some of their limitations. In *Proceedings of the Third PMA Seminar Program on Validation of Sterile Manufacturing Processes: Biological Indicators.* Lincolnshire, IL.

Pflug, I.J., and Schmidt, C.F. 1968. Thermal destruction of microorganisms. In *Disinfection, Sterilization and Preservation.* 1st Edition. Edited by C.A. Lawrence and S.S. Block. Lea & Febiger, Philadelphia.

Pflug, I.J., and Smith, G.M. 1977. The use of biological indicators for monitoring wet heat sterilization processes. In *Sterilization of Medical Products.* Edited by E.R.L. Gaughran and K. Kereluk. Johnson and Johnson, New Brunswick, NJ.

Pflug, I.J., Smith, G.M., and Christensen, R. 1981. Effect of soybean casein digest agar lot on number of *Bacillus stearothermophilus* spores recovered. Appl. Environ. Microbiol., *42*:226–230.

Pheil, C.G., and Pflug, I.J. 1964. Effect of heating temperature on the thermal resistance of *Bacillus subtilis.* Abstract No. 170, Institute of Food Technology Meeting Program.

Pheil, C.G., Pflug, I.J., Nicholas, R.C., and Augustin, J.A.L. 1967. The effect of various gas atmospheres on the destruction of microorganisms in dry heat. Appl. Microbiol., *15*, 120–124.

Pilcher, R.W. 1947. *The Canned Food Reference Manual.* 3rd Edition. New York, American Can.

Pivnick, H., Johnston, M.A., Thacker, C., and Loynes, R. 1970. Effect of nitrite on destruction and germination of *Clostridium botulinum* and putrefactive anaerobes 3679 and 3679h in meat and buffer. Can. Inst. Food Sci. Technol. J., *3*, 103–109.

Poole, G., and Malin, B. 1964. Some aspects of the action of tylosin on *Clostridium* species PA 3679. J. Food Sci., *29*, 475–478.

Prokop, A., and Humphrey, A.E. 1972. Mechanism of thermal death of bacterial spores. Electron microscopic observations. Folia Microbiol., *17*, 437–445.

Puleo, J.R., Favero, M.S., Oxborrow, G.S., and Herring, C.M. 1975. Method for collecting naturally occurring airborne bacterial spores for determining their thermal resistance. Appl. Microbiol., *30*, 786–790.

Rahn, O. 1928. Incomplete sterilization of food products due to heavy syrups. Canning Age, *8*, 705–706.

Rahn, O. 1945a. Physical methods of sterilization of microorganisms. Bacteriol. Rev., *9*, 1.

Rahn, O. 1945b. *Injury and Death of Bacteria.* Biodynamica Monograph No. 3. Normandy, MO, Biodynamica.

Read, R.B., Jr. 1963. Current status of instrumentation in milk and food research. Am. J. Public Health, *53*, 1579–1586.

Reed, J.M., Bohrer, C.W., and Cameron, E.J. 1951. Spore destruction rate studies on organisms of significance in the processing of canned foods. Food Res., *16*, 383–408.

Reynolds, H., Kaplan, A.M., Spencer, F.B., and Lichtenstein, H. 1952. Thermal destruction of Cameron's putrefactive anaerobe 3679 in food substrates. Food Res., *17*, 153.

Riemann, H. 1963. Safe heat processing of canned cured meats with regard to bacterial spores. Food Technol., *17*, 39–49.

Robach, M.C., Ivey, F.J., and Hickey, C.S., 1978. System for evaluating clostridial inhibition in cured meat products. Appl. Environ. Microbiol., *36*, 210–211.

Roberts, T.A., and Ingram, M. 1966. The effect of sodium chloride, potassium nitrate and sodium nitrite on the recovery of heated bacterial spores. J. Food Technol., *1*, 147–163.

Roberts, T.A., Gilbert, R.J., and Ingram, M. 1966. The effect of sodium chloride on heat resistance and recovery of heated spores of *Clostridium sporogenes* (PA 3679/S₂). J. Appl. Bacteriol., *29*, 549–555.

Robertson, A.H. 1928. Influence of age on the heat resistance of non-sporeforming bacteria. J. Bacteriol., *15*, 27.

Russell, A.D. (Ed.). 1982. *Destruction of Bacterial Spores.* London, Academic Press.

Sames, T. 1900. Zur Kenntnis der bei höher Temperatur wachsenden Bakterien und Streptococcusarten. Z. Hyg. Infektionsk., *33*, 313–362.

Schalkowsky, S., and Wiederkehr, R. 1968. Estimation of microbial survival in heat sterilization. In *Sterilization Techniques for Instruments and Materials as Applied to Space Research.* Edited by P.N.A. Sneath. Paris, Muray-Print, pp. 87–108. (COSPAR Techn. Man. No. 4.)

Schmidt, C.F. 1950. A method for determination of the thermal resistance of bacterial spores. J. Bacteriol., *59*, 433.

Schmidt, C.F. 1954. Thermal resistance of microorganisms. In *Antiseptics, Disinfectants, Fungicides and Sterilization.* Edited by G.F. Reddish. Philadelphia, Lea & Febiger, pp. 720–759.

Schmidt, C.F. 1955a. The effect of subculture media upon the apparent thermal resistance of spores of members of the genus *Bacillus.* Bacteriol. Proc., p. 40.

Schmidt, C.F. 1955b. The resistance of bacterial spores with reference to spore germination and its inhibition. Annu. Rev. Microbiol., *9*, 387–400.

Schmidt, C.F. 1957. Thermal resistance of microorganisms. In *Antiseptics, Disinfectants, Fungicides and Sterilization.* 2nd Edition. Edited by G.F. Reddish. Philadelphia, Lea & Febiger, pp. 831–884.

Schmidt, C.F., and Nank, W.K. 1958. Cultural factors influencing the thermal resistance of a strain of *Bacillus subtilis.* Bacteriol. Proc., p. 42.

Schmidt, C.F., Bock, J.H., and Moberg, J.A. 1955. Thermal resistance determinations in steam using thermal death time retorts. Food Res., *20*, 606.

Scott, W.J. 1957. Water relations of food spoilage microorganisms. Adv. Food Res., *7*, 83.

Sebranek, J.G., and Cassens, R.G. 1973. Nitrosamines: a review. J. Milk Food Technol., *36*, 76–91.

Segmiller, J.L., Xenones, H., and Hutchings, I.J. 1965. The efficiency of nisin and tylosin lactate in selected heat sterilized products. J. Food Sci., *30*, 166–171.

Senhaji, A.F. 1977. The protective effect of fat on the heat resistance of bacteria II. J. Food Technol., *12*, 217–230.

Senhaji, A.F., and Loncin, M. 1975. Protection des microorganismes par les matiéres grasses au cours des traitements thermiques. Premiere partie. Industries Alimentaires et Agricoles, *92*, 611–617.

Senhaji, A.F., and Loncin, M. 1977. The protective effect of fat on the heat resistance of bacteria I. J. Food Technol., *12*, 203–216.

Senhaji, A.F., Bimbenet, J.J., and LeMaguer, M. 1976. Protection des microorganismes par les matiéres grasses au cours des traitements thermiques. 2ᵉ partie. Industries Alimentaires et Agricoles, *93*, 13–20.

Sherman, J.M., and Albus, W.R. 1923. Physiological youth in bacteria. J. Bacteriol., *8*, 127–138.

Sherman, J.M., and Cameron, G.M. 1934. Lethal environmental factors within the natural range of growth. J. Bacteriol., *27*, 341–348.

Shull, J.J., Cargo, G.T., and Ernst, R.R. 1963. Kinetics of heat activation and of thermal death of bacterial spores. Appl. Microbiol., *11*, 485–487.

Silliker, J.H. 1959. The effect of curing salts on bacterial spores. In *Proc. 11th Res. Conf. Am. Meat Inst. Found.* Chicago, pp. 51–60.

Silverman, G.J. 1968. *The Resistivity of Microorganisms to Inactivation by Dry Heat.* Contract Ns G-691. Massachusetts Institute of Technology, Cambridge, Mass.

Simko, G.J., Devlin, J.D., and Wardle, M.D. 1971. Dry-heat resistance of *Bacillus subtilis* var. *niger spores* on mated surfaces. Appl. Microbiol., *22*, 491–495.

Smith, G., Kopelman, M., Jones, A., and Pflug, I.J. 1982. Effect of environmental conditions during heating on commercial spore strip performance. Appl. Environ. Microbiol., *44*:12–18.

Skillinglaw, C.A., and Levine, M. 1943. Effects of acid and sugar on viability of *Escherichia coli* and *Eberthella typhosa*. Food Res., *8*, 464–476.

Smith, G., and Pflug, I.J. 1972. Dry heat destruction rates of microorganisms on surfaces. In *Progress Report No. 8. Environmental Microbiology as Related to Planetary Quarantine.* NASA NGL 24-005-160, University of Minnesota. Minneapolis, MN.

Smith, G., Pflug, I.J., Gove, R., and Thun, Y. 1971. Survival of microbial spores under several temperature and humidity conditions. In *Progress Report No. 6. Environmental Microbiology as Related to Planetary Quarantine.* NASA NGL 24-005-160, University of Minnesota. Minneapolis, MN.

Sobernheim, G., and Mündel, O. 1936. Grundsätzliches zur Technik der Sterilisationsprüfung. Z. Hyg. Infektionsk., *118*, 328–345.

Sobernheim, G., and Mündel, O. 1938. Grundsätzliches zur Technik der Sterilisationsprüfung. II. Verhalten der Erdsporen bei der Dampfsterilisation. Ihre Eignung als Testsporen. Z. Hyg. Infektionsk, *121*, 90–112.

Sofos, J.N., Busta, F.F., and Allen, C.E. 1979a. Sodium nitrite and sorbic acid effects on *Clostridium botulinum* spore germination and total microbial growth in chicken frankfurter emulsions during temperature abuse. Appl. Environ. Microbiol., *37*, 1103–1109.

Sofos, J.N., Busta, F.F., and Allen, C.E. 1979b. Botulism control by nitrite and sorbate in cured meats: a review. J. Food Prot., *42*, 739–770.

Sognefest, P., and Benjamin, H.A. 1944. Heating lag in thermal death-time cans and tubes. Food Res., *9*, 234.

Sognefest, P., Hays, G.L., Wheaton, E., and Benjamin, H.A. 1948. Effect of pH on thermal process requirements of canned food. Food Res., *13*, 400–416.

Sommer, E.W. 1930. Heat resistance of the spores of *Clostridium botulinum*. J. Infect. Dis., *46*, 85–114.

Stark, C.N., and Stark, P. 1929. The relative thermal death rates of young and mature bacterial cells. J. Bacteriol., *18*, 333–337.

Stern, J.A., and Proctor. B.E. 1954. A micro-method and apparatus for the multiple determination of the rates of destruction of bacteria and bacterial spores subjected to heat. Food Technol., *8*, 139.

Stumbo, C.R. 1948a. Bacteriological considerations relating to process evaluation. Food Technol., *2*, 115.

Stumbo, C.R. 1948b. A technique for studying resistance of bacterial spores to temperatures in the higher range. Food Technol., *2*, 228.

Stumbo, C.R. 1973. *Thermobacteriology in Food Processing.* 2nd Edition. New York, Academic Press.

Stumbo, C.R., Gross, C.E., and Viton, C. 1945. Bacteriological studies relating to thermal processing of canned meats. Food Res., *10*, 260.

Stumbo, C.R., Murphy, J.R., and Cochran, J. 1950. Nature of thermal death time curves for P.A. 3679 and *Clostridium botulinum*. Food Technol., *4*, 321.

Sugiyama, H. 1951. Studies of factors affecting the heat resistance of spores of *Clostridium botulinum*. J. Bacteriol., *62*, 81.

Sundararaj, N. 1971. The Biometric Analysis of Non-linear Models with Applications to Disinfection. Ph.D. thesis, University of Minnesota.

Tanaka, N., Worley, N.J., Sheldon, E.W., and Goepfert, J.M. 1977. Effect of sorbate and sodium acid pyrophosphate on the toxin production by *Clostridium botulinum* in pork macerate. Ann. Rep. Food Res. Inst. University of Wisconsin, Madison, Wisconsin, pp. 366–368.

Theophilus, O.R., and Hammer, B.W. 1938. Influence of growth temperature on the thermal resistance of some bacteria from evaporated milk. Iowa State Coll. Agric. Exp. Stat. Res. Bull., 244.

Thuillot, M.L., Bossard, J., Thomas, G., and Cheftel, H. 1968. A propos de la thermorésistance de *S. aureus* dans l'huile. Ann. Inst. Pasteur-Lille, *19*, 153–157.

Tompkin, R.B., Christiansen, L.N., Shaparis, A.B., and Bolin, H. 1974. Effects of potassium sorbate on salmonellae, *Staphylococcus aureus*, *Clostridium perfringens*, and *Clostridium botulinum* in cooked uncured sausage. Appl. Microbiol., *28*, 262–264.

Townsend, C.T., Esty, J.R., and Baselt, F.C. 1938. Heat resistance studies on spores of putrefactive anaerobes in relation to determination of safe processes for canned foods. Food Res., *3*, 323–346.

Townsend, C.T., Yee, L., and Mercer, W.A. 1954. Inhibition of the growth of *Clostridium botulinum* by acidification. Food Res., *19*, 536–542.

Townsend, C.T., Somers, I.I., Lamb, F.C., and Olson, N.A. 1956. *A Laboratory Manual for the Canning Industry.* 2nd Edition. Washington, D.C., National Canners Association Research Laboratories, Chapters 4, 6, and 7.

Viljoen, J.A. 1926. Heat resistance studies. II. The protective effect of sodium chloride on bacterial spores heated in pea liquor. J. Infect. Dis., *39*, 286–290.

Von Angerer, K., and Küster, E. 1939. Über die Verzögerung des Hitzetodes von Bakterien und Sporen durch hochkonzentrierte als Funktion Medien des Tyndalleffectes. Arch. Hyg. Bakteriol., *122*, 57–97.

Wada, S. et al. 1975. The preservative effects of sorbic acid for fish sausage. J. Food Hyg. Soc. Jpn., *17*, 95–100.

Wallace, G.I., and Tanner, F.W. 1931. The effect of concentrated salt and sugar solutions on the thermal death time of molds. J. Bacteriol., *21*, 32.

Wang, D. I-C, Schorer, J., and Humphrey, A.E. 1964. Kinetics of death of bacterial spores at elevated temperatures. Appl. Microbiol., *12*, 451–454.

Weil, R. 1899. Zur Biologie der Milzbrandbazillen. Arch. Hyg. Bakteriol., *35*, 355–408.

Weiss, H. 1921. The heat resistance of spores with special reference to the spores of *B. botulinus*. J. Infect. Dis., *28*, 70–92.

Wheaton, E., and Hays, G.L. 1964. Antibiotics and the control of spoilage in canned foods. Food Technol., *18*, 549.

Wilder, C.J., and Nordan, H.C. 1957. A micromethod and apparatus for the determination of rates of destruction of bacterial spores subjected to heat and bactericidal agents. Food Res., *22*, 462–467.

Williams, C.C., Merrill, C.M., and Cameron, E.J. 1937. Apparatus for determination of spore-destruction rates. Food Res., *2*, 369.

Williams, F.T. 1936. Attempts to increase the heat resistance of bacterial spores. J. Bacteriol., *32*, 589.

Williams, O.B. 1929. The heat resistance of bacterial spores. J. Infect. Dis., *44*, 421.

Williams, O.B., and Robertson, W.J. 1954. Studies on heat resistance. VI. Effect of temperature of incubation at which formed on heat resistance of aerobic thermophilic spores. J. Bacteriol., *67*, 377.

Wolf, I.A., and Wasserman, A.E. 1972. Nitrates, nitrites and nitrosamines. Science 177, 15–19.

Yesair, J., and Cameron, E.J. 1942. Inhibitive effect of curing agents on anaerobic spores. Canner, *94*, 89–92.

Yesair, J., Bohrer, C.W., and Cameron, E.J. 1946. Effect of certain environmental factors on heat resistance of micrococci. Food Res., *11*, 327–331.

Yesair, J., Cameron, E.J., and Bohrer, C.W. 1944. Comparative resistance of desiccated and wet micrococci heated under moist and dry conditions. J. Bacteriol., *47*, 437–438 (abstr).

Zakula, R. 1969. Results on investigations of thermoresistance of some bacteria suspended in meat, lard, and tallow. In *Proceedings of European Meeting of Meat Research Workers.* 15th. Helsinki.

Zaleski, S., Sobolewska-Ceronik, K., and Ceronik, E. 1971. Influence de l'hydratation de l'huile de soja sur la résistance du staphylocoque enterotoxique a la chaleur. Ann. Inst. Pasteur-Lille, *22*, 263–267.

ZoBell, C.E., and Johnson, F.H. 1949. The influence of hydrostatic pressure on the growth and viability of terrestrial and marine bacteria. J. Bacteriol., *57*, 179–190.

Zuccaro, J.B., Powers, J.J., Morse, R.E., and Mills, W.C. 1951. Thermal death times of yeast in oil and movement of yeast between the oil and water phases of French dressing. Food Res., *16*, 30–38.

Disinfectants and Antiseptics
A. By Chemical Type

CHAPTER 7

CHLORINE AND CHLORINE COMPOUNDS

G.R. Dychdala

Although chlorine is one of the most widely distributed elements on earth, it is not found in a free state in nature. Instead, it exists mostly in combination with sodium, potassium, calcium, and magnesium. Elemental chlorine is a heavy gas of greenish-yellow coloration with a characteristic irritating and penetrating odor. According to Mellor (1927), chlorine must have been known to alchemists for many centuries, but only in 1809 did Sir Humphrey Davy conclude that chlorine gas was an element, and because of its characteristic yellow-green color, propose the name.

Observations of the bleaching properties of chlorine gas in water solution led to its first practical application in textile bleaching, with subsequent commercial production in 1785. Development of sodium and calcium hypochlorites for more convenient use followed shortly thereafter.

It was not until the first half of the nineteenth century that the disinfecting and deodorizing properties of chloride of lime were first recognized. Chlorinated lime was applied in the treatment of sewage in London as early as 1854 and also used for disinfection and deodorization of hospital wards. In 1846, Semmelweis used chloride of lime to combat and control puerperal fever in his clinic in Vienna. Finally, in 1881, a German bacteriologist, Koch, demonstrated under controlled laboratory conditions that pure cultures of bacteria may be destroyed by the use of hypochlorites. Five years later, the American Public Health Association issued a favorable report on the use of hypochlorites as disinfectants (Hadfield, 1957).

Traube, in 1894, established the purifying and disinfecting properties of hypochlorites in water treatment. Chloride of lime was first introduced to the North American continent by Johnson in 1908 for purification of water. Within a short period of time, many plants throughout the United States installed the chlorination process for water purification, alone or in combination with filtration, so that by 1911 an estimated 800,000,000 gallons of water were purified by the chlorination process

(Race, 1918). Today, it is rare to find municipal water that is not treated by chlorination. Later, the introduction of elemental chlorine as a commercial product supplemented the already existing hypochlorite process for the treatment of water and sewage. The use of chlorine* as a disinfectant gained wide acceptance later in other industries.

Wide use of chlorine as a disinfectant began during World War I when Dakin (1915) introduced a 0.45 to 0.50% sodium hypochlorite solution for disinfection of open and infected wounds. The original Dakin's solution was prepared by mixing chlorinated lime and sodium carbonate with boric acid. Because of the irritating properties then attributed to boric acid, the solution was modified to contain a mixture of sodium carbonate and sodium bicarbonate, replacing boric acid and sodium carbonate and resulting in greater stability of the hypochlorite and lesser irritation to the open wounds. Up to 1963, Dakin's solution was a standard product of the British Pharmacopeia (1958).

Treatment of wounds with hypochlorite necessitated information regarding solvent action, irritation, and toxicity, as well as the rate of reaction on the necrotic tissue. Various toxicity studies were reported by Taylor et al. (1918 a,b,c) and Cullen et al. (1918).

PRINCIPLES, MECHANISMS, AND OTHER ASPECTS OF CHLORINE DISINFECTION

Definitions of Chemical Terms

Available Chlorine

"Available chlorine" may be defined as a measurement of oxidizing capacity and is expressed in terms of the

---

*Following common practice in the industry, the word "chlorine" is broadly used to signify "active chlorine compounds." Generally, what is intended is "aqueous solution of active chlorine compounds, consisting of a mixture of OCl⁻, Cl₂, HOCl and other active chlorine compounds." Where "elemental chlorine" is intended, it will be referred to as such or as "liquid" or "gaseous chlorine."

equivalent amount of elemental chlorine. The concentration of hypochlorite (or any other oxidizing disinfectant) may be expressed as available chlorine by determining the electrochemical equivalent amount of Cl_2 to that compound. By Equation 1, it can be seen that one mole of elemental chlorine is capable of reacting with two electrons to form inert chloride:

$$Cl_2 + 2e^- = 2 Cl^- \qquad (1)$$

From Equation 2, it can also be noted that one mole of hypochlorite (OCl^-) may react with two electrons to form chloride:

$$OCl^- + 2e^- + 2H^+ = Cl^- + H_2O \qquad (2)$$

Hence, one mole of hypochlorite is equivalent (electrochemically) to one mole of elemental chlorine, and may be said to contain 70.91 grams of available chlorine (identical to the molecular weight of Cl_2).

Since calcium hypochlorite $(Ca(OCl)_2)$ and sodium hypochlorite $(NaOCl)$ contain two and one moles of hypochlorite per mole of chemical, respectively, they also contain 141.8 g and 70.91 g available chlorine per mole. The molecular weights of $Ca(OCl)_2$ and $NaOCl$ are, respectively 143 and 74.5, so that pure preparations of the two compounds contain 99.2 and 95.8 weight percent available chlorine; hence they are effective means of supplying chlorine for disinfection purposes.

Chlorine Demand

In chlorination of water, a certain part of this chlorine will be consumed by water impurities, and any unconsumed chlorine will remain as residual available chlorine. The difference between the chlorine applied and the chlorine remaining in the water may be referred to as the "chlorine demand" of this water. Because of its electronic configuration, chlorine possesses a strong tendency to acquire extra electrons, changing to inorganic chloride ions. This affinity for electrons makes the chlorine a strong oxidizing agent. Hence, chlorine in water reacts quickly with (1) inorganic reducing substances, such as ferrous iron (Fe^{++}), manganous manganese (Mn^{++}), nitrites (NO_2^-), and hydrogen sulfide (H_2S), and (2) organic material (other than amines) wherein the chlorine atom ceases to contain oxidizing properties by reduction to chloride and is lost as a disinfectant (Weidenkopf, 1953). The reactions with the inorganic reducing substances are quite rapid and stoichiometric, whereas those with organic material are generally slow and depend largely on the concentration of the free available chlorine.

Free and Combined Available Chlorine

When chlorine survives the chlorine demand of the water, the chlorine measured may be reported as free, combined, or total residual chlorine depending upon the analytical method used. According to Weidenkopf (1953), the term "free" available chlorine is usually applied to three forms of chlorine that may be found in water: (*a*) elemental chlorine (Cl_2), (*b*) hypochlorous acid $(HOCl)$, and (*c*) hypochlorite ion (OCl^-). These forms may be found in water, provided there is no ammonia or other nitrogenous compounds to form chloramines and there is enough chlorine to satisfy the organic and inorganic water demands.

During a chlorination process, a certain portion of chlorine combines with ammonia and other nitrogenous compounds

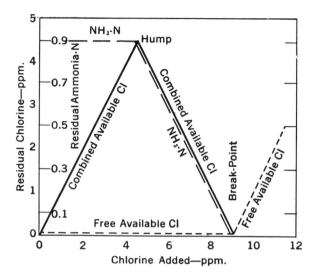

Fig. 7–1. Ideal residual chlorine curve (ammonia solution). (After Butterfield, C.T. 1948. Bactericidal properties of free and combined available chlorine. J. Am. Water Works Assoc., *80*:1305–1312.)

present in natural water to form chloramines or *N*-chloro compounds. This combination of chlorine with ammonia or with other nitrogenous compounds is referred to as "combined" available chlorine. The free and combined available chlorine, when present in the water, are collectively described as total residual (available) chlorine.

Breakpoint Chlorination

Under "breakpoint chlorination," a sufficient amount of chlorine is applied to satisfy the initial water demand, and an extra quantity of chlorine is added to provide a slight residual of free available chlorine. Prior to establishing this free residual, additions of chlorine (or hypochlorites) will oxidize all the inorganic and organic material, until at some "breakpoint," demand is fully satisfied. Any further additions of available chlorine will result in a constant rise of "free" available chlorine in proportion to the dose (Fig. 7–1).

Other Terms

"Marginal chlorination" is referred to as the addition of sufficient chlorine to water to just overcome the chlorine demand consumption and to obtain an initial level of available chlorine regardless of the type of residual produced. "Superchlorination" is a further step in which chlorine is added beyond the level that is needed to yield an initial residual without regard to the type of residual produced. If too much chlorine is added and a lower chlorine level is desired, a dechlorinating chemical (e.g., sodium thiosulfate) may be added, and this process is referred to as "dechlorination." The terms pre- and post-chlorination generally relate to a position of chlorination prior to or subsequent to filtration, respectively (Griffin, 1944).

Analysis of Available Chlorine

There are several methods to determine the available chlorine in solution or in products. In the iodometric method, the free chlorine liberates iodine in the acidified test solution containing potassium iodide (KI), and the liberated iodine is titrated with a standard sodium thio-sulfate solution to a starch end point. In the sodium arsenite method, the free chlorine is titrated with a standard sodium arsenite solution using KI-starch paper as the external indicator. In the orthotolidine (OT) method (Standard Methods of the Examination of Water and Wastewater, 1976), the colorless OT reagent, when added to dilute chlorine solution (at the ppm level), will turn to yellow-orange-red, depending on the chlorine concentration. The intensity of yellow-orange-red determines the amount of available chlorine present and is compared to previously prepared color standards. Palin's DPD method (Palin, 1969) employs N,N-diethyl-p-phenylene-diamine (DPD) reagent, and the dilute chlorine solution will turn the reagent pink to red, depending on the concentration of chlorine (at the ppm level). There are modifications in the OT and Palin methods distinguishing free available chlorine, total available chlorine, combined available chlorine and chloramines. The amperometric method consists of electrometric titration in which the current passes through a titration cell containing a dilute chlorine solution as the oxidizing agent and the standard phenylarsene oxide (PAO) as titrating reducing agent. The volume of PAO consumed determines the free available chlorine (at the ppm level) in solution, and the end point is indicated electrically. This titrating detection unit is composed of an indicator electrode, a reference electrode, and a microammeter (White, 1972).

Presently, chlorine measurements can be accurately made by employing polarographic membrane techniques. The probe is a plastic structure containing an anode and electrolyte, and is terminated by a membrane-covered noble metal cathode. When the probe is immersed in a chlorinated solution, the chlorine is reduced to chloride at the cathode; the generated current, being linear with chlorine concentration, is displayed on the meter of the analyzer. The probe lead is the only connection between the analyzer and the sample being measured. There is no need for reagents of any kind. This probe can be installed in a pipeline or any other desirable location and requires virtually no maintenance. One of the more important features of the probe analysis is the capability to distinguish between different forms of chlorine that may be present, thus yielding maximum efficiency at minimum cost. This application is widely accepted by various industries guaranteeing their users safety, performance, and economy.

Methods for Determining the Germicidal Activity of Chlorine

Many test methods have been devised during the past half century to demonstrate the antimicrobial activity of chlorine compounds. Initially, chlorine was evaluated for bactericidal effectiveness by the phenol coefficient method. This test has been a good procedure for evaluating phenols or phenolic compounds, but it was found unsuitable for testing chlorine compounds, always giving lower than true results for chlorine.

Johns (1934), working with hypochlorites and other chlorine compounds, developed his own technique, known as the glass slide method. Weber and Black (1948) developed a laboratory procedure to evaluate the effectiveness of germicides intended for sanitizing food utensils, which was later modified by Chambers (1956). To test the chlorine compound for fungicidal activity, the Association of Official Analytical Chemists Fungicidal Test method may be used (Official Methods of Analysis, 1980). All chlorinated compounds may be evaluated in the AOAC Available Chlorine Germicidal Equivalent Concentration Test (Ortenzio, 1957). To examine the effectiveness of swimming-pool sanitizers, another method has been proposed in which the unknown chemical compounds are compared to the effectiveness of standard sodium hypochlorite solution (Ortenzio et al., 1964). For determining algicidal properties of chlorine compounds, Palmer et al. (1955) developed a method suitable for screening potential algicides. (For more information on testing sanitizers, see Chapter 48.)

Mechanism of Chlorine Disinfection

Chlorine, in an aqueous solution, even in minute amounts, exhibits fast bactericidal action. The mechanism of this activity has not been fully elucidated, despite much research done in this field.

Andrewes et al. (1904) were among the early workers suggesting that hypochlorous acid was responsible for the destruction of microorganisms. When elemental chlorine or hypochlorites are added to water, they undergo the following reactions:

$$Cl_2 + H_2O \rightarrow HOCl + H^+ + Cl^- \qquad (3)$$

$$Ca(OCl)_2 + H_2O \rightarrow Ca^{++} + H_2O + 2OCl^- \qquad (4)$$

$$Ca(OCl)_2 + 2H_2O \rightarrow Ca(OH)_2 + 2HOCl$$

$$HOCl \rightleftharpoons H^+ + OCl^- \qquad (5)$$

The dissociation of hypochlorous acid depends on pH, and the equilibrium between HOCl and OCl$^-$ is maintained, even though HOCl is constantly consumed through its germicidal function (Baker, 1959) (Fig. 7–2). It appears that the disinfecting efficiency of chlorine decreases with an increase in pH and vice versa, which is parallel to the concentration of undissociated hypochlorous acid. This indicates that HOCl must be far stronger in bactericidal action than OCl$^-$. From our experience, we know that alkaline solutions of both sodium and calcium hypochlorite with small amounts of HOCl and larger amounts of OCl$^-$ definitely possess bactericidal properties. This suggests that OCl$^-$ ions may be a contributing factor in disinfection. However, Chang (1944), in his work with *Endamoeba histolytica* cysts, found OCl$^-$ to be non–cyst-penetrating and noncysticidal. An explanation may be that as traces of HOCl are consumed in the germicidal process, the hydrolysis equilibrium (equation 5 preceding) will be shifted to the left and HOCl will be formed continuously to effect the bactericidal

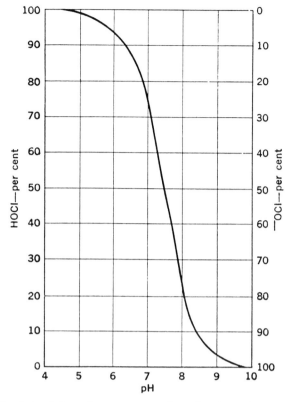

Fig. 7–2. Relationships among HOCl, ⁻OCl, and pH. (After Baker, R.J. 1959. Types and significance of chlorine residuals. J. Am. Water Works Assoc., *51*:1185–1190.)

action. Because the OCl⁻ ion contains active chlorine, it may well be that it has a germicidal power. Fair et al. (1948) and Morris (1966) calculated a theoretic curve for relative disinfecting efficiency of HOCl and OCl⁻ to produce 99% kill of *Escherichia coli* at 2° to 5°C at various pH levels within 30 minutes and found that the OCl⁻ ion possesses about 1/80 of the germicidal potency of HOCl under these conditions.

Exactly how HOCl destroys microorganisms has never been demonstrated experimentally. There have been speculations, however, that HOCl liberates nascent oxygen, which in turn supposedly combines with components of cell protoplasm, destroying the organism. This theory could not be substantiated, because other oxygen-producing compounds such as H_2O_2 and $KMnO_4$, despite larger amounts of nascent oxygen produced, would not kill so fast as chlorine, and because chlorine will kill even under conditions that exclude direct oxidation of protoplasm within the bacterial cell (Chang, 1944).

Baker (1926) advanced a theory that chlorine destroys bacteria by combining with proteins of cell membranes, forming N-chloro compounds, which in turn interfere with cell metabolism, causing eventual death of the organism. Other theories stipulated that chlorine action changes the cell membranes to allow diffusion of cell contents outward or that mechanical disruption of cell membranes exists due to chlorine disinfection.

According to Rudolph et al. (1941), the bactericidal

effect of hypochlorites is completed in two successive phases: (1) the penetration of an active germicidal ingredient into the bacterial cell and (2) the chemical reaction of this ingredient with the protoplasm of the cell to form toxic complexes (N-chloro compounds) that destroy the organism.

Green et al. (1946) advanced the enzyme trace substance theory. They postulated that, because of the low chlorine level required for bactericidal action, chlorine must inhibit some key enzymatic reactions within the cell. They found a correlation between the effect of chlorine on bacterial growth and its effect on the rate of glucose oxidation by the bacterial cell. Inhibition of glucose oxidation was measured by the percentage of bacteria killed.

Later, Knox et al. (1948) confirmed that the bactericidal effect of chlorine is produced by the inhibition of certain enzyme systems essential to life, and that mechanism here is the result of oxidative action of chlorine on the SH groups of vital enzymes or other enzymes sensitive to oxidation by chlorine. This reaction is apparently irreversible, because attempts to cause reversion of the reaction by addition of cysteine or glutathione were not successful (Ingols et al., 1953). The inhibition of essential cytoplasmic metabolic reactions is largely responsible for the destruction of the bacterial cell.

Friberg (1956), using radioactive ³⁵Cl, studied quantitatively whether or not and to what extent free available chlorine will combine with bacteria. He reported that no free available chlorine could be located at the end of a 5-minute chlorination period and that chlorine combination with bacteria increased with increasing exposure time and with increasing chlorine concentration. There was no chlorine uptake by bacteria from combined available chlorine. He concluded that chlorine combining chemically with bacterial protoplasm to form chloramines does not seem to contribute to the initial bactericidal effect and that the first contact oxidation reactions of chlorine with bacterial cells, prior to its accumulation, are responsible for the bactericidal action. His general postulations agreed closely with previous works of Green et al. (1946) and Knox et al. (1948) showing that chlorine, even at low concentration, can lead to certain and rapid destruction of bacterial substance prior to the formation of N-chloro compounds within the protoplasm. Friberg (1957), also using radioactive phosphorus (³²P), demonstrated that chlorine, in minute amounts, results in a destructive permeability change in the bacterial wall, as evidenced by leakage of ³²P from nucleoproteins of the bacterial cells.

According to Johns (1934) and Chang (1944), chloramines hydrolyze in water to form HOCl, and HOCl in trace amounts is the killing agent. Charlton et al. (1937) believed that the germicidal action of chloramines is due to a direct chlorination action by the active chlorine atoms of undissociated chloramine molecules. Later, Chang (1944) indicated that some chloramines (halazone, dichloramine) hydrolyzed to HOCl and then exhibited

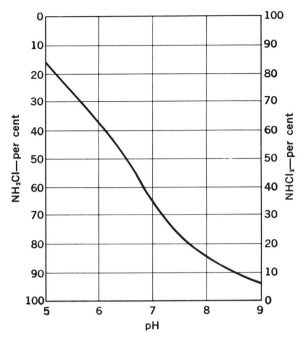

Fig. 7–3. Relationships among NH₂Cl, NHCl₂, and pH. These relationships are based on a weight ratio of 5:1 between chlorine and ammonia nitrogen. (After Baker, R.J. 1959. Types and significance of chlorine residuals. J. Am. Water Works Assoc., *51*:1185–1190.)

good cyst-penetrating power, whereas monochloramine and succinchlorimide did not produce a detectable amount of HOCl in hydrolysis within 2 hours and thus were poor penetrators of cysts. Marks et al. (1945) agreed with Chang (1944) and indicated that two different mechanisms of germicidal action occur with *N*-chloro compounds: (1) the undissociated chloramine molecule acts directly on bacteria and (2) HOCl formed via hydrolysis of *N*-chloro compound is the killing agent. As pH becomes an important factor in the germicidal activity of hypochlorous acid, it also exhibits an important influence on the rate of chloramine formation and on the antibacterial action of the chloramine. Fair et al. (1948) showed calculated relative percentages of monochloramine and dichloramine at different pH levels in solution, with a chlorine-to-ammonia weight ratio of 5:1 (Fig. 7–3).

Stability of Chlorine in Solution

The stability of free available chlorine in solution depends largely on the following factors: (1) chlorine concentration, (2) presence and concentration of catalysts, (3) pH of the solution, (4) temperature of the solution, (5) presence of organic material, and (6) ultraviolet irradiation. Any of these factors, alone or in combination, may greatly affect the stability of free available chlorine in solution. Iron and aluminum seem to have only a slight effect on the stability of chlorine solution, whereas copper, nickel, or cobalt are powerful catalysts of decomposition. The most stable free available chlorine solutions are those having the following characteristics: (1) low chlorine concentration, (2) absence of low contents of copper, cobalt, nickel, or other catalysts, (3) high alka-

linity, (4) low temperature, and (5) absence of organic material, and (6) are stored in dark and in closed containers, i.e., shielded from ultraviolet light. The stability of chlorine in solution or products may be rated by its half-life, which denotes the number of days required for the available chlorine content to be reduced to half its initial value (Chlorine Bleach Solutions, 1957).

Organic chloramines are considerably more stable in solution than free chlorine compounds, because they release chlorine rather slowly into solution, with delayed bactericidal action. Solutions of chloramine-T are quite stable, and a moderate exposure to high temperature, sunlight, or organic material does not seem to cause any appreciable decomposition (Dakin et al., 1916). To ensure a free chlorine stability in solution, chlorine stabilizers are often employed that will combine with chlorine to form *N*-chloro compounds, prolonging the life of chlorine considerably, but at the same time producing a slower germicidal effect.

Factors Affecting Chlorine Biocidal Activity

A long history and wide use of chlorine compounds have yielded much laboratory and field evaluation data, mostly concerning hypochlorites, but with application to all active chlorine compounds to some extent. Germicidal effectiveness will largely depend on the concentration of undissociated hypochlorous acid in water solution and the relationship between pH and the degree of dissociation of HOCl, as shown in Figure 7–2. In addition to pH, various other environmental factors, alone or in combination, will determine the antimicrobial action of chlorine. A full understanding of these environmental factors and manipulation thereof will enable the user of chlorine compounds to make proper adjustments for best results.

Effect of pH

pH has perhaps the greatest influence on the antimicrobial activity of the chlorine in solution. An increase in pH substantially decreases the biocidal activity of chlorine, and a decrease in pH increases this activity. Early work by Rideal et al. (1921) and Johns (1934) showed this pH dependency on hypochlorite effectiveness. Charlton et al. (1937), using *Bacillus metiens* and calcium hypochlorite solutions, showed that 100 ppm available chlorine at pH 8.2 would exhibit about the same kill of spores as a 1000 ppm solution at pH 11.3, demonstrating the controlling effect of pH. Later, Rudolph et al. (1941) showed the effect of pH on 25 ppm available chlorine solution to produce 99% kill of *B. metiens* spores. The results were: 2.5 minutes for pH 6, 3.6 minutes for pH 7, 5 minutes for pH 8, 19.5 minutes for pH 9, 35.5 minutes for pH 9.35, 131 minutes for pH 10, and 465 minutes for pH 12.86. The authors attributed the striking changes in killing time to changes in concentrations of undissociated hypochlorous acid and concluded that the concentration of HOCl is closely related to the speed of kill by hypochlorites in solution.

Mercer (1957), using *B. macerans* spores, showed that 15 ppm hypochlorite solution would effect 99% reduction of organisms within 8.5 minutes at pH 6, and that approximately 42 minutes were required at pH 8 for the same reduction. He also found no significant difference in the sporicidal activity with chlorine gas, sodium hypochlorite, and calcium hypochlorite. Friberg et al. (1956), in their work with bacteria and viruses, concluded that the virucidal effect of free available chlorine is affected by the pH in much the same manner as in the bactericidal action. Watkins et al. (1957) reported on the virucidal activity of NaOCl solution that, at 12.5 ppm available chlorine completely inactivated phage of *Streptococcus cremoris* within a 30-second interval; as pH was lowered from 9 to 4.4, progressively faster phase destruction occurred. This increased activity at lower pH levels was somewhat similar to results obtained with hypochlorites against bacterial spores and non spore-forming bacteria.

Bactericidal activity of chloramines is also influenced by pH. With a decrease in pH there is a corresponding increase in dichloramine formation, which is a more effective bactericide than the monochloramine. Chang (1944), in his work using cysts of *Endamoeba histolytica*, verified this point by showing that dichloramine was a considerably more powerful cyst-penetrating agent than monochloramine. He attributed this faster penetration power to one of the hydrolysis products of dichloramine, namely, to HOCl.

Effect of Concentration

It would be logical to assume that an increase in concentration in available chlorine in a solution would bring a corresponding increase in the antibacterial activity. This supposition may hold true as long as other factors, such as pH, temperature, and organic content, are held constant. Mallman et al. (1932), in their experiments with *Staphylococcus aureus* and at a constant pH value of 9, showed that by increasing the available chlorine in the hypochlorite solutions from 0.3 through 0.6, 1.2, to 2.0 ppm, the killing time was shortened or the bactericidal rate increased. The 2 ppm available chlorine produced complete kill in 5 minutes and 1.2 ppm in 10 minutes, whereas 0.3 ppm did not completely kill the organism even in 30 minutes.

Rudolph et al. (1941) tested hypochlorite solutions at concentrations of 25, 100, and 500 ppm of available chlorine at a constant pH of 10 and temperature of 20°C. The times required to provide the 99.9% kill of the resistant *Bacillus metiens* spores were 31 minutes for 500 ppm, 63.5 minutes for 100 ppm, and 121 minutes for 25 ppm available chlorine solutions. They concluded that a fourfold increase in the concentration of hypochlorite solution will result in a 50% reduction in killing time, and a twofold increase in only 30% reduction (see also Weber et al., 1944).

Effect of Temperature

The effect of temperature was demonstrated by Costigan (1936) on *Mycobacterium tuberculosis*; the author, using 50 ppm available chlorine hypochlorite solution at pH 8.35, obtained complete kill in 30 seconds at 60°C, in 60 seconds at 55°C, and in 2½ minutes at 50°C. Under the same test conditions, 200 ppm available chlorine solutions at pH 9 destroyed the organism in 60 seconds at 50°C and in 30 seconds at 55°C.

A temperature effect on the bactericidal activity of Ca(OCl)$_2$ solution was observed by Rudolph et al. (1941) at 20°, 30°, 35°, and 50°C. The 25 ppm hypochlorite solution at a constant pH of 10 killed in 121, 65, 38.7, and 9.3 minutes, respectively. These workers observed a 60 to 65% reduction in killing time with a 10°C rise in temperature. Later, Weber et al. (1944), in other related work with hypochlorite solutions at 25 ppm available chlorine and three different pH levels (10, 7, 5), concluded that a rise of 10°C produced a reduction of 50 to 60% in killing time, and that a drop of 10°C increased the necessary exposure time by about 2.1 to 2.3 times. This work also revealed that temperature coefficients were only slightly affected by pH.

Collins (1955), in his work with *Pseudomonas*, showed that Ca(OCl)$_2$ at 3 ppm available chlorine produced a 99.99% kill in 4 minutes at 21°C, but, on the average, in 10 minutes at 4.4°C. The effects of temperature on the bactericidal action of free available chlorine are especially evident at a pH higher than 8.5, and also when the chlorine residuals are low (0.02 to 0.03 ppm available chlorine) (Butterfield et al., 1943).

With respect to temperature effect on chloramines, it has been reported that 2½-times-higher concentrations of chlorine and 9-times-longer exposure times are necessary to produce the same kill at 3° as at 20°C (Weidenkopf, 1953). From all this work, it is evident that an increase in temperature produces an increase in bactericidal activity.

Effect of Organic Material

Organic material in chlorine solution consumes available chlorine and reduces its capacity for bactericidal activity; this is evident especially in solutions with low levels of chlorine. It has been reported that hypochlorites are selective in their attack on various types of organic material. There seems to be a difference of opinion among various workers on this subject.

Guiteras et al. (1934) showed that among different sugars, only levulose consumed chlorine, and that the chlorine loss with other non-nitrogenous substrates (lipids and alcohols) was negligible. They observed also that sodium hypochlorite was more reactive with organic substrates than either chloramine T or Azochloramid. Prucha (1927) reported early on the effect of 1 to 5% skim milk on chlorine losses in solution. Later, Loveless (1934) studied the amount of available chlorine loss in hypochlorite solution in the presence of 1.5% whole milk at a temperature range of 21° to 100°C for a period of 60 minutes, and observed that all solutions showed some loss in available chlorine at 21°C and that the rate of loss increased with rising temperatures. The control solutions with no milk, however, did not seem to lose any available chlorine during the 60 minutes, except for a small loss at 100°C. However, according to Mudge et al. (1935), the presence of milk in the tests with hypochlorite solutions did not seem to adversely affect the bactericidal action of chlorine.

If the organic matter contains proteins, the chlorine reacts and forms chloramines, retaining some of its antibacterial activity, even though the available chlorine levels are reduced considerably. This explains some questionable results in the early literature regarding the disappearance of anthrax spores from chlorinated tannery wastes in the absence of measurable free available chlorine (Tilley et al., 1930) or that hypochlorite solution of 130 ppm of available chlorine completely killed *Salmonella pullorum* in the presence of 5% organic matter in the form of chicken manure. Similar results were reported with *typhosa* and human feces (McCulloch, 1945).

Later, Johns (1948), using a modification of glass slide technique and *Escherichia coli* and *Staphylococcus aureus* as test organisms, reported no evidence of germicidal reduction due to the presence of skim or whole milk in the freshly prepared hypochlorite solutions. This reported feature may be significant for the use of hypochlorites as sanitizers on milk farms and in dairy plants, because minute amounts of milk may be encountered with no particular adverse effect on the germicidal activity of hypochlorites. However, Lasmanis et al. (1953) found, in their work with hypochlorite solutions employing strains of staphylococci (coagulase positive and negative), that with 3% of skim milk they did not obtain complete kill of organisms, although smaller amounts of milk exhibited progressively lesser effect on the bactericidal action.

It appears that sugars and starches do not affect the germicidal activity of chlorine. Shere (1948) reported that 500 ppm of alkyl aryl sulfonate did not exhibit any slowing action on the germicidal effectiveness of the hypochlorite solutions. Other organic materials such as tyrosine, tryptophan, cystine, egg albumin, peptone, body fluids, tissues, microbes, and vegetable matter, when present in a sanitizing solution, will consume chlorine to satisfy the organic water demand; in this case, the chlorine may lose its function as a germicidal agent unless it forms chloramines or unless the chlorine dosage is adjusted to overcome this demand. This loss of chlorine due to organic matter may be significant in cases in which minute amounts of chlorine are employed. Higher levels of chlorine, however, tend to produce a safety reserve for performing the desired bactericidal action.

Effect of Hardness

Water hardness components such as Mg^{++} and Ca^{++} ions do not exhibit any slowing effect on the antibacterial action of hypochlorite solution. Shere (1948) evaluated 5 ppm available chlorine sodium hypochlorite solution at 0 and 400 ppm hardness at 20°C. He obtained a complete kill of bacterial organisms at the two examined levels of hardness, indicating that raising the hardness from 0 to 400 ppm did not have any inhibitory action on the bacterial kill by hypochlorite solution.

Effect of Addition of Ammonia or Amino Compounds

The bactericidal activity of free chlorine is considerably diminished when chlorine is added to water containing ammonia or amino compounds and the concentration of chlorine is plotted against residual chlorine (Fig. 7–1). Part of the chlorine reacts immediately with ammonia to form mono- and di-chloramines. As more chlorine is added to the ammonia solution, to a ratio of chlorine to ammonia of 5:1, formation of chloramines continues until all the ammonia has been converted. Up to this point, chlorine remains in the form of combined available chlorine. After the so-called "hump" has been obtained, added amounts of chlorine will oxidize the chloramines, slowly reducing the residual chlorine and ammonia, until they both drop practically to zero. Increase of chlorine beyond this point (breakpoint) will produce an increase in free available chlorine (Butterfield, 1948). The available chlorine curves for different N-chloro compounds formed from amino acid or proteins vary due to variability of reactions and varying stabilities of the products of the reactions.

Weber et al. (1944) concluded that if the ammonia concentration is less than one eighth of the total available chlorine added, the ammonia will be destroyed and the excess chlorine will remain as free available chlorine, exhibiting fast bactericidal action. However, if the concentration of ammonia is greater than one fourth that of free chlorine, the available chlorine will exist in the form of chloramines and thus will be slow in bactericidal activity. Water temperature has an effect on the antibacterial action of the ammonia-chlorine treatment, the efficiency decreasing with lowering of the temperature. According to studies of Geiger et al. (1952), an excess of ammonium salt in the presence of high organic material enhanced the bactericidal effectiveness of hypochlorite solution.

From the information available, it appears that the killing time of chlorine is extended considerably in chloramines or N-chloro compounds, and the higher the concentration of ammonia or nitrogenous compounds, the greater is the lag in bactericidal time.

Effect of Addition of Iodine or Bromine (Halogen Mixture)

There is considerable evidence that small additions of bromine or iodine to chlorine solutions greatly enhance the bactericidal activity of chlorine. Houghton (1946) reported on improvement of bactericidal results in solutions containing chlorine, plus a small amount of ammonia salt and bromide ions. Kristoffersen et al. (1958) demonstrated that addition of NaBr to hypochlorite solution resulted in a 33 to 1000% increase in bactericidal effectiveness against a variety of bacteria at pH 11. Farkas (1964) reported that chlorine-bromine mixtures at various ratios increased the germicidal activity in purified and natural waters containing low and high amounts of nitrogenous growth-promoting material in a pH range of 5.4 to 8.6. He also demonstrated that chlorine reinforced by 5 to 10% bromide was effective in decreasing the number of chlorine- and bromine-resistant bacteria. Kamlet (1953), employing equimolecular mixtures of bromine and chlorine, obtained superior germicidal effects against *Escherichia coli* as compared to either chlorine or bromine alone. Darragh et al. (1954) claimed an advantage in using germicidal mixtures containing iodine with chlorine.

Paterson (1964) demonstrated that a halogen-substituted mixture, such as *N*-bromo-*N*-chlorodimethyl hydantoin, exhibited bactericidal activity against test bacteria superior to that obtained for either *N,N*-dibromo- or *N,N*-dichlorodimethyl hydantoin. Zsoldos (1964) produced a germicidal mixture by introducing dichlorodimethyl hydantoin and KI into aqueous solution, thereby generating a hypoiodous acid and chloramine combination.

ORGANISMS RESISTANT TO CHLORINE

Various types of bacteria, viruses, fungi, and algae exhibit different resistance to hypochlorites under diverse practical conditions (Table 7–1). This selective resistance of organisms to chlorine may be compensated for either by increased concentration, by lowering of pH, or by raising of temperature. Tonney et al. (1928 and 1930), in their studies with vegetative and spore-forming bacteria, concluded that various strains of cultures exhibit different resistances to chlorine. Generally, they have found that vegetative cells are less resistant to chlorine than the spore-forming group, and that 0.15 to 0.25 ppm available chlorine was sufficient to destroy the vegetative group within 30 seconds. Because *E. coli* was found to be generally more resistant to chlorine than other organisms of the vegetative bacteria, it was selected as the test organism for determining the effectiveness of disinfection by chlorine. The spore-forming organisms were about 10 to 1000 times more resistant to chlorine than vegetative forms.

Heathman et al. (1936) established variations in resistance of freshly isolated strains of *Salmonella typhosa* and members of the coli-aerogenes group to disinfection by chlorine. Kabler et al. (1939) reported that freshly isolated strains of *S. typhosa* are considerably more resistant than those that were grown on artificial media for some time. Phillips (1952) and Odlang (1981), in comparing the relative resistance of spores versus vegetative bacterial organisms, attributed this resistance of spores to changes in molecular configuration of proteins protecting the sulfhydryl groups of essential enzymes, whereas in the case of vegetative forms, these groups seemed to be unprotected. Clarke et al. (1954, 1959) disclosed that some viruses, being more resistant to chlorine, would require considerably higher chlorine levels to inactivate them.

Working with *Aspergillus niger* and *Trichophyton rosaceum*, Costigan (1931, 1941) showed that mold spores are considerably more resistant to chlorine and that 135 to 500 ppm of hypochlorite solution was necessary to inactivate a high density of spores in several minutes. Palmer et al. (1955), in screening algicides, found that different species of algae showed varying resistances to $Ca(OCl)_2$.

ANTIMICROBIALLY ACTIVE CHLORINE COMPOUNDS

A great number of antimicrobially active chlorine compounds are commercially available. Table 7–2 presents only a partial list. In the following sections, the special characteristics of some of the more important chlorine-bearing compounds will be discussed.

Liquid Chlorine

One of the most important commercial chlorine preparations is liquid chlorine. Although elemental chlorine is a gas (about $2\frac{1}{2}$ times as heavy as air), it is supplied, by compressing and cooling it, as an amber liquid ($1\frac{1}{2}$ times as heavy as water) and shipped in steel cylinders or tank cars. When released to atmospheric conditions, liquid chlorine reverts immediately to a gaseous form. It is highly reactive in the presence of moisture and possesses a great tendency to combine with organic compounds. Another characteristic of chlorine and chlorine compounds is their unique ability to displace bromine or iodine from their respective salts by metathesis. This chemical mechanism is frequently employed in practice for the controlled release of iodine and bromine in solution.

Hypochlorites

Hypochlorites are the oldest and most widely used of active chlorine compounds in the field of chemical disinfection. They are: (1) proven and powerful germicides controlling a wide spectrum of microorganisms, (2) deodorizers, (3) nonpoisonous to man at use concentrations, (4) free of poisonous residuals, (5) colorless and nonstaining, (6) easy to handle, and (7) most economical to use (Lesser, 1949).

Hypochlorites are available as powders or liquids. Calcium hypochlorite, lithium hypochlorite, and sodium hypochlorite, combined with hydrated trisodium phosphate (chlorinated TSP) make up the powder line; however, sodium and potassium hypochlorite is sold in solution form. Calcium hypochlorite dihydrate is a 65% available chlorine free-flowing powder, granulated material or tablet, having a strong chlorine odor (Dychdala, 1970). It may be blended with compatible inorganic diluents to produce lower available chlorine compounds (15 to 50%). Calcium hypochlorite products are soluble in water and fairly stable upon prolonged storage. Lithium hypochlorite is a 35% available chlorine free-flowing white granulated material with a strong chlorine odor. It is readily soluble in water and fairly stable. On exposure to air, the powdered hypochlorites attract moisture and become less stable. The sodium hypochlorite solutions range in concentration from 1 to 15%, with 1 to 5% available chlorine products employed for domestic use

Table 7–1. *Biocidal Effect of Free Available Chlorine on Various Organisms*

Organism	pH	Temp. (°C)	Exposure Time	ppm Av. Cl_2	Biocidal Results	References
ALGAE						
Chlorella variegata	7.8	22	—	2.0	Growth controlled	Palmer et al., 1955
Gomphonema parvulum	8.2	22	—	2.0	Growth controlled	Palmer et al., 1955
Microcystis aeruginosa	8.2	22	—	2.0	Growth controlled	Palmer et al., 1955
BACTERIA						
Achromobacter metalcaligenes	6.0	21	15 seconds	5.0	100%	Hays et al., 1963
Bacillus anthracis	7.2	22	120 minutes	2.3–2.4	100%	Brazis et al., 1958
B. globigii	7.2	22	120 minutes	2.5–2.6	99.99%	Brazis et al., 1958
Clostridium botulinum toxin type A	7.0	25	30 seconds	0.5	100%	Brazis et al., 1959
Escherichia coli	7.0	20–25	1 minute	0.055	100%	Butterfield et al., 1943
E. typhosa	8.5	20–25	1 minute	0.1–0.29	100%	Butterfield et al., 1943
Mycobacterium tuberculosis	8.4	50–60	30 seconds	50	100%	Costigan, 1936
Listeria monocytogenes	9.5	20	30 seconds	100	99.999%	Lopes, 1986, El-Kest et al., 1988
Pseudomonas fluorescens IM	6.0	21	15 seconds	5.0	100%	Hays et al., 1963
Shigella dysenteriae	7.0	20–25	3 minutes	0.046–0.055	100%	Butterfield et al., 1943
Staphylococcus aureus	7.2	25	30 seconds	0.8	100%	Dychdala, 1960, Bolton, 1988
Streptococcus faecalis	7.5	20–25	2 minutes	0.5	100%	Stuart et al., 1964
All vegetative bacteria	9.0	25	30 seconds	0.2	100%	Snow, 1956
Yersinia enterocolytica	9.0	20	5 minutes	100	99.99%	Orth et al., 1989
BACTERIOPHAGE						
S. cremoris phage strain 144F	6.9–8.2	25	15 seconds	25	100%	Hays et al., 1959
FISH						
Carassius auratus	7.9	Room	96 hours	1.0	Killed	Davis, 1934
Daphnia magna	7.9	Room	72 hours	0.5	Killed	Davis, 1934
FROGS						
Rana pipiens	8.3	21	4 days	10	100%	Kaplan, 1962
FUNGI						
Aspergillus niger	10–11	20	30–60 minutes	100	100%	Dychdala, 1961
Rhodotorula flava	10–11	20	5 minutes	100	100%	Dychdala, 1961
NEMATODES						
C. quadrilabiatus	6.6–7.2	25	30 minutes	95–100	93%	Chang et al., 1960
D. nudicapitatus	6.6–7.2	25	30 minutes	95–100	97%	Chang et al., 1960
PLANTS						
Cabomba caroliniana	6.3–7.7	Room	4 days	5	100%	Zimmerman et al., 1934
Elodea canadensis	6.3–7.7	Room	4 days	5	100%	Zimmerman et al., 1934
PROTOZOA						
Endamoeba histolytica cysts	7.0	25	150 minutes	0.08–0.12	99–100%	Clarke et al., 1956
VIRUSES						
Purified adenovirus 3	8.8–9.0	25	40–50 seconds	0.2	99.8%	Clarke et al., 1956
Purified Coxsackie A_2	6.9–7.1	27–29	3 minutes	0.92–1.0	99.6%	Clarke et al., 1959
Purified Coxsackie B_1	7.0	25	2 minutes	0.31–0.40	99.9%	Kelly et al., 1958
Purified Coxsackie B_5	7.0	25–28	1 minute	0.21–0.30	99.9%	Clarke et al., 1959
Infectious hepatitis	6.7–6.8	Room	30 minutes	3.25	Protected all 12 volunteers	Clarke et al., 1959 Grabow, et al., 1984
Purified poliovirus (Mahoney)	7.0	25–28	3 minutes	0.21–0.30	99.9%	Clarke et al., 1959
Purified poliovirus (Lensen)	7.4–7.9	19–25	10 minutes	1.0–0.5	Protected all 164 inoculated mice	Clarke et al., 1959
Purified poliovirus III (Sankett)	7.0	25–28	2 minutes	0.11–0.2	99.9%	Clarke et al., 1959
Purified Theiler's	6.5–7.0	25–27	5 minutes	4–6	99%	Clarke et al., 1959
Simian rotavirus	6.0	5	15 seconds	0.5	99.99%	Berman et al., 1984

Table 7–2. *Commercially Produced Chlorine Compounds*

		INORGANIC		
Commercial Name	*Chemical Name*	*Active Ingredient Chemical Formula*	*% Av. Cl₂*	*CAS Registry No.*
Sentry	Calcium hypochlorite dihydrate	$Ca(OCl)_2 \cdot 2H_2O$	65–70	[7778-54-3]
H T H	"	"	"	"
Pittchlor	"	"	"	"
Chloryte	"	"	"	"
Lithium hypochlorite	Lithium hypochlorite	$LiOCl$	30–35	[13840-33-0]
B K Powder	Calcium hypochlorite dihydrate	$Ca(OCl)_2 \cdot 2H_2O$	50–52	[7778-54-3]
Dakin's solution	Sodium hypochlorite	$NaOCl$	0.4–0.5	[7681-52-9]
Liquid bleach	"	"	12–15	
B K Liquid	"	"	5.25	
Clorox	"	"	5.25	
Liquid bleach	Potassium hypochlorite	$KOCl$	12–14	
Chlorinated T S P	Chlorinated trisodium phosphate	$4(Na_3PO_4 \cdot 11H_2O)NaOCl$	3.25	[56802-99-4]
Chlorine dioxide	Chlorine dioxide decahydrate	$ClO_2 \cdot 10H_2O$	17	[10049-04-4]

		ORGANIC		
Chloroazodin	N, N'-dichloroazodicarbonamidine	(structure)	77.8	—
Chloramine T	Sodium p-toluene sulfonchloramide	(structure)	24–26	[127-65-1]
Dichloramine T	p-Toluene sulfondichloramide	(structure)	56–60	[473-34-7]
Chloramine B	Sodium benzene sulfonchloramide	(structure)	29.5	—
Succinchlorimide	Succinchlorimide	(structure)	50–54	—
Halazone	p-Sulfondichloramidobenzoic acid	(structure)	48–52.8	[80-13-7]
Halane	1,3-Dichloro-5,5-dimethylhydantoin	(structure)	66	[118-52-5]
Antibac	"	"	16	[118-52-5]

Table 7–2. *Commercially Produced Chlorine Compounds* Continued

ORGANIC

Commercial Name	Chemical Name	Active Ingredient Chemical Formula	% Av. Cl₂	CAS Registry No.
ACL 85 (or CDB 90)	Trichloro-isocyanuric acid (trichloro-*s*-triazinetrione)		89–90	[87-90-1]
ACL 66	[(Monotrichloro)-tetra-(monopotassium dichloro)] penta-isocyanurate		66	[34651-95-1]
ACL 60 (or CDB 63)	Sodium dichloro-isocyanurate		60–63	[2893-78-9]
CDB Clearon (or ACL 56)	Sodium dichloro-isocyanurate dihydrate		55	[51580-86-0]
ACL 59 (or CDB 59)	Potassium dichloro-isocyanurate		59.0	[2244-21-5]
TCM	Trichloromelamine		70–129	[7673-09-8]

and stronger solutions sold to industrial customers. Sodium hypochlorites in water solution are less stable, especially in products with higher chlorine concentrations. Potassium hypochlorites are available as liquids at 10 to 12% available chlorine concentration. Chlorinated TSP is a fine white crystalline material, containing about 3.25% available chlorine. In addition to producing hypochlorite ion for sanitizing properties, it also contains alkaline phosphate for detergency.

Because of their wide acceptance as disinfectants in many industries, hypochlorite solutions serve as standards for testing of other sanitizers. Today hypochlorites are employed as sanitizers in most households, hospitals, schools, and public buildings. They are also widely used for microbial control in restaurants, soda fountains, and other public eating places, and for sanitizing food processing plants, dairies, canneries, breweries, wineries, and beverage bottling plants. Hypochlorites are sold for treatment of pool and drinking water, sewage, and wastewater effluents.

Chlorine Dioxide

Chlorine dioxide has received more attention in recent years. This chlorinated compound is employed with greater frequency for drinking water disinfection, for wastewater treatment and for slime control in cooling tower waters. It has a unique ability to break down phenolic compounds and remove phenolic tastes and odors from the water. Another favorable feature is said to be its lack of reaction with ammonia. Finally, chlorine dioxide does not form trihalomethanes or chlorophenols. That characteristic is of great importance to man and the environment. Chlorine dioxide is used in the chlorination of drinking water as well as in wastewater, and for elimination of cyanides, sulfides, aldehydes, and mercaptans. Ingols et al. (1948) showed the oxidation capacity of ClO_2 in terms of available chlorine to be about $2\frac{1}{2}$ times that of chlorine. Its oxidation-reduction potential is close to that of chlorine. The analysis for chlorine dioxide is similar to that of chlorine but with some modification. As in the case of chlorine detection, chlorine dioxide can be continuously measured by chlorine dioxide analyzer and transmitter systems based on amperometric sensing devices.

Chlorine dioxide at room temperature is soluble in water at 2.9 g/L at 30 mm partial pressure. In aqueous solution, the product is decomposed by light. It undergoes a valence change of 5 in the reduction reaction to chloride and does not pass through a hypochlorous acid phase during this reduction, but rather follows a different reaction path.

According to Ridenour et al. (1947), chlorine dioxide activity equals that of chlorine. The bactericidal efficiency of chlorine dioxide was found to be unaffected at pH levels of 6 to 10. In further work, Ridenour et al. (1949a) found that chlorine dioxide's bactericidal activity decreases with lowering of temperature. Later, in additional work with spores, the authors demonstrated greater sporicidal activity for chlorine dioxide than for chlorine. The greater sporicidal activity of chlorine dioxide is explained by greater utilization of its oxidation capacity involving a full change of five electrons. Vegetative bacteria do not activate this full oxidation potential (Ridenour et al., 1949b).

Harakeh et al. (1985) evaluated solutions of chlorine dioxide against *Yersinia enterocolitica* and *Klebsiella pneumoniae*. The authors showed that when test organisms were grown in natural aquatic environment of low temperature and lower nutrient contents, they were more resistant to chlorine dioxide than were the same microorganisms grown under optimum laboratory conditions. Berman et al. (1984) showed good antiviral activity by chlorine dioxide at pH 10 in less than 15 seconds.

Chlorine dioxide is an extremely reactive compound and consequently cannot be manufactured and shipped in bulk, but is prepared at the place of consumption. In practice, this consists of mixing a solution of chlorine with a solution of sodium chlorite; the product is then applied to a water supply. The chlorine dioxide is formed according to the equation:

$$Cl_2 + 2NaClO_2 \rightarrow 2ClO_2 + 2NaCl \qquad (6)$$

Chlorine dioxide may also be produced by the following reactions:

1. Acidification of chlorates with hydrochloric or sulfuric acid
2. Reduction of chlorates in acid medium
3. Reacting acids with chlorites
4. Electrolytically by using sodium chloride, sodium chlorite, and water

By combining separate solutions of sodium chlorite and acid, Alliger (1978) developed a germ-killing composition resulting in the production of chlorine dioxide at the site of application. Chlorine dioxide decahydrate may be prepared commercially, but it must be kept refrigerated, because it decomposes at room temperature and can be dangerously explosive under some conditions.

De Guevara (1955) prepared stable antiseptic solutions using inorganic boron compounds such as sodium tetraborate, boric acid, and sodium perborate to stabilize chlorine dioxide in aqueous solutions, forming a labile complex.

Anthium Dioxcide is manufactured by International Dioxcide, Inc., Clark, N.J. Here ClO_2 is generated and all traces of chlorine are removed by passing through the column of sodium carbonate peroxide. The final product contains 5% of stabilized ClO_2 complex. To make this material biologically active, one needs to release ClO_2 in solution by either acidification or introduction of chlorine. The manufacturer's instructions for use recommend that an adjustment of pH be made with either acetic acid, citric acid, or phosphoric acid, or by adding 2.5 g of "Activator K" to each gallon of solution (International Dioxcide, Inc., 1966). Presently, this type of stabilized ClO_2 is being used in the paper industry for removing slimes from paper-mill white water systems. The use of chlorine dioxide has been extended to the food industry in providing sanitation for different food products under a variety of situations (Masschelein, 1979; Field Report, 1977).

Inorganic Chloramines

When ammonia combines with chlorine in water solution, it forms monochloramine (NH_2Cl), dichloramine ($NHCl_2$), nitrogen trichloride (NCl_3), or nitrogen. The residual amine tends to suppress the release of hypochlorous acid. In monochloramine, the chlorine is not sufficiently active to demonstrate any antimicrobial activity. It has a low hydrolysis constant, which is too low for hypochlorous acid to be released in sufficient amounts. The activity of chloramines depends on the pH of the solution (Fig. 7–3). Because of a high degree of instability, inorganic chloramines are not produced for sale as such. The instability of $NHCl_2$ is important in breakpoint chlorination (Sheltmire, 1962).

Inorganic chloramine treatment of water supplies was used in the 1930s and early 1940s to improve tastes and odors of water. Race (1918) showed that the most efficient ratio of chlorine to ammonia is 2:1 by weight. The reason for ammonia use in water chlorination was to provide prolonged stability of chlorine. However, the work of Wattie et al. (1944) pointed to inferior kills with combined available chlorine compared to the effects produced by free available chlorine. It will take approximately 25 times as much chloramine as free available chlorine to effect a rapid bactericidal action; for chloramines, the contact time is about 100 times longer than that required for the same residual of free available chlorine to produce the same kill. As a result of this work, the chloramine water treatment was gradually discontinued in the United States. Chloramines are being considered for chlorination of water to prevent trihalomethane formation (Norman et al., 1980). Additionally, Kereluk et al. (1983), working with 5 to 10 ppm monochloramine solutions, demonstrated antimicrobial activity against bacteria and fungi.

Organic Chloramines

Chloramines are produced by the reaction of HOCl with an amine, amide, imine, or imide. The organic chloramines are the N-chloro derivatives of the following four groups: (1) sulfonamides (chloramine-T, dichloramine-T, chloramine-B, halazone), (2) heterocyclic compounds with nitrogen in the ring (hydantoin, succinchlorimide, dichloro- and trichloro-isocyanurates, trichloromelamine), (3) condensed amines from guanidine derivatives (chloroazodin), and (4) anilides (Sheltmire, 1962).

Chloramine-T

Sodium p-toluene sulfonchloramide is a white crystalline powder containing about 25% available chlorine. It has a slight chlorine odor and is soluble in water up to 12% at 25°C. This compound was applied in practice by Dakin et al. (1916) during World War I for treating infected wounds. It was favored over hypochlorites, because it was found less irritating, held chlorine longer, did not react as rapidly with organic material, was slightly less corrosive, and was stable to heat or light.

Many early workers (Dakin et al., 1917; Tilley, 1920; Myers, 1930; Beseman, 1928; Holwerda, 1930) generally disagreed on the merits of bactericidal action of chloramine-T when compared to hypochlorites. Most of them indicated, however, that chloramine-T was slow in germicidal action. There were also many opinions expressed on the mechanism of the bactericidal action. Johns (1934) reported that chloramine-T hydrolyzes to form hypochlorous acid, and that, as in the case of hypochlorites, HOCl is responsible for the germicidal activity of chloramine-T. Holwerda (1928) was unable to detect any HOCl in solutions containing chloramine-T equivalent to 10 ppm available chlorine. Charlton et al. (1937), in their bacteriologic studies of hypochlorite versus chloramine-T, using *Bacillus metiens* and *Bacillus subtilis*, showed that activity of chloramine-T was considerably slower than that of hypochlorites and that its bactericidal kill is significantly affected by pH, concentration, and temperature in the same way as hypochlorites (see also Johns, 1930; Weber, 1950; Ortenzio et al., 1959; and Trueman, 1971).

The Grade A Pasteurized Milk Ordinance (1985) and Ordinance and Code for Restaurants (1948), both prepared by the U.S. Public Health Service, permitted the use of chloramine-T, provided it was equivalent to the bactericidal activity of 50 ppm available chlorine hypochlorite solution within 1 minute of exposure time. Because of the slow bactericidal action attributed to chloramine-T solutions at more alkaline pH levels, its use in practice as a sanitizer is limited to only special applications, where low pH or long exposure is practical.

Dichloramine-T

Chemically, dichloramine-T is p-toluene sulfondichloramide and is prepared by the action of calcium hypochlorite solution on p-toluene sulfonamide followed by acidification with acetic acid. It is a pale yellow crystalline material with a strong chlorine odor and has a melting point of about 80°C. Upon exposure in air, it decomposes with loss of chlorine. Also, it decomposes in alcohol and turpentine. Because it is almost insoluble in water, its use as a germicide is limited to only a few antiseptic medicinal preparations (Leech, 1923).

Dichlorodimethylhydantoin

1,3-Dichloro-5,5-dimethyl hydantoin is a white free-flowing powder with a slight chlorine odor and a slight solubility in water. Several commercial cleaner-sanitizer products available are based entirely on this active ingredient or blends of it with other components. Work of Ortenzio et al. (1959) showed that, at a pH of 6, a 65 ppm hydantoin solution gave germicidal results comparable to 200 ppm hypochlorite solution; however, at a pH of 7, 8, or 9, hydantoin solutions of 175, 400, and

2000 ppm of available chlorine, respectively, were required to give results equivalent to 200 ppm hypochlorite solution.

Johns (1951), working with a dichlorodimethylhydantoin-based product and employing the glass slide and Weber and Black techniques, concluded that in spite of the tested pH (4.5 to 6.7) the product is often a slower-acting germicide than hypochlorites when examined against *Escherichia coli*, *Staphylococcus aureus*, and *Pseudomonas aeruginosa*. Bacon et al. (1953) showed that dichlorodimethylhydantoin solution, in a pH range of 5.8 to 7.0, was found similar in germicidal activity to hypochlorite.

In general, under acid conditions, the dichlorodimethylhydantoins are more effective as bactericides than hypochlorites, while less effective under alkaline conditions. Their effectiveness depends largely on specific formulation, concentration, and above all, specific pH.

Halazone

Halazone, or *p*-sulfondichloramidobenzoic acid, is prepared by chlorination of p-sulfonamidobenzoic acid in alkaline solution. The commercially available product consists of a mixture of mono- and di-chloramidobenzoic acid, with the dichloro compound predominating. Halazone is a white crystalline powder with a chlorine odor, melting at 195°C with decomposition. Because it is slightly soluble in water, its solubility may be increased by the use of sodium chloride, sodium carbonate, or borax, and in blends with one or more of these it is tableted for water disinfection use. Dakin et al. (1917) prepared 4-mg halazone tablets in this fashion, stabilizing them with small amounts of sodium chloride and sodium carbonate, and these were sufficient to treat 1 liter of water. The authors also reported that dilution of halazone at approximately 1:300,000 was satisfactory to kill *Salmonella typhosa*, *Escherichia coli*, and *Vibrio comma* in about 30 minutes.

Chang (1944), in his studies with cysts of *Endamoeba histolytica*, demonstrated that halazone, under similar test conditions of pH, had a cyst-penetrating power about two fifths that of free chlorine. These tests also revealed that halazone in solution hydrolyzes to form HOCl, which has strong cyst-penetrating power. He compared the behavior of halazone to that of hypochlorite-chloramine mixture. One half of the chlorine in the halazone molecule reacts rapidly with ammonium ion to form chloramine, whereas the other chlorine reacts rather slowly. Although halazone is similar to hypochlorite in its mode of action, it was found to be much inferior in germicidal effect under identical test conditions.

A definite effect of the ammonium ion toward increasing the bactericidal activity of halazone solution in the presence of organic material has been demonstrated by Geiger et al. (1952). The authors explained that ammonia seems to provide a "buffer" action and to form simple chloramines, thus preventing the chlorine from being completely inactivated by organic contamination. Work of these authors has shown that organic matter has an inhibiting effect on the bactericidal activity of halazone solution. One ppm available chlorine as halazone, in the absence of organic material, showed complete kill of *Escherichia coli* in 3 minutes, whereas in the presence of organic material, only partial bacterial destruction was observed in 1 hour.

There are some applications for halazone in the cleaning and sanitizing of equipment and utensils in the food and dairy industry, for water and sewage treatment, and for bleaching and sanitizing in commercial laundries.

Succinchlorimide

Succinchlorimide, a heterocyclic chlorine compound, is a white crystalline powder with a chlorine odor. Its solubility in water is about 1.4% at 25°C, and special water-solubilizing formulations are therefore prepared to make it more soluble at various temperatures. This chemical has been proposed as a germicidal agent for purification of water supplies (Wood, 1928). In bacteriologic work by Reddish et al. (1945), a two-grain tablet of 10% succinchlorimide per quart of polluted water of high chlorine demand killed high densities of test organisms (*Salmonella typhosa*, *Shigella dysenteriae*, and *Escherichia coli*) within 5 to 10 minutes at 2°, 23°, and 27°C. In separate work with *Endamoeba histolytica*, Chang (1944) showed that succinchlorimide at 50 ppm of titratable chlorine exhibited weak cyst-penetrating power and that 89 ppm of chlorine was needed to destroy the cysts, thus revealing succinchlorimide to be much inferior to hypochlorite in the cyst-penetrating and cysticidal activities. He also demonstrated that succinchlorimide in solution did not hydrolyze to give any detectable amount of HOCl, even during the 2-hour reaction period. According to Chang's conclusions, even though succinchlorimide is inferior in cysticidal properties, it is strongly bactericidal when compared to hypochlorites and is less affected by organic material.

Chlorinated Cyanuric Acid Derivatives

This class of organic available chlorine compounds consists of three commercial products: (1) the sodium salt of dichloroisocyanuric acid, (2) the potassium salt of dichloroisocyanuric acid, and (3) trichloroisocyanuric acid. The sodium and potassium salts of dichloroisocyanuric acid (60% and 59% available chlorine) are soluble in water, 25% and 9%, respectively, and the pH of a 1% solution of either salt is 5.9. Trichloroisocyanuric acid is also a white crystalline material with a strong chlorine odor, and its solubility in water is 1.2% at 25°C; the available chlorine content is 90%, and the pH of a 1% solution is 2.7 to 2.9. CDB-Clearon is a dihydrate form of sodium dichloroisocyanurate containing 55% available chlorine.

Chloroisocyanurates may be used in the field of sanitation by themselves or formulated into various products. The carefully formulated products based on chloroisocyanurates may be used as: (1) household and commercial laundry dry bleaches, (2) machine dishwashing compounds, (3) scouring powders, and (4) industrial sanitizing compounds (food, dairy, restaurant, swimming pool). In the preparation of these products, the specially selected ingredients must be moisture free, because moisture content adversely affects the stability of available chlorine in the finished product. Small amounts (1 to 5%) of dodecylbenzene sodium sulfonate may be incorporated into products, but nonionic surfactants generally should be avoided, because they will react rapidly and decompose the chloroisocyanurates (Industrial Uses of ACL, 1979; Thompson, 1964).

According to work of Ditzel et al. (1956), in evaluating trichloroisocyanuric acid at 100 and 50 ppm available chlorine in the Weber and Black method and against *Escherichia coli* and *Staphylococcus aureus*, acceptable results were obtained when compared at equivalent active chlorine concentration to sodium hypochlorite solution. The authors commented that the effectiveness of the trichloroisocyanuric acid will vary with pH. Further work of Petrie et al. (1958) confirmed the results just described in the Chambers method. Recently, Ortenzio et al. (1959) demonstrated the effect of pH on the bactericidal activity of dichloro- and trichloroisocyanuric acid. The authors concluded that both dichloro- and trichloroisocyanuric acid would give satisfactory results comparable to hypochlorites at pH 6.0 to 9.5.

When chloroisocyanurates are added to aqueous solution, they hydrolyze to form HOCl and cyanuric acid. In swimming-pool sanitation, using the potassium or sodium salt of dichloroisocyanurates, it was necessary to establish whether accumulation of cyanuric acid in the pool water would exhibit any influence on bactericidal activity. Ortenzio et al. (1964) showed that sodium dichloroisocyanurate at approximately 0.6 ppm available chlorine exhibited comparable results to hypochlorite within 30 seconds against *Escherichia coli*. However, against *Streptococcus faecalis*, twice the concentration (1.35 ppm available chlorine) was required to effect the same kill (within 30 to 60 seconds) produced by 0.59 ppm available chlorine sodium hypochlorite standard. In separate works of Andersen (1964) and Stuart et al. (1964), the effect of cyanuric acid in combination with NaOCl was demonstrated. Robinton et al. (1967) confirmed these findings and found a pronounced retardation of bactericidal activity of Ca(OCl)$_2$ in the presence of cyanuric acid. The three papers agree that cyanuric acid at 25, 50, and 100 ppm did slow down the bactericidal action of NaOCl solution (0.6 ppm) from 2 to about 10 minutes against *Streptococcus faecalis*, and that higher chlorine levels were required to restore action equal to that of NaOCl solution. Against *Escherichia coli*, the slowing effect of germicidal action was not as pronounced as it was in the case with *Streptococcus faecalis* and *Staphylococcus aureus*. However, Kowalski et al. (1966), in their pool studies, showed that chlorine was an effective bactericide independent of the presence of cyanuric acid.

Chloroazodin

Chloroazodin, or Azochloramid, is a *N,N'*-dichloroazodicarbonamidine and is a bright yellow flaky material with a faint chlorine odor. It decomposes explosively at about 155°C, and its decomposition is accelerated by contact with metals. It is slightly soluble in water, but its solubility increases considerably in solvents. Solutions of chloroazodin decompose on exposure to light.

Chloroazodin exerts a mild but sustained germicidal activity, while manifesting relatively low toxicity to tissues. Guiteras et al. (1934) showed that chloroazodin at different pH levels was far less reactive with amino acids and slightly less reactive with other organic matter (tissues and body fluids) than either chloramine-T or hypochlorites. Because Azochloramid is light sensitive, it should be protected from prolonged exposure to light. Various preparations containing Azochloramid with different combinations of surface-active agents, saline and sulfanilamide once found wide therapeutic use for irrigation of infected wound surfaces or other topical applications.

Trichloromelamine

Trichloromelamine (TCM) is prepared by chlorinating melamine. It is a whitish powder and is slightly soluble in water. Having three chlorine atoms, it hydrolyzes to release HOCl, depending on temperature and pH. TCM is quite a stable chlorine compound; heating the powder at 100°C for a day and boiling it briefly in solution resulted in small chlorine losses. According to Chang et al. (1959), TCM in aqueous solution releases HOCl in increasing amounts as the pH decreases, with a maximum at a pH of 3.0. TCM at 200 ppm available chlorine and at an acid pH produced good bactericidal results against *Streptococcus pyogenes*, *Streptococcus faecalis*, *Staphylococcus aureus*, and *Escherichia coli*. They concluded that TCM, being stable, moderately soluble, and slightly affected by organic material, is one of the more suitable germicides among the *N*-chloro compounds. However, the bactericidal, cysticidal, and virucidal activities of TCM fell short of those to be desired, especially when evaluated at 5°C.

Experimental New Products

The development of new biocides has been limited in the last decade because of the high cost of research, stringent regulations governing biocides, and excessive costs for the necessary toxicity data. It appears that, in the future, new biocides most likely may come only from large companies that are in a better position to afford these large expenditures. Even some of these large corporations are currently cutting costs for the basic research (Layman, 1978).

PRACTICAL APPLICATION OF CHLORINE SANITATION

In Water Treatment

Drinking Water

The chlorination practices for sanitizing drinking water to make it safe and palatable for human consumption have been long established in North America. Elemental chlorine or calcium hypochlorite has been used successfully for over half a century to treat drinking water, with or without subsequent filtration. Continuous chlorination of drinking water has practically eliminated various waterborne pathogens, such as those responsible for cholera, dysentery, and typhoid, thereby preventing the epidemics due to drinking water of previous times. Drinking waters are protected by Public Health standards, implemented by periodic checks to ensure the safety and complete physical, chemical, and microbiologic quality.

Swimming-Pool Water

In the case of pool water, the contact time of microorganisms with chlorine may be rather short, and a greater spectrum of organisms is constantly introduced into pool water by various swimmers. Environment also contributes to contamination and higher chlorine consumption in the pool water. When chlorinating the pool water, sufficient chlorine must be added to provide an adequate residual chlorine level to ensure rapid (15 to 30 seconds) kill of microorganisms and to prevent the spread of pathogens from one swimmer to another. In the most recent trend, regulatory agencies officially connected with swimming-pool standards have indicated that a level of 0.6 to 1.0 ppm of free chlorine residual (stabilized pools 1 to 2 ppm) should be maintained at all times when a swimming pool is in operation (see also Chapter 28).

Spas and Hot Tubs

Recently, spas and hot tubs have grown in popularity, and their sanitation has become an integral part of this fast-growing industry. Spas and hot tubs have been chlorinated on a daily basis to keep these relatively small volumes of water free from pollution and infection. Chlorine and chlorinated compounds are recommended mainly for use in this industry. These products not only satisfy the large chlorine demand of the water, but also provide a residual available chlorine to render this water sanitary for reuse. When spas and hot tubs are chlorinated, usually a level of 1 to 3 ppm (ideally 1.0 to 1.5 ppm) of free available chlorine must be continuously maintained, as required by the industry standards for spas and hot tubs. Also, superchlorination must be practiced frequently to keep the spa and hot tub waters free of pathogenic and low-chlorine-resistant microorganisms, thus ensuring a safe and continuous use of these facilities (Minimum Standard For Residential Spas, 1980).

Ice

Ice intended for human consumption or used in contact with water, food, food equipment, and utensils should be free of pathogenic organisms and should conform to the Public Health Service standards. Quite often, ice is chlorinated so that on melting it will not only produce a cooling effect but will also exhibit a simultaneous antibacterial action. Such chlorinated ices have been used often in food processing plants (poultry or fish), where microbial contamination is high (Tanner, 1944) and also for iced drinks and for icing other foods. Chlorinating ice at 2 ppm, Moore et al. (1953) reported low bacterial counts and no odor or flavor complaints noted in iced drinks.

In-Plant Chlorination

Plant chlorination of water supply beyond the breakpoint level is referred to as "in-plant chlorination." It is employed in many food industry plants involved with canning, freezing, poultry dressing, and fish processing. Somers (1951) reported that a 4 to 5 ppm chlorine level was sufficient for normal operating conditions and that a higher chlorine level (10 to 25 ppm) was recommended for cleanup operations.

In canneries and freezing plants, the bacteria, slimes, and foul odors are practically eliminated from plant premises as a result of in-plant chlorination. In poultry dressing plants, the use of in-plant chlorination of water at 10 to 20 ppm chlorine level produced improvement in the sanitary quality of processed birds. It reduced bacterial density and eliminated slime development and odors from equipment, pipelines, and other plant locations. About 30% of the time usually devoted to the cleanup operation of the plant was saved because of in-plant chlorination (Mercer et al., 1957).

In Food Handling and Processing Equipment

Chlorine in various forms, and hypochlorites in particular, have been successfully used to sanitize utensils and equipment in dairy and food handling and processing industries. Prucha (1929) was one of the early workers who studied extensively the chlorine compounds for sanitizing dairy farm and milk plant equipment. He made many practical recommendations: (1) Utensils and equipment should be clean before employing a sanitizing solution effectively, (2) freshly prepared chlorine solution should be applied to utensils or equipment always just before their use, (3) 50 to 100 ppm available chlorine should be employed for sanitizing large equipment and utensils and 200 ppm for spraying application of large equipment, (4) the contact time for an effective sanitation should be long enough to produce complete kill of bacteria, usually 10 seconds or longer, and (5) chlorine compounds or solutions should not be added directly to products, e.g., milk, in an attempt to reduce the number of organisms there. Loveless (1934), in later work with hypochlorites on farms, indicated definite improvement in bacteriologic quality of milk, as shown by plate counts and methylene blue reduction tests.

According to the Grade A Pasteurized Milk Ordinance, 1985 Recommendations of the U.S. Public Health Service, a hypochlorite solution of at least 50 ppm of available chlorine should be employed for sanitizing of utensils and equipment with a minimum of 1-minute exposure time at a minimum of 75°F (24°C). In spraying applications, the chlorine level should be doubled. Other chlorine compounds may be used as sanitizers, provided they will effect a fast bactericidal action equivalent to 50 ppm hypochlorite at a pH of 10 and a temperature of 75°F (24°C) with a 1-minute exposure time. Food Service Sanitation Manual (1962) Recommendation of U.S. Public Health Service recommends a sanitizing rinse of at least 50 ppm of available chlorine at a minimum of 75°F (24°C) for a time sufficient to provide fast kill of organisms.

In Sewage and Wastewater Treatment

Chlorine or hypochlorites have been used effectively in the field of sewage and wastewater treatment. Chlorination may be a continuous process or may be employed intermittently or seasonally. The benefits of chlorination include (1) general disinfection, (2) control of odors, (3) reduction of BOD (biochemical oxygen demand), (4) chemical precipitation, (5) color reduction (Laubusch, 1958a and b) and (6) cyanide treatment. Recently, there appears to be a concern that chlorination of sewage and wastewater may result in the formation of toxic chlorinated organic compounds capable of contaminating drinking water. Therefore, the effluents from sewage plants and industrial plants, if not treated properly, can contribute to contamination of drinking water, bathing water, wells, rivers, lakes, and oceans with adverse effect on animal and plant life. Because of the public health hazard, the sewage and wastewater disposal is regulated by federal, state, and local water pollution control commissions.

In Sanitizing of UF/RO/MF Membranes

A great number of different sanitizers are available on the market, but because of required chemical compatibilities, only a few sanitizers can safely be used on membranes. Cleaning of membranes is only the first step to sanitation. Soils or films may be instrumental in harboring bacteria or other microorganisms that are responsible for microbiologic fouling of membrane surfaces. Usually these soils or films cannot be removed by sanitizers alone; they have to be cleaned first. Once the surface is clean, the use of a suitable sanitizer will complete the job. Extreme care must be taken in the proper selection of the sanitizer for any specific membrane. The use of an incompatible sanitizer may result in irreversible damage to the membrane surface, usually requiring costly replacement of these membranes.

Ultrafiltration (UF), reverse osmosis (RO), and microfiltration (MF) membranes are used in many fields: food industry, water treatment, pharmaceuticals, biotechnology, and wastewater treatment. Sodium and potassium hypochlorites are often used for cleaning and sanitizing of certain polymeric and inorganic metallic membranes. Oxidizers such as chlorine are also helpful in the removal of protein during the cleaning process. Chlorinated compounds are not compatible with spiral-wound, cellulose acetate, polyamide, or thin film composite membranes, and therefore cannot be used for their disinfection. Even chlorinated water should not be used on these membranes. However, the use of chlorine on polysulfone, fluoropolymeric, or ceramic membranes is recommended. Even some polysulfone membranes do have limitations regarding the use of chlorine, chemical concentration, pH, and temperature, and they are usually regulated by strict manufacturer's specifications.

A number of manufacturers of membranes, including DDS, Rhone-Poulenc, Osmonics, Romicon, Desalination, and Dorr-Oliver, recommend sodium or potassium hypochlorite as a sanitizer on some of their membranes. Bragulla et al. (1987) discussed the use of chlorine on different membranes and alluded to the chemical limitations of these units. Smith et al. (1987) and Whittaker (1984) pointed to some problems associated with cleaning and sanitizing of UF/RO membranes. Wirth et al. (1961) showed the effects of oxidants on ion exchange resins that can adversely affect their performance.

In Treatment of Environment-Contaminated Foods

Chlorine disinfection of different foods is an established practice. Fish and shellfish caught in polluted waters may be carriers of pathogens, and hypochlorite treatment makes them safer for consumption (Wells, 1929). Because fish and shellfish contain a large amount of organic contamination, higher chlorine levels (200 to 6000 ppm) are necessary to reduce their bacterial content to safe levels (Tanner, 1944).

Fruits and vegetables may be decontaminated by washing in chlorine solution (4 to 5 ppm available chlorine) without damaging their quality (Somers, 1951). Because eggs are contaminated by their environment and may be carriers of pathogens, they too are treated with chlorine compounds. Chlorination of food, when carefully controlled, checks the microbial population and makes the foods safer for consumption, without adversely affecting the original nutritional value and palatability.

In Medicine and Allied Sciences

Chlorine compounds have been successfully employed for a long time in medicine and related fields to control infections or for the treatment of wounds. Dakin's solution has been used since World War I to disinfect open wound infections in the so-called Carrel-Dakin surgical irrigation treatment. In fungicidal foot baths, hypochlorite solutions (0.1 to 1.25%) have been used extensively in combating and controlling the spread of the athlete's foot infections (Costigan, 1941). During World War II, hypochlorite solutions were employed to treat trench mouth and burns, as well as wounds. Another application of sodium hypochlorite solution was in the irrigation of urinary bladders.

Chloramine-T was employed for general skin and wound disinfection, contributing greater stability of chlorine and lesser reactivity with organic material, including body fluids. Preparations containing chloramine-T were also applied by dentists to disinfect root canals, although recently this has been replaced by using sulfa drugs and antibiotics. Dichloramine-T has been used as an antiseptic for treatment of mucous membranes (Taub et al., 1954).

Bunyan (1960) reported that rinsing with 0.2% hypochlorite solution stops postoperative bleeding within 1 minute after a tooth extraction or other oral operation. The hypochlorite solution functions also to contract and harden the blood clots and makes them more resistant to infection. In addition to the effective hemostasis and the change in the character of the clot, the author reported a reduction of swelling of traumatized gingival tissues and diminution of the postoperative pain. Other organic chloramines, formulated into either liquid, paste, or ointment preparations, are used in the sterilization of wound surfaces or other topical applications (Leech, 1923). Chlorine compounds are widely employed in hospitals to disinfect equipment, instruments, laundry, and hands or for other applications (Sykes, 1963). In veterinary medicine, both hypochlorites and organic chloramines serve in treating wounds or combating infection in animals.

EFFECTS OF CHLORINE ON UNIQUE MICROBES

Biofilm Formation

Caldwell (1990), in his work with biofilms, showed that low levels of sodium hypochlorite (0.5 and 5 ppm Av. Cl_2) are only inhibitory to biofilms and their cells. He found that the cells will grow immediately when chlorine solution is removed and stop growing when exposed to chlorine. However, 50 ppm Av. Cl_2 solution resulted in the reduction of the biofilm and temporarily stopped the growth of cells, even after the chlorine solution was no longer in contact. Bolton et al. (1988) showed that endemic strains of *Staphylococcus aureus* isolated from poultry equipment were eight times more resistant to chlorine than the organisms grown on natural skin flora. This resistance was due to their ability to form macroclumps embedded in the extracellular slime layer.

Specific Pathogens

Orth et al. (1989), Lopes (1986), and El-Kest et al. (1988) conducted antimicrobial evaluations to determine the effectiveness of sodium hypochlorite against *Listeria monocytogenes*, *Campylobacter jejuni*, *Yersinia enterocolytica*, *Staphylococcus aureus*, *Enterococcus faecium*, *Proteus vulgaris*, or combinations thereof. The authors showed that different pathogens displayed varying degrees of resistance to chlorine and concluded that all organisms can be controlled by chlorine including those that are feared by all food processors, namely *Listeria*, *Campylobacter*, and *Yersinia*.

CHLORINE GENERATORS AND CHLORINATORS

In the last decade, a number of suppliers have offered electrolytic chlorine generators for the production of chlorine gas at the site of application. In these chlorine generators, a low current passes between electrodes, converting the brine solution to chlorine gas and sodium hydroxide. The electrodes for these generators can be made of a number of materials such as carbon, iron, and titanium. In the most recently built units, the anode is made of titanium coated with platinum and is located in the center of the salt cell. The cathode is constructed of stainless steel and surrounds the salt cell. Some of the advantages of these chlorine generators are: (1) semi-automation, (2) less chemical handling, (3) economy of operations once installed, and (4) relative safety. Some of the disadvantages associated with these units are high initial equipment cost, limited chlorine production capacity, corrosion of electrodes, and need for water circulation.

Chlorinators, on the other hand, are relatively new precision instruments that feed chlorine gas automatically from the source to its intended use. Some of these units are equipped with unique pressure checks and vacuum regulators that provide continuous chlorination and relative operating safety. Other smaller liquid chlorinators are merely feeding devices that automatically inject the concentrated chlorine solutions to their intended application site via proportioning pumps.

ACUTE ORAL TOXICITY AND OTHER TOXIC EFFECTS OF CHLORINATION

Acute Oral Toxicity

Over the years extensive toxicity studies were conducted on a great number of chlorinated compounds. Some of the data are published (RTECS, 1988; Wei et al., 1985), but the majority are kept in confidence by different manufacturers of these materials. Listed below are comparative acute oral toxicity data collected on various chlorinated compounds.

Chemical Name	Acute Oral Toxicity in Rats (LD_{50}/kg)
Calcium hypochlorite dihydrate 65% Av. Cl_2	1.3 g
Sodium hypochlorite 5.25% Av. Cl_2	6.4 g
Lithium hypochlorite	674 mg
Chlorine dioxide	292 mg
Chloramine T	1.64 g
Dichloroisocyanuric acid, sodium salt 50% Av. Cl_2	1.400 g
Dichloroisocyanuric acid, potassium salt 63% Av. Cl_2	1.215 g
Trichloroisocyanuric acid	406 mg
1,3 Dichloro-5,5-dimethyl hydantoin	542 mg
Succinchlorimide	256 mg
Trichloromelamine	490 mg

Trihalomethane Formation by Chlorination

There is general concern that our drinking water may contain substances that are believed to be potentially carcinogenic. On Dec. 16, 1974, the Safe Drinking Act became law, requiring the EPA to promulgate national drinking water standards. To do this, the EPA was to undertake a comprehensive study of public water supplies and drinking water sources in order to determine the nature, extent, sources, and controls of contaminating substances suspected of being carcinogenic. Tests, sponsored by the EPA, were conducted at numerous locations. Testing of new water sources and water treatment practices for suspected organic and inorganic carcinogens in drinking water were carried out. Trihalomethanes are organic contaminants present in drinking water, which include chloroform, bromodichloromethane, dibromochloromethane, and bromoform. Carbon tetrachloride and 1,2 dichloroethane are chlorinated solvents that were also investigated in the study. The objectives of the study were:

1. To find the types and amounts of these compounds in the water and determine whether or not they were formed by chlorination
2. To substantiate the effects on new water sources and water treatment practices and find out whether chlorination or any other treatment was responsible for the formation of these compounds
3. To check for the organic content of 10 finished drinking water supplies using existing analytical procedures
4. To find a way of removing these compounds from drinking water

This study was done on 80 different water supply locations, representing the continental United States. Based on this survey it was concluded that the presence of trihalomethanes in drinking water was the result of chlorination. Only very small amounts of carbon tetrachloride and 1,2-dichloroethane were detected in these finished waters. The maximum concentrations found in drinking water as a result of this study were chloroform—54 mg/L; bromodichloromethane—20 mg/L; dibromomethane—13.3 mg/L; and bromoform—10 mg/L. Subsequent water studies were made and confirmed the presence of trihalomethanes in a variety of finished drinking waters in Ohio, Indiana, and Alabama. Some of these studies indicated that other chlorination byproducts can occur during the chlorination process, and that naturally occurring substances were identified as precursors to the formation of the trihalomethanes.

In addition to the EPA, the National Academy of Sciences was involved to provide health hazard criteria by setting maximum concentrations of trihalomethane in drinking water. All carcinogenic contaminants that may be present in drinking water were considered from a vast range of toxic materials, both organic and inorganic. The organic sources of contamination were identified as coming from wastewater treatment plants, chlorination of water supplies, land fills, or other treatment processes.

A procedure for the removal of organic compounds from drinking water was developed by selecting the use of granular activated carbon columns. This procedure removes trihalomethanes, chlorinated hydrocarbons, and other precursors that may form trihalomethanes. The idea to effectively remove trihalomethane precursors from the water would be to preclude the formation of trihalomethanes during the chlorination of drinking water.

Many governmental, industrial, and technical people came to realize that there is no acceptable substitute for chlorination, the most suitable disinfectant for drinking water at the present time. Without chlorination, consequences derived from contamination and health hazards would be enormous. Simultaneously, there is concern about chlorination of organic materials found in natural water and wastewaters, and the need for their removal from our drinking water (Preliminary Assessment of Suspected Carcinogens in Drinking Water, 1975; Manual of Individual Water Supply Systems, 1982).

REFERENCES

Alliger, H. 1978. Germ killing composition and method. U.S. Patent 4,084,747.
Anderson, J.R. 1964. A study of the influence of cyanuric acid on the bactericidal effectiveness of chlorine. Paper presented at NSPI Convention, Chicago.
Andrewes, F.W., and Orton, K.S.P. 1904. Disinfectant action of hypochlorous acid. Zentrabl. Bakteriol. (Orig. A) 35, 645–651; 811–815.
Bacon, L.R., Sotier, A.L., and Roth, A.A. 1953. Field experience with Antibac. A new type of chlorine sanitizer. J. Milk Food Technol., 16, 61–65.
Baker, J.C. 1926. Chlorine in sewage and waste disposal. Can. Engr., Wtr. Sew., 50, 127–128.
Baker, R.J. 1959. Types and significance of chlorine residuals. J. Am. Water Works Assoc., 51, 1185–1190.
Berman, D., and Hoff, J.C. 1984. Inactivation of simian rotavirus SA 11 by chlorine, chlorine dioxide, and monochloramine. Appl. Environ. Microbiol., 48(2), 317–323.
Besemann, F. 1928. The chlorine absorption capacity of water. Vom. Wasser, (German), 2, 64.
Bolton, K.J., Dadd, C.E.R., Mead, G.C., and Waites, W.M. 1988. Chlorine resistance of strains of Staphylococcus aureus isolated from poultry processing plants. Appl. Microbiol., 6, 31–34.
Bragulla, S., and Lintner, K. 1987. Basics of cleaning and disinfection for ultrafiltration, reverse osmosis and electrodialysis. Henkel Technical Information, March, 1–4.
Brazis, A.R., Leslie, J.E., Kabler, P.W., and Woodward, R.L. 1958. The inactivation of Bacillus globigii and Bacillus anthracis by free available chlorine. Appl. Microbiol., 6, 338–342.
Brazis, A.R., et al. 1959. Effectiveness of halogens or halogen compounds in detoxifying Clostridium botulinum toxins. J. Am. Water Works Assoc., 51, 902–912.
British Pharmacopea. 1958. London, The Pharmaceutical Press, pp. 150–151.
Bunyan, J. 1960. The use of hypochlorite for the control of bleeding. Oral Surg., 13, 1026–1032.
Butterfield, C.T. 1948. Bactericidal properties of free and combined available chlorine. J. Am. Water Works Assoc., 60, 1305–1312.
Butterfield, C.T., Wattie, E., Megregian, S., and Chambers, C.W. 1943. Influence of pH and temperature on the survival of coli-forms and enteric pathogens when exposed to free chlorine. Public Health Rep., 58, 1837–1866.
Caldwell, D.R. 1990. Analysis of biofilm formation: confocal laser microscopy and computer image analysis. Abstracts of Papers to be Presented at the 77th Annual Meeting of the International Association of Milk, Food and Environmental Sanitarians, Inc., p. 11.
Chambers, C.W. 1956. A procedure for evaluating the efficiency of bactericidal agents. J. Milk Food Technol., 19, 183–187.
Chang, S.L. 1944. Destruction of micro-organisms. J. Am. Water Works Assoc., 36, 1192–1206.
Chang, S.L., and Berg, G. 1959. Chlormelamine and iodized chlormelamine germicidal rinse formulations. U.S. Armed Forces Med., J., 10, 33–49.
Chang, S.L., Berg, G., Clarke, N.A., and Kabler, P.W. 1960. Survival and protection against chlorination of human enteric pathogens in free-living nematodes isolated from water supplies. Am. J. Trop. Med. Hyg., 9, 136–142.
Charlton, D., and Levine, M. 1937. Germicidal properties of chlorine compounds. Bull. 132, Engr. Exp. Sta., Iowa State College.
Chlorinators. 1979. Philadelphia, Wallace & Tiernan, Pennwalt Corporation, pp. 1–8.

Chlorine Bleach Solutions. 1957. Solvay Tech. Eng. Service Bull. No. 14, pp. 6–7.

Chlorine Dioxide: The Dioxolin Process and Food Processing. 1978. A Technical Bulletin from Olin Corporation, pp. 1–4.

Clarke, N.A., and Chang, S.L. 1959. Enteric viruses in water. J. Am. Water Works Assoc., *51*, 1299–1317.

Clarke, N.A., and Kabler, P.W. 1954. The inactivation of purified Coxsackie virus in water by chlorine. Am. J. Hyg., *59*, 119–127.

Clarke, N.A., Stevenson, R.E., and Kabler, P.W. 1956. The inactivity of purified type 3 Adenovirus in water by chlorine. Am. J. Hyg., *64*, 314–319.

Collins, E.B. 1955. Factors involved in the control of gelatinous curd defects of cottage cheese. II. Influence of pH and temperature upon the bactericidal efficiency of chlorine. J. Milk Food Technol., *18*, 189–191.

Costigan, S.M. 1941. Fungicidal studies of some products commonly used in foot baths. Paper presented at 59th Annual Convention of Proprietary Association of America, New York City.

Costigan, S.M. 1936. Effectiveness of hot hypochlorites of low alkalinity in destroying *Mycobacterium tuberculosis*. J. Bacteriol., *32*, 57–63.

Costigan, S.M. 1931. Germicidal test of B-K using *Aspergillus niger* as the test organism. Pennwalt Corp., unpublished.

Cullen, G.E., and Taylor, H.D. 1918. Relative irritant properties of the chlorine group of antiseptics. J. Exp. Med., *28*, 681–699.

Dakin, H.D. 1915. The antiseptic action of hypochlorites. Br. Med. J., *2*, 809–810.

Dakin, H.D., and Cohen, J.B. 1916. On chloramine antiseptics. Br. Med. J., *1*, 160–162.

Dakin, H.D., and Dunham, E.K. 1917. The disinfection of drinking water. Br. Med. J., *1*, 682–684.

Darragh, J.L., and House, R. 1954. Addition products of halogen and quaternary ammonium germicides and method for making the same. U.S. Patent 2,679,533.

Davis, H.W. 1934. Discussion. Trans. Am. Fish. Soc., *64*, 1–280.

Ditzel, R.G., Arvan, P.G., and Symes, W.F. 1956. Bleaching and sanitizing agents. Soap Chem. Spec., *32*, 125–129; 137–139.

Dychdala, G.R. 1970. Calcium hypochlorite product and process for producing same. U.S. Patent 3,544,267.

Dychdala, G.R. 1961. Evaluation of yeasts and molds against different fungicides. Pennwalt Corp., unpublished.

Dychdala, G.R. 1960. Studies on bactericidal effectiveness of calcium hypochlorite stabilizers for swimming pool use. Pennwalt Corp., unpublished.

El-Kest, S.E., and Marth, E.H. 1988. Inactivation of *Listeria monocytogenes* by chlorine. J. Food Protect., *51*(7), 520–524, 530.

Fair, G.M., et al. 1948. The behavior of chlorine as a water disinfectant. J. Am. Water Works Assoc. *40*, 1051–1061.

Farkas-Himsley, H. 1964. Killing of chlorine-resistant bacteria by chlorine-bromine solutions. Appl. Microbiol., *12*, 1–6.

Field Report. 1977. Chlorine dioxide gains favor as effective sanitizer. Food Eng., *49*, 143.

Food Service Sanitation Manual. 1962. Food Service Sanitation Ordinance and Code. Recommendations of U.S. Public Health Service. Government Printing Office, Washington, p. 54.

Friberg, L. 1957. Further quantitative studies on the reaction of chlorine with bacteria in water disinfection. Acta Pathol. Microbiol. Scand., *40*, 67–80.

Friberg, L. 1956. Quantitative studies on the reaction of chlorine with bacteria in water disinfection. Acta Pathol. Microbiol. Scand., *38*, 135–144.

Friberg, L., and Hammerstrom, E. 1956. The action of free available chlorine on bacterial viruses. Acta Pathol. Microbiol. Scand., *38*, 127–134.

Geiger, K.H., and Moloney, P.J. 1952. Enhanced effectiveness of chlorination. Can. J. Public Health, *43*, 359–367.

Grabow, W.O.K., Gauss-Muller, V., Prozensky, O.W., and Deinhard, F. 1983. Inactivation of hepatitis A virus and indicator organisms in water by free chlorine residuals. Appl. Environ. Microbiol., *46*(3), 619–624.

Grade A Pasteurized Milk Ordinance. 1985. Recommendations of the U.S. Public Health Service, Appendix F. Government Printing Office, Washington, D.C., pp. 133–137.

Green, D.E., and Stumpf, P.K. 1946. The mode of action of chlorine. J. Am. Water Works Assoc., *38*, 1301–1305.

Griffin, A.E. 1944. Chlorination—a five-year review. J. N. Engl. Water Works Assoc., *58*, 322–332.

de Guevara, M.L. 1955. Aqueous chlorine dioxide compositions and production thereof. U.S. Patent 2,701,781.

Guiteras, A.F., and Schmelkes, F.C. 1934. The comparative action of sodium hypochlorite, chloramine-T, and azochloramid on organic substrate. J. Biol. Chem., *107*, 235–239.

Hadfield, W.A. 1957. Chlorine and chlorine compounds. In *Antiseptics, Disinfectants, Fungicides, Chemical and Physical Sterilization.* 2nd edition. Philadelphia, Lea & Febiger, pp. 558–580.

Harakeh, M.S., Berg, J.D., Hoff, J.C., and Matin, A. 1985. Susceptibility of chemostat-grown *Yersinia enterocolitica* and *Klebsiella pneumoniae* to chlorine dioxide. Appl. Environ. Microbiol., *49*(1), 69–72.

Hays, H., and Elliker, P.R. 1959. Virucidal activity of a new phosphoric acid-wetting agent sanitizer against bacteriophage of *Streptococcus cremoris.* J. Milk Food Technol., *22*, 109–111.

Hays, H., Elliker, P.R., and Sandine, W.E. 1963. Effect of acidification on stability and bactericidal activity of added chlorine in water supplies. J. Milk Food Technol., *26*, 147–149.

Heathman, L.S., Pierce, G.O., and Kabler, P. 1936. Resistance of various strains of *E. typhi* and *coli aerogenes* to chlorine and chloramine. Public Health Reports, *51*, 1367–1387.

Holwerda, K. 1928. Control and degree of reliability of chlorination process of drinking water in connection with chloramine procedure and chlorination of ammoniacal water. Mededeel. Dienst Volksgezondheid Nederland.–Indië, pt. II, 251–297.

Holwerda, K. 1930. Control and degree of reliability of chlorinating process of purifying drinking water, in relation to the use of chloramine, and chlorine process as applied to water containing ammonia in solution. Mededeel. Dienst Volksgezondheid Nederland.Z-Indië, pt. II, 325–385.

Houghton, G.U. 1946. Bromide content of underground waters. II. Chlorination of water containing free ammonia and naturally occurring bromide. J. Soc. Chem. Ind., *65*, 304–328.

Industrial uses of ACL—chlorinated s-triazine triones. 1979. St. Louis, Monsanto Tech. Bull., pp. 1–20.

Ingols, R.S., and Ridenour, G.M. 1948. Chemical properties of chlorine dioxide in water treatment. J. Am. Water Works Assoc., *40*, 1207–1227.

Ingols, R.S., et al. Bactericidal studies of chlorine. Ind. Eng. Chem., *45*, 996–1000.

International Dioxide, Inc. 1966. Technical properties of anthium dioxide, a chlorine dioxide complex. Bulletin 50.

Johns, C.K. 1951. The germicidal effectiveness of a new chlorine compound. J. Milk Food Technol., *14*, 134–136.

Johns, C.K. 1948. Influence of organic matter on the germicidal efficiency of quaternary and hypochlorite compounds. Can. J. Res., *26*, 91–104.

Johns, C.K. 1934. Germicidal power of sodium hypochlorite. Ind. Eng. Chem., *26*, 787–788.

Johns, C.K. 1930. The speed of germicidal action of chlorine compounds upon bacteria commonly found in milk. Sci. Agric., *10*, 553–563.

Kabler, P., Pierce, G.O., and Michaelson, G.S. 1939. Comparative resistance of recently isolated and older laboratory strains of *E. typhosa* to the action of chloramine. J. Bacteriol., *37*, 1–9.

Kamlet, J. 1953. Microbiocidal treatment of water with bromine chloride. U.S. Patent 2,662,855.

Kaplan, H.M. 1962. Toxicity of chlorine for frogs. Proc. Anim. Care Panel, *12*, 259–262.

Kelly, S., and Sanderson, W. 1958. The effect of chlorine in water on enteric viruses. Am. J. Public Health, *48*, 1323–1334.

Kereluk, K., and Borisenok, W.S. 1983. The antimicrobial activity of monochloramine. Dev. Ind. Microbiol., *24*, in press.

Knox, W.E., Stumpf, P.K., Green, D.E., and Auerbach, V.H. 1948. The inhibition of sulfhydryl enzymes as the basis of the bactericidal action of chlorine. J. Bacteriol., *55*, 451–458.

Kowalski, X., and Hilton, T.B. 1966. Comparison of chlorinated cyanurates with other chlorine disinfectants. Public Health Reports, *81*, 282–288.

Kristoffersen, T., and Gould, I.A. 1958. Effect of sodium bromide on the bactericidal effectiveness of hypochlorite sanitizers of high alkalinity. J. Dairy Sci., *41*, 950–955.

Lasmanis, J., and Spencer, G.R. 1953. The action of hypochlorite and other disinfectants on *Micrococci* with and without milk. Am. J. Vet. Res., *14*, 514–516.

Laubusch, E.J. 1958a. State practices in sewage disinfection. Sewage Ind. Wastes, *30*, 1233–1240.

Laubusch, E.J. 1958b. Chlorination of waste-water. Water Sewage Works, *105*, 12–18.

Layman, P.L. 1978. The search for new biocidal actives. Chemical Times & Trends, *1*, No. 3, 334–336.

Leech, P.N. 1923. Examination of American-made Chloramine-T, Dichloramine-T, Halazone and preparation. J. Am. Pharm. Assoc., *12*, 592–602.

Lesser, M.A. 1949. Hypochlorites as sanitizers. Soap Sanit. Chem., *25*, 119–125, 139.

Lopes, J.A. 1986. Evaluation of dairy and food plant sanitizers against *Salmonella typhimurium* and *Listeria monocytogenes.* J. Dairy Sci., *69*, 2791–2796.

Loveless, W.G. 1934. The use of chlorine products as germicides on dairy farms. Bull. 369, Vermont Agric. Exp. Sta.

Mallmann, W.L., and Schalm, O. 1932. The influence of the hydroxyl ion on the germicidal action of chlorine in dilute solution. Bull. No. 44, Michigan Eng. Exp. Sta., pp. 3–17.

Manual of Individual Water Supply Systems. 1982. U.S. Environmental Protection Agency, Office of Drinking Water, Washington, D.C.

Marks, H.C., Wyss, O., and Strandskov, F.B. 1945. Studies on the mode of action of compounds containing available chlorine. J. Bacteriol., *49*, 299–305.

Masschelein, W.J. 1979. Chlorine dioxide: chemistry and environmental impact of oxychlorine compounds. Ann Arbor, Science Publishers, Inc., p. 172.

McCulloch, E.C. 1945. *Disinfection and Sterilization*. 2nd edition. Philadelphia, Lea & Febiger, pp. 327–353.

Mellor, J.W. 1927. *Comprehensive Treatise on Inorganic and Theoretical Chemistry*. New York, Longmans Green & Co., p. 20.

Mercer, W.A., and Somers, I.I. 1957. *Chlorine in Food Plant Sanitation. Advances in Food Research*. Volume 7. New York, Academic Press, pp. 129–160.

Minimum Standard for Residential Spas. 1980. Washington, D.C., National Swimming Pool Institute, pp. 11–13.

Moore, E.W., Brown, E.W., and Hall, E.M. 1953. Sanitation of crushed ice for iced drinks. Am. J. Public Health, 43, 1265–1269.

Morris, J.C. 1966. Future of chlorination. J. Am. Water Works Assoc., 58, 1475–1482.

Mudge, C.S., and Smith, F.R. 1935. Relation of action of chlorine to bacterial death. Am. J. Public Health, 25, 442–447.

Myers, R.P. 1930. What chemicals are best adapted for the sterilization of dairy equipment? I. Milk bottles. Proc. Inst. Assoc. Milk Dealers, 23, 75–85.

Norman, T.S., Harms, L.L., and Looyenga, R.W. 1980. The use of chloramines to prevent trihalomethane formation. J. Am. Water Works Assoc., 72, 176–180.

Odlang, T.E. 1981. Antimicrobial activity of halogens. J. Food Protect., 44(8), 608–613.

Official Methods of Analysis of the Association of Offical Analytical Chemists. 1980. 14th edition. Washington, Assoc. Off. Anal. Chem., pp. 56–68.

Ordinance and Code Regulating Eating and Drinking Establishments. 1948. Public Health Service Bull. 280. Government Printing Office, Washington, p. 29.

Ortenzio, L.F. 1964. A standard test for efficacy of germicides and acceptability of residual disinfecting activity in swimming pool water. J. Assoc. Off. Agric. Chem., 47, 540–547.

Ortenzio, L.F. 1957. Available chlorine germicidal equivalent concentration test. J. Assoc. Off. Agric. Chem., 40, 755–759.

Ortenzio, L.F., and Stuart, L.S. 1964. A standard test for efficacy of germicides and acceptability of residual disinfecting activity in swimming pool water. J. Assoc. Off. Agric. Chem., 47, 540–547.

Orth, R., and Mrozek, H. 1989. Is the control of Listeria, Campylobacter and Yersinia a disinfection problem? Fleischwirtshaft, 69(10), 1575–1576.

Palin, A.T. 1967. Methods for the determination in water of free and combined available chlorine, chlorine dioxide, and chlorite, bromine, iodine, and ozone, using diethyl-p-phenylene diamine (DPD). J. Inst. Water Eng., 21, 537–547.

Palmer, C.M., and Maloney, T.E. 1955. Preliminary screening for potential algicides. Ohio J. Sci., 55, 1–8.

Paterson, L.O. 1964. Process of disinfecting water. U.S. Patent 3,147,219.

Petrie, E.M., and Roman, D.P. 1958. Chlorine sanitizing compounds. Soap Chem. Spec., 34, 67–68; ibid., 99.

Phillips, C.R. 1952. Relative resistance of bacterial spores and vegetative bacteria to disinfectants. Bacteriol. Rev., 16, 135–143.

Preliminary Assessment of Suspected Carcinogens in Drinking Water. 1975. Interim Report to Congress, U.S. Environmental Protection Agency, Washington, D.C., pp. 1–33.

Prucha, J.J. 1929. Chemical sterilization of dairy utensils. Circular 332, Illinois. Agric. Exp. Sta.

Prucha, J.J. 1927. Chemical sterilization in the dairy industry. Proc. Int. Assoc. Dairy Milk Inspectors, 16, 319–328.

Race, J. 1918. *Chlorination of Water*. New York, John Wiley & Sons, pp. 1–132.

Reddish, G.F., and Pauley, A.W. 1945. Succinchlorimide as a water decontaminant. Bull. Natl. Formulary Comm., 13, 11–18.

Rideal, E.K., and Evans, U.R. 1921. The effect of alkalinity on the use of hypochlorites. J. Soc. Chem. Ind., 40, 64R-66R.

Ridenour, G.M., and Armbruster, E.H. 1949a. Bacterial effect of chlorine dioxide. J. Am. Water Works Assoc., 41, 537–550.

Ridenour, G.M., Ingols, R.S., and Armbruster, E.H. 1949b. Sporicidal properties of chlorine dioxide. Water Sewer Works, 96, 279–283.

Ridenour, G.M., and Ingols, R.S. 1947. Bactericidal properties of chlorine dioxide. J. Am. Water Works Assoc., 39, 561–567.

Robinton, E.D., and Mood, E.W. 1967. An evaluation of the inhibitory influence of cyanuric acid upon swimming pool disinfection. Am. J. Public Health, 57, 301–310.

RTECS. 1988. Registry of Toxic Effects of Chemical Substances. Edited by Doris V. Sweet. U.S. Government Printing Office, Washington, D.C. 5 Volumes.

Rudolph, A.S., and Levine, M. 1941. Factors affecting the germicidal efficiency of hypochlorite solutions. Bull. 150, Eng. Exp. Sta., Iowa State College.

Sheltmire, W.H. 1962. *Chlorine, Its Manufacture, Properties and Uses*. New York, Rheinhold Publishing Corp., pp. 512–542.

Shere, L. 1948. Some comparisons of the disinfecting properties of hypochlorites and quaternary ammonium compounds. Milk Plant Monthly, 37, 66–69.

Smith, K.E., and Brandley, R.L., Jr. 1987. Efficacy of sanitizers using unsoiled spiral-wound polysulfone ultrafiltration membranes. J. Food Protect., 50, 567–572.

Snow, W.B. 1956. Recommended chlorine residuals for military water supplies. J. Am. Water Works Assoc., 48, 1510–1514.

Somers, I.I. 1951. Studies on in-plant chlorination. Food Technol., 5, 46–51.

Standard Methods of the Examination of Water and Wastewater. 1976. New York, 14th edition. American Public Health Association, pp. 309–328.

Stuart, L.S., and Ortenzio, L.F. 1964. Swimming pool chlorine stabilizers. Soap Chem. Spec., 40, 79–82; 112–113.

Sykes, J.H. 1963. Calcium hypochlorite for disinfection of hydrotherapy equipment. J. Am. Phys. Ther., 43, 345–347.

Tanner, F.W. 1944. *The Microbiology of Foods*. 2nd edition. Champaign, Garrard Press, pp. 780–794.

Taub, A., Hart, F., and Kassimir, S. 1954. Stability of some bactericidal chlorine-liberating compounds in special ointment bases. J. Am. Pharm. Assoc., 43, 178–181.

Taylor, H.D., and Austin, J.H. 1918a. The solvent action of antiseptics on necrotic tissue. J. Exp. Med., 27, 155–164.

Taylor, H.D., and Austin, J.H. 1918b. Behavior of hypochlorite and of Chloramine-T solutions in contact with necrotic and normal tissues in vivo. J. Exp. Med., 27, 627–633.

Taylor, H.D., and Austin, J.H. 1918c. Toxicity of certain widely used antiseptics. J. Exp. Med., 27, 635–646.

Thompson, J.S. 1964. Formulating with dichloroisocyanurates. Soap Chem. Spec., 40, 45–48; 122–123.

Tilley, F.W. 1920. Investigations of the germicidal value of some of the chlorine disinfectants. J. Agric. Res., 20, 85–110.

Tilley, F.W., and Chapin, R.M. 1930. Germicidal efficiency of chlorine and the N-chloro derivatives of ammonia, methylamine and glycine against *anthrax* spores. J. Bacteriol., 19, 295–302.

Tonney, F.O., Greer, F.E., and Danforth, T.F. 1928. The minimal "chlorine death points" of bacteria. Am. J. Public Health, 18, 1259–1263.

Tonney, F.O., Greer, F.E., and Liebig, G.F., Jr., 1930. The minimal "chlorine death points" of bacteria. II. Vegetative forms. III. Sporebearing organisms. Am. J. Public Health, 20, 503–508.

Trueman, J.R. 1971. The halogens. In *Inhibition and Destruction of the Microbial Cell*. London, Academic Press, pp. 137–183.

Watkins, S.H., Hays, H., and Elliker, P.R. 1957. Virucidal activity of hypochlorites, quaternary ammonium compounds and iodophors against bacteriophage of *Streptococcus cremoris*. J. Milk Food Technol., 20, 84–87.

Wattie, E., and Butterfield, C.T. 1944. Relative resistance of *Escherichia coli* and *Eberthella typhosa* to chlorine and chloramines. Public Health Reports, 59, 1661–1671.

Weber, G.R. 1950. Effect of concentration and reaction (pH) on the germicidal activity of Chloramine-T. Public Health Reports, 65, 503–512.

Weber, G.R, and Black, L.A. 1948. Laboratory procedure for evaluating practical performance of quaternary ammonium and other germicides proposed for sanitizing food utensils. Am. J. Public Health, 38, 1405–1417.

Weber, G.R., and Levine, M. 1944. Factors affecting germicidal efficiency of chlorine and chloramine. Am. J. Public Health, 32, 719–728.

Wei, C.I., Cook, D.L., and Kirk, J.R. 1985. Use of chlorine compounds in the food industry. Food Technol., 53(8), 107–115.

Weidenkopf, S.J. 1953. Water chlorination. U.S. Armed Forces Med. J., 4, 253–261.

Wells, W.F. 1929. Chlorination as a factor of safety in shellfish production. Am. J. Public Health, 19, 72–79.

White, G.C. 1972. *Handbook of Chlorination*. New York, Van Nostrand Reinhold Company, pp. 259–273.

Whittaker, C., Ridgway, H., and Olson, B.H. 1984. Evaluation of cleaning strategies for removal of biofilms from reverse-osmosis membranes. Appl. Environ. Microbiol., 48(3), 395–403.

Wirth, L.F., Jr., Feldt, C.A., and Odlaud, K. 1961. Effect of oxidants on ion exchangers. Ind. Eng. Chemistry, 52, 638–641.

Wood, C.B. 1928. Succinchlorimide for the treatment of small quantities of potable water. J. Am. Water Works Assoc., 20, 535–549.

Zimmerman, P.W., and Berg, R.O. 1934. Effects of chlorinated water on land plants, aquatic plants, and goldfish. Contrib. Boyce Thompson Inst., 6, 39–49.

Zsoldos, F.P., Jr. 1964. Procedure for water treatment. U.S. Patent 3,161,588.

CHAPTER 8

IODINE AND IODINE COMPOUNDS

W. Gottardi

Iodine, a nonmetallic, essential element discovered in 1812 by the French scientist Courtois, was named by Gay-Lussac in 1814 after the Greek word meaning violet, which is the color of iodine vapor.

It is not found in elemental form in nature but occurs sparingly in the form of iodides in seawater from which it is assimilated by seaweeds, in Chilean saltpeter and nitrate-bearing earth, known as *caliche*, in brines from old sea deposits, and in brackish waters from oil and salt wells.

Besides the one stable isotope ^{127}I, there exist more than 30 artificial isotopes with half-life periods between 0.2 s and 1.57×10^7 years. Some of them form a dangerous constituent part of the uncontrolled emissions during nuclear accidents, whereas others are used in nuclear medicine (mainly ^{131}I (8.04 d) and ^{123}I (13.2 h)).

So far as is known, the first use of iodine in medical practice was as a remedy for bronchocele (Halliday, 1821). The first specific reference to the use of iodine in wounds was made in 1839 (Davies, 1839; Boinet, 1865). Iodine was officially recognized by the Pharmacopeia of the United States in 1830, specifically as *tinctura iodini* (tincture of iodine). The first fundamental papers with a scientific basis about the degerming efficiency of iodine were published from 1874 to 1881 by Davaine (Vallin, 1882). In 1874, he found iodine to be one of the most efficacious antiseptics, a notion that is still valid 120 years later. On the basis of Davaine's experiences, Koch experimented with the disinfecting effect of iodine against anthrax spores. His results are contained in a comprehensive paper entitled "Desinfektion" (Koch, 1881). In the meantime, the literature about the use of iodine as a disinfectant has expanded markedly. Clinicians and microbiologists described a great number of experimental data and clinical applications, which can be found in numerous surveys (Reddish, 1957; Sykes, 1972; Bolek et al., 1972; Horn et al., 1972, 1974; Knolle, 1975; Gershenfeld, 1977).

Despite the successes that have been achieved with iodine, it was ascertained early that it also possesses properties unsuitable for practical application. Goebel (1906) referred to the fact that iodine has an unpleasant odor; in addition, it stains the skin with an intense yellow-brownish color, causes blue stains in the laundry in the presence of starch, and combines with iron and other metals. Furthermore, its solutions are not stable, it irritates animal tissue, and it is a poison. The adverse side effects of iodine, its painfulness on open wounds, and the possibility of allergic reactions have in the past 100 years led to the production of a great many iodine compounds (and iodine preparations), with the aim of avoiding these incompatibilities without a significant loss of germicidal efficiency. In this connection, the iodophors finally succeeded as ideal forms of application.

CHEMISTRY

Iodine, the halogen with the highest atomic weight (126.9) of the common halogens, forms grayish-black metallic scales that melt at 113.5°C to a black mobile liquid. Iodine boils at 184.4°C at atmospheric pressure to produce the characteristic violet-colored vapor. In spite of the high boiling point, it already has an appreciable vapor pressure at room temperature and sublimes before it melts if it is not heated too fast and with too high a degree of heat.

Elemental iodine is only slightly soluble in water (0.334 g, i.e., 1.315×10^{-3} M/L at 25°C), forming a brown solution. Its solubility in water is increased with the addition of alkali iodides by which triiodides (and higher polyiodides) are formed (see Equation 5 following). In polar organic solvents (alcohols, ketones, carbonic acids), iodine dissolves with a brown color, in apolar solvents (CCl_4, benzene, hydrocarbons) with a violet color. Whereas in the violet solutions, iodine is present as I_2 molecules (as in the gas phase), the brown color is explained by the formation of a compound between iodine and the solvent molecule (charge transfer complexes).

Iodine in Aqueous Solution

Compared with chlorine and bromine, the system I_2-H_2O is much more complex. One of the reasons is the disproportionation of the hypohalous acid (see Equation 4 following), which, in the case of HOI, occurs at room temperature with appreciable speed, whereas in the case of HOCl and HOBr, elevated temperatures are necessary. Another reason is the high affinity of molecular iodide to iodide, resulting in the formation constant of the triiodide ion (see Equation 5 following) being considerably higher than those of Cl_3^- and Br_3^- ($K_{Cl_3^-} = 0.12$; $K_{Br_3^-} = 19$; $K_{I_3^-} = 800$ at 20°C). In aqueous iodine solutions, therefore, the formation of the triiodide ion (and to a small extent also of the pentaiodide ion, $I_3^- + I_2 \rightleftharpoons I_5^-$) is an important reaction that greatly affects the chemical behavior of this halogen. Finally, in iodine solutions the cationic species H_2OI^+ is present, whereas the corresponding chlorine and bromine cations are not able to exist (Bell and Gelles, 1951).

The chemistry of aqueous iodine solutions is usually described with the following equations:

$$I_2 + H_2O \rightleftharpoons H_2OI^+ + I^- \text{ (hydrolytic ionization)} \quad (1)$$

$$H_2OI^+ \rightleftharpoons HOI + H^+ \text{ (dissociation of } H_2OI^+) \quad (2)$$

$$HOI \rightleftharpoons OI^- + H^+ \text{ (dissociation of HOI)} \quad (3)$$

$$3\ HOI \rightleftharpoons IO_3^- + 2\ I^- + 3\ H^+ \text{(disproportionation of HOI)} \quad (4)$$

$$I_2 + I^- \rightleftharpoons I_3^- \text{ (formation of triiodide)} \quad (5)$$

Whereas Equations 1, 2, 3, and 5 describe well defined and investigated elementary reactions, Equation 4 is an empiric formula that says nothing about the reaction mechanism and the iodous acid, HIO_2, which is to be expected as an intermediate reaction product and whose chemical and bactericidal behaviors are not known. Equations 1 and 2, as well as 1, 2, and 4, are usually combined and written as 6 and 7, respectively:

$$I_2 + H_2O \rightleftharpoons HOI + H^+ + I^- \text{ (iodine hydrolysis)} \quad (6)$$

$$3\ I_2 + 3\ H_2O \rightleftharpoons IO_3^- + 5\ I^- + 6\ H^+ \text{ (iodate formation)} \quad (7)$$

In pure aqueous iodine solutions, therefore, at least seven different ions or molecules are present, of which molecular iodine (I_2), the hypoiodic acid (HOI), and the iodine cation (H_2OI^+) are supposed to have strong germicidal properties (Black et al., 1968; Krusé et al., 1970). However, the concentration of the iodine cation is so low—at conditions relevant to disinfection more than four powers below the HOI concentration—that it plays virtually no role in disinfection processes (Chang, 1971; Gottardi, 1978a).

The same is the case with the hypoiodite ion, which becomes important only at pH >9 and in the absence of iodide. Because at these conditions the disproportiona-

tion of iodate takes place very fast and therefore is avoided in disinfections, hypoiodite can be neglected as a contribuent to microbicidal processes.

The tri-iodide ion (I_3^-), a major constituent in all iodide-containing preparations such as Lugol's solution, iodine tincture, and iodophor preparations is, compared to the free molecular iodine, only a weak oxidant and exhibits therefore only an inferior antibacterial activity, whereas the iodide ion (I^-) is without any effect (Kramer et al., 1952). Iodate (IO_3^-) is an oxidant only at pH values less than 4 and therefore has no effect on conditions where disinfections normally are carried out.

Calculations on the equilibrium concentrations show that at pH values less than 9 and at a total iodine concentration $\leq 10^{-4}$ M/L (25.4 mg/L), the sum $[I_2] + [HOI]^*$ of freshly prepared pure iodine solutions comes to over 97% of the total concentration (Table 8–1). The amount of OI^- and I_3^- ions can thus be neglected, with an oxidation capacity nearly present in the form of the bactericidal species I_2 and HOI (Gottardi, 1978a).

Although a differing behavior of I_2 and HOI has been observed against certain germs (Chang, 1971), in the pH range of 3 to 9 a more or less constant bactericidal activity of iodine in aqueous solution can generally be expected. This is in contrast to chlorine and bromine, where already at pH 8 the weak disinfecting hypohalite ions are present in appreciable amounts (Table 8–2). However, the ratio of [HOI] to $[I_2]$ at a certain temperature (25°C), as recorded in Tables 8–1 and 8–2, is governed not only by the pH value and total concentration, but also by the presence of substances that can interfere with the equilibria of Equations 1 through 7. In this latter connection, the iodide ion, I^-, is of primary importance: It emerges on the one hand at the hydrolysis of iodine (See Equations 1 and 6) and on the other hand at the reaction of iodine with organic material (except the addition to olefinic double bonds):

$$R—H + I_2 \longrightarrow R—I + H^+ + I^-$$

This additional I^- is always present in disinfecting solutions containing iodine and organic material and, as is seen in Table 8–3, may influence the ratio as well as the sum of [HOI] and $[I_2]$, the sum however being rather constant in the selected pH-range.

Table 8–3 shows that the stabilizing effect of the iodide (as to the pH dependence of the percentual proportion of the different iodine species) increases with its concentration. Therefore in Lugol's solution ($C_{I_2} = 0.197$ M/L, $C_{I^-} = 0.602$ M/L) the portion of $[I_2]$ and $[I_3^-]$ (0.34 resp. 99.66%) remains constant even up to pH 10, indicating that this disinfectant is virtually pH-independent. The values of Table 8–3 can be summarized as is done in Figure 8–1, which shows that only at iodide concentrations greater than 10^{-4} M/L a noticeable decrease of the sum $[I_2] + [HOI]$ is to be expected. In spite of the wide range of iodine concentration ($10^{-6} – 10^{-3}$ M/L) and pH (3 to 9) there is only a small variation

---

*[ ] means equilibrium concentration of the bracketed species.

Table 8–1. *Equilibrium Concentrations* of I_2, HOI, OI- and I_3^- in 10^{-6} to 10^{-3} M Iodine Solutions at pH 3 to 9 and 25°C (in % of the Total Concentration)*

pH	10^{-6}				10^{-5}				10^{-4}				10^{-3}			
	I_2	HOI	OI-	I_3^-	I_2	HOI	OI-	I_3^-	I_2	HOI	OI-	I_3^-	I_2	HOI	OI-	I_3^-
3.0	97.7	2.3	—	—	99.3	0.7	—	—	99.7	0.3	—	—	99.9	0.1	—	—
4.5	87.7	12.3	—	—	95.9	4.1	—	—	98.6	1.4	—	—	99.2	0.5	—	0.3
6.0	48.7	51.3	—	—	79.1	20.8	—	0.1	92.2	7.3	—	0.5	95.8	3.0	—	1.2
7.5	5.2	94.7	0.1	—	29.2	70.6	0.1	0.1	64.4	34.1	—	1.5	79.8	14.8	—	5.4
9.0	0.2	97.6	2.2	—	1.7	96.0	2.2	—	13.2	84.0	1.9	0.8	37.1	50.7	1.2	11.0

*Calculated after Gottardi, 1980.

Table 8–2. *Comparison of the Equilibrium Concentrations* of Aqueous Solutions of Chlorine, Bromine, and Iodine ($C = 4 \times 10^{-6}$ M/L, i.e., 0.3 PPM Chlorine, 0.64 PPM Bromine, 1 PPM Iodine) at pH 3 to 9 and 25°C (in % of the Total Concentration)*

pH	Iodine				Bromine			Chlorine		
	I_2	HOI	OI-	I_3^-	Br_2	HOBr	OBr-	Cl_2	HOCl	OCl-
3.0	98.8	1.2	—	—	32.1	67.9	—	—	100.0	—
4.5	93.7	6.3	—	—	2.1	97.9	—	—	100.0	—
6.0	69.3	30.5	—	0.1	0.1	99.7	0.2	—	97.1	2.8
7.5	16.4	83.5	0.1	—	—	93.5	6.5	—	52.0	48.0
9.0	0.7	97.0	2.2	—	—	31.4	68.6	—	3.3	96.7

*Calculated after Gottardi, 1980.

Table 8–3. *Equilibrium Concentrations* of I_2, HOI, OI- and I_3 in 10^{-6}, 10^{-5}, 10^{-4} and 10^{-3} M Iodine Solutions Containing Additional Iodide (10^{-5}, 10^{-3}, and 10^{-1} M/L) at pH 3 to 9 and 25°C (in % of the Total Concentration)*

C_{I2}	C_I- pH	0				10^{-5}				10^{-3}				10^{-1}			
		I_2	HOI	OI-	I_3^-	I_2	HOI	OI-	I_3^-	I_2	HOI	OI-	I_3^-	I_2	HOI	OI-	I_3^-
10⁻⁶ M/L (0.25 ppm)	3	97.7	2.3	—	—	99.3	—	—	0.7	58.0	—	—	42.0	1.4	—	—	98.6
	4.5	87.7	12.3	—	—	99.1	0.2	—	0.7	58.0	—	—	42.0	1.4	—	—	98.6
	6.0	48.7	51.3	—	—	94.2	5.1	—	0.7	58.0	—	—	42.0	1.4	—	—	98.6
	7.5	5.2	94.7	0.1	—	38.0	61.6	—	0.4	57.4	1.1	—	41.5	1.4	—	—	98.6
	9	0.2	97.6	2.2	—	1.9	95.8	2.2	—	43.1	25.0	0.6	31.3	1.4	—	—	98.6
10⁻⁵ M/L (2.5 ppm)	3	99.3	0.7	—	—	99.3	—	—	0.7	58.1	—	—	41.9	1.4	—	—	98.6
	4.5	95.9	4.1	—	—	99.1	0.2	—	0.7	58.1	—	—	41.9	1.4	—	—	98.6
	6	79.1	20.8	—	0.1	94.3	4.9	—	0.7	58.1	—	—	41.9	1.4	—	—	98.6
	7.5	29.2	70.6	0.1	0.1	46.6	52.8	—	0.5	57.5	1.0	—	41.5	1.4	—	—	98.6
	9	1.7	96.0	2.2	—	0.3	94.4	2.2	—	43.5	24.5	0.6	31.4	1.4	—	—	98.6
10⁻⁴ M/L (25.4 ppm)	3	99.7	0.2	—	—	99.3	—	—	0.7	59.0	—	—	41.0	1.4	—	—	98.6
	4.5	98.6	1.4	—	—	99.1	0.2	—	0.7	59.0	—	—	41.0	1.4	—	—	98.6
	6	92.2	7.3	—	0.5	95.1	4.0	—	0.9	59.0	—	—	41.0	1.4	—	—	98.6
	7.5	64.4	34.1	—	1.5	67.7	30.4	—	1.9	58.3	1.1	—	40.6	1.4	—	—	98.6
	9	13.1	84.1	2.0	0.8	14.2	82.9	1.9	1.0	43.5	24.7	0.6	31.3	1.4	—	—	98.6
10⁻³ M/L (254 ppm)	3	99.9	0.1	—	—	99.6	—	—	0.4	67.3	—	—	32.7	1.4	—	—	98.6
	4.5	99.2	0.5	—	0.3	99.2	0.2	—	0.5	67.3	—	—	32.7	1.4	—	—	98.6
	6	95.8	3.0	—	1.2	96.0	2.5	—	1.5	67.2	0.1	—	32.7	1.4	—	—	98.6
	7.5	79.8	14.8	—	5.4	80.0	14.4	—	5.6	65.6	1.7	—	32.7	1.4	—	—	98.6
	9	37.1	50.7	1.2	11.0	37.3	50.3	1.2	11.2	43.5	25.6	0.6	30.2	1.4	—	—	98.6

*Calculated after Gottardi, 1980.

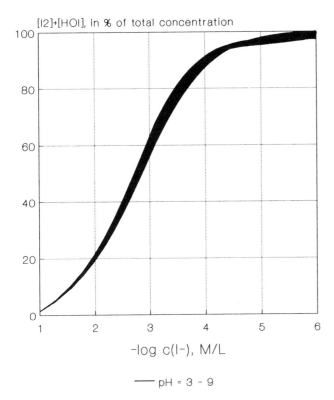

Fig. 8–1. Influence of the iodide concentration on the sum $[I_2]$ + $[HOI]$ in aqueous iodine solutions. $C(I_2) = 10^6 - 10^{-3}$ M resp. 0.254 – 254 mg/L; pH = 3.0 to 9.0.

in the calculated percentual equilibrium concentrations, causing a slight broadening of the curve, so that Figure 8–1 allows one to estimate the percentual amount of the sum $[I_2]$ + $[HOI]$ at a given iodide concentration and, because the concentration of OI^- can be neglected (it is only of importance at pH >9), the amount of triiodide, I_3^-, being the difference to 100%.

Stability of the Iodine-Water System

Iodine, like other disinfectants based on halogens in the oxidation states 0 or + 1, as far as they are not present as pure substances (i.e., without a solvent), can gradually lose a part of their degerming properties (e.g., during storage). This is due to (1) substitutions of covalent hydrogen, e.g., O-H, N-H, C-H (as a result of the reaction with solvent molecules like H_2O, EtOH, and others), (2) additions to olefinic double bonds, and (3) the disproportionation of the hypohalous acid to halate in aqueous preparations (Equations 4 and 7, respectively), which has no degerming properties (see previous section). Although substitutions, which in the case of iodine are considered to be fewer than with chlorine and bromine, and additions can be avoided by an appropriate composition, the equilibria 1 through 7 are established in any case if water is present; as a consequence the inactive iodate also can be formed.

On the basis of calculated equilibrium concentrations and reaction times, the following conclusions have been

drawn concerning the stability (with regard to iodate formation) of iodine-containing disinfecting agents (Gottardi, 1981):

1. Below pH 6, a decrease of disinfecting effectiveness due to the formation of iodate can be excluded.
2. Above pH 7, the formation of iodate, whose extent largely depends on the pH value as well as on the iodide concentration, must be regarded carefully. Raising the pH value lowers the stability (iodate formation increases), whereas raising the iodide concentration improves the stability (iodate formation is reduced).
3. Because of the stabilizing effect of the iodide ion, provided that its concentration is high enough, the opposite effect of the pH value can be overcompensated for, and as a result of this, iodine-containing agents can also exhibit sufficient stability for practice in the weak alkaline range (pH less than 9).

In highly diluted iodine solutions (less than 10^{-5} M/L, resp. 2.54 mg/L) which are present in disinfections of potable water or swimming-pool water, only a slow iodate formation can be expected even at pH 9 (Gottardi, 1978a). In accordance with this, in disinfection plants on an iodine basis, no significant iodate amounts have been detected (Black et al., 1968).

Effect of Organic Material

Iodine (like chlorine and bromine) reacts not only with living microorganisms but also with dead ones and with dissolved proteins. In the course of these complex reactions, halogen compounds emerge that have either a weaker degerming activity than the halogen originally used or none at all. The former are mainly compounds with N-halogen bonds, whereas the latter are those with C-halogen bonds and the halide ions.

With in-vitro experiments using peptone solutions, it was shown that iodine reacts with proteins at least three times slower than chlorine and nearly four times slower than bromine (Gottardi, 1976). Hence, in disinfection under conditions occurring in practice, i.e., in the presence of dissolved proteins (blood, serum, sputum), iodine is much more efficient than chlorine and bromine because the share of the employed halogen concentration that is available for the actual degerming reaction is considerably greater. The comparatively low reactivity with proteins, which is sufficient, however, to kill a living germ, and the virtual independence of the disinfecting activity of the pH value are the main reasons for the excellent degerming properties of iodine.

Mode of Action of Iodine as a Microbicide

Iodine, mainly in its molecular form, is able to penetrate the cell wall of microorganisms rapidly (Chang, 1971). Although exact details about the killing of a living cell by the I_2 molecule (or one of the reaction products occurring in aqueous solution) are not known, it can be assumed that iodine reacts

1. With basic N-H functions that are parts of some

amino acids (e.g., lysine, histidine, arginine) and the bases of nucleotides (adenine, cytosine, and guanine) forming the corresponding N-iododerivatives. By this reaction, important positions for hydrogen bonding are blocked, and a lethal disorder of the protein structure may occur.

2. By oxidizing the S-H group (Krusé et al., 1970) of the amino acid cysteine, through which the ability of connecting protein chains by disulfide (—S—S—) bridges, as an important factor in the synthesis of proteins, is lost.

3. With the phenolic group of the amino acid tyrosine, forming monoiododerivates or diiododerivates. In this case, the bulk of the iodine atom(s) in the ortho position may cause a form of steric hindrance in the hydrogen bonding of the phenolic OH group.

4. With the carbon-carbon double bond (C=C) of the unsaturated fatty acids. This could lead to a change in the physical properties of the lipids and membrane immobilization (Apostolov, 1980).

Annotation: Of these four points the second might be the most important, both because of the ubiquitous SH-groups and because of the very fast and irreversible reaction with iodine. The first point however is only of importance under alkaline conditions, which on grounds of stability (see previous section) are unusual at disinfections.

PREPARATIONS CONTAINING OR RELEASING FREE IODINE

Solutions of Iodine and Iodide

To this group belongs a great variety of preparations containing elemental iodine and potassium (or sodium) iodide in water, ethyl alcohol, and glycerol, or in mixtures of these solvents. They rank with the oldest disinfectants and have survived nearly 150 years on the basis of efficacy, economy, and stability. The following are official preparations according to USP XXI: (1) Iodine Topical Solution, an aqueous solution containing 2.0% iodine and 2.4% sodium iodide; (2) Strong Iodine Solution (Lugol's Solution), an aqueous solution containing 5% iodine and 10% potassium iodide; (3) Iodine Tincture containing 2.0% iodine and 2.4% sodium iodide in aqueous ethanol (1:1); and (4) Strong Iodine Tincture containing 7% iodine and 5% potassium iodide in 95% ethanol. Because all of these preparations contain large amounts of iodide (0.16 to 0.6 moles/L) the equilibria 1, 4, 6, and 7, which all contain iodide, are displaced far to the left side so that only the triiodide equilibrium 5 becomes important. As a result of this, these solutions virtually contain only iodine, iodide, and triiodide and are therefore very stable because there is no HOI or OI⁻ present that can undergo disproportionation to iodate (Equation 4). Because of their high content of free molecular iodine (e.g., Lugol's solution: $[I_2] = 170$ ppm) they are powerful disinfectants with the disadvantage of staining—and in some cases irritation—of living tissues.

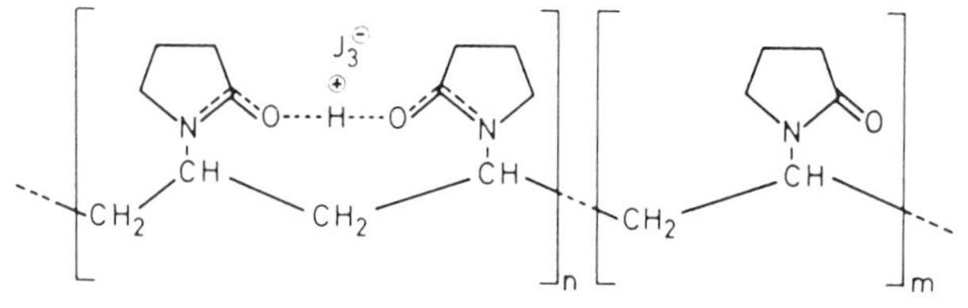

Fig. 8–2. Structure of solid povidone-iodine. After Schenck, H.U., Simak, P., and Haedicke, E. 1979. Structure of polyvinylpyrrolidone-iodine (povidone-iodine). J. Pharm. Sci., 68, 1505–1509.

Preparations Containing Iodine, Iodide, and Organic Complexing Agents

Besides preparations with complexing agents of low molecular weight, such as tetraglycine hydroperiodide (Gershenfeld, 1977) or the inclusion compound iodine-maltosylcyclodextrin (Kawakami et al., 1988), this group includes the important "iodophors," whose name indicates generally the combination of iodine with a carrier (as these complexing agents usually are called) of high molecular weight. In aqueous solution, iodophors form the same iodine species as do the pure iodine solutions; however, the polymer carriers, because of their complexing properties, partly reduce the equilibrium concentrations of the iodine species and give the iodophor preparations properties that make them superior in some respects to solutions containing only iodine and iodide.

Iodophors

An iodophor is a complex of elemental iodine or triiodide with a carrier that has at least three functions: (1) to increase the solubility of iodine, (2) to provide a sustained-release reservoir of the halogen, and (3) to reduce the equilibrium concentration of free molecular iodine. The carriers are neutral polymers, such as polyvinyl pyrrolidone, polyether glycols, polyvinyl alcohols, polyacrylic acid, polyamides, polyoxyalkylenes, and polysaccharides.

In the solid state iodophors form crystalline powders of a deep brown to black color, which in general do not smell of iodine, indicating a tight bonding with the carrier molecules. Their solubility in water is good but depends on the chain length of the polymeric molecules and varies in the case of povidone-iodine between 5% (type 90/04, average molecular weight near 1,000,000) and more than 20% (type 17/12, average molecular weight near 10,000). The best known iodophor is povidone-iodine, a compound of 1-vinyl-2-pyrrolidinone polymer with iodine, which according to USP XXI contains not less than 9.0% and not more than 12.0% available iodine. On the basis of spectroscopic investigations (Schenck et al., 1979), it was found that povidone-iodine (in the solid state) is an adduct not with molecular iodine (I_2) but with hydro-triiodic acid (HI_3), where the proton is fixed via a short hydrogen bond between two carbonyl groups of two pyrrolidinone rings and the triiodide anion is bound ionically to this cation (Fig. 8–2).

Aqueous Solutions of Iodophores. The chemistry of the aqueous solutions of iodophores is still more complex than that of pure iodine solutions, because the polymeric organic carrier molecules interact with the iodine species created by the reactions of Equations 1 through 5, which can cause a considerable change in their equilibrium concentrations.

As far as the chemistry of aqueous disinfectant solutions containing iodophors is understood today, both electronic and steric effects are responsible for this interaction (Gottardi, 1985). Thus, taking the known interactions with low molecular oxygen compounds such as amide, ester, ketone, and ether (Haruka Yamada and Kunio Kozima, 1960; Schmulbach and Drago, 1960) as an analogy, it can be assumed that, between molecular iodine and the iodophor molecules, which without exception contain such functional oxygen-containing groups (e.g., povidone: carbonyl oxygen of the amide function in the pyrrolidone ring), donor-acceptor complexes are formed, with iodine playing the part of the acceptor:

$$\text{>C} = \text{O} + \text{I}_2 \rightleftharpoons \text{>C} = \overset{\delta+}{\text{O}} \cdots \text{I} - \overset{\delta-}{\text{I}} \qquad (8)$$

Furthermore, the iodophors, especially when in high concentrations, because of the spatial arrangement of the dissolved polymer molecules (near regions with helix-like structure) (Horn and Ditter, 1984), are obviously able to surround the free iodine forms in the manner of clathrates and withdraw it from the equilibrium (Equations 9 through 11). This interaction must be of importance for the iodide ion and above all for the large-mass triiodide ion, because in this case the formation of a donor-acceptor complex is not possible on grounds of the negative charge.

$$\text{R} + \text{I}^- \longrightarrow \text{R} \cdot \text{I}^- \qquad (9)$$

$$\text{R} + \text{I}_2 \longrightarrow \text{R} \cdot \text{I}_2 \qquad (10)$$

$$\text{R} + \text{I}_3^- \longrightarrow \text{R} \cdot \text{I}_3^- \qquad (11)$$

R = structural regions of the iodophor molecule capable of forming complexes by steric effects

These two effects, together with the equilibria 1 through 5, result in the content of the free molecular iodine being greatly reduced in disinfection preparations containing iodophor molecules (10% aqueous solution of povidone-iodine: $C_{I_2} \approx C_I \approx 0.04$ M/L, $[I_2] \approx 10^{-5}$ M/L, resp. 2.54 ppm), in comparison with pure aqueous solutions with the same total iodine and total iodide content (aqueous iodine solution, $C_{I_2} = C_{I_-} = 0.04$ M/L, pH 5: $[I_2] = 6.8 \times 10^{-3}$ M/L, resp. 1727 ppm*). The high content of free iodide (which varies between 10^{-3} and 10^{-1} M/L, according to the preparation) also means that HOI can be disregarded (see equilibrium), and only I_2

*Because the solubility of iodine lies at 334 ppm (25°C), the calculated value of 1727 ppm does not correspond with the actual equilibrium concentration. Therefore an aqueous solution of this composition will contain undissolved iodine.

is responsible for disinfection. For the description of the chemical conditions existing in aqueous iodophor solutions, therefore, besides the triiodide equilibrium (5), at least the equilibria 8 through 10 are necessary. Because in the latter case no thermodynamic constants are known, these conditions can be ascertained only in an empirical way.

The virtual absence of HOI means also that iodophor preparations are not impaired by a decrease of micro-biocidal power owing to the formation of iodate (see Equation 4). In spite of this, iodophor preparations are not fully stable because iodine attacks the organic carrier (and other components), a reaction ($\text{>C—H} + \text{I}_2 \longrightarrow \text{>C—I} + \text{I}^- + \text{H}^+$) which, by consuming iodine, reduces not only the reservoir of the available iodine, but also the concentration of the free molecular iodine, the latter being reduced to a greater extent, because iodide is produced too (see Equation 5; Gottardi, 1985). However, these iodine-consuming reactions occur at room temperature only very slowly, and can be compensated for by the addition of iodate in the form of the potassium salt, which, at an appropriate pH, oxidizes iodide to iodine (see Equation 7) at such a rate that the available and free molecular iodine of this preparation virtually remains unchanged for a long time.

The concentration of free iodine is largely independent of the pH value (pH 3 to 6), but changes considerably with the degree of dilution, when it passes through a maximum of $[I_2] \approx 10^{-4}$ M/L in the 0.1% solution.

As can be seen in Figure 8–2, the concentration of free iodine in a 10% povidone-iodine solution comes to approximately 2.0 mg resp. 8×10^{-6} M/L and rises in a 1:100 dilution nearly tenfold. On further dilution, after passing the maximum the free iodine behaves more and more "normally"—i.e., it decreases—and below 0.01% the povidone-iodine solution can be regarded as a simple aqueous solution of iodine. This "anomalous" behavior (which is a consequence of the different equilibria combined together), mainly the fact that the more concentrated an iodophore solution is, the less free iodine and therefore the less disinfecting power it has, must always be kept in mind when making experiments with this class of disinfectant. The low content of free molecular iodine in concentrated povidone preparations was obviously also the reason for the unexpected observation that some preparations didn't fulfill the requirement of auto-sterility. The isolated germs were of the species *Pseudomonas*, organisms that are known to be protected by matrices of biofilms, exhibiting in this way an extraordinary resistance against degerming agents. (For more details on this topic, see the chapter "Disinfection of Medical and Surgical Materials").

Another important feature of aqueous povidone-iodine solutions, shown by Figure 8–3, is that there exists a maximum concentration of nearly 10^{-4} M/L, resp. 25.4 mg/L of "free iodine" that arises in the approximately 0.1% solution and that can never be exceeded.

Because $[I_2]$ not only depends on the concentration of

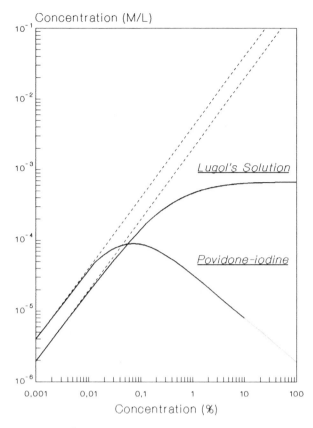

Concentration (M/L)

Fig. 8–3. Total available iodine (– – –) and free molecular iodine (——) in aqueous povidone-iodine (determined potentiometrically; Gottardi, 1983) and in Lugol's solution (calculated after Gottardi, 1980). Horn, D., and Ditter, W. 1984. Physikalisch-chemische Grundlagen der mikrobiziden Wirkung wässriger PVP-Iod-Lösungen. In *PVP-Iod in der Operativen Medizin*. Edited by G. Hierholzer and G. Görtz. Berlin, Springer.

povidone-iodine, but also on its total content of iodine and iodide which, as the specifications of the standard commercially available povidone-iodine show, undergoes considerable variations. Figure 8–3 only shows the typical course of $[I_2]$ as a function of the povidone-iodine concentration. Therefore the ordinate of the maximum (and to a lesser degree also its abscissa) in Figure 8–3 is not a constant for different iodophors and preparations containing iodophores.

Also in Figure 8–3 the behavior of Lugol's solution on dilution is shown, exhibiting the drastic reduction of free iodine caused by the complexing properties of the povidone molecules.

Influence of Temperature on the Concentration of Free Iodine. In a study about the concentration of free molecular iodine and its variation with temperature, nine commercial povidone-iodine preparations, as well as pure povidone-iodine solutions of different types and concentrations, have been investigated, setting forth the following results (Gottardi and Koller, 1986a): (1) The commercial products showed a remarkably great spread in the concentration of free iodine (0.2 to 10 ppm at 25°C), which may be attributed to their different compositions, especially the ratio of total iodine to iodide as

well as the kind and quantity of organic-pharmaceutical constituents. (2) All tested povidone-iodine systems showed a significant—and unexpectedly similar—change of the concentration of free iodine by the temperature. (3) The results concerning its relative alteration fit to an exponential function of the form

$$\Delta\% \ [I_2]_{\Delta t} = 100 \ [10^{(0.023 \ \pm \ 0.0026)\Delta t} - 1],$$

which is valid from 10 to 40°C. Following this equation $[I_2]$ increases about 5.4 resp. 100% if the temperature rises about 1.0 resp. 13.1°C. (4) This increase of $[I_2]$ must be considered in the application of povidone-iodine preparations as disinfectants or antiseptics on living tissues. Because of their higher temperature (c. 30 to 36°C) the applicated povidone-iodine preparations exhibit a significant higher $[I_2]$ than they do at room temperature ($\Delta t = 10$–16°C: $\Delta\% \ [I_2] = 70$ to 130%). Therefore, a significant higher degerming efficiency also can be expected compared to in-vitro experiments, which are conducted in general at room temperature.

The Relevance of Free Molecular Iodine to the Efficiency of Iodophor Preparations. Although the iodophores as important pharmaceutical base materials in the solid state represent more or less defined chemical compounds (the main qualm for this statement concerns the variation in the chain length of the polymeric carrier molecules), they cannot be, strictly speaking, called bactericidal agents. The real bactericidal agent (Gottardi, 1991) is the free molecular iodine, because it is this species alone for which a correlation between concentration and bactericidal activity has been proved (and not for the total iodine resp. iodophor concentration) (Berkelmann et al., 1982, Pinter et al., 1983, Gottardi and Puritscher, 1985).

The differing composition of pharmaceutical additives (such as detergents and back fatting agents), which all usually have iodine complexing properties, as well as the ratio of total iodine to total iodide (Pinter et al., 1983) that the preparations of the various manufacturers exhibit, result in great differences in the concentration of free molecular iodine in spite of the fact that the actual iodophor concentration resp. the concentration of the total (titrable) iodine might be the same. In this connection the determination of the free iodine—which can be done in three different ways: (1) by extraction with a nonpolar solvent, e.g., heptane (Pollack, 1985), (2) by dialysis (Horn and Ditter, 1984), and (3) by a potentiometric method (Gottardi, 1983)—is an important measure to get an indication of the bactericidal potency of the preparation. The total available iodine, however, which follows from the specification of preparation or simply can be assayed by titration, is a measure of the disinfection capacity. It comprises *all* oxidizing iodine species and should, therefore, not be mixed up with the free molecular iodine, which (except in highly diluted solutions) (see Table 8–3) amounts only to a small fraction of the total available iodine.

However, the importance of the concentration of the free iodine should not be overemphasized, because the commercially available iodophor preparations frequently contain other degerming constituents (e.g., alcohols) besides the iodine species; and on the other hand the pharmaceutical ingredients (e.g., detergents) may influence the susceptibility of a living germ for iodine, so that the bactericidal rate does not always exactly correlate with the concentration of free iodine. Nevertheless, for preparations of similar composition the determination of free iodine is a reliable and simple means to make predictions of the bactericidal properties (Gottardi and Puritscher, 1986). (See also the chapter on disinfection of medical and surgical materials.)

Forms of Application. According to USP XXI the following application forms of povidone-iodine are approved: Povidone-Iodine Topical Solution, Povidone-Iodine Cleansing Solution, Povidone-Iodine Ointment, and Povidone-Iodine Topical Aerosol Solution. Concerning the available iodine, they have to contain not less than 85% and not more than 120% of the labeled amount. In general povidone-iodine preparations contain 1 to 10% povidone-iodine, which is equivalent to 0.1 to 1.0% available iodine. They may contain a small amount of alcohol (Topical and Cleansing Solution); the cleansing solutions contain one or more surface-active agents. The aerosol solution, however, is a povidone-iodine solution under nitrogen in a pressurized container.

The Influence of the Halogen Consumption on the Efficacy of Povidone Iodine Preparations. Because iodophores are mainly used as medical antiseptics the influence of iodine-consuming body fluids is a very important feature concerning bactericidal capacity and rate.

Although iodine, as mentioned above, is less likely to be consumed by proteinaceous substrates than bromine and chlorine are, its efficacy as a disinfectant is still reduced in certain antiseptic applications, where great quantities of reducible constituents (e.g., blood) are present, and which leads to the conversion of iodine into nonbactericidal iodide. Thus, not only is the reservoir of available iodine diminished, but the equilibrium of triiodide is influenced as well. Both of these effects cause a decrease in the proportion of free molecular iodine, the actual antimicrobial agent (Gottardi and Koller, 1986b).

When povidone-iodine preparations are contaminated with liquid substrata (e.g., blood) there is, in addition, the dilution effect characteristic of povidone-iodine systems that causes an increase in the equilibrium concentration of free molecular iodine (Fig. 8–3). To what extent this effect compensates for the other two effects depends on the content of reducing substances. Thus with whole blood, a large decrease in the concentration of free molecular iodine occurs, whereas in the presence of plasma, this concentration remains practically unchanged if the ratio is not too high (Gottardi and Koller, 1987).

The consumption phenomena that can be seen with whole blood, such as (1) the strong and practically spontaneous iodine reduction, (2) a decrease of the specific iodine consumption along with the increase of the blood volume, and (3) the poor reproducibility can, among other things, be attributed to the high content of reduced protein sulfure (-SH) of whole blood, and to the possibility of different reactions of iodine with SH-groups (oxidation to disulfides resp. sulfenic, sulfinic, and sulfonic

acids). It is important to note that in practice no substantial decrease of the bactericidal efficacy of 10% povidone-iodine preparations is likely to occur with body fluids having a composition similar to plasma (volume substrate/volume povidone-iodine 10% ≤ 0.6). However, with whole blood this is indeed the case; therefore contamination by $>25\%$ full blood should be avoided.

Solid Microbicidal Compositions on Iodine Basis

To this group belong resins containing quaternary ammonium groups loaded with triiodide and higher polyiodide ions (e.g., pentaiodide). In contrast to the "classic" disinfectants, which contain antimicrobial agents that are dispersed in a liquid (or gas) phase, these resins rank among the "nonclassical chemical disinfectants" (NCCD), which consist of active moieties attached to, associated with, or stored (or a combination thereof) in a solid phase (Kril, Fitzpatrick, and Janauer, 1986). Their mode of action is explained either by direct, physical contact with their surface or by slowly releasing a disinfecting agent (in this case iodine) into the bulk phase being disinfected. Because the residuals of total iodine (I_2 and HOI) washed out by the water flowing through the resin are very low, the resins seem to be ideally suited for application in point-of-use and point-of-entry water purification units.

Preparations Producing Iodine in Connection with Water

Preparations of this kind do not contain elemental iodine, but rather iodide, and produce the former in a chemical reaction, which is started when iodide and an oxidant come in contact with water. "Heliogen," for example, is a mixture of chloramine-T, potassium iodide, and certain inert ingredients. The releasing of iodine can be generalized as

$$\rangle N\!-\!Cl + 2\,I^- + H^+ \rightarrow \rangle N\!-\!H + Cl^- + I_2$$

Preparations of this kind are marketed in the form of tablets or a powder, which can be used effectively as sanitizers. Other examples are the "Hio-Dine" process, which is used in swimming pool disinfection, with 1,3-dichloro-5,5-dimethylhydantoin as an oxidant (White, 1972), and a disinfection method published by Kinman and Layton (1976) using NH_2Cl as an oxidant.

N-Iodo Compounds

Because nearly all organic disinfectants on the basis of chlorine and bromine are N-chloro or N-bromo compounds, it is surprising that N-iodo compounds, which in aqueous solution release hypoiodic acid ($\rangle N\!-\!I + H_2O \rightarrow \rangle N\!-\!H + HOI$), are not used in practice. In a study on the usability of N-iodo compounds as disinfectants, the following conclusions were drawn (Gottardi, 1978b).

Fresh and diluted aqueous solutions of N-iodo compounds exhibit HOI concentrations corresponding to the sum of $[HOI] + [I_2]$ in pure iodine solutions of the same molarity, which let us expect similar bactericidal behavior of this class of compounds. Compared with iodine solutions, however, a higher rate of iodate formation and therefore less stability of this solution can be established, which is caused by the higher HOI concentration throughout. Under certain conditions (pH less than or equal to 7, concentration less than 10^{-5} M/L, normal interacting time), the stability should be sufficient for disinfecting purposes. Of particular interest is the possibility of investigating, in the virtual absence of molecular iodine, the bactericidal action of the HOI. Common practical use will depend on the costs, which are high as far as the purchasable N-iodo-succinimide is concerned. Hence, the N-iodo compounds should not be considered at present as an alternative to the more inexpensive elemental iodine.

Synopsis of Composition and Active Iodine Forms in Disinfectant Solutions Containing Iodine

Table 8–4 gives a synopsis of the different preparations containing resp. applications using iodine. Besides the total concentration of iodine and iodide, the presumable active species and their calculated, measured, or estimated equilibrium concentrations are shown. Furthermore a tentative description of the conditions in alcoholic solutions is given. In contrast to pure alcoholic solutions (containing only iodine and an alcohol), where iodine practically only occurs in the solvated molecular form, $I_2 \cdot ROH$, alcoholic preparations used in practice (Tincture and Strong Tincture of Iodine, USP XXI) also contain iodide and water, with the result that the equilibria 1 through 5 are established also. However, because of the iodide content, only the solvated iodine molecules ($I_2 \cdot ROH$ and $I_2 \cdot H_2O$, the latter being the "free mo-

lecular iodine"*)—apart from the alcohol itself—might be responsible as the active forms for disinfection. A differentiation between the two forms according to relative reactivity should turn out in favor of the hydrate complex because of the greater stability of the I_2-alcohol-solvate complex (inductive effect of the alkyl group increases the electron-donating properties of the oxygen).

HOI as a virtual contribuent to the microbicidal process is to be expected only in iodine/water systems of high dilution and low iodide concentration, as is the case of disinfection of drinking and swimming pool water (see also Table 8–3) on an iodine basis.

TOXICITY OF PREPARATIONS CONTAINING FREE IODINE

All preparations that contain elemental iodine have similar modes of action, not with qualitative but rather with quantitative differences. Preparations such as Strong Iodine Solution (Lugol's Solution, USP XXI), in which free molecular iodine is present in high quantities (170 ppm), of course have better degerming properties than an iodophor preparation that is designed to reduce, by complexing, the concentration of free molecular iodine, which normally comes to 2 to 10 ppm.

On the other hand, the toxicity of the free iodine for living tissue has to be considered. Impregnating healthy skin with Lugol's solution has no unpleasant effect, whereas the same agent applied to a large area of burned skin causes painful irritation. In this case, the application of a weaker disinfecting agent, e.g., an iodophor preparation, is preferred. With an increasing concentration of free iodine and an increasing capability of resorption of the treated body surface, the amount of iodine ab-

*The real *free* iodine (in the form of bare I_2-molecules) occurs only in the gasphase, or in apolar solvents like CCl_4, and is violet in colour, in contrast to $I_2 \cdot H_2O$ (and $I_2 \cdot ROH$), which causes a brown colour.

Table 8–4. *Composition and Active Iodine Form in Disinfectant Solutions Containing Iodine*

Components	Solvent	Examples	Total Iodine Content (total iodide content)	Iodine Form Mainly Responsible for the Microbicidal Effect (concentration proportion of the total iodine concentration)
I_2	Ethanol	Solution of iodine in alcohol	1%	$I_2 \cdot ROH$ (10,000 ppm*; 100%)
	H_2O	Drinking water, swimming pool iodination	$10^{-5} - 10^{-6}$ M/L	$I_2 \cdot aq$, HOI ($[I_2] + [HOI]$: 0·25 − 2·5 ppm†; 98−100%)
I_2, I^-	H_2O	Lugol's solution	5% (10% KI)	$I_2 \cdot aq$ (170 ppm†; 0·34%)
	Ethanol/H_2O	Iodine tincture	2% (2·4% NaI)	$I_2 \cdot ROH$, $I_2 \cdot aq$
I_2, I^-, polym. org. complexing agents§, additives‖	H_2O	Mucosal disinfectant and washing concentrates based on PVP-I	1−0·75% (iodide content varies greatly depending on the preparation)	$I_2 \cdot aq$ (0·2−10 ppm‡; 0·003−0·1%)
	Propanol/H_2O	Skin disinfectants (sprays)	0·1% (0·05%)	$I_2 \cdot ROH$, $I_2 \cdot aq$

*Estimated.
†Calculated (see Gottardi, 1981).
‡Measured potentiometrically (see Gottardi, 1983) in commercially available products.
§Povidone, polyoxyalkylenes, polyetherglycols etc.
‖Buffers, detergents, foam stabilizers, artificial colourings etc.

sorbed by the body also increases and manifests itself in the serum level of iodide. In general, therefore, the serum level rises less from the application of an iodophor than with iodine tincture or Lugol's solution (Knolle, 1975). On treating burns, Hunt et al. (1980) found that the amount of absorbed iodine was directly related to the size of the burn, and although clinical evidence of cell or organ toxicity is as yet undetermined, it seems that high serum levels of iodide imply toxicity. Kuhn et al. (1987) also state that on treating burns with a povidone-iodine preparation, plasma iodine (i.e., iodide) sharply increased; from 6.4 ± 0.4 to 20.7 ± 4.7 µg/100 mL, however, the authors hold that the thyroid function does not seem to be modified by plasma iodine overload.

In a large-scale study at an obstetric ward it was found that the iodine overload of the mothers, caused by skin disinfection prior to delivery using an iodophor preparation, induces a transient impairment of thyroid function of the infants, especially if breast fed. Because this situation is detrimental to screening for congenital hypothyroidism iodophor preparations are not recommended in obstetrics (Chanoine et al., 1989). High doses of free iodine, e.g., in form of iodine tincture, are highly toxic if brought into body cavities and cause swelling and bleeding of mucous membranes. Consumption of 30 g of iodine tincture can be fatal (Wirth et al., 1967). As an antidote for such accidents 10 to 20 g sodium thiosulfate (reduction of iodine to iodide) or starch (formation of inclusion compounds) per os are recommended (Kuschinsky and Lüllmann, 1984). Concerning the incorporation of iodine the following generalizations can be made:

1. Because the horny layer of the intact skin is an effective barrier against electrolytes (Goldsmith, 1983) it is penetrated by iodine in the form of molecular iodine and not of iodide.
2. In body cavities (at the treatment of mucous membranes, perineal wash, etc.) which are not protected by a stratum corneum, however, also the incorporation of iodide becomes important all the more that iodine preparations always contain iodide.
3. Depending on the chemical nature of the tissue iodine penetrates (dry skin with low, resp. surfaces of body cavities with high content of reducing substances), the absorbed iodine will be reduced more or less fast to iodide.
4. The amount of total iodine (I_2 and I^-) absorbed by the body mainly depends on
   a. The concentration of free molecular iodine (and of iodide) of the preparation
   b. The time of application
   c. The treated area
   d. The nature of the treated area.
5. As long as not reduced, i.e., free, iodine is present in the skin it will diffuse not only into deeper regions but also back (out of the skin), performing for a certain time a residual bactericidal activity on the skin surface. The reduced portion, however, remains for some time in the body and gives rise to an increase of the level of serum-iodide.
6. The incorporated iodine in the form of iodide and organic bound iodine (which comes to ~75% of the total resorbed iodine) leaves the body by urinary excretion with a biologic half-life of approximately 2 days (Gloebel et al., 1984).

The main restraints against iodine preparations are based upon the suspicion of a possible disorder of thyroid functions caused by the iodine uptake. Gloebel et al. (1984) investigated iodine uptake after use of povidone-iodine preparations (Betaisodona) as mouth antiseptic, vaginal gel, and liquid soap in subjects with normal thyroid function. By measuring serum I^-, T_3, T_4, TSH, and urinary iodide excretion (as an index of thyroid function), the authors observed an increase in iodine supply of up to 2 mg daily, but in no case the developing of hyperthyroidism or hypothyroidism. Because the test conditions were drastic (e.g., hands and forearms were washed 10 times for 2½ minutes with povidone iodine liquid soap within 5 hours) one would tend to think that povidone iodine preparations are nontoxic. However, taking into account that, as mentioned above, the iodine uptake depends—among other factors—on the concentration of free iodine of the used preparation, which in this case was not ascertained, the notion of nontoxicity strictly speaking applies only to the preparations used by the authors and the given application. Because the content of free molecular iodine at present needs not be specified and, what is more, varies considerably in commercially available preparations (Gottardi and Koller, 1986a), one should be careful in making generalizations.

RESIDUAL EFFECTS OF IODINE PREPARATIONS

The above-mentioned backdiffusion of the not-reduced portion of the absorbed iodine, which takes place much slower than the uptake, interestingly, has not been recognized until now. By means of a new photometric method this iodine flux ([dim] = mass/area · time) has been ascertained on the skin after application of Lugol's solution and povidone iodine preparations with various concentrations of free iodine. The most important findings are the following: The intensity of the iodine flux depends on the amount of iodine absorbed by the skin, which as far as it is concerned depends on the concentration of free iodine of the applied solution and the time of application. Applying Lugol's solution (170 ppm free iodine) for only 1 minute, the flux could be detected for approximately 24 hours (range: 50 to 0.005 µg I_2/cm² · min), whereas after application of a povidone iodine preparation (10 ppm) for 3 to 5 minutes the flux was detectable ½ to 1 hour (range: 0.2 to 0.005 µg I_2/cm² · min) (Gottardi, 1989).

The latter result suggests that even the application of iodophor preparations could give rise to a persistent (residual) microbicidal action. This has been proved by comparing the surviving CFUs of *Micrococcus luteus* (applied to the skin by artificial contamination) on normal skin as well as on skin that has been treated for 5 min with a povidone-iodine preparation (10 ppm free iodine) immediately before contamination. A logarithmic reduction rate of 0.4 was found, a result that confirmed the bactericidal action of the iodine diffusing out of the skin (Gottardi, in preparation).

As long as iodine diffuses out of the skin, so to speak, an active disinfection from the inner regions of the skin takes place; therefore an effective action on the residential germs can be expected, a feature that seems to be unique in the field of skin disinfection.

Regarding this, Hartmann (1985) found by a special method that the reduction of the total resident flora was significantly higher using povidone-iodine than it was with isopropanol. This is in contrast to the usual findings, mainly in testing preparations for surgical hand scrub, which exhibit in general a better degerming activity of alcohols.

ORGANIC IODINE COMPOUNDS

Compounds of this class contain iodine that is bound to a carbon atom. With regard to properties and mode of action as disinfectants, they differ from the previously described disinfectants in that they contain neither free iodine nor other oxidizing iodine species. In the case of iodoform (CHI_3), however, there exist contrary opinions, because on the one hand iodoform is supposed to produce elemental iodine and formaldehyde in connection with water (Knolle, 1975), while, on the other hand, it was impossible to detect any free iodine in an aqueous slurry of CHI_3 at 37°C and pH 7 with a method that is sensitive down to 5×10^{-8} M/L (Gottardi, unpublished).

Iodoform (triiodomethane), probably the oldest pharmaceutically used iodine compound, forms yellow crystals with a characteristic anesthetic odor. It came into extensive use as dusting powder, especially as a local anti-infective agent to promote granulation and diminish infections of open wounds (Gershenfeld, 1977). Because of its toxicity (it can cause such effects as sleeplessness, hallucinations, and spasms) it has been replaced by other preparations, especially those containing iodophors. The compound is not specified in the USP XXI.

Iodine derivatives of quinoline exhibit protozoacide and metazoacide properties and have shown excellent results in prophylactic and therapeutic use (Gershenfeld, 1977). Iodoquinol (USP XXI, 5,7-diiodo-8-quinolinol) and Clioquinol (USP XXI, 5-chloro-7-iodo-8-quinolinol) are the best known active substances of this type and serve as the basis for creams, ointments, powders, and tablets. To this class of compounds belong also the iodine-containing x-ray contrast media. Examples are Iocetamic Acid, Iopanoic Acid, and Iothalamic Acid (all USP XXI). They contain a benzene ring system with three iodine atoms in meta-position, and are used as such but also in form of their derivatives. The radioactive compounds Iodohyppurate Sodium I 123 resp. I 131 (both USP XXI)

should also be mentioned, which are used for nuclear medical purposes.

Iodonium Compounds

This class has the general formula $[R_2I^+]X^-$ (where R is an organic radical and X^- an inorganic or organic anion) and is of more theoretic than practical interest. The structure resembles the onium compounds (e.g., quaternary ammonium), and the active part of these compounds is iodine in the oxidation state +3. Diphenyliodonium chloride, whose degerming properties have been investigated by Gershenfeld and Witlin (1948), appears to be the most generally effective substance.

PRACTICAL APPLICATIONS

Iodine as a Disinfectant in Human Medicine

The most important application of iodine in human medicine is the disinfection of skin, which has been in use since the mid-nineteenth century (Reddish, 1954). Besides prophylactic actions (e.g., the preoperative preparations of the skin, the surgical disinfection of hands, the disinfection of the perineum prior to infections and transfusions), iodine preparations are also used for therapeutic purposes, e.g., the treatment of infected and burned skin. The previously used aqueous iodine and tincture nearly 30 years ago have been replaced, to a great extent, by the iodophors, which cause less unwanted side reactions, such as staining, irritation of tissue, and resorption of iodine. Among the investigated iodophors, povidone-iodine has been described as the compound of choice (Knolle, 1975). However, attempts are made to replace the povidone carrier by other macromolecules, which might be still more harmless than povidone, which after all has been used as a blood substitute. In this connection polymers built up of sugar molecules (e.g., polydextrose) are of great interest. When rigid aseptic precautions are required and no painful irritations are to be expected, however, iodine tincture is still in use as the strongest disinfectant based on iodine. A detailed review of the use of iodine in human medicine is given by Knolle (1975), and a good historical account and information on aqueous solutions of iodine and tincture is given by Reddish (1957).

Iodine has also been used for the disinfection of medical equipment, such as catgut, catheters, knife blades, ampules, plastic items, rubber goods, brushes, multiple-dose vials, and thermometers (Gershenfeld, 1977). It should be mentioned, however, that disinfection with iodine is not appropriate for every sort of material. Many metal surfaces in particular are not resistant to oxidation and can be altered. Furthermore, some plastics absorb elemental iodine, which causes a brownish staining.

Disinfection of Water

Drinking Water

The first known field use for iodine in water treatment was in World War I by Vergnoux (White, 1972), who reported rapid sterilization of water for troops. Since that time, several studies have been made (White, 1972) showing that iodination is suitable for the disinfection of drinking water, especially in case of emergency. Of considerable importance is the work of Chang and Morris (1953), which led to the development of tetraglycine hydroperiodide tablets ("Globaline"), which have been successfully used to disinfect small or individual water supplies in the U.S. Army. This method of water purification (addition of iodine tablets or calcium hypochlorite to the water, followed by a 25- or 30-minute disinfectant contact period, respectively, before drinking) is still in use in the U.S. Army. However one became also aware that this method of purification involves some health risks since the chemicals carrying out the disinfection are not removed at these procedures (Schaub, 1986). Black et al. (1965) have demonstrated, in two prison water systems, that iodine in doses up to 1.0 ppm is sufficient for disinfection, does not produce any discernible color, taste, or odor, and has no adverse effect upon the general health or thyroid function. Thomas et al. (1978) reported a pilot project with a 15-year duration in which they observed no instances of ill effect caused by the use of iodine for water disinfection. The authors found that iodination is an effective and economic means of water purification, of particular advantage in rural and underdeveloped countries.

Lately the iodine resins have been successfully used as a basis for purifier units, which, as long as they are not exhausted, work very well, bringing about a kill of 4 logs. For emergency and for travelers "pocket purifiers" have been developed whose performance was officially approved by being registered by the EPA (Regunathan and Beauman, 1986).

Swimming-Pool Water

The application of iodine to the treatment of swimming pools is an entirely different process from that of potable water treatment, because in the former, elemental iodine is applied directly to the water in crystal or possibly in tablet form, whereas in the latter, iodine is generally applied in the inert iodide form and later released as elemental iodine by coming in contact with an oxidant such as chlorine (White, 1972), as follows:

$$HOCl + 2I^- \longrightarrow I_2 + Cl^- + OH^-$$

1,3-Dichloro-5,5-dimethylhydantoin, whose combination with iodide is known as "Hio-Dine" process (designed especially for the disinfection of swimming pools), may also serve as an oxidant. It became apparent, however, that this N-chloro compound is not ideal because it decomposes in aqueous solution, forming undesirable end products (White, 1972).

Compared with chlorine, the use of iodine has the advantage that it reacts only to a small extent with ammonia or other nitrogenous compounds and therefore produces no compounds that are likely to contribute to swimmers' discomfort in the form of eye irritation or obnoxious odors (Black, 1961). The use of iodine in swimming-pool disinfection has the following advantages (Putnam, 1961): (1) approximately one third saving on chemical cost, (2) no disagreeable odor or taste, (3) no irritation of the mucous membranes, (4) good disinfection of swimming-pool waters, (5) no danger in storage or use, because material is in crystalline form, (6) residual is stable and does not fluctuate quickly, (7) pH is stable after balance is reached, and (8) swimmers' comfort is protected.

On the other hand, iodine is a notoriously poor algicide, and the control of algae growth requires additional measures. Probably the most serious flaw in the use of iodine is the difficulty in controlling the color of the pool water, mainly in the presence of a large amount of iodide, which causes the development of yellowish-brown I_3^- ions. The problem of color control plus the inability of iodine to control algae all but eliminate it from use by the swimming-pool industry (White, 1972).

Wastewater

Only few contributions deal with the use of iodine in the disinfection of waters that, in contrast to drinking and swimming-pool water, do not come in direct contact with man, e.g., wastewater and industrial waters. Because these waters in general are highly charged with dissolved nitrogenous substances (proteins and their hydrolysis products), the use of iodine, with its only slight tendency to react with nitrogen compounds, should be of great advantage.

In applications, however, which range in technical dimensions, the question of cost also has to be considered, and because iodine is nearly three times as expensive as chlorine in price per mole, the advantages and disadvantages of iodine must be weighed carefully. In a study about a new method of disinfection with a mixture of I^- and NH_2Cl that generates elemental iodine Kinman and Layton (1976) find that this system offers considerable potential for use in water disinfection for potable waters, industrial waters, and waters that must be discharged to shellfish areas. Investigating alternatives to wastewater disinfection, Budde et al. (1977), in pilot plant studies, compared the disinfectants chlorine, ozone, and iodine, finding that for the same level of fecal coliform destruction, iodine was most costly under all conditions studied.

Disinfection of Air

Since Lombardo (1926) first advocated the use of iodine as an aerial disinfectant, experiments on the disinfection of air have been carried out, mainly during World War II. Plesch (1941) recommended the aerial disinfection of air-raid shelters with iodine vapors as a prophylactic measure against influenza. White et al. (1944) reported iodine to be effective as an aerial disinfectant at concentrations much below its saturation vapor pressure, and Raymond (1946) found a "relatively tolerable" concentration of 0.1 mg/ft³ (3.5 mg/M³) to be sufficient for a rapid kill of freshly sprayed salivary organisms. Since that time, however, no more publications have appeared concerning iodine as an air disinfectant.

Obviously, one is aware of the danger that iodine vapors pose to the respiratory organs, documented by the fact that the maximum allowed concentration of iodine comes to 1.0 mg/M³ (threshold limit value; Lewis and Sweet, 1986), which is less than one-third of the concentration recommended by Raymond (1946).

RANGE OF ACTION

Iodine is an excellent prompt effective microbicide with a broad range of action that includes almost all of the important health-related microorganisms, such as enteric bacteria, enteric viruses, bacterial viruses, and protozoan cysts (Hoehn, 1976). Mycobacteria and the spores of bacilli and clostridia can also be killed by iodine (Wallhäusser, 1978). Furthermore, iodine also exhibits a fungicidal and trichomonacidal activity (Knolle, 1975). As is expected, varying amounts of iodine are necessary to achieve complete disinfection of the different classes of organisms. Within the same class, however, the published data on the disinfecting effect of iodine correspond only to a small extent. In particular, the published killing times of spores (Wallhäusser, 1978) and viruses (Knolle, 1975) are widely disparate. One reason for this might be the non-uniform sensitivity of microorganisms to iodine, which applies not only to the type of organism but also to the growth conditions. Pyle and McFeters (1989) could demonstrate that bacterial isolates (predominantly *Pseudomonas sp.*) from water systems disinfected by iodine showed differences (which had, however, not always the same sign) of up to 4 logs decrease after contact with iodine (1 mg/L, pH 7, 1 min) if grown in brain heart infusion or after cultivation in phosphate buffer.

As mentioned by Hoehn (1976), comparison of previously published references concerning effectiveness in disinfection processes of different microorganisms are difficult because of the myriad of different environmental conditions existing when experiments are conducted, e.g., pH value, temperature, concentration and type of iodine preparation, time of exposure to the disinfectant,

Table 8–5. *Practical Applications of Iodine as a Disinfectant: Concentration, Exposure Time, Disinfective Result*

Scope of Application	Concentration	Conditions	Exposure Time (Min)	Disinfective Result	References
Drinking water	8 ppm	—	10	"Kill of water-borne pathogens"	Committee on Medical Research, 1948
	3–4 ppm	25°C	12	"Reduces 10⁶ bacterial/mL to less than 10 bacterial/mL"	Chang and Morris, 1952
	3–4 ppm	3°C	22		
Drinking water in emergency	5–6 ppm	20–25°C	10	"Excellent disinfectant for water supplies under emergency conditions"	
	5–6 ppm	near 0°C	20		
	5 drops I₂-tincture to a quart of water	Clear water	30	"Water safe for drinking"	United States Public Health Service, 1940
	10 drops I₂-tincture to a quart of water	Cloudy water	30		
	4.0–8.0 mg/L	Turbid water of low quality	30	"Water of virtual potable quality"	Ellis and van Voce, 1989
Swimming-pool water	0.2 (0.1) ppm	—		"Provides water of satisfactory quality"	Black et al., 1959
	0.2 ppm	—		"Maintains the water at a satisfactory bacteriological quality"	U.S. Public Health Service, 1962
General germicidal action	1:20,000	Absence of organic matter	1	"Most bacteria are killed"	Goodman and Gilman, 1980
	1:20,000	Absence of organic matter	15	"Wet spores are killed"	Goodman and Gilman, 1980
	1:200,000	Absence of organic matter	15	"Will destroy all vegetative forms of bacteria"	Goodman and Gilman, 1980
Disinfection of skin	1% tincture	—	90 sec	"Will kill 90% of the bacteria"	Goodman and Gilman, 1980
	5% tincture	—	60 sec	"Will kill 90% of the bacteria"	Goodman and Gilman, 1980
	7% tincture	—	15 sec	"Will kill 90% of the bacteria"	Goodman and Gilman, 1980
	1% aqueous I₂-solution	Skin of hands	20 min	"Inactivation of rhenovirus"	Carter et al., 1980
	2% aqueous I₂-solution	Skin of hands	3 min	"Inactivation of rhenovirus"	Carter et al., 1980

and amount and type of dissolved organic and inorganic substances. Another problem is the fact that, in general, most of these conditions are not described in detail, and an exact comparison of the germicidal effectiveness of iodine against different organisms, as well as a comparison with the other halogens, is therefore virtually impossible. In spite of these difficulties, some authors have tried to summarize the disinfecting properties of iodine and the other halogens by reviewing the literature and analyzing the existing data. The most important conclusions are:

1. A standard destruction (i.e., a 99.999% kill in 10 minutes at 25°C) of enteric bacteria, amoebic cysts, and enteric viruses requires I_2 residuals of 0.2, 3.5, and 14.6 ppm, respectively (Chang, 1971).

2. On a weight basis, iodine can inactivate viruses more completely over a wide range of water quality than other halogens (Krusé, 1970).

3. In the presence of organic and inorganic nitrogenous substances, iodine is the cysticide of choice because it does not produce side reactions that interfere with its disinfecting properties (Krusé, 1970).

4. Iodine would require the smallest mg/L dosage compared to chlorine or bromine to "break any water" to provide a free residual (Krusé, 1970).

5. I_2 is two to three times as cysticidal and six times as sporocidal as HOI, whereas HOI is at least 40 times as virucidal as I_2. This behavior is explained on the one hand by the higher diffusibility of molecular iodine through the cell walls of cysts and spores and on the other hand by the higher oxidizing power of HOI (Chang, 1971).

6. For some microorganisms an iodine resistance also has been ascertained, e.g., *Pseudomonas alcaligenes* and *Alcaligenes faecalis*, which can account for the bulk of the microbial flora in iodinated swimming pools (Favero and Drake, 1966).

7. Because disinfection is a chemical reaction, the influence of temperature on reaction speed—as a rule of thumb lowering the temperature about 10° halves the speed—has to be considered at microbicidal events in such a way that either the contact time or the concentration of the disinfectant have to be increased if cold water has to be treated. The lack of efficiency at low temperatures was demonstrated by Regunathan and Beauman (1986), showing that some iodine preparations designated to purify canteen water worked well against Giardia at 20°C but not at 3°C if used according to the instructions.

A survey of concentration, exposure time, and disinfective result in practical applications of iodine is given in Table 8–5.

REFERENCES

Apostolov, K. 1980. The effects of iodine on the biological activities of myxoviruses. J. Hyg., *84*, 381–388.

Bell, R.P., and Gelles, E. 1951. The halogen cations in aqueous solution. J. Chem. Soc., *73*, 2734.

Berkelmann, R.L., Holland, B.W., and Anderson, R.L. 1982. Increased bactericidal activity of dilute preparations of povidone-iodine solutions. J. Clin. Microbiol., *15*, 635.

Black, A.P. 1961. Swimming pool disinfection with iodine. Water Sewage Works, *108*, 286.

Black, A.P., Lackey, J.B., and Lackey, E.W. 1959. Effectiveness of iodine for the disinfection of swimming pool water. Am. J. Public Health, *49*, 1060–1068.

Black, A.P., et al. 1968. Iodine for the disinfection of water. J. Am. Water Works Assoc., *60*, 69–83.

Black, A.P., et al. 1965. Use of iodine for disinfection. J. Am. Water Works Assoc., *57*, 1401.

Boinet, A.A. 1865. *Iodotherapie*. 2nd edition. Paris, Masson.

Bolek, S., Boleva, V., and Schwotzer, H. 1972. Halogene und Halogenverbindungen. In *Handbuch der Desinfektion und Sterilisation*. Volume I. Edited by H. Horn, M. Privora, and W. Weuffen. Berlin, Verlag Volk und Gesundheit, p. 132.

Budde, P.E., Nehm, P., and Boyle, W.C. 1977. Alternatives to wastewater disinfection. J. Water Pollut. Control Fed. (USA), *49*, 2144–2156.

Carter, C.H., et al. 1980. Rhinovirus inactivation by aqueous iodine in vitro and on skin. Proc. Soc. Exp. Biol. Med., *165*, 380.

Chang, S.L. 1971. Modern concept of disinfection. J. Sanit. Eng. Div. Proc. ASCE, *97*, 689.

Chang, S.L. and Morris, J.C. 1953. Elemental iodine as a disinfectant for drinking water. Ind. Eng. Chem., *45*, 1009.

Chang, S.L., and Morris, J.C. 1952. Use of elemental iodine as disinfectant for water supplies. Abstract, 122nd Meeting, 6-S-7S; 1953. Ind. Eng. Chem., J. Am. Chem. Soc., *45*, 1009–1012.

Chanoine, J.P., et al. 1988. Increased recall rate at screening for congenital hypothyroidism in breast fed infants born to iodine overloaded mothers. Arch. Dis. Child., *63*, (10), 1207–1210.

Committee on Medical Research, 1948. *Advances in Military Medicine*. Volume II. Boston, Little, Brown, p. 527.

Davies, J. 1839. *Selections in Pathology and Surgery*. Part II. London, Longmans, Orme, Brown, Green & Longmans.

Favero, M.S., and Drake, C.H. 1966. Factors influencing the occurrence of high numbers of iodine-resistant bacteria in iodinated swimming pools. Appl. Microbiol., *14*, 627–635.

Gershenfeld, L. 1977. Iodine. In *Disinfection, Sterilization and Preservation*. 2nd edition. Edited by S.S. Block. Philadelphia, Lea & Febiger.

Gershenfeld, L., and Witlin, B. 1948. Iodonium compounds and their antibacterial activity. Am. J. Pharm., *12*, 158–169.

Gilman, A.G., Goodman, L.S., and Gilman, A. 1980. *The Pharmacological Basis of Therapeutics*. 6th edition. New York, Macmillan.

Glöbel, B., Glöbel, H., and Anders, C. 1984. Resorption von Iod aus PVP-Iod-Präparaten nach Anwendung beim Menschen. Dtsch. Med. Wochenschr., *109*, 1401–1404.

Goebel, W. 1906. On the disinfecting properties of Lugol's solutions. Zentralbl. Bakt., *42*, 86, 176.

Goldsmith, L.A. 1983. *Biochemistry and Physiologie of the Skin*. Oxford, Oxford University Press.

Gottardi, W. 1976. On the reaction of chlorine, bromine, iodine and some N-chloro and N-bromo compounds with peptone in aqueous solution. Zentralbl. Bakt. Hyg., I. Abt. Orig. B, *162*, 384–388.

Gottardi, W. 1978a. Aqueous iodine solutions as disinfectants: composition, stability, comparison with chlorine and bromine solutions. Zentralbl. Bakt. Hyg., I. Abt. Orig. B, *167*, 206–215.

Gottardi, W. 1978b. On the usability of N-iodo-compounds as disinfectants. Zentralbl. Bakt. Hyg., I. Abt. Orig. B, *167*, 216–223.

Gottardi, W. 1980. Redoxpotential and germicidal action of aqueous halogen solutions. Zentralbl. Bakt. Hyg., I. Abt. Orig. B, *170*, 422–430.

Gottardi, W. 1981. The formation of iodate as a reason for the decrease of efficiency of iodine containing disinfectants. Zentralbl. Bakt. Hyg., I. Abt. Orig. B, *172*, 498–507.

Gottardi, W. 1983. Potentiometric evaluation of the equilibrium concentrations of free and complex bound iodine in aqueous solutions of Polyvinylprrolidone-iodine (Povidone-iodine). Fresenius Z. Anal. Chem., *314*, 582–585.

Gottardi, W. 1985. The influence of the chemical behaviour of iodine on the germicidal action of disinfectant solutions containing iodine. J. Hosp. Infect., *6* (Suppl.), 1–11.

Gottardi, W. and Koller, W. 1986a. The concentration of free iodine in aqueous PVP-iodine containing systems and its variation with temperature. Monatschefte für Chemie, *117*, 1011–1020.

Gottardi, W., and Koller, W. 1986b. The decrease of efficiency of povidone-iodine preparations by blood: Model experiments on the reaction of iodine containing disinfectants with protein constituents. 3rd Conference on Progress in Chemical Disinfection. Binghampton, NY.

Gottardi, W., and Puritscher, M. 1986. Degerming experiments with aqueous Povidone-iodine containing disinfecting solutions: Influence of the concentration of free iodine on the bactericidal reaction against Staphylococcus Aureus. Zentralbl. Bakt. Hyg., B, *182*, 372–380.

Gottardi, W., and Koller, W. 1987. The influence of the consumption on the efficacy of Povidone-iodine preparations. Hyg. Med., *12*, 150–154.

Gottardi, W. 1989. Residual effects on the skin caused by povidone-iodine preparations. Hyg. Med., *14*, 228–233.

Gottardi, W. 1991. Povidone iodine: Bactericidal agent or pharmaceutical base material. Reflections on the term active agent in disinfecting systems containing halogens. Hyg. Med., *16*, 346.

Halliday, A. 1821. Observations on the use of the different preparations of iodine as a remedy for bronchocele, and in the treatment of scrofula. London Med. Repos., *16*, 199.

Harakuda Yamada, and Kunio Kozima. 1960. The molecular complexes between iodine and various oxygen-containing organic compounds. J. Am. Chem. Soc., *82*, 1543.

Hartmann, A.A. 1985. A comparison of povidone-iodine and 60% n-propanol on the resident flora using a new test method. J. Hosp. Infect., *6*(Suppl. A), 73–78.

Hoehn, R.C. 1976. Comparative disinfection methods. J. Am. Water Works Assoc., *68*, 302–308.

Horn, D., and Ditter, W. 1984. Physikalisch-chemische Grundlagen der mikrobiziden Wirkung wässriger PVP-Iod-Lösungen. In *PVP-Iod in der Operativen Medizin*. Edited by G. Hierholzer and G. Görtz. Berlin, Springer.

Horn, H., Privora, M., and Weuffen, W. 1972. *Handbuch der Desinfektions und Sterilisation*. Volume I. Edited by W. Weuffen. Berlin, VEB Verlag Volk und Gesundheit.

Horn, H., Privora, M. and Weuffen, W. 1974. *Handbuch der Desinfektion und Sterilisation*. Volume III. Edited by W. Weuffen. Berlin, VEB Verlag Volk und Gesundheit.

Hunt, J.L., Sato, R., Heck, E.L., and Baxter, C.R. 1980. A critical evaluation of povidone-iodine absorption in thermally injured patients. J. Trauma, *20*, 127–129.

Kawakami, M., Sakamoto, M., and Kumazawa, T. 1986. Mouthwashes containing iodine-maltosylcyclodextrin inclusion compound as a microbicid with high water-solubility. Japan Patent 297473. CA, *109*(16), 134972w.

Kinman, R.N., and Layton, R.F. 1976. New method for water disinfection. J. Am. Water Works Assoc., *68*, 298–302.

Knolle, P. 1975. Alt und aktuell—Keime und Jod. Hospital–Hygiene 67, 389–402.

Koch, R. 1881. Über Desinfektion. In *Mitteilungen aus dem Kaiserlichen Gesundheitsamte*. 1st edition. Struck, Berlin, Struck, p. 234.

Kramer, H.P., Moore, W.A., and Ballinger, D.G. 1952. Determination of microquantities of iodine in water solution by amperometric titrations. Anal. Chem., *24*, 1892–1894.

Kril, M.B., Fitzpatrick, T.W., and Janauer, G.E. 1986. Toward a protocol for testing solid microbial compositions. 3rd Conference on Progress in Chemical Disinfection. Binghampton, NY.

Krusé, W.C., et al. 1970. Halogen action on bacteria, viruses and protozoan. Proc. Natl. Spec. Conf. Disinfection, ASCE, Amherst, MA, pp. 113–137.

Kuhn, J.M., et al. 1987. Thyroid function of burned patients: Effect of iodine therapy. Rev. Med. Interne, *8*(1), 21–26.

Kuschinsky, G., and Lüllmann, H. 1984. *Kurzes Lehrbuch der Pharmakologie und Toxikologie*. 10th edition. Stuttgart-New York, Georg Thieme.

Lombardo, F. 1926. Vapori di soluzione iodoiodurata come profilassi e terapia della influenza. Riforma Med., *42*, 1011–1012.

O'Connor, A.F.F., Freeland, A.P., Heal, D.J., and Rossouw, D.S. 1977. J. Laryngol. Otol., *91*, 903–907.

Pinter, E., Rackur, H., and Schubert, R. 1983. Die Bedeutung der Galenik für die mikrobizide Wirksamkeit von Polyvidon-Iod-Lösungen. Pharmazeutische Industrie, *46*, 3–8.

Plesch, J. 1941. Methods of air disinfection. Br. Med. J., *1*, 798.

Pollack, W., and Iny, O. 1985. A physicochemical study of PVP-I solutions leading to the reformulation of 'Betadine' preparation (5% PVP-I). J. Hosp. Infect., *6*(Suppl. A), 25–30.

Putnam, E.V. 1961. Iodine vs chlorine treatment of swimming pools. Parks and Recreations, April.

Pyle, B.H., and McFeters, G.A. 1989. Iodine sensitivity of bacteria isolated from iodinated water systems. Can. J. Microbiol., *35*, 520–523.

Raymond, W.F. 1946. Iodine as an aerial disinfectant. J. Hyg., *44*, 359–361.

Reddish, G.F. 1957. *Antiseptics, Disinfectants, Fungicides, and Chemical and Physical Sterilization*. 2nd edition. Philadelphia, Lea & Febiger, pp. 223–225.

Regulations, recommendations and assessments extracted from the registry of toxic effects of chemical substances, 1986. Edited by R.J. Lewis, and D.V. Sweet. Cincinnati, US Department of Health and Human Services NIOSH.

Regunathan, P., and Beauman, W.H. 1986. A comparison of point-of-use disinfection methods. 3rd Conference on Progress in Chemical Disinfection. Binghampton, NY.

Schaub, A.S. 1986. Preventive medicine considerations for army individual soldier water purification. 3rd Conference on Progress in Chemical Disinfection. Binghampton, NY.

Schenck, H.U., Simak, P., and Haedicke, E. 1979. Structure of polyvinylpyrrolidone-iodine (povidone-iodine). J. Pharm. Sci., *68*, 1505–1509.

Schmulbach, C.D., and Drago, R.S. 1960. Molecular addition compounds of iodine III. J. Am. Chem. Soc., *82*, 4484.

Sykes, G. 1972. *Disinfection and sterilization*. 2nd edition. London, Chapman and Hall.

Thomas, W.C., Jr., Malagodi, M.H., Oates, T.W., and McCourt, J.P. 1978. Effects of an iodinated water supply. Trans. Am. Clin. Climatol. Assoc. (USA), *90*, 153–162.

Vallin, E. 1882. Traitè des dèsinfectants et de la dèsinfection. Paris, Masson.

Wallhäusser, K.H. 1978. *Sterilisation, Desinfektion. Konservierung*. Stuttgart, Georg Thieme.

White, G.C. 1972. *Handbook of Chlorination*. New York, Van Nostrand Reinhold.

White, L.J., Baker, A.H., and Twort, C.C. 1944. Aerial disinfection. Nature, *153*, 141–142.

Wirth, W., Hecht, G., and Gloxhuber, C. 1967. *Toxikologie-Fibel*. Stuttgart, Georg Thieme.

CHAPTER 9

PEROXYGEN COMPOUNDS

Seymour S. Block

Research efforts in chemical disinfection research and development have taken many turns over the years. Where are we now headed? Our future guideline seems clear, and although it is not as simple as ABC it is as simple as two other three-letter combinations, namely, EPA and FDA. We will concentrate on chemicals that (1) will be effective against microorganisms when highly diluted, (2) will be low in toxicity to people and animals, and (3) will not injure the environment.

One such chemical, which will be considered in this chapter was appraised many years ago. Dr. Samuel S. Wallian in an address to the New York State Medical Society in 1892 said:

> One can hardly refer to the medical journals without finding enthusiastic recommendations of it as a disinfectant of rare efficiency, an antiseptic of recognized merit and a germicide of decided potency . . . It is also a reliable sporicide, and at the same time it is non-toxic and non-corrosive—qualities possessed by few if any of the other sporicides yet brought to notice.

The chemical Dr. Wallian referred to was then known as oxidized water; we know it as hydrogen peroxide. Although first reported in 1818 by the French chemist Thenard, it was the English physician B.W. Richardson who noted in 1858 its ability to do away with foul odors and thereby proposed its use as a disinfectant. It should be recognized that this was before Pasteur had published his famous work associating bacteria with disease, and since disease often produced unpleasant odors, it was thought that chemicals that reduced or masked these odors would serve as disinfectants. Richardson's proposal led to the early commercial use of hydrogen peroxide as a disinfectant under the trade name *Sanitas*. (It should be noted that this trade name has been used in more recent times but contains other chemicals as the active ingredient.)

HYDROGEN PEROXIDE

Hydrogen peroxide (HP) has had a rocky road in its acceptance as a disinfectant; first popular, then unpop-

ular, and now finding special application where it serves particular functions of great value. It is considered so safe that it has been approved for use in foods in many countries (Schumb et al., 1955). One of the major, new applications is in sterilizing containers for aseptically preserved foods like fresh milk and fruit juices (see Chapter 48). Hydrogen peroxide can be easily destroyed by heat or the enzymes catalase and peroxidase to give the innocuous end products, oxygen and water.

In wound application, low concentrations of unstable preparations of HP to tissues containing inactivating levels of catalase led to unfavorable results and general abandonment of this agent as an antiseptic. Examination of the early literature reveals, however, that hydrogen peroxide was satisfactory when used as a disinfectant for inanimate materials. For example, used in low concentrations, HP was considered ideal for the preservation of milk and water (Heinemann, 1913) and for the sterilization of cocoa milk beverage (Wilson et al., 1927). By 1950, an electrochemical process had been developed that produced pure preparations in high concentrations that were stable even at elevated temperatures and that had long shelf-lives (Schumb et al., 1955).

There has been an upsurge of interest in HP during the last 20 years. Yoshpe-Purer and Eylan (1968) used low concentrations for the sterilization of drinking water. Naguib and Hussein (1972) showed that 0.1% HP at 54°C for 30 minutes reduced the total bacterial count in raw milk by 99.999%, and the coliform, staphylococcal, salmonellae, and clostridial counts by 100%. Rosensweig (1978), investigating 3% HP to control contamination of hospital water sources, demonstrated that a final concentration of 0.03% in water killed 1 million colony-forming units per milliliter of seven bacterial strains overnight, with an 80% kill in 1 hour. The rapid virucidal activity of HP against rhinovirus, tested both in suspension and on carriers, was demonstrated in studies by Mentel and Schmidt (1973).

HP in relatively high concentrations (10 to 25%) was also a promising sporicidal agent. Toledo et al. (1973)

167

obtained D values of 0.8 to 7.3 minutes at 24°C with four aerobic spore strains and one anaerobic spore strain. Work in the USSR indicated the practicability of this agent for sterilization of spacecraft; this view was supported by the studies of Wardle and Renninger (1975) in the United States. These latter workers, using aerobic bacterial isolates from spacecraft, achieved a complete kill of spore suspensions at the level of 100 million colony-forming units per milliliter by a 10% concentration at 25°C in 60 minutes.

Pure HP is very stable. Discovery of factors that cause its decomposition led to the development of effective stabilizers that deactivate contaminating materials and do not act on hydrogen peroxide itself (Schumb et al., 1955). Thus, the stability of concentrated HP can be retained when diluted to 3% if this step is carried out with clean equipment and a good grade of deionized water in clean bottles of inert material.

The grade of HP (Super D) used chiefly for the drug and cosmetic trade is highly stabilized. In the presence of added catalytic decomposition ions of aluminum, iron, copper, manganese, and chromium, a 6% solution retains 98% of its original active oxygen after being subjected to 100°C for 24 hours (Technical Bulletin No. 42, *Super D Hydrogen Peroxide*, F.M.C. Corporation, Philadelphia, PA). The ordinary in-use stability of 3% HP (Parke-Davis) was checked, and there was no decrease in concentration when bottles (120 ml) were opened and 10 ml was discarded each day for 12 days. Seven randomly selected shelf samples of various brands were tested according to the USP XVIII, and all were found to meet the standards for nonvolatile residues, heavy metals, and H_2O_2 concentration.

The stability of a 3% HP solution that had been heated was also examined in terms of biocidal activity. The time required for an unheated 3% hydrogen peroxide solution to eliminate a 1×10^5 per milliliter inoculum was compared to that of a solution that had previously been subjected for 8 hours daily to 45°C for a total of 7 days. There was no significant difference in the killing times between these two preparations for seven bacterial strains and one fungus (Turner, 1974). Commercial HP is available in a number of strengths, namely, 3%, 30%, 35%, 50%, 70%, and 90% (FMC Corp.). A special food-grade HP in 35% and 50% strengths, which meets FDA safety regulations, is also available.

Mechanism of Action of Hydrogen Peroxide

HP may be regarded as nature's own disinfectant and preservative. It is naturally present in milk and in honey, which it helps to preserve from spoilage, and it is a normal resident of tissues as a result of cellular metabolism. Further, it protects us from infections by invading pathogenic microorganisms. In the mouth, where it is present in the mucous membranes, it acts as a powerful oxidant either alone or in combination with thiocyanate and peroxidase in the saliva, as follows (Thomas and Aune, 1978):

$$H_2O_2 + SCN^- \xrightarrow{\text{peroxidase}} OSCN^- + H_2O$$

$$OSCN^- + RSH \longrightarrow RS\overset{\overset{\displaystyle O}{\|}}{S}CN + H^+$$
$$\text{sulfenyl thiocyanate}$$

HP works in another, even more important way to protect us from infection. It is the germicide that kills those microorganisms that penetrate the outer defenses of the body and gain entrance to the bloodstream. The phagocytes, the specialized white blood cells, scavenge and absorb foreign invaders. But they don't absorb living cells; the cells must first be killed, and it is hydrogen peroxide in the phagocytes that kills the bacteria.

HP is produced in cells by the reduction of oxygen. Although oxygen is required by respiring cells it is also toxic to them; cells are protected because they have a system for disposing of the oxygen by reducing it to water. This may be performed in a series of enzymatic steps (Fridovich, 1975):

$$O_2 + e^- \rightarrow O_2^- \quad \text{superoxide ion}$$

$$O_2 + 2e^- + 2H^+ \rightarrow H_2O_2 \quad \text{hydrogen peroxide}$$

$$O_2 + 3e^- + 3H^+ \rightarrow H_2O + OH\cdot \quad \text{hydroxyl radical}$$

$$O_2 + 4e^- + 4H^+ \rightarrow 2H_2O$$

It is seen that HP, the superoxide ion, and the hydroxyl radical are intermediate products in this scheme for the reduction of oxygen to water. In the presence of myeloperoxidase enzyme, chloride in the bacteria may be oxidized by HP to hypochlorite (Klebanoff, 1968):

$$Cl^- + H_2O_2 \xrightarrow{\text{myeloperoxidase}} OCl^- + H_2O$$

Hypochlorite is a well known oxidant and germicide. Another proposed mechanism by which HP partcipates in the destruction of bacteria involves the reaction of the superoxide ion with hydrogen peroxide to produce the hydroxyl radical (Haber and Weiss, 1934; Fridovich, 1978):

$$O_2^- + H_2O_2 \rightarrow OH\cdot + OH^- + O_2$$

The hydroxyl radical is said to be the strongest oxidant known (Fridovich, 1975); and by this mechanism HP is believed to do the actual killing of the bacteria. The hydroxyl radical, being highly reactive, can attack membrane lipids, DNA, and other essential cell components. Transition metals are believed to catalyze the formation of the hydroxyl radical; Dittmer et al. (1930) found that a nontoxic quantity of iron, copper, chromium, cobalt, or manganese salts would increase the phenol coefficient of HP toward *Staphylococcus aureus* and *Escherichia coli* 100 times. Yoshpe-Purer and Eulan (1968) suggested that in the case of water free of metal ions the bacteria themselves provide the necessary metal ions. Colobert (1962) reported that in the absence of metal ions in the culture medium, or if these ions are chelated with ethylene diaminetetracetic acid, there is no bactericidal action on *Escherichia coli*. Gould and Hutchins (1962) suggested that the antimicrobial action of HP is due to its oxidation of sulfhydryl groups and double bonds in proteins, lipids, and surface membranes. The hydroxyl radical is also thought to account for most of the biologic damage done by ionizing radiation.

A question that might be asked is what protects the phagocytes against the hydrogen peroxide? An enzymatic glutathione (GSH) detoxification system has been proposed (Voetman et al., 1980).

$$H_2O_2 + GSH \xrightarrow{\text{glutathione peroxidase}} GSSH + 2H_2O$$

Although catalase produced by respiring cells may adequately protect the cell from damage by steady-state levels of metabolically produced HP, this defense is overwhelmed by concentrations (3% and greater) used for practical disinfection.

Antimicrobial Activity of Hydrogen Peroxide

HP is active against a wide range of organisms: bacteria, yeasts, fungi, viruses, and spores (Tables 9–1 through 9–3; Fig. 9–1). Anaerobes are even more sensitive, since they do not produce catalase to break down the peroxide. As seen in Table 9–4, 25 ppm or less will prevent growth of vegetative bacteria. As the 3% solution, HP is rapidly bactericidal (Table 9–3; Fig. 9–1). It is less rapid in its action against yeasts, some viruses, and especially bacterial spores (Tables 9–1 through 9–5). In general, HP has greater activity against gram-negative

than gram-positive bacteria. Although its activity is affected by changes in pH, with greater activity on the acid side (Tables 9–4 and 9–5), it is less affected than are many other disinfectants such as phenols and organic acids. Curran et al. (1940) found the greatest killing power against spores at pH 3 and the least at pH 9, when testing bacillus spores at pH 3, 6, and 9; however, the difference was only between 6, 7.5, and 8 hours with 1% peroxide at 50°C.

Destruction of spores is greatly increased both with rise in temperature and increase in concentration, making HP an effective sporicide under these conditions. In the 40 to 70°C range, the time for 1% peroxide to kill half the spores decreased from one-half to one-third for each 10°C temperature rise (Curran et al., 1940). Experiments by Leaper (1984a) (Table 9–2) showed that an increase in temperature from 20 to 45°C reduced the time to kill spores 10 to 20 times, and an increase in concentration from 17.7 to 35.4% caused a time reduction of 3 to 4 times. In practical sporicidal applications with HP, high concentrations combined with high temperatures are used together to produce sterile conditions. In aseptic packaging, 35% HP at up to 80°C for 3 to 9 seconds are employed.

Applications of Hydrogen Peroxide

When used as an antiseptic for open wounds HP serves not only to arrest microbial growth, but cleans the wound by oxidation of organic debris. The release of gaseous oxygen also helps in the mechanical removal of dirt. HP has been used in swimming pools in conjunction with other disinfectants such as Baquacil, a polymeric biguanidine, where it helps to prevent bacterial growth,

Table 9–1. *Antimicrobial Activity of Hydrogen Peroxide toward Bacteria, Yeasts, and Viruses*

Organism	Concentration (ppm)	Lethality (minutes)	Temperature (°C)	Reference
Bacteria				
Staphylococcus aureus	1000	60	—	Kunzmann, 1934
Staphylococcus aureus	25.8×10^4	0.2	24	Toledo et al., 1973
Escherichia coli	1000	60	—	Kunzmann, 1934
Escherichia coli	500	10–30	37	Nambudripad et al., 1949
Eberthella typhi	1000	60	—	Kunzmann, 1934
Aerobacter aerogenes	500	10–30	37	Nambudripad et al., 1949
Sarcina spp.	500	150	37	Nambudripad et al., 1949
Streptococcus lactis	500	150	37	Nambudripad et al., 1949
Streptococcus liquefaceus	500	240	37	Nambudripad et al., 1949
Micrococcus spp.	30	10	—	Wardle and Renninger, 1975
Staphylococcus epidermidis	30	10	—	Wardle and Renninger, 1975
Yeasts				
Torula spp.	500	180–210	37	Nambudripad and Iya, 1951
Oidium spp.	500	180–210	37	Nambudripad and Iya, 1951
Viruses				
Orthinosis virus	3.0×10^4	180	—	Nikolov and Papova, 1965
Rhinovirus types 1A, 1B, 7	0.75×10^4	50–60	37	Mentel and Schmidt, 1973
Rhinovirus types 1A, 1B, 7	1.5×10^4	18–20	37	Mentel and Schmidt, 1973
Rhinovirus types 1A, 1B, 7	3.0×10^4	6–8	37	Mentel and Schmidt, 1973
Poliovirus type 1	1.5×10^4	75	20	Kline and Hull, 1960
Poliovirus type 1	3.0×10^4	75	20	Kline and Hull, 1960

Table 9–2. *Sporicidal Activity of Hydrogen Peroxide toward Spore-forming Bacteria and Bacterial Spores*

Organism	Concentration (ppm)	Lethality (minutes)	Temperature (°C)	pH	Comment	Reference
Bacillus subtilis	500	420–1080	37	—	b.c.	Nambudripad et al., 1949
Bacillus cereus	500	420–1080	37	—	b.c.	Nambudripad et al., 1949
Bacillus megatherium	500	420–1080	37	—	b.c.	Nambudripad et al., 1949
Bacillus subtilis ATCC 15411*	3.0×10^4	1440	37	4.3	spores	Baldry, 1983
Bacillus subtilis SA 22	25.8×10^4	7.3	24	3.8	s.s.	Toledo et al., 1973
Bacillus coagulans	25.8×10^4	1.8	24	3.8	s.s.	Toledo et al., 1973
Bacillus stearothermophilus	25.8×10^4	1.5	24	3.8	s.s.	Toledo et al., 1973
Clostridium sporogenes	25.8×10^4	0.8	24	3.8	s.s.	Toledo et al., 1973
Bacillus subtilis var. *globigii*	25.8×10^4	2.0	24	3.8	s.s.	Toledo et al., 1973
Bacillus subtilis var. *globigii*	35×10^4	1.5	24	3.8	s.s.	Toledo et al., 1973
Bacillus subtilis var. *globigii*	41×10^4	0.75	24	3.8	s.s.	Toledo et al., 1973
Bacillus subtilis SA 22	17.7×10^4	9.4	20	—	s.s.	Leaper, 1984a
Bacillus subtilis SA 22	17.7×10^4	0.53	45	—	s.s.	Leaper, 1984a
Bacillus subtilis SA 22	29.5×10^4	3.6	20	—	s.s.	Leaper, 1984a
Bacillus subtilis SA 22	29.5×10^4	0.35	45	—	s.s.	Leaper, 1984a
Bacillus subtilis SA 22	35.4×10^4	2.3	20	—	s.s.	Leaper, 1984a
Bacillus subtilis SA 22	35.4×10^4	0.19	45	—	s.s.	Leaper, 1984a

b.c., bacterial cultures; s.s., spore suspension.
*Carrier test

Table 9–3. *Lens Disinfection—D Values with 3% H₂O₂ Solution*

	Minutes	
Microorganism	D Value*	Standard Error
Neisseria gonorrhoeae	†	—
Hemophilus influenzae	0.29	0.07
Pseudomonas aeruginosa	0.40	0.05
Bacillus subtilis	0.50	0.15
Escherichia coli	0.57	0.07
Proteus vulgaris	0.58	0.24
Bacillus cereus	1.04	0.12
Proteus mirabilis	1.12	0.33
Streptococcus pyogenes	1.50	0.25
Staphylococcus epidermidis	1.82	0.14
Staphylococcus aureus	2.35	0.18
Herpes simplex	2.42	0.71
Serratia marcescens	3.86	0.53
Candida albicans	3.99	0.54
Fusarium solani	4.92	0.54
Aspergillus niger	8.55	1.32
Candida parapsilosis	18.30	3.44

*Contamination level—700,000 organisms per lens, 7 ml of H₂O₂ solution.

†Too rapid to measure.

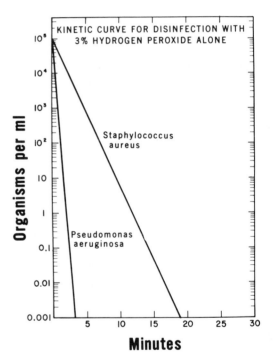

Fig. 9–1. Kinetic curves for disinfection with 3% hydrogen peroxide alone.

control algae, and keep the filters clean. It does this without producing harmful products, unpleasant odors, or irritation to the eyes. It is used in ultrasonic disinfectant cleaning baths for dental and medical instruments. HP is employed for odor control in sewage and sewage sludges (Sims, 1980). Another application is to treat landfill leachates. These nutrient-laden leachates support undesirable microbial growths in waters that receive these discharges (Mather, 1977; Holmes, 1980). Application of HP to these discharges into a stream re-

moved a slime mass for a distance of over 600 meters. In industrial effluent treatment its use is well documented (Sims, 1983). In the horticulture industry, capillary feed systems for nutrient supply to plants get plugged up because of algal growth. Mechanical cleaning is time-consuming and difficult, but HP as an oxidant serves to remove the debris and as a disinfectant to prevent further algal growth. At 700 ppm or less it is effective and not phytotoxic (Baldry and Fraser, 1988). For infor-

Table 9–4. *Effect of pH on the Bacteriostatic Activity of Hydrogen Peroxide (minimum inhibitory concentration in ppm)*

pH	Pseudomonas aeruginosa ATCC 15442	Klebsiella pneumoniae ATCC 4352	Streptococcus faecalis ATCC 10541	Staphylococcus aureus ATCC 6538
5.0	5	25	25	no growth
6.5	10	25	25	5
8.0	50	25	25	5

Baldry, M.C.G. 1983. The bactericidal, fungicidal, and sporacidal properties of hydrogen peroxide and peracetic acid. J. Appl. Bacteriol., *54*, 417–423.

mation on HP as a disinfectant for contact lenses see Turner (1983), and on its important application in aseptic packaging see Chapter 48 of this volume.

Synergistic Activity with Hydrogen Peroxide

HP shows synergism with both chemical and physical agents. Bayliss and Waites (1976) treated spores of *Clostridium bifermentans* with 100 μm copper sulfate and 0.28 M HP at 25°C. The copper alone permitted 95% colony formation; the peroxide alone 87%. When used together the colony formation was 0.028%, a 3000-fold reduction. Since HP is known to remove protein from spore coats, they tested it with dithiothreitol, which also possesses that property. Treatment with HP alone gave 93% colony formation, and with dithiothreitol alone 40%. Together they gave 0.082%, a 500-fold reduction. It was proposed that dithiothreitol removes the protein in the spore coat that protects the spore from HP, and that copper increases the rate of breakdown of HP and the rate of cleavage of peptide bonds by HP.

It has already been noted that heat sharply increases the activity of HP. One explanation is that HP makes spores more sensitive to heat, so heat may be the actual cause of death. HP also acts synergistically with ultraviolet radiation. Bayliss and Waites published a series of three papers on the subject (1979a, 1979b, 1982). They found that 0.3% HP plus ultraviolet radiation (UV) gave 2000 times greater increase of spore kill than radiation alone, and 4000 times greater than HP alone. Less than 1% HP in the presence of UV produced a synergistic

Table 9–5. *Effect of pH on the Sporicidal Activity of Hydrogen Peroxide and Peracetic Acid (time required in minutes to kill Bacillus subtilis ATCC 15441 spores)*

Peroxygen Compound	Concentration (ppm)	pH 5	pH 6.5	pH 8.0
Hydrogen peroxide	10,000	>360	>360	>360
	30,000	180	360	360
Peracetic acid	83	>360	>360	>360
	830	60	180	>360
	8300	<30	<30	<30

Baldry, M.C.G. 1983. The bactericidal, fungicidal, and sporicidal properties of hydrogen peroxide and peracetic acid. J. Appl. Bacteriol., *54*, 417–423.

kill, but the effect diminished as the concentration increased. The absorption of UV by HP was postulated as the cause for the loss of synergism. When high-intensity ultraviolet light (20 seconds) plus 2.5% HP was combined with heat up to 80°C for 60 seconds, a 5-$\log_{10}$ inactivation of *Bacillus subtilis* was obtained. The authors attribute the killing to the formation of hydroxyl radicals from HP within the spores, but explain that at higher concentrations the decrease in activity is due to reaction of breakdown products with HP molecules outside of the spore. The major drawback of UV with peroxide, as with UV alone, is that UV is not penetrating and is limited to surface action or to clear solutions that do not absorb UV.

The process for sterilization by a combination of UV and HP used sequentially was patented for the commercial sterilization of packaging before filling with ultrahigh-temperature processed foods (Peel and Waites, 1979). A later development by Waites et al. (1988) employed a synchronotron radiation source to produce a narrow band of radiation, showing the greatest kill of *B. subtilis* spores in the presence of HP with radiation close to 270 nm in wavelength. These results suggested that the action of the UV light is not directly on the spore DNA but is related to the free hydroxyl radicals produced from HP that are close to or within the spores.

Another physical agent that has shown synergism with hydrogen peroxide is ultrasonic energy. Ahmed and Russell (1975) conducted experiments using ultrasonic waves in conjunction with hydrogen peroxide and found that sonification of *Candida albicans* and *Bacillus cereus* spores with 6% HP was lethal in 10 minutes, whereas the agents separately did not kill the organisms in 30 minutes exposure at 35°C. Ultrasonic energy was thought to disperse and agitate the cell aggregates, increasing surface contact with the disinfectants, increasing the permeability of the cell membrane to the disinfectant, and accelerating the rate between the disinfectant and the cell components.

Vapor Phase Hydrogen Peroxide

Although HP has been used as a disinfectant for almost 150 years, vapor phase hydrogen peroxide (VPHP) is a development of just the last few years. It came about because of the pressure to find a cold gaseous sterilant that could be used in place of the toxic or carcinogenic gases, ethylene oxide and formaldehyde, presently used to decontaminate laboratory equipment and supplies that are not amenable to heat. Rickloff and Orelski (1989) reported on a use of VPHP that might offer a rapid turnaround time for sterilizing hard-surfaced dental instruments. In their experiment they vaporized a 30% HP solution into a flowing airstream at 35°C to achieve about 4 mg/L VPHP. They tested bacteria and fungi, finding that *Bacillus stearothermophilus* spores, which were the most resistant to VPHP, had an LD_{50} of 1 minute. Klapes (1990) noted the rapid inactivation of pathogenic bacteria, yeast, fungal spores, viruses, and bacterial spores with extremely low concentrations of VPHP. The D-values of *B. stearothermophilus*, *B. subtilis globigii*, and *Clostridium sporogenes* spores (dried onto stainless-steel coupons) were 0.3, 0.17, and 0.2 minutes, respectively. She noted that temperature appeared to have no significant impact on VPHP inactivation rates, except that higher temperatures permit higher concentrations of HP in the vapor phase. Further, the presence of organic soil (5% fetal calf serum) did not appear to adversely affect sterilization efficiency.

She observed that VPHP decontamination processes do not require a pressurized vessel and can be performed efficiently at temperatures as low as 4°C. HP vapor may be delivered via a carrier gas or by means of a vacuum. VPHP exhibits incompatibility with certain materials. However, residuals and corrosion are said to be minimal compared to chemical germicide wash or soak techniques. VPHP penetrates plastics such as polyethylene, polypropylene, PVC, and polypropylene/polyester composites. VPHP diffusion is a function of sample thickness and cycle time. Liquids and highly porous cellulose materials are said to be restricted from VPHP use. Although HP vapor is absorbed by the above plastics, its removal might be accelerated by vacuum and higher temperatures. The rapid spore inactivation rate suggests the possible use of VPHP as a high-level disinfectant and chemisterilant. Klapes foresees potential application of VPHP technology for health-care products, pharmaceuticals, foodstuffs, processing equipment, packaging materials, fermentors, dialyzers, and poultry hatcheries, as well as for the surface decontamination of centrifuges, incubators, lyophilizers, and similar items. In another paper (Klapes and Vesley, 1990), the experimental use of VPHP for surface decontamination and sterilization of an ultracentrifuge was presented. Spores were inactivated in 8 minutes at 4°C at the inner gap on the centrifuge and in 32 minutes at 27°C at the outer gap. It was proposed that the higher temperature and higher surface area exposed at the outer gap served to decompose the gas more rapidly, resulting in reduced sporicidal efficiency.

The use of VPHP for space decontamination of rooms and biologic safety cabinets was explored by Suen et al. (1990). In their experiments they used 30% HP solution in a prototye VPHP generator (American Sterilizer Co.) with air as the carrier gas, allowing the sterilization process to take place at or near atmospheric pressure. The VPHP concentration was determined by the temperature and humidity in the contained environment. The test site was a sealed room of 923 cubic feet. Coupons with *Bacillus stearothermophilus* spores were suspended in different parts of the room and in the VPHP return line. With an HP injection of 7.409 g per minute the spores on all the coupons in the room were killed in 37 minutes; in the return line, with an injection rate of 6.762 g per minute, the spores were killed in 45 minutes.

Another interesting development employing HP vapor (Jacobs and Lin, 1987) is described in an invention in which material to be sterilized is first treated with HP vapor and then with a low-temperature (below 100°C)

gaseous plasma. In the process, a solution of 3 to 20% HP is injected into an evacuated chamber to produce 0.05 to 10 mg/L of HP vapor, with a preferred concentration of 0.208. The material to be sterilized is held in the chamber from 5 to 30 minutes or longer, depending on the concentration of HP, to allow the HP vapor to penetrate the material. The object is then subjected to sufficient radio frequency (RF) energy at 2.49 MHz for 5 to 60 minutes to complete the sterilization. The RF energy dissociates the VPHP and other gases present into free radicals, ions, electrons, excited atoms, and excited molecules, which react with the microorganisms. In their trials, the inventors observed that O_2, H_2O, and glutaraldehyde in the chamber killed no more than a third of the test spores of *B. subtilis* var. *globigii*, whereas HP killed them all under the same conditions. In another test, plasma plus a water control killed no spores, nor did VPHP below 0.625 mg/L, but 0.416 mg/L HP plus plasma killed all the spores in the same period.

PERACETIC ACID

It would be desirable to have a chemical with the attributes of hydrogen peroxide—effective germicidal and sterilizing capabilities, no harmful decomposition products, and infinite water solubility—but with greater lipid solubility and freedom from deactivation by catalase and peroxidases. Such a compound exists. It is the peroxide of acetic acid, peroxyacetic acid, or peracetic acid (PAA). As an effective biocide with no toxic residuals, it has been the subject of considerable interest with recent reviews by Turner (1983), Schroeder (1984), Block (1986), and Baldry and Fraser (1988).

PAA is a more potent antimicrobial agent than HP (Eggensberger, 1979; Baldry, 1983), being rapidly active at low concentration against a wide spectrum of microorganisms. It is sporicidal even at very low temperatures and remains effective in the presence of organic matter. As a weak acid it is more active on the acid side but is germicidal with higher concentration in the alkaline range. Like HP it is useful both in solution and as a vapor. These properties make it a remarkably valuable compound. Sprossig (1975) stated that it has advantages for disinfection and sterilization not found in any other agent.

Surprising as it may seem, the excellent germicidal properties of PAA were reported in 1902 by Freer and Novy, who noted "the excellent disinfecting and cold sterilization actions of peracetic acid," but it was not until years later with the development of a commercial process for the production of 90% HP, necessary for PAA's manufacture, that it became generally available. Hutchings and Xezones in 1949 showed PAA to be the most active of 23 germicides tested against spores of *Bacillus thermoacidurans*. Greenspan and MacKellar in 1951 found it to be bactericidal at 0.001%, fungicidal at 0.003%, and sporicidal at 0.3%. It found early application as a disinfecting agent in gnotobiotics, the production of germ-free animals (see Chapter 40) at the Lobund Institute of the University of Notre Dame (Reyniers, 1946). Developments in Europe followed; back again in the United States, PAA is of special interest to the food processing industry, because its residuals are only acetic acid, oxygen, water, HP, and dilute sulfuric acid.

Antimicrobial Activity of Peracetic Acid

PAA will inhibit and kill gram-positive and gram-negative bacteria, fungi, and yeasts in 5 minutes or less, at less than 100 ppm (Tables 9–6 through 9–11). In the presence of organic matter, 200 to 500 ppm is required. For viruses (Tables 9–9, 9–12) dosage range is wide, with phages inactivated by 12 to 30 ppm in 5 minutes and enteric viruses requiring as much as 2000 ppm (0.2%) for 10 to 30 minutes. Poliovirus required 750 to 1500 ppm for 15 minutes for inactivation in demineralized water, but 1500 to 2250 ppm in the same time with yeast extract. Phage MS2 in demineralized water required 12 to 15 ppm for 5 minutes; in yeast extract, 75 to 94 ppm. With bacterial spores, 500 to 30,000 ppm (0.05 to 3%) inactivates spores in 15 minutes to 15 seconds at room temperature (Tables 9–13, 9–14). PAA remains effective at slightly increased concentrations in the presence of organic matter (Tables 9–13, 9–15, 9–16). This is one of the qualities of PAA, that it does function in the presence of organic matter. Another is that it can function at low temperatures (Tables 9–8, 9–14). Table 9–14 shows that at 30,000 ppm (3%) it is active at even −40°C, kills spores in 1 minute at 0°C, and in 0.5 minutes at 4°C. It is active as well at the high temperature of 85°C (Table 9–15).

PAA is affected by pH (Tables 9–5, 9–7 through 9–9), with greater activity at lower pH. With bacteria (Tables 9–7, 9–9), the difference is not great through pH 5 to 8, but the decrease in activity is demonstrated at pH 9. The same effect is noted with yeasts (Table 9–8) at 20°C but not at 4°C. With phage (Table 9–9) the pH effect of greater activity at low pH is evident. In the case of spores (Table 9–6), the pH effect is also demonstrated.

The germicidal activity of PAA is best appreciated when it is compared with other disinfectants (Tables 9–10, 9–11, 9–15 through 9–17). It is the most active in all these comparisons by different workers. Closest to it are chlorine and iodine, which also act as oxidizing agents.

The sporicidal effect of PAA in combination with al-

Table 9–6. *Antimicrobial Activity of Peracetic Acid toward Bacteria, Yeasts, and Fungi (pH = 7.0, Temperature = 20°C)*

Organisms	Concentration (ppm)	Lethality (minutes)	Comments	Reference
Bacteria				
Pseudomonas aeruginosa	50	—	Phosphate buffer	Greenspan and MacKellar, 1951
Pseudomonas aeruginosa	250	—	Nutrient broth	Greenspan and MacKellar, 1951
Escherichia coli	10	—	Phosphate buffer	Greenspan and MacKellar, 1951
Escherichia coli	200	—	Nutrient broth	Greenspan and MacKellar, 1951
Micrococcus pyogenes var. *aureus*	10	—	Phosphate buffer	Greenspan and MacKellar, 1951
Micrococcus pyogenes var. *auerus*	200	—	Nutrient broth	Greenspan and MacKellar, 1951
Escherichia coli	10–15	—		Baldry et al., in press
Streptococcus faecalis	75–100	—		Baldry et al., in press
Staphycoccus aureus ATCC 6538	90	5		Orth and Mrozek, 1989
Enterococcus faecium DSM 2918	90	5		Orth and Mrozek, 1989
Listeria monocytogenes	90	5		Orth and Mrozek, 1989
*Legionella pneumophila**	6	<5		Baldry and Fraser, 1988
Yeasts				
Saccharomyces cerevisiae NCYC 762†	83	<5		Baldry, 1983
Saccharomyces cerevisiae NCYC 1026†	42	<5		Baldry, 1983
Zygosaccharomyces baillii NCYC 580†	25	<5		Baldry, 1983
Fungi				
Aspergillus niger	50	—	Fungistatic, buffer	Greenspan and MacKellar, 1951
Aspergillus niger	500	—	Fungistatic, nutrient broth	Greenspan and MacKellar, 1951
Penicillium roquefortii	50	—	Fungistatic, buffer	Greenspan and MacKellar, 1951
Penicillium roquefortii	500	—	Fungistatic, nutrient broth	Greenspan and MacKellar, 1951

*pH = 5.0, Temp. = 25°C
†pH = 6.5, Temp. = 25°C

Table 9–7. *Effect of pH on Antibacterial Activity of Peracetic Acid*

pH	Pseudomonas aeruginosa ATCC 15442	Klebsiella pneumoniae ATCC 4352	Streptococcus faecalis ATCC 10541	Staphylococcus aureus ATCC 6538
Bacteriostatic (minimum inhibitory concentration in ppm)				
5.0	21	21	21	no growth
6.5	21	21	21	21
8.0	42	42	42	21
Bactericidal (lethality in less than 1 minute at concentration in ppm)				
5.0	42	42	42	42
6.5	42	42	42	84
8.0	42	42	84	84

Baldry, M.C.G. 1983. The bactericidal, fungicidal, and sporicidal properties of hydrogen peroxide and peracetic acid. J. Appl. Bacteriol., *54*, 417–423.

cohols has been studied. Werner and Wewalka (1973) observed the sporicidal effect of 0.05% PAA in 70% ethanol and of 0.025% PAA in 60% isopropanol, even in the presence of large amounts of garden soil. Using the resistant spores, *B. sublitis* SA22, Leaper (1984b) reported a synergistic effect of PAA with alcohols. With 0.08% PAA alone the D-value was 47.2 minutes, whereas with the combination of 0.08% PAA and 9.9% methanol, ethanol, or propanol-1, the D-values were 17.3, 4.7, and 1.6 minutes, respectively. Synergistic effects were observed with 0.04% and 0.08% PAA when up to 20% ethanol was used. Higher concentrations of ethanol or peracetic acid did not improve the sporicidal action. The simultaneous use of PAA and ethanol in aseptic packaging was suggested.

Table 9–8. *Effect of pH on the Cidal Activity of Peracetic Acid on Yeasts (ppm for complete kill in less than 5 minutes) at 25° and 4°C*

pH	Saccharomyces cerevisiae NCYC 762 25°C	Saccharomyces cerevisiae NCYC 762 4°C	Saccharomyces cerevisiae NCYC 1026 25°C	Saccharomyces cerevisiae NCYC 1026 4°C
5.0	83	830	42	415
6.5	83	415	42	415
8.0	415	830	83	415

Baldry, M.C.G. 1983. The bactericidal, fungicidal, and sporicidal properties of hydrogen peroxide and peracetic acid. J. Appl. Bacteriol., *54*, 417–423.

Table 9–9. *Effect of pH on Antimicrobial Activity of Peracetic Acid (minimum concentration to kill in ppm)*

Organism	pH 5	pH 7	pH 9
E. coli	20–25	10–15	100–150
Streptococcus faecalis	10–15	75–100	500–1000
Phage MS2	11–15	30–53	225–300
Phage φ_x 174	15–23	53–75	525–750

Baldry, M.G.C., French, M.S., and Slater, D. The activity of peracetic acid on sewage indicator bacteria and viruses. Water Sci. Tech.

Table 9–10. *Comparison of Peracetic Acid with Other Disinfectants Against Food-poisoning Bacteria: Effect of Temperature and Concentration in ppm to Obtain Lethality in 5 Minutes*

Organism	Peracetic acid	Active Chlorine	Benzalkonium Cl
20°C			
Listeria monocytogenes	45	100	200
Staphylococcus aureus ATCC 6538	90	860	500
Enterococcus faecium DSM 2918	45	300	250
5°C			
Listeria monocytogenes	90	860	500
Staphylococcus aureus ATCC 6538	90	1100	750
Enterococcus faecium DSM 2918	90	450	500

Orth, R., and Mrozeck, H. 1989. Is the control of Listeria, Campylobacter, and Yersinia a disinfection problem? Fleischwirtsch, *69*(10), 1575–1576.

Peracetic Acid Vapor

Compared to HP, peracetic acid vapor (PAAV) has some possible drawbacks. It is volatile (boiling point of 103°C, vapor pressure at 25°C 20 mm Hg); it has a sharp pungent odor; it has a flash point of 56°C, heated above which it is a possible fire and explosion hazard. It decomposes as the temperature is raised, and it is corrosive and toxic. Nevertheless its potent biocidal action captures our attention. Table 9–18 demonstrates the superiority of this vapor to other disinfectants in both speed of action and concentration required. Table 9–19 presents the data of Portner and Hoffman (1968), who found rapid reduction in number of spores in cold sterilization with PAAV. They found PAAV most effective at 80% relative humidity, lessening as the humidity was reduced, with very little activity at 20%. Spores on paper gave better results than spores on glass, apparently because of better penetration of the vapor into the paper. Doskocil and Fiser (1979) investigated PAAV for continual disinfection of air in rooms holding swine with

Table 9–11. *Bacteriostatic Activity of Disinfectants on* Streptococcus lactis *and* Streptococcus cremoris *in Cheese Vat (ppm for total inhibition of acid production)*

Disinfectant	ppm
Peracetic acid	5–35
Iodophor	75–200
Quaternary	>200
NaOCl	>400
Acid anionic	>600

Dunsmore, D.G., Makin, D., and Arkins, R. 1985. Effect of residues on five disinfectants in milk on acid production by strains of lactic starters used for cheddar cheesemaking and on organoleptic properties of the cheese. J. Dairy Res., *52*, 287–297.

Table 9–12. *Inactivation of Viruses by Peracetic Acid (temperature = 20°C)*

Organisms	Concentration (ppm)	Lethality (minutes)	Comments	Reference
Poliovirus 1	400	5	7.5 log$_{10}$ reduction	Kline and Hull, 1960
Cocksackievirus B-3	1280	5	5.5 log$_{10}$ reduction	Kline and Hull, 1960
Cocksackievirus B-5	325	30	7.25 log$_{10}$ reduction	Kline and Hull, 1960
Echovirus 10	1280	5	6.5 log$_{10}$ reduction	Kline and Hull, 1960
Adenovirus 3,4,7	1280	5	4, 1.5, 3.5 log$_{10}$ reductions	Kline and Hull, 1960
B virus	1280	5	7 log$_{10}$ reduction	Kline and Hull, 1960
Herpes simplex	1280	5	3 log$_{10}$ reduction	Kline and Hull, 1960
Enteric viruses	2000	10		Sprossig, 1975
Enteric viruses	2000	30		Harakeh, 1984
Human rotavirus	140	30		Harakeh, 1984
Simian rotavirus	20	30		Harakeh, 1984
Poliovirus 1	150–375,	60	DM	Baldry et al., in press
	> 750	30	DM	
	750–1500,	15	DM	
	1500–2250	10	DM	
Cocksackievirus	100–375	60	DM	Baldry et al., in press
	250–500	15	DM	Baldry et al., in press
Echovirus	100–375	60	DM	Baldry et al., in press
Phage MS2	12–15	5	DM	Baldry et al., in press
Phage φ$_x$ 174	25–30	5	DM	Baldry et al., in press
Poliovirus 1	375–750,	60	YE	Baldry et al., in press
	750–1500,	30	YE	Baldry et al., in press
	1500–2250,	15	YE	Baldry et al., in press
	> 2250	10	YE	Baldry et al., in press
Cocksackievirus	100–375	60	YE	Baldry et al., in press
	500–1000	15	YE	Baldry et al., in press
Echovirus	100–375	60	YE	Baldry et al., in press
Phage MS2	75–94	5	YE	Baldry et al., in press
Phage φ$_x$ 174	94–113	5	YE	Baldry et al., in press

DM, demineralized water; YE, yeast extract

Table 9–13. *Sporicidal Activity of Peracetic Acid Against Spore-forming Bacteria and Bacterial Spores*

Organisms	Concentration (ppm)	Lethality (minutes)	Temperature (°C)	Comments	Reference
Bacillus stearothermophilus	100	15	20	BC	Gershenfeld and Davis, 1952
Bacillus stearothermophilus	2000	1	20	BC	Gershenfeld and Davis, 1952
Bacillus stearothermophilus	500	15	20	SS	Gershenfeld and Davis, 1952
Bacillus stearothermophilus	3000	1	20	SS	Gershenfeld and Davis, 1952
Bacillus coagulans 43-P	100	15	20	BC	Gershenfeld and Davis, 1952
Bacillus coagulans 43-P	2000	1	20	BC	Gershenfeld and Davis, 1952
Bacillus coagulans 43-P	500	10	20	SS	Gershenfeld and Davis, 1952
Bacillus coagulans 43-P	2000	1	20	SS	Gershenfeld and Davis, 1952
Bacillus subtilis	3000	10	20	BC, buffer	Greenspan and MacKellar, 1951
Bacillus subtilis	5000	10	20	BC, nutrient broth	Greenspan and MacKellar, 1951
Bacillus subtilis var. niger ATCC 9372	10,000	0.25	20	SS	Han et al., 1980
Bacillus stearothermophilus oxoid code BR 23	10,000	0.25	20	SS	Han et al., 1980
*Bacillus subtilis** ATCC 15441	25,000	1440	37	Carrier test	Baldry, 1983

BC, bacterial culture; SS, spore suspension
*Same results at pH 4, 7, and 9

Table 9–14. *Sporicidal Activity of Peracetic Acid: Effect of Temperature and Concentration*

Temperature (°C)	Minutes for Lethality at Concentration in ppm				Organism	Reference
	5000	10,000	20,000	30,000		
37	10	10	<0.5	<0.5	*Bacillus anthracis*	Hussaini and Ruby, 1976
20	20	10	5	<0.5	*B. anthracis*	Hussaini and Ruby, 1976
4	>60	20	20	<0.5	*B. anthracis*	Hussaini and Ruby, 1976
0	—	—	—	1	*B. subtilis* var. *niger*	Jones et al., 1967
−30	—	—	—	6	*B. subtilis* var. *niger*	Jones et al., 1967
−40	—	—	—	600	*B. subtilis* var. *niger*	Jones et al., 1967

Table 9–15. *Sporicidal Activity of Disinfectants to* Bacillus thermoacidurans *at 85°C—Effect of Solids*

Disinfectant	(ppm for Kill with % Solids)	
	0	1
Peracetic acid	25	200
Chlorine-containing	50	400
Quaternaries	100	>400

Hutchings, I.J., and Xezones, H. 1949. Comparative evaluation of the bactericidal efficiency of peracetic acid, quaternaries and chlorine containing compounds. Proc. 49th Ann. Mfg. Soc. Am. Bacteriol. [Abstract], pp. 50–51.

atrophic rhinitis and obtained 91 to 94% kill of *Bordetella bronchiseptica* in 48 hours. Other workers showed that plastic tubing and medical instruments were sterilized in 2 hours at 22°C with PAAV.

Stability of Peracetic Acid

Peroxides in general are high-energy-state compounds, and as such can be considered thermodynamically unstable. PAA is considerably less stable than HP. 40% PAA loses 1 to 2% of its active ingredients per month, as compared with HP (30 to 90%), which loses less than 1% per year. The decomposition products of PAA are acetic acid, HP, oxygen, and water. Dilute PAA solutions are even more unstable: a 1% solution loses half its strength through hydrolysis in 6 days (Greenspan et al., 1955). PAA is produced by the reaction of acetic acid or acetic anhydride with HP in the presence of sulfuric acid, which acts as a catalyst, as shown:

$$CH_3C\!\!\underset{OH}{\overset{O}{\diagup}} + H_2O_2 \rightleftharpoons CH_3C\!\!\underset{OOH}{\overset{O}{\diagup}} + H_2O$$

Table 9–16. *Sporicidal Activity of Disinfectants to* Bacillus anthracis *Spores with 4% Horse-Serum at 20°C*

Disinfectant	ppm	Time (Hours)
Peracetic acid	2500	0.5
Glutaraldehyde	20,000	2
Formaldehyde	40,000	2

Lensing, H.H. and Oei, H.L. 1984. Study of the efficiency of disinfectants against anthrax spores. Tijdschr. Diergeneeskd, *109*, (13), 557–563.

To prevent the reverse reaction, the PAA solution is fortified with acetic acid and HP. In addition a stabilizer is employed. This may be a sequestering agent (sodium pyrophosphate) or a chelating agent (8-hydroxyquinoline) that removes trace metals, which accelerate the decomposition of peroxides. (For a good discussion of stabilizers for peroxides, see Schumb et al., 1955.) A patented process employing anionic surfactants with dilute PAA solutions shows not only greater stability but greater antimicrobial activity (Bowing et al., 1977). Greenspan et al. (1955) demonstrated that although a 1% PAA solution at pH 2.5 lost 13.4% PAA in 1 day, at pH 7.0 it lost 84% in 1 day. On the other hand a formulation of 1% PAA, 14.5% acetic acid, 5.0% HP, 78.5% water, and 1% sulfuric acid lost only 2.7% in 84 days. To maintain stability, solutions must be made up with especially pure chemicals and deionized water, and kept free of dust and other contaminants. Commercial preparations with excellent stability are offered as shown in Table 9–20.

For stability PAA should be stored at ordinary, preferably cool temperatures in original containers. It is unaffected by glass and most plastics. It may extract the plasticizer from some vinyl formulations used as gaskets and will attack natural and synthetic rubbers (Dychdala, 1988). Pure aluminum, stainless steel, and tin-plated iron are resistant to PAA but plain steel, galvanized iron, copper, brass, and bronze are susceptible to reaction and corrosion (Schroeder, 1984).

Mechanism of Action of Peracetic Acid

Little work has been done to probe the mechanism of action of PAA as an antimicrobial agent. One can only speculate that it functions much as other peroxides and oxidizing agents. It is likely that sensitive sulfhydryl and sulfur bonds in proteins, enzymes, and other metabolites are oxidized and that double bonds are reacted. It is suggested that PAA disrupts the chemiosmotic function of the lipoprotein cytoplasmic membrane and transport through dislocation or rupture of cell walls (Baldry and Fraser, 1988). Its action as a protein denaturant may help to explain its action as a sporicide and ovicide.

Applications of Peracetic Acid

The powerful antimicrobial action of PAA at low temperatures along with the absence of toxic residuals has led to a wide range of applications. It has been accepted worldwide in the food processing and beverage industries, which include meat and poultry processing plants,

Table 9–17. *Bactericidal Activity of Disinfectants Against Test Bacteria in 10 Minutes by the Use Dilution Method—Based on 100% Active Ingredient*

Disinfectant	Composition	Bactericidal Concentration (ppm) against			
		S. aureus	E. coli	P. vulgaris	P. aeruginosa
Persteril	40% peracetic acid	1,000	500	500	1,000
Chloramin	25% available chlorine	2,500	2,500	2,500	2,500
Wescodyne	1.6% available iodine	1,600	1,600	1,600	1,600
Jodoseptan	1.9% available iodine	1,520	950	1,520	1,900
Laurosept	25% laurylpyridinium bromide	2,500	2,500	2,500	25,000
Sterinol	10% dimethyl-lauryl-benzyl ammonium bromide	8,000	10,000	10,000	>10,000
Phenol	phenol	20,000	15,000	15,000	15,000
Lysol	50% cresol	40,000	40,000	40,000	40,000
Septyl	7.5% o-phenylphenol + 3.2% p-tert. amyl phenol	2,139	2,139	2,139	10,965
Formalin	37% formaldehyde	52,000	30,000	30,000	30,000
Alhydex	2% glutaraldehyde	6,000	5,000	5,000	5,000

Krzywicka, H., Jaszczuk, E., and Janowska, J. 1975. The range of antibacterial activity and the use concentrations of disinfectants. In *Resistance of Microorganisms to Disinfectants: Second International Symposium, Poznan.* Edited by W.B. Kedzia. Warsaw, Polish Academy of Sciences, pp. 89–91.

canneries, dairies, breweries, wineries, and soft drink plants (Dychdala, 1988), where it is said to be ideal for clean-in-place (CIP) systems. It is used as terminal disinfectant or sterilant for stainless steel and glass tanks, piping, tank trucks, and railroad tankers (Interox Chemicals Ltd., undated). Its non-rinse feature, where its breakdown products in high dilution are not objectionable from the taste, odor, or toxicity standpoints, saves time and money. Schroder (1984) presented data on the breakdown time in water, beer, lemonade, and milk. Teuber (1978, 1979) studied the virucidal effectiveness on bacteriophages that are specific for *Streptococcus lactis* and *Streptococcus cremoris* and the sporicidal effectiveness against *Clostridium tyrobutyricum*. Binder and Foissy (1979) examined the fungicidal effect of the disinfectant containing peracetic acid with regard to its use as a room disinfectant in dairies. Jager and Puesopoek (1980) investigated PAA for the beverage industry and reported that all bacteria, yeasts, and fungi tested with 2500 ppm (0.25%) PAA were inactivated in 30 minutes, and with 5000 ppm in 15 minutes. A preparation of PAA (P-3-oxonia active) was approved by the FDA in 1986, giving clearance for its ingredients as indirect food additives in sanitizing solutions. Subsequently, EPA registration was issued and USDA authorization granted (Dychdala, 1988). In the food industry, plastic food con-

Table 9–18. *Resistance of Spores to Chemicals*

Chemical	Organism	Kill	Time (h)	Concentration (% w/v)	Temperature (°C)	Reference
Peracetic acid vapour	B. subtilis var. niger	10^5	0.02	0.0001	25	Portner and Hoffman (1968)
HCl vapour	B. subtilis	10^3	0.08	31*	20	Tuynenberg Muys et al. (1978)
Ethylene oxide	B. subtilis	10^2	0.7	0.07	40	Marletta and Stumbo (1970)
Hydrogen peroxide	B. subtilis var. globigii	10^3	0.17	25.8	24	Toledo et al. (1973)
Hypochlorous acid	B. subtilis	10^3	2.0	0.01†	10	Dye and Mead (1972)
Glutaraldehyde	B. pumilis	10^3	0.5	2.0	37	Thomas and Russell (1974)
Formaldehyde	B. subtilis var. niger	10^3	1.5	1.0	40	Trujillo and David (1972)
Propylene oxide	B. subtilis var. niger	10^3	17.0	0.1	37	Bruch and Koesterer (1961)
Sodium hydroxide	B. subtilis	10^3	24.5	5.0	40	Whitehouse and Clegg (1963)
Iodine (as an iodophor)	B. subtilis	10^2	>4.0	0.08	21	Cousins and Allan (1967)

*0.25 ml in a 300 ml bottle.
†Free chlorine.

Waites, W.M. 1982. Resistance of bacterial spores. In *Principles and Practice of Disinfection, Preservation, and Sterilization.* Edited by A.D. Russell and G.A.J. Ayliffe. Oxford, Blackwell Scientific Publications, p. 221.

Table 9–19. *The Effect of Peracetic Acid Vapor on* Bacillus subtilis *var.* niger *Spores at 80% Relative Humidity and 25°C; Spores on Paper and Glass; 1 mg/L Peracetic Acid*

Exposure (Minutes)	Paper		Glass	
	Active spores	Sterile samples	Active spores	Sterile samples
0	816,000	—	813,000	—
1.25	676	0	5	7
2.5	1	5	2	7
5	< 1	12	< 1	13
10	< 1	14	< 1	13
20	0	16	< 1	10

Portner, D.M., and Hoffman, R.K. 1968. Sporicidal effect of peracetic acid vapor. Appl. Microbiol., *16*, 1782.

tainers were treated with a solution containing 0.1% PAA and 20% HP. They were sprayed on a conveyor belt using hot air to activate the solution and dry it off. Polyethylene strips with *Bacillus subtilis* spores were killed after treatment for 12 seconds at 65°C (Dallyn, 1980).

The properties of PAA have also been recognized by the medical community. The Centers for Disease Control of the United States have listed it as a chemical sterilant and high-level disinfectant (see Table 35–3). Application in the production of germ-free animals, where sterility is paramount, came very early (Greenspan et al., 1955). Wewalka and Werner (1973) found that 0.2% PAA killed *Mycobacterium tuberculosis* for the disinfection of respirators. Rubber tubes impregnated with *Staphylococcus aureus, Escherichia coli, Pseudomonas aeruginosa,* and *Proteus mirabilis* were disinfected with 0.5 or 1.0% PAA in 10 or 15 minutes, respectively. They recommended 0.5% PAA for 30 minutes for the disinfection of respirators, and stated that the large antimicrobial spectrum, short exposure time, and nontoxic decomposition products make peracetic acid a suitable disinfectant for medical machines. An automated machine to chemically sterilize medical, surgical, and dental instruments was developed using buffered PAA as the liquid sterilant (Steris System, 1988). It circulates the solution of PAA in a water bath at 50°C with an exposure time of 12 minutes. The tests reported showed spores of *Bacillus subtilis* and *Clostridium sporogenes* were all killed on 900 carriers in the AOAC carrier type test, and Steris System was granted FDA clearance to market the product. An interesting and novel application was described by Wutzler et al. (1975). They recommended 0.05 to

0.1% PAA to be used to sterilize serum and yeast-extract additions to mycoplasma-culture media, having found it to be as good as filtered components but less time- and equipment-intensive. Merka and Koubalik (1976) reported that a 5-minute immersion of rubber, steel, and plastic objects in 0.5% PAA provided sterilization, whereas 2% glutaraldehyde required 30 minutes immersion. Vashkov and co-workers (1974) found that 1% PAA took 20 to 45 minutes to sterilize medical instruments made of polymers and rubber, whereas 1% iodonate, 2% glutaraldehyde, or 6% hydrogen peroxide required more time.

In the preparation of pharmaceuticals, PAA permits the cold sterilization of emulsions, hydrogels, ointments, and powders. An oil-in-water emulsion contaminated with *Aspergillus* was sterilized in 10 minutes with 0.1% peracetic acid (Kuehn, 1978). Skin preparations containing zinc oxide and talc were preserved with 0.05 to 0.2%, yielding the same microbiocidal purity as hot-air–sterilized products (Kryzwicka et al., 1975). Zinc oxide lotions with 0.05 to 0.1% peracetic acid were tested on 26 patients for 1 year and did not cause skin irritation.

In industrial application, von Ballmoos and Soldavini (1959) reported on long-term experience with PAA in the disinfection of ion exchangers. They recommended the use of a 0.2% PAA solution for 1 hour to achieve complete disinfection. They found that the capacity of the respective cation and anion exchangers was not changed under the conditions used (0.2 to 1% PAA).

Microorganisms are now recognized as causing many problems in industrial water systems. These include microbially induced corrosion (see Chapter 53), plugging and fouling of heat exchangers, sprinklers, and cooling towers, and disease caused by the *Legionella* bacteria.

Table 9–20. *Commercial Peracetic Acid Equilibrium Solution—Approximate Chemical Composition (% by Weight)*

Ingredient	FMC Corporation Philadelphia, PA 35% Peracetic Acid	FMC Corporation Philadelphia, PA 15% Peracetic Acid	Interox Chemicals England Proxitane 1507	Economics Lab. St. Paul, MN P3 Oxonia Active	Diversey Wyandotte Ontario S.T. 201 H
Peracetic acid	35.5	15.0	15	5	14
H_2O_2	6.8	23.0	14	25	22
Acetic acid	39.3	16.0	28	6	28
H_2O	17.4	45.0	42	63	35
H_2SO_4	1.0	1.0	—	—	—
Stabilizer	0.05	0.05	< 1.0	1.0	1.0

Baldry and Fraser (1988) reported on site trials for Legionella with 10 mg/L PAA on five cooling towers. In all cases the organism was eradicated in 20 minutes. Algae was controlled with 20 mg/L PAA twice a year, but a slug dose of 30 mg/L with 10 mg/L thereafter was better when there was heavy algae accumulation.

The effectiveness of PAA against bacteria and viruses led Baldry and French (1989) to investigate the use of PAA as a disinfectant for sewage and sewage effluents in laboratory and field trials. They found PAA to be an effective disinfectant for secondary effluent and stated that the ease of implementing PAA treatment without expensive equipment, the broad-spectrum activity even in the presence of organic matter, and the lack of environmentally undesirable byproducts make PAA appear favorable for sewage treatment processes. Baldry and Fraser (1988) reported on experiments with the disinfection of sewage sludge. They noted that 35 million wet tons of sewage sludge are distributed on grazing land each year in the United Kingdom. The sludge serves as a fertilizer but carries pathogens including Salmonella bacteria and ova of the beef tapeworm *(Taenia saginata)*. Disinfection of the sludge can eliminate it as a vehicle of transmission of infection to farm animals and also reduce the no-grazing interval of the land to which the sludge has been applied. Levels of 300 to 500 mg/L PAA reduced *Salmonella* levels below the limits of enumeration in all treated sludges, and even at 150 mg/L, the level has been reduced so that the sludge was considered safe for distribution to pasture land.

PAA functions against the cestode (tapeworm) oncospheres in sewage sludges producing lack of motion, dark coloration, granulation, and ovoid shrunken appearance (Fraser, 1986). In a digested sludge, 250 mg killed 99% of the embryos.

OTHER PEROXYGEN COMPOUNDS

In addition to PAA, other organic peroxy acids have been examined. Performic and perpropionic acids are similar in antibacterial activity to PAA, but performic is volatile and unstable, and perpropionic is more costly (Greenspan, 1946). Baldry and Fraser (1988) report that peroxyheptanoic and peroxynonanoic acids have higher activity on a molar basis than PAA. The perlauric acid has limited aqueous solubility but an antimicrobial spectrum somewhat like the quaternaries because of the long hydrocarbon chain. Monoperglutaric and diperglutaric acids and succinylperoxide are active, the latter having been marketed for disinfecting medical instruments. Derivatives of perbenzoic acid have been claimed in patents for sporicidal action. The magnesium salt of peroxyphthalate is a commercial product. It is a water-soluble solid effective against bacteria, yeasts, and spores (Baldry, 1984). Its activity is increased in acid solution, and with alcohol and with heat. It has been formulated as a sanitizer for bathrooms, kitchens, and diapers. As a powder with anionics it can be used for walls and floors in hospitals and is said to control hepatitis B and AIDS

viruses. Eggensberger (1979) describes peracid powder disinfectants made in situ by adding water to mixtures of organic acid reservoirs (anhydrides, amides, and esters) to HP reservoirs such as sodium peroxide. Products based on this procedure are on the market in Germany for treating dentures and general hospital disinfection. Benzoyl peroxide is in general use in skin formulations for treating acne, and t-butyl hydroperoxide with phenols has been suggested for preventing microbial attack on engine fuels, cutting oils, and timber.

Inorganic peroxides have also been used to combat microbes. Perborates have been used in toothpastes and powders. Permanganate is antibacterial, antifungal, and antiviral; it was used as an antiseptic but its intense purple color is a disadvantage. It is said to be superior to copper sulfate as an algicide; 0.01% $KMnO_4$ kills algae in 4 to 6 hours in cooling towers (Fitzgerald, 1964, 1965). Calcium peroxide is reported to protect seed from microbial inhibition during sprouting. The alkali metal perdisulphates are strong oxidants but demonstrate little antimicrobial activity. However, monoperoxyysulfuric acid made from sulfuric acid and HP and partially neutralized with potassium hydroxide gives Caro's acid triple salt, which is used as a bleaching agent in toilet bowl and denture cleaners and as a swimming pool disinfectant. When investigated (Baldry, 1985), it showed activity against bacteria and viruses but none toward yeasts and fungi. However, with isopropanol it is synergistic and active toward yeast. With chloride or bromide it generates the hypohalite useful for slime control, pool disinfection, and sanitation of baby diapers (Gaya, 1979).

TOXICITY AND HAZARDS OF PEROXYGEN COMPOUNDS

Hydrogen peroxide is a clear, colorless liquid with a characteristic slightly acidic odor. It has low toxicity and is not a systemic poison because it is decomposed in the bowel before absorption (Gleason et al., 1969). Concentrated solutions are irritating to the skin, mucous membranes, and particularly to the eyes. The vapors can cause inflammation of the respiratory tract. It is not a carcinogen or a mutagen. Rubber gloves, safety goggles, and protective clothing should be worn when handling concentrated HP, PAA, or any liquid peroxygen compound or solution. They should be washed off immediately with large quantities of water if splashed on the skin or in the eyes. If swallowed, give milk or lukewarm water and call a physician (FMC Corp., undated).

PAA is a clear, colorless solution with a pungent odor, containing 40% or less of peracetic acid. The 40% solution has an LD_{50} to rats of 1540 mg per kilogram (National Institute of Safety and Health, 1974). Busch and Werner (1974) give LD_{50} values for rats of 315 for PAA and 263 for Wolfasteril, a preparation containing 36 to 40% PAA. For a 4% formulation (P-3 oxonia active) a value of 3.4 g per kilogram is given, which compares favorably to other common sanitizers (Dychdala, 1988). The subchronic oral feeding studies with this formulation showed no change in growth of the animals in 8 weeks. The acute inhalation toxicity, LC 50, was 13,439 mg per cubic meter. For the 35% PAA solution the vapor is lachrymatory and inhalation results in a stinging sensation in the nasal passages. Busch and Werner (1974) tested PAA on skin and stated that 0.4 to 0.8% PAA can be used directly as a body disinfectant for swine. According to the work of Bock et al. (1975) PAA is a potent tumor promoter and a weak carcinogen. At 3% and 1% PAA was a tumor promoter, but not at 0.3%. With 2% PAA in water, 10% of the animals developed skin tumors in 6 months; none did in the following 6 months. No tumors were produced by 1% PAA in acetone. PAA was considered a weak complete carcinogen, but decomposed PAA was inactive as a tumor promoter. HP, 3% in water, and 5% urea peroxide were not tumor producers and did not cause skin cancers. Perbenzoic acid, 0.1%, and 1% m-chloroperbenzoic acid in acetone promoted tumors and produced cancers.

Employing the Ames test, Yamaguichi and Yamashita (1980) studied the mutagenicity of peroxygen compounds. They found that HP and PAA were not mutagenic, and neither was m-chloroperbenzoic acid, which was found to be tumorogenic and carcinogenic by Bock et al. (1975). The only peroxygen compounds mutagenic by the tests of Yamaguichi and Yamashita were t-butylhydroperoxide and cumene hydroperoxide.

By their chemical nature the peroxygen compounds are powerful oxidizers. They appear to present no danger from toxicity or other hazards when diluted in water to their effective concentration as disinfectants and sterilants. However, in concentrated solution they must be treated with caution, as is the case with any strong oxidant. They should be stored in a cool place, not over 30°C, in the original containers provided, with vents and flame resisters. Spills or leaks should be covered with weak reducing agents such as sodium thiosulfate. Organic materials and heavy metals ions of copper, iron, and manganese should be avoided, because they can cause decomposition so rapid as to cause ignition and produce fires.

REFERENCES

Ahmed, F.I.K. and Russell, C. 1975. Synergism between ultrasonic waves and hydrogen peroxide in the killing of microorganisms. J. Appl. Bacteriol., 39, 31–40.

Baldry, M.G.C. 1984. The antimicrobial properties of magnesium monoperoxyphthalate hexahydrate. J. Appl. Bacteriol., 57, 499–503.

Baldry, M.G.C. 1983. The bactericidal, fungicidal, and sporicidal properties of hydrogen peroxide and peracetic acid. J. Appl. Bacteriol., 54, 417–423.

Baldry, M.G.C., and Fraser, J.A.L. 1988. Disinfection with peroxygens. In *Industrial Biocides*. Edited by K.R. Payne. New York, John Wiley & Sons, pp. 91–116.

Baldry, M.G.C., and French, M.S. 1989. Activity of peracetic acid against sewage indicator organisms. Wat. Sci. Tech., 21, Brighton, 1747–1749.

Baldry, M.G.C., French, M.S., and Slater, D. (In Press). The activity of peracetic acid on sewage indicator bacteria and viruses. Water Sci. Tech.

Bayliss, C.E., and Waites, W.M. 1982. Effect of simultaneous high intensity ultraviolet irradiation and hydrogen peroxide on bacterial spores. J. Food Technol., 17, 467–470.

Bayliss, C.E., and Waites, W.M. 1979a. The combined effect of hydrogen peroxide and ultraviolet irradiation on bacterial spores. J. Appl. Bacteriol., 47, 1658.

Bayliss, C.E., and Waites, W.M. 1979b. The synergistic killing of spores of *Bacillus subtilis* by hydrogen peroxide and ultra-violet light irradiation. FEMS Microbiol. Lett., 5; 331.

Bayliss, C.E., and Waites, W.M. 1976. The effect of hydrogen peroxide on spores of *Clostridium bifermentans*. J. Gen. Microbiol., 96, 401–407.

Binder, W., and Foissy, H. 1979. Test information on the fungicidal activity of "P3 oxonia aktiv." Institut fur Michwirtschaft und Mikrobiologie, Univers. fur Bodenkultur, Wien, 26, 2.

Block, S.S. 1986. Disinfection, where are we headed. A discussion of hydrogen peroxide and peracetic acid. Proc. 3rd Conf. Prog. Chem. Disinfection, Binghamton, NY, pp. 1–28.

Bock, F.G., Meyers, H.K., and Fox, H.W. 1975. Carcinogenic activity of peroxy compounds. J. Natl. Cancer Inst., 55, 1359–1361.

Bowing, W.G., et al. 1977. Stable peroxy-containing microbiocides. U.S. Patent 4,051,058.

Bruch, C.W. and Koesterer, M.G. 1961. The microbicidal activity of gaseous propylene oxide and its application to powdered or flaked foods. Journal of Food Science, 26, 428–435.

Busch, A., and Werner, F. 1974. Animal tolerance to peracetic acid. 1. Experimental results following the application of peracetic acid solutions on the skin of pigs. Monatsh. Veterinaermed., 29, (13), 494–498.

Colobert, L. 1962. Mechanism of bactericidal activity of hydrogen peroxide and ascorbic acid on Escherichia coli. Rev. Corps. Sante Armees Suppl., 3, 495–500.

Cousins, C.M. and Allan, C.D. 1967. Sporicidal properties of some halogens. Journal of Applied Bacteriology, 30, 168–174.

Curran, H.R., Evans, F.R., and Leviton, A. 1940. The sporicidal action of hydrogen peroxide and the use of crystalline catalase to dissipate residual peroxide. J. Bacteriol., 40, 423–434.

Dallyn, H. 1980. Sterilization of articles. British Patent No. GB-1570492.

Dittmer, H.R., Baldwin, I.L., and Miller, S.P. 1930. The influence of certain inorganic salts on the germicidal activity of hydrogen peroxide. J. Bacteriol., 17, 203.

Doskocil, O., and Fiser, A. 1979. Devitalization of *Bordetella bronchiseptica* in vitro with Persteril and triethylene glycol vapors. Vet. Med. (Prague), 24, 343–350.

Dunsmore, D.G., Makin, D., and Arkins, R. 1985. Effect of residues on five disinfectants in milk on acid production by strains of lactic starters used for cheddar cheesemaking and on organoleptic properties of the cheese. J. Dairy Res., 52, 287–297.

Dychdala, G.R. 1988. New hydrogen peroxide-peroxyacetic acid disinfectant. Proc. 4th Conf. Prog. Chem. Disinfection, Binghamton, NY, pp. 315–342.

Dye, M. and Mead, G.C. 1972. The effect of chlorine on the viability of clostridial spores. Journal of Food Technology, 7, 173–181.

Eggensberger, H. 1979. Disinfectants based on peracid splitting compounds. Zentralbl. Bakteriol. Mikrobiol. Hyg. [B], 168, 517–524.

Fitzgerald, G.P. 1965. Evaluation of potassium permanganate as an algicide in water cooling towers. Ind. Eng. Chem. Prod. Res. Dev., 3, 82–85.

Fitzgerald, G.P. 1964. Laboratory evaluation of potassium permanganate as an algicide in water reservoirs. S.W. Waterworks J., 45, 16–17.

FMC Corp. Technical Bulletin 4. Peracetic Acid, 35%. FMC Corp. Industrial Chemicals Group, 2000 Market St., Philadelphia.

Fraser, J.A.L. 1987. Novel applications of peracetic acid in industrial disinfection. Specialty Chemicals, 7, (3), 178, 180, 182, 184, 186.

Freer, P.C., and Novy, F.G. 1902. On the formation, decomposition and germicidal action of benzoylacetyl and diacetyl peroxides. Am. Chem. J., 27, 161–193.

Fridovich, I. 1978. The biology of oxygen radicals. Science, 201, 875–879.

Fridovich, I. 1975. Oxygen: Boon and bane. Am. Sci., 63, 54–60.

Gaya, H., Thirlwall, J., Shaw, E.J., and Hassam, Z. 1979. Evaluation of products for treating babies' napkins. J. Hyg., 82, 463–471.

Gershenfeld, L., and Davis, D.E. 1952. The effect of peracetic acid on some thermoaciduric bacteria. Amer. J. Pharm., 124, 337–341.

Gleason, M.N., Gosselin, R.E., Hodge, H.C., and Smith, R.P. 1969. *Clinical Toxicology of Commercial Products*. 3rd Ed. Baltimore, Williams & Wilkins.

Greenspan, F.P., Johnsen, M.A., and Trexler, P.C. 1955. Peracetic acid aerosols. Proc. 42nd Ann. Mtg. Chem. Special Mfctrs. Assoc., pp. 59–64.

Greenspan, F.P., and MacKellar, D.G. 1951. The application of peracetic acid germicidal washes to mold control of tomatoes. Food Technol., 5, 95–97.

Haber, F., and Weiss, J. 1934. The catalytic decomposition of hydrogen peroxide by iron salts. Proc. R. Soc. Lond. [A], 147, 332–351.

Han, B., Schornick, G., and Loncin, M. 1980. Destruction of bacterial spores on solid surfaces. J. Food Process Preserv., 4, (1–2), 95–110.

Harakeh, M.S. 1984. Inactivation of enteroviruses, rotaviruses, and bacteriophages by peracetic acid in a municipal sewage effluent. FEMS Microbiol. Lets., 23, 27–30.

Heinemann, P.G. 1913. The germicidal efficiency of commercial preparations of hydrogen peroxide. JAMA, 60, 1603–1606.

Holmes, R. 1980. The water balance method of estimating leachate production from landfill sites. Solid Wastes, 70, (1), 20–33.

Hussaini, S.N., and Ruby, K.R. 1976. Sporicidal activity of peracetic acid against *B. anthracis* spores. Vet. Rec. *98*, 257–259.

Hutchings, I.J., and Xezones, H. 1949. Comparative evaluation of the bactericidal efficiency of peracetic acid, quaternaries and chlorine containing compounds. Proc. 49th Ann. Mtg. Soc. Am. Bacteriol. [Abstract], 50–51.

Interox Chemicals Ltd. Oxymaster Peacetic Acid 12%. Marketing Dept. Warrington, Cheshire, England.

Jacobs, P.T., and Lin, S.M. 1987. Hydrogen peroxide plasma sterilization system. U.S. Patent 4,643,876.

Jaeger, P., and Puespoek, J. 1980. Peracetic acid as a disinfectant in breweries and soft drink factories. Mitt. Versuch. Gaerung. Wien, *34*, 32–36.

Jones, L.A., Hoffman, R.K., and Phillips, C.R. 1967. Sporicidal activity of peracetic acid and beta propiolactone at subzero temperatures. Appl. Microbiol., *15*, 357–362.

Klapes, N.A. 1990. New applications of chemical germicides: hydrogen peroxide. Am. Soc. Microbiol. Int. Symp. Chem. Germicides, Atlanta. Abstract *20*, pp. 14–15.

Klapes, N.A., and Vesley, D. 1990. Vapor-phase hydrogen peroxide as a surface decontaminant and sterilant. Appl. Env. Microbiol., *56*, (2), 503–506.

Klebanoff, S. 1968. Myeloperoxidase-halide-hydrogen peroxide antibacterial system. J. Bacteriol., *95*, 2131.

Kline, L.B., and Hull, R.N. 1960. The virucidal properties of peracetic acid. Am. J. Clin. Pathol., *33*, (1), 30–33.

Kryzywicka, H., Jaszczuk, E., and Janowska, J. 1975. The range of antibacterial activity and the use concentrations of disinfectants. In *Resistance of Microorganisms to Disinfectants: Second International Symposium, Poznan*. Edited by W.B. Kedzia. Warsaw, Polish Academy of Sciences, pp. 89–91.

Kuehn, H. 1978. Experiments with the antimicrobic treatment of dermatological preparations by peracetic acid. Parts 1, 2. Pharmazie, *33*, 292–293.

Kunzmann, T. 1934. Investigations on the disinfecting action of hydrogen peroxides. Fortschr. Med., *52*, 357.

Leaper, S. 1984a. Comparison of the resistance to hydrogen peroxide of wet and dry spores of *Bacillus subtilis* SA22. J. Food Technol., *19*, 695.

Leaper, S. 1984b. Synergistic killing of spores of *Bacillus subtilis* by peracetic acid and alcohol. J. Food Technol., *19*, 355.

Lensing, H.H., and Oei, H.L. 1984. Study of the efficiency of disinfectants against anthrax spores. Tijdschr Diergeneeskd, *109*, (13), 557–563.

Marletta, J. and Stumbo, C.R. 1970. Some effects of ethylene oxide on *Bacillus subtilis*. Journal of Food Science, 35, 627–631.

Mather, J.D. 1977. Attenuation and control of landfill leachates. Solid Wastes, 67, 362–378.

Mentel, R., and Schmidt, J. 1973. Investigations on rhinovirus inactivation by hydrogen peroxide. Acta Virol., *17*, 351–354.

Naguib, K., and Hussein, L. 1972. The effect of hydrogen peroxide on the bacteriological quality and nutritive value of milk. Milchwessenschaft, *27*, 758–762.

Nambudripad, V.K.N., and Iya, K.K. 1951. Bactericidal efficiency of hydrogen peroxide. 2. Influence of different concentrations of peroxide on the rate and extent of destruction of additional bacteria of dairy importance. Indian J. Dairy Sci., *4*, 38–44.

Nambudripad, V.K.N., Laxminarayana, I.I., and Lya, K.K. 1949. Bactericidal efficiency of hydrogen peroxide. 1. Influence of different concentrations on the rate and extent of destruction of bacteria of dairy importance. Indian J. Dairy Sci., *4*, 38–44.

Nikolov, Z.V., and Popova, O.M. 1965. Action of chemical disinfectants on the orthinosis virus. Kongr. Bulg. Mikrobiol. Inst., Sofia, 757–761. Published 1967.

National Institute of Safety and Health. 1974. Toxic Substances List. Rockville, MD.

Orth, R., and Mrozek, H. 1989. Is the control of Listeria, Compylobacter, and Yersinia a disinfection problem? Fleischwirtsch, *69*, (10), 1575–1576.

Peel, J.L., and Waites, W.M. 1979. Improvement in methods of sterilisation. U.K. Patent Applic. 791091.

Portner, D.M., and Hoffman, R.K. 1968. Sporicidal effect of peracetic acid vapor. Appl. Microbiol., *16*, 1782.

Reyniers, J.A. 1946. Germ-free life applied to nutrition studies. Lobund Report No. 1, (1), 87–120, Univ. Notre Dame Press.

Richardson, B.W. 1891. On peroxide of hydrogen, or ozone water, as a remedy. Lancet, *1*, 707, 760.

Rickloff, J., and Orelski, P. 1989. Resistance of various microorganisms to vapor phase hydrogen peroxide in a prototype dental handpiece/general instru-

ment sterilizer. 89th Ann. Mtg. Am. Soc. Microbiol., New Orleans, Abstract Q-59.

Schroder, W. 1984. Peracetic acid. Disinfectant for the food industry. Brauwelt Internat., Jan., pp. 115–120.

Schumb, W.C., Satterfield, C.N., and Wentworth, R.L. 1955. In *Hydrogen Peroxide*. New York, Van Nostrand Rheinhold, pp. 813–816.

Sims, A.F.E. 1983. Industrial effluent treatment with hydrogen peroxide. Chem. Ind., *27*, 555–558.

Sprossig, M. 1975. Peracetic acid and resistant microorganisms. In *Resistance of Microorganisms to Disinfectants: Second International Symposium*. Edited by W.B. Kedzia. Warsaw, Polish Academy of Sciences, pp. 89–91.

Steris System, 1988. Tech. Data Monograph. Steris Corp., Painesville, OH.

Suen, J. 1990. Personal communication.

Suen, J., Alderman, L., and Kiley, M.P. 1990. Use of vapor phase hydrogen peroxide (VPHP) as a space decontaminant. Am. Soc. Microbiol. Int. Symp. Chem. Germicides. Atlanta, Abstract 33, p. 21.

Teuber, M. 1979. Testing of the sporicidal properties the peracetic acid containing preparation "P-3 oxonia aktiv" and "P-3/VR 2828-20" against *Clostridium tyrobutyricum*. Institute for Microbiologie, Federal Institution for Dairy Investigations, Kiel, 11,2.

Teuber, M. 1978. Testing of peracetic acid containing preparation "P-3 oxonia aktiv" on bacteriophage specifically for *Streptococcus lactis*, *S. cremoris*, and *S. lactis* subsp. *diacetilactis*. Institute for Microbiology and Dairy Investigations, Kiel, 13, 10.

Thomas, E., and Aune, T. 1978. Lactoperoxidase, peroxide, thiocyanate antimicrobial system: Correlation of sulfhydryl oxidation with antimicrobial action. Infect. Immun., *20*, 456–463.

Thomas, S., and Russell, A.D. 1974. Studies on the mechanism of the sporicidal action of glutaraldehyde. Journal of Applied Bacteriology, 37, 83–92.

Toledo, R.T., Escher, F.E., and Ayers, J.C. 1973. Sporicidal properties of hydrogen peroxide against food spoilage organisms. Appl. Microbiol., 26, 592–597.

Trujillo, R., and David, T.J. 1972. Sporostatic and sporicidal properties of aqueous formaldehyde. Applied Microbiology, 23, 618–622.

Turner, F.J. 1983. Hydrogen peroxide and other oxidant disinfectants. In *Disinfection, Sterilization and Preservation*. 3rd Edition. Philadelphia, Lea & Febiger, pp. 240–250.

Tuynenberg Muys, G., Van Rhee, R., and Lelieveld, H.L.M. 1978. Sterilization by means of hydrochloric acid vapour. Journal of Applied Bacteriology, 45, 213–217.

Vashkov, V.I., Ramkova, N.V., Krivonosov, A.I., and Limanov, V.E. 1974. Sterilization of medical instruments from thermally-labile materials with solutions of chemical preparations. Med. Tekh., *6*, 9–11.

Voetman, A., Loos, J., and Roos, D. 1980. Changes in the level of glutathione in phagocytosing human neutrophils. Blood, *55*, 741.

Waites, W.M. 1982. Resistance of bacterial spores. In *Principles and Practice of Disinfection, Preservation, and Sterilization*. Edited by A.D. Russell, W.B. Hugo, and G.A.J. Ayliffe. Oxford. Blackwell Scientific Publications, p. 211.

Waites, W.M., et al. 1988. The destruction of spores of *Bacillus subtilis* by the combined effects of hydrogen peroxide and ultraviolet light. Appl. Microbiol., *7*, 139–140.

Wallian, S.S. 1892. Studies in aerotherapeutics. III. Hydrogen dioxide. N.Y Med. J., 56, 594.

Wardle, M.D., and Renninger, G.M. 1975. Biocidal effect of hydrogen peroxide in spacecraft bacterial isolates. Appl. Microbiol., *30*, 710–711.

Werner, H.P., and Wewalka, G. 1973. Destruction of spores in alcohol by peracetic acid. Zentralbl. Bakteriol. Mikrobiol. Hyg. [B], *157*, 387–391.

Wewalka, G., and Werner, H.P. 1973. Disinfection of medical machines by peracetic acid-aerosol. Zentralbl. Bakteriol. Mikrobiol. Hyg. [B], *156*, 557–563.

Whitehouse, R.L. and Clegg, L.F.L. 1963. Destruction of *Bacillus subtilis* spores with solutions of sodium hydroxide. Journal of Dairy Research, 30, 315–322.

Wilson, J.B., Turner, W.R., and Sale, J.W. 1927. Studies on bottled cocoa beverages. II. Efficiency of hydrogen peroxide in preserving cocoa-milk beverages. Am. Food J., *22*, 347–348.

Wutzler, P., Sprossig, M., and Peterseim, H. 1975. Suitability of peracetic acid for sterilization of media for mycoplasma cultures. J. Clin. Microbiol., *1*, 246–249.

Yamaguchi, T., and Yamashita, Y. 1980. Mutagenicity of hydroperoxides of fatty acids and some hydrocarbons. Agric. Biol. Chem., *44*, 1675–1678.

Yoshpe-Purer, Y., and Eylan, E. 1968. Disinfection of water by hydrogen peroxide. Health Lab. Sci., *5*, 233–238.

CHAPTER 10

DISINFECTION AND STERILIZATION BY OZONE

G.B. Wickramanayake

Ozone, an unstable three-atom allotrope of oxygen, is formed by the excitation of molecular oxygen into atomic oxygen in an energizing environment that allows the recombination of atoms into O_3. Ozone is a powerful oxidizing agent, with an oxidation-reduction potential of +2.7 volts. Pure ozone melts at a temperature of $-192.5 \pm 0.4°C$ and boils at $-111.9 \pm 0.3°C$ (Manley and Niegowski, 1967). At ambient temperatures ozone is a blue-colored gas, but at the low concentrations at which it is generated commercially for disinfection purposes, this color is not noticeable (Rice, 1986). Ozone was first introduced as a chemical disinfectant in drinking water treatment in 1893 at Oudshourn, Netherlands (Rice et al., 1981). Although used primarily for disinfection, it performs other functions such as color reduction, odor and taste removal, algae control, and oxidation of inorganic and organic compounds in water and wastewater treatment practice. At present, several thousands of plants worldwide employ ozone in water and wastewater treatment.

In addition to disinfection of drinking water and municipal wastewater, following are some other applications of ozone for disinfection and sterilization purposes (Rice, 1986):

Aquaculture: sea water disinfection in shellfish depuration stations (Fauvel, 1977) and influent water disinfection at freshwater hatcheries and fish farms (Monroe and Key, 1980)

Marine aquaria: disinfection of waters for recycle and reuse in large marine aquaria (Ramos and Ring, 1980)

Fish disease labs: treatment of discharges from these facilities (Thompson, 1976)

Heating and cooling units: treatment of cooling water to prevent biofouling (Edwards, 1981)

Process water treatment: sterilization of ultrapure water used in integrated circuit processing (Zomlek, 1977)

Oil treatment: recovery and reuse of spent lubricants and oils (Anonymous, 1973 and 1974)

Pharmaceutical processing waters: sterilization of high purity waters used in pharmaceutical industry (Nebel, 1983)

OZONE GENERATION

The corona discharge method is widely used in generation of ozone for commercial applications. In this technique, as shown in Figure 10–1, dry air or oxygen is passed between two electrodes separated by a ceramic dielectric medium. Concentrations ranging from 1 to 3% ozone are produced if the feed gas is air and 2 to 6% if the feed gas is pure oxygen (Rice, 1986). The ozone generation process is more efficient at low temperatures. More details on ozone generation can be found in literature published by Carlins and Clark (1982) and Masschelein (1982).

STABILITY OF OZONE

Ozone is more stable in gas phase than in aqueous phase. For example, the half-life of gaseous ozone in ambient atmosphere is 12 hrs. As shown in Figure 10–2, the half-life of aqueous ozone is less than 30 min. Rate of ozone decomposition in aqueous solutions increases with turbulence, temperature, pH, and ozone concentration. Gurol and Singer (1982) developed the following empirical equation to incorporate these parameters to express the rate of decrease of ozone concentration in the pH range of 2 to 9.5:

$$-\frac{d[O_3]}{dt} = K\,[OH^-]^{0.55}\,[O_3]$$

where, $[O_3]$ and $[OH^-]$ are ozone and hydroxide ion concentrations, respectively, and K is the rate constant which is a function of temperature and extent of turbulence.

Because of the instability of gaseous and aqueous ozone, it cannot be generated and stored for later ap-

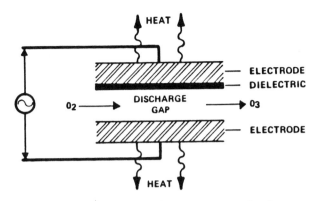

Fig. 10–1. Schematic diagram of ozone generation by the corona discharge procedure. From Rice, R.G. 1986. Application of ozone in water and wastewater treatment. In *Analytical Aspects of Ozone: Treatment of Water and Wastewater.* Edited by R.G. Rice, et al. Chelsea, MI, Lewis Publishers, 413.

plications. Consequently, ozone needs to be generated on-site as needed for disinfection and sterilization.

ANALYTICAL METHODS

Determination of residual ozone in aqueous solutions is rather difficult because of rapid decomposition of ozone, volatility from solution, and reactivity with many organic and inorganic chemicals. It is important to note that most of the ozone analytical methods, which are the modifications of chlorine residual methods, are based on the determination of total oxidants in the solution. Most of the ozone disinfection and sterilization data reported in the literature are based on such analytical techniques as iodometric methods, which do not necessarily measure the ozone alone. Therefore, ozone disinfection data should be carefully interpreted, especially when differ-

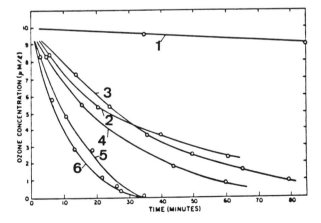

Fig. 10–2. Decomposition of ozone in various types of water at 20°C (1 = double-distilled water; 2 = distilled water; 3 = tap water; 4 = low hardness ground water; 5 = filtered water from Lake Zurich; 6 = filtered water from the Bodensee). From Rosenthal, H. 1974. Selected bibliography on ozone, its biological effects and technical applications. Fisheries Research Board of Canada Technical Report No. 456. Mamaimo, BC, Fisheries and Marine Service, Pacific Biological Station.

ent analytical techniques are used during the generation of inactivation data.

Grunwell et al. (1983) identified the indigo method and the arsenic (III) oxidation method as the methods of choice for aqueous ozone analyses. In the indigo method, ozone adds across the carbon-carbon double bond of sulfonated indigo dye and decolorizes it. The change in absorbance is determined spectrophotometrically (Bader and Hoigne, 1981). The indigo method is subject to fewer interferences than most of the colorimetric methods and all iodometric procedures (Gordon et al., 1988).

In the arsenic (III) direct oxidation method, ozone reacts with inorganic arsenic (III) at pH values ranging from 4 to 7. Then the excess As (III) species is back-titrated with standard iodine to a starch end point (Smart et al., 1979). A listing of all the ozone analytical methods for aqueous ozone is given in Table 10–1. Brief descriptions of some of these methods are presented in Table 10–2. More details of these methods can be found in publications by Rice et al. (1986) and Gordon et al. (1988) and in the Handbook of Ozone Technology and Applications (Rice and Netzer, 1982).

An accurate analysis of gas-phase ozone measurement is important, especially in the determination of cost, efficiency, safety, and improvement in the design and construction of ozone generators and contacting units or diffusers for water and wastewater disinfection. Therefore, precise and accurate analytical methods are necessary to measure ozone in gas-phase as well. The most commonly used gas-phase analytical methods include iodometry, UV absorption, and chemiluminescence, according to Gordon et al. (1988). An additional method that can be used for ozone analysis includes gas-phase titration with excess nitric oxide and ozone (Rehme et al., 1986). Most of the currently available gas-phase ozone analytical techniques are listed in Table 10–3. Based on the available information, Gordon et al. (1988) concluded that only the UV spectrophotometric method can be recommended for accurate determination of gas-phase ozone.

INACTIVATION OF MICROORGANISMS

Bacteria

Ozone is an effective inactivation agent for bacteria. Farooq and Akhlaque (1983) performed experiments on a number of bacteria, viruses, and yeasts to determine the response of these organisms to ozonation. The organisms tested include *Mycobacterium fortuitum, Escherichia coli, Salmonella typhimurium,* poliovirus 1 (Mahoney), along with the yeast, *Candida parapsilosis.* They conducted experiments on two different media at pH 7.0, and 24°C. The first experiment was performed in deionized water with the dissolved ozone residual levels maintained between 0.23 and 0.26 mg/L. The second experiment was performed on an activated sludge effluent with the ozone residuals level maintained between 0.29 and 0.36 mg/L. Contact time for both systems was

Table 10–1. *Analytical Methods for Ozone in Aqueous Solutions*

Analytical Method	Detection Limit (mg/L)	Working Range (mg/L)	Expected Accuracy (*%)	Expected Precision (*%)	Interferences	pH Range	Current Status
Ideal	0.01	0.01–10	0.5	0.1	None	Independent	Recommended
Iodometric	0.002	0.5–100	1–35	1–2	All ozone by-products and oxidants	<2	Abandon
Arsenic back titration	0.002	0.5–65	1–5	1–2	Oxidizing species	6.8	Continued study
FACTS	0.02	0.5–5	5–20	1–5	Oxidizing species	6.6	Not recommended
DPD	0.1	0.2–2	5–20	5	Oxidizing species	6.4	Not recommended
Indigo spectrophotometric	0.001	0.01–0.1	1	0.5	Cl_2, Mn ions, Br_2, I_2	2	Recommended
	0.006	0.05–0.5	1	0.5	Cl_2, Mn ions, Br_2, I_2	2	Recommended
	0.1	>0.3	1	0.5	Cl_2, Mn ions, Br_2, I_2	2	Recommended
	0.01	0.01–0.1	5	5	Cl_2, Mn ions, Br_2, I_2	2	Recommended
		>0.1	5	5	Cl_2, Mn ions, Br_2, I_2	2	Recommended
GDFIA	0.03	0.03–0.4 Other ranges possible	1	0.5	Cl_2 at >1 mg/L	2	Comparison studies needed
LCV	0.005	NR	NR	NR	S^{2-}, SO_3^{3-}, Cr^{6+}	2	Continued study
ACVK	0.25	0.05–1	NR	NR	Mn >1 mg/L Cl_2 >10 mg/L	2	Continued study
o-Tolidine	Not quantitative		NR	NR	Metal ions, NO_2^-	2	Abandon
Bisterpyridine	0.004	0.05–20	2.7	2.1	Cl_2	<7	Recommended (lab test)
Carmine indigio	<0.5	NR	NR	NR	NR	2	Continued study
Electrochemical amperometric	~1	NR	5	5	Oxidizing species	2	Relative monitoring
Amperometric iodometric	~0.5	NR	5	5	Oxidizing species	4–4.5	Not recommended
Bare electrode	0.2	NF	5	5	NR	NR	Continued study
Membrane electrode	0.062	NF	5	5	NR	NR	Continued study
Differential pulse dropping mercury	NR	NR	NR	NR	NR	NR	Research lab
Differential pulse polarography	0.003	NR	NR	NR	NR	4	Continued study
Potentiometric	NR	NR	NR	NR	NR	NR	Continued study
UV	0.02	>0.02	0.5	0.5	Other absorber	Independent	Establish molar absorptivity
Isothermal pressure change	4×10^{-5}	$4 \times 10^{-5} - 10$	0.5	0.5	None	Independent	Comparison study

From Gordon, G., Cooper, W.J., Rice, R.G., and Pacey, G.E. 1988. Methods for measuring disinfectant residuals. J. Am. Water Works Assoc., 80(9), 94–108.

Table 10–2. *Review of Some Analytical Methods for Ozone*

Method	Principle	Advantages/Limitations
Iodometric oxidation	Oxidation of I⁻ to I₂; detection of I₃⁻ by electrometric titration or photometric methods	High detection sensitivity approaching 2 μg/L; most oxidants interfere; reaction stoichiometry questioned; ozone losses probable, due to sample collection and handling
Ultraviolet spectrophotometry	Ozone molecule absorbs UV light at 254 nm; molar extinction coefficient approx. 2900 L/mole-cm	High detection sensitivity to 20 μg/L with 50-cm cell path length; can be used as a continuous process analyzer; potential interferences include organics and inorganics that absorb at 240- to 300-nm range, suspended solids and color
Leuco crystal violet (LCV)	Oxidation of leuco crystal violet to crystal violet; measure absorbance of crystal violet at 592 nm; molar absorptivity ca. 10⁶ L/mole-cm	Detection sensitivity approaching 1 μg/L; some oxidants interfere, notably manganese dioxide; major problem is test-kit staining due to use of dye
Diethyl-p-phenylene-diamine (DPD)	Oxidation of DPD; detection by titration or photometric methods	Detection sensitivity at sub-mg/L level, available for use in kit form; suffers interference from some oxidants, notably halogens and manganese; a major problem is reagent and product stability
FACTS (Syringaldazine)	Oxidation of iodide to iodine; iodine oxidizes syringaldazine; photometric detection at 530 nm	Moderate sensitivity; requires addition of two reagents; subject to interference from other oxidizing agents
Syringaldazine (glycine)	Glycine added to scavenge O₃; determination based on oxidation of I⁻ and syringaldazine; titrimetric detection	Sensitivity at sub-mg/L level; requires separate determinations of total oxidant and (oxidant-ozone)
Indigo-blue	Ozone bleaching of indigo dye measured spectrophotometrically at 600 nm	Good sensitivity at sub-mg/L level; peroxide does not interfere; manganese and chlorine do interfere, but can be corrected
Acid chrome violet K (ACVK)	Bleaching of ACVK dye measured spectrophotometrically at 550 nm	Moderate detection sensitivity
Amperometric bare electrodes	Reduction of O₃ to O₂ directly in solution; either solution of electrode rotated to establish diffusion layer; current directly proportional to concentration	Good sensitivity; applicable as continuous monitor; interferences from electrode fouling agents and other strong oxidants
Amperometric steady-state	Diffusion through films of O₃ to be reduced to O₂ in a thin electrolyte film between electrode and membrane; current controlled by rate of membrane diffusion is directly proportional to concentration	Very good selectivity for molecular ozone in presence of other oxidants; membrane limits effects of fouling agents, but can be fouled itself; good sensitivity; applicable for continuous monitoring; strong temperature dependence
Amperometric pulsed	Diffusion through membrane limits interferences but does not control current; O₃ in electrolyte film reduced to O₂; current directly proportional to concentration	Same advantages as above; membrane fouling and temperature dependence not as significant as with steady-state electrodes

From Stanley, J., and Johnson, J.D. 1986. Analysis of ozone in aqueous solution. In *Proceedings of the Second International Symposium on Ozone Technology.* Edited by R.G. Rice, P. Pichet, and M.A. Vincent. Norwalk, CT, International Ozone Association, pp. 682–693.

Table 10–3. *Analytical Methods for Ozone in Gas-Phase*

Analytical Method	Detection Limit (mg/L)	Working Range (mg/L)	Expected Accuracy (*%)	Expected Precision (*%)	Interferences	pH Range	Current Status
Ideal	1	1–50,000	1	1	None	Independent	Recommended
UV	0.5	0.5–50,000	2	2.5	None	NA	Recommended
Stripping absorption iodometry	0.002	0.5–100	1–35	1–2	SO₂, NO₂	NA	Abandon
Chemiluminescence	0.005	0.005–1	7	5	None	NA	Recommended
Gas-phase titration	0.005	0.005–30	8	8.5	None	NA	Not recommended
Rhodamine B-gallic acid	0.001	NR	NR	5	NR	NA	Not recommended
Amperometry	NR	NR	NR	NR	NR	NA	Not recommended

From Gordon, G., Cooper, W.J., Rice, R.G., and Pacey, G.E. 1988. Methods for measuring disinfectant residuals. J. Am. Water Works Assoc., *80*(9), 94–108.

1.67 minutes. As shown by the data presented in Tables 10–4, 10–5, and 10–6, the resistance of these organisms to inactivation was found to be in the following order: *M. fortuitum* > poliovirus type 1 > *C. parapsilosis* > *E. coli* > *S. typhimurium* for both systems. Edelstein et al. (1982) used concentrations of 0.1 mg/L to 0.63 mg/L to effect inactivation of *Legionella pneumophila*. A contact time of 20 minutes yielded log reduction values of 4.6 to 5.2. Joret et al. (1982) found no linear relation between bacterial inactivation rate and contact time. They used contact times ranging from 2.67 minutes to 19 minutes, at applied ozone concentrations of 0.45 mg/L to 4 mg/L. The most effective levels for inactivation of *E. coli* present in wastewater appeared to range from 2.2 to 4.0 mg/L for a 19-minute contact time. This yielded

an inactivation percentage of 99.9, leaving residual ozone concentrations of 0.06 to 0.35 mg/L.

Viruses

Ozone is also an effective virucide. As shown in Table 10–5, it requires only relatively low concentrations and contact times for the inactivation of viruses. For example, Harakeh and Butler (1985) observed that exposure of poliovirus type 1 to 0.25 mg/L of ozone for 5 minutes at pH 7.2 and 20°C caused 99% inactivation. Exposure of the same organisms to 0.4 mg/L of chlorine for 15 minutes in more favorable environmental conditions (pH 6 and temperature 25°C) resulted in only 38% inactivation (Alvarez and O'Brien, 1982).

The C·t value (concentration and time product) for 4-

Table 10–4. *Inactivation of Bacteria by Ozone*

Organism	Percent Reduction	Time (min)	Concentration* (mg/L)	pH	Temp. (°C)	Medium	Reactor Type	Comments	References
Escherichia coli	99.99	1.67	0.23–0.26	7	24	Ozone demand free water	Completely mixed continuous flow-through		Farooq and Akhlaque (1983)
Legionella pneumophila E221ADP	>99.997	20	0.32	7	24	Sterile distilled water	Batch		Edelstein et al. (1982)
	>99.999	20	0.47	7	24	Sterile distilled water	Batch		Edelstein et al. (1982)
Legionella pneumophila E102A₃DP	>99.999	20	0.32	7	24	Sterile distilled water	Batch		Edelstein et al. (1982)
	>99.999	20	0.47	7	24	Sterile distilled water	Batch		Edelstein et al. (1982)
Mycobacterium fortuitum	90	1.67	0.23–0.26	7	24	Ozone demand free water	Completely mixed continuous flow-through		Farooq and Akhlaque (1983)
Salmonella typhimurium	99.995	1.67	0.23–0.26	7	24	Ozone demand free water	Completely mixed continuous flow-through		Farooq and Akhlaque (1983)
Escherichia coli	17	19	Init. 0.85, res. 0	7.5	16	Raw wastewater	Continuous flow-through	TSS 85 mg/L COD 100 mg/L	Joret et al. (1982)
	97	19	Init. 1.4, res. 0	7.5	16	Raw wastewater	Continuous flow-through	TSS 85 mg/L COD 100 mg/L	Joret et al. (1982)
	99.9	19	Init. 2.2, res. 0.06	7.5	16	Raw wastewater	Continuous flow-through	TSS 85 mg/L COD 100 mg/L	Joret et al. (1982)
Fecal streptococci	17	19	Init. 0.85, res. 0	7.5	16	Raw wastewater	Continuous flow-through	TSS 85 mg/L COD 100 mg/L	Joret et al. (1982)
	93	19	Init. 1.4, res. 0	7.5	16	Raw wastewater	Continuous flow-through	TSS 85 mg/L COD 100 mg/L	Joret et al. (1982)
	99.6	19	Init. 2.2, res. 0.06	7.5	16	Raw wastewater	Continuous flow-through	TSS 85 mg/L COD 100 mg/L	Joret et al. (1982)
Escherichia coli	99.9998	0.16	0.51	7.0	20	Water	Continuous flow-through		Boyce et al. (1981)
	99.9995	0.16	0.18	7.0	20	Water	Continuous flow-through		Boyce et al. (1981)
	99	0.33	0.065	7.2	1	Water	Batch		Katzenelson et al. (1974)

*Some concentrations are reported as initial and residual levels.

Table 10–5. Inactivation of Viruses by Ozone

Organism	Percent Reduction	Time (min)	Concentration* (mg/L)	pH	Temp. (°C)	Medium	Reactor Type	Comments	References
Poliovirus type 1 (Mahoney)	99.7	1.67	0.23–0.26	7	24	Ozone demand free water	Completely mixed continuous flow-through		Farooq and Akhlaque (1983)
Coxsackie-virus B5	90	4.9	0.18	7.2	20	Activated sludge reactor effluent	Batch	TSS 12.5 mg/L NH₃ 1.55 mg/L BOD₅ 10.6 mg/L COD 37.2 mg/L	Harakeh and Butler (1985)
	0	10	0.1				Batch		
	99	5.5	0.25				Batch		
	99	2.0	0.32				Batch		
	99.99	2.5	0.40				Batch		
Poliovirus type 1	90	5	0.2	7.2	20	Activated sludge reactor effluent	Batch	TSS 12.5 mg/L NH₃ 1.55 mg/L BOD₅ 10.6 mg/L COD 37.2 mg/L	Harakeh and Butler (1985)
	99	5	0.25				Batch		
	99	10	0.2				Batch		
Poliovirus type 1 (Mahoney)	90	0.53	0.51	7.2	20	Water	Completely mixed continuous flow-through		Roy et al. (1981a)
		0.50	0.32	7.2	22	Water			
		0.75	0.32	4.3	N.R.	Water			
Poliovirus type 1	99	<0.3	0.13	7.2	5	N.R.	N.R.		Drinking Water and Health (1980)
	99	0.245	0.50	7.0	24	N.R.	N.R.		
	99	0.042	10	7.0	25	N.R.	N.R.		
Enteric virus	92	19	Init. 1.4, res. 0	7.5	16	Raw wastewater	Continuous flow-through	TSS 85 mg/L COD 100 mg/L	Joret et al. (1982)
	92	19	Init. 2.2, res. 0.06	7.5	16	Raw wastewater	Continuous flow-through	TSS 85 mg/L COD 100 mg/L	Joret et al. (1982)
Enteric virus	>98	19	Init. 4.10, res. 0.02	7.8	18	Raw wastewater	Continuous flow-through	TSS 103 mg/L COD 231 mg/L	Joret et al. (1982)
Echo virus type 1	99	10	0.26	7.2	20	Activated sludge effluent	Batch	TSS 12.5 mg/L NH₃ 1.55 mg/L BOD₅ 10.6 mg/L COD 37.2 mg/L	Harakeh and Butler (1985)
Bacteriophage f₂	80	10	0.1	7.2	20	Activated sludge effluent	Batch	TSS 12.5 mg/L NH₃ 1.55 mg/L BOD₅ 10.6 mg/L COD 37.2 mg/L	Harakeh and Butler (1985)
Simian rotavirus SA11	96	10	0.26	7.2	20	Activated sludge effluent	Batch	TSS 12.5 mg/L NH₃ 1.55 mg/L BOD₅ 10.6 mg/L COD 37.2 mg/L	Harakeh and Butler (1985)
Human rotavirus	80	10	0.31	7.2	20	Activated sludge effluent	Batch	TSS 12.5 mg/L NH₃ 1.55 mg/L BOD₅ 10.6 mg/L COD 37.2 mg/L	Harakeh and Butler (1985)
Poliovirus type 1	99	9	0.2	4	20	Activated sludge effluent	Batch	TSS 12.5 mg/L NH₃ 1.55 mg/L BOD₅ 10.6 mg/L COD 37.2 mg/L	Harakeh and Butler (1985)
	75	10	0.2	7.2	20		Batch		
	80	10	0.2	9	20		Batch		
Poliovirus type 1 sabin	>96	0.16	0.21	7.0	20	Water	Continuous flow-through	1TU, bentonite	Boyce et al. (1981)
	>97	0.16	0.21	7.0	20	Water	Continuous flow-through	5TU, bentonite	Boyce et al. (1981)
Coxsackie A9	>98	0.16	0.144	7.0	20	Water	Continuous flow-through	5TU, bentonite	Boyce et al. (1981)
	>98	0.16	0.035	7.0	20	Water	Continuous flow-through	5TU, bentonite	Boyce et al. (1981)
Bacteriophage f₂	>99.97	0.16	0.40	7.0	20	Water	Continuous flow-through	5TU, bentonite	Boyce et al. (1981)
	>99.995	0.16	0.41	7.0	20	Water	Continuous flow-through	5TU, bentonite	Boyce et al. (1981)

*Some concentrations are reported as initial and residual levels.

Table 10–6. Inactivation of Fungi and Yeasts by Ozone

Organism	Percent Reduction	Time (min)	Concentration (mg/L)	pH	Temp. (°C)	Medium	Reactor Type	References
Candida parapsilosis	99.8	1.67	0.23–0.26	7	24	Demand free water	Completely mixed continuous flow-through	Farooq and Akhlaque (1983)
Candida tropicalis	99	0.30 0.08	0.02 1	7.2	20	Demand free water	Completely mixed continuous flow-through	Kawamura et al. (1986)

log inactivation of coxsackievirus B5 at neutral pH and room temperature is estimated to be only 1 mg-min/L (Table 10–5). Under similar environmental conditions and C·t values, poliovirus inactivation was only 1 log. These data indicate that significant variation of resistance among viruses exists for ozone inactivation.

Inactivation of microorganisms in wastewaters required longer contact time and larger doses than inactivation in demand-free systems. A comparison of data from Joret et al. (1982) or Harakeh and Butler (1985) with other data in Table 10–5 will show the effects of suspended solids and organic matter on the virucidal effectiveness of ozone. As with chlorine and other oxidants, a portion of the applied ozone will react with any oxidizable materials present in the medium. The fraction of ozone, or any disinfectant, that does not inactivate microorganisms is often difficult to predict for these systems.

Fungi

Kawamura et al. (1986) studied the effect of ozone on *Candida tropicalis* at pH 7.2 and 20°C with 99% kill times ranging from 18 seconds at 0.02 mg/L ozone to approximately 5 seconds at 1 mg/L ozone (Table 10–6). *Candida tropicalis* was 10 or more times as resistant as *Escherichia coli*, *Salmonella typhimurium*, or *Staphy-*

lococcus aureus but approximately 15 times more sensitive than the spores of *Bacillus* spp. As has been found with most other microorganisms, ozone appears to be an effective fungicide.

Protozoa

Ozone inactivation data for protozoan cysts are limited. Wickramanayake (1986) studied the inactivation of three different organisms under different pH and temperatures. These three organisms are (1) cysts of nonpathogenic soil and water amoeba *Naegleria gruberi* (NEG), (2) parasite of mice *Giardia muris*, and (3) human pathogen *Giardia lamblia*. The inactivation data generated during these studies are summarized in Table 10–7. Based on the concentration-time data (C·t), *N. gruberi* appears to be the most resistant. *G. lamblia* is slightly less resistant than *G. muris*.

Subcellular Components

When poliovirus 1 (Mahoney) was exposed to ozone, Roy et al. (1981b) observed that the damage to the viral nucleic acid is the major cause of the inactivation of organism. RNA was observed to be damaged by ozone concentrations less than 0.3 mg/L within 2 min of contact times. Also, ozone altered two of the four polypeptide chains present in the viral protein coat.

Table 10–7. Inactivation of Protozoan by Ozone

Organism	Percent Reduction	Time (min)	Concentration (mg/L)	pH	Temp. (°C)	Medium*	Reactor Type	$C \cdot t'\left(\dfrac{mg-min}{L}\right)$[†]
Naegleria gruberi	99	7.8	0.55	7	5	Water	Batch	4.23
	99	2.1	2.0	7	5	Water	Batch	4.23
	99	4.3	0.3	7	25	Water	Batch	1.29
	99	1.1	1.2	7	25	Water	Batch	1.29
Giardia muris	99	12.9	0.15	7	5	Water	Batch	1.94
	99	2.8	0.7	7	5	Water	Batch	1.94
	99	9.0	0.03	7	25	Water	Batch	0.27
	99	1.8	0.15	7	25	Water	Batch	0.27
Giardia lamblia	99	5.3	0.1	7	5	Water	Batch	0.53
	99	1.1	0.5	7	5	Water	Batch	0.53
	99	5.5	0.03	7	25	Water	Batch	0.17
	99	1.2	0.15	7	25	Water	Batch	0.17

*Medium is 0.01 M ozone demand-free phosphate buffer solution.

†C·t' = concentration-time data averaged for a given pH and temperature for each organism.

From Wickramanayake, G.B. 1984. Kinetics and Mechanism of Ozone Inactivation of Protozoan Cysts. Ph.D. Dissertation, Dept. of Civil Engineering, The Ohio State University, Columbus, OH.

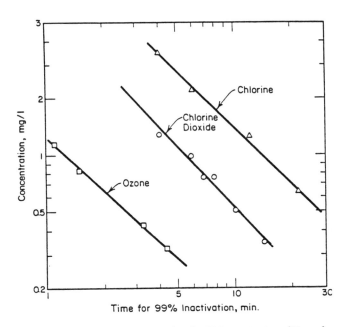

Fig. 10–3. Concentration-time plots for 99% inactivation of *N. gruberi* cysts with chlorine, chlorine dioxide, and ozone. From Wickramanayake, G.B. 1984. Kinetics and mechanism of ozone inactivation of protozoan cysts. Ph.D. Dissertation, Dept. of Civil Engineering, The Ohio State University, OH.

Kim et al. (1980) studied the kinetics and mechanism of ozone inactivation of bacteriophage f$_2$ and reported that the RNA enclosed in the phage coat was inactivated less by ozone than were whole phages, but was inactivated more than naked RNA. Important findings of this study are that the subcellular components of a microorganism can be more resistant than the whole organism, and that the inactivation of a microorganism does not necessarily denature the genetic materials in it.

COMPARISON WITH OTHER DISINFECTANTS

To compare the effectiveness of ozone with other disinfectants, tests need to be performed with the same organism and same environmental conditions such as pH, temperature, and reactor type for all the disinfectants that need to be compared. The results reported for inactivation of *Naegleria gruberi* (strain NEG) by chlorine (Rubin et al., 1983), chlorine dioxide (Chen et al., 1985), and ozone (Wickramanayake et al., 1984) at pH 7 and 25°C are presented in Figure 10–3. Based on this figure, ozone appears to be the most effective in cyst inactivation, then chlorine dioxide, followed by chlorine. When the respective concentration-time (C·t) values are compared, ozone is about 9 times more effective than free chlorine and 4 times more effective than chlorine dioxide in the inactivation of *N. gruberi* cysts at pH 7 and 25°C. Generally, ozone is known to be a more effective bactericide and virucide than chlorine and chlorine dioxide.

REFERENCES

Alvarez, M.E., and O'Brien, R.T. 1982. Effects of chlorine concentration on the structure of poliovirus. Appl. Environ. Microbiol., *43*, 237.

Anonymous. 1973. Ozone cleans bug-ridden oil. New Scientist, 8 March, p. 548.

Anonymous. 1974. Disposal, regeneration, and recovery of used industrial oils. Machine Moderne, Nov., p. 38–45.

Bader, H., and Hoigne, J. 1981. Determination of ozone in water by the indigo method. Water Res., *15*, 449–454.

Carlins, J.J., and Clark, R.G. 1982. Ozone generation by corona discharge. In *Handbook of Ozone Technology and Applications.* Edited by R.G. Rice and A. Netzer. Butterworth Publishers, p. 41–76.

Chen, Y.S.R., Sproul, O.J., and Rubin, A.J. 1985. Inactivation of *Naegleria gruberi* cysts by chlorine dioxide. Water Res., *19*(6), 783–789.

Edelstein, P.H., Whittacker, R.E., Kreiling, R.L., and Howell, C.L. 1982. Efficacy of ozone in eradication of *Legionella pneumophila* from hospital plumbing fixtures. Appl. Environ. Microbiol., *44*, 1330–1334.

Edwards, H.B. 1981. Treatment of cooling tower water with ozone in lieu of chemicals. In *Ozone Treatment of Water for Cooling Applications.* Edited by R.G. Rice. Norwalk, CT, Intl. Ozone Assoc., p. 21–30.

Farooq, S., and Akhlaque, S. 1983. Comparative response of mixed cultures of bacteria and virus to ozonation. Water Res., *17*, 809.

Fauvel, Y. 1977. Utilization of ozone in oyster culture and in connected industries. Paper presented at Third Ozone World Congress, Paris, France. Zurich, Intl. Ozone Assoc.

Gordon, G., Cooper, W.J., Rice, R.G., and Pacey, G.E. 1988. Methods for measuring disinfectant residuals. J. Am. Water Works Assoc., *80*(9), 94–108.

Grunwell, J., Benga, J., Cohen, H., and Gordon, G. 1983. A detailed comparison of analytical methods for residual ozone measurement. Ozone: Sci. Eng., *5*(4), 203–223.

Gurol, M.D., and Singer, P.C. 1982. Kinetics of ozone decomposition: A dynamic approach. Environ. Sci. Technol., *16*, 377.

Harakeh, M.S. 1984. The combined effects of various disinfectants against poliovirus 1 in a municipal wastewater effluent. FEMS Microbiol. Lett., *23*, 21.

Harakeh, M.S., and Butler, M. 1985. Factors influencing the ozone inactivation of enteric viruses in effluent. Ozone: Sci. Eng., *6*, 235–243.

Joret, J.C., Block, J.C., Hartemann, P., and Richard, Y. 1982. Wastewater disinfection: Elimination of fecal bacteria and enteric viruses by ozone. Ozone: Sci. Eng., *4*, 91–99.

Katzenelson, E., Kletter, B., and Shuval, H.I. 1974. Inactivation of kinetics of viruses and bacteria in water by use of ozone. J. Am. Water Works Assoc., *66*, 725.

Kawamura, K., Kaneko, M., Hirata, T., and Taguchi, K. 1986. Microbial indicators for the efficiency of disinfection processes. Water Sci. Technol., *18*, 175–184.

Kim, C.K., Gentile, D.M., and Sproul, O.J. 1980. Mechanism of ozone inactivation of bacteriophage f$_2$. Appl. Environ. Microbiol., *39*, 210.

Manley, T.C., and Niegowski, S.J. 1967. Ozone. In *Encyclopedia of Chemical Technology.* 2nd edition. Volume 14. New York, John Wiley and Sons, pp. 410–432.

Masschelein, W.J. (ed). 1982. *Ozonization Manual for Water and Wastewater Treatment.* New York, John Wiley and Sons.

Monroe, D.W., and Key, W.P. 1980. The feasibility of ozone for purification of hatchery waters. Ozone Sci. Eng., *2*, 203–224.

Nebel, C. 1983. Ozone in high purity water systems. In *Proceedings of the Sixth Ozone World Congress.* Norwalk, CT, Intl. Ozone Assoc., p. 139.

Ramos, N.G., and Ring, J.F. 1980. The practical use of ozone in large marine aquaria. Ozone Sci. Eng., *2*, 225–228.

Rehme, K.A., et al. 1981. Evaluation of Ozone Calibration Procedures. Project Summary, EPA-600/S4-80-050. US Environmental Protection Agency.

Rice, R.G. 1986. Application of ozone in water and wastewater treatment. In *Analytical Aspects of Ozone: Treatment of Water and Wastewater.* Edited by R.G. Rice, et al. Chelsea, MI, Lewis Publishers, pp. 7–26.

Rice, R.G., Bollyky, L.J., and Lacy, W.J. (eds.) 1986. *Analytical Aspects of Ozone: Treatment of Water and Wastewater.* Chelsea, MI, Lewis Publishers, p. 413.

Rice, R.G., and Netzer, A. (eds.) 1982. *Handbook of Ozone Technology and Applications.* Volume 1. Ann Arbor, Science Publishers.

Rice, R.G., Robson, C.M., Miller, G.W., and Hill, A.G. 1981. Use of ozone in drinking water treatment. J. Am. Water Works Assoc., *73*, 44–56.

Rosenthal, H. 1974. Selected bibliography on ozone, its biological effects and technical applications. Fisheries Research Board of Canada Technical Report No. 456. Fisheries and Marine Service. Pacific Biological Station, Nanaimo, BC.

Roy, D., Chian, E.S.K., and Engelbrecht, R.S. 1981a. Kinetics of enteroviral inactivation by ozone. J. Environ. Eng., Am. Soc. of Civil Eng., *107*, 887.

Roy, D., Wong, P.K.Y., Engelbrecht, R.S., and Chian, E.S.K. 1981b. Mechanism of enteroviral inactivation by ozone. Appl. Environ. Microbiol., *41*, 718.

Rubin, A.J., Engel, R.P., and Sproul, O.J. 1983. Disinfection of amoebic cysts in water with free chlorine. J. Water Poll. Cont. Fed., 55, 1174–1182.

Safe Drinking Water Committee. 1980. Drinking Water and Health. Volume 2. Washington, D.C., National Academy Press.

Smart, R.B., Lowry, J.H., and Mancy, K.H. 1979. Analysis for ozone and residual chlorine by differential pulse polarography of phenylarsine oxide. Environ. Sci. Technol., *13*, 89–92.

Stanley, J., and Johnson, J.D. 1986. Analysis of ozone in aqueous solution. In *Analytical Aspects of Ozone: Treatment of Water and Wastewater.* Edited by R.G. Rice, et al. Chelsea, MI, Lewis Publishers, pp. 71–90.

Thompson, G.E. 1976. Ozone applications in Manitoba, Canada. In *Proceedings of the Second International Symposium on Ozone Technology.* Edited by R.G. Rice, P. Pichet, and M.A. Vincent. Norwalk, CT, Intl. Ozone Assoc., pp. 682–693.

Wickramanayake, G.B. 1984. Kinetics and Mechanism of Ozone Inactivation of Protozoan Cysts. Ph.D. Dissertation. Dept. of Civil Engineering, The Ohio State University, Columbus, OH.

Wickramanayake, G.B., Rubin, A.J., and Sproul, O.J. 1984. Inactivation of *Naegleria* and *Giardia* cysts in water by ozonation. J. Water Pollut. Control Fed., *56*, 983–988.

Zomlek, C.R. 1977. Ultra pure water for integrated circuits processing. Ind. Water Eng., December, pp 6–11.

CHAPTER 11

ALCOHOLS

E.L. Larson and H.E. Morton*

The alcohols have been appreciated for centuries for their antiseptic qualities (Beck, 1984). As a chemical group, the alcohols possess many features desirable for a disinfectant or antiseptic. They have a bactericidal rather than a bacteriostatic action against vegetative forms; they are relatively inexpensive, usually easily obtainable, and relatively nontoxic with topical application. They have a cleansing action and evaporate readily. They are colorless, but if this property is undesirable, a coloring substance may be added. Like chemical disinfectants in general, their destructive action against spore forms is much less than that against vegetative forms. Although studied extensively as a group, their mode of action is not clearly understood. The greatest amount of work has been done with ethyl alcohol.

Wirgin (1904) pointed out that the bactericidal action of the aliphatic alcohols (methyl, ethyl, propyl, butyl, and amyl) increased with the increase in the molecular weights of the alcohols, with the exception of the tertiary alcohols. Testing alcohols in a liquid environment against *Salmonella typhosa*, Tilley and Schaffer (1926) observed an increase in the phenol coefficients from 0.026 for methyl to 21.0 for octyl alcohol. For *Staphylococcus aureus*, the phenol coefficients varied from 0.03 for methyl to 0.63 for amyl alcohol.

Tanner and Wilson (1943) tested alcohols containing from 1 to 11 carbon atoms by the agar cup-plate method. Methyl alcohol had no noticeable effect on the test organisms. The size of the zones in which no growth of the test organisms took place increased in size from that for ethyl alcohol to that for amyl alcohol, then decreased in size for the primary-normal alcohol series. The size of the zone of inhibition for primary-normal undecyl alcohol, the last alcohol in the series to be tested, was comparable to that for ethyl alcohol. In the case of *Pseudomonas aeruginosa* growth was stimulated rather than inhibited by the sample of undecyl alcohol. The bactericidal action varied from greatest to least in the following order: primary-normal > primary-iso > secondary-nor-

*Deceased

mal > tertiary alcohols, as was observed by Tilley and Schaffer (1926). Nine months' contact with 100% primary-normal methyl, ethyl, propyl, butyl, amyl, hexyl, heptyl, octyl, nonyl, and undecyl alcohols did not kill *Bacillus subtilis* and *Bacillus megatherium* spores.

Molinas and Brewer (1949) studied 27 compounds for their ability to reduce the number of bacteria on rabbit, guinea pig, and human skins. Solutions of 50% methyl alcohol and 10% acetone or 50% ethyl alcohol and 10% acetone or 50% isopropyl alcohol and 10% acetone were used as controls. These investigators concluded that the action of proprietary preparations designated for disinfecting the skin depends largely upon the alcoholic solutions in which they are incorporated. The results of in vitro tests with fewer compounds reported by Simmons in 1928 were similar. The addition of chlorhexidine and hexachlorophene to alcohols of 95 and 75% concentrations did not improve the immediate antibacterial effect of the alcohols, and 95% was preferable to 75% concentration (Kuipers, 1947). An alcoholic solution of cetrimide appeared clinically more effective than an aqueous solution of cetrimide for preoperative skin preparation (Noone, 1970). The length of time the alcohol is in contact with the skin is important (Lowbury et al., 1960). In quantitative tests, Novak and Hall (1939) observed the 50% alcohol–10% acetone mixture to be highly germicidal. It killed 96% of the organisms on the skin over the abdomen, whereas no disinfectant tested was able to kill 100% of the organisms.

MODE OF ACTION OF ALCOHOLS

Denaturing Action

The most plausible explanation for the antibacterial action of the alcohols is their denaturing of proteins. In the absence of water, proteins are not denatured as readily as when water is present. This affords an explanation of why absolute ethyl alcohol, a dehydrating agent, is less bactericidal than mixtures of alcohol and water.

Interference with Metabolism

Dadley et al. (1950) observed that a 0.41 molar concentration of ethyl alcohol increased the lag phase of *Enterobacter aerogenes*. This effect was decreased by the presence of the amino acids: DL-methionine, L-leucine, L-glutamic acid, L-histidine, and DL-tryptophane. The lag was increased by L-proline, glycine, DL-alanine, DL-serine, and DL-aspartic acid. The authors concluded that the bacteriostatic action was due to the inhibition of the production of metabolites essential for rapid cell division.

After being exposed to various chemical and physical agents, bacterial cells are often judged to be killed when they fail to multiply in suitable growth medium. When incubated in special media, however, these supposedly killed cells frequently can be rendered viable and capable of growth. Heinmets et al. (1954) reported that *Escherichia coli* B/r failed to grow after being exposed to 20% ethyl alcohol for 10 minutes, but grew after being treated with various metabolites. Best results in demonstrating viable cells in the "sterilized" suspensions of treated cells were obtained with cis-aconitic acid, a-ketoglutaric acid, and a mixture of 11 metabolites that included the two already mentioned. The concentration of 20% approaches the borderline of effectiveness of ethyl alcohol and represents a concentration much lower than that used for the purpose of disinfection. Such reactivation of "inactivated" cells needs to be studied under conditions that more nearly approach those in actual practice. The work indicates that it is possible to reverse the action of weak concentrations of ethyl alcohol.

The inhibition of spore germination by ethyl and other alcohols may be due to the inhibition of enzymes necessary for germination. This inhibition is reversible, because only the removal of the alcohol from the environment is necessary for germination to take place (Trujillo and Laible, 1970).

Lytic Action

Pulvertaft and Lumb (1948) reported that lysis of microorganisms occurred with many antiseptics when used at a concentration approximately double that of the minimum concentration producing bacteriostasis. Lysis was observed with formalin, mercuric chloride, thimerosal, phenol, and sodium hypochlorite, as well as with the antibiotic penicillin. Lysis was most marked with staphylococci, pneumococci, *Bacillus subtilis*, and *Escherichia coli*, less marked with *Shigella flexneri* and *sonnei*, and only slight with streptococci. The organisms were most susceptible to lysis when the antiseptic was added to the culture during its logarithmic phase, and lysis usually began about the third hour thereafter. The lytic action was thought to be due to using the antiseptic in a concentration that inhibited growth of the microorganisms without inhibiting the autolytic enzymes.

Leece (1953) observed that a suspension of the Campo strain of mycoplasma isolated from humans, estimated to contain 140 μg nitrogen per ml, was lysed within a few minutes by tertiary-butyl and isoamyl alcohols in a concentration of 0.1%. The organisms were not lysed under similar conditions by methyl, ethyl, propyl, isopropyl, and normal butyl alcohols. *Escherichia coli* in a suspension estimated to contain 500 μg dry weight per ml was lysed in the presence of 33% propyl and tertiary-butyl alcohols. Razin and Argaman (1963) found that *Acholeplasma laidlawii* and mycoplasma were lysed by ethyl alcohol in concentrations between 4.3 and 5.4 mol, by propyl alcohol in concentrations greater than 0.84 mol, and by normal butyl alcohol in concentrations greater than 0.24 mol.

TYPES OF ALCOHOLS: EARLY IN-VITRO WORK

Methyl Alcohol

Methyl alcohol has the weakest bactericidal action of the alcohols and thus is seldom considered for use as an antibacterial agent. Its slight antibacterial action was noted by Wirgin (1904) and Tilley and Schaffer (1926), but Tanner and Wilson (1943) reported no detectable activity. It apparently does not noticeably affect the bactericidal action of ethyl alcohol when used as a denaturant (Olivo, 1948). Kolb et al. (1952) reported that methyl alcohol in concentrations of 0.004 to 95% has no killing action on the spores of *Bacillus anthracis*. Although strains of influenza virus A and B are completely precipitated by 31% methanol, continued contact for even 10 hours produced no loss of infectivity (Cox et al., 1947).

Ethyl Alcohol (Ethanol)

Alcohol* is widely used for the destruction of the vegetative forms of microorganisms preceding such procedures as venipunctures, hypodermic injections, finger pricks, and other procedures that break the intact skin. It is also widely used in some European countries as a surgical hand scrub, and in the U.S. and Europe as a hand rinse.

During the latter part of the nineteenth century, it was common practice to test disinfectants against microorganisms dried on threads or beads. This demonstrated the fact that some water must be present for alcohol to exert its most effective bactericidal action. It also gave the erroneous impression that alcohol is a poor disinfectant because it failed to readily kill the dried organisms, and, like chemical disinfectants in general, it possessed poor killing action against bacterial spores. The erroneous perception was perpetuated in many textbooks that 95% alcohol was practically worthless as a disinfectant, possibly because 70% alcohol possessed a stronger killing action. In 1939, Price attempted to correct the

---

*In this section, the word alcohol, when used alone, refers to ethyl alcohol.

erroneous impression that alcohol was a poor disinfectant.

Effect of Ethyl Alcohol on Vegetative Bacteria

Harrington and Walker (1903) tested organisms on moist and dry threads against various concentrations of alcohol. *Escherichia coli* on moist threads was killed after exposure of less than 5 minutes to alcohol at 60 to 99% concentrations, whereas only the concentrations of 50 and 60% killed within 5 minutes when the organisms were dried on threads. Concentrations of 94 and 99% did not kill *E. coli, Pseudomonas aeruginosa, Staphylococcus epidermidis*, and *Staphylococcus aureus* in an exposure of 24 hours when the organisms were dried on threads. *Pseudomonas aeruginosa* on moist threads was killed in 5 minutes by concentrations of 40 to 99%, but on dried threads only the concentrations of 40 to 70% killed in the same period of time. *Staphylococcus epidermidis* on moist threads was killed in less than 1 minute by 50% alcohol. Concentrations of 40 to 99% killed in 5 minutes, but when the organisms were dried on threads, only the concentrations of 40 to 70% killed in the same period. Essentially the same results were obtained with *Staphylococcus aureus*. On moist threads, *Salmonella typhosa* was killed in 5 minutes by concentrations of 30 to 99%, but on dried threads only by concentrations of 30 to 80%. *Corynebacterium diphtheriae* on moist threads was killed in 5 minutes by concentrations of 40 to 99% and dried threads by concentrations of 40 to 90%. Thus, authors concluded more than three fourths of a century ago that against some common, nonspore-forming bacteria in a moist condition, any strength of alcohol above 40% by volume is effective within 5 minutes, and certain preparations are effective within an exposure

time of 1 minute. Against organisms in the dry state, concentrations of 60 to 70% are the most effective, and the same concentrations are equally effective against the organisms in the moist state. Typical results are reproduced in Table 11–1. Ethyl alcohol in a concentration of 70% was observed by Hare et al. (1963) to kill in an exposure of 30 seconds microorganisms of 10 species when dried on glass surfaces. This indicates it is possible for an aqueous alcoholic solution to exert its bactericidal action on even dried organisms before it evaporates.

By adding a loopful of suspension of microorganisms to the solution, Post and Nicoll (1910) found that 70 and 50% concentrations of alcohol killed *Streptococcus pyogenes, Streptococcus pneumoniae, Neisseria gonorrhoeae*, and *Salmonella typhosa* in less than 1 minute. Even 30% alcohol killed *Neisseria gonorrhoeae* in less than 1 minute.

Morton (1950) tested various concentrations of alcohol against a variety of microorganisms in exposure periods beginning with 10 seconds. To avoid altering the concentrations of the alcohol, the test organisms in 0.5-ml amounts of broth culture were placed in sterile tubes and centrifuged. The supernatant was removed, and the alcoholic solution was thoroughly mixed with the moist cells. One drop of the culture-cell mixture was subcultured at stated intervals. *Pseudomonas aeruginosa* was killed in 10 seconds by all concentrations of alcohol from 100 to 30% by volume. The lowest concentration of alcohol tested, 20%, killed in 30 minutes. *Serratia marcescens, Escherichia coli*, and *Salmonella typhosa* were killed in 10 seconds by all concentrations of alcohol from 100 to 40% (Table 11–2). Nathanson (1951) stated that 2% alcohol added to sulfonated vegetable oils prevented

Table 11–1. *The Killing Action of Various Concentrations of Alcohol against* Staphylococcus Aureus *on Moist and Dried Threads*

	Exposure Time																	
	Moist Threads									Dried Threads								
	Minutes					Hours				Minutes					Hours			
Alcohol %	5	10	15	30	45	1	2	7	24	5	10	15	30	45	1	2	7	24
15	+	+	+	+	+	+	+	+	+	+	+	+	+	+	+	+	+	+
20	+	+	+	+	+	+	+	+	−	+	+	+	+	+	+	+	+	+
25	+	+	+	+	+	+	+	−	−	+	+	+	+	+	+	+	+	−
30	+	+	+	+	+	+	−	−	−	+	+	+	+	+	+	+	−	−
40	−	−	−	−	−	−	−	−	−	+	+	−	−	−	−	−	−	−
50	−	−	−	−	−	−	−	−	−	+	−	−	−	−	−	−	−	−
60	−	−	−	−	−	−	−	−	−	−	−	−	−	−	−	−	−	−
70	−	−	−	−	−	−	−	−	−	−	−	−	−	−	−	−	−	−
75	−	−	−	−	−	−	−	−	−	−	−	−	−	−	−	−	−	−
80	−	−	−	−	−	−	−	−	−	+	−	−	−	−	−	−	−	−
85	−	−	−	−	−	−	−	−	−	+	+	−	−	−	−	−	−	−
90	−	−	−	−	−	−	−	−	−	+	+	+	−	−	−	−	−	−
94	−	−	−	−	−	−	−	−	−	+	+	+	+	+	+	+	+	−
99	−	−	−	−	−	−	−	−	−	+	+	+	+	+	+	+	+	+

+, growth; −, no growth

From Harrington, C., and Walker, H. 1903. The germicidal action of alcohol. Boston Med. Surg. J., *148*, 548–522.

the growth of *Serratia marcescens* and *Pseudomonas aeruginosa* in most cases. Ethyl or isopropyl alcohol in concentrations of 4 to 7% are used for preservatives of certain disinfectant solutions. The gram-positive vegetative organisms *Staphylococcus aureus* and *Streptococcus pyogenes* were a little more resistant, being killed in 10 seconds by concentrations of 60 to 95%. Exposures of 50 and 90 seconds, respectively, were required to kill the two organisms with absolute alcohol at room temperature. At higher temperatures, the killing action would be expected to be more rapid (Tilley, 1942).

Price (1939) employed an original technique in which the alcohol-culture mixture was diluted with water to stop the germicidal action, aliquot portions seeded into plates, and colonies from surviving organisms counted. He observed *Escherichia coli* to be killed in less than 60 seconds by 60% alcohol (by weight), in less than 30 seconds by 80% alcohol. *Staphylococcus epidermidis* was killed in less than 60 seconds by either 50 or 70% alcohol. *Staphylococcus aureus* was killed in less than 15 seconds by 70% alcohol. However, by employing essentially the same technique, Price (1950) reported that *Escherichia coli* required an exposure of 5 minutes to be killed by 60% alcohol. *Staphylococcus epidermidis* was not killed in 10 minutes by any concentration of alcohol. Hayes (1949) reported that *Escherichia coli, Proteus vulgaris, Pseudomonas aeruginosa,* and *Staphylococcus aureus* were killed in less than 5 minutes when exposed to concentrations of ethanol ranging from 50 to 100%. A concentration of 25% ethanol did not kill these organisms during an exposure of 30 minutes.

To test the capability of a germicide to penetrate deeper layers of skin, Seelig and Gould (1911) made a pouch of celloidin or living animal tissue at the end of a glass tube, placed the culture under study inside of the pouch, and immersed it in the disinfectant solution. After varying periods, subcultures were made of the culture within the pouch. *Salmonella typhosa* within celloidin pouches was killed within 6 minutes by 95 and 99.8% alcohol concentrations. Concentrations of 50%, 70%, and

80% did not kill in 1 hour. In a pouch of living rabbit omentum immersed in 95% alcohol, the organisms were alive after 5 minutes but dead after 10 minutes. When placed in a pouch of dried rat intestine and immersed in 99 and 95% alcohols, the organisms were still alive after 18 hours. An important incidental observation was that when the organisms lost their motility they were no longer viable. By making microscopic observations of the organisms inside the pouches, the authors could determine if the organisms had been killed, and the results of subculturing verified this in every case. In celloidin pouches, *Escherichia coli* was killed in 20 but not in 10 minutes by 95% alcohol, in 60 but not in 30 minutes by 80%, in 18 hours but not in 2 hours by 70%; 50% alcohol did not kill in an exposure of 18 hours. Comparable results were obtained with a staphylococcal culture. When certain germicides were dissolved in alcohol, their germicidal action was increased. An alcoholic solution of iodine killed microorganisms within the pouches quicker than 95% alcohol or aqueous solution of iodine alone.

Alcohol in the body may suppress the normal clearing mechanism of the body for bacteria. The retention of *Staphylococcus aureus* by the lungs of mice was 3.6 times greater when the mice were given an intraperitoneal injection of alcohol (Laurenzi et al., 1963). When 8% alcohol was supplied in the drinking water and the mice were challenged by intravenous injection of the organisms, the survival time was shorter and the number of staphylococci in the liver greater than in the control group. When the mice were given 5% alcohol in their drink for 3 weeks prior to challenge, the number of staphylococci in the liver was greater, but there was no significant difference between the number of organisms in the spleens and kidneys of the mice in the ethanol and control groups, and the mortality rates were comparable (Wasz-Hockert et al., 1959).

In testing the effect of ethyl alcohol against *Mycobacterium tuberculosis*, Smith (1947) observed that 95% alcohol killed the tubercle bacilli in sputum within 15 seconds, absolute and 70% alcohol required 30 seconds, and

Table 11–2. *The Killing Action of Various Concentrations of Alcohol Against* Streptococcus Pyogenes

Alcohol		Seconds					Exposures of Test Organism to Germicide											
							Minutes											
% by vol.	% by wt.	10	20	30	40	50	1	1½	2	3	3½	4	5	10	15	30	45	60
100	100	+	+	+	+	+	+	−	−	−	−	−	−	−	−	−		
95	92	−	−	−	−	−	−	−	−	−	−	−	−	−	−	−		
90	85	−	−	−	−	−	−	−	−	−	−	−	−	−	−	−		
70	62	−	−	−	−	−	−	−	−	−	−	−	−	−	−	−		
60	52	−	−	−	−	−	−	−	−	−	−	−	−	−	−	−		
50	42	+	+	−	−	−	−	−	−	−	−	−	−	−	−	−		
40	33	+	+	+	+	+	+	+	+	+	+	−	−	−	−	−		
30	24						+	+	+	+	+	+	+	+	+	+	−	−
25	20						+	+	+	+	+	+	+	+	+	+	+	−
20	16						+	+	+	+	+	+	+	+	+	+	+	−

+, growth; −, no growth

From Morton, H.W. 1950. Relationship of concentration and germicidal efficacy of ethyl alcohol. Ann. N.Y. Acad. Sci., 532, 191–196.

50% alcohol required 60 seconds. Tubercle bacilli in water suspensions were killed in 15 seconds by 95% alcohol, in 30 seconds by absolute alcohol, and in 60 seconds by 70% alcohol. When tuberculous sputum was allowed to dry on cover slips and then subjected to the action of the alcohols, 50% alcohol killed the tubercle bacilli in 1 or 2 minutes, depending on the thickness of the smears. In thin smears, 70% alcohol killed the organisms in 1 minute, but in thick smears, 95% alcohol killed the organisms in 20 minutes and absolute alcohol did not kill in an exposure of 60 minutes. Smith concluded that 95% ethyl alcohol was best for wet surfaces, 50% for dry surfaces, and 70% for either wet or dry surfaces.

The number of tubercle bacilli has an effect upon the killing action of 95% alcohol. When 0.0001 or 0.1 mg of bacilli were used, some of the subcultures were sterile after the organisms had been exposed for 2 minutes, and all subcultures from the longer exposures were sterile (Cohn, 1934). Of course, inoculum size has an important influence on efficacy of any germicide. Frobisher and Sommermeyer (1953) observed that 80 to 100% concentrations of ethanol were effective in killing tubercle bacilli only if precautions were taken to ensure intimate contact, such as violent shaking, between organisms and alcohol before the sputum became coagulated.

Like most chemical disinfectants, alcohol appears to be more toxic for certain tissue cells than for bacterial cells. Welch and Brewer (1942) found absolute alcohol to be 7.5 times more toxic for the phagocytic cells of human and guinea pig blood than for *Staphylococcus aureus*.

Effect of Ethyl Alcohol on Spiroplasmas

Using a microtiter technique, it was found that various species of *Spiroplasma* (microorganisms lacking walls) varied in their susceptibility to ethanol as well as to other antibacterial agents, such as formalin, glutaraldehyde, and phenol. A strain of *Spiroplasma* of tick origin, designated SMCA (suckling mouse, cataract agent), and two strains of honey-bee origin were comparable to *Staphylococcus aureus* and *Escherichia coli* (cell-wall bacteria) in susceptibility to the antibacterial action of alcohol; the 5 cultures survived in 30% alcohol for as long as 40 minutes. *Spiroplasma citri* was the most susceptible of the strains tested, surviving 20% ethanol for only 5 minutes. Against phenol, one of the honey-bee strains was comparable to *Staphylococcus aureus* and *Escherichia coli* in susceptibility, whereas the remaining strains of spiroplasma were more susceptible (Stanek et al., 1981).

Effect of Ethyl Alcohol on Bacterial Spores

Several investigators (Heuzenroeder and Johnson, 1958; Hare et al., 1963) have demonstrated that ethyl alcohol has little effect against bacterial spores. The greater killing action of alcohol for vegetative cells as compared to that for spores has been employed to facilitate the isolation of *Clostridium botulinum* type E (Johnson et al., 1964). Coulthard and Sykes (1936) demonstrated that the bactericidal action of ethyl alcohol was greatly increased by the addition of 10% amylmetacresol, or 1% hydrochloric, nitric, phosphoric, or sulfuric acid, or sodium or potassium hydroxide. They stated that the bactericidal action of methyl and isopropyl alcohols could be similarly enhanced. Samples of alcohols of various concentrations have been reported to occasionally contain bacterial spores. Gershenfeld (1938) tested 100 samples of 95% alcohol and 25 samples of absolute alcohol obtained on the open market from many different sources in the United States and found all to be free of bacteria and bacterial spores.

Alcohol may become contaminated with spores from having contaminated materials immersed in it. Kuhn and Dombrowsky (1932) reported half of the samples of alcohols tested to be contaminated. Fatal infections with *Clostridium* were reported by Nye and Mallory (1923) when alcohol was used for sterilization of surgical instruments contaminated with bacterial spores. Saegesser (1941) demonstrated gas gangrene bacilli in 70% alcohol in which syringes were stored and emphasized that alcohol was not an adequate method for disinfection.

Effect of Ethyl Alcohol on Fungi and Fungal Spores

The spores of *Tricophyton gypseum* were not killed by 50% alcohol but were killed by 85% alcohol in an exposure of 30 minutes (Emmons, 1933). Seventy percent alcohol inhibited the growth of *Microsporum audouini* from 40% of naturally infected hairs after an exposure of 1 to 2 minutes, and the inhibition was increased to 100% by an exposure of 1 hour (Loewenthal, 1961). Spaulding (1939) observed that *Candida albicans* was completely inhibited by a 1-minute exposure to 70% ethanol, even when the fungus was contained in pus and blood.

Seventy percent was the most effective concentration of ethyl alcohol for killing the tissue phase of *Cryptococcus neoformans*, *Blastomyces dermatidis*, *Coccidioides immitis*, and *Histoplasma capsulatum*, and for killing the culture phase of the latter three organisms when aerosolized onto painted wood, glass, stainless steel, neoprene, and asphalt floor tile surfaces (Kruse et al., 1963, 1964). Against the conidia of *Penicillium tardum*, Luthi (1954) observed that, within the range of 70 to 96%, the concentration of 90% ethanol exerted the greatest sporicidal effect.

Denatured Alcohol

Ethyl alcohol (96%) denatured by the addition of 10% methyl alcohol was found by Olivo (1948) to have practically the same bactericidal power as ethyl alcohol. His tests were made with *Staphylococcus aureus* and *Escherichia coli*.

Phenylethyl Alcohol

Phenylethyl alcohol (benzylcarbinol) was discovered by Lilley and Brewer (1953) to have a unique property among the alcohols in that it has a greater inhibitory effect against gram-negative than against gram-positive organisms. By incorporating 0.25% phenylethyl alcohol in the culture medium, it is possible to isolate gram-positive organisms from material containing troublesome contaminating gram-negative organisms such as *Proteus* species.

Mycoplasmas have been observed to be totally inactivated within 20 minutes by exposure to 1% phenylethyl alcohol, but enveloped viruses resisted such treatment (Staal and Towe, 1974). The stable L-form of *Streptococcus faecium*, but not the parent *S. faecium*, was lysed by 0.5 to 0.6% (v/v) phenylethyl alcohol (King, 1974).

Isopropyl Alcohol

The propyl alcohols (normal-propyl and isopropyl) are the alcohols of the highest molecular weight that are miscible with water in all proportions. Tanner and Wilson (1943) found normal-propyl alcohol to be the strongest bactericide of the water-soluble alcohols. In a review of the literature on isopropyl alcohol, Grant (1923) pointed out that it had no noticeable harmful effect on the human skin although it is slightly more toxic than ethyl alcohol. However, isopropyl alcohol vapors may be absorbed through the lungs and produce narcosis. Senz and Goldfarb (1958) stated that isopropyl was twice as toxic as ethyl alcohol and produced greater and longer-lasting toxic effects. Toxic reactions have been reported in children who were given alcohol sponge baths to reduce fever (Garrison, 1953; Wise, 1969).

The bactericidal action of isopropyl alcohol is slightly greater than that of ethyl alcohol. By making counts of surviving organisms after 30 seconds of exposure to varying concentrations of alcohols, Coulthard and Sykes (1936) found isopropyl alcohol slightly more bactericidal than either ethyl or methyl alcohol for *Escherichia coli* and *Staphylococcus aureus*.

Powell (1945) reported that *Staphylococcus aureus* was killed by a 1-minute exposure at 20° C to 50%, 60%, 70%, 80%, and 91% isopropyl alcohol solutions, but not by 20%, 30%, and 40% solutions. Other tests showed that the same organisms were killed in 5 minutes by 40% and greater concentrations of isopropyl alcohol, but not by 10%, 20%, or 30% solutions. *Escherichia coli* was killed in 5 minutes at 20° C by 30% and greater concentrations of isopropyl alcohol but not by 10 or 20% solutions. Well spored cultures of *Bacillus subtilis* and *Clostridium novyi* were not killed in 60 minutes at 20° C by any concentration of isopropyl alcohol ranging from 20 to 91%. In tests performed some 10 years earlier, Powell stated that the stocks of isopropyl alcohol were contaminated with a saprophytic spore-forming organism, which further substantiates its ineffectiveness against bacterial spores. The sporicidal activity of isopropyl alcohol can be greatly increased by adding 5% propylene oxide and maintaining a temperature of 30° C (Hart and Ng, 1975).

Tainter et al. (1944) reported that *Staphylococcus aureus* was killed in less than 10 seconds by a 50% aqueous solution of isopropyl alcohol. A 90% solution failed to kill the organisms in an exposure of 2 hours, thus emphasizing the importance of the presence of water for effective bactericidal action, as in the case of ethyl alcohol.

Against tubercle bacilli in dried sputum smears, Smith (1947) observed that the bactericidal activity of isopropyl alcohol paralleled that of ethyl alcohol in the upper and middle ranges of concentrations, but surpassed that of ethyl alcohol in the range of lower concentrations. Frobisher and Sommermeyer (1953) obtained results with 70 to 50% isopropyl alcohol that were comparable to those obtained with 80 to 100% ethanol against tubercle bacilli and other bacilli in sputum when precautions were taken to ensure intimate contact between the bacteria and alcohol before the sputum became coagulated. For a comparison of the ability of isopropyl alcohol to disinfect clinical thermometers with that of ethyl alcohol, the publications of Gershenfeld et al. (1951) and Sommermeyer and Frobisher (1952) should be consulted.

Aromatic Alcohols

Of the aromatic alcohols, benzyl alcohol appears to be the only one tested in recent years. It is soluble in water with difficulty, which perhaps explains its limited use. Prombo and Tilden (1950) found 4% benzyl alcohol by weight less effective than 70% ethyl alcohol (either by weight or by volume) or isopropyl alcohol (99%) in preventing infection in mice with *Streptococcus pneumoniae*. Benzyl alcohol, 4% by weight, was slightly better than ethyl alcohol (70% by weight) or isopropyl alcohol (99%) in protecting mice against infection with *Streptococcus pyogenes*.

The fate of *Pseudomonas aeruginosa* was determined in saline alone, 0.9%, and in saline, 0.9%, containing 0.9% benzyl alcohol. One ml of a 1:100 dilution of an overnight culture of *P. aeruginosa* in broth was added to 150-ml bottles of saline and saline plus 0.9% benzyl alcohol. The contents of the bottles were thoroughly mixed by shaking, and the bacterial concentrations were determined immediately and at 24-hour intervals by making pour plate preparations of appropriate dilutions of the contents of each bottle. It cannot be overemphasized that "bacteriostatic" preparations are not necessarily sterile preparations.

Long-Chain Alcohols

Maximum inhibition of growth of *Mycoplasma gallisepticum* and *M. pneumoniae* was obtained by the saturated primary alcohols varying in chain length from 16 to 19 carbon atoms at 64-μm concentration. The unsaturated alcohols, oleyl, linoleyl, and linolenyl, were less effective as inhibitors. The inhibitory effect of 48-μm concentrations of stearyl alcohol was not significantly mitigated by a concentration of 128 μm cholesterol (Fletcher et al., 1981).

EFFECT OF ALCOHOLS ON VIRUSES

Vaccinia virus was reported by Gordon (1925) to be inactivated by 50% ethyl alcohol in 1 hour but not by 20% alcohol in 24 hours. Methyl alcohol appeared to be slightly more effective in that a 20% concentration had a noticeable effect in 1 hour and inactivated the virus in

24 hours. Groupe et al. (1955) likewise reported a strong virucidal action of ethanol on chick embryo material during an exposure at 25° C for 10 minutes. The virus of Newcastle disease was observed by Cunningham (1948) to be inactivated by 70 and 95% alcohols in an exposure period of 3 minutes. Alcohol of 40 and 25% concentrations did not inactivate the virus under similar conditions. The results with 25% ethyl alcohol were comparable to those with isopropyl alcohol in a report by Tilley and Anderson (1947). When mixed with an equal volume of saline filtrate of the virus of hoof-and-mouth disease and held at room temperature, ethyl alcohol did not inactivate the virus in 3 days but did so in 6 days (Stockman and Minett, 1926). Ethyl alcohol in a dilution of 1 in 6, formalin 1 in 15, eosin (yellowish) 1 in 300, sodium oleate 1 in 50, and liquor cresolis compositus 1 in 200 were reported by Frobisher (1930) to inactivate the virus of yellow fever (Asibi strain) contained in monkey serum. Bichloride of mercury 1 in 7500, phenol 1 in 150, hexylresorcinol 1 in 1500, and sodium oleate 1 in 150 did not inactivate the virus of yellow fever. The virus of eastern equine encephalomyelitis (1% aqueous suspension of chick embryo material) was reduced in activity 4 logs or more after 1 hour of exposure at 18 to 20° C to 50% ethyl alcohol (Bucca, 1956).

Ethyl alcohol in a final concentration of 20% brought about a loss in activity exceeding 95% of the virus of mouse encephalomyelitis, in mouse brain suspension, after 45 minutes' exposure in refrigerator (Theiler and Gard, 1940), but ether had no apparent effect. Two strains of the virus of rabbit fibroma (Shope) were inactivated in 1 hour at 0° C by 30 and 40% concentrations of ethyl alcohol (Pontier and Chaumont, 1954). Against the Lansing strain of poliomyelitis virus, ethyl alcohol in concentrations of 63 and 70% had little virucidal action (Faber and Dong, 1953). Influenza virus, type A, in chick embryo material, was exposed to varying concentrations of ethyl alcohol for 10 minutes at 25° C. A concentration of 14% ethanol exerted no action, 35% exerted a weak action, and 70% completely inactivated the virus under the conditions of the test (Groupe et al., 1955).

Ethyl alcohol in the concentrations of 70 to 90% inactivated all viruses tested that were representative of seven general types of viruses (Klein and Deforest, 1963). The greatest virucidal action was against those viruses with a lipid envelope. For general virucidal activity, ethanol was stronger than isopropyl alcohol. Isopropyl alcohol in concentrations of 48.5 and 99% showed a strong inactivating effect on vaccinia virus and influenza virus, type A (Groupe et al, 1955). In a concentration of 49.5%, it reduced the activity of eastern equine encephalomyelitis virus 4 logs or more after 1-hour exposure at 18 to 20° C (Bucca, 1956).

Tilley and Anderson (1947) mixed equal volumes of 50% isopropyl alcohol and suspension of the virus of Newcastle disease. After varying periods of exposure up to 60 minutes at 20° C, portions of the mixtures were diluted with distilled water, and portions of this diluted mixture inoculated into chick embryos. All the embryos died, but it must be pointed out that a 25% solution is much weaker than that which gives maximum bactericidal action.

Isopropyl alcohol was less active than ethyl alcohol against the enteroviruses, but slightly more active than ethanol against the viruses with a lipid envelope (Klein and Deforest, 1963). A comparison of the activities of the two alcohols against viruses is summarized in Table 11–3.

Caspo et al. (1962) reported that the serum from individuals with hepatitis B infection still contained active virus, although it was attenuated, after treatment with 40% ethyl alcohol for 14 days at −5° C. Horst et al. (1972) reported that exposure to 80% ethanol for 3 hours did not inactivate the immunologic reactivity of hepatitis B surface antigen. On the other hand, Bond et al. (1983) noted inactivation of the virus by isopropyl alcohol, and Kobayashi et al. (1984), using chimpanzee inoculation as an assay method, found that a 2-minute exposure to 80% ethyl alcohol at 11° C was effective in preventing transmission of hepatitis B in treated plasma.

Even though animal rotaviruses have been shown to be relatively resistant to a number of common disinfectants and antiseptics (Tan and Schnagl, 1981; Snodgrass and Herring, 1977), Sattar et al. (1983) reported that a formulation of 70% isopropyl alcohol and 0.1% hexachlorophene produced a 3 or greater $\log_{10}$ (99.9%) reduction in human rotavirus plaque titer, even in the

Table 11–3. *The Virucidal Action of Ethyl and Isopropyl Alcohols on Seven Viruses*

Virus	Lowest Concentration Inactivating in 10 Minutes		Lipid Envelope	Lipophilic
	Ethyl	Isopropyl		
Poliovirus, type 1	70%	95% (Negative)		
Coxsackie B-1	60%	95% (Negative)		
ECHO 6	50%	90%		
Adenovirus, type 2	50%	50%		+
Herpes simplex	30%	20%	+	+
Vaccinia	40%	30%	+	+
Influenza, Asian	30%	30%	+	+

From Klein, M., and Deforest, A. 1963. Antiviral action of germicides. Soap Chem. Spec., *39*, 70–72, 95–97.

presence of organic matter, after a 1-minute contact time. In a suspension test, both ethyl and isopropyl alcohol were effective in inactivating human rotavirus at concentrations of 70% or greater, again in the presence of organic matter (Springthorpe et al., 1986). In another study designed to simulate conditions in nature, human rotavirus was suspended in diluted fecal samples and placed on inanimate surfaces. Using this protocol, Lloyd-Evans et al. (1986) reported that 70% (v/v) ethyl and isopropyl alcohol did not inactivate the virus, whereas these alcohols in concentrations over 40% had marked virucidal activity when combined with other active ingredients such as chlorhexidine gluconate.

In contrast to the rotavirus, the retrovirus, human immunodeficiency virus (HIV), is readily inactivated by most chemical disinfectants, including alcohols. Using reverse transcriptase as an indicator of viral inactivation, Spire et al. (1984) reported a 99% reduction in activity after 5 minutes of treatment with 19% ethanol, and complete inactivation of HIV with concentrations greater than 20%. They recommend 25% ethanol or 1% glutaraldehyde as effective means to disinfect instruments contaminated with HIV. Using a microculture assay to calculate the infectious HIV titer (ID_{50}), defined as the reciprocal of the dilution at which 50% of the cultures were positive, Martin et al. (1985) tested isopropyl, ethyl, and absolute alcohol with exposure times of 2 to 10 minutes. HIV was inactivated in 50% ethyl alcohol and in 35% isopropyl alcohol. Likewise, Resnick et al. (1986) reported complete loss of HIV infectivity (a reduction of more than 7 log_{10} tissue culture infectious dose) after 1-minute exposure to 70% alcohol. Respiratory syncytial virus has also been shown to be rapidly destroyed by 70% isopropanol (Platt and Bucknall, 1985).

ALCOHOLS FOR CHEMICAL DISINFECTION

The availability of more reliable alternatives such as ethylene oxide and glutaraldehyde makes the use of alcohol for instrument disinfection unnecessary and inadvisable. Indeed, the inability of alcohols, like other chemical disinfectants, to destroy bacterial spores makes their use as a disinfectant hazardous. Nevertheless, in the absence of bacterial spores, alcohol is better than many substances. Spaulding (1939) observed that 70% ethyl alcohol killed *Candida albicans*, *Escherichia coli*, *Streptococcus pyogenes*, and *Pseudomonas aeruginosa* on knife blades contaminated with pus or blood within 1 minute; rarely was exposure of 2 minutes required. *Staphylococcus aureus* was slightly more resistant when the pus and blood were dried. Exposures of 10 minutes were required to kill the organisms in dried pus and 5 minutes in dried blood. *Clostridium tetani*, *Clostridium perfringens*, and *Bacillus anthracis* were not killed after an exposure of 18 hours, except *B. anthracis* in wet pus, which was killed in that period. Although Ziegler and Jacoby (1956) reported that soaking in 70% ethyl alcohol completely destroyed vegetative bacteria on airways, endotracheal tubes, and cuffs within 15 minutes, Winge-

Heden (1962) reported that such soaking did not always sterilize rubber tubing. Force and Kerr (1920) reported that an exposure of 4 minutes to 50% ethyl alcohol adequately disinfected oral glass thermometers if they were wiped with a cotton sponge wet with water to free them of mucus before placing them in the alcohol.

Sommermeyer and Frobisher (1952) contaminated glass rods or unfilled oral thermometers with a thin film of tuberculous sputum that was strongly positive for acid-fast bacilli by direct smear examination. Cultures of *Corynebacterium diphtheriae* were added to the samples of sputum, which contained staphylococci, streptococci, and other bacteria in addition to the acid-fast bacilli. The contaminated thermometers were then allowed to dry for 30 minutes. This level of contamination probably exceeded that encountered in ordinary practice, so the results erred on the side of safety. These authors found that wiping the thermometers with cotton and a mixture of equal parts of 95% ethyl alcohol and tincture of green soap before placing in the disinfectant decreased the number of viable organisms in practically every case. After the cleaning procedure, immersion of the thermometers for 10 minutes in 70% ethyl or isopropyl alcohol containing 0.5 or 1% iodine reduced the number of viable organisms to a low number. Aqueous iodine solutions or 70% solutions of ethyl or isopropyl alcohol were nearly as effective as the alcoholic iodine solutions. The importance of wiping the thermometers was emphasized by Ryan and Miller (1932).

Gershenfeld et al. (1951) tested various agents for their ability to disinfect 2-inch segments of thermometers contaminated with bacterial cultures. Ethyl alcohol in 95%, 70%, and 50% concentrations, isopropyl alcohol in 70 and 50% concentrations, and 2% iodine, aqueous solution and tincture, were tested. *Streptococcus pneumoniae* was killed by all disinfectants within 20 seconds. *Streptococcus pyogenes* was killed by all disinfectants within 20 seconds, except 95% ethyl alcohol, which required 60 seconds. Cultures of these two organisms were used to contaminate the thermometer segments and, without drying, the segments were transferred to the disinfectants. This may be one factor that accounts for the fast killing action in the experiments. Ecker and Smith (1937) reported that thermometers contaminated with sputum from cases of lobar pneumonia were not sterilized by exposures for as long as 30 minutes to 70 and 95% solutions of ethyl alcohol. This is difficult to interpret in light of the findings of Sommermeyer and Frobisher (1952) and of Gershenfeld et al. (1951) with pure cultures of *Streptococcus pneumoniae*. The sputum may have exerted a protective action, as Gershenfeld et al. observed for plasma.

The activity of alcohols in the presence of organic material, particularly blood, pus, or feces, deserves additional study. Although some researchers have reported continued activity of the alcohols in the presence of organic material (Spaulding, 1939; Smith, 1947; Springthorpe et al., 1986), others report reduced effectiveness

(Gershenfeld et al., 1951). Wallbank (1985) stated that 80% (v/w) ethanol was neutralized by rabbit blood in his laboratory, but study methods were not described.

ALCOHOLS IN SKIN DEGERMING

It is probably not possible to sterilize the skin; the best one can hope to accomplish is to reduce the number of viable organisms on or in the skin and to destroy the pathogenic organisms that may be on the skin as transients. Price (1939) pointed out that, in the surgical scrub, immersion of the hand and arms in a 65.5% solution of alcohol by weight for 1 minute was as effective as scrubbing for 4.2 minutes in reducing the number of bacteria on the skin. This effectiveness of alcohol has been amply confirmed (Pohle and Stuart, 1940; Pillsbury et al., 1942; Hatfield and Lockwood, 1943; Gardner and Seddon, 1946; Gardner, 1948; Story, 1952; Rotter, 1984; Ayliffe, 1984; Larson et al., 1986).

Employing a testing procedure similar to that of Price, Hatfield and Lockwood (1943) concluded that ethyl alcohol in strengths of 95 or 70% by weight was preferable to any of a group of commercially prepared agents available for skin degerming at that time. The ideal concentration was 95%, but for economy the concentration could be reduced to 70%. Pillsbury et al. (1942) also observed that 80% or more by volume produced a satisfactory decrease in the number of viable bacteria remaining on or in the skin. They expressed doubt about the necessity of alcohol of an exact concentration for clinical use so long as the concentration exceeds 70% by volume.

Skin bacteria have been described as "transients" and "residents" (Price, 1938). The transient bacteria lie free on the skin or are loosely attached by lipoidal substances. Their removal is relatively easy compared to removal of the resident bacteria, which are a relatively stable population in size and kinds. The terms exposed and sheltered flora, in place of transient and resident flora, were proposed by Evans et al. (1980). They observed that in 15 individuals with a sparce flora in the antecubital fossa, no surviving bacteria were detected after alcohol treatment (60 seconds), but in 10 individuals with a more abundant flora, viable bacteria remained, and their number bore no quantitative correlation with the surface flora. Following scrubbing of the skin after alcohol treatment, sheltered or resident bacteria could be demonstrated in each of the individuals studied. Lacey (1968) cleaned the skin on the forearm with alcohol, applied *Staphylococcus aureus*, and covered it with an occlusive dressing for 5 hours. The degree of decrease in bactericidal activity of the skin was about the same as for soap and was thought to be due to the removal of bactericidal substances from the skin. On the other hand, Lowbury et al. (1979) noted that the bacterial counts on alcohol-scrubbed hands continued to drop for several hours after gloving and concluded that this was probably a result of the continued death of damaged organisms. Likewise, Larson et al. (1988) found that regrowth of colonizing flora after 4 hours of gloving was minimal after a 5-minute scrub with a formulation of 70% ethyl alcohol and 0.5% chlorhexidine gluconate.

Studies of skin antiseptics are generally divided into those which assess the effects on transient, artificially contaminating flora, and those which assess effects on colonizing or resident flora. Many of these studies vary in design and with regard to important variables such as contact time and method of product application. Sebben (1983) noted that 70% ethanol destroyed 90% of cutaneous bacteria after 2 minutes of contact, but emphasized the necessity of maintaining moist conditions throughout the entire time of application.

Effect of Alcohols on Contaminating Flora

In 1977 Rotter et al. developed a test method for the evaluation of health care personnel handwash products. The method, with some modifications, has been adopted by the German and Austrian governments for testing health care personnel handwashing products (Deutsche Gessellschaft fur Hygiene und Pravenventivmedizin, 1981). The method includes artificial contamination of the hands with *Escherichia coli*, decontamination with two 30-second applications of 3 ml of 60% (by volume) isopropanol as a standard, compared with any test product applied according to manufacturer's directions. He has reported (Rotter, 1981; Rotter, 1984; Rotter et al., 1986) 4 or greater $\log_{10}$ reductions with all alcohols tested, in comparison with 2 to 3 $\log_{10}$ reductions with soaps containing phenolic, chlorhexidine, or povidone-iodine. Efficacy in those studies was greatest for 50 to 60% n-propanol, and comparable for 60% isopropanol and 70 to 80% ethanol.

Ulrich (1982) contaminated hands with *Micrococcus roseus* and used a glove-fluid sampling protocol to test products containing 7.5% povidone-iodine and a combination of 70% isopropyl alcohol and 0.5% chlorhexidine gluconate. He reported 2 to 3 $\log_{10}$ reductions after 5, 10, 15, 20, and 25 repetitive contamination and degerming cycles, with the alcohol-based product significantly better at each test point. Aly and Maibach (1980), using a similar contamination/treatment procedure and sampling protocol, reported the same combination of 70% alcohol and 0.5% chlorhexidine to be significantly superior to 70% isopropyl alcohol in reducing counts of *Serratia marcescens*. Marples and Towers (1979) developed a model to assess the transfer of organisms by contact. They contaminated a fabric-covered bottle with *Staphylococcus saprophyticus*. Subjects grasped the contaminated bottle, then a sterile fabric-covered bottle, and the numbers of organisms transferred were counted. Washing hands with plain soap reduced transfer by 95%, whereas washing in 500 ml of 70% ethanol for 30 seconds reduced transfer by 99.9%. Fifteen minutes after testing, the contaminating organism was still present on the hands of subjects who washed with soap, but was undetectable on alcohol-treated hands. An alcohol-impregnated towelette and a small volume (0.2 ml) of 80% ethanol resulted in reductions of a lesser magnitude, 80 and

93% respectively. Casewell et al. (1988) demonstrated complete removal of an epidemic multiply-resistant strain of *Klebsiella* using 0.5% chlorhexidine in isopropyl alcohol. Butz et al. (1990) reported reductions in colonizing flora following use of 30% ethyl alcohol-impregnated towelettes to be comparable to reductions following plain soap. This emphasizes the importance of the volume of alcohol to its antimicrobial efficacy.

Effects of Alcohols on Colonizing Flora

In a series of studies conducted by a group of British investigators (Lilly and Lowbury, 1971; Lowbury and Lilly, 1973; Lowbury et al., 1974; Lilly et al., 1979), plain soap, 4% chlorhexidine in detergent base, 10% povidone-iodine detergent, and 70% isopropyl alcohol with 0.5% chlorhexidine were compared in a surgical scrub protocol. The alcoholic chlorhexidine produced the greatest initial reduction in bacterial flora (98% as compared with 87% for chlorhexidine detergent, 68% for povidone-iodine, and 13% for soap), but the chlorhexidine and povidone-iodine detergents had almost identical effects to the alcoholic product (greater than 99% reductions in flora) after six applications. Ayliffe (1984) reported continued reductions in bacterial counts following hand degerming with 70% isopropyl alcohol as well as alcoholic chlorhexidine and chlorhexidine detergent after wearing gloves for 3 hours. Alcoholic preparations are efficacious as surgical scrubs, perhaps in part because of their superior activity in reducing bacterial populations under the fingernails (Gross et al. 1979; McGinley et al. 1988; Larson et al. 1990).

Several investigators have evaluated the effectiveness of alcohols as hand rinses after short contact times. Morrison et al. (1986) compared three alcohol-based hand rinses, including 70% isopropanol, 0.5% chlorhexidine in 70% isopropanol, and a 60% isopropanol formulation containing evaporative retardants, in 14 subjects. The 60% isopropanol with evaporative retardants was associated with significantly greater reductions after each of four consecutive handwashes. Similarly, Larson et al. (1986) reported significant reductions over baseline counts among subjects using this formulation of isopropanol after a single 15-second application. After use 15 times per day for 5 consecutive days, subjects using either one of two alcoholic hand rinses, 70% isopropyl alcohol, or 4% chlorhexidine in detergent all had significant reductions in their colonizing flora, but the two alcoholic hand rinses continued to be associated with the greatest reductions. There was no significant change in bacterial counts among subjects using a nonmedicated control soap.

In another study, Larson et al. (1987) demonstrated a significant dose response with two alcohol hand rinses: subjects using 3-ml hand rinse had significantly greater reductions in bacterial flora counts than did subjects using 1-ml rinse. Contrary to popular opinion, alcoholic products seem to be quite acceptable to users, and newer formulations containing emollients reduce the drying effects of alcohol on skin (Gross et al. 1979; Larson et al.,

Table 11–4. *Mean Log Reductions in Bacterial Counts with Various Products*

Product	Transient Flora: After 30-sec wash*	Normal Flora: After Surgical Scrub†
Plain, unmedicated soap	2.1	<1.0
7.5% povidone-iodine liquid soap	2.5	<1.0
4.0% chlorhexidine gluconate liquid soap	2.9	<1.0
70% isopropyl alcohol (v/v) + 0.5% chlorhexidine gluconate	3.1	~2.5
70% isopropyl alcohol (v/v)	3.3	~2.5
60% n-propanol (v/v)	3.4	~3.0

*Data from Rotter, 1981
†Data from Ayliffe et al., 1988

1986; Larson et al., 1987; Nystrom, 1984; Mitchell and Rawluk, 1984; Jones et al., 1986). Based on these data, alcohols deserve serious consideration for use as surgical scrubs and hand cleansing (Table 11–4).

The use of alcohol-based products for preoperative patient skin preparation has been evaluated by several investigators. Davies et al. (1978) reported greater than 99% immediate reductions in bacterial counts from skin of the abdomen when using 70% isopropanol, 70% alcoholic chlorhexidine, or povidone-iodine. Geelhoed et al. (1983) randomly assigned 173 patients to one of three skin preparation methods: a traditional 5-minute iodophor scrub followed by painting and draping of the skin; the same 5-minute scrub followed by alcohol cleansing (type and percentage of alcohol was unspecified) and application of an iodophor-impregnated drape; or a 1-minute alcohol cleansing followed by application of the antimicrobial drape. The bacterial kill after the 1-minute alcohol cleansing was significantly better than that of the 5-minute iodophor scrub. Johnston et al. (1987) studied the rate of bacterial recolonization of the skin of the abdomen in 15 volunteers after treatment with chlorhexidine or povidone-iodine in 70% alcohol for 3 minutes; 70% isopropyl alcohol for 1 minute and application of a plastic adhesive drape; or 70% isopropyl alcohol and application of an iodophor-impregnated drape. Although all methods were initially comparable, with bacterial reductions of greater than 99%, recolonization of the site was significantly reduced after 60 minutes at the site prepared with the alcohol and iodophor drape when compared to the other methods.

ABILITY OF ALCOHOLS TO PREVENT INFECTION

The crucial test of any disinfectant is the ability of the substance to prevent infection in a susceptible animal with the test organism. Neufeld and Schiemann (1938) demonstrated by intraperitoneal injection in mice that a culture of *Streptococcus pneumoniae*, type 1, was killed by treatment with 80% alcohol. Not all of the pneumococci were destroyed when 96% alcohol was used.

Nungester and Kempf (1942) devised a test in which the tail of a mouse was scrubbed with 4 or 5 strokes of a swab that had been moistened with a broth culture of the test organism. The tail was then dipped for 2 minutes into a tube containing disinfectant. At the end of this time, a half-inch portion of the tail was cut off and implanted in the peritoneum of the same animal. In the case of *Streptococcus pneumoniae*, type 1, 100% of the mice died following treatment with either physiologic salt solution, which served as a control, or aqueous thimerosal (Merthiolate), 1:1000. The mortality rate was 69% among the mice when a mixture of 50% alcohol and 10% acetone was used; the mortality rate was 63% when 70% alcohol (by volume) was employed. Employing 2% aqueous iodine solution resulted in a mortality rate of only 5%, but when a 2% iodine solution in 95% alcohol was employed, the mortality rate was 0%. When using a hemolytic streptococcus, none of the animals was protected by the use of the alcohol-acetone mixture.

Employing the technique of Nungester and Kempf, Prombo and Tilden (1950) reported a mortality rate of slightly more than 10% when using 70% alcohol by weight, and slightly less than 20% when using 70% ethyl alcohol by volume. With *Streptococcus pyogenes* and 70% alcohol by weight, mortality was 20% in the mice. In preventing infection in mice with *Streptococcus pneumoniae*, the authors found 99% isopropyl alcohol as effective as ethyl alcohol, 70% by weight, and nearly as effective as ethyl alcohol, 70% by volume. It was less effective than ethyl alcohol, 70% by weight, in preventing infection in mice with *Streptococcus pyogenes*.

Murie and Macpherson (1980) compared postoperative wound infection rates associated with two hand-scrub techniques in the operating room. They alternated each month for a period of 6 months between 0.5% chlorhexidine in 95% methanol and 4% chlorhexidine in detergent. Among 226 patients studied (117 in one group, 109 in the other), there was no difference in infection rates. Additionally, the alcoholic preparation was five times less expensive, less time-consuming, and more acceptable to users.

Dorff et al. (1985) compared the use of triple dye versus alcohol (type not specified) for umbilical cord care in neonates and the impact on staphylococcal infections in a newborn nursery over a 1-year period. There was no significant difference in infection rates (0.4% for newborns receiving triple dye and 0.6% for those receiving alcohol treatments). The alcohol-treated infants had fewer cord complications and better healing of umbilical stumps. Butz et al. (1989) evaluated the effect of use of a 60% ethyl alcohol hand rinse by day-care providers in 12 centers in reducing transmission of infection among preschool children. When compared with 12 control centers over a 19-month period (8840 child days), children in 12 test centers had fewer fever days (69 versus 122,

$p < .001$), vomiting days (11 versus 62, $p < .001$), and diarrhea days (77 versus 102, $p = .09$).

REFERENCES

Aly, R., and Maibach, H.I. 1980. A comparison of the antimicrobial effect of 0.5% chlorhexidine (Hibistat) and 70% isopropyl alcohol on hands contaminated with *Serratia marcescens*. Clin. Exp. Dermatol., 5, 197–201.

Ayliffe, G.A.J. 1984. Surgical scrub and skin disinfection. Infect. Control, 5, 23–27.

Ayliffe, G.A.J., Bobb, J.R., Davies, J.G., and Lilly, H.A. 1988. Hand disinfection: A comparison of various agents in laboratory and ward studies. J. Hosp. Infect., 11, 226–243.

Beck, W.C. 1984. Benefits of alcohol rediscovered. AORN J., 40, 172–176.

Bond, W.W., Favero, M.S., Petersen, N.J., and Ebert, J.W. 1983. Inactivation of hepatitis B virus by intermediate-to-high-level disinfectant chemicals. J. Clin. Microbiol., 18, 535–538.

Bucca, M.A. 1956. The effect of various chemical agents on eastern equine encephalomyelitis virus. J. Bacterial., 71, 491–492.

Butz, A., Laughon, B.E., Gullette, D.L., and Larson, E.L. 1990. An alternative for hand hygiene in community health settings. Am. J. Infec. Contr. 18, 70–76.

Butz, A., Fosarelli, P., and Larson E. 1989. Reduction of infectious disease symptoms in day care homes. Am. J. Dis. Child., 143, 426.

Casewell, M.W., Law, M.M., and Desai, N. 1988. A laboratory model for testing agents for hygienic hand disinfection: Handwashing and chlorhexidine for the removal of Klebsiella. J. Hosp. Infect., 12, 163–175.

Caspo, J., et al. 1962. Studies on the active immunization against epidemic hepatitis. II. The role of the relative amounts of virus and gamma globulin in the inocula: The effect of ethanol treatment on the virus. Acta Paediatr. Acad. Sci. Hung., 3, 167–172.

Cohn, M.L. 1934. The antiseptic effect upon tubercle bacilli of certain recently-advocated compounds. J. Bacteriol., 27, 517–526.

Coulthard, C.E., and Sykes, G. 1936. Germicidal effect of alcohol. Pharm. J., 137, 79–81.

Cox, H.R., van der Scheer, J., Aiston, S., and Bohnel, E. 1947. The purification and concentration of influenza virus by means of alcohol precipitation. J. Immunol., 56, 149–166.

Cunningham, C.H. 1948. The effect of certain chemical agents on the virus of Newcastle disease of chickens. Am. J. Vet. Res., 9, 195–197.

Dagley, S., Dawes, E.A., and Morrison, G.A. 1950. Inhibition of growth of *Aerobacter aerogenes*: The mode of action of phenols, alcohols, acetone and ethyl acetate. J. Bacteriol., 60, 369–379.

Davies, J., et al. 1978. Disinfection of the skin of the abdomen. Br. J. Surg., 65, 855–858.

Deutsche Gesellschaft fur Hygiene und Mikrobiologie. 1981. Richtlinien fur die prufung und bewertung chemischer disinfektionsverfahren—erster Teilabschnitt. Zentralbl. Bakteriol. Mikrobiol. Hyg. [B], (I. Abteilung Orginale, Reihe B), 172, 528–556.

Dorff, G., Warshauer, D., Roth, M., and Land, G. 1985. Use of triple dye vs. alcohol in newborn and care for prevention of *Staphylococcus aureus* infections. Proceedings of the 1985 Interscience Conference on Antimicrobial Agents and Chemotherapy, Washington DC: American Society for Microbiology, p. 185.

Ecker, E.E., and Smith, R. 1937. Disinfecting clinical thermometers. Mod. Hosp., 48, 86–87.

Ellner, P.D., Stoessel, C.J., Drakeford, E., and Vasi, F. 1966. A new culture medium for medical bacteriology. Am. J. Clin. Pathol., 45, 502–504.

Emmons, C.W. 1933. Fungicidal action of some common disinfectants on two dermatophytes. Arch. Dermatol., 28, 15–21.

Evans, C.A., and Mattern, K.L. 1980. The bacterial flora of the antecubital fossa: The efficacy of alcohol disinfection of this site, the palm and the forearm. J. Invest. Dermatol., 75, 140–143.

Faber, H.K., and Dong, L. 1953. Poliocidal activity of some common antiseptics with special reference to localized paralysis. Pediatrics, 12, 657–663.

Fletcher, R.D., Gibertson, J.R., Albers, S.C., and White, J.D. 1981. Inactivation of Mycoplasmas by long-chain alcohols. Antimicrob. Agents Chemother., 19, 917–921.

Force, J.N., and Kerr, W.J. 1920. The efficient disinfection of hospital clinical thermometers. Mod. Hosp., 15, 156–158.

Frosbisher, M., Jr., 1930. Properties of yellow fever virus. Am. J. Hyg., 11, 300–320.

Frosbisher, M., Jr., and Sommermeyer, L. 1953. A study of the effect of alcohols on tubercle bacilli and other bacteria in sputum. Am. Rev. Tuberc., 68, 419–424.

Gardner, A.D. 1948. Rapid disinfection of clean unwashed skin. Lancet, 2, 760–763.

Garrison, R.F. 1953. Acute poisoning from use of isopropyl alcohol in tepid sponging. JAMA, 152, 317–318.

Geelhoed, G.W., Sharpe, K., and Simon, G.L. 1983. A comparative study of surgical skin preparation methods. Surg. Gynecol. Obstet., 157, 265–268.

Gershenfeld, L. 1938. The sterility of alcohol. Am. J. Med. Sci., 195, 358–361.

Gershenfeld, L., Greene, A., and Witlin, B. 1951. Disinfection of clinical thermometers. J. Am. Pharm. Assoc., Sci. Ed., 40, 457–460.

Gordon, M.H. 1925. Studies of the viruses of vaccinia and variola. Privy Council, Medical Research Council, Special Report Series No. 98, London.

Grant, D.H. 1923. Antiseptic and bactericidal properties of isopropyl alcohol. Am. J. Med. Sci., 166, 261–265.

Gross, A., Cutright, D.E., and D'Alessandro, S.M. 1979. Effect of surgical scrub on microbial population under the fingernails. Am. J. Surg., 138, 463–465.

Groupe, V., Engle, G.G., Gaffney, P.E., and Manaker, R.A. 1955. Virucidal activity of representative antiinfective agents against influenza A and vaccinia viruses. Appl. Microbiol., 3, 333–336.

Hared, R., Raik, E., and Gash, S. 1963. Efficiency of antiseptics when acting on dried organisms. Br. Med. J., 1, 496–500.

Harrington, C., and Walker, H. 1903. The germicidal action of alcohol. Boston Med. Surg. J., 148, 548–552.

Hart, A., and Ng, S.N. 1975. Effect of temperature on the sterilization of isopropyl alcohol by liquid propylene oxide. Appl. Microbiol., 30, 483–484.

Hatfield, C.A., and Lockwood, J.S. 1943. Evaluation of some materials commonly used for preoperative preparation of skin. Surgery, 13, 931–940.

Hayes, W. 1949. The bactericidal properties of some disinfectants in common use. Br. J. Urol., 21, 198–208.

Heinmets, F., Taylor, W.W., and Lehman, J.J. 1954. The use of metabolites in the restoration of the viability of heat and chemically inactivated Escherichia coli. J. Bacteriol., 67, 5–12.

Heuzenroeder, M., and Johnson, K.D. 1958. Sterilization of chemical agents. Aust. J. Pharm., 40, 944–948.

Hortst, H., Tripatzis, I., and Konstantinidis, I. 1972. Australia antigen: Effect of chemical and physical measures upon antigenicity. Zentralbl. Bakteriol. Mikrobiol. [A], 219, 1–6.

Jones, M.V., Rowe, B.G., Jackson, B., and Prichard, N.J. 1986. The use of alcoholic paper wipes for routine hand cleansing: Results of trials in two hospitals. J. Hosp. Infect., 8, 268–274.

Johnston, D.H., Fairclough, J.A., Brown, E.M., and Morris, R. 1987. Rate of bacterial recolonization of the skin after preparation: Four methods compared. Br. J. Surg., 74, 64.

Johnston, R., Harmon, S., and Kautter, D. 1964. Method to facilitate the isolation of Clostridium botulinum type E. J. Bacteriol., 88, 1521–1522.

King, J.R. 1974. Lysis of enterococcal L-forms by phenylethyl alcohol. Antimicrob. Agents Chemother., 5, 98–100.

Klein, M., and Deforest, A. 1963. Antiviral action of germicides. Soap Chem. Spec., 39, 70–72, 95–97.

Kobayashi, H., et al. 1984. Susceptibility of hepatitis B virus to disinfectants or heat. J. Clin. Microbiol., 20, 214–216.

Kolb, R.W., Schneiter, R., Floyd, E.P., and Byers, D.H. 1952. Disinfective action of methyl bromide, methanol, and hydrogen bromide on anthrax spores. Arch. Ind. Hyg. Occupat. Med., 5, 354–364.

Kruse, R.H., Green, T.D., Chambers, R.C., and Jones, M.W. 1964. Disinfection of aerosolized pathogenic fungi on laboratory surfaces. II. Culture phase. Appl. Microbiol., 12, 155–160.

Kruse, R.H., Green, T.D., Chambers, R.C., and Jones, M.W. 1963. Disinfection of aerosolized pathogenic fungi on laboratory surfaces. I. Tissue phase. Appl. Microbiol., 11, 436–445.

Kuhn, P., and Dombrowsky, K.H. 1932. Ueber die Sterilitat bei Operationen. MMW, 79, 790–793.

Kuipers, J.S. 1974. Skin disinfection with ethanol, without and with additives. Arch. Chir. Neerl. 26, 15–25.

Lacey, R.W. 1968. Antibacterial action of human skin. In vivo effect of acetone, alcohol, and soap on behaviour of Staphylococcus aureus. Br. J. Exp. Pathol., 49, 209–215.

Larson, E.L., Eke, P.I., and Laughon, B.E. 1986. Efficacy of alcohol-based hand rinses under frequent-use conditions. Antimicrob. Agents Chemother., 30, 542–544.

Larson, E.L., Eke, P.I., Wilder, M.P., and Laughon, B.E. 1987. Quantity of soap as a variable in handwashing. Infect. Control, 8, 271–375.

Larson, E.L., Butz, A.M., Gulette, D.L., and Laughon, B.A. 1990. Alcohol for surgical scrubbing? Infec. Contr. Hosp. Epidemiol., 11, 139–143.

Laurenzi, G.A., Guarneri, J.J., Endriga, R.B., and Carey, J.P. 1963. Clearance of bacteria by the lower respiratory tract. Science, 142, 1572–1573.

Leece, J.B. 1954. Personal communication to Dr. Morton.

Lilly, B.D., and Brewer, J.H. 1953. The selective antibacterial action of phenylethyl alcohol. J. Am. Pharm. Assoc., 52, 6–7.

Lilly, H.A., and Lowbury, E.J.L. 1971. Disinfection of skin: An assessment of new preparations. Br. Med. J., 3, 674–676.

Lilly, H.A., Lowbury, E.J.L., and Wilkins, M.D. 1979. Detergents compared with each other and with antiseptics as skin degerming agents. J. Hyg., Camb., 82, 89–93.

Lloyd-Evans, N., Springthrope, V.S., and Sattar, S.A. 1986. Chemical disinfection of human rotavirus-contaminated inanimate surfaces. J. Hyg., Camb., 97, 163–173.

Lowbury, E.J.L., and Lilly, H.A. 1973. The use of 4% chlorhexidine detergent solution (Hibiscrub) and other methods of skin disinfection. Br. Med. J., 1, 510–515.

Lowbury, E.J.L., Lilly, H.A., and Ayliffe, G.A.J. 1974. Preoperative disinfection of surgeons' hands: Use of alcoholic solutions and effects of gloves on skin flora. Br. Med. J., 4, 369–374.

Lowbury, E.J.L., and Lilly, H.A. 1975. Gloved hand as applicator of antiseptic to operation site. Lancet, 2, 15–156.

Lowbury, E.J.L., Lilly, H.A., Wilkins, M.D., et al. 1979. Delayed antimicrobial effects of skin disinfection by alcohol. J. Hyg., Camb., 32, 497–500.

Lowenthal, K. 1961. The antifungal effect of 70% ethyl alcohol. Arch. Dermatol., 83, 803–805.

Lowbury, E.J.L., Lilly, H.A., and Bull, J.P. 1960. Disinfection of the skin of the operation sites. Br. Med. J., 2, 1039–1044.

Luthi, H. 1954. The resistance of conidia of Penicillium to alcohol. Mitt. Lebensm. Hyg., 45, 26–33.

Marples, R.R., and Towers, A.G. 1979. A laboratory model for the investigation of contact transfer of micro-organisms. J. Hyg., Camb., 82, 237–249.

Martin, L.S., McDougal, J.S., and Loskoski, S.L. 1985. Disinfection and inactivation of the human T lymphotropic virus type III/lymphadenopathy associated virus. J. Infect. Dis., 152, 400–403.

McGinley, K.J., Larson, E.L., and Leyden, J.J. 1988. Composition and density of microflora in the subungual space of the hand. J. Clin. Microbiol., 26, 950–953.

Mitchell, K.G., and Rawlulk, D.J.R. 1984. Skin reactions related to surgical scrub-up results of a Scottish survey. Br. J. Surg., 71, 223–224.

Morrison, A.J., Gratz, J., Cabezudo, I., and Wenzel, R.P. 1986. The efficacy of several new handwashing agents for removing non-transient bacterial flora from hands. Infect. Control, 7, 268–272.

Morton, H.W., 1950. Relationship of concentration and germicidal efficacy of ethyl alcohol. Ann. N. Y. Acad. Sci., 532, 191–196.

Murie, J.A., and Macpherson, S.G. 1980. Chlorhexidine in methanol for the preoperative cleansing of surgeons' hands: a clinical trial. Scott. Med. J., 25, 309–311.

Nathanson, C. 1951. Personal communication to Dr. Morton.

Neufeld, F., and Schiemann, O. 1938. Ueber die Wirkung des Alkohols bei der Handedesinfektion. Z. Hyg. Infekt., 121, 312–333.

Noone, P. 1970. Water or alcohol? Lancet, 2, 982.

Novak, M., and Hall, H. 1939. Efficiency of preoperative skin sterilization. Surgery, 5, 560–566.

Nungester, W.J., and Kempf, A.H. 1942. An "infection prevention" test for the evaluation of skin disinfectants. J. Infect. Dis., 71, 174–178.

Nye, R.N., and Mallory, T.B. 1923. Fallacy of using alcohol for sterilization of surgical instruments. Boston Med. Surg. J., 189, 561–563.

Nystrom, B. 1984. Scandinavian experience differs (letter). Infect. Control, 5, 211.

Olivio, R. 1948. Richerche sul potere batericida dell'alcool denaturats. Riv. Ital. Igiene, 8, 430–436.

Osterreichische Gesellschaft fur Hygiene, Mikrobiologie und Praventivmedizin. 1981. Richtlinie vom 4 November 1980 fur die Bewertung der Disinfektionswirkung von Verfahren fur die Hygienische Handedesinfektion. Osterreichische Krankenhauszeitung, 22, 23–31; Hygiene Medizin, 6, 4–9.

Pillsbury, D.M., Livingood, C.S., and Nichols, A.C. 1942. Bacterial flora of the normal skin. Arch. Dermatol., 45, 61–80.

Platt, J., and Bucknall, R.A. 1985. The disinfection of respiratory syncytial virus by isopropanol and a chlorhexidine-detergent handwash. J. Hosp. Infect., 6, 89–94.

Pohle, W.D., and Stuart, L.S. 1940. Germicidal action of cleaning agents. J. Infect. Dis., 67, 275–281.

Pontier, G., and Chaumont, L. 1954. Action of different antiseptics on the virus of Shope fibroma. Ann. Inst. Pasteur, 86, 532–534.

Post, W.E., and Nicoll, H.K. 1910. Comparative efficiency of some common germicides. JAMA, 55, 1635–1639.

Powell, H.M. 1945. The antiseptic properties of isopropyl alcohol in relation to cold sterilization. J. Indiana State Med. Assoc., 38, 303–304.

Price, P.B. 1950. Reevaluation of ethyl alcohol as a germicide. Arch. Surg., 60, 492–502.

Price, P.B. 1939. Ethyl alcohol as a germicide. Arch. Surg., 38, 528–542.

Price, P.B. 1938. The bacteriology of normal skin; a new quantitative test applied to a study of the bacterial flora and the disinfectant action of mechanical cleansing. J. Infect. Dis., 63, 301–318.

Prombo, M.P., and Tilden, E.B. 1950. Evaluation of disinfectants by tests in vivo. J. Dent. Res., 29, 108–122.

Pulvertaft, R.J.V., and Lumb, G.D. 1948. Bacterial lysis and antiseptics. J. Hyg., 46, 62–64.

Razin, S., and Argaman, M. 1963. Lysis of mycoplasma, bacterial protoplasts, spheroplasts and L-forms by various agents. J. Gen. Microbiol., 30, 155–172.

Resnick, L., Veren, K., Salahuddin, S.Z., Tondreau, S., and Markham, P.D.

1986. Stability and inactivation of HTLV-III/LAV under clinical and laboratory environments. JAMA, 255, 1887–1981.

Rotter, M., Koller, W., and Kundi, M. 1977. Eignung dreier Alkohole fur eine Standard-Desinfektiosmethode in der Wertbestimmung von Verfahren fur die Hygienische Handedesinfektion. Zentrabl. Bakteriol. Mikrobiol. Hyg. [B], 164, 428–438.

Rotter, M.L. 1981. Povidone-iodine and chlorhexidine gluconate containing detergents for disinfection of hands (letter). J. Hosp. Infect., 2, 273–280.

Rotter, M.L. 1984. Hygienic hand disinfection. Infect. Control, 5, 18–22.

Rotter, M.L., et al. 1986. Evaluation of procedures for hygienic hand-disinfection: Controlled parallel experiments on the Vienna test model. J. Hyg., Camb., 96, 27–37.

Ryan, V., and Miller, V.B. 1932. Disinfection of clinical thermometers. Am. J. Nurs., 32, 197–206.

Saegesser, M. 1941. Die Gasbrandinfektion nach Injektione. Schweiz. Med. Wochenschr., 71, 552–554. (Abst. In JAMA, 117, 1049, 1941).

Sattar, S.A., Raphael, R.A., Lochnan, H., and Springthrope, V.S. 1983. Rotavirus inactivation by chemical disinfectants and antiseptics used in hospitals. Am. J. Microbiol., 29, 1464–1469.

Sebben, J.E. 1983. Surgical antiseptics. J. Am. Acad. Dermatol., 9, 759–763.

Seelig, M.G., and Gould, C.W. 1911. Osmosis as an important factor in the action of antiseptics. Surg. Gynecol. Obstet., 12, 262–267.

Senz, E.H., and Goldfarb, D.L. 1958. Coma in a child following use of isopropyl alcohol in sponging. J. Pediatr., 53, 322–323.

Simmons, J.S. 1928. Bactericidal action of Mercurochrome-220 soluble and iodine solutions in skin disinfection. JAMA, 91, 704–708.

Snodgrass, D.R., and Hevring, J.A. 1977. The action of disinfectants on lamb rotavirus. Vet. Rec., 101, 81.

Sommermeyer, L., and Frobisher, M., Jr. 1952. Disinfection of oral thermometers. Nurs. Res., 1, 32–35.

Spaulding, E.H. 1939. Chemical sterilization of surgical instruments. Surg. Gynecol. Obstet., 69, 738–744.

Springthrope, V.S., Grenier, J.L., Lloyd-Evans, N., and Sattar, S.A. 1986. Chemical disinfection of human rotaviruses: Efficacy of commercially available products in suspension tests. J. Hyg., Camb., 97, 139–161.

Spire, B., Barre-Sinoussi, F., Montagnier, L., and Chermann, J.C. 1984. Inactivation of lymphadenopathy associated virus by chemical disinfectants. Lancet, 2, 899–901.

Staal, S.P., and Rowe, W.P. 1974. Differential effect of phenethyl alcohol on mycoplasmas and enveloped viruses. J. Virol., 14, 1620–1622.

Stanekk, G., Hirchl, A., and Laber G. 1981. Sensitivity of various spiroplasma strains against ethanol, formalin, glutaraldehyde, and phenol. Zentralbl. Bakteriol. Mikrobiol. Hyg. [B], 174, 348–354.

Stockman, S., and Minett, F.C. 1926. Researches on the virus of foot-and-mouth disease. J. Comp. Pathol. 39, 1–30.

Story, P. 1952. Testing of skin disinfectants. Br. Med. J., 2, 1128–1130.

Tainter, M.L., Throndson, A.H., Beard, R.R., and Wheatlake, R.J. 1944. Chemical sterilization of instruments. J. Am. Dent. Assoc., 31, 479–489.

Tan, J.A. and Schnagl, R.D. 1981. Inactivation of rotavirus by disinfectants. Med. J. Austr., 1, 19–23.

Tanner, F.W., and Wilson, F.L. 1943. Germicidal action of aliphatic alcohols. Proc. Soc. Exp. Biol. Med., 52, 138–140.

Theiler, M., and Gard S. 1940. Encephalomyelitis of mice. I. Characteristics and pathogenesis of the virus. J. Exp. Med., 72, 49–67.

Tilley, F.W. 1942. Influence of temperature of bactericidal activities of alcohols and phenols. J. Bacteriol., 43, 521–555.

Tilley, F.W., and Anderson, W.A. 1947. Germicidal action of certain chemicals on virus of Newcastle disease (avian pneumoencephalitis). Vet. Med., 42, 229–230.

Tilley, F.W., and Schaeffer, J.M. 1926. Relation between the chemical constitution and germicidal activity of monohydric alcohols and phenols. J. Bacteriol. 12, 303–309.

Trujillo, R., and Laible, N. 1970. Reversible inhibition of spore germination by alcohols. Appl. Microbiol., 20, 620–623.

Ulrich, J.A. 1982. Clinical study comparing Hibistat (0.5% chlorhexdine gluconate in 70% isopropyl alcohol) and Betadine surgical scrub (7.5% povidone-iodine) for efficacy against experimental contamination of human skin. Curr. Therap. Res., 31, 27–30.

Wasz-Hockert, O., Kosunen, T., and Kohonen, J. 1959. Effect of ethyl alcohol on the susceptibility of mice to staphylococcal infection. Ann. Med. Exp. Biol. Fenn., 37, 121–127.

Wallbank, A.M. 1985. Disinfectant inactivation of AIDS virus in blood or serum (letter). Lancet, 1, 642.

Welch, H., and Brewer, C.M. 1942. Toxicity-indices of some basic antiseptic substances. J. Immunol., 43, 25–30.

Winge-Heden, K. 1962. Bacteriologic studies on anaesthetic apparatus. Acta Chir. Scand., 124, 294–303.

Wirgin, G. 1904. Vergleichende Untersuchung ueber die keimtoedtenden und die entwickelungshemmenden Wirkungen von Alkoholen der Methyl-Aethyl-, Propyl, Butyl-und Amnylreihen. Z. Hyg. Infektions, 46, 149–168.

Wise, J.R. 1969. Alcohol sponge baths. N. Engl. J. Med., 280, 840.

Ziegler, C., and Jacoby, J. 1956. Anesthetic equipment as a source of infection. Anesth. Analg., 35, 451–459.

CHAPTER 12

PHENOLIC COMPOUNDS

D.O. O'Connor and J.R. Rubino

Phenol (carbolic acid) no longer plays a significant role as an antibacterial agent, although its use has not been abandoned entirely. Phenol is still used today in drug formulations such as cold-sore creams and liquids, throat lozenges, and washes. Today phenol derivatives make up one of the major classes of disinfectants used institutionally and commercially. Phenol derivatives are also used as preservatives and antibacterial agents in germicidal soaps and lotions.

Since its adoption by Lister as the germicide par excellence, phenol has been the subject of extensive study over a period of many years. The variations in the antibacterial behavior of phenol solutions as a function of concentration, temperature, pH, and other physical and chemical factors are the subjects of numerous papers. Kronig and Paul (1897) published the first well documented laboratory study of disinfectants. They established test conditions and criteria for evaluating germicidal activity of various compounds.

The sum accumulation of biologic data has, however, permitted a reasonable assessment of the relationship between structure and activity in the phenol series (Suter, 1941). Very briefly the main conclusions from this survey were as follows:

1. Parasubstitutions to the phenolic ring of an alkyl chain up to six carbons in length increases the antibacterial action of phenolics, presumably by increasing the surface activity and ability to orient at an interface. Activity falls off after this because of decreased water solubility. Because of the polarity enhancement of polar properties, straight chain parasubstituents confer greater activity than branched-chain substituents containing the same number of carbon atoms.
2. Halogenation increases the antibacterial activity of phenol. The combination of alkyl and halogen substitution, which confers the greatest antibacterial activity, is that where the alkyl group is ortho to the phenolic group and the halogen para to the phenolic group.

3. Nitration, while increasing the toxicity of phenol to bacteria, also increases the systemic toxicity to other, higher species. Specific biologic properties are confered to the molecule, enabling it to interfere with oxidative phosphorylation. This is due to the ability of nitrophenols to act as uncoupling agents.
4. In the bisphenol series, activity is found with a direct bond between the two C_6H_5-groups or if they are separated by —CH_2—, —S—, or —O—. If a —CO—, —SO—, or —CH(OH)— group separates the phenyl groups, activity is low. In addition, maximum activity is found with the hydroxyl group at the 2,2′ position of the bisphenol. Halogenation of the bisphenol confers additional biocidal activity.

Richardson and Reid (1940) showed that the observed action of phenol derivatives could be correlated with their partition ratio of oil to water. This was confirmed subsequently by Fogg and Lodge (1945), with *Aerobacter* (i.e., *Enterobacter*) *aerogenes* serving as the test organism; preferential solubility in olive oil was found to be associated with greater antibacterial activity

HALOGENATED PHENOL DERIVATIVES

Halogenation of phenolic compounds leads to a potentiation of their antibacterial effectiveness. As early as 1906 (Bechhold and Ehrlich), it was observed that polychloro and polybromo derivatives of phenol and of betanaphthol had considerable effectiveness against *Corynebacterium diphtheriae* and *Straphylococcus aureus*, and that this effectiveness was not retained in the presence of serum. Polyhalogen compounds, however, displayed considerable toxicity (Bechhold, 1909, 1914). Laubenheimer (1909) showed that monohalogen-substituted alkyl derivatives of phenol, although considerably more active than the unsubstituted compounds, were only partly inactivated in the presence of serum. Wolf and Westveer (1952) showed that, in the case of phenol itself, potentiation by chlorine substitution occurs only until the trichloro derivatives have been reached. The tetrachloro isomers are considerably less active than any other trichloro isomers. Pentachorophenol is about as effective as the phenol itself against *Salmonella typhosa*, although more effective than the phenol against *Staphylococcus aureus*. There is considerable difference in the germicidal activity between five (of six possible) trichlorophenol isomers tested; thus, at a constant pH of 6.7, the killing dilution for *Salmonella typhosa* of 2,3,6-trichlorophenol is 1:500, and that of the 2,4,5-isomer is 1:4200. On the other hand, the activity of the trichlorophenols depends to an extraordinary degree on pH variations. 2,3,4-trichlorophenol kills *S. typhosa* at pH 7.2 in 1:2400, but at pH 8.2 only in the eight-times-stronger concentration of 1:300. Similar responses were obtained with the other trichloro isomers.

Klarmann et al. (1929) refer to the influence of a stepwise substitution of halogen in the phenol nucleus on bactericidal effectiveness. The paper shows that the impairment of bactericide effectiveness by organic matter also is a function of the extent of the halogen substitution. Monosubstituted phenol derivatives suffer a lower reduction in the presence of organic matter, comparable to that of phenol itself. However, the loss of potency in the presence of organic matter shown by 2,4,6-trichlorophenol is on the order of 50% with respect to both *Salmonella typhosa* and *Staphylococcus aureus*. In almost all studies dealing with the effect of nuclear substitution on antibacterial action of phenol derivatives, the quantitative data reported by the various investigators need not be regarded necessarily as indicative of the practical germicidal effectiveness of the compounds studied. As a rule, these data are mostly of a theoretic interest in that they illustrate the relationships between the chemical structure of the phenol derivatives and their antibacterial potential. They do not usually assure a given compound's superiority or even fitness for practical use,

i.e., use in the presence of one or more of the interfering factors encountered in the practice of disinfection or antisepsis, such as organic and inorganic soil, pus, serum, blood, and mucus.

A systematic examination of the relationships between the chemical structure and the microbiocidal action of aliphatic and aromatic substitution derivatives of *p*- and *o*-chlorophenol was carried out by Klarmann et al. (1933). Tables 12–1 and 12–2 illustrate the conditions found in the case of ortho-alkyl derivatives of *p*-chlorophenol and of para-alkyl derivatives of *o*-chlorophenol. Tables 12–3 and 12–4 deal with ortho-alkyl derivatives of *p*-bromophenol and with para-alkyl derivatives of *o*-bromophenol, respectively. The general trends are summarized as follows:

1. Halogen substitution intensifies the microbiocidal potency of phenol derivatives; the presence of halogen in the para position to the hydroxyl group is more effective in this respect than in the ortho position.

2. Introduction of aliphatic or aromatic groups into the nucleus of halogen phenols increases the bactericidal potency (up to certain limits). The increase depends in the case of alkyl substitution on the number of carbon atoms present in the substituting group or groups.

3. As a rule, the intensifying effect on the bactericidal potency of a normal aliphatic chain with a given number of carbon atoms is greater than that of a branched chain, or of two alkyl groups with the same total of carbon atoms.

4. Ortho-alkyl derivatives of *p*-chlorophenol are more actively germicidal than para-alkyl derivatives of *o*-chlorophenol.

5. In the case of the higher homologs, the germicidal action manifests a "quasispecific" character. Beginning with a definite point (which is different in the

Table 12–1. *Microbicidal Action of Ortho-Alkyl Derivatives of Para-Chlorophenol (Phenol Coefficients, 37°C)*

Name	a	b	c	d	e	f	g
p-Chlorophenol (II)	4.3	4.3	4.3	4.4	3.9	3.3	4.0
Methyl II	12.5	12.9	12.5	11.1	11.1	7.1	11.1
Ethyl II	28.6	28.6	34.4	31.1	27.8	25.0	32.5
n-Propyl II	93.3	714.0	93.8	77.8	66.7	714.0	100.0
n-Butyl II	141.0	114.0	257.0	250.0	178.0	156.0	178.0
n-Amyl II	156.0	100.0	500.0	556.0	389.0	278.0	389.0
*sec*Amyl II	46.7	42.9	312.0	312.0	222.0	229.0	182.0
n-Hexyl II	23.2*	21.4*	1250.0	1333.0	333.0	357.0	556.0
Cyclo-Hexyl II	<26.7	<14.3	438.0	361.0	278.0	222.0	300.0
n-Heptyl II	20.0*	14.3*	1500.0	2222.0	>400.0	175.0	>363.0
n-Octyl II	—	—	1750.0	>312.0	—	—	—

*Approximate

a = *Salmonella typhosa*
b = *Salmonella schotmuelleri*
c = *Staphylococcus aureus*
d = *Streptococcus pyogenes (hemol.)*
e = *Mycobacterium tuberculosis*
f = *Trichophyton schoenleni*
g = *Candida albicans*

Table 12–2. *Microbicidal Action of Para-Alkyl Derivatives of Orthochlorophenol (Phenol Coefficients, 37°C)*

Name	a	b	c	d	e	f
o-Chlorophenol (III)	2.5	2.1	2.9	2.0	2.2	2.2
Methyl III	6.3	5.4	7.5	5.6	5.6	8.3
Ethyl III	17.2	25.0	15.7	15.0	17.8	22.2
n-Propyl III	40.0	35.7	32.1	33.3	33.3	44.4
n-Butyl III	86.7	66.7	93.8	88.9	77.8	88.9
n-Amyl III	80.0	40.0	286.0	222.0	222.0	278.0
tert Amyl III	32.1	21.4	125.0	122.0	111.0	100.0
n-Hexyl III	23.3	—	500.0	555.0	178.0	278.0
n-Heptyl III	16.7	—	375.0	350.0	77.8	70.0

a = *Salmonella typhosa*
b = *Salmonella schotmuelleri*
c = *Staphylococcus aureus*
d = *Streptococcus pyogenes (hemol.)*
e = *Mycobacterium tuberculosis*
f = *Candida albicans*

Table 12–3. *Microbicidal Action of Ortho-Alkyl Derivatives of Para-Bromo-Phenol (Phenol Coefficients, 37°C)*

Name	a	b	c	d
p-Bromophenol (IV)	6.0	5.0	5.6	6.3
Methyl IV	12.5	11.3	13.3	13.3
Ethyl IV	31.3	25.0	27.8	27.8
n-Propyl IV	62.5	62.5	77.8	77.8
n-Butyl IV	156.0	313.0	278.0	222.0
n-Amyl IV	62.5	571.0	444.0	278.0
sec Amyl IV	>33.0	150.0	156.0	150.0
n-Hexyl IV	—	1250.0	778.0	278.0
cycloHexyl IV	>23.0	429.0	278.0	222.0

a = *Salmonella typhosa*
b = *Staphylococcus aureus*
c = *Mycobacterium tuberculosis*
d = *Candida albicans*

Table 12–4. *Microbicidal Action of Para-Alkyl Derivatives of Ortho-Bromophenol (Phenol Coefficients, 37°C)*

Name	a	b	c	d
o-Bromophenol (V)	3.3	3.1	3.9	3.8
tert Amyl V	33.3	150.0	100.0	77.8
n-Hexyl V	>20.0	625.0	556.0	222.0
n-Propyl-m,m-dimethyl V	—	357.0	220.0	138.0

a = *Salmonella typhosa*
b = *Staphylococcus aureus*
c = *Mycobacterium tuberculosis*
d = *Candida albicans*

A comparison of the substituted *p*-chlorophenol derivatives with a total of four substituting carbon atoms illustrates the effect on the germicidal action of the distribution of the added weight over several substituting radicals. It shows that substitution of *p*-chlorophenol by one alkyl group generally leads to a more effective compound than substitution by two or three alkyl groups with the same total number of carbon atoms; similarly, dialkyl-substituted derivatives are considerably more germicidal than trialkyl-substituted ones.

Iso-alkyl-substituted compounds are less effective than the corresponding normal alkyl derivatives. This follows from the comparison of 6-*n*-propyl-3-methyl-4-chlorophenol and 6-isopropyl-3-methyl-4-chlorophenol (chlorothymol). Thus the *n*-propyl derivative is distinctly more potent than chlorothymol. Polyalkyl compounds of equal molecular weight, containing iso-alkyl groups, may show considerable variation in their germicidal action, depending on their structure.

In the case of the normal monoalkyl derivatives, the maximum effect on *Salmonella typhosa* is shown by a compound with five carbon atoms in the side chain, although in the case of the polyalkyl derivatives, this maximum is reached by a compound with a total of four substituting carbon atoms. In Table 12–5, the derivatives with a total of seven carbon atoms generally show the greatest microbiocidal efficacy against the other test organisms. The effect of steric isomerism is illustrated by

case of the various test organisms), a further increase in the weight of the substituting groups causes the germicidal capacity to drop sometimes to almost total inactivity with respect to certain microorganisms, e.g., *Salmonella typhosa*, and at the same time to rise to comparatively enormous values with respect to others, e.g., *Staphylococcus aureus*. Klarmann et al. (1934) proposed the term "quasispecific" to describe this effect; that is a compound that is extremely active against one organism and yet not very effective against a second.

Figure 12–1 illustrates this "quasispecific" behavior, and indicates the difference in the order of magnitude of the bactericidal potencies with respect to the several groups of microorganisms under discussion.

In addition to the homologous series of alkyl derivatives of *p*- and *o*-chlorophenol, and of *p*- and *o*-bromophenol, a series of polyalkyl and aromatic derivatives of *p*-chlorophenol were studied for their microbiocidal potency. The former are referred to in Table 12–5, the latter in Table 12–6. As in the mono alkyl series, the weight of the substituting groups determines the selective quasispecific action.

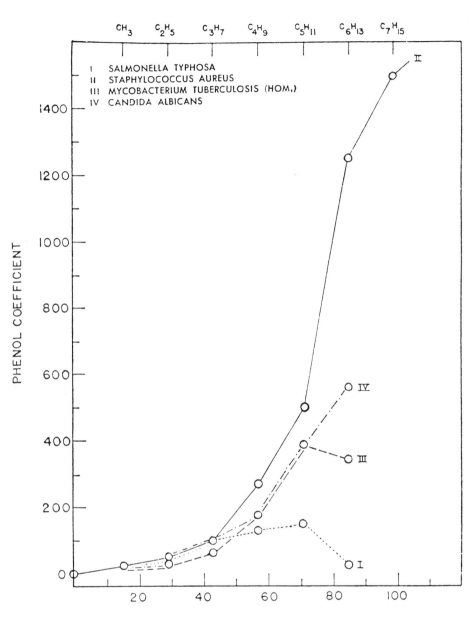

Fig. 12–1. The "quasispecific" effect in the case of the homologous series of *o*-alkyl *p*-chlorophenol derivative.

the findings of Heicken (1939). This author found the chlorine and bromine derivatives of the 1,2,3-, 1,3,5-, and 1,4,2-xylenols to be 50 to 70 times more effective than phenol (against *Escherichia coli* and *Staphylococcus aureus*), whereas those of the 1,2,4-, 1,3,2-, and 1,3,4-xylenols showed an effectiveness only 15 to 20 times greater than phenol. These studies were extended by Lockemann and Heicken (1939).

Among the aromatic derivatives of *p*-chlorophenol are some potent germicides (Klarmann et al., 1932b) (Table 12–6). It is noteworthy that the step from the benzyl derivative to the next one with a higher molecular weight

is accompanied by different results, depending on the place in the molecular structure to which the additional weight is attached. Thus, 5-methyl-2-benzyl-4-chlorophenol is much less effective than 2-benzyl-4-chlorophenol against the four test organisms, whereas 2-phenylethyl-4-chlorophenol is a more effective germicide than the former. The difference in the germicidal potencies of the methyl-benzyl and the phenyl-ethyl derivatives is less pronounced against other organisms. A further increase in the molecular weight lowers the germicidal action with reference to the test bacteria, as shown by the figures obtained with 3,5-dimethyl-2-benzyl-4-chlo-

Table 12–5. *Bactericidal Action of Polyalkyl Derivatives of Parachlorophenol (Phenol Coefficients, 37°C)*

Name	a	b	c	d
p-Chlorophenol (II)	4.3	4.3	4.4	3.9
3-Methyl II	10.7	11.3	11.3	11.1
3,5-Dimethyl II	30.0	25.7	27.5	28.1
6-Ethyl-3-methyl II	64.3	50.0	55.6	55.6
6-n-Propyl-3-methyl II	133.0	200.0	178.0	156.0
6-iso-Propyl-3-methyl II	107.0	150.0	138.0	138.0
2-Ethyl-3,5-dimethyl II	46.4	106.0	94.4	122.0
6-sec Butyl-3-methyl II	50.0	500.0	361.0	389.0
2-iso-Propyl-3,5-dimethyl II	81.3	313.0	313.0	325.0
6-Diethylmethyl-3-methyl II	23.3	625.0	611.0	777.0
6-iso-Propyl-2-ethyl-3-methyl II	56.7	200.0	175.0	200.0
2-sec Butyl-3,5-dimethyl II	28.6	563.0	556.0	556.0
2-sec Amyl-3,5-dimethyl II	15.6*	750.0	889.0	700.0
2-Diethylmethyl-3,5-dimethyl II	<13.0	1143.0	1000.0	667.0
6-sec Octyl-3-methyl II	21.4*	>89.0	122.0	>70.0

*Approximate
a = *Salmonella typhosa*
b = *Staphylococcus aureus*
c = *Mycobacterium tuberculosis*
d = *Candida albicans*

Table 12–6. *Bactericidal Action of Aromatic Derivatives of Para-Chlorophenol (Phenol Coefficients, 37°C)*

Name	a	b	c	d	e
p-Chlorophenol (II)	4.3	4.3	4.3	4.4	4.0
o-Benzyl II	71.4	71.4	200.0	225.0	178.0
o-Benzyl-m-methyl II	18.3	28.6	375.0	389.0	—
o-Benzyl-m,m-dimethyl II	—	—	750.0	778.0	—
o-Phenylethyl II	100.0	71.4	375.0	500.0	333.0
o-Phenylethyl-m-methyl II	—	—	375.0	250.0	178.0

a = *Salmonella typhosa*
b = *Salmonella schottmuelleri*
c = *Staphylococcus aureus*
d = *Staphylococcus pyogenes (hemol.)*
e = *Mycobacterium tuberculosis*

rophenol. However, the germicidal potency is increased considerably with regard to the other four organisms. Curiously, 3-methyl-6-phenylethyl-4-chlorophenol, which is isomeric with 3,5-dimethyl-2-benzyl-4-chlorophenol, is not only less effective than the latter, but also, in most instances, weaker than the 2-phenylethyl derivative. The aliphatic and aromatic derivatives of the chlorophenols and bromophenols studied display good bacteriostatic action. This is illustrated by the results shown in Table 12–7, obtained respectively with o-n-amyl and with o-n-heptyl p-chlorophenol.

A series of halothymols (6-chloro-, 6-bromo-2,6-dibromo-, and 6-iodothymol) were tested by Cross et al. (1955) for their antifungal action, by means of the FDA serum agar cup-plate method. Generally speaking, the iodo derivative was found to be most effective, as determined by the diameter of the area in which inhibition of growth took place.

Mention may be made here of the series of 2-alkyl-4-fluorophenol derivatives prepared by Suter et al. (1939). The following phenol coefficients were determined for the individual members of this series: ethyl 10, propyl 21, butyl 66, amyl 69, hexyl less than 62. Suter and Schuetz (1951) prepared and described a series of alkyl iodophenols.

It is significant that the increase in the molecular weight of the phenol derivatives, which is accompanied by an increase in antibacterial potency, is also accom-

Table 12–7. *Bacteriostatic Dilutions of Ortho-n-Amyl and Ortho-n-Heptyl Para-Chlorophenol*

Name	Staphylococcus aureus	Mycobacterium smegmatis	Mycobacterium tuberculosis
n-Amyl II	1:150,000	1:200,000	1:150,000
n-Heptyl II	1:200,000	1:200,000	1:200,000

Table 12–8. *Oral LD₅₀ Grams/Kilo*

	Rats	*Rabbits*
Phenol	0.53	—
2-Phenylphenol	8.0 ± 1.1	4.7 ± 0.9
2-Benzyl-4-chlorophenol	6.4 ± 1.1	5.4 ± 1.1
4-*tert*-Amylphenol	6.9 ± 1.0	5.4 ± 1.2

panied by decreasing toxicity. There is a tenfold difference in oral toxicity between phenol itself and commonly used phenol derivatives, as shown in Table 12–8.

BISPHENOLS

Bisphenols are composed of two phenolic groups connected by various linkages. A large number of such compounds are known. Certain members of this group possess high bacteriostatic or fungistatic properties. The most important linkage is methylene and, when named according to Chemical Abstracts nomenclature, results in:

2,2'-methylenebis (4,6-dichlorophenol)

The antibacterial action of bisphenols was first observed by Bechhold and Ehrlich (1906), who found a great increase in effectiveness of phenols when connected directly or by an alkylene group. Particularly effective were the halogenated compounds.

A large number of compounds were prepared and described as moth-proofing agents by Weiler et al. (1929). Dunning and associates (1931) prepared a series of 2,2'-thiobisphenols and showed the halogenated members to be active against *Staphylococcus aureus*.

Beginning in 1937, halogenated bisphenols were studied intensively in the laboratories of the Givaudan Corporation. Out of this long series, two compounds found important commercial applications. One is 2,2'-methylene-bis (4-chlorophenol), first prepared by Weiler (1929) and later by the improved method of Gump and Luthy (1943). Although active against bacteria, its special value is in mildew-proofing under the trade names G-4 and Preventol G D. The other compound is 2,2'-methylene-bis (3,4,6-trichlorophenol), synthesized by Gump (1941) and named G-11 or hexachlorophene. The outstanding usefulness of this substance was in the formulation of antiseptic soaps and detergents, its substantivity to the skin providing continuing bacteriostatic activity against gram-positive organisms. Halogenated 2,2'-thiobisphenols, particularly 2,2'-thiobis (4,6-dichlorophenol), have been used in soaps and cosmetics (Schetty, 1956). Development of photosensitivity caused these uses to be discontinued.

The more halogens are substituted into phenols, the more effective the compound. A similar pattern is found in the bisphenols in regard to gram-positive organisms. When tested in soap against *Staphylococcus aureus*, the superiority of the highly chlorinated members of a series becomes evident (Kunz, 1950).

In addition to the requirement that bisphenols must contain halogen, the phenols must be linked at the position ortho(2,2'-) to the hydroxyls for maximum activity.

The toxicity of both phenols and bisphenols increases with the degree of halogenation. Florestano (1949) found that oral toxicity in mice increased with increased chlorination of the rings. Hexachlorophene was the most toxic in the series, with an LD₅₀ of 80 mg/kg, but was also the most effective bacteriologically. Gump (1969) gives pertinent references on the human toxicity of hexachlorophene. Vaterhaus and Hostynek (1973) found no teratogenic effect in rats and guinea pigs.

The absorption of hexachlorophene through the skin, its retention, and its excretion were studied by a number of investigators. Hexachlorophene accumulated on the skin during the first 3 or 4 days and remained constant thereafter (Isikow and Gump, 1952; Compeau, 1960; Stoughton, 1965; Taber et al., 1971). Blood levels in infants and operating room personnel regularly using the 3% emulsion were found to be 0.1 to 0.6 ppm. A complete review of hexachorophene toxicity was made by Kimbrough (1973).

After considering the neurotoxicity and the potential absorption through the skin, the Food and Drug Administration banned over-the-counter sales of all soaps, drugs, and cosmetics containing more than 0.1% hexachlorophene. All products containing higher amounts were restricted to sale by prescription only (Federal Register, 1972, 20160–20164). Use was limited to surgical scrubbing as a bacteriostatic hand cleanser, handwashing as a part of patient care, or topical application to control the outbreak of gram-positive infection where other procedures had been unsuccessful. Its use on burned or denuded skin or mucous membrane or for routine prophylactic total body bathing is contraindicated.

Although the proprietary use of hexachlorophene for deodorant soaps and cosmetics is no longer allowed in the United States, several foreign countries still permit it.

BIS(HYDROXYPHENYL) ALKANES

Bis(hydroxyphenyl) alkanes can also be discussed under the heading of phenol derivatives. Harden and Reid (1932) and, subsequently, Richardson and Reid (1940), studied two groups of compounds of the types $HOC_6H_4CH(R)C_6H_4OH$ and $HOC_6H_4(CH_2)_nC_6H_4OH$. In both groups, the hydroxyl is in the para position. In the former, R may be hydrogen or an alkyl group from methyl to *n*-hexyl; in the latter, *n* may vary from 1 to 10. Increasing the length of the aliphatic chain in the alpha,alpha-group resulted in an increase of the germicidal effect on the same test organism only in the case of the first four members of the series.

A large number of bis(hydroxyphenyl) alkanes were

studied by Heinemann (1944). These compounds derived from bis(hydroxyphenyl) propane are of the type $HOC_6H_4CH(R_1)CH(R_2)CH(R_3)C_6H_4OH$, where R_1, R_2, R_3 may be hydrogen or an organic radical. Another variant is introduced by the relative position of the hydroxyl radicals in both benzene rings. Structure-activity correlation shows that

1. Increasing the length of the aliphatic chain attached to a hydroxyphenyl ring results in increased antibacterial activity.
2. A given number of carbon atoms contributes a greater effectiveness in a single chain than when distributed between two or more chains.
3. Branching of the aliphatic chain lowers the activity below that of the normal straight chain compound.
4. The position of the hydroxyl group on the rings does not materially influence bactericidal activity in unsubstituted isomeric compounds.
5. The susceptibility of *Salmonella typhosa* reaches a maximum with an alkyl chain containing four carbon atoms, whereas homologs of high molecular weight, up to an alkyl chain of nine carbon atoms, are effective against *Staphyloccus aureus*.

In a group of 23 compounds, only 3 were found to be active against *Salmonella typhosa*, the most effective being 1,3-bis(*p*-hydroxyphenyl) butane, which was bactericidal in a dilution of 1:8000. With respect to *Staphylococcus aureus*, the most effective homolog is 1,3-bis(*p*-hydroxyphenyl) octane with a bactericidal dilution of 1:150,000. Less effective but still potent is 4,6-bis(*p*-hydroxyphenyl) nonane with a bactericidal dilution of 1:90,000.

A series of 38 halogen-, nitro-, arseno-, carboxy-, and alkyl-substituted derivatives of bis(hydroxyphenyl) methane was prepared and tested by Florestano and Bahler (1953). In vitro activity appeared to be more or less specific for gram-positive bacteria; it was markedly inhibited in the presence of bovine albumin. Eleven of these compounds were tested in vivo and found to be relatively ineffective against streptococcal infection in mice. The functional variants of diethylstilbestrol investigated by Rubin and Wishinsky (1944) belong in this chapter. Although diethylstilbestrol itself inhibits *Staphylococcus aureus* in a dilution of less than 1:10,000, the monohydroxylated, i.e., phenolic, derivative $C_6H_5C(C_2H_5)=C(C_6H_4OH)$ inhibits multiplication of this organism in a dilution of 1:640,000, and its monobromo derivative does it in one of 1:1,000,000. This generally agrees with the information available for substituted phenol derivatives.

NITROPHENOLS

The introduction of the nitro group into the nucleus of phenol and cresol enhances the antimicrobial action (Cooper, 1913; Glaser and Prufer, 1923; Glaser and Wulwek, 1924; Ishiware, 1924). Although the work of these authors credits the *m*-nitrophenol isomer with the highest potency (about three times that of phenol itself), Mazzetti (1928) found *p*-nitrophenol to be the most effective with respect to *Salmonella typhosa* and *o*-nitrophenol the most active against *Staphylococcus aureus*. According to Beutner et al. (1941), *o*-nitrophenol is a comparatively active bactericide, whereas Cains et al. (1927) found it comparable to phenol with respect to *Pasteurella* (i.e., *Yersinia*) *pestis*. The antiseptic action of 2,4-dinitrophenol was found to be weaker than that of phenol with respect to *Pasteurella* (i.e., *Yersinia*) *pestis* (Cains, 1929). Woodward et al. (1933) compared the effect of the three nitrophenol isomers on *Monilia tropicalis* and assigned the following phenol coefficients to them: to the ortho-isomer, 6.6; to the meta-isomer, 5.3; and to the para-isomer, 5.1.

A comparison of the inhibitory effect on fermentation produced by 4-hydroxybenzoic acid and 3-nitro-4-hydroxybenzoic acid, as well as by several esters of each, points to a greater activity of the latter series. A comparison of six dinitrophenol isomers with regard to their inhibitory capacity was carried out by Lecoq et al. (1949). Of these, the 2,5-dinitrophenol was found to be the most active isomer. Its action on streptococci and tubercle bacilli is particularly pronounced, the respective inhibitory dilutions being 1:200,000 and 1:1,000,000. It is effective also against other microorganisms such as *Salmonella typhosa*, *Escherichia coli*, and *Staphylococcus aureus*, but in higher concentrations is comparable to those in which the other isomers show an inhibitory effect.

Picric acid (2,4,6-trinitrophenol) is more active than either phenol or mononitrophenol against both *Salmonella typhosa* and *Staphylococcus aureus* (Cooper, 1913). A phenol coefficient of 6 was ascribed to it by Tidy (1915); its activity against *Pasteurella* (i.e., *Yersinia*) *pestis* was noted by Cains (1929). Woodward et al. (1933) found it to be moderately effective against *Monilia tropicalis* (when brought into solution with the aid of sodium carbonate); the phenol coefficient with respect to the latter microorganism was determined at 5.3.

AMINOPHENOLS

The effect on *Pasteurella* (i.e., *Yersinia*) *pestis* of *p*-aminophenol is greater than that of *o*-aminophenol (Cains et al., 1928), whereas 2,4-diaminophenol is more active than either, and more active than phenol itself. The inhibitory action of a series of para-alkyl derivatives of *o*-aminophenol on a number of organisms (*Salmonella typhosa*, *Staphylococcus aureus*, *Pseudomonas aeruginosa*) was studied by Barber and Haslewood (1944, 1945). No substantial enhancement of the bacteriostatic effect was observed over that of the unsubstituted *o*-aminophenol.

NAPHTHOL AND DERIVATIVES

Of the two isomers, alpha- and beta-naphthol, the latter has been explored more thoroughly as an antibacterial agent because of its greater economy and stability. It is no longer commonly used in disinfectants. Thalhimer and Palmer (1911) assign to beta-naphthol a phenol coefficient of 12.5. A mutual potentiation of the antibacterial effects of beta-naphthol and formaldehyde has been claimed by Frei and Krupski (1915). Of the several polybromonaphthols studied, the tribromo and tetrabromo derivatives are particularly effective against staphylococci and streptococci, whereas their activity with respect to *Escherichia coli* and *Salmonella paratyphi* is low (Bechhold, 1909).

RESORCINOL DERIVATIVES

An extensive study of the antibacterial properties of resorcinol derivatives began with the basic findings of Johnson and his co-workers (Johnson and Hodge, 1913; Johnson and Lane, 1921). Additional data were contributed by investigators entering this field subsequently (Dohme et al., 1926; Schaffer and Tilley, 1926, 1927; Hampil, 1928; Rettger et al., 1929). Klarmann et al. (1931) prepared and studied the series of monoethers of resorcinol. They reported high activity for the 4-alkyl resorcinols and little activity for the monoethers. Also reported are data on aromatic substituted resorcinol derivatives, which show some activity.

The data justify the conclusion that the bactericidal effectiveness of substituted resorcinol derivatives is practically the same regardless of whether the substituting radical is in the nucleus in the ortho or para position to the two hydroxyl groups or attached to one of the oxygen atoms. It follows also that one hydroxyl group of the resorcinol molecule is sufficient to bring about the antibacterial action.

As with the phenol derivatives, in the case of the resorcinol derivatives, a quasispecific effect is in evidence. With respect to the test organism *Staphylococcus aureus*, the bactericidal efficacy increases with the increasing weight of the radical, whereas with respect to *Salmonella typhosa*, maximum is reached by the *n*-hexyl derivatives, followed by a sharp decline.

Klarmann et al. (1932a) studied also the monoethers of the other two dihydric phenols: hydroquinone and pyrocatechol. Among the hydroquinone and pyrocatechol monoethers are a number of effective antibacterial agents, although in general the monoethers of resorcinol appear to show a greater efficacy than those of the other two dihydric phenols.

As with resorcinol, in the case of pyrocatechol, a comparison is possible between the monoalkyl ethers and the corresponding nucleus-substituted alkyl derivatives, because several of the latter were prepared and studied by Rawlins and Hamilton (1938). Contrary to the situation found in the case of the resorcinol derivatives, the 4-alkyl derivatives of pyrocatechol yield substantially higher phenol coefficients than their monoether isomers; in fact, their antibacterial potency appears to compare favorably with that of the corresponding 4-*n*-alkyl resorcinols. The phenyl ethers of the three dihydric phenols, which may be regarded also as isomeric hydroxyphenyl oxides, permit a comparison with the corresponding isomeric sulfides prepared by Hilbert and Johnson (1929).

It appears that with respect to *Salmonella typhosa* as a test organism, the three hydroxydiphenyl sulfides are more effective than the corresponding oxides.

A number of symmetric dyhydroxydiphenyl sulfides were prepared and studied by Dunning et al. (1931). These sulfides were derived from the following initial compounds: phenol, resorcinol, *m*-cresol, *p*-chloro- and *p*-bromophenol, and thymol. The antibacterial potency of the sulfides is several times that of the initial phenol derivatives.

Of the several nucleus-substituted alkyl resorcinol derivatives studied, 4-*n*-hexyl resorcinol has acquired considerable practical significance. Although in the early stages of its investigation, it seemed possible that the combination of high antibacterial potency with low toxicity might yield a drug of chemotherapeutic utility, it was found soon that such a hope was not justified. Nevertheless, 4-*n*-hexyl resorcinol became an important antiseptic for topical use. It was accepted into the U.S. Pharmacopeia; a solution of 4-*n*-hexyl with low surface tension is employed widely as a popular antiseptic for first aid and other uses.

DERIVATIVES OF TRIHYDRIC PHENOLS

Phloroglucinol is not an effective germicide. Its phenol coefficient with respect to *Salmonella typhosa* is only 0.35 (Cooper, 1912). However, introduction of alkyl or aralkyl radicals into its nucleus potentiates its antibacterial efficacy. Klarmann and Figdor (1926) prepared the *n*-hexyl derivative with a phenol coefficient of 8. This is over three times that of the isomeric triethyl phloroglucinol with a phenol coefficient of 2.5. The *Salmonella typhosa* phenol coefficients of the three aralkyl phloroglucinols tested, i.e., the benzyl, phenylethyl, and phenylprophyl derivatives, are also around 8 (Klarmann, 1926b).

Pyrogallol is a comparatively weak bactericide, although somewhat more effective than phloroglucinol. Its *Salmonella typhosa* phenol coefficient is 2.77. However, the series of 4-*n*-alkyl derivatives of pyrogallol contains several comparatively potent bactericides (Hart and Woodruff, 1936). The quasispecific phenomenon is shown here. The maximum effectiveness against *Escherichia coli* is reached by the 4-*n*-hexyl compound (phenol coefficient: 38), whereas with respect to *Staphylococcus aureus*, such a maximum may not have been attained with the 4-*n*-heptyl derivative (phenol coefficient 50). The 4-*n*-heptenyl pyrogallol has a phenol coefficient of 120 against *Staphylococcus aureus* (Hard and Parrish, 1935).

The third isomeric trihydric phenol is hydroxydroquinone. Neither this compound nor its derivatives appears to have been examined for any antibacterial properties.

HYDROXYCARBOXYLIC ACIDS AND ESTERS

Orthohyroxybenzoic, or salicylic acid, has been the subject of several studies. Two investigators have found very different results, however, Cains (1929) found salicylic acid less effective than phenol against *Pasteurella* (i.e., *Yersinia*) *pestis*. Woodward (1933) found it to have a high phenol coefficient of 13.3. Monochloro, dichloro, and dibromo derivatives of salicylic acid were prepared and investigated for both their killing and inhibitory action on bacteria, fungi, and yeasts (Delauney, 1937; Rochaix and Pinet, 1927).

The phenol coefficient of *m*-hydroxybenzoic acid is approximately 2.7 with *Salmonella typhosa* and 2.1 with *Staphylococcus aureus* (Wyss and Poe, 1945). The esters of *p*-hydroxybenzoic acid hold a position of considerable importance, notably in the field of preservation. They are used to preserve carbohydrates, gums, proteins, and other organic materials of industrial, pharmaceutical, and cosmetic significance. The bulk of the original data has been contributed by Sabalitschka and his co-workers over a period of several years (Sabalitschka, 1924a, 1924b, 1931, 1932; Sabalitschka and Liedge, 1934; Sabalitschka and Tietz, 1931). Gershenfeld and Perlstein (1939) regarded these esters as among the most useful preservatives available at the time of the publication of their report. A tabulation indicating the proper concentration of the several esters required for preservation was prepared by Suess (1936). Sokol (1952) investigated the antibacterial and antifungal properties of the methyl, ethyl, propyl, and butyl *p*-hydroxybenzoates. Table 12–9 indicates the concentration of these four esters required to effect complete inhibition of growth.

Esters other than the four listed in Table 12–9 were tested for their inhibitory action upon *Aspergillus niger*. Among them were the hexyl, cyclohexyl, *p*-chlorobenzyl, tetrahydrofurfuryl, glyceryl, and pentaerithrytyl derivatives. None was found to be more effective than the propyl and butyl *p*-hydroxybenzoates. The data on inhibition of bacterial and fungal growth published later by Aalto et al. (1953) agree with those obtained by Sokol. Aalto and associates also studied other subjects of practical interest, such as the additive action of mixtures of certain *p*-hydroxybenzoates, the preservation of antibiotic solutions and suspensions, the methods of incorporation, detection, and determination, and others.

The esters of *p*-hydroxybenzoic acid display a low order of acute (Schubel and Manger, 1929; Schubel, 1930) and subacute (Cremer, 1935) toxicity. The average lethal doses for cats, dogs, and rabbits (in grams per kilogram of body weight) of the methyl, ethyl, and propyl esters are 3, 5, and 6, respectively. (Benzoic acid, which is used widely as a food preservative, yields a lethal dose of 2, thereby appearing to be more toxic than any of three *p*-hydroxybenzoates tested.) The methyl ester appears to be only one-fourth as toxic as the free *p*-hydroxybenzoic acid when administered intraperitoneally. Two to 20 mg/kg per day of the lower esters given to rabbits, guinea pigs, and rats for a period of 120 days appeared to be entirely harmless. Three times this quantity given to rats for 30 days also failed to produce any ill effects. Sokol (1952) concluded that the esters of *p*-hydroxybenzoic acid approximate the requirements of an "ideal" pharmaceutical preservative as formulated by Gershenfeld and Perlstein (1939). This was based on irritation, absorption, and excretion studies carried out with animals and humans. These conclusions agree with those reached later by Mathews et al. (1956).

The physiologic disposition of *p*-hydroxybenzoic acid and of its esters is the subject of a paper by Jones et al. (1956). Both the methyl and propyl esters are described in the U.S. Pharmacopeia. For an extensive review of the literature on the esters of *p*-hydroxybenzoic acid, the paper by Neidig and Burrell (1944) should be consulted.

8-HYDROXYQUINOLINE AND DERIVATIVES

8-Hydroxyquinoline is the only one of seven possible isomers displaying antimicrobial properties. This quality is attributed to its capacity to form freely dissociated chelate complexes in which the metal becomes a part of a heterocyclic ring system.

8-Hydroxyquinoline and its salts (sulfate, benzoate) are used as an ingredient of antiseptics, particularly those claiming fungitoxic action, because of their capacity to produce microbial stasis rather than microbiocidal action. Older studies by Post and Nicoll (1910) showed that a 25% solution of the sulfate (Chinosol, Quinosol) is not

Table 12–9. *Inhibition of Bacterial and Fungal Growth by Esters of* p-*Hydroxybenzoic Acid (Percentages)*

Microorganism	Methyl	Ethyl	Prophyl	Butyl
Salmonella typhosa	0.2	0.1	0.1	0.1
Escherichia coli	0.4	0.1	0.1	0.4
Staphylococcus aureus	0.4	0.1	0.05	0.0125
Proteus vulgaris	0.2	0.1	0.05	0.05
Pseudomonas aeruginosa	0.4	0.4	0.8	0.8
Aspergillus niger	0.1	0.04	0.02	0.02
Rhizopus nigricans	0.05	0.025	0.0125	0.00625
Chaetomium globosum	0.05	0.025	0.00625	<0.003125
Trichophyton interdigitale	>0.008	0.008	0.004	0.002
Candida albicans	0.1	0.1	0.0125	0.0125
Saccharomyces cerevisiae	0.1	0.05	0.0125	0.00625

germicidal in 30 minutes for gonococci, pneumococci, hemolytic streptococci, and typhoid bacilli. Inhibitory action is seen with staphylococci and streptococci, but much less so against typhoid and coli bacilli (Heubner and Siege, 1926). According to Liese (1927), a 1:50,000 dilution is inhibitory for streptococci, and 1:100,000 for staphylococci; by contrast, a 1:5000 dilution is required to inhibit the growth of *Salmonella schottmuelleri*, and 1:10,000 to produce this effect in the case of *Salmonella typhosa* and *Escherichia coli*. A 1% solution does not kill staphylococci in less than 10 hours. Streptococci and coli bacilli require an exposure period of 30 hours. Vapors of 8-hydroxyquinoline were shown to inhibit the growth of staphylococci and coli bacilli exposed in petri dishes for 24 hours (Lebduska and Pidra, 1922).

Albert and associates (1947) found that 8-hydroxyquinoline inhibits the growth of mycobacteria in high dilutions. Its bacteriostatic action on tubercle bacilli is intensified in the presence of copper ions and reduced by cobalt ions (Sorkin et al., 1951).

Oster and Golden (1947) reported that 8-hydroxyquinoline benzoate was the most active antifungal agent in a series of 24 derivatives of quinoline tested. The same authors reported successful treatment of dermatophytosis with the aid of a preparation containing 2.5% of 8-hydroxyquinoline benzoate (1949).

According to Uri and Szabo (1952), 8-hydroxyquinoline is fungistatic in a concentration of 4 to 5 µg per milliliter in liquid, and 5 to 10 µg per milliliter in solid media. A 0.5% solution is claimed to be fungicidal within 30 to 60 minutes, the effect being more marked on pathogenic than on nonpathogenic strains. The character of the fungitoxicity of 8-hydroxyquinoline and of its copper chelate (i.e., whether fungistatic or fungicidal) is the subject of an investigation by Block (1956), who concludes that both compounds are fungistatic in action.

Only brief mention can be made in this context of the extensive series of interesting studies by Albert and his associates (1947, 1950, 1952, 1953). Zentmeyer (1943, 1944) found that the antifungal action of 8-hydroxyquinoline was due to the formation of chelates with trace metals essential to the functioning of certain vital cellular enzymes. Albert et al. (1947) showed that this ability to form chelate complexes with divalent metals was also the basis of its antibacterial activity. The addition of certain metal salts, however, could neutralize the antimicrobial effect of 8-hydroxyquinoline and stimulate bacterial growth. The addition of cobalt salt in the presence of inhibitory concentrations of 8-hydroxyquinoline produces growth of gram-positive bacteria. Zinc and iron salts reverse the inhibitory effect on gram-negative bacteria. Later, Albert et al. (1950) found that the presence of iron or copper in the medium was essential for antibacterial action; they advanced the hypothesis that the chelates formed produced their effect by catalytically promoted oxidative destruction of certain essential cell elements, whereas a metal, such as cobalt, protected the essential cell constituent. In the case of a total absence

of iron or copper, 8-hydroxyquinoline exhibits no antibacterial activity at any concentration (Albert et al., 1952). Anderson and Swaby (1951) found that the fungistatic action of 8-hydroxyquinoline also depends on the presence of cupric or ferrous ions; the ratio between the concentrations of iron and of 8-hydroxyquinoline is critical with respect to the bactericidal action of the combination.

2-Methyl-5,7-dichloro-8-hydroxyquinoline is a halogen derivative of 8-hydroxyquinoline. It is used to treat cutaneous fungus infections (Jadassohn et al., 1944, 1947; Sigg, 1947). 5-Chloro-7-iodo-8-quinolinol (iodochlorhydroxyquin USP), although used chiefly for amebic dysentery, is also employed in dermatologic therapy because of its antibacterial and antifungal properties. It is applied by insufflation (in a powder vehicle) to treat *Trichomonas vaginalis* infections. 5,7-Dibromo- and 5,7-diiodo-8-hydroxyquinoline (diiodohydroxyquin USP, BP) are less effective against staphylococci, coli bacilli, and fungi than the corresponding dichloro compound. Sodium 7-iodo-8-hydroxyquinoline-5-sulfonate (chiniofon USP, BP) is used in the treatment of amebiasis, but also has a record of use as an antibacterial agent.

COAL-TAR DISINFECTANTS

Whereas phenols and cresols are slightly soluble in water, the higher homologs display a decreasing solubility with the increasing weight of their substituting radicals. Other things being equal, this solubility depends on the structure of the substituent, i.e., whether it is a normal or a branched chain alkyl radical, or a cycloalkyl, aralkyl, aryl radical, etc.

In the case of the poorly soluble phenol homologs, and in the case of other phenol derivatives of low solubility, advantage is taken often of the "solubilizing" effect of soaps when easy and rapid miscibility with water is desired. However, considerable care must be exercised in arriving at the optimal ratio of soap to phenol derivative. A deficiency of soap will affect the stability of the "solution," whereas an excess of soap will act like a "lipoid phase," tending to reduce the proportion of the phenolic compound available for antibacterial action. Indeed, the antibacterial effect in this class of compounds may be said to depend, among other things, on the tendency of the phenolic agent to migrate from the aqueous to the "lipoid" phase; the latter is represented in the absence of any interfering factors by the totality of the bacterial cells exposed to the action of the particular phenolic compound. When an interfering factor is present—i.e., in the form of another definite lipoid phase (oil), an added water-miscible solvent (alcohol, ethylene glycol, glycerol), or an excessive proportion of soap (also of certain other emulsifying agents)—a minor or major proportion of the phenolic compound is rendered unavailable for antibacterial action owing to its engagement by such an interfering factor (Tilley and Schaffer, 1931; Gershenfeld and Miller, 1933; Cooper, 1947, 1948, 1949).

The composition of soap as well as the proportion plays

a determining role in antimicrobial activity of the formulation. Thus, in compounding disinfectants of the type of saponated cresol solution, coconut oil soap used in the correct proportion appears to enhance the antibacterial effect of cresol (against *Salmonella typhosa*, though not against *Staphylococcus aureus*). Soaps derived from linseed oil or soybean oil have no such action (Tilley and Schaffer, 1925). A substantial excess of soap may deprive the phenol derivative of most if not all of its germicidal power (Tilley and Schaffer, 1931). These findings agree with those of Cade (1935), who showed that phenol, as well as phenol derivatives (thymol, chlorothymol, betanaphthol, *o*-phenylphenol, resorcinol, hexyl resorcinol), are aided in their antibacterial action by the addition of certain soaps, and within certain concentration ranges. An optimal range appears to exist for a given soap (sodium ricinoleate, coconut oil soap, castile soap). Sodium palmitate and stearate are essentially ineffective as synergists.

The appearance on the market of synthetic phenolic disinfectants is a newer development. Prior to this, the phenolic disinfectants employed in the practice of disinfection were almost exclusively of the category of coal-tar disinfectants. Within this category there are two different groups of disinfectants, each with definite characteristics: the "soluble" and the "emulsifiable" groups. The former comprises preparations containing as the active principle phenol derivatives of low molecular weight, such as the isomeric cresols or xylenols. The saponated cresol solution of the National Formulary (formerly at the U.S. Pharmacopeia) is the outstanding example of this class. The products of the emulsifiable group contain, in addition to phenolic constituents, varying proportions of coal-tar hydrocarbons and other constituents of the so-called neutral oil. Soaps made from vegetable oils or resins form an essential part of the formulas of both groups. Their miscibility with water is due to the presence of soap. Physically, the two classes may be distinguished by the appearance of their mixtures with distilled water. In low concentrations, the soluble disinfectants form practically clear solutions, while those of the emulsifiable group show a milky turbidity.

The regularities in antibacterial behavior referred to in the case of the lower homologs of the alkyl phenol series are observed also with the usual variety of the soluble coal-tar disinfectants. As a rule, they contain the cresol or the xylenol isomers. The *Salmonella typhosa* phenol coefficient may be expected to give a reasonable idea of their general germicidal potency. This is borne out by the results obtained with three commercial "soluble" disinfectants of different germicidal strengths (cresol compound N.F. and cresylic disinfectants A and B) (Klarmann and Shternov, 1936). These authors also give the results obtained with six commercial emulsifiable tar oil disinfectants. Here the picture is entirely different. There appears to be no relationship between the *Salmonella typhosa* phenol coefficients and those obtained with the other microorganisms. The three disinfectants

of the "soluble" group showed that the ratio of *Salmonella typhosa* and *Staphylococcus aureus* phenol coefficients is not in excess of approximately 2 to 1 for any given product. Ratios of 8 to 1 or 20 to 1 occur in the emulsifiable group.

Brewer and Ruehle (1931) found that the *Salmonella typhosa* phenol coefficient is unable to adequately describe the germicidal potency of all coal-tar disinfectants. These authors list certain products with comparatively high *Salmonella typhosa* phenol coefficients of over 3 that would conceal the fact that they are about 10 to 30 times less effective against *Streptococcus pyogenes* (hemol.), thus tending to misrepresent their germicidal value. This contrasts with earlier work done by Philbrick (1929).

Emulsifiable coal-tar disinfectants contain varying proportions of "neutral oil." This consists mostly of methyl and dimethyl naphthalenes, other hydrocarbons (fluorene, acenaphthene), organic bases (quinoline, pyridine) and their alkyl derivatives, certain oxygenated compounds, and organic sulfur compounds. Neutral oil itself is practically free from phenol or phenol derivatives. Obviously, therefore, the antibacterial action of disinfectants containing considerable proportions for neutral oil hydrocarbons cannot be expected to show the functional regularity encountered in the case of phenolic compounds.

There is additional experimental information relevant to this matter. Klarmann and Shternov (1936) found that gradual replacement by neutral oil or cresol does not reduce the *Salmonella typhosa* phenol coefficient of an emulsifiable disinfectant formulated with such a mixture. On the other hand, the effect on *Staphylococcus aureus, Streptococcus pyogenes* (hemol.), and *Mycobacterium tuberculosis* (hom.) decreases as the proportion of cresol goes down and that of the neutral oil goes up. Substantially the same results were obtained when the replacement of cresol was made respectively with alpha- and beta-methyl naphthalene.

The *Salmonella typhosa* phenol coefficient was at one time used extensively as an index of the germicidal potency of coal-tar and related disinfectants. The experimental data just described shows this has some limitations. Similar limitations apply to other classes of disinfectants bearing no relation to phenol., i.e., pine oil compounds and quaternary ammonium salts. The germicidal effect on *Salmonella typhosa* of the pure alkyl phenol derivatives of lower homologs parallels that of other vegetative pathogenic microorganisms to such a degree that the *Salmonella typhosa* phenol coefficient might be regarded as a relative index of the germicidal potency of these compounds. Because soluble coal-tar disinfectants contain certain lower phenol homologs as the active principle, the same consideration would apply in these cases.

However, in the case of the emulsifiable disinfectants, no quantitative relationship exists between the effect on *Salmonella typhosa* and that on other microorganisms.

Some disinfectants of this type, with high *Salmonella typhosa* phenol coefficients, actually may be less effective against other pathogenic microorganisms than disinfectants with lower *Salmonella typhosa* coefficients. Also, of two products with the same phenol coefficient, one may be a much better general germicide than the other. This condition arises mainly from the indefiniteness of the composition of the emulsifiable disinfectants, and its quantitative expression is affected particularly by the variability in the ratio of phenolic to nonphenolic constituents.

GERMICIDAL ACTION OF PHENOLIC DERIVATIVES

Table 12–10 gives the phenol coefficients of a series of simple phenol homologs against *Salmonella typhosa*, *Staphylococcus aureus*, *Mycobacterium tuberculosis* (hom.), and *Candida albicans* (Klarmann and Shternov, 1936). The germicidal potency against these test organisms increases with increasing molecular weight. After the *n*-amyl derivative, a further increase of the molecular weight produces an increase in the germicidal action on *Staphylococcus aureus*, *Mycobacterium tuberculosis* (hom.), and *Candida albicans*. However, effectiveness against *Salmonella typhosa* declines, becoming rather indefinite in the case of the heptyl phenol, which nevertheless shows considerable activity against the other three test organisms. The three isomeric cresols and the four isomers of xylenol, which are coal-tar disinfectants, show increases in activity of up to five times that of phenol.

The bactericidal action of the homologous *p*-alkyl phenol derivatives was studied by other investigators. Coulthard et al. (1930) observed an increasing potency against *S. typhosa* resulting from the lengthening of the substituting alkyl radical up to the amyl, and a subsequent drop of this potency in the case of the hexyl and heptyl

radicals. The phenol coefficients of *n*-amyl cresol were reported by Coulthard and Pyman (1931).

Rettger et al. (1929) showed that the three isomers of normal butyl phenol yielded approximately the same phenol coefficient of 51. On the other hand, Bartz et al. (1935) found the isobutyl phenols to be less effective. The highest germicidal power of several isobutyl derivatives was displayed by 2-isobutyl-4,5-dimethyl phenol, which killed *Staphylococcus aureus* in a dilution of 1:5000.

"Octyl cresol" is a mixture of "octylated" *m*- and *p*-cresol. It and octyl phenol are inhibitory for *S. aureus* in a dilution of 1:128,000. *E. coli* is not inhibited by a dilution of 1:1000 of either, however (Boocock, 1951). The same source gives the following bacteriostatic dilutions for a number of other phenol derivatives: thymol, 1:4000 with both test organisms (growth at 1:8000); *p*-chloro-*m*-cresol, 1:2000 with *Staphylococcus aureus* (growth at 1:4000), and 1:4000 with *E. coli* (growth at 1:8000); *p*-chloro-*sym.m*-xylenol 1:8000 (growth at 1:16,000) with both organisms. For additional data on alkyl phenols and their antimicrobial potency, refer to the papers by Read and Mullin (1928), Read and Miller (1932), Schaffer and Tilley (1926, 1927), and Woodward et al. (1933).

Phenol and its derivatives exhibit several types of bactericidal action. At higher concentrations these compounds act as a gross protoplasmic poison, penetrating and disrupting the cell wall and precipitating the cell proteins (Cooper, 1912, 1913). However, at lower concentrations phenol and its derivatives inactivate essential enzyme systems. Very small amounts of phenolic antibacterial agents result in bacteriostatic action.

In general, gram-negative bacteria show a greater resistance to phenolics than do gram-positive bacteria. This is not entirely true for phenol, which in the AOAC Phenol Coefficient Test shows *Staphylococcus aureus* with a greater resistance than *Pseudomonas aeruginosa* and *Salmonella choleraesuis*.

Table 12–10. *Microbicidal Action of Phenol Derivatives (Phenol Coefficients, 37°C)*

Name	Salmonella typhosa	Staphylococcus aureus	Mycobacterium tuberculosis	Candida albicans
Phenol (I)	1.0	1.0	1.0	1.0
2-Methyl I	2.3	2.3	2.0	2.0
3-Methyl I	2.3	2.3	2.0	2.0
4-Methyl I	2.3	2.3	2.0	2.0
4-Ethyl I	6.3	6.3	6.7	7.8
2,4-Dimethyl I	5.0	4.4	4.0	5.0
2,5-Dimethyl I	5.0	4.4	4.0	4.0
3,4-Dimethyl I	5.0	3.8	4.0	4.0
2,6-Dimethyl I	3.8	4.4	4.0	3.5
4-*n*-Propyl I	18.3	16.3	17.8	17.8
4-*n*-Butyl I	46.7	43.7	44.4	44.4
4-*n*-Amyl I	53.3	125.0	133.0	156.0
4-*tert*-Amyl I	30.0	93.8	111.1	100.0
4-*n*-Hexyl I	33.3	313.0	389.0	333.0
4-*n*-Heptyl I	16.7*	625.0	667.0	556.0

*Approximate

Gram-positive and gram-negative bacteria both are surrounded by a cell wall made of peptidoglycan. Gram-negative bacteria contain an additional cell wall structure—the outer membrane. It is believed that this cell membrane acts as a barrier, selectively allowing nutrients in and keeping other agents out. Moreover, this membrane contains channels called porins. These porins normally allow the passage of low-molecular-weight nutrients such as amino acids, sugars, and salts, and keep out higher-molecular-weight compounds.

Pulvertaft and Lumb (1948) studied the effect of antiseptics on the lysis of bacterial cultures. They found that *Escherichia coli* underwent complete lysis at a phenol concentration of 0.45%. No lysis took place at a concentration of 0.54%.

The effect of antibacterial agents on the leakage of amino acids from the bacterial cell is the subject of a study by Gale and Taylor (1947). A 1% solution of phenol caused a leak of glutamic acid, almost as intensive as that produced by boiling with *Streptococcus faecalis*. From this and other findings, it was concluded that the bactericidal action of phenol depends on its rendering the cell wall permeable to certain essential cell constituents. This appears to agree with the observations of Maurice (1952). He reported that the presence of phenol promotes the penetration of basic dyes through the cell wall of *E. coli*. Haydon (1956) showed that phenol causes leakage of essential metabolites from the cell. By measuring the release of radioactivity from *E. coli* grown on various labeled compounds, Judis (1963) concluded that the lethal action of phenolic disinfectants is due to physical damage to the permeability barrier in the cell wall.

The action of phenol on bacterial enzymes was studied by Bach and Lambert (1937). A 1:1000 dilution of phenol acting for 30 minutes on *Staphylococcus aureus* destroyed the systems activating succinate, fumarate, pyruvate, and glutamate, whereas the lactate, glucose, formate, and butanol systems were partially inactivated. According to Sykes (1939), the concentrations of phenol, *p*-butyl phenol, amyl-*m*-cresol, and hexyl resorcinol required to inactivate the succinic dehydrogenase of *E. coli* is slightly higher than the minimum killing concentration.

The free hydroxyl group constitutes the reactive entity of the phenol molecule. Introduction of the different substituents into the nucleus of phenol (and of polyphenols) modifies this reactivity in different respects. Thus alkyl substitutions affect such significant qualities as the distribution ratio between the aqueous and the nonaqueous (including bacterial) phases, the capacity for reducing surface tension, and, in some instances, species selectivity, all of which determine the antibacterial action of a given phenol derivative. Halogen substitution probably has a similar effect. It also affects the electrolytic dissociation of the phenol derivative, intensifying the acid character of the compound with the increase in the number of substituting halogen atoms (Klarmann et al., 1929).

Table 12–11. *Dilutions Tuberculocidal in 10 Minutes at 20°C*

Phenolic Combinations	Dilutions
A,J	1:100
B,J	1:60
C,J,L	1:150
C,K	1:150
C,D,K	1:300
E,F,J	<1:20
G,H,I,J	<1:20
G,H,I,J	1:150

A = Coal tar nertal oils and phenols
B = Cresol
C = *o*-Hydroxydiphenyl
D = *p*-tert-Amylphenol
E = *o*-Benzyl-*p*-chlorophenol
F = Sodium *o*-phenylphenate
G = Potassium *p*-tert-Amylphenate
H = Potassium *o*-Phenylphenate
I = Potassium *o*-Benzyl-*p*-chlorophenate
J = Solubilized by soap
K = Solubilized by potassium ricinoleate
L = Cresylic acid

Phenol and phenolic compounds are considered to be highly effective tuberculocidal agents. Tilley et al. (1931) found a 1:200 solution of *o*-phenylphenol to be effective against *Mycobacterium tuberculosis* in the presence of organic matter. Klarmann et al. (1934) studied a series of homologous *p*-chlorophenol derivatives and found them to be highly effective against several strains of mycobacteria. Using a modified phenol coefficient test, Wright and Shternov (1958) showed that phenol and various combinations of phenolic derivatives demonstrated good tuberculocidal activity (Table 12–11). Hegna (1977) found *o*-phenylphenol with soap to be more effective than a mixture of *p*-chloro-*m*-cresol and *o*-benzyl-*p*-chlorophenol in a detergent system against *M. tuberculosis*. This work also showed that 1% and 2% *o*-phenylphenol solutions with soap were more effective than a 3.5% solution with soap. It was concluded that the higher concentration of soap in the 3.5% solution reduced its tuberculocidal activity.

A comprehensive study of disinfectants for tuberculosis hygiene was made by Smith (1951), in which he observed that tubercle bacilli were more difficult to kill than other bacteria. He concluded that phenolic disinfectants had great practical value. In a study of the disinfection of clinical thermometers from a tuberculosis sanitarium, it was found that alcohol and phenolic disinfectants disinfected thermometers harboring *M. tuberculosis*, whereas the quaternary ammonium compound and the iodophor tested did not (Wright and Mundy, 1961). The mycobacterial cell wall consists of lipid-rich hydrophobic layers, which is more or less similar to the content of waxy material. It is the content of this cell wall that is probably responsible for the resistance of this organism to so many chemical disinfectants. The ability of phenol and phenolic derivatives to dissolve

Table 12–12. *Survival and Growth of Fungi after 15, 30, and 60 Minutes of Exposure to Phenolic Disinfectant (15% o-Phenylphenol and 6.3% p-tert-Amylphenol) at 1:50 Dilution*

Fungus	Exposure Time		
	15 Min	30 Min	60 Min
Candida albicans	−	−	−
Trichophyton rubrum	−	−	−
Trichophyton mentagrophytes	−	−	−
Epidermophyton floccosum	−	−	−
Microsporum canis	−	−	−
Microsporum gypseum	−	−	−
Scopulariopsis brevicaulis	±	−	−
Aspergillus niger	±	−	−
Aspergillus fumigatus	+	+	+
Mucor spp.	−	−	−
Fusarium spp.	−	−	−

− : No growth on three replicate agar slants
+ : Growth on three repicate agar slants
± : Growth on one of three replicate agar slants

this lipid material probably gives them their tuberculocidal capabilities. Phenolic compounds are generally regarded as fungicidal or fungistatic agents. A 2% phenolic was shown to exhibit fungicidal action over a wide spectrum of clinically important fungi (Terlecky and Axler, 1987) (Table 12–12). Hegna (1977) showed that o-phenylphenol in linseed oil and soya oil soap had greater fungicidal activity than did a combination of p-chloro-m-cresol and o-benzyl-p-chlorophenol in a detergent system.

Zentmyer (1943, 1944) found that the action of 8-hydroxyquinoline in fungi was due to the formation of chelates with trace metals essential to the functioning of certain vital cellular enzymes. When applied to surfaces, phenolics leave residuals that often inhibit the growth of mold.

VIRUCIDAL ACTION OF PHENOLIC DERIVATIVES

Viruses are not alike in their susceptability to phenol or a given phenolic derivative. The chemical makeup and structure of the virus accounts for this. Viruses can be divided into three broad categories:

1. Lipophilic—those surrounded by a lipid envelope that combines with lipids
2. Hydrophilic—those that do not have a lipid envelope (naked virus) and do not combine with lipids
3. Intermediate—those that do not have a lipid envelope but do have some lipophilicity in the capsomere (Prince, 1982)

Klein and Deforest (1963) found that 5% phenol inactivated both hydrophilic and lipophilic viruses, but that o-phenylphenol was only effective against lipophilic viruses and not hydrophilic viruses. Moreoover, o-phenylphenol was approximately 10 times as active against these viruses as was phenol (Table 12–13). The additional

carbon atoms of o-phenylphenol makes it much more lipophilic than phenol. This accounts for its greater activity against lipophilic viruses and its loss of activity against hydrophilic viruses.

During the 1980s a new disease, acquired immunodeficiency syndrome (AIDS), was discovered. It was found that the principal agents responsible for this disease are human immunodeficiency virus (HIV) types 1 and 2. These viruses are lipophilic by nature. As expected, phenolic disinfectants show a high degree of virucidal activity against them. Martain et al. (1985) showed that Lysol brand disinfectant (2.8% o-phenylphenol and 2.7% o-benzyl-p-chlorophenol) at 0.5% produced a >4.71-log reduction in HIV-1 within 10 minutes. Today, numerous phenolic disinfectants are registered with the EPA as HIV-1 virucidal agents.

In summary, one can expect phenolic derivatives to show virucidal action against lipophilic viruses. Activity against hydrophilic viruses is less certain.

SURVEY OF ANTIMICROBIAL APPLICATIONS FOR PHENOLICS

Phenolic compounds have a variety of antimicrobial applications. They are used as the active ingredient in hard-surface disinfectants, germicidal soaps and lotions, and antiseptics, and as preservatives in toiletries and household and institutional products.

The only phenolic derivatives found in hospital, institutional, and household disinfectants in the United States today are o-phenylphenol, o-benzyl-p-chlorophenol, and p-tert-amylphenol. They possess the following characteristics:

Broad-spectrum antimicrobial activity, including gram-negative and gram-positive bacteria; fungicidal, tuberculocidal, and virucidal activity against lipophilic viruses
Tolerance for organic load and hard water
Residual activity
Biodegradable

Phenolic disinfectants are considered to be low to intermediate level disinfectants. They are appropriate for general disinfection of noncritical and semicritical areas. They are not sporicidal and should not be used when sterilization is required.

Phenolic compounds are appropriate for use in aqueous or aqueous/alcohol formulations. Levels of 400 ppm to 1300 ppm in the diluted formulation are typical.

Christensen (1989) showed that o-phenylphenol in high levels of ethanol exhibited extraordinary antimicrobial action against *Pseudomonas aeruginosa, Staphylococcus aureus, Salmonella choleraesuis, Mycobacterium tuberculosis*, and poliovirus within 3 minutes in the presence of 50% whole human blood.

Two incidents of hyperbilirubinemia in newborns in the early 1970s were attributed to the use of phenolic disinfectants in hospital nurseries (Morbidity and Mortality, 1975). Upon further investigation, it was deter-

Table 12–13. *Lowest Virucidal Concentration in 10 Minutes*

Virus	Classification	Phenol	o-Phenylphenol
Poliovirus type 1	Hydrophilic	5%	12% inactive
Coxsackie B-1	Hydrophilic	5%	12% inactive
Echo 6	Hydrophilic	5%	12% inactive
Adenovirus type 2	Intermediate	5%	0.12%
Herpes simplex	Lipophilic	1%	0.12%
Vaccinia	Lipophilic	2%	0.12%
Asian influenza	Lipophilic	2%	0.12%

mined that the phenolic disinfectants were used at two to four times the recommended dilution, and that they were used repeatedly on bassinet and other surfaces in the nursery. It was also reported, but not confirmed, that cloths used with these underdiluted products were laundered with the nursery linen. No further incidents have been recorded.

Parachlorometaxylenol (PCMX) and 2,4,4'-trichloro-2'-hydroxydiphenol (Triclosan, Irgasan) are common phenolic derivatives used in antibacterial soaps. They are also sometimes used as preservatives in household and institutional products and cosmetics.

PCMX was developed in Europe and brought to the United States in 1948. Since then, it has dominated the nonsurgical scrub antimicrobial hand soap category. PCMX has a broad spectrum of antimicrobial activity including gram-negative and gram-positive vegetative bacteria, and fungi. As a preservative PCMX is found in printing ink, cosmetics, adhesives, cutting fluids, photographic emulsions, shoe polishes, and wood pulp. PCMX is effective in acids, alkalis, and neutral media.

Irgasan is a broad-spectrum antimicrobial agent used in deodorant soaps, underarm deodorants, and liquid soaps. In recent years, it has become increasingly popular as the active ingredient in antibacterial soaps, replacing PCMX. Irgasan prevents the uptake of essential amino acids at bacteriostatic concentrations. Bactericidal concentration causes disorganization of the cytoplasmic membrane and leakages of low-molecular-weight cellular contents. It is less active against *Pseudomonas aeruginosa* than other bacteria. Thymol is 2-iso-propyl-3-methylphenol. It is a more potent germicide than phenol. Thymol is soluble only at a dilution of 1:1000 in water, but is much more soluble in organic solvents such as ethanol and glycerol. Thymol formulations are used as disinfectants, antiseptics, and embalming fluid, and in mouthwash preparations. Chlorothymol is made by the action of sulfuryl chloride on thymol in CCl_4. It is used as a preservative in cosmetics, antiseptic formulations, and mouthwash preparations. The optimal pH range is 4 to 9.

According to Schaffer and Tilley (1927), thymol and carvacrol show comparable antibacterial properties; their respective phenol coefficients to *Salmonella typhosa* are 28.5 and 27.5, and to *Staphylococcus aureus*, 45 and 44. This close similarity in bactericidal efficacy is understandable on the grounds of chemical constitution, both compounds being isomeric methyl isopropyl phenols.

Chlorothymol makes a satisfactory antiseptic when applied in the form of a solution in alcohol and glycerine (Beck, 1933). It has a phenol coefficient of 106.6 (Woodward et al., 1933–1934). Monochloro and dichloro derivatives of carvacrol were found to be particularly effective against *Staphylococcus aureus* (Kuhn, 1931), comparing favorably with the corresponding thymol derivatives. "Carvasept" is a combination of chlorocarvacrol with soap; its phenol coefficient is 45 (Hoder, 1931).

p-Chloro-*m*-cresol (3-methyl-4-chlorophenol) has gained considerable importance as a component of an industrial preservative, under the name of Collatone. *p*-Chloro-*sym.m*-xylenol (3,5-dimethyl-4-chlorophenol) is used, among other things, in liquor chloroxylenolis of the British Pharmacopeia.

4-Hexyl-6-chloro-*m*-cresol (2-hexyl-5-methyl-4-chlorophenol) makes a clinically acceptable antiseptic because of high bactericidal potency coupled with low tissue toxicity, according to Hartman and Schelling (1939).

The germicidal action of 2,6-dichloro-4-*n*-alkyl phenol derivatives was studied by Blicke and Stockhaus (1933). 2,4-Dichloro-*m*-xylenol gained some prominence as an ingredient of "degerming" soap formulations (Gemmell, 1952; Innes, 1953; Lewis, 1954).

The formulation of disinfectants with benzyl phenols and their halogen-substitution products is the subject of a study by Carswell and Doubly (1936). A liquid soap properly formulated with *p*-chloro-*o*-benzylphenol (5-chloro-2-hydroxydiphenyl methane) compared favorably with one containing the same proportion of hexachlorophene in regard to degerming effectiveness (Bowers, 1950).

Direct chlorination of phenol or phenol derivatives results in chlorophenol. Examples of these, in addition to PCMX and *o*-benzyl-*p*-chlorophenol, are pentachlorophenol, 2,4,5,trichlorophenol, chlorophene, 2-chlorophenol, and 4-chlorophenol.

Pentachlorophenol is used to control slime-forming bacteria, algae, fungi, and sulfate-reducing bacteria in oil fields. 2,4,5,Trichlorophenol, 2-chlorophenol, and 4-chlorophenol are used as preservatives. Chlorophene (*o*-benzyl-*p*-chlorophenol), also known by the trade name Santophen, is used for disinfection and preservation.

Other noteworthy phenolic compounds used as preservatives or antiseptics are hexylresorcinol, parachlorometacresol, and dichloroxylenol.

PRODUCT FORMULATION USING PHENOLICS

The ratio of soap to *p*-chloro-*o*-benzylphenol is critical with regard to the bactericidal effectiveness of the combination. Bean and Berry (1951), working with *p*-chloro-*o*-benzylphenol and potassium laurate, showed that the bactericidal activity of the solutions is related to the concentration of the benzylchlorophenol in the micelles of the potassium laurate, and independent of the overall concentration in the solutions. An increase in the proportion of benzylchlorophenol to potassium laurate produces an increase in bactericidal activity. Similarly, the bactericidal activity of systems containing chloroxylenol solubilized by potassium laurate was found to be a function of the concentration of chloroxylenol in the soap micelles (Bean and Berry, 1953). A wide variety of synthetic detergents are available. Of the three general classes, anionic, nonionic, and cationic, only the anionic detergents are generally usable in formulating phenolic disinfectants. The nonionic detergents reduce or completely destroy the antimicrobial activity of the phenols, and the cationic detergents are generally incompatible.

Phenolic dispersions made with natural soaps are sensitive to hard water and readily precipitate calcium and magnesium soaps when diluted. Most synthetic detergents have much greater hard-water tolerance. Properly formulated phenolic disinfectants can be diluted with hard water of 400 ppm total hardness and maintain complete clarity and germicidal activity. Wallhausser (1980) reported that highest activity was found when using phenols with secondary alkane sulfonates as solubilizing agents.

The ratio of synthetic detergent to phenolic or natural soap to phenolic compound plays a role in germicidal activity. As ratios and pH are changed, activity changes also. This allows the formulator to design his product to meet the desired germicidal criteria and solution properties. Certain synthetic detergents even greatly increase the activity of the disinfectant against *Staphylococcus aureus*. In recent years, several phenylphenols and benzylphenols and their monohalogenated derivatives have been widely used in commercial formulations. Also, 2-cyclopentyl-4-chlorophenol found a use in disinfectant formulating. Its properties were similar to 2-benzyl-4-chlorophenol, showing high activity against gram-positive organisms. It is no longer commercially available.

A commercial detergent-disinfectant using *o*-phenylphenol and *o*-benzyl-*p*-chlorophenol reveals broad-spectrum activity against both gram-positive and gram-negative organisms, as shown in Table 12–14 (Lehn and Fink Products Group, unpublished data). These data are obtained with the product at use dilution. For many of the organisms listed, greater dilutions are germicidal, because the use dilution is determined by the activity against the most resistant strains.

A simple formulation of two parts dodecyl-benzene sulfonate and one part of substituted phenol at pH 8.5 shows considerable variation in activity against types of microorganisms (Table 12–15). Combinations of phenols

Table 12–14. *Broad-Spectrum Activity of a Commercial Disinfectant AOAC Use-Dilution Method*

Microorganism	Number of "Positives" in 60 Tests
Salmonella typhosa	0
Salmonella choleraesuis	0
Salmonella schottmuelleri	0
Salmonella paratyphi	0
Shigella dysenteriae	0
Shigella sonnei	0
Aerobacter aerogenes	0
Escherichia coli	0
Proteus vulgaris	0
Pseudomonas aeruginosa	0
Klebsiella pneumoniae	0
Staphylococcus aureus	0
Staphylococcus epidermidis	0
Streptococcus pyogenes	0
Streptococcus mitis	0
Mycobacterium tuberculosis	0
Candida albicans	0
Trichophyton mentagrophytes	0

Dilution: 1 oz. to 1 gallon, resulting in 800 ppm phenols.
From Lehn and Fink Products Group, unpublished data.

and other anionic surfactants will show other variations, and the optimal combination must be determined by experiment. Synthetic detergents of high detergency have provided great latitude in formulating phenolic disinfectants. Careful selection of builders and control of pH can result in highly efficient preparations with excellent disinfectant and detergent properties.

The addition of detergents, builders, and appropriate solvents to the basic formulation gives products that clean and disinfect in one step. Such products have found widespread use in hospitals when reduction of labor costs has been a highly important consideration.

The development of pressurized spray packaging was a logical extension for disinfectants, and this type of formulation simplifies use in small areas. When sprayed wet, a surface is readily and conveniently disinfected. A large number of such products are found on the market. The active microbiologic ingredient is frequently a substituted phenol, particularly *o*-phenylphenol. Normal aerosol packaging requires an anhydrous system, but because the biologic activity of a disinfectant depends on the presence of water, an effective aerosol product must contain a significant amount of water. Suitable corrosion inhibitors must be incorporated to provide package stability. U.S. Patent 3,287,214 was granted to Taylor and Prindle in 1966, covering such a system.

Disinfectants formulated with phenolic compounds of low volatility have a noteworthy point in their favor, compared to solutions of cresol. They impart an enduring antibacterial potential to disinfected surfaces (Klarmann et al., 1953; Lester and Dunklin, 1955). This is in contrast to the comparatively fleeting effect of hypochlorites.

Properly formulated phenolic disinfectants are substantially nonspecific in regard to their bactericidal and

Table 12–15. *Germicidal Activity of Some Commercial Phenols AOAC Use-Dilution Method*

	PPM Germicidal in 10 Minutes		
	Salmonella choleraesuis	*Staphylococcus aureus*	*Pseudomonas aeruginosa*
2-Phenylphenol	400	600	800
2-Benzyl-4-cholorphenol	400	400	>1000
2-Cyclopentyl-4-chlorophenol	400	400	>1000
4-*t*-Amylphenol	400	500	>1000
4-*t*-Butylphenol	500	1000	1000
4 and 6-chloro-2-pentylphenol	400	400	>1000

fungicidal action, and are thereby qualified for use in disinfecting practice that is directed logically against pathogenic vegetative microorganisms in general rather than against any species or class in particular. In this connection, it is noteworthy that bacterial strains of staphylococci that have become resistant to antibiotics did not, at the same time, acquire a greater resistance to phenol or to phenolic disinfectants (Klarmann, 1957).

Klarmann (1934, 1937) has observed that combinations of certain alkyl and aryl phenols with other phenol derivatives or with terpineol may display a considerable potentiation of antibacterial power as compared with the theoretic effectiveness derived on an additive basis. However, systematic studies of combinations showed the effects to be only additive, refuting claims of synergism (Hugbo, 1976).

Generally speaking, the addition of alkali to phenol and to phenol derivatives decreases the germicidal action until a point is reached where this action is no longer in evidence (Lundy, 1938; Ordal et al., 1942); however, in the presence of the proper amount and kind of soap, a distinct germicidal effect can be produced at a pH and in a concentration at which the phenol-alkali combination alone shows no such effect to any appreciable degree (Cade, 1935; Ortenzio et al., 1961).

The conversion of phenol and of the phenol derivatives to the corresponding sodium or potassium phenates causes a reduction in bactericidal power. However, these phenates are much more soluble in water than the phenols from which they are derived. Moreover, in certain cases, the phenates may act as "solubilizing" agents for the free phenols. To effect solution of a phenolic compound by means of alkali, in some instances, half the proportion needed for complete neutralization is sufficient. The advantage of this property is that, other things being equal, the resulting compound displays a greater microbiocidal power than it would in the case of complete neutralization.

Whether or not this property may be used depends on the individual phenol derivative. In fact, some phenols require an excess of alkali over that calculated on a stoichiometric basis. They still may be useful under certain conditions directly in the form of their solutions (with a high pH), or the alkaline solutions may serve as a means of depositing such phenols in the form of poorly soluble precipitates on surfaces (fabrics, leather, paperboard)

that are to be protected against attacks by airborne microorganisms (bacteria, molds, and yeasts). Often, exposure to the carbon dioxide of the atmosphere suffices to liberate the phenol from its phenate combination, with attendant fixation of the "insoluble" phenol on the surface to which it has been applied as the soluble phenate.

The effect of pH is particularly noticeable when phenols are solubilized with alkyl aryl sulfonates. Greater latitude in pH adjustment is possible because the alkyl aryl sulfonic acids have much greater water solubility than fatty acids. Highly active phenolic disinfectants can be made having high acidity (as low as pH 3). In some cases, activity against *Staphylococcus aureus* is greatly increased (Prindle, 1959; Rosein, 1960).

For example, 2,4,5-trichlorophenol shows a phenol coefficient of 40 when tested at pH 6 against *Salmonella typhosa*; at pH 10 or above, the phenol coefficient drops to about 1. To protect a given suitable material against microbial action, one could apply either the free trichlorophenol in a volatile solvent (e.g., acetone) or as the corresponding sodium salt in aqueous solution. As a matter of fact, in spite of the wide divergence in the phenol coefficients, both forms furnish approximately equal protection against microbial spoilage to the material to be preserved. 2-Chloro-4-phenyl phenol gives a phenol coefficient against *Salmonella typhosa* of 120 to 130; 2-bromo-4-phenyl phenol gives one of 140 to 160. The phenol coefficients of the corresponding sodium salts are 73 to 80 and 128 to 147, respectively. It is evident that in these cases, unlike that of 2,4,5-trichlorophenol, conversion into the sodium salts, although causing a distinct reduction in bactericidal potency, did not bring about anything like an almost complete abolition of this potency.

Undoubtedly, this phenomenon depends on the difference in the dissociation constants of the two phenol derivatives under consideration. It is known that the acidic character of phenol derivatives is a function of their degree of halogenation. Thus, a trichloro derivative, being distinctly acidic in character and therefore having a comparatively high dissociation constant, will yield an almost completely dissociated sodium salt. In contrast, a monochloro derivative representing a weak acid (with a low dissociation constant) will yield a sodium compound with a tendency toward hydrolysis. Its aqueous solution will contain some of the free phenolic substance and, therefore, the apparent degree of impairment of the antibacterial effect will be less in this case than in that of a polyhalogen phenol derivative.

No noteworthy germicidal activity was encountered by Cole et al. (1941) among several substituted naphthol derivatives. Thus, 4-bromo-2-naphthol, 2-butyro-1-naphthol, 4-bromo-2-propionyl naphthol, and 2-propyl-1-naphthol ethyl ether were practically ineffective against *Salmonella typhosa*, *Escherichia coli*, *Bacillus subtilis*, and *Staphylococcus aureus*; however, 2-ethyl-1-naphthol killed all test organisms in 30 minutes, and 2-propyl-1-naphthol all but *Escherichia coli*.

ENVIRONMENTAL PROTECTION AGENCY REGULATIONS

The Federal Insecticide, Fungicide and Rodenticide Act of 1947 (FIFRA), which has been amended several times (most recently in 1989), is the basic law requiring the formal registration of disinfectant products. The FIFRA regulates ecologic poisons to ensure effectiveness, safety, and no significant adverse effect on the environment. Enforcement now is the responsibility of the Environmental Protection Agency.

Previously, the Association of Official Analytical Chemists (AOAC) Phenol Coefficient Method was the determining test for efficacy of a disinfectant. Most of the earlier investigations used this procedure as a measure of activity. The Phenol Coefficient Method has been replaced by the AOAC Use-Dilution Method. All registered bactericidal claims must be supported by data using this method. Tuberculocidal, fungicidal, and virucidal claims are supported by AOAC or EPA methods.

Antimicrobial products are further divided into several classes, each requiring specific test procedures, number of samples, and designated organisms. Although a concise review of regulations was given by Brown (1973), these regulations are constantly changing, with the latest complete revision in 1982; the reader must obtain current regulations from the Office of Pesticides Regulation, Environmental Protection Agency, Washington, D.C., to be assured of conformation to the law.

The requirements for establishing safety when used as directed have also undergone many revisions. At the present time, minimum data to support an application for registration must include skin, eye, dermal, and oral toxicity. Other data may be required, and current regulations must be obtained from the EPA.

Chemical analysis is done on the disinfectant formulation after it has been aged, usually 1 year, to assure that the level of active ingredient or ingredients remains at the specified concentrations.

The subject of biodegradation of phenolic compounds has received much attention and is particularly important in current considerations of environmental contamination and its ecologic impact. Biodegradation of phenols has been reported by many investigators, beginning as early as 1914. Tabak et al. (1964) made a survey of the earlier literature and reported the degradation of a large number of chlorophenols, hydroxyphenols, and alkylphenols and arylphenols. They concluded that all types are decomposed by adapted strains of bacteria, although major differences in rates occur depending on degree and type of substitution. The widely used *o*-phenylphenol was 50% degraded in 3 hours by natural mixed cultures from soil, compost, or a refinery waste lagoon. Chu and Kirsch (1972) have shown that a bacterial isolate from a continuous-flow enrichment culture can metabolize pentachlorophenol as the sole source of organic carbon. The characteristics of the bacterium suggest a relationship to the saprophytic coryneform bacteria. Swisher and Gledhil (1973) find that *o*-benzyl-*p*-chlorophenol is degraded by sewage sludge in 1 day and by unacclimated river water in 6 days. It has been reported that fluorescent group *Pseudomonas* readily metabolized cresol at concentrations of 1450 ppm in wastewater (Cobb et al., 1976). French patent 2,311,759 (French patent, 1976) describes the degradation of phenols in concentrations equal to or greater than 1 g/L in waste water. A *Nocardia* species isolated from a soil sample and adapted to increasing levels of phenols on nutrient agar and neutral pH was used. It appears that phenolic materials can be removed from the environment by normal biologic means and should present no significant problem of accumulation.

REFERENCES

Aalto, T.R., Firman, M.C., and Rigler, N.E. 1953. *p*-Hydroxybenzoic acid esters as preservatives. I. Uses, antibacterial and antifungal studies, properties, and determination. J. Am. Pharm. Assoc., *42*, 449–457.

Albert, A. 1952. Quantitative studies of the avidity of naturally occurring substances for trace metals II. Biochem. J., *50*, 690–697.

Albert, A., Gibson, M.I., and Rubbo, S.D. 1953. The influence of chemical constitution on antibacterial activity. VI. The bactericidal action of 8-hydroxyquinoline (Oxine). Br. J. Exp. Pathol., *34*, 119–130.

Albert, A., Gibson, M.I., and Rubbo, S.D. 1950. The influence of chemical constitution on anti-bactericidal activity. VI. The bactericidal action of 8-hydroxyquinoline (Oxine). Br. J. Exp. Pathol., *31*, 425–441.

Albert, A., Rubbo, S.D., Goldacre, R.J., and Balfour, B. 1947. The influence of chemical constitution on antibacterial activity. III. A study of 8-hydroxyquinoline (Oxine) and related compounds. Br. J. Exp. Pathol., *28*, 69–87.

Anderson, B.J., and Swaby, R.J. 1951. Factors influencing the fungistatic action of 8-hydroxyquinoline (Oxine) and its metal complexes. Aust. J. Sci. Res. B., *4*, 275–282.

Association of Official Analytical Chemists. 1984. Official Methods of Analysis of the Association of Official Analytical Chemists. 14th edition. Washington, D.C., AOAC, pp. 67–68.

Bach, D., and Lambert, J. 1937. Action de quelques antiseptiques sur la lactico-deshydrogenase du staphylocoque dore. C.R. Soc. Biol. (Paris), *126*, 209–300; Action de quelques antiseptiques sur les deshydrogenases du staphylocoque dore; systemes activants le glucose, l'acide formique et un certain nombre d'autres substrates. Ibid., *126*, 300–302.

Barber, M., and Haslewood, G.A.D. 1945. Antibacterial activity of simple derivatives of 2-aminophenol. Biochem. J., *39*, 285–287.

Barber, M., and Haslewood, G.A.D. 1944. Antibacterial action of 2-aminophenol. Br. Med. J., *2*, 754–755.

Bartz, Q.R., Miller, R.F., and Adams, R. 1935. The introduction of isobutyl groups into phenols, cresols, and homologous compounds. J. Am. Chem. Soc., *57*, 371–376.

Bean, H.S., and Berry, H. 1953. The bactericidal activity of phenols in aqueous solutions of soap. III. The bactericidal activity of chloroxylenol in aqueous solutions of potassium laurate. J. Pharm. Pharmacol., *5*, 632–639.

Bean, H.S., and Berry, H. 1951. The bactericidal activity of phenols in aqueous solutions of soap. II. The bactericidal activity of benzylchlorophenol in aqueous solutions of potassium laurate. J. Pharm. Pharmacol., *3*, 639–655.

Beck, A.C. 1933. Chlorothymol as an antiseptic in obstetrics. Am. J. Obstet. Gynecol., *26*, 885–889.

Bechhold, H. 1914. Halbspezifische Desinfektionsmittel. Munch. Med. Wochenschr., *61*, 1929.

Bechhold, H. 1909. Halbspezifische chemische Desinfektionsmittel. H. Hyg. Infektionskrank., *63*, 113–142.

Bechhold, H., and Ehrlich, P. 1906. Beziehungen zwischen chemischer Konstitution und Desinfektionswirkung. Z. Physiol. Chem., *47*, 173–199.

Beutner, R., Cohen, A., and Beutner, K.R. 1941. Nitrophenol as an antiseptic. J. Pharmacol. Exp. Ther., *72*, 4.

Blicke, F.F., and Stockhaus, R.P. 1933. The germicidal action of 2-chloro-4-n-alkyl phenols. J. Am. Pharm. Assoc., *22*, 1090–1092.

Block, S.S. 1956. Examination of the activity of 8-quinolinol to fungi. Appl. Microbiol., *4*, 183–186.

Boocock, D. 1951. Octyl cresol—A new germicide. Mfg. Chem., *22*, 308–310.

Bowers, A.G. 1950. Germicidal liquid soaps. Soap Sanit. Chem., *26*, 36–38.

Brewer, C.M., 1944. Report on (analysis of) disinfectants. J. Assoc. Off. Anal. Chem., *27*, 554–556.

Brewer, C.M., and Ruehle, G.L.A. 1931. Limitations of phenol coefficients of coal tar disinfectants. Ind. Eng. Chem., *23*, 150–152.

Brown, H. 1973. Disinfectant registration. Soap Chem. Spec., *49*, 45–47.

Cade, A.R. 1935. Germicidal detergents—The synergistic action of soaps on the germicidal efficiency of phenols. Soap, *11*, 27–30, 115–117.

Caius, J.F., Naidu, B.P.B., and Jang, S.J. 1928. The bactericidal action of the common phenols and some of their derivatives on B. pestis. Indian J. Med. Res., *15*, 117–134.

Carswell, T.S., and Doubly, J.A. 1936. Germicidal action of formulation with sulphonated oil. Ind. Eng. Chem., *28*, 1276–1278.

Christensen, R.P., et al. 1989. Antimicrobial activity of environmental surface disinfectants in the absence and presence of bioburden. J. Am. Dent. Assoc., *119*, 493–505.

Chu, J.P., and Kirsch, E.J. 1972. Metabolism of pentachlorophenol by an axenic bacterial culture. Appl. Microbiol., *23*, 1033–1035.

Clark, W.A., and Sessions, L.W. 1951. Development and application of copper 8-quinolinolate as an industrial preservative. Proc. Chem. Spec. Mfr. Assoc., Dec., 55–60.

Cobb, H., Olive, W., and Atherton, R., 1976. Waste water treatment. Gov. Rep. Announce. Index, *76*, 154.

Cole, H.L., Prouty, C.C., and Meserve, E.R. 1941. Germicidal activity of certain organic compounds. J. Am. Chem. Soc., *63*, 3523–3524.

Compeau, G.M. 1960. The absorption of dodecylbenzene-sulfonate and hexachlorophene on the skin. J. Am. Pharm. Assoc., *49*, 574–580.

Cooper, E.A., 1949. The influence of organic solvents on the bactericidal power of aliphatic and aromatic compounds. Chem. Ind., *47*, 805–806.

Cooper, E.A. 1948. The influence of ethylene glycol and glycerol on the germicidal power of aliphatic and aromatic compounds. J. Soc. Chem. Ind., *67*, 69–70.

Cooper, E.A. 1945, 1947. The influence of organic solvents on the bactericidal action of the phenols. J. Soc. Chem. Ind., *64*, 51–53; *66*, 48–50.

Cooper, E.A. 1913. Relations of phenols and their derivatives to proteins. Biochem. J., *7*, 175–185.

Cooper, E.A. 1912. The bactericidal action of cresols and allied compounds. Br. Med. J., *1*, 1234, 1293, 1359.

Coulthard, C.E., and Pyman, F.L. 1931. The disinfectant and antiseptic properties of amyl-m-cresol. Br. J. Exp. Pathol., *12*, 331.

Cremer, H.F. 1935. Biologische Versuche mit den Estern der p-Oxybenzoesaure. Z. Untersuch. Lebensm., *70*, 136–150.

Cross, J.M., Discher, C.A., and Iannarone, M. 1955. Synthesis and antifungal properties of 6-halothymols. J. Am. Pharm. Assoc., *44*, 637–638.

Delauney, P. 1937. Action sur les microbes, des substances phenoliques. Influence de la constitution chimique. J. Pharm. Chim., *25*, 254–260.

Dohme, A.R.L., Cox, E.H., and Miller, E. 1926. The preparation of aryl and alkyl derivatives of resorcinol. J. Am. Chem. Soc., *48*, 1688–1693.

Dunning, F., Dunning, B. Jr., and Drake, W.E. 1953. Preparation and bacteriological study of some symmetrical organic sulphides. J. Am. Chem. Soc., *53*, 3466–3469.

Florestano, H.J., and Bahler, M.E. 1953. Antibacterial activity of a series of diphenylmethanes. J. Am. Pharm. Assoc., *42*, 576–578.

Fogg, A.H., and Lodge, R.M. 1945. The mode of antibacterial action of phenols in relation to drugfastness. Trans. Faraday Soc., *41*, 359–365.

Frei, W., and Krupski, A. 1915. Ueber die Wirkung von Giftkombination auf die Bakterien. Int. Z. Phusik. Chem. Biol., *2*, 118–196.

French patent 2,311,759, 1976.

Gale, E.F., and Taylor, E.S. 1947. Action of tyrocidin and some detergent substances in releasing aminoacids from the internal environment of Streptococcus faecalis. J. Gen. Microbiol., *1*, 77–84.

Gemmell, J. 1952. A new British base for germicidal soaps. Soap Perfum. Cosmet., *25*, 1160–1163.

Gershenfeld, L., and Miller, R.E. 1933. Ointment bases for bacterial agents. Am. J. Pharm., *105*, 194–198.

Gershenfeld, L., and Miller, R.E. 1933. Bactericidal efficiency of 2% phenol ointments. Am. J. Pharm., *105*, 186–194, 194–198.

Gershenfeld, L., and Perlstein, D. 1939. Preservatives for preparations containing gelatin. Am. J. Pharm., *111*, 227–287.

Glaser, E., and Prufer, H. 1923. Ueber die Synthese des Metanitrokresolglucoside and uber die Desinfektionskraft des Metanitrokresols. Biochem. Z., *137*, 429–438.

Glaser, E., and Wulwek, W. 1924. Ueber neue synthetisch dargestellte. Nitrophenolglucoside nebst Beitragen zur Desinfektionskraft und Giftigkeit der Nitrophenole. Biochem. Z., *145*, 514–534.

Gump, W.S. 1969. Toxicological properties of hexachlorophene. J. Soc. Cosmet. Chem., *20*, 173–184.

Gump, W.S., and Luthy, M. 1943. Process for making chlorinated phenolaldehyde condensation products. U.S. Patent No. 2,334,408.

Hampil, B. 1928. Bactericidal properties of the aryl and alkyl derivatives of resorcinol. J. Infect. Dis., *43*, 25–40.

Harden, W.C., and Brewer, J.H. 1937. Condensation products of 2-hydroxy-3,5-dibromobenzyl bromide with phenols and their germicidal power. J. Am. Chem. Soc., *59*, 2379–2380.

Harden, W.C., and Reid, E.E. 1932. Condensation of certain phenols with some aliphatic aldehydes. J. Am. Chem. Soc., *54*, 4325–4334.

Hart, M.C., and Woodruff, E.H. 1936. Alkyl phenols 1. The 4-n-Alkylpyrogallols. J. Am. Chem. Soc., *58*, 1957–1959.

Hartman, F.W., and Schelling, V. 1939. Studies on hexylchloro-m-cresol and other carbocyclic antiseptics. Am. J. Surg., *46*, 460–467.

Haydon, D.A. 1956. Surface behaviour of Escherichia coli. II. Interaction with phenol. Proc. R. Soc. Lond. [Biol], *145*, 383–391.

Hegna, I.K. 1977. A comparative investigation of the bactericidal and fungicidal effect of three phenolic disinfectants. J. Appl. Bact. *43*, 179–181.

Hegna, I.K. 1977. An examination of the effect of three phenolic disinfectants on Mycobacterium tuberculosis. J. Appl. Bact., *43*, 183–187.

Heicken, K. 1939. Keimtotende Wirkung und chemische Konstitution der isomeren Xylenole und ihrer Monohalogenderivate. Angew. Chem. 52, 263–265.

Heinemann, B. 1944. The bactericidal activity of some bis-(hydroxyphenyl) alkanes. J. Lab. Clin. Med., *29*, 254–258.

Heubner, W., and Siegel, R. 1926. Bemerkung Chinosol. Klin. Wochenschr., *5*, 1709.

Hilbert, G.C., and Johnson, T.B. 1929. Germicidal activity of diarylsulphide phenols. J. Am. Chem. Soc., *51*, 1526–1536.

Hoder, F. 1931. Wirkung von Carvasept (Chlorkarvakrol) and Dichlorkarvakrol auf Syphilisspirochaten. Dtsch. Med. Wochenschr., *57*, 1108–1109.

Hugbo, P.G., 1976. Additivity of effects in combination of some chemically related preservative compounds. Can. J. Pharm. Sci., *11*, 66–68.

Hard, C.D., and Parrish, C.I. 1935. Unsaturated ethers of pyrogallol. J. Am. Chem. Soc., *57*, 1731–1734.

Ishiwara, F. 1924. Baktericide Kraft und chemische Struktur. Z. Immunitaetsforsch., *40*, 429–452.

Isikow, H.M., and Gump, W.S. 1952. The synthesis of bis (2-hydroxy-3,5,6-trichlorophenyl)-methane-C14 (hexachlorophene). J. Am. Chem. Soc., *74*, 2434–2435.

Jadassoh, W., Fierz, H.E., and Pfanner, E. 1944. Ein neues Mittel zur Behandlung von Pyodermien. Schweiz. Med. Wochenschr., *74*, 168–170.

Jadassoh, W., Fierz, H.E., Pfanner, E., and Hausmann, W. 1947. Weitere Untersuchungen uber die Wirkung von Chinolinderivaten auf pathogene Mikroorganismen in vitro. Schweiz. Med. Wochenschr. 77, 987–989.

Johnson, T.B., and Hodge, W.W. 1913. A new method of synthesizing the higher phenols. J. Am. Chem. Soc., *35*, 1014–1023.

Johnson, T.B., and Lane, F.W. 1921. The preparation of some alkyl derivatives of resorcinol and the relation of their structure to antiseptic properties. J. Am. Chem. Soc., *43*, 348–360.

Jones, P.S., Thigpen, D., Morrison, J.L., and Richardson, A.P. 1956. p-Hydroxybenzoic acid and its esters. J. Am. Pharm. Assoc., *45*, 268–273.

Judis, J. 1963. Mechanism of action of phenolic disinfectants. II. Patterns of release of radioactivity from E. coli labeled by growth on various compounds. J. Pharm. Sci., *52*, 126–131.

Kimbrough, R.D. 1973. Review of the toxicity of hexachlorophene, including its neurotoxicity. J. Clin. Pharmacol., *13*, 439–451.

Klarmann, E.G. 1957. Environmental disinfection factor in the control of staphylococcal hospital sepsis. Am. J. Pharm., *129*, 42–52.

Klarmann, E.G. 1956. Some aspects of chemical "sterilization" of instruments. Am. J. Pharm., *128*, 4–18.

Klarmann, E.G. 1937. Germicidal compositions. U.S. Patent No. 2,085,318.

Klarmann, E.G. 1934. Germicidal composition. U.S. Patent No. 1,953,413.

Klarmann, E.G. 1926a. The preparation of 2,4-dihydroxydiphenylmethane and of 2,4-dihydroxydiphenylmethane. J. Am. Chem. Soc., *48*, 791–794.

Klarmann, E.G. 1926b. Further studies on the introduction of alkyl and aryl groups into the nucleus of polyphenols. J. Am. Chem. Soc., *48*, 2358–2367.

Klarmann, E.G., and Figdor, W. 1926. The preparation of some alkyl and aryl derivatives of phloroglucinol. J. Am. Chem. Soc., *48*, 803–805.

Klarmann, E.G., Shternov, V.A. 1936. Bactericidal value of coal-tar disinfectants. Limitations of the B. typhosus phenol coefficient as a measure. Ind. Eng. Chem., *8*, 369–372.

Klarmann, E.G., and Von Wowern, J. 1929. The preparation of certain chloro- and bromo-derivatives of 2,4-dihydroxydiphenylmethane and -ethane and their germicidal action. J. Am. Chem. Soc., 51, 605–610.

Klarmann, E.G., Gates, L.W., and Shternov, V.A. 1932a. Bactericidal properties of monoethers of dihydric phenols. II. The monoethers of hydroquinone. II. The monoethers of pyrocatechol. J. Am. Chem. Soc., 54, 298–305, 1204–1211.

Klarmann, E.G., Gates, L.W., and Shternov, V.A. 1932b. Halogen derivatives of monohydroxydiphenylmethane and their antibacterial action. J. Am. Chem. Soc., 54, 3315–3328.

Klarmann, E.G., Gates, L.W., and Shternov, V.A. 1931. Bactericidal properties of monoethers of dihydric phenols. I. The monoethers of resorcinol. J. Am. Chem. Soc., 53, 3397–3407.

Klarmann, E.G., Shternov, V.A., and Gates, L.W. 1934. The bactericidal and fungicidal action of homologous halogen phenol derivatives and its "quasi-specific" character. J. Lab. Clin. Med., 19, 835–851; 20, 40–47.

Klarmann, E.G., Shternov, V.A., and Gates, L.W. 1933. The alkyl derivatives of halogen phenols and their bactericidal action. I. Chlorophenols. J. Am. Chem. Soc., 55, 2576–2589.

Klarmann, E.G., Shternov, V.A., and Von Wowern, J. 1929. The germicidal action of halogen derivatives of phenol and resorcinol and its impairment by organic matter. J. Bacteriol., 17, 423–442.

Klarmann, E.G., Wright, E.S., and Shternov, V.A. 1953. Prolongation of the antibacterial potential on disinfected surfaces. Appl. Microbiol., 1, 19–23.

Klarmann, E.G., Gates, L.W., Shternov, V.A., and Cox, P.H., Jr. 1933. The alkyl derivatives of halogen phenols and their bactericidal action. Bromo-phenols. J. Am. Chem. Soc., 55, 4657–4662.

Klein, M., and Deforest, A. 1963. The inactivation of viruses by germicides. Proc. Chem. Spec. Mfr. Assoc., May, 116–118.

Kronig, B., and Paul, T.H. 1897. Die Chemischen Grundlegen der Lehre von der Giftwirkung und Desinfektion. Z. Hyg., 25, 1–112.

Kuhn, P. 1931. Ueber die Desinfektionswirkung von Thymol und Karvakrol-praparate. Arch. Hyg., 1051, 18–27.

Kunz, E.C. 1950. Germicidal soaps containing halogenated dihydroxydiphen-ylmethanes. U.S. Patent No. 2,535,077.

Laubenheimer, K. 1909. Phenol und seine Derivate als Desinfektionsmittel. Berlin, Urban Schwarzenberg.

Lebduska, J., and Pidra, J. 1922. Antiseptic action of vapors from solid sub-stances. Zentralbl. Bakteriol., 145, 425–438.

Lecoq, R., Landrin, P., and Solomides, J. 1949. Mesure comparative du pouvoir bacteriostatique des six nitrophenols isomeres. Compt. Rend. Soc. Biol., 228, 1385–1387.

Lester, W., Jr., and Dunklin, E.W. 1955. Residual surface disinfection I. The prolonged action of dried surfaces treated with orthophenylphenol. J. Infect. Dis., 96, 40–53.

Liese, W. 1927. Der Einfluss von chinosol auf Bakterien und Protozoen in Re-agenzglass und im Tierkorper. Zentralbl. Bakteriol., 105, 137–141.

Lockeman, G., and Heicken, K. 1939. Ueber kie Keimtotende Wirkung der 6 isomeren Xylenole und ihrer Monochlor- und Monobromderivate. Zen-tralbl. Bakteriol., 145, 61–71.

Lundy, H.W. 1938. The effect of salts upon the germicidal action of phenol and sec. amyltricresol. J. Bacteriol., 35, 633–639.

Martain, L.S., McDougal, J.S., Likoski, S.L. 1985. Disinfection and inactivation of human t lymphotropic lymphadenopathy-associated virus. J. Infect. Dis. 152, 400–403.

Mathews, C., et al. 1956. p-Hydroxybenzoic acid esters as preservatives. II. Acute and chronic toxicity in dogs, rats and mice. J. Am. Pharm. Assoc., 45, 260–267.

Maurice, P. 1952. A substitute for measuring viability in the evaluation of dis-infectants. Proc. Soc. Appl. Bacteriol., 15, 144–154.

Mazzetti, G. 1928. Isomeria e Potere battericida. II. potere battericida dell'orto-meta-e paranitrofenolo. Boll. Soc. Ital. Biol. Sper., 3, 1198–1201.

Morbidity and Mortality, U.S. Department of Health, Education and Welfare, Centers for Disease Control, Atlanta, GA, September 5, 1975.

Neidig, C.P., and Burrell, H. 1944. Esters of p-hydroxybenzoic acid as preser-vatives. Drug Cosmet. Ind., 54, 408–410, 481–489.

Ordal, E.J., Wilson, J.L., and Borg, A.F. 1942. Studies on the action of wetting agents on microorganisms. I. The effect of pH and wetting agents on the germicidal action of phenolic compounds. J. Bacteriol., 42, 117–126.

Ortenzio, L.F., Opalsky, C.D., and Stuart, L.S. 1961. Factors affecting the activity of phenolic disinfectants. Appl. Microbiol., p. 562–566.

Oster, K.A., and Golden, M.J. 1949. Treatment of Dermatophytosis pedis with 8-hydroxyquinoline. Exp. Med. Surg., 7, 37–45.

Oster, K.A., and Golden, M.J. 1947. Evaluation of the antifungal properties of quinones and quinolines. J. Am. Pharm. Assoc., 37, 283–288.

Philbrick, B.G. 1929. The variation of the phenol coefficients of coal tar disin-fectants with the use of different test organisms. J. Bacteriol., 17, 45.

Post, W.E., and Nicoll, H.K. 1910. The comparative efficiency of some common germicides. JAMA, 55, 1635–1639.

Prince, H.N. 1983. Disinfectant activity against bacteria and virus: A hospital guide. Particulate and Microbial Control, March/April.

Prindle, R.F. 1958. Practical aspects of interaction of surfactants and disinfec-tants. Soap Chem. Spec., 34, 11, 81–89.

Pulvertaft, R.J.V., and Lumb, G.D. 1948. Bacterial lysis and antiseptics. J. Hyg. 46, 62–64.

Rawlins, A.L., and Hamilton, H.C. 1938. Polyhydroxy poly-sec-alkyl phenol germicides. U.S. Patent No. 2,107,307.

Read, R.R., and Miller, E. 1932. Some substituted phenols and their germicidal activity. J. Am. Chem. Soc., 54, 1195–1199.

Read, R.R., and Mullin, D.B. 1928. Derivatives of normal butylbenzene. J. Am. Chem. Soc., 50, 1763–1765.

Rettger, L.F., Valley, G., and Plastridge, W.N. 1929. Disinfectant properties of certain alkyl phenols: Normal butyl resorcinol. Zentralbl. Bakteriol. Mi-krobiol. Hyg. [A], 110, 80–92.

Richardson, E.M., and Reid, E.E. 1940. Alpha, gamma-Di-p-Hydroxyphenyl-alkanes. J. Am. Chem. Soc., 62, 413–415.

Rochaix, A., and Pinet, L. 1927. Sur l'action microbicide de quelque derives halogenes de l'acide salicylique. Bull. Sci. Pharmacol., 34, 486–487.

Roesin, M., Pilz, I., and Olerin, G. 1960. The synergism between disinfectants and surface-active substances. Farmatsiia, 8, 629–631.

Rubin, M., and Wishinsky, H. 1944. Functional variants of diethyl stilbestrol. J. Am. Chem. Soc., 66, 1948–1950.

Sabilitschka, Th. 1932. Die konservierende Wirkung einiger Paraoxybenzoesau-reester. Pharm. Monatsh., 13, 225–228.

Sabalitschka, Th. 1931. Preservatives for pharmaceuticals and cosmetics. Mfg. Chem., 2, 5–7.

Sabalitschka, Th. 1924a. Chemische Konstitution und Konservierungsvermogen. Pharm. Monatsh., 5, 235–237.

Sabalitschka, Th. 1924b. Chemische Konstitution und konservierungsvermogen. A. Angew. Chem., 37, 811.

Sabilitschka, Th., and Tietz, H. 1931. Synthetische Studien uber die Beziehung zwischen chemischer Konstitution und antimikrober Wirkung. XI. Zwei und derifach hydroxylierte oder oxyalkylierte Benzoesauren und deren Ester. Arch. Pharm., 269, 545–566.

Sabilitschka, Th., and Liedge, K.H. 1934. Synthetische Studien uber die Be-ziehung zwischen chemischer Konstitution und antimikrober Wirkung. XII. 3-Nitro and 3-amino-4-hydroxylierte oder oxalkylierte Benzoesauren und deren Ester. Arch. Pharm., 272, 383–394.

Schaffer, J.M., and Tilley, F.W. 1927. Further investigations on the relation between the chemical constitution and the germicidal activity of alcohols and phenols. J. Bacteriol., 14, 259.

Schaffer, J.M., and Tilley, F.W. 1926. Relation between the chemical consti-tution and germicidal activity of alcohols and phenols. J. Bacteriol., 12, 307.

Schetty, G., and Stammbach, W. 1956. Bis (2-hydroxy-4, 5-dichlorophenyl) sul-fide. U.S. Patent No. 2,760,988.

Schubel, K. 1930. Zur Toxikologie einiger neuerer Konservierungsmittel; p-chlor-ester der p-Oxybenzoesaure. MMWR, 77, 13–14.

Schubel, K., and Manger, J. 1929. Pharmacology of some p-hydroxybenzoesaure acid esters: Their fate in the organism and toxicity. Arch. Exp. Pathol. Pharmakol., 146, 208–222.

Sigg, K. 1947. Behandlung der Fussmykose und mykotischer Ekzeme mit Ster-osan. Schweiz. Med. Wochenschr., 77, 123–125.

Smith, C.R. 1951. Disinfectants for tuberculosis hygiene. Soap Sanit. Chem., 27, 130–134.

Sokol, H. 1952. Recent developments in the preservation of pharmaceuticals. Drug Stand., 20, 89–106.

Sorkin, E., Roth, W., Kocher, V., and Erlemmeyer, H. 1951. The effect of metallic ions on the tuberculostatic action of 8-hydroxyquinoline and p-aminosalicylic acid. Experientia, 7, 257–258.

Stoughton, R.B. 1965. Hexachlorophene deposition in human stratum corneum. Arch. Dermatol., 94, 646–648.

Suess, A. 1936. Preservatives for cosmetics. Am. Perfum. Essent. Oil Rec., 32, 55–57.

Suter, C.M. 1941. Relationships between the structure and bactericidal prop-erties of phenols. Chem. Rev., 28, 269–299.

Suter, C.M., and Schuetz, R.D. 1951. Synthesis and properties of some alky-liodophenols. J. Org. Chem., 16, 1117–1120.

Suter, C.M., and Smith, P.G. 1939. Synthesis of 4- and 5-phenylresorcinols. The "positive" bromine of the dibromobiphenyls. J. Am. Chem. Soc., 61, 166–168.

Swisher, R.D., and Gledhill, W.E. 1973. Biodegradation of o-benzyl-p-chloro-phenol. Appl. Microbiol., 26, 394–398.

Sykes, G. 1939. Influence of germicides on dehydrogenase of Bacterium coli; Succinic acid dehydrogenase of Bacterium coli. J. Hyg., 59, 463–469.

Tabak, H.H., Chambers, C.W., and Kabler, P.W. 1964. Microbial metabolism of aromatic compounds. I. Decomposition of phenolic compounds and ar-omatic hydrocarbons by phenol-adapted bacteria. J. Bacteriol., 87, 910–918.

Taber, D., Lazanas, J.C., Fancher, O.E., and Calandra, J.C. 1971. The accu-mulation and persistence of antibacterial agents in human skin. J. Soc. Cosmet. Chem., 22, 369–377.

Taylor, F.G., and Prindle, R.F. 1966. U.S. Patent No. 3,287,214.

Terleckyj, B., and Axler, D.A. 1987. Quantitative neutralization assay of fungicidal activity of disinfectants. Antimicrob. Agents Chemother., 794–798.

Thalhimer, W., and Palmer, B. 1911. A comparison of the bactericidal action of quinone with that of some of the commoner disinfectants. J. Infect. Dis., 9, 181–189.

Tilley, F.W., and Schaffer, J.M. 1931. Germicidal efficiency of mixtures of phenols with sodium hydroxide, with glycerin, and with ethyl alcohol. J. Agric. Res., 43.

Tilley, F.W., and Schaffer, J.M. 1925. Germicidal efficiency of coconut oil and linseed oil soaps and of their mixtures with cresols. J. Infect. Dis., 37, 359–367.

Tilley, F.W, McDonald, A.D., and Schaffer, J.M. 1931. Germicidal efficiency of o-phenyl-phenol against Mycobacterium tuberculosis. J. Argric. Res., 42, 653–656.

Uri, J., and Szabo, G. 1952. The inhibition of the growth of dermatophytes by 8-hydroxyquinoline. Acta Physiol., 3, 425–429, 611–617.

Vaterlaus, B.P., and Hostynek, J.J. 1973. Die Vertraglichkeit von Hexachlorophen. J. Soc. Cosmet. Chem., 24, 291–305.

Wallhausser, K.H., 1980. Compatibility of surfactants with disinfectants. Seifen, Oele, Fette. Wocheschr., 106, 107–111.

Watson, H.E. 1908. Variations of the rate of disinfection with change in the concentration of the disinfectant. J. Hyg., 8, 536–542.

Weiler, M., Wenk B., and Stotter, H. 1929. Condensation products from p-halogenated phenolic compounds and aldehydes. U.S. Patent No. 1,707,181.

Wolf, P.A., and Westveer, W.M. 1952. The relation of chemical structure to germicidal activity as evidenced by chlorinated phenols. Arch. Biochem-Biophysics, 40, 306–309.

Woodward, C.J., Kingery, L.B., and Williams, R.J. 1935. Fungicidal power of pheno derivatives. II. Strength in presence of proteins. J. Lab. Clin. Med., 20, 950–953.

Woodward, C.J., Kingery, L.B., and Williams, R.J. 1933. The fungicidal power of phenol derivatives. I. The effect of alkyl groups and halogens. J. Lab. Clin. Med., 19, 1216–1223.

Wright, E.S., and Mundy, R.A. 1961. Studies of disinfection of clinical thermometers II. Oral thermometers from a tuberculosis sanatorium. Appl. Microbiol., 9, 508–510.

Wright, E.S., and Shternov, V.A. 1958. An adaption of the phenol coefficient method to Mycobacterium tuberculosis. Proc. Chem. Soc. Mfg. Assoc., September, 95–99.

Wysonski, D.K. et al. 1975. Epidemic neonatal hyperbilirubinemia and use of a phenolic disinfectant detergent. Pediatrics, 2, 61.

Wyss, A.P., and Poe, C.F. 1945. Germicidal values of benzoic acid and benzoates. Proc. Inst. Food Technol., 21–28.

Zentmeyer, G. 1944. Inhibition of metal catalysts as a fungistatic mechanism. Science, 100, 294–295.

Zentmeyer, G. 1943. Mechanism of action of 8-hydroxyquinoline [Abstract]. Phytopathology, 33, 1121.

CHAPTER 13

QUATERNARY AMMONIUM ANTIMICROBIAL COMPOUNDS

John J. Merianos

The quaternary nitrogen moiety is an essential component for many biologically active compounds. Quaternary ammonium compounds play an important role in the living process. From vitamins (vitamin B complex and thiamine) to enzymes carboxylase, which participates in the carbohydrate metabolism, to choline, which is involved in transmethylation reaction of the fat metabolism, and to acetylcholine, a mediator in the transmission of nerve impulses (Burger, 1960), all play a fundamental function.

There are at least four types of physiologic actions (Burger, 1960) associated with quaternary ammonium compounds: (1) Curare-like (curaremimetic or curareform) action, a muscular paralysis with no involvement of central nervous system or heart, produced by d-tubocurarine chloride used to induce muscular relaxation during surgery; (2) muscarinic-nicotinic action, which is a direct stimulation of smooth muscles, and is a primary transient stimulation and secondary persistent depression of sympathetic and parasympathetic ganglia; (3) ganglia-blocking action; and (4) neuromuscular blockade. Table 13–1 illustrates the chemical structures of representative compounds responsible for these physiologic actions.

Medicinal chemists using the principle of structure activity relationships (Goldstein, 1974) have synthesized many quaternary ammonium compounds that will mimic certain biologic effects. Thus a very complex structure of d-tubocurarine chloride can be reduced to a much simpler decamethonium structure, a neuromuscular blocking agent. Hexamethonium acts as a ganglionic blocker by preventing the receptor from responding to acetylcholine. The decamethonium is too long to fit the ganglionic receptor but would act as a neuromuscular blocker by preventing the combination of acetylcholine with muscle end plate receptors. When the number of carbon atoms separating the quaternary nitrogens is increased above 12 carbons, the autonomic nervous activity

disappears and the compounds become surface active and antimicrobial. However, there are exceptions to this rule, as we will discuss later on in the case of bis-quaternary and polymeric quaternary ammonium compounds, where two and four carbon atoms separate the quaternary nitrogen, and the products have antimicrobial properties. This chapter is concerned exclusively with antimicrobial quaternary ammonium compounds.

DISCUSSION

Although there are many stages in the historical development of quaternary ammonium germicides, there is general agreement on at least two truly historical milestones. The first is the work of Jacobs et al., which examined structure, preparation, and antimicrobial activity. Jacobs and Heidelberger, in 1915, published a number of papers describing the preparation of various different series of the quaternary ammonium salts of hexamethylenetetramine. In 1916 Jacobs and his coworkers published three papers describing the antimicrobial activity of many of the quaternary ammonium compounds they had previously synthesized and of additional derivatives prepared therefrom. In these publications, they related structure to antimicrobial activity. Although some reviews have challenged the work of Jacobs et al. as the earliest investigations of quaternary ammonium germicides, their preeminence is assured by their quality, quantity, and treatment, which included antimicrobial activity and correlation between structure and antimicrobial activity. The only valid criticism of the work of Jacobs may be the fact that some of the antimicrobial activity of his products may be due to the release of formaldehyde from hexamethylenetetramine. Jacobs reported that the antimicrobial activity is due to the presence of hexamethylenetetramine nucleus. Methenamine mandelate USP is used as a urinary tract anti-infective

Table 13–1. *Quaternary Structures with Physiological Actions*

[1] d-Tubocurarine Chloride USP

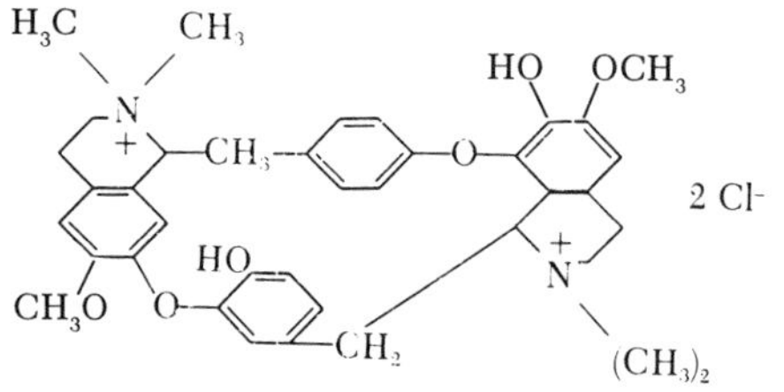

[2] Choline Chloride

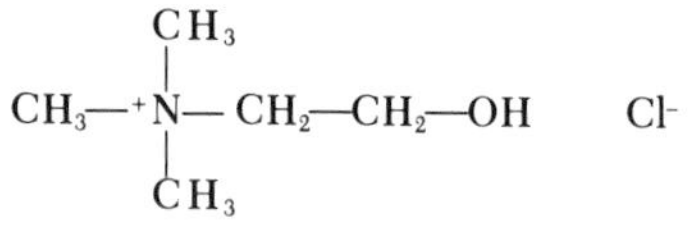

$$CH_3-^+N-CH_2-CH_2-OH \quad Cl^-$$

[3] Muscarine Hydroxide

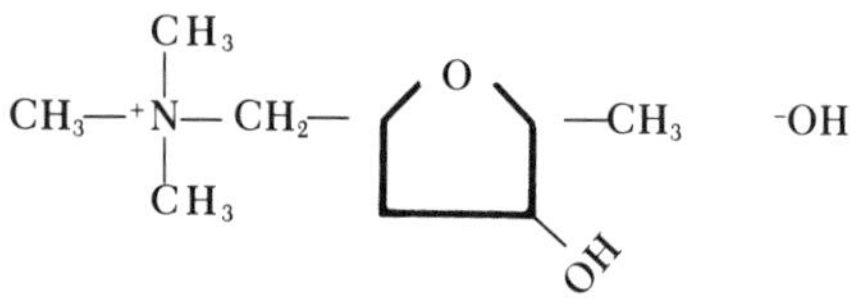

[4] Acetylcholine Hydroxide

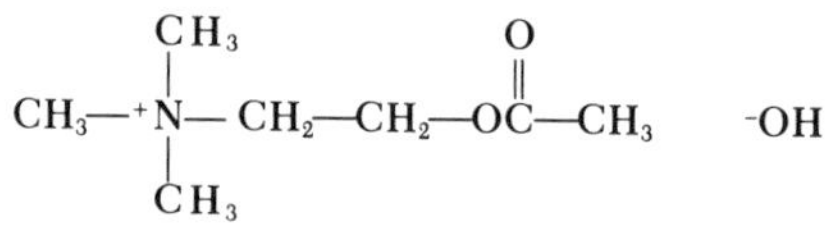

$$CH_3-^+N-CH_2-CH_2-OC-CH_3 \quad ^-OH$$

[5] Betaine

$$CH_3-^+N-CH_2-C-O^-$$

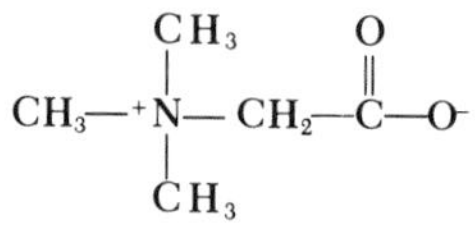

[6] Decamethonium Chloride

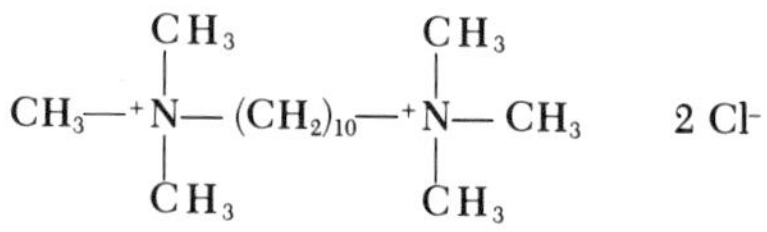

$$CH_3-^+N-(CH_2)_{10}-^+N-CH_3 \quad 2\ Cl^-$$

[7] Hexamethonium Chloride

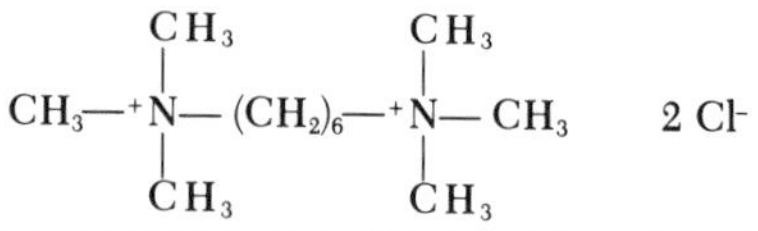

$$CH_3-^+N-(CH_2)_6-^+N-CH_3 \quad 2\ Cl^-$$

even today, acting by releasing formaldehyde in an acid medium (Gennaro, 1985).

In any consideration of earlier investigations, the reader is reminded that our interests are solely with the various aspects of the antimicrobial activity of the quaternary ammonium compounds. Consequently, we may exclude those early publications dealing completely with synthesis of these compounds and in addition refute the role attributed by other reviews to the nineteenth century research on curare (Cucci, 1949).

Not until the 1920s did any additional information appear, at which time Browning et al. (1922, 1926) and Browning (1926) described the bacterial activity of quaternary derivatives of pyridine, quinoline, and other ring structures. Hartmann and Kagi, in 1928, reported on the antibacterial activity of quaternary ammonium compounds of acylated alkylene diamines. It was not until 1935, when Domagk disclosed the antibacterial activity of the long-chain quaternary ammonium salts, that the second and most important milestone in the development of antimicrobial quaternary ammonium compounds took place. The improved germicidal activity that occurred when a large aliphatic residue was attached to the quaternary nitrogen atom established the practicability and utility of these compounds, first in medicine and later in many other applications. This important disclosure stimulated research in synthesis and antimicrobial testing of quaternary ammonium compounds, with the consequent frequent publications and patents issued from 1935 to the present. After Domagk's discovery of the biocidal properties of cationic surface active agents several generations of structurally variable quaternary ammonium antimicrobials of commercial importance were developed.

The first generation is the standard benzalkonium chloride of specific alkyl distribution, namely C_{12}—40%, C_{14}—50%, C_{16}—10%. Another version of equally commercially successful alkyl distribution in the benzalkonium series is C_{12}—5%, C_{14}—60%, C_{16}—30%, C_{18}—5% as shown in Table 13–2. The official United States Pharmacopeia recognizes the benzalkonium chloride as a pharmaceutical aid (antimicrobial preservative). The USP specification for the C_{12}/C_{14} homologs components is 70% minimum of the total alkylbenzyldimethyl ammonium chloride content. This broad specification does not always give the most efficacious product. The major determining factor for biocidal efficacy is the hydrophilic-lipophilic balance of the products. The peak for biocidal activity of the homolog series is illustrated on Table 13–3, with a carbon chain of 14 offering the best activity (Cutler et al., 1966; Daoud et al., 1983; Hansch et al., 1973, 1964; Lien et al., 1976, 1968).

Modifications in the first-generation quaternaries by substitution of the aromatic ring hydrogen with chlorine, methyl, and ethyl groups resulted in the second generation of the substituted benzalkonium compounds. Out

Table 13–2. *Commercial Antimicrobial Quaternary Ammonium Compounds*

Chemical Structure	Trade Names	Manufacturers
Benzalkonium Chlorides:		
$R_1 = C_{12}$—40%, C_{14}—50%, C_{16}—10% $R_1 = C_{12}$—5%, C_{14}—60%, C_{16}—30%, C_{18}—5%	BTC 835, BTC 824 BTC 50 USP Barquat MB-50 Variquat 50 MC Zephiran Chloride Hyamine 3500 Maquat MC 1412 Maquat MC 1416	Stepan (Onyx) " Lonza Sherex Winthrop Lonza Mason Mason
Substituted Benzalkonium Chlorides:*		
$R_2 = C_{12}$—50%, C_{14}—30%, C_{16}—17%, C_{18}—3% $R_2 = C_{12}$—68%, C_{14}—32%	BTC 471 BTC 2125M Barquat 4250 Maquat MQ-2525M	Stepan (Onyx) " Lonza Mason
*See Text and Brochures		
Twin Chain Quaternaries:		
Dioctyl 25%, Didecyl 25%, Octyldecyl 50% R_1 = Octyl. R_2 = Dodecyl	BTC 818, BTC 812 BTC 1010 Bardac 2050 Bardac 205M Bardac 2250	Stepan (Onyx) " Lonza " "
Cetylpyridinium Chloride:		
	Cepacol Chloride Ceepryn Chloride	Merrell Labs. "
N-(3-Chloroallyl)Hexaminium Chloride:		
	Dowicide Q Dowicil 200 Dowicil 75	Dow Dow Dow
Domiphen Bromide:		
	Bradosol Oradol Modicare	Proctor & Gamble Ciba "
Benzethonium Chloride:		
	Phemerol Chloride Hyamine 1622	Parke-Davis Rohm & Haas Lonza
Methylbenzethonium Chloride:		
	Diaparene Chloride Hyamine 10X	Rohm & Haas Rohm & Haas

Table 13–3. *Effect of Length of Carbon Chain on Bactericidal Activity of Benzalkonium Chloride*

	Bactericidal Test (Minimum Concentration That Kills in 10 Minutes but Not in 5 Minutes in ppm)		
Long-Chain Length	Staphylococcus aureus #6538	Salmonella typhosa #6539	Pseudomonas aeruginosa #15,442
8	3000	4500	6000
9	800	1400	2500
10	450	300	1200
11	160	130	400
12	45	40	120
13	25	20	50
14	15	12	40
15	25	20	70
16	30	25	200
17	170	15	360
18	450	60	1000
19	330	90	1300

of this group the product with commercial significance is the alkyldimethylethylbenzyl ammonium chloride under the trade name BTC 471 with alkyl distribution C_{12}—50%, C_{14}—30%, C_{16}—17%, C_{18}—3%. Another product with high biocidal activity in this group is alkyldimethyl-3,4-dichlorobenzyl ammonium chloride under the trade names of Tetrosan 3,4D, and Riseptin with same alkyl distribution as above.

By far the product of greatest commercial significance today is of the third generation of quaternary ammonium compounds, the *dual quats*, developed in 1955 under the trade name BTC 2125M. This product is a mixture of equal proportions of alkyldimethylbenzyl ammonium and alkyldimethylethylbenzyl ammonium chlorides of specific alkyl distribution, as shown in Table 13–2.

This combination of benzalkonium chloride with alkyl distribution (C_{12}—5%, C_{14}—60%, C_{16}—30%, C_{18}—5%) and alkyldimethylethylbenzyl ammonium chloride with alkyl distribution (C_{12}—68%, C_{14}—32%) is BTC 2125M, with superior microbiologic performance (Onyx or Stepan brochures). This synergistic combination of the third generation of quaternaries not only had an increased biocidal activity, it reduced the acute oral LD_{50} from 0.3 g/kg of benzalkonium chloride to an acute oral LD_{50} of 0.750 g/kg for BTC 2125M.

In summary, the third generation—the dual quats—offer improved biocidal activity, stronger detergency, and a relatively lower level of toxicity. In the early 1950s the nonionic detergents were being developed with far greater cleaning power than natural soaps. The compatibility of quaternary ammonium compounds with nonionic detergents resulted in superior formulations that helped overcome the environmental factors, such as hard water, anionic residues of soap, and proteinaceous soils, which were found to weaken their effectiveness (Greene and Petrocci, 1980).

A continual change and improvement in advancing and broadening the spectrum of biocidal activity enabled disinfectants to work under the most adverse conditions and produced safer, more economical products. In 1965 an-

other technological development, catalytic amination of long-chain alcohols, made commercially feasible the production of dialkylmethyl amines, which in turn can be quaternized with methyl chloride to give us the *twin chain quats*, the fourth generation of quaternaries antimicrobials with high performance, unusual properties, and tolerances (Ditoro, 1969; Petrocci et al., 1974). The twin chain quats, like dioctyl dimethyl ammonium bromide and didecyldimethyl ammonium bromide were first introduced by the British Hydrological Corporation (BHC, 1947. "DECIQUAM 222") for the British food industry.

These products displayed outstanding germicidal performance; unusual tolerance for anionic surfactants, protein loads, and hard water; and even low-foaming characteristics. Table 13–4 illustrates the cidal activities and pseudomonicidal, fungicidal, and hard-water tolerance of five of the most active twin chain quats, out of 20 as measured by the official AOAC procedure reported by Petrocci et al. (1974). The product of choice in this series is C_8/C_{12}DMAC because of its superior water solubility and germicidal activity. However, the odd number chain C_9/C_{11}DMAC is an equally active product, although its commercial feasibility has not been explored because of high cost of the odd carbon chain alcohols. Recently several odd carbon chain alcohols have been offered in semicommercial quantities. The concept of synergistic

Table 13–4. *Antimicrobial Activity of Twin-Chain Quaternary Ammonium Compounds*

Compounds	Pseudomonicidal	Fungicidal	HWT
1. C_{10}/C_{10}DMAC	500 PPM	210 PPM	1100 PPM
2. C_8/C_{12}DMAC	500 PPM	200 PPM	1200 PPM
3. C_9/C_{11}DMAC	500 PPM	190 PPM	1400 PPM
4. C_9/C_{12}DMAC	550 PPM	235 PPM	1300 PPM
5. C_{10}/C_{11}DMAC	550 PPM	210 PPM	1300 PPM

HWT = Hard Water Tolerance; DMAC = Dimethylammonium Chloride combination in the dual quats has been applied to twin chain quats dialkyldimethyl ammonium chlorides (dioctyl—25%, didecyl—25%, octyldecyl—50%) was combined with benzalkonium chlorides (R=C_{12}—40%, C_{14}—50%, C_{16}—10%). According to the work of Schaeufele (1984), a 60/40 blend of the above quaternaries proved to be superior to the individual components tested via the AOAC Use-Dilution Test (Official Methods of Analysis of the AOAC, 1984). This newest blend of quaternaries represents the fifth generation of quaternary ammonium compounds. The blend remained active under the most hostile conditions, was less toxic and less costly, and provided more convenient disinfectants.

In the 1980s the toxicity of quaternaries underwent scrutiny by the EPA and other U.S. regulatory agencies. The safety of the biocides in general received top priority over their efficacy. A new class of biocides, the polymeric quaternaries, has emerged, which are less toxic than the standard benzalkonium chlorides and less powerful than the dual quats or twin chain quats. The polymeric quaternaries are milder and have found applications in pharmaceuticals as preservatives (Stark, 1985; Merianos, 1988). The polymeric quaternary ammoniums are polyelectrolytes, representing the sixth generation of quaternary ammonium compounds. They are milder and safer than all other classes based on LD_{50} and cytotoxicity (Stark, 1985). More recently another synergistic combination, which may be considered the seventh generation of quaternary blends of bis-quats and polymeric quaternary (Polyionenes), offer excellent antimicrobial activity against oral flora bacteria, namely *Bacteroids gingivalis* 318, A7A128, *Actinomyces viscosus*, and *Streptococcus mutans* in the level of 1 to 5 ppm in a pharmaceutically accepted polymer formulation (MerPan Chemical Consultants Brochures, MerPanocide L. and MerPanocide LHD) (Merianos, 1988). Reduction of toxicity in the bis-quats without compromising efficacy is not an easy task. These preliminary results required further testing to confirm safety and true synergism in this series of polymeric quaternaries with bis-quats blends (Merianos, 1986).

CHEMISTRY

The quaternary ammonium compounds are the products of a nucleophilic substitution reaction of alkyl halides with tertiary amines. Chemically, they have four carbon atoms linked directly to the nitrogen atom through covalent bonds, while the anion in the original alkylating agent becomes linked to the nitrogen by an electrovalent bond. The general formula for the quaternary ammonium compounds is represented as follows:

$$R_1-\overset{\overset{\displaystyle R_2}{|}}{\underset{\underset{\displaystyle R_4}{|}}{N^+}}-R_3 \quad X^-$$

R_1, R_2, R_3, and R_4 are alkyl groups that may be alike or different, substituted or unsubstituted, saturated or unsaturated, branched or unbranched, and cyclic or acyclic, and that may contain ether or ester or amide linkages; they may be aromatic or substituted aromatic groups. The nitrogen atom plus the attached alkyl groups forms the positively-charged cation portion, which is the functional part of the molecule. The portion attached to the nitrogen by an electrovalent bond may be any anion, but is usually chloride or bromide to form the salt.

Depending on the nature of the R groups, the anion, and the number of quaternary nitrogen atoms present, the antimicrobial quaternary ammonium compounds may be classified as follows.

Monoalkyltrimethyl Ammonium Salts

In this instance, one R group is a long-chain alkyl group, and the remaining R groups are short-chain alkyl groups, such as methyl or ethyl groups. All of the quaternary compounds in this group are prepared from the reaction of a tertiary amine with an alkyl halide (Domagk, 1935; Shelton et al., 1946; Hartmann, 1929). The tertiary amine may be the long-chain alkyldimethylamine or the short-chain trimethylamine, which react with methyl halide or with the long-chain alkyl halide, respectively. Examples of commercially available products in this group are cetyltrimethylammonium bromide as CTAB, alkyltrimethyl ammonium chloride as Arquad 16, alkylaryltrimethyl ammonium chloride as Gloquat C, cetyldimethyl, ethylammonium bromide as Cycloton D256B, Ammonyx DME, and Bretol.

Monoalkyldimethylbenzyl Ammonium Salts

In this group, one R is a long-chain alkyl group, a second R is a benzyl radical, and the two remaining R groups are short-chain alkyl groups, such as methyl or ethyl groups. These compounds are prepared by the reaction of a long-chain alkyldimethylamine with the benzyl halide (Wakeman and Tesoro, 1954; Domagk, 1938; Dunn, 1936).

Examples of commercially available products in this group are alkyldimethylbenzyl ammonium chlorides, as BTC 824, Hyamine 3500, Cyncal Type 14, and Catigene.

In addition, there are substituted benzyl quaternary ammonium compounds such as dodecyldimethyl-3,4-dichlorobenzyl ammonium chloride, sold under the trade name of Riseptin. There are also mixtures of alkyldimethylbenzyl and alkyldimethyl substituted benzyl (ethylbenzyl) ammonium chlorides, such as BTC 2125M, Barquat 4250 (Stepan; Lonza Brochures).

Dialkyldimethyl Ammonium Salts

In this instance, two R groups are long-chain alkyl groups, and the remaining R groups are short-chain alkyl groups, such as methyl groups. These compounds are prepared by the reaction of the long-chain alkyldimethylamine with a long-chain alkyl halide or dialkylmethylamine with methyl halide (Kirby and Frick, 1963; Tonaka, 1944; Kuhn et al., 1940).

Examples of commercially available products in this

group are didecyldimethyl ammonium halides, such as Deciquam 222 and Bardac 22, and octyldodecyldimethyl ammonium chloride, such as BTC 812 (Stepan; Lonza Brochures).

Heteroaromatic Ammonium Salts.

In this group, one R chain is a long alkyl group, and the remaining three R groups are provided by some aromatic system. Thus, the quaternary nitrogen to which these three R groups are attached is part of an aromatic system such as pyridine, quinoline, or isoquinoline.

These compounds are prepared by reaction of the aromatic amine with a long-chain alkyl halide (Browning et al., 1922; Shelton et al., 1946; Mosher and Howard, 1948). Examples of commercially available products in this group are cetylpyridinium halide (CPC and Ceepryn), reaction product of hexamethylenetetramine with 1,3-dichloropropene to give cis-isomer 1-[3-chloroallyl]-3,5,7-triaza-1-azoniaadamantane (Dowicil 200), alkyl-isoquinolinium bromide (Isothan Q), and alkyldimethyl-naphthylmethyl ammonium chloride (BTC 1100).

Polysubstituted Quaternary Ammonium Salts

In this group, the cation portion of the molecule is the same as that described for any of the aforementioned groups. However, the anion portion is not a small inorganic ion as previously described, but a large, high-molecular-weight organic ion. These compounds are prepared by reaction of the quaternary ammonium halides with the sodium, potassium, or calcium salt of a high-molecular-weight organic moiety, so that an exchange of the anions is effected (Wakeman et al., 1971; Shibe et al., 1955).

Examples of commercially available products in this group are alkyldimethylbenzyl ammonium saccharinate (Onyxide 3300 and Loroquat QA 100), and alkyldimethylethylbenzyl ammonium cyclohexylsulfamate (Onyxide 172).

Bis-Quaternary Ammonium Salts

In this group of compounds, there are two symmetric quaternary ammonium moieties arranged in the general formula:

$$R_1—N^+—(Z)—N^+—R_4 \quad 2X^-$$

with R_2, R_3 attached to the first nitrogen and R_5, R_6 attached to the second nitrogen.

Here the R groups are as described for any of the aforementioned groups, Z is a carbon-hydrogen chain, and an anion is attached to each quaternary nitrogen via an electrovalent bond. These compounds are prepared by reaction of a bis-tertiary amine with alkyl halide or of a di-halo compound with a tertiary amine (Hwa, 1963; DeBenneville and Bock, 1950; Babbs et al., 1956).

An example of a commercially available product in this group is 1,10-bis(2-methyl-4-aminoquinolinium chloride)-decane, sold under the trade name of Dequadin or

Sorot. Another example of bis-quat is 1,6-Bis [1-methyl-3-(2,2,6-trimethyl cyclohexyl)-propyldimethylammonium chloride] hexane or triclobisonium chloride sold by trade name Triburon. Another commercially available bis-quat is CDQ (Buckman Brochures), used for industrial water treatment for controlling sulfate-reducing bacteria (*Desulfovibrio* sp.). The CDQ is prepared by reaction of alkyl[C_{12}—40%, C_{14}—50%, C_{16}—10%] dimethylamine with dichloroethyl ether. Also, reaction of 1,4-dichloro-2-butene with two moles of alkyldimethyl-amines or hexamethylenetetramine offer another example of bis-quats with broad spectrums of biocidal activity.

Polymeric Quaternary Ammonium Salts

Many different types of polymeric quaternary ammonium salts have been reported to have antimicrobial activity (Ghosh, 1988, 1986; Ikeda and Tazuke, 1983, 1984, 1985; Samour, 1978; Rembaum, 1973, 1975, 1977). The methods of preparation of these polymers are also many, from free radical polymerization of monomers containing quaternized nitrogen, to cationic, anionic polymerization, polycondensation of diamines with dihalides, or polycondensation of haloamines. The last method was used by Rembaum for the preparation of ionenes, which are polyelectrolytes with positively-charged nitrogen atoms located in the backbone of polymeric chain. This type of polycation was first reported in 1941 and is formed by the Menchutkin reaction from ditertiary amines and dihalides (Rembaum, 1973). Although a number of patents were published since 1941 concerning the applications of ionene polymers (Fush and Stamberger, 1965; Boyer and Santiago, 1974; Walker and Cambre, 1970), little information was available on the mechanism and kinetics of their formation, or their solution properties. The scope of this polycondensation reaction, the effect of concentration and solvent on rates and molecular weight of ionenes, and a proposed mechanism were first reported by Rembaum in 1968, when it was realized that under well defined conditions relatively high molecular weight (3,3 ionene chloride 65,000) ionenes were obtainable. The polymerization conditions for the formation of ionenes involves a total concentration of 3.0 mol [1.5 mol of each monomer] in a mixture of DMF/MEOH solvent [1:1 or 4:1] and 5 to 7 days of reaction time at room temperature to give polyionenes with molecular weight of about 65,000. In condensation polymerization the purity of the condensing species and stoichiometry are critical in obtaining high-molecular-weight polymer. Rembaum (1973) reported that polyionenes exhibit the following biologic effects: (1) *Bactericidal action*, (2) *Formation of insoluble complexes with DNA and heparin*, (3) *Neuromuscular blocking action*, (4) *Cell lysis and aggregation*, and (5) *Cell adhesion*. The antimicrobial and antifungal properties of ionenes were studied by the zone of inhibition method against *Staphylococcus aureus*, *Escherichia coli, Pseudomonas aeruginosa, Bacillus subtilis, Candida sporogenes, S. typhimurium, M. smegmatis, Pseudomonas mirabilis, Pseudomonas vulgaris*,

Table 13–5. *Minimum Inhibitory Concentration of Polyionenes*

Polyionene	MIC (ppm)	
	S. aureus	E. coli
1. 3, 3-ionene bromide	>128	>128
2. 6, 6-ionene bromide	16	16
3. 6, 10-ionene bromide	4	4
4. 2, 10-ionene bromide	4	8
5. 6, 16-ionene bromide	4	32

Candida globosum, M. verrucaris, F. oxysporum and *Alternaria sp.* The MIC for five of the most active ionenes bromides against *S. aureus* and *E. coli* are listed in Table 13–5.

The 6,10 ionene bromide is the most active in these series, and at concentrations up to 4 ppm stimulated the growth of normal cells while this range showed inhibition and death of the transformed human cells W138, possibly by electrostatic cytotoxic interaction (Rembaum et al., 1975). It has been suggested that malignant cells are more electronegative than normal cells. If so, malignant cells should demonstrate a greater affinity for the electropositive ionene polymer. This hypothesis has been supported by experimental work. However, this preliminary study appears to warrant more extensive studies to evaluate this class of polymers as chemotherapeutic agents. Rembaum concluded that polyionenes and their low-molecular-weight analogues constitute a unique model system for a molecular probe of the living cell machinery, because their structure, their positive charge densities, their counterions, and their molecular weights can be varied systematically. These considerations apply not only to the study of toxicity or antimicrobial activity, but also to the understanding of the interaction of the polyionenes with DNA or as molecular probes to elucidate the properties of cell membranes.

The high charge density of polyionenes is responsible for their bactericidal and fungicidal activities, for the prolonged duration of the curarizing action, and for the formation of complexes with DNA and heparin. The differences in the biologic properties or stability of the complexes may be explained on the basis of electrostatic association between the negative and the positive moieties of the interacting molecules.

Because the normal and neoplastic cells show an array of different surface properties, including an increase in anodic mobility after transformation, some polyionenes (e.g., 6,10 ionene bromide) may preferentially bind to cancer cells and inactivate them. This differential binding and toxicity to transformed cells conforms with topologic changes of membrane binding sites in the transformed cells. All four products in Table 13–6 are ionenes containing the quaternary nitrogen atom on the backbone of the polymer chain. The main difference is the molecular weight, which is due to reactivity of the alkylating monomer, reaction time, solvent, temperature, and

method of preparation. The ionene bromides (MW 65,000) reported by Rembaum, however, are not commercially available, despite their many biologic effects and potential applications, perhaps due to poor yields, incomplete reaction (65 to 75% conversion), long reaction time, and toxicity. The other three products listed in Table 13–6 are items of commerce. The WSCP or Busan 77 from Buckman Laboratories, which is chemically identified as poly[oxyethylene(dimethyliminio)-ethylene (dimethyliminio)-ethylenedichloride] is made by condensation of N,N″ tetramethylethylenediamine with dichloroethyl ether in water to give molecular weight 2000 to 3000. The molecular weight was measured by Gel Permeation Chromatography (GPC) using polyethyleneglycol standard according to Levy and Dubin's reported method (Merianos, 1986).

The manufacturer has provided brochures and data sheets describing minimum inhibitory concentration (MIC of 10 to 50 ppm) levels indicating a broad spectrum of antimicrobial activity, with dual functionality as microbicide and polymer clarifier for swimming pools. The material is registered with the Environmental Protection Agency as a swimming-pool algicide, with 2 ppm of active product used as a maintenance dose, and 5 to 8 ppm of active product used to rid pools of heavy, objectionable algae growth. The presence of WSCP at only 2 ppm can reduce by 80% or more the chlorine needed to kill the bacteria. In general, WSCP enhances the activity of all oxidizers used in the swimming pools. In addition, the material is registered with the Environmental Protection Agency as a cooling water treatment biocide at 20 to 40 ppm of active product. WSCP microbicide formulations can be used to control the growth of algae, bacteria, and fungi on cooling towers and other parts of commercial and industrial recirculating cooling water systems.

Another polymeric quaternary ammonium compound is the product Mirapol A-15 from the Miranol Chemical Company, which is chemically identified as poly[N-3-dimethylammonio)propyl]N-[3-ethyleneoxyethylenedimethylammonio)propyl]urea dichloride] or by the CTFA name Polyquaternium 2. This product is made by reacting a symmetrically substituted urea ditertiary amine with dichloroethylether in water to give MW 2000 to 3000.

The manufacturer, who is primarily concerned with hair care products, reports a static level of 80 ppm and a destruction level of 100 ppm against *Pityrosporum ovale*. Additional examination of this structure demonstrates inhibitory levels at 100 ppm against both *Staphylococcus aureus* and *Escherichia coli*. By a time/kill water treatment screening procedure, the product demonstrates a high-percentage kill of *Pseudomonas aeruginosa* and *Enterobacter aerogenes* at 10, 15, and 20 ppm of active product following a 30-minute contact period. Although unpublished reports by Petrocci have demonstrated antimicrobial activity for this product, attempts to repeat these results with current production of this product failed to confirm biocidal activity. This product is not sold as an antimicrobial but as a hair conditioning agent for shampoos.

The last structure on Table 13–6 of the polymeric quaternary ammonium compound, from Onyx (Stepan) Chemical Company, is chemically identified as α-4-[1-tris(2-hydroxyethyl)ammonium chloride-2-butenyl] poly[1-dimethyl ammonium chloride-2-butenyl]-W-tris(2-hydroxyethyl)ammonium chloride, or Onamer M or Polyquat or with the CTFA name Polyquaternium 1. The Onamer M is made by reacting 1,4-bis[dimethylamino]-2-butene (0.9 mol), triethanolamine (0.2 mol), and 1,4-dichloro-2-butene (1.0 mol) in water to give an average molecular weight of 5000 to 10,000 (Green et al., 1975, 1977, 1978, 1982; Good et al., 1987). The purpose of the triethanolamine in the preparation was to randomly terminate the polymeric chain, so that we obtained a low-molecular-weight product by design. The 1,4-dichloro-2-butene alkylating agent is very reactive and gave us a 98% conversion of organic chloride to ionic within 6 to 8 hours in water. Polyquaternium 1 was originally intended for hair conditioning applications (Merianos et al., 1977); however, with the good anti-microbial activity combined with excellent toxicologic data, it emerges as an excellent preservative candidate for ophthalmic preparations (Stark, 1985). Today this product is registered with FDA as a preservative for contact lens solutions (Opti-Tears, Opti-Clean, Opti-Soft, Opti-Free, Polyflex Tears-Naturale II—all are trade names of Alcon Labs, Fort Worth, TX 76134). Table 13–7 lists the comparative cytotoxic response of Onamer M at various concentrations and other solutions by in-vitro testing of Mouse L929 cells (Stark, 1985). The most common ophthalmic preservatives are thimerosal, benzalkonium chloride, and chlorhexidine. These compounds are toxic to the eye and may cause corneal erosion and corneal ulceration resulting in pain. This problem is particularly severe with quaternary ammonium compounds that are concentrated more than 400 times by hydrophilic lenses. Chlorhexidine is concentrated as much as 100-fold by hydrophilic contact lenses, which results in the potential for injury to the eye. The comparative cellular toxicity of soft contact lenses soaked in Onamer M at various concentrations and other solutions was determined by in-vitro testing. Mouse L929 cells were grown

Table 13–6. *Polymeric Polyquaternary Ammonium Compounds*

A. Ionenes A. Rembaum Applied Polymer Symposium No. 22 299-317 (1973)

B. Poly[oxyethylene(dimethyliminio)ethylene(dimethyliminio)ethylene dichloride] (WSCP or Busan 77)

C. Polyquaternium 2 CTFA-adapted name (Mirapol-A15)

n = 6 (average)

D. Polyquaternium 1 CTFA-adapted name (Onamer M)

plus triethanolamine hydrochloride

Table 13–7. *Comparative Cytotoxicity of Soft Contact Lenses Soaked in Preserved Solutions on Mouse L929 Cells*

| | Cytotoxic Response | | |
Lens Soaked	Cell Lysis	Zone of Cell Death (mm)	Cytotoxicity Conclusion†
Saline	−	0	None
0.001% Onamer M	−	0	None
0.01% Onamer M	−	0	None
0.01% Onamer M	−	0	None
0.01% Onamer M	−	0	None
0.1% Onamer M	−	0	None
0.3% Onamer M	−	0	None
1.0% Onamer M	+	31	Moderate
Alkyltriethanol ammonium*			
Chloride [0.03%] + thimerosal [0.002%]*	+	16	Minimal
Chlorhexidine [0.005%] + thimerosal [0.001%]*	+	25	Moderate
Thimerosal [0.001%]*	+	10	Minimal
Sorbic acid [0.1%]*	+	16	Minimal
0.01% Benzalkonium chloride	+	48	Severe
0.01% Benzalkonium chloride	+	64	Severe

*Commercially available marketed solutions.

†Cytotoxicity was rated as follows: Minimal zone of decoloration was 20 mm; Moderate zone of decoloration was 20–40 mm; Severe zone of decoloration was 40 mm.

on a basal salts medium using standard tissue culture techniques. The cells were grown until confluent growth was obtained. HEMA soft contact lenses were cycled through seven 8-hour cycles of fresh solution prior to exposure to the mouse cells. After soaking, the lenses were rinsed in water. The mouse cells were then exposed to each respective lens for 24 hours, whereupon the cell growth was examined microscopically and with staining procedures. The cytotoxic response cell lysis and zone of cell death was reported as in Table 13–7. The results from Table 13–7 conclusively show that Onamer M is not cytotoxic to Mouse L929 cells. This cytotoxic response may be related to the acute oral LD_{50} of these compounds listed on Table 13–8. Additional work is needed to prove if there is a correlation of cytotoxicity and acute oral LD_{50} of the biocides within the same class or different ones. This seems to be the case, if one compares Onamer M with the benzalkonium chloride and

Table 13–8. *Acute Oral LD_{50}: Commercial Antimicrobial Quaternary Ammonium Compounds*

Compounds	LD_{50}
1. Cetylpyridinium chloride	0.20 g/kg
2. Benzalkonium chloride	0.30 g/kg
3. Domiphen bromide	0.32 g/kg
4. Methylbenzethonium chloride	0.35 g/kg
5. Benzethonium chloride	0.42 g/kg
6. Didecyldimethylammonium chloride	0.53 g/kg
7. Octyldodecyldimethylammonium chloride	0.72 g/kg
8. BTC 2125M	0.75 g/kg
9. Dowicil 200	2.20 g/kg
10. 6,10-ionene bromide	1.00 g/kg
11. WSCP or Bussan 77	2.77 g/kg
12. Mirapol A-15 (not sold as antimicrobial)	2.85 g/kg
13. Onamer M or Polyquat or Polyquaternium-1	4.47 g/kg

Chem. Pharm. Bull., *34*, 4215–4224.

the other products. All are more toxic than Onamer M, as can be seen from LD_{50} reported in the literature. Petrocci et al. in 1979 examined this compound and determined that the product was bacteriostatic against *Staphylococcus aureus*, *Escherichia coli*, *Pseudomonas aeruginosa*, and *Streptococcus faecalis* at 50 ppm of active product.

In addition, Onamer-M, when tested by the EPA-required Use-Dilution method, demonstrated efficacy as a hard surface disinfectant at 300 ppm of active product against *Salmonella choleraesuis*, at 350 ppm of active product against *Staphylococcus aureus*, and at 800 ppm of active product against *Pseudomonas aeruginosa*. The product demonstrated excellent activity by a time/test at 10 and 15 ppm of active product against *Pseudomonas aeruginosa* and *Enterobacter aerogenes* following a 30-minute contact period.

At least two characteristics are common to the WSCP and Onamer-M polymeric quaternaries, making them uniquely different from the ordinary biocidal quaternary ammonium compound. One is the absence of foaming, even at high aqueous concentrations. The other is the remarkably low toxicity shared by these polymeric quaternary products. As an example, for Onamer-M at 30% active material, primary abraded and intact skin irritation scores were zero for all observation periods. Draize eye irritation studies recorded a mild conjunctival irritation with scores of 2 or 4 in each rabbit, which cleared on the second day of observation. The acute oral LD_{50} in rats was determined to be 4470 mg/kg. The product was described as nonmutagenic by the mouse lymphoma forward mutation assay and by the sex-linked recessive lethal test in *Drosphila melanogaster*. In addition, it was not considered carcinogenic by the in-vitro transformation of Balb/3T3 cells assay.

For reasons of structure, size, foaming, and toxicity, these polymeric quaternary compounds must be considered uniquely different from the biocidal quaternary ammonium compounds heretofore utilized. The results obtained to date should encourage synthesis within this structure group to produce additional compounds for consideration. Besides the polyionenes quaternary polymers there are other classes of antimicrobial polymers in which the quaternary nitrogen is pendant away from the backbone chain of the polymer (Table 13–9). Samour and coworkers (1978) reported a number of quaternary monomers, homopolymers, and copolymers of N-vinyl-pyrrolidone and 2-methacryloxyethyl-N,N,N-triethyl ammonium bromide and iodide with antimicrobial activity. This activity increases as the content of quaternary ammonium moiety increases. The quaternary nitrogen is pendant away from backbone chain and requires the proper lipophilic groups and proper charge density of the quaternary nitrogen for biocidal activity. In Table 13–9 are listed the most common polymers made by free radical polymerization. None of these polymers is used as an antimicrobial, but they are commercially available as hair conditioning agents for shampoos and other cosmetic products. Examples are Gafquats (Polyquaternium 11) and Merquats (Polyquaternium 7). These products are made by the free radical polymerization of diallyl quaternary monomer, and their molecular weight is over 100,000 (Butler et al., 1966—U.S. Patent No. 3,288,770).

However, more recently Andrews et al. (1981—U.S. Patent No. 4,304,894) reported related Terpolymer, with molecular weight 10,000 to 20,000, to have surprisingly effective sterilizing activity against *Candida albicans* at 0.1%, when it was used as a preservative for soft contact lenses without accumulation into the lenses.

Table 13–9. *Free Radical Polymeric Quaternary Ammonium Compounds*

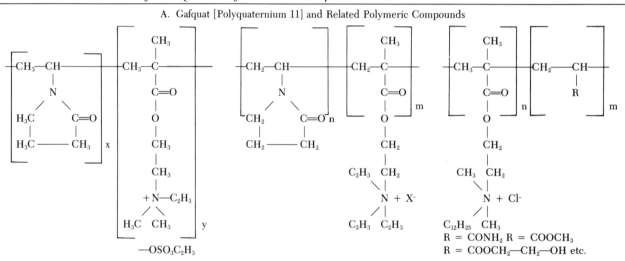

A. Gafquat [Polyquaternium 11] and Related Polymeric Compounds

B. Merquat (Polyquaternium 7)

Diallyl Dimethyl Ammonium Chloride

Poly(Dimethyl Diallyl Ammonium Chloride) (DMDAAC)

Ikeda and Tazuke (1983) reported that antimicrobial activities (MIC) of poly[trialkyl(vinylbenzyl)ammonium chloride] type of polycations against bacteria and fungi were more active than the corresponding monomers; however, the absolute activity is low compared to commercially used quaternaries. The antibacterial assessment was based only on the conventional spread plate method, which has been widely used to evaluate the antibacterial activity of ordinary antibiotics and disinfectants. However, the antibacterial activity of the polycations can not be determined precisely by this method on account of the adsorption of the polycations by some constituents in the culture media. The activity must be evaluated in the absence of any interfering material. More recently, Ikeda and Tazuke (1984, 1985) obtained peculiar results for poly[dodecyldimethyl{vinylbenzyl}ammonium chloride] and its monomer using the conventional spread plate method for evaluation. The MIC of the monomer was 10 to 100 ppm against *Escherichia coli*, *Aerobacter aerogenes* and *Pseudomonas aeruginosa*, whereas the MIC of the polymer product was greater than 1000 ppm against the same organisms.

The poly[dodecyldimethyl{vinylbenzyl}ammonium chloride interacted with the negatively charged species (such as sodium caseinate of the agar plate) and produced an insoluble complex, leading to inactivation of the polymer. In order to evaluate the antibacterial activity of such disinfectants correctly, it is preferred that the products come in contact with bacterial cells in sterile water or saline, and then that the surviving cells be counted after being cultivated on agar plates. Using this viable counting method the antibacterial activity of poly-[dodecyldimethyl{vinylbenzyl}ammonium chloride] was determined against *Staphylococcus aureus*, and at a concentration of 0.5 ppm all the bacterial cells were killed within 30 minutes of contact, whereas the corresponding monomer was inactive. Compounds with the longest alkyl chain studied (dodecyl) were found to exhibit high activity, and this was ascribed to the contribution of the increased hydrophobicity of the compounds to the activity.

In conclusion, the most significant finding was that the polymers are more active than the corresponding monomers, particularly against gram-positive bacteria. The higher activity of the polymers was interpreted as due to favored adsorption onto the bacterial cell surface and the cytoplasmic membrane with subsequent disruption of its integrity, although they have the disadvantage of diffusing through the cell wall, especially with the gram-negative bacteria.

Sheldon et al. (1985—U.S. Patent No. 4,532,128) reported that polymeric quaternary ammonium compounds having repeat vinylbenzylammonium units were antimicrobial and particularly useful for preserving ophthalmic solutions.

Ikeda and Tazuke in 1985 reported an optimal MW region of 14,300 for the 6,6-ionene bromide with antibacterial activity minimum bactericidal concentrations

(MBC) of 6.6 ppm to 10 ppm against *Staphylococcus aureus*. The same workers reported that polymeric biguanides of MW 11,900 and poly{alkyl[C_2–C_{12}]-dimethyl[vinylbenzyl]ammonium chloride} of similar MW exhibit better bactericidal action against gram-positive than gram-negative bacteria. The poly{dodecyldimethyl[vinylbenzyl]ammonium chloride} was the most active with 0.5 ppm against *Staphylococcus aureus*, which suggests that hydrophobicity plays an important role in bactericidal action.

In conclusion, in all three types of polymers reported by Ikeda and Tazuke (1985), there is a clear MW dependence of the biocidal activity—that is, polymers with low MW as well as high MW exhibit lower bactericidal activity—and there exists an optimal MW region for the biocidal action. This MW dependence was confirmed in my work with Onamer M analogues (Merianos, 1986). It is my belief that a fine balance exists in the polymeric biocides between MW, biocidal activity (cytotoxicity), and (toxicity) acute oral LD_{50} as seen in Tables 13–8 and 13–7.

ANALYSIS

The chemical structure of quaternary ammonium compounds permits a variety of quantitative procedures to determine their concentration. Recently various analytical methods have been reported for the determination of benzalkonium chlorides by high-performance liquid chromatography (HPLC) (Marsh et al., 1983; Sato et al., 1984) and gas chromatography (GC) (Suzuki et al., 1989; Cybulski, 1984; Ng et al., 1986). Chemical ionization mass spectroscopy (MS) has been used to identify and determine the proportions of various alkyl chain lengths in commercial mixtures of benzalkonium chlorides (Dauod et al., 1983). The diphasic or the dye transfer method or the Epton method (1947) cannot be used for the determination of polymeric quaternary ammonium compounds. Recently, two methods for determination of low concentration of Onamer-M or polyquaternium 1 antimicrobial preservative in ophthalmic solutions (Good et al., 1987; Stevens and Eckardt, 1987) were reported. A direct titration technique for the accurate, quantitative determination of cationic and anionic polyelectrolytes has been reported by Wang and Shuster (1975). The technique is based on a direct neutralization reaction between cationic and anionic forms of the polymers. Modification of poly[vinylsulfuric acid] potassium salt (PVSAK) method has been used for determination of high concentration of Onamer-M (Merianos et al., 1977). The cationic polyelectrolytes show a light blue color in the presence of toluidine blue O dye, and the blue color turns to bluish purple when the titration end point is reached. With the many methods available, the method of choice is usually dictated by the level of quaternary ammonium compound anticipated in the sample. For solutions estimated to contain 0.5% or more quaternary ammonium compound, the chemist may employ a diphasic or direct titration procedure.

STRUCTURE-ACTIVITY RELATIONSHIPS

Jacobs and Heidelberger in 1916 were the first to report correlation between chemical structure and antimicrobial activity of benzyl and substituted benzyl hexamethylenetetrammonium salts. The results obtained with some 40 substances upon *Bacillus typhosus* demonstrated the existence of direct relationships between chemical constitution and bactericidal action within the series. The degree of the bactericidal action, however, is determined by the position, character, and number of groups substituted in the benzene nucleus. By introduction of the methyl, chlorine, bromine, iodine, cyano, and nitro groups into the benzene nucleus of the parent benzylhexamethylenetetrammonium salt, the bactericidal power of this compound was notably enhanced. The substitution of these groups in the ortho position almost invariably resulted in substances that were more active than their meta or para isomers; the introduction of the methoxy group was without marked effect.

Several substances in which two hexamethylenetetrammonium groups on the same aromatic nucleus (namely bis-quats 1,2-xylylenebis[hexamethylenetetrammonium chloride and mesitylenebis[hexamethylenetetrammonium chloride]) were found to be the most active of the substances of this series when tested against *Bacillus typhosus*. Comparative tests with other bacterial types demonstrated that these compounds possessed a marked degree of specificity for *Bacillus typhosus*. The bactericidal character is directly attributable to the presence of the hexamethylenetetramine nucleus.

The same general principle of increased antimicrobial activity was observed with benzalkonium and substituted benzalkonium chlorides, as illustrated in Table 13–10. The AOAC germicidal and detergent sanitizers test was used, and the hard water tolerance in ppm as $CaCO_3$ was measured. The test organism was *Escherichia coli* ATCC No. 11229; a 99.999% reduction in 30 seconds is required with quaternary level of 200 ppm to pass.

A synergistic blend of alkyl[C_{12}/C_{14} 70/30] 2,4,6-trimethylbenzyldimethyl ammonium chloride [C] has the highest hard water tolerance (HWT) of 1300 ppm, with the 2,4,5 isomer [D] having the next best HWT of 1200 ppm, which is twice as high as the corresponding benzalkonium chloride [A]. The mesitylenyl and pseudocuminyl quaternary compounds are highly crystalline nonhygroscopic materials with excellent microbiocidal properties; however, economics favors alkyl[C_{12}/C_{14} 70/30] ethyl[15% ortho, 85% para]benzyldimethylammonium chloride[B]. The HWT of the alkyl[C_{12} and C_{14}] ethylbenzyldimethylammonium chloride is reported in U.S. Patent Nos. 3,472,939 and 3,525,793.

Synergistic blends of microbiocidal quaternary ammonium compounds with dodecyl to tetradecyl proportion 85/15 to 55/45 are listed in Table 13–11.

Kourai and coworkers (1985) have reported on quantitative structure-activity relationships of antimicrobial N-laurylpyridinium iodides (Table 13–12). The antimicrobial activities of N-laurylpyridinium iodides (19 compounds) having various substituents (methyl, ethyl, propyl, amino, carboxyl, and carbomoyl groups) on the pyridine nuclei were studied against *Escherichia coli* K12, *Bacillus subtilis var. niger*, *Aspergillus niger*, and *Candida utilis* with respect to their chemical structures. The N-lauryl-2,4,6-trimethylpyridinium iodide had the highest antimicrobial activity, whereas N-lauryl-2-carboxylpyridinium iodide had the lowest activity.

In general it can be seen from Table 13–12 that electron-releasing groups on the pyridine nucleus such as amino or methyl group markedly enhanced the activities, and the electron-attracting groups such as carboxyl or carbamoyl group highly reduced them. There was a clearly linear relationship between the antimicrobial activities and the acidic dissociation constant (pK_a) for the corresponding pyridines, and the same relationships exist between the pK_a and both bacteriolytic and bactericidal activities.

In conclusion the findings obtained suggest that the antimicrobial activities of the N-laurylpyridinium iodides are linearly dependent on the electron density of the ammonium moiety. It needs to be mentioned here, however, that the authors did not report on the stability of the iodide salts. It is well known that iodides under acidic conditions in the presence of oxygen and light can be oxidized to iodine, which is a well known biocide (Merianos, 1988). The only commercially used pyridinium quaternary is cetylpyridinium chloride, as the active ingredient in mouthwash (Cepacol), and in preservatives in pharmaceutical preparations. Economic considerations have prevented the commercialization of the substituted N-laurylpyridinium iodide quaternaries.

Kourai and coworkers (1989) reported on the relationship between hydrophobicity of bacterial cell surface and drug susceptibility to alkylpyridinium iodides. The value of antimicrobial activity (log 1/MIC) of quaternary iodides having long alkyl chains (hexyl, octyl, decyl, dodecyl, tetradecyl, hexadecyl, octadecyl) against each bacterium was regarded as the drug susceptibility. The partition coefficient of bacterial cells between n-hexadecane and physiologic saline was regarded as representing their hydrophobicity of the cell surface.

The logarithm of the coefficient was employed as a measure of the hydrophobicity at 37°C. The hydrophobicity of the gram-negative bacteria was always higher than that of the gram-positive bacteria. The susceptibility of the bacteria to each of the alkylpyridinium iodides was analyzed by use of the hydrophobicity, and a quantitative relationship between the susceptibility and their hydrophobicity was found. These findings eventually lead to a conclusion that the first step of the antimicrobial action of the iodides is a hydrophobic interaction between the cell surface and the iodide, and that the magnitude of the drug-susceptibility of the bacteria depends upon the hydrophobicity of the cell surface. Daoud et al. (1983) investigated the relationships between physicochemical properties and the antimicrobial activity of a homologous series of alkyldimethylbenzyl ammonium chlorides

Table 13–10. *AOAC Germicidal and Detergent Sanitizers Test Method* Escherichia Coli ATCC No. 11229 200 ppm Active Quat to Give 99.999% Reduction of E. Coli in 30 Seconds

	Hard Water Tolerance (ppm) $CaCO_3$			
Alkyl	A	B	C	D
R_{12}	100	400	900	1250
R_{14}	700	700	1000	700
R_{16}	400	400	600	500
R_{18}	100	300	550	350
$R_{12-(70)}$	650	1000	1300	1200
14 (30)				

U.S. Patents 3,525,793, 3,472,939

against a variety of microorganisms, and considered whether benzalkonium chloride mixtures could be improved as antimicrobial agents through a more rational choice of alkyl chain length composition. The minimum growth inhibitory concentrations (MIC) of various members of the homologous series of alkyldimethylbenzyl ammonium chlorides were determined against 12 strains of microorganisms, representative of gram-positive and gram-negative bacteria, yeast, and fungi.

The critical micelle concentrations and octanol-water partition coefficient (P) were measured for alkyldimethylbenzyl ammonium chlorides. The partition coefficients were calculated as the ratio of the concentration in the aqueous and oil (alcohol) phases expressed as the means of the replicate determination. Physicochemical data such as log P and log 1/MIC were subjected to multiple regression analysis to produce quadratic equations of the general form:

$$\text{Log 1/MIC} = a + b \log P + C [\log P]^2$$

The log P values were plotted against biologic activity for a series of compounds, and a parabolic relationship was obtained. Log P_o would in this instance be the value of log P for compounds with optimal biologic activity. This value of log P_o will vary between different types of organisms. Many such parabolic relationships have been demonstrated, including several for quaternary ammonium compounds (Hansch and Clayton, 1973; Hansch and Fujita, 1964). The levels of antimicrobial activity

were observed to be parabolically related to the alkyl chain length, and thereby to log P. The chain lengths with optimal activity varied from organism to organism, reflecting differences in their cell-wall structures. The lower chain lengths [C_{10} to C_{12}] were more active against yeast and fungi, whereas gram-negative organisms were most susceptible towards the more lipophilic C_{16} compounds. This was probably a consequence of the lipophilic nature of the gram-negative cell wall and of the difficulties often encountered by hydrophilic molecules to traversing it. As result gram-negative microorganisms were the least sensitive towards all of the homologues, MIC values being approximately 10 times greater than those towards the gram-positive organisms and the fungi. The possibility of dual binding sites has experimental support from the observations of Salt and Wiseman (1968) working with cetyltrimethyl ammonium bromide, which binds in two stages, representing high- and low-affinity binding sites for the drug. Such a mechanism implies potential synergy in combination of benzalkonium chlorides and might influence the choice of alkyl chain components for preservative mixture. Hansch and Fujita (1964) and Lien et al. (1968) reported that the differences in the biologic activity of chemically related antimicrobials, acting at similar sites within the cell, would reflect their relative ease of penetration through the various liquid barriers of the cells and their ability to react at that site. The outer components of the cells were considered as a series of aqueous and lipophilic layers. Sub-

Table 13–11. *AOAC Germicidal and Detergent Sanitizers Test* Escherichia Coli *ATCC No. 11229 200 PPM Active Quat to Give 99.999% Reduction of* E. Coli *in 30 Seconds*

$$
\left[R-\underset{\underset{CH_3}{|}}{\overset{\overset{CH_3}{|}}{N}}-CH_2-\!\!\left\langle\!\!\!\bigcirc\!\!\!\right\rangle\!\!-Et \right]^{\oplus} \quad Cl^{\ominus}
$$

U.S. Patent 3,525,793

R		Hard Water Tolerance PPM	
C_{12}	C_{14}	Calculated	Determined
100	0	400	400
95	5	415	500
90	10	430	750
85	15	445	1000
82.5	17.5	453	1050
80	20	460	1110
77.5	22.5	468	1000
75	25	475	1050
70	30	490	1000
65	35	505	1000
60	40	520	900
55	45	535	1000
50	50	550	900
45	55	565	1000
40	60	580	900
35	65	595	800
30	70	610	750
25	75	625	800
20	80	640	800
10	90	670	800
5	95	685	600
0	100	700	700

stances of low water solubility would be unable to penetrate these aqueous layers and would accumulate within the lipid regions; similarly, those with low oil solubility would be unable to cross the lipophilic barriers. Compounds between these two extremes must exist that possess the optimum balance between hydrophilicity and lipophilicity for traversing the cell barriers.

In summary, antimicrobial activity of the compounds was found to be a parabolic function of their lipophilicity and maximized with n-alkyl chain length of between C_{12} and C_{16}. Generally yeast and fungi were most sensitive towards C_{12}, gram-positive bacteria towards C_{14}, and gram-negative bacteria towards C_{16}. The gram-negative cells were the most resistant towards all the compounds, and gram-positive cells the least.

Tomlinson and coworkers in 1977 reported on the effect of colloidal association on the measured activity of alkyldimethyl benzylammonium chlorides (ADBAC) homologous series C_8 to C_{18} against *Pseudomonas aeruginosa* (ATCC 9027). The critical micelle concentrations (CMC) is an important factor in the study of antimicrobial

activity of cationics; at high concentrations of ADBAC, formation of a micellar state of the salt is interfering with the cationics' antibacterial action. Tomlinson et al. (1977) questioned the normally accepted parabolic relationship reported to exist between the lipophilicity of many quaternary ammonium salts and their antibacterial activities. The high concentration of nutrient salts, which is used in screening, would alter the concentration of monomeric quaternary ammonium salt. This may be responsible for some of the parabolic relationships, rather than the intrinsic antibacterial activity of the compounds. As early as 1953 it was reported that for the homologous series of cationic surface active agents, a parabolic relationship could exist between their antibacterial properties and their hydrophobic character. Thus, there is a linear relationship between activity and alkyl chain length with increased carbon number up to a maximum of between C_{12} and C_{14}, at which region there is observed a decrease in activity. In Table 13–3, the work of Cutler et al. (1967) showed that with broth dilution tests a peak activity against various microorganisms could be observed at an alkyl chain length of 14 carbon atoms. The turndown in activity is probably related to more than one physical property of the compounds: (a) The longer the chain the greater the tendency for the molecule to be adsorbed at the surface of a bacterium; (b) There is a reduction of aqueous solubility of the molecule as the carbon number is increased. These workers failed to discuss the relevance of micellization to the thermodynamic state of the ADBAC molecule in the test system. Salt additives are known to increase the tendency of ionic surface active agents to micellize in water. In some instances the micellar molecular weights can increase, indicating a change in micellar type.

In conclusion, Tomlinson et al. (1977) have measured the antibacterial activities of ADBAC homologous by the minimum inhibitory concentration procedure and by a sterilization kinetics test carried out in deionized water. There was a log-linear relationship between activity measured by kinetics test and carbon number. With the MIC method there was a log-linear relationship up to C_{14}, then there was a turndown in activity. So consideration of the colloidal association of ADBAC in deionized water and in a simple salts growth media led these authors to suggest that use of high concentrations of nutrient salts in MIC tests will lower the effective concentration of the surface active agents. This change may be responsible for the turndown in activity observed in MIC tests, and that in such circumstances the MIC test does not give a true reflection of the intrinsic activity of the compounds.

Jono and coworkers (1986) investigated the effect of alkyl chain length of benzalkonium chloride (BAC) on the bactericidal activity and binding to organic materials during a short contact time (10 s, 30 s, 1 min, 10 min) by counting survivors. Table 13–13 lists the results. The effect of human serum and dried yeast on the bactericidal activity of ADBAC standard blend OSN Alkyl[C_{12}—59

Table 13–12. *Minimum Inhibitory Concentration of N-Laurylpyridinium Iodides Against* Escherichia Coli *K12,* Bacillus Subtilis *Var.* Niger, Candida Utilis, *and* Aspergillus Niger

							MICs(M)*			
No.	2	3	4	5	6	Abbreviation	E. coli K12	B. subtilis var. niger	C. utilis	A. niger
1.	H	H	H	H	H	Py	53	5.6	61	85
2.	CH_3	H	H	H	H	2-Me-Py	21	3.6	26	26
3.	H	CH_3	H	H	H	3-Me-Py	51	4.9	59	82
4.	H	H	CH_3	H	H	4-Me-Py	31	4.6	45	72
5.	CH_3	H	CH_3	H	H	2,4-Me-Py	20	4.0	32	35
6.	CH_3	H	H	H	CH_3	2,6-Me-Py	20	5.0	30	40
7.	H	CH_3	CH_3	H	H	3,4-Me-Py	40	2.7	20	35
8.	H	CH_3	H	CH_3	H	3,5-Me-Py	74	5.5	17	69
9.	CH_3	H	CH_3	H	CH_3	2,4,6-Me-Py	2.6	0.39	0.49	29
10.	H	$CONH_2$	H	H	H	3-$CONH_2$-Py	71	20	210	67
11.	H	H	$CONH_2$	H	H	4-$CONH_2$-Py	84	24	220	77
12.	COOH	H	H	H	H	2-COOH-Py	1100	380	640	460
13.	H	COOH	H	H	H	3-COOH-Py	780	280	430	400
14.	H	H	COOH	H	H	4-COOH-Py	1000	350	700	460
15.	NH_2	H	H	H	H	2-NH_2-PY	44	10	13	23
16.	H	NH_2	H	H	H	3-NH_2-PY	29	1.8	3.8	35
17.	H	H	NH_2	H	H	4-NH_2-PY	10	1.6	7.0	23
18.	C_2H_5	H	H	H	H	2-C_2H_5-Py	45	12	160	130
19.	C_3H_7	H	H	H	H	2-C_3H_7-Py	24	6.3	53	120

*MICs against bacteria and yeast were measured by a Hitachi Recording Incubator, and MICs against mold by the test-tube dilution method.

to 63%, C_{14}—29 to 34%, C_{16}—6.8 to 7.2%]dimethylbenzyl ammonium chloride and pure C_{12}BAC, C_{14}BAC, C_{16}BAC was compared against 13 strains of bacteria.

It was concluded that from the practical point of view C_{12} benzalkonium chloride was the most effective component of the homologues series in the presence of organic materials. The bactericidal activity of BAC was inhibited by both dried yeast and human serum. The inhibition by 2.5% dried yeast was stronger than that by 10% human serum. As the carbon chain was increased, the inhibition increased. The C_{12}BAC was bactericidal against *Pseudomonas cepacia, Pseudomonas aeruginosa, Achromobacter guttatis, Alcaligenes faecalis,* and *Serratia marcescens* at 5000 ppm in a suspension of 2.5% dried yeast and at 2500 ppm in a 10% solution human serum at 1 min of contact, but C_{14}BAC and C_{16}BAC could not kill them at 10,000 ppm at 10 min. Many factors might be affected by the alkyl carbon length of BAC, producing changes in the bactericidal activity; for example, (1) aqueous solubility; (2) aqueous critical micelle concentration; (3) lipophilicity; and (4) the cell surface characteristics of the microorganisms used. The C_{12}BAC and C_{14}BAC were effectively bactericidal with all bacteria tested, even at a short contact time (30 s to 1 min). The inhibition of bactericidal activity by organic materials was least for the C_{12}BAC (Table 13–13). To clarify the relationship between inhibition of bactericidal activity of BAC by organic materials and binding of BAC to them, the authors assayed unbound C_{12}BAC and C_{14}BAC in a solution of bovine serum albumin by HPLC. As the carbon chain was lengthened, aqueous solubility decreased.

When the carbon chain is longer than C_{14}, the solubility and the critical micelle concentration of BAC are extremely low. The binding to bovine serum albumin is increased with increase in the carbon chain; the C_{14}BAC bound to bovine serum albumin 2.5 to 3.7 times more than C_{12}BAC did. The bactericidal activity of BAC in a solution of bovine serum albumin depended on the amount of unbound BAC. The results in Table 13–13 show that other factors in human serum also inhibited the activity. Human serum tended to stimulate bactericidal activity against *Staphylococcus aureus* and *Pseudomonas cepacia* when the contact time was short. Human serum may make the surface of some bacteria more sensitive to BAC. These results suggest that C_{12}BAC is the most effective component of the homologous series of BAC in the presence of organic materials. The greater the content of C_{12}BAC in the blends, the more effective the mixture will be as a sanitizer from the practical point of view.

ANTIMICROBIAL ACTIVITY

The assessment of the antimicrobial activity of the quaternary ammonium compounds has, in some recent instances, demonstrated a lack of scientific objectivity. Those statements about antimicrobial quaternary ammonium compound testing that, by the selection of the

Table 13–13. *Effect of Human Serum and Dried Yeast on Bactericidal Activity of Homologues of the Long-Chain Alkyl Benzalkonium Chlorides*

Bactericidal Concentration ($\times 10^3$ µg/ml)[a]

Organism		OSN 10s	OSN 30s	OSN 1 min	OSN 10 min	C₁₂-BAC 10s	C₁₂-BAC 30s	C₁₂-BAC 1 min	C₁₂-BAC 10 min	C₁₄-BAC 10s	C₁₄-BAC 30s	C₁₄-BAC 1 min	C₁₄-BAC 10 min	C₁₆-BAC 10s	C₁₆-BAC 30s	C₁₆-BAC 1 min	C₁₆-BAC 10 min
S. aureus FDA 209P	DW	0.5	0.5	0.2	0.05	5	1	0.5	0.1	1	0.4	0.1	0.025	0.4	0.2	0.025	0.01
	HS	1	0.5	0.5	0.5	1	1	0.5	0.5	5	1	0.5	0.5	0.5	0.5	0.5	0.5
	DY	5	5	2.5	2.5	5	5	2.5	2.5	5	5	2.5	2.5	>10	2.5	2.5	2.5
S. epidermidis IFO 3762	DW	0.2	0.1	0.0125	0.006	1	0.4	0.4	0.025	0.8	0.025	0.025	0.006	0.05	0.006	< 0.006	< 0.006
	HS	0.5	0.5	0.5	0.5	2.5	1	0.5	0.5	0.5	0.5	0.5	0.5	2.5	0.5	0.5	0.5
	DY	2.5	2.5	2.5	2.5	2.5	1	2.5	2.5	2.5	2.5	2.5	2.5	2.5	2.5	2.5	1
P. cepacia ATCC 17774	DW	5	1	1	0.4	1	0.8	0.5	0.2	2.5	0.5	0.2	0.1	>10	>10	0.2	0.05
	HS	2.5	0.5	0.5	0.5	2.5	1	0.5	0.5	0.5	0.5	2.5	0.5	>10	>10	>10	2.5
	DY	10	5	5	2.5	5	5	5	2.5	>10	5	2.5	0.5	>10	>10	>10	>10
P. cepacia H130	DW	5	5	0.2	0.1	5	1	1	0.5	10	5	10	5	>10	>10	>10	2.5
	HS	5	1	0.5	0.5	5	1	1	0.5	5	5	5	0.2	>10	>10	>10	2.5
	DY	>10	5	5	2.5	>10	5	5	5	>10	>10	2.5	1	>10	>10	>10	5
P. aeruginosa IFO 13736	DW	0.05	0.05	0.025	0.01	0.1	0.1	0.05	0.025	0.05	0.5	0.025	0.001	0.1	0.025	0.025	0.01
	HS	2.5	1	0.5	0.5	10	5	0.5	0.5	10	5	2.5	1	>10	>10	5	1
	DY	10	10	5	5	5	5	5	5	>10	>10	10	5	>10	>10	10	5
P. aeruginosa 82-2-32	DW	0.1	0.1	0.025	0.01	0.2	0.1	0.1	0.025	0.2	0.2	0.025	0.01	10	0.1	0.05	0.01
	HS	2.5	2.5	0.5	0.5	5	5	2.5	1	10	5	2.5	1	5	5	0.5	0.5
	DY	>10	10	10	10	10	5	5	5	>10	>10	10	10	>10	>10	>10	>10
P. mirabilis ATCC 21100	DW	0.2	0.2	0.05	0.05	0.4	0.2	0.01	0.01	0.2	0.05	0.05	0.025	0.1	0.05	0.01	0.01
	HS	5	2.5	0.5	0.5	5	1	1	0.5	10	2.5	2.5	1	>10	5	5	1
	DY	>10	5	5	2.5	10	5	5	2.5	>10	>10	5	1	>10	>10	>10	>10
P. mirabilis 82-1-4	DW	5	5	0.1	0.01	1	0.4	0.2	0.05	1	0.1	0.05	0.05	>10	0.2	0.05	0.025
	HS	5	1	0.5	0.5	10	2.5	1	1	10	2.5	2.5	0.1	>10	>10	2.5	0.5
	DY	>10	5	5	5	5	5	5	5	>10	>10	5	5	>10	>10	>10	5
P. morganii 82-2-11	DW	0.5	0.2	0.1	0.05	1	0.2	0.05	0.05	1	0.05	0.01	0.01	1	0.05	0.05	0.025
	HS	2.5	1	0.5	0.5	10	1	0.5	0.5	10	5	1	1	>10	5	5	1
	DY	5	5	5	5	10	5	5	5	10	10	5	5	>10	>10	>10	10
S. marcescens 82-2-52	DW	5	0.4	0.2	0.05	>10	0.4	0.4	0.025	>10	0.4	0.2	0.025	>10	0.2	0.025	0.025
	HS	5	2.5	1	0.5	5	1	0.5	0.5	5	5	1	2.5	>10	>10	2.5	2.5
	DY	>10	>10	5	5	5	2.5	2.5	1	>10	>10	5	5	>10	>10	5	5
Flavobacterium sp. 82-1-98	DW	0.1	0.05	0.05	0.025	0.2	0.05	0.05	0.025	0.2	0.05	0.025	0.025	0.2	0.1	0.025	0.01
	HS	2.5	0.5	0.5	0.5	5	1	0.5	0.5	5	5	1	0.5	10	5	2.5	0.1
	DY	2.5	2.5	2.5	2.5	10	2.5	2.5	1	10	>10	5	1	10	5	5	2.5
A. guttatis A-39	DW	5	5	1	0.2	>10	>10	1	1	>10	>10	10	1	>10	>10	>10	0.5
	HS	5	5	1	0.5	5	5	1	1	>10	>10	>10	1	>10	>10	>10	>10
	DY	>10	>10	>10	2.5	>10	5	5	1	>10	>10	>10	>10	>10	>10	>10	>10
A. faecalis 572	DW	1	1	0.2	0.1	1	0.4	0.2	0.2	>10	0.2	0.2	0.2	>10	>10	>10	>10
	HS	10	2.5	1	0.5	10	5	2.5	0.5	>10	10	10	0.5	>10	>10	>10	0.2
	DY	>10	>10	10	5	10	10	5	5	5	10	10	5	>10	>10	>10	10

[a] Killed from 10^6 to <10 cfu/ml at 25 C. DW, deionized water; HS, 10% human serum; DY, 2.5% dried yeast. OSN, alkyl(59–63% C₁₂H₂₅-, 29–34% C₁₄H₂₉-, 6.8–7.2% C₁₆H₃₃-) dimethylbenzylammonium chloride.

Joyo, K., et al. 1986. Chem. Pharm. Bull., 34, 4215–4224.

proper test method, the compounds may appear as good disinfectants (Mallman et al., 1946), or that the phenol coefficient test cannot be used to test quaternary ammonium compounds (Sykes, 1965), or that disinfection end points obtained via inoculated carrier tests require much larger amounts of compound over those observed from phenol coefficient testing (Mallman and Hanes, 1945; Stuart et al., 1953), or that tests with quaternary ammonium compounds measure bacteriostatic activity instead of bactericidal activity (Klarmann and Wright, 1946) are grossly misleading unless some additional interpretive and qualifying information is provided. Unfortunately, a large amount of the experimental work of the middle 1930s, immediately following Domagk's publication (1935), did indeed indicate a widespread spectrum of antimicrobial activity, including sporicidal and tuberculocidal activity at extremely low concentrations of quaternary ammonium compounds. There is little doubt that this was a result of inadequate neutralization of the test material carried over to the subculture medium, so that a static condition produced in the subculture was mistaken for destructive activity.

However, it must be remembered that the entire area of neutralization to prevent carryover stasis was inadequately dealt with at the time. A firm distinction between the biostatic and biocidal activities of an antimicrobial was not always determined. The necessity to obviate stasis from the subculture medium was not always demanded as a requisite of antimicrobial testing, and the neutralization with specific chemical moieties used for individual classes of antimicrobials was not always insisted upon. Any neutralization that occurred utilized dilution of the carryover antimicrobial from the aliquot sample to the volume of subculture medium to obtain a less than static concentration of the antimicrobial in the subculture medium.

More recently, the successful identification of discrete chemicals as specific quaternary ammonium compound neutralizers, which may be incorporated into subculture media or into diluents, has made it mandatory that antimicrobial testing be performed only in the presence of such neutralizers (Quisno et al., 1946). Consequently, the more recent experimental results with quaternary ammonium compounds cannot be discredited as static instead of destructive. The statement that the quaternary ammonium compounds may be made to look good by the proper test selection (Mallman et al., 1946) may be applied to any antimicrobial chemical.

Certainly, a manipulation of the various test parameters such as type and amount of soil, selection of test organisms, and many others will bias the results, so that any chemical product will appear as a good or poor antimicrobial agent. Of the many inadequacies attributed to the phenol coefficient test method (Klarmann and Wright, 1946; McCulloch, 1947), the most pertinent objection was its use as an index of actual disinfection levels for quaternary ammonium compounds (Sykes, 1965). However, this same objection may be raised for the entire spectrum of modern disinfectant products, because extrapolation from the phenol coefficient to recommended use-dilution for a product by way of some arbitrary factor is invalid and untenable in any and every instance (Klarmann, 1959; Ortenzio et al., 1961). If the in-use characterization of a disinfectant is divorced from the phenol coefficient test, the method becomes entirely useful to describe the antimicrobial activity of a substance as the concentration that will destroy a bacterial suspension in 5-, 10-, or 15-minute contact periods. The method, which fixes many independent variables such as operation equipment, media, temperature, and volumes of test solution and inoculum, may be applied with some minor reservations to any species of microorganism. That carrier type test methods provide lower dilution end points than the phenol coefficient method has already been stated for quaternary ammonium products (Mallman and Hanes, 1945; Stuart et al., 1953) and, more importantly, for other kinds of chemical products (Klarmann, 1959; Ortenzio et al., 1961). The dynamics of testing carriers prepared with inocula as dried films of microorganisms provide a more severe test than the liquid inoculum system of the phenol coefficient method. This feature of carrier-type tests has led to the development and use of these tests by the United States regulatory agencies to measure bactericidal, sporicidal, tuberculocidal, and sanitizing activity (Official Methods, AOAC, 1984).

Of special note are the efforts to determine the validity and accuracy of product-label statements and claims made by manufacturers of disinfectant products for sale in the United States. This regulation of antimicrobials intended for treatment of inanimate surfaces was formerly exercised by the United States Department of Agriculture and currently by the United States Environmental Protection Agency. It includes deliberate scrutiny of a product for antimicrobial efficacy and toxicologic and chemical properties in compliance with the product-label claims and other attendant information—all prior to the initial sale of the product. Further, the agency is required to monitor future production obtained on a periodic inspection schedule. To facilitate the antimicrobial examination, a number of testing protocols are prescribed to examine specific antimicrobial activity (Greene and Petrocci, 1980).

For those catalogued as AOAC methods, the reader is referred to the AOAC publications (Official Methods of Analysis of the AOAC, 1984) for the purpose, scope, precise methods, and application areas served by these tests. In addition to the AOAC methods, the Environmental Protection Agency recommends methods to determine the sanitizing activity on inanimate, nonfood contact surfaces, the initial and residual bactericidal and bacteriostatic activity of treated laundry fabric, the sanitizing activity on carpeting, the virucidal activity on environmental surfaces, and the initial and residual fungicidal and fungistatic activity on inanimate surfaces. This requirement to test products by specified protocols provides a useful means to collect data that may be compared, and so to more accurately characterize the antimicrobial activity of a substance. The recent installations of prescribed test methods by other agencies and in other countries is a most salutary development to eliminate the confusing conclusions developed heretofore from many different kinds of experimental studies.

Quaternary ammonium compounds have been tested by a multitude of different procedures, which may be generally classified as (1) In vitro static or minimum inhibitory level tests, usually as broth dilution tests; (2) In vitro or killing dilution tests, with phenol coefficient as an example; (3) Simulated use-dilution tests, including inoculated carriers of representative surfaces such as stainless steel, unglazed porcelain, and fabric; and (4) In-use tests, which use the product in the actual environment (Greene and Petrocci, 1980). The results of such testing with quaternary ammonium compounds may be summarized as follows: the active quaternary ammonium compounds sold as items of commerce are algistatic, bacteriostatic, tuberculostatic, sporostatic, and fungistatic at low concentration levels of 0.5 to 5 ppm (Hueck et al., 1966; Freelander, 1940; Schneider, 1935); they are algicidal, bactericidal, fungicidal, and virucidal against lipophilic viruses at medium concentration levels of 10 to 50 ppm (Lawrence, 1950; Petrocci et al., 1974; Klein and Deforest, 1963); they are not tuberculocidal or spo-

ricidal or virucidal against hydrophilic viruses at high concentration levels (Klein and Deforest, 1963; Smith et al., 1950; Davies, 1949). They are bactericidal to both gram-positive and gram-negative bacteria, with some evidence for greater activity against the gram-positive bacteria (Quisno and Foter, 1946). In this regard, it should be remembered that the gram-negative bacteria as a group, and especially the pseudomonas species, are more resistant to all the antimicrobial compounds currently available.

The quaternary ammonium compounds are bactericidal agents in acid and alkaline environments, with some evidence for greater activity in the alkaline range (Gershenfeld and Perlstein, 1941). The following descriptions of antimicrobial results are presented as representative data for quaternary ammonium compounds. They are compiled and prepared from the published scientific literature, from Onyx (Stepan) unpublished work, from brochures and data sheets supplied by the quaternary ammonium compound manufacturers, and from patents issued for quaternary ammonium compounds. It is important to recognize the absence of bias in information supplied by the manufacturers' literature that is carefully scrutinized by the regulatory agencies in advance of the sale of the chemical. The bacteriostatic, fungistatic, and algistatic activities of fatty nitrogen compounds, including quaternary ammonium compounds, were described

Table 13–14. *Inhibiting Concentrations (in PPM) of Fatty Nitrogen Compounds For Some Bacteria, Fungi, and Algae*

| | Bacteria | | | |
| | G–N | | G–P | |
Compound	Escherichia coli	Pseudomonas fluorescens	Bacillus subtilis	Staphylococcus aureus
Benzethonium chloride	1,000	300	3	3
Benzalkonium chloride	200	300	3	4
Dodecyltrimethyl ammonium chloride	500	500	5	5
Dodocylbenzyldimethyl ammonium chloride	750	750	2	2
Cocobenzyldimethyl ammonium chloride	225	225	2	2
Didecyldimethyl ammonium chloride	225	750	0.7	7

| | Fungi | | | |
Compound	Aspergillus niger	C. globosum	M. verrucaria	T. viridae
Benzethonium chloride	300	30	300	200
Benzalkonium chloride	60	10	40	80
Dodecyltrimethyl ammonium chloride	500	50	500	500
Dodocylbenzyldimethyl ammonium chloride	75	7	150	75
Cocobenzyldimethyl ammonium chloride	20	7	20	20
Didecyldimethyl ammonium chloride	75	7	20	20

| | Algae | | | |
Compound	Ch. vulgaris	Stigeoclonium species	A. cylindrica	Os. tenuis
Benzethonium chloride	3	1	1	1
Benzalkonium chloride	1	0.7	1	0.6
Dodecyltrimethyl ammonium chloride	50	5	5	0.5
Dodocylbenzyldimethyl ammonium chloride	0.2	0.2	0.2	0.2
Cocobenzyldimethyl ammonium chloride	2	0.5	2	0.7
Didecyldimethyl ammonium chloride	2	0.7	0.2	0.7

by Hueck et al. (1966); data selected therefrom for the quaternary ammonium compounds are presented in Table 13–14. The killing dilutions for some chemically different, commercially available quaternary ammonium compounds after a 10-minute contact period at 20°C by the phenol coefficient method against the recommended test organisms *Staphylococcus aureus* and *Salmonella typhosa* are compiled from the manufacturers' brochures (e.g., Brochure: Hyamine, Brochure: Roccal, BTC 2125M BTC, Brochure: Bardac) as Table 13–15.

These are at high dilutions against both organisms, and they are at significantly different dilutions depending on the specific chemical structure of the quaternary compound. The effect of the size of the quaternary molecule on the antimicrobial activity of a homologous series of alkyldimethylbenzyl ammonium chlorides is well documented by Cutler et al. (1966). They demonstrated a maximum activity as the highest 10-minute killing dilution against *Staphylococcus aureus* and *Salmonella typhosa* and *Pseudomonas aeruginosa* for the C_{14} member compound tested. Their results are shown in Table 13–3. Additional evidence for the structure and antimicrobial activity relationship is offered by the work of Petrocci et al. (1974), who evaluated the interference of hard water with the sanitizing activity against *Escherichia coli* of a group of dialkyldimethyl ammonium chloride compounds of varying long-chain lengths. This comparison of the hard-water tolerances, which are defined as the maximum concentrations of synthetic hard water (as $CaCO_3$), in which 200 ppm of active quaternary compound will continue to effectively sanitize (at 99.999% reduction) a suspension of *Escherichia coli* after a 30-second contact period, are displayed in Table 13–16.

Quisno's work with cetyl pyridinium chloride (Quisno and Foter, 1946) illustrates several characteristics of quaternary ammonium compounds, such as the greater activity for gram-positive bacteria over gram-negative bacteria (Table 13–17), and the positive effect of temperature

and the negative effect of organic matter on antimicrobial activity (Table 13–18).

Lawrence (1950) described the effect of pH on the antibacterial activity of an alkyldimethylbenzyl ammonium chloride at 5-, 10-, and 15-minute contact periods against *Staphylococcus aureus*. A portion of these data is available as Table 13–19. Over many years, Petrocci has examined the fungicidal activity of many quaternary structures against *T. interdigitale* (Petrocci, unpublished). Some of these data are available as Table 13–20. This small section of antimicrobial activity is only a minute portion of the total information that has been published and is available for examination. The space limitations of this chapter do not permit a complete listing of this information; instead, I have attempted to select and present representative data that are compatible with the bulk of current opinions in the field.

TOXICOLOGY

On March 4, 1987, the EPA issued a Data Call-In Notice requiring all registrants of antimicrobial active ingredients to submit subchronic and chronic toxicologic data to support the continued registration of their products. The EPA will permit registrants to select among several options for ways to comply with the data requirements of this notice. The EPA has concluded that it should be possible to evaluate risk by acquiring exposure data and by acquiring toxicity data under a tiered approach. The three-tier studies may be summarized as follows:

A. *The first-tier studies:*
1. 90-days dermal
2. 90-days inhalation
3. Teratogenicity 1st
4. Mutagenicity

B. *The second-tier studies:*
1. Subchronic feeding

Table 13–15. *Killing Dilutions of Commercially Available Quaternary Ammonium Germicides for 10-Minute Contact Periods at 20°C from Phenol Coefficients in Manufacturers' Brochures*

| | Killing Dilutions vs. | |
Chemical	Staphylococcus aureus	Salmonella typhosa
Di-isobutylphenoxyethoxyethyl dimethyl benzyl ammonium chloride	1/25,000	1/25,000
40% Methyldodecylbenzyl trimethyl ammonium chloride, 10% methyl-dodecylxylylene bis (trimethyl ammonium chloride)	1/24,000	1/22,500
N-alkyl (50%C$_{14}$, 40%C$_{12}$, 10%C$_{16}$) dimethyl benzyl ammonium chlorides	1/45,000	1/45,000
Benzyldimethyltetradecyl ammonium chloride	1/42,800	1/67,500
N-alkyl (60%C$_{15}$, 30%C$_{16}$, 5%C$_{12}$, 5%C$_{18}$) dimethylbenzyl ammonium chlorides	1/44,000	1/39,600
25% N-alkyl (68%C$_{12}$, 32%C$_{14}$) dimethylethylbenzyl ammonium chlorides	1/55,500	1/54,300
N-alkyl (98%C$_{12}$, 20%C$_{14}$) dimethyl 1-naphthylmethyl ammonium chlorides	1/60,000	1/58,500
N-alkyl (50%C$_{12}$, 30%C$_{14}$, 17%C$_{16}$, 3%C$_{18}$) isoquinolinium bromides	1/38,000	1/40,000
Octyldodecyldimethyl ammonium chlorides	1/61,800	1/57,500
Alkyl (50%C$_{14}$, 40%C$_{12}$, 10%C$_{16}$) dimethylbenzyl ammonium saccharinates	1/43,500	1/40,500
Didecyldimethyl ammonium chlorides	1/63,000	1/84,000

Table 13–16. *Hard Water Tolerances (PPM CaCO₃) of Dialkyldimethyl Quaternary Ammonium Compounds with Long-Carbon Chains (R₁ + R₂) that Total 19 to 22 Carbons*

Totals Carbons (R₁ + R₂)*	Hard Water Tolerance (ppm CaCO₃)						
19	700	800	500	550			
20	500	900	1200	1400	1100		
21	300	700	900	1300	1300		
22	400	550	750	900	800	650	R₁ carbon
	6	7	8	9	10	11	length

*R₂ carbon chain length obtained by subtracting R₁ carbon chain length from the R₁ + R₂ total carbon chain length.

Table 13–17. *Germicidal Activity of Cetyl Pyridinium Chloride Aqueous Solution*

Organism	No. Strains Tested	Average Critical Killing Dilution In Terms of Active Ingredients at 37°C No serum
Staphylococcus aureus	5	1:83,000
Staphylococcus albus	1	1:73,000
Streptococcus viridans	1	1:42,500
Streptococcus hemolyticus	2	1:127,500
Neisseria catarrhalis	2	1:84,000
Diplococcus pneumoniae I	1	1:95,000
Pseudomonas aeruginosa	2	1:5,800
Klebsiella pneumoniae	2	1:49,000
Corynebacterium diphtheriae	1	1:64,000
Mycobacterium phlei	1	1:1,500
Eberthella typhosa	5	1:48,000
Escherichia coli	2	1:66,000
Proteus vulgaris	2	1:34,000
Shigella dysenteriae	1	1:60,000
Shigella paradysenteriae (Flexner)	2	1:52,000
Shigella paradysenteriae (Hiss)	1	1:49,000
Shigella sonne	2	1:68,000

2. Teratogenicity 2nd
3. Dermal absorption
4. 90-days neurotoxicity

C. *The third-tier studies:*
   1. Chronic feeding, two species
   2. Oncogenicity, two species
   3. Reproduction
   4. Metabolism to clarify issues concerning structure activity relationships

On February 26, 1988, the EPA clustered the quaternary ammonium compounds into four groups, so that the toxicity study would be facilitated by selecting one member from each group for testing.

Group I: The straight-chain alkyl or hydroxyalkyl quaternaries; the most common product in this group is the twin chain quats. The EPA will allow a full set of subchronic and chronic toxicity studies on didecyldimethyl ammonium chloride and teratology studies on alkyltrimethyl ammonium chloride.

Group II: The nonhalogenated substituted benzyl and alkyldimethylbenzyl ammonium compounds (ADBAC); namely benzalkonium chlorides. The EPA will allow a full set of subchronic and chronic studies on alkyl[C_{12}—40%, C_{14}—50%, C_{16}—10%] dimethylbenzyl ammonium chloride. The EPA notes that after evaluating the data it expects to receive on the Group I and II compounds, it may also require one or more studies on alkyl[C_{12}—68%, C_{14}—32%]dimethylethylbenzyl ammonium chloride, to determine whether the Group I and ADBAC data is representative of the toxicity of the ethylbenzyl quats.

Group III: The alkyl[di- and tri- chlorobenzyl]dimethyl ammonium compounds. The EPA will allow a full set of subchronic and chronic studies on alkyl[C_{12}—5%, C_{14}—90%, C_{16}—5%] dimethyl 3,4-dichlorobenzyl ammonium chloride.

Group IV: The heterocyclic ammonium compounds with unusual substituents. In this group the EPA was unable to reach a conclusion in testing a small subset of quats. Each chemical in this category must be tested separately, unless registrants can develop a testing scheme using representative compounds that is acceptable to the EPA. Representative compounds in *Group IV* are (a) alkyl[C_{12}/C_{16}] substituted Picolinium compounds; (b) alkyl[C_8/C_{18}] imidazolinium compounds; (c) alkyl[C_{14}/C_{18}] N-ethyl-morpholinium compounds; and (d)

Table 13–18. *Effect of Temperature and Serum Upon Germicidal Activity of Cetyl Pyridinium Chloride*

Organisms	Critical Killing Dilutions Expressed in Terms of Active Ingredients			
	37°C		20°C	
	No Serum	10% Bovine Serum	No Serum	10% Bovine Serum
Staphylococcus aureus	1:110,000	1:11,500	1:67,500	1:6,750
Eberthella typhosa	1:83,500	1:4,000	1:62,500	1:1,300

Table 13–19. *Effects of pH on the Antiseptic Efficiency of a Quaternary Ammonium Germicide Against* Staphylococcus Aureus

Quaternary Ammonium Compound Conc.	Acid or Alkali per 100 ml	pH	Bacterial Growth after Minutes of Exposure		
			5	10	15
1:15,000	0.10 ml N/10 HCl	4.3	−	−	−
1:15,000	0.25 ml N/10 HCl	3.8	−	−	−
1:15,000	0.50 ml N/10 HCl	3.5	+	+	+
1:15,000	1.00 ml N/10 HCl	3.2	+	+	+
Control (no quaternary ammonium compound)	1.00 ml N/10 HCl	3.2	+	+	+
1:25,000	0	6.7	+	+	+
1:25,000	0.10 ml N/10 NaOH	9.4	+	+	+
1:25,000	0.25 ml N/10 NaOH	10.0	+	+	−
1:25,000	0.50 ml N/10 NaOH	10.2	+	+	−
1:25,000	1.00 ml N/10 NaOH	10.5	+	−	−
1:25,000	1.25 ml N/10 NaOH	10.6	+	−	−
Control (no quaternary ammonium compound)	1.25 ml N/10 NaOH	10.6	+	+	+

alkyl[C_{12}/C_{18}] isoquinolinium compounds and other heterogeneous structures.

A knowledge of the toxicologic properties of quaternary ammonium compounds is important so that the safety, health, and well-being of man and animals are not compromised by contact with these chemicals as they are manufactured, shipped, compounded, or used. Although these specific investigations are not germane, the studies to characterize the general toxicologic properties of antimicrobial quaternary ammonium compounds and the studies of the harmful consequences of these chemicals at concentrations simulating their use patterns are of primary importance. Toxicologic effect is measured at three levels: (1) at the amount necessary to bring about the response with 100% of the experimental animals, LD_{100}; (2) at the amount that will cause the response with 50% of the animals, LD_{50}; and (3) at the amount that does not produce the response with any of the animals, LD_0. The LD_{50} level is most frequently used to characterize toxicity. In addition, the methods of administering the chemical are also identified using descriptions such as oral, subcutaneous, intraperitoneal, intravenous,

Table 13–20. *Critical Killing Dilution (10-Minute Contact Period) Required for Aqueous Dilutions of Quaternary Compounds to Kill Spores of* Trichophyton Interdigitalis; *Dilutions are Based on Anhydrous Germicide*

Chemical Structure	Avg. Killing Dil.
40% methyldodecylbenzyltrimethyl ammonium chloride, 10% methyldodecylxylylene bis (trimethyl ammonium chloride)	1/2000
25% n-alkyl (60%C_{14}, 30%C_{16}, 5%C_{12}, 5%C_{18}) dimethylbenzyl ammonium chloride, 25% n-alkyl (68%C_{12}, 32%C_{14}) dimethylethylbenzyl ammonium chlorides	1/800
Octyldodecyldimethyl ammonium bromide	1/5000
Didecyldimethyl ammonium chloride	1/4750

and dermal. Also, the toxicity is determined as an acute response following a single administration of the chemical, as a short-term or subacute response following a multiple, periodic administration of the chemical over a short period such as 30 or 90 days, and finally as a chronic response following a multiple, periodic administration over a long period, such as the animal's life span. The LD_{50} amounts of quaternary ammonium compound depend on the route of administration. A notable example of this is the work of Nelson and Lyster (1946), who examined myristal picolinium chloride and reported an LD_{50} of 250 mg/kg by oral administration, 200 mg/kg for subcutaneous injection, 7.5 mg/kg for intraperitoneal injection, and 30 mg/kg for intravenous injection. Using the acute oral LD_{50}, which is the toxicologic characteristic most frequently described, one may compare the toxicities of different quaternary compounds. When this is done with the work of Shelanski (1949) and Finnegan and Dienna (1954), we observe acute oral LD_{50} values in white rats of 445 mg/kg for alkyldimethylbenzyl ammonium chloride, 500 mg/kg for alkenyldimethylethyl ammonium bromide, 730 mg/kg for alkyldimethyl 3,4-dichlorobenzyl ammonium chloride, 420 mg/kg for diisobutylphenoxyethoxyethyldimethylbenzyl ammonium chloride, and 389 mg/kg for alkyltolymethyltrimethyl ammonium chloride. These and similar data obtained from studies with man and laboratory animals have led to the generalized conclusion that the antimicrobial quaternary ammonium compounds examined to date exhibit similar toxicologic and pharmacologic properties.

Dermal toxicity was also examined by Shelanski (1949) and Finnegan and Dienna (1954), who concluded from animal and human testing that 0.1% was the maximum concentration of the aforementioned compounds that would not produce primary irritation on intact skin or act as a sensitizer. The conjunctival mucous membrane obviously requires special consideration, which was undertaken by a number of investigators. Nelson and Lyster (1946) observed that a 1:3000 (333 ppm) solution of myristal picolinium chloride produced a slight irritation of the conjunctival mucosa of rabbits. Walter (1938) reported that a 1:1000 dilution (1000 ppm) of alkyldimethylbenzyl ammonium chloride instilled into the eyes of human subjects produced burning and stinging reactions, whereas a 1:5000 dilution (200 ppm) produced no unpleasant sensations. Whitehill (1945) determined that the maximum nonirritating concentrations of alkyldimethylbenzyl ammonium chloride and cetylpyridimium chloride in the eyes of rabbits were 1:3000 (333 ppm) and 1:2000 (500 ppm), respectively. Finnegan and Dienna (1954) observed comparable irritation levels for diisobutylphenoxyethoxyethyldimethyl benzyl ammonium chloride and for alkyltolymethyltrimethyl ammonium chloride (Shelanski, unpublished); in Shelanski's investigation of laurylisoquinolinium bromide, he observed that the compound at 0.5% produced moderate to severe corneal involvement of the rabbit eye, which cleared up in 5 days. However, rabbit eyes similarly exposed and washed at 2 or 4 seconds after instillation produced only a slight conjunctival involvement, which cleared up after 2 days. A most important toxicologic consideration arising from the widely encountered application area of sanitizing food contact surfaces is the cumulative effect in animals and man of the ingestion of food contacted by the small residues of the quaternary sanitizer. The laboratory study simulating this situation is the daily oral administration of quaternary ammonium compound in the food or drinking water of test animals over a considerable period of time, including the normal life span of the animal. Such studies were made early by Nelson and Lyster (1946), who determined that myristal picolinium chloride at 0.1% in the diet of rats did not interfere with their normal growth rate, but this concentration produced death when administered as a sole source of fluid and required reduction to 0.05% to permit a normal growth rate of the test animal.

Fitzhugh and Nelson (1948) summarized the results of a 2-year chronic feeding study of rats on a diet containing 0.5, 0.25, 0.125, or 0.063% alkyldimethylbenzyl chloride; they found that all the quaternary compound concentrations were toxic to rats, as evidenced by lower growth rates over an untreated control group and as determined by the histopathologic lesions present in the treated animals. Alfredson et al. (1951), however, using a significantly larger number of experimental animals and a more randomized statistical design, demonstrated that alkyldimethylbenzyl ammonium chloride at 0.25% in the diet of rats over a 2-year feeding period did not demonstrably affect the growth, food consumption, blood picture, or histopathology of the treated animals. Dogs that were fed over a 15-week period a diet containing 0.12% or less quaternary compound demonstrated similar nontoxic effects. Shelanski (1949) noted a minimal toxicologic effect, evidenced by weight loss, a depressed growth rate, and an abnormal blood or histopathology, for dogs that were allowed a 1:5000 aqueous dilution of either alkyldimethylbenzyl ammonium chloride, alkenyl-

dimethylethyl ammonium bromide, laurylisoquinolinium bromide, or alkyldimethyl 3,4-dichlorobenzyl ammonium chloride as their sole source of drinking water over a 6-month period, for guinea pigs administered 25, 12.5, or 5 mg/kg of the aforementioned quaternary ammonium compounds daily for a 1-year period, and for rats similarly treated daily over a 2-year period. Finnegan and Dienna (1954) demonstrated that a concentration of 2500 ppm of alkyltolylmethyltrimethyl ammonium chloride or diisobutylphenoxyethoxyethyldimethyl benzyl ammonium chloride in the diet of rats produced minimal deleterious toxicologic effects over a 2-year period, whereas a concentration of 1000 ppm produced no undesirable toxicologic effects over the same period.

The concern of the Food and Drug Administration over the unsafe adulteration of food, especially of milk, with residues from quaternary sanitizers led to label statements for these products requiring a potable water rinse following the quaternary compound sanitization and reuse of the food equipment. Recently, a careful scrutiny by the FDA of additional chronic feeding studies supplied by manufacturers of quaternary ammonium compounds has concluded that the food additive regulations should be amended to provide for the safe use of a sanitizing solution on food processing equipment and utensils and on food contact surfaces in bars and restaurants if the solution does not exceed 200 ppm of quaternary compound and if the quaternary compound solution contains equal amounts of n-alkyl $[C_{12}-C_{18}]$ benzyldimethyl ammonium chloride and n-alkyl $[C_{12}-C_{14}]$dimethylethylbenzyl ammonium chloride having an average molecular weight of 384. In this instance, safe use does not require a potable water rinse of treated food contact surfaces and equipment prior to reuse (Federal Register, 1969).

A short time later, the same statement was made for an aqueous solution containing n-alkyl $[C_{12}C_{18}]$ benzyldimethyl ammonium chloride having an average molecular weight of between 351 and 380 and consisting principally of alkyl groups with 12 to 16 carbon atoms with or without, but not over, 1% each of groups with 8 and 10 carbon atoms (Federal Register, 1969).

Most recently, the same statement was made for a detergent-sanitizer solution containing the first sanitizing product described as a mixture of benzyl and ethylbenzyl quaternary compounds, with the optional adjuvant substances tetrasodium ethylenediaminetetraacetate or a(p-nonylphenyl)-w-hydroxypoly(oxyethylene) (or both) having an average poly(oxyethylene) content of 11 moles (Federal Register, 1974). Gleason (1969) points out that at least 10 human fatalities implicating quaternary ammonium compounds are medically recorded as resulting from alkyldimethylbenzyl ammonium chloride solutions of 10 or 15% that were introduced into the victims via oral ingestion, intramuscular or intravenous administration, or intrauterine instillation. The reader is referred to Gleason's work for a complete description of the medical and clinical symptoms of quaternary ammonium compound poisoning and also for the recommended treatment, including first aid, for the same. One symptom should be mentioned: namely, the ingestion of concentrated solution leads to immediate burning pain in the mouth, throat, and abdomen.

The toxicologic information presented is generalized as follows: quaternary ammonium compound germicides as concentrated solutions of 10% or more are toxic, causing death if taken internally and severe irritation to the skin and conjunctival mucosa when applied externally. With normal precautions and operating procedures, the probability of such contact is extremely remote, because the effective use-dilutions of these materials are well below the concentrated level causing death and severe injury. In addition, oral ingestion, the most likely route of accidental internal administration, is self-limiting for concentrated quaternary ammonium solutions, because the immediate burning in the mouth and throat acts as a signal. At the dilute solutions of the use levels of quaternary ammonium compound germicides, which range from several to about 1000 ppm, only the most deliberate distortions of normal operating procedures could offer acute toxicity problems. Finally, chronic toxicity, as from the cumulative effect of food adulterated with quaternary ammonium compound germicides via residues from dilute sanitizing solutions used on food processing equipment, is not a problem.

Aursnes (1982) studied the ototoxic effects of quaternary ammonium compounds (QAC), benzethonium chloride, and benzalkonium chloride, frequently used for skin disinfection. The disinfectant QACs, at concentrations of 0.1% in water solution or in 70% alcohol, were introduced into the tympanic cavity (middle ear) of guinea pigs for exposure times of 10, 30, or 60 minutes. The animals were sacrificed 2 or 9 weeks after the exposure, and the organ of Corti and vestibular neuroepithelia were studied as surface preparations with phase contrast microscopy. It was found that most of the ears exposed to the disinfectants had suffered damage, affecting both the vestibulum and the perilymphatic and endolymphatic spaces of the cochlea of the inner ear. The extent of the damage was related both to the duration of exposure and to the length of the animal's survival after the exposure. Furthermore it was found that the tympanic cavity and the perilymphatic spaces of vestibulum and cochlea were pathologically changed.

The final report on the safety assessment of benzethonium chloride and methylbenzethonium chloride has been issued by CTFA (1985) in the journal of the American College of Toxicology. It was concluded that both compounds are safe at concentrations of 0.5% in cosmetics applied to the skin. A maximum concentration of 0.02% is safe for cosmetics used in the eye area. Chronic and subchronic feeding studies indicated little or no toxic effects for both ingredients. In clinical studies, benzethonium chloride produced mild skin irritation at 5% but not at lower concentrations. Neither ingredient is considered to be a sensitizer.

APPLICATIONS

Following Domagk's publication in 1935, a large number of application areas were developed for the quaternary ammonium compounds. Initially, they were used as an adjunct to surgery, such as in preoperative patient skin treatment, degerming the hands of the surgical team preoperatively, and disinfection of surgical instruments. Wetzel, in 1935, described the superiority of 0.1% alkyldimethylbenzyl ammonium chloride over 60% alcohol for treatment of the surgeon's hands prior to surgery. Much additional evidence was provided for the treatment of the surgeon's hands with alkyldimethylbenzyl ammonium chloride by Caesar in 1935, Walter in 1938, Naegel in 1940, and Swan et al. in 1949. In 1938, both Walter and White et al. reported that the use of alkyldimethylbenzyl ammonium chloride as a skin preparation for a patient prior to surgery reduced the incidence of wound infection. Hagan et al., in 1946, compared the activity of cetylpyridinium chloride and alkydimethylbenzyl ammonium chloride to mercurials as skin preparation prior to surgery and found the quaternary compounds superior. However, Miller et al., in 1943, offered evidence that quaternary compounds applied to the skin formed a continuous residual sheet, beneath which bacteria survived.

Rahn (1946) proposed that the film is formed as an oriented adsorption of the quaternary compound on an organophilic surface, with the nontoxic ends directed toward the skin and the germicidally active ends directed toward the outside, which explained the favorable results obtained for quaternary compounds in many studies. Blank and Coolidge, in 1950, rejected the film concept and proposed instead that treatment with the quaternary compounds altered the charge of the skin to positive, which attracted and held the negatively charged bacteria, leading to the favorable, if inaccurate, results obtained in basin tests with quaternary compounds. In the same publication, they speculated that phospholipids present on the surface of the skin inhibited the antimicrobial activity of the quaternary compound.

These negative comments and the widespread popular use of hexachlorophene-based products should have seriously curtailed the use of quaternary compounds as skin degerming agents. Thus it is interesting to note that King and Zimmerman, in 1965, reporting on skin degerming practices in hospitals, did determine that 37% of hospitals were using quaternary compounds, compared to the 48% observed by Price in 1948. Walter, in 1965, described a hand degerming treatment for the surgeon as a mechanical soap hand scrubbing followed by application of a mixture of isopropyl alcohol, alkyldimethylbenzyl ammonium chloride, and cetyl alcohol. Verdon, in 1961, tested a number of skin degerming agents used in British hospitals and demonstrated the utility of quaternary compounds.

Caesar and Schmidt in 1935 and Walter in 1938 recommended the use of alkyldimethylbenzyl ammonium chloride for the disinfection of surgical instruments, Caesar specifying a 1:100 concentration of quaternary compound for a 10-minute contact period and Walter a 1:1000 concentration over a 30-minute contact period. Hornung (1935) recommended the addition of sodium carbonate to the quaternary solution to prevent rusting of the instruments; Post (1946) later proposed sodium nitrite for this purpose. The early investigators, with some few exceptions, did indeed subscribe to the idea of a total spectrum of germicidal activity for the quaternary compounds and thus endorsed them as surgical instrument sterilizers. Early exceptions were Zeissler and Gunther (1939), who pointed out that Zephirol would not kill spores from the soil.

Sommermeyer and Frobisher, in 1952, using glass rods inoculated with sputum containing tubercle bacilli to simulate contaminated thermometers, demonstrated that aqueous solutions of alkyldimethylbenzyl ammonium chloride and cetylpyridinium chloride at 1:1000 dilution did not kill the organism after a 10-minute contact period, whereas tinctures of the same compounds (50% alcoholic) did in fact kill the organism. The subsequent use of specific quaternary compound neutralizers as a requisite for testing has prevented additional instances of residual bacteriostasis that were interpreted as bactericidal activity, as in the case of tuberculocidal and sporicidal testing.

The inability of quaternary compounds to kill the tubercle bacillus or bacterial spores should seriously limit their use as surgical instrument sterilizers in the future. However, in some few special cases, they are still recommended for the disinfection of comparable devices (Kasper and Kirk, 1972).

The widespread use of quaternary ammonium compounds for environmental disinfection of floors, walls, and equipment surfaces in hospitals, nursing homes, public places, and gymnasia required the development of a detergent compatible with the quaternary compounds that would permit the combination of the two operations of cleaning and disinfection. Rahn and Eseltine (1947) pointed out the utility of such a system and indicated work in progress as described by Guiteras and Shapiro (1946), who combined cetyldimethylethyl ammonium bromide with the nonionic wetting agent alkylated aryl polyether alcohol and inorganic salts. The formulation prepared by Guiteras and Shapiro diluted as 1 oz/gal aqueous solution cleaned glass slides contaminated with heavy artificial soil inoculated with bacteria. When the contact period of the slide and diluted formulation was extended to 10 minutes, all the bacteria on the soiled slides were killed, as demonstrated by negative broth subcultures of the slides and by zero-count agar plates prepared from the broth subcultures.

The concept of a one-step operation to produce cleaning and antimicrobial activity, which made the treatment of large surface areas practical, met with success and furthered research to the present time toward the development of quaternary nonionic formulations with optimum cleaning and antimicrobial properties (Greene

and Petrocci, 1980). Publications (Kundsin and Walter, 1961; Lenhart et al., 1961) of both in-vitro laboratory tests and of field tests under actual conditions attest to the utility of these products. Treatment of large areas of environmental surface is accomplished by a mop-and-bucket operation, by mechanical flooding and vacuum pick-up, by sponge or cloth hand-wipe operation, and by liquid spray. As an additional treatment procedure for disinfection of surfaces, there is available liquefied gas, quaternary ammonium compound germicidal formulation discharges from pressurized containers as an aerosol spray that, according to Fulton et al. (1948), killed both *Escherichia coli* and *Staphylococcus aureus* as air-borne suspensions and surface contaminations. The patent issued to Taylor and Prindle (1966) is an instance of popular and widely used surface disinfectant and space deodorant aerosol spray composition.

Recently, treatment of surfaces is reported via a mist of quaternary ammonium compound germicide generated from commercial fogging devices that produce droplets of approximately 50 μm in diameter by the shearing action of air pressure on the liquid germicide solution. This procedure is suggested as an adjunct for terminal disinfection of hospital areas. The germicidal results obtained with 0.2% active aqueous solution of a 50:50 mixture of alkyldimethylbenzyl ammonium chloride and alkyldimethylethylbenzyl ammonium chloride in field tests and in simulated in-use tests are described by Friedman et al. (1968) and Hauser et al. (1963).

Treatment of food contact surfaces, i.e., those found on equipment in the food processing industries and on food and beverage utensils in eating and drinking establishments, in order to obtain sanitary conditions that will prevent transmission of disease through the food, is defined as a sanitizing treatment or as sanitation of such surfaces. Practicable sanitizing requires that any treatment residual will not in itself be harmful; it does not require a destruction of all the bacteria present on the treated surface. The utility of quaternary ammonium compounds in sanitizing such surfaces was suggested by Krog and Marshall (1940), who experimentally contaminated the rims of glass drinking tumblers, allowed them to air dry, and treated them with a 1:5000 aqueous dilution of alkyldimethylbenzyl ammonium chloride for various contact periods before swabbing and plating procedures were employed to enumerate the viable bacteria present; this demonstrated a reduction to less than 100 bacteria per rim after only a 1 minute contact period. Two years later they reported that the use of alkyldimethylbenzyl ammonium chloride at a 1:6000 dilution in a dairy pasteurizing plant caused a 60 to 98% reduction of the bacteria count on the milk handling and processing equipment (Krog and Marshall, 1942). Frayer (1943), Mueller et al. (1946), DuBois and Dibblee (1946), Puhle (1950), and Speck and Lucas (1957) are several of the many investigators who determined the utility of quaternary ammonium compounds as germicides for the dairy farm and dairy plant. Similar reports to demonstrate the advantage of quaternary compounds as germicides in other food processing industries have appeared, such as those of Penniston and Hedrick (1945) in the egg processing industry, Tressler (1947) in the fishing industry, Lehn and Vignolo (1946) and Resuggan (1951) in the brewing industry, and Casey (1972) in the sugar refining industry.

The treatment of large amounts of water to destroy and prevent the proliferation of disease-producing microorganisms, of industrial process-interfering microorganisms, and finally of noxious, esthetically undesirable microorganisms is an important application area of the quaternary ammonium compounds. The destruction of cysts of Entamoeba histolytica was reported by Fair et al. (1945) and by Kessel and Moore (1946). Kessel and Moore offered their opinion that quaternary ammonium compounds should be considered for the emergency sterilization of drinking water; this opinion was based on the high germicidal levels observed. Sotier and Ward (1947) observed that a product containing 0.5% of Hyamine 1622 was an effective disinfectant of new water mains and of hemp used to prepare joints on the mains. Quaternary ammonium compounds have been recommended for treating process water in paper mills (Erskine et al., 1958; Shema, 1966) to prevent the proliferation of microorganisms on the surface of equipment contacting the pulp solution. These proliferations form microbial slimes that become detached and are carried along to become spots in the paper, often causing paper breaks during the manufacturing process that result in expensive, time-delaying machine shutdowns. Quaternary compounds are used in cooling water systems (Darragh and Stayner, 1954; Berneschot et al., 1964) to prevent proliferation of bacteria in the circulating cooling water system that would form microbial slimes that may reach the heat exchange units and impair their operational efficiency. Prusick and Gregory (1956) recommended the use of dicocodimethyl ammonium chloride to prevent proliferation of bacteria in injection water or brine used in secondary oil recovery operations. The injection water is pumped under pressure into injection wells drilled around the producing well, so that as it spreads through the subterranean sand structures containing residual oil, it will displace the residual oil in the direction of the producing well and increase the productivity of the well. If there is a proliferation of microorganisms in the injection waters, the subterranean sand structures will become plugged, requiring greater pressures to be applied to the injection waters until the operation cannot function. Steinberger (1963) described the ability of N-alkyl crude tar base quaternary ammonium compounds at 5 to 20 ppm to inhibit the proliferation of Desulfovibrio desulfuricans, which with pseudomonas species are primarily involved in plugging the sand formation.

Outdoor swimming pools are regularly treated with quaternary ammonium compounds to prohibit growth of algae, an esthetic rather than a public health problem. Palmer and Maloney (1955) determined that 2 ppm of several different quaternary ammonium compounds did effectively inhibit the growth of various algae species. Antonides and Tanner (1961) recommended a formulation containing trimethylalkyl ammonium compound at 4.5 ppm as a swimming-pool algicide and bactericide. Shay et al. (1964) demonstrated that alkyldimethylisopropylbenzyl ammonium chloride at 7 ppm killed both Escherichia coli and Streptococcus faecalis at a 30-second contact time by the AOAC test method prescribed for swimming pool bactericides.

The positively charged functional portion of the quaternary molecule is attracted to and substantive to negatively charged fabric; it may be applied to the fabric from a quaternary solution by rinsing, padding, or spraying. Taking advantage of this phenomenon, Benson et al. (1947, 1949) proposed that diapers be treated with [methylbenzethonium chloride]p-diisobutylcresoxyethoxyethyldimethylbenzyl ammonium chloride monohydrate in the final rinse of the laundry cycle. Treated diapers would prevent the formation of ammonia from urine by the action of ammonia-producing bacteria found in the infant's feces; thus, ammonia dermatitis leading to diaper rash could be prevented. Lawrence (1950) pointed out the need to apply chemical treatment between the laundry loads of different customers using public automatic clothes-washing machines.

Although large commercial laundries could provide sufficient volumes of hot water at disinfecting temperatures, the small automatic installations could not. Lawrence used alkyldimethylbenzyl ammonium chloride to treat laundry in the final rinse cycle of automatic machines in a coin-operated self-service laundry. He determined that there were high bacteria counts in the first soak and wash cycle water, which following treatment with the quaternary compound at 1:5000 (200 ppm) or 1:10,000 (100 ppm) dilution, were reduced to zero counts in the deep rinse cycle.

McNeil and Choper (1962) treated naturally soiled wash loads at the warm or hot water setting and in the wash or rinse cycle with alkyldimethylbenzyl ammonium chloride to provide 200 ppm of active quaternary compounds in the presence of anionic or nonionic laundry detergent. Compared to untreated wash loads, the quaternary compound used with the warm or hot water setting consistently reduced the numbers of bacteria in the wash and rinse waters and on fabric swatches attached to laundry items. This occurred with the quaternary compound added to the rinse cycle, and to the wash cycle when a nonionic detergent was used. Utilizing the AOAC antimicrobial laundry additive test procedure (Petrocci and Clarke, 1969), a simulated use test, Shay and Petrocci (1968) demonstrated sanitization of fabric during the laundry cycle following addition of a 50:50 mixture of alkyldimethylbenzyl ammonium chloride and alkyldimethylethylbenzyl ammonium chloride at a 200 ppm level based on the weight of dry laundry fabric. In addition, fabric similarly treated and allowed to air dry demonstrated residual bacteriostatic activity against

Staphylococcus aureus, Escherichia coli, and *Brevibacterium ammoniagenes,* and also demonstrated residual self-sanitizing activity against *Staphylococcus aureus* and *Escherichia coli.* Some of the miscellaneous applications for quaternary ammonium compounds are as preservatives. Lawrence (1950) evaluated a large number of chemicals as preservatives for ophthalmic solution and selected benzalkonium chloride at 1:5000 and 1:10,000 as superior. More recently, Stark (1985) used Polymeric quaternary ammonium compounds, namely Polyquat, for disinfecting and preserving solution for contact lenses, ointments, and other ocular medicaments. The polyquaterium-1 (Onamer M) has been approved by the FDA as a preservative in several brands of contact lens soaking solutions at 0.01 to 0.001% [Opti-Soft, Opti-Clean, Opti-Tears, Opti-Free, and Tears-Natural II]. This product has replaced benzalkonium chloride and Thiomerosal in these preparations. Bernarducci and Harrison (1988) have discovered that water-soluble cationic polymers (Busan 77, WSCP, Onyxsperse 12S, Onamer M), when formulated in an aqueous medium with one or more nonionic surfactants, provide stable, isotropic liquid laundry detergent and sanitizer compositions having good detergency and bactericidal properties, and in addition are less irritating to the eye and practically non-irritating to the skin.

Like et al. (1975) examined a number of compounds, including a 50:50 mixture of alkyldimethylbenzyl ammonium and alkyldimethylethylbenzyl ammonium chlorides, as preservatives for cosmetic oil-in-water systems using amine oxides as emulsifiers. At 1000 or 2000 ppm, the quaternary ammonium compounds reduced the microbial count of the cosmetic system inoculated with bacteria and fungal spores from an initial count of several million per ml to less than 10 per ml over an 8-week incubation period, including a reinoculation after 4 weeks of incubation.

In another instance, as a fungistat for exterior latex paint films, Ramp et al. (1966) demonstrated that alkyldimethyl ethylbenzylammonium cyclohexylsulfamate at about a 1% level in exterior latex paints would produce a paint film resistant to attack by fungi. In another instance, as a moth-proofing agent for wool fabric, Tolygesi et al. (1971) concluded that tricaprylylmethyl ammonium chloride was superior to all other quaternary ammonium compounds tested for this purpose. Both compounds applied to wool fabric at 0.15 to 0.40% add-on levels protected the fabric from the black carpet beetle and the webbing clothes-moth larvae.

MODE OF ACTION

The earliest accounts of the quaternary ammonium compounds related antimicrobial activity to chemical structure by utilizing homologous series of quaternary compounds and noting the effect on antimicrobial activity offered by variations in structure (Jacobs, 1916). This method of collecting information on the antimicrobial attributes of a quaternary compound is constantly employed to determine the most effective structure that may be used as an item of commerce. Beyond this purpose, this method contributes little to our understanding of the basic mechanism of quaternary ammonium compounds as antimicrobial agents. Although the mode of action has not yet been completely or definitively described in detail, there are well defined and accepted steps explaining the mode of action of cationic disinfectants or antiseptics as reported by Ikeda and Tazuke (1985) and Franklin and Snow (1989). Many techniques have been used in elucidating the mode of action of antimicrobial agents. Once the primary site of action is established the overall effect of the drug on the metabolism of microbial cells can often be explained. The most important site of adsorption is the cytoplasmic membrane. Spheroplasts or protoplasts lacking the outer cell wall layers will bind the cationic antiseptic and may be lysed or damaged. Adsorption by isolated cell membranes can be demonstrated.

The extent of killing of the bacteria is governed by five principal factors: (a) Concentration of antiseptic or disinfectant; (b) nature of bacterial cells and density; (c) time of contact; (d) temperature of medium; (e) the pH; and (f) the presence of foreign matter.

The adsorption of a given amount of the compound per cell leads to the killing of a definite fraction of the bacterial population in the chosen time interval. The lowest concentration of the antiseptic that causes death of the bacteria also brings about leakage of cytoplasmic constituents of low molecular weight. The most immediately observed effect is loss of K^+ ions. The increased permeability is a sign of changes in the membrane that are initially reversible but become irreversible on prolonged treatment. The necessary characteristic of an antiseptic is its bactericidal action, but there is often a low and rather narrow concentration range in which its effect is bacteriostatic. At this low concentration, certain biochemical functions associated with the bacteria membrane may be inhibited. In the presence of a higher concentration of antiseptic and after prolonged treatment, the compound usually penetrates the cell and brings about extensive ill defined disruption of normal cellular functions. The primary effect of these antiseptics on the cytoplasmic membrane is thus established beyond doubt, but secondary actions on the cytoplasmic processes are less defined and may vary from one compound to another.

A review of the most reliable evidence on the mode of action of cationic antiseptics suggests the following generalizations:

1. Adsorption of compound on the bacterial cell surface
2. Diffusion through the cell wall
3. Binding to the cytoplasmic membrane
4. Disruption of the cytoplasmic membrane
5. Release of K^+ ions and other cytoplasmic constituents

6. Precipitation of cell contents and the death of the cells

It is well known that the bacterial cell surfaces are usually negatively charged, and then that adsorption of polycations on to the negatively charged cell surfaces (process 1) is expected to be enhanced with increasing molecular weight of the polymer due to the increasing charge density of the polycations. The binding of polymers to the cytoplasmic membranes and its disruption is expected to be facilitated by increasing the molecular weight of the polymer and by increasing the amount of the bound polymers to the bacteria cells. To examine this hypothesis Ikeda and Tazuke (1985) studied the effect of MW of the polymers on lysis of protoplasts, which are bacteria cells freed entirely of cell walls, so that the interactions processes 1 (adsorption) and 2 (diffusion) of the polymer with the protoplasts can be left out of consideration. The amount of cytoplasmic constituents released from protoplasts and from intact cells of *Bacillus subtilis* was measured at 260 nm after exposure to fractionated samples of polymers of various MW. Lysis of protoplasts was clearly enhanced with increase in MW of polymer[poly{n-butyldimethyl[vinylbenzyl]-ammonium chloride]}. A bell-shaped curve relationship of the activity to the MW of fractionated polymer was observed in the case of intact cells of *B. subtilis*. Because separate experiments have shown that release of cytoplasmic constituents from intact cells correlates well with the death of the cells, these results support the concept that the mode of action of the polymeric biocides is disorganization of cytoplasmic membrane followed by rupture of membrane, leading to the death of the bacteria (Franklin and Snow, 1989).

Ikeda and Tazuke in 1985 reported an optimal MW region of 14,300 for the 6,6-ionene bromide with antibacterial activity with minimum bactericidal concentration of 6.6 ppm to 10 ppm against *Staphylococcus aureus*. The same workers reported that polymeric biquanides of MW 11,900 and poly{alkyl[C_2–C_{12}]dimethyl[vinylbenzyl]ammonium chloride} of similar MW exhibit better bactericidal action against gram-positive than gram-negative bacteria. The poly{dodecyldimethyl[vinylbenzyl]-ammonium chloride} was the most active at 0.5 ppm against *Staphylococcus aureus*, which suggests that hydrophobicity plays an important role in bactericidal action.

A primary consideration in examining the mode of action is the characterization of quaternary compounds as surface-active agents, or surfactants. These are adequately defined by James (1965) as compounds with a structural balance between one or more water-attracting (hydrophilic) groups; depending on the nature of the charge or absence of ionization of the hydrophilic group, they may be classified as anionic, cationic, or nonionic. Quaternary ammonium compounds are cationic surface agents and possess such properties as a reduction of the surface tension at interfaces upon absorption; a ready attraction to an absorption on surfaces possessing a neg-ative charge such as wool, glass, protein, and bacteria; the formation of ionic aggregates or micelles with attendant changes in electrical conductivity, surface tension, and solubility; a precipitation, complex formation, and denaturing effect on proteins; and an inhibiting or stimulating effect on enzyme activity (James, 1946).

With these demonstrable properties for cationic surfactants, it was natural for some investigators (Cowles, 1938) to attribute the antimicrobial activity of quaternary ammonium compounds entirely to the presence and amount of surface activity. However, this obvious explanation has been refuted (Gershenfeld and Milanick, 1941; Hotchkiss, 1946).

An excellent presentation on the mode of action of cationic surface-active agents on microbial cells was given by Hugo (1965). The concepts concerning the mode of action of surface-active agents on microorganisms may be divided into five broad categories.

1. Effects on protein. See Putnam (1948) for protein-denaturing agents, Khun and Dann (1940) for enzyme-disrupting agents. Quaternary ammonium compounds are surface-active agents and will denature protein or cause dissociation of an enzyme from its prosthetic group. This effect is usually caused at concentrations much higher than those which are lethal to the microbial cells, and it is unlikely that this effect is the primary cause of the antibacterial activity of surface-active disinfectants except at high concentration.

2. Effects on metabolic reactions. See Baker et al. (1941) on the aerobic and anaerobic respiration of glucose by a variety of bacteria and Ordal and Borg (1942) on the oxidation of lactate by *Escherichia coli* and *Staphylococcus aureus*. Attempts have been made to relate inhibition of metabolism with inhibition of growth. Such a correlation has been observed at high concentration, and almost any degree of agreement or disagreement may be demonstrated depending upon the enzyme system chosen and the test organism. It can be expected that those enzymes located in the cytoplasmic membrane will be the first to be affected. Penetration of the cell will follow, and cytoplasmic enzymes will then be inhibited. The enzyme inhibition is not the primary or main lesion caused by these compounds. A specific detergent-sensitive enzyme does not exist or has not been discovered.

3. Effects on cell permeability. See Armstrong (1957) on cytolytic damage and phosphorus loss and Scharff and Maupin (1960) on membrane damage and loss of potassium. The cytoplasmic membrane is probably the organelle most sensitive to surface-active agents within the cell of bacteria and yeasts, and the alteration in the semipermeable properties of this structure can lead to leakage of metabolites and coenzymes and disturbance in the delicate balance of metabolite concentrations within the cell. This lesion may be a major contribution to the death of a cell and cause an apparent loss in enzymic activity due to the loss or dilution of coenzymes or substrates. There is a well established relationship between cytolytic action and surface tension. This lends support to the idea that cytolytic damage may in fact be the primary lesion caused by surface-active substances.

4. Stimulatory effect of the glycolysis reaction. This is suggested by the work of Strickland (1956) and Bihler et al. (1961). This reaction is of interest, but because the effect is elicited at concentrations well below those which are antibacterial, it cannot be considered of significance for the antibacterial action of surface-active agents.

5. Effect on an enzymatically-maintained dynamic membrane. This is offered as a speculative theory by Newton (1958). Results to support this interesting hypothesis are awaited. This concept of the dynamic cell membrane enzymatically maintained could well be the detergent-sensitive enzyme, which as it was stated before does not exist.

Hugo has selected the effect on the cytoplasmic membrane controlling the cell permeability as the mode of action for quaternary ammonium compound germicides. This, he feels, is most consistent with the data presented to date, and it is well accepted (Franklin and Snow, 1989; Ikeda and Tazuke, 1985).

REFERENCES

Alfredson B.V., et al. 1951. Toxicity studies on Alkyldimethylbenzylammonium Chloride in rats and dogs. J. Am. Pharm. Assoc., 40, 263–267.

Andrews, J.K., et al. 1981. Quaternary ammonium terpolymers. U.S. Patent 4,304,894.

Antonides, J.H., and Tanner, W.S. 1961. Algicidal and sanitizing properties of Armazide. Appl. Microbiol., 9(6), 572–580.

Armstrong, W.McD. 1957. Surface active agents and cellular metabolism. I. The effects of cationic detergents on the production of acid and of carbon dioxide by bakers yeast. Arch. Biochem., 71, 137.

Aursnes, J. 1982. Ototoxic effects of quaternary ammonium compounds. Acta Otolaryngol., 93, 421–433.

Babbs, M., et al. 1956. Salts of decamethylene-bis-4-aminoquinaldinium ("Dequadin"); a new antimicrobial agent. J. Pharm. Pharmacol., 8, 110–119.

Baker, Z., Harrison, R.W., and Miller, B.F. 1941. Action of synthetic detergents on the metabolism of bacteria. J. Exp. Med., 73, 249–271.

Benson, R.A., et al. 1949. Treatment of ammonia dermatitis with Diaperene. J. Pediatr., 34, 49.

Benson, R.A., et al. 1947. A new treatment for diaper rash. J. Pediatr., 31, 369–374.

Berenschot, D.J., King, E.G., Stubbs, R.K., and Babalik, G.R. 1964. Quaternary ammonium germicide. U.S. Patent 3,140,976.

Bernarducci, E., and Harrison, K.A. 1988. Isotropic laundry detergents containing polymeric quaternary ammonium salts. U.S. Patent 4,755,327.

Bihler, I., Rothstein, A., and Bihler, L. 1961. The mechanism of stimulation of aerobic fermentation in yeast by a quaternary ammonium detergent. Biochem. Pharmacol., 8, 289.

Blank, I.H., and Coolidge, M.H. 1950. Degerming the cutaneous surface. I. Quaternary ammonium compounds. J. Invest. Dermatol., 15, 249–256.

Boyer, J.W., and Santiago, E. 1974. Polymeric quaternary ammonium compounds and methods for making same. U.S. Patent 3,784,529.

Brochure, 1968. "Deciquam 222" British Hydrological Corporation, Deer Park Road, S.W. 19 London.

Brochure. 1987. Merpanocide L. LHD. MerPan Chem. Consultants. Middletown, NJ 07748.

Brochure. Bardac 22, Bardac 205M, Barquat 4250. Lonza, Inc., Fair Lawn, NJ 07410.

Brochure. BTC 824, BTC 2125M, BTC 1100, Isothan Q, BTC 812, Onamer M, Onyxide 3300. Stepan Co., Northfield, IL 60093.

Brochure. Hyamine 10-X, Hyamine 2389, Hyamine 3500. Lonza, Inc., Fair Lawn, NJ 07410.

Brochure. Roccal MC-14. Sterwin Chem., Inc., New York, NY.

Browning, C.H. 1926. Summary: experimental studies in tuberculosis. Br. Med. J., 1(2), 73.

Browning, C.H., Cohen, J.B., Ellingsworth, S., and Gulbransen, R. 1926. Antiseptic properties of the amino derivatives of styrl- and anilquinoline. Proc. R. Soc. Med., 100B, 293–325.

Browning, C.H., Cohen, J.B., Gaunt, R., and Gulbransen, R. 1922. Relationship between antiseptic action and chemical constitution with special reference to compounds of the pyridine, quinoline, acridine and phenazine series. Proc. R. Soc. Med., 93B, 329–366.

Buckman Laboratories Brochures. 1987, 1977, 1973. WSCP For Algae Control in Swimming Pools. WSCP For Cooling Water Treatment. CDQ, Busan 77. Buckman Labs, Inc., Memphis, TN 38108.

Burger, A. 1960. Medicinal Chemistry. Volumes 1 and 2. New York, Interscience.

Butler, G.B. 1966. Water soluble quaternary ammonium polymers. U.S. Patent 3,288,770.

Casey, J.A. 1972. Method and composition for sanitation of sugar factories. U.S. Patent 3,694,262.

Ceasar, F. 1935. Erfahrungen mit Zephirol. Fortschr. Ther., 4, 249–250.

Cowles, P.B. 1938. The germicidal power of some alcohols for Bacterium typhosum and Staphylococcus aureus, and its relation to surface tension. Yale J. Biol. Med., 11, 127–135.

CTFA. 1985. The final report on the safety assessment of benzethonium chloride and methylbenzethonium chloride. J. Am. Coll. Toxicol., 4(5), 65–106.

Cucci, M.W. 1949. Quaternary ammonium compounds, a review. Soap Sanit. Chem., 25(10), 129–134, 145.

Cutler, R.A., Cimijotti, E.B., Okolwich, T.J., and Wetterau, W.F. 1966. Alkylbenzyldimethylammonium chlorides—a comparative study of the odd and even chain homologues. C.S.M.A. Proceedings of the 53rd Annual Meeting, pp. 102–113.

Cybulski, Z.R. 1984. Determination of benzalkonium chloride by gas chromatography. J. Pharm. Sci., 73, 1700–1702.

Daoud, N.N., Dickinson, N.A., Gilbert, P. 1983. Antimicrobial activity and physico-chemical properties of some alkyldimethylbenzylammonium chlorides. Microbios, 37, 73–85.

Daoud, N.N., Crooks, P.A., Speak, R., and Gilbert, P. 1983. Determination of benzalkonium chloride by chemical ionization mass spectroscopy. J. Pharm. Sci., 72, 290–292.

Darragh, J.L., and Stayner, R.D. 1954. Quaternary ammonium compounds from dodecylbenzene algae control in industrial cooling systems. Ind. Eng. Chem., 46, 254–257.

Davies, G.E. 1949. Quaternary ammonium compounds. A new technique for the study of their bactericidal action and the results obtained with Cetayalon (cetyl trimethyl ammonium bromide). J. Hyg., 47, 271.

DeBenneville, P.L., and Bock, L.H. 1950. 1,4-but-2-yne bis-quaternary ammonium halides. U.S. Patent 2,525,778.

Ditoro, R.D. March 1969. New generation of biologically active quaternaries. Soap Chem. Specialties, 47–52, 86–88, 91–92.

Domagk, G. 1938. Preserving and disinfecting media. U.S. Patent 2,108,765.

Domagk, G. 1935. Eine neue Klasse von Disinfektionsmitteln. Dtsch. Med. Wochenschr., 61, 829–832.

Dubin P.I. and Levy I.J. 1981. High Performance Aqueous Exclusion Chromatography of polycations on a hydrophilic gel column. Polymer Reprints 22, 132–134.

Dubois, A.S., and Dibblee, D.D. 1946. The influence of surface active cationic germicides on the bacterial population of milk. J. Milk Technol., 9, 260–268.

Dunn, C.C. 1936. A mixture of high molecular alkyldimethylbenzyl-ammonium chlorides as an antiseptic. Proc. Soc. Exp. Biol. Med., 35, 427–429.

Epton, S.R. 1947. A rapid method of analysis for certain surface active agents. Nature, 160, 795–796.

Ereskine, A.M., Garin, M.H., Rosenstein, L., and Chesbro, R.M. 1958. Organic ammonium salts of lignin acids. U.S. Patent 2,850,492.

Fair, G.M., Chang, S.L., Taylor, M.P., and Wineman, M.A. 1945. Destruction of waterborne cysts of Entamoeba histolytica by synthetic detergents. Am. J. Public Health, 35, 228–232.

Federal Register, 1969. Part 121—Food additives; Subpart F—Food additives resulting from contact with containers or equipment and food additives otherwise affecting food. 11/26/1969; Fed. Reg. 34/117, 18556. 12/13/1969; Fed. Reg. 34/239; 19655. 8/9 1974; Fed. Reg. 39/155; 28627.

Finnegan, J.K., and Dienna, J.B. 1954. Toxicity of quaternaries. Soap Sanit. Chem., 30(2), 147–153, 157, 173, 175.

Fitzhugh, O.G., and Nelson, A.A. 1948. Chronic oral toxicities of surface active agents. J. Am. Pharm. Assoc., 37, 29–32.

Franklin, T.J., and Snow, G.A. 1989. Biochemistry of Antimicrobial Action. 4th Edition. London, Chapman and Hall.

Frayer, J.M. 1943. Non-chlorine materials for the germicidal treatment of dairy utensils. J. Milk Technol., 6, 110–119.

Freelander, B.L., 1940. Bacteriostatic action of various wetting agents upon growth of tubercle bacilli in vitro. Proc. Soc. Exp. Biol. Med., 44, 51–53.

Friedman, H., Volin, E., and Laumann, D. 1968. Terminal disinfection in hospitals with quaternary ammonium compounds by use of a spray-fog technique. Appl. Microbiol., 16(2), 223–227.

Fulton, J.D., et al. 1948. Germicidal aerosols: Discussion of investigations in development of a liquid gas germicidal aerosol formula. Soap Sanit. Chem., 24, 125, 157, 159.

Fush, W.M., and Stamberger, P. 1965. Polymeric quaternary ammonium salt compositions and method of making same. U.S. Patent 3,219,639.

Gennaro, A.R. (ed). 1985. Antimicrobial drugs. In *Remington's Pharmaceutical Sciences*. 17th edition. Easton, PA, Mack Publishing, pp. 1158–1169.

Gershenfeld, L., and Milanick, V.E. 1941. Bactericidal and bacteriostatic properties of surface tension depressants. Am. J. Pharm., *113*, 306–326.

Gershenfeld, L., and Perlstein, D. 1941. Significance of hydrogen ion concentration in the evaluation of the bactericidal efficiency of surface tension depressants. Am. J. Pharm., *113*, 306.

Ghosh, M. 1986. Effect of various parameters on the biological activities of polymeric drugs. Polymer Material Sci. Eng. ACS, *55*, 755–757.

Ghosh, M. 1988. Synthetic macromolecules as potential chemotherapeutic agents. Polymer News, *13*, 71–77.

Gleason, M.N. 1969. *Clinical Toxicology of Commercial Products*. Baltimore, Williams & Wilkins.

Goldstein, A., Aronow, L., and Kalman, S.M. 1974 Principles of drug action. In *Structure-Activity Relationships*. 2nd edition. New York, John Wiley & Sons.

Good, R.M., Liao, J.C., Hook, J.M., and Punko, C.L. 1987. Colorimetric determination of a polymeric quaternary ammonium antimicrobial preservative in an ophthalmic solution. J. Assoc. Off. Anal. Chem., *70*(6), 979–980.

Green, H.A., Merianos, J.J., and Petrocci, A.N. 1975. Microbiocidal polymeric quaternary ammonium compounds. U.S. Patent 3,874,870, U.S. Patent 3,929,990.

Green, H.A., Merianos, J.J., and Petrocci, A.N. 1977. Randomly terminated capped polymers. U.S. Patent 4,027,020, U.S. Patent 4,036,959.

Green, H.A., Merianos, J.J., and Petrocci, A.N. 1982. Antimicrobial, cosmetic and water treating ionene polymeric compounds. U.S. Patent 4,325,940.

Green, H.A., Merianos, J.J., and Petrocci, A.N. 1978. Randomly terminated capped polymers. U.S. Patent 4,091,113.

Greene, D.F. and Petrocci, A.N. 1980. Formulating quaternary cleaner disinfectants to meet EPA requirements. Soap Cosmet. Chem. Spec., *8*,33–35, 61.

Guiteras, A.F., and Shapiro, R.L. 1946. A bactericidal detergent for eating utensils. J. Bacteriol., *52*, 635–638.

Hagan, H.H., Maguire, C.H., and Miller, W.H. 1946. Cetyl pyridinium chloride as a cutaneous germicide in major surgery. Arch. Surg., *52*, 149–159.

Hansch, C., and Clayton, J.M. 1973. Lipophilic character and biological activity of drugs II: The parabolic case. J. Pharm. Sci., *62*, 1–21.

Hansch, C., and Fujita, T. 1964. A method of the correlation of biological activity and chemical structure. J. Am. Chem. Soc., *86*, 1616–1626.

Hartmann, M. 1929. Quaternary ammonium compound and process of making same. U.S. Patent 1,737,458.

Hartmann, M., and Kagi, H. 1928. Saure Seifen. Z. Agnew. Chem., *41*, 127–130.

Hauser, P.H., Crawford, R.H., and Clarke, P.H. 1963. Germicidal fogging of sick rooms. Soap Chem. Spec., *39*(2), 80–81, 84, 87, 106, 108, 110.

Hornung, H. 1935. Zephirol, ein neues Disinfektionsmittel. Z. Imminitaetsforsch., *84*, 119–135.

Hotchkiss, R.D. 1946. The nature of the bactericidal action of surface-active agents. Ann. N.Y. Acad. Sci., *46*, 478–483.

Heuck, H.J., Adema, D.M.M., and Weigmann, J.R. 1966. Bacteriostatic, fungistatic, and algistatic activity of fatty nitrogen compounds. Appl. Microbiol., *14*(3), 308–319.

Hugo, W.B., and Russell, A.D. 1980. *Pharmaceutical Microbiology*. Oxford, Blackwell Scientific.

Hugo, W.B. 1965. Some aspects of the action of cationic surface-active agents on microbial cells with special reference to their action on enzymes. S.C.I. Monograph No. 19, *Surface-Active Agents in Microbiology*. London, Soc. Chem. Ind., pp. 67–82.

Hwa, J.C.H. 1963. Bis-quaternary ammonium compounds. U.S. Patent 3,079,436.

Ikeda, T., Yamaguchi, H., and Tazuke, S. 1984. New polymeric biocides: Synthesis and antibacterial activities of polycations with pendant biguanide groups. Antimicrob. Agents Chemother., *26*, 139–144.

Ikeda, T., Tazuke, S., and Suzuki, Y. 1984. Biologically active polycations. 4. Synthesis and antimicrobial activity of poly[trialkylvinylbenzylammonium chlorides]. Macromol. Chem., *185*, 869–876.

Ikeda, T., and Tazuke, S. 1985. Biocidal polycations. Polym. Prepr., *26*, 226–227.

Ikeda, T., and Tazuke, S. 1983. Biologically active polycations: antimicrobial activities of poly[trialkylvinylbenzylammonium chlorides] type polycations. Macromol. Chem. Rapid Commun., *4*, 459–461.

Jacobs, W.A. 1916. The bactericidal properties of the quaternary salts of hexamethylenetetramine. I. The problem of the chemotherapy of experimental bacterial infections. J. Exp. Med., *23*, 563–568.

Jacobs, W.A., and Heidelberger, M. 1915. The quaternary salts of hexamethylenetetramine. I. Substituted benzyl halides and the hexamethylenetetrammonium salts derived therefrom. J. Biol. Chem., *20*, 659–683.

Jacobs, W.A., and Heidelberger, M. 1915. The quaternary salts of hexamethylenetetramine. II. Monohalogenacetylbenzylamines and their hexamethylenetetraminium salts. J. Biol. Chem., *20*, 685–694.

Jacobs, W.A., and Heidelberger, M. 1915. The quaternary salts of hexamethylenetetramine. III. Monohalogenacylated aromatic amines and their hexamethylenetetraminium salts. J. Biol. Chem., *21*, 103–143.

Jacobs, W.A., and Heidelberger, M. 1915. The quaternary salts of hexamethylenetetramine. IV. Monohalogenated simple amines, ureas, urethanes, and the hexamethylenetetraminium salts derived therefrom. J. Biol. Chem., *21*, 145–152.

Jacobs, W.A., and Heidelberger, M. 1915. The quaternary salts of hexamethylenetetramine. V. Monohalogenacetyl derivatives of amino-alcohols and the hexamethylenetetraminium salts derived therefrom. J. Biol. Chem., *21*, 403–437.

Jacobs, W.A., and Heidelberger, M. 1915. The quaternary ammonium salts of hexamethylenetetramine. VI. Halogenethyl esters and ethers and their hexamethylenetetraminium salts. J. Biol. Chem., *21*, 439–453.

Jacobs, W.A., and Heidelberger, M. 1915. The quaternary salts of hexamethylenetetramine. VII. Halogen derivatives of aliphatic aromatic ketones and their hexamethylenetetraminium salts. J. Biol. Chem., *21*, 455–464.

Jacobs, W.A., and Heidelberger, M. 1915. The quaternary salts of hexamethylenetetramine. VIII. Miscellaneous substances containing aliphatically bound halogen and the hexamethylenetratraminium salts derived therefrom. J. Biol. Chem., *21*, 465–475.

Jacobs, W.A., Heidelberger, M., and Amoss, H.L. 1916. The bactericidal properties of the quaternary salts of hexamethylenetetramine. II. The relation between constitution and bacterial action in the substituted benzylhexamethylenetraminium salts. J. Exp. Med., *23*, 569–576.

Jacobs, W.A., Heidelberger, M., and Bull, C.G. 1916. The bactericidal properties of the quaternary salts of hexamethylenetetramine. III. The relation between constitution and bactericidal action in the quaternary salts obtained from halogenacetyl compounds. J. Exp. Med., *23*, 577–599.

James, A.N. 1965. Surface activity and the microbial cell. S.C.I. Monograph No. 19. *Surface-Active Agents in Microbiology*. London, Soc. Chem. Ind., pp. 3–23.

Jono, K., Takayama, T., Kuno, M., and Higashide, E. 1986. Effect of alkyl chain length of benzalkonium chloride on the bactericidal activity and binding to organic materials. Chem. Pharm. Bull., *34*, 4215–4224.

Kaspar, H.H., and Kirk, P.F. 1972. Resterilizing contact lens solution. U.S. Patent 3,639,576.

Kessel, J.F., and Moon, F.J. 1946. Emergency sterilization of drinking water with heteropolar cationic antiseptics. I. Effectiveness against cysts of Entamoeba histolytica. Am. J. Trop. Med. Hyg., *26*, 345–350.

King, T.C., and Zimmerman, J.M. 1965. Skin degerming practices; chaos and confusion. Am. J. Surg., *109*, 695–698.

Kirby, A.H.M., and Frick, E.L. 1963. Greenhouse evaluation of chemicals for control of powdery mildews. Ann. Appl. Biol., *52*, 45–54.

Klarmann, E.G. 1959. Hospital infection and environmental disinfection. Soap Chem. Spec., *35*(3), 101–112.

Klarmann, E.G., and Wright, E.S. 1946. An inquiry into the germicidal performance of quaternary ammonium disinfectants. Soap Sanit. Chem., *22*, 125–137.

Klein, M., and Deforest, A. 1963. Antiviral action of germicides. Soap. Sanit., *39*, 70.

Klun, T.P., et al. 1987. Structure-property relationships of ionene polymers. J. Polymer Sci., Part A, *25*, 87–109.

Kourai, H., et al. 1985. The antimicrobial characteristics of quaternary ammonium salts. Part XI. Quantitative structure-activity relationship of antimicrobial n-laurylpyridinium iodides. J. Antibact. Antifung. Agents, *13*, 245–253.

Kourai, H., et al. 1985. Part X. Antimicrobial characteristics and a mode of action of N-alkylpyridinium iodides against Escherichia coli K12. Bokin Bobai, *13*, 3–10.

Kourai, H., et al. 1989. Part XIV. Relationship between hydrophobicity of bacterial cell surface and drug susceptibility to alkylpyridinium iodides. J. Antibact. Antifung. Agents, *17*, 119–128.

Krog, A.J., and Marshall, C.G. 1940. Alkyldimethylbenzyl-ammonium chloride for sanitization of eating and drinking utensils. Am. J. Public Health, *30*, 341–347.

Krog, A.J., and Marshall, C.G. 1942. Roccal in the dairy pasteurizing plant. J. Milk Technol., *5*, 343–347.

Kuhn, R., and Dann, O. 1940. Uber Invertseifen II; Butyl-Octyl-Lauryl-, and Cetyl-Dimethyl Sulfonium Iodide. Ber. Dtsch. Chem. Ges., *73*, 1092.

Kuhn, R., Jerchel, D., and Westphal, O. 1940. Uber Invertseifen. III. Dialkylmethyl-benzyl-ammonium-chlorid. Ber. Dtsch. Chem. Ges., *73*, 1095–1100.

Kundsin, R.B., and Walter, C.W. 1961. In-use testing of bactericidal agents in hospitals. Appl. Microbiol., *9*(2), 167–170.

Lawrence, C.A. 1950. *Surface Active Quaternary Ammonium Germicides*. New York, Academic Press.

Levy, I.J., and Dubin, P.L. 1982. Molecular weight distributions of cationic polymers by aqueous gel permeation chromatography. Ind. Eng. Chem. Prod. Res Dev., *21*, 59–63.

Lehn, G.J., and Vignolo, R.L. 1946. Applications of quaternary ammonium compounds in the brewing industry. Brewers Dig., *21*, 41–44.

Lenhart, E., Petrocci, A., and Gardon, R. 1961. Hospital evaluation of multipurpose and single-action disinfectants. Mod. Sanit. Build. Maint., *5*(12), 27–30.

Lien, E.J., and Anderson, S.M. 1968. Structure-activity correlations for antibacterial agents on gram-negative and gram-positive cells. J. Med. Chem., *11*, 430–441.

Lien, E.J., and Perrin, J.H. 1976. Effect of chain length upon critical micelle formation and protein binding of quaternary ammonium compounds. J. Med. Chem., *19*, 849–850.

Like, B., Sorrentino, R., and Petrocci, A. 1975. Utility of amine oxides in oil/water cosmetic systems. J. Soc. Cosmet. Chem., 26, 155–168.

Marsh, D.F., and Takahashi, L.T. 1983. Determination of benzalkonium chloride in the presence of interfering alkaloids and polymeric substrates by reverse-phase high-performance liquid chromatography. J. Pharm. Sci., 72, 521–525.

Mallman, W.L., and Hanes, M. 1945. The use dilution method of testing disinfectants. J. Bacteriol., 49, 526.

Mallman, W.L., Kivela, E.W., and Turner, G. 1946. Sanitizing dishes. Soap. Sanit. Chem., 22, 130–133.

McCulloch, E.C. 1947. False disinfection velocity curves produced by quaternary ammonium compounds. Science, 105, 480–481.

McNeil, E., and Choper, E.A. 1962. Disinfectants in home laundering. Soap Chem. Spec., 38(8), 51–54, 94, 97–100.

Merianos, J.J., Smith, L.R., and Weinstein, M. 1977. Onamer M—A new cosmetic ingredient. SCC Specialties, 12, 54–74.

Merianos, J.J. 1988. "Structure activity relationships in quaternary ammonium antimicrobial compounds." Abstracts. SIM NEWS Supplement, Vol. 38, No. 4, S-63. SIM 45th Annual Meeting, Chicago, IL.

Merianos, J.J. 1986. Unpublished report. Merpan Chemical Consultants, Middletown, NJ 07748, 201 6716925.

Miller, B.F., Abrams, R., Huber, D.A., and Klein, M. 1943. Formation of invisible, non-perceptible films on hands by cationic soaps. Proc. Soc. Exp. Biol. Med., 54, 174–176.

Miranol Chemical Company, Inc., Dayton, NJ. Brochure: 1987. Mirapol A-15.

Mosher, H.H., and Howard, F.L. 1948. Cationic isoquinoline pesticide. U.S. Patent 2,435,458.

Mueller, W.S., Bennett, E., and Fuller, J.E. 1946. Bactericidal properties of some surface active agents. J. Dairy Sci., 29, 751–760.

Nagel, A. 1940. Ueber die desinfizierende Wirkung des Blattzephirols. Munch. Med. Wochenschr., 36, 970–972.

Nelson, J.W., and Lyster, S.C. 1946. The toxicity of Myristyl-gamma-picolinium chloride. J. Am. Pharm. Assoc., 35, 89–94.

Ng, Lay-Keow, Hupe, M., and Harris, A.G. 1986. Direct gas chromatographic method for determining the homologue composition of benzalkonium chlorides. J. Chromatography, 351, 554–559.

Newton, B.A. 1958. The Strategy of Chemotherapy. Surface Active Bactericides; 8th Symposium Society General Microbiology. Cambridge, Cambridge University Press.

Official Methods of Analysis of the AOAC. 1984. Washington, D.C., Association of Official Analytical Chemists.

Official Methods of Analysis of the AOAC. 1984. Disinfectants. 11th edition. Washington, D.C., Association of Official Analytical Chemists, pp. 59–72.

Ordal, E.J., and Borg, A.F. 1942. Effect of surface active agents on oxidations of lactate by bacteria. Proc. Soc. Exp. Biol. Med., 50, 332–336.

Ortenzio, L.F., Opalsky, C.D., and Stuart, L.S. 1961. Factors affecting the activity of phenolic disinfectants. Appl. Microbiol., 9(6), 562–566.

Palmer, C.M., and Maloney, T.C. 1955. Preliminary screening for potential algicides. Ohio J. Sci., 55, 1–8.

Penniston, V.J., and Hedrick, L.R. 1945. The germicidal efficiency of Emulsept and of chlorine in washing dirty eggs. Science, 101, 362–363.

Petrocci, A.N. Unpublished report.

Petrocci, A.N., and Clarke, P. 1969. Proposed test method for antimicrobial laundry additives. J. Assoc. Off. Anal. Chem., 52(4), 836–842.

Petrocci, A.N., et al. 1969. Synergistic blends of microbiocidal quaternary ammonium compounds. U.S. Patent 3,472,939.

Petrocci, A.N., et al. 1970. Microbiocidal quaternary ammonium compounds containing synergistic blends of alkyl groups. U.S. Patent 3,525,793.

Petrocci, A.N., Clarke, P., Merianos, J., and Green, H. 1979. Quaternary ammonium antimicrobial compounds: old and new. Dev. Indust. Microbiol., 20, 11–14.

Petrocci, A.N., Green, H.A., Merianos, J.J., and Like, B. 1974. The properties of dialkyldimethyl quaternary ammonium compounds. C.S.M.A. Proceedings of the 60th Mid-Year Meeting, May 1974, pp. 87–89.

Post, M.H. 1946. Dust-borne infection in ophthalmic surgery. Am. J. Ophthalmol., 29, 1435–1443.

Price, P.B., and Bonnett, A. 1948. Antibacterial effects of G-5, G-11, and A-151. Surgery, 24, 542–554.

Prusick, J.H., and Gregory, V.P. 1956. Chemical treatment of flood waters used in secondary oil recovery. U.S. Patent 2,733,206.

Puhle, R.G. 1950. Quaternary-type detergent sanitizers on the dairy farm. Soap Sanit. Chem., 26, 133–139.

Putnam, F.W. 1948. The interaction of protein and synthetic detergents. Adv. Protein Chem., 4, 79.

Quisno, R., and Foter, M.J. 1946. Cetyl pyridinium chloride. J. Bacteriol., 52, 111–117.

Quisno, R., Gibby, I.W., and Foter, M.J. 1946. A neutralizing medium for evaluating the germicidal potency of quaternary ammonium salts. Am. J. Pharm., 118, 32–33.

Rahn, C. 1946. Protection of dry bacteria against cationic detergents. Proc. Soc. Exp. Biol. Med., 62, 2–4.

Rahn, C., and Eseltine, W.P. 1947. Quaternary ammonium compounds. Annu. Rev. Microbiol., 1, 173–192.

Ramp, J.A., Mancuso, C.G., and Huig, J.G. 1966. Dimethyl alkyl ammonium cyclohexysulfamate—a new paint mildewcide. VIII Congres FATIPEC, 1966, Verlag Chemie, GMBH, Weinbeim, Bergstrasse.

Rembaum, A. 1973. Biological activity of ionene polymers. Applied Polymer Symposium No. 22, pp. 299–317.

Rembaum, A., Senyei, A.E., and Rajaraman, R. 1977. Interaction of living cells with polyionenes and polyionene-coated surfaces. J. Biomed. Mater. Res. Symposium, 8, 101–110.

Rembaum, A., and Selegny, E. 1975. Polyelectrolytes and Their Applications. Boston, D. Reidel, pp. 187–195, 131–144, 163–174.

Resuggan, J.C.L. 1951. Quaternary Ammonium Compounds in Chemical Sterilisation. London, United Trade Press.

Russell, A.D., and Furr, J.R. 1987. Comparative sensitivity of smooth, rough and deep rough strains of Escherichia coli to Chlorhexidine, Quaternary Ammonium Compounds and Dibromopropamidine isethionate. Int. J Pharmaceut., 36, 191–197.

Salt, W.G., and Wiseman, D. 1968. The uptake of cetyltrimethylammonium bromide by Escherichia coli. J. Pharm. Pharmacol. Suppl., 20, 14–17.

Salt, W.G. and Wiseman, D. 1970. Relation between the uptake of Cetyltrimethylammonium bromide by Escherichia coli and its effects of cell growth and viability. J. Pharm. Pharmacol., 22, 261–264.

Samour, C.M. 1978. Polymer drugs. Chemtech., August, 494–501.

Sakai, T. 1983. Spectrophotometric determination of trace amounts of quaternary ammonium salts in drugs by ion-pair extraction with bromophenol blue and quinine. Analyst, 108, 608–614.

Sato, S., Tanaka, S. 1984. Determination of benzalkonium chlorides by high-performance liquid chromatography. Bunseki Kagaku, 338.

Schaeufele, P.J. 1984. Advances in quaternary ammonium biocides. JAOCS, 61, 387–389.

Scharff, T.G., with technical assistance of Maupin, W.C. 1960. Correlation of the metabolic effects of benzalkonium chloride with its membrane effects in yeast. Biochem. Pharmacol., 5, 79.

Schmidt, W. 1935. Praktische erfahrungen mit demneuen Desinfektionsmittel Zephirol. Med. Welt., 29, 1043–1044.

Schneider, G. 1935. Untersuchungen uber das disinfektionsmittel zephirol. Z. Immunitaetsforsch., 85, 194–199.

Shay, E.G., and Petrocci, A.N., 1968. New trends in fabric softener-sanitizers. Presented at 41st Annual Meeting of Soap and Detergent Assoc., 1968.

Shay, E.G., Clarke, P.H., and Crawford, R. 1964. An evaluation of some experimental chemicals for swimming-pool disinfection. C.S.M.A. Proceedings of the 51st Annual meeting, December, 1964, pp. 108–109.

Shelanski, H.A. Unpublished report.

Shelanski, H.A. 1949. Toxicity of quaternaries. Soap Sanit. Chem., 25(2), 125–129, 153.

Sheldon, B.G., et al. 1985. Quaternary Ammonium Group Containing Polymers Having Antimicrobial Activity. U.S. Patent 4,532,128.

Shelton, R.S., et al. 1946 Quaternary ammonium salts as germicides. I. Nonacylated quaternary ammonium salts derived from aliphatic amines. J. Am. Chem. Soc., 68, 753–755.

Shema, B.F. 1966. Slimicidal composition and method. U.S. Patent 3,231,509.

Shibe, W.J., Cohen, S., and Front, M.S. 1955. Quaternary ammonium saccharinates and process for preparing the same. U.S. Patent 2,725,326.

Smith, C.R., et al. 1950. The bactericidal effect of surface active agents on tubercle bacilli. U.S. Public Health Dept., No. 48, pp. 1588–1600.

Sommermeyer, L., and Frobisher, M., Jr. 1952. Laboratory studies on disinfection of oral thermometers. Nurs. Res., 1, 32–35.

Sotier, A.L., and Ward, H.W. 1947. Quaternary ammonium germicidal treatment for jute-packed water mains. J. Am. Water Works Assoc., 39, 1038–1045.

Speck, M.L., and Lucas, H.L. 1957. The performance of a detergent-sanitizer for milk utensil sanitation in unsupervised field tests. J. Milk Food Technol., 20(1), 3–6.

Stark, R.L. 1985. Aqueous antimicrobial ophthalmic solutions. U.S. Patent 4,525,346.

Stark, R.L. 1983. Ophthalmic solutions. U.S. Patent 4,407,791.

Steinberger, S. 1963. Chemical treatment of flood waters used in secondary oil recovery. U.S. Patent 3,111,492.

Stevens, L.E., and Eckardt, J.I. 1987. Spectrophotometric determination of polyquaternium-1 with trypan blue by a difference procedure. Analyst, 112, 1619–1621.

Stickland, L.M. 1956. The Pasteur effect in normal yeast and its inhibition by various agents. Biochem. J., 64, 503.

Stone, R.V. 1947. A paper test for quaternary compounds. Sanitarian, 9, 203–205.

Stuart, L.J., Ortenzio, L.F., and Freidl, J.L. 1953. Use dilution confirmation test for results obtained by phenol coefficient methods. J. Assoc. Off. Anal. Chem., 36(2), 466–480.

Suzuki, S., et al. 1989. Analysis of benzalkonium chlorides by gas chromatography. J. Chromatography, 463, 188–191.

Swan, H., et al. 1949. Use of a quaternary ammonium compound for the surgical scrub. Am. J. Surg., 77, 24–37.

Sykes, G. 1965. Disinfection and Sterilization. London, Chapman & Hall.

Taylor, G.F., and Prindle, R.F. 1966. Surface disinfectant and space deodorant aerosol spray composition. U.S. Patent 3,287,214.

Tolgyesi, E., Schwartz, A.M., Rader, C.A., and Bry, R.E. 1971. Mothproofing with ammonium quats. Chem. Technol., 1, 27–30.

Tomlinson, E., Brown, M.R.W., and Davis, S.S. 1977. Effect of colloidal association on the measured activity of alkyldimethylbenzylammonium chlorides against Pseudomonas aeruginosa. J. Med. Chem., 20, 1277–1282.

Tonaka, F. 1944. Invert soaps as disinfectants. IX. Relationship between bactericidal actions and molecular weight. J. Pharm. Soc. Jap., *64*, 35–36.

Tressler, D.K. 1947. Frozen sea food: Preliminary steps to freezing. Fishing Gaz., *Jan.*, 66.

Tsubouchi, M., and Yamamoto, Y. 1983. Determination of anionic surfactants in presence of cationic by two-phase titration. Anal. Chem., *55*, 583–584.

Tsubouchi, M., and Mallory, J.H. 1982. Differential determination of cationic and anionic surfactants in mixtures by two-phase titration. Analyst, *108*, 636–639.

Verdon, P.E. 1961. Efficiency tests on a series of common skin antiseptics under ward conditions. J. Clin. Pathol., *14*, 91–93.

Wakeman, R.L., and Coates, J.F. 1971. Quaternary ammonium compounds having a branched chain aliphatic acid anion. U.S. Patent 3,565,927.

Wakeman, R.L., and Tesoro, G.C. 1954. Ethylbenzyl, lauryl, dimethyl ammonium salts. U.S. Patent 2,676,986.

Walker, G.E., and Cambre, C.M. 1970. Antibacterial compositions containing polymeric quaternary ammonium salts. U.S. Patent 3,491,191.

Walter, C.W. 1938. The use of a mixture of coconut oil derivatives as a bactericide in the operating room. Surg. Gynecol. Obstet., *67*, 683–688.

Walter, C.W. 1965. Disinfection of hands [editorial]. Am. J. Surg., *109*, 691–693.

Wang, L.K., and Shuster, W.W. 1975. Polyelectrolyte determination at low concentration. Ind. Eng. Chem. Prod. Res. Dev., *14*, No. 4, 312–314.

Wetzel, U. 1935. Handedisinfektionsversuche mit Zephirol. Arch. Hyg. Bakteriol., *114*, 1.

White, C.S., Collins, J.L., and Newman, H.E. 1938. The clinical use of alkyldimethylbenzylammonium chloride (Zephiran): A preliminary report. Am. J. Surg., *39*, 607–609.

Whitehill, A.R. 1945. Evaluation of some liquid antiseptics. J. Am. Pharm. Assoc., *34*, 219–221.

Zeissler, J., and Gunther, O. 1939. Kann durch Kochen in Zephirol. Quartamon-Losungen sterilisiert werden? Zentralbl. Bakteriol., Orig., *144*, 402–407.

CHAPTER 14

SURFACE-ACTIVE AGENTS: ACID-ANIONIC COMPOUNDS

G.R. Dychdala and John A. Lopes

A great volume of information may be found in the literature describing the antimicrobial properties of cationic surfactants, and especially of the quaternary ammonium compounds. Considerably fewer data have been accumulated discussing the anionic surface-active agents and their biologic activities. It has been known for some time that anionic surfactants, under certain conditions, definitely exhibit antibacterial activity and that they are especially effective against gram-positive organisms and less effective against gram-negative bacteria (Cowles, 1938; Birkeland and Steinhaus, 1939; Baker et al., 1941a). Cowles (1938) also found that straight-chain alkyl sulfates in the 12- to 16-carbon chain range optimally inhibited *Staphylococcus aureus*. Klotz and Ayers (1953) have shown that anionic agents have greater ability to bind to proteins than do cationic agents.

The slow and selective activity of anionic surfactants may be partly attributed to higher pH levels employed in most of these experiments. Even in the aforementioned early investigation, Baker et al. (1941) had discovered a certain interdependence of anionic surfactant and acid pH for effective antimicrobial activity. A number of other investigators had reported that a decrease in pH enhanced the antimicrobial effectiveness of a variety of anionic surface-active agents (Baker et al., 1941b; Gainor, 1948; Gershenfeld and Milanick, 1941; Gershenfeld and Perlstein, 1941; Scales and Kemp, 1941; Prince and Prince, 1987).

Later, Lewandowski (1952) prepared formulations based on acid-anionic surfactants and demonstrated a rapid bactericidal action at low concentrations (about 200 ppm) of certain anionic surfactants in acid solution. Employing the Weber and Black method (1948), he showed that gram-negative as well as gram-positive microorganisms were rapidly inactivated by mixtures of acids and anionic surfactants at low pH levels (pH 2 to 3). In his extensive work, he tried many types of anionic surfactants in combination with different acids and found that

alkyl aryl sulfonates exhibited the best overall results. Food-grade phosphoric acid was selected as the most suitable acid, based on economic, toxicity, and corrosion considerations. This work led to a development of commercial sanitizers that were introduced to the food and dairy processing industries for disinfecting modern equipment and utensils.

MECHANISM OF BIOCIDAL ACTION

The precise mechanism of antimicrobial activity of anionic or other ionic surface-active agents at low pH is not properly understood. Several theories have been advanced, which are discussed in different reviews: Hotchkiss (1946), Glassman (1948), Lawrence (1950), Newton (1958), and Hugo (1965). James (1965) has discussed various theories with regard to antibacterial activity by anionic surfactants and showed their effects on the electrokinetic properties of bacteria. The anionic surfactants (except for acid unstable esters) are chemically stable at low pH. Other than the degree of ionization, these molecules do not undergo significant chemical change that can explain their enhanced microbicidal activity at low pH. Similarly pH alone does not show the magnitude of microbicidal activity exhibited by acid anionic sanitizers.

Investigations via the Weber and Black method against *E. coli* and *Staphylococcus aureus* revealed that neither acid nor anionic surfactant alone will kill in 5 minutes. However, the combination of agents will provide a 30-second kill, thereby suggesting a synergistic effect of acid and anionic surfactant (Lewandowski, 1952; Dychdala, 1962b). The most significant change pH can likely bring about is primarily the degree of ionization or charged groups on the microbial cell surface. Only those anionic surfactants that show certain structural features show microbicidal activity at low pH. To understand the mechanism of action of acid anionic sanitizers, it is necessary to relate the structure of active molecules to the changes in the microbial cell that occurs at low pH.

Rapid microbicidal action of acid-anionic sanitizers may be due to one or all of the following activities:

Disorganization of the cell membrane
Inhibition of key enzymic activities
Interruption of cellular transport and denaturation of cellular proteins

Anionic surfactants have been shown to possess these activities (Glassman, 1948; Salton, 1957; Newton, 1960; Swisher, 1987; Bartnik and Küenstler, 1987).

Of the multiple modes of antimicrobial action of the anionic surfactants, interaction with the cell membrane appears to be the leading cause of rapid microbicidal activity. A number of reports document injury to the bacterial cell membranes by anionic surfactants (Glassman, 1948; Salton, 1957; Rode and Foster, 1960). Disruption of cell membranes and leakage of intracellular components by the anionic surfactants can explain rapid cell death. However, a sudden surge of microbicidal activity of anionic surfactants at pH 2 to 3 and their relative ineffectiveness on gram-negative microorganisms above pH 3 has not been explained. Baker et al. (1941c) reported that phospholipids counteract inhibition of bacterial metabolic activity by surface active agents. Gilby and Few (1960) suggested that phospholipids in the protoplast membranes of *Micrococcus lysodeikticus* are suitable ionic groups for electrostatic interaction with ionic surfactants. The role of anionic surfactant, sodium dodecyl sulfate, in disruption of cell membranes of *Escherichia coli* and *Rhodospirillum rubrum* was demonstrated by Salton (1957).

Bilayer phospholipid matrix forms the basic framework of biologic membranes (Wallach and Winzler, 1974a; Jain and Wagner, 1980a). Anionic surfactants show structural similarity to phospholipids in having hydrophilic and hydrophobic domains and, like phospholipid molecules, partition at the surface of bilayer lipid membranes (Wallach and Winzler, 1974a,b). The interaction of anionic surfactants on both artificial and biologic phospholipid membranes is enhanced at pH < 3 (Feinstein et al., 1970; Vanderkooi and Martonosi, 1969). This has been demonstrated by using fluorescent membrane probe 8-anilino 1-naphthalene sulfonate (ANS). Like other anionic surfactants, ANS has both hydrophobic and hydrophilic domains. The molecule partitions on the surface of bilayer lipid membranes, with its aromatic region penetrating the hydrophobic core of the membrane.

The transfer of ANS from aqueous to hydrophobic environment is marked by increase in its fluorescence intensity. Membrane preparations treated with ANS showed increase in fluorescence with decreasing pH, indicating facilitated penetration of ANS into hydrophobic environment. The maximum fluorescence intensity was observed to be between pH 1.5 and 3 with preparations of different phospholipids (Flanagan and Hesketh, 1973; Feinstein et al., 1970). As the pH is lowered through their pKa, the phosphate groups of phospholip-

Table 14–1. pKa Values of Acidic Groups

Compound	pKa
Glycine	2.35
Glutamic acid	2.2
Tyrosine	2.2
Cysteine	2.0
Lysine	2.2
Arginine	2.2
Histidine	1.8
Glycylglycine	3.1
Pentaglycine	2.95
α-Glycerophosphate	1.4

Adapted from Netter, H. 1960. *Theoretical Biochemistry.* New York, Wiley—Interscience Division, pp. 190 and 462.

ids get protonated. This in turn reduces electrostatic repulsion between the negatively charged groups of anionic surfactants and phospholipid phosphate, resulting in facilitated binding of anionic surfactants to the membrane (Flanagan and Hesketh, 1973).

The negative charges on microbial cell membrane may arise from carboxylic groups of amino acids and sugar acids, as well as phosphate groups of phospholipids, teichoic acids, lipopolysaccharides, and other phosphorylated compounds. Table 14–1 shows that these groups have pKa below pH 3 and would be protonated below that pH. Thus, lowering the pH of microbial cell suspension below 3 would result in protonation or neutralization of negative charges and facilitate the interaction of anionic surfactants with membrane phospholipid matrix (Flanagan and Hesketh, 1973). The negative charges on anionic surfactants, especially sulfonates, remain ionized because they have pKa below pH 1.0. The negative groups of the anionic surfactants can remain solvated in the aqueous phase or salt linked to cationic charges on membrane surface (Flanagan and Hesketh, 1973).

Introduction of external molecules in the phospholipid matrix of the membrane can bring about changes from those of subtle intermolecular relationships to the most disruptive changes of disorganizing the membrane matrix. The addition of cholesterol apparently increases the separation between phospholipid molecules until intermolecular interaction between phospholipid headgroups can no longer take place (Yeagle, 1978). Introduction of 1-pyrenedecanoic acid can increase intermolecular separation by about 10 to 15% (Subramanian and Patterson, 1985). At higher concentration the anionic surfactants can disaggregate and solubilize the membrane components (Wallach and Winzler, 1974b).

A concentration of anionic surfactant in a sanitizer preparation required to reduce the viability of 10^8 cells by 99.999% in 30 seconds is around 0.02% (Lewandowski, 1952). It would be interesting to compare this concentration to the critical micelle concentration (CMC) of anionic surfactants below pH 3. Most physicochemical properties of surfactants like detergency, surface tension, osmotic pressure, and interfacial tension occur at the CMC because of micelle formation (Rosen, 1978).

Whether the microbicidal action of acid-anionic sanitizers correlates with the CMC of anionic surfactants remains to be investigated. Preliminary evidence indicates that the bactericidal activity of acid-anionic surfactants is enhanced by lowering the CMC (Lopes, 1990). Sands (1986) concluded that because cetyl trimethyl ammonium bromide inactivates viruses below the CMC, monomers of the surfactants interact with viral surface. Similar investigation about acid-anionic sanitizer would elucidate one aspect of its mode of action.

Enhancement of interaction of anionic surfactants with membranes by removing electrostatic repulsion through neutralization of negative charges can also be achieved by cations and cationic organic compounds. Flanagan and Hesketh (1973) reported that interaction of anionic fluorescent probe, ANS, with phospholipid membranes was enhanced by Ca^{2+}, Mg^{2+}, Sr^{2+}, and Ba^{2+}, as well as by stearylamine. Berg and Zimmerer (1987) found that Mg^{2+} and rare earth cation La^{2+} enhanced microbicidal activity of anionic surfactants against both gram-positive and gram-negative bacteria. Miller et al. (1942) reported that protamines increased susceptibility of gram-negative bacteria to anionic surfactants. These findings might be relevant in developing anionic sanitizers at less acidic pH or potentiating existing acid anionic sanitizers.

The elucidation of the mechanisms involved in the bactericidal activity of anionic surfactants is far from complete. The answer awaits revelation of the details of chemical composition and biochemical functions of the protoplast membrane, as well as more knowledge about the bacterial cell wall, structure, and metabolism.

ACID-ANIONIC SURFACTANTS AS GERMICIDES AND FACTORS AFFECTING THEIR ACTIVITY

The anionic surface active agents are the active chemical ingredients in acid-anionic sanitizers. Typically an anionic surface active agent has two distinct domains of hydrophilic and hydrophobic groups spacially separated from each other along the length of the molecule. The hydrophilic domain carries a negative charge at pH above its pKa. The chemical groups in the hydrophilic domain may include carboxylic acid. (–COO⁻), sulfonic acid (–SO₃⁻), sulfuric acid ester (–O-SO₃⁻), phosphoric acid ester (–O-PO₃⁻), or phosphonic acid (–PO₃⁻). The hydrophobic domain is made up of saturated or unsaturated straight or branched alkyl chains, which may be substituted with aromatic groups like benzene or naphthalene rings.

The structure of the hydrophobic domain and the nature of the hydrophilic group are important factors in determining antimicrobial activity of the anionic surfactants. Hydrophobic domain interacts with the bilayer lipid matrix, whereas the hydrophilic groups determine the interaction with ionic charges at the membrane interface. Structural requirements of anionic surfactants are thus determined by these factors in the membrane.

Nature of the Hydrophobic Functional Groups

It has been known that the antimicrobial activity of anionic surfactants is related to the length of the alkyl chain (Cowles, 1938; Klein et al., 1945). Cowles (1938) found a chain length of alkyl sulfates between 12 to 16 carbon atoms optimal for inhibition of *Staphylococcus aureus*. Hassinen et al. (1951) and Karabinos (1975) reported that C_{10} to C_{12} fatty aids possessed optimal antimicrobial activity. Similarly C_8 and C_{10} fatty acids were also found in natural antimicrobial systems in suckling rabbits by Canas-Rodriguez and William Smith (1966), and in leaf-cutting harvest ants by Schildknecht and Koob (1971).

The effective alkyl chain length of about C_{12} of anionic surfactants correlates with that of acyl residues in bilayer phospholipid matrix of cell membranes. Most common membrane phospholipids have fatty acids with chain lengths corresponding to C_{12} to C_{16} carbon atoms (Jain and Wagner, 1980b). Distance between two carbon atoms on an acyl chain is 0.127 nm (Jain and Wagner, 1980a), and as a result the length of alkyl chain with 12 carbon atoms is 1.5 nm. Anionic surfactants with equivalent chain length can easily integrate with cell membranes. Those with longer or shorter chains have no thermodynamic advantage of integration into the membrane (Cooper and Berner, 1985). A chain length greater than C_{12} reduces aqueous solubility and in turn reduces effective concentration of the anionic surfactants (Siebert and Boltersdorf, 1988). A chain length greater than C_{16} is less efficiently adsorbed at the interface because of its increase in cross-sectional area due to coiling of the long chain (Rosen, 1978b). Alkyl chain length of less than C_8 has low hydrophobicity and appreciably exchanges between lipid bilayers and the bulk aqueous phase (Jain and Wagner, 1980a). Thus for optimal antimicrobial activity the desired length of the hydrophobic domain appears to be about 1.5 nm.

Surfactants with alkyl chain length of 12 carbon atoms show maximum biologic activities (Bartnik and Küenstler, 1987; Siebert and Boltersdorf, 1988). Interestingly high levels of physicochemical properties like detergency, surface tension, and osmotic pressure are exhibited by anionic surfactants with alkyl chain lengths around 12 carbon atoms (Siebert and Boltersdorf, 1988). Because of superimposing physicochemical and biologic characteristics, some of the physicochemical parameters (i.e., the CMC and interfacial adsorption) are likely to be useful for selecting anionic surfactants for microbicidal activity. Anionic surfactants with lower CMC and higher interfacial adsorption would tend to have higher microbicidal activity. In case of substitution or branching of alkyl chain the effective length can be estimated by values for benzene ring or methyl branch (Rosen, 1978a,b). Substitution of benzene ring increases the length of alkyl chain by 3.5 methylene residues, or about 0.44 nm. Thus the length of octyl benzene, dodecyl and n-butylnaphthalene groups would be approximately equivalent. In case of a branched alkyl chain the effect of a carbon atom on the branch is one-half the effect on a straight chain. Nonterminal polar groups on the alkyl chain raise the CMC and put restrictions on intergration of the alkyl chain in lipid micelles. Double bonds in the alkyl chain and cis-isomers increase the CMC and therefore are less desirable than the saturated alkyl chain and trans isomers, respectively. However, these properties have to be balanced with other properties like solubility and stability of anionic surfactants in a sanitizer preparation.

Nature of the Hydrophilic Group

Aqueous solubility is an important requirement of the anionic surfactant for use in an acid anionic sanitizer preparation. Anionic groups like sulfates and especially sulfonates with pKa lower than pH 2 are most commonly used in acid-anionic sanitizer preparations. Acid esters like sulfates get hydrolyzed by the acid at low pH; the sanitizer preparation would have short shelf-life. Carboxylic groups with high pKa values get protonated at low pH and cannot be solubilized without hydrotroping agents.

Some of the hydrotropes used for solubilizing alkyl carboxylic acids in acid-anionic sanitizer preparations may also exhibit antimicrobial activity and complement sanitizing activity of the preparation. Alkyl, alkenyl, beta-hydroxy, or branched alkyl monocarboxylic acids like octanoic-decanoic, undecenylic, beta-hydroxydecanoic, and neodecanoic acids, respectively, have been used in mixed acid-anionic sanitizer preparations (Wang, 1983; Osberghaus et al., 1974; Karabinos and Andriole, 1975; Dychdala, 1987). The use of alkyl and alkenyl succinic acids by Lopes and Stanton (1987) marks the use of a new species of carboxylic acids in acid-anionic sanitizer preparations.

Terminal location of hydrophilic group on the alkyl chain has been found to increase surface activity (Rosen, 1978a,b). A terminal hydrophilic group facilitates partitioning of an anionic surfactant molecule at the membrane interface (Wallach and Winzler, 1974a,b). The acid-anionic sanitizers presently used generally contain anionic surfactants with terminal hydrophilic groups. However, acid-anionic sanitizers prepared with molecules, like sulfonated fatty acid or secondary alkane sulfonate, with nonterminal hydrophilic group have hydrophobic alkyl chains capable of interaction with the lipid matrix of membrane interior.

Table 14–2 shows different anionic surfactants presently employed in the acid sanitizers and used on food-processing equipment.

Germicidal Activity of Acid-Anionic Sanitizers

Most of the commercially available acid-anionic surfactant sanitizers are registered with the Environmental Protection Agency under the Federal Insecticide, Fungicide, and Rodenticide Act and exhibit acceptable antibacterial properties when examined by the Weber and Black (1948), Chambers (1956), or Official AOAC Germicidal and Detergent Sanitizing Test (1984) methods. Therefore, they fulfill the criteria established in Appendix F of the Grade A Pasteurized Milk Ordinance, 1965 Recommendation of the U.S. Public Health Service 1985 Revision. These sanitizers are formulated with low levels of anionic surfactant, with either organic or inorganic acid, with a solubilizer, and with or without a small amount of nonionic surfactant. Also, these antimicrobial compositions intended for food contact surface disinfection must have prior FDA clearance of ingredients as indirect food additives. FDA-cleared sanitizers do not require a potable water rinse after sanitizing, but only complete drainage of the sanitizing solution from surfaces before processing food products.

In extensive microbiologic studies, Lewandowski

Table 14–2. Typical Anionic Surfactants Used in Modern Acid Sanitizers

Chemical Name	Chemical Formula	CAS Reg. No.	% Activity
Dodecyl benzene sulfonic acid	$C_{18}H_{30}O_3S$	27176-87-0	96–98
Oleic acid, sodium salt sulfonated‡	$C_{18}H_{34}O_2SNa$	143-19-1	45–50
Dodecyl benzene sulfonic acid, sodium salt‡	$C_{18}H_{30}O_3SNa$	25155-30-0	30–90
Dodecyl benzene sulfonic acid, potassium salt‡	$C_{18}H_{30}O_3SK$	27177-77-1	30–60
Dodecyl benzene sulfonic acid, ammonium salt‡	$C_{18}H_{30}O_3SH_3N$	1331-61-9	50–60
1-octane sulfonic acid, monosodium salt*‡	$C_{10}H_{22}O_4SNa$	68845-22-7†	40–50
9-octadecenoic acid, sulfonated	$C_{18}H_{34}O_2S$	68988-76-1	30–50
Dodecyl diphenyloxidedisulfonic acid	$C_{36}H_{60}O_7S_2$	30260-73-2	40–70
Fatty acids, tall oil, sulfonated, sodium salts‡	$C_{18}H_{33}O_2SNa$	68369-27-3	40–45
Naphthalene sulfonic acid	$C_{10}H_7SO_3H \cdot H_2O$	68412-23-7	90–98

*Octane sulfonic acid, 1-hydroxy-3, 7-dimethyl-monosodium salt.
†5324-84-5.
‡The salts change to corresponding acids under acidic conditions.

(1952) determined that acid-anionic surfactant sanitizers displayed fast bactericidal action (within 30 seconds) on a number of gram-negative and gram-positive bacteria, including some thermoduric organisms that are of particular importance to the dairy industry. In another study, it was shown that an acid-anionic surfactant sanitizer gave an effective 30-second kill of organisms prevalent in mastitis cases, including *Streptococcus agalactiae*, *Streptococcus dysgalactiae*, *Streptococcus uberis*, *Staphylococcus aureus*, and *Pseudomonas aeruginosa* (Dychdala, 1962a). In limited sporicidal studies, Lewandowski (1952) showed that spores of *Bacillus subtilis* and *B. stearothermophilus* apparently were not affected in a 1-hour exposure by the normally used concentration of acid-anionic surfactants, suggesting considerably slower activity against bacterial spores.

Employing the Official AOAC Fungicidal Test Method in further studies with a number of fungal organisms, it was observed that an acid-anionic surfactant sanitizer was effective against most yeast strains, inactivating them in less than 10 minutes, and that mold spores were considerably more resistant, often requiring exposure longer than 60 minutes or higher concentrations of sanitizer for complete destruction (Dychdala, 1961). Hays and Elliker (1959) studied the virucidal effect of an acid-anionic surfactant sanitizer against *Streptococcus cremoris* phage strain 144F, which destroys the lactic acid streptococci used as starter cultures in the dairy industry. They concluded that an acid-anionic surfactant sanitizer inactivated the phage in 15 seconds in hard and distilled water, comparing favorably with other generic types of sanitizers.

Influence of Factors on Biocidal Activity

Various factors exhibit varying degrees of influence on the bactericidal kill by an acid-anionic surfactant sanitizer. A pH range of 1.5 to 3.0 offers the optimum acidity for an effective antimicrobial action. As the pH increases beyond the pH 3 level, the bactericidal activity decreases rapidly, reaching a minimum at neutral or slightly alkaline pH. Alkaline salts up to 900 ppm (as $NaHCO_3$) can be tolerated and do not raise the pH appreciably with typical acid concentrations, nor do they detract significantly from the 99.999% kill of *Staphylococcus aureus* and *E. coli*.

Organic material (0.05% skim milk or 0.05% peptone) and water hardness in excess of 1000 ppm (as $CaCO_3$) separately exhibited no significant slowing effect on the bactericidal effectiveness of an acid-anionic surfactant sanitizer against *E. coli* or *Staphylococcus aureus* (Weber and Black procedure). However, skim milk in combination with water hardness will delay bactericidal action, slowing it from a level of 30 to a level of 60 seconds for *E. coli* and from a total of 30 to as long as 120 seconds for *Staphylococcus aureus* for 99.999% kill. Increases in temperature enhanced the bactericidal activity, and decreases from room temperature resulted in slower germicidal action. The inclusion of about 1% of nonionic surface-active agent in the acid-anionic surfactant formulation did not result in a decrease of the bacterial kill of the composition (Lewandowski, 1952; Light, 1957; Dychdala, 1959). Similar synergism and corresponding increase in the antibacterial effectiveness were observed when anionic surfactants were added to phenols (Ordal and Deromedi, 1943).

If a phosphoric acid-alkyl aryl sulfonate sanitizer is not rinsed from treated equipment, it can provide a residual antibacterial effectiveness on stainless steel equipment surfaces for as long as 24 hours, as substantiated by microbiologic studies using *E. coli* and *Micrococcus caseolyticus* (Lewandowski, 1952).

After alkaline cleaning and thorough water rinse, acid-anionics will provide an acidified rinse as well as a sanitizing rinse in one step, thus eliminating acid treatment and subsequent water rinse steps.

APPLICATIONS IN PRACTICE

The introduction of acid-anionic surfactant sanitizers to the field of disinfection has presented a new sanitizing concept for the destruction of microbes and offers certain advantages to the user: (1) rapidity in antimicrobial activity, (2) effectiveness against a wide spectrum of microorganisms, (3) noncorrosion and nonstaining of stainless steel equipment, (4) absence of objectionable odor, (5) removal and control of milkstone and waterstone formation, (6) product stability in concentrated and diluted form, (7) short-duration residual sanitation on stainless steel surfaces, (8) complete water solubility, (9) acidified and sanitizing rinse in one step, and (10) good detergency in addition to excellent sanitizing activity. Some of their limitations are: (1) effectiveness at acid pH only, (2) generation of foam, and (3) slower activity against spore-forming organisms.

Acid-anionic surfactant sanitizers have relatively low toxicity and at the same time are powerful germicides employed in a variety of applications in different industries.

Dairy and Food Industry

Acid-anionic surfactant sanitizers have been successfully used for less than four decades in the dairy, beverage, and food processing industries in diverse applications. They are used to sanitize stainless steel equipment, utensils, or other surfaces to combat microbial contamination and spoilage, thereby preserving good food quality. By means of circulation, spraying, or fogging techniques, sanitizing with acid-anionic surfactant sanitizers of storage tanks, tank trucks, silos, and processing equipment has been practiced effectively in the dairy industry for many years. Also, in the manufacture of cheese, bacteriophage can be effectively controlled by acid-anionic surfactant sanitizers. On dairy farms, solutions of acid-anionic surfactant sanitizers are employed to disinfect cows' udders prior to milking as a precautionary measure for combatting contamination and mastitis-causing infections.

Lopes (1986) evaluated the activity of two acid-anionic

sanitizers, used in dairy and food plants, against food-borne pathogens by the Official AOAC Germicidal and Detergent Sanitizing Test. These sanitizers were effective at the recommended use concentration against both *Salmonella typhimurium* and *Listeria monocytogenes*. Schroeder and Orth (1987), in their laboratory studies, demonstrated that *Listeria monocytogenes* strains were effectively killed within 5 minutes with a recommended use-concentration of low-foaming acid-anionic surfactant sanitizer, even in the presence of organic contamination (skim milk).

Restaurants and Beverage Industries

The use of acid-anionic surfactant sanitizers has increased to include sanitation of equipment in eating and drinking establishments and for disinfection of premix vending machines in the soft drink industry. The recent introduction of low-foam acid-anionic surfactant sanitizers (Sedliar et al., 1972; Carandang and Dychdala, 1976; Wang, 1983) opened the door for the use of these products in spray and circulation applications in food processing, dairy, brewery, and beverage plants.

Other Industries, Institutions, and Homes

In hospitals, medical or dental laboratories, and other institutions such as schools and hotels, acid-anionic surfactant sanitizers are used for disinfecting hard surfaces, such as walls, floors, and other inanimate areas, provided these surfaces are not adversely affected by the acid environment produced by the sanitizer. A limited use of these sanitizers can be made in the household around the kitchen and the bathroom. Again, because of the acidity, these products should be used with care, guarded from accidental spills or splashes, and kept always out of reach of children. They should *not* be mixed with chlorinated compounds. Surgical and dental instruments or stainless steel equipment in offices and operating rooms can be sanitized effectively with acid-anionic surfactant sanitizers. Also, these compounds are excellent materials for the disinfection of stainless steel animal cages, walls and floors in animal experimental laboratories, animal breeding establishments, and zoos.

Freshly picked fruits and vegetables and some other environment-contaminated foods, such as fish and shell-fish caught in polluted waters, may be effectively washed and sanitized after harvesting. However, each sanitizing step should be followed with a potable water rinse.

Additional applications for this relatively new class of sanitizers will develop in the future as more field and laboratory data, as well as new equipment, become available.

REFERENCES

AOAC. 1984. *Official Methods of Analysis of the Association of Official Analytic Chemists*. 14th Edition. Washington, D.C., AOAC, pp. 65—77.

Baker, Z., Harrison, R.W., and Miller, B.F. 1941a. Action of synthetic detergents on the metabolism of bacteria. J. Exp. Med., 73, 249–271.

Baker, Z., Harrison, R.W., and Miller, B.F. 1941b. The bactericidal action of synthetic detergents. J. Exp. Med., 74, 611–620.

Baker, Z., Harrison, R.W., and Miller, B.F. 1941c. Inhibition by phospholipids of the action of synthetic detergents on bacteria. J. Exp. Med., 74, 621–637.

Bartnik, F., and Küenstler, K. 1987. Biological effects, toxicity and human safety. In *Surfactants in Consumer Products: Theory, Technology and Application*. Edited by J. Falbe. New York, Springer Verlag.

Berg, R.W., and Zimmerer, R.E. 1987. Effect of rare earth cations on bactericidal activity of anionic surfactants. J. Ind. Microbiol., 1, 377–381.

Birkeland,J.M., and Steinhaus, E.A. 1939. Selective bacteriostatic action of sodium lauryl sulfate and of "Dreft." Proc. Soc. Exp. Biol. Med., 40, 86–88.

Canas-Rodriguez, A., and William Smith, H. 1966. The identification of antimicrobial factors of the stomach contents of suckling rabbits. Biochem. J., 100, 79–82.

Carandang, C.M., and Dychdala, G.R. 1976. Low foaming acid-anionic surfactant sanitizer compositions. U.S. Patent 3,969,258.

Chambers, C.W. 1956. A procedure of evaluating the efficiency of bactericidal agents. J. Milk Food Technol., 19, 183–187.

Cooper, E.R., and Berner, B. 1985. Interaction of surfactants with epidermal tissues: physico-chemical aspects. In *Surfactants in Cosmetics*. Edited by M.M. Rieger. New York, Marcel Dekker, pp. 195–210.

Cowles, P.B. 1938. Alkyl sulfates: Their selective bacteriostatic action. Yale J. Biol. Med., 11, 33–38.

Dychdala, G.R. 1979. Antifungal activity of acid-anionics. Pennwalt Corporation (unpublished).

Dychdala, G.R. 1962a. Germicidal activity of Pennsan against mastitis-causing organisms. Pennwalt Corporation (unpublished).

Dychdala, G.R. 1962b. Effect of anionics on bactericidal activity. Pennwalt Corporation (unpublished).

Dychdala, G.R. 1961. Fungicidal time of Pennsan against fungi in the A.O.A.C. method. Pennwalt Corporation (unpublished).

Dychdala, G.R. 1959. Bactericidal effectiveness of Pennsan in relation to dilution, hard water, temperature and pH. Pennwalt Corporation (unpublished).

Dychdala, G.R., 1987. Sanitizer preparations with neodecanoic aid. Pennwalt Corporation (unpublished).

Feinstein, M.B., Sperro, L., and Felsenfeld, H. 1970. Interaction of a fluorescent probe with erythrocyte membrane and lipids: Effects of local anesthetics and calcium. FEBS Lett. 6, 245–248.

Flanagan, M.T., and Hesketh, T.R. 1973. Electrostatic interactions in the binding of fluorescent probes to lipid membranes. Biochim. Biophys. Acta, 298, 535–545.

Gainor, C. 1948. Effects of certain anionic, cationic and non-ionic agents on growth of Escherichia coli, Salmonella paratyphi B, and Staphylococcus aureus. Ph.D. Dissertation, Michigan State College, pp. 1–72.

Gershenfeld, L., and Milanick, V.E. 1941. Bactericidal and bacteriostatic properties of surface tension depressants. Am. J. Pharm., 113, 306–326.

Gershenfeld, L., and Perlstein, D. 1941a. Significance of hydrogen-ion concentration in the evaluation of the bactericidal efficiency of surface tension depressants. Am. J. Pharm. 113, 89–92.

Gilby, A.R., and Few, A.V. 1960. Lysis of protoplasts of Micrococcus lysodeikticus by ionic detergents. J. Gen. Microbiol., 23, 19–26.

Glassman, H.N. 1948. Surface active agents and their application in bacteriology. Bacteriol. Rev., 13, 105–148.

Grade A Pasteurized Milk Ordinance. 1985 Revision. Recommendations of the U.S. Public Health Service, Appendix F. Washington, D.C., U.S. Department of Health and Human Services, Food and Drug Administration, pp. 133–137.

Hassinen, J.B., Durbin, G.T., and Bernhart, F.W. 1951. The bacteriostatic effects of saturated fatty acids. Archiv. Biochem. Biophys., 31, 183–189.

Hays, H., and Elliker, P.R. 1959. Virucidal activity of a new phosphoric acid-wetting agent sanitizer against bacteriophage of Streptococcus cremoris. J. Milk Food Technol., 2, 109–111.

Hugo, W.B. 1965. Some aspects of the action of cationic surface-active agents on microbial cells with special reference to their action on enzymes. In *Surface Activity and the Microbial Cell*. New York, Gordon and Breach Science Publishers, pp. 67–80.

Jain, M.K., and Wagner, R.C. 1980a. The bilayer and related structures. In *Introduction to Biological Membranes*. New York, Wiley & Sons, pp. 53–86.

Jain, M.K., and Wagner, R.C. 1980b. Membrane components: isolation, composition and metabolism. In *Introduction to Biological Membranes*. New York, Wiley & Sons, pp. 25–52.

Karabinos, J.V., and Andriole, V.T. 1975. Bactericidal composition. U.S. Patent No. 3,867,300.

Klein, M., Kalter, S.S., and Mudd, S. 1945. The action of synthetic detergents upon certain strains of bacteriophage and virus. J. Immunol., 51, 389–396.

Klotz, I.M., and Ayers, J. 1953. Proteins interactions with organic molecules. Discuss. Faraday Soc., 13, 189–196.

Lawrence, C.A. 1950. Mechanism of action and neutralizing agents for surface-active materials upon microorganisms. Ann. N.Y. Acad. Sci., 53, 66–75.

Lewandowski, T. 1952. Bactericidal action of synthetic anionic detergents at low pH levels for gram positive and gram negative bacteria of possible significance in the dairy and food industries. Pennwalt Corporation (unpublished paper).

Light, D.G. 1957. Bactericidal effect of Pennsan on various organisms by Weber and Black method. Pennwalt Corporation (unpublished).

Lopes, J.A. 1986. Evaluation of dairy and food plant sanitizers against *Salmonella typhimurium* and *Listeria monocytogenes*. J. Dairy Sci., *69*, 2791–2796.

Lopes, J.A., and Stanton, J.H. 1987. Antimicrobial sanitizing composition containing n-alkyl and n-alkenyl succinic acid and methods for use. U.S. Patent No. 4,715,980.

Lopes, J.A. 1990. (In preparation).

Miller, B.F., Abrams, R., Dorfman, A., and Klein, M. 1942. Antibacterial properties of protamine and histone. Science, *96*, 428–431.

Netter, H. 1969. *Theoretical Biochemistry*. New York, Wiley—Interscience Division, pp. 190 and 462.

Newton, B.A. 1960. The mechanism of the bactericidal action of surface active compounds. A summary. J. Appl. Bacteriol., *23*, 345–349.

Newton, B.A. 1958. Surface-active bactericides. In *The Strategy of Chemotherapy*. Soc. Gen. Microbiol. Symposium No. 8. Cambridge University Press, pp. 62–93.

Ordal, E.J., and Deromedi, F. 1943. Studies on the action of wetting agents on microorganisms: II. The synergistic effect of synthetic wetting agents on the germicidal action of halogenated phenols. J. Bacteriol., *45*, 293–299.

Osberghaus, R., Krouch C., Kolaczaski, G., and Koppensteiner, G. 1974. Use of B-hydroxy carboxylic acids as antimicrobial substances. German Patent No. 2312280.

Prince, H.N., and Prince, R.N. 1987. Balancing animal rights and consumer safety: Progress to date. Chemical Times and Trends, July, p. 8.

Rode, L.J., and Foster, J.W. 1960. The action of surfactants on bacterial spores. Arch. Microbiol., *36*, 67–94.

Rosen, M.J. 1978a. Adsorption of surface-active agents at interfaces: the electrical double layer, In *Surfactants and Interfacial Phenomena*. Edited by M.J. Rosen. New York, John Wiley & Sons, pp. 27–82.

Rosen, M.J. 1978b. Micelle formation by surfactants, In *Surfactants and Interfacial Phenomena* Edited by M.J. Rosen, New York, John Wiley & Sons, pp. 83–122.

Salton, M.R.J. 1957. The action of lytic agents on the surface structures of the bacteria cell. Proc. Int. Congr. Surf. Activity, London. London, Butterworth, pp. 245–253.

Sands, J.A. 1986. Virucidal activity of cetyltrimethyl ammonium bromide below the critical micelle concentration. FEMS Microbiol. Lett., *36*, 261–263.

Scales, F.M., and Kemp, M. 1941. A new group of sterilizing agents for the food industries and a treatment for chronic mastitis. Int. Assoc. Milk Dealers Bull., *19*, 491–519.

Schildknecht, H., and Koob, K. 1971. Myrmicasin, the first insect herbicide. Angew. Chem. Int. Ed., *10*, 124–125.

Schroeder, W., and Orth, R. 1987. Antimicrobial studies of different disinfectants against *Listeria monocytogenes* strains with and without organic contamination. Henkel KGaA, Duesseldorf. (Personal communication.)

Sedliar, R.M., Garvin, D.F., and Aepli, O.T. 1972. Low foam anionic acid sanitizer compositions. U.S. Patent No. 3,350,964.

Siebert, K., and Boltersdorf, D., 1988. Magnesium surfactants—a contribution to mildness. Presented at the 2nd World Surfactant Congress. Paris, pp. 646–661.

Subramanian, R., and Patterson, K. 1985. Effects of molecular organization on photophysical behavior. Excimer kinetics and diffusion of 1-pyrenedecanoic acid in lipid monolayers at the nitrogen water interface. J. Am. Chem. Soc., *107*, 5820–5821.

Swisher, R.D. 1987. *Surfactant Biodegradation*. New York, Marcel Dekker, pp. 181–209.

Vanderkooi, J., and Martonosi, A. 1969. Sarcoplasmic reticulum VIII. Use of 8-anilino-1-naphthalene sulfonate as conformational probe on biological membranes. Arch. Biochem. Biophys., *133*, 153.

Wallach, D.F.H., and Winzler, R.J. 1974a. Fluorescence, fluorescent probes and optically absorbing probes. In *Evolving Strategies and Tactics in Membrane Research*. New York, Springer-Verlag, pp. 262–303.

Wallach, D.F.H., and Winzler, R.J. 1974b. Membrane macromolecules-anionic detergents. In *Evolving Strategies and Tactics in Membrane Research*. New York, Springer-Verlag, pp. 88–92.

Wang, Y. 1983. Short chain fatty acid sanitizing composition and methods. U.S. Patent No. 4,404,040.

Weber, G.R., and Black, L.A. 1948. Laboratory procedure for evaluating practical performance of quaternary ammonium and other germicides proposed for sanitizing food utensils. Am. J. Public Health, *38*, 1405–1417.

Yeagle, P.L. 1978. Headgroup conformation in phospholipid bilayers. In *Biomolecular Structure and Function*. Edited by P.F. Agris. New York, Academic Press, pp. 65–70.

CHAPTER 15

SURFACE-ACTIVE AGENTS: AMPHOTERIC COMPOUNDS

Seymour S. Block

The amphoteric surfactants, or ampholytes, differ from other ionic surfactants because in water they act as electrolytes by ionizing to give anions, cations, and zwitterions (ions with a positive and negative charge in the same molecule). The relationship between surface activity and germicidal action was aroused by the important development with quaternary ammonium germicides by Domagk in 1935 (Chapters 1, 13), and investigation of the amphoterics soon followed. Attention was drawn to their importance and practical value by McCutcheon at the first International Congress for Surface Activity in Paris in 1954. He introduced dodecyl-β-alanine, which was produced by General Mills under the name Deriphat. Armour and Co. marketed dodecyl-β-aminobutyric acid under the name Armeen Z, and Miranol Chemical Inc. made an imidazol ring derivative called Miranol. A group of related amphoteric disinfectants under the trade name Tego, or Tegol in some countries, was produced by Th. Goldschmidt AG (Schmitz, 1952, 1954). These were based on the ampholyte dodecyl-di(aminoethyl)-glycine. The composition of these products is given in Table 15–1. Tego 2000, the latest addition to this family, is a mixture of an amphoteric and a cationic amine surfactant. These products have been used extensively as biocides in Europe for the past 40 years; in 1980 their sales were said to be 3000 tons.

In preliminary studies it was observed that amphoteric surfactants with the same chain length and number of amine groups as cationic biocidal agents had a similar but somewhat lower antibacterial activity. It was learned, however, that the activity of the ampholytes could be greatly increased by increasing the number of amine nitrogens, which also increases the pH as shown in Figure 15–1 and Table 15–2. It will be noted that the mixture of ampholytes, as in Table 15–1, results in extending the microbiocidal activity over a wider pH range.

Although the ampholytes contain cationic groups, they appear to act differently than the cationic quaternary germicides. Figure 15–2 shows the difference between these agents in regard to their precipitation of protein and antibacterial activity as affected by pH. Dodecyl-di(aminoethyl)-glycine, dodicin, has a different pH for maximum bactericidal activity from that for protein precipitation, whereas the quat, dodecyl dimethylbenzylammonium chloride, has parallel curves for both pH and protein precipitation. The quats are more adversely affected in their antimicrobial activity by the presence of proteins than are the ampholytes. Further, quaternaries have greater activity toward gram-positive and less against gram-negative organisms, whereas ampholytes are not as selective in their activity. Quaternaries, on the other hand, are bacteriostatic at much lower concentrations than the ampholytes. This sometimes works in favor of the latter, as in cases of foods processed with microorganisms such as cheese, beer, and wine in which any residual biocide is detrimental to the growth of the culture and the process.

Table 15–1. *Composition of Tego Disinfectants*

Tego	Active Ingredient	Composition	pH
103S	RNH(CH$_2$)$_2$NH(CH$_2$)$_2$NHCH$_2$CO$_2$H·HCl	15% aqueous solution	~7.7
103G	RNH(CH$_2$)$_2$NH(CH$_2$)$_2$NHCH$_2$CO$_2$H·HCl + [RNH(CH$_2$)$_2$]$_2$NCH$_2$CO$_2$H·HCl	10% aqueous solution	~7.7
51	RNH(CH$_2$)$_2$NH(CH$_2$)$_2$NHCH$_2$CO$_2$H + RNH(CH$_2$)$_3$NHCH$_2$CO$_2$H	9% aqueous solution	~8.2
51B	RNH(CH$_2$)$_2$NH(CH$_2$)$_2$NHCH$_2$CO$_2$H + RNH(CH$_2$)$_3$NHCH$_2$CO$_2$H	22.5% aqueous solution	~8.2
2000	RNH(CH$_2$)$_3$NHCH$_2$CO$_2$H + RNH(CH$_2$)$_3$NH$_2$	20% aqueous solution	~8.0

*R = C$_{12}$H$_{25}$ and C$_{14}$H$_{29}$

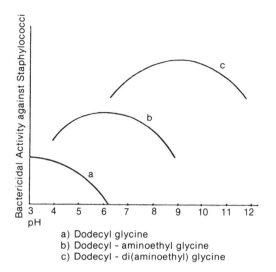

a) Dodecyl glycine
b) Dodecyl - aminoethyl glycine
c) Dodecyl - di(aminoethyl) glycine

Fig. 15–1. Bactericidal activity against staphylococci of three forms of amphoteric surfactants. From Schmitz, I.A., and Harris, W.S. 1958. Germicidal ampholytic surface-active agents. Manufact. Chem., 29, 51–54.

ANTIMICROBIAL ACTIVITY

Antibacterial tests on Tego 51, Tego 103, and phenol by the suspension method at 1% and 2% concentrations with *Salmonella enteritidis, Escherichia coli, Erysipelothrix rhusiopathiae, Staphylococcus albus, Staphylococcus citreus, Staphylococcus aureus, Corynebacterium pyogenes, Streptococcus agalactiae,* and *Brucella abortus* were run by Wagener (1954). Other tests on Tego 51 at 0.5%, 1%, and 10% concentrations with *Salmonella typhosa, Shigella dysenteriae, Coliaerogenes, Pseudomonas aeruginosa, Streptococcus pyogenes, Streptococcus viridans,* and *Streptococcus aureus* were

Table 15–2. *The Bactericidal Activities toward* Staphylococcus aureus *of Substituted Glycines (0.05% Solutions)*

Compound	Bactericidal Action in Minutes
$C_{12}H_{25}NHCH_2CO_2H$	10
$C_{12}H_{25}NH(CH_2)_2NHCH_2CO_2H$	5
$C_{12}H_{25}NH(CH_2)_2NH(CH_2)_2NHCH_2CO_2H$	1

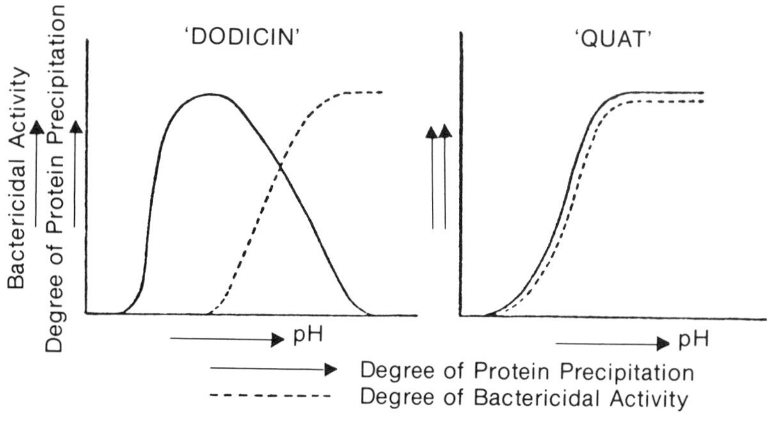

reported by Sorenson et al. (1969). With both Tego disinfectants, but not with phenol, a 1% solution acting for 30 minutes produced sterility with all of the bacteria, and with a 10% solution of Tego 51, the organisms were killed in 1 minute's contact. Wagener also compared the same disinfectants and organisms at 55° to 60°C rather than at room temperature. At this higher temperature, both disinfectants at 1% strength killed all the bacteria in 1 minute, whereas phenol in 1% strength took 8 minutes to kill all of the bacteria, although half of the species were killed in 1 minute. Bactericidal test data on a long list of microorganisms given by Goldschmidt (undated, *a*) show most organisms killed by 1% aqueous solutions of the Tego compounds in 1 minute. The molds and some bacteria were more resistant but, except for *Mycobacterium tuberculosis,* all were killed in 15 minutes. The latter was destroyed in 1 to 4 hours. Sykes (1965) stated that in his tests, 0.2% of Tego 51, 103G, and 103S killed *Staphylococcus aureus, Streptococcus pyogenes, E. coli,* and *Pseudomonas pyocyanea* in 1 to 3 minutes and solutions of 0.1% in 4 to 10 minutes. Tatewaki et al. (1981) reported that 0.00078 to 0.0125% Tego 51 inhibited 27 bacterial strains, but greater than 0.1% was necessary to inhibit *Serratia marcescens* and *Proteus vulgaris.* In their tests Tego 51 was more active than cresol soap (50% cresol). At 0.01 to 0.8% Tego 51 showed high bactericidal activity against *E. coli, Pseudomonas aeruginosa, Staphylococcus aureus, Streptococcus faecalis, Bacillus subtilis, Mycobacterium phlei,* and *Oospora lactis* (Andriasyan, 1983). At 0.5% it displayed good detergency and inhibited bacterial contamination by 99.8%. He suggested its use as a detergent and disinfectant for the sanitation of dairy equipment.

On the other hand, Dold and Gust (1957) isolated living *Pseudomonas fluorescens* from Tego solutions. This led to changes in the composition of the Tego preparations (Goldschmidt, 1967). Kuipers and Dankert (1970) compared the activity of 1% 103S on *Pseudomonas aeruginosa, Staphylococcus aureus,* and *Achromobacter anitratus* with 0.5% chlorhexidine in 70% ethanol and with 1% 103G with 0.3% Halamid (a quaternary ammonium salt). The germicides were tested in three ways: by a suspension test, a membrane filter test, and surface tests with swabs and agar cylinders. In all three tests, the

Fig. 15–2. Comparisons of protein precipitation and bactericidal activity by solutions of "docidin" and "quat" at different pH values. From Schmitz, I.A., and Harris, W.S. 1958. Germicidal ampholytic surface-active agents. Manufact. Chem., 29, 51–54.

'DODICIN'   'QUAT'

Degree of Protein Precipitation
Degree of Bactericidal Activity

chlorhexidine solution killed the bacteria in 0.5 to 2 minutes, whereas 103S did not kill in 10 minutes except in one test with one bacterium. In the comparison of 103G and Halamid, kill with 103G took place in 15 to more than 60 minutes, whereas Halamid took 10 to 60 minutes. Halamid was superior or equal to 103G with all bacteria in all tests. From their results, the experimenters concluded that the bactericidal properties of Tego 103S and 103G are slight.

These experiments raise two questions: (1) How long did it take 103S to kill the bacteria? All we know is that it took more than 10 minutes, and the authors say that "an antiseptic should have an immediate effect within a short time of contact and the reference antiseptic, chlorhexidine in ethanol, did." Yet there are applications in which effectiveness over a short period is not so important, and one wonders, therefore, how much longer than 10 minutes did it take 103S to be effective? (2) What part did the 70% ethanol play in the effect of the chlorhexidine solution, and what results would have been obtained if 103S were made up in 70% ethanol, since 70% ethanol is an effective antiseptic in its own right?

Sainclivier and Kerherve (1966), working with Tego 51 (1%), obtained results corresponding to those of Wagener, namely, that maximum disinfection toward *Staphylococcus aureus*, *Pseudomonas aeruginosa*, *E. coli*, and *Streptococcus lactis* was obtained in about 10 minutes' contact.

Kovats and Tamasi (1975), investigating Tego 51 for the disinfection of animal houses, reported it to be effective for controlling *E. coli*, *Staphylococcus pyogenes aureus*, and *Pseudomonas aeruginosa*. Working on the same type of problem, Kellett (1979) found 1% Tego 51 to be effective for only 1 to 2 days, but not for 7 days, because of resistance of the organisms in the animal quarters, which were identified as *Achromobacter* species, and gram-negative bacilli. The organisms were also resistant to Tego Diocto, a cationic amine salt, and to all antibiotics, but were controlled for over 2 months with 1% Tegodor, a mixture containing cationic agents and aldehydes. Sakagami et al. (1980) gave further evidence of bacteria developing resistance to Tego 51. They discovered that bacteria in river sludge that became acclimatized to 8-hydroxyquinoline were able to degrade not only 8-hydroxyquinoline but also other organic compounds, including some disinfectants like Tego 51 and paraformaldehyde. The bacteria in the river sludge were shown to be *Pseudomonas* and *Clostridium*.

Lee (1981) found that 10% saponified cresol killed *Mycobacterium tuberculosis* in 1 minute on slides and 5% in 10 minutes in sputum samples. Two ampholytes, Tego 51 and Vista 300, gave approximately parallel results, although the cresol was more potent in the short run, that is, 1 hour or less. Ten percent benzalkonium chloride and 5% chlorhexidine showed no bactericidal effect against the TB organism.

Vista 300 (now Anon 300) is alkyl bis(amino-

ethyl)glycine alkyldiethylenetriamine glycolate.* It was tested at 1% against *E. coli*, *Serratia marcescens*, *Pseudomonas aeruginosa*, *P. cepacia*, *Acinetobacter anitratus*, *S. aureus*, *Candida albicans*, and *Cryptococcus neoformans* showing antibacterial activity to all except *Serratia marcescens*. Bovine serum albumins (1 to 10%) lowered its activity (Nagai, 1979). Nada et al. (1980) evaluated Vista 300, chlorhexidine gluconate, cresol-soap solution, phenol, and benzethonium chloride against nonfermentative gram-negative rods at 50-fold dilution for 15 to 20 seconds. Vista 300 was second to chlorhexidine bacteriostatically, and first in effectiveness bactericidally.

Against bovine tuberculosis organisms, Thiel (1960) found Tego 51 at 5% to be highly bactericidal after 1 to 72 hours. Palvas (1967) reported that 10% Tego 51 inhibited *Mycobacterium bovis* in 10 to 20 minutes, as against the same results with 0.1% hexachlorophene.

Further data on the bactericidal effect of Tego 51 on *Mycobacterium tuberculosis* and *M. bovis* were provided by Ichikawa and Miyoshi (1980). They showed that a disinfectant composition containing Tego 51 as its active ingredient killed *M. tuberculosis* in 2.5 minutes and *M. bovis* in 10 minutes. With 2% phenol or 0.5% cresol, these organisms were killed in 2.5 minutes. Interestingly enough, chlorhexidine was inactive against these organisms unless mixed with 70% ethanol.

These disinfectants were also compared in tests made by Waller (1979) on spores of *Encephalitozoon cuniculi*. These spores were completely inactivated by 9 of 11 disinfectants, including 1% Tego 51, after 30 minutes' exposure. The two that were not effective were 0.1% chlorhexidine and 1% citric acid. Among those agents that were effective was 70% ethanol. Tests that led to a patent (Hesselgren et al., 1973) showed that at 10 or more ppm of Tego 51 inhibited *E. coli*, *Candida albicans*, and *Streptococcus faecalis* in vitro and inactivated bacteria in dental plaque; however, Tego 51 and chlorhexidine together exhibited greater inhibition than the additive effect of each alone.

In the presence of guinea pig feces, Tego 51 was ineffective. Trautwein and Nassal (1958) tested the bactericidal action of 33 disinfectants against *M. bovis*, *Staphylococcus aureus*, and *E. coli* by injecting the mixtures into guinea pigs. Of the 33 disinfectants, 15 were highly effective, including 7% Tego 51. The fungicidal activity of 2% Tego 51 was established at 0°C for 10 minutes (El-Bahay et al., 1968), whereas, under like conditions, 8% $CuSO_4$ and 3% of a disinfectant containing 22% chlorine were inactive. According to Devos et al. (1968), Tego 51 and two quaternary ammonium germicides were the most effective of 16 disinfectants tested against 17 bacterial and fungal species. Kamada (1964) tested Tego 51, a cationic surfactant (benzalkonium chloride) and an anionic surfactant (saponified cresol) disinfectant against *Paramecium caudatum*. After 10 minutes' contact, the order of activity was quaternary ammonium germicide > Tego > cresol but after 30 minutes the

---

*Inui Syoji Co., Ltd., Osaka, Japan

activity was quaternary ammonium germicide = Tego > cresol. As mentioned earlier (Waller, 1979), spores of *Encephalitozoon cuniculi* were inactivated by 1% Tego 51 in 30 minutes.

Work by Micheletti et al. (1978) on antiviral activity showed that 1% Tego 51 had no effect on the hydrophilic virus, poliovirus 1, but rapidly inactivated five lipophilic viruses, namely herpes simplex virus, vaccinia virus, influenza virus, adenovirus 2, and VSV (vesicular stomatitis virus). Cationic disinfectants also demonstrated the same activity against the viruses. Newcastle disease virus and Aujeszky's disease virus was controlled after 15 minutes' exposure with 0.5% of Tego 51 for use in disinfecting the animal house (Kovats and Tamasi, 1975). In the hydrochloride form, Tego 51 rapidly inactivated transmissible gastroenteritis (TGE) virus, but when this virus was dried onto wooden surfaces, it was ten times as resistant to disinfection as in aqueous suspension (Nakao et al., 1978).

As shown in Table 15–3, Tego 51 is least effective in terms of concentration against *Pseudomonas aeruginosa* but is more active than glutaraldehyde and chlorhexidine against *Salmonella* and *Staphylococcus* organisms. Its temperature profile in comparison to other disinfectants is shown in Table 15–4. It is superior to glutaraldehyde at most temperatures and exposure times and to the quaternary in 20 or 30 minutes exposure at 37° and 50°C. Sykes (1970), using Tego 103G and *Bacillus pumilus* spores, showed the effect of temperature on the sporicidal activity of this compound and a quaternary, domiphen bromide (Fig. 15–3). With the Tego at 25°C there was no inactivation in 5 hours; at 37°C there was a 4 log reduction in 5 hours; and at 50°C there was a 5 log reduction in 2 hours.

Gelinas and Goulet (1983a) also investigated the effect of the type of surface on the activity of disinfectants. Using *Pseudomonas aeruginosa* and the use-dilution method they obtained on steel the same results shown in Table 15–3 (since stainless steel cylinders were used in the AOAC use-dilution method). On plastic (polypropylene) and aluminum the effectiveness was much less for all disinfectants. Tego 51 required 1.25% on steel, more than 5% on plastic, and 10% on aluminum.

Effect of Protein

Proprietary literature on Tego compounds makes the categoric statement that the disinfectant efficiency is not decreased by the presence of protein. Sainclivier and Kerherve (1972) compared Tego 51 (1%), 51B (0.2%), and NaOCl (200 ppm available Cl) on *Streptococcus lactis, Staphylococcus aureus, E. coli,* and *Pseudomonas aeruginosa.* The activity of NaOCl was decreased by milk proteins, but the Tego compounds were not affected, maintaining their maximum activity after 5 to 10 minutes of contact. Other evidence on this effect was offered by Chen and Wu (1976). In water containing 0.03% powdered whole milk, Tego 51, but not NaOCl, inhibited *E. coli, Aeromonas hydrophila,* and *Staphylococcus aureus* within 5 minutes, although both were effective in the absence of the milk. Sorenson and colleagues (1971) reported, however, that milk protein inhibited the antibacterial activity of 0.5 to 1% Tego 51, as did gastrointestinal fluids; bovine blood or fish cleaning liquors did not.

Most of the reported investigations find a significant reduction in activity in the presence of proteins, but generally less than with most other disinfectants, particularly the quaternary nitrogen surfactants (Schmitz, 1952). For example, Kendereski and Ilic (1969) reported that Tego 51 was reduced 3 to 4 times in bactericidal activity in the presence of 10% milk, whereas the germicidal power of several quaternary compounds was reduced 20 to 50 times. Puhac and Hrgovic (1969) determined the activity of Tego 51 and 103S against *Staphylococcus aureus, E. coli,* and *Salmonella pullorum.* Bacteriostatic concentrations were 0.01 to 0.03%. Bactericidal activity was obtained for 0.3% solutions in 1 minute, but the bactericidal properties were reduced in the presence of proteins. Varga (1972) found 0.5% Tego 51 and several other disinfectants to be lethal to representative bacteria, *Candida albicans,* and *Aspergillus fumigatus* in 10 minutes' exposure. Blood protein reduced the effect in all cases except for Iosan, an organic iodine compound.

On the other hand Gelinas and Goulet (1983) found that an iodophor and hypochlorite, which were highly active against *Pseudomonas aeruginosa* by the use-di-

Table 15–3. *Comparison of Disinfectants by the AOAC Use-dilution Method—Critical Disinfection Point Values in mg/L at 20°C and 10-minute Contact Time*

Disinfectant	Pseudomonas aeruginosa ATCC 15442	Salmonella choleraesuis ATCC 10708	Staphylococcus aureus ATCC 6538
Tego 51	12,500	2,750	1,000
Glutaraldehyde	8,500	7,500	5,000
Chlorhexidine	5,500	6,500	8,500
Quaternary	2,250	1,000	550
Aldoquaternary complex	1,100	650	550
Acid-anionic	225	175	325
Sodium hypochlorite	175	125	110
Iodophor	40	40	40

Gelinas, P., Goulet, J., Tastayre, G.M., and Picard, G.A. 1984. Effect of temperature and contact time on the activity of eight disinfectants—A classification. J. Food Protection, 47(11), 841–847.

Table 15–4. *Comparative Effect of Temperature on Disinfectants—A.O.A.C. Use-dilution Test with* Pseudomonas aeruginosa; *Minimum Bactericidal Concentration in mg/L*

Disinfectant	Contact Time	Temperature (°C)			
		4	20	37	50
Tego 51	10	12,500	12,500	2,250	850
	20	11,000	7,500	275	125
	30	3,250	3,250	275	100
Glutaraldehyde	10	65,000	8,500	750	750
	20	32,500	2,000	750	550
	30	32,500	2,000	750	425
Chlorhexidine	10	12,500	5,500	250	150
	20	7,500	2,000	250	50
	30	7,500	2,000	225	50
Quaternary	10	4,250	2,250	1,000	275
	20	2,000	425	425	275
	30	1,500	425	325	275
Aldoquaternary	10	2,750	1,100	225	110
complex	20	1,000	650	225	110
	30	1,000	550	85	50
Acid anionic	10	375	225	50	20
	20	375	225	50	20
	30	175	150	40	20
Sodium hypochlorite	10	375	175	100	—*
	20	110	65	45	—
	30	50	50	25	—
Iodophor	10	110	40	40	—*
	20	40	40	40	—
	30	40	20	40	—

*Unstable at 50°
Gelinas, P., Goulet, J., Tastayre, G.M., and Picard, G.A. 1984. Effect of temperature and contact time on the activity of eight disinfectants—A classification. J. Food Protection, 47(11), 841–847.

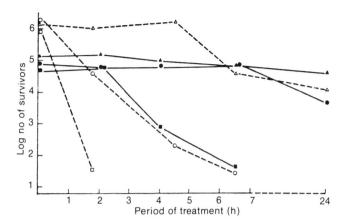

Fig. 15–3. Effect of Tego (2% w/v) and domiphen bromide (1% w/v) on *B. pumilis* at 25°, 37°, and 50°C. Black circles, domiphen bromide treated spores; clear circles, Tego treated spores; triangles, at 25°C; squares, at 50°C. From Sykes, G. 1970. The sporicidal properties of chemical disinfectants. J. Appl. Bacteriol., 33, 147–156.

lution method, did not tolerate high concentrations of organic matter in the form of milk powder, fish meal, or dried blood. Tego 51 retained disinfectant action with the protein, although not as well as glutaraldehyde, which was superior to seven other agents in withstanding protein.

According to DeMazza et al. (1970), 0.5% Tego 51 was inhibitory to a group of food-contaminating bacteria (1 to 5 × 10⁶/ml) in meat-tryptone broth at 37°C and was bactericidal at 1.8% concentration. With fewer organisms (1 to 5 × 10⁵/ml), it was bactericidal at 1%. With 1% Tego 51, low-bacterial-count milk at 20°C did not sour for 4 days after the addition, but there was growth of microorganisms and foaming. Pasteurized milk with a high bacterial count was coagulated 1 day after addition of 1% Tego 51.

In tests by Baumgarten (1968), 2% Tego 51 destroyed the trophozoites of *Toxoplasma gondii* as tested by subsequent intraperitoneal injections of the trophozoites in

mice. When 50% serum was used as the diluent, exposure of the trophozoites had to be prolonged by a factor of 5. Sykes (1965) noted that in the presence of blood, Tego 51, 103G, and 103S solutions, active at 0.2% in its absence, required an increase to 10%. In whole milk, an increase to 4% was necessary. Ayliffe (1966) gives data to show that 1% Tego 103G, which killed *Pseudomonas aeruginosa* in 1 minute, was not germicidal in 10 minutes with 20% serum. In his tests, phenols, a quaternary ammonium compound, and chlorhexidine were less affected by the serum. Yoh and colleagues (1984) reported that a combination of benzalkonium chloride and Tego 51 was effective in the presence of calf serum.

General Properties

The most obvious property of these compounds is their surface activity. Whether the germicidal activity depends on surface activity or not, the relationship between concentration and these activities is evident (Table 15–5), and certainly the wettability, detergency, and penetrating power resulting from surface activity would be expected to assist in antimicrobial effectiveness. Yet Yamada (1968), employing Tego 51 and 103G along with

Table 15–5. *The Effect of Concentration of Tego Compounds on Surface Activity (100% Surface Activity Equals Approximately 25 to 30 dynes/cm)*

Tego No.	Surface Activity (%) at Concentration (%)					
	0.05	0.1	0.2	0.3	0.4	0.6
103S	21	46	86	98	100	100
103G	31	49	70	80	90	100
51	60	88	98	100	100	100
51B	46	68	92	100	100	100

other surface-active disinfectants applied to bacterially contaminated glass rods and dental burs, concluded that there was no relationship between disinfection and the physiochemical properties of these compounds. According to his measurements, the degree of surface tension and the permeability of amphoteric surfactants at working concentrations were less than those of isopropanol and saponified cresol, but higher than those of other disinfectants. The Tego compounds were also found to be inferior to the saponified cresol in detergency.

T. Nakamura (1958) noted that pretreatment of bacteria with surface-active agents improved the action of some disinfectants since the surfactant made it easy for the disinfectants to penetrate the organism. He employed several surfactants, one of which, di-(octylaminoethyl)glycine·HCl, is chemically related to the Tego compounds. This surfactant and sodium alkylarene sulfonate in 0.1% or higher concentration, and a quaternary ammonium compound at 0.002% or higher, improved the disinfecting activity toward *Staphylococcus aureus* of phenol, mercuric chloride, Mercurochrome, and Acrinol (aminoacridine compound). Nonionic compounds, however, had no influence on activity. The hardness of water was found not to affect the bactericidal properties of Tego 51 (Puhac and Hrgovic, 1969), nor did alcohol (Herrmann and Preuss, 1949) affect Tego 103.

Another interesting property of the Tego compounds is their ability to adsorb onto solid surfaces and leave a film that resists removal by running water. This can be shown by a clear zone on seeded agar plates around pieces of material which had been put in 1% Tego solution for 5 minutes and thoroughly rinsed with water. Similar adsorption to the bacterial cell is no doubt functional in germicidal action. Adsorption on glass is greater than on metals and is equivalent to a maximum of 0.24 mg/L on a 0.5-L bottle with an area surface of 230 sq. cm (Goldschmidt, undated, *b*). This might be of concern in bottle washing disinfection, except for the fact of the low toxicity of the compounds. The quantity of adsorbed compound is determined by titration with guanidinium dodecylbenzenesulfonate on eosin, or colorimetrically after producing a blue color with ninhydrin (Cramer, 1958).

The toxicity of Tego compounds according to the manufacturer's data is low—a minimum lethal dose taken orally of 3 g/kg for the undiluted concentrate—which is slightly greater than that of table salt. Soerensen and coworkers (1969), conducting toxicity tests on Tego 51 with Swiss mice, observed that at the recommended concentrations of 0.5 to 1.0%, the compound did not influence the weight increase of the animals, and pathologic investigation did not reveal lesions due to the drug. With 1% Tego 51, there was no difference from the control, but with 3% and higher, the animals failed to gain weight in 18 days of testing. Table 15–6 gives the data on their survival tests when Tego 51 solution was used in place of drinking water. It is noted that toxicity was demonstrated between 1 and 3% and was progressively greater at concentrations of 5 and 10%.

Table 15–6. *Survival of Mice with Tego 51 in Drinking Water*

Tego Solution (%)	Number of Animals Alive After (Days)						
	0	3	6	9	12	15	18
0	20	20	20	20	20	20	20
0.5	20	20	20	20	20	20	20
1.0	20	18	18	18	18	18	18
3.0	20	20	18	18	18	18	18
5.0	20	18	18	18	18	18	16
10.0	20	18	16	12	12	12	10

With regard to skin compatibility of microbiocidal amphoterics, it is noted that skin reactions are rare, since only 0.3% of users show signs of any skin reaction. Herrmann and Preuss (1949) reported that solutions of Tego 103S did not damage skin when used as a detergent for a month. Sanderink and Singelenberg (1963) noted, in the nursing staff, several cases of contact dermatitis linked to Tego 103G. Patch tests were performed. It appeared to them that this dermatitis must be partly attributed to a toxic reaction and partly to sensitization.

Tego microbiocidal amphoterics have no odor, but it is claimed that they act as deodorizers when used in normal concentrations. It is said that when bowls filled with triethylamine, which smells somewhat like pickled herring, are rinsed with Tego solution, the bowls are deodorized, whereas those rinsed with water are not (Goldschmidt, undated, *c*).

As is well recognized, bacteria become resistant to some antibacterial substances. Tests were run to see if this occurred with Tego materials. Data are presented on germicidal tests of Tego on *E. coli* after 25 and 50 subcultures on sublethal concentrations of Tego biocides. The results indicate no difference in growth at different concentrations and exposed for different lengths of time for the tests prior to subculturing and after 50 subcultures. Results with *Staphylococcus aureus* were also reported to be negative in regard to induction of resistance. Further, from a practical standpoint, swabs taken from rooms treated with Tego materials did not show the presence of a predominant organism (Goldschmidt, undated, *d*). As already discussed in the section *Antimicrobial Activity*, some microorganisms developed resistance to Tego compounds.

It is claimed that the solutions of microbiocidal amphoterics resist deterioration in use and may be recovered and used again. Since the strength of the solution may be reduced due to adsorption on surfaces, this should be determined by one of the chemical methods and makeup concentrate added.

The heat and light stability of eight sanitizers was investigated by Gelinas and Goulet (1982). Solutions at 40°C at use concentration were exposed to fluorescent light of 50,000 lux for 6 days. The hypochlorite and iodophor lost antibacterial activity after 2 days, but Tego 51 retained full activity for the 6 days.

Tests on the corrosiveness of Tego 51 to metals were reported by Hurka (1961). A number of metals were exposed to 1% Tego 51 for 48 hours at 20° and 50°C. The results showed little effect on stainless steel, aluminum, or tinned iron, which are metals commonly used in dairies and food plants. Iron, copper, and brass, however, showed considerable pitting and corrosion. Tests on Tego 51, 103S, and three other commercial disinfectants were run by Puhac et al. (1969). They observed that aluminum was not corroded by any of the disinfectants. Unlike the findings of Hurka, the Tego compounds were the least corrosive for iron, but in agreement with Hurka, they were the most corrosive for copper and brass. Tego 103S and two non-ampholytic materials caused great corrosion of zinc.

APPLICATION IN HOSPITALS AND MEDICINE

Skin Disinfection

Use of Tego in disinfection of the hands for surgery or merely for hygienic purposes is one of the oldest applications, having been described by Herrmann and Preuss in 1949. They employed a disinfectant, di-(octylamino-ethyl)glycine lactate, in solution with an amphoteric detergent, alkyl-aminoethylglycine hydrochloride. This mixture was at that time called Tego 103, but the composition of Tego 103 has been changed over the years. By the Liesegang test, the detergency of a 10% solution was 6 to 10, compared to equal concentration of anion-active soap of 15 to 30, and cation-active quaternary compound of 20 to 25. In practical tests, thick suspensions of bacteria were swabbed on the back of the hand and underarm and rubbed in. After drying, 10% solutions of disinfectants were applied. None produced sterility in 1 minute, but in 5 minutes' contact with Tego and two other disinfectants (Kodan and Desderman), sterility was achieved with *E. coli* and *Staphylococcus aureus*. With Mercurochrome and dibromal, there was some growth.

Naumann (1952) conducted experiments on surgical hand disinfection using Tego 103S (at that time containing an octyl rather than a dodecyl group), a quaternary compound (Desogen), and an anion-active phenolic soap (Bactol). He found that, on the hands, Desogen formed a continuous antiseptic film and was able to block the transfer of bacteria completely. This protective film was destroyed by soap, serum, or mucous membranes. Bactol was without influence on the transmission of germs, whereas Tego had, in addition to its bactericidal properties, the ability to form a tight unimolecular film and thereby reduce the transmission of bacteria from washed and unwashed hands. The film, however, was destroyed by soap and protein. In another study on the disinfection of hands for surgery, Günther and Sprössig (1955) discovered that a high degree of hardness of the water, whether carbonate or noncarbonate, is advantageous. For ordinary hand washing and for instrument disin-

fecting, high noncarbonate hardness is somewhat disadvantageous and carbonate hardness advantageous. Tego 103S was found to be indifferent to the chemical composition of the water.

Frisby (1959) gave his results with Tego 103S in preoperative skin preparation. The shaved and washed skin was prepared just before the operation by being thoroughly swabbed twice with a 1% solution of the compound and then left wet. Of the 24 swabs taken from the skin before it was prepared, 5 gave no growth and the remaining 19 gave growth of micrococci. Further, 4 also gave growth of *Streptococcus viridans* and of *Bacterium anitratum*, and 1 of spore-bearing organisms. Of the 24 swabs taken from the closed wound at the end of the operation, 3 gave growth of micrococci and 21 no growth. In Frisby's opinion, these findings indicated that Tego 103S is a good skin-cleansing agent for preoperative use. Before the wounds were dressed, they were again swabbed with Tego 103S and then covered with Nobecutane (thiram). All wounds were swabbed on the third postoperative day at the time of the first dressing. Of 33 wounds swabbed, 8 gave no growth, 3 produced *Staphylococcus aureus* (but did not look infected), 17 yielded micrococci, 2 gave *Streptococcus viridans*, and 1 gave *E. coli* and *Bacterium anitratum*. Compared with the wound-infecting rate for two wards, Frisby concluded that this was an extremely good record. On the subject of hand cleansing with this agent, he noted three advantages: (1) the time for scrubbing up is much reduced, (2) the need for scrubbing of the skin is eliminated, (3) the skin usually remains free from viable organisms for long periods.

Studies mentioned earlier by Hesselgren et al. (1973) have shown that Tego 51 may have value as an antiseptic in the oral cavity. At concentrations exceeding 10 ppm, it inactivated bacteria in dental plaque material. The optimum effect was at neutral pH, but saliva decreased the inhibitions. Curti and Pagani (1977) investigated the use of Tego 51 to sterilize rubber ontologic dams. A 1% solution killed gram-negative bacteria on these objects, but not gram-positive bacteria or fungi.

Disinfection of Instruments, Walls, and Floors

Tego 103S is also recommended by the manufacturer for disinfection of surgical instruments and rubber articles (1% solution for 10 minutes' minimum contact) and for prophylactic foot baths (1% solution for 5 minutes' minimum contact). For disinfection of operating theaters, wards, sick rooms, toilets, and equipment, the related Tego 103G is recommended. Frisby (1959) employed it for such purposes in a hospital and recorded his findings. An operating theater was sprayed weekly and the walls and floors were mopped more often with 1% 103G. Twenty swabs taken biweekly for 6 months were negative for *Staphylococcus aureus* and *Clostridium welchii*. When 103G was replaced with 1% phenol, 6 of 32 and then 17 of 32 swabs were positive for *Clostridium welchii* in two periods. When 103G was started again, this organism disappeared. The surgeons' and nurses' changing rooms and sitting rooms were found to be rich sources of these two organisms, but 2 weeks after cleaning with 103G, all the swabs were negative. The contamination was found to be introduced on the shoes of the staff; 20 out of 24 were positive for *Clostridium welchii*. After washing the shoes with 1% 103G, none showed growth of the organism.

Jones et al. (1962) evaluated the control of wound sepsis in a badly overcrowded, old hospital. In the operating theaters, even after cleaning, swabs of the walls and floor gave profuse growth of *Staphylococcus aureus*, *Clostridium welchii*, and aerobic spore formers. After spraying with 1% 103G, check swabs were virtually sterile. Since the bed curtains were badly contaminated with *Staphylococcus aureus* and coliforms, an experiment was conducted with curtains made of Terylene that were dipped into Tego solution and dried overnight. Preliminary bacteriologic tests showed them to be virtually sterile. Since disinfecting the operating theaters had proven successful, Tego treatment of the wards by mopping the walls and floor once a week was attempted. It was reported that saline-moistened swabs from the floor yielded many fewer organisms than before. The overall results in this hospital in terms of number of cases of wound infection reported over 2.5 years indicated that, prior to the use of Tego, there was an average of ten cases, whereas after Tego treatment, the number of cases decreased to about two and the germicidal agent was considered to have been effective.

The treatment of floors with disinfectant to prevent the spread of infection is one that has engendered a great deal of controversy (see Jones et al., 1962, and Ayliffe et al., 1966, for discussion and references). As is seen above, the treatment of hospital floors with Tego 103G was found to be successful. Frisby (1961) also claimed success in the disinfection of hospital floors. In one experiment, the floor of the surgical ward with thermoplastic tiles was investigated for *Staphylococcus aureus*. For 7 weeks prior to using Tego 103G, the counts were from 2 to 5 million per gram of dust. For 4 weeks after mopping with 1% 103G, the count fell to low values, sometimes less than 100 per gram. The experiments were continued in other surgical wards with floors of terrazo, wood, linoleum, etc. After 18 weeks, the counts remained low except where overzealous maids mixed soap with the Tego and neutralized its bactericidal effect.

Opposed to such affirmative findings are those of Ayliffe and co-workers (1966). In their experiments, which included Tego 103G and 13 other disinfectants, impression plates showed little or no reduction of total bacteria or *Staphylococcus aureus* on exposed floors 1 hour after treatment. When the floor was covered with a box after treatment to prevent recontamination, however, the reduction with the disinfectants was 93 to 99%, and with just soap and water 80%. The difference in results between the soap and water and disinfectants was statistically significant, but the findings suggested that none of the treatments was practical because of rapid recon-

tamination. The differences between these findings and those of other workers would seem to be caused by the method of testing. However, whatever the explanation, the results with infection of patients, if sufficiently confirmed, would appear to be more convincing than laboratory tests.

Other possible medical applications of the Tego compounds that have received attention are as a vaginal antiseptic and as an antiseborrheic agent. Jones et al. (1962) refer to the former, having employed Tego 103G in vaginal operations and noting that preliminary findings indicated that this substance rendered the vaginal operation field completely sterile before operation. Tego Betaine, a detergent of related structure, has also been reported to be effective in vaginal deodorant douches (Nowak, 1968) and antidandruff shampoo bases. Tego 103S was among a list of 20 chemicals tested for antiseborrheic properties against the bacterial agents of infectious dandruff, *Staphylococcus aureus*, *Pityrosporum ovale*, and *Microsporum lanosum*, and showed appreciable antibacterial activity, though less against *Staphylococcus aureus* than several of the more active materials (Lubowe, 1957). There has also been some interest in Tego compounds for dental hygiene (Kamada, 1963, 1964).

APPLICATION IN FOOD AND BEVERAGE INDUSTRIES

In the food industries, the Tego compounds are employed as sanitizers and disinfectants, not as food preservatives to be incorporated in the food. The two preparations used most in this area are Tego 51, which is recommended for the food industry, especially milk, meat, and fish processing, and Tego 51B for use in the beverage industry, for soft drink manufacture and brewery application.

Dairy and Meat Industries

Perhaps the greatest application of Tego 51 in the food industries is in dairies, including the following: 1% solution for hand washing and cleaning of boots and rubber aprons; 0.5 to 1% for cleaning of milk tanks and cans; 0.2% in pipes, hoses, and pumps; 0.2% after cleaning heaters, coolers, separators, and homogenizers; 0.05 to 0.1% in ice water used for cooling; 0.2% rinse after cleaning butter churn; 0.5 to 1% spray following cleaning of cheese vats, presses, and sieves; circulation of warm 0.5% solution through freezers and other ice cream equipment (Goldschmidt, undated, *e*).

In both the dairy and meat industries, some types of bacteria are necessary in food processing; Tego 51 does not interfere with them as long as the concentration of Tego in the product is below 0.05%, and it should be much below this amount if there has been sufficient rinsing with water. In tests of 1% Tego 51 on milking equipment, Yablochkin (1971) found that Tego demonstrated high wetting and germicidal properties, causing neither skin irritation nor corrosion of aluminum; however, it was somewhat less effective than the Soviet product, Desmol. Wagner et al. (1971) preferred iodophores to Tego 51 for the milk industry since they reported the former solutions at 1% give complete sterility, killing *Pseudomonas aeruginosa* and schizomycetes instantly and hypomycetes in 1 hour and inhibiting fungi after 24 hours.

Tego 51 is claimed to provide overall protection against meat-decomposing bacteria and meat-inhabiting pathogenic microorganisms (see Goldschmidt, undated, *f*, for 48 references). It is reported that bacteria causing epidemic diseases and those putrefying food are killed in a few minutes by a 1% solution. With it, salmonellae on wooden surfaces are killed in 12 minutes and on aluminum in 3 to 5 minutes. Other organisms inactivated or killed are beef trichophyta, chicken aspergilli, live mycoplasma, swine fever virus, Newcastle disease virus, and the organisms causing enzootic pneumonia. Applications include disinfection of slaughtering rooms, instruments and machines, cattle transport vehicles and loading bays, postmortem areas, meat-cutting tables, slicers, mincing machines, poultry scalding and evisceration vats, meat canning equipment, and display cases in butcher shops.

According to Edelmeyer and Laqua (1978), Tego 51 is a safe, suitable disinfectant for use in the processed edible gelatin industry. The minimum inhibitory concentration of Tego 51 in gelatin was found to be 90 ppm. The nontoxic effect level was said to be 300 ppm, and an acceptable daily intake was 3 ppm or 9 mg per person per day.

The newest addition to the Tego line is Tego 2000, a mixture of an amphoteric surfactant and a cationic one, as shown in Table 15–1. It is made by the reaction of N-alkyl-propanediamine-1,3 with monochloroacetic acid. The alkyl group is of native origin. This product is a general disinfectant and sanitizer for the food and beverage industry, but is also used in hospitals and medical applications. Its antibacterial activity in hard water and in the presence of albumin is presented in Table 15–7 and its toxicity data are given in Table 15–8.

Soft Drink and Brewing Industries

Schara (undated) reported on extended experience with Tego 51B in the soft drink industry. In practice, 0.5% solution was effective for short-contact-time disinfection of tanks and equipment and 0.1% for longer contact time in pipes. In his factory Schara applied the disinfectant on Fridays after cleaning the system with caustic soda. A 0.1% solution in hot water was pumped through a closed circuit of pipes and vessels for one-half hour and then left in the system over the weekend before removal. Upon rinsing, water samples were filtered through a membrane filter and incubated on wort or orange juice agar. This medium was selective for yeasts, lactobacilli, spore-forming aerobes, *Achromobacter*, and molds—the types of organisms that infect such drinks. From the results of 734 samples taken during operation in his lemonade plant, Schara noted that about 50% of

Table 15–7. *Antimicrobial Activity of Amphoteric Microbiocide Tego 2000 (Th. Goldschmidt AG)—Suspension Test in Standard Hard Water and 0.2% Albumin*

Concentration (%)	Log reduction (minutes)					
	Hard Water			Albumin		
	5	30	60	5	30	60
Staphylococcus aureus						
0.75	—	—	—	5.4	5.2	5.3
0.50	—	—	—	4.7	5.0	5.0
0.25	5.0	5.4	5.2	4.0	5.0	5.5
0.10	4.3	5.3	5.1	2.8	5.0	5.5
0.05	3.6	5.0	4.9	1.1	2.4	3.1
0.025	1.7	4.2	4.9	0.2	0.5	0.6
0.0125	0.7	2.5	3.5	—	—	—
0.00625	0.08	0.5	0.5	—	—	—
Pseudomonas aeruginosa						
0.50	4.6	4.2	4.0	4.9	4.7	5.0
0.25	4.3	4.1	4.0	4.4	4.3	4.7
0.10	4.0	4.0	4.0	3.2	3.3	3.8
0.05	3.0	3.3	3.6	1.9	2.8	3.0
0.025	1.8	2.7	2.6	0.04	−0.05	0.0
0.0125	1.1	2.0	2.2	—	—	—

the counts in the table were completely acceptable, and the others were so low that they indicated no danger of infection of the lemonade. The organisms were ubiquitous, with only a few lemonade contaminants. In the circuit with the heater, 90% of the samples were sterile. Only 25% of the tanks were sterile since they were open-top tanks and became recontaminated. The filling machines and filling nozzles were difficult to disinfect because of faulty design that required improvement. Schara concluded that disinfection with Tego 51B was highly satisfactory.

The production of alcoholic beverages, beer, wine, and distilled beverages requires a high degree of sanitation because the condition of the medium for a considerable period of time must favor the growth of desired microorganisms, thus allowing also the growth of undesired organisms and their deleterious effects on yield and flavor. Cultured yeasts are the desired organisms; those undesired are wild yeasts, thermophilic bacteria, lactobacilli, sarcinae, and molds. Nikolov et al. (1970) studied the control of competing microorganisms in the fermentation of cane molasses to alcohol by the use of antiseptics such as ampholytes and quaternary ammonium compounds in the molasses. Tego 51B was effective at 0.05% in destroying the unwanted microflora. Adapting the yeast to the antiseptics was proposed to raise its resistance and to thereby not hinder the fermentation.

Table 15–8. *Toxicity of Amphoteric Microbiocide Tego 2000 (Th. Goldschmidt AG)*

LD_{50} oral (rat): 3783 mg/kg
LD_0 dermal (rat): 2000 mg/kg
Draize test 1% solution: no irritation
NOEL (no observed effect level): 12.5 mg/kg/day
ADI (Acceptable daily intake): 8.75 mg/person/day

In the brewing industry, the use of Tego 51B as a disinfectant has been of interest since it does not cause beer turbidity with less than 4 ml/L of a 0.1% solution in bottom fermented beer, does not produce chill haze with as much as 2 ml of 0.1% Tego 51B per liter of beer, and has no effect on head retention with as much as 16 ml/L of a 0.1% solution. Further, 8 ml/L of a 0.1% solution has no effect on taste or smell (Goldschmidt, undated, *g*). In the brewery, fermented beer is partially protected against infection by its alcohol and carbonic acid, but fresh wort is readily tainted and spoiled. Solutions of 0.1% and 0.5% Tego 51B are prescribed for use on brewery equipment in a manner similar to their use in the soft drink plant.

REFERENCES

Andriasyan, B.V. 1983. Bactericidal properties of Tego 51 ampholytic soap. Tr. Evevan Zoovet. Inst., *54*, 28–31.

Ayliffe, G.A., Collins, B.J., and Lowbury, E.J.L. 1966. Cleaning and disinfection of hospital floors. Br. Med. J., *2*, 442–445.

Baumgarten, H.J. 1968. Effect of Cialit and Tego 51 as disinfectants on trophozoites of *Toxoplasma gondii*. DTW, *75*, 598–600.

Chen, H.C., and Wu, C.Y. 1976. Studies on the disinfectants used in frozen baked eel processing factories. Taiwan Shui Chan Hseuh Hui Kan., *5*(1), 80–84.

Cramer, G. 1958. Adhesion of ampholyte soaps on surfaces of solid objects. Fette, Seifen, Anstrichmittel, *60*, 35–39.

Curti, A., Jr., and Pagani, C. 1977. Use of chemical agent Tego 51 in the disinfection of the odontological rubber dam as an integral part of the absolute isolation of an operating field. Rev. Fac. Odontol. Sao Jose dos Campos, *6*(1–2), 13–19.

DeMazza, D., Landolfi, M.R., and Leandro Montes, A. 1970. Determination of the antibacterial activity of Tego 51. An. Soc. Cient. Argent., *189*(1–2), 3–10.

Devos, A., Viaene, N., and Devriese, L. 1968. *In vitro* bactericidal activity of some disinfectants. Tijdschr. Diergeneeskd, *37*, 281–293.

Dold, H., and Gust, R. 1957. On the occurrence of living bacteria in a disinfectant solution. Arch. Hyg. Bakteriol., *141*, 321.

Domagk, G. 1935. A new class of disinfectants. Dtsch. Med. Wochenschr., *61*, 829–832.

Edelmeyer, H., and Laqua, A. 1978. The importance of traces of amphoteric disinfectants in edible gelatin. Arch. Lebensmittelhygiene, *29*(2), 62–65.

El-Bahay, G.M., Elmossalami, E., and Refai, M. 1968. Use of some disinfectants as fungicides. Mykosen, *11*, 807–810.

Frisby, B.R. 1961. Tego compounds in hospital practice. Lancet, *2*, 829.

Frisby, B.R. 1959. "Tego" compounds in hospital practice. Lancet, *2*, 57–58.

Gelinas, P., and Goulet, J. 1983a. Efficacy of eight disinfectants on three types of surface contamination by *Pseudomonas aeruginosa*. Can. J. Microbiol., *29*, 1715–1730.

Gelinas, P., and Goulet, J. 1983b. Neutralization of the activity of eight disinfectants by organic matter. J. Appl. Bacteriol., *54*(2), 243–247.

Gelinas, P., and Goulet, J. 1982. Heat and light stability of eight sanitizers. J. Food Protect., *45*, 1195–1196.

Gelinas, P., Goulet, J., Tastayre, G.M., and Picard, G.A. 1984. Effect of temperature and contact time on the activity of eight disinfectants—A classification. J. Food Protection, *47*(11), 841–847.

Goldschmidt, A.G. Th. 1967. On action of Tego disinfectant solution on bacteria. Ned. Tijdschr. Geneeskd., *3*, 234.

Goldschmidt, A.G. Th. Undated, *a*. Disinfection throughout the world. pp. 11–16.

Goldschmidt, A.G. Th. Undated, *b*. Disinfection throughout the world. p. 18.

Goldschmidt, A.G. Th. Undated, *c*. Disinfection throughout the world. p. 25.

Goldschmidt, A.G. Th. Undated, *d*. Disinfection throughout the world. p. 17.

Goldschmidt, A.G. Th. Undated, *e*. Tego 51. Factory hygiene with Tego disinfection.

Goldschmidt, A.G. Th. Undated, *f*. Tego 51. Disinfection in the food industry.

Goldschmidt, A.G. Th. Undated, *g*. Tego 51B. Disinfection in breweries.

Gonnert, R., and Bock, M. 1956. Chemical resistance of viruses. Arzneimittelforsch, *6*, 522–527.

Günther, G., and Sprössig, M. 1956. Bacteriological and chemical studies on the influence of the chemical composition of water on the practical disinfection of hands with quaternary ammonium salts. Z. Hyg. Infektionskrankh., *142*, 416–428.

Herrmann, W., and Preuss, H. 1949. A new principle for disinfection of hands. Dtsch. Med. Wochenschr., *74*, 928–931.

Hesselgren, S.G., Dahl, G.H., and Nedlich, V. 1973. Dodecyldiamino glycine as an inhibitor of bacteria, fungi, and dental plaques. Sv. Tandlaek. Tidskr., *66*(2), 181–196.

Ichikawa, M., and Miyoshi, Y. 1980. Bactericidal effect of several disinfectants against *Mycobacterium tuberculosis* and *Mycobacterium bovis*. Bokin Bobai, *8*(4), 143–147.

Ilic, M. 1968. Disinfectant properties of Meripol BQ, Omnisan, and Tego 51 preparations under laboratory conditions. Tehnol. Mesa, *9*(5), 136–140.

Jones, E.H., Howells, C.H.L., and Dickinson, C.W. 1962. Control of wound sepsis in an overcrowded hospital. Hospitals, *58*, 218–223.

Kamada, K. 1964. A dental-pharmacological study of surface-active agents. II. On the toxicity of a few amphoteric surface-active agents against *Paramecium caudatum*. Shika Igaku, *27*(1), 16–21.

Kamada, K. 1963. Dental pharmacological studies of surface-active agents. I. Antibiotic action of some amphoteric surface-active agents. Shika Igaku, *26*(4), 345–354.

Kellet, B.S. 1979. Bacterial growth in ampholytic disinfectant solutions. Lab. Anim., *13*(2), 135–138.

Kendereski, S., and Ilic, M. 1969. Comparative investigation of bactericidal power of some modern disinfectants important to the food industry. Hrana Ishrana, *10*, 433–438.

Kovats, J., and Tamasi, G. 1975. Factors affecting the efficiency of disinfection and a method for disinfectant evaluation. Prog. Anim. Hyg. 1st., 114–119.

Kuipers, J.S., and Dankert, J. 1970. Bactericidal properties of Tego 103S and Tego 103G. J. Hyg., *168*, 343–348.

Lee, Y. 1981. Bactericidal activities of various disinfectants against *Mycobacterium tuberculosis*. Kekkaku, *56*(12), 567–576.

Lubowe, I.I. 1957. Antiseborrheic agents. Drug Cosmet. Ind., *81*, 602–603, 674, 676.

Micheletti, P.G., Ponti, R., and Cantoni, C. 1978. Virucidal activity of some disinfectants containing amphoteric, cationic, and cationogenic surface-active compounds (Tego). Arch. Lebensmittelhygiene, *29*, 94–96.

Nada, T., Ito, H., Yamamoto, H., Imai, J., and Tamura, T. 1980. Bacteriostatic and bactericidal effects of ordinary disinfectants against glucose-nonfermenting gram-negative rods. Esei Kensa, *29*(7), 929–937.

Nagai, T. 1979. Antimicrobial activity of disinfectants. Naika Hokan, *26*(4), 155–160.

Nakamura, T. 1958. Effectiveness of disinfectants on *Staphylococcus aureus* treated by various surface active agents. Nagasaki Igakkai Zasshi, *33*, 1060–1076, 1086.

Nakao, J., Hess, R.G., Bachmann, P.A., and Mahnel, H. 1978. Tenacity and inactivation of transmissible gastroenteritis (TGE) virus of pigs. Berl. Muench Tieraerztl. Wochenschr., *91*(18), 353–357.

Naumann, P. 1952. Critique and experiments on surgical hand disinfection. Z. Hyg. Infektionskrankh., *135*, 161–190.

Nikolov, T., Kibarska, T., and Luchev, St. 1970. Possibilities for the use of certain surface-active substances as antiseptics in the processing of cane molasses into alcohol. Dokl. Akad. Nauk Bolg., *3*, 195–199.

Nowak, G.A. 1968. Amphotensides of betaine structure in cosmetics. Seifen-Oele-Fette-Wachse, *94*, 475–477.

Pavlas, M. 1967. The disinfectant effect of some preparations in tuberculosis contaminated environment. Cesk. Epidemiol. Mikrobiol. Immunol., *16*(4), 228–236.

Puhac, I., and Hrgovic, N. 1969. Comparative laboratory tests of the bactericidal properties of Tego surfactants and some other disinfectants. Tehnol. Mesa, *10*, 224–227.

Puhac, I., and Hrgovic, N. 1969. Effect of water hardness on disinfectant properties of Tego 51 (15DL) and Meripol BQ solutions. Tehnol. Mesa, *10*, 249–252.

Puhac, I., Gadanski, G., and Hrgovic, N. 1969. Corrosive effects of some modern disinfectants. Tehnol. Mesa, *10*, 274–275.

Sainclivier, M., and Kerherve, L. 1972. Activity of ampholytic disinfectant Tego 51 and 51B. Sci. Aliment., *18*(2), 60–71.

Sainclivier, M., and Kerherve, L. 1966. Effect of combined ampholytic disinfecting agents, Tego 51 and Tego 51B. Ind. Aliment. Agric., *83*, 127–136.

Sakagami, Y., Yokohama, H., and Ose, Y. 1980. Bacteria capable of utilizing commercial disinfectants in the river sludge. Degradation of anaerobic bacteria acclimatized to 8-hydroxyquinoline. Bokin Bobai, *8*(9), 377–383.

Sanderink, J.F.H., and Singelenberg, O. 1963. Contact dermatitis due to the disinfectant Tego 103G in nursing staff. Ned. Tijdschr. Geneeskd., *107*, 1902–1904.

Schara, A. Undated. Hygiene in the soft drinks industry is indispensable. Darmstadt, Germany, Döhler GmbH.

Schmitz, A. 1952. Amino acids having bactericidal properties. German Patent 845,941.

Schmitz, A. 1952. Ampholyte soaps as new disinfectants for dairy and food plants. Milchwissenschaft, *7*, 250–257.

Schmitz, A. 1954. Washing and disinfecting compounds. U.S. Patent 2,684,946.

Schmitz, I.A., and Harris, W.S. 1958. Germicidal ampholytic surface-active agents. Manufact. Chem., 29, 51–54.

Soerensen, B., Correa, H.S., and Neto, L.Z. 1969. Use of Tego 51 in meat products of the food industry. Toxicity and antibacterial action. Biologico, 35, 3–7.

Soerenson, B., Zezza Neto, L., Miyamota, A., and Yoshio, M.E. 1971. Inactivation of antibacterial action of dodecylbis (aminoethyl) glycine in the presence of bovine milk and gastrointestinal fluids. Ciencia, 1(3), 24–28.

Sykes, G. 1970. The sporicidal properties of chemical disinfectants. J. Appl. Bacteriol., 33, 147–156.

Sykes, G. 1965. Disinfection and Sterilization. 2nd Edition. Philadelphia, J.B. Lippincott, pp. 377–378.

Tatewaki, K., Moro, K., Sugiyama, S., and Yasunaga, K. 1981. Estimation of the disinfecting effect of Tego 51 toward various bacteria. Bokin Bobai, 9(10), 465–469.

Thiel, W. 1960. Tests with the disinfectant Tego 51 for freeing stalls of tuberculosis organisms. Monatsh. Tierheilkd., 12, 142–148.

Trautwein, K., and Nassal, J. 1958. The comparative bactericidal action of 33 disinfectants, especially on tubercle bacilli. Monatsh. Tierkeilkd., 10, Sonderteil 1–10.

Varga, J. 1972. Comparative study on several disinfectants. Magy. Allatorv. Lapja, 27, 627–628, 631–633.

Wagner, A., Fabian, A., Dobas Kovas, M., and Magyar, K. 1971. Comparative investigation of some disinfectants from the aspect of milk industry with particular respect to iodophors. Elelmiszervizsgalati Kozlem, 17, 71–82.

Wagener, K. 1954. Tests on Tego 51 as a disinfectant against animal disease bacteria. Hannover, Germany, Institute of Hygiene, College of Veterinary Science, July 17.

Waller, T. 1979. Sensitivity of Encephalitozoon cuniculi to various temperatures, disinfectants, and drugs. Lab. Anim., 13(3), 227–230.

Yablochkin, V.D. 1971. Comparative trials of detergent-disinfectants Tego 51 and Desmol. Tr. Vses. Nauch.-Issled. Inst. Vet. Sanit., 38, 115–119.

Yamada, Y. 1968. Relations between disinfectant action and physico-chemical properties of some amphoteric solutions. Shika Igaku, 31(5), 506–534.

Yoh, M., et al. 1984. Sterilization effect of some disinfectants in the concentration of common use. Especially sterilization effect of ampholytic surface active agents. Rinsho Saikin, 11(2), 205–211.

CHAPTER 16

CHLORHEXIDINE

Graham W. Denton

Chlorhexidine was first synthesized in 1950 in the laboratories of ICI England during antimicrobial research into synthetic antimalarial agents of the proguanil-type. It was found to possess a high level of antibacterial activity, low mammalian toxicity, and a strong affinity for binding to skin and mucous membranes. These properties led to the development of chlorhexidine principally as a topical antiseptic for application to such areas as skin, wounds, and mucous membranes, and for dental use. In addition, chlorhexidine has been used as a pharmaceutical preservative, particularly in ophthalmic solutions and as a disinfectant for items such as inanimate surfaces and instruments.

CHEMISTRY

Chlorhexidine is 1,6-di(4-chlorophenyl-diguanido) hexane, a cationic bisbiguanide of the following formula:

Chlorhexidine

Study of the related group of bisbiguanides demonstrated that this compound, with a single chlorine substituent in each phenol ring, was the most active (Davies, 1954). Chlorhexidine itself is a strong base, practically insoluble in water (0.008% w/v at 20°C), that reacts with acids to form salts of the RX_2 type. The water solubility of the different salts varies widely.

The very soluble chlorhexidine digluconate cannot be isolated as a solid and is manufactured as a 20% w/v aqueous solution (Chlorhexidine Gluconate Solution BP), higher concentrations being too viscous for convenient use. The diacetate salt has a solubility of 1.9% w/v (20°C), whereas the dihydrochloride and other inorganic salts are relatively insoluble (Table 16–1).

The low solubility of the inorganic salts may cause problems of precipitation if a water-soluble salt such as digluconate is formulated with, or diluted in, a solution containing inorganic anions such as sulphate or carbonate.

Generally, the solubility of chlorhexidine salts in alcohol is higher than that in water; however, chlorhexidine gluconate solution should not be added directly to neat alcohol, because precipitation may occur.

Solutions and powders of chlorhexidine are colorless or almost colorless and usually odorless, although formulations prepared from the diacetate salt occasionally have an odor of acetic acid. Solutions prepared from all salts have an extremely bitter taste that must be masked in formulations intended for oral use.

Chlorhexidine is moderately surface-active and forms micelles in solution; the critical micellar concentration of the acetate is 0.01% w/v at 25°C (Heard and Ashworth, 1968). Aqueous solutions of chlorhexidine are most stable within the pH range 5 to 8. Above pH 8.0 chlorhexidine base is precipitated, and in more acid conditions there is gradual deterioration of activity because the compound is less stable. Hydrolysis yields p-chloroaniline; the amount is insignificant at room temperature, but is increased by heating above 100°C, especially at alkaline pH (Goodall, 1968).

Chemical analysis of chlorhexidine preparations may be performed using a variety of different methods. Samples containing 1 g or more of chlorhexidine may be assayed by the method described in the British Pharmacopoeia, i.e., by dissolving the evaporated residue in glacial acetic acid (neutralized to crystal violet) and titrating against perchloric acid potentiometrically, using a glass electrode. For lower concentrations, a colorimetric method may be used, involving a reaction with alkaline sodium hypobromide, which produces a reddish-brown color (Holbrook, 1958). Chlorhexidine can also be analyzed by gas liquid chromatography (Siefert, 1975) and high-performance liquid chromatography (Huston, 1982; Richard, 1984).

Table 16–1. *Solubility of Chlorhexidine Base and Salts in Water at 20°C (% w/v)*

Chlorhexidine base	0.008
Diacetate	1.9
Dihydrobromide	0.07
Dihydrochloride	0.06
Dinitrate	0.03
Sulphate	0.01
Carbonate	0.02

PHARMACEUTICAL ASPECTS

Compatibility

Chlorhexidine is a cationic molecule and is thus generally compatible with other cationic materials such as quaternary ammonium compounds (e.g., cetrimide, benzalkonium chloride), although compatibility will depend on the nature and relative concentration of the second cationic species. It is, however, possible for a reaction to occur between chlorhexidine and the counter-ion of a cationic molecule, resulting in the formulation of a less-soluble chlorhexidine salt, which may then precipitate.

Nonionic substances such as detergents, although not directly incompatible with chlorhexidine salts, may inactivate the antiseptic to varying degrees, according to chemical type and concentration used. In many cases a suitable ratio of chlorhexidine to excipient can be chosen to give the required degree of bioavailability and hence activity, and this should be confirmed by suitable microbiologic tests.

Chlorhexidine is incompatible with inorganic anions in all but very dilute solutions (Table 16–1). This incompatibility may sometimes be overcome by adding a suitable solubilizing agent in formulations in which this is acceptable. Chlorhexidine is also incompatible with organic anions such as soaps, sodium lauryl sulphate, sodium carboxymethyl cellulose, alginates, and many pharmaceutical dyes. In certain instances there will be no visible signs of incompatibility, but the antimicrobial activity may be significantly reduced because of the chlorhexidine being incorporated into micelles.

Effect of pH on Activity

The antimicrobial activity of chlorhexidine is pH-dependent; the optimum range of 5.5 to 7.0 corresponds to the pH of the body surfaces and tissues. Within the pH range 5 to 8, however, antibacterial activity will vary with the organism and the type of buffer used. For example, activity against *Staphylococcus aureus* and *Escherichia coli* rises with increased pH, whereas the reverse is true for *Pseudomonas aeruginosa*.

Isotonicity

The use of sodium chloride to render chlorhexidine solutions isotonic with plasma should be regarded with caution because of the low solubility of chlorhexidine hydrochloride in physiologic saline (<1 mg/100 ml). Although solutions may be free from precipitate on prep-aration, the solutions (normally containing at least 0.02% chlorhexidine) will be supersaturated, and precipitation of the hydrochloride salt is likely to occur on standing.

Sodium acetate may be used to adjust the tonicity of chlorhexidine solutions without the problem of precipitation. However, the pH of the required solution (2.1% w/v Sodium Acetate Ph. Eur) may be as high as 8.0 and should not, therefore, be stored for prolonged periods.

Coloring Solutions

There are only a limited number of approved dyes that can be used to color chlorhexidine solutions, and even these are anionic in nature and therefore not fully compatible. They can usually be added at low concentrations to tint chlorhexidine solutions for identification purposes but are liable to form a precipitate when used at the higher concentrations necessary to give good skin-staining properties. For example, carmoisine (E122) at a concentration of 0.0005% provides sufficient coloring for identification purposes and will remain stable for long periods. At a concentration of 0.05% it has good skin-staining properties, but may precipitate on storage. This solution has a shelf-life of 7 days, after which it should be discarded.

Packaging

The nature and quality of containers for concentrates and use-dilutions is important. Glass, high-density polypropylene, and high-density polyethylene, are usually suitable. Low-density polyethylene may be unsuitable because of excessive absorption, and other packaging materials may interact with the antiseptic. Cork stoppers or cap-linings should never be used, because water-soluble tannins present may inactivate chlorhexidine (Linton, 1966).

Sterilization

Dilute solutions of chlorhexidine (<1.0% w/v) may be sterilized by autoclaving at 115°C for 30 minutes or at 121 to 123°C for 15 minutes. Autoclaving of solutions greater than 1.0% can result in the formation of insoluble residues and is therefore unsuitable. If sterile solutions are required at such high concentrations, then filtration through a 0.22 μm sterilizing-grade membrane filter is recommended; however, the first 10 ml should be discarded because adsorption may occur in the initial stage; fibrous and porcelain filters are unsuitable.

Chlorhexidine hydrochloride powder is stable to dry-heat sterilization at 150°C. The solid salts are stable to sterilizing doses of gamma radiation, but chlorhexidine in solution is decomposed.

Storage

Dilute chlorhexidine solutions may be stored at room temperature, and a shelf-life of at least 1 year can be expected, provided that the packaging is adequate. Prolonged exposure to high temperature or light is to be avoided because this can adversely affect the stability of chlorhexidine solutions. All dilute solutions to be stored should be either heat-treated (sterilized or pasteurized) or chemically preserved (4% isopropanol or 7% ethanol) to eliminate the possibility of microbial contamination.

For autoclaved solutions the choice of container material is important, best results being achieved with neutral glass or polypropylene. If soda glass is used with chlorhexidine solutions the resultant pH may be above that which is considered optimal for stability (pH 5 to 7) because of leaching of alkaline materials from the bottle.

Chlorhexidine and Laundering

Chlorhexidine is absorbed onto the fibers of certain fabrics, particularly cotton, and resists removal by washing. If a hypochlorite (chlorine-releasing) bleach is used during the washing procedure, a fast brown stain may develop because of a chemical reaction between the chlorhexidine and the bleach. This can be avoided by eliminating the use of a bleach or replacing the chlorine-releasing bleach with one based on peroxide, such as sodium perborate. Pretreatment of the fabrics with dilute (1%) hydrochloric acid or oxalic acid for 10 to 15 minutes reduces or eliminates staining when a chlorine bleach is subsequently used.

MICROBIOLOGY

The antimicrobial activity of chlorhexidine is directed mainly toward vegetative gram-positive and gram-negative bacteria. It is inactive against bacterial spores except at elevated temperatures. Acid-fast bacilli are inhibited but not killed by aqueous solutions. The infectivity of some lipophilic viruses (e.g., influenzavirus, herpesvirus, HIV) is rapidly inactivated by chlorhexidine. Yeasts (including *Candida albicans*) and dermatophytes are usually sensitive, although chlorhexidine's fungicidal action in general is subject to species variation, as are other agents.

Mechanisms of Antibacterial Action

The mechanism of action of chlorhexidine and related biguanides was recently reviewed by Woodcock (1988).

At relatively low concentrations, the action of chlorhexidine is bacteriostatic, whereas at higher concentrations the action is rapidly bactericidal, the actual levels varying somewhat from species to species.

The lethal process has been shown to consist of a series of related cytologic and physiologic changes, some of which are reversible, that culminate in the death of the cell. The sequence is thought to be as follows: (*1*) Rapid attraction towards the bacterial cell; (*2*) Specific and strong adsorption to certain phosphate-containing compounds on the bacterial surface; (*3*) Overcoming the bacterial cell wall exclusion mechanisms; (*4*) Attraction towards the cytoplasmic membrane; (*5*) Leakage of low molecular weight cytoplasmic components, e.g., potassium ions, and inhibition of certain membrane-bound enzymes, e.g., adenosyl triphosphatase; (*6*) Precipitation of the cytoplasm by formation of complexes with phos-

phated entities such as adenosine triphosphate and nucleic acids.

Characteristically, a bacterial cell is negatively charged, the nature of the ionogenic groups varying with bacterial species. It has been shown that, given sufficient chlorhexidine, the surface charge of the bacterial cell is rapidly neutralized and then reversed. The degree of charge reversal is proportional to the chlorhexidine concentration, and reaches a stable equilibrium within 5 minutes. The rapid electrostatic attraction of the cationic chlorhexidine molecules and the negatively charged bacterial cell undoubtedly contributes to the rapid rate of kill associated with chlorhexidine. However, surface charge reversal is secondary to cell death.

Electron microscopy and assay for characteristic outer-membrane components such as 2-keto-3-deoxyoctonate (KDO) demonstrate that sublethal concentrations of chlorhexidine bring about changes in the outer membrane integrity of gram-negative cells. An efflux of divalent cations, especially calcium ions, occurs prior to or during such outer-membrane changes. Chlorhexidine molecules are thought to compete for the negative sites on the peptidoglycan, thereby displacing metallic cations.

In terms of the lethal sequence, the bacterial cytoplasmic membrane appears to be the important site of action. Several changes indicative of damage to the cytoplasmic membrane have been observed in bacterial populations treated with bacteriostatic and bactericidal levels of chlorhexidine. Leakage of cytoplasmic contents is a classic indication of damage to the cytoplasmic membrane and this starts with low molecular weight molecules typified by potassium ions. Electron micrographs of these sublethally treated cells show a shrinkage or plasmolysis of the protoplast. Cells treated with bacteriostatic levels of compound can recover viability despite having lost up to 50% of their K^+. This is particularly true if the excess chlorhexidine is removed by a neutralizing agent, as happens in many in-vitro testing situations.

As the chlorhexidine concentration is increased, higher molecular weight cell contents, such as nucleotides, appear in the supernatant fluid around the cell. Bacterial cells showing more than a 15% increase in nucleotide leakage have been found to be irreversibly damaged; levels of chlorhexidine producing this effect are therefore bactericidal. The rate of membrane disruption and cell leakage increases with chlorhexidine concentration up to a maximum and then falls back and at concentrations that are rapidly bactericidal (100 to 500 mg/L) release of cell components does not occur. Electron microscopy shows the cytoplasm of these cells to be chemically precipitated, this precipitation having been caused by an interaction between the chlorhexidine and phosphated entities within the cytoplasm, such as adenosine triphosphate and nucleic acids.

Studies on membrane-associated enzyme systems have failed to reveal specific effects. Inhibition of ATPase and of the active transport systems for amino acids has been reported, whereas dehydrogenase activity is stimulated by a low concentration of chlorhexidine, possibly because the damaged membrane is more permeable to their substrates. The behavior of chlorhexidine at an oil-water interface suggests that the molecules may become oriented within the lipid component, causing general disruption of membrane structure and function.

Antimicrobial Spectrum

Although there are numerous publications that refer to the bacteriostatic and bactericidal properties of chlorhexidine against particular organisms, the methods used vary, and it is often difficult to compare results. A series of studies have therefore been performed to provide a comprehensive spectrum of activity for chlorhexidine using both microbiostatic and microbiocidal methods. The strains of organisms tested include clinical isolates, laboratory strains, and standard culture collection types. Each strain was tested to determine the MIC of chlorhexidine and its susceptibility to the bactericidal action of 0.05% aqueous chlorhexidine gluconate using a rate-of-kill method.

MIC Method

Two-fold dilutions of chlorhexidine gluconate were prepared in Isosensitest agar, the surface of which was then inoculated with a suspension of each test organism. After incubation at 37°C for 24 hours the agar was examined for distinct growth. The MIC was recorded as the lowest chlorhexidine concentration that prevented growth.

Molds and yeasts were tested on Sabouraud's agar incubated at 30°C for 24 to 72 hours. Anaerobes were incubated anaerobically for 2 to 3 days on agar containing 5% lysed blood. Fastidious organisms were incubated in CO_2 for 2 to 3 days (Tables 16–2 and 16–3).

Rate-of-Kill Test

The in-vitro bactericidal and fungicidal activity of 0.05% chlorhexidine gluconate was determined using a procedure based on British Standard 3286 (1960). One milliliter of a 24-hour broth culture of the test organism was added to 10 ml of aqueous 0.05% w/v chlorhexidine gluconate solution, which was maintained at ambient temperature (18 to 21°C). One-milliliter aliquots of the mixture were removed after 20 seconds, 1 minute, and 10 minutes, and transferred to inactivator broth containing 1.5% soya lecithin and 10% polysorbate 80. A viable count was performed on appropriate further dilutions and, by comparison with an untreated control, a 10-log reduction factor was calculated (Tables 16–4 and 16–5).

Bacterial Susceptibility

The susceptibility of individual bacterial strains to chlorhexidine has been shown to vary widely; however, few have been found capable of surviving concentrations of the antiseptic encountered in use (Pitt, 1983; Hammond, 1987). It has been suggested that prolonged use of the antiseptic may lead to reduced susceptibility and to the development of resistant bacteria. However, this is not supported by the work of Martin (1969) and Simpson (1989), who found that bacterial strains encountered in areas of prolonged and extensive use of the antiseptic have similar susceptibilities to strains of the same species encountered in areas where there is little or no chlorhexidine.

There is also no good evidence that the plasmid-mediated antibiotic resistance common amongst gram-negative bacteria is associated with resistance to chlorhexidine. Michel-Briand (1986), Ahonkai (1984), and Sykes (1976) were unable to find any increase in chlorhexidine-resistance amongst antibiotic-resistant strains of *Escherichia coli*, *Pseudomonas aeruginosa*, *Serratia marcescens*, or *Proteus mirabilis*.

Several workers claim to have demonstrated reduced-sensitivity to chlorhexidine amongst strains of methicillin-resistant *Staphylococcus aureus* (MRSA) compared to methicillin-sensitive strains of this organism (MSSA), using bacteriostatic MIC test procedures (Brumfitt, 1985; Mycock, 1985). However, this is considered to be of little clinical relevance, because the highest chlorhexidine MIC value quoted in these studies is 4 mg/L, and therefore all strains of *Staphylococcus aureus*, including MRSA, can be regarded as highly sensitive to user concentrations of chlorhexidine. Haley (1985) found the bactericidal activity of a 4% chlorhexidine handwash to be similar for strains of MRSA and MSSA. Cookson et al. (1989) examined both the bacteriostatic and bactericidal activity of chlorhexidine against these organisms. They confirmed that although certain strains of MRSA may have raised MIC values, these organisms are just as susceptible to the bactericidal action of the antiseptic as strains of MSSA. A number of clinical reports also support the use of chlorhexidine preparations as part of programs for the control of outbreaks with MRSA (Bradley, 1985; Lejeune, 1986; Jones, 1987).

Depathogenizing Effect

Although killing potentially pathogenic bacteria will certainly prevent them from causing infection, certain types of sublethal chemical treatment might also alter or damage bacterial cells in such a way as to reduce their ability to initiate the disease process. Thus the bacteria would still be alive, but less pathogenic. The ability of chlorhexidine to produce such a depathogenizing effect was first investigated by Holloway (1986) using a peritonitis model in mice. Pathogenic strains of *E. coli* and *Klebsiella aerogenes* were treated with sublethal concentrations of chlorhexidine, after which the antiseptic was neutralized and the test suspension injected into susceptible animals. The results of these studies demonstrated that the pathogenicity of bacteria surviving treatment with chlorhexidine was reduced by more than 90%. This was confirmed by Rotter (1988), who could not demonstrate a similar effect with alcohol. The depathogenizing effect of chlorhexidine must be considered secondary to the direct bactericidal activity of the anti-

Table 16–2. *Bacteriostatic Activity of Chlorhexidine Gluconate*

Test Organism	(No. of Strains)	MIC (mg/L) Mean	MIC (mg/L) Range
Gram-positive cocci			
Micrococcus flavus	(1)	0.5	
Micrococcus lutea	(1)	0.5	
Staphylococcus aureus	(16)	1.6	(1–4)
Staphylococcus epidermidis	(41)	1.8	(0.25–8)
Streptococcus faecalis	(5)	38	(32–64)
Streptococcus mutans	(2)	2.5	
Streptococcus pneumoniae	(5)	11	(8–16)
Streptococcus pyogenes	(9)	3	(1–8)
Streptococcus sanguis	(3)	9	(4–16)
Streptococcus viridans	(5)	25	(2–32)
Gram-positive bacilli			
Bacillus cereus	(1)	8	
Bacillus subtilis	(2)	1	
Clostridium difficile	(7)	16	(8–32)
Clostridium welchii	(5)	14	(4–32)
Corynebacterium sp.	(8)	1.6	(0.5–8)
Lactobacillus casei	(1)	128	
Listeria monocytogenes	(1)	4	
Propionibacterium acne	(2)	8	
Gram-negative bacilli			
Acinetobacter anitratus	(3)	32	(16–64)
Acinetobacter lwoffi	(2)	0.5	
Alkaligenes faecalis	(1)	64	
Bacteroides distastonis	(4)	16	
Bacteroides fragilis	(11)	34	(8–64)
Campylobacter pyloridis	(5)	17	(8–32)
Citrobacter freundii	(10)	18	(4–32)
Enterobacter cloacae	(12)	45	(16–64)
Escherichia coli	(14)	4	(2–32)
Gardnerella vaginalis	(1)	8	
Haemophilus influenza	(10)	5	(2–8)
Klebsiella aerogenes	(5)	25	(16–64)
Klebsiella oxytoca	(2)	32	
Klebsiella pneumoniae	(5)	64	(32–128)
Proteus mirabilis	(5)	115	(64–>128)
Proteus morganii	(5)	73	(16–128)
Proteus vulgaris	(5)	57	(32–128)
Providencia stuartii	(5)	102	(64–128)
Pseudomonas aeruginosa	(15)	20	(16–32)
Pseudomonas cepacia	(1)	16	
Pseudomonas fluorescens	(1)	4	
Salmonella bredeney	(1)	16	
Salmonella dublin	(1)	4	
Salmonella galinarum	(1)	8	
Salmonella montivideo	(1)	8	
Salmonella typhimurium	(4)	13	(8–16)
Salmonella virchow	(1)	8	
Serratia marcescens	(10)	30	(16–64)

Table 16–3. *Fungistatic Activity of Chlorhexidine Gluconate*

Organism (No. of Strains)		Mean MIC (mg/L)
Mould Fungi		
Aspergillus flavus	(1)	64
Aspergillus fumigatus	(1)	32
Aspergillus niger	(1)	16
Penicillium notatum	(1)	16
Rhizopus sp.	(1)	8
Scopulariopsis sp.	(1)	8
Yeasts		
Candida albicans	(2)	9
Candida guillermondii	(1)	4
Candida parapsilosis	(2)	4
Candida pseudotropicalis	(1)	3
Cryptococcus neoformans	(1)	1
Prototheca zopfii	(1)	6
Saccharomyces cerevissia	(1)	1
Torulopsis glabrata	(1)	6
Dermatophytes		
Epidermophyton floccosum	(1)	4
Microsporum canis	(2)	4
Microsporum fulvum	(1)	6
Microsporum gypseum	(1)	6
Trichophyton equinum	(1)	4
Trichophyton interdigitale	(2)	3
Trichophyton mentagrophytes	(1)	3
Trichophyton quinkeanum	(1)	3
Trichophyton rubrum	(2)	3
Trichophyton tonsurans	(1)	3

septic; however, it is believed to be an additional, clinically-relevant property that is not evident in conventional in-vitro studies concerned with viability alone.

Sporicidal Activity

Chlorhexidine will inhibit the growth of the vegetative cells of spore-forming bacteria at relatively low concentrations (Table 16–2), and will also inhibit spore germination. However, it is generally recognized that chlorhexidine has little sporicidal activity except at elevated temperatures. Shaker (1986) investigated the sporicidal activity of an aqueous solution of chlorhexidine gluconate (25 mg/L) against *Bacillus subtilis* spores at various temperatures. At 20°C, 30°C, and 37°C, the antiseptic had little effect on spore viability, even after 120 minutes exposure. At a temperature of 70°C, however, the antiseptic reduced the number of spores by 5 logarithms (i.e., a 99.999% reduction).

Virucidal Activity

Antiseptics act by destroying some part of a microorganism that is essential for its infectivity. In the case of bacteria, this may be the cell wall, the cell membrane, the internal metabolic processes, or the genetic material. Because viruses have no synthetic capability of their own, the action of antiseptics is restricted to either the nucleic acid core or the outer coat. Some have coats made entirely of protein, whereas others have significant amounts of lipoprotein or glycoprotein present. Other viruses have an outer envelope surrounding the coat; this is also mainly lipoprotein.

Chlorhexidine has been shown to have good activity against viruses with a lipid component in their coats or with an outer envelope. These include many respiratory viruses, herpes, and cytomegalovirus. Aqueous solutions of chlorhexidine do not, however, have any significant activity against the small protein-coat viruses, which include many of the enteric viruses, poliomyletis, and papilloma (warts) virus.

Human Immunodeficiency Virus (HIV), the organism responsible for Acquired Immunodeficiency Syndrome (AIDS), is known to be one of the enveloped viruses and can, therefore, be predicted to be sensitive to the action of chlorhexidine. This has been confirmed in a series of in-vitro studies performed at Vanderbilt University, Nashville. A 4% chlorhexidine handwash preparation and 0.5% chlorhexidine in 70% alcohol were both found to be 100% effective against HIV type I after a 15-second contact. Aqueous solutions of chlorhexidine down to a final test concentration of 0.05% were 100% effective within 1 minute (Montefiori, 1990).

Published data on the activity of chlorhexidine against a wide range of viral agents are summarized in Table 16–6.

CLINICAL APPLICATIONS AND EFFICACY

Skin Disinfection

Chlorhexidine formulated in a detergent base is used extensively for disinfection of the hands of surgeons and nurses and also for whole-body skin disinfection of patients undergoing surgery. Alcohol-based chlorhexidine solutions with emollients are also used by surgeons and nurses for hand disinfection. Alcohol-based chlorhexidine solutions are particularly suitable for final-stage skin preparation of the operation site; the area should be kept wet for at least 2 minutes to achieve the maximal effect. The immediate bactericidal action of chlorhexidine surpasses that of similar preparations containing povidone-iodine, triclosan, hexachlorophane or parachlorometaxylenol (PCMX). Its valuable persistent (residual) effect, which prevents regrowth of organisms on the skin, is comparable to that of hexachlorophane or triclosan, although chlorhexidine has a broader spectrum of activity, particularly against gram-negative bacteria.

The evidence for efficacy is derived from extensive laboratory testing on volunteers and hospital staff and is generally supported by clinical experience now extending over more than 25 years. Some of this evidence is presented, although differences such as experimental method inevitably make it difficult to compare data produced by different authors. Furthermore, because the efficacy of any formulation is significantly affected by the excipients present, trials demonstrating activity of one

Table 16–4. *Bactericidal Activity of 0.05% Chlorhexidine Gluconate*

Test Organism	(No. of Strains)	Mean $\log_{10}$ Reduction After:		
		1/3 min	1 min	10 min
Gram-positive cocci				
Micrococcus flavus	(1)	0.1	0.4	2.1
Micrococcus lutea	(1)	0.2	0.7	2.9
Staphylococcus aureus	(16)	0.4	0.7	2.5
Staphylococcus epidermidis	(41)	2.2	3.4	>5.1
Streptococcus faecalis	(5)	0.4	0.4	1.1
Streptococcus mutans	(2)	0.8	>4.6	5.8
Streptococcus pneumoniae	(5)	0.8	1.5	>3.5
Streptococcus pyogenes	(9)	1.2	1.8	>3.7
Streptococcus sanguis	(3)	1.1	2.2	>3.9
Streptococcus viridans	(5)	0.4	0.8	2.3
Gram-positive bacilli				
Bacillus cereus	(1)	2.0	2.0	4.7
Bacillus subtilis	(2)	0.5	0.5	0.3
Clostridium difficile	(7)	0.2	0.3	0.3
Clostridium welchii	(5)	2.1	3.1	>4.8
Corynebacterium sp.	(8)	1.1	1.4	3.7
Lactobacillus casei	(1)	0.2	0.2	4.1
Listeria monocytogenes	(1)	0.6	2.2	4.8
Propionibacterium acne	(2)	0.7	1.8	3.6
Gram-negative bacilli				
Acinetobacter anitratus	(3)	1.4	2.6	>5.3
Acinetobacter lwoffi	(2)	>4.0	>4.3	>4.8
Alkaligenes faecalis	(1)	1.5	2.7	4.1
Bacteroides distastonis	(4)	0.9	2.7	>4.9
Bacteroides fragilis	(11)	3.0	4.2	5.2
Campylobacter pyloridis	(5)	N.T.	2.8	>4.0
Citrobacter freundii	(10)	3.4	4.9	>6.0
Enterobacter cloacae	(12)	3.5	4.5	>6.3
Escherichia coli	(14)	3.2	5.0	>6.4
Gardnerella vaginalis	(1)	2.3	3.3	>5.8
Haemophilus influenza	(10)	>4.1	>4.1	>4.1
Klebsiella aerogenes	(5)	2.7	3.9	>5.9
Klebsiella oxytoca	(2)	3.2	5.2	>6.4
Klebsiella pneumoniae	(5)	3.0	4.8	>6.2
Proteus mirabilis	(5)	0.8	0.9	2.9
Proteus morganii	(5)	1.0	1.5	4.2
Proteus vulgaris	(5)	0.8	1.0	4.1
Providencia stuartii	(5)	0.6	0.9	1.8
Pseudomonas aeruginosa	(15)	1.7	2.7	4.9
Pseudomonas cepacia	(1)	1.1	1.3	>4.6
Pseudomonas fluorescens	(1)	3.8	5.0	>6.7
Salmonella bredeney	(1)	1.6	3.4	>6.4
Salmonella dublin	(1)	1.5	2.9	3.2
Salmonella galinarum	(1)	2.5	4.0	>6.2
Salmonella montivideo	(1)	2.4	3.8	>6.3
Salmonella typhimurium	(4)	2.0	3.7	>6.0
Salmonella virchow	(1)	1.9	3.9	>6.2
Serratia marcescens	(10)	1.5	3.7	>5.9

Table 16–5. *Fungicidal Activity of 0.05% Chlorhexidine Gluconate*

Test Organism	(No. of Strains)	Mean log_{10} Reduction After:		
		1/3 min	1 min	10 min
Mould Fungi				
Aspergillus flavus	(1)	0.4	0.8	1.7
Aspergillus fumigatus	(1)	0.7	1.2	2.4
Aspergillus niger	(1)	0.7	1.2	3.0
Penicillium notatum	(1)	0.6	2.0	3.5
Rhizopus sp.	(1)	0.4	0.4	0.5
Scopulariopsis sp.	(1)	0.6	1.1	2.3
Yeasts				
Candida albicans	(2)	2.8	>4.1	>4.2
Candida guillermondii	(1)	3.5	>4.3	>4.3
Candida parapsilosis	(2)	2.1	3.4	>4.2
Candida pseudotropicalis	(1)	3.6	>4.4	>4.4
Cryptococcus neoformans	(1)	4.0	>4.2	>4.2
Prototheca zopfii	(1)	3.3	>3.6	>3.6
Saccharomyces cerevissia	(1)	3.7	>3.7	>3.7
Torulopsis glabrata	(1)	1.3	2.2	>4.4
Dermatophytes				
Epidermophyton floccosum	(1)	0.7	0.5	>1.8
Microsporum canis	(2)	0.4	1.0	>2.0
Microsporum fulvum	(1)	0.2	0.6	>2.4
Microsporum gypseum	(1)	0.1	0.3	2.0
Trichophyton equinum	(1)	0.5	1.1	>2.1
Trichophyton interdigitale	(2)	0.4	0.9	>2.4
Trichophyton mentagrophytes	(1)	1.3	>2.1	>2.1
Trichophyton quinkeanum	(1)	0.2	0.9	>2.8
Trichophyton rubrum	(2)	0.3	0.6	>2.4
Trichophyton tonsurans	(1)	0.4	0.3	1.6

Table 16–6. *Virucidal Activity of Chlorhexidine Gluconate*

Virus	Viral Family	Activity	Conc. (%)	Reference
Respiratory syncytial virus	Paramyxovirus	+	0.25	Platt (1985)
Herpes hominis/simplex	Herpesvirus	+	0.02	Bailey (1972)
Polio virus type 2	Enterovirus	−	0.02	Bailey (1972)
Adenovirus type 2	Adenovirus	−	0.02	Bailey (1972)
Equine infectious anaemia virus	Retrovirus	+	2.0	Shen (1977)
Variola virus (smallpox)	Poxvirus	+	2.0	Tanabe (1976)
Herpes simplex type 1/type 2	Herpesvirus	+	0.02	Shinkai (1974)
Equine influenza virus	Orthomyxovirus	+	0.001	Eppley (1968)
Hog cholera virus	Togavirus	+	0.001	Eppley (1968)
Bovine viral diarrhoea	Togavirus	+	0.001	Eppley (1968)
Parainfluenza virus	Paramyxovirus	+	0.001	Eppley (1968)
Transmissible gastroenteritis virus	Coronavirus	+	0.001	Eppley (1968)
Rabies virus	Rhabdovirus	+	0.001	Eppley (1968)
Canine distemper virus	Paramyxovirus	+	0.01	Eppley (1968)
Infectious bronchitis virus	Coronavirus	+	0.01	Eppley (1968)
Newcastle virus	Paramyxovirus	+	0.01	Eppley (1968)
Pseudo rabies virus	Herpesvirus	+	0.01	Matishek (1978)
Cytomegalovirus	Herpesvirus	+	0.1	Faix (1986)
Coxsackie virus	Picornavirus	−	0.4	Narang (1983)
Echo virus	Picornavirus	−	0.4	Narang (1983)
Human Rota virus	Reovirus	−	1.5	Springthorpe (1986)
Human Immunodeficiency Virus Type I	Retrovirus	+	0.2	Harbison (1989)

+ = Active in vitro at the concentration stated

− = Not active in vitro at the concentration stated

formulation cannot be used as evidence for the efficacy of another.

When assessing the effectiveness of an agent for skin disinfection, several properties of the product must be taken into consideration: immediate bactericidal action against both the resident and transient flora, persistence of action preventing regrowth of skin organisms, and a cumulative effect resulting from regular use. The product must also retain its activity in the presence of blood and have good cosmetic acceptability for the user. The relative importance of these individual properties varies to some degree according to the particular application of the antiseptic.

Surgical Hand Disinfection

The objective of surgical hand disinfection is to render the skin free of bacteria, thus preventing the escape of organisms into the operation wound through the punctures in surgical gloves, which occur frequently during operation (Sebben, 1983; O'Connor, 1984). The procedure must eliminate the transient organisms that are likely to be present on the skin and reduce the resident flora to as low a level as is possible. The agent should also remain persistent on the skin in order to maintain the numbers of survivors at this low level throughout the course of the operation.

In a series of volunteer hand-disinfection studies, Lowbury and Lilly (1973) compared the effectiveness of a 4% chlorhexidine handwash with that of other antiseptic agents. A single 2-minute wash with chlorhexidine achieved an 86% reduction in the skin flora, whereas an iodophor preparation achieved a 68% reduction, and hexachlorophane only 47%. This was confirmed in a study from Denmark in which chlorhexidine handwash reduced numbers by 92%, compared to 57% with a hexachlorophane cream and 39% with a triclosan soap (Askgaard, 1975).

In the first in-use study involving a 4% chlorhexidine handwash, Smiley (1973) found this antiseptic to be at least as effective as hexachlorophane in reducing the numbers of bacteria on the hands of the surgical team, and in maintaining these low numbers for several hours under gloves. A povidone-iodine handwash was found to be less effective initially and to allow the numbers of survivors on the hands to increase dramatically during the course of an operation. The chlorhexidine handwash was also more acceptable to users than the other handwashes, undesirable side-effects occurring most frequently with the povidone-iodine preparation.

In a large volunteer study using the official FDA guidelines for assessing surgical hand scrubs, Peterson (1978) found that a chlorhexidine handwash produced significantly greater reductions in numbers of resident bacteria than either hexachlorophane or povidone-iodine preparations and maintained these low numbers for up to 6 hours under gloves. Povidone-iodine was not persistent—allowing a significant increase in bacterial numbers with time. This particular chlorhexidine handwash (Hibiclens) was also the first surgical hand-scrub to be approved as safe and effective (Category 1) by the Topical Antimicrobials Committee of the FDA.

Aly and Maibach (1983) examined the effectiveness of sponge brushes impregnated with either chlorhexidine or povidone-iodine handwashes in a volunteer surgical hand disinfection study. They compared the immediate and persistent effects of the agents and also the effect of blood, which commonly penetrates through punctured surgical gloves. Chlorhexidine proved to be significantly more effective than povidone-iodine in both the presence and absence of blood. This confirmed an earlier study by Lowbury and Lilly (1974), who found that blood significantly reduced the effectiveness of povidone-iodine, but not of chlorhexidine.

Hygienic Hand Disinfection

The major source of infectious organisms within the hospital is the infected or heavily colonized patient, and the principal route of transmission is via the hands of hospital personnel. Handwashing or disinfection is therefore considered to be the single most important measure to prevent nosocomial infection.

The primary objective of hygienic hand disinfection is therefore to eliminate the transient organisms that have been acquired on the hands, thus preventing transfer of these organisms between patients. The agent must act rapidly, because busy hospital staff wash for only a short time.

Persistence of antibacterial action on the skin is considered desirable to help prevent colonization with hospital pathogens and reduce the level of contaminants acquired between handwashes.

User acceptability of a formulation is of particular importance in the ward situation, where frequent handwashing is often necessary. Factors such as soreness and dryness of the hands can have more influence on the use of a product than its antimicrobial efficacy (Larson, 1986).

Rapidity of action of chlorhexidine against transient contaminants artificially applied to the skin was demonstrated by La Rocca et al. (1985). In a study designed to mimic a ward handwash, the hands of 47 subjects were contaminated with Serratia marcescens and washed with chlorhexidine skin cleanser for 15 seconds. Ten consecutive contamination/treatments were conducted in 2 hours. A 99.9% reduction of transient contaminants was demonstrated after a single 15 second wash with chlorhexidine. Progressively greater reductions of the contaminants were obtained following repeated washing, owing to the cumulative activity of residual chlorhexidine.

Larson (1986) compared the microbiologic and physiologic changes to skin brought about by frequent handwashing (15-second wash, 24 times daily). A chlorhexidine handwash significantly reduced the bacterial handflora when compared with all other agents tested and produced no more skin trauma than nonmedicated soap.

Maki (1979) compared the effectiveness of chlorhexidine skin cleanser with other handwash preparations in a controlled trial with nurses in a neurosurgical unit. Following a single 15-second wash, chlorhexidine significantly reduced both the total skin flora and gram-negative organisms acquired naturally during patient contact. There were no significant reductions in bacterial counts following washing with unmedicated soap or an iodophor-containing preparation. The effect of regular use of the agents was also investigated. Each agent was used exclusively on the neurosurgical unit for 4 weeks, during which period repeated hand samples were taken. Regular use of chlorhexidine produced the lowest total bacterial counts and lowest mean numbers of gram-negative bacilli and *Staphylococcus aureus*. This confirms the marked effectiveness of chlorhexidine skin cleanser in a single brief handwashing and demonstrates its persistent effect between repeated handwashes.

In a later study Maki (1982) investigated the effect of different handwash preparations on the incidence of nosocomial infection in a large intensive care unit. Lower rates of infection were obtained with both chlorhexidine and povidone-iodine handwash preparations than with unmedicated soap; however, chlorhexidine was found to be better tolerated and was considered more acceptable for routine use. Stanley (1989) also demonstrated that the rate of infection in an intensive care unit was significantly lower when hands were washed with a 4% chlorhexidine preparation than when liquid soap and an alcohol rinse were used.

Preoperative Whole-Body Disinfection

A significant proportion of postoperative wound infections are caused by microorganisms from the patient's own skin, which may be derived from sites remote from that of the operation. Reducing the level of the skin microflora over the whole body is, therefore, thought to be of benefit in reducing the incidence of infection from these sources.

Davies (1977) examined the effect of bathing, using different antiseptic detergent preparations, on the skin flora. Chlorhexidine skin cleanser was the only agent to achieve a significant reduction in numbers; bacterial counts remained at the pretreatment levels after bathing with povidone-iodine or hexachlorophane and increased significantly after bathing with unmedicated soap.

Brandberg and Anderson (1980) also demonstrated a significant reduction in total skin flora following a shower bath with chlorhexidine and found that this reduction was maintained for up to 1 week, emphasizing the persistent properties of the antiseptic. These results were confirmed by Kaiser (1988), who also demonstrated a beneficial cumulative effect with repeated application of chlorhexidine.

Following earlier microbiologic studies, Brandberg et al. (1980) performed a clinical investigation to determine the effect of preoperative showering with chlorhexidine skin cleanser on infection rates in patients undergoing vascular surgery. On admission, patients bathed daily with the antiseptic (three to eight baths, depending upon length of preoperative stay).

Immediately prior to surgery the operation site was washed with this same solution and finally prepared using 0.5% chlorhexidine in 70% alcohol. A control group of patients did not perform daily bathing but received the same operation-site preparation. All wound reactions in the groin were recorded, even those with minimal pus formation that resolved spontaneously. No prophylactic antibiotics were administered. The infection rate was reduced from 17.5% in the control group to 8% in the patients who showered preoperatively with chlorhexidine.

In a closely monitored clinical study involving over 2000 surgical patients Hayek (1987) demonstrated a significant reduction in infection rate in patients who bathed with chlorhexidine skin cleanser on two occasions in the 24 hours prior to surgery. The overall infection rate was 9% for those patients bathing with chlorhexidine, compared to 12.5% for those using unmedicated bar soap.

In addition to reducing patient morbidity, this infection control measure was considered to be of significant economic benefit to the hospital in terms of improved bed use and cost effectiveness. Hayek (1988) reported that the reduction in infection rate achieved by preoperative bathing with chlorhexidine would save 22 bed-days per 100 patients. Such a saving would allow almost 3% more patients to be admitted for elective surgery.

Other workers have investigated the effect of both pre- and post-operative bathing with chlorhexidine. Randall reported the results of two prospective studies in men undergoing vasectomy. In the first of these (Randall, 1983), preoperative bathing with chlorhexidine skin cleanser was found to be microbiologically effective, significantly reducing the flora of the scrotum and perineum, but it did not reduce the postoperative infection rate, which was found to be in excess of 30%. In the second study (Randall, 1985), preoperative bathing with chlorhexidine was retained and the effect of additional postoperative bathing on the days following operation was examined. This procedure, involving both pre- and post-operative bathing, was found to reduce the infection rate from 37.8 to 6.7%. Wound infection in this group of patients was considered to be largely a secondary phenomenon occurring after the patient left the hospital.

Some trials have failed to demonstrate a clinical benefit, although these either have not followed the recommended skin disinfection method or have included too few patients to show statistical significance. Brandberg (1989), who has reviewed all studies on the use of chlorhexidine for whole-body disinfection, concludes that the procedure is a valuable adjunct to existing antiseptic and aseptic measures that will contribute toward a reduction in infections caused by organisms derived from the patient's own skin.

Urology

There have been numerous reports demonstrating the effectiveness of chlorhexidine preparations in preventing urinary tract infections. A solution of 0.05% chlorhexidine in either glycerine (Miller, 1960) or ethylene glycol

(Gillespie, 1962) has been used successfully as a combined urethral antiseptic and lubricant. Intermittent bladder irrigation with 0.02% aqueous solution of chlorhexidine has been found to be effective in reducing the incidence of bacteria in catheterized patients (Ball, 1987; Kirk, 1979; Bruun, 1978). Solutions used in the urinary tract should be prepared from Chlorhexidine Gluconate Solution BP, which contains no additives. The inadvertent use of solutions containing surfactants has been found to cause hematuria in some patients.

Obstetrics and Gynecology

In one of the earliest reports involving chlorhexidine, Calman and Murray (1956) reported upon the suitability of several antiseptics for use in obstetrics. They considered that the most exacting test, and the one most relevant to practical obstetrics, was a 2½-minute bactericidal test in the presence of fresh blood. By this standard, only chlorhexidine achieved a complete kill of all organisms at its recommended user dilution of 1 in 2000 (0.05%). On the basis of this work and on the experience of 2½ years of clinical use, chlorhexidine was considered the most satisfactory antiseptic available for use in midwifery.

Byatt and Henderson (1973) compared the ability of different antiseptics to disinfect the perineum. The most effective aqueous preparation was a 4% chlorhexidine detergent preparation both undiluted and at a dilution of 1 in 80, which brought about reductions in recoverable bacteria of 98 and 82%, respectively. An equivalent concentration of chlorhexidine without added cleansing agents was less effective, suggesting that the mucus secretions and fatty acid exudates present in this situation prevent penetration of antiseptics to the bacteria.

Christensen (1985) investigated the effectiveness of vaginal washing with a 0.2% chlorhexidine solution for the prevention of neonatal colonization with Group-B streptococci. A significant reduction in colonization with this organism was noted in the infants of treated mothers, and the authors concluded that this procedure may prevent serious infection in the early neonatal period.

Wounds and Burns

Platt (1984), using a wound model in guinea pigs, demonstrated that irrigation with 0.05% chlorhexidine was highly effective in preventing wound sepsis. This was confirmed in the clinical situation by Colombo (1987), who demonstrated a significant reduction in postoperative infection in patients whose wounds were sprayed with 0.05% chlorhexidine during suturing. Groups of workers in France have also found irrigation with chlorhexidine to be effective for controlling existing wound infection (Carrier-Clerambault, 1978; Gerard 1979).

Chlorhexidine preparations have been used extensively in the management of burns for cleansing and antisepsis. In addition, several groups of workers have used the antiseptic for balneotherapy of major burns. The patients were immersed in baths containing aqueous solutions of chlorhexidine gluconate at concentrations ranging from 0.01 to 0.05%. This treatment was considered a valuable adjunct to the existing infection control measures (Collier, 1978; Jouglard, 1979).

Oral Disease

The role of chlorhexidine as an effective agent for the prevention and treatment of oral disease has been widely recognized for a number of years. With the exception of fluoride, no chemical agent for use in the mouth has been so extensively studied. The effectiveness of chlorhexidine stems from its ability to adsorb to negatively charged surfaces in the mouth (e.g., tooth, mucosa, pellicle, restorative materials) maintaining prolonged antimicrobial activity for many hours (Gjermo, 1974). Retention studies with radiolabeled chlorhexidine show that approximately one-third of the dose is retained after a 60-second mouth rinse with 10 ml of a 0.2% solution (Bonesvoll, 1977). Clinical studies demonstrate that this treatment applied twice daily produces optimum uptake and retention in the mouth (Cancro, 1974; Agerbaek, 1975).

Plaque formation is a continual process, and an agent showing persistence of effect offers an advantage over agents with only a limited duration of effect. At present, chlorhexidine is considered the agent of choice for supragingival plaque control (Addy, 1986; Kornman, 1986).

Treatment with chlorhexidine mouthwash or gel has been shown to reduce the duration of and discomfort from minor aphthous ulceration and increase the total number of ulcer-free days (Hunter and Addy, 1987; Addy et al., 1976).

Pre- and post-operative use of chlorhexidine mouthwash has been shown to reduce the oral microflora and the incidence of postextraction bacteremia (Martin and Nind, 1987; Field, 1988). Postoperative gingival healing has been shown to be enhanced by the use of chlorhexidine applied as either a mouthwash or a gel. The antiseptic is thought to achieve this by reducing the level of microbial contamination of the wound (Langebaek and Bay, 1976; Bakaeen and Strahan, 1980).

Oral hygiene can prove difficult to maintain in certain compromised groups. Individuals with mental or physical disabilities may be unable to either understand or perform adequate control measures. Immunocompromised patients are particularly susceptible to oral infections, especially with *Candida* spp., and the same is true of denture wearers. Chlorhexidine mouthwash, gel, and spray have been shown to be effective in helping maintain the oral hygiene of mentally and physically handicapped groups (Francis, 1987; Usher, 1975); the mouthwash and gel have been used successfully in immunocompromised patients to control candidiasis and mucositis (Ferretti, 1987; Jacobsen, 1979).

Soaking dentures in chlorhexidine has also been shown to be effective in reducing colonization with *Candida* species (Olsen, 1975; Budtz-Jorgensen, 1977). It is suggested that the antiseptic exerts both antifungal and antiadhesive effects, which may last for several days (McCourtie, 1986).

Individuals with an increased caries risk can be identified from the high salivary levels of *Streptococcus mutans*. Use of chlorhexidine gel (Zickert, 1982) or chlorhexidine fluoride mouthwash (Luoma, 1978), alongside other preventive measures such as fluoride treatment and diet control, has been shown to significantly reduce the incidence of caries in these individuals. Radiation caries have also been controlled by a chlorhexidine/fluoride mouthwash (Katz, 1982).

The most common side effect associated with oral use of chlorhexidine is extrinsic tooth staining. This seems to be an unavoidable consequence of having clinically effective chlorhexidine available at the tooth surface. The highly reactive molecule combines with dietary chromogens, which are then precipitated onto the tooth surface (Addy et al., 1985); it is this chlorhexidine/chromogen complex that forms the characteristic stain. Maximum staining occurs in vitro at 0.1% chlorhexidine (Prayitno and Addy, 1979); however, reducing the concentration in order to limit staining requires a corresponding increase in volume to maintain clinical efficacy. Thus, clinically equivalent doses of chlorhexidine have equivalent levels of stain.

The stain is extremely variable from individual to individual, and may be minimized by prior toothbrushing with a dentifrice (Kornman, 1986). Although tooth staining limits the longterm oral use of chlorhexidine, for some patient groups the benefits outweigh the disadvantages. Indeed, for the physically and mentally handicapped, chlorhexidine may be the only option for effective oral hygiene (Storhaug, 1977).

SAFETY IN USE

Chlorhexidine has been in use throughout the world for more than 30 years in a wide range of clinical situations; during this period, reports of adverse reactions have been relatively few. Extensive studies involving experimental animals and human volunteers, as well as observations of hospital staff and patients, have been carried out to determine the nature and probability of untoward reactions that may be associated with the varied applications of chlorhexidine to living tissues. These range from disinfection of intact adult skin to delicate mucous membranes (e.g., bladder and eye) and traumatic or surgical wounds. Systemic (oral, intramuscular, intravenous) and topical routes of administration have been investigated for short- and long-term adverse effects.

The acute effects of accidental ingestion or injection are associated only with high doses. Longterm effects of animal feeding and topical (human) use show that absorption from the alimentary tract or through the skin is negligible or absent. There is no evidence of carcinogenicity. The incidence of skin irritation and hypersensitivity is low when chlorhexidine is applied at its recommended concentrations. There is no deleterious effect on healing of wounds or grafting of burns. As with most disinfectants, a high probability of total deafness rules out the use of chlorhexidine during surgery on the inner or middle ear. Chlorhexidine has been shown to be toxic to nerve tissue, and therefore contact with the brain and meninges must be avoided. Strong solutions of chlorhexidine and preparations which are formulated with other excipients (such as alcohols and surfactants) should also be kept away from the eyes.

Acute Toxicity

Systemic administration of formulations of chlorhexidine by oral, intravenous, and subcutaneous routes has been performed in rats and mice. Oral LD_{50} values are high because chlorhexidine is poorly absorbed from the gut and is mainly excreted unchanged in the feces. Administration by the intravenous route results in greater toxicity than either the oral or subcutaneous routes because of a stromalytic effect on red blood cells due to its surfactant activity.

Subacute and Chronic Toxicity

In longer-term studies (up to 3 months), there is a dose-related decrease in body weight and a decrease in consumption of drinking water due to the unpalatable taste of chlorhexidine. Rats receiving 50, 100, or 200 mg/kg/day of chlorhexidine in their drinking water for 90 days produced only evidence of reactive histiocytosis of the mesenteric lymph nodes; however, this is known to occur in aging rats. The change was not neoplastic, and phagocytic function was normal. In longer-term tests, up to 2 years, the effect on the mesenteric lymph nodes was found to be nonprogressive.

The effect of chlorhexidine gluconate at doses of 5 and 50 mg/kg/day on the reproductive performance of male and female rats was also studied. Mating performance, pregnancy rate, duration of gestation, litter parameters, and the condition of the dams at terminal necropsy were unaffected by the treatment.

Oncogenicity

Carcinogenicity studies have been performed in both rats and mice given oral chlorhexidine plus artificially increased levels of its degradation product p-chloroaniline. No evidence of carcinogenicity was found in rats after 2 years of up to 40 mg/kg/day chlorhexidine plus 0.6 mg/kg/day p-chloroaniline.

There have been several reports of mutagenicity tests with chlorhexidine based on modifications of the microbiologic Ames test procedure. This type of microbiologic test is considered to be fundamentally inappropriate for use with known antimicrobial agents because it is difficult, if not impossible, to separate the legitimate lethal action of the drug on the bacterial cell from any toxicologic activity that the drug may possess. Although some reports claim to have demonstrated positive mutagenicity with chlorhexidine by this means (Ackermann-Schmidt, 1982), the significance of the findings is considered extremely doubtful, particularly in view of the complete lack of carcinogenicity demonstrated in more meaningful animal studies. From the evidence available it is concluded that chlorhexidine is not a carcinogen.

Dermal Absorption

All the available information on chlorhexidine suggests that the antiseptic is absorbed through skin to an extremely small degree, if at all.

Case (1980) reported on a series of studies to detect percutaneous absorption of chlorhexidine following application to the skin of volunteers. Radiolabeled chlorhexidine formulated as a 4% handwash or 5% aqueous solution was applied to forearm skin and left in contact for 3 hours. Levels ranging from 96 to 98% of the radioactivity were subsequently recovered from the skin. No radioactivity was detected in blood or urine. The equivalent of 0.007% of the administered dose was detected in only one of the fecal samples. In a further study subjects followed an exaggerated surgical scrub schedule using a 4% chlorhexidine handwash five times daily for 3 5-day weeks. Each treatment lasted 6 minutes and included 3 minutes of brush scrubbing. Blood samples were taken throughout the test period and analyzed for chlorhexidine using a gas liquid chromatography method with a sensitivity of 0.01 to 0.05 mg/L. No detectable blood levels were found in any of the volunteers at any time. Blood samples were also taken from hospital staff members who had been regular users of 4% chlorhexidine for surgical hand disinfection for at least 6 months. No detectable levels of chlorhexidine were found in any of the subjects.

Husak (1981), who used 4% chlorhexidine handwash for bathing infants, was unable to detect skin absorption of chlorhexidine on each of the 3 days following bathing. Cowen (1979), who also bathed infants with this preparation, did find significant levels of chlorhexidine in the blood when samples were taken by heel prick, but this was thought to be due to contamination from the treated skin. Samples of venous blood taken in an attempt to avoid this contamination showed very low levels of chlorhexidine in some babies and none in others.

Gongwer (1980) bathed neonatal rhesus monkeys for 90 days with an experimental handwash formulation containing 8% chlorhexidine gluconate. There were no adverse effects on the brain or other tissues. Minimal amounts of chlorhexidine were detected in a few tissues and in the feces, and it was suggested that the antiseptic had entered the body by oral ingestion following grooming.

From the results of all the studies listed, it is clear that percutaneous absorption of chlorhexidine, if it occurs at all, is minimal. There is no evidence that any chlorhexidine that may be absorbed will be toxic.

Skin Irritation and Sensitization

Primary dermal irritancy studies with aqueous chlorhexidine gluconate solutions (20%, 0.5%) or a 4% chlorhexidine handwash were performed in rabbits using the Draize test method. The results showed that none of the formulations was a primary skin irritant. A repeated-application dermal toxicity study was also performed in rabbits with aqueous chlorhexidine gluconate (20%) applied once daily, 5 days a week for 3 weeks. The concentrated solution caused damage to both intact and abraded skin, which healed within 2 weeks of stopping treatment.

Tests in human volunteers to detect allergic contact sensitization and photosensitization following repeated application of chlorhexidine formulations proved negative.

Longterm experience has demonstrated that an extremely low incidence of sensitization reactions occur in patients using chlorhexidine. There have been isolated reports of generalized allergic reactions, and in the most severe cases shock has occurred (fall in blood pressure, nausea, dizziness, dyspnea) (Ohtoshi, 1986; Okano, 1989). However, when considered against the extensive use of the antiseptic over more than 30 years, the incidence of such side effects must be considered extremely low.

Wound Healing

Saatman (1986) assessed the effects of 0.05% and 4% chlorhexidine gluconate solutions on the healing of surgically induced wounds in guinea pigs. Wounds were irrigated after surgery and daily thereafter until necropsy. Daily progress of the wound appeared normal in all treatment groups with no gross evidence of treatment effects. Upon histopathologic evaluation treated animals exhibited a slight delay in healing compared to saline-treated animals on days 3, 6, and 9. However, by days 14 and 21 no differences were detectable.

Hirst (1973) investigated the effect of chlorhexidine on gingival wound healing in dogs. Biopsy sites were treated with 20% chlorhexidine or saline for 42 days, after which the sites were graded for inflammatory response. Sites exposed to chlorhexidine had less evidence of inflammation than the control sites, and healing was judged as complete.

It has been reported that chlorhexidine is cytotoxic to exposed fibroblasts when assessed in vitro using tissue culture methods. However, Sanchez et al. (1988) demonstrated that this cytotoxicity observed in vitro does not occur in vivo. Using an infected-wound model they found that chlorhexidine actually accelerated the rate of healing compared with saline-treated controls.

Ototoxicity

Sensorineural deafness was found to occur in patients who had undergone vascular myringoplasty operations; the common factor was the use of 0.05% chlorhexidine in 70% alcohol for perioperative disinfection of the middle ear. It was thought that the solution had penetrated the membrane of the round window, entering the inner ear and causing damage to the cochlea, which resulted in permanent hearing loss (Bicknell, 1971). This has since been extensively investigated using animal models. Severe vestibular and cochlear damage has been found to occur, the extent of which is related to concentration and duration of exposure (Morizono, 1973; Igarashi, 1985). Other antiseptics have been found to be similarly ototoxic when administered in this way. Toxicity is significantly enhanced in the presence of high levels of alcohol or detergent (Morizono, 1974).

Neurotoxicity

The neurotoxicity of chlorhexidine was investigated by Henschen (1984) using a rat model. A dose-dependent degeneration of the adrenergic nerves was found to occur following application of chlorhexidine, and the authors suggested that neurotoxic effects on thin unmyelinated fibers should also be looked for in the central nervous system. In an earlier study, Hurst (1955) had found that chlorhexidine, along with most other antiseptics, was toxic when injected into the cerebrospinal fluid of monkeys.

Ocular Toxicity

Although dilute solutions of pure chlorhexidine have been used for eye irrigation (0.05%) and as a preservative for such preparations as eye drops (0.01%), higher concentrations and preparations containing other excipients may cause eye damage.

Following direct topical application of up to 2% chlorhexidine to the eye, no changes to the cornea were detected by either direct observation or light microscopy; however, superficial epithelial changes were noted by electron microscopy following application of 0.1% and 0.5% chlorhexidine (Browne, 1976; Dormans, 1982).

Multiple concentrations of chlorhexidine ranging from 0.1 to 4% were evaluated for their toxic effects on re-growth of corneal epithelium. Concentrations of greater than 2% were clearly toxic to both the corneal epithelium and conjunctiva; a concentration of 1% produced no significant delay in epithelial healing but did cause mild conjunctivitis. Concentrations of less than 1% were not statistically different from the control group either in re-epithelialization or visible toxic effects (Hamill, 1984).

Isolated reports have been received of injury resulting from accidental introduction into the eye of an antiseptic handwash containing 4% chlorhexidine in a detergent base. Accidental splashes entering the eye during normal handwashing cause irritation, which has resolved completely following prompt and thorough water washing of the affected eye. However, irreversible corneal damage occurred following more-prolonged ocular exposure. This has resulted from misuse of the antiseptic handwash on anesthetized patients for skin preparation of the periorbital area and eyelids. The product was found to have pooled on the eye surface and remained there for up to 1 hour (Hamed, 1987; Phinney, 1988). From the information available, it would appear that the excipients present in the handwash formulation, or possibly a synergistic interaction between the excipients and chlorhexidine, are a more likely cause of permanent ocular damage than the chlorhexidine alone.

REFERENCES

Ackermann-Schmidt, B., Suessmuth, R., and Lingens, F. 1982. Effects of 1.1'-hexamethylene-bis [(5-p-chlorophenyl)-biguanide] on the genome and on the synthesis of nucleic acids and proteins in the bacterial cells. Chem. Biol. Interact., 40, 85–96.

Addy, M. 1986. Chlorhexidine compared with other locally delivered antimicrobials. A short review. J. Clin. Periodontol., 13, 957–964.

Addy, M., Carpenter, R., and Roberts, W.R. 1976. Management of recurrent aphthous ulceration: A trial of chlorhexidine gluconate gel. Br. Dent. J., 141, 118–120.

Addy, M., Moran, J., Griffiths, A.A., and Wills-Wood, N.J. 1985. Extrinsic tooth discolouration by metal and chlorhexidine I. Surface protein denaturation or dietary precipitation? Br. Dent. J., 159, 281–285.

Agerbaek, N., Melsen, B., and Rolla, G. 1975. Application of chlorhexidine by oral irrigation systems. Scand. J. Dent. Res., 83, 284–287.

Akonhai, I., Pugh, W.J., and Russell, A.D. 1984. Sensitivity to antimicrobial agents of some mercury-sensitive and mercury-resistant strains of gram-negative bacteria. Curr. Microbiol., 11, 183–185.

Aly, R., and Maibach, H.I. 1983. Comparative evaluation of chlorhexidine gluconate ('Hibiclens') and povidone-iodine ('E-Z Scrub') sponge-brushes for presurgical hand scrubbing. Curr. Ther. Res., 34, 740–745.

Askgaard, K. 1975. A comparative trial of different antiseptic detergent preparations for surgical hand washing. Ugeskr. Laeger, 137, 2515–2518.

Bailey, A., and Longson, M. 1972. Virucidal activity of chlorhexidine in strains of Herpes virus hominis, Poliovirus and Adenovirus. J. Clin. Pathol., 25, 76–78.

Bakaeen, G.S., and Strahan, J.D. 1980. Effects of a 1% chlorhexidine gel during the healing phase after inverse level mucogingival flap surgery. J. Clin. Periodontol., 7, 20–25.

Ball, A.J., et al. 1987. Bladder irrigation with chlorhexidine for the prevention of urinary infection after transurethral operations: A prospective controlled study. J. Urol., 138(3), 491–494.

Bicknell, P.G. 1971. Sensorineural deafness following myringoplasty operations. J. Laryngol. Otol., 85, 957–961.

Bonesvoll, P. 1977. Oral pharmacology of chlorhexidine. J. Clin. Periodontol., 4(Extra issue), 49–65.

Bradley, J.M., Noone, P., Townsend, D.E., and Grubb, W.B. 1985. Methicillin-resistant Staphylococcus aureus in a London hospital. Lancet, 1, 1493–1495.

Brandberg, A., and Anderson, I. 1980. Whole-body disinfection by shower-bath with chlorhexidine soap. In Problems in the Control of Hospital Infection. Edited by S.W.B. Newsom and A.D.S. Caldwell. Royal Society of Medicine International Congress and Symposium Series, No. 23. London, RSM/Academic Press, pp. 65–70.

Brandberg, A., Holm, J., Hammarsten, J., and Shersten, T. 1980(a). Postoperative wound disinfection by shower bath with chlorhexidine soap. In Problems in the Control of Hospital Infection. Edited by S.W.B. Newsom and A.D.S. Caldwell. Royal Society of Medicine International Congress and Symposium Series, No. 23. London, RSM/Academic Press, pp. 71–75.

Brandberg, A. 1989. Preoperative whole body disinfection (Viewpoint Sweden). J. Chemotherapy, 1(Suppl. 1), 19–24.

Browne, R.K., Anderson, A.N., Charvez, B.W., and Azzarello, R.J. 1975. Ophthalmic response to chlorhexidine digluconate in rabbits. Toxicol. Appl. Pharmacol., 32, 621–627.

Brumfitt, W., Dixson, S., and Hamilton-Miller, J.M.T. 1985. Resistance to antiseptics in methicillin and gentamycin resistant Staphylococcus aureus. Lancet, 1, 1442–1443.

Bruun, J.N., and Digranes, A. 1978. Bladder irrigation in patients with indwelling catheters. Scand. J. Infect. Dis., 10, 71–74.

Budtz-Jorgensen, E. 1977. Hibitane in the treatment of oral candidiasis. J. Clin. Periodontol., 4, 117–128.

Byatt, M.E., and Henderson, A. 1973. Pre-operative sterilization of the perineum: A comparison of six antiseptics. J. Clin. Pathol., 26, 921–924.

Calman, R.M., and Murray, J. 1956. Antiseptics in midwifery. Br. Med. J., 2, 200–204.

Cancro, L.P., Paulovich, D.B., Bolton, S., and Picozzi, A. 1974. Dose response of chlorhexidine gluconate in a model in-vivo plaque system. J. Dent. Res., 53, 765.

Carrier-Clerambault, R., et al. 1978. Traitement des infections chirurgicales et urologiques par la chlorhexidine. Mediterrannee Medicale, 164, 61–63.

Case, D.E. 1980. Chlorhexidine. Attempts to detect percutaneous absorption in man. In Problems in the Control of Hospital Infection. Edited by S.W.B. Newsom and A.D.S. Caldwell. Royal Society of Medicine International Congress and Symposium Series, No. 23. London, RSM/Academic Press, pp. 39–43.

Christensen, K.K., Christensen, P., Dykes, A.-K., and Kahlmeter, G. 1985. Chlorhexidine for prevention of neonatal colonisation with Group B streptococci III. Effect of vaginal washing with chlorhexidine before rupture of the membranes. Eur. J. Obstet. Gynecol. Reproduct. Biol., 19(4), 231–236.

Collier, F., de Laet, M.H., and Deconinck, P.G. 1978. Anti-infection prophylaxis of infantile burns. Acta Chir. Belg., 77(5), 365–369.

Colombo, A.A., et al. 1987. Chlorhexidine in the prophylaxis of surgical wound infections. Minerva Chir., 42, 23–24.

Cookson, B.D., Bolton, M., Platt, J., and Phillips, I. 1989. Chlorhexidine resistance in methicillin-resistant S. aureus or just an elevated MIC? An invitro and in-vivo assessment. 4th Congr. Clin. Microbiol. Nice, Abstr. 476.

Cowen, J., Ellis, S.H., and McAinsh, J. 1979. Absorption of chlorhexidine from the intact skin of newborn infants. Arch. Dis. Child., 54, 378–383.

Davies, G.E., et al. 1954. 1:6-Di(4'chlorophenyl) diguanido-hexane ("Hibitane"). Laboratory investigations of a new antibacterial agent of high potency. Br. J. Pharmacol., 9, 192–196.

Davies, J., Babb, J.R., Ayliffe, G.A.J., and Ellis, S.H. 1977. The effect on the skin flora of bathing with antiseptic solutions. J. Antimicrob. Chemother., 3, 473–481.

Dormans, J.A., and van Logten, M.J. 1982. The effect of ophthalmic preservatives on the corneal epithelium of the rabbit: A scanning electron microscopical study. Toxicol. Appl. Pharmacol., 62, 251–261.

Eppley, J.R., Hayes, B.M., and Kucera, C.J. 1956. 'Nolvasan'—a virucide. Bio. Chem. Rev., 33, 9–13.

Faix, R.G. 1986. Comparative efficacy of handwashing agents against Cytomegalovirus. Pediatr. Res., 20(Abstr), 436.

Ferretti, G.A., et al. 1987. Therapeutic use of chlorhexidine in bone marrow transplant patients: Case studies. Oral Surg. Oral Med. Oral Pathol., 63, 683–687.

Field, E.A., Nind, D., Varga, E., and Martin, M.V. 1988. The effect of chlorhexidine irrigation on the incidence of dry socket: A pilot study. Br. J. Oral. Maxillofac. Surg., 26, 395–401.

Francis, J.R., Addy, M., and Hunter, B. 1987. A comparison of three delivery methods of chlorhexidine in handicapped children. 1. Effects on plaque, gingivitis and tooth staining. J. Periodontol., 58, 451–455.

Gerard, Y., Thirion, Y., Schernberg, F., and Desfachelles, J.L. 1979. Utilisation de la chlorhexidine dans le traitement des infections osseuses et articulaires. Ann. Med. Nancy, 18, 1385–1389.

Gillespie, W.A. 1962. Progress in the control of hospital cross-infection. Public Health, 77(1), 44–52.

Gjermo, P., Bonesvoll, P., and Rolla, G. 1974. Relationship between plaque inhibiting effect and retention of chlorhexidine in the human oral cavity. Arch. Oral Biol., 19, 1031–1034.

Gongwer, L.E., et al. 1980. The effects of daily bathing of neonatal rhesus monkeys with an antimicrobial skin cleanser containing chlorhexidine gluconate. Toxicol. Appl. Pharmacol., 52, 255–261.

Goodall, R.R., Goldman, J., Woods, J. 1968. Stability of chlorhexidine solutions. Pharm. J., 200, 33–34.

Haley, C.E., et al. 1985. Bactericidal activity of antiseptics against methicillin-resistant Staphylococcus aureus. J. Clin. Microb., 21(6), 991–992.

Hamed, L.M., et al. 1987. 'Hibiclens' keratitis. Am. J. Ophthalmol., 104, 50–56.

Hamill, M.B., Osato, M.S., and Wilhelmus, K.R. 1984. Experimental evaluation of chlorhexidine gluconate for ocular antisepsis. Antimicrob. Agents Chemother., 26, 793–796.

Hammond, S.A., Morgan, J.R., and Russell, A.D. 1987. Comparative susceptibility of hospital isolates of gram-negative bacteria to antiseptics and disinfectants. J. Hosp. Infect., 9(3), 255–264.

Harbison, M.A., and Hammer, S.M. 1989. Inactivation of human immunodeficiency virus by 'Betadine' products and chlorhexidine. J. Acquired Immun. Defic. Synd., 2(1), 16–20.

Hayek, L.J., Emerson, J.M., and Gardner, A.M.N. 1987. Clinical trial of 'Hibiscrub' whole-body disinfection in elective surgery. J. Hosp. Infect., 10, 165–172.

Hayek, L.J., and Emerson, J.M. 1988. Preoperative whole body disinfection—a controlled study. J. Hosp., Infect., 11(Suppl. B), 15–19.

Heard, D.D., and Ashworth, R.W. 1969. The colloidal properties of chlorhexidine and its interaction with some macromolecules. J. Pharm. Pharmacol., 20, 505–512.

Henschen, A., and Olson, L. 1984. Chlorhexidine-induced degeneration of adrenergic nerves. Acta Neuropathol., 63(1), 18–23.

Hirst, R.C., et al. 1973. Microscopic evaluation of topically applied chlorhexidine gluconate on gingival wound healing in dogs. J. South. California Dental Assoc., 41(4), 311–317.

Holbrook, A. 1958. The determination of small quantities of chlorhexidine in pharmaceutical preparations. J. Pharm. Pharmacol., 10, 370–374.

Holloway, P.M., Bucknall, R.A., and Denton, G.W. 1986. The effect of sub lethal concentrations of chlorhexidine on bacterial pathogenicity. J. Hosp. Infect., 8, 39–46.

Hunter, L., and Addy, M. 1987. Chlorhexidine gluconate mouthwash in the management of minor aphthous ulceration. A double-blind, placebo controlled cross-over trial. Br. Dent. J., 162, 106–110.

Hurst, W.E. 1955. Adhesive arachnoiditis and vascular blockage caused by detergents and other chemical irritants: An experimental study. J. Pathol. Bact., 70, 167–178.

Husak, M., et al. 1981. Effect of 'Hibiclens' bathing on neonatal bacterial colonisation. Am. Soc. Microbiol. (Conf.), Abstract 714.

Huston, C.E., Wainwright, P., Cooke, M., and Simpson, R. 1982. High-performance liquid chromatographic method for the determination of chlorhexidine. J. Chromatog., 237, 457–464.

Igarashi, Y., and Suzuki, J.I. 1985. Cochlear ototoxicity of chlorhexidine gluconate in cats. Arch. Otorhinolaryngol., 242, 167–176.

Jacobsen, S., Brynhni, I.-L., and Gjermo, P. 1979. Oral candidosis—frequency, treatment and relapse tendency in a group of psychiatric inpatients. Acta Odontol. Scand., 37, 353.

Jones, M.R., and Martin, D.R. 1987. Outbreak of methicillin-resistant Staphylococci in a New Zealand Hospital. N. Z. Med. J., 100, 369–373.

Jouglard, J.P., et al. 1979. La place de la balneotherapie dans le traitement des grands brules. Mediterranee Med., 192, 75–77.

Kaiser, A.B., Kernodle, D.E., Barg, N.L.B., and Petracek, M.R. 1988. Influence of preoperative showers on staphylococcal skin colonisation: A comparative trial of antiseptic skin cleansers. Ann. Thorac. Surg., 45, 35–38.

Katz, S. 1982. The use of fluoride and chlorhexidine for the prevention of radiation caries. JADA, 104, 164–170.

Kirk, D., et al. 1979. Hibitane bladder irrigation in the prevention of catheter-associated urinary infection. Br. J. Urol., 51(6), 528–531.

Kornman, K.S. 1986. The role of supragingival plaque in the prevention and treatment of periodontal diseases. A review of current concepts. J. Periodont. Res., 21(Suppl.), 5–22.

Langebaek, J., and Bay, L. 1976. The effect of chlorhexidine mouthrinse on healing after gingivectomy. Scand. J. Dent. Res., 84, 224–228.

La Rocca, M.A.K., La Rocca, P.T., and La Rocca, R. 1985. Comparative study of three handwash preparations for efficacy against experimental bacterial contamination of human skin. Adv. Therap., 2(6), 269–274.

Larson, E., et al. 1986. Physiologic and microbiologic changes in skin related to frequent handwashing. Infect. Control., 7, 59–63.

Lejeune, B., et al. 1986. Outbreak of gentamycin-methicillin-resistant Staphylococcus aureus infection in an intensive care unit for children. J. Hosp. Infect., 7(1), 21–25.

Linton, K.B., and George, E. 1966. Inactivation of chlorhexidine (Hibitane) by bark corks. Lancet, 1, 1353–1355.

Lowbury, E.J.L., and Lilly, H.A. 1973. Use of 4% chlorhexidine detergent solution and other methods of skin disinfection. Br. Med. J., 1, 510–515.

Lowbury, E.J.L., and Lilly, H.A. 1974. The effect of blood on disinfection of surgeon's hands. Br. J. Surg., 61, 19–21.

Luoma, H., et al. 1978. A simultaneous reduction of caries and gingivitis in a group of school children receiving chlorhexidine-fluoride applications. Results after 2 years. Caries Res., 12, 290–298.

Maki, D.G., Zilz, M.A., and Alvarado, C.J. 1979. Evaluation of the antibacterial efficacy of four agents for handwashing. Curr. Chemother. Infect. Dis., 11, 1089–1090.

Maki, D.G., and Hecht, J.A. 1982. Comparative study of handwashing with chlorhexidine, povidone-iodine, and non-germicidal soap for prevention of nosocomial infection. Clin. Res., 30(Abstr.), 303A.

Martin, M.V., and Nind, D. 1987. Use of chlorhexidine gluconate for pre-operative disinfection of apicectomy sites. Br. Dent. J., 162, 459–461.

Martin, T.D.M. 1969. Sensitivity of the genus Proteus to chlorhexidine. J. Med. Microbiol., 2, 101–108.

Matisheck, P. 1978. In-vitro activity of chlorhexidine gluconate against Pseudorabies virus. Vet. Med./Small Animal Clin., 73, 796–799.

McCourtie, J., MacFarlane, T.W., and Samaranayake, L.P. 1986. A comparison of the effects of chlorhexidine gluconate, amphotericin B, and nystatin on the adherence of Candida species to denture acrylic. J. Antimicrob. Chemother., 17, 575–583.

Michael-Briand, Y., Laporte, J.M., Bassignot, A., and Plesiat, P. 1986. Antibiotic resistance plasmids and bactericidal effects of chlorhexidine on Enterobacteriaeceae. Lett. Appl. Microbiol., 3, 65–68.

Miller, A., et al. 1960. Prevention of urinary tract infection after prostatectomy. Lancet, 2, 886–888.

Montefiori, D.C., Robinson, W.E., Modliszewski, A. and Mitchell, W.M. 1990. Effective inactivation of human immunodeficiency virus with chlorhexidine antiseptics containing detergents and alcohol. J. Hosp. Infect., 15, 279–282.

Morizono, T., Johnstone, B.M., and Hadjar, E. 1973. The ototoxicity of antiseptics (preliminary report). J. Otolaryngol. Soc. Aust., 3(4), 550–553.

Morizono, T., Johnstone, B.M., and Entjep, H. 1974. Sensorineural deafness caused by preoperative antiseptics. Otologia Fukuoka, 20(2), 97–99.

Mycock, G. 1985. Methicillin/antiseptic resistant Staphylococcus aureus. Lancet, 2, 945–950.

Narang, H.K., and Codd, A.A. 1983. Action of commonly used disinfectants against enteroviruses. J. Hosp. Infect., 4(2), 209–212.

O'Connor, A.G. 1984. Glove puncture during operation. Nurs. Times, 80(Suppl.), 5–6.

Ohtoshi, T., et al. 1986. IgE antibody-mediated shock reaction caused by topical application of chlorhexidine. Clin. Allergy, 15, 155–161.

Okano, M., et al. 1989. Anaphylactic symptoms due to chlorhexidine gluconate. Arch. Dermatol., 125(1), 50–52.

Olsen, I. 1975. Denture stomatitis. The clinical effects of chlorhexidine and amphotericin B. Acta Odontologica Scand., 33, 47–52.

Peterson, A.F., Rosenberg, A., and Alatary, S.D. 1978. Comparative evaluation of surgical scrub preparations. Surg. Gynecol. Obstet., *146*, 63–65.

Phinney, R.B., et al. 1988. Corneal edema related to accidental Hibiclens exposure. Am. J. Ophthalmol., *106*, 210–215.

Pitt, T.L., Gaston, M.A., and Hoffman, P.N. 1983. In-vitro susceptibilities of hospital isolates of various bacterial genera to chlorhexidine. J. Hosp. Infect., *4*(2), 173–176.

Platt, J., and Bucknall, R.A. 1984. An experimental evaluation of antiseptic wound irrigation. J. Hosp. Infect., *5*, 181–188.

Platt, J., and Bucknall, R.A. 1985. The disinfection of respiratory syncytial virus by isopropanol and a chlorhexidine-detergent handwash. J. Hosp. Infect., *6*, 89–94.

Prayitno, S., and Addy, M. 1979. An in-vitro study of factors affecting the development of staining associated with the use of chlorhexidine. J. Periodontol. Res., *14*, 397–402.

Randall, P.E., Ganguli, L., and Marcuson, R.W. 1983. Wound infection following vasectomy ('Hibiscrub'). Br. J. Urol., *55*, 564–567.

Randall, P.E., Ganguli, L.A., Keaney, M.G.L., and Marcuson, R.W. 1985. Prevention of wound infection following vasectomy (chlorhexidine gluconate). Br. J. Urol., *57*, 227–229.

Richard, A., Elbaz, M., and Andermann, G. 1984. Determination of 4-chloroaniline and chlorhexidine digluconate by ion-pair reversed-phase high-performance liquid chromatography. J. Chromatog., *298*, 356–359.

Rotter, M.L., Hirschl, A.M., and Koller, W. 1988. Effect of chlorhexidine-containing detergent, non-medicated soap or isopropanol and the influence of neutraliser on bacterial pathogenicity. J. Hosp. Infect., *11*(3), 220–225.

Saatmann, R.A., et al. 1986. A wound healing study of chlorhexidine digluconate in guinea pigs. Fundam. Appl. Toxicol., *6*(1), 1–6.

Sanchez, I., et al. 1988. Effects of chlorhexidine-diacetate and povidone-iodine on wound healing in dogs. Vet. Surg., *17*(6), 291–295.

Sebben, J.E. 1983. Dermatologic surgery: Surgical antiseptics. J. Am. Acad. Dermatol., *9*, 759–765.

Shaker, L.A., Russell, A.D., and Furr, J.R.. 1986. Aspects of the action of chlorhexidine on bacterial spores. Int. J. Pharm., *34*, 51–56.

Shen, D.T., Crawford, T.B., Gorham, J.R., and McGuire, T.C. 1977. Inactivation of equine infectious anemia virus by chemical disinfectants. Am. J. Vet. Res., *38*, 1217–1219.

Shinkai, K. 1974. Different sensitivities of type 1 and 2 Herpes simplex virus to sodium p-chloromercuribenzoate and chlorhexidine gluconate. Proc. Soc. Exptl. Biol. Med., *147*, 201–204.

Siefert, K., and Casagrande, D. 1975. Analysis of chlorhexidine via gas-liquid chromatography. J. Chromatog., *109*(1), 193–198.

Simpson, R.A., Hawkey, P.M., Woodcock, P.M. 1989. Antibiotic resistance and chlorhexidine susceptibility of Gram negative bacteria in the hospital and community. Program Abstr. 29th ICAAC, Sept. 17–20, 1989, Houston, pp. 212, 663.

Smylie, H.G., Logie, J.R.C., and Smith, G. 1973. From pHisoHex to Hibiscrub. Br. Med. J., *4*, 586–589.

Springthorpe, V.S., Grenier, J.L., Lloyd-Evans, N. and Sattar, S.A. 1986. Chemical disinfection of human rotaviruses: Efficacy of commercially-available products in suspension tests. J. Hygiene, *97*(1), 139–161.

Stanley, G., Sheetz, C., Pfaffer, M. and Wenzel, R. 1989. The comparative effect of alternative handwashing agents on nosocomial infection rates. Proc. 29th ICAAC, Houston, Abstr. 662.

Sykes, R.B. and Matthew, M. 1976. The β-lactamases of gram-negative bacteria and their role in resistance to β-lactam antibiotics. J. Antimicrob. Chemother., *2*, 115–157.

Tanabe, I., and Hotta, S. 1976. Effect of disinfectants on Variola virus in cell culture. Appl. Env. Microbiol., *32*, 209–212.

Usher, P.J. 1975. Oral hygiene in mentally handicapped children. A pilot study of the use of chlorhexidine gel. Br. Dent. J., *138*, 217–221.

Woodcock, P.M. 1988. Biguanides as industrial biocides. In *Industrial Biocides*. Edited by K.R. Payne. Chichester, John Wiley, pp. 19–36.

Zickert, I., Emilson, C.G., and Krasse, B. 1982. Effect of caries preventative measures in children highly infected with the bacterium Streptococcus mutans. Arch. Oral Biol., *27*, 861–868.

CHAPTER 17

NITROGEN COMPOUNDS

H.W. Rossmoore

In this chapter, the variety of compounds containing nitrogen is emphasized, and modes of action where suspected or known are cited, as are successful and unsuccessful applications. Although specific chapters deal in detail with several applications (e.g., industry, food, cosmetics, agriculture, antifungal, antiparasitic), for purposes of exemplification many compounds mentioned elsewhere will be treated here. In addition, where compounds are in actual (i.e., legal) use, mention will be made.

In this regard, a major change in EPA registration (U.S. EPA, 1987b) requirements and impending changes in Western Europe, especially regarding the testing for human safety and concerns for environmental impact, have slowed considerably the development of products based on new chemistry. Instead, the emphasis has been placed on finding new uses for established chemicals and combining several compounds of known activity. These latter concepts will be stressed when appropriate.

Nitrogen is the most electronegative of all Group-V elements; this tends to confer a high degree of reactivity on compounds containing covalently bound nitrogen. In addition, nitrogen contains five valence electrons (three unpaired, two paired), making valence states from 5+ to 3- theoretically possible. This propensity for both covalent and ionic bonding establishes an avidity for a wide variety of interacting compounds. Such chemical diversity is a basis for the formation of antimicrobial activity by nitrogenous compounds. For purposes of discussion, these can be divided into two groups: those that appear to react directly with some sensitive biologic molecule, resulting in an inactive (or nonfunctional) end product, and those adducts yielding starting reactants that combine with a sensitive site in the cell. This dichotomy is not always applicable because neither the sensitive site in the cell nor the active antimicrobial moiety is always known.

THE SIMPLEST COMPOUNDS

Certainly the simplest of N-containing compounds are those with nitrogen plus one other element. In this cat-

egory is sodium azide. This is one of several compounds that appear to function by tying up heme iron, e.g., cytochrome and catalase (Heim et al., 1956). Sodium azide was suggested by Snyder and Lichstein (1940) as an agent that selectively inhibits gram-negative species. It is used in a blood agar medium for the preferential isolation of hemolytic streptococci; however, the inhibitor also reacts with blood heme (catalase), permissively resulting in a greater hemolytic expression of microbial cell hydrogen peroxide (Rossmoore and Trubey, 1967). It is also used as a selective soil sterilant (Rozycki and Bartha, 1981) and for control of soil-borne plant diseases (Van Wambeke et al., 1985).

Other compounds shown to stimulate hemolysis (Rossmoore and Trubey, 1967) also inhibit heme-associated bacterial functions. These include cyanide and hydroxylamine. What all of these have in common is the highly electronegative nitrogen to act as a chelator to form bidentate coordination complexes with Fe^{++}. The reaction of N_2 with reduced ferredoxin may be the equivalent first step in nitrogen fixation.

It should be obvious that toxicity and instability both prevent the widespread use of these simple compounds as preservatives, disinfectants, or sanitizers. Nevertheless, their high activity, a reflection of coordination complex formation, is also a major interpretation of the mode of action of larger and more complex nitrogen-containing compounds (Albert, 1968; Repaske, 1958; Russell, 1971).

FORMALDEHYDE CONDENSATE COMPOUNDS

Among those compounds that have antimicrobial activity only after decomposition (Albert, 1968) are those based on putative formaldehyde release (Rossmoore and Sondossi, 1988). However, CH_2O has recently been investigated as a potential human carcinogen. A summary statement (U.S. EPA, 1987a) makes that a certainty for the regulatory record. This leaves open to speculation the useful future of compounds based on CH_2O. Nevertheless, because of differences in application and possible differences in how CH_2O is released and is available for human contact, CH_2O adducts will be covered in detail. These include a large number of compounds, both cyclic and acyclic, representing a diverse array of structures. Although a large majority of the compounds result from the reaction of NH_2R with formaldehyde, several are based on the methylolate derivations of nitroalkanes (Bennett et al., 1960; Trotz and Pitts, 1981; Bennett, 1973; Paulus et al., 1967; Paulus, 1980). The applications of these compounds are as widespread as their chemical variety, including urinary tract antisepsis (Mandell and Sande, 1980; Musher and Griffith, 1974), cosmetic preservation, metalworking fluids, secondary oil recovery, spin finishes, inks, latex paint, and textile impregnation (Trotz and Pitts, 1981). However, many suffer from the same ultimate shortcoming as does formaldehyde itself (Paulus, 1976; DeMare et al., 1972; Rossmoore and Holtzman, 1974; Rossmoore, 1979): differential quantitative inhibition between bacteria on the one hand and fungi on the other.

The formaldehyde-releasing compound with the longest history of use is hexamethylenetetramine (HTM, Hexamine, Urotropin) (Table 17–1), first synthesized in 1860 from the condensation of NH_3 and CH_2O and first used for cystitis in 1894 (Goodman and Gilman, 1958a). One notable property of this compound (and other cyclic adducts of the $CH_2O + NH_2R$ reaction) is its relative resistance to hydrolysis at alkaline pH. The elevation of urine pH by ammonia-producing *Proteus* specimens involved in bladder infections increases the need to compensate for alkaline stability of HTM used as therapy. Thus, standard treatment with HTM includes an organic acid, e.g., mandelic acid, administered with the HTM. Mandelamine lowers urine pH sufficiently to hydrolyse the producing formaldehyde in situ (Mandell and Sande, 1980). This pH dependency can be readily demonstrated stoichiometrically (Musher and Griffith, 1974; Scott and Wolf, 1962). The demonstration of in-vitro synergism between methenamine hippurate (another clinically acceptable ester of HTM) and trimethoprim against more than 14 bacterial isolates in urine depended on release of CH_2O at pH 5 (Raisenen et al., 1985). Although this combination may have advantages in treating urinary tract infections, no evidence is available to indicate that the interaction is anything more than the effect of CH_2O.

Jacobs et al. (1916a and b) examined a number of quaternary derivatives of HTM and attributed their bactericidal activity to the HTM cation as well as to the formaldehyde released. Scott and Wolf (1962), however, using traditional neutralizers (lecithin and tween), were unable to show decreased activity of quaternized derivatives. One important result of quaternization was the sensitivity to alkaline hydrolysis, with a subsequent yield of formaldehyde even at pH 10 (Table 17–2). Graymore (1938) depicts a mechanism for this reaction in which a quaternized hexahydrotriazine (HT) is hydrolyzed at pH 8 to yield 1 mole of CH_2O per mole of triazine, a theoretic

yield of approximately 30%; this is close to the level reported by Scott and Wolf for HTM.

This broadening of the hydrolysis spectrum of HTM has created useful niches for the quaternized products in metalworking fluids, cosmetics, and latex paints (Trotz and Pitts, 1981; Sharpell, 1980). Its instability, i.e., hydrolysis at alkaline pH, however, has conferred upon it a handicap in preservation requirements at (longterm) alkaline pH. Some innovations bridge this problem. Adducts of CH_2O and primary alkylamines are resistant to alkaline hydrolysis (DeMare et al., 1972), but nevertheless possess significant antimicrobial activity at those pH values (DeMare et al., 1972; Bennett, 1973).

A number of adducts based on CH_2O and NH_2R have achieved commercial success. The ethanolamine derivative introduced first in Europe (Schuelke and Mayr, 1963) and the ethyl derivative (Brooks and Harvey, 1973) have the bulk of the market. Because of their cost effectiveness, compatibility, and relative lack of toxicity, these compounds have approximately 50% of the metalworking fluid preservative market. Unfortunately, they have the same deficiency in their antimicrobial spectrum mentioned previously for CH_2O; i.e., a relative decreased activity against fungi for longer-term use in active field conditions (Sykes, 1958).

Fungal blooms are a common result of underdosing (with respect to fungi) metalworking fluid systems (Rossmoore and Holtzman, 1974; Rossmoore et al., 1972; Bennett, 1973). In this regard, it is difficult to accept the implications of a recent patent (Brazda et al., 1988), which claims specifically that 1,3,5-tris(2-hydroxyethyl) hexahydro-s-triazine is a fungicide against *Fusarium*. This is certainly contrary to the finding of DeMare et al. (1972) as well as my own practical experience. One has little choice between the ethanolamine and the ethylamine with regard to their antimicrobial activity (DeMare et al., 1972; Bennett, 1973). The ethanolamine is much less pungent and is therefore easier to mask at use-dilutions, whereas the ethylamine derivative has a much more advantageous partition coefficient, making it the triazine of choice for oil concentrates.

The importance of polar/nonpolar solubility was demonstrated in a water/jet fuel system preserved with a series of derivatives based on methylamine to amylamine/CH_2O condensations (Jones et al., 1972). Methyl and ethyl triazines were optimally active (Table 17–3), whereas activity decreased with increasing alkyl chain length, a phenomenon strictly dependent on water solubility.

Another innovative structure (Borchert, 1974) based on ethoxyethanolamine purportedly had greater activity in metalworking fluids than other known alkylamine/CH_2O condensates. However, none of the alkyl derivatives were specifically designed for, and thus lacked success in, controlling fungi. Grier and Witzel (1978, 1979) presented evidence that tetrahydrofuran derivatives condensed with CH_2O formed adducts with superior antifungal activity. This was exemplified (Grier et

Table 17–1. *Selected Structures of Nitrogen-Containing Antimicrobial Agents*
(See explanation of naming system at end of table, p. 300)

Name	Structure	CAS Registry No.
PUTATIVE FORMALDEHYDE-RELEASE AGENTS		
CN: 1,3,5,7-tetra-aza-adamantane hexamethylenetetramine		[100-97-0]
CN: 1-(3-chloroallyl)-3,5,7-triaza-1-azoniaadamantane TN: DOWICIL 75, DOWICIL 200		[4080-31-3]
CN: 1,3,5-tris(2-hydroxyethyl) hexahydro-s-triazine TN: GROTAN BK, ONYXIDE 200, TRIADINE 3, BUSAN 1060, BIOBAN GK		[4719-04-4]
CN: 1,3,5-tris(ethyl)hexahydro-s-triazine TN: VANCIDE TH		[7779-27-3]
CN: 1,3,5-tris(tetrahydro-2-furanyl-methyl)hexahydro-s-triazine		[69141-51-1]
CN: 3,5-dimethyltetrahydro-1,3,5(2H)-thiadiazine-2-thione TN: METASOL D3T, BIOCIDE-N-521		[533-74-4]
CN: 1,3(dihydroxymethyl)-5,5-dimethylhydantoin TN: DANTOIN DMDMH-55		[6440-58-0]
CN: methanebis[N,N¹-(5-ureido-2,4-diketotetrahydro-imidazole)-N,N-dimethylol] GN: Imidazolidinylurea TN: GERMALL 115		[39236-46-9]

Table 17–1. *Selected Structures of Nitrogen-Containing Antimicrobial Agents*
(See explanation of naming system at end of table, p. 300) Continued

Name	Structure	CAS Registry No.
CN: 4,4-dimethyloxazolidine* *1 of 2 oxazolidines in commercial mixture TN: BIOBAN CS-1135		[51200-87-4]
CN: 5-hydroxymethyl-1-aza-3,7-dioxabicyclo(3.3.0.)octane** **1 of 3 cyclo-octanes in commercial mixture TN: NUOSEPT 95		[56709-13-8]
CN: N-methylolchloroacetamide TN: GROTAN HD2		[2832-19-1]
CN: tris(hydroxymethyl)nitromethane TN: TRISNITRO		[126-11-4]
CN: 2(hydroxymethyl)aminoethanol TN: TROYSAN 174		[34375-28-5]
CN: 2(hydroxymethyl)amino-2-methylpropanol TN: TROYSAN 192		[522-99-20-4]
CN: bis(1,1-dioxoperhydro-1,2,4-thiadiazinyl-4)methane GN: Taurolin		[19388-87-5]

NITRILES

Name	Structure	CAS Registry No.
CN: methylenebisthiocyanate (MBT) TN: CYTOX 3552, BIOCIDE N948		[G317-18-6]

Table 17–1. *Selected Structures of Nitrogen-Containing Antimicrobial Agents*
(*See explanation of naming system at end of table, p. 300*) Continued

Name	Structure	CAS Registry No.
CN: 2,2-dibromo-3-nitrilopropionamide TN: DBNPA		[10222-01-2]
CN: 1,2-dibromo-2,4-dicyanobutane TN: TEKTOMER 38		[35691-65-7]

PYRIDINES

CN: 4-pyridinecarboxylic acid hydrazide GN: Isoniazid		[54-85-3]
CN: 2-acetylpyridine thiosemicarbazone †variations based on substitutions of the *N*-		representative formula
CN: 4-pyridinemethanol ‡variations based on *H* substitution		representative formula
CN: sodium 2-pyridinethiol-1-oxide TN: SODIUM OMADINE		[3811-73-2]
CN: bis(2-pyridylthio)zinc 1,1'-dioxide TN: ZINC OMADINE		[13463-41-7]

Table 17-1. *Selected Structures of Nitrogen-Containing Antimicrobial Agents*
(See explanation of naming system at end of table, p. 300) Continued

Name	Structure	CAS Registry No.
CN: *N-tert*-butylamino-2-pyridine-1-oxide TN: OMADINE TBAO		[33079-68-2]
CN: 2,3,5,6-tetrachloro-4-(methylsulfonyl)pyridine TN: DOWICIL S-13		[1308-52-6]
CN: 3,5,6-trichloro-4-(propylsulfonyl)pyridine TN: DOWICIL-A40		[38827-35-9]
CN: 2-chloro-6-(trichloromethyl)pyridine GN: Nitrapyrin		[1929-82-4]
CN: N,N'-(1,10 decanediyldi-1[4H]-pyridinyl-4-ylidene)bis- (1-octanamine)dihydrochloride GN: Octenidine Hydrochloride		[70775-75-6]
CN: bis[2,9-dimethyl-1,10-phenanthroline]copper(1)nitrate		[50725-40-1]

Table 17–1. *Selected Structures of Nitrogen-Containing Antimicrobial Agents*
(See explanation of naming system at end of table, p. 300) Continued

Name	Structure	CAS Registry No.
THIAZOLES/IMIDAZOLES		
CN: 5-(*p*-methoxyphenyl)imidazole(2,1b)thiazole		not available
CN: 2-(4-thiazolyl)benzimidazole TN: METASOL TK-100		[148-79-8]
CN: 2(*n*-lauroylamido)5-nitrothiazole		not available
CN: 2-mercaptobenzothiazole (MBeT)		[149-30-4]
CN: 1,2-benzisothiazoline-3-one TN: PROCEL CRL		[2634-33-5]
CN: 2-*n*-octyl-4-isothiazolin-3-one TN: SKANE, KATHON LP		[26530-20-1]
CN: 5-chloro-2-methyl-3(2*H*)-isothiazalone TN: KATHON 886MW, KATHON CT, KATHON CG		[26172-55-4]
	+	
CN: 2-methyl-3(2*H*)-isothiazalone Trade names above apply to a mixture of both isothiazalones.		[2682-20-4]

Table 17–1. *Selected Structures of Nitrogen-Containing Antimicrobial Agents*
(See explanation of naming system at end of table, p. 300) Continued

Name	Structure	CAS Registry No.
NITROS		
CN: 2-bromo-2-nitro-1,3-propanediol TN: BRONOPOL, ONYXIDE 500		[52-51-7]
CN: β-bromo-β-nitrostyrene TN: SLIME-TROL, GIV-GARD BNS		[7166-19-0]
CN: 4,4′(2-ethyl-2-nitrotrimethylene)dimorpholine		[1854-23-5]
CN: 4-(2-nitrobutyl)morpholine TN: BIOBAN P-1487 Trade name is for mixture of morpholines.		[2224-44-4]
CN: N[α(1,-nitroethyl)benzyl]ethylenediamine TN: METASOL J-26		[14762-38-0]
CN: N(5-nitro-2-furfurylidene)-1-amino-hydantoin GN: Nitrofurantoin		[67-20-9]
CN: 5-nitro-2-furaldehyde semicarbazone GN: Furacin		[59-87-0]
CN: 2-thiophenecarboxylic acid, 5-nitro-[3-(5-nitro-2-furanyl)-2-propenylidene]hydrazide TN: NIFURZIDE		[39978-48-2]

Table 17–1. *Selected Structures of Nitrogen-Containing Antimicrobial Agents*
(See explanation of naming system at end of table, p. 300) Continued

Name	Structure	CAS Registry No.
CN: 1-β-(hydroxyethyl)-2-methyl-5-nitroimidazole GN: Metronidazole		[433-48-1]
AMINES		
CN: *N*-Cocotrimethylenediamine	R—NHCH$_2$CH$_2$CH$_2$NH$_2$ [R = C$_8$ – C$_{18}$]	[61791-63-7]
CN: Dodecylmorpholine-*N*-oxide		[2530-46-3]
ANILIDES		
CN: 3,4,4′-trichlorocarbanilide GN: Triclocarban		[101-20-2]
CN: 3,4′,5-tribromosalicylanilide GN: Tribromsalan TN: TEMASEPT IV		[38848-67-8]
CN: salicylanilide TN: SHIRLAN		[87-17-2]
CN: 3-trifluoromethyl-4,4′-dichlorocarbanilide GN: Cloflucarban TN: IRGASAN CF$_3$		[369-77-7]

Table 17-1. *Selected Structures of Nitrogen-Containing Antimicrobial Agents*
(See explanation of naming system at end of table, p. 300) Continued

Name	Structure	CAS Registry No.
CN: 3'-trifluoromethyl-3,5-dibromosalicylanilide GN: Fluorosalan		[4776-06-1]

QUINOLINES

Name	Structure	CAS Registry No.
CN: 6-methoxy-β-(5-vinyl-2-quinuclidinyl)-4-quinoline methanol GN: Quinine		[130-95-0]
CN: 6-chloro-9-[[4-(diethylamino)-1-methylbutyl]amino]- 2-methoxyacridine dihydrochloride GN: Quinacrine HCl TN: ATABRINE		[69-05-6]
CN: dibenzpyridine GN: Acridine		[260-94-6]
CN: 8-hydroxyquinoline GN: Oxine		[1321-40-0]
CN: 1,4-quinoxaline-di-N-oxide		[2423-66-7]

Table 17–1. *Selected Structures of Nitrogen-Containing Antimicrobial Agents*
(See explanation of naming system at end of table.) Continued

Name	Structure	CAS Registry No.
CN: 2,4-diaminoquinazoline (R₁ and R₂ substitutions pyrrole/benzene derivatives)		representative formula
CN: 1-ethyl-1,4-dihydro-7-methyl-4-oxo-1,8-naphthyridine-3-carboxylic acid GN: Nalidixic acid		[389-08-2]
CN: 5-ethyl-5,8-dihydro-8-oxo-1,3-dioxolo[4,5-g]quinoline-7-carboxylic acid GN: Oxolinic acid		[14698-29-4]
CN: 3-quinolinecarboxylic acid, 1-cyclopropyl-6-fluoro-1,4-dihydro-4-oxo-7-(1-piperazinyl) GN: Ciprofloxacin		[85721-33-1]

The listings for generic/trivial names have the first letter capitalized, and trade names have the entire name capitalized. This listing is not meant to be all-inclusive. Some products are made or sold by several companies under different proprietary names. Frequently, proprietary compounds contain inert or stabilizing additives, and the trade name refers to the total mixture, not only to the active antimicrobial agents. For additional information, see Rossmoore (1979), Sharpell (1980), Trotz and Pitts (1981), Manowitz and Sharpell (Chapter 51 of this book), and Block (Chapter 52 of this book). CN, Chemical name; GN, generic name; TN, trade name.

Table 17–2. *Effect of pH on Formaldehyde Release From Hexamethylene Tetramine/Halohydrocarbons*

	% Recovery Based on 6 Moles Formaldehyde per Compound							
pH:	4		6		8		10	
Compound*	24 hr	1 wk	24 hr	1 wk	24 hr	1 wk	24 hr	1 wk
Formaldehyde	104	104	98	97	97	90	97	80
HTM†	17	44	4	21	0	0	0	0
HTM 3-chloropropene	74	105	52	86	46	66	35	35
HTM 1,3-dichloropropene	32	70	31	46	28	36	23	35
HTM chlorotoluene	31	64	31	43	26	39	24	38

*500 ppm
†Hexamethylene tetramine
Modified from Scott, C.R., and Wolf, P.A. 1962. Antibacterial activity of a series of quaternaries prepared from hexamethylenetetramine and halohydrocarbons. Appl. Microbiol., *10*, 211–216.

Table 17–3. *Percent Bacterial Survival in JP-4 Fuel/1% Bushnell-Haas (Contaminated) with 0.05% Hexahydro-S-Alkyltriazine Added*

R*	1 H	2 H	3 H	5 H	24 H
Me	9×10^{-1}	0	0	—	—
Et	0	0	0	—	—
Et$_2$n-Bu	2×10^{-3}	—	2.6×10^{-6}	0	0
n-Pr	5.2×10^{-2}	3.1×10^{-3}	0	0	0
Et (n-Bu)$_2$	7.8×10^{-2}	—	9×10^{-4}	2×10^{-6}	0
n-Bu	4.7×10^{-1}	3.4×10^{-1}	6.3×10^{-2}	3.7×10^{-2}	0
n-Am	5.7×10^{-1}	4.7×10^{-1}	2×10^{-1}	5.4×10^{-2}	4.9×10^{-5}

*Me = Methyl, Et = Ethyl, Pr = Propyl, B = Butyl, Am = Amyl

Modified from Jones D.G., Limaye, S.H., and Young, B.R. 1972. Biocides for the petroleum industry and allied trades. J. Inst. Petrol., *58*(563), 268–271.

al., 1980) by 1,3,5-tris(tetrahydro-2-furanylmethyl)hexahydro-s-triazine (Table 17–1). Over a 9-week period in two metalworking fluids, 0.1% of the furfural derivative controlled fungal populations of approximately 10^4 cfu/ml; at the same level, the 2-hydroxyethyl triazine allowed fungal levels to be at the same level as the control (Table 17–4).

One mechanism proposed (Grier et al., 1980) is based on the greater solubility of the furfural derivative in n-octanol, assuming a greater penetrability into the fungal cell membrane (Hansch and Lien, 1971). This untested hypothesis is based on the assumptions that (1) the intact triazine penetrates the fungal protoplast and hydrolyses in the cytoplasm to CH$_2$O and furfural, and (2) the furfural makes no contribution to the antimicrobial activity of the triazine. The differential effect could be due to the greater instability of hydroxyethyl derivative in the contaminated system. For the first 2 weeks, fungal populations were controlled equally with either triazine derivative. The condensation of CH$_2$O with an antifungal agent, released by hydrolysis, would appear to be the

most reasonable approach to fungal control with these products.

A compound that appears to combine CH$_2$O release with known or presumed antifungal activity is 3,5-dimethyltetrahydro-1,3,5(2H)-thiadiazine-2-thione (Table 17–1). According to Bennett (1973), this compound was the most active CH$_2$O releaser in experimental metalworking systems. It has also been suggested, however, that N-methyl dithiocarbamate is one product of alkaline hydrolysis (Ross and Hollis, 1976). This compound is a known antislime, antifungal agent used in a number of industrial systems (Trotz and Pitts, 1981; Sharpell, 1980).

No verification has been published of frank CH$_2$O release from cyclic formaldehyde condensates except after quaternization (Scott and Wolf, 1962; Graymore, 1938). The relative stability of HTs under alkaline conditions seems to preclude this event. No CH$_2$O was detected from ethyl, hydroxyethyl, and hydroxypropyl HT at pH 9, but it was detected at pH 5 using methone complexing (Fig. 17–1) as an aldehyde scavenger (DeMare et al., 1972).

Table 17–4. *Microbial Growth Inhibition by Triazine (I) in Cutting Fluids* Over A 9-Week Period*

Triazine (I) Conc. (%, w/v):		Bacteria (cfu/ml)†						Fungi (cfu/ml)‡					
		0.025		0.05		0.075		0.05		0.075		0.10	
Weeks	Metalworking Fluid:	A	B	A	B	A	B	A	B	A	B	A	B
1		<10	<10	<10	<10	<10	<10	2×10^3	8×10^2	<10	1×10^1	<10	<10
2		<10	<10	<10	<10	<10	<10	2×10^3	7×10^2	<10	9×10^2	<10	<10
3		3×10^2	<10	<10	<10	<10	<10	3×10^3	8×10^3	<10	8×10^3	<10	<10
4		3×10^4	<10	<10	<10	<10	<10	3×10^3	8×10^3	1×10^1	7×10^3	<10	<10
5		5×10^6	<10	3×10^4	<10	<10	<10	2×10^3	5×10^3	3×10^3	4×10^3	<10	<10
6		8×10^6	3×10^4	3×10^8	<10	<10	<10	4×10^3	7×10^3	7×10^3	5×10^3	<10	<10
7		2×10^7	2×10^7	1×10^7	<10	<10	<10	5×10^3	8×10^3	2×10^3	6×10^3	<10	<10
8		4×10^7	3×10^7	2×10^7	<10	<10	<10	5×10^3	8×10^3	5×10^3	6×10^3	<10	<10
9		3×10^7	2×10^7	2×10^7	<10	<10	<10	7×10^3	1×10^4	3×10^3	8×10^3	<10	<10

*Pennwalt oils: A—soluble oil, B—synthetic oil, each inhibitor-free and diluted 1:20 with tap water

†After inoculation, initial bacterial count: A. 6×10^7 cfu/ml; B. 5×10^7 cfu/ml. Control fluids, no triazine (I) addition: 1–9 Weeks: A. $3–7 \times 10^8$ cfu/ml. B. $5 \times 10^7 - 1 \times 10^8$ cfu/ml.

‡Initial fungal count: A. 5×10^3 cfu/ml; B. 8×10^4 cfu/ml. 1–9 Weeks: A. $3–9 \times 10^4$ cfu/ml; B. $3–8 \times 10^4$ cfu/ml.

From Grier, N., Witzel, B.E., Jakubowski, J.A., and Dulaney, E.L. 1980. A broad spectrum hexahydro-s-triazine inhibitor of microbial deterioration in cutting fluids. Dev. Indust. Microbiol., *21*, 411–418.

Methone   Formaldehyde   Dimethone (precipitates)

Fig. 17–1. Formation of an insoluble adduct from methone and formaldehyde.

This lack of responsiveness at alkaline pH did little to help explain the antimicrobial activity at those pH values. A series of reports (Neely, 1963a and b) suggested that low levels of CH_2O acted by blocking methionine biosynthesis via cyclization with homocysteine (Fig. 17–2). This was confirmed (Holtzman and Rossmoore, 1977) for CH_2O and was demonstrated also for 1,3,5-tris(2-hydroxyethyl) hexahydro-s-triazine. In this instance, the homocysteine was added externally as a neutralizer for CH_2O. At pH 9, homocysteine completely blocked the antibacterial activity of the triazine, whereas at pH 4, only partial neutralization occurred.

This apparent contradiction with regard to CH_2O presence and activity from alkaline treatment of HT and homocysteine neutralization must presume a region localized around the bacterial cell with a net negative charge sufficiently acidic to hydrolyse the HT. This assumption would help explain the decrease in activity of HT in hard water (Bennett, 1974). In this case, Ca^{++} and Mg^{++} could neutralize the free anionic charges on the peptidoglycan (Beveridge and Murray, 1976; Beveridge and Koval, 1981; Rayman and MacLeod, 1975). It would also help to explain in part the potentiation of HT by ethylenediaminetetraacetic acid (EDTA) (Izzat and Bennett, 1979). However, an extensive series of reports (Sondossi et al., 1984, 1985, 1986a, 1986b; Candal and Eagon, 1984; Eagon and Barnes, 1986; Rossmoore and Sondossi, 1988) have demonstrated that CH_2O is indeed the active moiety of most CH_2O condensates, and that this is a quantitative function dependent on the number of CH_2O moles in the adduct molecule.

Demonstration that cross resistance between select CH_2O adducts and CH_2O is also stoichiometric (Sondossi et al., 1986a) (Fig. 17–3) was verified chemically with the Nash reagent (Rossmoore et al., 1986b) (Table 17–5). Additional CH_2O adducts completely mimic CH_2O nei-

Fig. 17–2. Formation of 1,3-thiazane-1-carboxylic acid from formaldehyde and homocysteine. Modified from Neely, W.B. 1963b. Action of formaldehyde on microorganisms. II. Formation of 1,3-thiazane-4-carboxylic acid in *Aerobacter aerogenes* treated with formaldehyde. J. Bacteriol., *85*, 1420–1422.

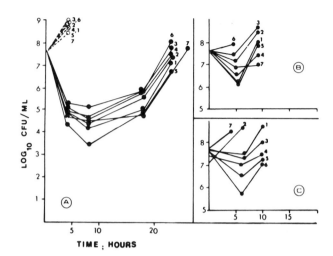

Fig. 17–3. *A*, Exponentially growing sensitive (solid lines) and resistant (dotted lines) strains of *Pseudomonas aeruginosa* were exposed to 3 mM of formaldehyde and equimolar concentration of biocides (3 mM available formaldehyde). 1, formaldehyde; 2, 1,3,5-tris-(ethyl)-hexahydro-s-triazine; 3, 1,3,5-tris-(2-hydroxyethyl)hexahydro-s-triazine; 4, 4,4-dimethyloxazolidine, a commercial mixture; 5, 2-(hydroxymethyl)aminoethanol; 6, 2-(hydroxymethyl)amino-2-methyl propanol; 7, a commercial mixture of 3 and 16 (in Table 17–1). *B*, The sensitive strain was induced with 3 mM of formaldehyde. Then cells were exposed to equimolar concentrations (3 mM available formaldehyde) of biocides. *C*, The sensitive strain was induced with biocides (3 mM available formaldehyde), then exposed to 3 mM of formaldehyde. From Sondossi, M., Rossmoore, H.W., and Wireman, J.W. 1986a. The effect of fifteen biocides on formaldehyde-resistant strains of *Pseudomonas aeruginosa*. J. Ind. Microbiol., *1*, 87–96.

ther biologically nor chemically. It appears that the stability of an CH_2O adduct with respect to the relative avidity of a specific reagent (e.g., Nash) determines the level of activity of that adduct. It should also be emphasized that pH may play an important role in adduct stability and subsequent availability of CH_2O. The electron deficiency of the carbonyl group makes it highly reactive with nucleophiles, especially amines and thiols (Paulus, 1988).

The most reactive adducts may in fact reflect the reactivity of mixtures rather than pure compounds. These mixtures would include untreated CH_2O in equilibrium with other components and potential end products (Eggensperger, 1971, personal communication; Rossmoore, 1979). The continual consumption of CH_2O by biologic molecules would shift equilibrium in that direction.

A contributing factor to both resistance development (Sondossi et al., 1985; Eagon and Barnes, 1986) and mode of action (Barnes and Eagon, 1986; Jacobson, unpublished data) is reaction of available CH_2O with essential thiol groups in the cell. Increase in glutathione levels in resistant isolates is related to increase in glutathione-dependent formaldehyde dehydrogenase (Table 17–5). Crosslinking of sulfhydryls from cysteine moieties, especially sulfhydryl-dependent essential enzymes (e.g., ATPase), is a most probable lethal target. Formaldehyde adducts readily donate CH_2O to both amines and thiols with the former readily able to act as temporary repos-

Table 17–5. *Specific Activity of Formaldehyde Dehydrogenase (FADH) in Cell-Free Extracts of* Pseudomonas Aeruginosa

Strain	Inducer	NAD⁺-Linked FADH (μmol NADH/min per mg protein)		DCPIP[a]-Linked FADH (nmol DCPIP/min per mg protein)	
		Glutathione-Independent	Glutathione-Dependent	PMS[b]-Independent	PMS-Dependent
ATCC 27853	None	ND[c]	11.20	ND	1.047
ATCC 27853	ET[d]	7.90	82.44	ND	0.71
Sensitive	None	ND	2.65	ND	ND
Sensitive	ET	4.08	47.19	ND	ND
Resistant	None	ND	219.59	2.26	9.86
Resistant	ET	11.79	200.23	5.94	26.49
Resistant	Methanol	2.375	260.13	3.5	13.48

[a]DCPIP = 2,6-dichlorophenolindophenol
[b]PMS = phenazine methosulfate
[c]ND = not detectable
[d]ET = 1,3,5-tris-(ethyl)hexahydro-s-triazine

From Sondossi, M., Rossmoore, H.W., and Wireman, J.W. 1986b. Induction and selection of formaldehyde-based resistance in *Pseudomonas aeruginosa*. J. Ind. Microbiol., *1*, 97–103.

itories (i.e., N-methylol) of CH_2O. Studies with Cu^{++} and CH_2O or CH_2O adducts reinforce the central role of sulfhydryls in mechanism of action and resistance because these mixtures show synergism (Rossmoore, 1986; Sondossi et al., 1990) and Cu^{++} alone reduces the level of free sulfhydryl (Jacobson, unpublished data).

The primary use of HTs in water-soluble metalworking fluids impacts these biocides with a large variety of metals, most of which are highly insoluble at alkaline pH. Several amphoteric elements, including aluminum and tin, however, are in solution at high enough levels to possibly interact with HT. Under dose-limiting conditions, aluminum chips reduce the effectiveness of hydroxyethyl HT but not ethyl HT. This result is related most probably to the highly electropositive character of aluminum as well as to the electronegative N-O zone that chelates Al^{+++}, eventually reducing or slowing hydrolysis of HT (Rossmoore, 1979).

Several highly electropositive cations (Mg^{+++}, Al^{+++}) also reduced the activity of hydroxyethyl HT (Rossmoore, 1979). The acyclic metholated nitrogen compounds are no less complex in their variety and include fairly unstable as well as highly stable adducts.

Methylolation of haloalkyl amines (Paulus et al., 1967) yields an active but readily hydrolyzable formaldehyde condensate. A commercially successful version is N-methylol chloroacetamide (Grotan HD). It has an extremely short half-life at alkaline pH values and therefore has limited application in longterm preservation. Because of this and other shortcomings, it has been withdrawn from the U.S. market by its manufacturers.

Mercaptobenzothiazole (MBeT) has an antimicrobial life of its own. However, methylolation (Paulus, 1980) of MBeT increases the activity of the adduct 15-fold against *Pseudomonas fluorescens* and *Pseudomonas aeruginosa* without reducing activity against 12 other species of bacteria and fungi. Other possible functions of MBeT will be discussed later.

All of the preceding formaldehyde condensates re-

sulted from the methylolation of amino nitrogen, covalently bonding nitrogen to the carbon of the methylol group. In addition, several methylolated compounds are based on nitromethane in which the formaldehyde alkylates the carbon atom (Wheeler and Bennett, 1956; Bennett and Hodge, 1961) (Table 17–1).

Wheeler and Bennett (1956) found tris(hydroxymethyl)nitromethane (TN) to be one of the most effective of a large group of antimicrobial additives for metalworking fluids. It was further described as a slow formaldehyde releaser. This is evidenced in the cross-resistance studies of Sondossi et al. (1986a) in which tris-nitro at more than 10 times the equivalent CH_2O levels not only did not reduce viable population levels but actually increased levels. Although survivors of CH_2O treatment were not resistant to TN, TN survivors were relatively resistant to CH_2O. However, this was at pH 7, whereas most effective applications of tris-nitro are above pH 8. TN is a highly cost-effective compound, and although it has the same shortcomings as all commercially used formaldehyde adducts, i.e., it is less effective against fungi than against bacteria, it has been used with confidence for 20 years.

An extensive number of additional compounds can, from their structures or method of synthesis, be assumed to release CH_2O to account for their antimicrobial activity. Many of these are nitroparaffin derivatives (Bennett et al., 1960); another group are heterocyclic, e.g., hydantoins or oxazolidines or imidazoles (Bennett, 1973; Sharpell, 1980; Sidi and Johnson, 1975; Rosen and Berke, 1973). Most of these latter structures are used as contaminant-limiting preservatives in closed systems such as in-can latex paint, adhesives, and cosmetics (Table 17–1).

In addition to HTM, three other CH_2O adducts have been used chemically with apparent success. The first, polyoxymethylurea (Haler and Aebi, 1961; Haler, 1963), was effective against gram-positive coccal infection but only minimally effective against vaginal moniliasis. The thiourea derivative, noxythiolin, was used favorably to treat fecal peritonitis (Browne and Staller, 1970). An initial assumption (Kingston, 1965) stating that activity of both compounds was directly related to CH_2O release was later substantiated (Gidley and Sanders, 1983).

The third of these compounds was first reported by Browne et al. (1976). Taurolin is based on the condensation of taurine, aminosulfonic acid, NH_3, and CH_2O. It was found effective against both *Ps. aeruginosa* and *Salmonella typhimurium* infections in mice (Browne et al., 1976), in mitigation of clinical bacterial peritonitis (Browne et al., 1978), and in neutralization of lipopolysaccharide (LPS) endotoxin from a number of gram-negative bacteria (Pfirrmann and Leslie, 1979).

A most interesting similarity between these compounds relates to activity ascribed to them and not to CH_2O. Gorman et al. (1987) concluded that, in fact, noxythiolin was superior to equivalent CH_2O as a candidicide, and Gidley et al. (1981) similarly concluded that taurolin activity was based on a methylimminium ion and was likewise superior to equivalent CH_2O. The authors either erroneously measured "free" CH_2O for noxythiolin or used one CH_2O equivalent rather than three for taurolin. After making corrections for this error, the activity of both compounds is seen to be related directly to CH_2O.

The LPS-neutralizing activity of taurolin was also demonstrated with CH_2O and several CH_2O adducts (Douglas et al., 1990), emphasizing that any activity ascribed to CH_2O condensates is most probably due to CH_2O. Recently, an extensive update of taurolin in-vitro bacteriology was published (Broadhage and Pfirrmann, 1985).

NITRITE

Perhaps no single reaction has achieved greater notoriety recently than the reaction of NO_2^- with a variety of environmentally available amines, forming presumably carcinogenic adducts (N-nitrosamines). Thus, the practicality of using an antimicrobial based on the nitrite radical is open to question. Several reports of activity and, indeed, one important use require, however, that a short discussion be included here.

The wisdom of nitrite use in cured meats has been debated (Ingram, 1976). Germane to this section, however, is an evaluation of a possible mode of action of NO_2^- on *Clostridium botulinum* metabolism. The net result of nitrite use, and the only rationale for that use, is the absence of botulinum toxin in the food being protected. Action can take place at four sites: (1) inhibition of germination, (2) inhibition of outgrowth, (3) inhibition of cell division, and (4) inhibition of toxigenesis. Current thinking (Sofos et al., 1979; Duncan and Foster, 1968a and b; Christiansen et al., 1974) concludes that nitrite does not inhibit germination and that possibly the germinated spore is particularly sensitive to nitrite, because in one report (Christiansen et al., 1978), death was proportional to residual nitrite.

An added safety factor to be noted in nitrite use is its anomalous lack of activity versus aerobic bacteria, permitting maximal population densities in the presence of 156 ppm NO_2^- (Bayne and Michener, 1975). However, *Salmonella* species are relatively resistant to 400 ppm NO_2^-, even after EDTA treatment (Page and Solberg, 1979). From a pragmatic viewpoint, contaminated prepared meat should show visible signs of spoilage while inhibiting botulinum toxin formation. Certainly the consumption of spoiled food is a less likely prospect, making botulism an even lesser possibility.

Other effects of nitrite have been reported: transient inhibition of CO_2 production from glucose (5 ppm) or protein hydrolysate (10 ppm in an acid forest soil) (Bancroft et al., 1979) and suppression (30%) of O_2 consumption by *Pseudomonas fluorescens* (Wodzinski et al., 1978) at 14 ppm. This latter fact is interesting because NO_2^- can be reductively assimilated by some *Pseudomonas* species. These separate and distinctive concerns with NO_2^- in foods and soils (artificial and natural ecosystems) emphasize the importance of control over disposition of putative antimicrobial residues.

NITRILES

The nitrile group is highly reactive, made more so by the presence of a halogen atom on the same or adjacent carbon atoms. The simplest derivative is the cyanide radical (CN^-), a well known inhibitor of oxidative phosphorylation (Wilson and Chance, 1967). Like many other highly electronegative radicals, CN^- forms complexes with Fe^{++}. Because of its toxicity, it is limited to research application. It may help ascertain sensitive enzyme sites in some organisms whose control is of economic importance.

Lactate metabolism, but not glucose or pyruvate, is sensitive to CN^- (Rossmoore et al., 1964). Subsequently (Czechowski and Rossmoore, 1990), heme iron (cytochrome C_3) was found as a component of the lactic dehydrogenase complex of *Desulfovibrio desulfuricans*. Historically, several naturally occurring oils (onion, garlic, mustard) containing allyl isothiocyanate have been used empirically for preservation, and more recently, antifungal activity has been demonstrated for a broad group of naturally occurring isothiocyanates and their derivatives (Drobnica et al., 1967a and b).

On a more practical level, during the past 20 years, a number of nitrile derivatives have been used with increasing frequency in a variety of industrial systems requiring antimicrobial protection. Wehner (1965, 1966, 1967) and Wehner and Hinz (1971) reported on the activity of thiocyanate derivatives (Table 17–6)—more specifically, bisthiocyanates. These were recommended for cooling waters, for drilling muds, and in some paper and pulp systems. This group of compounds is active at low levels but has minimal activity at alkaline pH. This fact makes it completely unsuitable for metalworking fluids, which are always poised above pH 7. It is unfortunate that methylenebisthiocyanate (MBT) has been suggested for metalworking fluids.

Table 17–6. *In Vitro Evaluation of Thiocyanates*

Structure	Aspergillus flavus	Bacillus mycoides	Chaetomium globosum	Fusarium moniliforme	Penicillium citrinum	Trichoderma viridae
NCS—CH₂—SCN (NCS—C(H)(H)—SCN)	2.5	2.5	2.5	2.5	2.5	
H SCN / NCS H C=C (vinyl dithiocyanate)	6.25	2.5	2.5	2.5	2.5	2.5
NCS—CH₂—CH₂—SCN	>50	>50	25	25	>50	50
Cl—CH₂—CH₂—SCN	50	>50	50	50	50	50
H—CH₂—NCS	>500	>500	250	250	500	500
NCS—CH₂(CH₂)₄CH₂—SCN	>500	>500	>125	>500	>500	>500
H—CH₂—SCN	>500	>500	125	500	500	500
O=S—(SCN)₂	>500	>500	>500	>500	>500	>500
Cl—C₆H₄—CO—CH₂—SCN	>50	>50	25	25	25	>50
Zn(SCN)₂	>50	>50	25	50	50	50

*Minimum inhibiting concentration in ppm
From Wehner, D.C., and Hinz, C.F. 1971. Organic thiocyanates as industrial antimicrobial agents. Dev. Indust. Microbiol., *12*, 404–410.

The potential for cyanide formation was explored from degradation of MBT. Only with strong reducing agents at alkaline pH is any CN⁻ produced, and even this is minimal (Wehner and Hinz, 1971). It has been used in fuel oil bottom water with modest success (Klemme and Leonard, 1971). Certainly, if alkaline pH is avoided, cyanide should be no trouble. Friend and Whitekettle (1980) have speculated that MBT may act as an uncoupler of oxidative phosphorylation. The thiocyanate radical may indeed inhibit that reaction as readily as cyanide.

Another nitrile derivative (Wolf and Sterner, 1972), 2,2-dibromo-3-nitrilopropionamide (DBNPA), was first introduced as a slimicide for cooling tower treatments as well as in paper manufacturing (pulp slurries). The compound currently is well accepted in these areas and also, in limited application, in metalworking fluids: namely, in the forming of two-piece aluminum cans. It is sold as a 5%, 10%, or 20% active compound in a polyglycol solution. Care must be taken in interpreting the dosage levels reported in the literature because most of DBNPA is sold under proprietary label that inclusively covers the concentration without so stating. In a laboratory evaluation (Friend and Whitekettle, 1980), both the formulated ^{14}C glucose 50% incorporating dose and the pure material dose were reported. Notice the variation in doses needed to control the eight different organisms (Table 17–7).

The performance of DBNPA is based on rapid action and dissipation. This is highly advantageous where continual discharge of treated process water is required, e.g., once-through cooling water, because the residue is without apparent toxicity (Meitz, 1984). In addition, it is compatible and possibly synergistic with chlorine in treating cooling waters (Walter et al., 1985).

Rapid dissipation (Exner et al., 1973), however, is not always favorable. DBNPA is severely affected by alkaline pH, temperatures above ambient temperature, and nucleophilic reagents. Above pH 8.5 and at elevated temperatures, the hydrolysis products can cause severe lacrimation. This is especially true if excessive levels (more than twice the recommended dose) of DBNPA are reached. Thus, slug doses in metalworking operations are to be avoided where operational temperatures are high. Nucleophilic reagents react readily, debrominating DBNPA and leaving an inactive adduct. Using DBNPA in areas containing high sulfide levels, e.g., drilling muds and metalworking fluids, could greatly decrease efficiency of the biocide.

The pH sensitivity and decomposition pathway may offer a clue to a potential mode of action. *Escherichia coli* quickly removed DBNPA from solution, but ^{14}C-DBNPA was not found in the cell, dead cells being more active in the removal than living cells (Friend and Whitekettle, 1980). Thus, adsorption to the cell surface could be blamed for inhibition of "C-glucose accumulation." Beta-galactoside permease activity was also inhibited (Wolf, 1974), but not without killing the cells.

A comparison of the preservative activity of a series of propenenitriles in two types of latex paint was made in which compounds were based on 2-methyl piperidine.

No cohesive hypothesis could be developed to explain the variation in bacterial growth in inoculated systems based on R-group structure (Dybas et al., 1978) (Fig. 17–3, Table 17–8). Possibly the mechanism proposed by Dybas et al. could explain how this absence of the olefin double bond (methylene group) decreases reactivity for the electron-rich nucleophile. Whether the adduct from Figure 17–4 is the basis for inhibition is partly speculative.

A nitrile derivative, 1,2-dibromo-2,4-dicyanobutane (Grier and Lederer, 1974, 1975), is recommended for a wide variety of preservative uses as disparate as latex paint emulsions and water-soluble metalworking fluids (Table 17–1). Effectiveness is claimed against bacteria, fungi, and algae associated with the deterioration of paints, adhesives, cements, and metalworking fluids. This is a proprietary compound of Merck Chemical (Tektomer 38), registered with both the EPA and the FDA (cleared for use in food contact adhesives). It is sufficiently stable at pH 9 to 10 to use in metalworking fluid concentrates at 10 to 30 times the use dosages (0.025 to 0.1%). Although no statements have been provided on the mode of action of this compound, it is composed of several highly electron-withdrawing centers, reminiscent of DBNPA. Possibly, they are strongly reactive with nucleophilic groups in the cell. This may be the basis for the synergism claimed with isothiazolones (Jakubowski and Bennett, 1987). Based on both acute and subchronic toxicity testing, claims are made for reduced hazards in applications of Tektomer 38 (Lederer et al., 1983).

DYES

No group of commercial compounds is so intimately tied to the history and the fabric of microbiology as the dye group (Rossmoore, 1983). Aside from their use as selective agents in stain and media, the triphenylmethane dyes have had a checkered, broad-spectrum career. Official preparations (e.g., USP) and others have been recommended for a wide variety of infections, from the top of the head (tinea capitis, i.e., ringworm of the scalp) to the bottom of the feet (tinea pedis, i.e., athlete's foot) and just about everything in between for bacteria, yeast, fungi, protozoans, and helminths.

Table 17–7. *Antimicrobial Activity of Biocide Active Ingredients*

Biocide	I_{30} (μg/ml)* Microorganisms							
	Klebsiella pneumoniae	*Bacillus megaterium*	*Candida krusei*	*Trichoderma viridae*	*Chlorella pyrenoidosa*	*Scenedesmus obliquus*	*Anacystis nidulans*	*Anabaena flos-aquae*
Methylene bis (thiocyanate) (MBT)	2.7	1.5	3.1	0.7	1.4	1.2	1.0	2.5
2,2-Dibromo-3-nitrilopropionamide (DBNPA)	26 (5.1)	6.3 (1.2)	80 (16)	50 (10)	55 (11)	100 (20)	5.5 (1.1)	7.5 (1.5)
β-Bromo-β-nitrostyrene (BNS)	3.6	2.5	2.0	0.6	0.85	5.0	1.5	0.7

*I_{30} values determined by inhibition of incorporation of ^{14}C-labeled carbon source after 4 hours. MBT = 95% active; BNS = 92% active; DBNPA = 20% active; ( ) = estimated I_{30} for DBNPA, 100% active.

From Friend, P.L., and Whitekettle, W.K. 1980. Biocides and water cooling towers. Dev. Indust. Microbiol., *21*, 123–131.

Table 17–8. *Preservative Action of 2-(Substituted Piperidinomethyl)-Propenenitriles in Acrylic Paint*

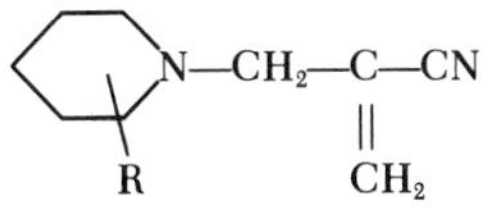

| | *Microbial Growth Rating** | | | | | | | | | | | | | | |
| Days of Incubation: | 1 | | | 2 | | | 3 | | | 7 | | | 14† | | |
Concentration, % by Weight	0.1	0.05	0.01	0.1	0.05	0.01	0.1	0.05	0.01	0.1	0.05	0.01	0.1	0.05	0.01
1. R = H	0	3	4	0	0	4	0	0	0	0	0	0	0	0	0
2. 4-HO	0	3	4	0	0	4	0	0	4	0	0	0	0	0	0
3. 3-HO	0	0	0	0	0	1	0	0	4	0	0	4	0	0	4
4. 3-HOCH$_2$	0	0	4	0	3	4	0	0	4	0	0	0	0	0	4
5. 4-CONH$_3$	0	0	0	0	0	4	0	0	4	0	0	4	0	0	4
6. 4-CONHC$_4$H$_9$	4	4	4	4	4	4	4	4	4	0	4	4	0	0	4
7. 4-COOC$_2$H$_5$	0	4	4	4	4	4	4	4	4	0	0	4	0	0	4
8. 4-COOH	2	3	4	3	3	4	0	1	4	0	0	0	0	0	0
9. 4-HO, 4-⟨phenyl⟩ 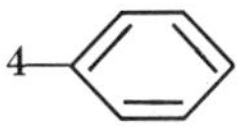	1	1	2	0	4	4	4	4	4	0	0	4	0	1	4
10. 4-N⟨cyclohexyl⟩ 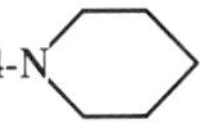	4	4	4	0	3	4	0	4	4	0	0	4	0	0	4
11. bis-4,4'-(—CH$_2$CH$_2$CH$_2$—)	4	4	4	4	4	4	4	4	4	0	3	4	0	4	4
12. 4-C(CH$_3$)$_3$	4	4	4	4	4	4	4	4	4	0	4	4	0	4	4
13. 4-CH$_2$—⟨cyclohexyl⟩ 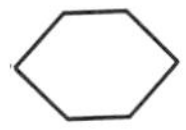	4	4	4	4	4	4	4	4	4	3	4	4	4	4	4
14. 4-F	4	4	4	4	4	4	4	4	4	4	4	4	4	4	4
15. 4-HO, benzyl bromide quat.	0	0	4	0	0	4	0	0	4	4	0	4	0	4	4
16. 4-HO, methyl iodide quat.	0	2	4	0	0	4	0	0	4	4	4	4	3	4	4
Phenylmercuric acetate	0	0	0	0	0	0	0	0	0	0	0	0	0	0	0

*0 = no growth; 1 = 1 to 5 colonies; 2 = 6 to 25 colonies; 3 = more than 25 isolated colonies; 4 = confluent growth

†After 7 days of paint incubation, a reinoculation with *Pseudomonas aeruginosa* is made, and samplings are taken on day 14.

From Dybas, R.A., et al. 1978. 2-(substituted piperidinomethyl) preopenenitriles and analogs as preservatives in aqueous systems. Dev. Indust. Microbiol., *19*, 347–353.

The use of gentian violet in vaginal gels and suppositories to treat moniliasis and trichomoniasis, although no longer in vogue, points out a fundamental shortcoming of the dyes and other antimicrobials that are also colorants (e.g., iodine, mercurochrome). They stain clothing, bedding, and noninfected body parts as well as the infected areas. One of the original topical dye antiseptics, Castellani's stain, was based on carbol-fuchsin and contained 0.3% fuchsin as well as boric acid and resorcinol (APhA, 1936).

Oxyuriasis (pinworm) and strongyloidiasis have been treated internally with gentian violet (Goodman and Gilman, 1958b). This therapy has passed from the scene. Later, two triphenyl methane dyes were used in jet fuel bottom water without much success (Klemme and Neihof, 1969).

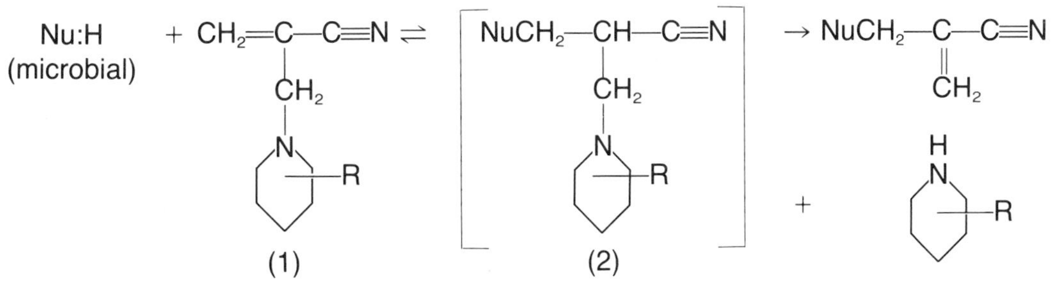

Fig. 17–4. Potential inhibition mechanism for propenenitriles. Modified from Dybas, R.A., et al. 1978. 2-(substituted piperidinemethyl) propenenitriles and analogs as preservatives in aqueous systems. Dev. Indust. Microbiol., *19*, 347–353.

PYRIDINES

Structures containing the pyridine moiety are potentially excellent candidates for antimicrobial agents if this presumption is based solely on their relationship to two critical metabolites, nicotinamide and pyridoxal. Activity against a broad spectrum of microorganisms has been reported in chemotherapy (Shipman et al., 1981; Schmidt et al., 1978; Fox, 1953; Casero et al., 1980; Priestly and Savin, 1976), preservative activity (Wolf and Bobalek, 1967; Rossmoore et al., 1972; DeMare et al., 1972; Rossmoore et al., 1978; Klemme and Leonard, 1971; Klemme and Neihof, 1976; Cooney and Felix, 1972; Edmonds and Cooney, 1968), and antiseborrheic activity (Imokawa, 1982).

Perhaps the first compound in this group with significant antimicrobial activity was isonicotinyl hydrazine (isoniazid) (INH) (Table 17–1). It has been an accepted part of the chemotherapeutic regimen for tuberculosis for almost 30 years; however, despite an extensive amount of research on its mode of action, no consensus appears to have been reached on a single metabolic site.

Davis and Weber (1977) report that INH competes with NAD^+ on a regulatory site in the electron transport pathway in *Mycobacterium phlei*. They present evidence that INH may function in destroying membrane activity. Similar qualitative effects were also reported for *Mycobacterium tuberculosis*, indicating that use of the saprophytic strain for antimicrobial evaluation is valid. A more recent report (Herman and Weber, 1980b) offers evidence that NAD^+ and INH have different binding sites in the electron transport system and that INH had no effect on binding affinity; it could neither block nor displace while interfering with NAD^+-dependent membrane dehydrogenase in *Mycobacterium*. Another potential mode of action (Herman and Weber, 1980a) is related to the in-vitro neutralization of INH by tyrosine. Tyrosine moieties in active sites of membrane LDH reacting with INH could lose their affinity for NAD^+ regulatory activity. Still another mechanism is proposed: inhibition of synthesis of long-chain fatty acids (Davidson and Takayama, 1979), interference with transaminase activity (Beggs and Jenne, 1967), and interference with nucleic acid synthesis (Gangadharam et al., 1963; Wimpenny, 1967). This latter activity has been partially verified with DNA gene probe studies (Kawa et al., 1989).

Another pyridine-derived group, 2-acetyl-pyridine thiosemicarbazones (Table 17–1), was reported by Domagk et al. (1946). These were primarily found to be inhibitory to *M. tuberculosis*, and it was during their synthesis that the activity of INH, an intermediate, was discovered (Fox, 1953). A postulated mechanism deduced from the structures of the most active compounds suggests ligand formation with an iron-containing parasite enzyme, blocking its activity (Casero et al., 1980). Other derivatives were found to inhibit *Staphylococcus aureus*, *Neisseria gonorrhoeae*, and *Neisseria meningitidis* while exhibiting minimal activity against gram-negative rods (e.g., enterobacteria) (Dobek et al., 1980).

Shipman et al. (1981) reported for the first time in-vitro inhibition of herpes simplex virus strains 1 and 2 by 2-acetylpyridine thiosemicarbazone derivatives. All of the compounds tested were differentially more active against the virus than the host cell culture was.

These selected reports emphasize the broad spectrum demonstrated for some pyridine derivatives. The thiosemicarbazones and INH have in common a potentially nucleophilic attraction site in the region of the $N=N, C=N$, also reminiscent of nitrilo compounds discussed previously.

Another interesting group of pyridine derivatives, 2,6-substituted 4-pyridinemethanol (Table 17–1), exhibited marked success in controlling the schizont stage of *Plasmodium falciparum* and otherwise resistant strains of *Plasmodium vivax* in owl monkeys (Schmidt et al., 1978). This finding is interesting because similar compounds were bypassed in the search for antimalarial agents during World War II.

One of the compounds described previously (Schmidt et al., 1978), enpiroline [DL-threo-alpha-(2-piperidyl)-2-trifluoromethyl-6-(4-trifluoromethylphenyl) 4-pyridinemethanol], successful against chloroquin-resistant *P. falciparum*, was found to have similar crystal and molecular structure to cinchona alkaloids (Karle and Karle, 1989). This is an excellent example of molecular design determining biologic activity.

Pyridine compounds have also been used extensively as antiseptics and preservatives as well as in chemotherapy. The compounds with the longest track record as well as the broadest diversity of application are derived from 2-pyridine-thiol-1-oxide (Table 17–1). Bernstein, the coauthor of the patent covering this discovery, also investigated INH derivatives against *Mycobacterium tuberculosis* (Bernstein et al., 1953). This affirms again the continuity among antimicrobial agents, whether they are used for chemotherapy or disinfection.

Exploitation of this compound began with use in shampoo, presumably to control seborrheic dermatitis (Tenenbaum and Opdyke, 1967; Orentreich, 1972). In this preparation, the zinc salt (Table 17–1) is used, giving some clue to a suggested mode of action. Albert (1968) stated that the activity of the pyridinethione depended on its coordinating property, i.e., the iron chelate being active, not the free pyridine compound. This was analogous to oxine (8-copper-hydroxyquinolate), the only oxyquinoline derivative with chelating properties and the only one with antimicrobial activity (Albert et al., 1956b). In studies on *Paracoccus denitrificans*, Smit et al. (1980) found similar results with several 2,2'-bipyridyl derivatives. Copper complexes of the bipyridyls or noninhibitory levels of $CuSO_4$ plus the bipyridyls, but not the free ligand, interfered with cell growth.

In addition to chelation, a number of mechanisms have been proposed for the pyridinethiols, beginning in 1953 (Pansy et al., 1953). Yale (1964) suggested that the similarity between pyridinethione and nicotinic acid and pyridoxal could be used to explain the antimicrobial activity. Chandler and Segel (1978) studied the effect of sodium pyridinethiol and related compounds on ATP levels, transport, and protein synthesis in *Penicillium chrysogenum* and *P. notatum*. There appears to be evidence showing impairment of all three functions in the *Penicillium* species. In addition, the interference with protein synthesis appeared related to a drop in transaminase activity. This, in part, was inferred previously (Cooney and Felix, 1972) when pyridoxine (cotransaminase) was shown to partially reverse pyrithione inhibition of *Cladosporium resinae*. Although even partial reversal of inhibition could be significant, in this case it was accomplished by using a ratio of antagonist to metabolite of 100:1, an inverse of the ratio normally expected of competitive inhibition.

The pyridinethiols are used in a wide number of preservative applications (Rossmoore, 1979; Sharpell, 1980; Trotz and Pitts, 1981), including adhesives, plastics, latex paints, and polyurethane foam. Perhaps the most notable success has been in controlling fungi in water-based metalworking fluids (Rossmoore et al., 1978), especially in combinations with some triazines. Recently, it has been increasingly necessary to control microbial growth in fuel-storage entrained water, especially of sulfate-reducing bacteria. The sodium salt of pyridinethiol was found effective in seawater/avgas (aviation fuel) mixtures of 20 ppm (Klemme and Leonard, 1971). A series of derivatives was tested in distillate fuel (Table 17–9). Notice that neither the tertiary butyl amine derivative nor the bispyridinethiol had any advantage over the parent compound.

The need for the presence of the 2-mercapto derivative of N-oxide pyridine seen earlier (Chandler and Segel, 1978) was confirmed by evaluation of the activity of the photodegradation products of pyrithiones (Neihof et al., 1979). In the presence of sunlight, the photodegradation products are noninhibitory and, by extension, also environmentally nontoxic. It has been claimed in a patent application (Eggensperger et al., 1975), however, that 2-mercapto pyridine is an active agent.

Wolf and Bobalek (1967) reported on the many uses and broad spectrum of two chlorinated pyridines. Effectiveness was claimed against bacteria, including *D. desulfuricans*, and fungi in cement, asphalt, metalworking emulsions, and paints. Both the tetrachloro and a propyl trichloro were commercially exploited for paint preservation, especially retardation of surface mildew, although it is reputed to be effective in protecting can contents as well as painted surfaces (Greminger, 1972). Keith (1971) stated that the tetrachloro compound was unstable in the presence of certain amines, even in some paint systems. For this reason and possibly others, the products are no longer available commercially.

Another tetrachloro pyridine derivative, nitrapyrin, is a well characterized inhibitor of ammonia oxidation by *Nitrosomonas europaea* (Table 17–1). This phenomenon is dose-dependent, low doses inhibiting NH_3 oxidation and higher doses preventing growth. This compound has useful application in agricultural practice as a control of nitrification to slow down leaching of oxidized nitrogen from fertilized soil. This inhibition was found in seven other strains from three genera of NH_3 oxidizers (Belser and Schmidt, 1981), improving the chances for practical success in a variety of soils.

Table 17–9. *Pyridine N-Oxide Derivatives Used on Sulfate-Reducing Bacteria Under Navy Distillate Fuel*

Inhibitor	Conc. (ppm)	Growth Response*		
		3 days	10 days	21 days
None	—†	2	4	4
	—	4	4	4
(A) Sodium pyridyl-N-oxide-2-thiolate	5	2	0	0
	10	2	0	0
(B) 2-(*t*-Butylamine)thio-pyridine-N-oxide	1	3	3	1
	1	4	4	4
	5	3	0	0
	5	1	0	0
	10	<1	0	0
	20	2	0	0
(C) Bis(2-pyridyl-N-oxide)disulfide	1	3	4	4
	5	1,2	0,3	0,3
	10	1	0	0
	20	<1	0	0

*Arbitrary scale based on visible blackening when tube is shaken: 1 = slight gray, 4 = intense opaque black. All assays were run in duplicate, and whenever the responses were the same, a single numerical rating is shown in the table; when the responses were different, both ratings are given.

†Data were gathered in several experiments, each having growth controls containing no inhibitor. These controls were intense black throughout except in the first experiment, designated by a †.

Modified from Klemme, D.E., and Leonard, J.M. 1971. Inhibitors for marine sulfate-reducing bacteria in shipboard fuel storage tanks. Naval Research Laboratory Memorandum Report 2324.

The number of effective and safe topical degerming agents is limited. Chlorhexidine gluconate (CHG) has been the benchmark in this area. Octenidine hydrochloride (Table 17–1), originally reported as a control agent for dental plaque (Slee and O'Connor, 1983), has been successfully evaluated as an in-vivo skin degerming agent using the so-called glove-juice technique (Sedlock and Bailey, 1985). It proved equal or superior to CHG in this study. However, both the antiplaque (in vitro) and the skin degerming studies (on macaque monkeys) exclude direct human contact, indicating that appropriate regulatory agency approval has not thus far been received. A related series of amine derivatives, although not based on pyridine, has also been found to have activity against dental plaque bacteria (Murata et al., 1989).

THIAZOLES

Much of the earlier interest in thiazoles was centered on antiparasitic activity (Cuckler et al., 1955; Brown et al., 1961). However, Staron and Allard (1964) demonstrated the activity of 2(4'thiazolyl) benzimidazole (TBZ) against a plant fungal infection. Currently TBZ has successful application as a paint surface mildewcide (Carter, 1973). Apparently this compound inhibits spore germination (Gottlieb and Kumar, 1970) but is even more effective after germination. Evidence for a more specific primary mode of action is presented by Allen and Gottlieb (1970). They showed that TBZ blocks electron transport before cytochrome C and somewhere between substrate and coenzyme Q; this block is reflected also in inhibition of exogenous respiration of *Penicillium atravenetum*, the test organism.

Another antimicrobial agent based on a thiazole/imidazole structure was reported by Weuffen et al. (1965). Of 33 derivatives tested against both gram-negative and gram-positive species, only 5-(p-methoxyphenyl)-imidazole (2, 1-b) thiazole was effective (Table 17–1). A similarity in structure exists between this compound and TBZ, although the target effect of TBZ was mitochondrial, and this has not been demonstrated in analogous systems in the bacteria used in this study.

A most interesting paper (Dymicky et al., 1977) lists 30 5-nitrothiazole derivatives extremely inhibitory to *C. botulinum*. The minimum inhibitory concentration (MIC) levels extend from 0.9 μg/ml for the parent compound to 0.0025 μg/ml for 2-lauroylamido derivative. Methylation or bromination in the 2 position reduced activity. Although toxicity is not mentioned, one could speculate that the lauroyl compound effective at approximately 10^{-7} M would be a good candidate to evaluate as a food additive.

A followup study (Huhtanen, 1984) on 2-substituted-5-nitrothiazoles demonstrated that several were more effective than $NaNO_2$, with 2-amido-5-nitrothiazole being most effective in preventing can swelling as well as inhibiting toxin formation. Unfortunately, available evidence suggests that these compounds may be carcinogenic.

MERCAPTOBENZOTHIAZOLE

Mercaptobenzothiazole has both antifungal and antibacterial properties, which have been attributed to its chelation qualities (Albert et al., 1947). In addition, it also has commercial popularity as a copper antioxidant (another example of dual utility of some compounds). Perhaps its effectiveness against *D. desulfuricans* (Lewis et al., 1973; Czechowski and Rossmoore, 1981) is due to its chelation of nonheme iron in the LDH complex. Although it is used alone as a slimicide, it is most frequently found in combination with dimethyldithiocarbamate.

Perhaps a more promising group of compounds for industrial control are those based on the isothiazole structure (Lewis et al., 1973; Czechowski and Rossmoore, 1981; Miller and Lewis, 1976; Hinton et al., 1961). The earliest of these is 1,2-benzisothiazolin-3-one, a product of Imperial Chemicals Limited, sold as Proxel. It is compatible with a large number of systems requiring preservation, including adhesives, paper coatings, metalworking fluids, and latex paints, although it is in latex paints that the compound has achieved major prominence. Evidence was presented showing photodegradation in adhesive formulations, probably limiting use under longterm exposure to light (Lugg, 1981).

Currently, a more extensively used group of isothiazoles is based on 4-isothiazolin-3-one. Essentially two types of derivatives have evolved: one primarily for water-based metalworking fluids, hydraulic fluids, and cooling towers (Rossmoore, 1979; Skaliy et al., 1980; Law et al., 1985) in which the population to be controlled includes bacteria, algae, and fungi; and another for paint surfaces (Dupont et al., 1974), fabrics, leather processing, and wood, essentially for mildew protection. The latter derivatives were rated not only for efficacy but also for persistence, an invaluable attribute when materials are exposed to cleaning and weathering. The most effective was found to be 2-n-octyl-3(2H)-isothiazolone, which is sold under a variety of trade names by Rohm and Haas (Skane M-8 for paint; Kathon LM for fabrics; Kathon LP for leather).

A series of N-substituted isothiazolones (ITs) was evaluated for the control of wood decay fungi (Preston et al., 1985), including the N-octyl and 4,5 dichloro N-octyl derivatives. The chlorinated octyl compound was by far the most active of the test organisms and also resisted leaching. This nonchlorinated derivative has also been applied successfully in metalworking fluids in which fungi and not bacteria are the major biodeteriogen (Lashen and Law, 1988).

The former derivatives found most effective are a combination of 5-chloro-2-methyl-3(2H)-isothiazolone and 2-methyl-3(2H)-isothiazolone. This mixture is available commercially as Kathon 886MW (metalworking) and Kathon WT (water treatment), and is also used for a variety of other products and applications.

Another successful application involves treatment of distillate fuel water bottoms and storage tanks (Dorris and Pitcher, 1988; Andrykovitch and Neihof, 1987). A recent patent (Jordan, 1988) makes disinfectant claims for a series of isothiazolin-3-ones, including the previously described compounds. Specifically, N-octyl isothiazolin-3-one is mentioned. In the context of the accepted definition of disinfectant, no evidence is available indicating that these compounds would qualify (i.e., achieve 100% kill in 10 minutes). In addition, the N-octyl derivative has minimal antibacterial activity, its utility being based on its fungicidal efficacy.

No reports have been published on the mode of action of this mixture, although related reports exist on the degradative fate in the environment (Krzeminski et al., 1975). In solution, these compounds are fairly unstable and must be stabilized by calcium and magnesium nitrates. The chloro derivative is first dechlorinated to the 2-methyl compound, after which the ring is opened before further degradation takes place (Table 17–1). Apparently, the loss of chlorine reduces antimicrobial activity considerably because the nonchlorinated compound has little or none. Appreciable loss in activity is also noticed in the presence of nucleophilic reagents (e.g., SH groups), suggesting the possible removal of Cl by such groups.

Czechowski and Rossmoore (1981) reported on a specific effect of several thiazoles, including the isothiazolones, against lactate metabolism in *D. desulfuricans*; only those with a thiazole or isothiazole moiety had any effect on lactate metabolism. Lactic dehydrogenase from *D. desulfuricans* has been characterized as an fe-S enzyme (Czechowski and Rossmoore, 1990) with the potential for interacting with the electrophilic ITs (Paulus, 1988). The reaction of IT with cell nucleophiles is undoubtedly related to mode of action. The use of copper salts has been suggested to protect IT from destructive environmental nucleophiles and nonlethal nucleophile targets in the cell (Piet and Rossmoore, 1985; Rossmoore, 1986; Law and Lashen, 1990; Riha et al., 1990). In addition, a number of synergists based on formaldehyde and glutaraldehyde are available as commercial (Rossmoore and Sondossi, 1988) and experimental (Becrens and Lepage, 1980) products.

Sondossi (unpublished data) showed that CH_2O alone effectively extended the activity of IT. In all of these studies, the mol ratio of Cu^{++} and CH_2O was greatly in excess of the IT levels, indicating that nonlethal target nucleophiles were tied up. This permitted the IT to be available for lethal sites.

The question of resistance selection to IT has also been investigated (Sondossi, unpublished data). Severe sequential underdosing by less than 1-ppm increments resulted in permanent resistance at each step. However, regardless of the level of resistance (1 to 30 ppm), the resistance dose plus about 2 ppm was sufficient to produce lethality.

NITRO DERIVATIVES

The addition of a nitro group to the structure of phenolic antimicrobials increases the activity of those com-

Table 17–10. *Nitroparaffin Compounds and Their Derivatives Effective Against Sulfate-Reducing Bacteria in a Concentration of 25 PPM*

3-chloro-3-nitro-2-butanol
2-chloro-2-nitro-1-butanol stearate
2-chloro-2-nitro-butyl acetate
4-chloro-4-nitro-3-hexanol
1-chloro-1-nitro-2-pentanol
3-chloro-3-nitro-2-pentanol
2-chloro-2-nitro-1-propanol

Modified from Bennett, E.O., Guynes, G.J., and Isenberg, D.L. 1960. The sensitivity of sulfate-reducing bacteria to antibacterial agents. III. The nitroparaffin derivatives. Producers Monthly, *24*(5), 26–27.

pounds. Two nitro groups (e.g., 2,4-dinitrophenol) produce well known inhibitors of oxidative phosphorylation. The trinitrophenol, picric acid, has a modest history of antimicrobial activity. It would appear that no real advantage is realized in the use of nitro derivatives of phenols, because for the small gain in activity an equal gain in toxicity may be seen. However, derivatives of 4-nitrophenol and 2-chloro-4-nitrophenol have been reportedly used as leather fungicides (Dahl and Kaplan, 1960).

In addition to the methylolated nitroparaffins, other derivatives, both aliphatic and aromatic, have demonstrated antimicrobial activity. More than 200 nitroparaffin derivatives were tested for their effect on *D. desulfuricans* (Bennett et al., 1960). More than 150 of these prevented growth at 0.1% or less. Seven were active at 0.0025% (Table 17–10). Notice that all have halogen substitution on the same carbon as the nitro group. This combination makes for a highly reactive molecule most certainly being drawn to nucleophilic groups.

Later, claims were made for two additional halogenated nitro compounds (Table 17–1) (Manowitz et al., 1971, 1975). These were stated to be effective against bacteria, yeasts, filamentous fungi, and algae in a variety of preservative systems, including latex paint, cosmetic lotions, metalworking fluids, cooling water, and pulp and paper waters. However, their major commercial application is in the latter two areas.

Huitric et al. (1956) had previously shown that beta-nitro styrenes had antifungal activity; Friend and Whitekettle (1980) reported similar activity for the bromineless compound against *Klebsiella pneumoniae*. The beta-nitro styrene was taken up by the bacteria, a process requiring energy that was self-limiting, probably due to inhibition of the transport system by nitrostyrene. The hydrolysis of beta-bromo-beta-nitrostyrene yields bromonitromethane and benzaldehyde (Friend and Whitekettle, 1980), environmentally more acceptable compounds than their predecessor. This conclusion is worthy of commentary. Toxicity of antimicrobials is a function of time and place (Ong and Rutherford, 1980; Fan et al., 1978). The production of bromonitromethane in cooling water is considered advantageous; in cosmetics, secondary and tertiary amines are part of the formulation and nitrosamines are produced, a decided disadvantage.

Another compound based partially on bromonitromethane is 2-bromo-2-nitropropanol-1,3-diol (Bronopol) (Table 17–1), which is formed by the bromination of tris-nitro (TN), a putative CH_2O releaser. Bronopol was discussed in the third edition of this book with CH_2O adducts, perhaps with the assumption that its mode of action was via CH_2O release. This was reported at neutral and alkaline pH with CH_2O, accompanied by mixed bromine compounds (Elder, 1980a; Rosen and Berke, 1973). However, these results are not compatible with those reported by Sondossi et al. (1986a), which failed to show cross resistance to CH_2O at stoichiometric equivalence. In addition, no more than 25% of structural CH_2O was detected by Nash reagent at neutral pH (Rossmoore and Sondossi, 1988). Actually, an alternative mechanism based on thiol oxidation (Stretton and Manson, 1973) was presented and reinforced (Shephard et al., 1988) with the caveat, however, that thiol oxidation may not be the only mode of action.

Elsmore (1989), in an efficacy study of Bronopol versus *Legionella pneumophila*, showed that Bronopol activity was greater at pH 8 and 9 than at neutral or acid pH. This is similar to the reactions of tris-nitro, a related nitromethane with presumed CH_2O activity at alkaline pH. Hurwitz and McCarthy (1985) found that μ values for Bronopol and CH_2O were about equal (1 ± 0.01), which implied similar modes of action. Bronopol is also a most effective nitrosating reagent (Fan and Tannenbaum, 1973; Ong and Rutherford, 1980). Triethanolamine, a component in many cosmetic formulas, is nitrosated by the nitro group, the presence of an electron-withdrawing group like bromine on the same carbon increasing its reactivity. Although this propensity for nitrosamine formation may limit its usefulness in some cosmetics, Bronopol still has widespread application in pharmaceutical products, toiletries, consumer products, cooling towers, and metalworking fluids.

Two morpholine derivatives (in Biosan P-1487) also belong to the class of nitroparaffins because one of the starting compounds in the synthesis is nitropropane. However, they could easily be included with formaldehyde condensates or with morpholines. The latter were found to inhibit marine pseudomonads in a diesel bottom-water preservative test (Rossmoore et al., 1988); the basis for the synthesis is reaction with formaldehyde (Hodge, 1965) (Table 17–1). This synthesis points out the necessity of clearly stating the conditions of formaldehyde-yielding adducts. For example, cyclic condensates, such as HTs, yield formaldehyde on sample hydrolysis, whereas acyclic adducts, such as TN, need an available methylol (hydroxymethyl) to yield formaldehyde.

How the morpholine derivatives work has not been fully investigated. The commercial product (Biosan P-1487) is a mixture of the two compounds and is used primarily in metalworking fluids and distillate fuels. It has the advantage of good nonpolar solubility and thus is of value in oil concentrates that are to be emulsified later in water. Equal effectiveness in these systems has been claimed against bacteria and fungi, although a mixture with greater broad-spectrum activity is claimed for a mixture with TN (Purcell and Selleck, 1978).

In a comparative study with other CH_2O adducts and CH_2O, cells induced with the nitromorpholine developed resistance to CH_2O, whereas the converse was not true (Sondossi et al., 1986a). Both nitropropane and morpholine, the other reactants along with CH_2O in nitromorpholine synthesis, whether alone or together, were ineffective (Sondossi, unpublished data).

Another industrial biocide directed toward slime control in paper and paperboard manufacture has a related structure, i.e., N[alpha-(1-nitroethyl)benzyl]ethylenediamine (Metasol J-26, Merck & Co.) (Table 17–1). As in the morpholine compounds, the nitro group and the amino-N are on adjacent carbons.

The last group of nitro compounds are distinctive for their use, both topically and systemically, to control a wide variety of pathogenic microorganisms.

The addition of a 5-nitro to 2-substituted furans was found to produce antimicrobial activity (Dodd and Stillman, 1944). The first compound clinically exploited is still recognized today, 5-nitro-2-furaldehyde semicarbazone (Nitrofurazone or Furacin) (Table 17–1). It is listed officially in USP XX (Furacin) as a broad-spectrum, topical antibacterial agent. It exerts bacteriostatic activity at levels as low as 1:200,000

A related compound is N-(5-nitro-2-furfurylidene)-1-aminohydantoin (Nitrofurantoin or Furadantin) (Table 17–1). Although still recognized as a urinary tract antiseptic (USP XX Nitrofurantoin), it is ineffective against many gram-negative species frequently involved in genitourinary tract infections (e.g., *Proteus* and *Klebsiella*, as well as *Pseudomonas* and *Enterobacter*). To its credit, it has displayed effectiveness against a number of strains of *E. coli*.

The nitrofurans have been a fertile area for antimicrobial research, more than 7000 publications having appeared on this subject before 1967 (Grunberg and Titsworth, 1973). However, little has been reported concerning their mode of action.

Herrlich and Schweigler (1976) demonstrated that nitrofurantoin inhibited inducible protein synthesis when used at low levels. A novel derivative, nifurzide, was found to produce elongation without septation in *E. coli*, whereas at higher doses (50 μg), growth stopped and was followed by cell death. No effects on cell structure were noted, but a large number of nifurzide molecules were bound per cell (7×10^7). Upon cell disruption, similar levels were found in cytoplasm, membrane, and wall, much of it protein bound (Delsarte et al., 1981).

Nifurzide was recently evaluated in vitro against 320 strains of enteropathogens, including *Campylobacter* sp., *Shigella*, *Salmonella*, and *Yersinia*. Best results were achieved for the former two, whereas lesser effects were noted for the latter two (Gavinet and Megraud, 1987).

A related group of 5-nitro heterocyclic compounds are those based on imidazole. One-beta(hydroxyethyl)-2-methyl-5-nitroimidazole was first introduced as an antitrichomoniasis compound and is active in both semen and urine when taken internally. However, it is specifically active against anaerobic and microaerophilic bacteria, and its selective activity and mode of action have been demonstrated (Edwards et al., 1973; Knight et al., 1978). In *Clostridia*, for example, the nitro group is reduced by cell ferredoxin, depriving the cell of reducing capacity. Subsequently, reduced metronidazole destabilizes cell DNA helical structure.

Not only does metronidazole appear to be selective for physiologic type, i.e., only against anaerobes, but in one study, the only surviving species in an ecologic experiment was an anaerobic coccus, *Peptostreptococcus productus* (Bracke et al., 1978). Oral feeding of the drug to *Periplaneta americana* drastically reduced methane production and eliminated bacillary forms from the colon. The survival of the coccal species has clinical implications because, in the treatment of protozoal vaginitis, these organisms may be responsible for post-treatment problems. Another application, far afield from medical use, was investigated by Littman (personal communication). Specific control of anaerobic sulfate reducers was achieved in oil field flood waters.

Nevertheless, metronidazole is widely used to treat anaerobic infections (Tally et al., 1975). In a survey of MICs against 15 anaerobic species of *Bacteroides* and *Clostridium* and including two facultative species (*E. coli* and *Propionibacterium acnes*), Tally et al. (1978) again verified the selectivity of metronidazole for anaerobes; anaerobic MICs ranged from 0.5 to 8.0 μg/ml, whereas the two nonanaerobes were not inhibited by 500 μg/ml.

A further substantiation of the mode of action and selectivity of metronidazole was reported by Hof et al. (1986). Deficiency in nitroreductase in mutants of normally susceptible *Salmonella typhimurium* reduces susceptibility drastically. The potential for susceptibility in facultative organisms exists, especially related to *E. coli* deficient in DNA repair (Yeung et al., 1984). Lethality is a result of DNA damage from a metronidazole reduction product. This conclusion was confirmed and reinforced more recently (Hof et al., 1987).

AMINE DERIVATIVES

These encompass a large and diverse group of compounds, mostly with unspecified modes of action lacking in dramatic and spectacular activities. What some seem to have in common are their capabilities to add alkaline reserve and lower surface tension. Thus, these compounds act secondarily as wetting agents and corrosion inhibitors.

One example that has achieved some commercial notice is produced by at least four companies for at least three stated purposes: recirculating cooling waters, secondary oil recovery water, and paper and pulp slime control. Because of the source of the alkyl chain, it is

Table 17-11. *Dependence of Cytolytic Activity of 4-Alkylmorpholine-N-Oxides on the Chain Length of the Hydrophobic Alkyl Group*

Amine oxide	Minimal Conc. (mM) Inducing Total Lysis of Yeast Protoplasts
4-Decylmorpholine-N-oxide	10.0
4-Dodecylmorpholine-N-oxide	0.5
4-Tetradecylmorpholine-N-oxide	0.15
4-Hexadecylmorpholine-N-oxide	0.07

From Subick, J., Takacsova, G., Psenak, M., and Devinsky, F. 1977. Antimicrobial activity of amine oxides: mode of action and structure-activity correlation. Antimicrob. Agents Chemother., *12*(2), 139–146.

referred to as a fatty amine (Table 17–1). The trivial name is N-cocotrimethylene diamine, and it represents the bulk of some 3.5×10^6 pounds of fatty amine derivatives used as microbial control agents. Only limited information is available in the literature on the specific efficacy of these compounds, although they are reputed to have activity against sulfate-reducing bacteria. However, a recent report states that *L. pneumophila*, a known cooling-tower isolate, was not susceptible to this amine at recommended dose levels (Grace et al., 1981).

Bennett (1978, 1979) and his coworkers (Bennett et al., 1979) examined for antimicrobial activity a large series of putative corrosion inhibitors based on diethylene triamine and amine alcohols. These studies were carried out in a number of metalworking fluids in the hope that the presumed corrosion inhibitors needed to replace the suspect nitrites (nitrosamines) could also serve as part of the antimicrobial package. The levels of these compounds needed to achieve modest success as antimicrobials may preclude their use for economic and compatibility reasons. Nevertheless, some of the more effective compounds should be mentioned.

Of 40 substituted monoethanolamines evaluated, only four or five could be considered active in most of the metalworking fluids in which they were evaluated. The most active derivative proved to be 2(N-amyl)ethanolamine, with 2-cyclohexyl ethanolamine and N-butyl ethanolamine second best. On the other hand, isoamyl was much less effective, whereas the tertiary butyl compound could not control fungi. It would appear that carbon chain length is an important factor in determining efficacy in this series, a fact well established previously with phenols and triazines.

An unusual group of amines is based on the N-oxides of tertiary amines. The potential antimicrobial activity of amine N-oxides has been noted (Mlynarcik et al., 1975). Similar structures with antimicrobial activity have also been described (e.g., pyridine N-oxides and quaternary ammonium cations) (Table 17–1).

The relationship between structure and activity of a series of amine oxides showed that the chain length of the hydrophobic alkyl substituent is most important in establishing activity (Subik et al., 1977) (Table 17–11). The compounds tested inhibited differentiation and outgrowth of *Bacillus subtilis* of several filamentous fungi, and induced lysis in *Saccharomyces* protoplasts.

Further, studies on 1-dodecylpiperidine N-oxide against *Staphylococcus aureus* showed that inhibition of growth was directly related to specific membrane function (i.e., proton uptake and subsequent loss of ATP synthesizing ability) (Mlynarcik, 1981). This membrane-specific targeting was shown to be related to micelle formation. Minimal inhibitory concentrations against *S. aureus*, *Candida albicans*, and *E. coli* were optimal only within critical micelle concentrations (Devinsky et al., 1985).

Structurally, EDTA and its salts qualify as amines. In a limited sense, they also qualify as antimicrobial agents. The first report on EDTA activity indicated that it sensitized gram-negative species to lysis and was a function of divalent cation level pH, buffer type, and age and species of organism (Repaske, 1958). These parameters and probable modes of action have been reviewed in general (Russell, 1971) and more specifically as they apply to *Pseudomonas aeruginosa* (Wilkinson, 1975). Two general effects of EDTA seem to be observable, resulting in either cell death or inhibition. The compound can act directly on sensitive species, causing autolytic death rapidly (within 2 minutes) or a delayed, more protracted death, or it can act indirectly by sensitizing cells to a wide variety of established antimicrobial agents. This latter activity results in true synergistic response.

Fundamentally, it appears that the direct effects as well as the potentiating effects can be related to the chelating ability of EDTA. Some of the results were achieved with other aminopolycarboxylic acids (Wilkinson, 1975), as well as with sodium hexametaphosphate. Levels of EDTA used with demonstrable effect range from 0.1 mM (Repaske, 1958) to 1.0 mM (Gray and Wilkinson, 1965), with the latter reporting 99.99% reduction in viable counts.

According to Wilkinson (1975), the disadvantage of EDTA resistance caused by magnesium limitation may be more apparent than real, because such cells still show increased sensitivity to other antimicrobials, also noted by Bennett (1979). In addition, it would be important to emphasize that controlled laboratory conditions may often fall short of the challenges imposed by actual situations in the field, Bennett's finding probably more closely approximating a field inoculum.

Extensive studies on mode of action reviewed by Wilkinson (1975) relate essentially to metal binding by EDTA, especially magnesium, for *Pseudomonas* species in general. It appears that the outer membrane of gram-negative cells, i.e., the lipopolysaccharide, is structurally stabilized by Mg^{++}. Removal of Mg^{++} by EDTA complexing disorients the outer membrane exposing the thin (one-molecular-layer) peptidoglycan sacculus to environmental insult, including increased permeability to many antimicrobial agents. It is most interesting that one of the more resistant of all prokaryotic species to antimicrobial agents, *Ps. aeruginosa*, is also the gram-negative

species most susceptible to EDTA. This is also true for some other members of the *Pseudomonadales*. In contrast to the pseudomonads whose EDTA sensitivity is related to outer membrane structure, *E. coli* seems affected at the intracellular level (Prasad and Chitnis, 1986).

It is apparent that the major mechanism against sensitive gram-negative species is based on outer-membrane disorientation by the sequestration of Mg^{++}. Effectiveness against gram-positive organisms in the absence of other antimicrobials has not been demonstrated. However, 20 mg/ml of disodium EDTA maintained potency of an infusion catheter lumen while reducing viable *Staphylococcus epidermidis* from 10^3 cfu/ml to about 10^1 cfu/ml. This level of EDTA is some hundred times higher than that needed for gram-negative control, but another anticoagulant, heparin, permitted *S. epidermidis* to exceed 10^8 cfu/ml. An antimicrobial mode of action for gram-positive species probably involves deprivation of some essential divalent or trivalent cation (Root et al., 1988).

Notwithstanding the variability of EDTA activity when used alone, which makes it difficult to classify it as a de facto antimicrobial, the Environmental Protection Agency, under the Pesticide Act of 1974, for purposes of disinfectant and sanitizer registration, has given EDTA *de jure* status as an antimicrobial by classifying it as an active ingredient in formulations.

ANILIDES

This group includes derivatives of salicylanilide and carbanilide (Table 17–1). The simplest of these is salicylanilide, which was introduced by The Shirley Institute in England in 1930 for preventing mildew in stored fabric sizing (Shirlan). Since then it has been used in leather, paper, plastics, paint, and MFP (moisture-fungus-proofing) treatment. This latter technique involved incorporating as much as 10% salicylanilide in organic coatings (e.g., lacquers) to protect surfaces susceptible to fungal attack (Greathouse and Wessel, 1954). It was evaluated in colored marker lacquers and varnishes used in the Jupiter and Redstone missiles. All of the coatings containing salicylanilide inhibited the test fungi after 90 days in a tropical chamber (Rossmoore and Jackson, 1959). Salicylanilide weathers poorly (Greathouse and Wessel, 1954), however, and probably would not be satisfactory for mildewproofing of outdoor surface coatings.

The three other compounds based on the anilide structure are all halogenated and have been used primarily as skin-degerming agents, although 3,4',5-tribromosalicylanilide has been promoted for use in paints and metalworking fluids. It was successfully demonstrated as an antifungal adjunct to a HT in metalworking fluid (Rossmoore et al., 1972). Chapter 14 in the second edition of this book gives an excellent review of the chemistry, pharmacology, and microbiology of the anilides, particularly with regard to their use as skin-degerming agents, and presents a strong case for the topical use of soaps and cosmetics containing the halogenated anilides (Stecker, 1977).

Pharmacologically, however, the anilides fall into two classes: the halogenated salicylanilides and the halogenated carbanilides. The salicylanilide derivatives are frank photosensitizers and are not recommended as safe or effective by the FDA OCT Panel No. 1 (Table 17–12). The carbanilides are given a little better treatment. They have been placed in Category III by the OTC Panel in three categories of use that apply only to incorporation into bar soap and use with water. This category states merely that data were insufficient at the time of the classification to make a more judgmental decision. A difference of opinion exists on the efficacy of these compounds, however, based on the published literature. Stecker (1977) believes they have been proven effective, whereas the FDA panel draws the opposite conclusion (U.S. Department of HEW, FDA, 1974, 1978). In addition, the primary manufacturer of one of the compounds in question, trifluoromethyldichlorocarbanilide, has discontinued production and distribution since that date. However, the trichlorocarbanilide was shown to be effective in an in-vivo occlusive protocol against *Staphylococcus aureus* and *Corynebacterium minitissimus*. The active agent was incorporated in a bar soap to simulate actual use (Finkey et al., 1984).

QUINOLINES AND RELATED COMPOUNDS

Certainly this group has been extensively exploited in all areas of antimicrobial application, beginning with the original empiric use of cinchona bark (quinine) as a prophylactic and therapeutic measure for malaria. Quinine is structurally related to many of the antiprotozoal compounds used in the past and currently in vogue (Table 17–1). These include chloroquine, diiodohydroxyquin (diodoquin), and primaquine.

Another group historically and somewhat structurally related are those based on acridine, which is actually benzquinoline. The antimalarial, quinacrine hydrochloride (Atabrine), is based on this structure, as are acriflavine and proflavine. Acriflavine has a long history as an antitrypanosomal agent first demonstrated by Paul Ehrlich in 1910. Quaternization of the acridines increases the activity of these dye derivatives, because the most highly ionized cationic species are the most active (Albert et al., 1945) (Table 17–13). This group of compounds has found widespread use as a mucous membrane antiseptic in the past, as well as limited application in urinary tract infections. Acridine itself is a powerful mutagenic agent, especially in "curing" bacterial cells of plasmid "infections" (the terms "curing" and "infection" are not being used in the traditional sense, i.e., of an antimicrobial effect on infectious disease, but are accepted genetic jargon). These antibacterial dyes and others are reviewed in detail by Foster and Russell (1971).

One of the more interesting quinoline derivatives is the 8-hydroxy compound (oxine). This was reported to have antifungal activity, but only as the copper chelate. Originally (Post and Nicoll, 1910), the parent compound was found to have only minimal activity; it was learned from the studies of Albert and coworkers (Albert et al., 1947), however, that coordination with divalent cation (e.g., Fe^{++} or Cu^{++}) produced extremely effective adducts. Of the seven possible hydroxyquinolines, only the 8-hydroxy is antibacterial and chelates metals as well. When the ring N is methylated, activity is impaired. The dual phenomenon of chelation and activity results in lipid solubility of the 1:2 complex, which passes through the cell membrane and dissociates into the toxic 8-hydroxy compound (Albert et al., 1956a). (For an extensive review, see Albert, 1968.)

The 8-hydroxyquinoline activity against fungi in the absence of metals has been reported (Block, 1956). However, the addition of Cu^{++} to fungal spores previously treated with oxine and washed free of inhibitory levels

Table 17–12. *Classification of Antimicrobial Agents for Use on Skin and Mucous Membrane**

Active Ingredient	Antimicrobial Soap	Health Care Personnel Hand Wash	Patient Preoperative Skin Preparation	Skin Antiseptic	Skin Wound Cleanser	Skin Wound Protectant	Surgical Hand Scrub
Cloflucarban	III	III	II	II	II†	II	II
Fluorosalan	II	II	II	II	II	II	II
Tribromsalan	II	II	II	II	II†	II	II
Triclocarban	III	III	II	II	II†	II	II

*Category definitions: I = Conditions under which antimicrobial products are generally recognized as safe and effective and are not misbranded. II = Conditions under which antimicrobial products are not generally recognized as safe and effective or are misbranded. III = Conditions for which the available data are insufficient to permit final classification at this time.

†Classified in Category III when formulated in a bar soap to be used with water.

Modified from U.S. Department of HEW, FDA. 1974. Certain halogenated salicylanilides as active ingredients in drug and cosmetic products. Fed. Reg., 39(179), 33102–33104.

Table 17–13. *Importance of Cationic Ionization for Bacteriostasis in the Acridine Series*

Substance	Minimum Bacteriostatic Concentration for Streptococcus pyogenes *after 48 Hrs.* Incubation at 37°C (Medium 10% Serum Broth; pH = 7.3)	% Ionized (pH 7.3; 37°C)			
		Cation	Anion	Zwitterion	Neutral Molecule
9-Aminoacridine	1 in 160,000	99	0	0	0
9-Aminoacridine-2-carboxylic acid	<5,000	0	0.2	99.8	0
Methyl ester of above	160,000	89	0	0	11
Acridine	5,000	0.3	0	0	99.7
Acridine-9-carboxylic acid	<5,000	0	99.3	0.7	0
Methyl ester of above	<5,000	0	0	0	100

From Albert, A., Rubbo, S., Goldacre, R., and Stone, J. 1945. The influence of chemical constitution on antibacterial activity. Part II. General survey of the acridine series. Br. J. Exp. Pathol., *26*, 160–192.

restored toxicity. This implies that antifungal activity may be potentiated by coordination in addition to the resultant increase in lipid solubility.

Halogenated derivatives of 8-hydroxyquinoline have been used both as preservatives (5,7-dibromo and 5,7-dichloro) and, more extensively, to treat protozoal infections systemically (diiodohydroxyquinoline) and topically (iodochlorhydroxyquinoline). The mode of action of several halogenated 8-hydroxyquinolines has been studied by Gershon et al. (1972). They found that activity was increased with an additional halogen atom and that the order was I>Br>Cl>F in the 5 substitution.

Two groups of compounds, both based on the benzdiazine structure (quinoline is benzpyridine) (Table 17–1), have been studied with unusual results. The first of these, derivatives of quinoxaline (Suter et al., 1978), especially quinoxaline-1,4-di-N-oxides, was found to inhibit various bacteria, *Chlamydia* and *Entamoeba histolytica*. It appears to be much more effective in inhibiting DNA synthesis in *E. coli* anaerobically than aerobically. In addition, DNA degradation was more pronounced anaerobically in both growing and resistant cells. This same phenomenon was not seen with either protein or RNA. From electron spin resonance (ESR) signals, it would appear that the active moiety is a free radical derived from quindoxin. A DNA repair process similar to that reported for nitrofurantoin or x-ray damage is suggested.

The other compounds structurally are quinazolines, in which the diazine nitrogens are in the 1 and 3 positions rather than the 1 and 4 positions, as in the quinoxolines (Table 17–1).

Castaldo et al. (1979) reported that derivatives based on 2,4-diamine quinazoline were effective in vitro against a number of *Candida* species. This study reiterated previous work that showed that these compounds were nontoxic in a mouse model, as well as showing in-vivo promise in similar infections. The diamine quinazolines also exhibit antifolate activity similar to the known mode of action of trimethoprim. What both have in common is a 1,3-diazine ring as part of their total structure. This is also the distal diazine in the pteridine portion of folic acid. Apparently, 1,4-diazines (quinoxoline) do not ex-

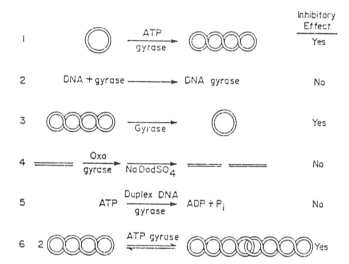

Fig. 17–5. Inhibitory activity of oxolinic and nalidixic acid versus ATP-gyrase. The reactions depicted are supercoiling (1), binding (2), relaxation (3), cleavage (4), ATPase (5), and catenation and uncatenation (6). The DNA substrate is shown as relaxed, duplex, circular DNA for reaction 1, as negatively supercoiled DNA for reactions 3 and 6, and as linear DNA for reaction 4. Modified from Cozzarelli, N.R. 1980. DNA gyrase and the supercoiling of DNA. Science, *207*(4434), 953–960.

hibit antifolate activity, despite the presence of this ring in pteridine also.

Another most interesting quinoline analog is based on a double pyridine (Lesher et al., 1962). It has found a therapeutic niche in treating infections involving the enterobacteriaceae (Mandell and Sande, 1980) and for selectively isolating resistant *Pseudomonas* species (Ito et al., 1980) (Table 17–1). Most recently, specific modes of action have been elucidated for nalidixic acid. It appears that it interferes with DNA synthesis, specifically with functions of the enzyme gyrase, which catalyses DNA supercoiling and catenation (Cozzarelli, 1980) (Fig. 17–5).

It appears that resistant strains and species may be less permeable to nalidixic acid, because EDTA potentiates the activity of nalidixic acid against *E. coli* (Nagate et al., 1980) and *Pseudomonas aeruginosa* (Nezval and Halacka, 1967). Structural changes can affect uptake without affecting mode of action. Oxolinic acid is 15 times more effective against *E. coli* than nalidixic acid (Table 17–1). The addition of EDTA has no effect on oxolinic acid activity, but it increases nalidixic acid action so that, with EDTA, oxolinic acid is only four times more effective than nalidixic acid. However, the actions of the two antimicrobials are qualitatively identical (Cozzarelli, 1980). In addition to their effect on gyrase function, they both inhibit glycyl and leucyl transfer RNA synthetases in yeast (Wright et al., 1981). It would appear that conformational changes produce an inactive form of the enzymes.

The addition of fluorine to the No. 6 position and a piperazine to the No. 8 position has produced a large number of clinically very active, broad-spectrum antimicrobial agents. They all have in common the ability to antagonize DNA gyrase (Topoisomerse II) (Wolfson and Harper, 1985). However, there is some indication that these quinolines may also have additional sites of action (Chu and Fernandes, 1989). The quinolines that specifically antagonize gyrase subunit A in eubacterial species and *Ciprofloxacin* (Table 17–1), a representative fluoroquinoline, also inhibited DNA replication in several archaebacterial species, a halophile, and a methanogen (Sioud et al., 1988).

PATENTED SYNERGISTIC COMBINATIONS

The lack of innovative, safe chemicals has resulted in the exploitation of existing successful molecules in putative synergistic combinations with each other and with other compounds. The reader should keep in mind that the patent process is not a peer review process and that issuance of a patent is not always a guarantee of repeatability of claims. The following have been selected as examples of some mixtures currently available for potential exploitation: Bronopol (Szabo et al., 1986; Donofrio and Whitekettle, 1988; Otokuni and Kitanishi, 1986); methylchloroisothiazalones (Law, 1979; Clifford and Birchall, 1985; Martin and LaMarre, 1987; Umekawa et al., 1987; Hahn, 1984; Okamoto, 1987); Nitromorpholines (Borovian, 1986; Beyme et al., 1988); Pyridinethiol (Odajima and Matsumoto, 1988); Dibromonitrilopropionamide (Okamoto, 1987; LaMarre and Martin, 1987; Jakubowski, 1986); 2-bromo-2-(bromoethyl) glutaronitrile (Jakubowski, 1986); Benzimidazoles (Odajima and Matsumoto, 1988; Beyme et al., 1988); and triazines (Rossmoore, 1977; Rossmoore, 1987).

A literature search since 1982 of the compounds treated in this chapter yielded over 4000 citations. By excluding the blatantly clinical contributions, the number was reduced to about 1300. Additional gatekeepers (e.g., patent applications) and new syntheses brought the number down to 459. These were scanned and those with greatest relevancy were included in this chapter.

REFERENCES

Albert, A. 1968. *Selective Toxicity: The Physico-Chemical Basis of Therapy.* 5th Edition. London, Chapman and Hall.

Albert, A., Rees, C.N., and Tomlinson, A. 1956a. Why are some metal binding substances antibacterial? Rec. Trav. Chim., 75, 819–834.

Albert, A., Rees, C.N., and Tomlinson, A.J.H. 1956b. The influence of chemical constitution on antibacterial activity. Part VIII. 2-mercaptopyridine-N-oxide and some general observations on metal-binding agents. Br. J. Exp. Pathol., 37, 500–511.

Albert, A., Rubbo, S., Goldacre, R., and Balfour, B. 1947. The influence of chemical constitution on antibacterial activity. Part III. A study of 8-hydroxyquinoline (oxine) and related compounds. Br. J. Exp. Pathol., 28, 69–87.

Albert, A., Rubbo, S., Goldacre, R., and Stone, J. 1945. The influence of chemical constitution on antibacterial activity. Part II. General survey of the acridine series. Br. J. Exp. Pathol., 26, 160–192.

Allen, P.M., and Gottlieb, D. 1970. Mechanisms of actions of the fungicide thiabendazole, 2-(4'-thiazolyl) benzimadazole. Appl. Microbiol., 20(6), 919–926.

Andrykovitch, G., and Neihof, R. 1987. Fuel-soluble biocides for control of *Cladosporium resinae* in hydrocarbon fuels. J. Ind. Microbiol., 2(1), 35–40.

APhA. 1936. *The Pharmaceutical Recipe Book.* 2nd Edition. American Pharmaceutical Association.

Bancroft, K., Grant, I.F., and Alexander, M. 1979. Toxicity of NO_2: effect of nitrite on microbial activity in an acid soil. Appl. Environ. Microbiol., 38(5), 940–944.

Barnes, C.P., and Eagon, R.G. 1986. The mechanism of action of hexahydro-1,3,5-triethyl-s-triazine. J. Ind. Microbiol., 1, 105–112.

Bayne, H.G., and Michener, H.D. 1975. Growth of *Staphylococcus* and *Salmonella* on frankfurters with and without sodium nitrite. Appl. Microbiol., 30, 844–849.

Becrens, H., Romand, C., and Lepage, C. 1980. The synergistic action of isothiazolone E + imidazolidynlurea. Parfums. Cosmet. Aromes., 36, 81–84.

Beggs, W.H., and Jenne, J.W. 1967. Mechanism for the pyridoxal neutralization of isoniazid action on *Mycobacterium tuberculosis*. J. Bacteriol., 94, 793–797.

Belser, L.W., and Schmidt, E.L. 1981. Inhibitory effect of nitrapyrin on three genera of ammonia-oxidizing nitrifiers. Appl. Environ. Microbiol., 41(3), 819–821.

Bennett, E.O. 1973. Formaldehyde preservatives for cutting fluids. Int. Biodetn. Bull., 9(4), 95–100.

Bennett, E.O. 1974. Water quality and coolant life. Lubr. Engg., 30, 549–555.

Bennett, E.O. 1978. The antimicrobial properties of diethylene triamines in metalworking fluids. Int. Biodetn. Bull., 14, 21–29.

Bennett, E.O. 1979. Corrosion inhibitors as preservatives for metalworking fluids—ethanolamines. Lubr. Engg., 35(3), 137–144.

Bennett, E.O., and Hodge, E.B. 1961. Process for the control of bacteria in water flooding operations. U.S. Patent No. 3,001,936

Bennett, E.O., Adams, M.C., and Tavana, G. 1979. Antimicrobial properties of butanolamines and propanolamines in metalworking fluids. J. Gen. Appl. Microbiol., 25, 63–69.

Bennett, E.O., Guynes, G.J., and Isenberg, D.L. 1960. The sensitivity of sulfate-reducing bacteria to antibacterial agents. III. The nitroparaffin derivatives. Producers Monthly, 24(5), 26–27.

Bernstein, J., et al. 1953. Chemotherapy of experimental tuberculosis. VI. Derivative of isoniazid. VII. Heterocyclic acid hydrazides and derivatives. Am. Rev. Tuberc., 67, 354–375.

Beveridge, T.J., and Koval, S.F. 1981. Binding of metals to cell envelopes of *Escherichia coli* K-12. Appl. Environ. Microbiol., 42(2), 325–335.

Beveridge, T.J., and Murray, R.G.E. 1976. Uptake and retention of metals by cell walls of *Bacillus subtilis*. J. Bacteriol., 127(3), 1502–1518.

Beyme, B., et al. 1988. Synergistic fungicide mixture comprising morpholine and benzimidazole derivatives. Ger. (East) Patent DD 256,448.

Block, S.S. 1956. Examination of the activity of 8-quinolinol to fungi. Appl. Microbiol., 4, 183–186.

Borchert, E.E. 1974. Bacterial spoilage inhibited by metalworking lubricant compositions. U.S. Patent No. 3,791,974.

Borovian, G.E. 1986. Preservative compositions employing antimicrobial morpholine derivatives. U.S. Patent No. 4,607,036.

Bracke, J.W., Cruden, D.L., and Markovetz, A.J. 1978. Effect of metronidazole on the intestinal microflora of the American cockroach, *Periplaneta americana* L. Antimicrob. Agents. Chemother., 13(1), 115–120.

Brazda, G., et al. 1988. Triazine derivative fungicide. Ger. (East) Patent DD 258,166.

Brodhage, H., and Pfirrmann, R.W. 1985. Taurolin—bacteriology *in vitro*. In *Taurolin.* Edited by W.L. Brueckner and R.W. Pfirrmann. Munich, FGR, Urbon & Schwartzenberg, pp. 38–45.

Brooks, L., and Harvey, A.M. 1973. Certain triazines used to control bacteria and fungi. U.S. Patent No. 3,755,590.

Brown, H.D., et al. 1961. Antiparasitic drugs. IV. 2-(4'thiazolyl) benzimidazole, a new anthelmintic. J. Am. Chem. Soc., 83, 1764–1765.

Browne, M.K., Leslie, G.B., and Pfirrmann, R.W. 1976. Taurolin, a new chemotherapeutic agent. J. Appl. Bacteriol., 41, 363–368.

Browne, M.K., Mackenzie, M., and Doyle, P.J. 1978. A controlled trial of taurolin in established bacterial peritonitis. Surg. Gynecol. Obstet., *146*, 721–724.

Browne, M.K., and Stoller, J.L. 1970. Intraperitoneal noxythiolin in faecal peritonitis. Br. J. Surg., *57*, 525–529.

Candal, F.J., and Eagon, R.G. 1984. Evidence for plasmid-mediated bacterial resistance to industrial biocides. Intl. Biodetn., *20*(4), 221–224.

Carter, G. 1973. Some aspects of the prevention of microbiological attack on emulsion paint systems. J. Oil Colour Chem. Assoc., *56*(7), 302–306.

Casero, R.A., Jr., et al. 1980. Activity of 2-acetyl-pyridine thiosemicarbazones against *Trypanosoma rhodesiense in vitro*. Antimicrob. Agents Chemother., *18*(2), 317–322.

Castaldo, R.A., Gump, D.W., and McCormack, J.J. 1979. Activity of 2,4-diaminoquinazoline compounds against *Candida* species. Antimicrob. Agents Chemother., *15*(1), 81–86.

Chandler, C.J., and Segel, I.H. 1978. Mechanism of the antimicrobial action of pyrithione: effects on membrane transport, ATP levels, and protein synthesis. Antimicrob. Agents Chemother., *14*(1), 60–68.

Christiansen, L.N., et al. 1974. Effect of sodium nitrite on toxin production by *Clostridium botulinum* in bacon. Appl. Microbiol., *27*, 733–737.

Christiansen, L.N., Tompkin, R.B., and Shaparis, A.B. 1978. Fate of *Clostridium botulinum* in perishable canned cured meat at abuse temperature. J. Food Protect., *41*, 354–355.

Chu, D.T.W., and Fernandes, P.B. 1989. Structure-activity relationships of the fluoroquinolones. Antimicrob. Agents Chemother., *33*(2), 131–135.

Clifford, R.P., and Birchall, G.A. 1985. Biocide. U.S. Patent No. 4,539,071.

Cooney, J.J., and Felix, J.A. 1972. Inhibition of *Cladosporium resinae* in hydrocarbon-water systems by pyridinethiones. Int. Biodetn. Bull., *8*(2), 59–63.

Cozzarelli, N.R. 1980. DNA gyrase and the supercoiling of DNA. Science, *207*(4434), 953–960.

Cuckler, A.C., Kupferberg, A.B., and Millman, N. 1955. Chemotherapeutic and tolerance studies on aminonitrothiazoles. Antibiot. Chemother., *5*, 540–550.

Czechowski, M., and Rossmoore, H.W. 1981. The effect of selected industrial biocides on lactate metabolism in *Desulfovibrio desulfuricans*. Dev. Indust. Microbiol., *22*, 797–804.

Czechowski, M., and Rossmoore, H.W. 1990. Purification and partial characterization of a D(−) lactate dehydrogenase from *Desulfovibrio desulfuricans* (ATCC 7757). J. Ind. Microbiol., in press.

Dahl, S., and Kaplan, A.M. 1960. 4-nitrophenyl esters, including mixed carbonates and bis carbonates, as leather fungicides. J. Am. Leath. Chem. Assoc., *55*, 480–500.

Davidson, L.A., and Takayama, K. 1979. Isoniazid inhibition of the synthesis of monounsaturated long-chain fatty acids in *Mycobacterium tuberculosis* H37Ra. Antimicrob. Agents Chemother., *16*(1), 104–105.

Davis, W.B., and Weber, M.M. 1977. Specificity of isoniazid on growth inhibition and competition for an oxidized nicotinamide adenine dinucleotide regulatory site on the electron transport pathway in *Mycobacterium phlei*. Antimicrob. Agents Chemother., *12*(2), 213–218.

Delsarte, A., et al. 1981. Nifurzide: a nitrofuran antiinfectious agent: interaction with *Escherichia coli* cells. Antimicrob. Agents Chemother., *19*(3), 477–486.

DeMare, J., Rossmoore, H.W., and Smith, T.H.F. 1972. Comparative study of triazine biocides. Dev. Indust. Microbiol., *13*, 341–347.

Devinsky, F., et al. 1985. Relationship between critical micelle concentrations and minimum inhibitory concentrations for some non-aromatic quaternary ammonium salts and amine oxides. Tenside Deterg., *22*, 10–15.

Dobek, A.S., et al. 1980. Inhibition of clinically significant bacterial organisms *in vitro* by 2-acetylpyridine thiosemicarbazones. Antimicrob. Agents Chemother., *18*(1), 27–36.

Dodd, M.C., and Stillman, W.B. 1944. The *in vitro* bacteriostatic action of some simple furan derivatives. J. Pharmacol. Exp. Ther., *82*, 11–18.

Domagk, G., Behnisch, R., Mietzsch, F., and Schmidt, H. 1946. New compound active against tuberculosis bacilli *in vitro*. Naturwissenschaften, *33*, 315–320.

Donofrio, D.K., and Whitekettle, W.K. 1988. Synergistic bactericidal mixture of 2-bromo-2-nitropropane-1,3-diol and tetradecylmethyl-sulfonium methosulfate for control of slime-forming microorganisms in aqueous systems. U.S. Patent No. 4,753,961.

Dorris, M.M., and Pitcher, D. 1988. Effective treatment of microbially contaminated fuel storage tanks. In *ASTM Special Technical Publication 1005, Distillate Fuel: Contamination, Storage and Handling*. Edited by H.L. Chesneau and M.M. Dorris. Philadelphia, Am. Soc. for Testing and Materials, pp. 146–156.

Douglas, H., Rossmoore, H.W., Passman, F.A., and Rossmoore, L.A. 1990. Evaluation of endotoxin-biocide interaction by the *Limulus* ameobocyte lysate assay. Dev. Ind. Microbiol., in press.

Drobnica, L., et al. 1967a. Antifungal activity of isothiocyanates and related compounds. Appl. Microbiol., *15*(4), 701–709.

Drobnica, L., et al. 1967b. Antifungal activity of isothiocyanates and related compounds. II. Mononuclear aromatic isothiocyanates. Appl. Microbiol., *15*(4), 710–717.

Duncan, C.L., and Foster, E.M. 1968a. Effect of sodium nitrite, sodium chloride, and sodium nitrate on germination and outgrowth of anaerobic spores. Appl. Microbiol., *16*, 406–411.

Duncan, C.L., and Foster, E.M. 1968b. Nitrite-induced germination of putrefactive anaerobe 3679h spores. Appl. Microbiol., *16*, 412–416.

Dupont, J.A., Lashen, E.S., and Scott, J.D. 1974. Isothiazalones as paint film mildewcides. AES Organic and Plastic Preprint, *34*(2), 149–155.

Dybas, R.A., et al. 1978. 2-(substituted piperidinomethyl) propenenitriles and analogs as preservatives in aqueous systems. Dev. Indust. Microbiol., *19*, 347–353.

Dymicky, M., Huhtanen, C.N., and Wasserman, A.E. 1977. Inhibition of *Clostridium botulinum* by 5-nitrothiazoles. Antimicrob. Agents Chemother., *12*(3), 353–356.

Eagon, R.G., and Barnes, C.P. 1986. The mechanism of microbial resistance to hexahydro-1,3,5-triethyl-s-triazine. J. Ind. Microbiol., *1*, 113–118.

Edmonds, P., and Cooney, J.J. 1968. Microbial growth in a fuel-water system containing polyesterurethane foam. Appl. Microbiol., *16*, 426–427.

Edwards, D.I., Dye, M., and Carne, H. 1973. The selective toxicity of antimicrobial nitroheterocyclic drugs. J. Gen. Microbiol., *76*, 135–145.

Eggensperger, H. Personal communication, 1971.

Eggensperger, H., Diehl, K.-H., and Ramlau, P. 1975. Preservative and disinfectant. German OLS Patent No. 2,337,755.

Elder, R.L. 1980. Final report on the safety assessment for 2-bromo-2-nitropropane-1,3-diol [52-51-7]. J. Environ. Pathol. Toxicol., *4*, 47–61.

Elsmore, R. 1989. The activity of BNPD against *Legionella pneumophila*-Serogroup I. The interaction of pH, inoculum level and test media. Intl. Biodetn., *25*, 107–113.

Exner, J.H., Burk, G.A., and Kryiacou, D. 1973. Rates and products of decomposition of 2,2-dibromo-3-nitrilopropionamide. J. Agric. Food Chem., *21*, 838–842.

Fan, T.Y., and Tannenbaum, S.R. 1973. Factors influencing the rate of formation of nitrosomorpholine from morpholine and nitrite: acceleration by thiocyanate and other anions. J. Agric. Food Chem., *21*, 237–240.

Fan, T.Y., Vita, R., and Fine, D.H. 1978. C-nitro compounds: A new class of nitrosating agents. Toxicol. Lett., *2*, 5–10.

Finkey, M.B., et al. 1984. *In vivo* effect of antimicrobial soapbars containing 1.5% and 0.8% trichlorocarbanilide against two strains of pathogenic bacteria. J. Soc. Cosm. Chem., *35*(7), 351–355.

Foster, J.H.S., and Russell, A.D. 1971. Antibacterial dyes and nitrofurans. In *Inhibition and Destruction of the Microbial Cell*. Edited by W.B. Hugo. New York, Academic Press, pp. 185–208.

Fox, H.H. 1953. The chemical attack on tuberculosis. Tr. N.Y. Acad. Sci., *15*, 234–242.

Friend, P.L., and Whitekettle, W.K. 1980. Biocides and water cooling towers. Dev. Indust. Microbiol., *21*, 123–131.

Gangadharam, P.R.J., Harold, F.M., and Schaefer, W.B. 1963. Selective inhibition of nucleic acid synthesis in *Mycobacterium tuberculosis* by isoniazid. Nature, *198*, 712–714.

Gavinet, A.M., and Magraud, F. 1987. Susceptibility of enteropathogenic bacteria to nifurzide. Pathol. Biol., *35*(5), 542–544.

Gershon, H., Parmegiani, R., and Godfrey, P.K. 1972. Antifungal activity of 5-,7-, and 5,7-substituted 2-methyl-8-quinolinols. Antimicrob Agents Chemother., *1*(5), 373–375.

Gidley, M.J., et al. 1981. The mode of antibacterial action of some "masked" formaldehyde compounds. FEBS Lett., *127*(3), 225–227.

Gidley, M.J., and Sanders, J.K.M. 1983. Mechanisms of antibacterial formaldehyde delivery from noxythiolin and other masked-formaldehyde compounds. J. Pharm. Pharmacol., *35*(11), 712–717.

Goodman, L.S., and Gilman, A. 1958a. Antiseptics, germicides, fungicides, virucides, and ectoparasiticides. In *The Pharmacological Basis of Therapeutics*. 2nd Edition. New York, Macmillan, p. 1086.

Goodman, L.S., and Gilman, A. 1958b. Drugs used in the chemotherapy of helminthiasis. In *The Pharmacological Basis of Therapeutics*. 2nd Edition. New York, Macmillan, p. 1145.

Gorman, S.P., McCafferty, D.F., Woolfson, A.D., and Jones, D.S. 1987. Reduced adherence to human mucosal epithelial cells following treatment with taurolin, a novel antibacterial agent. J. Appl. Bacteriol., *62*(4), 315–320.

Gottlieb, D., and Kumar, K. 1970. The effect of thiabendazole on spore germination. Phytopathol., *60*(10), 1451–1455.

Grace, R.D., DeWar, N.E., Barnes, W.G., and Hodges, G.R. 1981. Susceptibility of *Legionella pneumophila* to three cooling tower microbicides. Appl. Environ. Microbiol., *41*(1), 233–236.

Gray, G.W., and Wilkinson, S.G. 1965. The action of ethylenediamine-tetraacetic acid on *Pseudomonas aeruginosa*. J. Appl. Bacteriol., *28*, 153–164.

Graymore, J. 1938. The cyclic methenamines. Hydrolysis of quaternary compounds. I. Preparation of aliphatic secondary amines. Chem. Soc. J., (trans.) *1938*, 1311–1313.

Greathouse, G.A., and Wessel, C.J. (eds.) 1954. *Deterioration of Materials. Causes and Preventive Techniques*. New York, Reinhold Publishing.

Greminger, G.K., Jr. 1972. Recent developments in additives for water-based paints. Pitture e Vernici, *48*(2), 45–50.

Grier, N., and Lederer, S.J. 1974. Dihalomethylglutaronitriles used as antibacterial and antifungal agents. U.S. Patent No. 3,833,731.

Grier, N., and Lederer, S.J. 1975. Algicidal dihalomethylglutaronitriles. U.S. Patent No. 3,877,922.

Grier, N., and Witzel, B.E. 1978. 1,3,5-s-hexahydrotrisubstituted triazines. U.S. Patent No. 4,119,779.

Grier, N., and Witzel, B.E. 1979. 1,3,5-s-hexahydrotrisubstituted triazines and hydrocarbon metalworking fluids containing same. U.S. Patent No. 4,159,254.

Grier, N., Witzel, B.E., Jakubowski, J.A., and Dulaney, E.L. 1980. A broad spectrum hexahydro-s-triazine inhibitor of microbial deterioration in cutting fluids. Dev. Indust. Microbiol., 21, 411–418.

Grunberg, E., and Titsworth, E.H. 1973. Chemotherapeutic properties of heterocyclic compounds: monocyclic compounds with five-membered rings. Ann. Rev. Microbiol., 27, 317–346.

Hahn, W. 1984. Germicidal mixtures. German Patent Spec. 2,800,737.

Haler, D. 1963. Polynoxylin. Nature, 198, 400–401.

Haler, D., and Aebi, A. 1961. A new, highly effective but non-toxic antibacterial substance. Nature, 190, 734–735.

Hansch, C., and Lien, E.J. 1971. Structure-activity relationships in antifungal agents. J. Med. Chem., 14, 653–670.

Heim, W.G., Appleman, D., and Pyrofrom, H.J. 1956. Effects of 3-amino 1,2,4-triazole on catalase and other compounds. Am. J. Physiol., 186, 19–23.

Herman, R.P., and Weber, M.M. 1980a. Isoniazid interaction with tyrosine as a possible mode of action of the drug in mycobacteria. Antimicrob. Agents Chemother., 17(2), 170–178.

Herman, R.P., and Weber, M.M. 1980b. Site of action of isoniazid on the electron transport chain and its relationship to nicotinamide adenine dinucleotide regulation in Mycobacterium phlei. Antimicrob. Agents Chemother., 17(3), 450–454.

Herrlich, P., and Schweigler, M. 1976. Nitrofurans, a group of synthetic antibiotics with a new mode of action: discrimination of a new class of messenger RNA. Proc. Natl. Acad. Sci. U.S.A., 73, 3386–3390.

Hinton, A.J., Turner, J.N., and Morley, J.S. 1961. Process for the control of micro-organisms. London Patent Specification 884,541.

Hodge, E.B. 1965. Process for the stabilization of petroleum lubricants. U.S. Patent No. 3,192,163.

Hof, H., Chakrabarty, T., Royer, R., and Buisson, J.P. 1987. Mode of action of nitro-heterocyclic compounds on Escherichia coli. Drugs Exp. Clin. Res., 13(10), 635–639.

Hof, H., Stroeder, J., Buisson, J.P., and Royer, R. 1986. Effect of different nitroheterocyclic compounds on aerobic, microaerophilic and anaerobic bacteria. Antimicrob. Agents Chemother., 30(5), 679–683.

Holtzman, G.H., and Rossmoore, H.W. 1977. Evaluation of action of a formaldehyde condensate germicide. Dev. Indust. Microbiol., 18, 753–758.

Huhtanen, C.N. 1984. Nitrite substitutes for controlling Clostridium botulinum. Dev. Ind. Microbiol., 25, 349–362.

Huitric, A.C., Pratt, R., Okano, Y., and Kumler, W.D. 1956. Antifungal activity of B-nitrostyrenes and some cyclohexane derivatives. Antibiot. Chemother., 6, 290–293.

Hurwitz, S.J., and McCarthy, T.J. 1985. Dynamics of disinfection of selected preservatives against Escherichia coli. J. Pharm. Sci., 74(8), 892–894.

Imokawa, G., Shimizu, H., and Okamoto, K. 1982. Antimicrobial effect of zinc pyrithione. J. Soc. Cosmet. Chem., 1982, 33(1), 27–37.

Ingram, M. 1976. The microbial role of nitrite in meat products. In Microbiology in Agriculture, Fisheries, and Food. Edited by F.A. Skinner and J.G. Carr. New York, Academic Press, pp. 1–18.

Ito, A., et al. 1980. In vitro antibacterial activity of AM-715, a new nalidixic acid analog. Antimicrob. Agents Chemother., 17(2), 103–108.

Izzat, I.N., and Bennett, E.O. 1979. Potentiation of the antimicrobial activities of cutting fluid preservatives by EDTA. Lubr. Engg., 35(3), 153–159.

Jacobs, W.A., Heidelberger, M., and Amoss, H.L. 1916a. The bactericidal properties of the quaternary salts of hexmethylene tetramine. II. The relation between constitution and bactericidal action in the substituted benzylhexamethylene tetraminium salts. J. Exp. Med., 23, 569–576.

Jacobs, W.A., Heidelberger, M., and Bull, C.G. 1916b. The bactericidal properties of the quaternary salts of hexamethylenetetramine. III. The relation between constitution and bactericidal action in the quaternary salts obtained from halogenacetyl compounds. J. Exp. Med., 23, 577–599.

Jakubowski, J. 1986. Admixtures of 2-bromo-2-bromomethyl-glutaronitrile and 2,2-dibromo-3-nitrilopropionamide. U.S. Patent No. 4,604,405.

Jakubowski, J.A., and Bennett, E.O. 1987. A novel biocide combination with potentiated activity in cutting fluids. Lub. Eng. 43(7), 568–571.

Jones, D.G., Limaye, S.H., and Young, B.R. 1972. Biocides for the petroleum industry and allied trades. J. Inst. Petrol., 58(563), 268–271.

Jordan, U. 1988. Medical disinfectants containing isothiazolin-3-ones. Ger. Offen (Patent) DE 3,702,546.

Karle, J.M., and Karle, I.L. 1989. Crystal and molecular structure of the antimalarial agent empiroline. Antimicrob. Agents Chemother., 38(7), 1081–1089.

Kawa, D.E., Pennell, D.R., Kubista, L.N., and Schell, R.F. 1989. Development of a rapid method for determining the susceptibility of Mycobacterium tuberculosis to isoniazid using the gene-probe hydridization system. Antimicrob. Agents Chemother., 33(7), 1000–1007.

Keith, J.R. 1971. Non-mercurial antimicrobial agents for the paint industry. Am. Paint J., 55, 28–30.

Kingston, D. 1965. Release of formaldehyde from polynoxylin and noxythiolin. J. Clin. Pathol., 18, 666–667.

Klemme, D.E., and Leonard, J.M. 1971. Inhibitors for marine sulfate-reducing bacteria in shipboard fuel storage tanks. Naval Research Laboratory Memorandum Report 2324.

Klemme, D.E., and Neihof, R.A. 1969. Control of marine sulfate-reducing bacteria in water-displaced shipboard fuel storage tanks. Naval Research Laboratory Memorandum Report 2069.

Klemme, D.E., and Neihof, R.A. 1976. An evaluation in large-scale test systems of biocides for control of sulfate-reducing bacteria in shipboard fuel tanks. Naval Research Laboratory Memo Report 3212.

Knight, R.C., Skolimowski, I.M., and Edwards, D.I. 1978. The interaction of reduced metronidazole with DNA. Biochem. Pharmacol., 27, 2089–2093.

Krzeminski, S.F., Brackett, C.K., Fisher, J.D., and Spinnler, J.F. 1975. Fate of microbicidal 3-isothiazolone compounds in the environment: products of degradation. Agric. Food Chem., 23(6), 1075.

LaMarre, T.M., and Martin, C.H. 1987. Synergistic biocide of 2-(p- hydroxyphenyl) glyoxylohydroximoyl chloride and 2,2-dibromo-3-nitrilo propionamide for treating industrial process water. U.S. Patent No. 4,661,518.

Lashen, E.S., and Law, A.B. 1988. Fungicidal efficacy of octhilinone preservative in metalworking fluids. Lub. Eng., 44(5), 447–452.

Law, A.B. 1979. Synergistic microbicidal compositions. U.S. Patent No. 4,173,643.

Law, A.B., Donnelly, T.W., and Lashen, E.S. 1985. Evaluation of methylchloroisothiazolone/methylisothiazolone and other antimicrobial agents for home and industrial products. In Biodeterioration 6, Proceedings of the Sixth International Biodeterioration Symposium. Edited by S. Barry and D.R. Houghton. C.A.B. Intl. Mycological Inst., The Biodetn. Soc., United Kingdom, pp. 111–118.

Law, A.B., and Lashen, E.S. 1990. Microbicidal efficacy of a methylchloro/methylisothiazolone copper preservative in metalworking fluids. Lub. Eng., in press.

Lederer, S.J., Jakubowski, J.A., and Birnbaum, H.A. 1983. Biocides for industry. An effective preservative for adhesives with reduced health hazards. Spec. Chem., 3(3), 19–20, 22–23.

Lesher, G.Y., et al. 1962. 1,8-naphtyridine derivatives. A new class of chemotherapeutic agents. J. Med. Pharm. Chem., 5, 1063–1065.

Lewis, S.N.A., Miller, G.A., and Law, A.B. 1973. 3-isothiazolones. U.S. Patent No. 3,761,488.

Lugg, M.J. 1981. Photodegradation of the biocide, 1,2 benzisothiazolin-3-one used in a paper jointing material. Intl. Biodetn. Bull., 17, 11–13.

Mandell, G.L., and Sande, M.A. 1980. Antimicrobial agents: sulfonamides, trimethoprim-sulfamethoxazole, and urinary tract antiseptics. In The Pharmacological Basis of Therapeutics. 6th Edition. Edited by A.G. Gilman, L.S. Goodman, and A. Gilman. New York, Macmillan, pp. 1119–1122.

Manowitz, M., Walter, G.R., and Foris, S.A., Jr. 1971. Preservatives for aqueous systems. U.S. Patent No. 3,629,465.

Manowitz, M., Walter, G.R., and Foris, S.A., Jr. 1975. Preservatives for aqueous systems. U.S. Patent No. 3,871,860.

Martin, C.H., and LaMarre, T.M. 1987. Synergistic biocide of dodecylguanidine hydrochloride and a mixture of 5-chloro-2-methyl-4-isothiazolin-3-one for industrial process waters. U.S. Patent No. 4,661,503.

Meitz, A.K. 1984. Efficacy and decomposition of DBNPA in two cooling systems. In Proceedings of 45th International Water Conference. Philadelphia, Engineering Soc., pp. 293–298.

Miller, G.A., and Lewis, S.N. 1976. 3-alkoxyisothiazoles. U.S. Patent No. 3,957,808.

Mlynarcik, D., Denyer, S.P., and Hugo, W.B. 1981. A study of the action of a bisquaternary ammonium salt, an amine oxide and an alkoxy phenylcarbomic acid ester on some metabolic functions in Staphylococcus aureus. Microbios, 30, 27–35.

Mlynarcik, D., Georch, D., Figurova, M., and Lacko, I. 1975. Antimicrobial effect of some amine oxides. Folia Microbiol., 20, 60–77.

Murata, Y., Mita, K., Miyamota, E., and Ueda, M. 1989. Antimicrobial activity of N,N'-dialkylpolymethynediamines against some dental plaque bacteria. Antimicrob. Agents Chemother., 33(9), 1636–1638.

Musher, D.M., and Griffith, D.P. 1974. Generation of formaldehyde from methenamine: effect of pH and concentration, and antibacterial effect. Antimicrob. Agents Chemother., 6, 708–711.

Nagate, T., et al. 1980. Mode of action of a new nalidixic acid derivative, AB206. Antimicrob. Agents Chemother., 17(5), 763–769.

Neely, W.B. 1963a. Action of formaldehyde on microorganisms. I. Correlation of activity with formaldehyde metabolism. J. Bacteriol., 85, 1025–1031.

Neely, W.B. 1963b. Action of formaldehyde on microorganisms. II. Formation of 1,3-thiazane-4-carboxylic acid in Aerobacter aerogenes treated with formaldehyde. J. Bacteriol., 85, 1420–1422.

Neihof, R.A., Bailey, C.A., Patouillet, C., and Hannan, P.J. 1979. Photodegradation of mercaptopyridine-N-oxide biocides. Arch Environ. Contam. Toxicol., 8, 355–368.

Nezval, J., and Halacka, K. 1967. The enhancing effect of EDTA on the antibacterial activity of nalidixic acid against *Pseudomonas aeruginosa*. Experientia, 23, 1043–1044.

Odajima, O., and Matsumoto, K. 1988. Synergistic industrial microbicides containing 2-pyridinethiol-1-oxide (salts) and 2-(4-thiazolyl)benzimidazole. Jpn. Kokai Tokkyo Koho. Japanese Patent 63,196,502 [88,196,502].

Okamoto, K. 1987. Microbicides containing isothiazolone derivatives 2,2-dibromo-3-nitrilopropionamide and/or hexachlorodimethylsulfone. Jpn. Kokai Tokkyo Koho JP 62,70301 [87,70301].

Ong, J.T.H., and Rutherford, B.S. 1980. Some factors affecting the rate of N-nitrosodiethanolamine formation from 2-bromo-2-nitropropane-1,3-diol and ethanolamines. J. Soc. Cosmet. Chem., 31, 153–159.

Orentreich, N. 1972. A clinical evaluation of two shampoos in the treatment of seborrheic dermatitis. J. Soc. Cosmet. Chem., 23, 189–194.

Otokuni, T., and Kitanishi, Y. 1986. Industrial microbicides and preservatives. Jpn. Kokai Tokkyo Koho JP 61,210,004 [86,210,004].

Page, G.V., and Solberg, M. 1979. Redox potential-dependent nitrite metabolism by *Salmonella typhimurium*. Appl. Environ. Microbiol., 37(6), 1152–1156.

Pansy, F.E., Slander, H., Koerber, W.L., and Donovich, R. 1953. *In vitro* studies with 1-hydroxy-2-(1H) pyridinethione. Proc. Soc. Exp. Biol. Med., 82, 122–124.

Paulus, W. 1976. Problems encountered with formaldehyde-releasing compounds used as preservatives in aqueous systems, especially lubricoolants—possible solutions to the problems. Proc. 3rd Intl. Biodegr. Sympos., 1975. London, Applied Science.

Paulus, W. 1980. Formaldehyde releasing compounds and their utility as microbicides. Biodetn. Proc. IV Intl. Sympos. Berlin. London, Pitman Publishing.

Paulus, W. 1988. Developments in microbicides for the protection of materials. In *Proceedings of the 7th International Biodeterioration Symposium*. Edited by H.O.W. Eggins, D. Houghton, and R.N. Smith. London, Elsevier Applied Science, pp. 1–19.

Paulus, W., Pauli, O., and Genth, H. 1967. Disinfectants and preservatives. U.S. Patent No. 3,328,240.

Pfirrmann, R.W., and Leslie, G.B. 1979. The antiendotoxin activity of taurolin in experimental animals. J. Appl. Bacteriol., 46, 97–102.

Piet, L., and Rossmoore, H.W. 1985. A further study on the use of monocopper (II) citrate as an antimicrobial agent in metalworking fluid. Lubr. Engg., 41(2), 103–105.

Post, W.E., and Nicoll, H.K. 1910. The comparative efficiency of some common germicides. JAMA, 55, 1635–1639.

Prasad, K.S., and Chitnis, S.M. 1986. Transcription but not translation is required for EDTA-induced autolysis in *Escherichia coli*. Biochem. Biophys. Res. Commun., 134, 338–343.

Preston, A.F., et al. 1985. Efficacy of N-substituted isothiazolones for the control of wood decay fungi. In *Biodeterioration 6, Proceedings of the 6th International Biodeterioration Symposium*. Edited by S. Barry and D.R. Houghton. C.A.B. Intl. Mycological Inst., The Biodetn. Soc., United Kingdom, pp. 100–107.

Priestly, G.C., and Savin, J.A. 1976. The microbiology of dandruff. Br. J. Dermatol., 94, 469–471.

Purcell, R.F., and Selleck, J.R. 1978. Composition (of antimicrobial agents useful for controlling the growth of microorganisms). U.S. Patent No. 4,101,433.

Raisanen, S., Ylitalo, P., Topenen, A., and Seppanen, J. 1985. Trimethoprim and methenamine hippurate, a new theoretical combination for the treatment of urinary tract infections. Scand. J. Infect. Dis., 17(2), 211–218.

Rayman, M.K., and MacLeod, R.A. 1975. Interaction of Mg^{2+} with peptidoglycan and its relation to the prevention of lysis of a marine Pseudomonad. J. Bacteriol., 122(2), 650–659.

Repaske, R. 1958. Lysis of gram-negative organisms and the role of versene. Biochimica et Biophysica ACTA, 30, 225–232.

Riha, V.F., Sondossi, M., and Rossmoore, H.W. 1990. The potentiation of industrial biocide activity with Cu^{++}. II. Synergistic effects with 5-chloro-2-methyl-4-isothiazolin-3-one. Intl. Biodetn., in press.

Root, J.L., McIntyre, O.R., Jacobs, N.J., and Daghlian, C.P. 1988. Inhibitory effect of disodium *Staphylococcus epidermidis in vitro*: relation to prophylaxis of Hickman catheters. Antimicrob. Agents Chemother., 32(1), 1627–1630.

Rosen, W.E., and Berke, P.A. 1973. Modern concepts of cosmetic preservation. J. Soc. Cosmet. Chem., 24, 663–675.

Ross, R.T., and Hollis, C.G. 1976. The microbiological deterioration of pulpwood, paper and paint. In *Industrial Microbiology*. Edited by B. Miller and W. Litsky. New York, McGraw-Hill.

Rossmoore, H.W. 1977. Antimicrobial compositions and methods. British Patent No. 1,476,862.

Rossmoore, H.W. 1979. Heterocyclic compounds as industrial biocides. Dev. Ind. Microbiol., 20, 41–71.

Rossmoore, H.W. 1983. Nitrogen compounds. In *Disinfection, Sterilization and Preservation*. 3rd Edition. Edited by S.S. Block. Philadelphia, Lea & Febiger, pp. 271–306.

Rossmoore, H.W. 1986. Synergistic antimicrobial or biocidal mixtures including isothiazolones. U.S. Patent No. 4,608,183.

Rossmoore, H.W. 1987. Synergistic antimicrobial or biocidal mixtures. U.S. Patent No. 4,666,616.

Rossmoore, H.W., DeMare, J., and Smith, T.H.F. 1972. Anti- and pro-microbial activity of hexahydro-1,3,5 tris (2-hydroxyethyl)-2-triazine in cutting fluid emulsion. In *Biodeterioration of Materials*. Volume 2. Edited by A.H. Walters and E.H. Hueck-Van Der Plas. London, Applied Science, pp. 286–293.

Rossmoore, H.W., and Holtzman, G.H.M. 1974. Growth of fungi in cutting fluids. Dev. Indust. Microbiol., 15, 273–280.

Rossmoore, H.W., and Jackson, J.R. 1959. Fungus resistance test on selected non-metallics from the Jupiter and Redstone missiles. Technical Report U.S. Army Ord. RN-23428B, 2DA-20-Ord. 14800.

Rossmoore, H.W., Shearer, M.E., and Shearer, C. 1964. Growth studies on *Desulfovibro desulfuricans*. Dev. Indust. Microbiol., 5, 334–342.

Rossmoore, H.W., Sieckhaus, J.F., Rossmoore, L.A., and DeFonzo, D. 1978. The utility of biocide combinations in controlling mixed microbial populations in metalworking fluids. Lubr. Engg., 35(10, 559–563.

Rossmoore, H.W., and Sondossi, M. 1988. Applications and mode of action of formaldehyde condensate biocides. Adv. Appl. Microbiol., 33, 223–277.

Rossmoore, H.W., and Trubey, J.D. 1967. The role of catalase in the hemolytic reaction. Rev. Latinoam. Microbiol., 8(2), 61–73.

Rozycki, M., and Bartha, R. 1981. Problems associated with the use of azide as an inhibitor of microbial activity in soil. Appl. Environ. Microbiol., 4(3), 833–836.

Russell, A.D. 1971. Ethylenediaminetetra-acetic acid. In *Inhibition and Destruction of the Microbial Cell*. Edited by W.B. Hugo, New York, Academic Press, pp. 209–224.

Schmidt, L.H., Crosby, R., Rasco, J., and Vaughan, D. 1978. Antimalarial activities of various 4-pyridinemethanols with special attention to WR-172,435 and WR-180,409. Antimicrob. Agents Chemother., 14(3), 420–435.

Schuelke and Mayr Gesellschaft Mit Beschrankter Haftung. 1963. Disinfectants and methods of disinfecting. London Patent Specification 920,301.

Scott, C.R., and Wolf, P.A. 1962. Antibacterial activity of a series of quaternaries prepared from hexamethylenetetramine and halohydrocarbons. Appl. Microbiol., 10, 211–216.

Sedlock, D.M., and Bailey, D.M. 1985. Microbicidal activity of octenidine hydrochloride, a new alkanediylbis[pyridine] germicidal agent. Antimicrob. Agents Chemother., 28(6), 786–790.

Sharpell, F. 1980. Industrial uses of biocides in processes and products. Dev. Indust. Microbiol., 21, 133–140.

Shepherd, J.A., Waigh, R.D., and Gilbert, P. 1988. Antibacterial action of 2-bromo-2-nitropropane-1,3-diol(bronopol). Antimicrob. Agents Chemother., 32(11), 1693–1698.

Shipman, C., Jr., Smith, S.H., Drach, J.C., and Klayman, D.L. 1981. Antiviral activity of 2-acetylpyridine thiosemicarbazones against *Herpes simplex* virus. Antimicrob. Agents Chemother., 19(4), 682–685.

Sidi, H., and Johnson, H.R. 1975. Surface coating compositions containing substituted oxazolidines. U.S. Patent No. 3,905,928.

Siond, M., et al. 1988. Coumarin and quinoline action in archaebacteria; evidence for a gyrase-like enzyme. J. Bacteriol., 170(2), 1946–1953.

Skaliy, P., et al. 1980. Laboratory studies of disinfectants against *Legionella pneumophila*. Appl. Environ. Microbiol., 40(4), 697–700.

Slee, A.M., and O'Connor, J.R. 1983. *In vitro* anti-plaque activity of octenidine dihydrochloride (WIM 41464-2) against preformed plaques of selected oral plaque-forming microorganisms. Antimicrob. Agents Chemother., 23(3), 379–384.

Smit, H., et al. 1980. Mode of action of copper complexes of some 2,2'- bipyridyl analogs on *Paracoccus denitrificans*. Antimicrob. Agents Chemother., 18(2), 249–256.

Snyder, M.L., and Lichstein, H.C. 1940. Sodium azide as an inhibiting substance for gram negative bacteria. J. Infect. Dis., 67, 113–115.

Sofos, J.N., Busta, F.F., and Allen, C.E. 1979. Sodium nitrite and sorbic acid effects on *Clostridium botulinum* spore germination and total microbial growth in chicken frankfurter emulsions during temperature abuse. Appl. Environ. Microbiol., 37(6), 1103–1109.

Sondossi, M., Riha, V.F., and Rossmoore, H.W. 1990. The potentiation of industrial biocide activity with Cu^{++}. I. Synergistic effect of Cu^{++} with formaldehyde. Intl. Biodetn., in press.

Sondossi, M., Rossmoore, H.W., and Wireman, J.W. 1984. Regrowth of *Pseudomonas aeruginosa* following treatment with a formaldehyde condensate biocide. Dev. Ind. Microbiol., 25, 515–522.

Sondossi, M., Rossmoore, H.W., and Wireman, J.W. 1985. Observations of resistance and cross-resistance to formaldehyde and a formaldehyde-condensate biocide. Intl. Biodetn., 21(2), 105–106.

Sondossi, M., Rossmoore, H.W., and Wireman, J.W. 1986a. The effect of fifteen biocides on formaldehyde-resistant strains of *Pseudomonas aeruginosa*. J. Ind. Microbiol., 1, 87–96.

Sondossi, M., Rossmoore, H.W., and Wireman, J.W. 1986b. Induction and selection of formaldehyde-based resistance in *Pseudomonas aeruginosa*. J. Ind. Microbiol., *1*, 97–103.

Staron, T., and Allard, C. 1964. Proprietes antifongique de 2-(4'-thiazolyl) benzimidazole ou thiabendazole. Phytiat. Phytopharm., *13*, 163–168 (Rev. Appl. Mycol., *44*, 1965).

Stecker, H.C. 1977. The salicylanilides and carbanilides. In *Disinfection, Sterilization, and Preservation*. 2nd Edition. Edited by S.S. Block. Philadelphia, Lea & Febiger, pp. 282–300.

Stretton, R.J., and Manson, T.W. 1973. Aspects of the mode of action of the antibacterial compound bronopol(2-bromo-2-nitropropan-1,3-diol). J. Appl. Bacteriol., *36*, 61–76.

Subick, J., Takacsova, G., Psenak, M., and Devinsky, F. 1977. Antimicrobial activity of amine oxides: mode of action and structure-activity correlation. Antimicrob. Agents Chemother., *12*(2), 139–146.

Suter, W., Rosselet, A., and Knusel, F. 1978. Mode of action of quindoxin and substituted quinoxaline-di-N-oxides on *Escherichia coli*. Antimicrob. Agents Chemother., *13*(5), 770–783.

Sykes, G. 1958. *Disinfection and Sterilization*. New York, D. Van Nostrand Co.

Szabo, J., et al. 1986. Hung. Teljes HU 38,833.

Tally, F.P., et al. 1978. Antimicrobial activity of metronidazole in anaerobic bacteria. Antimicrob. Agents Chemother., *13*(3), 460–465.

Tally, F.P., Sutter, V.L., and Finegold, S.M. 1975. Treatment of anaerobic infections with metronidazole. Antimicrob. Agents Chemother., *7*, 672–675.

Tenenbaum, S., and Opdyke, D.L. 1967. Antimicrobial properties of antiseborrheic agents. V. A standard method for comparing zinc pyrithione to other compounds. Proc. Scient. Sect. Toilet Goods Assoc., *47*, 20–23.

Trotz, S.I., and Pitts, J.J. 1981. Industrial antimicrobial agents. In *Encyclopedia of Chemical Technology*. 3rd Edition. Volume 13. Edited by Kirk-Othmer. pp. 223–253.

U.S. Department of HEW, FDA. 1974. Certain halogenated salicylanilides as active ingredients in drug and cosmetic products. Fed. Reg., *39*(179), 33102–33140.

U.S. Department of HEW, FDA. 1978. OTC topical antimicrobial products: over-the-counter drugs generally recognized as safe, effective, and not misbranded. Fed. Reg., *43*(4), 1210–1253.

U.S. EPA. 1987a. *Formaldehyde Health Risk Assessment—Office of Toxic Substances, April 16, 1987*. Washington, D.C.

U.S. EPA. 1987b. Toxicology Data Call-In for Antimicrobial Pesticides. Fed. Reg., *52*(4), 595–596.

Umekawa, O., Yosuke, I., and Katayama, S. 1987. Industrial bactericides and algicides containing aliphatic nitroalcohols and isothiazolones. Jpn. Kokai Tokkyo Koho JP, *62*, 10,003 [87, 10,003].

Van Wambeke, Vanachter, E.A., and Van Assche, C. 1985. Fungicidal treatment with azides. Monograph Br. Crop Prot. Counc., *31*, 253–256.

Walter, R.W., Mills, J.F., and Relenyi, A.C. 1985. Compatibility of DBNPA with chlorine as water treatment biocides. In *Proceedings of 46th International Water Conference*. Philadelphia, Engineering Soc., pp. 434–443.

Wehner, D.C. 1965. Trans-dithiocyanoethylene and its derivatives as industrial preservatives. U.S. Patent No. 3,212,963.

Wehner, D.C. 1966. Method of controlling algal growth. U.S. Patent No. 3,252,855.

Wehner, D.C. 1967. Process water treatment and method of controlling sulfate reducing bacteria. U.S. Patent No. 3,300,375.

Wehner, D.C., and Hinz, C.F. 1971. Organic thiocyanates as industrial antimicrobial agents. Dev. Indust. Microbiol., *12*, 404–410.

Weuffen, W., Pyl, T., Gruebner, W., and Juelich, W.D. 1965. Relations of chemical constitution and bacteriostatic activity. X. Bacteriostatic properties of certain thiazole and thiadiazole derivatives. Pharmazie, *20*, 629–633.

Wheeler, H.O., and Bennett, E.O. 1956. Bacterial inhibitors for cutting oil. Appl. Microbiol., *4*, 122–126.

Wilkinson, S.G. 1975. Sensitivity to ethylenediaminetetraacetic acid. In *Resistance of Pseudomonas aeruginosa*. Edited by M.R.W. Brown. New York, John Wiley & Sons, pp. 145–188.

Wilson, D.F., and Chance, B. 1967. Azide inhibition of mitochondrial electron transport. I. The aerobic steady state of succinate oxidation. Biochim. Biophys. Acta, *131*, 421–430.

Wimpenny, J.W.T. 1967. Effect of isoniazid on biosynthesis in *Mycobacterium tuberculosis* var. bovis BCG. J. Gen. Microbiol., *47*, 379.

Wodzinski, R.S., Labeda, D.P., and Alexander, M. 1978. Effects of low concentrations of bisulfite-sulfite and nitrite on microorganisms. Appl. Environ. Microbiol., *35*, 718–723.

Wolf, P.A. 1974. The antimicrobial activity of several types of bactericides as related to beta-D-galactoside transport. Dev. Indust. Microbiol., *15*, 353–357.

Wolf, P.A., and Bobalek, F.J. 1967. Antimicrobial performance of tri- and tetrachloro-4-(methylsulfonyl) pyridines as industrial preservatives. Appl. Microbiol., *15*(6), 1376–1381.

Wolf, P.A., and Sterner, P.W. 1972. 2,2-dibromo-3-nitrilopropionamide, a compound with slimicidal activity. Appl. Microbiol., *24*(4), 581–584.

Wolfson, J.S., and Harper, D.C. 1985. The fluoroquinolmers: structures, mechanisms of action, and resistance, and spectra of action *in vitro*. Antimicrob. Agents Chemother., *29*(4), 581–586.

Wright, H.T., Nurse, K.C., and Goldstein, D.J. 1981. Nalidixic acid, oxolinic acid, and novobiocin inhibit yeast glycyl- and leucyl-transfer RNA synthetases. Science, *213*(4506), 455–456.

Yale, H.L. 1964. Sulfur and selenium compounds of pyridine. In *Pyridine and Its Derivatives, Part IV*. Edited by E. Klingsberg. New York, Interscience Publishers, pp. 345–437.

Yeung, T.C., Beaulieu, B.B., Jr., McLafferty, M.A., and Goldman, P. 1984. Interaction of metronidazole with DNA repair mutants of *Escherichia coli*. Antimicrob. Agents Chemother., *25*(1), 65–70.

CHAPTER 18

POLYMERIC ANTIMICROBIAL AGENTS

Oscar W. May

Certain synthetic polymers as well as some modified natural polymers possess antimicrobial properties that make them potentially useful as microorganism control agents. Such polymers include those in which a biocidal moiety is chemically bonded as a pendant group on the polymeric backbone and is subsequently released through hydrolysis or other chemical breakdown mechanisms. With this type, the polymer itself, which is often not water-soluble, serves only as a type of controlled-release vehicle for the active antimicrobial agent. Another class of antimicrobial polymers is made up of compounds that have antimicrobial groups as integral parts of the main polymer structural chains. These polymers are usually water-soluble, and their activity does not depend on the hydrolysis of the molecule or other degradative reactions. It is this latter type of polymer that is the main focus of this chapter.

Although a thorough discussion of the first type of antimicrobial polymer is beyond the scope of this chapter, some examples of uses of this type can be given. One example of the first type is represented by the tributyltin methacrylate-methyl methacrylate polymers that are used in marine antifouling coatings to prevent the biologic fouling of ship bottoms and other underwater marine structures. The biocidal tributyltin group is chemically bound as a pendant group that is released slowly by hydrolysis in the sea water, as shown in Figure 18–1. The effect is to inhibit the growth of bacteria, algae, barnacles, and other organisms that tend to foul submerged surfaces in sea water. In this case, the initial polymer is not water-soluble but becomes soluble because of the slow hydrolysis by the sea water and the formation of the water-soluble salt forms of the polymer (Sghibartz, 1984).

This approach of chemically anchoring biocides to polymers has also been used as a way to prepare fungicidal paints, with pentachlorophenol being the most frequently used biocide (Pittman, 1976; Pittman and Stahl, 1981; Pleurdeau et al., 1985). Another application is in

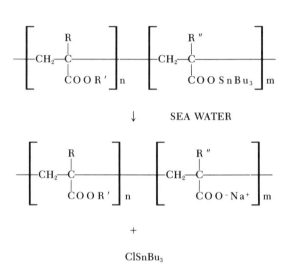

↓ SEA WATER

+

ClSnBu₃

Fig. 18–1. Hydrolysis of organotin polymers. From Sghibartz, C.M. 1984. Antifouling paints—present and future. Congr. FATIPEC, *17*(4), 145–164.

the preparation of controlled-release agricultural biocides (Akelah and Selim, 1987).

Polymers with pendant biocidal groups have also been found useful in food packaging materials to provide extended food shelf-life. For example, Halek and Garg (1989) chemically coupled the fungicide benomyl* to an ionomeric packaging film prepared from an ethylene-methacrylic acid copolymer. The coupled film was tested for its effectiveness against two strains of fungi, *Aspergillus flavus* and *Penicillium notatum*, employing potato dextrose agar in Petri dish "zone of inhibition" tests. After 21 days of incubation, there was a zone of inhibition around the film coupled with benomyl, but the untreated film did not show any inhibition of microbial growth. The results showed that the plastic coupled with fungicide

---

*[1-[(butylamino)carbonyl]-1H-benzimidazol-2-yl]carbamic acid, methyl ester (CAS Reg. No. 17804-35-2).

was effective against the growth of microorganisms, or if the fungicide was being released, it remained effective after coupling.

Although controlled-release products based on the chemical bonding of biocides to polymer molecules are becoming increasingly important, the polymers that have found the widest variety of uses as antimicrobial agents in disinfection, sterilization, and preservation applications are those of the second type, that is, those in which the antimicrobial groups are integral parts of the main polymer chain. Of these, two types have so far achieved the greatest economic importance. These are the biguanide polymers and the quaternary ammonium polymers, particularly that class called "ionene polymers."

BIGUANIDE POLYMERS

Biguanides have long been used as antimicrobial agents in the preservation of cosmetics and pharmaceuticals and as antiseptics (Curd and Rose, 1946; Rose and Swain, 1956). The prime example is chlorhexidine,* a bis(biguanide) that is the subject of Chapter 16 in this book. When it was found that this bis(biguanide) had a much greater bactericidal activity than did the monomeric biguanides, investigators became interested in developing the polymeric biguanides as antimicrobial agents, particularly polyhexamethylene biguanide (PHMB) hydrochloride (Davies et al., 1968; Davies and Field, 1969). Today a number of antimicrobial agents based on these polymers are commercially available under such trademarks as Vantocil, Cosmocil, and Baquacil, and are used in a variety of antimicrobial applications.

Chemistry

A process for the preparation of polymeric biguanides of the unit formula

$$-X-NH-\underset{\underset{NH}{\|}}{C}-NH-\underset{\underset{NH}{\|}}{C}-NH-Y-NH-\underset{\underset{NH}{\|}}{C}-NH-\underset{\underset{NH}{\|}}{C}-NH-$$

was described in 1954 in a British patent issued to Rose and Swain. The process involved reacting a bis(dicyandiamide) of the formula

$$CN-NH-\underset{\underset{NH}{\|}}{C}-NH.X.NH-\underset{\underset{NH}{\|}}{C}-NH-CN$$

with a diamine of the formula NH_2-Y-NH_2, or with the salt of such a diamine, where X and Y were bridging groups such as polymethylene chains. Improvements in the mechanical details of the process were later described in a U.S. patent issued in 1969 (Dickinson et al.). From the beginning, the preferred reactants were hexamethylene bis(dicyandiamide) and hexamethylenediamine (or preferably its hydrochloride salt), yielding a polymer in

*1,6-Bis[5-(p-chlorophenyl)biguanidino]hexane (CAS Reg. No. 55-56-1).

Table 18–1. *Bacteriostatic Activity of Cosmocil CQ*

Organism	MIC (ppm)
Staphylococcus aureus	20
Streptococcus faecalis	<5
Proteus vulgaris	250
Escherichia coli	20
Aerobacter aerogenes	20
Salmonella typhi	5
Pseudomonas aeruginosa	100
Saccharomyces cerevisiae	25
Saccharomyces ellipsodeus	25
Saccharomyces turbidans	25

From ICI Americas Inc. 1986. Cosmocil CQ. Polyhexamethylene biguanide hydrochloride solution. Company brochure.

which both X and Y were hexamethylene chains and with a general formula that could be written as follows:

$$-\left[(CH_2)_6-NH-\underset{\underset{NH}{\|}}{C}-NH-\underset{\underset{NH}{\|}}{C}-NH-\right]_n$$

The polymer chains are terminated by either an amino or aminohydrochloride group or a dicyandiamide group, and the value of n reportedly may range as high as 500 or more. This is equivalent to a molecular weight near 100,000, but most commercial products based on the polyhexamethylene biguanide have much lower molecular weights, typically in the 1000 to 3000 range (Carter and Hinton, 1977; Ogunbiyi et al., 1989).

Antimicrobial Activity

In their 1954 patent on the composition and manufacture of polymeric biguanides, Rose and Swain reported that these polymers possessed good antibacterial activity against *Streptococcus* spp., *Staphylococcus* spp., *Escherichia coli*, *Clostridium perfringens*, and *Pseudomonas aeruginosa*. They also stated that they strongly inhibited the growth of many fungi, including *Fusarium graminearum* and *Aspergillus niger*. That document contained no supporting data, but more-recently published information (ICI, 1986b) provided the figures shown in Tables 18–1 and 18–2 as examples of the bacteriostatic

Table 18–2. *Fungistatic Activity of Cosmocil CQ*

Organism	MIC (ppm)
Chaetomium globosum	125
Polystictus versicolor	1250
Trichoderma viride	250
Cladosporium resinae	1250
Alternaria tenuis	375
Cladosporium sphaerospermum	375
Aspergillus niger	375
Penicillium notatum	1250
Fusarium solani	1250
Candida albicans	250

From ICI Americas Inc. 1986. Cosmocil CQ. Polyhexamethylene biguanide hydrochloride solution. Company brochure.

and fungistatic activity of a 20% solution of polyhexamethylene biguanide hydrochloride (PHMB) with a molecular weight of 1000 to 1400 and sold under the tradename Cosmocil CQ.* The same publication states that the bactericidal activity of the product was established by tests conforming with British Standard 3286 and using five organisms: *Staphylococcus aureus, Escherichia coli, Pseudomonas aeruginosa, Saccharomyces cerevisiae,* and *Saccharomyces turbidans.* The activity is said to be high even in the presence of organic matter such as blood, milk, or peptone.

In a study with *E. coli,* Broxton et al. (1983) showed that the bactericidal efficacy of polyhexamethylene biguanides was related to the molecular weight or degree of polymerization of the polymers. In tests with an amine-ended dimer (AED) (n = 2), Vantocil IB (a polydisperse mixture of PHMB with n = 5.5), and a high-molecular-weight fraction (n ≥10) of PHMB, they found that the Vantocil and the high-molecular-weight fraction could totally inhibit the growth and motility of *E. coli* in liquid culture, whereas the AED never totally inhibited either function regardless of concentration. Growth inhibition and bactericidal activity increased with increasing levels of biocide polymerization. Extrapolation of the data gave estimates of minimum growth inhibitory concentrations of 1.25 μg/ml and 0.29 μg/ml, respectively, for the Vantocil and the high-molecular-weight PMHB. For the AED, concentrations between 0.5 and 3 μg/ml gave progressive reductions in growth rate, but the level of growth rate inhibition never exceeded 70%, and it was not possible to extrapolate to a minimum inhibitory concentration.

PHMB has been shown to be effective in killing pathogenic free-living amoebae (PFLA), both in axenic conditions (Dawson et al., 1983a) and in simulated natural conditions (Dawson et al., 1983b). The studies by Dawson and his coworkers in New Zealand were undertaken because of concern by public health authorities over the finding of PFLA in chlorinated swimming pool waters and the possible contraction of amoebic meningoencephalitis from these waters. Baquacil, a 20% solution of PHMB used as an antimicrobial in the treatment of swimming pools, was tested against four strains of *Naegleria* and two of *Acanthamoeba* in axenic conditions at 25°, 30°, and 37°C. The axenically cultured amoebae of each strain were centrifuged from the culture media, resuspended in a sterile phosphate buffer (pH 7.0), washed three times in the same buffer, counted, and again resuspended. For each test, a measured amount of the amoebae suspension was diluted with sterile buffer containing the required concentration of Baquacil. Following incubation for a period of between 30 and 240 minutes at the specified temperature, a viable count was done in each case using a plaque formation method on a bacterial lawn plate. In the control dilutions (containing no Baquacil), all of the strains grew equally well at 30°C,

*Cosmocil, Vantocil, and Baquacil are all trademarks used by ICI for aqueous solutions of poly(hexamethylene biguanide) hydrochloride, usually 20% active.

whereas the nonpathogenic strains of *Naegleria (N. gruberi* P1200f) and *Acanthamoeba (A. castellanii* 1501) grew best at 25°C, and the pathogenic strains of *Naegleria (N. fowleri* MsM, MsT, and Northcott) and *Acanthamoeba (A. culbertsoni* A–1) showed stimulated growth at 37°C. At the latter temperature, MsM, MsT, and Northcott showed 2.25%, 1.5%, and 0.0% survival, respectively, after 30 minutes exposure to 50 mg/l of Baquacil, and the survival rates for P1200f, A–1, and 1501 were, respectively, 0.0%, 1.5%, and 0.75%. At 30°C, the survival rates at the same concentration were MsM, 7.5%; MsT, 3.0%; Northcott, 0.0%; P1200f and A–1, 3.0%; and 1501, 3.0%. At 25°C, all survival rates were zero except for MsT (2.25%) and 1501 (1.5%). When the exposure time was increased to 240 minutes against strains with high survival rates at 30 minutes, *N. fowleri* MsM proved to have the greatest potential to survive Baquacil. However, all strains were killed in a maximum time of 2½ hours.

In the second series of tests with Baquacil and PFLA, simulated natural conditions were established by adding bacteria, bovine fecal matter, or both to the water to create a biochemical oxygen demand. The experiments were run with both axenically and monoxenically cultured amoebae. Although there was the expected increase in disinfectant demand, it was shown that the Baquacil was amoebicidal to PFLA in conditions similar to those likely to be encountered in swimming pools. However, the disinfectant was not amoebicidal at 50 mg/l in simulated heavily polluted conditions.

Mechanism of Action

The mechanism of antimicrobial action of PHMB has been studied by a number of researchers (Davies et al., 1968, 1969; Ikeda et al., 1983, 1984, 1985a, 1985b; Broxton et al., 1983, 1984a, 1984b, 1985a, 1985b). Based on the work of these investigators, the proposed bactericidal sequence (ICI, 1986c) begins with a rapid attraction of the cationic PHMB to the negatively charged bacterial surface, its binding to a receptive site on that surface, and a breaking down of the cell-wall exclusion and defense mechanisms. The PHMB is attracted to the cytoplasmic membrane, where it causes leakage of low-molecular-weight cytoplasmic components such as K^+ ions and inhibition of membrane bond enzymes such as ATPase. Subsequent extensive disruption of the cytoplasmic membrane then can lead to leakage of macromolecular components (e.g., nucleotides) and precipitation of cell contents. The experimental evidence suggests that the lethal action is from the irreversible loss of essential cellular components due to cytoplasmic membrane damage and that the cytoplasmic precipitation is a secondary event to the death of the cell. These mechanisms are, of course, similar to those of monomeric cationic agents such as the monomeric quaternary ammonium compounds.

Applications

Polymeric biguanides, particularly the poly (hexamethylene biguanide) hydrochloride (PHMB), have been sold as disinfectants for over 20 years (Boardman, 1969). Since their introduction, a large variety of applications have been developed or have been proposed for these antimicrobials. For example, a 20% solution of PHMB (Cosmocil CQ) is used for the preservation of cosmetics and pharmaceuticals at concentrations of 0.2 to 1.0%, and it has been suggested for use in the preparation of surgical scrubs at concentrations of 2 to 4% (ICI, 1986b). The same active ingredient is registered with the U.S. Environmental Protection Agency (EPA) under the name Vantocil IB for the control of pathogenic gram-positive and gram-negative bacteria in bottle washer water, cannery cooling canal water, synthetic adhesives, leather processing liquors, and metalworking fluids (EPA Reg. No. 10182-128). Under the name Baquacil, it is registered for the control of pathogenic bacteria and algae in swimming pools (EPA Reg. No. 10182-19), an application discussed in more detail below.

PHMB has been claimed to be useful for the preservation of foods. Strandskov and Bocklemann (1975) obtained a patent on its use for preserving fruit and vegetable juices, soft drinks, and light alcohol beverages during storage. It was shown that by the addition of about 1 to 10 ppm of PHMB to a beverage the growth of the spoilage organisms could be inhibited, a procedure that could eliminate the need for more costly procedures to preserve the beverages, such as pasteurization, microfiltration, or constant refrigeration.

Islam and Islam (1979a) evaluated PHMB for the extension of the shelf-life of fresh poultry. Freshly processed poultry carcasses were immersed for 2 hrs at $2 \pm 0.5°C$ in distilled water solutions containing varying amounts of PHMB and then were drained, packaged in polyethylene bags, and stored at $2 \pm 0.2°C$. Shelf-life determinations were made by a sensory panel checking for off-odors beginning on the eighth day of storage. Birds treated with 200, 300, and 400 ppm PHMB had average shelf-lives of 22.9, 25.9, and 26.0 days, respectively, compared to 10.5 days of shelf-life for water-treated controls. In a later study, these same investigators did comparative studies with PHMB, glutaraldehyde, and iodacetamide as poultry preservatives (Islam and Islam, 1979b). In this case, the carcasses were dipped in 500 ppm solutions of the preservatives, and it was found that the PHMB provided the greatest shelf-life improvement, and glutaraldehyde the least.

In another study on the use of PHMB to treat broiler carcasses (Thomson et al., 1981), the effectiveness of adding the antimicrobial agent to the prechilling water in order to minimize *Salmonella* contamination was investigated. Broiler carcasses, each inoculated with 30 cells of marker *S. heidelberg*, were prechilled and chilled together with uninoculated carcasses in a simulated commercial chilling system. When either 10 or 25 ppm PHMB was added to the prechill water, cross contamination of uninoculated carcasses was prevented and no viable *Salmonella* were found on the inoculated carcasses. With 60,000 cells of marker *Salmonella* and 10 ppm PHMB, cross contamination was not prevented, and viable *Salmonella* cells were found on the inoculated carcasses. With 25 ppm PHMB and 60,000 cells, cross contamination was prevented, but viable *Salmonella* remained on the inoculated carcasses.

Rosenthal et al. (1982) investigated the use of PHMB in foods and food processing equipment because of concerns about development of reliable methods for determining PHMB residues, its toxicity to animals, and its effectiveness in the presence of organic matter. A colorimetric method based on the reaction with nitro-prusside reagent was found suitable for the dosimetry. In a bacteriologic medium, PHMB was inhibitory at 20 μg/ml to *E. coli* but was less effective against *Staphylococcus aureus* and practically ineffective against *Pseudomonas aeruginosa*. The bactericidal activity was impaired in the presence of milk but not affected much by the addition of blood. In an in-vitro toxicologic test, PHMB was toxic to Chinese hamster cells at doses comparable to the antibacterial doses.

A number of patents have been issued for the use of PHMB in ophthalmic compositions and contact lens disinfecting compositions. Hydrophilic soft contact lenses tend to absorb and concentrate low-molecular-weight bactericides used for disinfection; when placed in the eye, these lenses can release the concentrated solution and irritate the eyes. Drain and Simmonite (1976) claimed that polymeric biguanides would alleviate this problem. Their preferred compositions were isotonic with tear fluid, generally phosphate-buffered, and contained from 0.0005 to 0.0025% of the polymer. These polymeric bactericides were also said to be suitable for use in compositions for hard contact lenses and for eye drops. Stockel and Jelling (1985) claimed that the addition of an oxidizing agent such as stabilized chlorine dioxide or hydrogen peroxide would potentiate the bactericidal effect of polymeric biguanides as well as that of certain other polymeric microbicides. Ogunbiyi et al. (1988, 1989) found that when they used a borate buffer system, the bactericidal activity was greatly improved over that obtained by Drain and Simmonite (1976) with the phosphate buffer system. This increased activity made it possible to use PHMB concentrations in the range of 0.000001 to 0.0003%. The lower amounts of PHMB were said to reduce a lens-staining problem associated with higher concentrations of the polymer.

Another type of application for biguanide polymers for which patents have been issued or applied for recently is the treatment of nonwoven fabrics used in disposable diapers, incontinence pads, feminine hygiene pads, and similar articles. Fawkes (1986) claimed that by applying a polymeric biguanide to the nonwoven material bacterial activity would be inhibited when the article became contaminated with body emissions, which would help control odors, skin irritation, and other problems caused by microorganisms. Related applications include coating surgical dressings or incise drape material with an adhesive containing PHMB in order to prevent infection during and after surgery (Brown, 1987; Feld and Soto, 1987), and producing antimicrobial wet wiper products by applying PHMB to nonwoven fabrics during the web-forming process (Quantrille and Johnson, 1989).

Smith and Singer (1977) obtained a British patent on the use of PHMB as a dual-purpose additive for purification of natural waters, particularly water intended for drinking. The PHMB was said to be effective in replacing chlorine and other sanitizers for the control of harmful bacteria and other microorganisms, and at the same time it was said to be effective in flocculating and precipitating suspended solids in the water. This sanitizer is also reported to destroy aquatic mollusks that transmit the debilitating disease bilharziasis. These mollusks are found in water supplies in many parts of Africa, the Middle East, and the Far East and constitute a major public health problem in some areas.

An important commercial use of PHMB for water treatment is as a swimming pool sanitizer and algistat. A U.S. patent was issued in 1977 covering its application for algae control in swimming pools (Carter and Hinton), and it is sold in this country and others under the name of Baquacil for the control of both pathogenic bacteria and algae. Its advantages are said to be that it can replace chlorine (with which it is not compatible) and that it can be used much less frequently and still maintain an effective residual level of the sanitizer. The manufacturer recommends an initial dose of 50 ppm of the Baquacil and maintenance of the concentration between 30 and

mers in 1968. The general structure of the simple aliphatic ionenes can be illustrated as follows:

$$\left[\begin{array}{c} R^1 \\ | \\ -N^+ - R^2 - N^+ - R^3 - \\ | \quad\quad\quad | \\ R^1 \quad Z^- \quad R^1 \quad Z^- \end{array} \right]_n$$

where R^1, R^2, and R^3 are alkyl groups, Z is a halogen, and n is the degree of polymerization. R^1 is typically a methyl group, and R^2 and R^3 may be identical or different alkyl groups.

Because monomeric compounds containing quaternary nitrogen atoms possess antimicrobial activity, it could have been assumed that the ionene polymers would also have such activity. This, of course, proved to be true, and a large number of such polymers have been synthesized by various workers and shown to be active, particularly against bacteria and algae. However, to date only a few of these have been developed commercially for microorganism control.

Chemistry

Although most of the research and development work with ionenes has taken place in the past 20 years or so, the history of these polymers goes much further back. For example, Gibbs et al. reported in 1933 that by allowing 3-chloro-N,N-dimethyl-propylamine to react with itself in aqueous solution, a linear quaternary ammonium polymer was formed with a molecular weight of 1500 or greater and the following structure:

$$ClCH_2CH_2CH_2-\overset{\overset{\displaystyle CH_3}{|}}{\underset{\underset{\displaystyle Cl^-}{|}}{N^+}} \quad \left[-CH_2CH_2CH_2-\overset{\overset{\displaystyle CH_3}{|}}{\underset{\underset{\displaystyle CH_3}{|}}{N^+}} \right]_n \overset{Cl^-}{} -CH_2CH_2CH_2-N\overset{\diagup CH_3}{\diagdown CH_3}$$

50 ppm for bacterial control, and the supplementation of this with an algicide and a periodic treatment with a hydrogen peroxide solution to clarify the water (ICI, 1986a).

McLeod and Webb (1981) patented the method of using alkali metal perborates along with the polymeric biguanides to control pathogenic organisms in water. The perborates, of course, produce hydrogen peroxide when dissolved in water.

IONENE POLYMERS

Although polymers containing quaternary nitrogens in their backbones had long been known, Rembaum et al. first proposed the name "ionenes" for these ionic poly-

However, these authors reported that this same reaction had been carried out by other workers as early as 1906, but that these earlier workers (Knoor and Roth) had postulated that what was formed was an eight-membered cyclic structure, and had not recognized it as a polymer. Gibbs and Marvel (1934) found that when an amine such as Br-(CH₂)₃-NR₂ reacts with itself, linear polymerization occurs when R is methyl, but when R is ethyl, n-propyl, or n-butyl, then cyclization occurs and a four-membered ring is formed.

During the course of research on proteins and protein models, Kern and Brenneisen (1941) investigated polymeric bases, and among the compounds they synthesized were the polymeric products already described by Gibbs and coworkers. Kern and Brenneisen found that the reaction of the dihalides 1,3-dibromopropane, 1,5-dibromopentane, or 1,10-dibromodecane with the ditertiary amines N,N,N',N'-tetramethylethylenediamine or N,N,N',N'-tetramethylpropylenediamine led to the formation of linear quaternary ammonium polymers that were water-soluble and had molecular weights from about 3000 to 10,000. The structure assigned to these polymers was that suggested by Gibbs and coworkers, with a covalent halogen as one end group and a tertiary amine group at the other end of the chain.

In 1942, Searle of E.I. duPont de Nemours and Co. was issued one of the earliest patents on ionene polymers as agents for the control of bacteria and fungi. The general structure of the polymers claimed was as follows:

$$\left[-R^1 \underset{\underset{A}{|}}{\overset{\overset{R^2 \quad R^3}{\diagdown \diagup}}{N}} - R^4 - \underset{\underset{A}{|}}{\overset{\overset{R^5 \quad R^6}{\diagdown \diagup}}{N}} - \right]_x$$

where x is an integer representing the number of repeating units, A is the anion of an acid, and R^1, R^2, R^3, R^4, R^5, and R^6 are all organic radicals joined to the nitrogen by carbon. The preparation of these polymers had been described in an earlier patent (Ritter, 1941) that covered both the composition of the polymers and the process of their manufacture. The process of making these polymers is, of course, analogous to the quaternization process used in the manufacture of conventional, nonpolymeric quaternary ammonium compounds. The difference is that difunctional tertiary amines are reacted with difunctional halides, making possible the formation of a chain of repeating quaternary ammonium units.

The polymers said by Searle to be the most effective bactericides were those prepared from the reaction of a dibromide in which the bromines were attached to aliphatic hydrogen-bearing carbon atoms and a ditertiary diamine in which the nitrogens are separated by an aliphatic chain of at least six carbon atoms, or a ditertiary diamine in which the radical between the nitrogens contained one or more arylene groups. Examples included polymers made by reacting decamethylene dibromide with N,N,N',N'-tetramethylhexamethylenediamine and one made from the same dibromide and N,N,N',N'-tetramethyl-p,p'-diaminophenylmethane.

Many other dihalides and ditertiary diamines were listed in the Searle patent as reactants for the preparation of quaternary ammonium polymers with antimicrobial activity. However, there are no publications showing that much was ever done to develop these polymers for commercial or practical microorganism control applications. The existence of these patents and the broad range of polymers covered by the claims would certainly have discouraged development of these polymers by others, and little more was published on them until the mid- and late-1960s.

Many of the advances later made with ionene polymers derived from the pioneering work of Rembaum and his coworkers at the Jet Propulsion Laboratory, California Institute of Technology, Pasadena, California. In 1968, they reported that the synthesis of a variety of aliphatic ionenes with molecular weights of 10,000 to 15,000 and yields of over 90% could be achieved at room temperature by the condensation of diamines with dihalides in a number of solvents, and they noted that these polymers were bacteriostatic and bactericidal. A typical synthesis used N,N,N',N'-tetramethylhexamethylenediamine and 1,5-dibromopentane to yield a polymer of the following structure:

$$\sim\!\!-\!\!\underset{\underset{CH_3}{|}}{\overset{\overset{CH_3}{|}}{N^+}}\!\!-\!\!(CH_2)_6\!\!-\!\!\underset{\underset{CH_3 \ Br^-}{|}}{\overset{\overset{CH_3}{|}}{N^+}}\!\!-\!\!(CH_2)_5\!\!-\!\!\underset{\underset{CH_3 \ Br^-}{|}}{\overset{\overset{CH_3}{|}}{N^+}}\!\!-\!\!(CH_2)_6\!\!-\!\!\underset{\underset{CH_3 \ Br^-}{|}}{\overset{\overset{CH_3}{|}}{N^+}}\!\!-\!\!(CH_2)_5\!\!-\!\!\!\!\sim$$

To specify the pendant group on the nitrogen atom, the length of the chains between the nitrogens, and the counterion, Rembaum suggested calling this "tetramethyl-6,5-ionene bromide." Because the pendant groups are generally methyl, the general practice became to call these simple aliphatic ionenes "x,y-ionene halides," where x and y are the numbers of CH_2 groups in the diamine and dihalide, respectively (Rembaum, 1973).

Rembaum and his associates extensively investigated the chemistry and biologic properties of ionene polymers prepared by the condensation of tertiary diamines and dihalides (Rembaum et al., 1968, 1970; Rembaum, 1973). The biologic activity they found for these polymers went beyond their antimicrobial properties and indicated that they should be useful in chemotherapeutic applications as well. For example, the ionenes combine with nerve cell receptors and act as ganglionic blockers, an effect that suggests they might be useful in increasing the duration of action of drugs; ionenes also have antiheparin and antihemorrhagic properties (Rembaum, 1973). It has been shown that these polymers exhibit selectivity toward malignant mammalian cells. In animal tests, they demonstrated antitumor activity, and in in-vitro tests with a mixture of normal and malignant cells showed growth of normal cells while exhibiting toxic effects on malignant cells (Rajaraman et al., 1975; Rembaum, Senyei, and Rajaraman, 1977; Rembaum, 1977).

Green, Merianos, and Petrocci are some other researchers that have done a lot of work with ionene polymers, and they have obtained numerous patents on both the composition and use of ionene polymers as antimicrobial agents (1975a, 1975b, 1976a, 1976b, 1976c, 1976d, 1977a, 1977b, 1977c, 1977d, 1977e, 1977f, 1978b). Many of the polymers they synthesized were based on the condensation reaction of 1,4-dichloro-2-butene with various difunctional tertiary amines.

Another process for the manufacture of ionene polymers starts with the reaction of a secondary amine with an epihalohydrin or a diepoxide, the most common reactants being dimethylamine and epichlorohydrin. The preparation of polymers of this type was described by Panzer and Dixon in a U.S. patent issued to them in 1973, a patent that was later split and published with some changes as two reissue patents in 1976. Panzer and Dixon cited some earlier patents for polyquaternaries prepared from dimethylamine and epichlorohydrin, including one as early as 1948. However, they claimed differences that distinguished the polymers made by their process from those of the prior method and thus made their polymers new and patentable compositions of matter. One difference claimed was the higher viscosity and hence higher molecular weight obtained, which made the polymers more effective as flocculants in the water and effluent treatment applications that were apparently of primary interest to the inventors at the time. They made no mention of possible antimicrobial efficacy, but others would later obtain patents for the antimicrobial use of polymers prepared from dimethylamine and epichlorohydrin.

For example, in 1978 Shair et al. obtained a patent on a method of controlling microorganisms in cooling water systems with polymers prepared as described by Panzer and Dixon. In another patent, Green, Merianos, and Petrocci (1978a) described the preparation of an antimicrobial polymer by the reaction of equimolar proportions of the intermediates 1,3-bis-dimethylamino-2-propanol and 1,3-dichloro-2-propanol at 40 to 90°C, the intermediates having been prepared previously from the basic reactants dimethylamine and epichlorohydrin. These same workers were later issued another patent (Merianos et al., 1979) on a method of inhibiting microorganisms with a polymer made by the direct condensation of equimolar proportions of dimethylamine and epichlorohydrin under certain specific conditions of time and temperature.

Other processes of interest for the preparation of ionene polymers with microbicidal properties are described by Bauman (1975), Buckman et al. (1977), Fenyes and Pera (1985, 1986, 1988, 1989), and Pera (1989).

Antimicrobial Activity

As mentioned earlier, the antimicrobial activity of ionene polymers could have been anticipated, because they are polymeric quaternary ammonium compounds. The monomeric compounds of this type are, of course, widely used for sanitation, disinfection, and other microbicidal applications and have been for many years. These polymeric quaternaries, however, do exhibit certain differences in properties from most of the conventional monomeric products. These differences in characteristics can affect both the efficacy and utility of the ionenes.

Ionene polymers generally are not surface-active and do not cause foaming, even in high concentrations. This is a definite advantage in applications such as water sanitation in swimming pools, air-washer systems, and cooling water systems. Another advantage of ionene polymers is that they generally have much lower toxicity and tissue irritation tendencies to mammals and other higher animals than do the conventional quaternaries. These properties increase the potential usefulness of the polymers in applications involving human or animal contact, including not only the treatment of water intended for swimming or bathing but also treatment of potable water,

chemotherapeutic applications, and preservation of cosmetics, pharmaceuticals, and food substances.

Most ionene polymers have other properties, however, that limit their use in some antimicrobial applications. First of all, these compounds tend to be relatively slow acting in killing microorganisms. Other drawbacks are that their effect against some organisms is more biostatic than biocidal, and they generally have very little activity against mold-type fungi. For these reasons, most ionene polymers are not generally suited for uses requiring a quick kill of essentially all microorganisms. For example, ionenes ordinarily do not perform well in typical use-dilution tests with brief contact times, which are commonly used to evaluate disinfectants.

One ionene polymer with antimicrobial properties that received attention in the 1950s was prepared by the reaction of 1,3-dibromo propane and N,N,N',N'-tetramethylhexanediamine. This polymer, which was introduced by Abbott Laboratories in 1959 as a "heparin antagonist" drug with the generic name hexadimethrine bromide and tradename of Polybrene,* has the following structure:

$$\left[\begin{array}{c} CH_3 \\ | \\ N^+ ——(CH_2)_6—N^+ —(CH_2)_3 \\ | \\ CH_3 \end{array} \begin{array}{c} CH_3 \\ | \\ \\ | \\ CH_3 \end{array} \right]_n \cdot 2nBr^-$$

Hexadimethrine bromide has a molecular weight of 5000 to 10,000, is soluble in water to about 10%, and is stable in solution after being autoclaved. Its main medical use has been to restore the normal coagulability of blood when needed after a patient has been receiving the anticoagulant heparin. However, the polymer does possess strong antimicrobial properties. Maruzzella, Handler, and Robbins (1958) tested polybrene in vitro against a number of bacteria and fungi. They found that bacterial growth was completely inhibited at 0.5 mg/ml against *Bacillus subtilis*, 0.25 mg/ml against *E. coli*, 5 mg/ml against *Neisseria perflava*, and 1 mg/ml against *Serratia marcescens*. Against fungi, the lowest concentration tested, 0.01 mg/ml, completely inhibited the growth of *Saccharomyces cereviseae*, *Ustilago avenae*, and *Phycomyces blakesleeanus*. On the other hand, *Staphylococcus aureus* was not completely inhibited in these tests even at 10 mg/ml. In a more recent paper, Mulholland and Mellersh (1987), using culture media and test conditions different from those of Maruzzella et al., determined the minimum concentrations of polybrene necessary to obtain at least a 99.9% kill of the inoculum for various laboratory stock strains and clinical isolates of a number of bacteria. The minimum concentrations of polybrene required varied, depending on species, from 4 to 32 mg/l.

Rembaum (1973) demonstrated that the antimicrobial

---

*Polybrene is no longer a proprietary name and is used, mostly outside the U.S., as a common name for hexadimethrine bromide.

Table 18–3. *Minimum Inhibitory Concentrations of Some Ionene Polymers*

	S. aureus (ppm)	E. coli (ppm)
3,3-ionene bromide	>128	>128
6,6-ionene bromide	16	16
6,10-ionene bromide	4	4
2,10-ionene bromide	4	8
6,16-ionene bromide	4	32

From Rembaum, A. 1973. Biological activity of ionene polymers. Applied Polymer Symposium, J. Wiley & Sons, No. 22, pp. 299–317.

efficacy of the ionene polymers was significantly greater than that of the corresponding monomeric quaternary ammonium salts and that the structure of the ionene plays an important role in its activity. Table 18–3 shows the minimum inhibitory concentrations (MIC) that Rembaum found for some ionene polymers against two representative bacteria, *Staphylococcus aureus* and *E. coli*. Similar MIC values were reportedly found for *Pseudomonas aeruginosa, Bacillus subtilis, Clostridium sporogenes,* and *Mycobacterium smegmatis*. None of the corresponding low-molecular-weight ammonium salts inhibited bacterial growth even at 1000 ppm, but some of the polymers had MIC values as low as 4 ppm. The ionenes were also found to inhibit the growth of several species of fungi at low concentration. For example, the 3,3- and 6,10-ionene bromides had MIC values of 4 ppm against *Alternaria* spp. Rembaum in the same report also presented data showing that the intraperitoneal and oral toxicity to mice of the low-molecular-weight diammonium salts was higher than that of most of the ionene polymers.

The antimicrobial efficacy of several ionene polymers against some of the pathogenic organisms found in water supplies is illustrated by the data in Table 18–4 (Buckman, 1987). The tests were run in deionized water and in artificial pond water at pH 6.8 and 37°C, and the inoculum in each case was 10×10^6 cfu/ml. Recovery was on nutrient agar after 24 hours contact. These ionene polymers are all commercially available products that are being manufactured and sold in several countries as antimicrobial agents, including one (Ionene A in Table 18–4) that is currently registered in the U.S.A. for preservation and for the control of bacteria and algae in various water systems.

Ionene polymers typically have good activity against algae. For example, Pera and Johnson (1973) demonstrated the efficacy of the polymer called "Ionene A" in Table 18–4 against green and blue-green algae. In each case, the sterile algae medium was treated with appropriate concentrations of the ionene polymer, inoculated with the appropriate algal culture, and then incubated at $28 \pm 2°C$ under fluorescent illumination of 250-foot-candle intensity (8 hours light, 16 hours darkness) for a period adequate for good growth in the controls. Observations of growth were made at 7-day intervals, and the results after 28 days are shown in Table 18–5. These data indicate that 1 to 4 ppm of the polymer provided complete inhibition of growth for all four species under these test conditions. Buckman and Mercer (1977) ran similar tests with the polymer called "Ionene B" in Table 18–4 and with this product obtained complete inhibition of *Chlorococcum hypnosporum* at 0.5 ppm, *Chlorella pyrenoidosa* at 2.0 ppm, and *Phormidium inundatum* at 8.0 ppm.

Mechanism of Action

The mechanism of antimicrobial action of ionene polymers has not been studied as extensively as has that of other commonly used chemical agents. Because they are polymeric quaternary ammonium compounds, ionenes could be expected to interact with bacteria and other microorganisms in ways similar to those of the conventional, nonpolymeric quats and other cationic agents. That is, like these other compounds, ionenes are strongly attracted to negatively charged surfaces such as bacteria and their adsorption onto cell membrane surfaces would be expected to interfere with cell permeability and transport across the membrane. Subsequent disruption of the cytoplasmic membrane and leakage of cell components could also be expected.

However, the ways in which ionene polymers differ from the nonpolymeric cationic agents would certainly affect the interaction of these compounds with microbial cells. Their higher molecular weight and multiple positively charged nitrogen groups would increase their attraction to negatively charged surfaces and bind them more tightly to these surfaces. The larger molecules of the polymers also could present a greater barrier to cell membrane transport processes. Another important difference is that most of the ionenes that have been investigated as antimicrobial agents are not surface-active, that is, they generally have little if any effect on surface or interfacial tension. Thus any of the effects of other, nonpolymeric quaternary ammonium compounds that are due to their surfactant properties would not be observed with the ionenes.

Rembaum (1973) postulated that the first step in microbial growth inhibition by ionene polymers might be either a flocculation phenomenon or adsorption of the ionenes onto the bacterial membranes. Ionenes, like other positively charged polyelectrolytes, are widely used in various applications to flocculate colloidal suspensions of organic and inorganic materials. So they could also be expected to flocculate, for example, a bacterial suspension. However, Rembaum found that this did not happen when an inhibitory concentration of 6,10-ionene bromide was added to a *Pseudomonas* suspension. Four hours after the addition of the polymer, even though further growth of the organism had been stopped, the optical density (OD) of the medium had not changed significantly and only slowly decreased to 50% of the original value after 12 hours. If flocculation of the bacteria had occurred, a rapid decrease of the OD to near zero would be expected.

In some cases, of course, flocculation of the organisms by ionene polymers does occur, as I and others have

Table 18–4. *Antimicrobial Activity of Ionene Polymers Against Some Pathogenic Organisms in Deionized (DI) Water and Artificial Pond Water*

| | Concentration (ppm) of Polymer Required to Give 99.9% Kill | | | | | | | |
| | Ionene A | | Ionene B | | Ionene C | | Ionene D | |
Organism	DI	Pond	DI	Pond	DI	Pond	DI	Pond
Bacteria:								
Escherichia coli	2.5	5	10	5	2.5	5	10	10
Yersinia enterocolitica	2.5	5	2.5	5	2.5	5	2.5	5
Salmonella typhi	2.5	5	2.5	5	2.5	5	10	10
Shigella dysenteriae	2.5	5	2.5	5	2.5	5	2.5	5
Campylobacter jejuni	2.5	5	2.5	5	2.5	5	2.5	5
Vibrio parahemolyticus	2.5	5	2.5	10	2.5	10	2.5	5
Mycobacterium bovis	2.5	5	10	5	2.5	5	2.5	5
Staphylococcus aureus	2.5	5	2.5	5	10	5	2.5	5
Pseudomonas aeruginosa	2.5	5	2.5	5	2.5	5	2.5	5
Yeast:								
Candida albicans	2.5	5	2.5	5	2.5	5	2.5	5
Protozoa (trophozoites):								
Entamoeba histolytica	2.5	5	2.5	5	2.5	5	2.5	5
Giardia intestinalis	2.5	5	2.5	5	2.5	5	2.5	5

Notes:

1. Ionene A is a 60% active solution of N,N,N′,N′-tetramethyl-1,2-ethanediamine polymer with 1,1′-oxybis[2-chloroethane], CAS Reg. No. 31075-24-8, molecular weight ca. 3500.

2. Ionene B is a 60% active solution of N,N,N′,N′-tetramethyl-1,2-ethanediamine polymer with (chloromethyl)oxirane, CAS Reg. No. 25988-98-1, molecular weight ca. 3000.

3. Ionene C is a 50% active solution of N-methylmethanamine polymer with (chloromethyl)oxirane, CAS Reg. No. 25988-97-1, molecular weight ca. 5000.

4. Ionene D is a 25% active solution of 1,1′-(methylimino)bis[3-chloro-2-propanol) polymer with N,N,N′,N′-tetramethyl-1,2-ethanediamine, CAS Reg. No. 68140-76-1, molecular weight ca. 50,000.

From Buckman Laboratories International, Inc.

Table 18–5. *Inhibition of Green and Blue-Green Algae by Ionene A after 28 Days*

| Polymer Concentration (ppm) | Growth | | | |
	Volvox carteri	*Oscillatoria prolifera*	*Chlorococcum hypnosporum*	*Chlorella pyrenoidosa*
0	4	4	4	4
0.5	1	3	1	4
1.0	0	3	0	4
2.0	0	4	0	4
4.0	0	0	0	0
8.0	0	0	0	0
10.0	0	0	0	0
15.0	0	0	0	0

NOTES:

1. See notes in Table 18–4 for description of Ionene A.

2. Growth Key: 4 = Excellent
        3 = Good
        2 = Poor
        1 = Very poor, scant, questionable
        0 = No growth

From Pera, J.D., and Johnson, B.S. 1973. Method of controlling the growth of algae. U.S. Patent No. 3,771,989.

often observed. However, this phenomenon probably is not generally a major mechanism for the antimicrobial action of these compounds. Rembaum concluded that the adsorption of the polyelectrolyte onto the cell membrane surfaces and interference with transport across the membranes or with the replicative system were more likely mechanisms of inhibition. He also suggested that chemical interaction with microbial DNA was a remote possibility that should not be overlooked, based on his work that showed that ionenes form strong water-insoluble complexes with DNA.

A published study that indirectly supports the proposed mechanism of cell membrane disruption was one made on the interaction of various chemical agents on single cells of plant leaves (Towne et al., 1978). Included in this study was the commercial product WSCP, which contains 60% of poly[oxyethylene(dimethyliminio)-ethylene(dimethyliminio)ethylene dichloride].* Enzymatically isolated mesophyll cells of soybean and cotton were treated with the nonionic surfactants Sterox SK (polyoxyethylene thioether) or Renex 36 (polyoxyethylene-6-tridecylether) or the cationic ionene WSCP—alone or in combination with two herbicides—to determine, among other things, the effects of these substances on cell permeability. The greatest amount of efflux of ^{14}C-labeled material from soybean cells was caused by WSCP, whereas the other chemical agents gave only slightly higher effluxes than the controls. All of the chemicals caused considerable leakage on cotton cells. WSCP also caused extensive disorganization of the cellular membranes, whereas the two nonionic surfactants disrupted only grana-intergrana thylakoids, causing abnormal grana. The authors observed that the results with WSCP agreed with earlier findings that cationic surfactants (alkylbenzyl quaternary ammonium halides) caused a greater efflux of intracellular material from isolated plant cells than did nonionic surfactants.

Applications

As indicated in the foregoing discussion, the literature, particularly the patent literature, shows that many ionene polymers have been synthesized and shown to be effective as antimicrobial agents. However, only a few have been developed commercially for microorganism control applications. Probably the major product of this type is the ionene polymer WSCP manufactured by Buckman Laboratories and used as the active ingredient in microorganism-control products sold under a great variety of tradenames by Buckman as well as other chemical suppliers. (The chemical nature of the WSCP polymer has been described earlier in this chapter.) Products containing WSCP are registered with the U.S. EPA for a number of applications. These include the control of algae, bacteria, and fungi in industrial fresh water systems; the control of bacteria in industrial air-washing systems; and the control of algae in swimming pools (both

heated and unheated), exterior whirlpools, and hot tubs as well as in decorative fountains and ponds that do not contain fish. The recommended concentration range for these applications is from 2 to 20 ppm of a 60% active product. WSCP-containing products are also registered as preservatives for some aqueous products. To protect aqueous metalworking fluids against microbial degradation, it is used at concentrations that provide 60 to 600 ppm of the polymer at maximum dilution of the fluid. Similar concentrations are used for the preservation of cooked starch solutions used in paper manufacture. A typical metalworking fluid preservative application has been discussed by Zabik et al. (1988).

Two other ionene polymers that are manufactured and sold in countries outside the U.S. for antimicrobial applications similar to those of WSCP are the polymers designated "Ionene B" and "Ionene C" in the notes to Table 18–4. The efficacy of each of these two products against bacteria, algae, and fungi varies somewhat from that of WSCP, but it is close, particularly when compared on a cost-effectiveness basis (Buckman Laboratories).

Work has been done in New Zealand that indicates WSCP could be effective in controlling bovine mastitis and possibly other dermal diseases of animals. Hayward and Webster (1977) carried out trials on milk cows using a teat sanitizer formulated for spraying and consisting of a 1% emulsion of WSCP along with emollients. They found that regular sanitizing of teats by spray application of this sanitizer during the lactation period reduced the level of subclinical mastitis. At least a 45% reduction in the incidence of new intramammary infection was obtained, and a large reduction in the number of organisms on the teat skin area was observed during the trial period when the sanitizer was being applied. When the spraying was stopped for more than two milkings, a large increase in the number of organisms present on the skin was seen.

Ionene polymers have also been found useful as components of liquid laundry detergent-sanitizer products. Bernarducci and Harrison (1988) found that formulating one of these polymeric quaternary ammonium compounds in an aqueous medium with one or more nonionic surfactants provided stable, isotropic liquid laundry detergent compositions with good detergency and bactericidal properties. These products were only moderately irritating to the eyes and practically nonirritating to the skin. The ionenes claimed to be suitable for use in these compositions include WSCP and some of its analogs as well as polymers of the type synthesized by Green et al. (1976a, 1977a, 1977b, 1977c, 1978). An example of the latter polymers is poly(dimethylbutenylammonium chloride)-alpha, omega-bis(triethanolammonium chloride),* which is sold under the trade names Onyxsperse 12S and Onamer M. Nonionic surfactants used in the formulations included polyethylene glycol long-chain alkyl ethers, polyethylene glycol alkylphenol ethers, and N-alkyl-N,N-di-lower-alkylamide-N-oxides. The formulations of the invention were tested for cleaning efficacy

---

*Manufactured by Buckman Laboratories, Inc. This is the same ionene polymer that is designated "Ionene A" in Table 18–4.

*CAS Reg. No. 75345-27-6.

and germicidal efficacy against *Klebsiella pneumoniae* and *Staphylococcus aureus* and were evaluated for eye irritation and dermal irritation in rabbits. In comparison to formulations based on the nonionic surfactants and a monomeric quaternary ammonium compound, the compositions with the ionene polymers provided superior detergency and equal or better sanitizing and had lower eye and skin irritancy.

A recently developed use of the ionene WSCP that could achieve importance in the future is as a molluskicide to control two troublesome species of freshwater macrofouling bivalves (McMahon and Lutey, 1988; McMahon et al., 1989). Although this is not an antimicrobial application, it is of interest because this use of the ionene could involve public health concerns in the treatment of drinking water. The Asian clam *(Corbicula fluminea)* was introduced from southeast Asia into North American freshwater drainage systems in the early 1900s and has since spread to 35 of the 48 contiguous states and continues to spread into northern and central Mexico. It also is now found in many other areas of the world. This organism has long been a major source of macrofouling problems of freshwater systems, for example, in the service water systems of nuclear and fossil-fuel electric power stations. The Zebra mussel *(Dreissena polymorpha)* is another exotic bivalve species that was introduced into North America more recently, apparently around 1985 by the dumping into the Great Lakes of ship ballast water carried from freshwater ports in Europe or western Asia. It is now a highly troublesome fouling organism not only in municipal and industrial water systems but also on ship and boat hulls, buoys, piers, and marine structures. It has been demonstrated, however, that WSCP can kill these organisms at relatively low concentrations and contact times. It has been shown to be 100% toxic to *Corbicula fluminea* at concentrations as low as 0.5 ppm. LT_{50} values (estimated time for death of 50% of individuals in the sample) ranged from 44.8 hrs at 8.0 ppm to 255.7 hrs at 0.5 ppm. This ionene polymer was also shown to be effective against the *Dreissena polymorpha*, with LT_{50} values of 146.9 hrs at 8 ppm and 714.3 hrs at 0.5 ppm. The potential value of the ionene polymer for the control of these bivalves is particularly enhanced by the fact that it is not only effective in killing these freshwater organisms but its toxicologic characteristics are such that it most likely can be used even in potable water systems.

REFERENCES

Akelah, A., and Selim, A. 1987. Applications of functionalized polymers for controlled release formulations of agrochemicals and related biocides. La Chimica e l'Industria, 69(1–2), 62–67.

Bauman, R.A. 1975. Anti microbial compositions containing unsymmetrical oligoquaternary ammonium compounds. U.S. Patent No. 3,925,556.

Bernarducci, E., and Harrison, K.A. 1988. Isotropic laundry detergents containing polymeric quaternary ammonium salts. U.S. Patent No. 4,755,327.

Boardman, G. 1969. A polymeric biguanide for industrial disinfection. Food Technol. New Zealand, 4(12), 421, 423, 425.

Broxton, P., Woodcock, P.M., and Gilbert, P. 1983. A study of the antibacterial activity of some polyhexamethylene biguanides towards *Escherichia coli* ATCC 8739. J. Appl. Bacteriol., 54, 345–353.

Broxton, P., Woodcock, P.M., and Gilbert, P. 1984a. Injury and recovery of

Escherichia coli ATCC 8739 from treatment with some polyhexamethylene biguanides. Microbios, 40, 187–193.

Broxton, P., Woodcock, P.M., and Gilbert, P. 1984b. Binding of some polyhexamethylene biguanides to the cell envelope. Microbios, 41, 15–22.

Broxton, P., Woodcock, P.M., Heatley, F., and Gilbert, P. 1984c. Interaction of some polyhexamethylene biguanides and membrane phospholipids in *Escherichia coli*. J. Appl. Bacteriol., 57, 115–124.

Brown, C.C. 1987. Antimicrobial dressing or drape material. U.S. Patent No. 4,643,181.

Buckman, S.J., and Mercer, G.D. 1977. Method of controlling the growth of algae. U.S. Patent No. 4,018,592.

Buckman, J.D., Buckman, S.J., Mercer, G.D., and Pera, J.D. 1977. Amine-epichlorohydrin polymeric compositions. U.S. Patent No. 4,054,542.

Buckman Laboratories International, Inc. Unpublished internal reports used by permission of the company.

Carter, G., and Hinton, A.J. 1977. Water treatment for controlling the growth of algae employing biguanides. U.S. Patent No. 4,014,676.

Curd, F.H.S., and Rose, F.L. 1946. Synthetic antimalarials. Part X. Some aryl-diguanide ("-biguanide") derivatives. J. Chem. Soc., 1946, 729–737.

Davies, A., Bentley, M., and Field, B.S. 1968. Comparison of the action of Vantocil, cetrimide and chlorhexidine on *Escherichia coli* and its spheroplasts and protoplasts of Gram positive bacteria. J. Appl. Bacteriol., 31, 448–461.

Davies, A., and Field, B.S. 1969. Action of biguanides, phenols and detergents on *Escherichia coli* and its spheroplasts. J. Appl. Bacteriol., 32, 233–243.

Dawson, M.W., Brown, T.J., and Till, D.G. 1983a. The effect of Baquacil on pathogenic free-living amoebae (PFLA). 1. In axenic conditions. N. Z. J. Marine Freshwater Res., 17, 305–311.

Dawson, M.W., Brown, T.J., Biddick, C.J., and Till, D.G. 1983b. The effect of Baquacil on pathogenic free-living amoebae (PFLA). 2. In simulated natural conditions—in the presence of bacteria and/or organic matter. N. Z. J. Marine Freshwater Res., 17, 313–320.

Dickinson, J.D., Fowkes, F.S., and Rose, T.J. 1969. Manufacture of polymeric diguanides. U.S. Patent No. 3,428,576.

Drain, D.J., and Simmonite, D. 1976. Ophthalmic compositions and contact lens disinfecting compositions. British Patent 1,432,345.

Fawkes, D.M. 1986. Treated non-woven material. Eur. Pat. Appl. 174,128.

Feld, D., and Soto, T.A. 1987. Antimicrobial dressing. U.S. Patent No. 4,643,180.

Fenyes, J.G., and Pera, J.D. 1985. Polymeric quaternary ammonium compounds and their uses. U.S. Patent No. 4,506,081.

Fenyes, J.G., and Pera, J.D. 1986. Polymeric quaternary ammonium compounds and their uses. U.S. Patent No. 4,581,058.

Fenyes, J.G., and Pera, J.D. 1988. Polymeric quaternary ammonium compounds, their preparations and use. U.S. Patent No. 4,778,813.

Fenyes, J.G., and Pera, J.D. 1989. Ionene polymeric compositions, their preparation and use. U.S. Patent No. 4,851,532.

Gibbs, C.F., Littmann, E.R., and Marvel, C.S. 1933. Quaternary ammonium salts from halogenated alkyl dimethylamines. II. The polymerization of gamma-halogenopropyldimethylamines. J. Am. Chem. Soc., 55, 753–757.

Gibbs, C.F., and Marvel, C.S. 1934. Quaternary ammonium salts from bromopropyldialkylamines. IV. Formation of four-membered rings. J. Am. Chem. Soc., 56, 725–727.

Green, H.A., Merianos, J.J., and Petrocci, A.N. 1975a. Microbicidal polymeric quaternary ammonium compounds. U.S. Patent No. 3,874,870.

Green, H.A., Merianos, J.J., and Petrocci, A.N. 1975b. Anti-microbial quaternary ammonium co-polymers. U.S. Patent No. 3,928,323,

Green, H.A., Merianos, J.J., and Petrocci, A.N. 1976a. Capped polymers. U.S. Patent No. 3,931,319.

Green, H.A., Merianos, J.J., and Petrocci, A.N. 1976b. Certain 1,4-bis-(morpholino)-2-butene-containing condensation products and their preparation. U.S. Patent No. 3,933,812.

Green, H.A., Merianos, J.J., and Petrocci, A.N. 1976c. Quaternary ammonium co-polymers for controlling the proliferation of bacteria. U.S. Patent No. 3,961,042.

Green, H.A., Merianos, J.J., and Petrocci, A.N. 1976d. Quaternary ammonium co-polymers for controlling the proliferation of bacteria. U.S. Patent No. 3,966,904.

Green, H.A., Merianos, J.J., and Petrocci, A.N. 1977a. Method of inhibiting the growth of bacteria by the application thereto of capped polymers. U.S. Patent No. 4,001,432.

Green, H.A., Merianos, J.J., and Petrocci, A.N. 1977b. Capped polymers. U.S. Patent No. 4,012,446.

Green, H.A., Merianos, J.J., and Petrocci, A.N. 1977c. Anti-microbial quaternary ammonium co-polymers. U.S. Patent No. 4,026,945.

Green, H.A., Merianos, J.J., and Petrocci, A.N. 1977d. Randomly terminated capped polymers. U.S. Patent No. 4,027,020.

Green, H.A., Merianos, J.J., and Petrocci, A.N. 1977e. Microbiocidal capped polymers. U.S. Patent No. 4,036,959.

Green, H.A., Merianos, J.J., and Petrocci, A.N. 1977f. Method of preparing capped polymers. U.S. Patent No. 4,055,712.

Green, H.A., Merianos, J.J., and Petrocci, A.N. 1978a. Polymeric antimicrobial agent. U.S. Patent No. 4,089,977.

Green, H.A., Merianos, J.J., and Petrocci, A.N. 1978b. Randomly terminated capped polymers. U.S. Patent No. 4,091,113.

Halek, G.W., and Garg, A. 1989. Fungal inhibition by a fungicide coupled to an ionomeric film. J. Food Safety, 9, 215–222.

Hayward, P.J., and Webster, A.N. 1977. Reduction in mastitis by use of a teat spray sanitizer. N.Z. J. Dairy Sci. Technol., 12, 78–82.

ICI Americas Inc. 1986a. Baquacil chlorine-free swimming pool sanitizer and algistat pool care guide. Company brochure.

ICI Americas Inc. 1986b. Cosmocil CQ. Polyhexamethylene biguanide hydrochloride solution. Company brochure.

ICI Americas Inc. 1986c. Poly(hexamethylene biguanide): a review of the mechanism of antimicrobial action. Company bulletin.

Ikeda, T., Tazuke, S., and Watanabe, M. 1983. Interaction of biologically active molecules with phospholipid membranes. I. Fluorescence depolarization studies on the effect of polymeric biocide bearing biguanide groups in the main chain. Biochim. Biophys. Acta, 735, 380–386.

Ikeda, T., Ledwith, A., Bamford, C.H., and Hann, R.A. 1984. Interaction of a polymeric biguanide biocide with phospholipid membranes. Biochim. Biophys. Acta, 769, 57–66.

Ikeda, T., Tazuke, S., Bamford, C.H., and Ledwith, A. 1985a. Spectroscopic studies on the interaction of polymeric in-chain biguanide biocide with phospholipid membranes as probed by 8-anilinonaphthalene-1-sulfonate. Bull. Chem. Soc. Japan, 58, 705–709.

Ikeda, T., Tazuke, S., and Bamford, C.H. 1985b. Interaction of membrane-active biguanides with negatively charged species. A model for their interaction with target sites in microbial membranes. J. Chem. Research (S), 6, 180–181.

Islam, M.N., and Islam, N.B. 1979a. Extension of poultry shelf-life by poly(hexamethylenebiguanide hydrochloride). J. Food Protection, 42(5), 416–419.

Islam, M.N., and Islam, N.B. 1979b. Comparison of the efficacy of three potential poultry preservatives: glutaraldehyde, iodacetamide, and poly(hexamethylenebiguanide hydrochloride). J. Food Process. Preserv., 2(1978), 1–9.

Kern, W., and Brenneisen, E. 1941. Über heteropolare Molekülkolloide, III. Polymere Amine als Modelle des Eiweißes. J. Prakt. Chem., 159, 193–218.

Knoor, L., and Roth, P. 1906. Synthese und Abbau eines dem Dimethyl-piperazin-dichlormethylat kerenhomologen Achtringes. Berichte der Deutschen Chemischen Gesellschaft, 39(6), 1420–1429.

Maruzzella, J.C., Handler, D., and Robbins, A.L. 1958. The in vitro antimicrobial properties of polybrene. Drug Standards, 26, 122–123.

McLeod, N.A., and Webb, C.P.N. 1981. Water treatment. U.S. Patent No. 4,253,971.

McMahon, R.F., and Lutey, R.W. 1988. Field and laboratory studies of the efficacy of poly[oxyethylene(dimethyliminio)ethylene-(dimethyliminio)ethylene dichloride] as a biocide against the Asian clam, Corbicula fluminea. Paper presented at Electric Power Research Institute Service Water System Reliability Improvement Seminar, Oct. 17–19, 1988, Charlotte, N.C.

McMahon, R.F., Shipman, B.N., and Ollech, J.A. 1989. Effects of two molluscicides on the freshwater macrofouling bivalves Corbicula fluminea and Dreissena polymorpha. Buckman Laboratories Bulletin No. W115US, Oct. 1989.

Merianos, J.J., Green, H.A., and Petrocci, A.N. 1979. Method of inhibiting microorganisms. U.S. Patent No. 4,140,798.

Mulholland, B., and Mellersh, A.R. 1987. The antimicrobial activity of protamine and polybrene. J. Hosp. Infect., 10, 305–307.

Ogunbiyi, L., Smith, F.X., and Riedhammer, T.M. 1988. Disinfecting and preserving systems and methods of use. U.S. Patent No. 4,758,595.

Ogunbiyi, L., Smith, F.X., and Riedhammer, T.M. 1989. Disinfecting and preserving systems and methods of use. U.S. Patent No. 4,836,986.

Panzer, H.P., and Dixon, K.W. 1973, 1976. Polyquaternary flocculants. U.S. Patent No. 3,738,945. (U.S. Reissue Patent No. 28,807 and No. 28,808.)

Pera, J.D., and Johnson, B.S. 1973. Method of controlling the growth of algae. U.S. Patent No. 3,771,989.

Pera, J.D. 1989. Polymeric quaternary ammonium compounds, their preparation and use. U.S. Patent No. 4,851,532.

Pittman, Jr., C.U. 1976. Chemical anchoring of mildewcides in paint. Analysis of the literature. J. Coatings Technol., 48(617), 31–37.

Pittman, Jr., C.U., and Stahl, G.A. 1981. Copolymerization of pentachlorophenyl acrylate with vinyl acetate and ethyl acrylate. Polymer-bound fungicides. J. Appl. Polymer Sci., 26, 2403–2413.

Pleurdeau, A., Potin, C., and Bruneau, C.M. 1985. Biocide macromolecules, Proc. 11th Intl. Conf. Organic Coatings, Sci. Technol., pp. 293–301.

Quantrille, T.E. 1989. Antimicrobially active, non-woven web used in a wet wiper. U.S. Patent No. 4,837,079.

Rajaraman, R., Round, D.E., Yen, S.P.S., and Rembaum, A. 1975. Effects of ionenes on normal and transformed cells. In Polyelectrolytes and Their Applications. Edited by A. Rembaum and E. Sélégny. Dordrecht, Holland, D. Reidel Publishing, pp. 163–174.

Rembaum, A., Baumgartner, W., and Eisenberg, A. 1968. Aliphatic ionenes. J. Polym. Sci., Polym. Lett. Ed., 6(3), 159–171.

Rembaum, A., Yen, S.P.S., Landel, R.F., and Shen, M. 1970. Synthesis and properties of a new class of potential biomedical polymers. J. Macromol. Sci.-Chem., A4(3), 715–738.

Rembaum, A. 1973. Biological activity of ionene polymers. Applied Polymer Symposium, J. Wiley & Sons, No. 22, pp. 299–317.

Rembaum, A., Senyei, A.E., and Rajaraman, R. 1977. Interaction of living cells with polyionenes and polyionene-coated surfaces. J. Biomed. Mater. Res., 11(1), 101–110.

Rembaum, A. 1977. Ionene polymers for selectively inhibiting the vitro growth of malignant cells. U.S. Patent No. 4,013,507.

Ritter, D.M. 1941. Organic nitrogen compounds. U.S. Patent No. 2,261,002.

Rose, F.L., and Swain, G. 1954. Polymeric diguanides. British Patent No. 702,268.

Rose, F.L., and Swain, G. 1956. Bisdiguanides having antibacterial activity. J. Chem. Soc., 1956, 4422–4425.

Rosenthal, I., Juven, B.J., and Ben-Hur, E. 1982. Evaluation of poly(hexamethylene biguanide.HCl) as a biocide in the food industry. J. Food Safety, 4, 191–197.

Searle, N.E. 1942. Pest control. U.S. Patent No. 2,271,378.

Sghibartz, C.M. 1984. Antifouling paints—present and future. Congr. FATIPEC, 17(4), 145–164.

Shair, S.A., Paul, S.N., and Cairns, J.E. 1978. Polyquaternary compounds for the control of microbiological growth. U.S. Patent No. 4,111,679.

Smith, M.R., and Singer, M. 1977. Purification of water. British Patent No. 1,460,626.

Stockel, R.F., and Jelling M. 1985. Anti-microbial compositions and associated methods for preparing the same and for the disinfecting of various objects. U.S. Patent No. 4,499,077.

Strandskov, F.B., and Bocklemann, J.B. 1975. Preservation of beverages with poly(hexamethylenebiguanide hydrochloride). U.S. Patent No. 3,860,729.

Thomson, J.E., Cox, N.A., Bailey, J.S., and Islam, M.N. 1981. Minimizing Salmonella contamination on broiler carcasses with poly(hexamethylenebiguanide hydrochloride). J. Food Protection, 44(6), 440–441.

Towne, C.A., Bartels, P.G., and Hilton, J.L. 1978. Interaction of surfactant and herbicide treatments on single cells of leaves. Weed Science, 26(2), 182–188.

Zabik, M.J., Wildman, J.L., Moran, C., and Lukanich, J.T. 1988. Unique use of a cationic microbicide for extending the life of a synthetic metalworking fluid in a manufacturing environment—a case history. Lubr. Eng., 44(8), 677–679.

CHAPTER 19

MERCURY—INDUSTRIAL USES AS PRESERVATIVES

Robert A. Oppermann

The final paragraph of the extensive chapter by Grier, "Mercurials—Inorganic and Organic," in the third edition of *Disinfection, Sterilization, and Preservation* (1983), predicts a major decrease in the use of mercurial compounds in coming years:

> The voluminous scientific literature dealing with the inhibitory properties, utility, and limitations of mercury compounds reflects the widespread interest and importance formerly given to them. In medicine and allied fields, the continuous effort to develop effective and relatively safe agents for prophylaxis and chemotherapy practically eliminates mercurials for further consideration. The apparent universal presence of mercury-resistant pathogenic microorganisms contributes to such decisions. Potential environmental toxicity hazards have curtailed nearly all industrial and agricultural antimicrobial uses of these compounds. However, the unique and valuable attributes that, for millennia, aided man's survival and sustenance and that still find application in research, in the future may be refitted to special problems of disease control.

Indeed, this prediction has come true and the noted events continue to restrict uses for mercury and its compounds. A survey of *Chemical Abstracts* for the last 10 years shows that no new mercurial antimicrobials have been produced in useful volumes, and that there has been little or no research to develop new mercurial compounds as biocides for medical, agricultural, or industrial uses.

However, one large area of mercury's use as a preservative still accounts for the use of at least 5722 flasks of mercury per year (U.S. Bureau of Mines, 1988). The paint and coatings industry is the largest user of mercury products for their antimicrobial effects.

HISTORICAL PERSPECTIVE

Paints and coatings have been in existence for thousands of years. The manufacture of paint or coatings

for decorative and protective effects has been known from ancient times. The major increased use of paints for protective purposes developed during the Industrial Revolution as a method of protecting metal machinery from corrosion.

Industrial and house paints were based on drying oils until the 1920s. About this time inexpensive water-based paints were introduced for interior use but did not command much of the industry sales.

All paints have two objectives: protection and appearance. The "oil-based" paints initially accomplished these easily, but if the material was used outside rather than inside a building, weathering and fungal disfigurement occurred. The recognition that "mildew" (fungal) growth contributed to the deterioration of the coating was reported often during the period 1910 to 1920. About the same time fungicides began making an appearance as paint "preservatives." Mercury in the form of phenylmercury salts, either as oil-soluble compounds or as phenylmercury acetate (PMA), was introduced in the late 1930s, and by the end of the 1960s phenylmercury salts were the prime fungicides used by the paint and coatings industry.

Since the 1920s there had been experimentation with inexpensive water-based paints. These were indoor house paints usually purchased as a dry powder that was mixed with water. The binder (film-forming agent) was casein, a milk protein.

The combination of water and an organic material, such as protein, meant that these paints were liable for microbial degradation. The microbes most likely to be involved were bacteria, because they require the presence of liquid water and have such a fast growth rate they would out-compete other microorganisms. The early water-based paints were made from dry materials, so there was usually no biodeterioration of the product until it was combined with water, and then it was used rapidly. When these water-based mixtures were not used quickly or stored for some reason, they quickly became malodorous and unusable. For those few products that were made in a liquid condition, an antibacterial preservative was necessary. It wasn't until the late 1930s that mercury compounds began to be used as this preservative.

The introduction of synthetic resin emulsion, latex, paints, in approximately 1958, was a major opportunity for the use of mercury products. The advantage of organomercurials was that they furnished both bacterial and fungal protection. The addition of phenylmercuric acetate (PMA) as a fungicide to prevent mildew automatically provided protection from growth of bacteria in the product. The amount of PMA used for mildew protection was 1000 to 3000 parts per million (ppm). The amount required for protection from bacterial growth was 60 to 100 ppm. So the use of mercury compounds as fungicides furnished all the antimicrobial protection the paint required.

The level of mercury microbicides used in paint increased steadily from 1959 to 1970 (Fig. 19–1) (U.S. Bureau of Mines). The period of greatest usage was just before the time of environmental concern of "mercury pollution of the environment," 1969 to 1975. Several sad and unfortunate events fueled this concern. The Minamata tragedy, the consumption of treated seed in Iraq, the Huckleby family in the U.S.A., and other incidents have been reviewed in the past (Grier, 1983; Mann, 1971).

The publication of a request for submission of "views"

with respect to the uses of mercurial pesticides in the Federal Register in December 1970 was the real beginning of an attempt by the Environmental Protection Agency (EPA) to cancel all registrations of mercury-containing pesticides. The notice asked interested parties to comment on why mercury products should not be prohibited. The original notice was aimed at *alkyl* mercury products used as seed treatments (to prevent fungal decay and damping off), as algaecides, as slimicides (reduction of microbial growth in pulp and paper mills), and in laundries.

This was followed in March 1972 with an EPA notice (PR Notice 72–5) canceling the registration of *all* pesticides containing mercury. Included in the notice was the following: "In addition, registrations for alkyl compounds and nonalkyl uses on rice seed, in laundry, and marine antifouling paint create an imminent hazard and these registrations are hereby suspended"!

Several registrants requested a hearing, which initiated a lengthy formal hearing starting October 1974 and lasting almost a year. As Levinson (1975) says, "The taking of evidence was completed on September 10, 1975 after 89 witnesses had testified during 41 hearing days resulting in 4466 pages of transcript." This resulted in several interesting "Findings of Fact," a few of which follow:

1. "Mercury from man-made sources is released into the environment by direct discharge into the atmosphere or waterways, or by indirect discharge through volatilization, runoff, or leaching. There is

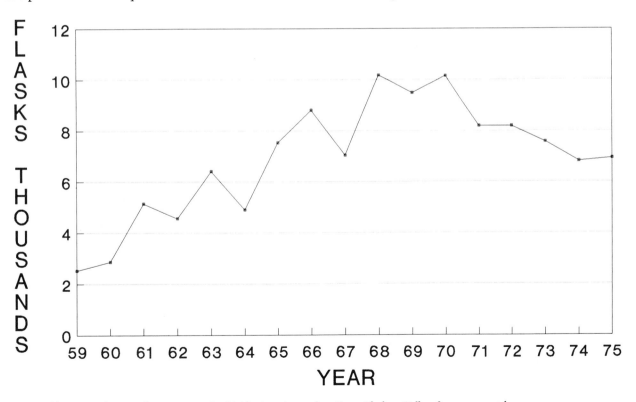

Fig. 19–1. Changes in the use of mercury as microbicides in paints and coatings. Flasks—76 lbs of mercury metal.

no direct discharge of mercury into the atmosphere or waterways from pesticidal use.

2. "The hazards to the environment with respect to mercury are related primarily to the presence of methylmercury in aquatic environments. Methylmercury is a highly toxic compound of mercury. Methylmercury is not used in pesticides.

3. "Mercury levels in fish consumed by man are not significantly different today from levels in the past 30 to 40 years, except in locations immediately below industrial plants discharging mercury directly into the aquatic environment.

4. "Methylmercury poisoning can cause very severe neurological impairments in man. Methylmercury can cross the placental barrier and result in the birth of children with methylmercury poisoning even though the mother appears unaffected.

5. "The very serious adverse effects shown in the studies of man and other forms of life from the use of methylmercury and other mercury compounds do not necessarily establish that such or similar adverse effects will result from such mercury as may be introduced into the environment by use of pesticides.

6. "Phenylmercurials are used in biocides in paint. Mercury is slowly released from painted surfaces through volatilization and is widely dispersed in the general environment. The total amount of mercury that is volatilized does not increase the background levels of mercury in the atmosphere significantly. The volatilized mercury is returned to earth by natural process and is tightly bound to the soil. It does not move freely from soil to water. Such mercury as reaches a natural aquatic environment is tightly bound to the silt.

7. "Such small amounts of mercury as may be leached from paints have no significant effect on the environment.

8. "Water-based paints require an effective and broad spectrum in-can preservative to control the growth of bacterial organisms. Phenylmercuric compounds are effective for this purpose. The substitutes put forth by respondent may be adequate and effective in some paint formulations but they do not have the broad-spectrum and long-lasting bactericide effect in all of the water-based paints as do the phenylmercurials and are not effective and adequate substitutes.

9. "A mildewcide is generally not necessary in paints used in interiors. A mildewcide is necessary for water-based paints for exterior application. The substitutes put forth by respondent may be adequate and effective in some paint formulations but they do not have the long-lasting effectiveness against mildew in all of the great variety of water-based paint formulations used in the exterior paints and are not effective and adequate substitutes for phenylmercurials."

The following conclusions were drawn after considering the evidence:

The use of mercury-containing pesticides for the following purposes, when used in accordance with widespread and commonly accepted practice, will not generally cause unreasonable adverse effects on the environment within the meaning of section 2 (bb) of FIFRA and the registration for such uses should not be canceled:

1. As an in-can preservative in water-based paints and coatings

2. As a fungicide in water-based paints and coatings used for exterior application

3. As a fungicide on golf course greens for the control of fungi of the snow mold complex

4. As a fungicide in the treatment of textiles and fabrics for out-of-door use

5. As a fungicide to control brown mold (*Cephaloascus fragrans*) on freshly sawn lumber

Russell Train, EPA Administrator, confirmed the allowed use of mercury in water-based paints and coatings on May 22, 1976. The other recommendations of the administrative law judge were decided by other hearings, and only the limited use of mercurials on golf turf also survived.

The decision saved the paint and coatings industry from much spoiled or defaced paint. It had been shown during the proceedings before Judge Levinson that phenylmercury salts were more efficient as microbicides for water-based paint than any of the other products available at that time.

The general use of mercury was reduced during the early years of the 1970s. This was due to the apprehension that all registrations of mercury containing antimicrobials would be canceled by the EPA. The level dropped to 60% of its 1970 high (Fig. 19–2). However, as soon as it appeared as though there might be a favorable decision in the appeal against cancellation, the rate of mercury use increased. In the 3 to 4 years after the decision not to cancel mercury registration, the use of mercury almost reached its 1970 high (U.S. Bureau of Mines). From 1980 to the present the number of flasks of mercury used as "fungicides" as reported by the Bureau of Mines decreased (Fig. 19–3). This apparent reduction was the result of three factors. During that time several useful nonmercurial mildewcides made an impact on the industry. Secondly, the environmental concern that engendered the mercury cancellation hearings—although reduced—never faded. From time to time this concern would resurface with renewed vigor, with a drop in the use of mercury-based pesticides. And third, and perhaps most important, the numbers used by the Bureau of Mines are furnished only by U.S. producers.

There has always been importation of mercury compounds as well as of metallic mercury. With the introduction of the phenylmercuric compounds as microbicides some of this importation changed from simple mercuric salts to the forms most useful to the antifungal market. As the market increased so did the amount of phenylmercuric compounds produced overseas. This was

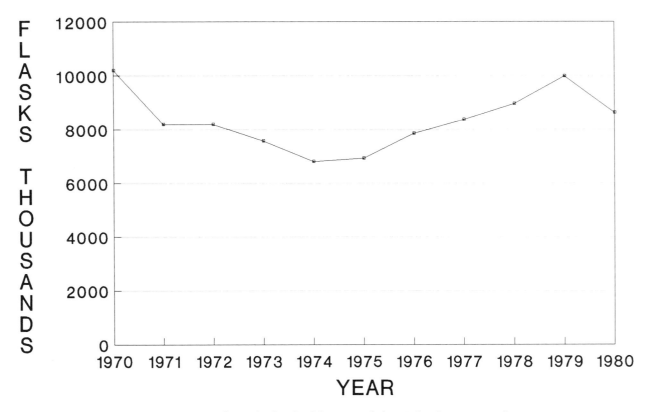

Fig. 19–2. Loss and recovery of mercury usage during the decade of the 1970s. Flasks—76 lbs of mercury metal.

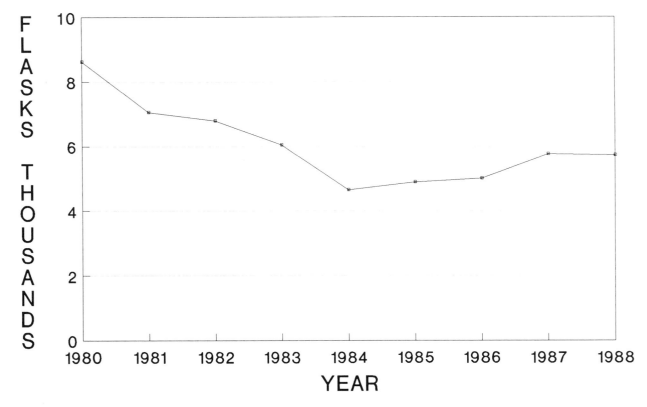

Fig. 19–3. Decrease in mercury biocide use after 1980. Flasks—76 lbs of mercury metal.

Table 19–1. *Pounds of Phenylmercuric Acetate (PMA) Sold in the State of California*

Year	Pounds of PMA
1980	132,230
1981	111,259
1982	178,091
1983	179,217
1984	227,429
1985	247,318
1986	424,104
1987	246,018

especially true as the price of foreign material became less compared to the U.S. price.

The importation of phenylmercuric acetate had another effect—the loss of domestic producers of mercury compounds. As the competitive pressure became greater one after another of the domestic producers stopped production and bought the finished product to be used as a raw material for their own production or for selling to their customers directly. This continued until 1986, when there was (and is) only one U.S. producer of PMA.

There is still a major market for mercurial pesticides. The size of that market is not known at this time but can be estimated. It can be said that the use in California is typical of national use. There has been an increase in California of PMA use in the last 8 years of approximately 1.5% per year (Table 19–1) (California D.F.A. 1980–1987). This is half of the presumed growth of the paint and coatings industry of 3.0% annually. There is no way of knowing if this PMA use is an expansion of old lines already using mercury or if some of the increase reflects addition of new formulas using PMA. In any case there appears to be a slight yearly increase in the total sales of mercury compounds.

Although there still exists a market for mercurial fungicides in paint, several other uses of mercury have been lost. In the cancellation hearings, mention was made of mercurial use in pulp and paper as "slimicides"; in agriculture as seed treatments, sod fungicides, and treatments for Dutch Elm disease; for textiles and fabrics as a fungicide; and to prevent "brown mold" on green lumber. All these except a limited use on golf course greens for "snow mold" have been canceled.

Large amounts of mercury are not going into the environment because of these cancellations. Figure 19–4 shows the amounts of mercury used as pesticides for 10 years before the cancellation of these uses. To the abovementioned uses, the figure adds mercury's use as an antifoulant. All these uses either stopped or decreased markedly with the onset of the attempt to cancel mercury pesticide registrations in 1972. The "agricultural" use decreased until 1982, the last year listed; it was then only 36 flasks (U.S. Bureau of Mines, 1982). In the other two categories, other compounds could be used effectively, so use of mercury was discontinued.

PHYSIOLOGIC PROPERTIES

The mercury compounds still used by the paint and coatings industries belong to the Aryl or Alkyloxy classes of organometallic compounds. These compounds are:

Phenylmercuric acetate
Phenylmercuric oleate or benzoate
Di (phenylmercuric) dodecenyl succinate
Chloromethoxypropylmercuric acetate

Earlier, there were a great many other compounds used in the industry, but by 1970 they had been reduced to the above plus their liquid formulations (Mann, 1971). This was primarily because of two papers produced in 1953 and 1957 that showed that the activity of mercurial compounds was due to the quantity of mercury present in the compound (Hopf, 1953; Stewart and Klens, 1957). The effects of the acidic radical was more for solubility or other physical properties, unless it had some antimicrobial activity of its own. Since that time the quantity of a mercury-based biocide has often been expressed in parts per million as mercury rather than as the compound.

The reason the phenylmercuric salts were used rather than the alkyl mercury compounds has to do with the greater human toxicity of the alkyl compounds. Alkyl mercury salts (e.g., methyl, ethyl) were found to cause central-nervous-system lesions because they pass through the neural sheath, the brain-blood barrier, and the placenta. Such damage is not reversible. Alkyl mercury salts are distinctly more toxic than aryls, alkoxyalkyl, or inorganic salts. The aryl (phenyl) mercury salts, on the other hand, do not pass through the neural sheaths, nor do they deposit mercury in the tissues, so such compounds are easily "washed" out of the body.

Arylmercuric and alkoxyalkyl compounds are considered to possess the toxicologic characteristics of inorganic mercurial salts. Their mammalian toxicity is considerably less than that of alkyl mercurials (Goldwater, 1973). The ecological hazard from the use of the alkoxyalkyl mercurials is also considerably less, according to Swedish experience (Johnels, 1971).

For human exposure there is apparently no significant difference between the toxicities of the various phenylmercury compounds. (The same was noted at an earlier time for microbial toxicity.) Most importantly, poisoning due to the phenylmercurials is rare and *chronic occupational poisoning is unknown* (Ladd et al., 1964). In studies done for the National Paint Varnish and Lacquer Association, Goldwater and Jacobs found that although there was exposure to mercury from paint, "painters using mercury-bearing paints showed no evidence of absorption or effects of inhaling the concentrations of mercury found in the workroom air." Also, "no evidence was found of mercury exposure or absorption in a degree that would constitute a hazard to the painters or the occupants of the painted room" (Goldwater and Jacobs, 1964; Jacobs and Goldwater, 1965). A later study agreed with earlier findings of no hazard (Taylor and Unter, 1972).

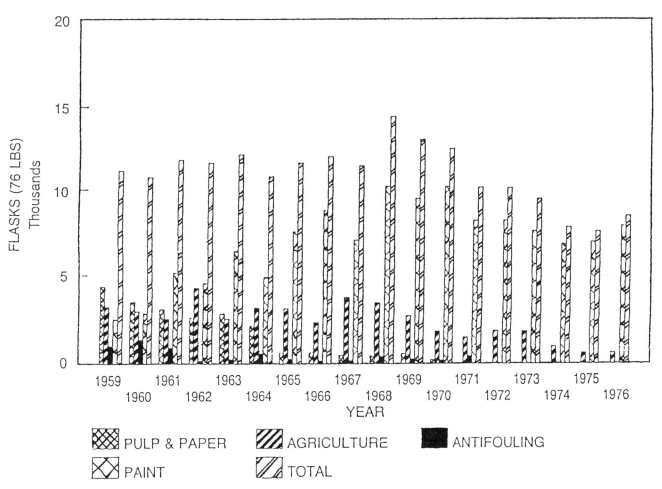

Fig. 19–4. Consumption of mercury by industries.

GENETIC AND TOXATOGENIC EFFECTS

Experimentally, in certain systems of plants and in *Drosophila* organomercurials (primarily methyl mercury), mercury may produce genetic mutations and some chromosomal aberrations, but such changes have not been shown in test mammals.

Mutagenic effects of mercurials were studied in mammalian systems while testing for dominant lethals using male CBA mice. Methyl mercury dicyanamide was the test compound at a dose of 3 mg of mercury/kg I.P. No significant increase in the dominant lethals was found (Ramel, 1967).

A second series was examined by Khera (1971) using methylmercuric chloride. Male rats were treated with 0.1 to 5.0 mg of mercury/kg for 7 days. A slight increase in dominant lethals was noted, as was a reduction in litter size when the rats were bred.

Examination of PMA for mutagenic characteristics in 1981 by the Ames Assay and Escheriches DNA Repair Suspension Assay showed no significant effects. This

Table 19–2. *The LD$_{50}$ For Phenylmercurials on Rat (Oral)*

Phenylmercurial	LD$_{50}$
Phenlymercuric acetate	35 mg/kg
Chloromethoxypropylmercuric acetate	324 mg/kg
Di (phenylmercuric) dodecenyl succinate	0.25 mg/kg

again showed the greater safety of the phenylmercurics. In the 1988 to 1989 tests for continued registration in California, PMA used as a type compound for all the mercurics showed no mutation or teratogenic effects.

TOXIC EFFECTS

The LD$_{50}$ values for the phenylmercurials have been determined as noted in Table 19–2; the skin absorption is shown in Table 19–3.

There is no doubt of the phenylmercuric acute toxicity. In this case the bad reputation of mercury works to its advantage. Industrial workers who use the material are

Table 19–3. *Dermal Toxicity for Rabbits*

Phenylmercurial	LD_{50}
Phenylmercuric oleate	880 mg/kg (male); 780 mg/kg (female)
Di (phenylmercuric) dodecenyl succinate	0.98 ml/kg (male)
Di (phenylmercuric) dodecenyl succinate, abraded	1.51 ml/kg (combined)
Phenylmercuric acetate	204 mg/kg (combined)

cautious and careful to follow the handling instructions for the products. The paint and coatings industry has been using mercury products for 30 years or more and knows how to treat the antimicrobial safely. In the more modern paint plants, with the use of large-volume liquid shipping containers (300 gallons or more), potential contact with the mercury-containing biocide has been drastically reduced. Usually only one man, properly fitted with the required safety equipment, is needed to connect the tank to the automated transfer system, and that may occur at 7- to 20-day intervals (Anonymous, 1983; Simpson, 1984). The required cautionary label on each container tells what steps are needed for the safe use of the product.

A method of "double bagging" has been used to protect workers from exposure to solid PMA for approximately 20 years. The outer bag is waterproof plastic; the inner bag contains a pre-weighed quantity of PMA (from ounces to pounds) and is water soluble. The outer bag is opened and the inner bag is allowed to slip into the batch of paint. In this way there is no exposure to the mercurial itself. This simple system has been accepted by the EPA as constituting "no exposure" to the pesticide. The State of California has likewise agreed with the no-exposure argument and has required minimal toxicology testing of PMA.

From the above one might think that the nonmercurial biocides that were devised to replace mercury-based products would be safer. Although this is true as far as acute animal toxicity (oral LD_{50}) is concerned, most nonmercurial biocides have problems with chronic toxicity, compatibility with paints, or cost-effectiveness. For example, some of the fungicides used after 1972 cause allergic reactions or are sensitizers or suspect carcinogens. An exterior paint not using a mercury-based fungicide must use both a fungicide for film mildew resistance *and* a bactericide for preservation of the liquid paint. Also, many of the currently used in-can preservatives for paint are formaldehyde-releasing compounds with the problems of that material.

PHENYLMERCURY COMPOUNDS IN THE PAINT INDUSTRY

It is precisely because of PMA's general microbial toxicity that it has found broad use in the paint and coatings industry. In 1976 use of PMAs was limited to water-based latex paints by the EPA. Prior to that time the mercurials

had been used in all products of the industry. In 1976, 7845 flasks of mercury were used. In 1977, even with the change in product type in which mercury could be used, the amount of mercury use in the paint industry increased by almost 500 flasks and averaged an increase of approximately 600 flasks per year until 1980. If mercury has remained useful, it is because of its unique properties.

Mercurial antimicrobials possess four useful properties for the paint and coatings industry:
1. Low levels act as general bactericides.
2. At even lower levels they can act as cellulase inhibitors. Mercury will not inhibit all cellulases but will stop the activity of a majority of these enzymes.
3. Higher levels of mercurials act as broad-spectrum fungicides and are used to prevent mildew growth.
4. The cost effectiveness of mercurials is greater than non-mercurial fungicides (Table 19–4).

Liquid paint is subject to biodeterioration before and during use by bacteria. The dried film is prone to surface disfiguration from mildew (fungus) growth. Because of the high activity of the mercurials, only 60 to 100 parts per million of PMA are used in the liquid paint as an antibacterial and only 0.1 to 0.2% is used as a fungicide (mildewcide) for the final dried film.

The highest level of biocide in paints is required for mildew protection, and this is *used only for exterior paints*. The graying of a white painted house is most often mildew growth rather than a wearing of the paint or an accumulation of "dirt." The use of a fungicide (mildewcide) prevents or inhibits this growth for years.

It has been shown that some, if not most, of the mercurials used in painting wood surfaces either stay in the paint film or migrate into the wood, where they are bound (Sibbett, 1972; Broome and Lowrey, 1970). Any mercury compound lost from the film ultimately is bound into insoluable complexes with humic acids in the soil (Ross and Stewart, 1962).

One of the prime requirements for a water-based latex paint is an optimum viscosity, which is necessary for proper application and covering. Loss of this viscosity accounts for the most commonly seen paint spoilage. Most paints use a modified cellulose (e.g., hydroxyethyl cellulose, carboxymethyl cellulose) as a thickening-leveling agent. Unfortunately, this thickener is degraded by bacteria and fungi by means of cellulase to produce a paint of water-like consistency. The prevention of microbial growth usually protects these thickeners. How-

Table 19–4. *Average Cost of Film Mildewcides*

Fungicide	Manufacturer's Recommended Use Level	Approximate Cost (1988)
A	0.3–1.2%	$0.66/gallon
B	0.5–1.0	0.49/gallon
C	.2% + 75# ZnO/100gal.	0.40/gallon
D	0.7–1.2%	0.63/gallon
PMA-100	0.1–0.2%	0.20/gallon

ever, the cellulytic enzyme(s) may have already been produced because of microbial growth in one or more raw materials that are later incorporated into the paint. In that case, loss of viscosity could occur in a sterile paint.

The protection of the paint film from mildew growth requires more biocide than in-can preservation. This is because the fungus is growing on the surface of the film or is deriving its nutrients from something other than the protected film. The nature of the fungal organism also gives it a greater resistance to most antimicrobials. It is not unusual to find that many antibacterial compounds are without effect on fungi or require much higher levels for antifungal effects.

The effectiveness of phenylmercury compounds was paramount in allowing the continued registration of these microbicides. Their high profile also made them a prime target for competing nonmercurial fungicides. It is worth noting that several of the nonmercurial alternatives on the market at the time of the cancellation hearings are no longer used.

There was a long history of searching for nonmercurial fungicides. These were supplied and tested by the paint-additive supply houses. The various technical committees of the paint industry provided a test market for the products. The data from the testing formed a series of papers starting in the mid-1960s (C.D.I.C. Society, 1967, 1968, 1970, 1973; Louisville Society for Coating Technology, 1976; Kansas City Society for Coating Technology, 1976; Post et al., 1976; Mark, 1978). The number of these papers dropped off quickly after 1976, but occasionally one is still seen today. In each case a mercury antimicrobial was the standard to surpass. In most cases the mercury compound held its own. And so even today, on the introduction of a new fungicide PMA is usually used as the "positive control" to beat or at least equal (Lewis and Alderman, 1976; Smith and Rizoff, 1977; Dalton, 1988).

In the years since 1976, a dramatic portion of the sales of fungicides has been captured by nonmercurial compounds. This was greatly propelled by the possible cancellation of organomercurial registrations in 1975. Many companies stopped using these cost-effective products on the assumption that (1) organomercurial compounds would no longer be permitted and (2) there would be a benefit in public relations by the claim that no heavy-metal biocides were used in the products. However, after the allowance of mercury compounds in water-based paints and coatings, there was an increase in use until 1980, when the apparent drop seen in Figure 19–3 occurred. A large segment of the market is still strongly opposed to the use of mercury-based antimicrobials. When new paints are formulated, more than half the time nonmercurial fungicides are now used. As the paint industry grows, it would seem that the amount of mercury remains stable or slightly increases in total pounds, but decreases in relation to the total amount of antimicrobials in use.

RECENT ACTIVITY

Since 1976 there have been few papers published dealing with the organomercurials as biocides. Much of the literature was published earlier or during the time of the EPA cancellation hearings.

There have been attempts to reduce the amount of mercury by using mercury compounds and zinc oxide or another biocide (Engelhardt, 1969; Mark, 1978; Abbott Laboratories, 1977). The concept was to reduce the amount of toxic mercury used as mildewcide and still have an active fungicide. The concept is good, but it did not hold up except in a few paints. Few, if any, paints are made with combinations of fungicides. The industry is consistently trying to simplify its raw material supply. Usually one compound is preferred to obtaining two different materials. This becomes particularly true now that zinc has become a toxic metal that should be removed from the environment. Zinc oxide is being used today with organomercurials, but whether this is to enhance the effect of the biocide is moot. In any case both cost and "environmental pressure" are reducing the amount of zinc in use.

In the late 1970s Crang and Perchak (1977 and 1978) examined the effect of PMA on *Aureobasidium pullulans*, the prime cause of paint mildew. This was an attempt to define the toxic level and mechanism of toxicity of mercury on this organism. Major changes in structure of the organism could be caused by levels of mercury much lower than those used to prevent the growth of *A. pullulans* on a paint film. However, in the experiments of Crang and Perchak, the fungus was immersed in the mercury-containing medium—not growing on the surface of a polymer film as it would in a paint. Their papers show that the action of mercury was diffuse, targeting several structures. Any one of the damaged areas could cause the death of the cell. There were indications of some detoxification of PMA, but the methods did not allow verification.

The only work to appear dealing with the use of mercury *and* the paint and coatings industry was that of Machemer (1979). The possibility that mercury-containing products could still be banned if an effective, cost-efficient alternative was found caused him to examine the new possible substitutes, which he compared to mercury compounds in paints, a clay slurry, and a water-based adhesive. The characteristics studied were antibacterial and fungicidal effects. The results indicated that " . . . mercurial candidates offer the most efficient in-can preservation." However, in the other systems examined, mercury was only moderately effective because of the type of materials preserved. For example, one was already contaminated with a hydrogen sulfide producer. The H_2S reacted to inactivate the organomercury additive.

This paper did not add much to the existing literature but did show that some nonmercurial compounds have utility in some materials and conditions. It could well have been an enforcing argument for those interested in not using organomercurials in paint products.

From 1979 to the present, there have been no publications recording industrial mercury biocide use. The majority of the world's literature was more interested in mercury transformation or detection in the environment or in the nature of resistance to mercury toxicity.

Mercury is a part of the environment. In some areas it is concentrated and recovered as an important product, but it is a small part of the general background of the planet. These facts were made known at the time of the EPA hearings on the mercury compound's cancellation. At the time, there were mercury findings in important lakes, rivers, and land areas. The defendant's contention was that except for areas of known dumping, mercury was ubiquitous, as are most elements if the analyses are sensitive enough. The findings of mercury were not due to new contamination; the areas simply had not been examined so closely before (Buhler, 1973; Taylor, 1975).

The transformation of mercury from other organic or inorganic compounds to methylmercury or to elemental mercury had been shown earlier. The researches done in the last decade were attempts to quantitate the natural reactions (Barkay et al., 1979; Kazak and Forsberg, 1979; Pan-Hou and Imurs, 1981; Trevors, 1986). The results of the research seems to be that both processes occur simultaneously, with the production of mercury vapor (metallic mercury) being more general in a bacteria population. The rates of reaction seem about the same, with the methylation slightly faster but with the demethylation being accomplished by greater numbers in a population. The finding of methylmercury or mercury vapor in any one area depends on the transfer rate of the products in the environment (Letunona et al., 1984; Brown, 1985).

The sensitivity and detoxification of microbes was also investigated with an eye to determining the mechanism of resistance to mercury. A series of geographic area surveys showed the presence of many microbes with a mercury resistance (Berland et al., 1981; Timoney and Port, 1982; Chen, 1983; Reha et al., 1983; Nuto et al., 1987). In Japan, Porter et al. (1982) showed large decreases in the mercury resistance of *Escherichia coli* and *Staphylococcus aureus* cultures obtained in hospitals. The findings were attributed to the "termination of the use of organomercurials (largely phenyl mercuries and Themersol) in hospital disinfectants and detergents." The highest concentration of resistant organisms, partially bacteria, was found in or near deposits of mercury (Reha et al., 1983; Thriene and Hellwig, 1985).

Based on some of the earlier papers and their own research, Hansen et al. (1984) suggested a method for the bacterial removal of mercury from sewage using bacterial cultures capable of volatilizing mercury.

The actual genetic mechanism of mercury resistance was examined and found to be produced by both chromosomes and plasmids (Silver, 1981; Yoshio and Imura,

1981; Kelly, 1984). The translocatable elements of resistance were recognized early on, and continuing research fully disclosed the extent of heavy-metal resistances (Radford et al., 1981; Olson et al., 1979). The reviews of Summers (1986) and Silver and Mesra (1988) provide a good overall view of the pertinent research.

The most recent investigations are now examining cell-free reactions or preparation of DNA probes for detection of specific genes (Barkay et al., 1989; Ji et al., 1989).

Finally, late in October 1989, a 4-year-old child in Detroit, Michigan, became ill with a rare form of mercury poisoning after the interior of his home was freshly painted. The paint used was shown to contain 930 ppm of mercury, several times the accepted limit of a mercury-based biocide for an interior paint.

The federal EPA examined the exposures resulting from the use of mercury containing preservatives in interior latex paints, meanwhile noting the availability of other efficient biocides. The EPA concluded that the use of mercurial compounds in interior paints and coatings presented an unreasonable risk. After this finding, the registrants of mercury-containing products agreed to delete the use of their products in interior paints and coatings; also some registrations for mercury-based biocides were voluntarily withdrawn. These changes were published in the Federal Register, June 29, 1990, pp. 26754–26756.

Mercury biocides are still allowed in exterior paints and coatings, but registrants are required to develop and submit additional data regarding their effect and use. The ban for interior use will undoubtedly influence the final determination of the acceptability of mercury-based antimicrobials when they are re-registered.

FUTURE CONSIDERATIONS

Because of the currently required re-registration of all pesticides before 1997, the eventual fate of phenylmercury compounds as antimicrobials for industry is in doubt. However, because of the high rate of removal from the human body, any "chronic" testing of these compounds must be done at, or extremely close to, toxic levels. It may turn out to be a case of either kill or have no chronic effect. This reaction would be compared to other biocides now known to be possible carcinogens, sensitizers, or irritants, and so may very well show chronic toxicity. The paint and coatings industry has a 30-year history of "safe" handling of organomercurials that may be used to illustrate how materials can be used without problems. Therefore, it is possible that phenylmercuric antimicrobials will survive where other, newer products may be canceled. This is because of the current belief that we can cope with acutely toxic materials, but that materials showing problems of chronic toxicity must be removed from the environment.

For a more complete discussion of mercury compounds and their effect, the reader is referred to Chapter 17 by Grier (1983) in the 3rd edition of this book.

REFERENCES

Abbott Laboratories. 1977. Amical 50 as a cobiocide in latex paint systems. North Chicago, IL.

Anonymous. 1983. A new chapter in paint production. Modern Paint Coatings, 73(5), 42.

Barkay, T., Olson, B.H., and Colwell, R.R. 1979. Heavy metal transformations mediated by estuarine bacteria. Manage. Control Heavy Metal Environment Int. Conf. 1979, pp. 356–363.

Barkay, T., Liebert, C., and Gillman, M. 1989. Hybridization of DNA probes with whole-community genome for detection of genes that encode microbial responses to pollutants: mer genes and Hg^{2+} resistance. Appl. Environ. Microbiol., 55(6), 1574–1577.

Berland, B., Chretiennot-Dinet, M.J., Ferrara, R., and Arlhec, D. 1981. Short term action of mercury on the natural phytoplankton and bacterial population of coastal waters in the northwestern Mediterranean. J. Etud. Pollut. Mar. Mediterranean, 5, 721–733.

Broame, T.T., and Lowrey, E.J. 1970. Mechanism for film preservation by phenyl mercurials on wood substrates. J. Paint Tech., 42(543), 227–236.

Brown, N.L. 1985. Bacteria resistance to mercury—reducto ad absurdum? Trends Biochem. Sci. (Pers. Ed.), 10(10), 400–403.

Buhler, D.R. 1973. Mercury in the Western environment. Workshop Proc., Oregon State University, Cornallis, OR.

California Department of Food and Agriculture Report of Pesticides Sold in California for 1980–1987. 1981–1988.

C.D.I.C. Society for Paint Technology. 1967. Investigation of some factors in mildew-growth on coated surfaces. J. Paint Technol., 39(514), 650–654.

C.D.I.C. Society for Paint Technology. 1968. Some further observations on mildew growth. J. Paint Technol., 40(527), 582–585.

C.D.I.C. Society for Paint Technology. 1970. Three-year study of mildew-growth on coated surfaces. J. Paint Technol., 43(554), 76–80.

C.D.I.C. Society for Paint Technology. 1973. Continued search for nonmercurial fungicides for exterior latex house paints. J. Paint Technol., 46(588), 54–61.

Chen, H. 1983. Mercury-tolerant bacteria in the intertidal and coastal zone of the Jeaozhow Bay: I. Distribution of mercury-tolerant bacteria. Huanjing Kexue, 4(1), 15–20.

Crang, R.E., and Pechak, D.G. 1977. The effects of phenyl mercuric acetate (PMA) on the ultrastructure of the paint mildew, Aureobasidium pullulans. Ann. EMSA Meet., 35th, pp. 654–655.

Crang, R.E., and Pechak, D.G. 1978. The effects of threshold levels of phenylmercuric acetate (PMA) on the paint mildew Aureobasedium pullulans. Can. J. Bot., 56(9), 1177–1185.

Dalton, D.L. 1988. Introduction of a novel, nonmetallic fungicide for the coatings industry. J. Coatings Technol., 60(761), 45–53.

Engelhardt, C.L. 1969. Phenylmercury-zinc oxide. Paint Varnish Prod., November, 1969.

Goldwater, L.J. 1973. Aryl and Alkoxyalkyl mercurials. In Mercury, Mercurials and Mercaptans. Springfield, IL, C.C Thomas, pp. 56–58.

Goldwater, L.J., and Jacobs, M.B. 1964. Mercury Exposure from Use of a Mercury-Bearing Paint. Washington, D.C. Natl. Paint, Varn. and Lacquer Assoc.

Grier, N. 1983. Mercurials—inorganic and organic. In Disinfection, Sterilization and Preservation. 3rd Edition. Edited by S. Block. Philadelphia, Lea & Febiger, pp. 346–374.

Hansen, C.L., Zuolinski, G., Martin, D., and Williams, J.W. 1984. Bacterial removal of mercury from sewage. Biotechnol. Bioeng., 26(11), 1330–1333.

Hopf, P.P. 1953. Comparative activity of phenyl mercury compounds. Manufact. Chem., 24, 444–445.

Jacobs, M.B., and Goldwater, L.J. 1965. Absorption and excretion of mercury in man: VIII, mercury exposure from house paint. Arch. Environ. Health, 11, 582–587.

Ji, G., Zalzberg, S.P., and Silver, S. 1989. Cell-free mercury volatilization activity from three marine caulobacter strains. Appl. Environ. Microbiol., 55(2), 523–525.

Johnels, A.G. 1971. Observed levels and their dynamics in the environment; results from Sweden. In Mercury in Man's Environment. Ottawa, Royal Society of Canada, p. 66.

Kansas City Society for Coatings Technology. 1976. Nonmercurial preservatives as supplements to mercury in latex paints. J. Coatings Technol., 48(615), 58–62.

Kelly, W.J. 1984. Mercury resistance among soil bacteria: ecology and transferability of genes encoding resistance. Soil Biol. Biochem., 16(1), 1–8.

Khera, K.S. 1971. The effect of methylmercury on male fertility. A comparative study in rats and mice. Presented 2nd Ann. Meet. Environ. Mut. Soc., Washington, D.C.

Kozak, S., and Forsberg, C.W. 1979. Transformation of mercuric chloride and methylmercury by the rumen microflora. Appl. Environ. Microbiol., 38(4), 626–636.

Ladd, A.C., Goldwater, L.J., and Jacobs, M.B. 1964. Absorption and excretion of mercury in man: V. Toxicity of phenylmercurials. Arch. Environ. Health, 9, 43–52.

Letunova, S.V., Ermakor, V.V., and Alekseera, S.A. 1984. Role of soil microflora in the biogenic migration of mercury and antimony. Agrokhimiya, 4, 77–82.

Levinson, B.D. Initial decision of Bernard D. Levinson. FIFRA Docket No. 246 et al., 1975.

Lewis, W.M., and Alderman, J. 1976. Nonmercurial mildewcide. Mod. Paint Coatings Technol., June, 1976, 33–34.

Louisville Society for Coating Technology. 1976. Continuing study of nonmercurial mildewcides in alkyd and acrylic house paints. J. Coatings Technol., 48(618), 62–67.

Machemer, W.E. 1979. Use of mercury in protective coatings. Dev. Ind. Microbiol., 20, 25–39.

Mann, A. (ed). Mercurial biocides: paints problem material. Paint Varnish Production, March, 1971, 26–36.

Mark, S. 1978. Zinc oxide/nonmercurial biocide combinations in alkyd house paints. J. Coatings Technol., 50(644), 62–65.

Nieto, J.J., Ventosa, A., and Ruiz-Berraquero, F. 1987. Susceptibility of halobacteria to heavy metals. Appl. Environ. Microbiol., 53(5), 1199–1202.

Olson, B.H., et al. 1979. Plasmid mediation of mercury volatilization and methylation by etuarine bacteria. Dev. Ind. Microbiol., 20, 275–284.

Pan-Hou, H.S.K., and Imura, N. 1981. Biotransformation of mercurials by intestinal microorganisms isolated from yellowfin tuna. Bull. Environ. Contam. Toxicol., 26(3), 359–363.

Porter, F.D., Silver, S., Ong, C., and Nakahara, H. 1982. Selection for mercurial resistance in hospital settings. Antimicrob. Agents Chemother., 22(5), 852–858.

Post, M.A., Iverson, W.P., and Campbell, P.G. 1976. Non-mercurial fungicides. Mod. Paint Coatings, September, 1976.

Radford, A.J., Oliver, J., Kelly, W.J., and Renney, D.C. 1981. Translocatable resistance to mercury and phenylmercuric ions in soil bacteria. J. Bacteriol., 174(3), 1110–1112.

Ramel, C. 1967. Genetic effects of organic mercury compounds. Hereditas, 57, 445.

Riha, V., Cerna, L., and Nymburska, K. 1983. The frequency of mercury and cadmium resistant bacteria in ponds polluted predominantly from agricultural sources. Heavy Met. Environ. Int. Conf. 4th., 1, 369–379.

Ross, R.G., and Stewart, D.R. 1962. Movement and accumulation of mercury in apple trees and soil. Can. J. Plant Sci., 42, 280–283.

Sibbett, D.J. 1972. Emission of mercury from latex paints. Am. Chem. Soc., Div. Water, Air, Waste Chem., 12(1), 20–26.

Silver, S. 1981. Mechanisms of bacterial resistance to toxic heavy metals: arsenic, antimony, silver, cadmium and mercury. NBS Spec. Publ. (U.S.), 1981, 618, 301–324.

Silver, S., and Misra, T.K. 1988. Plasmid-mediated heavy metal resistances. Ann. Rev. Microbiol., 42, 717–743.

Simpson, D.J. 1984. Automated processing and recordkeeping system for paint manufacturers. Paint Coatings, 74(2), 45–48.

Smith, R.A., and Rizoff, W.J. 1976. Latex paint mildewcides: mercurials vs. nonmercurials. J. Coatings Technol., 48(617), 61–64.

Stewart, W.J., and Klens, P.F. 1957. Comparative fungicidal performance of phenylmercury compounds. Am. Paint J., August 12, 1957.

Summers, A.O. 1986. Organization, expression and evolution of genes for mercury resistance. Ann. Rev. Microbiol., 40, 607–634.

Taylor, D. 1975. Mercury as an Environmental Pollutant; A Bibliography. 5th Edition. Birmingham, U.K., Kynoch Press.

Taylor, C.G., and Unter, G.H. 1972. Radiometric studies of mercury loss from fungicidal paints: III. Loss from three paints with various mercury contents. J. Appl. Chem. Biotechnol., 22(6), 711.

Thriene, B., and Hellwig, A. 1985. Bacterial resistance to heavy metals in the environment. Z. Gesamte Hyg. Grenzgeb., 31(2), 109–111.

Timoney, J.F., and Port, J.G. 1982. Heavy metal and antibiotic resistance in Bacillus and Vibrio from sediments of New York bight. Ecol. Stress N.Y. Bight Sci. Manage. (Proc. Symp.), pp. 235–248.

Trevors, J.T. 1986. Mercury methylation by bacteria. J. Basic Microbiol., 26(8), 499–504.

Yoshio, N., and Imura, N. 1981. Mechanism of acquisition of mercury resistance in microorganisms. Menamatabyo ni Kanauru Sogotki Kenkyu 1980, p. 19.

U.S. Bureau of Mines. 1959–1988. Minerals Yearbook, Volume I. Metals, Minerals and Fuels. Washington, D.C., U.S. Govt. Printing Office.

CHAPTER 20

ORGANOTIN COMPOUNDS

M.H. Gitlitz and C.B. Beiter

Tin and its oxide, the mineral cassiterite, have been known and valued since the Bronze Age. Along with copper and mercury, tin accompanied early man's progress towards a civilized society. Unlike copper and mercury, however, inorganic tin compounds are generally physiologically inert by ingestion. Stannous fluoride and stannous pyrophosphate have been used in dentifrice preparations as anticaries agents, and stannous chloride was, for many years, used as a preservative and antioxidant in foods and beverages.

Like many other metals and metalloids, tin forms stable compounds called organotins with direct tin-carbon bonds. Organotins can be represented by the formula R_nSnX_{4-n} where n = 1 to 4, R = alkyl or aryl, and X is an anionic group, commonly halide, carboxylate, oxide, or hydroxide. Organotin compounds have at least one tin-carbon bond and, in these compounds, tin is tetravalent.

The first organotin compounds were prepared in the mid-19th century, but it was not until the early 1950s that van der Kerk and Luijten (1954, 1956) at TNO in the Netherlands systematically explored the biocidal properties of organotin compounds.

van der Kerk found that compounds with four tin-carbon bonds (tetraorganotins) and those with one tin-carbon bond (monoorganotins) were essentially devoid of biologic activity. Of the remaining triorganotin and diorganotin compounds, the triorganotins showed the highest antimicrobial activity. The lower trialkyltins (tripropyl, tributyl, and tripentyl) showed the highest fungicide and bactericide activity within this class. The dialkyltin compounds are substantially less active than the trialkyltins. The typical relationship between chain length of di- and tri-substituted organotin compounds and their minimum inhibitory concentrations for a particular bacteria, *Mycobacterium phlei*, are shown in Figure 20–1.

The response of fungi to triorganotins is generally similar to that exhibited by bacteria in the foregoing example and is illustrated as it is seen typically in Figure 20–2 for the fungus *Aspergillus niger*. Although the lower tri-alkyltins show high fungicide activity, they are unlikely candidates for agricultural fungicide use because of their high phytotoxicity.

Various studies have shown that the nature of the anion group has little influence on the spectrum of biologic activity provided that the anion is not biologically active in its own right and that it confers a sufficient minimal solubility on the compound. Except for trimethyltin and triethyltin compounds, short-chain trialkyltin compounds have only slight solubility in water. Substantial evidence exists that, in dilute aqueous solution, the lower trialkyltin compounds exist as hydrated cations, and these are the biologically active species. Triorganotins with alkyl groups longer than pentyl (C_5) are practically insoluble in aqueous media, perhaps accounting for their lack of biocidal properties.

The work at TNO laid the foundation for the commercial application of organotin compounds as biocides and led, even if indirectly, to their use in the control of a wide variety of pests. Table 20–1 shows the diversity of biocidal applications for which organotins are being used or for which they have been suggested.

AGRICULTURAL APPLICATIONS

Although the patent literature is replete with many examples of triorganotin compounds with agriculturally useful pesticidal activity, only a handful of compounds have been developed commercially.

In the early 1960s, the first organotin agricultural chemical, the fungicide triphenyltin acetate (common name: fentin acetate) was introduced commercially in Europe by Hoechst AG as Brestan. Fentin acetate was recommended for the control of *Phytophthora* (late blight) on potatoes and *Cercospora* on sugar beets at rates of a few ounces per acre (Hartel, 1962). Fentin acetate is a nonsystemic fungicide that is recommended for the control of *Ramularia spp.* on celery and sugar beets and *Phytophthora infestans* on potatoes at 160 to 260 g a.i./ha. It is claimed to be nonphytotoxic to sugar

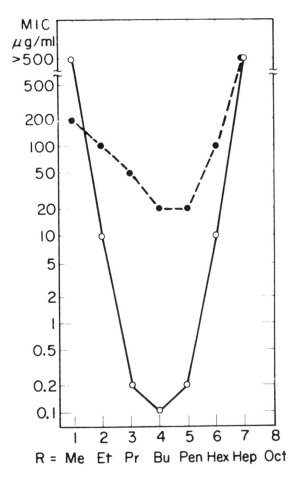

Fig. 20–1. Influence of chain length of di- and tri-substituted tin compounds on minimum concentration inhibitory to *Mycobacterium phlei*. From Sijpesteijn, A.K., Luijten, J.G.A., and van der Kerk, G.J.M. 1969. Organometallic fungicides. In *Fungicides*. Volume 2. Edited by D.C. Torgeson. New York, Academic Press, p. 352.

beets, celery, cocoa, potatoes, and rice at recommended use levels (Worthing, 1983).

Shortly after the introduction of Brestan, triphenyltin hydroxide (fentin hydroxide) was introduced as Du-Ter by Philips-Duphar N.V. with about the same spectrum of disease control as the acetate. Fentin hydroxide is a nonsystemic protectant fungicide that has been recommended for the control of early and late blights of potato at 250 to 350 g a.i./ha, of leaf spot on sugar beets at 350 to 400 g/ha, of blast diseases of rice at 220 to 450 g/ha, of coffee berry disease at 1 kg/ha, and of brown spot disease of tobacco at 200 to 350 g/ha (Worthing, 1983). The hydroxide is presently registered in the United States as a fungicide for potatoes, sugar beets, and pecans.

Both triphenyltin hydroxide and acetate exhibit the unusual property of deterring insects from feeding (Ascher, 1965). They have been proposed for the control of certain leaf-eating larvae, including *Spodoptera spp.*, on the basis of this activity (Worthing, 1983). Several triphenyltin compounds, including the hydroxide, have

been shown to be effective fly sterilants at sublethal concentrations (Kenaga, 1965).

In 1968, tricyclohexyltin hydroxide (common name: cyhexatin), the result of a joint research effort by M&T Chemicals Inc. and Dow Chemical Co., was introduced as an acaricide under the name Plictran. Allison et al. (1968) reviewed the properties of Plictran. It was recommended for the control of phytophagous (plant-feeding) mites on apples and pears and was also registered for use on citrus, stone fruit, strawberries, almonds, walnuts and hops. Cyhexatin is a nonsystemic acaricide effective by contact against the motile stages of a wide range of phytophagous mites, the usual dosage being 20 to 30 g a.i./100 L. It is nonphytotoxic to deciduous fruit, most ornamentals grown in the open, wind-break tree species, vegetables, and vines. Citrus (immature foliage and fruit in the early stages of development), as well as the seedlings and immature foliage of some greenhouse-grown ornamentals and vegetables, are susceptible to possible injury, usually in the form of localized spotting (Worthing, 1983). Cyhexatin is selective and provides good control of harmful arachnids, with little toxicity towards honey bees and most predacious mites and insects at the recommended use rates. The compound also shows antifeedant activity against some insect larvae

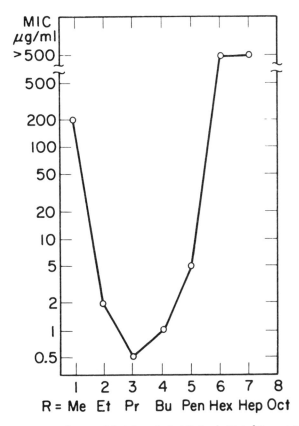

Fig. 20–2. Influence of chain length of trialkyl-substituted tin acetates on minimum concentration inhibitory to *Aspergillus niger*. From Sijpesteijn, A.K., Luijten, J.G.A., and van der Kerk, G.J.M. 1969. Organometallic fungicides. In *Fungicides*. Volume 2. Edited by D.C. Torgeson. New York, Academic Press, p. 340.

Table 20–1. *Biocidal Applications of Organotin Compounds*

Fungicidal
    Control of fungi on potatoes and sugar beets*
    Control of scab on pecans and peanuts*
    Control of rice blast and pine needle blight
    Preservation of wood (from fungi and insects)*
    Paint additive to prevent mold growth

Bacteriostatic
    Control of fouling in cooling water systems*
    Fabric disinfectant
    Antimicrobial in synthetic fibers

Insecticidal
    Antifeedant against insect larvae
    Chemosterilant (preventing reproduction)
    Aracnidicide against phytophagous mites*

Other
    Tapeworm and helminthes eradication in poultry*
    Protection of surfaces (e.g., ships and piers) from attack by
        marine organisms*
    Plankton control in reservoirs
    Molluscicide for bilharzia control
    Rodent repellent for wire and cable

*Commercially significant use

(Ascher et al., 1970). Plictran was withdrawn from the marketplace by Dow in 1987 based on interim results of a dermal teratology study in rabbits which showed fetal hydrocephaly. Details of the Dow study have not been published.

A derivative of cyhexatin, tricyclohexytin 1,2,4-triazole (common name, azocyclotin), is sold as Peropal in Europe by Bayer AG. Its activity spectrum is similar to that of cyhexatin. It is hydrolyzed by aqueous acids to cyhexatin and 1,2,4-triazole (Worthing, 1983).

Hexakis(2-methyl-2-phenylpropyl)distannoxane, (bis [trineophyltin]oxide), (common name: fenbutatin oxide) was introduced as acaricide in the U.S. and abroad as Vendex and Torque, respectively, in the mid-1970s. In the U.S., the product is now marketed by Du Pont. Fenbutatin oxide gives effective and long-lasting control, at 20 to 50 g a.i./100 L of spray, of the mobile stages of a wide range of phytophagous mites on citrus, greenhouse crops, ornamentals, top fruit, vegetables, and vines. No phytotoxicity has been seen on these crops at concentrations twice those recommended. It is relatively nontoxic to predacious arthropods, including *Stethorus punctum* and *Amblyseius finlandicus* (Worthing, 1983). Water causes conversion of fenbutatin oxide to tris(2-methyl-2-phenylpropyl)tin hydroxide, which is reconverted to the parent compound slowly at room temperature and rapidly at 98°C. The structures of these organotin acaricides are shown in Figure 20–3.

The lower trialkyltins, from trimethyltin to tripentyltin, show high biologic activity, but none are used in agriculture. Trimethyltin compounds are highly insecticidal but their high mammalian toxicity and neurotoxic effects make them unlikely candidates for commercial

use. Tripropyltin, tributyltin, and tripentyltin compounds have a high degree of fungicide and bactericide activity, but their high phytotoxicity does not allow their use on living plants. While the higher (C_8 and above) trialkyltins are nonphytotoxic, they are neither fungicidal nor insecticidal. Tricyclohexyl and tricycloheptyltins are also essentially nonphytotoxic. Attempts to moderate the phytotoxicity of the trialkyltins with asymmetric oganotins of the form R_2CySnX or RCy_2SnX where R = lower alkyl group, Cy = cyclohexyl, and X = chloride, hydroxide, or acetate have met with only limited success. Although these compounds are less phytotoxic than the trialkyltins, this quality is attained at the expense of fungicidal activity (Reifenberg and Gitlitz, 1974). Attempts to combine the good acaricidal properties of the tricyclohexyltins with the high fungicidal activity of the triphenyltins in one molecule have been successful to a degree. Dicyclohexylphenyltin hydroxide is almost as good an acaricide as tricyclohexyltin hydroxide, and slightly poorer than triphenyltin hydroxide as a fungicide (Gitlitz, 1975). Asymmetric triorganotin compounds show the same biologic activity as a physical mixture of the two parent symmetric triorganotins that constitute them.

The nature of the organic groups bonded to tin through carbon and their number govern the biologic activity of organotins. Both the number and arrangement of carbon atoms around tin have a profound effect on the acaricidal and fungicidal activity. The activity of the molecule is sensitive to even the slightest change in the environment around the tin atoms.

Tricyclohexyltin hydroxide is an extremely good acaricide. The insertion of a methylene group between the cyclohexyl ring and tin causes a marked diminution in miticidal activity. A propylene group between the ring and tin renders the compound inactive as a miticide. Although interposing a methylene group between the cyclohexyl ring and tin leads to a decrease in acaricidal and fungicidal activity, the internally methylene-bridged compound, tris(2-norbornyl)tin hydroxide, is comparable in activity to the tricyclohexyltin compound (Gitlitz, 1976). Another striking example of the importance of steric effects was provided by Horne (1972). Bis[tris(3-

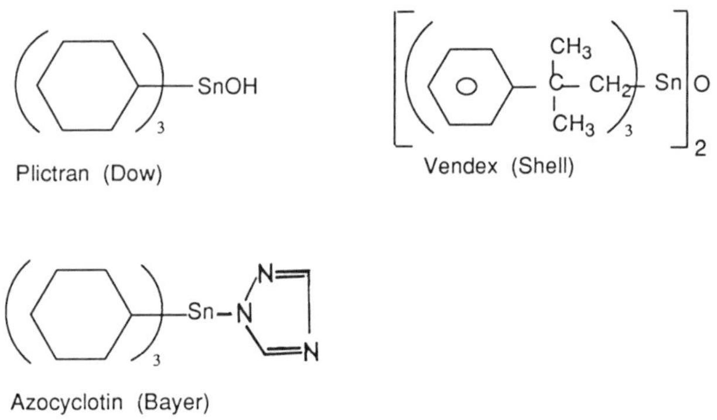

Plictran (Dow)

Vendex (Shell)

Azocyclotin (Bayer)

Fig. 20–3. Organotin acaricides.

phenylpropyl)tin] oxide shows no acaricidal activity; however, the homologous 2,2-dimethyl-3-phenylpropyl-tin derivative is the active ingredient in the commercial acaricide, Vendex. The thiophene analogue of Vendex, with which it is isoelectronic, also is acaricidal (Foster and Soloway, 1973).

Most reports confirm the initial observation by van der Kerk of the relative unimportance of the nature of the anionic portion of the triorganotin molecule to the overall biologic activity (Ison et al., 1971; McIntosh, 1971). Given the facile anion exchange in aqueous media described earlier, this is not surprising.

ANTIFOULING SYSTEMS

Growth of marine organisms on shipbottoms and sub-merged structures causes economic losses resulting from higher fuel consumption, loss of speed due to additional drag, and collapse of structures due to corrosion. In the 1970s, the increased size of vessels and requirements for extended operating times between dry-dockings placed severe demands on the conventional copper-based an-tifouling systems that offered at most a service life of 2 to 3 years.

With some conventional paint systems, the service life could be extended with underwater scrubbing to delay dry-docking an additional 6 months. However, the in-troduction of organotin copolymer paints has made the 3 to 5 year system a reality.

A description of marine fouling and the early history of its prevention prior to the introduction of the organo-tins in the early 1950s is presented in the excellent book *Marine Fouling and Its Prevention*, prepared by the Woods Hole Oceanographic Institute (1952). Gitlitz (1981) provided an overview of the state of the art in antifouling coatings through 1981 and reviewed the his-tory of the organotins as antifoulants. The potential of organotins, primarily tributyltin and triphenyltin deriv-atives, was first recognized in the 1950s, and commer-cialization occurred in the 1960s. Their acceptance was based on broad-spectrum control of marine fouling forms, including the following:

Barnacles
  Acorn
  Goose
Algae
  Enteromorpha sp.
  Ectocarpus sp.
Tube worms
Bryozoans
Tunicates
Hydroids
Wood borers
  Mollusks, teredos
  Crustaceans, limnoria

Antifouling systems function by slowly releasing a tox-icant such as copper or triorganotin so that it is readily available at the surface to prevent attachment of marine organisms.

The organotins, particularly bis(tributyltin) oxide, found acceptance in the pleasurecraft market because of their broad-spectrum activity, compatibility with alu-minum (which corrodes in the presence of copper), and ability to allow the preparation of bottom paints with a wide range of attractive colors. Other triorganotin de-rivatives, such as tributyltin fluoride and triphenyltin compounds, gained acceptance because of their pigment-like physical properties, which permitted higher loadings than the oxide (a liquid) in paints, thus extending the service life.

There are three classes of paints in which organotins are used:

1. *Free association*, in which the antifoulant is phys-ically mixed into the paint and its release depends on diffusion from the paint film.
2. *Copolymer*, in which the tributyltin moiety is chemically bonded to the paint polymer matrix (usually an acrylate polymer) and is released by slow hydrolysis when exposed to seawater (Figure 20–4).
3. *Ablative*, in which the antifoulant is mixed into the paint, which is designed to soften and ablate or slough off when exposed to seawater to release the antifoulant (Figure 20–5).

The efficacy of antifouling paints is established using the following:

Antifoulant performance tests
  Static panel tests attached to rafts or fixed piers
    (by ASTM Method D3623-78a, 1982)
  Panels attached to the bilge keel of vessels
  Patch tests on vessels
Erosion rate determinations
  To measure the erosion rate (polishing rate) of co-polymer antifouling paints under specified condi-tions.
Antifoulant release rate determinations
  ASTM Draft Method: "Organotin Release Rates of Antifouling Coating Systems in Seawater" to meas-ure the release of tributyltin from coatings as re-quired by the U.S. EPA (ASTM Subcommittee D01.45)

The conventional free-association fouling control coat-ings employ a soluble matrix consisting of a vinyl or chlorinated rubber resin modified with water-soluble components (e.g., rosin) to obtain release of the toxicant in water. The ratio of resin to rosin is critical for proper release of the antifoulant, as illustrated in Table 20–2 for tributyltin fluoride. At too low a rosin content, the an-tifoulant will be held in the film or released at a rate too slow to control fouling; at too high a rosin content, the release will be too fast, depleting the antifoulant in the surface layers of the paint, which then becomes suscep-tible to fouling. Cuprous oxide, tributyltin compounds, and triphenyltin compounds are the primary antifoulants in these systems.

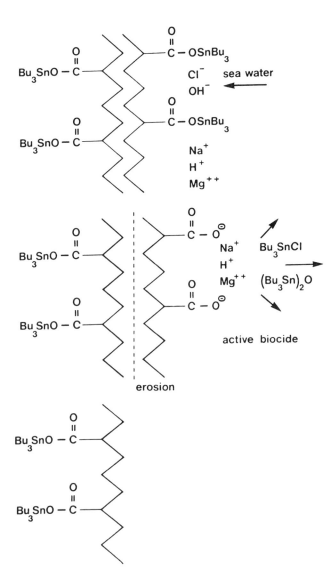

Fig. 20–4. Schematic diagram of antifoulant release from tributyltin acrylate copolymers. From Gitlitz, M.H. 1981. Recent developments in marine antifouling coatings. J. Coat. Tech., 53, p. 50.

Tributyltins that have been used commercially are the following:

Compound	Form
bis(tributyltin) oxide (TBTO)*	Liquid
bis(tributyltin) adipate	Semisolid
bis(tributyltin) dodecylsuccinate	Waxy solid
bis(tributyltin) sulfide	Liquid
Tributyltin acetate	Waxy solid
Tributyltin resinate	Waxy solid
Tributyltin fluoride (TBTF)	Solid

Of these, bis(tributyltin) oxide and tributyltin fluoride received the widest acceptance and are the only non-polymeric organotins still registered with the EPA.

Except for some pleasurecraft bottom paints and paints

*Registered trademark of Elf Atochem NA Inc.

Table 20–2. *Influence of Rosin on Leaching Rate of Tributyltin Fluoride (TBTF) in Vinyl Ship-Bottom Paints Exposed in Biscayne Bay, Miami, FL*

	Vinyl/Rosin ratio (by wt.)					
	3:1		1.5:1		1:2	
Exposure Months	Residual TBTF (%)*	F.R.	Residual TBTF (%)	F.R.	Residual TBTF (%)	F.R.
0	100	—	100	—	100	—
3	82.5	100	37.5	100	18.9	100
6	71.0	100	18.5	100	10.2	35
10	70.0	90	18.3	80	3.5	0
14	64.3	90	—	55	—	0
16	67.0	85	—	40	—	0

F.R. = Fouling rating; 100 = No fouling; 0 = Complete fouling
*Percent of original paint content

From Englehart, J., Beiter, C.B., and Freiman, A. 1974. Recent developments in slow release organotin antifoulants. Proc. 1st Int. Contr. Rel. Symp., Akron, OH. Sept. 18, 1974.

for aluminum-hulled vessels, tributyltins are always used in combination with cuprous oxide. Other antifoulants used as cotoxicants are zinc dimethyldithiocarbamate, thiuram, and copper thiocyanate. The formula for a typical conventional antifouling paint system based on tributyltin fluoride is shown in Table 20–3. Such systems inevitably foul before all the antifoulant is exhausted from the paint film. The residual film must be cleaned thoroughly or removed prior to being recoated.

The full potential of the organotins as antifoulants was not realized until the introduction of organotin polymers such as the tributyltin methacrylate/methyl methacrylate copolymers, which serve as both the paint binder and antifoulant source. A general description of a coating formulation based on organotin copolymers is given in Table 20–4.

The tributyltin moiety is released by hydrolysis when exposed to seawater, as illustrated earlier in Figure 20–4. This hydrolysis and erosion of the film surface as the vessel moves through the water not only controls toxicant release but also smooths the coating surface to provide savings in fuel costs while maintaining the vessel's speed (Fig. 20–6). In dry dock, the residual paint retains its effectiveness and can be recoated with a minimum of surface preparation (Table 20–4).

Because of environmental concerns, new regulations have recently been placed on antifouling paints containing organotins in the U.S. by the Organotin Antifouling Paint Control Act of 1988:

1. Organotin paints are restricted to use on vessels 25 meters (82 feet) or larger, with the exception of aluminum-hulled vessels.
2. A maximum tributyltin (TBT) release rate of 4 μg/cm²/day is permitted.

This action, which eliminates the use of organotin paints on most pleasurecraft, has been taken to reduce tributyltin levels in coastal waters. Their presence has been associated with adverse chronic effects on nontarget

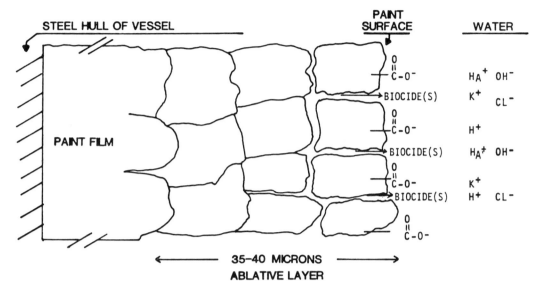

Fig. 20–5. Pattern of tributyltin release from conventional ablative antifoulant coatings. From Anderson, C.D., and Dalley, R. 1988. Use of organotins in antifouling paints. Proceedings of Oceans 86 Conference. Volume 4. Organotin Symposium, Marine Tech. Soc., Washington, D.C., Sept. 23–25, 1986. New York, IEEE, p. 1109.

aquatic organisms (see Federal Register Vol. 52, No. 194, pp. 37510–37519, Oct. 7, 1987). The adoption of the EPA-specified maximum release rate and existing shipping traffic patterns will control any adverse environmental effects from the use of organotin paints on commercial vessels.

WOOD PRESERVATION

Wood is subject to biodeterioration from fungi, termites, and insects, which reduces market value and service life by staining fresh-cut timbers and weakening or destroying existing structures.

The common forms of attack by fungi are characterized as:

Brown rot, which occurs when the cellulose is the primary food source. It includes *dry rot,* typified by brown powdery growth produced by basidiomycetes such as *Merulius lacrymans,* and *wet rot,* produced by *Coniophora puteana* and *Poria vaporaria,* which tolerate more moisture than the dry rot fungi.

White rot is produced by *Coriolus versicolor* and results from digestion primarily of the lignin, whereas *soft rot* is produced by fungal attack on the surface of very wet or water-logged wood.

Table 20–3. *Conventional Organotin Antifoulant Paint Systems*

Components (Wt. %)	Vinyl bioMet TBTF	Chlorinated Rubber bioMet TBTF
Binder resin	11.2 VAGH[1]	13.7 (50% Parlon S-20)[2]
Red iron oxide	15.1	20.0
Talc	11.2	8.4
Zinc oxide	7.1	9.4
WW gum rosin	3.7	23.0 (60% in xylene)
bioMet TBTF[3]	11.9	15.6
Methyl isobutyl ketone	20.3	—
Xylene	18.8	9.0
Bentone 27[4]	0.5	0.7
Methanol	0.2	0.2
Totals	100.0	100.0

[1]Union Carbide Co.
[2]Hercules Inc.
[3]Elf Atochem NA Inc.
[4]Spencer-Kellogg Products

Table 20–4. *Formulation Parameters for Antifouling Paints Based on bioMet 300 Series* Organotin Polymers*

Ingredients	Parts by Weight (range)
Binder	
Tributyltin methacrylate/methyl methacrylate copolymer (50% solids)	30–40
Pigment (30–40 PVC)	
Inert: e.g., iron oxide, titanium dioxide, organic pigment	15–30
Reactive: zinc oxide	0–25
Cotoxicants	
Cuprous oxide	16–30
or	
TBTF	2–4
Thixotrope	
Fumed silica	1–2
Solvent	
MIBK/xylene	25–35

*Elf Atochem NA Inc. trademark for its tributyltin methacrylate/methyl methacrylate copolymers.

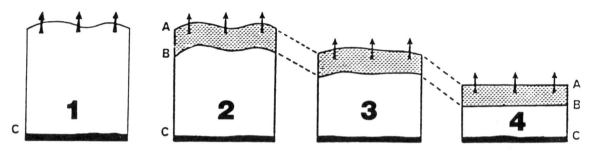

Fig. 20–6. Erosion and polishing in antifouling coatings based on tributyltin acrylate copolymers. *1.* Freshly applied paint. Surface is saponifying, and the tributyltin cation is being released to create a hydrolyzed layer. *2.* A and B is a hydrophilic hydrolyzed layer approximately 5 to 20 μm thick, releasing tributyltin. B is the interface at which copolymer reacts with water to release tributyltin. B to C is a hydrophobic zone 100 to 300 μm thick that makes up the bulk of available paint. *3,* As the biocide release continues at a constant rate, the surface of the paint becomes smoother. *4.* Biocide release continues at a constant rate until the paint is eroded down to the anticorrosive coating or underlying hull. From Anderson, C.D., and Dalley, R. 1986. Use of organotins in antifouling paints. Proceedings of Oceans 86 Conference. Volume 4. Organotin Symposium, Marine Tech. Soc., Washington, D.C., Sept. 23–25, 1986. New York, IEEE p. 1110.

Sap stain, the primary cause of disfigurement of wood, is a blue-gray stain produced in the wood by *Pullaria pullulans* or other common molds.

Soil block tests have been the standard method for determining the threshold values for wood preservatives. In an effort to obtain data quickly, accelerated tests, such as soil beds or mold chambers, are often used for screening of new preservative systems. This is followed by field and in-service tests such as stake tests in which rot and termite control is established in outdoor ground contact. More recently, tests employing wood L or T joints and fences are being employed to identify more selective preservatives for use in above-ground applications.

The major heavy-duty wood preservatives, creosote, coal tar, pentachlorophenol, and arsenicals—e.g., CCA (chromated copper arsenate), ACA (ammoniacal copper arsenate), and FCAP (fluor chrome arsenate phenol)—have come under increased scrutiny in recent years, because of environmental and toxicologic concerns. This has resulted in the increasing use of alternative preservatives in some critical applications. Triorganotins have proven to be viable alternatives in many above-ground applications, e.g., millwork, posts and fences, lumber, and home and farm use.

The activity of the tributyltins is demonstrated by TBTO in soil block tests against a broad spectrum of wood rot fungi (Table 20–5).

Table 20–5. *Toxic Values for TBTO on Unleached Scots Pine Blocks Against Basidiomycete Fungi, According to BS 838*

Fungus	Toxic Values (kg/m³)
Poria vaporaria	0.013–0.03
Coriolus versicolor	0.15–1.33
Coniophora puteana	0.12–0.81
Merulius lacrymans	0.02–0.06
Poria monticola	0.02–0.06

From Hill, R., and Killmeyer, A.J. 1988. Chemical and biological investigations of organotin compounds as wood preservatives. Proc. 84th Ann. Mtg. AWPA, Minneapolis, MN.

The tributyltins are used at concentrations as low as 0.3% in retail brush-on solutions and up to 2% in industrial solutions for pressure or vacuum treatment of joinery or millwork. They are characterized by low volatility, low water solubility, and solubility in organic solvents. They do not discolor, nor do they affect the dimensional stability of the wood; they are compatible with glue, caulking, and glazing compounds.

The organotins used commercially are:

TBTO
Tributyltin naphthenate
Tris(tributyltin) phosphate

Treatment of wood is accomplished by:

Pressure
Double vacuum
Immersion
Flooding
Spraying
Brushing

Dip, brush, and spray treatments generally give less penetration and shorter-term performance than pressure or vacuum treatments.

Tributyltin compounds have a proven record of performance in treatment of joinery in Europe. Products such as TBTO, tributyltin naphthenate, and tributyltin phosphate are used alone and also formulated with insecticides. TBTO is employed in wood-preservation solutions designed for brush, dip, and pressure treatment of wood, imparting resistance to a wide spectrum of wood-rot fungi and reduced susceptibility to termites (Table 20–6) and wood-boring beetles. These products are employed primarily in treatment of lumber, in mill work, and in above-ground use. Surface mold control in pigmented stains is enhanced with use of cotoxicants, e.g., fungicides such as:

Folpet	N-(trichloromethylthio)phthalimide
Chlorothalonil	tetrachloroisophthalonitrile
Azaconazole	1-[[2-(2,4-dichlorophenyl)-1,3-dioxolan-2-yl]methyl]-1*H*-1,2,4-triazole

Table 20–6. *Resistance of Dip-Treated[1] Southern Yellow Pine Blocks to the Subterranean Termite* Reticulitermes Flavipes, *After Water Leaching*

Preservative	Treating Solution Conc. (% a.i.)	Weight Solution Pickup (g)	% Wt. Loss	Block Ratings[2]
TBTO	0.75	0.42	0.2 ± 0.5	9.0
TBTO	1.0	0.41	0.8 ± 0.5	9.6
Polyphase[3]	1.0	0.44	29.7 ± 4.9	3.2
Pentachlorophenol	5.0	0.46	1.9 ± 0.6	9.2
Control	—	—	35.0 ± 6.4	0.0

[1]Dip treatment 1 minute
[2]Block rating: 10 = Sound—surface nibbles permitted; 9 = Light attach; 8 = Moderate attach; 4 = Heavy attach; 0 = Failure
[3]Registered trademark of Troy Chemical Co., Newark, NJ, for their 3-iodo-2-propynylbutyl carbamate

Dichlofluanid   IUPAC name: N-dichlorofluoromethylthio-N′,N′-dimethyl-N-phenyl-sulphamide
C.A. use: 1,1-dichloro-N-[(dimethylamino)sulfonyl]-1-fluoro-N-phenylmethanesulfenamide

The longterm performance of the tributyltins has been questioned because of reports of dealkylation attributed to fungal action, free-radical reactions, or both in the wood. It has been suggested by Richardson and Lindner (1979) that the enzymatic action of the fungi responsible for deterioration is blocked by the organotin moieties, which are bound at the active sites on the cellulose rather than by direct fungal inhibition. Any breakdown of the tributyltins in wood to dibutyltin, monobutyltin, and inorganic tin is not reflected in the good service history of treated wood. This is supported by 25 years of performance without significant failures of organotin-treated wood in Europe.

Water-based wood preservatives have been achieved with TBTO formulated in combination with quaternary ammonium compounds at a ratio of 1 to 8, e.g., "Permapruf T" offered by Wykamol Ltd. (U.K.). Water-soluble tributyltin alkanesulfonates have been described by the International Tin Research Institute and show promise in early evaluations.

Solvents do not have a significant influence on performance of the organotins, although Richardson (1988) has reported improved activity when moisture is present.

WATER TREATMENT

Biocides are necessary to control microbial growth responsible for slime that can clog piping, hinder heat transfer, or otherwise interfere with the proper functioning of equipment. Three principal groups of organisms are responsible for problems in cooling water recirculating systems:

1. *Algae*   Blue-green, green, and diatoms
2. *Bacteria*   Gram-negative, gram-positive spore-forming rods, iron and sulfate-reducing
3. *Fungi*   Molds, yeasts, wood rot

Table 20–7. *Control Advantages Using TBTO Plus QUAT** *(Broth Dilution Test)*

Organism	Concentration Necessary for Complete Inhibition of Growth		
	Bis(Tributyltin) Oxide Plus Quat* (1:5)	Bis(Tributyltin) Oxide	Quat*
B. mycoides	2	0.1	2
A. aerogenes	8	> 500	31
P. aeruginosa	16	> 500	63
C. albicans	2	1.0	4
A. flavus	2	0.5	63
P. funiculosum	2	3.0	4

*Alkyldimethylbenzylammonium chloride

TBTO was first introduced into the U.S. for control of slime in process waters, especially in pulp and paper manufacture. Because of its low water solubility, lack of control of gram-negative bacteria, and substantiveness to cellulose, initial performance was poor. Investigations to overcome these deficiencies led to the development of TBTO/Quat combinations, which provide water dispersibility while complementing the activity of the tributyltins (Table 20–7).

Tributyltin compounds in combination with quaternary ammonium compounds are used in industrial water treatment for the control of slime produced by bacteria, algae, and fungi.

MISCELLANEOUS BIOCIDAL APPLICATIONS

Additional biocidal applications of organotin compounds that have never achieved significant commercial use include the following:

Paint additives: For mold resistance and in-can preservation. The activity of organotins is selective at an unfavorable cost/performance level.

Disinfectants and sanitizers: Products based on organotin/quat formulations provide a good spectrum of activity but at a higher cost than phenolics.

Rodent repellent: Excellent control of rodent attack on field wire and cable, but difficulties in handling treated wire precluded their general acceptance.

Schistosomiasis (Bilharizia) control: Very effective in controlling the intermediate host—the snail; however, broadcast treatment of water is not environmentally acceptable with organotins.

TOXICOLOGY AND HUMAN HEALTH EFFECTS

The toxicology of organotin compounds has recently been reviewed by Nicklin and Robson (1988) and Saxena (1987). For the purposes of this summary, we will concentrate on the toxicologic properties of those triorganotins that have achieved commercial importance, including the tributyltins, the triphenyltins, and the tricyclohexyltins. For information on other triorganotin compounds, the interested reader is referred to the Nicklin and Robson paper, the Saxena review, or the earlier review prepared by the International Tin Research Institute (1978). The human health and safety aspects of tributyltin compounds were recently updated by Schweinfurth (1987).

Biocides are by definition toxic, and triorganotin compounds are no exception. These compounds are powerful metabolic inhibitors that interfere with mitochondrial respiration. In industrial antibacterial and antifungal applications, tributyltin derivatives provide the best balance of efficacy and spectrum of control along with mammalian toxicity effects that are manageable with proper precautions. In agricultural applications, triphenyltin, tricyclohexyltin, and trineophyltin compounds have commercially significant usage and have been manufactured and used safely for almost 20 years. Therefore, the most data exist on these four classes of triorganotin compounds.

Triorganotins like bis(tributyltin) oxide and triphenyltin hydroxide cause irritation, vesication, and corrosion—depending on length of contact—when applied to the skin as neat or moderately concentrated organic solutions if not promptly removed. They are also corrosive to the eye. Aerosols and dusts of triorganotin compounds are irritating to the respiratory tract, and can cause a variety of effects depending on concentration, from lung edema to death. Aqueous suspensions of triphenyltin and tricyclohexyltin compounds such as are used in agriculture can cause irritation or more severe skin reaction with prolonged contact.

Schweinfurth and Gunzel (1987) reviewed the inhalation toxicity of tributyltins and pointed out the difference in the results from aerosol studies, which show an LC_{50} of 65 to 200 mg/m³ for tributyltin compounds, and studies conducted on the saturated vapors of tributyltin compounds that, because of their very low vapor pressures, caused only minor clinical signs (nasal discharge).

The quantitative determination of the dermal toxicity of triorganotins is complicated by their irritative and corrosive properties, especially in occlusive testing where prolonged exposure takes place with no remediation.

Table 20–8 lists the acute dermal toxicity of the common tributyltin derivatives.

Table 20–8. *Acute Dermal Toxicity of Tributyltin Derivatives*

Derivative	Species	LD_{50} (mg/kg)	Reference
Oxide	Rabbit	11,700	Elsea (1959)
	Rat	605	Klimmer (1969)
Benzoate	Rat	505	Klimmer (1969)
Naphthenate	Rat	4600	Schweinfurth (1987b)
Fluoride	Rabbit	680	Sheldon (1975)

It is interesting to note that the dermal LD_{50} values for these TBT compounds have a broader range than the oral LD_{50} values (Schweinfurth, 1987b; also see Table 20–9). However, these differences may be due to the formulation or method of testing. In all cases, however, the acute dermal toxicity is less than the acute oral toxicity. In tests on rats, a maximum dose of 300 mg/kg TBTO as a 10% emulsion was sprayed onto the skin, covered for 24 hrs, then washed off. At necropsy after 10 days, dry necrosis was noted in the area of application but no indication of systemic organ damage could be detected macroscopically (Schweinfurth and Gunzel, 1987). Nevertheless, because of their potential irritative effects on the skin and respiratory system and their corrosivity to the eyes, spraying of organotins in solution or suspension should only be carried out by workers in protective gear (gloves, face-mask, and goggles at the minimum).

The acute oral LD_{50} of a material is recognized as a useful measure of its relative toxicity, although alone it gives no indication of mechanism of action and its meaning is complicated by corrosive effects and the method and medium of administration. Table 20–9 provides a listing of acute oral LD_{50} values from the literature for

Table 20–9. *Acute Oral Toxicities of Selected Triorganotin Compounds*

Compound	LD_{50} (mg/kg⁻¹)	Species	Reference
Bis(tributyltin) oxide	150–234	Rat	ITRI* (1978)
Tributyltin benzoate	130–140	Rat	ITRI (1978)
Tributyltin fluoride	200	Rat	ITRI (1978)
Tributyltin naphthenate	224	Rat	ITRI (1987b)
Tributyltin methacrylate copolymer	> 800	Rat	Lin (1985)
Tributyltin acetate	140–300	Rat	Worthing (1983)
Triphenyltin hydroxide	110–171	Rat	Worthing (1983)
Tricyclohexyltin hydroxide	540	Rat	Worthing (1983)
Tricyclohexyltin 1,2,4-triazole	99	Rat	Worthing (1983)
Bis(trineophyltin) oxide	2630	Rat	Worthing (1983)

*International Tin Research Institute

some of the commercially significant triorganotin compounds.

Chronic animal studies with repeated dietary or inhalation exposure reported in the literature have shown effects on the kidneys, liver, and immune system including the thymus, spleen, lymph nodes, and blood. For valid testing on organotins, appropriate test levels must be determined prior to the study by rangefinding experiments to avoid confounding the results by acute effects of these chemicals, which can be highly irritating or corrosive to the gastrointestinal tract of the test animals. In dietary studies on organotins, the compound or its metabolites is found in the liver, kidneys, spleen, and blood; at high doses the animals do not gain weight. When incorporated as part of a polymer, however, tributyltin becomes much less bioavailable. In studies by Lin et al. (1985) no excess tin could be found by neutron activation analysis in the kidney, liver, stomach, or brain tissue of rats fed up to 800 mg/kg/day of powdered trialkytin methacrylate–methyl methacrylate copolymer suspended in propylene glycol. Although the organotin polymer is not characterized, it presumably is representative of the commercially available tributyltin methacrylate copolymers that serve as the basis for modern self-polishing antifouling paints (see previous section).

The effect of tributyltin oxide on the immune system of rats was studied by Vos (1984). At concentrations of 20 ppm in the diet and above, a suppression of thymus-dependent immune responses was seen. The practical consequences of these observations are not well understood, and research in this area is continuing. It is significant that in one study on the immunotoxic effects of tributyltin compounds, in which the test animals were not overwhelmed, the toxic responses disappeared after the cessation of the exposure (Snoeij et al., 1985).

Although some of the early (and even recent) literature promoted concern about possible neurotoxic, mutagenic, carcinogenic, or teratogenic effects from tributyltin compounds or other commercially significant triorganotins, recent work and critical examination of the existing literature provides no evidence that these compounds are such hazards in humans at practical exposure levels encountered in their normal manufacture or use. Animal studies on triphenyltin acetate and hydroxide, tricyclohexyltin hydroxide, and bis(trineophyltin) oxide, have shown these compounds to be noncarcinogenic (Blunden and Chapman, 1986). In recent repeated dose studies on rats with tributyltin oxide (Kranjnc et al., 1984) and tributyltin acetate (Mushak et al., 1982), no neurotoxic effects were reported.

It should be noted here that trimethyltin and triethyltin compounds are powerful neurotoxins, but these materials are not manufactured commercially although they may be encountered in the research laboratory. Saxena (1987) summarized the literature on the CNS effects of these compounds.

Laboratory workers, process workers, and applicators accidentally exposed to triorganotin compounds provide the most useful documentation of adverse effects produced by accidental exposure. Contact with neat or concentrated solutions of tributyltin compounds was reported as early as 1958 to cause skin burns in the form of an itching erythematous reaction that becomes apparent between 1 and 8 hours after exposure. Cessation of contact with the material resulted in rapid and complete healing (Lyle, 1958). In contact studies on the back of the hands of volunteers, skin lesions were produced by a single application of tributyltin oxide and acetate. Irritation was apparent after 8 hrs, and sterile pustules appeared on the second day. These discrete lesions gradually healed over the course of 1 week (Nicklin and Robson, 1988). If the material is washed off with soap and water immediately after contact, such lesions do not appear, in our experience. Schweinfurth (1987) reported that in studies on human volunteers, a single exposure of both 1% bis(tributyltin) oxide and 2% tributyltin naphthenate in a vehicle composed of 90% hydrocarbon solvent plus 10% alkyd resin (a model wood preservative system), the organotin solutions gave the same skin response as the vehicle alone after up to 4 hours. No systemic effects were reported.

Incidents involving accidental occupational exposure to triphenyltin acetate, used as an agricultural fungicide, are reported in the literature and have been summarized by Nicklin and Robson (1988). Effects include malaise, nausea, vomiting, headache, visual disturbances, dizziness, gastric distress, and anorexia. Unfortunately such reports are anecdotal and of limited scientific value. In all cases, however, there was complete recovery.

Only one fatality in which accidental occupational exposure to an organotin compound may be implicated has been reported in the literature. The incident involved a plant worker who was accidentally drenched in a hot organic solvent mixture containing diphenyltin and triphenyltin chlorides. The worker suffered extensive third-degree burns, and death occurred from renal failure 12 days after the accident (NIOSH, 1976).

The U.S. National Institute for Occupational Safety and Health has recommended a maximum allowable concentration of organotin in the workplace of 0.1 mg (measured as tin) per cubic meter of air determined as a time-weighted average concentration for up to a 10-hr work shift in a 40-hr work week (NIOSH, 1976).

ENVIRONMENTAL IMPACT

As the commercial use of organotin agricultural chemicals and biocides has increased, there has been some concern about their possible environmental effects. These environmental effects have been reviewed by Blunden et al. (1984), Blunden and Chapman (1986), and Maguire (1987). Recent attention has focused on their use in ship-bottom antifouling paints, which, next to agricultural uses, is the major source of triorganotins entering the environment. The industrial preservative uses in wood preservation and slime control do not have a significant impact on the environment, not only because the use of organotins in these areas is relatively small, but also because of their chemical properties and methods of use. Tributyltin compounds are strongly bound to wood, and commercial wood treatment operations are usually conducted in a closed system to control solvent losses. Industrial water treatment systems that use biocides are usually of the closed-loop, recirculating type. In neither case should there be any significant release to the environment.

In antifoulant applications, however, environmental concerns center on the effect of tributyltin leachates from antifouling paints on nontarget marine organisms. There is no question that tributyltins are toxic to certain forms of marine life. That is their function as antifoulants. Their high toxicity to fish in artificial laboratory environments has been documented (Table 20–10). Some higher toxicities to fish have been noted by the U.S. EPA (EPA, 1987).

In poorly exchanged natural marine environments, a high concentration of ship-bottoms painted with heavily loaded conventional leaching-type organotin-based antifouling paints could present some risk to nontarget organisms. There is no evidence to suggest that such lethal concentrations are reached in a well flushed embayment, marina, or harbor, however, and there have been no reports of fish or shellfish kills in the 20+ years that organotins have been used (mostly in conjunction with cuprous oxide as the primary toxicant) in industrial and recreational marine paint applications. Some recent studies (Jackson et al., 1982; Maguire et al., 1982) have concluded that elevated levels of butyltin compounds are present in sea water in certain areas as a result of widespread use of these compounds in antifouling paints. Alzieu (1986) suggested a strong correlation between the high levels of organotin in the Arcachon Bay of France and abnormal shell growth of Pacific oysters, although such effects are known to be caused by many types of environmental stress, including other pollutants. Nevertheless, concern about possible effects of TBT compounds from antifouling paints on commercial shellfish cultivation led to government action in the U.S. and some European countries even while scientific evidence on the nature and extent of the risk was being developed.

In the U.S., the Organotin Antifouling Paint Control Act of 1988 (OAPCA) established a maximum tributyltin (TBT) release rate of 4 μg TBT/cm²/day, a total ban of tributyltin paints on nonaluminum vessels under 25 meters in length, and a certification program for all tributyltin paints sold in this country. Similar measures are in place or under consideration in other countries. These measures were taken to reduce tributyltin in the environment to levels deemed safe for marine life.

In 1986 and 1987 the EPA issued data call-in notices to all producers of tributyltin antifouling paints and active ingredients in order to gather information on their acute, chronic, and behavioral toxicity along with their bioavailability and bioaccumulation characteristics in the marine environment. Data on use patterns, sources, and economic benefits of these compounds is also being collected in order to develop a risk assessment. This review process, which encompasses a variety of indicator organisms including fish, bivalves, gastropods, crustaceans, and algae, is ongoing and will take at least an additional 3 to 5 years to complete. The growing acceptance around the world of erodible organotin polymer

Table 20–10. *Toxicity of Organotin Compounds to Fish*

Compound	Fish Species	LC_{50}* (ppm)	Reference
$((C_4H_9)_3Sn)_2O$	*Lecuciscus idus melanotus* (Golden Orfe)	0.05 (48 hrs)	Plum (1981)
$(C_4H_9)_3SnOAc$	*Lebistes reticulatus* (Guppy)	0.026 (48 hrs)	Polster (1974)
$(C_4H_9)_3SnF$	*Alburnus alburnus* (Bleak)	0.06–0.08 (96 hrs)	Linden (1979)
$(C_4H_9)_3Sn$ naphthenate	*Leuciscus idus melanotus* (Golden Orfe)	0.07 (48 hrs)	Plum (1981)
$(C_6H_5)_3SnOH$	*Salmo gairdneri* (Rainbow Trout Fry)	0.015 (96 hrs)	Tooby (1975)
$(C_6H_5)_3SnOAc$	*Lebistes reticulatus* (Guppy)	0.034 (48 hrs)	Linden (1979)
$(C_6H_5)_3SnF$	*Alburnus alburnus* (Bleak)	0.40 (96 hrs)	Linden (1979)
$(c\text{-}C_6H_{11})_3SnOH$	*Microterus salmonoides* (Large Mouth Bass)	0.06 (24 hrs)	Anonymous (Dow, 1979)
$(c\text{-}C_6H_{11})_3Sn$ 1,2,4-triazole	*Carassius auratus* (Goldfish)	0.01–0.1 (96 hrs)	Hammann (1978)

*LC_{50} is the initial concentration of a compound killing 50% of the test organisms during the time denoted in parentheses.

From Blunden, S.J., and Chapman, A. 1986. Organotin compounds in the environment. In *Organometallic Compounds in the Environment.* Edited by P.J. Craig. London, Longman Group, pp. 111–159.

systems as the standard against which other antifouling systems are judged provides a strong argument for a market-driven effort to reduce risk to the marine environment. As the older, conventional, high-leaching-rate paints are replaced with the lower-release-rate organotin polymer systems, we can expect that the influx of tributyltin from marine paints will decrease as a consequence and that the concentrations in harbors and marinas will be significantly reduced.

It is well established that triorganotin compounds are not persistent in the environment. The evidence was summarized by Blunden and Chapman (1968). Degradation of tributyltin to less toxic species in the marine environment has been reported most recently by Seligman et al. (1988), who found that the half-life of TBT in San Diego Bay marina water was 6 days. The principal degradation product was a dibutyltin species. The degradation was attributed to microbial action. Maguire (1987), in a recent review of the environmental aspects of tributyltin compounds, concluded that biologic degradation of tributyltins in water and sediment is the most important factor limiting the persistence of these compounds in aquatic environments. Additionally, because triorganotins bind strongly to soils and sediments, their bioavailability and toxicity in the presence of these media should be considerably lower than is demonstrated by laboratory bioassays in aquaria using seawater artificially laced with tributyltin compounds.

Triorganotin compounds are readily dealkylated or dearylated to less-toxic species by ultraviolet (UV) light because of the relatively weak nature of the tin-carbon bond. This is a strong mitigating factor in any description of their environmental persistence. Barnes et al. (1973) demonstrated that triphenyltin acetate was dearylated to inorganic tin on exposure to UV light, and Chapman and Price (1972) also identified and quantitatively determined diphenyltin and monophenyltin species as intermediate degradation products.

The UV-induced breakdown of tributyltins to dibutyltin and less-alkylated species on a variety of substrates has been studied by a number of workers. Their results were summarized by Blunden and Chapman (1986). Maguire et al. (1983) found that the UV degradation of tributyltins in water involved sequential debutylation to inorganic tin and showed that a similar reaction occurred more slowly in natural sunlight. Soderquist and Crosby (1980) reported that UV irradiation under simulated environmental conditions caused dephenylation of triphenyltin hydroxide in water to a diphenyltin species that underwent further breakdown, possibly to a polymeric monophenyltin species.

It is significant that modern tin copolymer antifouling paints provide very localized control of fouling within a painted area. Less than a centimeter outside this treated area, lush growth of marine organisms continues unabated (Fig. 20–7). Such observations provide strong evidence for little translocation of triorganotins from antifouling paints in normal marine environments.

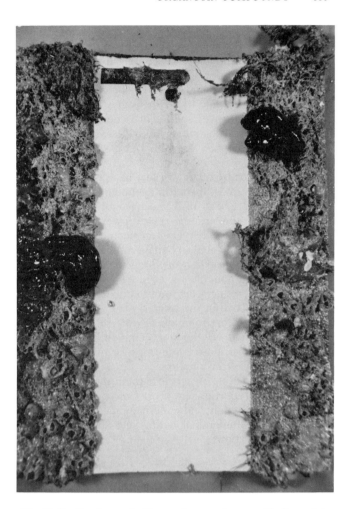

Fig. 20–7. Panel coated with a modern copolymer antifouling paint, mounted on an untreated fiberglass panel after 24 months of immersion in Miami, FL.

The gradual replacement of conventional leaching-type organotin paints by controlled-release tin copolymer paints together with the restrictions placed on the use of all organotin paints on pleasurecraft will allow the safe use of organotin-based antifouling paints on commercial and naval vessels, where their superior performance is most critically needed, without endangering the environment.

The largest potential route for the direct entry of triorganotins into the environment results from their use as agricultural pesticides. Because of agricultural chemical application procedures, which usually involve aerial spraying, the possibility exists that not only the soil but also the air and adjacent waterways could be contaminated. The physical and chemical characteristics of the triorganotins used in agriculture, however, considerably reduce the environmental impact these chemicals could produce if misused.

Because almost all the triorganotins used as agricultural chemicals are highly polymeric via intermolecular association in the solid state or in aqueous suspension (as in spray formulations), their vapor pressures are exceedingly low or nonexistent. Thus, volatilization after application is unlikely to be a concern.

Triorganotin compounds are strongly absorbed on soil, so translocation from the site of application is unlikely. Barnes et al. (1973) found that ^{14}C-labeled triphenyltin acetate was not leached by water from a 25-cm layer of an agricultural loam over a period of 6 weeks. Subsequent analysis of the soil for radioactivity showed that more than 75% of the triphenyltin compound remained in the top 4 cm.

Similar studies by other workers have confirmed the nonleachability of triphenyltin compounds in various soils (Suess and Eben, 1973; Leeuwangh et al., 1976). Because of their similar, exceedingly low water-solubility and polymeric nature, tricyclohexyltin and trineophyltin compounds are expected to behave similarly.

Although a handicap in many fungicide and insecticide applications, the nonsystemicity of triorganotin agricultural chemicals reduces any environmental risk related to translocation within the treated plant. It also means that food residues are minimized, especially from foliar applications, which are the most common. Residues can be further reduced on treated crops by simple washing or peeling before consumption.

In all, triorganotins, by virtue of their unique chemical and physical properties, are a class of compounds that have been used safely and effectively for over 20 years in a variety of antimicrobial, antifoulant, and agricultural pesticide applications.

REFERENCES

Allison, W.E., et al. 1968. Laboratory evaluations of Plictran miticide against two-spotted spider mites. Econ. Entomol., 61, 1254–1257.

Alzieu, C., San Juan, J., Deltreil, J.P., and Borel, M. 1986. Tin contamination in Arcachon Bay; effects on oyster shell. Mar. Pollut. Bull., 17, 494–498.

Anderson, C.D., and Dalley, R. 1986. Use of organotins in antifouling paints. Proc. Oceans 86 Conf. Vol. 4, Organotin Symposium, Marine Tech. Soc., Washington, D.C., Sept. 23–25, 1986. IEEE N.Y., pp. 1101–1330.

Anonymous. 1979. Plictran Miticide Tech. Inf. Bull. Dow Chemical Co., Midland, MI.

Ascher, K.R.S., Avdat, J., and Kamhi, J. 1970. Further antifeeding studies with two novel organotins, TD-5032 and Plictran. Int. Pest. Control., 12(2), 11–13.

Ascher, K.R.S., and Nissim, S. 1965. Quantitative aspects of antifeeding: comparing "antifeedants" by assay with P. litura. Intl. Pest. Control, 7(4), 21–24.

Barnes, R.D., Bull, A.T., and Poller, R.C. 1973. Studies on the persistance of the organotin fungicide, triphenyltin acetate, in soil and on surfaces exposed to light. Pestic. Sci., 4, 305–317.

Beiter, C.B. 1988. Considerations for the effective use of tributyltins in wood preservation. Proc. Ninth Ann. Can. Wood Preserv. Assoc. Mtg., Nov. 2, 1988, Toronto, Canada.

Blunden, S.J., and Chapman, A. 1986. Organotin compounds in the environment. In Organometallic compounds in the environment. Edited by P.J. Craig. London, Longman Group, 1986, pp. 111–159.

Blunden, S.J., Hobbs, L.A., and Smith, P.J. 1984. The environmental chemistry of organotin compounds. In Environmental Chemistry. Edited by H.J.M. Bowen. Spec. Per. Rep., 3, 49–77. London, Royal Society of Chemistry.

Chapman, A.H., and Price, J.W. 1972. The degradation of triphenyltin acetate by U.V. light. Int. Pest Control, 14, 11–12.

Elsea, J.R., and Paynter, O.E. 1958. Toxicological studies on bis(tributyltin) oxide. AMA Arch. Ind. Health, 18, 214–217.

Engelhart, J., Beiter, C.B., and Freiman, A. 1974. Recent developments in slow release organotin antifoulants. Proc. 1st Int. Contr. Rel. Symp. Akron, Ohio, Sept. 18, 1974.

EPA (John A. Moore), 1987. Preliminary determination to cancel certain registrations of tributyltin products used as antifoulants. Federal Register, 52, (194), 37510–37519.

Foster J.P., and Soloway, S.B. 1973. Thienylalkyltin compounds. U.S. Patent No. 3,736,333.

Gitlitz, M.H. 1981. Recent developments in marine antifouling coatings. J. Coat. Tech., 53, 46–52.

Gitlitz, M.H. 1975. Certain triorganotin compounds used to combat plant fungi. U.S. Patent No. 3,923,998.

Hammann, I., Buchel, K.L., Bungarz, K., and Born, L. 1978. Peropal, a new acaricide. Pflanzenschultz-Nachr Bayer Engl. Ed., 31, 61–83.

Hartel, K. 1962. A new fungicidal group of active substances—their biological properties and their application to agriculture. Agr. Vet. Chem., 3, 19–24.

Hill, R., and Killmeyer, A.J. 1988. Chemical and biological investigations of organotin compounds as wood preservatives. Proc. 84th Ann. Mtg. AWPA, Minneapolis, MN.

Horne, C.A. 1972. Use of organotin compounds as acaricidal agents. U.S. Patent No. 3,657,451.

Ison, R.R., Newbold, G.T., and Saggers, D.T. 1971. Biocidal activities of some heterocyclic organotin sulphides. Pesticide Sci., 2, 152–159.

Kenega, E.E. 1965. Triphenytin compounds as insect reproduction inhibitors. J. Econ. Entomol., 58(1), 4–8.

Jackson, J.A., Blair, W.R., Brinckman, F.E., and Iverson, W.P. 1982. Gas chromatographic speciation of methylstannanes in the Chesapeake Bay using purge and trap sampling with a tin selective detector. Environ. Sci. Technol., 16, 110–119.

Klimmer, O.R. 1969. Die-Anwendung von organozinn-verbindungen in experimentell-toxikologischer sicht. Arzneim-Forsch., 19(6), 934–939.

Krajnc, E.I., et al. 1984. Toxicity of bis(tri-n-butyltin) oxide in the rat. I. Short term effects on general parameters and on the endocrine and lymphoid systems. Toxicol. Appl. Pharmacol., 75(3), 363–386.

Leeuwangh, P., et al. 1976. Toxicity of triphenyltin fungicides in the aquatic environment. Med. Fac. Landbouww Rijkuniv. Ghent, 41, 1483–1490.

Linden, E., Bentsson, B.E., Svanberg, O., and Sundstrom, G. 1979. The acute toxicity of 78 chemicals and pesticide formulations against two brackish water organisms, the Bleak (Alburnus alburnus) and the Harpacticoid (Nitocra spinipes). Chemosphere, 8, 834–851.

Lin, S.M., Chiang, C.H., Tseng, C.L., and Yang, M.H. 1985. Instrumental neutron activation analysis in study of the toxicity of trialkyltin-methacrylate copolymer as an antifouling agent. J. Radioanalyt. Nuc. Chem., Articles, 90(1), 123–128.

Lyle, W.H. 1958. Lesions of the skin in process workers caused by contact with butyl tin compounds. Br. J. Ind. Med., 15, 193–196.

Maguire, R. 1987. Environmental aspects of tributyltin. Appl. Organometal. Chem., 1, 475–496.

Maguire, R.J., Carey, J.H., and Hale, E.J. 1983. Degradation of the tri-n-butyltin species in water. J. Agric. Food Chem., 31, 1060–1065.

Maguire, R.J., et al. 1982. Occurrence of organotin compounds in Ontario lakes and rivers. Environ. Sci. Technol., 16, 698–702.

McIntosh, A.H. 1971. Tests of aryl tin compounds as potato blight fungicides. Ann. Appl. Biol., 69, 43–46.

Mushak, P., Krigman, M.R., and Mailman, R.B. 1982. Comparative organotin toxicity in the developing rat, somatic and morphological changes and relationship to accumulation of total tin. Neurobehav. Toxicol. Teratol., 4, 209–215.

Nicklin, S., and Robson, M.W. 1988. Organotins; toxicology and biological effects. Applied Organomet. Chem., 2, 487–508.

NIOSH, 1976. Criteria for a recommended standard. . . Occupational exposure to organotin compounds. Washington, D.C., U.S. Government Printing Office, DHEW (NIOSH) Publ. No. 77–115.

Plum, H. 1981. The environmental effects of organotin compounds. Inf. Chim., 220, 135–139.

Polster, M., and Halacka, K. 1974. Action of triphenyltin acetate residues of some aquatic organisms. Tag. Ber. Akad Landwertsch-Wiss DDR, Berlin, 126, 117–122.

Richardson, B.A., and Lindner, G.H. 1979. Organotin wood treatments; effectiveness and reliability. Proc. Second Penarth Conference, Cambridge, England. 26th June, 1979.

Reifenberg, G.H., and Gitlitz, M.H. 1974. A process for preparing asymmetrical triorganotin halides. U.S. Patent No. 3,789,057.

Saxena, A.K. 1987. Organotin compounds: Toxicology and biomedical applications. Appl. Organomet. Chem., 1, 39–56.

Schweinfurth, H. 1987. Tributyltin compounds in wood preservatives: An update of health and safety aspect. Presented at the British Wood Preserving Assoc. Convention, Cambridge, 30 June–3 July, 1987.

Schweinfurth, H., and Gunzel, P. 1987. The tributyltins: Mammalian toxicity and risk evaluation for humans. Proceedings Oceans 87 Conference, Halifax, NS. Vol. 4, 1422–1428. Sept. 28–Oct. 1, 1987, Marine Technology Society, IEEE, NY.

Seligman, P.F., Valkirs, A.O., Stang, P.M., and Lee, R.F. 1988. Degradation of tributyltin in San Diego Bay, California. Mar. Pollut. Bull., 19(10), 531–534.

Sheldon, A.W. 1975. Effects of organotin antifouling coatings on man and his environment. J. Paint Technol., 47(600), 54–58.

Sijpesteijn, A.K., Luijten, J.G.A., and van der Kerk, G.J.M. 1969. Organometallic fungicides. In *Fungicides*. Edited by D.C. Torgeson, Vol. 2, pp 340, 352, New York, Academic.

Snoeij, N.J., van Iersel, A.A.J., Penninks, A.H., and Seinen, W. 1985. Toxicity of triorganotin compounds: comparative in vivo studies with a series of trialkyltin compounds and triphenyltin chloride in male rats. Toxicol. Appl. Pharmacol., *81*, 274–286.

Soderquist, C.J., and Crosby, D.G. 1980. Degradation of triphenyltin hydroxide in water. Agric. Food Chem., *28*, 111–117.

Suess, A., and Eben, C. 1973. Fate of triphenyltin acetate in soil and the uptake by plants from treated soils. Z. Pflanzenkrankh Pflanzenshultz, *80*, 288–294.

Tooby, T.E., Hursey, P.A., and Alabaster, J.J. 1975. The acute toxicity of 102 pesticides and miscellaneous substances to fish. Chem. Ind., 523–526.

van der Kerk, G.J.M., and Luijten, J.G.A. Organotin compounds. II. Biocidal properties of organotin compounds. J. Appl. Chem., *4*, 314–319.

van der Kerk, G.J.M., and Luijten, J.G.A. 1956. Organotin compounds. V. Preparation and antifungal properties of unsymmetrical tri-n-alkyltin acetates. J. Appl. Chem., *6*, 56–60.

Vos, J.G., et al. 1984. Toxicity of bis(tri-n-butyltin) oxide in rat. II. Suppression of thymus dependent immune responses and of parameters of nonspecific resistance after short term exposure. Toxicol. Appl. Pharmacol., *75*, 387–408.

Worthing, C.R. (ed.) 1983. The Pesticide Manual. 7th Edition. Lavenham, Suffolk, U.K., British Crop Protection Council, Lavenham Press.

Wood's Hole Oceanographic Institute. 1952. Marine Fouling and Its Prevention. U.S. Naval Institute, Annapolis, MD.

Zuckerman, J.J. (ed.) 1976. Organotin compounds: New chemistry and applications. Advances in Chemistry Series, No. 157, American Chemical Society, Washington, D.C.

CHAPTER 21

COPPER AND ZINC PRESERVATIVES

Charles C. Yeager

In ancient times, it was well known that copper-clad ship bottoms resisted the growth of barnacles and algae. In more recent times, the use of Bordeaux Mixture for controlling certain fungal diseases of crops was a common practice among farmers. It was therefore understandable that man would turn to the products that he was most familiar with to protect susceptible material from deterioration by fungal organisms. Copper salts became the preferred antimicrobials. Copper oxides were widely used as antifouling treatments for boat bottoms but were found to be unsatisfactory for preserving textiles and wood against fungal attack. Attention was turned to more soluble systems such as copper-oleate, copper tallate and, finally, copper naphthenate.

Copper naphthenate was first adopted for the preservation of textiles at the beginning of World War II. Because most of the fabrics to be protected were either olive drab or khaki in color, the pale green color imparted to the fabrics was of little consequence. Because most of the fabrics treated were to be used in tents, tarpaulins, and other heavy-duty items, any stiffening that resulted from the treatment was of little concern.

Copper naphthenate is made from naphthenic acids derived from petroleum and a mixture of salts of other fatty acids. Although it imparts a rather unpleasant odor to the item treated, it is stable and long-lasting enough that the odor is ignored. It is low in human toxicity and effective in preserving any susceptible substrate to which it is applied.

Naphthenic acid is derived from crude oils from California and Venezuela. The copper salt is soluble in most organic solvents such as mineral spirits, kerosene, aromatic solvents, and other petroleum oils. It prevents rotting of cotton fabrics and wood products at lower concentrations than other copper soaps such as copper oleate and copper tallate (Marsh et al., 1944). This is probably due to the lower solubility in water of the naphthenic acid derivative. Naphthenic acid itself is somewhat fungitoxic, whereas tall oil fatty acid and oleic acid are susceptible (Block, 1949). A fabric treated with 0.1 to 0.5%

metallic copper as copper naphthenate would resist deterioration even after exposure to Gulf Coast weather for 2 years (Bayley and Weatherburn, 1947). Copper-tolerant organisms, such as the penicillia and aspergilli, could solubilize most copper but they could not solubilize copper naphthenate.

Copper napthenate, unlike other soaps, has excellent leach resistance. It is therefore used often without water repellents. Government specifications have listed copper naphthenate as one of the preferred textile treatments for 50 years. Millions of yards of fire, water, and mildew-resistant fabrics were purchased by the military during and after World War II, many containing copper naphthenate. Military standards called for 0.6 to 0.8% copper as metal, and specifications required analysis for copper content.

Copper salts have long been known to accelerate photodidation. Sunlight alone will deteriorate cotton; the addition of many copper salts will accelerate that deterioration. One can distinguish between photooxidation and microbial deterioration by measuring cupra-ammonium fluidity. The fluidity is higher in the case of photooxidation (Shanor et al., 1949). Some copper-accelerated oxidation has been noticed in copper naphthenate–treated fabrics, but it is far less than what one finds when other copper salts are used (Benignus, 1948).

The few drawbacks of copper naphthenate, such as color, odor, its stiffening effect, and its photochemical effect on cellulosics, encouraged researchers to search for other, less objectionable copper salts. In 1947, a product known as copper 8-hydroxyquinoline (copper 8-quinolinolate, or copper oxinate) was found to have outstanding properties as a textile, paint, and wood preservative.

For 50 years prior to 1947, 8-hydroxyquinoline (oxine) was known as a heavy metals extractor that worked by chelating them to form highly insoluble metal salts. Long known as an excellent antibacterial, its copper salt was found to be more effective in the preservation of textiles than any other copper salt. Its solubility was less than 0.8 ppm in water and thus showed remarkable antileaching qualities. It is less toxic than other copper salts and, because of its low solubility, does not tender delicate fibers. It will provide maximum protection at much lower levels.

Its low solubility presented an immediate problem—how to apply the product to fabrics or wood. The first application developed was the two-bath treatment for textiles. The fabric was first passed through an 8-hydroxyquinoline water bath and then passed through a copper acetate solution. Early dispersions of copper 8-quinolinolate were primitive and caused considerable dusting or loss of active ingredient. Further, it was impossible to effect an even or controlled application. These early procedures were soon discarded as impractical.

In 1951, Kalberg developed a solubilization process by which the copper 8-quinolinolate was dissolved in a mixture of a metal octoate and nonyl phenol (Kalberg, 1951a, b). For the first time, this interesting new product was easily and evenly applied to any type of textile, wood, and paint system. Control of the application was now possible or practical.

There have been many theories to explain why copper 8-quinolinolate is a superior fungicide. It is well known that many chemicals have the ability to penetrate the cell wall and membrane of a fungal cell, but only a few of these will kill or retard fungal growth. One theory first proposed had the 8-hydroxyquinoline chelating the essential metals within the cell, thus removing essential elements for growth (Zentmeyer, 1943). This was reinforced by the discovery that any change in the structure of the 8-hydroxyquinoline would destroy its fungitoxicity (Albert, 1951). Another theory called "The Shaped Charge Theory" claimed that the amino acids in the cell were stronger chelators than 8-hydroxyquinoline. The 8-hydroxyquinoline served only to get the copper into the cell. Once there, the amino acids of the cell chelated the copper, thus poisoning the cell. A modification of that theory was the idea that the iron and copper chelates were the cause of toxicity, and not the 8-hydroxyquinoline. The statement was made that "the toxic effect is undoubtedly initiated by chelation, and is completed by the subsequent poisoning effect of the metal, either in combination with 8-hydroxyquinoline or as free ferrous or copper ions liberated, after transfer through the cell wall in the chelated condition" (Albert, 1951). This poisoning apparently takes place through catalysis of the oxidation of an essential enzyme or metabolite. This destructive oxidation can be prevented by lowering the oxidation-reduction potential (Albert, 1951). The fact that only a few of the more toxic metals in the form of the metal 8-hydroxyquinoline chelate are toxic to microorganisms seems to emphasize that 8-hydroxyquinoline is merely a mechanism for getting the metal through the complex cell wall and membrane barriers, after which it combines with enzyme systems or metabolites and poisons the cell.

Other copper salts such as tallate, stearate, resinate, and oleate will provide protection against cellulose-de-

stroying fungi, but their durability leaves much to be desired, and the amounts required prevent wide use.

It is interesting to note that, of all effective and durable paint preservatives on the market today, copper 8-quinolinolate is the only one allowed by the Food and Drug Administration for wide food-plant use. This is due to its extremely low water solubility and exceptionally low human toxicity.

Several years ago, debilitated patients at the University of Maryland hospital in Baltimore were dying prematurely. Autopsies showed that they were dying from aspergillosis, a disease that can be better described as suffocation from *Aspergillus* spores too numerous to count. A search of the hospital revealed that the air ducts in the spaces above the patients' rooms were covered with a heavy growth of *Aspergillus* spp. The fire-retardant coating over the duct was a natural medium for encouraging the growth of the organism. The only fungicide that could be safely used without harm to the patients was copper 8-quinolinolate. Two thorough sprayings with this product dropped the fungal spore count from "too numerous to count" to zero. The product has since been used in other hospitals and apartment houses.

Some months later, another interesting problem came to light. In New York City, easily seen from the Triborough Bridge, is a large parabolic building. This is the site where, for many years, asphalt for the New York streets was made. This building was crammed to the top with rusting equipment. Around the building were some 12 acres of property. This complex, called Asphalt Green, had been given to a pathologist at Cornell University Medical School. It was planned to be used for New York City children as a playground and activity center. There was one big problem. Through the years, pigeons had used the building as a roosting place, getting in through a number of openings. The floor was covered 6 inches to a foot deep with pigeon droppings. Inspectors from the New York City Department of Health found that the filth in the building was teeming with a *Cryptococcus* organism that was the cause of meningitis in debilitated patients. They refused to permit the building to be used until it was cleaned up and the *Cryptococcus* destroyed.

It was decided to spray a solution of copper 8-quinolinolate over everything in the building, including the pigeon droppings on the ground. The spraying took place at 9:00 A.M. one morning and was followed by a second spraying at 4:00 P.M. that afternoon. Two days later, a spore count was taken and, amazingly, the spore count had dropped from too numerous to count to zero. The city permitted work to commence on clearing out the building. Several months later, a party was held on the lawn for those who had been concerned about the new facility, with offices and game rooms on the first floor and a basketball court on the second floor—a fine demonstration of how effective this excellent copper compound can be.

The only other copper compounds that can still be used for textile treatments today are the cupra-ammonium complexes. These are basic copper compounds dissolved in aqueous ammonia to give complexes stable in aqueous solution. When the ammonia is given off upon drying, the fabric becomes resistant to leaching and weathering. Care must be taken, though, to prevent stiffening and a glazed finish. The finish provides excellent resistance to soil burial against cellulose-destroying organisms, but provides little protection against surface-growing organisms, such as *Aspergillus* spp. and *Penicillium* spp. (Goodavage, 1943).

Zinc salts of various organic acids provide varying degrees of protection, although none of them are as effective as the copper derivatives of the same acids. Zinc naphthenate is the most widely used, and military specifications call for approximately twice as much zinc as copper. Another well known product is a mixture of zinc dimethyldithiocarbamate and zinc 2-mercaptobenzothiazole. This product has been widely used in the treatment of fabrics to be subsequently coated with polyvinylchloride. This mixture has good weathering characteristics and good fungitoxicity, but should not be used on dyed goods. It has a tendency to "bloom" on the surface, interfering with the aesthetic quality of the goods. It is interesting to note that there has never been a market for zinc 8-quinolinolate chelation. This was undoubtedly due to the fact that, unlike other zinc compounds, zinc 8-quinolinolate is a bright yellow salt. It therefore discolored any substrate almost as much as did the copper salt and, like other zinc salts, is not as effective.

Copper compounds have long been used in the treatment of wood. Copper naphthenate was introduced in Denmark in 1911 and after World War II was widely used as partial replacement for creosote, then in short supply. When creosote became more plentiful, the use of copper naphthenate decreased because of its relatively high cost. Today, with the demise of pentachlorophenol, its use is again growing. It is now used primarily for dip, spray, or brush treatment of lumber, boat timbers, and wood used around homes for such applications as decks and roofs. It is toxic to many wood-destroying fungi, insects, and marine borers. It is normally used at levels of 1 to 3% copper as metal (12.5 to 37.5% of copper naphthenate) in aliphatic hydrocarbon solvents.

Copper 8-quinolinolate is used more and more in specialty wood items. It is effective against most decay fungi and surface growers, is odorless, and has very low human toxicity. It is specified for such items as railroad car interiors, greenhouse benches and flats, foodstuff containers, floors and walls of food plants, wood house shingles, and decks. It has even been used widely in food plants with tile walls to protect the grout between the tiles.

One of the fastest-growing uses for copper compounds is as a waterborne fungicide. The most important of such fungicides are acid copper chromate, chromated copper arsenate (CCA), and ammoniacal copper arsenate (ACA). In 1928, acid copper chromate was first discovered. The chromate is used for two reasons. It reduces the corrosiveness of the copper and precipitates insoluble copper chromate to make an unleachable preservative in the wood.

Chromated copper arsenate was developed in 1933. It is particularly effective against decay and wood-destroying fungi, but is ineffective against surface growers. It is widely used on wood to be used in ground contact. Specifications in the United States call for retentions from 0.25 lbs/cubic foot (4.0 kg/m³) for wood above ground to 2.5 lbs/cubit foot (40 kg/m³) in the outer ½ inch of wood to be used in salt water. Because of reactions that take place within the wood fibers and between the compound and the wood, the final products are determined to be basic copper arsenate, tertiary chrome arsenate, and chromic acid (Dahlgren and Hartford, 1972). The resultant CCA complex is distributed throughout the cell walls and forms a protective barrier within the lumen (Chou et al., 1973).

Ammoniacal copper arsenate was also developed in 1928. Consisting of copper and arsenic salts dissolved in an ammoniacal solution, it is used for vacuum pressure treatment of dry wood. The ammonia is allowed to evaporate, leaving an unsoluble copper arsenate in the wood (Clarke and Rak, 1954). This product can be used interchangeably with CCA, although some believe that deeper penetration can be achieved with ACA than with CCA.

Wood treated with any of these arsenate products is odorless and clean and can be painted. They may be used in buildings where people or animals may come into contact with the wood. Recently, it was suggested that some children playing on playground equipment treated with CCA were showing signs of arsenic poisoning, and some cities now require that any playground equipment treated with ACA or CCA must be painted before it can be used.

Here again, the copper in these complexes is the important factor in the control of the organism. Its ability to penetrate the cell wall and membrane is determined by its ability to be absorbed by the fungal organism. It is thought by some that, if sufficient preservative is present, it will arrest the growth before decay starts.

A study by Chou et al. (1974) clearly points out that, in explaining the mode of action of fungicides, it is essential to consider not only the effect of the preservative on fungi but also the effect of fungi on preservatives.

Copper octoate (copper 2-ethylhexanoate) was introduced in 1985. It serves most of the same uses as copper naphthenate. Available in a variety of 2% (copper content) formulations, and in 6%, 8%, 10%, and 12% formulations, it is recommended at the same levels as recommended for copper naphthenate. It provides a light blue discoloration to any substrate to which it is applied. Wood block and stake tests indicate that it is fungitoxic at about the same levels as copper naphthenate. Unlike copper naphthenate, it is odorless and is considered useful in any area where odor is a problem. It is reported, though, not to be as leach-resistant as copper naphthenate, although the work in this area is far from being finished. Claims for the product indicate that it is a better textile treatment than copper naphthenate because it causes less stiffening, less odor, and less discoloration. It is not yet accepted by wood treaters for below-ground wood applications, whereas copper naphthenate is acceptable. Copper octoate is available for both solvent and water-based applications.

REFERENCES

Albert, A. 1951. *Selective Toxicity.* New York, Wiley, p. 109.
Bayley, C.H., and Weatherburn, M.W. 1947. Can. J. Ris., 25, 209.

Benignus, P.G. 1948. Ind. Eng. Chem., *40*, 1946.
Block, S.S. 1949. Ind. Eng. Chem., *41*, 1783.
Chou, C.K., Chandler, J.A., and Preston, R.D. 1973. Wood Sci. Technol., 7, 151.
Chou, C.K., Preston, R.D., and Levi, M.P. 1974. Phytopathology, *64*, 335.
Clarke, M.R., and Rak, J.R. 1954. Forest. Chron., *50*, 114.
Dahlgren, S.E., and Hartford, W.H. 1972. Holzforshung, *26*, 142.
Goodavage, J.E. 1943. Am. Dyestuff Reptr., *32*, 265.
Kalberg, V.N. 1951a. U.S. Patent 2,561,379.
Kalberg, V.N. 1951b. U.S. Patent 2,561,380.
Marsh, P.B., Greathouse, G.A., Bollenbacher, K., and Butler, M.L. 1944. Ind. Eng. Chem., *36*, 176.
Shanor, L., and The Sub-Committee on Textiles and Cordage, National Defense Research Committee. 1949. *Office of Scientific Research and Development Report No. 4513.* Washington, D.C.
Zentmeyer, G.A. 1943. Phytopathology, *33*, 1121.

Disinfectants and Antiseptics

B. By Type of Microorganisms

CHAPTER 22

CHEMICAL SPORICIDAL AND SPOROSTATIC AGENTS

A. D. Russell

Bacterial spores are highly resistant to most chemical and physical agents, although the degree of insensitivity fluctuates considerably during the process of sporulation on the one hand and of germination and outgrowth on the other. It is hardly surprising, therefore, that a vast amount of data has accumulated about spores, mainly of the genera *Bacillus* and *Clostridium* (Russell, 1982a,b, 1983; Waites, 1982, 1985; Gould, 1983, 1985), although information about two other genera of spore-formers, *Desulfomaculum* and *Sporolactobacillus*, is also increasing (Doores, 1983).

The responses of spores of the first two genera to a range of biocides will be considered, together with the possible reasons for the high level of insensitivity shown by these organisms. In addition, the possible mechanisms of sporicidal activity will be discussed and areas for future research highlighted.

SPORE STRUCTURE AND COMPOSITION

Any attempt at explaining the mechanisms of sporicidal action of, or the mechanisms of spore resistance to, antibacterial agents must consider the complex structure and composition of the bacterial spore. A diagrammatic representation of a "typical" bacterial spore is presented in Figure 22–1, from which it can be seen that a spore is a considerably more complex entity than is a vegetative bacterial cell. The germ cell (protoplast) and germ cell wall are surrounded by the cortex, around which are the spore coats, of which the outer is more dense. In some spores, e.g., *Bacillus polymyxa*, a layer (the exosporium) external to the spore coats is found. In other spores, e.g., *B. cereus*, an exosporium is also present but surrounds only one dense spore coat.

The spore core (protoplast) is, in terms of its macromolecular constituents, a relatively normal cell (Warth, 1978). The core is the location of ribonucleic (RNA) and deoxyribonucleic (DNA) acids, as well as of dipicolinic

acid (DPA) and most of the calcium, potassium, magnesium, manganese, and phosphorus present in the spore. The spore cores also contain a substantial amount of low-molecular-weight, basic proteins that are rapidly degraded during germination (Setlow, 1988).

The cortex is a zone present between the spore core and the spore coats (Figure 22–1). A dense inner layer (primordial cell wall, cortical membrane, germ cell wall) develops into the cell wall of the emergent cell when the cortex is broken down during germination. The cortex consists largely of peptidoglycan (Figure 22–2), an interesting feature of which is that some 45 to 60% of the muramic acid residues do not have either a peptide or an N-acetyl substituent but instead form an internal amide, muramic lactam. The sites of action of lysozyme and nitrous acid/sodium nitrite on spore peptidoglycan are also depicted in Figure 22–2.

During sporulation, two membranes surround the forespore. These are the inner (IFSM) and outer (OFSM) forespore membranes, which have opposite structural polarity to each other. The IFSM eventually becomes the cytoplasmic membrane of the germinating spore, whereas the OFSM persists in the spore integuments. Initially, both the IFSM and OFSM are extensions of the mother cell membrane, but they are later differentiated in both function and composition, with the specialized spore integument being formed between them.

The spore coats make up a major portion of the spore, occupying about 50% of the spore volume (Murrell, 1969). They consist mainly of protein with smaller amounts of complex carbohydrates and lipid and possibly large amounts of phosphorus. The inner (ISC) and outer (OSC) spore coats differ considerably, however, in the type of protein material that they contain. The alkali-resistant fraction resides in the OSC and is associated with the presence of cystine-rich protein, i.e., protein rich in disulphide (-S-S-) bonds. The alkali-soluble fraction is found in the ISC, and consists predominantly of

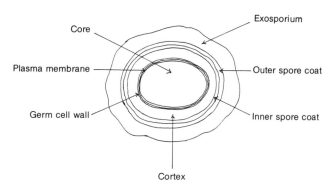

Fig. 22–1. Structure of a "typical" bacterial spore.

Table 22–1. *Chemical Composition of Bacterial Spores*

Spore Component	Composition	Comment
Outer spore coat	Mainly protein	Alkali-resistant, removed by DTT
Inner spore coat	Mainly protein	Alkali-soluble fraction
Cortex	Mainly peptidoglycan	Presence of internal amide (muramic lactam); see Fig. 22–2
Core	Protein, DNA, RNA, DPA, divalent metals	Unique spore proteins are associated with DNA

DTT, dithiothreitol; DNA, deoxyribonucleic acid; RNA, ribonucleic acid; DPA, dipicolinic acid

acidic polypeptides that can be dissociated to their unit components by treatment with sodium dodecyl sulfate (SDS). The spore coats play a major role in the resistance of spores to biocides.

A summary of the chemical composition of spore components is presented in Table 22–1.

ACTIVITY OF ANTIBACTERIAL AGENTS AGAINST SPORES

A wide variety of antibacterial agents is available for different purposes (Hugo and Russell, 1982; Simmons, 1983; Russell and Hugo, 1987; Rutala, 1987; Scott and Gorman, 1987; Russell, 1990a,b), but not all of these act as sporicides. On the other hand, many of them are effective sporostatic agents at concentrations similar to those that inhibit the growth of gram-positive nonsporing bacteria such as staphylococci (Table 22–2). Gram-negative rods tend to be less sensitive to antimicrobials such as quaternary ammonium compounds (QACs). The fact that a substance acts sporostatically means that it prevents a spore from producing a vegetative cell, but whether the inhibitor acts on either or both of the germination and outgrowth stages (or indeed merely on vegetative cell growth) and why it is sporostatic rather than sporicidal cannot be deduced from determinations of minimum inhibitory concentrations (MICs).

In contrast to the similarity between bacteriostatic and sporostatic concentration for a particular compound, bac-

tericidal and sporicidal concentrations usually show marked differences. Table 22–3. lists several important antibacterial agents, only some of which (glutaraldehyde, formaldehyde, and hypochlorite) are actively sporicidal, and even with these the concentrations necessary to destroy bacterial spores are consistently higher than those which are lethal to nonsporing bacteria. It must be pointed out that some compounds, e.g., chlorocresol, lack sporicidal activity at their maximum water solubility at ambient temperatures, but that many compounds are sporicidal at high temperatures (Russell, 1982a,b, 1990b; Shaker et al., 1986).

Sporostatic activity can be determined in several ways, e.g., by conventional MIC estimation in liquid or solid nutrient media or microscopically by agar slide technique (Russell et al., 1990). Sporicidal activity can be assessed by rate-of-kill tests (Forsyth, 1972; Waites and Bayliss, 1980; Russell et al., 1990) or by a carrier technique utilizing spores standardized in their resistance to 2.5 N hydrochloric acid (Ortenzio et al., 1953; AOAC, 1980; Reybrouck, 1982).

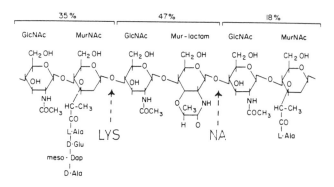

Fig. 22–2. Chemical structure of spore peptidoglycan and sites of action of lysozyme (LYS) and nitrous acid (NA, or sodium nitrite).

Table 22–2. *Bacteriostatic and Sporostatic Concentrations*

Inhibitor	Bacteriostatic Concn.* (% w/v)	Sporostatic Concn.† (% w/v)
Benzalkonium chloride	0.0004–0.0016	0.0005
Cetylpyridinium chloride	0.0005–0.01	0.00025
Chlorhexidine diacetate	0.0001	0.0001
Chlorocresol	0.02	0.02
Cresol	0.08	0.1
Phenol	0.2	0.2
Phenylmercuric nitrate (PMN)	0.00001–0.0001	0.00002

*Higher figure, where stated, refers to gram-negative bacteria, which are less susceptible than gram-positive nonsporeformers to quaternary ammonium compounds and PMN.
†Based on data provided by Russell (1982a).

Table 22–3. *Bactericidal and Sporicidal Concentrations of Some Disinfectants*

Antibacterial Agent	Bactericidal Concn. (% w/v)	Sporicidal Concn. (% w/v)
Chlorhexidine diacetate	0.002	>0.05
Cetylpyridinium chloride	0.002	>0.05
Chlorocresol	0.1	>0.4
Cresol	0.3	>0.5
Phenol	0.5	>5
Phenylmercuric nitrate (PMN)	0.002	>0.02
Glutaraldehyde	<0.1	2
Formaldehyde	<1	8
Sodium hypochlorite	1–2 ppm	20 ppm

Individual Sporicides

Properties of the most important sporicidal agents are considered below.

Glutaraldehyde (Pentanedial)

Of several mono- and di-aldehydes tested, glutaraldehyde has been found to be the most active (Gorman et al., 1980; Russell, 1982a,b). It is most stable in an acid formulation but most highly sporicidal at alkaline pH. Most glutaraldehyde (2%) formulations are thus activated to alkaline pH before use and retain stability when stored at room temperature for approximately two weeks (Power and Russell, 1989), although longer-life preparations are also available commercially. Glutaraldehyde is not particularly pleasant to use, and various toxic effects have been reported (Russell and Hopwood, 1976). The dialdehyde is most widely employed for its sporicidal and bactericidal properties in the disinfection of heat-sensitive equipment such as endoscopes, although the treatment time is considerably less than that (up to 3 to 10 hours) recommended by the AOAC for a sporicidal action.

Formaldehyde (Methanal)

Formaldehyde is used in both the liquid and vapor phases. Ortenzio et al. (1953) claimed that formaldehyde solution was rapidly lethal to *B. subtilis* but not to *Clostridium sporogenes* spores. Spaulding (1939) had earlier found the monoaldehyde to be sporicidal but did not use neutralizing agents in the subculture medium. Failure to control sporostasis in these media may lead to incorrect findings: Klarmann (1950) observed a lack of sporicidal action in his experiments. Formaldehyde is a useful gaseous disinfectant, especially in the newer process of low temperature steam with formaldehyde (LTSF).

Chlorine Compounds

Chlorine-releasing agents can be most conveniently considered as being of two types (Trueman, 1971):

Hypochlorites. These possess bactericidal and sporicidal properties, but their activity is greatly reduced in the presence of organic matter. They are more active at acid than alkaline pH, the active moiety being HClO.

Organic Chlorine Compounds. N-chloro compounds, containing the $=N\text{-}Cl$ group, show microbicidal activity. Examples include chloramine T, dichloramine T, dichloroisocyanuric acid, and salts and trichloroisocyanuric acid. All appear to hydrolyze in water to produce an imino ($=NH$) group. Their sporicidal activity is slower than that of the hypochlorites.

Iodine Compounds

Iodine itself is bactericidal, fungicidal, and sporicidal (Russell, 1982a,b). It is most active at acid pH, the active moiety being diatomic iodine (I_2), although hypoiodous acid (HI) plays some contributory role. Iodine is most usually employed as iodophors (iodine carriers) in which iodine is solubilized by means of an appropriate surface-active agent. Disinfectant-strength iodophor solutions retain the sporicidal, but not the undesirable, properties of iodine and are active over a wide pH range. The bactericidal activity of povidone-iodine solutions is determined by the concentration of noncomplexed iodine. Antiseptic-strength iodophors are not usually sporicidal.

Peroxygens

Peroxygen compounds are assuming greater importance as disinfectants. Hydrogen peroxide, H_2O_2, is a bactericidal and sporicidal agent (Toledo et al., 1973; Baldry, 1983; Baldry and Fraser, 1988), probably acting through the formation of free hydroxyl radicals ($\cdot OH$). Peractic acid, CH_3COOOH, decomposes ultimately to hydrogen peroxide, acetic acid, and oxygen which, at the recommended in-use concentrations, are toxologically safe (Baldry and Fraser, 1988). It is, nevertheless, a more potent sporicide than hydrogen peroxide, and its activity is reduced only slightly in the presence of organic matter. Unlike peroxide, its activity is unaffected by the presence of the enzyme catalase.

Gaseous Sporicidal Agents

The most important gaseous sporicides are ethylene oxide (EtO), beta-propiolactone (BPL), and formaldehyde. Formaldehyde was considered above. EtO and BPL are slow sporicidal agents, and their activity depends upon concentration, temperature, and, especially, relative humidity. It is not so much the relative humidity of the environment that is important, however, but rather the microenvironment and the water content of the spores themselves. Spores dehydrated beyond a certain point are extremely difficult to kill by EtO or BPL: see Russell (1982a,b, 1990b).

Combined Procedures

As can be seen from the foregoing, comparatively few agents are actively sporicidal. It is, however, possible to achieve a sporicidal effect by using combinations of chemicals or by judicious use of a chemical combined with a physical process. Glutaraldehyde, for example, is claimed to have a potentiated effect in the presence of surface-active agents (Gorman et al., 1980) and of phenate (Isenberg, 1985). The low activity of acid glutaraldehyde is enhanced by high temperatures and ultrasonic radiation (Boucher, 1974). Chlorhexidine, chlorocresol, and phenylmercuric nitrate are not sporicidal but have this ability at high temperatures (Russell, 1982a,b; Shaker et al., 1986, 1988b; Gorman et al., 1987). An increased sporicidal effect is observed when hydrogen peroxide is employed in conjunction with ultraviolet radiation (Bayliss and Waites, 1979; Waites, 1985). Sykes (1965) cites the example of two nonsporicidal agents, acid and alcohol, possessing this activity in combination. In the food industry, acid-heat treatment is an effective sterilization procedure (Sofos and Busta, 1982). Methanol, which is most certainly not sporicidal, has been found to improve the sporicidal activity of hypochlorites (Coates and Death, 1978). Despite the apparent use at an incorrect pH, the efficacy of hypochlorites is increased considerably in the presence of alkali which, by virtue of its effect on the inner spore coat, renders the spore more permeable to these agents (Cousins and Allan, 1967).

Clearly, there are several examples of improved sporicidal activity, although the underlying reasons for this enhancement have not always been provided.

Revival of Disinfectant-Injured Spores

The revival of bacteria, including spores, sublethally injured as a result of exposure to physical processes such as heat and x-ray or ultraviolet radiation has received extensive coverage (Adams, 1978; Foegeding and Busta, 1981; Andrew and Russell, 1984; Gould, 1984; Waites and Bayliss, 1984). In contrast, the revival of chemically injured bacterial spores has received scant attention, although this is undoubtedly an area of importance, both in food (or other) preservation and in disinfection. A few authors have considered the revival of B. subtilis spores treated with disinfectants such as glutaraldehyde, formaldehyde, povidone-iodine, and hypochlorites. Their findings (summarized in Table 22–4) demonstrate that it is possible to revive spores even after prolonged exposure to these disinfectants. Spicher and Peters (1981a,b), for example, claimed that a post-treatment heat shock at temperatures between 50 and 90°C enabled the majority of spores treated with formaldehyde (methanal) to produce colonies in an appropriate recovery medium. They therefore concluded that formaldehyde was considerably

less potent as a sporicide than had originally been thought. These findings do not, as yet, appear to have been confirmed by other, independent, workers. If they are substantiated, then a reappraisal of the role of formaldehyde as a sporicidal agent is necessary.

Table 22–4 also provides evidence to show that the revival of glutaraldehyde-treated spores of B. subtilis is possible by means of subsequent alkali (NaOH or KOH) treatment. It must be emphasized that only a comparatively small number (about 5×10^2 cfu) can be revived by such a method following treatment of a large inoculum (about 5×10^8 cfu) for 3 hours with 2% alkaline glutaraldehyde (Dancer et al., 1989). It was also found that (a) alkali acted at the germination rather than the outgrowth stage, and (b) lysozyme or coat removing agents were unable to revive glutaraldehyde-treated spores. Post-treatment heating at 57°C had some revival effect but less than that of alkali (Power et al., 1989). Other work from this laboratory has demonstrated that alkali-induced revival is found after spore treatment with some, but not all, aldehydes studied to date. These studies are proceeding.

THE SPORULATION PROCESS AND ANTIBACTERIAL AGENTS

Sporulation is a complex, multiphase process, in which the stages occur in a fairly synchronous manner. There are seven stages in this process, and these will be considered briefly (see also Figure 22–3).

Stage 0 is the vegetative cell, and represents the time at the end of logarithmic growth of the vegetative cell culture. There appears to be a link between the induction of sporulation and a specific stage in the DNA replication cycle; the amount and rate of sporulation in starting cultures depends on DNA replication, and the successful termination of existing rounds of DNA replication is essential for sporulation to occur (Keynan et al., 1976).

Stage I is the pre-septation stage, in which DNA is present as an axial filament in Bacillus spp. (although rarely observed in Clostridium spp.). Stage I terminates when a septum starts to form asymmetrically in the

Table 22–4. *The Revival of Disinfectant-Injured Bacterial Spores*

Antibacterial Agent	Post-Treatment Revival Procedure	Reference
Glutaraldehyde	(1) UDS ± sonication, incubation in GML, plating in TSA	Gorman et al., 1983, 1984a,b
	(2) Heat (50–90°C), dilution in GM or GML, plating in TSA	Gorman et al., 1983, 1984a,b
	(3) NaOH or KOH, plating	Dancer et al., 1989
Formaldehyde	Heat activation (60–90°C), plating	Spicher and Peters, 1981
Povidone-iodine	Incubation in GML, plating in TSA	Gorman et al., 1983, 1984a,b

UDS = urea + dithiothreitol + sodium lauryl sulfate
GM = germination medium
GML = germination medium + lysozyme
TSA = tryptose soy agar

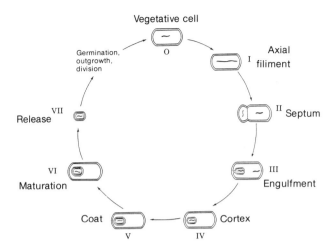

Fig. 22–3. Stages in the sporulation process.

mother cell, resulting in the synthesis of the forespore membranes and the compartmentalization of DNA in Stage II. In Stage III, the forespore is engulfed, the result of which is the existence of the forespore as a discrete cell, bounded by two membranes, within the mother cell. The IFSM later becomes the cytoplasmic membrane of the germinating spore (Ellar, 1978), whereas the OFSM persists in the spore integuments.

Cortex synthesis occurs in Stage IV, in which peptidoglycan is laid down between the IFSM and OFSM in two phases: in the first, vegetative cell-type polymer is produced, and in the second the spore-specific peptidoglycan. Synthesis of the spore coats takes place in Stage V, although deposition of at least part of the coat layers occurs during earlier stages. In this stage, DPA accumulates and there is an uptake of calcium. In Stage VI (maturation), the coat material becomes more dense in appearance, and spore refractility increases. Liberation of the spore takes place in Stage VII.

It is apparent from the above that there are several stages at which an antibacterial agent might act or, alternatively, at which resistance might develop. Techniques for studying these aspects have thus tended to take the following forms: (a) using wild-type cultures and sampling during the sporulation process for development of resistance to chemical and physical agents (Milhaud and Balassa, 1973); and (b) employing sporulation (Spo⁻) mutants, which are incapable of proceeding beyond specific stages in sporulation, and relating their final development to sensitivity or resistance (Russell et al., 1990). Useful markers in such studies are toluene and lysozyme, to which resistance develops early and late, respectively, in the sporulation process. By means of such procedures it has been found that resistance to chlorhexidine in *B. subtilis* develops later than toluene and at roughly the same time as heat resistance (Shaker et al., 1988a), whereas resistance to glutaraldehyde is a later event, occurring after lysozyme (Power et al., 1988). In fact, resistance to glutaraldehyde appears to be the latest event in sporulation that is currently known. Some

12 or so polypeptides are found in the spore coat of *B. subtilis*. These are synthesized at different times and are incorporated into the spore at Stages V and VI (Jenkinson, 1981, 1983; Jenkinson et al., 1980, 1981; Hill, 1983). It has been suggested that one polypeptide, molecular weight 36,000 (36K), which is formed very late in sporulation, may have a direct role in conferring lysozyme resistance upon the spores (Jenkinson, 1981). The development of glutaraldehyde resistance is, however, unlikely to be due to the deposition of specific spore coat proteins because of the highly reactive nature of the dialdehyde molecule (Power et al., 1988).

Disinfectant-induced changes in fully developed spores have been described (Kulikovsky et al., 1975), but these have not been adequately related to the biochemical effects of these agents on sporulating cells. In consequence, the mechanism of action of many of these biocides on spores and sporulating cells is often poorly understood, as indeed is the mechanism of resistance.

VEGETATIVE CELL DEVELOPMENT AND ANTIBACTERIAL AGENTS

Three sequential phases are involved in the transformation of a bacterial spore into a vegetative cell: activation, germination, and outgrowth (Halvorson and Szulmajster, 1973).

Activation is a treatment that results in a spore that is poised for germination but that still retains most spore properties. It is thus a process for the breaking of dormancy in spores, but is reversible (Keynan and Sandler, 1983). Methods of activating bacterial spores include heat shock (the procedure usually used), calcium dipicolinate, ethanol, and pH changes (Russell, 1982a).

Unlike activation, *germination* is an irreversible process that results in a change of activated spores from a dormant to a metabolically active state within a short time. Germination may be determined experimentally by a variety of techniques, the most rapid of which utilizes decreases in the optical density (O.D.) of spore suspensions. This O.D. method is not, however, a suitable technique for measuring commitment to germination, the trigger reaction (Stewart et al., 1981).

Outgrowth is a process resulting from the development of a vegetative cell from a germinated spore, and occurs in a synchronous and orderly manner when germination takes place in a medium that can support vegetative growth.

Several antibacterial agents, either sporicidal or sporostatic in nature, have been studied for their effects on germination and outgrowth. This aspect is considered below.

Inhibition of Germination

Specific chemical agents trigger the rapid germination of bacterial spores. This initiation process can be induced by metabolic or nonmetabolic means, although it is now generally believed that the trigger reaction is allosteric in nature rather than metabolic, because the inducer

Table 22–5. *Inhibitors of Spore Germination, Outgrowth, or Both*

Process	Inhibitors	Comment
Trigger mechanism	Glutaraldehyde	Does not inhibit L-alanine binding
	Alcohols? Sorbate? Chlorocresol }	Exact action unclear
Germination	Phenols & cresols Parabens Alcohols }	More effective than against outgrowth
	Hg²⁺	Compare with organomercury compounds
	Formaldehyde	
Outgrowth	QACs Chlorhexidine }	Little effect on germination
	Organomercury compounds	Compare with Hg²⁺
	Glutaraldehyde	Has more than one site of action

does not need to be metabolized to induce germination. The most widely studied nutrient germinant is L-alanine (Prasad, 1974). Non-nutrient germinants include bicarbonate and calcium dipicolinate (CaDPA); enzymatic germinants are exemplified by lysozyme and spore lytic enzyme, and physical germinants by hydrostatic pressure. Initiation of germination is followed rapidly by various degradative changes in the cell, leading to outgrowth. Inhibition and control of spore germination are important considerations in many fields, including food preservation (Smoot and Pierson, 1982).

Many antibacterial compounds are known to inhibit germination (Table 22–5). They include preservatives such as phenols and cresols, parabens, and sorbic acid, as well as sporicides acting at concentrations well below those which are sporicidal, e.g., glutaraldehyde (Russell, 1983; Dancer et al., 1988). It is interesting to note that the inhibitory concentrations are similar to the MICs of these agents for nonsporulating bacteria, and usually considerably below those which might be sporicidal (Table 22–3). Most antibiotics, such as those inhibiting cell wall peptidoglycan synthesis (penicillins, cephalosporins), protein synthesis (chloramphenicol, tetracyclines), and RNA (rifampicin) or DNA (mitomycin, nalidixic acid) synthesis, are without effect on germination (Russell, 1982a,b; Russell et al., 1985).

The action of many germination-inhibiting compounds is reversible; i.e., when the agents are removed, either by (a) washing the spores with water or a neutralizing chemical, or (b) by membrane-filtering the treated suspension and washing the spores in situ on the membrane, the spores will germinate as rapidly as control (untreated) spores. This is clearly apparent from studies on phenols (Parker and Bradley, 1968; Lewis and Jurd, 1972; Yasuda et al., 1982; Russell et al., 1985), formaldehyde (Trujillo and David, 1972), alcohols (Trujillo and Laible, 1970; Yasudi-Yasaki et al., 1978), and parabens (Watanabe and

Takesue, 1976; Yasuda-Yasaki, et al. 1978). These findings suggest a fairly loose binding of these agents to a site (or sites) on the spore surface, because mere washing is sufficient to dislodge the inhibitors.

An interesting exception to the property of decreased biocide resistance during germination is found with *B. brevis* Nagano, a gramicidin S-producing organism. Germination-initiated spores are almost as resistant to heat and 70% alcohol as dormant spores, and considerably more so than vegetative cells (Daher et al., 1985).

The effects of inhibitors of germination have been widely reported, but as pointed out by Smoot and Pierson (1982), it is often not known at what stage of germination an inhibitor is effective. Because of the nature of the germination process, the only types of antibacterial agents that are effective inhibitors are those which inhibit the trigger reaction or those which prevent the degradative processes. Known inhibitors of germination (Table 22–5) include phenols and cresols, parabens, alcohols, glutaraldehyde, and Hg²⁺ (Russell, 1982a,b). Unfortunately, many of the studies investigating germination-inhibitory aspects have used an optical density (O.D.) method. A decrease in O.D. is a late event in germination and is thus not suitable for studying the initial reactions (Stewart et al., 1981). The above antibacterial agents are thus likely to prevent the degradative processes, but it is unclear whether they affect the trigger reaction. Even a procedure involving short exposure to an inducer, such as L-alanine, followed by measurement of O.D. fall is inappropriate, as is one detecting release of ⁴⁵Ca (Stewart et al., 1981). A suitable method is to expose spores to L-alanine for a short period, stop the reaction with an excess of D-alanine, and determine the commitment to germinate by counting how many phase-dark spores are produced from phase-bright ones. This technique was employed by Sofos et al. (1986) in their studies with sorbic acid, from which it was concluded that sorbate did not compete with L-alanine for a common binding site on the bacterial spore.

Yasudi-Yasaki et al. (1978) showed that alcohols inhibited the L-alanine-initiated germination of *B. subtilis* spores, and proposed that inhibition resulted from an interaction of a hydrophobic region in or near the L-alanine receptor site on the spore with the hydrophobic group on the alcohol itself. This interaction is presumably of a weak nature, because the inhibition of germination by alcohols (or phenols, cresols, and parabens) is reversible.

Glutaraldehyde is another antibacterial agent that prevents germination, although this is irreversible, but it also inhibits the outgrowth of germinated spores (Power et al., 1989). A problem in studying these aspects of glutaraldehyde action is the fact that the dialdehyde interacts strongly with L-alanine (used in germination studies) and with nutrient broth (employed in measuring outgrowth). This problem has been overcome by pretreating cells with glutaraldehyde, washing them, and then exposing them to the appropriate menstruum. The results of germination studies suggested that the aldehyde could be inhibiting germination of *B. subtilis* spores by one or more of the following mechanisms: (a) inhibition of uptake of L-alanine by competition for binding sites on the spore, (b) prevention of passive diffusion of L-alanine into the spore, (c) sealing of the spore surface by the dialdehyde, akin to its fixative properties so widely employed in electron microscopy, or (d) a later, unexplained inhibition of the L-alanine–stimulated trigger effect.

Accordingly, experiments were undertaken with ¹⁴C-L-alanine in the presence and absence of D-glucose to obtain further information about these hypotheses. It was concluded that glutaraldehyde was, at low concentrations, an effective inhibitor of the trigger mechanism, but that it did not achieve this by preventing L-alanine uptake, but rather by its sealant effect on the spore surface (Power and Russell, 1990). In their studies on the uptake of ³H-L-alanine to *B. subtilis* spores, Downing and Dawes (1977) showed that the spores did not concentrate L-alanine and that uptake proceeded rapidly without the necessity for an energy-dependent active transport system. They concluded that the dormant spore was freely permeable to L-alanine, which entered by simple diffusion.

An examination of a series of analogs of L-alanine for their ability to initiate germination revealed that both –NH– and –COO– groups are important for germinant activity (Kanda et al., 1988). Glucose appears to stimulate L-alanine-induced germination by means of a cooperative effect, which disappears during heat activation (Yasuda and Tochikubo, 1984, 1985a,b). The apparent binding constant of L-alanine to spores was found by these authors to be some 3 to 4 times higher in the presence of glucose. However, binding was calculated solely on the loss of heat resistance and of turbidity of germinated spores, rather than on direct binding studies.

Germination (Ger) mutants of *B. subtilis* 168 (Moir et al., 1979; Sammons et al., 1981) could be of value in studying the mode of action of antibacterial agents on germination but do not, as yet, appear to have been widely used in this context.

The effect of sorbic acid deserves further comment. This organic acid appears to exert multiple modes of inhibition of germination and outgrowth, which may contribute to its broad degree of effectiveness (Blocher and Busta, 1985; Sofos et al., 1986). Sorbic acid inhibits germination of spores triggered to germinate by L-alanine, but inhibition occurs after germinant binding.

An excellent account of germination inhibition by sorbic acid and other agents is provided by Cook and Pierson (1983).

Inhibition of Outgrowth

Mercuric chloride is a powerful inhibitor of the germination of spores of *Cl. botulinum* type A (Ando, 1973) and of *Bacillus* spp. (Gould and Sale, 1970; Vinter, 1970). It inhibits some reactions in germination before the loss in heat resistance but not the subsequent release of peptidoglycan (Hsieh and Vary, 1975). In contrast, the organomercury compound phenylmercuric nitrate (PMN) has little effect on germination of *B. subtilis* spores but a pronounced effect on their outgrowth (Parker, 1969; Russell et al., 1975). It is difficult to reconcile these apparently contradictory findings other than to state that the studies with PMN utilized an optical density method of measuring germination and outgrowth. As pointed out above, a fall in optical density is a late event in germination (Stewart et al., 1981), and it is possible that any inhibition by PMN of an early stage in germination might have been missed.

Other agents acting at the outgrowth rather than the germination level include QACs and chlorhexidine (Lund, 1962; Chiori et al., 1965; Russell et al., 1985; Shaker et al., 1986). QACs, like chlorhexidine, are sporostatic and not sporicidal. They bind strongly to spores, and simple washing procedures will not remove them; it is necessary to use a neutralizing medium consisting of lubrol plus lecithin (Chiori et al., 1965). QAC-treated spores that are membrane-filtered are still prevented from undergoing outgrowth when transferred to an appropriate medium (Russell et al., 1985).

As mentioned previously, the parabens and similar substances inhibit germination. Higher concentrations are needed to inhibit outgrowth. High concentrations of chlorine are necessary to prevent germination of spores, whereas moderate concentrations markedly retard outgrowth, and low concentrations have only slight effects on either (Wyatt and Waites, 1975).

Sublethal concentrations of ethylene oxide (EtO) inhibit outgrowth but not germination (Reich, 1980). The resistance of spores to this gaseous disinfectant is not lost rapidly during germination (Dadd and Daley, 1982), so that hydration of the spore coat and alteration of spore coat layers do not appear to be linked to sensitivity. Even spores exposed to high concentrations of EtO can germinate freely under a variety of conditions but will not outgrow (Dadd and Rumbelow, 1986). Interestingly, however, asparagine acts as a germinant for unexposed but not for EtO-treated spores.

Sodium nitrite is a particularly interesting compound, and several theories have been published about its antimicrobial activity (reviewed by Russell, 1982a). It does not affect spore germination and in fact induces germination, but only at high concentrations (Labbe and Duncan, 1970; Ando, 1980). Nitrite inhibits postheating germination, outgrowth, or both, heat-injured spores being rendered more sensitive to the salt (Ingram and Roberts, 1971).

Table 22–5 lists those agents that are effective at the outgrowth stage.

MECHANISMS OF SPORICIDAL ACTION

A considerable amount of information is available as to how antibacterial agents kill nonsporulating bacteria (see Russell, 1982b). In contrast, mechanisms of sporicidal action are poorly understood. The major reason for this paucity of knowledge is undoubtedly the complex nature of the bacterial spore, allied to the fact that an antibacterial compound may have several actual or potential sites of action, some or all of which might contribute to its overall lethal effect (Russell, 1990b).

Several techniques are available for studying the effects of biocides on spores; the theoretic concepts and practical considerations have recently been discussed in detail (Russell et al., 1990). Uptake studies of biocide with spores and decoated forms might provide useful, preliminary evidence, especially if radiolabeled biocides are available. It must be borne in mind, however, that sporostatic agents may also be taken up by spores. Surface changes can also be studied, for example, by use of microelectrophoresis data and hydrophobicity studies. Bacterial spores are only slightly hydrophobic, but changes occur during germination and outgrowth (Shaker et al., 1988b) and when cells are exposed to agents such as glutaraldehyde (Power and Russell, 1989a).

The spore coat(s) may play an important role in spore resistance to chemical agents. Some disinfectants themselves alter the spore coat(s). Chlorine removes coat protein (Waites and Bayliss, 1979a). Hydrogen peroxide also removes protein (presumably from the coat) in *Cl. bifermentans* (Bayliss and Waites, 1976; Stevenson and Shafer, 1983), sublethal levels of peroxide increasing the germination rate in this organism.

Interaction of an antibacterial agent with spore cortex may be inferred from a knowledge of the chemical properties of the agent, of the cortex, and of the effects of the compound—e.g., glutaraldehyde (Russell, 1982a)—on spores. Studies with coatless forms exposed to glutaraldehyde and then to peptidoglycan-affecting agents such as lysozyme or sodium nitrite have yielded useful information about the mechanism of action of the dialdehyde (Gorman et al., 1980, 1984).

Fitz-James (1971) described a method of producing spore protoplasts, the procedure involving the use of lysozyme, which digests both the cortex and the germ cell wall. These protoplasts have been used in studying the mechanism of action of glutaraldehyde (Gorman et al., 1984).

The release of DPA from bacterial spores is indicative of membrane damage. Spores exposed to hypochlorites leak DPA (Kulikovsky et al., 1975). Pretreatment of spores with alkaline, but not acid, glutaraldehyde reduces, but does not eliminate, leakage when spores are subsequently exposed to high temperatures. Glutaraldehyde also reduces the loss of DPA during germination, a process itself inhibited by the dialdehyde (Russell et al., 1990). In contrast, chlorhexidine increases the thermally-induced DPA loss but decreases the amount leaked during germination, although the biguanide predominantly inhibits outgrowth (Russell et al., 1990).

Direct interaction of biocides with spore proteins and DNA or RNA is also known (Russell, 1982a).

From the above and other data (see Russell, 1982a,b,

Table 22–6. *Mechanisms of Action of Antibacterial Agents*

Sporicidal Action	Site of Mechanism of Action	Comment
Alkali	Inner spore coat	Outer spore coat resistant
Hypochlorites	Cortex	Effect on coats also
Ethylene oxide	Alkylation of core protein and DNA	
Glutaraldehyde	Cortex	pH-dependent action; action on coats also
Hydrogen peroxide	Spore core?	Effect on coats also
Lysozyme	Cortex	Beta,1–4 links in peptidoglycan
Nitrous acid	Cortex	At muramic acid residues

1983), the following conclusions may be reached about the mechanism(s) of action of sporicidal agents:

1. Glutaraldehyde at both acid and alkaline pH interacts strongly with the spore surface, but at alkaline pH the aldehyde penetrates more extensively into the spore, where it fixes the cortex.

2. Formaldehyde is believed to penetrate into the spore, where it combines with protein, RNA, and DNA.

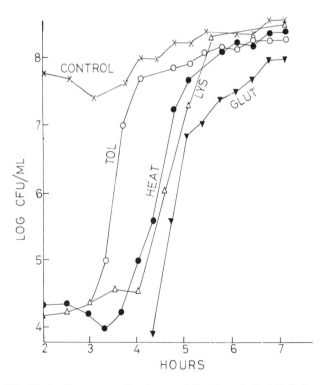

Fig. 22–4. Emergence of resistance of *Bacillus subtilis* 168 during sporulation. X, viable count, untreated (control) cells; Open circles, exposure to toluene (1 min); Filled circles, heat (80°C, 10 min); Triangles, lysozyme (250 units/ml, 10 min, 37°C); Inverted filled triangles, glutaraldehyde (2%, pH 7.9, 22°C, 10 min). Based on Power, E.G.M., Dancer, B.N., and Russell, A.D. 1988. Emergence of resistance to glutaraldehyde in spores of *Bacillus subtilis* 168. FEMS Microbiol. Lett., 50, 223–226.

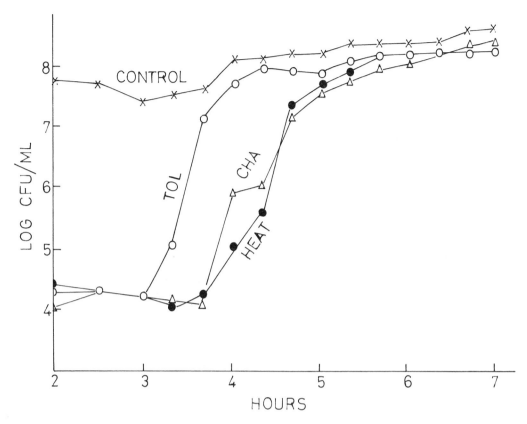

Fig. 22–5. Emergence of resistance of *Bacillus subtilis* 168 during sporulation. X, viable count, untreated (control) cells; Open circles, exposure to toluene (1 min); Filled circles, heat (80°C, 10 min); Triangles, chlorhexidine diacetate (CHA, 200 μg/ml, 10 min). Based on Shaker, L.A., Dancer, B.N., Russell, A.D., and Furr, J.R. 1988a. Emergence and development of chlorhexidine resistance during sporulation of *Bacillus subtilis* 168. FEMS Microbiol. Lett., *51*, 73–76.

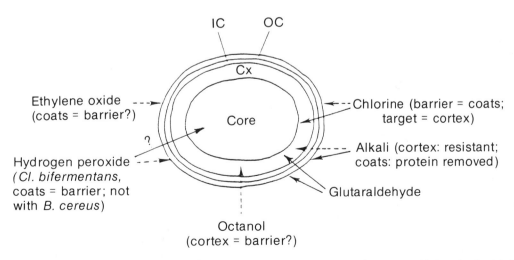

Fig. 22–6. Possible sites of action of sporicidal agents and spore barriers. The most important barriers are likely to be disulphide-rich protein, alkali-soluble protein, and cortex. Cx, cortex; IC, inner coat; OC, outer spore coat; dotted arrow, barrier; solid arrow, target. Modified from Russell, A.D. 1982a. *The Destruction of Bacterial Spores*. London, New York, Academic Press.

Table 22–7. *Mechanisms of Bacterial Spore Resistance to Antibacterial Agents*

Antibacterial Agent	Spore Component(s) Conferring Resistance
Alkali	Cortex
Lysozyme Hypochlorites Glutaraldehyde Iodine	Coat(s): UDS-spores highly sensitive
Hydrogen peroxide	Coat(s): but varies with strain
Chlorhexidine	Coat(s): UDS-spores more sensitive
Ethylene oxide	Coat(s)? Exact relationship unclear
Octanol Xylene	Cortex: conclusions based on findings with Dap⁻ mutants of *B. sphaericus*

UDS = urea + dithiothreitol + sodium lauryl sulfate
Dap = diaminopimelic acid

3. Alkylating agents, such as ethylene oxide and beta-propiolactone, are considered to kill spores by combining with specific groups in proteins and by alkylation of guanine in DNA.
4. Hypochlorites have an effect on spore coats, but their major action appears to be on the cortex. They increase spore permeability.
5. Hydrogen peroxide affects both the outer spore layers and the spore core (protoplast).
A summary is provided in Table 22–6.

MECHANISMS OF SPORE RESISTANCE

During sporulation, cells develop resistance to many chemically unrelated antibacterial agents (Figs. 22–4 and 22–5). Conversely, significant changes occur during these processes that lead to considerable increases or decreases in resistance. The possible mechanisms of spore resistance will be considered here, although they are still poorly understood.

Generally, penetration of the outer spore layers is necessary for an antibacterial agent to achieve a sporicidal action. Little is known, however, about the manner in which this permeation is achieved, and indeed in at least one case, ethylene oxide, the role of the spore coats in resistance is equivocal (Dadd and Daley, 1982).

The cortex has been suggested as being a contributing factor in spore resistance expressed to certain agents (Imae and Strominger, 1976a,b). However, changes in the cortex could also result in changes elsewhere in the spore (Waites, 1982), and it is therefore difficult to reach a firm conclusion about the role of the cortex in biocide resistance.

The spore coats are more likely to participate in the intrinsic resistance shown by spores, although the extent of this resistance varies with different types of spores (Waites and Bayliss, 1979). Coatless spores retain their viability; thus, an invaluable method for studying the role of the coats in resistance is to remove one or both of the coats and compare the response to biocides of these and "normal" spore forms. One of the most useful meth-

ods for achieving such spores is by treatment with UDS (urea + dithiothreitol + sodium lauryl sulfate at alkaline pH), as described by Nishihara et al. (1980, 1981a,b). The outer spore coat is alkali-resistant, unlike the inner coat. UDS-treated spores are highly sensitive to glutaraldehyde, iodine, hydrogen peroxide, chlorine, and ozone (Gorman et al., 1980; Foegeding, 1983, 1985; Foegeding and Busta, 1983a–d; Stevenson and Shafer, 1983; Ando and Tsuzuki, 1986a,b). Thus, the spore coats must have an important role to play in rendering intact spores less susceptible to these disinfectants. It must be added, however, that the spore coat is much less effective in presenting a barrier against peroxide in *B. cereus* than in *Cl. bifermentans* (Waites and Bayliss, 1979). Furthermore, chlorine will itself remove protein from spore coats, although it tends to lose some activity in consequence, allowing lysozyme to initiate germination by virtue of the effect of the latter on cortical peptidoglycan (Waites et al., 1976).

As described earlier, the use of Spo⁻ mutants of *B. subtilis* strain 168 can also yield useful information about mechanisms of spore resistance. These mutants are unable to develop beyond a genetically determined stage in the sporulation process and are clearly of value in correlating structural changes, biochemical characteristics, and response to antibacterial agents. Studies with glutaraldehyde (Power et al., 1988) and chlorhexidine (Shaker et al., 1988) have already been undertaken in these laboratories, and further investigations with other biocides are currently in progress.

A summary of the above is provided in Figure 22–6 and Table 22–7.

REFERENCES

Adams, D.M. 1978. Heat injury of bacterial spores. Adv. Appl. Microbiol., 23, 245–261.

Ando, Y. 1973. Studies on germination of spores of clostridial species capable of causing food poisoning. II. Effects of some chemicals on the germination of spores of *Clostridium botulinum* Type A [in Japanese]. J. Food Hyg. Soc. Japan, 14, 462–466.

Ando, Y. 1980. Mechanism of nitrite-induced germination of *Clostridium perfringens* spores. J. Appl. Bacteriol., 49, 527–535.

Ando, Y., and Tsuzuki, T. 1986a. The effect of hydrogen peroxide on spores of *Clostridium perfringens*. Lett. Appl. Microbiol., 2, 65–68.

Ando, Y., and Tsuzuki, T. 1986b. Changes in decoated spores of *Clostridium perfringens* caused by treatment with some enzymatic and non-enzymatic systems. Lett. Appl. Microbiol., 3, 61–64.

Andrew, M.H.E., and Russell, A.D. (eds). *The Revival of Injured Microbes*. Society for Applied Bacteriology Symposium Series, No. 12. London and New York, Academic Press.

AOAC. 1980. *Official Methods of Analysis*. 13th Edition. Washington, D.C., Association of Official Analytical Chemists.

Baldry, M.G.C. 1983. The bactericidal, fungicidal, and sporicidal properties of hydrogen peroxide and peracetic acid. J. Appl. Bacteriol., 54, 417–423.

Baldry, M.G.C., and Fraser, J.A.L. 1988. Disinfection with peroxygens. In *Industrial Biocides: Critical Reports on Applied Chemistry*. Volume 23. Edited by K.R. Payne. Chichester, John Wiley & Sons, pp. 91–116.

Bayliss, C.E., and Waites, W.M. 1976. The effect of hydrogen peroxide on spores of *Clostridium bifermentans*. J. Gen. Microbiol., 96, 401–407.

Bayliss, C.E., and Waites, W.M. 1979. The synergistic killing of spores of *Bacillus subtilis* by hydrogen peroxide and ultraviolet light irradiation. FEMS Microbiol. Lett., 5, 331–333.

Blocher, J.C., and Busta, F.F. 1983. Bacterial spore resistance to acid. Food Technol., 37(11), 87–99.

Blocher, J.C., and Busta, F.F. 1985. Multiple modes of inhibition of spore germination and outgrowth by reduced pH and sorbate. J. Appl. Bacteriol., 59, 469–478.

Boucher, R.M.G. 1974. Potentiated 1,5-pentanedial, a breakthrough in chemical sterilizing and disinfecting technology. Am. J. Hosp. Pharm., *31*, 546–557.

Chiori, C.O., Hambleton, R., and Rigby, G.J. 1965. The inhibition of spores of *Bacillus subtilis* by cetrimide retained on washed membrane filters and on the washed spores. J. Appl. Bacteriol., *28*, 322–330.

Coates, D., and Death, J.E. 1978. Sporicidal activity of mixtures of alcohol and hypochlorites. J. Clin. Pathol., *31*, 148–152.

Cook, F.M., and Pierson, M.D. 1983. Inhibition of bacterial spores by antimicrobials. Food Technol., *37*(11), 115–126.

Cousins, C.M., and Allan, C.D. 1967. Sporicidal properties of some halogens. J. Appl. Bacteriol., *30*, 168–174.

Dadd, A.H., and Daley, G.M. 1982. Role of the coat in resistance of bacterial spores to inactivation by ethylene oxide. J. Appl. Bacteriol., *53*, 109–116.

Dadd, A.H., and Rumbelow, J.E. 1986. Germination of spores of *Bacillus subtilis* var. *niger* following exposure to gaseous ethylene oxide. J. Appl. Bacteriol., *60*, 425–433.

Daher, E., Rosenberg, E., and Demain, A.L. 1985. Germination-initiated spores of *Bacillus brevis* Nagano retain their resistance properties. J. Bacteriol., *161*, 47–50.

Dancer, B.N., Power, E.G.M., and Russell, A.D. 1989. Alkali-induced revival of *Bacillus* spores after inactivation by glutaraldehyde. FEMS Microbiol. Lett., *57*, 345–348.

Doores, S. 1983. Bacterial spore resistance-species of emerging importance. Food Technol., *37*(11), 127–134.

Downing, R.G., and Dawes, I.W. 1977. L-Alanine binding during initiation of germination in *Bacillus subtilis*. In *Spore Research 1976*. Edited by A.N. Barker, et al. London and New York, Academic Press, pp. 711–719.

Ellar, D.J. 1978. Spore-specific structures and their functions. In *Relations between Structure and Function in the Prokaryotic Cell*. Edited by R.Y. Stanier, H.J. Rogers, and J.B. Ward. 28th Symposium of the Society for General Microbiology. Cambridge, Cambridge University Press, pp. 295–325.

Fitz-James, P.C. 1971. Formation of protoplasts from resting spores. J. Bacteriol., *105*, 1119–1136.

Foegeding, P.M. 1983. Bacterial spore resistance to chlorine compounds. Food Technol., *37*(11), 100–104, 110.

Foegeding, P.M. 1985. Ozone inactivation of *Bacillus* and *Clostridium* spore populations and the importance of the spore coat to resistance. Food Microbiol., *2*, 123–134.

Foegeding, P.M., and Busta, F.F. 1981. Bacterial spore injury—an update. J. Food Prot., *44*, 776–786.

Foegeding, P.M., and Busta, F.F. 1983a. Hypochlorite injury of *Clostridium botulinum* spores alters germination responses. Appl. Environ. Microbiol., *45*, 1360–1368.

Foegeding, P.M., and Busta, F.F. 1983b. Proposed role of lactate in germination of hypochlorite–treated *Clostridium botulinum* spores. Appl. Environ. Microbiol., *45*, 1369–1373.

Foegeding, P.M., and Busta, F.F. 1983c. Proposed mechanism for sensitisation by hypochlorite treatment of *Clostridium botulinum* spores. Appl. Environ. Microbiol., *45*, 1374–1379.

Foegeding, P.M., and Busta, F.F. 1983d. Differing L-alanine germination requirements of hypochlorite-treated *Clostridium botulinum* spores from two crops. Appl. Environ. Microbiol., *45*, 1415–1417.

Forsyth, M.P. 1975. A rate of kill test for measuring sporicidal properties of liquid sterilizers. Dev. Ind. Microbiol., *16*, 37–47.

Gorman, S.P., Jones, D.S., and Loftus, A.M. 1987. The sporicidal activity and inactivation of chlorhexidine gluconate in aqueous and alcoholic solution. J. Appl. Bacteriol., *63*, 183–188.

Gorman, S.P., Scott, E.M., and Hutchinson, E.P. 1984a. Interaction of the *Bacillus subtilis* spore protoplast, cortex, ion-exchange and coatless forms with glutaraldehyde. J. Appl. Bacteriol., *56*, 95–102.

Gorman, S.P., Scott, E.M., and Hutchinson, E.P. 1984b. Emergence and development of resistance to antimicrobial chemicals and heat in spores of *Bacillus subtilis*. J. Appl. Bacteriol., *57*, 153–163.

Gorman, S.P., Scott, E.M., and Russell, A.D. 1980. Antimicrobial activity, uses and mechanism of action of glutaraldehyde. J. Appl. Bacteriol., *48*, 161–190.

Gorman, S.P., Hutchinson, E.P., Scott, E.M., and McDermott, L.M. 1983. Death, injury and revival of chemically treated *Bacillus subtilis* spores. J. Appl. Bacteriol., *54*, 91–99.

Gould, G.W. 1983. Mechanisms of resistance and dormancy. In *The Bacterial Spore*, Volume 2. Edited by A. Hurst and G.W. Gould. London and New York, Academic Press, pp. 173–209.

Gould, G.W. 1984. Injury and repair mechanisms in bacterial spores. In *The Revival of Injured Microbes*. Edited by M.H.E. Andrew and A.D. Russell. Society for Applied Bacteriology Symposium Series No. 12. London and New York, Academic Press, pp. 199–220.

Gould, G.W. 1985. Modification of resistance and dormancy. In *Fundamental and Applied Aspects of Bacterial Spores*. Edited by G.J. Dring, D.J. Ellar, and G.W. Gould. London and New York, Academic Press, pp. 371–382.

Gould, G.W., and Sale, A.J.H. 1970. Initiation of germination of bacterial spores by hydrostatic pressure. J. Gen. Microbiol., *60*, 335–346.

Halvorson, H.O., and Szulmajster, J. 1973. In *The Biochemistry of Bacterial*

Growth, 2nd Edition. Edited by J. Mandelstam and K. McQuillen. Oxford, Blackwell Scientific Publications, pp. 494–516.

Hill, S.H.A. 1983. *spoVH* and *spoVJ*—new sporulation loci in *Bacillus subtilis* 168. J. Gen. Microbiol., *129*, 293–302.

Hsich, L.K., and Vary, J.C. 1975. Germination and peptidoglycan solubilization in *Bacillus megaterium* spores. J. Bacteriol., *123*, 463–470.

Hugo, W.B., and Russell, A.D. 1982. Types of antimicrobial agents. In *Principles and Practice of Disinfection, Preservation and Sterilisation*. Edited by A.D. Russell, W.B. Hugo, and G.A.J. Ayliffe. Oxford, Blackwell Scientific Publications, pp. 8–106.

Imae, Y., and Strominger, J.L. 1976a. Relationship between cortex content and properties of *Bacillus sphaericus* spores. J. Bacteriol., *126*, 907–913.

Imae, Y., and Strominger, J.L. 1976b. Conditional spore cortex-less mutants of *Bacillus sphaericus* 9602. J. Biol. Chem., *251*, 1493–1499.

Ingram, M., and Roberts, T.A. 1971. Application of the 'D-concept' to heat treatments involving curing salts. J. Food Technol., *6*, 21–28.

Isenberg, I. 1985. Clinical laboratory studies of disinfection with Sporicidin. J. Clin. Microbiol., *22*, 735–739.

Jenkinson, H.F. 1981. Germination and resistance defects in spores of a *Bacillus subtilis* mutant lacking a coat polypeptide. J. Gen. Microbiol., *127*, 81–91.

Jenkinson, H.F. 1983. Altered arrangement of proteins in the spore coat of a germination mutant of *Bacillus subtilis*. J. Gen. Microbiol., *129*, 1945–1958.

Jenkinson, H.F., Kay, D., and Mandelstam, J. 1980. Temporal dissociation of late events in *Bacillus subtilis* sporulation from expression of genes that determine them. J. Bacteriol., *141*, 793–805.

Jenkinson, H.F., Sawyer, W.D., and Mandelstam, J. 1981. Synthesis and assembly of spore coat proteins in *Bacillus subtilis*. J. Gen. Microbiol., *123*, 1–16.

Kanda, K., Yasuda, Y., and Tochikubo, K. 1988. Germination-inducing activities for *Bacillus subtilis* spores of analogues of L-alanine derived by modification at the amino or carboxy group. J. Gen. Microbiol., *134*, 2747–2755.

Keynan, A., and Sandler, N. 1983. Spore research in historical perspective. In *The Bacterial Spore*, Volume 2. Edited by A. Hurst and G.W. Gould. London and New York, Academic Press, pp. 1–48.

Keynan, A., et al. 1976. Resporulation of outgrowing *Bacillus subtilis* spores. J. Bacteriol., *128*, 8–14.

Klarmann, E.G. 1950. The role of antagonisms in the evaluation of antiseptics. Ann. N. Y. Acad. Sci., *53*, 123–147.

Kulikovsky, A., Pankratz, H.S., and Sadoff, H.L. 1975. Ultrastructural and chemical changes in spores of *Bacillus cereus* after action of disinfectants. J. Appl. Bacteriol., *38*, 39–46.

Labbe, R.G., and Duncan, C.L. 1970. Growth from spores of *Clostridium perfringens* in the presence of sodium nitrite. Appl. Microbiol., *19*, 353–359.

Lewis, J.C., and Jurd, L. 1972. Sporostatic action of cinnamylphenols and related compounds on *Bacillus megaterium*. In *Spores V*. Edited by H.O. Halvorson, R. Hanson, and L.L. Campbell. Washington D.C., American Society for Microbiology, pp. 384–389.

Lund, B.M. 1962. Ph.D. Thesis, University of London, England.

Milhaud, P., and Balassa, G. 1973. Biochemical genetics of bacterial sporulation. IV. Sequential development of resistances to chemical and physical agents during sporulation of *Bacillus subtilis*. Mol. Gen. Genet., *125*, 241–250.

Moir, A., Lafferty, E., and Smith, D.A. 1979. Genetic analysis of spore germination mutants of *Bacillus subtilis* 168: the correlation of phenotype with map locations. J. Gen. Microbiol., *111*, 165–180.

Murrell, W.G. 1969. Chemical composition of spores and spore structures. In *The Bacterial Spore*. Edited by G.W. Gould and A. Hurst. London, Academic Press, pp. 215–273.

Nishihara, T., et al. 1980. Studies on the bacterial spore coat. 7. Properties of alkali-soluble components from spore coat of *Bacillus megaterium*. Microbiol. Immunol., *24*, 105–112.

Nishihara, T., Yutsodo, T., Ichikawa, T., and Kondo, M. 1981a. Studies on the bacterial spore coat. 8. On the SDS-DTT extract from *Bacillus megaterium* spores. Microbiol. Immunol., *25*, 327–331.

Nishihara, T., Yoshimoto, I., and Kondo, M. 1981b. Studies on the bacterial spore coat. 9. The role of surface charge in germination of *Bacillus megaterium* spores. Microbiol. Immunol., *25*, 763–771.

Ortenzio, L.F., Stuart, L.S., and Friedl, J.L. 1953. The resistance of bacterial spores to constant boiling hydrochloric acid. J. Assoc. Off. Agric. Chem., *36*, 480–484.

Parker, M.S. 1969. Some effects of preservatives on the developments of bacterial spores. J. Appl. Bacteriol., *32*, 322–328.

Parker, M.S., and Bradley, T.J. 1968. A reversible inhibition of the germination of bacterial spores. Can J. Microbiol., *14*, 745–746.

Power, E.G.M., and Russell, A.D. 1989. Glutaraldehyde: its uptake by sporing and non-sporing bacteria, rubber, plastic and an endoscope. J. Appl. Bacteriol., *67*, 329–342.

Power, E.G.M., and Russell, A.D. 1990. Uptake of L-(^{14}C)-alanine to glutaraldehyde-treated and untreated spores of *Bacillus subtilis*. FEMS Microbiol. Lett., *66*, 271–276.

Power, E.G.M., Dancer, B.N., and Russell, A.D. 1988. Emergence of resistance to glutaraldehyde in spores of *Bacillus subtilis* 168. FEMS Microbiol. Lett., *50*, 223–226.

Power, E.G.M., Dancer, B.N., and Russell, A.D. 1989. Possible mechanisms for the revival of glutaraldehyde-treated spores of *Bacillus subtilis* NCTC 8236. J. Appl. Bacteriol., *67*, 91–98.

Prasad, C. 1974. Initiation of spore germination in *Bacillus subtilis*: relationship to inhibition of L-alanine metabolism. J. Bacteriol., *119*, 805–810.

Reich, R. 1980. Effect of sublethal ethylene oxide exposure on *Bacillus subtilis* spores and biological indicator performance. J. Parent. Drug. Assoc., *34*, 200–211.

Reybrouck, G. 1982. The evaluation of the antimicrobial activity of disinfectants. In *Principles and Practice of Disinfection, Preservation and Sterilisation*. Edited by A.D. Russell, W.B. Hugo, and G.A.J. Ayliffe. Oxford, Blackwell Scientific Publications, pp. 134–157.

Russell, A.D. 1982a. *The Destruction of Bacterial Spores*. London and New York, Academic Press.

Russell, A.D. 1982b. Factors influencing the efficacy of antimicrobial agents. In *Principles and Practice of Disinfection, Preservation and Sterilisation*. Edited by A.D. Russell, W.B. Hugo, and G.A.J. Ayliffe. Oxford, Blackwell Scientific Publications, pp. 107–133.

Russell, A.D. 1983. Mechanisms of action of chemical sporicidal and sporistatic agents. Int. J. Pharm., *16*, 127–140.

Russell, A.D. 1990a. The effects of chemical and physical agents on microbes: disinfection and sterilization. In *Topley and Wilson's Principles of Bacteriology, Virology and Immunity*, 8th Edition. Volume 1. Edited by H.M. Dick and A.H. Linton. London, Edward Arnold.

Russell, A.D. 1990b. The bacterial spore and chemical sporicidal agents. Clin. Microbiol. Rev., *3*, 99–119.

Russell, A.D., and Hopwood, D. 1976. The biological uses and properties of glutaraldehyde. Progr. Med. Chem., *13*, 271–301.

Russell, A.D., and Hugo, W.B. 1987. Chemical disinfectants. In *Disinfection in Veterinary and Farm Animal Practice*. Edited by A.H. Linton, W.B. Hugo, and A.D. Russell. Oxford, Blackwell Scientific Publications, pp. 12–42.

Russell, A.D., Dancer, B.N., and Power, E.G.M. 1990. Effects of chemical agents on bacterial sporulation, germination and outgrowth. Society for Applied Bacteriology Technical Series (in press).

Russell, A.D., Jones, B.D., and Milburn, P. 1985. Reversal of the inhibition of bacterial spore germination and outgrowth by antibacterial agents. Int. J. Pharm., *25*, 105–112.

Rutala, W.A. 1987. Disinfection, sterilization and waste disposal. In *Prevention and Control of Nosocomial Infections*. Edited by R.P. Wenzel. Baltimore, Williams & Wilkins, pp. 257–282.

Sammons, R.L., Moir, A., and Smith, D.A. 1981. Isolation and properties of spore germination mutants of *Bacillus subtilis* 168 deficient in the initiation of germination. J. Gen. Microbiol., *124*, 229–241.

Scott, E.M., and Gorman, E.P. 1987. Chemical disinfectants, antiseptics and preservatives. In *Pharmaceutical Microbiology*. 4th Edition. Edited by W.B. Hugo and A.D. Russell. Oxford, Blackwell Scientific Publications, pp. 226–252.

Setlow, P. 1988. Small, acid-soluble spore proteins of *Bacillus* species: Structure, synthesis, genetics, function and degradation. Ann. Rev. Microbiol., *42*, 319–338.

Shaker, L.A., Russell, A.D., and Furr, J.R. 1986. Aspects of the action of chlorhexidine on bacterial spores. Int. J. Pharm., *34*, 51–56.

Shaker, L.A., Dancer, B.N., Russell, A.D., and Furr, J.R. 1988a. Emergence and development of chlorhexidine resistance during sporulation of *Bacillus subtilis* 168. FEMS Microbiol. Lett., *39*, 73–76.

Shaker, L.A., Furr, J.R., and Russell, A.D. 1988b. Mechanism of resistance of *Bacillus subtilis* spores to chlorhexidine. J. Appl. Bacteriol., *64*, 531–539.

Simmons, B.P. 1983. CDC Guidelines for the Prevention and Control of Nosocomial Infections. Guidelines for hospital environmental control. Am. J. Infect. Control, *11*, 96–115.

Smoot, L.A., and Pierson, M.D. 1982. Inhibition and control of bacterial spore germination. J. Food Prot., *45*, 84–92.

Sofos, J.N., and Busta, F.F. 1982. Chemical food preservatives. In *Principles and Practice of Disinfection, Preservation and Sterilisation*. Edited by A.D. Russell, W.B. Hugo, and G.A.J. Ayliffe. Oxford, Blackwell Scientific Publications, pp. 306–342.

Sofos, J.N., Pierson, M.D., Blocher, J.C., and Busta, F.F. 1986. Mode of action of sorbic acid on bacterial cells and spores. Int. J. Food Microbiol., *3*, 1–17.

Spaulding, E.H. 1939. Chemical sterilization of surgical instruments. Surg. Gynecol. Obstet., *69*, 738–744.

Spicher, G., and Peters, J. 1981a. Hitzeaktivierung von bakteriellen sporen nach inaktivierung durch formaldehyd. Abhängigkeit der hitzeaktivierung von der temperatur und ihrer einwirkungsdauer. Zentralbl. Bakteriol. Mikrobiol. Hyg. [B], 188–196.

Spicher, G., and Peters, J. 1981b. Resistenz mikrobieller Keime gegenüber formaldehyd. II. Abhängigkeit des mikrobiziden effektes von der konzentration und der einwirkungsdauer des formaldehyds. Zentrabl. Bakteriol. Mikrobiol. Hyg. [B], 133–150.

Stevenson, K.E., and Shafer, B.D. 1983. Bacterial spore resistance to hydrogen peroxide. Food Technol., *37*(11), 111–114, 126.

Stewart, G.S.A.B., Johnstone, K., Hagelberg, E., and Ellar, D.J. 1981. Commitment of bacterial spores to germinate. A measure of the trigger reaction. Biochem. J., *198*, 101–106.

Sykes, G. 1965. *Disinfection and Sterilization*. 2nd Edition. London, F. & N. Spon.

Toledo, P.T., Escher, S.E., and Ayres, J.C. 1973. Sporicidal properties of hydrogen peroxide against food-spoilage organisms. Appl. Microbiol., *26*, 592–597.

Trueman, J.R. 1971. The halogens. In *Inhibition and Destruction of the Microbial Cell*. Edited by W.B. Hugo. London and New York, Academic Press, pp. 135–183.

Trujillo, P., and David, T.J. 1972. Sporostatic and sporicidal properties of aqueous formaldehyde. Appl. Microbiol., *23*, 618–622.

Trujillo, P., and Laible, N. 1970. Reversible inhibition of spore germination by alcohols. Appl. Microbiol., *20*, 620–623.

Vinter, V. 1970. Germination and outgrowth: effect of inhibitors. J. Appl. Bacteriol., *33*, 50–59.

Waites, W.M. 1982. Microbial resistance to non-antibiotic antimicrobial agents: Resistance of bacterial spores. In *Principles and Practice of Disinfection, Preservation and Sterilisation*. Edited by A.D. Russell, W.B. Hugo, and G.A.J. Ayliffe. Oxford, Blackwell Scientific Publications, pp. 207–220.

Waites, W.M. 1985. Inactivation of spores with chemical agents. In *Fundamental and Applied Aspects of Bacterial Spores*. Edited by G.J. Dring, D.J. Ellar, and G.W. Gould. London and New York, Academic Press, pp. 383–396.

Waites, W.M., and Bayliss, C.E. 1979. The effect of changes in the spore coat on the destruction of *Bacillus cereus* spores by heat and chemical agents. J. Appl. Biochem., *1*, 71–76.

Waites, W.M., and Bayliss, C.E. 1980. The preparation of bacterial spores for evaluation of the sporicidal activity of chemicals. In *Microbial Growth and Survival in Extremes of Environment*. Edited by G.W. Gould and J.E.L. Corry. Society for Applied Bacteriology Technical Series No. 15. London and New York, Academic Press, pp. 159–172.

Waites, W.M., and Bayliss, C.E. 1984. Damage to bacterial spores by combined treatments and possible revival and repair processes. In *The Revival of Injured Microbes*. Edited by M.H.E. Andrew and A.D. Russell. Society for Applied Bacteriology Symposium Series No. 12. London and New York, Academic Press, pp. 221–240.

Waites, W.M., Wyatt, L.R., King, N.R., and Bayliss, C.E. 1976. Changes in spores of *Clostridium bifermentans* caused by treatment with hydrogen peroxide and cations. J. Gen. Microbiol., *93*, 388–396.

Warth, A.D. 1978. Molecular structure of the bacterial spore. Adv. Microb. Physiol., *17*, 1–45.

Watanabe, K., and Takesue, S. 1976. Selective inhibition of the germination of *Bacillus megaterium* spores by alkyl *p*-hydroxybenzoates. Chem. Pharm. Bull., *24*, 224–229.

Wyatt, L.R., and Waites, W.M. 1975. The effect of chlorine on spores of *Clostridium bifermentans*, *Bacillus subtilis* and *Bacillus cereus*. J. Gen. Microbiol., *89*, 327–334.

Yasuda, Y., and Tochikubo, K. 1985a. Germination-initiation and inhibitory activities of L- and D-alanine analogues for *Bacillus subtilis* spores. Microbiol. Immunol., *29*, 229–241.

Yasuda, Y., and Tochikubo, K. 1985b. Disappearance of the cooperative effect of glucose on L-alanine binding during heat activation of germination of *Bacillus subtilis* spores. Microbiol. Immunol., *29*, 1011–1017.

Yasuda, Y., et al. 1982. Quantitative structure-inhibitory relationships of phenols and fatty acids for *Bacillus subtilis* spore germination. J. Med. Chem., *25*, 315–320.

Yasuda-Yasaki, Y., Namie-Kanie, S., and Hachisuka, Y. 1978. Inhibition of *Bacillus subtilis* spore germination by various hydrophobic compounds: Demonstration of hydrophobic character of the L-alanine receptor site. J. Bacteriol., *136*, 484–490.

Yasuda, Y., and Tochikubo, K. 1984. Relation between D-glucose and L- and D-alanine in the initiation of germination of *Bacillus subtilis* spore. Microbiol. Immunol., *28*, 197–207.

CHAPTER 23

MYCOBACTERIAL DISINFECTION AND CONTROL

Jeffrey Rubin

Mycobacterium tuberculosis and *Mycobacterium leprae* are historically the causative agents of two devastating diseases in man, tuberculosis and leprosy, respectively. More recently, "atypical" or "environmental" mycobacteria have been identified as causing significant disease in man. Leprosy (Hansen's disease) is still endemic in Texas and Louisiana. *M. leprae*, the infectious agent, has not been cultured in bacteriologic media or tissue culture. Our knowledge of the effects of disinfecting agents are surmised from other mycobacteria tested.

For many years, advances in living conditions, our understanding of the epidemiology of tuberculosis, and increasingly effective drug therapy greatly reduced the incidence of this disease, as well as its morbidity and mortality. From 1963 to 1985, the annual incidence rate of tuberculosis declined an average of 5.9% (Centers for Disease Control, 1988). Since 1985, however, this downward trend has stoppped, with marked increases in many areas, especially among individuals infected with the human immunodeficiency virus (HIV), the causative agent of AIDS (Centers for Disease Control, 1987c). There were 22,768 cases of tuberculosis reported to the Centers for Disease Control (CDC) in 1986, an increase of 2.6% over 1985 and the first substantial increase since 1953 (Centers for Disease Control, 1988). McEuen (1988), in her article, "Tuberculosis—threshold of an epidemic," emphasizes her concern about marked future increases in tuberculosis incidence in areas of high HIV prevalence. She states that tuberculosis is the only life-threatening disease that HIV-infected individuals develop that can be readily spread through casual contact to others.

Although tuberculosis, in most cases, is treated on an outpatient basis, it nonetheless is the cause of often severe and occasionally fatal disease. It remains today a major public health problem, especially among the poor, the elderly, and nonwhites. Cases among nonwhites increased from 23% in 1953 to 48% in 1985 (Centers for Disease Control, 1987b).

The decline of tuberculosis incidence prior to 1985 was associated with the closing of specialty hospitals and the concomitant loss of tuberculosis specialists (Edsall, 1977; Gunnels and Bates, 1977; Danboy and Elman, 1972). This decline, coupled with the great new epidemic of HIV and associated tuberculosis, has forced many new cases of tuberculosis to be diagnosed and initially treated in general hospitals and clinics, so more widespread understanding of mycobacterial disinfection and infection control procedures is becoming increasingly important.

PATHOLOGY

Tuberculosis in the United States today is caused by the tubercle bacillus, *Mycobacterium tuberculosis*, in most cases. The "atypical" or "environmental" mycobacteria, though not communicable from person to person, may cause disease clinically indistinguishable from tuberculosis. These organisms frequently demonstrate significant resistance to drug therapy and, as we see later, show some differences in their susceptibility to disinfecting agents. Large percentages of AIDS patients with mycobacterial disease are infected with the "environmental" mycobacteria, especially *M. avium* complex (Young, 1988; Grange, 1987). Grange states that these organisms are among the most difficult bacterial diseases to manage, representing "a growing concern, particularly in the developed world."

Drug resistance to *M. tuberculosis* is also a serious problem, with reports of transmission of resistant strains within households, shelters for the homeless, and even community outbreaks (Centers for Disease Control, 1987a, 1985, 1977, 1983b).

Tuberculosis is characterized by its chronicity and clinical variability. Initial or primary infection is usually subclinical; tuberculin sensitivity and pulmonary lymph node calcification are the only signs. The initial infection may progress to clinical pulmonary tuberculosis, which may begin as a pneumonia, may heal on its own with minimal or no symptoms, or may progress to the characteristic pulmonary lesions of tuberculosis. These consist of a nonliquefying "caseous" necrosis with epithelioid and giant cells, the classic tubercle. The tubercle may calcify and heal, or it may cavitate, the cavity representing the highly contagious form of the disease. The cavity may rupture into a bronchus, extruding large quantities of bacilli, or it may ulcerate into a blood vessel producing hematogenous spread. Disease may then localize in lymph nodes, kidneys, and bones or spread to the meninges, causing tuberculous meningitis, the major cause of death from tuberculosis in children. Patients with laryngeal tuberculosis give off large numbers of infective particles to the air and are considered highly infectious (Riley et al., 1962).

BACTERIOLOGY AND VIABILITY

The tubercle bacilli are acid-fast, nonmotile, obligate aerobes characterized by peculiar colonial morphology and lack of pigmentation on solid agar, inability to grow at room temperature, virulence for man, monkeys, and guinea pigs, susceptibility to drugs, and capacity to remain dormant in human tissue for decades. They are considered to have unusual resistance to conditions destructive to other vegetative bacteria, but are also susceptible to specific physical and chemical agents.

The bacillus is relatively resistant to heat, but is killed by boiling for 2 minutes. It is not killed by freezing and is highly resistant to desiccation. Smith (1942a) found that dried tubercle bacilli survived in unfiltered room light from 4 hours to 5 days under varying conditions and retained their viability in the dark for "less than 40 days to between 3½ to 5 months." Sunlight kills the tubercle bacillus and thus has been an important factor in sterilizing infected material (Long, 1958). The organisms are susceptible to ultraviolet light; the practical application of this is discussed later.

The bacilli survive for unusually long periods under certain conditions. Twelve-year-old cultures maintained at 37°C remained both viable and virulent after storage for this period of time (Corper and Cohn, 1933). Tubercle bacilli deposited in books and magazines were recoverable alive for 2 weeks to 3½ months (Smith, 1942b).

The environment in which the bacilli are found appears to be an extremely important factor in their viability, especially in the presence of chemical agents. Bacilli in sputa are surrounded by proteinaceous material. Smith (1968) cultured the organism from a tuberculous pulmonary cavity embalmed for about 24 hours and stated that formaldehyde, though ordinarily mycobactericidal, "cannot be depended upon to kill mycobacteria in the presence of large amounts of organic material." Other studies (Frobisher et al., 1953; Frobisher and Sommermeyer, 1953) suggest that disinfectant agents vary in their potency in the presence of organic material, and this factor must be carefully considered in their selection.

TRANSMISSION AND INFECTIOUSNESS

Tuberculosis in the United States today is spread almost exclusively by airborne transmission of the residues of tiny droplets produced by infectious individuals during the course of coughing, speaking, laughing, etc. These small particles of moisture quickly evaporate, leaving "droplet nuclei" that float freely, carried by air currents. Larger particles fall to the ground or, if inhaled, are removed by the bronchi and nasal passages and eliminated (Wells et al., 1948). The small particles are capable of reaching the susceptible deep lung tissues, where they multiply and produce infection. An analysis of major epidemics shows that tubercle bacilli that fall on clothing, furniture, floors, and walls do not constitute a significant hazard (Olsen, 1967). An excellent review and historical perspective of the airborne mode of transmission of tuberculosis is presented by Riley (1970).

Epidemiologic evidence for the spread of tuberculosis by the airborne route is abundant in the literature (Ehrenkranz and Kicklighter, 1972; Lincoln, 1967; Hardy and Schmidek, 1968; Bates et al., 1965; Houk et al., 1968). Airborne transmission in hospitals and nursing homes is also well documented (Catanzaro, 1982; Stead et al., 1985; Welty et al., 1985). Tuberculosis resulting from exposure to infected autopsy material (Barrett and Rentein, 1981), ingestion of infected milk, venereal transmission from prostatic tuberculosis (McClement, 1972), and even a case of primary cutaneous tuberculosis of the lip resulting from mouth-to-mouth resuscitation of a dying patient (Heilman and Muschenheim, 1965) all represent extremely rare modes of transmission.

Live tubercle bacilli were found in 33.3% of anesthetic masks removed from active tuberculosis patients in 1940. Fifteen percent of the masks were still positive after the "routine washing in water and were potential sources for the spread of tuberculosis." No masks were positive after immersing them in a formaldehyde-alcohol solution for 1 hour (Livingstone et al., 1941).

The flexible fiberoptic bronchoscope is an important diagnostic tool in pulmonary disease, its use associated with few complications. Transmission of tuberculosis and other pathogens by improperly disinfected instruments is a risk, however, and reports of transmission of tuberculosis by bronchoscopes are found in the literature (Nelson, 1983; Leers, 1980; George, 1988). Gastroscopy may also be a hazard because tuberculous sputum is swallowed (Ayliffe, 1988).

Heycock and Noble (1961) described four infants who developed tuberculous abscesses following injection of penicillin given by a nurse with open pulmonary tuberculosis. Although fomites and objects are considered extremely rare sources of infection, McLean (1963) believed that infants must be carefully protected from objects that may be contaminated by sputum-positive patients.

In a fascinating article, Notlebart (1980) describes a number of hospital employees awarded compensation after developing tuberculosis. The types of exposure cited in their cases included exposure to autopsy material and to machines that suctioned secretions from tuberculosis patients, the adjusting of tuberculosis patients' beds, and the application of an ointment to a tuberculous ulcer on a few occasions.

Nosocomial infections due to "environmental" mycobacteria have been reported in hospitals and clinics. In 2 outpatient hemodialysis centers in Louisiana in 1982, 27 of 140 patients were found to be infected with nontuberculous mycobacteria, mostly *Mycobacterium chelonei*, an organism frequently found in soil and water. The source was attributed to water used in processing the dialyzers and associated with "inconsistent and inadequate disinfection procedures" (Centers for Disease Control, 1983a). Elsewhere, three children with cystic fibrosis had positive sputa infected with *M. chelonei* (one developed clinical disease) after using a hydrotherapy pool later found to be growing this organism. The polymeric biguanide used to disinfect the pool water was later changed to chlorine (Begg et al., 1986). Endocarditis with *M. chelonei* and *M. fortuitum* probably resulting from infected ice used in surgery has been reported (George, 1988).

The infectiousness of the individual patient depends on a variety of factors. Among these are the extent of disease, the presence of cavities, and the amount of bacteria produced in the sputum. Treatment with drugs rapidly renders the patient noninfectious (Olsen, 1967) by reducing the number of organisms in the sputum, by the very presence of drugs in the sputum, and by decreasing the frequency of coughing (Loudon and Spohn, 1969). A cough may produce up to 3500 droplets, but a sneeze is estimated to produce up to 1 million particles (Johnson and Wildrick, 1974). Evidence that the culture positivity of the sputum in tuberculosis patients receiving drug therapy is not important in their infectivity has been presented (Gunnels et al., 1974).

Age is another important factor. Children with primary uncomplicated tuberculosis produce no sputum, have little or no cough, and are considered noninfectious (Report of the Committee on Infectious Diseases, 1974). In a survey of 109 epidemics of tuberculosis in 12 countries, there was no epidemic in which a child with primary tuberculosis was shown to be the source (Lincoln, 1967).

In conclusion, except for some rare instances described, tuberculosis is transmitted almost exclusively by inhalation by susceptible persons of air contaminated by "droplet nuclei" containing the tubercle bacillus. These particles are produced by diseased persons, who, in almost all instances, are undiagnosed and under no treatment. Such individuals giving off infectious airborne particles into areas of closed ventilation represent the greatest hazard. Obviously, location of active cases and administration of chemotherapy are the most critical aspects of control.

CONTROL OF MYCOBACTERIA IN THE MEDICAL ENVIRONMENT

Estimates of the frequency of undiagnosed tuberculosis in hospital patients range from 0.03 to 0.3% of ad-

missions (Craven et al., 1975). Excellent guidelines exist for tuberculosis control and surveillance programs in hospitals (AHA, 1979a; George, 1988).

The risk of acquiring tuberculosis in a medical environment is almost exclusively a function of the concentration of infectious particles in the air. Rare but real risks include instruments and equipment infected with *Mycobacterium tuberculosis* and "environmental" mycobacteria as described in the previous section. In areas occupied by known or suspected producers of infectious airborne particles, air control is necessary. This is accomplished by ventilation, high-efficiency air filtration, and the use of ultraviolet irradiation.

To prevent the rarer instances of infection from medical equipment requires sterilization and appropriate disinfecting agents. Carefully prepared procedures for handling these agents must be readily available (Fereres, 1988).

Special problems exist in the various medical specialties. The risks of patient-to-patient spread of mycobacterial infection by inadequately disinfected instruments has been presented earlier. Bronchoscopy, intubation, and mechanical ventilation of infected patients "may increase the rate of generation of infectious particles to very high levels" (Catanzaro, 1982), requiring control measures suggested in the following section.

In the dental office, the greatest risk is the unrecognized case. A tuberculosis patient regularly taking adequate medication can be safely treated in the dental office within a few weeks of the onset of treatment, although efforts should be taken to minimize the risk of droplet spread by the use of the rubber dam and avoidance of the high-speed handpiece (Rowe and Brooks, 1978). Periodic surveillance of dental personnel with skin testing and appropriate chemoprophylaxis of converters is extremely important.

VENTILATION, AIR FILTRATION, AND ULTRAVIOLET LIGHT RADIATION

Good ventilation is of obvious importance in diluting infectious airborne particles. Six air changes per hour reduce the concentration of infectious particles to 1% of the initial level (Gunnels and Bates, 1977). It is important that contaminated air not be recirculated or rerouted to other areas of the hospital or clinic. In high-risk areas, air should be ventilated to the outside whenever possible. Care should be taken that such exhausted air not re-enter through adjacent windows or air-intake vents (AHA, 1979b). If air must be recirculated, then high-efficiency filters or ultraviolet radiation should be used (Catanzaro, 1982).

Ultraviolet light has long been known to be effective in destroying infectious airborne particles. In a well-designed study, Lurie (1947) showed that ultraviolet light is highly effective in killing tubercle bacilli suspended in the air. Ultraviolet irradiation of air completely protected rabbits from an " . . . air-borne contagion of tuberculosis of such intensity which killed 73 percent of rabbits, of the same genetic constitution, exposed to the same contagion within the period of one year."

Riley et al. (1962) showed that ultraviolet light effectively kills airborne tubercle bacilli in hospital wards. Huber et al. (1970) showed that an ultraviolet chamber was effective in greatly reducing mycobacteria on contaminated paper, and *Mycobacterium tuberculosis* was the most sensitive of the strains of mycobacteria tested. David (1973) confirmed the relatively greater sensitivity of *M. tuberculosis* to other mycobacteria tested, but believed the difference to be small.

The effectiveness of ultraviolet light in controlling airborne dissemination of tuberculosis is supported by work with other pathogens (McLean, 1961; Perkins et al., 1947). Riley (1972) believes that "a UV installation throughout a hospital will . . . control most of the airborne infections" and strongly advocates this as a major method of control of tuberculosis and other respiratory diseases in areas of high hazard. Catanzaro (1982) reports that ultraviolet light can kill mycobacteria, providing a reduction of infectious units to the equivalent of 50 air changes per hour.

Nevertheless, ultraviolet light is not widely used for infection control. Disadvantages of its use include eye irritation and extensive maintenance requirements; tubes must be scrupulously cleaned and emission levels frequently monitored (Editorial Notes, J. Am. Hosp. Assoc., 1972). It is generally believed, however, that ultraviolet lighting, properly installed and maintained, destroys airborne infectious particles and is protective. An interesting article (Burk et al., 1978) describes a case of 528 highly susceptible newborn infants exposed to a nurse who had smear- and culture-positive pulmonary tuberculosis and a productive cough for over 3 months before her disease was diagnosed. Two protective measures were used in the nursery: a high-flow ventilation system and wall-mounted ultraviolet light serviced monthly. In spite of this highly infectious exposure, none of 514 infants available for skin testing had been infected. Adequate ventilation, coupled with the ultraviolet radiation used in the nursery, may have had significant protective value for these infants.

Good ventilation systems (including high-efficiency air filtration) and ultraviolet radiation should not create a sense of false security and are not a substitute for, but rather a supplement to, important other measures for infection control, such as surveillance of patients and staff and chemoprophylaxis of converters. Covering the mouth and nose during coughing and sneezing and the use of well-fitted masks capable of filtering particles as small as one micron have been stressed for potentially infectious individuals (Bennett and Brachman, 1979).

CHEMICAL AGENTS

The importance of adequate disinfection of various medical instruments has been stressed, and controversy concerning adequate disinfection of endoscopes, the subject of numerous articles (Working Party of the British Society of Gastroenterology, 1988; Babb, 1988; Hanson et al., 1988; Aliberti, 1987; Spector, 1987; Gerding et al., 1982), is further discussed under specific agents. The value of disinfecting agents in various housekeeping procedures, such as their application to floors in hospitals, as opposed to the use of water and detergents alone, is controversial (Spaulding, 1964b; Finegold et al., 1962).

No one disinfectant is satisfactory for all purposes. Differences in organisms likely to be encountered, the physical nature of the item to be disinfected, acceptable levels of toxicity and allergenicity, the amount of time needed for disinfection, the expense, and the accessory equipment required are all factors in choosing a disinfectant.

The mycobacteria are generally more resistant to chemical disinfection than other vegetative bacteria. The results of studies of disinfectants and their potency against mycobacteria are not conclusive. Although general agreement exists with regard to most agents, results by different workers vary. Hanson et al. (1988) state that discrepancies regarding the mycobactericidal properties of disinfectants results "from the use of different assays and an initial failure to account for important variables that influence the mycobactericidal properties of disinfectants in clinical practice."

The following is a discussion of various commonly used agents and their potency and practical uses against the mycobacteria. Recommendations for microbiologic surveillance of disinfection procedures are presented by Simmons et al. (1981).

Alcohols

Ethyl and isopropyl alcohols in high concentrations are generally accepted to be excellent mycobactericidal agents. Concentration is of considerable importance, and an aqueous solution of less than 50% of either ethyl or isopropyl shows markedly decreased activity, whereas ethanol in a concentration above 95% contains too little water to be effective (Spaulding, 1964a).

It is generally accepted that the germicidal effect of alcohols is increased when they are added to other agents, such as iodine and formaldehyde.

A distinct disadvantage of alcohols appears to be their relative inactivity in the presence of organic matter. Although earlier studies (Smith, 1947) suggested that the effect of alcohol was not reduced by sputum except "where the smears were very thick," the studies of Frobisher and Sommermeyer (1953) showed that 70% ethanol and isopropanol were not effective as disinfectants against the tubercle bacillus in sputum.

Alcohol is useful as a disinfectant for skin, thermometers, and metal instruments. It is damaging to some rubber and plastic materials and cannot be used with lensed instruments containing shellac mountings. Prior wiping or cleaning of articles contaminated with organic materials is important.

Axon et al. (1974) compared 70% ethyl alcohol with 2.5% glutaraldehyde in disinfection of endoscopes and found the former inadequate in a 10-minute soaking procedure. Cleaning of bronchoscopes with 70% alcohol and periodic ethylene oxide gas sterilization was found to be inadequate and responsible for an outbreak of pulmonary infection due to *Serratia marcescens* (Webb and Vall-Spinoza, 1975).

Babb (1988) believes that 70% alcohol is useful on items that cannot be immersed, such as electrical and x-ray equipment and external monitors.

Phenolic Compounds

Phenolic compounds for many years have been considered highly effective against *Mycobacterium tuberculosis*. Tilley et al. (1931) noted their usefulness in this regard, but also acknowledged their great disadvantages, toxicity and a strong odor that was likely to be absorbed by food and other products. These workers tested the derivative orthophenylphenol because it was found to be practically odorless. They found that a 1:200 solution of *o*-phenylphenol was "uniformly effective in mixtures containing tubercle bacilli and in the presence of a high percentage of organic matter." Klarmann et al. (1934) studied a series of homologous *p*-chlorophenol derivatives and demonstrated "remarkable" potency against several acid-fast strains tested, accompanied by a low toxicity to mice. Lester and Dunklin (1955) found a residual effect up to 30 days after an application of *o*-phenylphenol to dry surfaces (wood, wool, and cotton). Smith (1968) tested a number of phenol derivatives in his laboratory and found 20 to be more effective than *o*-phenylphenol.

More recent studies by Bergan and Lystad (1971) with various commercial products consisting of a mixture of alkylated and arylated phenolic compounds, chlorophenols, *o*-phenylphenol in various soap and alcoholic solutions concluded that the "phenolic disinfectants on the whole are more effectively tuberculocidal than are most other disinfectants."

Phenolic compounds are useful in disinfecting glassware, metal instruments, linens, wash bowls, toilets, furniture, and floors (Smith, 1968). They are stable and are not inactivated by soap or organic matter (Spaulding, 1967).

Formaldehyde

Formaldehyde is generally accepted to have good mycobactericidal activity. Smith (1968), however, reports studies in which *M. tuberculosis* was cultured from embalmed (formalin 10%) tuberculous tissues stored for as long as 1 year. In an older study, on the other hand, guinea pigs inoculated with tuberculous embalmed autopsy material (embalmed 3 months to 4 years before) did not develop tuberculosis (Meade and Steenken, 1949). Epidemiologic evidence for the spread of tuberculosis from embalmed autopsy material suggests that formalin solutions cannot be depended upon to protect individuals working with this material (Albert and Levison, 1964; Meade, 1948).

Some more recent studies have suggested the use of formaldehyde vapors in disinfection. Benn et al. (1972) used 2-hour exposure of formaldehyde vapors to sterilize all inocula of *Mycobacterium smegmatis* placed in a ventilator system. Formaldehyde solutions can be used for disinfection of certain metal objects, but the agent is generally corrosive, irritating, and toxic.

A study of an outbreak of nontuberculous mycobacterial infections in hemodialysis patients described in a previous section (Centers for Disease Control, 1983a) showed that "an *M. chelonei*-like organism" survived exposure to 2% formaldehyde for 24 hours, although none of the mycobacteria isolates survived 4% formaldehyde for 24 hours. Two percent formaldehyde solution was the concentration routinely used for disinfection of the dialyzers.

Glutaraldehyde

Unlike formaldehyde, glutaraldehyde has two active carbonyl groups, is noncorrosive, and is much less irritating. When alkalinized, a 2% aqueous solution of glutaraldehyde shows a wide range of bactericidal and sporicidal activity. Alkalinized solutions of glutaraldehyde between pH 8 to 9 show greatest bactericidal activity (Rubbo et al., 1967; Collins and Montalbine, 1976). A number of studies have shown 2% alkalinized glutaraldehyde to have considerable mycobactericidal activity (Stonehill et al., 1963; O'Brien et al., 1966; Borick et al., 1964; Snyder and Cheatle, 1965; Spaulding, 1967), and the agent is generally highly regarded in this respect. Bergan and Lystad (1971), however, were disappointed and surprised in their studies with 2% alkalinized glutaraldehyde against *Mycobacterium tuberculosis* and believed that the agent was "not adequately effective." Gorman et al. (1980) reported that a French worker, Ralyveld, found glutaraldehyde to be less effective than hypochlorite against mycobacteria. Collins and Montalbine (1976) reported variations in the activity of glutaraldehyde against different species of mycobacteria but believed the differences "not sufficiently large to be of practical importance." Pappas et al. (1983) suggested that the original source of *Mycobacterium chelonei* isolated from numerous bronchoscopy-derived specimens may have been contaminated glutaraldehyde "because *M. chelonei* is known to persist in this material." The article he cites as support for this (Laskowski et al., 1977) describes *M. chelonei* cultured from porcine heart valves packed in a 0.2% solution of glutaraldehyde at a pH of 7.4, a concentration and pH known to be nonmycobactericidal.

Glutaraldehyde does not have deleterious effects on lensed instruments and is widely regarded as an agent of choice in disinfecting endoscopes (Axon et al., 1974; Spector, 1987; Working Party of British Society of Gastroenterology, 1988; Nelson et al., 1983; Gerding et al., 1982; Babb, 1988; O'Connor and Axon, 1983; and Aliberti, 1987). It is effective in the presence of serum and protein (Borick et al., 1964) and is noncorrosive (O'Brien et al., 1966).

Hanson et al. (1988), however, stress the importance of thorough cleaning of instruments prior to disinfection with glutaraldehyde, especially if prolonged soaking is not practical. In a survey of 52 large endoscopy units in Britain, Axon and Cotton (1983) noted that "less than half were using effective disinfecting schedules." After describing a case of "almost certain" transmission of hepatitis B virus at endoscopy, Birnie et al. (1983) believed it imperative that "cleaning and sterilization of endoscopes be carried out only by staff specially trained to do these specialized tasks."

Bageant et al. (1981) studied four commercially available glutaraldehyde preparations and found wide variations in effective use-life when tested against mycobacteria (*M. smegmatis*). These workers found that the only one of the four disinfectants to perform as claimed by its manufacturer was Cidex. Cidex remained effective against *M. smegmatis* for 2 weeks.

Whereas older studies indicated glutaraldehyde to be relatively nontoxic and nonallergenic (O'Brien et al., 1966), Mallison (1979) reported skin contact with glutaraldehyde over a period of months may cause serious allergenic reactions. Stonehill et al. (1963) studied the effects of 2% glutaraldehyde on the skin and eye of rabbits showing inflammation after repeated applications.

Trigg (1984) found that 91% of hospitals surveyed used glutaraldehyde, and 55% reported reactions among staff to this agent. These included irritation of eyes and skin, sore, dry throats, and dry, itching nasal passages. Babb (1988) reports glutaraldehyde to be "highly irritant and sensitizing." Valpela et al. (1971) found that glutaraldehyde was absorbed in detectable amounts by rubber and plastic parts during disinfecting, but concluded, by virtue of their inhalation tests on mice, that the amounts absorbed "seem to constitute no danger to patients."

Iodine and Iodophors

Iodine and iodophors are considered to be effective agents against the tubercle bacillus. Knaysi (1932) and Gershenfeld (1954) showed the tuberculocidal effect of low concentrations of iodine in solution. Frobisher and Sommermeyer (1953), in their studies with clinical thermometers contaminated with tubercle bacilli, considered a 1.0% solution of iodine in 70% alcohol to be effective. Wright and Mundy (1961) found an iodophor solution (nonionic detergent with 1.6% iodine) not to be effective on thermometers contaminated with tubercle bacilli. Iodine combined with alcohol (0.2 to 0.5% and 70 to 80%, respectively) is considered to be a treatment of choice for thermometer disinfection (Taylor et al., 1966; Spaulding, 1967).

Iodine and iodophors stain fabrics and are corrosive to some materials. They are relatively nontoxic and are useful in disinfecting metal and glass instruments and as presurgical skin disinfectants (Postlethwait and Dillon, 1964).

Nelson et al. (1983) showed that several available iodophor compounds were ineffective in killing two strains of *Mycobacterium tuberculosis*, "whether they were used diluted or undiluted, even after 30 minute exposures." The authors believed that these compounds

should not be used for disinfection of fiberoptic bronchoscopes. O'Connor and Axon (1983) disagree, believing povidone-iodine to be "an effective disinfectant for endoscopic equipment."

Ethylene Oxide

Ethylene oxide is a relatively nontoxic, highly diffusible gas that is considered a good tuberculocidal agent. Kereluk et al. (1970) found the cells of *Mycobacterium phlei* to be less resistant to ethylene oxide than other nonspore-forming species tested. The gas is not injurious to most materials and is useful in disinfection of leather, fabrics, paper, plastic, wood, metals, cellophane, and rubber (Newman et al., 1955). Although treatment with this gas appears to be most satisfactory, the major disadvantage is the expense of the equipment required for its use (Sanford and Pierce, 1979). Exposure to ethylene oxide gas, 10% concentration in CO_2 at 55 to 69°C for 8 to 10 hours, is a recommended method for disinfection of dental instruments (Rowe and Brooks, 1978).

Ethylene oxide is highly regarded for use with instruments, especially fiberoptic endoscopes, that would be damaged by autoclaving (Nelson, 1983; O'Connor and Axon, 1983; Leers, 1980). The lengthy exposure time, however, is considered a major disadvantage in many busy endoscopic units (Gerding et al., 1982). Routine exposure and aeration time is 24 hours (O'Connor and Axon, 1983), and although these authors believe this to be a disadvantage, they stress that ethylene oxide is the best available treatment for endoscopes used on patients with known infection due to hepatitis B virus, tuberculosis, and typhoid fever.

Chlorine Compounds

Smith (1968) reports various studies with chlorine compounds and feels that sodium hypochlorite is a "potent mycobactericide and a good digestant of sputum and other exudate." He suggests the advantages of availability and low cost along with the disadvantages of corrosiveness, odor, bleaching action, and lack of persistence. Chlorine compounds are not recommended for disinfection of instruments and equipment (Babb, 1988).

Alkylamines

N-Dodecyl-1,3-propanediamine (referred to as diamine) was shown by Hoyt et al. (1956) to be an effective mycobactericidal disinfectant of tuberculous exudate. The addition of sodium hydroxide was found to increase the activity of this agent. Diamine was found to be nonirritating. These authors suggest various concentrations depending on suspected degree of contamination and feel the agent can be used for specimen bottles, floors, bed-frames, and laboratory surfaces. Smith (1968) believes that diamine cannot be depended upon in the presence of masses of sputum.

Miscellaneous Agents

Numerous disinfectants that are effective against other vegetative bacteria are not effective against the mycobacteria. Hexachlorophene, a bisphenol, although more or less effective against gram-positive organisms, is not effective against gram-negative organisms (Miller et al., 1962) and mycobacteria (Smith, 1951). Quaternary ammonium compounds are generally believed to be of little value as tuberculocidal agents (Spaulding, 1967), although Ritter (1956) found cetylpyridinium chloride (1:1000 in 50% ethanol) to be effective in sterilizing glass rods contaminated by *Mycobacterium tuberculosis*. Exceptions are the alkylamines, discussed separately.* Benzalkonium chloride (Zephiran) is not effective in killing tubercle bacilli in moderate concentrations, whereas even low concentrations were found to be rapidly bactericidal to other microorganisms (Hirsch, 1954). In fact, by adding this agent to culture media, the resistance of *M. tuberculosis* to Zephiran is put to advantage in the selective isolation of the organism (Patterson et al., 1956; Wayne et al., 1962).

Mercurial compounds are considered to be ineffective against the mycobacteria.

Hanson (1988) states that quaternary ammonium compounds are being used in many endoscopy units for disinfection, "although they have poor activity against viruses and mycobacteria." O'Connor and Axon (1983) agree that these compounds do not reliably disinfect endoscopes.

REFERENCES

Albert, M.E., and Levison, M.E. 1964. An epidemic of tuberculosis in a medical school. N. Engl. J. Med., 272, 718.

Aliberti, L.C. 1987. The flexible sigmoidoscope as a potential vector of infectious disease, including suggestions for decontamination of the flexible sigmoidoscope. Yale J. Biol. Med., 60, 19–26.

American Hospital Association (AHA). 1979a. Appendix E: Guidelines on tuberculosis control programs for hospital employees. In *Infection Control in the Hospital.* 4th Edition. Chicago, American Hospital Association.

American Hospital Association (AHA). 1979b. Appendix A: Guidelines on care of pulmonary tuberculosis patients in general hospitals. In *Infection Control in the Hospital.* 4th Edition. Chicago, American Hospital Association.

Axon, A.T.R., and Cotton, P.B. 1983. Endoscopy and infection. Gut, 24, 1064–1066.

Axon, A.T.R., Phillips, I., Cotton, P.B., and Avery, S.A. 1974. Disinfection of gastrointestinal fibre endoscopes. Lancet, 1(859), 656–658.

Ayliffe, G.A.J. 1988. Equipment related infection risks. J. Hosp. Infect., 11(Suppl. A), 279–284.

Babb, J.R. 1988. Methods of reprocessing complex medical equipment. J. Hosp. Infect., 11(Suppl. A), 285–291.

Bageant, R.A., et al. 1981. In-use testing of four glutaraldehyde disinfectants in the Cidematic washer. Respir. Care, 26, 1255.

Barrett, T., and Rentein, H.A. 1981. Tuberculosis infection associated with tissue processing—California. MMWR, 30, 73.

Bates, J.H. 1974. Ambulatory treatment of tuberculosis—an idea whose time is come. Am. Rev. Respir. Dis., 109, 317.

Bates, J.H., Potts, W.E., and Lewis, M. 1965. Epidemiology of primary tuberculosis in an industrial school. N. Engl. J. Med., 272, 714.

Begg, N., et al. 1986. *Mycobacterium chelonei* associated with a hospital hydrotherapy pool. Community Med., 8, 348.

Benn, R.A., Dutton, A.A., and Tully, M. 1972. Disinfection of mechanical ventilators—an investigation using formaldehyde in a cape ventilator. Anaesthesia, 27, 265.

Bennett, J.V., and Brachman, P.S. (eds.) 1979. *Hospital Infections.* Boston, Little, Brown.

Bergan, T., and Lystad, A. 1971. Antitubercular action of disinfectants. J. Appl. Bacteriol., 34, 751.

Birnie, G.G., et al. 1983. Endoscopic transmission of hepatitis B virus. Gut, 24, 171.

Borick, P.M., Dondershine, F.H., and Chandler, V.L. 1964. Alkalinized glutaraldehyde, a new antimicrobial agent. J. Pharm. Sci., 53, 1273.

Burk, J.R., et al. 1978. Nursery exposure of 528 newborns to a nurse with pulmonary tuberculosis. South. Med. J., 71, 7.

Catanzaro, A. 1982. Nosocomial tuberculosis. Am. J. Respir. Dis., 125, 559.

Centers for Disease Control. 1977. Drug-resistant tuberculosis—Mississippi. MMWR, 26, 417.

Centers for Disease Control. 1983a. Nontuberculous mycobacterial infection in hemodialysis patients—Louisiana. MMWR, 32, 244.

Centers for Disease Control. 1983b. Interstate outbreak of drug-resistant tuberculosis involving children—California, Montana, Nevada, Utah. MMWR, 32, 516.

Centers for Disease Control. 1985. Drug-resistant tuberculosis among the homeless—Boston. MMWR, 34, 429.

Centers for Disease Control. 1987a. Multi-drug-resistant tuberculosis—North Carolina. MMWR, 35, 785.

Centers for Disease Control. 1987b. Tuberculosis in minorities—United States. MMWR, 36, 77.

Centers for Disease Control. 1987c. Tuberculosis and acquired immunodeficiency syndrome—New York City. MMWR, 36, 785.

Centers for Disease Control. 1988. Tuberculosis, final data—United States, 1986. MMWR, 36, 817.

Collins, F.M., and Montalbine, V. 1976. Mycobactericidal activity of glutaraldehyde solutions. J. Clin. Microbiol., 4, 408.

Corper, H.J., and Cohn, M.L. 1933. The viability and virulence of old cultures of tubercle bacilli. Am. Rev. Tuberc., 28, 856.

Craven, R.B., Wenzel, R.P., and Nuhzet, O.A. 1975. Minimizing tuberculosis risk to hospital personnel and students exposed to unsuspected disease. Ann. Intern. Med., 82, 628.

Dandoy, S., and Elman, S. 1972. Current status of general hospital use for tuberculous patients in the United States. Am. Rev. Respir. Dis., 106, 580.

David, H.L. 1973. Response of mycobacteria to UV light radiation. Am. Rev. Respir. Dis., 108, 1175.

Editorial Notes. 1972. TB and ultraviolet irradiation. N. Am. Hosp. Assoc., 46, 45.

Edsall, J.R. 1977. Tuberculosis in a general hospital. Bull. N.Y. Acad. Med., 53, 513.

Ehrenkranz, N.J., and Kicklighter, J.L. 1972. Tuberculosis outbreak in a general hospital: evidence for airborne spread of infection. Ann. Intern. Med., 77, 377.

Fereres, J. 1988. Equipment-related infections—national policies. J. Hosp. Infect., 11(Suppl. A), 292.

Finegold, S.M., et al. 1962. Hospital floor decontamination: controlled blind studies in evaluation of germicides. Antimicrob. Agents Chemother., 250.

Frobisher, M., and Sommermeyer, L. 1953. A study of the effect of alcohols on tubercle bacilli and other bacteria in sputum. Am. Rev. Tuberc., 68, 419.

Frobisher, M., Sommermeyer, L., and Blackwell, M.J. 1953. Studies on the disinfection of clinical thermometers. Appl. Microbiol., 1, 187.

George, R.H. 1988. The prevention and control of mycobacterial infections in hospitals. J. Hosp. Infect., 11(Suppl. A), 386.

Gerding, D.N., Peterson, L.R., and Vennes, J.A. 1982. Cleaning and disinfection of fiberoptic endoscopes: evaluation of glutaraldehyde exposure time and forced-air drying. Gastroenterology, 83, 613.

Gershenfeld, L., Flagg, W., and Witlin, B. 1954. Iodine as a tuberculocidal agent. Milit. Surg., 114, 172.

Gorman, S.P., Scott, E.M., and Russell, A.D. 1980. A review. Antimicrobial activity, uses and mechanism of action of glutaraldehyde. J. App. Bacteriol., 48, 161–190.

Grange, J.M. 1987. Infection and disease due to the environmental mycobacteria. Trans. R. Soc. Trop. Med. Hyg., 81, 179.

Gunnels, J.J., and Bates, J.H. 1977. Shifting tuberculosis care to the general hospital. J. Am. Hosp. Assoc., 51, 133.

Gunnels, J.J., Bates, J.H., and Swindoll, H. 1974. Infectivity of sputum-positive tuberculosis patients in chemotherapy. Am. Rev. Respir. Dis., 109, 323.

Hanson, P.V.J., Jeffries, D.J., Batten, J.C., and Collins, J.V. 1988. Infection control revisited: dilemma facing today's bronchoscopists. Br. Med. J., 297, 185.

Hardy, M.A., and Schmidek, H.H. 1968. Epidemiology of tuberculosis aboard a ship. JAMA, 203, 109.

Heilman, K.M., and Muschenheim, C. 1965. Primary cutaneous tuberculosis resulting from mouth-to-mouth respiration. N. Engl. J. Med., 273, 1035.

Heycock, J.B., and Noble, T.C. 1961. Four cases of syringe-transmitted tuberculosis. Tubercle, 42, 25.

Hirsch, J.G. 1954. The resistance of tubercle bacilli to the bactericidal action of benzalkonium chloride (Zephiran). Am. Rev. Tuberc., 70, 312.

Houk, V.N., Baker, J.H., Sorensen, K., and Kent, D.C. 1968. The epidemiology of tuberculosis infection in a closed environment. Arch. Environ. Health, 16, 26.

Hoyt, A., Djang, A.H.K., and Smith, R.C. 1956. Tuberculosis disinfection with diamine. Public Health Rep., 71, 1097.

Huber, T.W., Reddick, R.A., and Kubica, G.P. 1970. Germicidal effect of ultraviolet irradiation on paper contaminated with mycobacteria. Appl. Microbiol., 19, 383.

Johnson, R.F., and Wildrick, K.H. 1974. "State of the Art." Review, the impact of chemotherapy on the care of patients with tuberculosis. Am. Rev. Respir. Dis., 109, 636.

Kereluk, K., Gammon, R.A., and Lloyd, R.S. 1970. Microbiological aspects of ethylene oxide sterilization—microbial resistance to ethylene oxide. Appl. Microbiol., 19, 152.

Klarmann, E., Shternov, V.A., and Gates, L.W. 1934. The bactericidal and fungicidal action of homologous halogen phenol derivatives and its quasi-specific character. J. Lab. Clin. Med., 19, 835.

Knaysi, G. 1932. The toxicity of iodine for the cells of Mycobacterium tuberculosis. J. Infect. Dis., 50, 253.

Laskowski, L.F., et al. 1977. Fastidious mycobacteria grown from porcine prosthetic-heart-valve cultures. N. Engl. J. Med., 297(2), 101–102.

Leers, W. 1980. Disinfecting endoscopes: how not to transmit mycobacterium tuberculosis by bronchoscopy. Can. Med. Assoc. J., 123, 275.

Lester, W., and Dunklin, E.W. 1955. Residual surface disinfection. J. Infect. Dis., 96, 40.

Lincoln, E.M. 1967. Epidemics of tuberculosis. Arch. Environ. Health, 14, 473.

Livingstone, H., Heidrick, F., Holicky, I., and Dack, G.M. 1941. Cross infections from anesthetic face masks. Surgery, 433.

Long, E.R. 1958. The Chemistry and Chemotherapy of Tuberculosis. 3rd Edition. Baltimore, Williams & Wilkins.

Loudon, R.G., and Spohn, S.K. 1969. Cough frequency and infectivity in patients with pulmonary tuberculosis. Am. Rev. Respir. Dis., 99, 109.

Lurie, M.B. 1947. Experimental airborne infection and its control. Am. Rev. Tuberc., 55, 124.

McClement, J.H. 1972. Chapter 14. In Bronchopulmonary Diseases and Related Disorders. Volume 1. Edited by C.W. Holman and C. Muschenheim. New York, Harper and Row.

McEuen, M. 1988. Tuberculosis—threshold of an epidemic. J. Fla. Med. Assoc., 75, 355.

McLean, R.L. 1963. How contagious is tuberculosis? N.T.A. Bull. Department of Health, Education, and Welfare. Washington, Public Health Service.

McLean, R.L. 1961. The effect of ultraviolet radiation upon the transmission of epidemic influenza in long-term hospital patients. Am. Rev. Respir. Dis., 83, 36.

Mallison, G.F. 1979. The inanimate environment. In Hospital Infections. Edited by J.V. Bennett and P.S. Brachman. Boston, Little, Brown.

Meade, G.M. 1948. The prevention of primary tuberculosis infections in medical students. Am. Rev. Tuberc., 58, 675.

Meade, G.M., and Steenken, W. 1949. Viability of tubercle bacilli in embalmed human lung tissue. Am. Rev. Tuberc., 59, 429.

Miller, J.M., Jackson, D.A., and Collier, C.S. 1962. The microbial property of pHisohex. Milit. Med., 127, 576.

Nelson, K.E., Larson, P.A., Schraufnagel, D.E., and Jackson, J. 1983. Transmission of tuberculosis by flexible fiberbronchoscopes. Am. J. Respir. Dis., 127, 97.

Newman, L.B., Colwell, C.A., and Jameson, E.L. 1955. Decontamination of articles made by tuberculosis patients in physical medicine and rehabilitation (a study using carboxide gas). Am. Rev. Tuberc., 71, 272.

Notlebart, H.C. 1980. Nosocomial infections acquired by hospital employees. Infect. Control, 1, 257.

O'Brien, H.A., et al. 1966. The use of activated glutaraldehyde as a cold sterilizing agent for urological instruments. J. Urol., 95, 429.

O'Conner, H.J., and Axon, A.T.R. 1983. Gastrointestinal endoscopy: infection and disinfection. Gut, 24, 1067.

Olsen, A.M. (committee chairman) 1967. Infectiousness of tuberculosis–a statement by the Ad Hoc Committee on the Treatment of Tuberculosis Patients in General Hospitals. Am. Rev. Respir. Dis., 96, 836.

Pappas, S.A., et al. Contamination of flexible fiberoptic bronchoscopes. Am. Rev. Respir. Dis., 127, 391.

Patterson, R.A., Thompson, T.L., and Larsen, D.H. 1956. The use of Zephiran in the isolation of M. tuberculosis. Am. Rev. Tuberc., 74, 284.

Perkins, J.E., Bahlke, A.M., and Silverman, H.F. 1947. Effect of ultraviolet irradiation of classrooms on the spread of measles in large rural central schools. Am. J. Public Health, 37, 529.

Postlethwait, R.W., and Dillon, M.L. 1964. Iodophor for presurgical skin antisepsis. Arch. Surg., 89, 462.

Report of the Committee on Infectious Diseases. 1974. American Academy of Pediatrics.

Riley, R.L. 1970. Airborne transmission. In Therapy and Control of Tuberculosis. Edited by J. Johnson, Gainesville, University of Florida Press.

Riley, R.L. 1972. The ecology of indoor atmospheres—airborne infection in hospitals. J. Chronic Dis., 25, 421.

Riley, R.L., et al. 1962. Infectiousness of air from a tuberculosis ward. Am. Rev. Respir. Dis., 85, 511.

Ritter, H.W. 1956. Germicidal effect of a quaternary ammonium compound (cetylpyridinium chloride) on M. tuberculosis. Appl. Microbiol., 4, 114.

Rowe, N.H., and Brooks, S.L. 1978. Contagion in the dental office. Dent. Clin. North Am., 22, 491.

Rubbo, S.D., Gardiner, J.F., and Webb, R.L. 1967. Biocidal activities of glutaraldehyde and related compounds. J. Appl. Bacteriol., 30, 78.

Sanford, J.P., and Pierce, A.K. 1979. Chapter 15. Lower Respiratory Infections. In Hospital Infections. Edited by J.V. Bennett and P.S. Brachman. Boston, Little, Brown.

Simmons, B.P., Hooton, T.M., and Mallison, G.F. 1981. Guidelines for hospital environmental control. Infect. Control, 2, 131.

Smith, C.R. 1942a. Survival of tubercle bacilli. Am. Rev. Tuberc., 45, 334.

Smith, C.R. 1942b. Survival of tubercle bacilli in books. Am. Rev. Tuberc., 46, 549.

Smith, C.R. 1947. Alcohol as a disinfectant against the tubercle bacillus. Public Health Rep., 62, 1285.

Smith, C.R. 1951. Disinfectants for tuberculosis hygiene. Soap Sanit. Chem., Sept–Oct., 2.

Smith, C.R. 1968. Chapter 31. In Disinfection, Sterilization and Preservation. 1st Edition. Edited by C.A. Lawrence and S.S. Block. Philadelphia, Lea & Febiger.

Snyder, R.W., and Cheatle, E. 1965. Alkaline glutaraldehyde—an effective disinfectant. Am. J. Hosp. Pharm., 22, 321.

Spaulding, E.H. 1964a. Alcohol as a surgical disinfectant. Assoc. Oper. Rm. Nurses J., 2, 67.

Spaulding, E.H. 1964b. Evaluation of hospital germicides. Soap. Chem. Specialties, 40, 71.

Spaulding, E.H. 1967. Recommendations for chemical disinfection of medical and surgical materials. Public Health Service Publication 930-C-15. Washington, Department of Health, Education, and Welfare.

Spector, G.J. 1987. Cleaning of endoscopic instruments to prevent spread of infectious disease. Laryngoscope, 97, 887.

Stead, W.W., Lofgren, J.P., Warren, E., and Thomas, C. 1985. Tuberculosis as an endemic and nosocomial infection among the elderly in nursing homes. N. Engl. J. Med., 312, 1483.

Stonehill, A.A., Krop, S., and Borick, P.M. 1963. Buffered glutaraldehyde—a new chemical sterilizing solution. Am. J. Hosp. Pharm., 20, 458.

Taylor, J.W., Smith, V.M., and Zacher, J.L. 1966. For effective thermometer disinfection. Nurs. Outlook, 14, 2.

Tilley, F.W., MacDonald, A.D., and Schaeffer, J.M. 1931. Germicidal efficiency of o-phenylphenol against Mycobacterium tuberculosis. J. Agric. Res., 42, 653.

Trigg, J.A. 1984. A sensitive issue. Nursing Mirror (N.A.T.N. Suppl.), 6.

Valpela, E., Otterstrom, S., and Hackman, R. 1971. Liberation of alkalinized glutaraldehyde by respirators after cold sterilization. Acta Anaesthesiol. Scand., 15, 291.

Wayne, L.G., Krasnow, I., and Kidd, G. 1962. Finding the "hidden positive" in tuberculosis eradication programs. Am. Rev. Respir. Dis., 86, 537.

Webb, S.F., and Vall-Spinoza, A. 1975. Outbreak of Serratia marcescens associated with the flexible fiberbronchoscope. Chest, 68, 703.

Wells, W.F., Ratcliff, H.L., and Crumb. C. 1948. On the mechanics of droplet nuclei infection. II. Quantitative experimental airborne tuberculosis in rabbits. Am. J. Hyg., 47, 11.

Welty, C., Burstin, S., Muspratt, S., and Tager, I.B. 1985. Epidemiology of tuberculosis infection in a chronic care population. Am. Rev. Respir. Dis., 132, 133.

Working Party of the British Society of Gastroenterology. 1988. Cleaning and disinfection of equipment for gastrointestinal flexible endoscopy: interim recommendations of a working party of the British Society of Gastroenterology. Gut, 29, 1134.

Wright, E.S., and Mundy, R.A. 1961. Studies on disinfection of clinical thermometers. II. Oral thermometers from a tuberculosis sanatorium. Appl. Microbiol., 9, 508.

Young, L.S. 1988. Mycobacterium avium complex infection. J. Infect. Dis., 157, 863.

CHAPTER 24

FUNGISTATIC AND FUNGICIDAL COMPOUNDS FOR HUMAN PATHOGENS

Ernest M. Walker, Jr. and Glen R. Gale

Fungi make up a diverse group of microorganisms occupying a position intermediate between that of bacteria on the one hand and protozoa on the other. They are eukaryotic, contain mitochondria, are devoid of chlorophyll, and are totally dependent upon external carbon sources for growth and replication. They can live as saprophytes on nonliving organic matter, either natural or synthetic, or as parasites on or in the living cells of plants, animals, and man. The vegetative fungus body, the thallus, is totally undifferentiated and forms a plectenchymatic aggregate of cells in culture. Hyphae of the vegetative mycelium penetrate the growth medium and absorb nutrients. Aerial mycelia bear reproductive structures in the form of motile or nonmotile spores; however, a minute fragment of mycelium can initiate new growth containing all the inherent organic material of the parent colony.

Microscopically, fungi grow on agar or in broth as discrete cells (yeasts) or as multinucleated filaments (molds). These later forms typically possess septa, or cross-walls, which confer compartmentalization, but these structures are absent in the Phycomycetes (e.g., species of *Mucor* and *Rhizopus*). Certain fungi, including some human pathogens, are dimorphic and can grow as yeasts or molds, depending upon cultural conditions. Both forms of pathogenic fungi can cause serious mycoses in man (e.g., *Coccidioides immitis, Blastomyces dermatitidis, Paracoccidioides brasiliensis, Histoplasma capsulatum*). Observation with the light microscope usually yields sufficient information to allow an approximation of the classification of a given fungus when considered along with gross growth characteristics of the organism, although examination with the electron microscope of appropriately fixed, sectioned, and stained specimens is necessary to visualize the nuclear and cytoplasmic membranes, mitochondria, vacuoles, and ribosomes. The cytoplasmic membrane of the yeast and mycelial forms of fungi is surrounded by a rigid cell wall that determines cell morphology and confers mechanical strength to constrain the osmotically labile protoplast. This cell wall is typically composed of complex insoluble, crystalline polysaccharides such as beta-glucans, cellulose, and chitin. These are usually bonded together with amorphous heteropolysaccharides and proteins that have been identified as the immunodeterminant groups of cell wall antigens.

Although the emphasis in this chapter is on those agents active against fungi that are important human pathogens, a number of fungi pathogenic to plants have had devastating effects worldwide. Perhaps the most notable of these were the epiphytotics of late blight in potatoes in 1843 to 1845 in northern Europe and the British Isles. The destruction of the potato crop was so extensive that in Ireland alone approximately a quarter of a million persons died of famine. Other fungal diseases of plants that have had large economic impacts include tobacco downy mildew, wheat rusts, chestnut blight, and blister rust of white pines; the various leaf spots of beets, soybeans, and tomatoes; and a number of Deuteromycete infections involving peas, cotton, watermelons, beans, corn, barley, cabbage, and celery. Of unique significance were the outbreaks of downy mildew on grapes in Europe, especially in the vineyards of France and Italy. The causal fungus, *Plasmopora viticola*, indigenous to the United States, had been introduced into Europe in 1878. To prevent pilfering of his grapes, a grower sprinkled his vines with a mixture of lime and copper sulfate. The subsequent observation that the grapes so treated remained free from downy mildew led to the development of Bordeaux mixture, once proclaimed as the world's best-known fungicide. Contemporary agricultural antifungal agents are described elsewhere in this book.

Medical mycology as a distinct discipline may be said to have begun with Schoenlein, who in 1839 implicated a fungus in the lesions of flavus, a form of ringworm characterized by depilation and formation of yellow crusts composed of small, cup-like scales. The organism was assigned the binomial *Achorion schoenleini* a few years later, but the generic name *Trichophyton* was subsequently applied. The suppurative form of ringworm known as kerion was shown in 1856 to be induced by *Trichophyton* originating from animals, and further work demonstrated that ringworm could be transmitted to man from horse, cow, dog, or cat. A period of relative inactivity ensued until Sabouraud began his studies in the last decade of the nineteenth century. The early decades of the twentieth century were a period of rapid development of medical mycology as a recognized component of medical microbiology, with documentation of the natural history and pathogenesis of each of the major deep-seated mycoses, along with detailed descriptions of the causative microorganisms. In more recent decades, it has been recognized that many of the fungi once characterized as harmless saprophytes (e.g., species of *Aspergillus, Mucor, Rhizopus, Absidia, Cryptococcus,* and *Candida*) are indeed capable, given the appropriate opportunities presented by a compromised host, of causing a variety of serious and often fatal infections in man.

The history of the development of pharmacologic treatment of fungus infections can be followed by reference to selected major pharmacology textbooks published over the past 40 years. Krantz and Carr's *Pharmacological Principles of Medical Practice,* published in 1949, was devoid of any allusion to fungi or antifungal agents. The second edition (1956) of Goodman and Gilman's *Pharmacological Basis of Therapeutics* devoted part of a chapter to descriptions of fungicidal fatty acids—propionic, caprylic, and undecylenic—in treatment of superficial dermatophyte infections, the use of Bordeaux mixture as a plant fungicide, and the salutary actions of sulfur in the treatment of ringworm infections. The next few years were extraordinary in that, for the first time, rational treatment of both deep systemic mycoses and disseminated dermatophytic infections became a reality. For example, in the mid-1960s *Drill's Pharmacology in Medicine,* in addition to giving brief mention of Whitfield's ointment, resorcinol, salicylic acid, selenium sulfide, gentian violet, hydroxyquinoline, and potassium iodide, described in detail the pharmacologic properties of hydroxystilbamidine, amphotericin B, nystatin, and griseofulvin (Hildick-Smith, 1965). Since that time the major advances have been the development of tolnaftate, ciclopirox olamine, haloprogin, and certain imidazoles (miconazole, clotrimazole, and econazole) as antidermatophytic agents (Harvey, 1985), and flucytosine and ketoconazole for the treatment of certain systemic mycoses (Sande and Mandell, 1985).

In this chapter we present a brief description of the fungi pathogenic to humans, those that are considered opportunistic, and the pathogenic actinomycetes. Primary emphasis is on clinical characteristics, gross and microscopic morphology, and epidemiology. For detailed descriptions of antigenic structure, immunity, and laboratory diagnosis, the reader is referred to one of the major texts (e.g., Braude, 1986). The drugs currently used in treatment of the various infections are presented in detail. For information on older drugs or those of limited clinical utility, the reader is referred to the corresponding chapter in the previous edition of this work (Oster and Woodside, 1983).

DERMATOPHYTES AND DERMATOMYCOSES

The dermatophytes are a group of closely related fungi that parasitize the superficial keratinized layers of the body: skin, hair, and nails. They only rarely invade subcutaneous tissues. Infections caused by these organisms are called *tinea* infections, which, from the Latin, literally means "gnawing worm." The term ringworm has persisted as a lay designation. Although infections with dermatophytes are not associated with mortality, such conditions are cosmetically disfiguring and can cause much discomfort from severe itching, which accompanies involvement of all areas except the nails. The major causative organisms are species of *Trichophyton* and *Microsporum,* as well as one species of *Epidermophyton.* Table 24–1 shows the organisms most commonly associated with infections of specific anatomic sites. Over 30 species have been identified as etiologic (Ajello, 1968).

Clinical appearance of infection varies with the site involved. In tinea pedis (athlete's foot), intensely itching vesicles develop between the toes or on the dorsal, plantar, or lateral aspects of the feet. Spontaneous healing seldom occurs, but symptoms may be reduced by going barefoot or by wearing sandals without socks. Secondary infections with bacteria can lead to lymphadenitis and lymphangitis. Some persons infected with species of *Trichophyton* become extremely sensitive to the fungus and have distant, sterile vesicular lesions, particularly on the palms of the hands. These are called dermatophytids, or simply ids. Lesions of tinea cruris show a well-demarcated, scaling border. The advancing inflammatory margin is the site of the most intense itching. In severe childhood tinea capitis, in which the scalp and scalp hair are involved, alopecia is often widespread as a consequence of hair breakage and involvement of follicles. Dermatophyte infection of the nails may involve any fingernail, but particularly the big toenails. One sees marked discoloration and distortion of nail growth. The nail is usually brittle and breaks erratically upon trimming. This type of infection is particularly distressing to women who wear open-toed sandals.

Presumptive diagnosis of tinea infections is usually made on the basis of the appearance of the lesions and the presence of itching. Microscopic examination of hair or skin scrapings in a 10% KOH solution reveals clear outlines of branching filaments. Identification of the causative organisms is based upon gross cultural characteristics and microscopic morphology of the fungus after growth on Sabouraud agar. Dermatophytes grow slowly at room temperature and form colonies of various colorations. Microscopic visualization of conidiophores

Table 24–1. *Dermatomycoses: Anatomic Sites and Usual Causative Fungi*

Designation	Anatomic Site	Microorganism
Tinea capitis	Scalp and hair	*Trichophyton schoenleini, T. violaceum, T. tonsurans, Microsporum canis,* or *M. audouini*
Tinea glabrosa (Tinea corporis)	Glabrous body skin	*M. audouini, M. canis,* or *T. mentagrophytes*
Tinea barbae	Bearded region of face	*T. mentagrophytes, T. verrucosum,* or *M. gypseum*
Tinea unguium (Onychomycosis)	Nails	*T. rubrum* or *T. mentagrophytes*
Tinea cruris (Jock itch)	Inguinal region	*T. rubrum, T. mentagrophytes,* or *Epidermophyton floccosum*
Tinea pedis (Athlete's foot)	Feet	*T. mentagrophytes* or *T. rubrum*

and macroconidia usually allows species identification. Because all dermatophytes typically respond in a similar fashion to antimycotic agents, initiation of treatment need not be delayed until the genus and species are identified.

Transmission of dermatophytes occurs from animals to man and from man to man. This is the only group of pathogenic fungi transmitted from man to man. Various species can be recovered from used shoes, common shower facilities, and swimming pool areas, and some have been isolated directly from soil.

SYSTEMIC MYCOSES

Diseases caused by fungi that invade various organs and tissues of otherwise healthy individuals and cause severe morbidity and often a high rate of mortality are referred to as systemic mycoses. These infections are not transferred from man to man or from animals to man, but animals may be concomitantly infected from a natural source. The portal of entry is usually the respiratory tract, except for the fungus causing sporotrichosis, which is usually introduced into the subcutaneous tissues by accidental inoculation. Fungi causing four of these infections have unique geographic distributions; travelers from nonendemic areas may be at higher risk than the native population for development of disease. Some degree of acquired resistance probably develops through acquisition of subclinical infections and spontaneous resolution in the native population. Investigators who work with these organisms in a laboratory setting or with experimentally infected animals should be fully cognizant of the biohazard levels assigned to each organism and should undertake no experimental manipulations unless the appropriate degree of biologic containment can be achieved.

Blastomyces dermatitidis

This fungus is the etiologic agent of blastomycosis. Although this infection was once referred to as North American blastomycosis to distinguish it from a disease in South America caused by a related organism, cases have now been reported from Europe and Africa. Nonetheless, most cases originate in the Mississippi and Ohio Valleys, along the Appalachian Mountain chain from the middle Atlantic states to the Carolinas, in the southeastern Piedmont region, and in the areas surrounding the Great Lakes.

Following entry of the organism through the respiratory tract, a relatively rare form of pulmonary blastomycosis that is benign and resolves without treatment may ensue. In typical progressive blastomycosis, however, the onset is insidious and usually mimics a "chest cold," with low-grade fever, weight loss, and progressive lethargy. Pneumonia, usually of a cavitary nature, may involve any segment of the lung. Progressive disease is characterized by chest pain, production of purulent and hemorrhagic sputum, and dyspnea. Metastatic extrapulmonary lesions occur in bones, skin, and various viscera. Skin lesions are initially nodular, but progress to extensive ulcerations. The prostate, testes, and brain can also be involved. About 90% of untreated cases terminate fatally, with survival varying from 6 months to about 2 years from the onset of symptoms.

In tissues and on appropriate laboratory media at 37°C, the dimorphic organism grows in a budding yeast form, but grows as a mold in culture at room temperature. The yeast cells are about 9 to 16 μm in diameter and often have a single bud with a large connecting pore. The cell wall is thick and refractile. The thick wall with the wide pore connecting the adjacent single bud is characteristic among the fungal pathogens. Mycelial phase cultures on Sabouraud agar are almost white when young, but become buff colored with a yellow-brown underside. Gross morphology is floccose or glabrous and may be smooth or furrowed. The septate hyphae bear pyriform conidia on lateral or terminal branches. A presumptive diagnosis of blastomycosis can usually be made by microscopic observation of yeast cells in clinical materials such as sputum or biopsy sections. Yeast cells are stained black with methenamine silver. Diagnosis is confirmed by the typical appearance of the yeast phase culture on brain-heart infusion broth agar at 37°C. Cultures at room temperature should be incubated for at least 3 weeks, but growth often occurs within 1 week.

Soil is the probable source of *B. dermatitidis*, although it has seldom been cultured directly from suspected areas. The disease occurs primarily in rural inhabitants who have close contact with soil, however, and there is a report of one epidemic in northern Minnesota involving members of several families after they cleared a large area of wooded undergrowth (Tosh et al., 1974). The disease can occur in dogs, but dog-to-man transfer is not thought to occur. Bird droppings are a probable source of infection following inhalation of conidia from the mycelial phase of the fungus.

Paracoccidioides brasiliensis

Paracoccidioidomycosis, caused by *Paracoccidioides brasiliensis*, is a chronic granulomatous infection of a number of organs. The disease has been described in South America, Costa Rica, Guatemala, Honduras, and Mexico, with the greatest number of cases reported from Brazil. Cases reported outside Latin America have invariably been patients who at one time lived in an endemic region. The initial infection occurs primarily in young rural inhabitants, whereas most cases of the progressive form of the disease are seen in patients between the ages of 30 and 50. The disease is about 15 times as prevalent in males as in females.

The fungus enters the body by way of the respiratory tract and initially invades the pulmonary lymph nodes. These initial lesions are typically quiescent until the third to fifth decade of life, when recrudescence may occur spontaneously or through the influence of disease-induced or iatrogenic immunosuppression. Reactivation of the lesions leads to progressive pulmonary infection as well as hematogenous dissemination to other organs. The mucocutaneous areas are most frequently involved, with ulcerations and granuloma formation. Other organs frequently affected are the skin, spleen, adrenal glands, intestine, and liver.

In highly endemic areas, a variation of the disease may occur that has been termed the acute juvenile form. Almost all organs are involved, but most of the symptoms are referred to the gastrointestinal tract. This form of the disease often presents a perplexing differential diagnosis in view of the multiple organ involvement.

When examined in a 10% KOH smear, exudates of active lesions frequently show the typical yeast form of the dimorphic fungus. The cells are relatively large, ranging from 10 to about 40 μm in diameter, and appear to possess a double wall. The presence of multiple buds on a single cell is characteristic. Materials such as pus, spu-

tum, or biopsy aspirates should be cultured on Mycosel agar at both 25 and 35°C. Inoculation of sputum and feces intratesticularly into guinea pigs often yields large numbers of organisms when pus from these lesions is cultured. In the mycelial phase at 25°C, the organism is indistinguishable from *Blastomyces dermatitidis*. Unequivocal diagnosis depends upon microscopic observation of the multiple budding yeast cells from growth at 37°C after about 5 days of incubation.

There is no evidence of man-to-man transmission of paracoccidioidomycosis. Because the disease occurs primarily in males from rural areas, it is assumed that acquisition is from some source in nature that has not yet been identified. No evidence indicates that bird or bat manure is a natural reservoir.

Coccidioides immitis

Coccidioides immitis, the etiologic agent of coccidioidomycosis, is a dimorphic soil fungus normally found in the highly restricted geographic areas (Lower Sonoran Life Zone) of the southwestern United States, contiguous regions of northern Mexico, specific areas of Central America, and Argentina and other specific areas of South America (Zinsser, 1988; Kirkland, 1986). The mycelia, found several inches below the surface of the alkaline soil of high salinity in endemic regions of semiarid climate, are brought to the soil surface after spring rains. The subsequent hot and dry climate converts mycelia into infectious arthroconidia; this explains the summer peak rates of infection (Zinsser, 1988) following inhalation of the airborne arthroconidia by man and animals. The risk of infection is particularly high among construction workers or others who disrupt the soil in endemic areas. Severe windstorms may spread infected soil to regions nonendemic for the disease (Zinsser, 1988; Kirkland, 1986).

Inhaled arthroconidia develop within the lungs into thick-walled 30- to 60-μm spherules; these spherules may contain hundreds of 2- to 5-μm endospores, each of which may be released when the parent spherule ruptures and form additional mature spherules. The spherules, as well as hyphae, may be found in the host tissue. In most cases, the inhaled infectious arthroconidia produce primary coccidioidomycosis, which is asymptomatic or mild without complications. In a few cases hematogenous dissemination may occur and may be fulminant or chronic, with periods of remission or exacerbation (Zinsser, 1988). Extrapulmonary dissemination may lead to a generalized systemic infection of most tissues and organs, most often the meninges, skin, and bone. Arthroconidia and spherules are engulfed by phagocytes, but early in most infections are resistant to phagocytic destruction and replicate freely within these cells. In most cases, an acquired immunity develops, cell-mediated immunity improves, and phagosomes are activated to kill ingested fungi. In a minority of cases, cell-mediated immunity is defective, delayed, or absent, so the infection may persist or disseminate from the lungs to other tissues or organs (Kirkland, 1986). Dissemination is more likely in immunocompromised individuals or in those receiving immunosuppressive drugs or agents. It is more common in men, older people, and in the third trimester of pregnancy, possibly because of a stimulation in the in vivo growth of the fungus by high levels of circulating steroid hormones. Dissemination to the central nervous system is associated with an almost 100% mortality rate in untreated patients.

Skin tests are available for coccidioidomycosis, and they usually become positive within 2 weeks of the appearance of symptoms and remain positive for a lifetime in over 90% of those who have been infected (presence of F and/or HL bands) (Zinsser, 1988).

Transmission among humans and animals is unusual (Zinsser, 1988), and the few cases developing may result from animal bites, accidental percutaneous inoculations of research or laboratory personnel working with the organism, or contact with the mycelial phase in body fluids (Zinsser, 1988; Kirkland, 1986). The spherule and its endospores released from lesions appear to be killed by the external environment, so the disease is not contagious, and isolation procedures of infected patients are not necessary (Kirkland, 1986).

Colonies grown at room temperature on Sabouraud agar are white, gray, or brown, with a powdery, woolly, or cottony texture. Dry cultures contain numerous infective arthroconidia that can be aerosolized, easily creating a hazard for laboratory workers who should be protected by the use of safety hoods and other laboratory precautions. The production of arthroconidia in hyphae is the diagnostic feature of these cultures, along with the presence of spherules or endospores in sputum, exudate, or tissue specimens stained by PAS and silver stains and delayed hypersensitivity responses to coccidioidin or other *C. immitis* antigens (Zinsser, 1988; Kirkland, 1986). Serologic tests are useful for detecting antibodies to the TP, HL, or F (CF) exoantigens of *C. immitis* (Zinsser, 1988; Kirkland, 1986).

Histoplasma capsulatum

Histoplasma capsulatum is the causative agent of histoplasmosis (Starling's disease), the most common pulmonary mycosis of humans and animals. This thermally dimorphic soil fungus grows as a white or brown mold at temperatures below 35°C and as a budding yeast at 37°C (Zinsser, 1988). The mold form below 35°C has both single, 1- to 5-μm microconidia on each short conidiophore and tuberculate, mature, thick-walled, spheric macroconidia with projections radiating from their cell walls (Zinsser, 1988). At 37°C, hyphal cells or microconidia may convert to budding yeast cells, as found in the tissues of infected hosts. Irreversible inhibition of this conversion at 37°C is prevented by *p*-chlormercuriphenylsulfonic acid (PCMS), a sulfhydryl blocking agent, while mycelial growth is allowed to continue (Zinsser, 1988). Microconidia in dried mold cultures may be dislodged by air currents, and the aerosols produced may be important in disease transmission.

H. capsulatum grows in soil having a high nitrogen content, especially in regions of avian or bat habitats. Soils from various areas of the world contain different concentrations of the organism, with a high prevalence in the Ohio-Mississippi Valley, an area having a large population of starlings (Zinsser, 1988; Sarosi and Davies, 1986; Rippon, 1988), which tend to roost together in large numbers. The organism survives best in moist nitrogenous soil at 37°C or less. As soil temperature increases, the vegetative forms and then the microconidia are destroyed, so only the macroconidia survive for any appreciable time at 40°C or higher.

Airborne microconidia are inhaled and reach the alveoli of the lungs where they develop into budding yeasts that may be phagocytized by alveolar macrophages (Zinsser, 1988; Sarosi and Davies, 1986; Rippon, 1988). The disease may localize in the lung or may spread by the hematogeneous or lymphatic system (Zinsser, 1988). Classic tissue response begins as an infiltrate of neutrophils and lymphocytes, but eventually evolves to the formation of epithelioid cell granulomas with concentric rings of fibrosis and calcification (Zinsser, 1988; Sarosi and Davies, 1986; Rippon, 1988). Patients with acute pulmonary histoplasmosis may initially have a mild, flu-like illness that is self-limited and resolves, or they may progress to moderate-to-severe disease. Chronic cavitary pulmonary histoplasmosis is most often seen in adult male long-term smokers who have underlying chronic obstructive lung disease with emphysema, especially men beyond the fifth decade of life. It is commonly associated with tuberculosis or bronchogenic carcinoma. In disseminated histoplasmosis, the yeast cells may spread throughout the body inside macrophages unable to destroy them. Total acute progressive histoplasmosis may occur in patients with compromised cell-mediated immunity such as AIDS patients, patients receiving immunosuppressive drugs, or patients with neoplasms associated with immune deficiencies (Zinsser, 1988; Sarosi and Davies, 1986; Rippon, 1988). Primary cutaneous histoplasmosis is rare and is associated with wound contamination, animal bites, or accidental percutaneous inoculation of research or laboratory personnel.

About 40 million people in the United States are estimated to have been exposed to *H. capsulatum*, with 500,000 new infections each year. From 10 to 40% are symptomatic, and about 100 deaths occur among approximately 4000 associated hospitalizations annually (Zinsser, 1988; Sarosi and Davies, 1986; Rippon, 1988).

The laboratory diagnosis is not always easy. It includes the finding of *H. capsulatum* yeasts in clinical body fluids or tissues, yeast-laden macrophages in blood buffy coats, or bone marrow with samples fixed with methanol and stained with Wright or Giemsa stains. Cultures of *H. capsulatum* may require up to 12 weeks to mature into the usual sporulating mold with characteristic macroconidia.

Conversion of the organism to the yeast form is encouraged by use of an enriched medium such as brain-heart infusion agar with 5% sheep blood without cycloheximide at 37°C (Zinsser, 1988). Skin testing with histoplasmin is of limited value in most patients unless a recent conversion of seronegativity to seropositivity has occurred (Zinsser, 1988; Sarosi and Davies, 1986; Rippon, 1988). Two available serologic tests, the measurement of complement-fixation (CF) antibodies and the immunodiffusion (ID) test for precipitins, are often of value in the diagnosis and prognosis of histoplasmosis (Zinsser, 1988; Sarosi and Davies, 1986; Rippon, 1988).

Sporothrix schenckii

This organism of worldwide distribution lives as a saprophyte on vegetation and a variety of other materials and is introduced into any part of the body upon traumatic contact. The areas initially affected most frequently are the hands, arms, feet, and legs. From 2 to 10 months after the injury, the fungus produces a reddish-purple nodule at the injured site; this has been termed the sporotrichotic chancre. The infection occasionally remains fixed at the original site, possibly because of acquired immunity from previous contact. More typically, the fungus spreads along lymphatics from the chancre, producing a "cord" of nodular lesions. This form of the disease usually causes no pain, fever, or related symptoms.

Disseminated sporotrichosis may take various forms. In one, multiple red skin nodules may occur anywhere, accompanied by bone and joint lesions. Symptoms are suggestive of arthritis. Some patients develop deep abscesses of the striated muscles. Mucous membranes may be invaded, producing ulcerations, suppurating nodules, and regional lymphadenopathy. Invasion of the bone may result in bone destruction, with draining sinuses from bone through the skin. Evidence indicates that strains of *S. schenckii* involved in this type of disseminated disease are more thermotolerant than those isolated from fixed lesions (Kwon-Chung, 1979).

Another type of dissemination occurs as a single metastatic focus that involves a joint, the orbit, bone, or genitourinary tract. Because contiguous skin lesions are not present, spread is assumed to be by the hematogenous route.

Some evidence indicates that some cases of disseminated sporotrichosis may have an opportunistic component. In one study of four patients with multifocal systemic sporotrichosis, underlying disease was present: alcoholism, Hodgkin's disease, or multiple myeloma (Lynch et al., 1970). Those authors reviewed the literature describing this form of disseminated multifocal disease and suggested a new classification that would recognize the opportunistic aspect of the infection in immunocompromised patients.

Microscopic examination of smears of pus or sputum seldom shows the yeast phase of the dimorphic fungus, but occasionally cells are abundant. Cultural isolation is usually accomplished by aspiration of pus from a closed nodule or ulcer and plating this on Sabouraud agar for incubation at room temperature. Early mycelial growth is cream colored and resembles bacterial colonies. This is followed by wrinkling and development of a brown-to-black coloration. Thin septate hyphae with hyaline conidia are seen microscopically. When the fungus is grown at 37°C under CO_2 on a blood agar base, yeast-like creamy colonies that resemble bacterial colonies appear. Microscopically, the yeast-like cells from culture are ovoid to globose to elongate and measure 2.5 to 5.0 by 3.5 to 6.5 μm. Inoculation of pus from a lesion into mice results in growth of the yeast form in the peritoneal cavity or testicles. These appear as gram-positive, cigar-shaped rods within polymorphonuclear leukocytes. Growth is rapid, permitting prompt differentiation from other chronic subcutaneous infections.

S. schenckii has been recovered from many sources in nature throughout the world. Most cases occur following a penetrating injury from a thorn or splinter. Sphagnum moss is a major source of infection. Primary pulmonary infection occasionally occurs after inhalation of the fungus. The ubiquitous nature of the organism mandates precautions to be taken by persons at high risk by virtue of outdoor vocations or avocations, coupled with awareness of development of primary lesions secondary to traumatic injuries incurred in pursuit of these activities.

OPPORTUNISTIC YEASTS AND FUNGI

A number of fungi and yeasts that usually exist as either saprophytes in the environment or as innocuous cohabitants of the body's microflora can cause debilitating disease and death under certain predisposing conditions. Although these predisposing circumstances are usually referred to as immunodeficiencies, they actually include endocrinopathies, neoplastic and hematological diseases, organ transplantation with its attendant immunosuppressive treatment, antimicrobial antibiotic administration, corticosteroid therapy, antineoplastic chemotherapy, infancy, pregnancy, and AIDS. Virtually any organ and system can be affected. Because these infections are secondary processes, they either may have no influence on the primary disease process or may aggravate it. In many cases these mycotic overgrowths become the predominant disease and overshadow the significance of the underlying pathologic process. Unlike the systemic fungus infections acquired by otherwise healthy individuals that usually run a chronic course, certain opportunistic infections can run a rampant, fulminating course and cause death within a few days of the onset of signs and symptoms. In certain infections of this type, an unequivocal deficiency in cell-mediated (T lymphocyte) immunity can be demonstrated and is presumed to represent the underlying deficit. In other cases, a clinically predisposing condition such as diabetic acidosis is often associated with the infection, but the mechanism by which these metabolic changes favor invasion by the fungus has not been fully clarified. Constant surveillance of individuals known to be at risk is mandatory to detect the onset of these infections as early as possible.

The number of microorganisms implicated as etiologic in opportunistic infections is increasing constantly. In this section, we present descriptions of four types of infection in which fungi once considered to be harmless can have devastating effects on the compromised host. We hope that this discussion will serve to acquaint the reader with the wide spectrum of invasion patterns that these organisms may display, as well as the consequences of the ensuing infections if aggressive treatment is not instituted in a timely fashion.

Mucormycosis

Mucormycosis is the term applied to invasion by any of the three genera of fungi known as *Mucor, Rhizopus,* or *Absidia* within the order Mucorales. The cerebral form of the disease was first described in 1943 (Gregory et al., 1943) and the pulmonary form in 1948 (see Baker, 1957). Bauer et al. (1955) reviewed the literature and presented 2 new cases in patients who had episodes of diabetic acidosis, one of which was the first antemortem diagnosis of this infection. Baker (1957) subsequently reviewed 13 cases and described 2 additional cases. Berk et al. (1961) described the typical rhinomucormycosis that occurs primarily in leukemic patients and in patients with poorly controlled diabetes. Various other forms of the disease have now been reported, including infections of the head and neck (nasal, rhino-orbital, or rhinocerebral), bronchopulmonary tree, and digestive tract. Focal infections may also occur in the kidney, spleen, or liver. Acute suppurative superficial lesions may be present, in addition to chronic ulcers and granulomas.

A typical case of rhinomucormycosis as it occurs in a poorly controlled diabetic with acidosis, with or without ketosis, serves to demonstrate the acute course of infection. Initially, the patient typically has orbital pain and proptosis, associated with swelling and induration of the periorbital tissues. Mucopus and bloody crusting are noted in the ipsilateral nasal cavity. The fungus then extends via the blood vessels to the internal carotid artery, cavernous sinus, meninges, and brain. Without treatment, death usually occurs within 1 week. Regulation of the diabetic acidosis alone seldom retards progression of disease. At autopsy, cerebral vessels contain numerous thrombi with hyphal elements. The dura may be roughened and adherent to the meninges of the frontal lobe, and the underlying bone may be necrotic. There may be pulmonary involvement through hematogenous spread, but some cases of the primary pulmonary form have been described. The organism penetrates the walls of bronchi in the primary form of the disease, after which it invades the pulmonary artery and vein and causes thrombosis, resulting in pulmonary infarction.

The three important pathogenic organisms in the order Mucorales are *Mucor, Rhizopus,* and *Absidia.* They grow rapidly on Sabouraud agar, producing a woolly appearance that varies from white to gray. The fluffy growth represents aerial hyphae that are nonseptate, with the mass resembling one enormous branching, multinucleate cell. The mycelia bear conidiophores, which in turn bear sporangia filled with asexual spores. In *Rhizopus* and *Absidia,* other specialized branches of the hyphae bear stolons or "runners." The stolons produce the rhizoids that firmly anchor the growth to the underlying substrate. *Mucor* is devoid of stolons and rhizoids and thus is less firmly bound to the grown medium. Biopsy or autopsy sections of infected tissues show typical nonseptate hyphal elements in, for example, nerves of the cavernous sinus, the wall of the internal carotid artery, and lung tissue, where they stain intensely with silver stain. Thrombi within vessels are usually rich in such elements. Species identification cannot be made from such preparations, but the organisms grow rapidly when subcultured on common fungal media.

All the fungi that produce mucormycosis are ubiquitous in soil and dust and are invariably found on bread and fruit. They are not considered to be part of the normal human microflora, although inhalation of airborne spores is substantially unavoidable. Nosocomial infections have occurred in association with or as a consequence of progress in management of seriously ill patients, and these hospital-acquired infections have been attributed to airborne spores as well as to contact with contaminated items such as surgical dressings (Walsh and Pizzo, 1988).

Aspergillosis

Aspergillosis is an infection caused by several of the many members of the genus *Aspergillus,* most frequently *A. fumigatus.* Other species that may be etiologic include *A. niger, A. clavatus,* and *A. flavus.* Although uncompromised hosts can develop local skin infections with *Aspergillus,* such as external otitis, the most serious forms of the disease are seen in patients with underlying pathologic processes. Virtually any organ may be affected.

Allergic bronchopulmonary aspergillosis, which occurs in some asthmatics, is characterized by dilated bronchi containing fungal elements embedded in mucus. No invasion of the bronchial wall occurs, but some of the smaller bronchioles are obliterated by granulation tissue, and the alveoli show eosinophilic pneumonia. An arthustype of reaction from antigens in the fungal hyphae may be partially responsible for damage to bronchi. A *colonizing type of aspergillosis* may occur in patients with preexisting pulmonary cavities secondary to tuberculosis, carcinoma, or bronchiectasis. Radiologic evidence of thickening of the cavity wall and a distinctive fungus ball composed of masses of hyphae are present. In *chronic necrotizing pulmonary aspergillosis,* the fungus causes progressive tissue destruction with upper-lobe fibrocavitary disease. There is usually a concomitant centrilobular emphysema, malnutrition, or diabetes mellitus, but patients are not deeply immunosuppressed. *Invasive aspergillosis* occurs in profoundly immunosuppressed patients and can affect almost any organ. Multiple areas of bronchopneumonia occur when invasion of blood vessels leads to thrombi and infarction. Metastatic spread occurs to the brain, liver, and heart. *Aspergillus endocarditis* as an occasional consequence of cardiac surgery is characterized by large, friable lesions that can be disseminated hematogenously and produce distant emboli in critical arteries. Invasive pulmonary aspergillosis almost always involves A. fumigatus, whereas the allergic bronchopulmonary form may be caused by A. flavus, A. niger, A. fumigatus, and probably other species. Pulmonary aspergillomas typically are composed of A. fumigatus or A. niger, whereas the widely disseminated form is usually caused by A. fumigatus or A. flavus.

Species of Aspergillus are septate fungi of the class Hyphomycetes. A differentiated section of hypha, the foot cell, gives rise to a conidiophore bearing a terminal vesicle. The sterigmata are arrayed peripherally around the vesicle and bear the chains of conidia, or spores. The overall appearance of this structure is strikingly similar to that of the aspergillum, a short-handled brush used for sprinkling holy water. All species grow readily at room temperature on Sabouraud agar and frequently appear as contaminants in specimens from patients not infected with the fungus. In contrast, sputum from patients with pulmonary aspergilloma or blood from patients with disseminated aspergillosis seldom yields positive cultures. Biopsy of invaded tissue is most likely to be effective in isolating the causative organisms, yielding material that grows readily when cultured. Histologic examination of the tissue shows the organism after staining with hematoxylin and eosin or with methenamine silver. Species identification depends upon examination of cultures after several days of incubation to allow development of the characteristic pigments and the conidial structures. A means of rapid identification of medically important species has been presented by Braude (1986a).

Aspergilli have a ubiquitous, worldwide distribution, making prophylaxis substantially impractical. Grain stores that become moldy are a particularly rich source of spores. The most pathogenic species, A. fumigatus, is thermophilic and thus grows well in the relatively warm environment of compost piles of manure, leaves, and wood chips. In the hospital setting, nonfiltered and nonventilated air are important sources of spores. Involvement of hospital air-handling systems in nosocomial aspergillosis has been reviewed by Walsh and Pizzo (1988).

Candidiasis

Candidiasis is the term applied to invasion of organs and tissues by any of several species of the genus Candida. By far the most important species is C. albicans, although C. tropicalis, C. krusei, C. guilliermondi, C. parapsilosis, C. pseudotropicalis, and C. stellatoidea are sometimes involved. These organisms are virtually innocuous in uncompromised individuals; they cause infection only when appropriate underlying conditions prevail. Major predisposing conditions that lead to Candida invasion are endocrinopathies (diabetes and hormonal changes secondary to pregnancy or use of oral contraceptives), attenuation of cell-mediated immunity, and administration of antibacterial antibiotics that alter the normal microbial flora. With the rare exception of a few instances of hospital-acquired infections (Walsh and Pizzo, 1988), candidiasis arises from the endogenous mi-

croflora of the skin, gastrointestinal tract, and genitalia. In this regard, it stands in marked contrast to mucormycosis, aspergillosis, and cryptococcosis, which derive from exogenous foci. No proclivity exists for any particular race, sex, or age group.

Acute pseudomembranous candidiasis, also referred to as thrush, is characterized by white to blue-white patches on the oral mucosa. These lesions are typically asymptomatic until removed, when the denuded surface is raw and prone to bleeding. The presenting signs of chronic oral candidiasis are firm, white plaques on the cheek, lips, and tongue. These are accompanied by microabscess formation, epithelial edema, and chronic inflammatory cell infiltration of the corneum. Cutaneous sites affected include the genitalia, perianal area, the diaper distribution area of infants, and the nails. Candida albicans esophagitis is a frequent occurrence in AIDS patients. Disseminated candidiasis can occur via a contaminated intravenous line; the organs predominantly affected are the kidney and brain, with death ensuing from renal failure or encephalitis. Patients with prosthetic heart valves who are receiving broad-spectrum antibacterial antibiotics are particularly susceptible to Candida endocarditis. Hematogenous Candida endophthalmitis is a common complication associated with vascular catheters and may lead to blindness in the involved eye if not treated vigorously. Granulocytopenic patients may develop a hepatosplenic form of candidiasis that should be suspected in susceptible patients who develop fever and abdominal pain and who have elevated serum alkaline phosphatase levels in the presence of normal serum transaminase values (Thaler et al., 1988).

Various species of Candida grow readily as gram-positive yeast-like cells and as pseudohyphae. The most pathogenic species, C. albicans, develops true hyphae. The pseudohyphae are chains of budding cells that remain adherent. Terminal chlamydospores that develop at the ends of hyphae when cultured on cornmeal agar distinguish C. albicans from other species. This species, as well as some strains of C. stellatoidea, also produce short germ tubes when suspended in serum at 37°C. A probable relationship exists between germ tube formation and virulence because polymorphonuclear leukocytes that have ingested cells of C. albicans are penetrated by the developing germ tubes with ensuing release of the cells (Braude, 1986b). Gross and microscopic features that permit species differentiation are summarized by Braude (1986b).

Human infections with C. albicans are exclusively endogenous in origin. The carrier incidence in young, healthy individuals is 10 to 15%, as assessed by oral or rectal cultures. This rate tends to increase to almost 50% with both age and antibacterial antibiotic administration. The skin isolation rate is about 5%. The endogenous habitat of Candida thus poses a diagnostic dilemma when cultures are positive; it must be determined whether the presence of C. albicans in a clinical specimen is due to a focus of infection or whether it is merely a contaminant.

Sputum cultures should be particularly suspect because *C. albicans* hardly ever causes pulmonary infections. Prophylactic measures to be taken in patients at risk are obviously different from the procedures used to guard against other opportunists and may include administration of antifungal agents.

Cryptococcosis

Cryptococcosis is an infection primarily of the lungs or central nervous system (CNS) caused by *Cryptococcus neoformans*, a yeast-like organism distributed widely in nature and found in extraordinarily large numbers in bird droppings. Although the disease can occur in seemingly otherwise healthy individuals, it is usually considered a harbinger of an underlying deficit of cell-mediated immunity. Indeed, individuals who have recovered from cryptococcal meningitis and have no known immunologic impairment produce normal antibody to pneumococcal polysaccharide, but fail to respond to cryptococcal capsule antigen (Henderson et al., 1982). Cryptococcosis of the CNS is a significant cause of morbidity and mortality in patients with AIDS (McCutchan and Mathews, 1986).

Cryptococci enter the body via the lungs by inhalation of airborne infectious particles found in dried pigeon droppings. The primary infection in the lungs is usually subclinical. Even if symptoms occur, resolution generally occurs without treatment. Whereas infectious foci may occur subsequently in skeletal muscle or various viscera, CNS involvement by hematogenous spread is by far the most frequent and serious form of the disease. Once this occurs, the disease is consistently fatal if not treated. Progressive disease in the CNS may be a result of diminished cellular or phagocytic response (Henderson et al., 1982; Diamond et al., 1974), because infection of the CNS provides little inflammatory reaction. If meningeal disease progresses to encephalitis, many cystic spaces may be present in the brain. Patients show typical signs and symptoms of meningitis or a bulky lesion. The course is usually subacute or chronic, varying from a few months to several years, but most untreated patients die within 6 months of onset of symptoms. Mortality may be reduced to about 40% by appropriate treatment, but survivors have permanent brain damage with associated deficits, including cranial dysfunction, and may require placement of a shunt if hydrocephalus is present. Patients who have only the pulmonary stage of the infection are generally placed on close observation and are treated only if there is evidence of dissemination.

Colonies of *C. neoformans* are creamy white, becoming yellow to tan with age. The mucoid appearance is attributed to the large amount of capsular polysaccharide. Individual cells are about 4 to 7 μm in diameter, surrounded by a capsule with a thickness varying from 2 to 30 μm. The capsule may be lost or markedly diminished in subcultures. The cells are gram positive and urease positive. They have no germ tubes, chlamydospores, or hyphae, but buds are usually present. *C. neoformans* is distinguished from nonpathogenic cryptococci by its ability to grow at 37°C. The large capsule usually seen surrounding the cells in clinical specimens and early cultures is demonstrated best by a wet India ink preparation, which reveals the capsule as a clear area excluding the ink around the cell. The perfect (sexual) stage has been identified and designated *Filobasidiella neoformans* (Kwon-Chung, 1975), but this stage is not present in clinical materials. Conversion to the perfect state may contribute to survival of the species in nature because some free-living amebae can ingest and kill numerous cryptococci when the latter are in the asexual stage (Ruiz et al., 1982).

Diagnosis of cryptococcal disease of the CNS can be made presumptively on the basis of the large capsular forms observed in India ink preparations of spinal fluid sediments. These forms are seen in just over half of all proved cases. Isolation of *C. neoformans* in culture is essential for a final diagnosis, and at least three negative cultures should be obtained before an alternate diagnosis is considered. Urine cultures are occasionally positive. Cerebrospinal fluid obtained by cisternal tap is sometimes positive when fluid obtained by lumbar puncture yields negative cultures. The latex agglutination test for detection of cryptococcal antigen in most body fluids has about a 95% detection rate (Gordon and Vedder, 1966) and is a highly reliable diagnostic tool.

There is no evidence of man-to-man or direct animal-to-man transmission of cryptococcosis. The fungus can be isolated from the skins of fruit, from fruit juices, and from soil, but it is particularly prevalent in pigeon droppings. Although the capsule is an important virulence factor, its size would seem to preclude its entry into the terminal bronchioles. In nature the capsule is diminished in size, however, and the basidiospores of the sexual stage of the fungus are only about 1 μm in diameter. Even though only a few hundred cases of cryptococcal meningitis are reported each year in the United States, Ajello (1969) estimated that several thousand cases of subclinical respiratory infections occurred each year in New York City alone. Individuals who are susceptible to more serious CNS cryptococcal infections by virtue of an impaired immune status should be made fully aware of the possible consequences of exposure to environments likely to harbor the organism.

ACTINOMYCETES

The Actinomycetes are gram-positive bacilli having features in common with the classic fungi in their tendency to form simple or branching filaments or, in some cases, spores (Zinsser, 1988; Pine, 1986; Rippon, 1988a). The Actinomycetes include the infectious causative agents of actinomycetoma, actinomycosis, and nocardiosis.

Streptomycetes

The Streptomycetes are useful aerobic bacteria that produce long, branched, nonfragmenting filaments and sometimes spores. These pharmaceutically and medically useful organisms are found a few inches beneath the soil, in water, and associated with organic debris (Zinsser, 1988). As a group, they produce about 85% of the available antibacterial and antifungal antibiotics plus antiparasitic, antiviral, and antitumor agents (Zinsser, 1988). *Streptomyces somaliensis* has been reported to be the causative agent in about 7% of worldwide cases of actinomycetoma, a localized swollen skin, subcutaneous, fascial or bone lesion, most often associated with pus-draining sinus tracts containing characteristic, hard, yellow-to-brown grains or granules up to 2 mm in diameter; *S. griseus* and *S. albus* have been reported rarely as causative agents of actinomycetoma (Pine, 1986; Rippon, 1988a).

Actinomycosis

Actinomycosis is a chronic suppurative granulomatous infection with pyogenic lesions or abscesses interconnected by draining sinus tracts (Conant et al., 1971c). Characteristic 100- to 300-μm mycelial grains or sulfur granules may be found in the lesions, sinus tracts, or areas of drainage in these tracts and may appear as dense rosettes of club-shaped, gram-positive terminal ends of filaments of the causative agent in radial arrangement (Braude, 1986). These granules may become calcified. Four clinical forms of actinomycosis have been described and, in decreasing order of distribution, are: (1) cervicofacial; (2) thoracic; (3) abdominal; and (4) genital in women with intrauterine devices (Braude, 1986c). Cervicofacial is the most common type (about 56% of the cases) and has the best prognosis (Conant et al., 1971). The causative agents of actinomycosis, often seen as normal flora of the human mouth and gastrointestinal tract, in order of decreasing association with infection, are: *Actinomyces israelii*, *Arachnia propionica*, and *Actinomyces naeslundii*, with *Bifidobacterium dentium* rarely implicated and usually in the age range of 15 to 35. *Actinomyces bovis*, the causative agent of lumpy jaw in cattle, has not been shown to produce human actinomycosis. Actinomycosis is twice as common in males and occurs usually in the age range of 15 to 35.

Tissue, body fluids, or grains rinsed with sterile saline can be used to inoculate brain-heart infusion blood agar or chocolate agar plates that are incubated aerobically or anaerobically, with or without antibacterial agents (Braude, 1986c). Colonial morphology is characteristic enough to differentiate *Actinomyces* from contaminants or from one another (Braude, 1986c).

Nocardiosis

Nocardiosis is a worldwide acute or chronic suppurative disease caused by the inhalation or inoculation of the aerobic, soil-inhabiting, gram-positive, partially acid-fast *Nocardia asteroides* and, less often, by *N. brasiliensis* or *N. caviae*, which have highly developed branched filaments (Rippon, 1988c). Four distinct clinical forms of the disease are: (1) primary cutaneous (actinomycotic mycetoma); (2) primary subcutaneous; (3) primary pulmonary; and (4) systemic (Rippon, 1988c). The last form is usually caused by hematogenous dissemination to any organ, commonly the central nervous system (Rippon, 1988c). The disease can be treacherous because the patient may appear to recover completely from the disease, only to display later metastatic sites or abscesses of infection in the central nervous system. Nocardiosis is increasingly frequently encountered, especially in immunocompromised, usually male, individuals and is often a terminal event in chronic progressive disease states (Rippon, 1988c). The prognosis of nocardiosis even with present antibiotics is not good in cases of metastatic or systemic infections.

N. asteroides differs from *Actinomyces sp.* in that it grows readily on ordinary laboratory media without antibiotics aerobically or anaerobically and best at 37°C, but also at temperatures as high as 45°C (Rippon, 1988; Conant et al., 1971). The organisms grow well on Sabouraud glucose agar or 7 H 11 medium to form a glabrous, irregularly folded, wrinkled or granular, commonly yellow to orange-red colony. Microscopically, the organisms appear as long, delicate, gram-positive, partially acid-fast filaments that demonstrate multiple branches at long intervals and at right angles to the main mycelial axis. These filaments may sporulate to form bead-like chains or may fragment into bacillary forms of various lengths (Rippon, 1988c). As in the case of *Actinomyces*, soft, variously colored granules may be found in pus from draining sinuses in patients with subcutaneous nocardial infections. Granules are apparently not usually formed in systemic nocardiosis (Rippon, 1988c). Unlike fungal infections, nocardiosis may be highly infectious.

At present, no reliable serologic tests are available for the detection of nocardiosis. Approximately 1000 cases of nocardiosis occur each year in the United States (Rippon, 1988c).

Actinomycotic mycetoma

Actinomycotic mycetoma characteristically consists of localized suppurating abscesses and granulomata with associated draining sinuses in which characteristic granules or grains may be found (Rippon, 1988b). In fact, mycetoma refers to the triad of tumefaction, draining sinuses, and grains. Mycetoma may involve cutaneous and subcutaneous tissue, fascia, and bone and most often occurs after traumatic implantation of soil-containing causative organisms usually into tissues of a foot or hand. The resulting lesion gradually increases in size and may eventually progress to cause great deformation of the infected hand or foot. The condition is caused by several species of *Nocardia*, *Actinomadura*, and at least one species of *Streptomyces*. It is relatively rare in the United States and Europe, but more common in Mexico, Central and South America, India, and tropical Africa (Conant et al., 1971a; Rippon, 1988). Sudan may have as many as 400 new cases per year, the highest number of cases per capita of any country in the world (Rippon, 1988b). The condition occurs most often in the 20- to 50-year age range and is 3 to 5 times as common in men as in women. Actinomycotic mycetoma of the foot is also known as Madura foot, to differentiate it from maduro-mycosis caused by true fungi, because the subcutaneous infections are clinically indistinguishable (Conant et al., 1971a). At least 8 actinomyces may be involved in acti-nomycotic mycetoma: *Nocardia asteroides, N. brasilien-sis, N. caviae, N. transvalensis, Nocardiopsis dassonvil-lei, Actinomadura madurae, A. pelletierii* and *Streptomyces somaliensis* (Rippon, 1988b).

TREATMENT OF SUPERFICIAL FUNGAL INFECTIONS

In spite of recent advances in drug therapy of mycoses with the development of the new imidazole analogs, the state of the art of treatment of superficial and systemic fungus infections leaves much to be desired. A few ex-amples serve to justify this statement; details are pre-sented in the subsequent sections of this chapter:

1. Griseofulvin, the major drug for treatment of der-matomycoses, was discovered and isolated 50 years ago (Oxford et al., 1939) and was originally used as an agricultural fungicide (Brian, 1960). Effective treatment requires administration over a period of several months.

2. The effectiveness of potassium iodide in treatment of sporotrichosis was described by Davis in 1919 and it remains the drug of choice for treatment of the primary lymphocutaneous form of this disease. Few drugs have retained a rational place in ther-apeutics for three score and ten years. The mode of action of iodide has yet to be clarified fully.

3. Amphotericin B, which has long been the drug of choice for certain of the systemic mycoses and op-portunistic fungus infections, must be administered daily or intermittently over a period of weeks or months. The requisite hospitalization imposes a se-vere economic impact, and the drug is extremely toxic to the kidneys. No amphotericin B analogs with altered pharmacologic properties have been forthcoming, unlike the situation with the amino-glycosides, cephalosporins, and penicillins.

There seems little doubt that much of the lack of prog-ress in development of more effective and less toxic an-timycotic agents stems from economic considerations. For example, the annual incidence of certain of the sys-temic mycoses numbers in the hundreds, not hundreds of thousands. Consequently, little incentive exists for development and testing of new compounds that may lead to a marketable product. Within this context, we hope that recent changes in the licensing procedures for orphan drugs may overcome some of the previous re-luctance of firms to enter into this field more aggressively. Although the impact on Wall Street may prove to be negligible, the benefits to affected individuals could be enormous.

Undecylenic Acid

The antifungal action of fatty acids was first reported late in the nineteenth century (Clark, 1899). Kiesel (1913) subsequently undertook the first study of the structure-activity relationships of this group of compounds. He found that inhibitory action increased with the length of the carbon chain up to 11 carbon atoms, the branched chain acids were less active than those with straight chains and an equal number of carbon atoms, and sub-stitution of hydrogen atoms with hydroxyl groups de-creased activity.

$$H_2C=CH(CH_2)_8-COOH$$

Undecylenic Acid

Prince (1959) subsequently examined the relationship between concentration of undissociated acid and inhi-bition. The minimal inhibitory concentration of unde-cylenic acid to *Trichophyton mentagrophytes* varied from 3.0 μg/ml at pH 4.5 to 1500 μg/ml at pH 9.0. When calculated as the actual concentration of undissociated acid at each hydrogen ion concentration tested, however, the amount required for complete inhibition of the test organism remained remarkably constant at about 2.2 μg/ml between pH 4.5 and pH 6.0, but dropped abruptly to a value of approximately 0.2 μg/ml at pH 9.0. Although the results of such studies do not permit a determination of the precise mechanism of action against fungi, they do suggest that activity is associated with the nonionized molecule rather than the dissociated anion. The major mode of action of undecylenic acid is most likely a com-promise of integrity of the cytoplasmic membrane, with resulting loss of low-molecular-weight intracellular com-ponents. The action is primarily fungistatic, but a fun-gicidal effect can be detected after prolonged exposure to high concentrations.

Nonprescription preparations of undecylenic acid are available in several formulations: 20% cream, 22% oint-ment, 19% powder, 10% liquid, and 10% foam. A zinc undecylenic preparation, also available, combines the mild astringent action of zinc with the antifungal action of the fatty acid. Such formulations are unequivocally effective in ameliorating symptoms of tinea pedis due to *Trichophyton mentagrophytes*, and the cure rate may approach 50%, but infections due to *Microsporum rub-rum* may not respond readily to treatment. Cutaneous infections with *Candida albicans* do not respond to treat-ment with any of these products. The formulations that are currently widely available over the counter are sub-stantially free of toxic or sensitizing properties.

As a corollary to the foregoing, tinea capitis caused by *Microsporum audouini*, virtually epidemic in the United States in the 1940s, is still seen sporadically in children, but hardly ever in adults. Rothman et al. (1945) observed that hair of children contained only fractions of the amounts of fatty acids found in adult hair and postulated that the infection in children was due to the absence of fatty acids. This simplistic explanation persists as an ar-ticle of faith, even though the total amounts of these acids in adult hair and sebum are well below those nec-essary to inhibit the growth of dermatophytes (Kligman and Ginsberg, 1950).

Tolnaftate

Tolnaftate (*m*,N-dimethylthiocarbanilic acid 0-2-naphthyl ester) is a thiocarbamic acid analog with a high degree of activity against the dermatophytic fungi but with lesser activity against other Hyphomycetes and yeast-like fungi such as *Candida albicans*. It is effective in the topical treatment of infections due to *Trichophyton sp.*, *Microsporum sp.*, and *Epidermophyton floccosum*, and the cure rate is about 93% (Keczkes et al., 1975). Minimum inhibitory concentrations for most strains are in the range of 0.1 to 0.4 μg/ml (Georgopoulos et al., 1981). Tinea infections due to *Trichophyton rubrum*, which tend to be unresponsive to undecylenic acid, usually respond well to tolnaftate treatment. When first introduced into the United States, the drug was available only by prescription, but is now obtained over the counter. It is formulated at a 1% concentration as a gel, spray liquid, powder, spray powder, cream, and solution. When used daily on washed and dried areas, it usually resolves most tinea infections of the skin within 2 to 4 weeks. Tinea unguium (onychomycosis) is unresponsive, owing to the inaccessibility of the fungi within the nails. No significant toxic or sensitizing responses have been reported following the use of this agent.

Tolnaftate

Recent studies of the biochemical mode of action of tolnaftate have shown that it is a potent inhibitor of de novo sterol biosynthesis from acetate in susceptible fungi (Morita and Nozawa, 1985; Ryder et al., 1986; Barret-Bee et al., 1986). Squalene is one intermediate in this multistep metabolic process. When tolnaftate was added to a culture of *Trichophyton mentagrophytes* at a final concentration of only 0.003 μg/ml, the ergosterol concentration was reduced 45%, accompanied by a 1700% increase in squalene accumulation. At a concentration of 0.03 μg/ml, the rate of ergosterol synthesis was reduced 92%, and squalene accumulated to a level 3400% greater than the control level. Ergosterol synthesis in intact cells of *Candida albicans* was relatively resistant to the action of the drug, whereas marked inhibition was evident in a cell-free system prepared from this organism (Ryder et al., 1986). This suggests that the relative insensitivity of *Candida* infections to tolnaftate treatment is a consequence of a permeability or transport barrier to the drug. Sterol biosynthesis in a cell-free extract of mammalian liver was not inhibited. Because ergosterol is a vital component of the fungal cytoplasmic membrane, selective inhibition of its synthesis disrupts assembly of the cellular organelle responsible for selective partitioning of intracellular and extracellular nutrients and ions. Additional examples of the critical nature of ergosterol in fungal cell membranes are described later in this chapter, in the sections on amphotericin B and nystatin.

Haloprogin

Haloprogin (HaloTex) was first synthesized in Japan as a halogenated phenolic ether and is currently prepared by Meiji Seka Kaisha of Tokyo. The agent is fungicidal against a number of dermatophytes including some species of *Trichophyton*, *Microsporum*, *Epidermophyton*, and *Pityrosporum*, and also active against *Candida*, *Streptococcus*, and *Staphylococcus* (Seki et al., 1963).

Haloprogin

Several clinical investigations have shown haloprogin to be superior to placebo and equally effective as tolnaftate (Hermann, 1972; Katz and Cahn, 1972; Carter, 1972; Kessler, 1978). The largest study included 556 patients in a well-controlled, double-blind study and showed good response rates of tinea pedis, tinea corporis, tinea versicolor, and dermal candidiasis (Hermann, 1972; Smith, 1976). Haloprogin cream produced cures of infants with diaper rash (Montes and Hermann, 1978). Haloprogin is not well absorbed through the skin, but that which is absorbed is metabolized to trichlorethanol, which is excreted in the urine. The poor skin absorption may explain the common resistance of thick-skin infections, such as on the palms, soles, and nails, to topical application. The agent is available as a 1% solution (HaloTex) and is usually applied to the infected area twice daily for 2 to 4 weeks. No systemic adverse effects have been reported, and the rare localized adverse effects include local irritation with erythema, itching, or burning sensations, vesiculation, increased maceration, exacerbation of the preexisting lesion, and uncommon allergic contact hypersensitivity. Contact with the eyes should be avoided (Robertson and Maibach, 1987). The mechanism of antifungal action of haloprogin is not known, but may be disruption of yeast-cell membranes or respiratory inhibition.

Ciclopirox olamine

Ciclopirox olamine (Loprox) was the first hydroxypyridone to be developed as a topical antifungal agent (Hanel et al., 1988). This nonimidazole drug has activity against a broad spectrum of dermatophytes, yeasts, actinomycetes, molds, and other fungi, as well as against a variety of gram-positive and gram-negative bacteria (Jue et al., 1985). It inhibits the growth of dermatophytes, yeasts, dimorphic fungi, and actinomycetales, usually at concentrations of 4 μg/ml or less, in vitro. Concentrations ranging from 0.25 to 15.6 μg/ml inhibit some strains of *Aspergillus* and many different bacterial species and strains; concentrations of 31.3 to 125 μg/ml inhibit *Proteus mirabilis*, *Pseudomonas aeruginosa*, *Mycoplasma spp.*, *Trichomonas vaginalis*, and other microorganisms (Jue, 1985; Yamaguchi, 1986). After topical application, the therapeutic efficacy of this agent is similar or superior to that of clotrimazole with a similar frequency of associated adverse reactions (Jue et al., 1985; Cullen et al., 1985). Use of carbon-14 labeled ciclopirox olamine, applied in the form of 1% aqueous cream, showed penetration into healthy torso skin in about 6 hours, with 1.3% of the dose absorbed percutaneously and excreted by the kidney as a glucuronide with a biologic half-life of 1.7 hours. The agent exhibited its highest levels in the horny layer of skin, but attained minimum inhibition concentrations or higher in the skin corium (Kellner et al., 1981).

Ciclopirox Olamine

Ciclopirox olamine penetrated average or thick horny layers of skin, as well as fingernails (Dittmar, 1981). After vaginal application of ^{14}C-labeled ciclopirox olamine, 42 to 97% of the dose was recovered in feces and urine, usually as a glucuronide in urine. Absorbed radiolabeled agent appeared to bind to serum proteins in humans and was poorly absorbed across placental barriers in rats (Kellner et al., 1981). The highest concentrations of ciclopirox olamine were detected in the liver, kidney, and smooth muscle of the stomach.

Ciclopirox olamine, 1% cream, has shown clinical activity against *Trichophyton rubrum*, *Trichophyton mentagrophytes*, *Microsporum canis*, *Epidermophyton floccosum*, and tinea (pityriasis) versicolor caused by *Pityrosporum orbiculare (Malassezia furfur)* (Torres et al., 1981; Dittmar, 1981; Cullen et al., 1985). It has also been used successfully in treatment of vulvovaginal candidiasis (Peil, 1981) and onychomycoses (Qadripur et al., 1981). Ciclopirox olamine at 1% solutions exhibited antifungal efficacy similar to that produced by a 1% solutions of tolnaftate or clotrimazole, and a 1% cream gave similar results to a 1% clotrimazole cream (Beyer, 1981). The 1% cream is applied to the infected skin twice daily, and treatment may be continued 2 to 4 weeks for clinical improvement. Side effects are rare and include local irritation, redness, pruritus at the injection site, occasional hypersensitivity, and rare worsening of the clinical disease signs or symptoms (Jue, 1985). Eye contact with 1% ciclopirox olamine cream should be avoided. The mechanism of action is not completely understood, but the agent appears to concentrate in cell membranes of sensitive organisms and block the cellular uptake of amino acids and other precursors needed for macromolecular synthesis. Higher concentrations of the agent may disrupt the cell membrane and may thereby allow leakage of these precursors and other intracellular materials from cells of the microorganism (Jue, 1985). Ciclopirox olamine (1%) cream (Loprox) is available in the United States for the treatment of dermatomycosis (tinea corporis, cruris, pedis, and versicolor) and cutaneous or vaginal candidiasis.

Griseofulvin

Griseofulvin was first isolated from *Penicillium griseofulvum* by Oxford and associates in 1939, but it was not investigated vigorously in view of its lack of activity against bacteria. In 1946 Brian and colleagues isolated from a strain of *Penicillium janczewski* a substance that produced stunting of hyphae of susceptible fungi with induction of coils and curls; this product was later found to be identical to griseofulvin described earlier by Oxford et al. (1939). This antibiotic was initially used in Great Britain against a number of plant pathogens and for treatment of ringworm in cattle. Soon after Gentles (1958) demonstrated its effectiveness by the oral route in treating experimental dermatomycoses in guinea pigs, it was subjected to clinical trials that established its utility in treating tinea infections in man (Williams et al., 1958; Blank and Roth, 1959).

Griseofulvin

Blank and Smith (1960) published a report of the first patient treated at the University of Miami with griseofulvin. A 27-year-old white male was admitted with a history of rheumatoid arthritis for which he had received oral cortisone treatment for 7 years. Four years prior to admission, he had developed pruritic eruptions, many of which became nodular and ulcerated. Cultures from scaly areas and purulent material from abscesses repeatedly grew *Trichophyton rubrum*. One abscess contained 300 ml pus. Initial therapy included blood transfusions and many topical antifungal agents, all to no avail. The patient's serum failed to inhibit fungal growth at a concentration of 80%, and biopsies of granulomas revealed numerous fungal hyphae. Intravenous amphotericin B effected some improvement, but was discontinued when renal toxicity supervened. Ten months after admission, the patient was started on griseofulvin, 5.0 g/day orally. Marked improvement occurred in 1 week. Discontinuance of the drug after 1 month resulted in recurrence of cutaneous lesions, so maintenance therapy was instituted, 1.0 g/day for life. No toxic effects were noted after several months, and there was no evidence that the organism became resistant. The drug was probably life-saving in this patient.

Chemically, griseofulvin is 7-chloro-2′,4,6-trimethoxy-6′-methylspiro-[benzofuran-2(3H),1′-(2)-cyclohexene]-3,4′-dione. It is a white, thermostable powder almost insoluble (10 μg/ml) in water, slightly soluble in ethanol, methanol, acetone, benzene, chloroform, ethyl acetate, and acetic acid, but soluble to the extent of 14 g/100 ml in dimethylformamide. Of the fungi important in human infections, griseofulvin is active only against the dermatophytes: *Trichophyton, Microsporum,* and *Epidermophyton.* When transported into actively growing cells, it exerts a fungicidal action (Foley and Greco, 1960) and is concentrated up to 100-fold in *Microsporum gypseum* (El-Nakeeb and Lampen, 1965). Morphologic changes include production of multinucleate cells, indicative of mitotic inhibition (Gull and Trinci, 1973), and disruption of the mitotic spindle (Malawista et al., 1968; Weber et al., 1976). Current evidence points to the microtubules in the mitotic spindle apparatus as the major site of griseofulvin action. These organelles are polymers composed of a 120,000-dalton protein called tubulin (Bryan, 1974). Griseofulvin can interact with purified tubulin and prevent its polymerization into microtubules (Wehland et al., 1977; Keates, 1981; Sloboda et al., 1982). The actual site on tubulin that is bound by griseofulvin differs from the sites bound by colchicine or the *Vinca* alkaloids (Wilson, 1970).

The absorption of griseofulvin after oral administration is dependent upon the size of the particles in the various preparations. Up to 50% of a micronized powder may be absorbed, and this is increased slightly by administration of the ultramicrocrystalline form (Davies, 1980). The rate of absorption is decreased by barbiturates. A single dose of 500 mg in an adult yields a blood level of about 1.0 μg/ml after 4 hours. The half-life in plasma is about 24 hours. Approximately 50% of an oral dose is recovered in the urine within 5 days, primarily as the metabolite, 6-demethylgriseofulvin. Upon repetitive administration, the drug binds to keratin, with highest concentrations in the stratus corneum. Microbial keratin-digesting enzymes may have a role in the pathogenesis of certain dermatomycoses (Collins et al., 1973), and some evidence indicates that keratin that is bound by griseofulvin is more resistant to digestion (Yu and Blank, 1973). Uptake of the drug into keratin is achieved by both passive diffusion and secretion in sweat (Shah et al., 1974). Concentrations finally attained in the skin and palm surfaces range from 12 to 22 μg/g tissue (Epstein et al., 1972), well in excess of the minimal inhibitory concentrations for susceptible fungi. Treatment is usually given for 4 to 6 weeks for most skin infections, except those of the soles and palms, which may require up to 8 weeks of treatment; infections of the nails are typically treated for 3 to 6 months. Griseofulvin does not penetrate readily into intact nails and must be deposited in keratin at the site of new nail growth. Similarly, deposition in hair occurs only in the follicle at the site of new hair growth; proximal hair shafts may be free of fungi, whereas distal portions remain infected.

Strains of dermatophytes resistant to griseofulvin have been selected in vitro, and these resistant strains are characterized by a reduced uptake of the drug (El-Nakeeb and Lampen, 1965). Development of clinical resistance during treatment has occurred only infrequently, and sensitivity testing is not considered necessary prior to initiation of therapy.

Griseofulvin is readily taken up by mammalian cells and can cause similar abnormalities in the mitotic structures, but the drug is remarkably free of side effects at the doses used clinically. The major complaint is of headaches, by about 10% of patients receiving the drug. These are seldom severe enough to indicate withdrawal and may actually subside during treatment. Gastrointestinal symptoms, paresthesias, and skin rashes are the next most common group of untoward symptoms. Leukopenia has been reported, and most practitioners recommend occasional blood counts during the first weeks of administration. A griseofulvin-induced increase in porphyrin excretion is without significance, except in patients with porphyria, who may show acute exacerbations of symptoms. Although the drug has been reported to produce some relief in patients with gouty arthritis, presumably as a consequence of its colchicine-like action, it is not currently indicated for this condition. A number of animal studies indicated that griseofulvin is both teratogenic (Klein and Beall, 1972; Scott et al., 1975) and tumorigenic (Epstein et al., 1967; Rustia and Shubik, 1978), but there is no evidence of such actions in humans. There is also no evidence that spermatogenesis is impaired in patients taking the customary doses of 500 mg/day. Many years of clinical use have established that griseofulvin is a safe drug for treatment of tinea infections that cannot be treated with topical agents, but it is probably prudent to withhold the drug during pregnancy.

Griseofulvin is available in tablets of 125, 250, 330, and 500 mg from various manufacturers. Grisactin (Ayerst), Gris-Peg (Herbert), and Fulvicin (Schering) are available in ultramicrosize tablets. The daily dose recommendations are 330 mg or 375 mg/day for adults in a single or in divided doses, and 3.3 mg/lb for children over the age of 2 years. Grifulvin V (Ortho) microsize tablets are also available; the suggested dose is 500 mg/day for adults and 5 mg/lb for children. Doses up to 1000 mg/day in adults are recommended for extensive involvement.

TREATMENT OF SYSTEMIC MYCOSES

Amphotericin B

The discovery of amphotericin B in the mid-1950s (Gold et al., 1956) was an outstanding contribution to the treatment of systemic fungus infections. The earliest (and perhaps crudest) preparations had antifungal potency far greater than that of any antimycotic drug then in use. The minimal inhibitory concentrations ranged from 0.07 μg/ml for the yeast phase of *Sporothrix schenckii* to about 0.5 μg/ml for most isolates of *Candida albicans.* Although its clinical application has been supplanted to some degree by some of the newly developed imidazole analogs, amphotericin B remains a mainstay in the treatment of progressive or disseminated systemic infections due to *Blastomyces dermatitidis, Histoplasma capsulatum,* and *Coccidioides immitis,* as well as opportunistic infections due to *Cryptococcus neoformans* and species of *Candida, Aspergillus, Mucor, Rhizopus,* and

Absidia. It is an alternate drug (to ketoconazole) for treatment of South American blastomycosis due to *Paracoccidioides brasiliensis* and for treatment of the disseminated stages of sporotrichosis due to *Sporothrix schenckii.*

Structure

Amphotericin B is one of a large group of antibiotic compounds known as polyenes, a generic term applied to structures one portion of which contains several conjugated double bonds that confer lipophilic properties and a hydroxylated portion that is hydrophilic. Amphotericin B contains seven double bonds. The unsaturated chromophore is sensitive to photo-oxidation, which leads to inactivation of the molecule. Of the many polyenes that have been described, only amphotericin B is sufficiently nontoxic to be used parenterally (see Korzybski et al., 1967, for review). Because the compound is insoluble in aqueous media, it is formulated with sodium deoxycholate for intravenous administration. The resulting product is a fine colloidal dispersion that appears grossly to be a clear, yellow solution.

Amphotericin B

Mechanism of Action

The first suggestion that the mode of antifungal action of amphotericin B may involve an interaction with the fungal cytoplasmic membrane was made by Gale (1960), who noted that anaerobic glycolysis in intact cells of *Candida albicans* was inhibited by the drug at 5.0 $\mu g/ml$, but was unaffected in a cell-free system at drug concentrations up to 100 $\mu g/ml$. In addition, pyruvate was neither oxidized nor anaerobically decarboxylated by control cells, but both these events occurred in cells exposed to amphotericin B. It was concluded that the drug abolished the natural barrier to entry of pyruvate into the cell.

A decade later, Kinsky (1970) reviewed the literature regarding polyene actions on membranes. The presence of sterol in the membrane was an absolute requirement for antibiotic action, because organisms devoid of sterols were unaffected. This feature accounts for the selective antimicrobial toxicity of polyenes for fungi, as compared with bacteria, which do not have sterol-containing membranes. A consequence of the drug-membrane interaction is a loss of selective membrane permeability with entry of H^+ ions and loss of intracellular K^+ ions. Over long exposure times or with higher drug concentrations, leakage of higher-molecular-weight components including proteins and nucleic acids ultimately occurs. Other

sterol-containing cell types lacking a cell wall (fungal protoplasts, protozoa, mammalian erythrocytes) undergo lysis as a result of permeability alterations. The action of amphotericin B as well as other polyenes on membranes of nongrowing (resting) cells indicates that the events induced, principally loss of K^+ and Mg^{++} ions, are rapidly fungicidal rather than merely fungistatic, and cell death occurs without the requirement that the cells be actively dividing.

In an elegant presentation, Pratt and Fekety (1986) drew upon the work of Andreoli (1974) to summarize the actions of amphotericin B and other polyenes on bilayered membrane models at the molecular level. In the membrane-bound configuration, two or more molecules of amphotericin B are aligned along their long axes (length = 24 A) and are, in turn, aligned along the long axes of the phospholipid membrane components, closely associated with the interspersed sterol molecules. The hydroxylated hydrophilic portion of each drug molecule extends to the water surface of the membrane, whereas the lipophilic conjugated portion orients toward the center of the membrane bilayer. On the opposite side of the membrane a similar process occurs, with the nonpolar ends of the polyene molecules in juxtaposition near the center of the membrane to form a polyene aggregate about 48 A in overall length. This cluster of abutting antibiotic molecules, polarity-oriented in respect to the encompassing membrane components, serves as a 4- to 5-A diameter channel through which essential intracellular components pass to the exterior with attendant loss of cell viability.

In spite of the evidence to support the sterol hypothesis as the key biochemical lesion in the antifungal action of amphotericin B, the hypothesis is not without its critics. Medoff et al. (1983) noted that the presence of sterols in membranes is not absolutely essential for the binding of amphotericin B to those membranes (granted that "binding" may not be tantamount to disturbances in permeability), and the presence of sterol in the membranes is not necessary for amphotericin B-induced permeability changes. Medoff (1987) subsequently strengthened his position by pointing out that the lytic and lethal effects of amphotericin B on red blood cells and yeasts are dependent on incubation in an oxygen environment, are inhibited by catalase, and are accelerated by ascorbate. In contrast, none of these variables influences the effects of amphotericin B on cell membrane permeability. These findings are interpreted as indicating that oxidative damage is involved in amphotericin B-induced lysis and lethality, but not in permeability aberrations.

Parenteral administration of amphotericin B leads to a number of toxic events, many of which are due to interactions with host membranes in much the same manner as its interactions with fungal membranes. Thus, in regard to the host, the degree of selective toxicity is low. The basis of the limited selective toxicity of amphotericin B resides in the differences in sterol composition of animal and fungal membranes. Ergosterol is the principal sterol in fungal membranes, whereas cholesterol predominates in animal membranes. Amphotericin B binds to ergosterol with a greater affinity than to cholesterol (Readio and Bittman, 1982). Further, ergosterol is much more effective than cholesterol in antagonizing K$^+$ efflux and growth inhibition induced in fungus cultures by amphotericin B (Kotler-Brajtburg et al., 1974; Gale, 1974).

Fungal Sensitivity

Virtually all fungi that cause systemic infections are sensitive to amphotericin B at levels lower than those attainable in plasma. Mean minimal inhibitory concentrations range from a low of 0.04 μg/ml for *Histoplasma capsulatum* up to 3.5 μg/ml for *Candida tropicalis* (Rippon, 1982). Emergence of resistant fungal strains during treatment has not been a major problem. When relapse has occurred following a course of treatment, the organism usually is approximately as sensitive to the drug as was the original isolate. A survey of 1372 yeasts from 308 patients revealed that only 55 isolates were resistant, as defined by the ability to grow at amphotericin B concentrations at or over 2.0 μg/ml (Dick et al., 1980). All the resistant organisms were from only 6 seriously ill patients who had received long-term treatment with the drug. The resistant strains isolated from clinical sources had lowered levels of ergosterol in the membranes (Dick et al., 1980; Woods et al., 1974), similar to resistant strains selected in vitro (Fryberg et al., 1974; Pierce et al., 1978).

Drug Combinations

The use of drug combinations, a practice used for years in almost all cancer chemotherapy and in treatment of some bacterial infections, has emerged as a rational intervention in treatment of certain fungus infections. Studies using in vitro culture systems and animal models have shown varying degrees of summation or true synergy when amphotericin B was used with rifampin, an inhibitor of microbial RNA-directed DNA polymerase (Kobayashi et al., 1972); tetracycline, an inhibitor of bacterial protein synthesis (Huppert et al., 1974); or flucytosine (Medoff et al., 1971). Flucytosine, a fluorinated pyrimidine analog with activity against some strains of *Candida albicans* and *Cryptococcus neoformans*, is described in detail in a subsequent section of this chapter. When amphotericin B was added to cultures of *Candida albicans* along with flucytosine, the uptake of flucytosine into cells was enhanced significantly (Medoff et al., 1972). Synergism with the two drugs in growth inhibition was observed at amphotericin B levels well below its minimal inhibitory concentration. Because flucytosine enters the cell via an active transport mechanism, it is conceivable that amphotericin B facilitates the uptake.

The first controlled, multicenter study of the use of amphotericin B with flucytosine in treatment of cryptococcal meningitis was reported by Bennett et al. (1979). Amphotericin B alone was used in 27 courses of treatment, whereas a combination of amphotericin B plus flucytosine was used in 24 courses; 50 patients were enrolled in the study. The combination regimen, given for 6 weeks, as opposed to 10 weeks for amphotericin B alone, cured more patients (16 vs. 11), resulted in fewer treatment failures or relapses (3 vs. 11), produced significantly more rapid sterilization of the cerebrospinal fluid, and evoked less nephrotoxicity. A later multicenter study using a larger number of patients (Dismukes et al., 1987) was designed to determine if the duration of combined therapy could be reduced even further to 4 weeks. Results were consistent with the view that such a regimen may be used for patients with meningitis without neurologic complications, underlying disease, or immunosuppressive therapy, and cerebrospinal fluid white cell count above 20 mm^2, but patients who do not meet these criteria should be treated for 6 weeks or more. Current recommendations are that flucytosine should be combined with amphotericin B in treatment of cryptococcal meningitis or disseminated candidiasis (Sarosi et al., 1988; Medical Letter, 1988).

Medoff (1987) discussed the controversy surrounding the reported use of drug combinations in antifungal chemotherapy and cited the anecdotal nature of many of the reports on the use of amphotericin B and flucytosine against other fungal infections and on use of amphotericin B with rifampin or tetracycline. Nonetheless, one authoritative source (Medical Letter, 1988) recommends amphotericin B, with or without flucytosine or rifampin, as first-choice treatment for disseminated aspergillosis.

The development of new antifungal agents may lead to evaluation of other drug combinations for treatment of serious mycoses. Amphotericin B seems likely to remain the major drug in such combinations in view of its high degree of potency and its probable immunoadjuvant properties (Little et al., 1983; Medoff, 1987). Such studies should be undertaken only after the biochemical mechanism of action of each new drug has been clarified, however, to avoid the risk of possible drug antagonism. For example, the combination of amphotericin B and the imidazole analog, miconazole, is antagonistic against *Candida albicans* in vitro and in vivo (Schacter et al., 1976; Dupont and Drouhet, 1979), probably because miconazole inhibits the de novo synthesis of ergosterol, the major drug receptor for amphotericin B.

Prophylactic Use

Another emerging area of importance in control of fungal infections is the possibility of prophylactic treatment of patients who are highly susceptible to opportunistic infections by virtue of underlying disease or immunosuppressive therapy. For example, candidiasis and aspergillosis are common in neutropenic patients with cancer, and many attempts have been made to evaluate potential prophylactic procedures. Published reports have been reviewed critically by Meunier (1987). No single regimen was recommended for preventing invasive candidiasis, but further evaluation of amphotericin B aerosols or nasal sprays for prevention of invasive aspergillosis was encouraged.

An initial intravenous infusion of 1 to 5 mg/day of amphotericin B, gradually increased to 0.65 mg/kg/day, produces peak plasma concentrations of 2 to 4 μg/ml. These levels tend to be persistent, because the plasma half-life is about 24 hours. More than 90% of the drug is bound to plasma proteins and is poorly dialyzable. Cerebrospinal fluid levels are only 2 to 5% of serum levels, and concentrations in aqueous humor and in peritoneal, pleural, and joint fluids are only about half of those in plasma (Polak, 1979). The drug is excreted slowly by the kidneys, but only a small fraction is excreted in a biologically active form. It can be detected in the urine for up to 7 or more weeks after discontinuance of therapy, and in one case was detected in renal tissue from a patient who had received the drug a year earlier (Reynolds et al., 1963).

Dosage

The American Thoracic Society has recently issued a revised statement of dosage recommendations for amphotericin B (Sarosi et al., 1988). Intravenous doses of 20 to 50 mg/day are suggested; after 1 week they can be given either daily or on alternate days. Some authorities recommend a test dose of 1, 5, or 10 mg, followed by 10-mg increments until the optimal dose is reached. When the patient is critically ill or when the disease is caused by *Aspergillus* or by a phycomycete, the schedule should be accelerated. Chills and fever, which often accompany the initiation of therapy, can be controlled by aspirin, codeine, meperidine, or hydrocortisone, depending upon severity. Thrombophlebitis may be avoided by alteration of infusion sites or by infusion of heparin. Most practitioners begin treatment in the hospital, but continue treatment on an outpatient basis or at home after implantation of a cannula. Recommended doses for other routes of administration are as follows: intraventricular or intracisternal, 50 μg initially followed by 200 to 500 μg given 1 to 3 times a week; intra-articular, 5 to 15 mg per administration; intraocular, up to 10 μg; and bladder, irrigation with 50 μg/ml.

Side Effects

Intravenous infusion of amphotericin B leads to a number of toxic effects. In addition to the chills and fever previously mentioned, severe abdominal pain or frank anaphylaxis may occur. The major organ affected, however, is the kidney. In addition to a direct effect on renal blood flow (Butler et al., 1964), the drug alters the renal tubule by interaction with tubular membrane sterols. Hypokalemia, which requires potassium replacement, can ensue. Sodium loading often improves renal function despite continuance of the drug. Baseline hematocrit, creatinine, and potassium levels should be obtained, followed by weekly or biweekly determinations during therapy. The normochromic, normocytic anemia frequently seen is due to a direct effect on the marrow; hemolysis of circulating erythrocytes does not occur at therapeutic plasma levels. Potentially fatal pulmonary reactions can occur in patients receiving amphotericin B

concurrently with leukocyte infusions (Wright et al., 1981). No evidence of teratogenicity has been reported. For a detailed description of polyene toxicity, see Pratt and Fekety (1986).

Availability

Amphotericin B for intravenous use is available as Fungizone (Squibb), a sterile, lyophilized cake containing 50 mg amphotericin B and 41 mg sodium deoxycholate with 20.2 mg sodium phosphates as buffer. It is indicated for treatment of cryptococcosis, North American blastomycosis, disseminated candidiasis, coccidioidomycosis, and histoplasmosis; mucormycosis caused by any of the phycomycetes; disseminated sporotrichosis; and aspergillosis. It is cautioned that a total daily dose of 1.5 mg/kg should not be exceeded. Amphotericin B is also supplied as Fungizone (Squibb), a cream, lotion, and ointment at 3% concentration in an aqueous vehicle for treatment of cutaneous and mucocutaneous candidiasis. Capsules containing a fixed dose combination of amphotericin B and tetracycline, Mysteclin-F (Squibb), designed to provide simultaneous antibacterial therapy and anticandidal prophylaxis, have been declared ineffective by a panel of the National Academy of Science, National Research Council.

Nystatin

Nystatin is a polyene antibiotic with a structure similar to that of amphotericin B. It was first described by Hazen and Brown (1951) under the name fungicidin, but the name was subsequently changed to nystatin to reflect that much of its early development took place in the laboratories of the New York State Health Department in Albany. Its structure is similar to that of amphotericin B, except it contains only four conjugated double bonds. Its mode of action against susceptible fungi is considered to be virtually identical to that of amphotericin B. Although nystatin has a broad antifungal spectrum, its systemic toxicity limits its use to topical and oral preparations and vaginal inserts for treatment of candidiasis. At concentrations attained at sites of infection, the action of the drug is predominantly fungicidal. Because all pharmaceutic formulations are mixtures in which the nystatin component predominates, doses of all products are expressed on a unit basis rather than as micrograms. No notable toxicity has been reported from extended use of nystatin by any age group, even though detectable blood levels can occur following oral administration of large doses. Diarrhea, nausea, and vomiting sometimes occur after oral ingestion. Severe hypersensitivity reactions have not been a major problem associated with its use. Various formulations are available from eight pharmaceutical firms in the United States (Squibb, Savage, Lederle, Fougera, Pharmaderm, Geneva, Paddock, and Par).

Flucytosine

Flucytosine was originally synthesized and evaluated as a potential antineoplastic agent (Duschinsky et al.,

1957; Wempen et al., 1961). Although it was without remarkable effect on experimental tumors, Grunberg et al. (1963) subsequently demonstrated its effectiveness in the treatment of experimental cryptococcosis in mice, and clinical trials initiated shortly thereafter proved its value in treatment of candidiasis and cryptococcosis in man (Steer et al., 1972; Utz et al., 1968; Vandevelde et al., 1972).

Chemically, flucytosine is 5-fluorocytosine, a fluorinated analog of the naturally occurring pyrimidine common to all cells. This white to off-white crystalline powder has a molecular weight of 129.1.

Flucytosine

The minimal inhibitory concentrations of flucytosine in vitro for most strains of *Candida albicans* range from 0.1 to 1.0 μg/ml, with a few strains requiring up to 20 μg/ml for complete inhibition. *Candida tropicalis* is slightly more resistant; most strains are inhibited by 6.0 μg/ml, but an occasional isolate is resistant to over 100 μg/ml. Most strains of *Cryptococcus neoformans* are inhibited by less 2.0 μg/ml, whereas most isolates of *Aspergillus fumigatus* are inhibited by 1.0 to 12 μg/ml (Scholer, 1980). The apparent sensitivities of these organisms can be influenced by the composition of the growth medium in which the test is conducted because cytosine antagonizes the action of the drug, as discussed in the next paragraph. Interlaboratory assessments of sensitivities of pretreatment isolates of *Candida* or *Torulopsis glabrata* were found to be frequently in disagreement, because the populations sampled for testing contained subpopulations of a few resistant cells that predominated ultimately in tube dilution assays (Normark and Schönebeck, 1972; Block et al., 1973). When assay conditions were modified to suppress growth of these subpopulations, it was found that over 80% of *Candida* isolates were sensitive to concentrations less than 20 μg/ml (Shadomy, 1969). Primary resistance of *Cryptococcus neoformans* has been rare, but resistance arising during therapy has been a major cause of treatment failure when flucytosine was used alone (Fass and Perkins, 1971; Lewis and Rabinovich, 1972). As a consequence of the rapid emergence of resistance in originally sensitive organisms during treatment, few indications exist for use of this drug alone. Its use in combination with amphotericin B is described in a preceding section of this chapter.

The biochemical mode of antifungal action of flucytosine is unique in that the compound is actually a prodrug that remains pharmacologically inert until it is metabolized by the very fungal cell that is its ultimate victim. The drug is first transported into the cell by cytosine permease, a process that can be antagonized by cytosine (Polak and Scholer, 1973a). It is then deaminated by intracellular cytosine deaminase to form 5-fluorouracil, a compound used extensively in cancer chemotherapy for many years. 5-Fluorouracil can also be considered a prodrug, because it too is pharmacologically inactive until it is converted to 5-fluorouridine monophosphate by the action of the uridine monophosphate pyrophosphorylase system (Grenson, 1969). At this point, the compound enters into two distinct metabolic pathways. On the one hand, it undergoes stepwise phosphorylation to the di- and then the triphosphate, when it is actually incorporated into fungal RNA by the action of RNA polymerase. This phosphorylated product can replace as much as 50% of the uracil in RNA (Polak and Scholer, 1973b, 1975). The erroneous pyrimidine confers inappropriate base-pairing properties to the RNA polymer, such that the fidelity of protein synthesis is compromised and "nonsense" proteins are synthesized. On the other hand, some of the 5-fluorouridine monophosphate undergoes reduction to 5-fluoro-2'-deoxyuridine monophosphate (Diasio et al., 1978a). This step, which can be termed a "lethal synthesis," yields a potent inhibitor of thymidylate synthetase, the enzyme that converts deoxyuridine monophosphate to thymidine monophosphate via donation of a methyl group from methylenetetrahydrofolate to the 5- position of uridine monophosphate. This results in a block in the synthesis of DNA via substrate (thymidine monophosphate) depletion. The actual mechanism of inhibition appears to be a covalent interaction of 5-fluoro-2'-deoxyuridine monophosphate with a cysteinyl group in the active site of thymidylate synthetase (Bellisario et al., 1976; Pagolotti et al., 1976), with the consequent formation of a stable ternary complex composed of the inhibitor, the enzyme, and the methylenetetrahydrofolate cofactor that donates the methyl group (Langenbach et al., 1972; Santi et al., 1974).

Selective toxicity of flucytosine is based upon the virtual absence in mammalian cells and cells of naturally resistant fungi of cytosine deaminase, the enzyme that carries out the first step in converting the drug to a pharmacologically active compound. Traces of 5-fluorouracil that have been detected in sera of patients receiving the drug probably arise through the action of microbial cytosine deaminases present in the gut microflora and may be present in sufficient quantities to account for some of the clinical toxicity of the drug (Diasio et al., 1978b).

A number of biochemical aberrations have been defined in strains of fungi that emerged as resistant to flucytosine during the course of treatment or were selected for resistance in vitro. One of these is a decreased activity of cytosine permease, which is required for transport of the drug into the cell (Block et al., 1973). Other resistant strains have a reduced level of cytosine deaminase activity (Hoeprich et al., 1974), which is required for conversion of the drug to 5-fluorouracil, whereas yet others have reduced levels of uridine monophosphate pyrophosphorylase activity (Block et al., 1973; Normark and Schönebeck, 1972), which converts 5-fluorouracil formed from deamination of the drug to 5-fluorouridine monophosphate. A fourth type of biochemical defect related to resistance is the absence in some organisms of the feedback inhibition of pyrimidine synthesis (Jund and Lacrute, 1970). This is the mechanism by which the levels of uridine triphosphate regulate the activity of aspartate transcarbamylase, the first enzyme in the de novo pyrimidine synthesis pathway. Without this mode of inhibition, endogenous pyrimidine biosynthesis proceeds unchecked, producing elevated levels of uridine nucleotides that compete with flucytosine-derived fluorinated uridine analogs and antagonize their antifungal actions.

The usual dose of flucytosine is 50 to 150 mg/kg/day, given in 4 to 6 divided doses. Absorption from the gastrointestinal tract is rapid and virtually complete. Peak serum levels of 35 to 50 μg/ml are reached in about 2 hours. The steady-state concentration after repeated administration should not exceed 100 μg/ml. Flucytosine is not bound significantly to plasma proteins. The volume of distribution approximates total body water, which allows fungistatic levels to be attained in about all body fluids. Concentrations in the cerebrospinal fluid are about 75% of plasma levels. Excretion is by glomerular filtration, with most of a given dose appearing in the urine within 48 hours. The half-life in patients with nor-

mal renal function is about 4 hours, but it is increased markedly in the presence of renal insufficiency. Most of the drug is excreted unchanged. The small amount of 5-fluorouracil detected is likely a consequence of the action of the intestinal microflora.

Flucytosine is usually well tolerated, with only about a 5% reported incidence of nausea, vomiting, and diarrhea. Occasional skin rashes have also been reported. Hepatic disturbances as signaled by elevations in serum transaminases are usually reversible. Bone marrow depression, which manifests as reversible neutropenia, is associated with serum levels of the drug greater than 100 μg/ml and is probably due to the presence of 5-fluorouracil (Diasio et al., 1978b). Because flucytosine is usually given with amphotericin B, which is nephrotoxic, it is important to monitor blood levels of flucytosine at least twice weekly. Patients receiving both drugs can also develop enterocolitis with a fatal outcome.

Flucytosine is available as Ancobon (Roche), capsules of 250 and 500 mg, for use in combination with amphotericin B for the treatment of cryptococcosis and disseminated candidiasis. It has been reported that flucytosine used alone is effective in treatment of chromomycosis, but the drug is not approved by the United States Food and Drug Administration for this purpose.

Azoles

The antifungal azoles consists of a five-member azole ring bound by a carbon nitrogen bond to other aromatic rings. Those agents with two nitrogen atoms in the azole ring are triazoles (Dismukes, 1988).

AZOLES

IMIDAZOLES

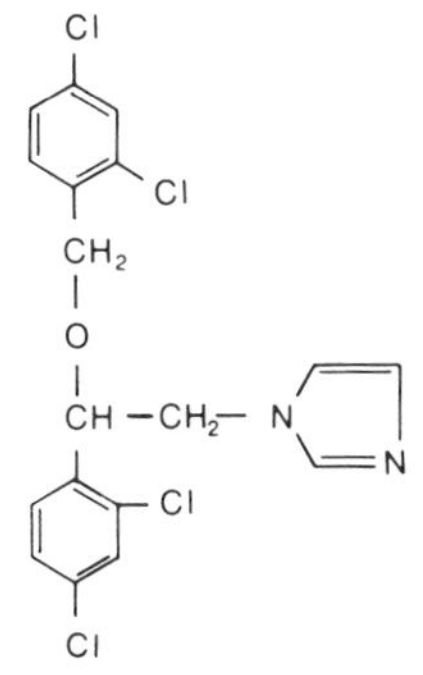

Miconazole

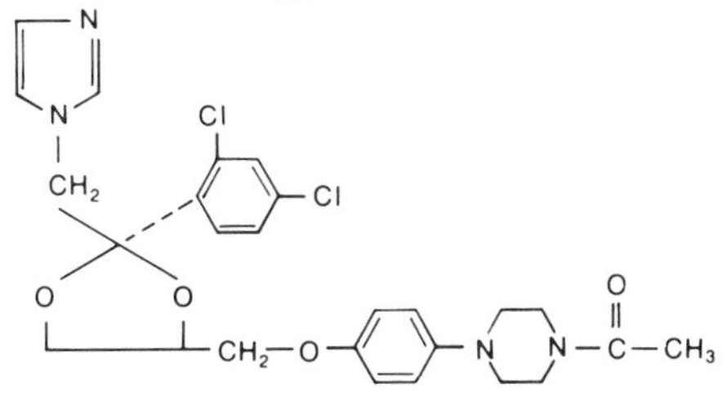

Ketoconazole

TRIAZOLES

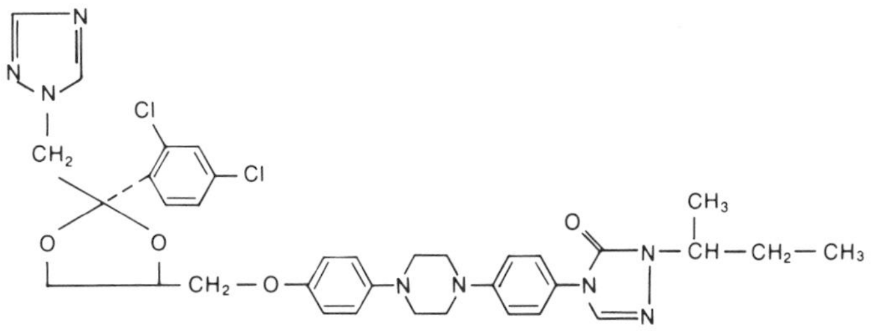

Itraconazole

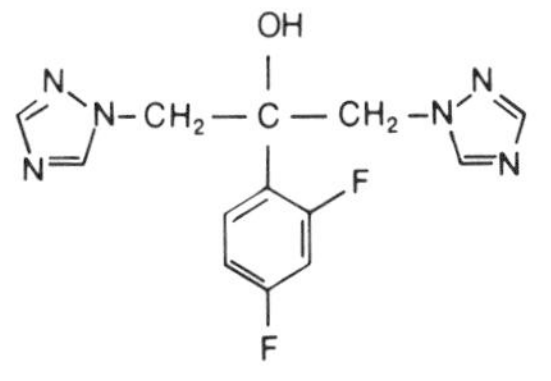

Fluconazole

Reports of the antifungal potential of azole compounds first appeared about 45 years ago with the imidazole compound, benzimidazole (Woolley, 1944) but intensive evaluation of these antifungal agents was delayed for nearly 30 years. Clotrimazole, the first orally effective imidazole against animal and human fungal infections, was shown to stimulate its own hepatic metabolism during chronic usage, so it is currently used only as a topical or troche agent (Saag and Dismukes, 1988). Another imidazole, micronazole, was found to be slowly metabolized and proved to be an effective intravenous agent against a wide spectrum of systemic or topical fungal agents and is probably the drug of choice in the treatment of a pseudoallescheriosis, an infection sometimes seen in immunocompromised patients (Bodey, 1988). Miconazole is not an effective oral agent. Experience with intravenous administration revealed multiple toxic effects, especially to the hematologic and cardiovascular systems and the skin (Dismukes, 1988); the drug is currently used primarily in the treatment of cutaneous mycoses or against systemic fungal infections when amphotericin B or ketoconazole is not effective or contraindicated (Saag and Dismukes, 1988). As miconazole began to lose its popularity in the late 1970s, another imidazole, ketoconazole, appeared as an orally active agent and soon became the best azole antifungal agent available.

Ketoconazole

Oral ketoconazole, was first synthesized in 1976 and appeared to present a breakthrough in antifungal therapeutics (Cauwenbergh and Van Cutsem, 1988). This agent, a synthetic imidazole, has proved to be effective against most pathogenic fungi except many isolates of *Candida tropicalis, Aspergillus sp., Zygomyces,* and *Microsporum canis* (Bodey, 1988).

Ketoconazole is effective in most systemic human mycoses including paracoccidioidomycosis, coccidioidomycosis, blastomycosis, and histoplasmosis. It is less effective in cases of chromoblastomycosis and pseudoallescheriosis. Ketoconazole is effective against dermatophytoses, such as *Trichophyton rubrum, Trichophyton mentagrophytes, Epidermophyton floccosum,* and *Microsporum canis,* pityriasis versicolor, onychomycoses, and most forms of candidiasis (Stevens, 1988). Relapses have been reported, especially in patients receiving ketoconazole in the treatment of deep or systemic fungal infection. Its oral effectiveness depends upon its proper gastrointestinal absorption, which is impaired by reduced gastric acidity and conditions such as drug-induced mucositis that damage the absorption mechanism. Ketoconazole appears to lose most of its therapeutic efficacy in neutropenic patients with systemic fungal infections; restoration of normal neutrophil counts usually improves the antifungal response (Bodey, 1988).

Ketoconazole is associated with a low frequency of serious side effects. The most common are the gastrointestinal effects of nausea, vomiting, and anorexia, which are lessened or prevented by administering the drug with food (Bodey, 1988). In one study involving ketoconazole treatment of 160 patients with coccidioidomycosis, toxic effects were reversible and consisted of nausea and vomiting (50%), gynecomastia (21%), decreased libido (13%), alopecia (8%), elevated liver function tests (5%), pruritus (5%), and rash (4%) (Sugar et al., 1988).

In a second study including the ketoconazole treatment of 52 patients with systemic fungal infections, the drug was most effective in patients with histoplasmosis and nonmeningeal cryptococcosis, less effective against blastomycosis and nonmeningeal coccidioidomycosis, and least effective against sporotrichosis (Dismukes et al., 1983). It does not appear to be useful in aspergillosis or meningeal cryptococcosis (Heel, 1982). The drug is about 100 times as potent as miconazole in inhibiting pseudomycelium formation of *Candida albicans;* this is important because pseudomycelial forms may dominate in infections (Borgers et al., 1979; Kucers et al., 1987a, 1987b).

Problems with ketoconazole have become apparent after several years of widespread use. It has a relatively short half-life, and it is difficult to achieve adequate drug levels in some tissues when compared to plasma levels. Use of the agent has been associated with rare but serious side effects such as hepatic toxicity and endocrine dysfunction. The mechanism of ketoconazole action is probably a selective inhibition of fungal ergosterol biosynthesis over that of mammalian cholesterol (Van den Bossche et al., 1980). More specifically, ketoconazole inhibits fungal and, at higher concentrations, mammalian cytochrome P-450-dependent enzymes of steroidogenesis. Unfortunately, ketoconazole in these high doses inhibits testicular, ovarian, and adrenal steroidogenesis in humans (De Coster et al., 1986). The major site of inhibition appears to be 17- to 20-desmolase, with a moderate inhibition of 17-hydroxylase, and a marked inhibition of 21- and/or 11-hydroxylase (Trachtenberg and Zadra, 1988; Medda et al., 1987; DeCoster et al., 1986). The suppressive effects appear to be reversible within at least 5 days after discontinuing the drug (Bradbrook et al., 1985).

Ketoconazole is a potent inhibitor of cholesterol biosynthesis, probably by blocking the conversion of lanosterol to cholesterol (Kraemer and Pont, 1986). As a consequence of these findings, this agent is under evaluation as a new endocrine drug in suppressing the production of excess cortisol and other glucocorticoids in the various forms of Cushing's syndrome (Delkers et al., 1986; Farwell et al., 1988), control of hyperaldosteronism (Benito et al., 1987), and suppression of androgen production in prostate cancer patients who have not undergone orchiectomy (Tapazoglou et al., 1986). Ketoconazole has been shown to reduce low-density lipoprotein (LDL) cholesterol levels up to 38%, but without concomitant changes in high-density lipoprotein (HDL) cholesterol levels (Kraemer and Pont, 1986).

Hepatotoxicity has been documented during ketoconazole treatment, as shown by transient, asymptomatic increases in serum transaminase or alkaline phosphatase levels. The estimated incidence of symptomatic hepatic reactions is about 1 in 10,000 (Janssen and Symoens, 1983). A 3-year evaluation of ketoconazole usage in the United Kingdom (1981 to 1984) associated the drug with 64 episodes of possible hepatotoxicity, including 3 deaths. It was concluded that periodic clinical and laboratory evaluations of patients for hepatitis should be conducted during long-term therapy with ketoconazole (Lake-Bakaar et al., 1987). Other rare but reported side effects of ketoconazole include hypothyroidism (Kitching, 1986; Tanner, 1987), potentiation of oral anticoagulants (Smith, 1984), drug-drug interactions with cyclosporin resulting in increased, prolonged serum levels of cyclosporin, increased toxicity and immunosuppression of cyclosporin (Shepard et al., 1986; Anderson et al., 1987), drug-drug interaction with rifampicin resulting in reduced ketoconazole levels (Doble et al., 1988), immune hemolytic anemia (Umstead et al., 1987), inhibition of drug N-demethylase activity and hepatic oxidative drug metabolism (Brown et al., 1985; Heusner et al., 1987; Meredith et al., 1985; Sheets and Mason, 1984), and a disulfiram-like reaction when taken with alcohol (Magnasco and Magnasco, 1986). Other associated side effects have been reported, but they are rare. In at least one case, ketoconazole was effective in the control of disseminated intravascular coagulation in a patient with underlying metastatic cancer of the prostate (Lowe and Somers, 1987). Ketoconazole, therefore, in spite of its wide spectrum of antifungal activity, has several disadvantages. First, even though its toxicity is considerably less than that of miconazole, its potential for toxicity remains. Second, a number of pathogenic fungi are not sensitive to ketoconazole. Third, the agent has a relatively short serum elimination half-life of about 3 to 4 hours after the oral administration of 200 mg to long-term users (Badcock et al., 1987; Stockley et al., 1986; Brass et al., 1982). Fourth, peak serum concentrations 2 to 3 hours after the oral administration of 200 mg ketoconazole are approximately 2.0 to 4.0 µg/ml, but there are no correlations between serum concentration and clinical efficacy, or between minimal inhibitory concentration and clinical efficacy, or between inhibitory concentrations (MICs) and therapeutic efficacy in animals or man (Saag and Dismukes, 1988; Drouhet and Dupont, 1987; Shadomy et al., 1985). Fifth, ketoconazole does not penetrate well into the central nervous system. These disadvantages of ketoconazole have caused the serious search for better azole antifungal agents to continue.

Itraconazole and Fluconazole

The need for new azole antifungal agents with increased therapeutic potential without the numerous associated adverse reactions and with superior therapeutic profiles led to the synthesis of itraconazole and fluconazole. These triazole antifungal agents have an equal or better spectrum of antifungal activity with the same mechanism of action as the imidazole antifungal agents. They share in common the mechanism of disrupting sterol biosynthesis within the fungal cell wall by inhibiting the fungal cytochrome P-450-associated enzymes. When compared to ketoconazole, they appear to have an increased affinity for fungal rather than mammalian cytochrome P-450 enzymes; this feature explains their lack of interference with adrenal or gonadal steroidogenesis and with metabolism of drugs via cytochrome P-450 enzymes (Garrison and Rotschafer, 1988; Eckhoff et al., 1988).

Itraconazole is a highly lipophilic, orally effective triazole that is tightly bound to plasma proteins, extensively metabolized by the liver, and excreted in the feces (Van Cauteren et al., 1987). In contrast, fluconazole is minimally bound by plasma proteins, is excreted by the kidney, and is probably effective when given either orally or intravenously (Humphrey et al., 1985; Perfect et al., 1986). Both new triazoles share with the older triazoles the problem of poor correlation between in vitro and in vivo activity.

Itraconazole and fluconazole appear to possess a greater spectrum of antimicrobial activity than ketoconazole with greater reduced adverse effects to the host (Van Cursem et al., 1987). These agents are active against most dermatophytoses, paracoccidioidomycosis, coccidioidomycosis, chromoblastomycosis, blastomycosis, histoplasmosis, and cryptococcosis, as well as *Alternaria spp.*, *Candida* and *Torulopsis spp.* (Stevens, 1988). Itraconazole is superior to ketoconazole in its effectiveness against meningeal cryptococcosis, sporotrichosis, and, surprisingly, aspergillosis (Van Cauteren et al., 1987; Longman and Martin, 1987; Ganer et al., 1987; Garrison and Rotschafer, 1988). Itraconazole possesses greater antifungal activity than fluconazole at equivalent doses (Perfect et al., 1986) but fungicidal serum or tissue concentrations of itraconazole are difficult to achieve by the oral route. Absorption and bioavailability of oral itraconazole are improved by administration with food (Stevens, 1988). Serum levels of 0.1 to 0.3 µg/ml are obtained about 4 hours after a 100-mg dose; then serum concentrations decline biexponentially, with an average terminal half-life of 19 hours (Garrison and Rotschafer, 1988). The steady state is reached in 1 to 2 weeks after the daily administration of 100 mg itraconazole (Stevens, 1988), with the drug accumulating in the liver, skin, and body fat.

Oral fluconazole is almost completely absorbed with the 1-mg/kg dose, producing average 4-hour serum levels of 1.4 µg/ml and an average half-life of 22 hours (Brammer and Tarbilt, 1987; Humphrey et al., 1985), so serum fungicidal levels are more easily obtainable than with itraconazole. Both agents distribute well to tissues (Van Cauteren et al., 1987), but fluconazole has the advantage over other azole antifungal agents in its ability to cross the blood-brain barrier and penetrate into the cerebrospinal fluid. Serum urine and tissue levels of azole antifungal agents are easily monitored by gas chromatographic methods or by high-performance liquid chromatography (HPLC) (Alton, 1980; Riley and James,

1986; Warnock et al., 1988; Woestenborghs et al., 1987; Wood and Tarbilt, 1986).

The use of both triazole agents is associated with only few and usually transient adverse reactions including gastrointestinal complaints, headaches, dizziness, increased urinary frequency, and mild elevations in hepatic enzyme levels (Garrison and Rotschafer, 1988). Unlike miconazole and ketoconazole, there are no reported instances of adverse interactions with anticoagulants, although interactions between itraconazole and cyclosporin have been reported (Shaw et al., 1987; Novakova et al., 1987; Kwan et al., 1987).

Most studies of itraconazole and fluconazole antifungal activity have been done in animal models, but results of some human itraconazole clinical studies have been reported (First International Symposium on Itraconazole). More recent reports of the results of clinical trials are available (Cauwenbergh et al., 1987; Hay, 1988; Tucker et al., 1988; Restrepo et al., 1988; Graybill, 1988). Fewer clinical studies have been completed with fluconazole but some are available (Stern et al., 1988; Sugar and Saunders, 1988; Dupont and Drouhet, 1988; Brammer and Feczko, 1988; Tucker et al., 1988; Van't Wout et al., 1988).

Current conclusions are that the new triazole antifungal agents offer equal or superior antifungal activity in comparison with other antifungal agents, with fewer adverse effects and improved pharmacokinetic profiles. Itraconazole and fluconazole are proving to be of superior importance in treating systemic fungal infections. Both agents are awaiting approval by the Food and Drug Administration for more extensive use in the United States.

Potassium Iodide

Seventy years ago, Davis (1919) wrote that the experience accrued with the use of iodide in treatment of sporotrichosis showed that ". . . the iodids (sic) in sporotrichosis furnish one of the best examples of a specific therapeutic agent known." Davis went on to note the impressive difference between the prompt reaction to potassium iodide (KI) of sporotrichitic patients and the effect of KI in other infections such as blastomycosis, actinomycosis, and tuberculosis, in which cases ". . . the reaction is irregular and uncertain and may be beneficial, indifferent, or possibly harmful." Davis (1919) also reviewed the then prevailing concepts regarding the salutary action of KI in lymphocutaneous sporotrichosis, including contentions of some of his contemporaries that I- was converted to free iodine (I_2) by leukocytes through which the antifungal activity was then expressed. He stressed that KI was curative and not preventive and demonstrated the inactivity of I- in vitro, compared with the high degree of antifungal activity of I_2.

Whereas KI remains the drug of choice for treatment of nondisseminated sporotrichosis (Pratt and Fekety, 1986), its mode of antifungal action is still not known. The general concept that I- has some inherent "antigranulomatous" action has been explored by few investigators. For example, Mielens et al. (1968) reviewed the

admittedly vague literature in this field and examined in some detail the action of KI against granuloma pouch formation, cotton granuloma formation, carrageenan and croton oil edema, and turpentine abscess formation using rats and monkeys. Oral administration of KI inhibited granuloma pouch formation in rats, but was without effect on the other four study parameters.

Hiruma and Kagawa (1987) recently studied structural changes induced in yeast cells of *Sporothrix schenckii* after in vitro exposure of the cells to dilute solutions of iodine-KI. Germination was inhibited totally at I_2 concentrations of 1.25 to 5.0 μg/ml. The accompanying ultrastructural changes were characterized as coagular changes with development of lomosomes.

Although evidence is still far from conclusive, some data implicate the myeloperoxide-peroxide-halide system in the mechanism of action of KI against fungi. This enzyme, a hemoprotein with a molecular weight of about 150,000, occurs in azurophilic granules of neutrophils and granulocytes and catalyzes the oxidation of halide ions to hypohalite ions by H_2O_2. This system and other oxygen-dependent microbicidal mechanisms of phagocytes were reviewed in detail by Babior (1978). Diamond and his colleagues studied the action of this system on standardized cell suspensions of *Candida albicans* (Diamond et al., 1980), *Rhizopus oryzae*, and *Aspergillus fumigatus* (Diamond and Clark, 1982) and found that hyphal damage to all organisms occurred in an in vitro system containing myeloperoxidase and 10^{-4} M concentrations of NaCl, H_2O_2, and NaI. It is clear that a detailed study of this neutrophil system is needed to define its possible role in the antisporotrichal action of KI.

Lymphocutaneous sporotrichosis is the only fungal disease for which iodide is indicated, but for this indication it is the drug of choice. The drug is usually given as a saturated solution of potassium iodide (SSKI, Upsher-Smith) that contains approximately 1.0 g KI/ml. The usual adult dose is 3.0 ml/day given in 3 divided doses, with slow escalation to 9 to 12 ml/day. The most common side effects are a bitter taste, gastrointestinal discomfort, excessive lacrimation, swelling of salivary glands, and an acneiform rash. These problems seldom necessitate discontinuance of the drug. Treatment should be continued about 6 weeks after healing of the lesions is evident. The usual total course of treatment may thus extend over a period of several months.

Investigational Antifungal Agents

Tioconazole, the most potent topical and in vitro anticandidial imidazole yet described, is highly effective in the treatment of dermal and vaginal candidiasis; a single treatment or brief exposure produces a lethal anticandidal effect. It is effective against dermatophytosis, onychomycosis, pityriasis versicolor, *Trichomonas*, *Gardnerella*, and several bacteria. An incidence of about 7% adverse effects of local itching and burning is associated with use as a topical agent (Stevens, 1988).

Terbinafine acts in vitro against superficial and systemic fungi, but apparently not in vivo against systemic fungal infections after oral administration of the agent. Topical activity has been noted in humans against pityriasis versicolor, dermatophytes, and candidiasis and activity after oral administration against dermatophytes, dermal candidiasis, and onychomycosis. Terbinafine, like the azole antifungal agents, inhibits fungal sterol synthesis, but at an earlier biosynthetic step, the squalene epoxidation step. Combinations of terbinafine and azoles act antagonistically against fungi. The lipophilic terbinafine is estimated to be 1000 to 10,000 times more active against fungal than mammalian enzymes in squalene epoxidation. Resistant fungi may possess a pool of sterol precursors distal to squalene. Oral doses of terbinafine are well absorbed, with peak serum concentrations noted 1.2 to 2.7 hours after dosing, and a serum half-life of about 12 hours.

TREATMENT OF ACTINOMYCOSIS AND NOCARDIOSIS

Benzyl penicillin (penicillin G) is the drug of choice for all forms of actinomycosis. The usual dose is up to 20 million U/day intravenously for at least 6 weeks. Some practitioners continue treatment for several months with oral penicillin V, 500 mg given 4 times a day. In patients who have a history to hypersensitivity to penicillin, the alternate drug is a tetracycline, usually tetracycline hydrochloride. In severe infections, the drug is usually given intravenously for 1 week, followed by oral administration for at least 1 month. Surgical drainage of accessible sites improves the therapeutic response.

Nocardiosis is treated initially with a sulfonamide or with the trisulfapyrimidine mixture; the latter preparation reduces the risk of crystalluria. The trimethoprim-sulfamethoxazole formulation is also effective, but as yet it is not approved for this indication by the United States Food and Drug Administration. In patients who are hypersensitive to sulfonamides or who are deficient in glucose-6-phosphate dehydrogenase, a favorable outcome may be obtained with minocycline, ampicillin, or erythromycin, although these drugs are not approved for this indication.

REFERENCES

Ajello, L. 1968. A taxonomic review of the dermatophytes and related species. Sabouraudia, 6, 147.

Ajello, L. 1969. A comparative study of the pulmonary mycosis of Canada and the United States. Public Health Rep., 84, 869.

Alton, K.B. 1980. Determination of the antifungal agent, ketoconazole, in human plasma by high-performance liquid chromatography. J. Chromatogr., 221, 337.

Anderson, J.E., Morris, R.E., and Blaschke, T.F. 1987. Pharmacodynamics of cyclosporin-ketoconazole interaction in mice: combined therapy potentiates cyclosporin immunosuppression and toxicity. Transplantation, 43, 529.

Andreoli, T.E. 1974. The structure and function of amphotericin B-cholesterol pores in lipid, bilayer membranes. Ann. N.Y. Acad. Sci., 235, 448.

Babior, B.M. 1978. Oxygen-dependent microbial killing by phagocytes. N. Engl. J. Med., 298, 659.

Badcock, N.R., et al. 1987. The pharmacokinetics of ketoconazole after chronic administration in adults. Eur. J. Clin. Pharmacol., 33, 531.

Baker, R.D. 1957. Mucormycosis—a new disease? JAMA, 163, 805.

Barrett-Bee, K.J., Lane, A.C., and Turner, R.W. 1986. The mode of antifungal action of tolnaftate. J. Med. Vet. Mycol., 24, 155.

Bauer, H., Ajello, L., Adams, E., and Hernandez, D.U. 1955. Cerebral mucormycosis: pathogenesis of the disease. Am. J. Med., 18, 822.

Bellisario, R.L., Maley, G.F., Gahvan, J.H., and Maley, F. 1976. Amino acid sequences at the FdUMP binding site of thymidylate synthetase. Proc. Natl. Acad. Sci. U.S.A., 73, 1848.

Benito, P., Corpas, M.S., Quesada, J.M., and Jimienez, J.A. 1987. Control of hyperaldosteronism by ketoconazole. Drug Intell. Clin. Pharm., 21, 752.

Bennett, J.E., et al. 1979. A comparison of amphotericin B alone and combined with flucytosine in the treatment of cryptococcal meningitis. N. Engl. J. Med., 301, 126.

Berk, M., Fink, G.I., and Uyeda, C.T. 1961. Rhinomucormycosis: report of a case diagnosed by clinical signs. JAMA, 177, 121.

Beyer, M. 1981. Selected double-blind comparative studies on the efficacy and tolerance ciclopiroxolamine solution and cream. Arzneimittelforschung, 31, 1378.

Blank, H., and Roth, F.J., Jr. 1959. The treatment of dermatomycoses with orally administered griseofulvin. Arch. Dermatol., 79, 259.

Blank, H., and Smith, J.G. 1960. Widespread Trichophyton rubrum granulomas treated with griseofulvin. Arch. Dermatol., 81, 779.

Block, E.R., and Bennett, J.E. 1973. The combined effort of 5-fluorocytosine and amphotericin B in the therapy of murine cryptococcosis. Proc. Soc. Exp. Biol. Med., 142, 476.

Block, E.R., Jennings, A.E., and Bennett, J.E. 1973. 5-Fluorocytosine resistance in Cryptococcus neoformans. Antimicrob. Agents Chemother., 3, 649.

Bodey, G.P. 1988. Fungal infections in cancer patients. Ann. N.Y. Acad. Sci., 544, 431.

Borgers, M., DeBrabander, M., Van Den Bossche, H., and Van Cutsem, J. 1979. Promotion of pseudomycelium formation of Candida albicans in culture: a morphological study of the effects of miconazole and ketoconazole. Postgrad. Med. J., 55, 687.

Bradbrook, I.D., et al. 1985. Effects of single and multiple doses of ketoconazole on adrenal function in normal subjects. Br. J. Clin. Pharmacol., 20, 163.

Brammer, K.W., and Feczko, J.M. 1988. Single-dose oral fluconazole in the treatment of vaginal candidosis. Ann. N.Y. Acad. Sci., 554, 561.

Brammer, K.W., and Tarbilt, M.H. 1987. A review of the pharmacokinetics of fluconazole (UK-49, 858) in laboratory animals and man. In Recent Trends in the Discovery, Development and Evaluation of Antifungal Agents. Edited by R.A. Fromptling. Barcelona, J.R. Prous, p. 141.

Brass, C., et al. 1982. Disposition of ketoconazole, an oral antifungal, in humans. Antimicrob. Agents Chemother., 22, 151.

Braude, A.I. 1986a. The aspergilli. In Infectious Diseases and Medical Microbiology. Edited by A.I. Braude, C.E. Davis, and J. Fierer. Philadelphia, W.B. Saunders, p. 592.

Braude, A.I. 1986b. Candida. In Infectious Diseases and Medical Microbiology. Edited by A.I. Braude, C.E. Davis, and J. Fierer. Philadelphia, W.B. Saunders, p. 571.

Braude, A.I. 1986c. Actinomycosis. In Infectious Diseases and Medical Microbiology. 2nd Edition. Edited by A.I. Braude, C.E. Davis, and J. Fierer. Philadelphia, W.B. Saunders, p. 740.

Brian, P.W. 1960. Griseofulvin. Br. Mycol. Soc. Trans., 43, 1.

Brian, P.W., Curtis, P.J., and Hemming, H.J. 1946. Biologic assay, production, and isolation of "curling factor." Br. Mycol. Soc. Trans., 29, 173.

Brown, M.W., Maldonado, A.L., Meredith, C.G., and Speeg, Jr., K.V. 1985. Effect of ketoconazole on hepatic oxidative drug metabolism. Clin. Pharmacol. Ther., 37, 290.

Bryan, J. 1974. Biochemical properties of microtubules. Fed. Proc., 33, 152.

Butler, W.T., Hill, G.J., Szwed, C.F., and Knight, V. 1964. Amphotericin B renal toxicity in the dog. J. Pharmacol. Exp. Ther., 143, 47.

Carter, V.H. 1972. A control study of haloprogin and tolnaftate in tinea pedis. Curr. Ther. Res. Clin. Exp., 14, 307.

Cauwenbergh, G., and Van Cutsem, J. 1988. Role of animal and human pharmacology in antifungal drug design. Ann. N.Y. Acad. Sci., 544, 264.

Cauwenbergh, G., et al. 1987. Experience with itraconazole in treatment of fungal infections. Ann. Inst. Super. Sanita, 23, 865.

Clark, J.F. 1899. On the toxic effects of certain deleterious agents on the germination and development of certain filamentous fungi. Botan. Gaz., 28, 289.

Collins, J.P., Grappel, S.F., and Blank, F. 1973. Role of keratinases in dermatophytosis. II. Fluorescent antibody studies with keratinase II of Trichophyton mentagrophytes. Dermatologica, 146, 95.

Conant, N.F., Smith, D.T., Baker, R.D., and Callaway, J.L. 1971a. Actinomycotic mycetoma. In Manual of Clinical Mycology. 3rd Edition. Philadelphia, W.B. Saunders, p. 62.

Conant, N.F., Smith, D.T., Baker, R.D., and Callaway, J.L. 1971b. Nocardiosis. In Manual of Clinical Mycology. 3rd Edition. Philadelphia, W.B. Saunders, p. 38.

Conant, N.F., Smith, D.T., Baker, R.D., and Callaway, J.L. 1971c. Actinomycosis. In Manual of Clinical Mycology. 3rd Edition. Philadelpha, W.B. Saunders, p. 1.

Cullen, S.I., et al. 1985. Treatment of tinea versicolor with a new antifungal agent, ciclopirox olamine cream 1%. Clin. Ther., 7, 574.

Davis, D.J. 1919. The effect of potassium iodide on experimental sporotrichosis. J. Infect. Dis., 25, 124.

Davies, R.R. 1980. Griseofulvin. In *Antifungal Chemotherapy*. Edited by D.C.E. Speller. New York, John Wiley & Sons, p. 149.

De Coster, R., et al. 1986. Effects of high-dose ketoconazole therapy on the main plasma testicular and adrenal steroids in previously untreated prostatic cancer patients. Clin. Endocrinol., 24, 657.

Delkers, W., Bahr, V., Hensen, J., and Pickartz, H. 1986. Primary adrenocortical micronodular adenomatosis causing Cushing's syndrome: effects of ketoconazole on steroid production and *in vitro* performance of adrenal cells. Acta Endocrinol., 113, 370.

Diamond, R.D., and Clark, R.A. 1982. Damage to *Aspergillus fumigatus* and *Rhizopus oryzae* hyphae by oxidative and nonoxidative microbicidal products of human neutrophils in vitro. Infect. Immun., 38, 487.

Diamond, R.D., Clark, R.A., and Haudenschild, C.C. 1980. Damage to *Candida albicans* hyphae and pseudohyphae by the myeloperoxidase system and oxidative products of neutrophil metabolism *in vitro*. J. Clin. Invest., 66, 908.

Diamond, R.D., et al. 1974. The role of the classical and alternate complement pathways in host defenses against *Cryptococcus neoformans* infection. J. Immunol., 112, 2260.

Diasio, R.B., Bennett, J.E., and Myers, C.E. 1978a. Mode of action of 5-fluorocytosine. Biochem. Pharmacol., 27, 703.

Diasio, R.B., Lakings, D.E., and Bennett, J.E. 1978b. Evidence for conversion of 5-fluorocytosine to 5-fluorouracil in humans: possible factor in 5-fluorocytosine clinical toxicity. Antimicrob. Agents Chemother., 14, 903.

Dick, J.D., Merz, W.G., and Saral, R. 1980. Incidence of polyene-resistant yeasts recovered from clinical specimens. Antimicrob. Agents Chemother., 18, 158.

Dismukes, W.E. 1988. Azole antifungal drugs: old and new. Ann. Intern. Med., 109, 177.

Dismukes, W.E., et al. 1983. Treatment of systemic mycoses with ketoconazole: emphasis on toxicity and clinical response in 52 patients. National Institute of Allergy and Infectious Diseases Collaborative Antifungal Study. Ann. Intern. Med., 98, 13.

Dismukes, W.E., et al. 1987. Treatment of cryptococcal meningitis with combination amphotericin B and flucytosine for four as compared with six weeks. N. Engl. J. Med., 317, 334.

Dittmar, W. 1981a. Penetration and antifungal activity of ciclopiroxolamine in hornified tissues. Arzneimittelforschung, 31, 1353.

Dittmar, W. 1981b. Non-European open clinical studies on the efficacy and tolerance of ciclopiroxolamine in dermatomycoses. Arzneimittelforschung, 31, 1381.

Doble, N., et al. 1988. Pharmacokinetic study of the interaction between rifampicin and ketoconazole. J. Antimicrob. Chemother., 21, 633.

Drouhet, E., and Dupont, B. 1987. Evolution of antifungal agents: past, present, and future. Rev. Infect. Dis., 9, 54.

Dupont, B., and Drouhet, E. 1979. *In vitro* synergy and antagonism of antifungal agents against yeast-like fungi. Postgrad. Med. J., 55, 683.

Dupont, B., and Drouhet, E. 1988. Fluconazole for the treatment of fungal diseases in immunosuppressed patients. Ann. N.Y. Acad. Sci., 554, 564.

Duschinsky, R., Pleven, E., and Heidelberger, C. 1957. The synthesis of 5-fluoropyrimidines. J. Am. Chem. Soc., 79, 4559.

Eckhoff, C., Oelkers, W., and Bahr, V. 1988. Effects of two oral antimycotics, ketoconazole and fluconazole, upon steroidogenesis in rat adrenal cells in vitro. J. Steroid Biochem., 31, 819.

El-Nakeeb, M.A., and Lampen, J.O. 1965. Uptake of griseofulvin by microorganisms and its correlation with sensitivity to griseofulvin. J. Gen. Microbiol., 39, 285.

Epstein, S.S., Andrea, J., Joshi, S., and Mentel, N. 1967. Hepatocarinogenicity of griseofulvin following parenteral administration to infant mice. Cancer Res., 27, 1900.

Epstein, W.L., Sheb, V.P., and Riegelman, S. 1972. Griseofulvin levels in stratum corneum: study after oral administration in man. Arch. Dermatol., 106, 344.

Farwell, A.P., Devlin, J.T., and Stewart, J.A. 1988. Total suppression of cortisol excretion by ketoconazole in the therapy of the ectopic adrenocorticotropic hormone syndrome. Am. J. Med., 84, 1063.

Fass, R.J., and Perkins, R.L. 1971. 5-Fluorocytosine in the treatment of cryptococcal and Candida mycoses. Ann. Intern. Med., 74, 535.

First International Symposium on Itraconazole. 1987. Oaxaca, Mexico, October 7–8, 1985. Rev. Infect. Dis., 9, S1–S152.

Foley, E.J., and Greco, G.A. 1959–1960. Studies on the mode of action of griseofulvin. Antibiotic. Ann., p. 670.

Fryberg, M., Oehlschlager, S.C., and Unrau, A.M. 1974. Sterol biosynthesis in antibiotic-resistant yeast: nystatin. Arch. Biochem. Biophys., 160, 83.

Gale, E.F. 1974. The release of potassium ions from *Candida albicans* in the presence of polyene antibiotics. J. Gen. Microbiol., 80, 451.

Gale, G.R. 1960. The effects of amphotericin B on yeast metabolism. J. Pharmacol. Exp. Ther., 129, 257.

Ganer, A., Arathoon, E., and Stevens, D.A. 1987. Initial experience in therapy

for progressive mycoses with itraconazole, the first clinically studied triazole. Rev. Infect. Dis., 9, 577.

Garrison, M.W, and Rotschafer, J.C. 1988. Itraconazole and fluconazole. Hosp. Ther., 13, 68.

Gentles, J.C. 1958. Experimental ringworm in guinea pigs: oral treatment with griseofulvin. Nature, 182, 476.

Georgopoulos, A., Petranyi, G., Mieth, H., and Drews, J. 1981. In vitro activity of naftifine, a new antifungal agent. Antimicrob. Agents Chemother., 19, 386.

Gold, W., Stout, H.A., Pagano, J.F., and Donovick, R. 1955–1956. Amphotericins A and B, antifungal antibiotics produced by a streptomycete. I. *In vitro* studies. Antibiot. Ann., p. 579.

Gordon, M.A., and Vedder, D.K. 1966. Serologic tests in diagnosis and prognosis of cryptococcosis. JAMA, 197, 961.

Graybill, J.R. 1988. Treatment of coccidioidomycosis. Ann N.Y. Acad. Sci., 544, 481.

Gregory, J.E., Golden, A., and Haymaker, W. 1943. Mucormycosis of central nervous system: Report of 3 cases. Bull. Johns Hopkins Hosp., 73, 405.

Grenson, M. 1969. The utilization of exogenous pyrimidines and the recycling of uridine-5'-phosphate derivatives in *Saccharomyces cerevisiae*, as studied by means of mutants affected in pyrimidine uptake and metabolism. Eur. J. Biochem., 11, 249.

Grunberg, E., Titsworth, E., and Bennett, M. 1963. Chemotherapeutic activity of 5-fluorocytosine. Antimicrob. Agents Chemother., 3, 566.

Gull, K., and Trinci, A.P.J. 1973. Griseofulvin inhibits fungal mitosis. Nature, 244, 292.

Hanel, H., Raether, W., and Dittmar, W. 1988. Evaluation of fungicidal action in vitro and in a skin model considering the influence of penetration kinetics of various standard antimycotics. Ann. N.Y. Acad. Sci., 544, 329.

Harvey, S.C. 1985. Antiseptics and disinfectants; fungicides; ectoparasiticides. In *Goodman and Gilman's The Pharmacological Basis of Therapeutics*. Edited by A.G. Gilman, L.S. Goodman, T.W. Rall, and F. Murad. New York, Macmillan, p. 959.

Hay, R.J. 1988. New oral treatments for dermatophytosis. Ann. N.Y. Acad. Sci., 544, 580.

Hazen, E.L., and Brown, R. 1951. Fungicidin, an antibiotic produced by a soil actinomycete. Proc. Soc. Exp. Biol. Med., 76, 93.

Heel, R.C. 1982. *Ketoconazole in the Management of Fungal Disease*. Sydney, Adis Press, p. 84.

Henderson, D.K., Bennett, J.E., and Huber, M.A. 1982. Long-lasting specific immunologic unresponsiveness associated with cryptococcal meningitis. J. Clin. Invest., 69, 1185.

Hermann, H.W. 1972. Clinical efficacy studies of haloprogin, a new topical antimicrobial agent. Arch. Dermatol., 106, 839.

Heusner, J., et al. 1987. Effect of chronically administered ketoconazole on the elimination of theophylline in man. Drug Intell. Clin. Pharm., 21, 514.

Hildick-Smith, G. 1965. Chemotherapy of fungus infections. In *Drill's Pharmacology in Medicine*. Edited by J.R. Di Palma. New York, McGraw-Hill, p. 1363.

Hiruma, M., and Kagawa, S. 1987. Ultrastructure of *Sporothrix schenckii* treated with iodine-potassium iodide solution. Mycopathologia, 97, 121.

Hoeprich, P.D., Ingraham, J.L., Kleker, E., and Winship, M.J. 1974. Development of resistance to 5-fluorocytosine in *Candida parapsilosis* during therapy. J. Infect. Dis., 130, 112.

Humphrey, M.J., Jevons, S., and Tarbit, M.H. 1985. Pharmacokinetic evaluation of UK-49, 858, a metabolically stable triazole antifungal drug, in animals and humans. Antimicrob. Agents Chemother., 28, 648.

Huppert, M., Sun, S.H., and Vukovich, K.R. 1974. Combined amphotericin B-tetracycline therapy for experimental coccidioidomycosis. Antimicrob. Agents Chemother., 5, 473.

Janssen, P.A., and Symoens, J.E. 1983. Hepatic reactions during ketoconazole treatment. Am. J. Med., 74, 80.

Jue, S.G., Dawson, G.W., and Brogden, R.N. 1985. Ciclopirox olamine 1% cream: a preliminary review of its antimicrobial activity and therapeutic use. Drugs, 29, 330.

Jund, R., and Lacrute, F. 1970. Genetic and physiological aspects of resistance to 5-fluoropyrimidines in *Saccharomyces cerevisiae*. J. Bacteriol., 102, 607.

Katz, S., and Cahn, B. 1972. Haloprogin therapy for dermatophyte infections. Arch. Dermatol., 106, 837.

Keates, R.A.B. 1981. Griseofulvin at low concentration inhibits the rate of microtubule polymerization *in vitro*. Biochem. Biophys. Res. Commun., 102, 746.

Keczkes, K., Leighton, I., and Good, C.S. 1975. Topical treatment of dermatophytoses and candidoses. Practitioner, 214, 412.

Kellner, H.M., et al. 1981. Pharmacokinetics and biotransformation of the antimycotic drug ciclopiroxolamine in animals and man after topical and systemic administration. Arzneimittelforschung, 31, 1337.

Kessler, H.J., Buitrago, B., and Strauss, E. 1978. Investigations of the fungicidal activity of haloprogin. Mykosen, 21, 138.

Kiesel, A. 1913. Recherches sur l'action de divers acides et sels acides sur le developpement de l'*Aspergillus niger.* Ann. Inst. Pasteur Microbiol., *27*, 391.

Kinsky, S.C. 1970. Antibiotic interaction with model membranes. Annu. Rev. Pharmacol., *10*, 119.

Kirkland, T.N. 1986. Coccidioidomycosis. In *Infectious Diseases and Medical Microbiology.* 2nd Edition. Edited by A.I. Braude, C.E. Davis, and J. Fierer. Philadelphia, W.B. Saunders, p. 867.

Kitching, N.H. 1986. Hypothyroidism after treatment with ketoconazole. Br. Med. J. (Clin. Res.), *293*, 993.

Klein, M.F., and Beall, J.R. 1972. Griseofulvin: a teratogenic study. Science, *175*, 1483.

Kligman, A.M., and Ginsberg, D. 1950. Immunity of the adult scalp to infection with *Microsporum audouini.* J. Invest. Dermatol., *14*, 345.

Kobayashi, G.S., et al. 1972. Amphotericin B potentiation of rifampicin as an antifungal agent against the yeast phase of *Histoplasma capsulatum.* Science, *177*, 709.

Korzybski, T., Kowszk-Gindifer, Z., and Kurylowicz, W. 1967. *Antibiotics.* Oxford, Pergamon Press.

Kotler-Brajtburg, J., et al. 1974. Molecular basis for the selective toxicity of amphotericin B for yeast and filipin for animal cells. Antimicrob. Agents. Chemother., 5, 377.

Kraemer, F.B., and Pont, A. 1986. Inhibition of cholesterol synthesis by ketoconazole. Am. J. Med., *80*, 616.

Kucers, A., Bennett, N. McK., and Kemp, R.J. 1987a. Ketoconazole. In *The Use of Antibiotics: A Comprehensive Review with Clinical Emphasis.* 4th Edition. Philadelphia, J.B. Lippincott, p. 1505.

Kucers, A., Bennett, N. McK., and Kemp, R.J. 1987b. Miconazole. In *The Use of Antibiotics: A Comprehensive Review with Clinical Emphasis.* 4th Edition. Philadelphia, J.B. Lippincott, p. 1491.

Kwan, J.T., Foxall, P.J., Davidson, D.G., and Eisinger, A.J. 1987. Interaction of cyclosporin and itraconazole. (Letter.) Lancet, *2*, 282.

Kwon-Chung, K.J. 1975. A new genus, *Filobasidiella,* the perfect state of *Cryptococcus neoformans.* Mycologia, *67*, 1197.

Kwon-Chung, K.J. 1979. Comparison of isolates of *Sporothrix schenckii* obtained from fixed cutaneous lesions with isolates from other types of lesions. J. Infect. Dis., *139*, 424.

Lake-Bakaar, G., Scheuer, P.J., and Sherlock, S. 1987. Hepatic reactions associated with ketoconazole in the United Kingdom. Br. Med. J. (Clin. Res.), *294*, 419.

Langenbach, R.J., Danenberg, P.V., and Heidelberger, C. 1972. Thymidylate synthetase: mechanism of inhibition by 5-fluoro-2'-deoxyuridylate. Biochem. Biophys. Res. Commun., *48*, 1565.

Lewis, J.L., and Rabinovich, S. 1972. The wide spectrum of cryptococcal infections. Am. J. Med., *53*, 315.

Little, J.R., Abegg, A., and Plut, E. 1983. The relationship between adjuvant and mitogenic effects of amphotericin methyl ester. Cell Immunol., *78*, 224.

Longman, L.P., and Martin, M.V. 1987. A comparison of the efficacy of itraconazole, amphotericin-B and 5-fluorocytosine in the treatment of *Aspergillus fumigatus* endocarditis in the rabbit. J. Antimicrob. Chemother., *20*, 719.

Lowe, F.C., and Somers, W.J. 1987. The use of ketoconazole in the emergency management of disseminated intravascular coagulation due to metastatic prostatic cancer. J. Urol., *137*, 1000.

Lynch, P.J., Vorhees, J.J., and Harrell, E.R. 1970. Systemic sporotrichosis. Ann. Intern. Med., *73*, 23.

Magnasco, A.J., and Magnasco, L.D. 1986. Interaction of ketoconazole and ethanol. Clin. Pharm., *5*, 522.

Malawista, S.E., Sato, H., and Bensch, K.G. 1968. Vinblastine and griseofulvin reversibly disrupt the living mitotic spindle. Science, *160*, 770.

McCutchan, J.A., and Mathews, W.C. 1986. Acquired immunodeficiency syndrome. In *Infectious Diseases and Medical Microbiology.* Edited by A.I. Braude, C.E. Davis, and J. Fierer. Philadelphia, W.B. Saunders, p. 1568.

Medda, F., et al. 1987. Short-term treatment with ketoconazole: effects on gonadal and adrenal steroidogenesis in women. Clin. Exp. Obstet. Gynecol., *14*, 161.

Medical Letter on Drugs and Therapeutics. 1988. *Handbook of Antimicrobial Therapy 1988.* New Rochelle, NY, Medical Letter, p. 106.

Medoff, G. 1987. Controversial areas in antifungal chemotherapy: short-course and combination therapy with amphotericin B. Rev. Infect. Dis., *9*, 403.

Medoff, G., Comfort, M., and Kobayashi, G.S. 1971. Synergistic action of amphotericin B and 5-fluorocytosine against yeast-like organisms. Proc. Soc. Exp. Biol. Med., *138*, 571.

Medoff, G., Brajtburg, J., Kobayashi, G.S., and Bolard, J. 1983. Antifungal agents useful in therapy of systemic fungal infections. Annu. Rev. Pharmacol. Toxicol., *23*, 303.

Medoff, G., et al. 1972. Potentiation of rifampicin and 5-fluorocytosine as antifungal antibiotics by amphotericin B. Proc. Nat. Acad. Sci. U.S.A., *69*, 196.

Meredith, C.G., Maldonado, A.L., and Speeg, Jr., K.V. 1985. The effect of ketoconazole on hepatic oxidative drug metabolism in the rat in vivo and in vitro. Drug Metab. Dispos., *13*, 156.

Meunier, F. 1987. Prevention of mycoses in immunocompromised patients. Rev. Infect. Dis., *9*, 408.

Mielens, Z.E., Rozitis, J., Jr., and Sansome, V.J., Jr. 1968. The effect of oral iodides on inflammation. Texas Rep. Biol. Med., *26*, 117.

Montes, L.F., and Hermann, H.W. 1978. Clinical and antimicrobial effects of haloprogin cream in diaper dermatitis. Cutis, *21*, 410.

Morita, T., and Nozawa, Y. 1985. Effects of antifungal agents on ergosterol biosynthesis in *Candida albicans* and *Trichophyton mentagrophytes:* differential inhibitory sites of naphthiomate and miconazole. J. Invest. Dermatol., *85*, 434.

Normark, S., and Schönebeck, J. 1972. In vitro studies of 5-fluorocytosine resistance in *Candida albicans* and *Torulopsis glabrata.* Antimicrob. Agents Chemother., *2*, 114.

Novakova, I., et al. 1987. Itraconazole and cyclosporin nephrotoxicity. (Letter.) Lancet, *2*, 920.

Oster, K.A., and Woodside, R. 1983. Fungistatic and fungicidal compounds. In *Disinfection, Sterilization and Preservation.* 3rd Edition. Edited by S.S. Block. Philadelphia, Lea & Febiger, p. 435.

Oxford, A.E., Raistrick, H., and Simonart, P. 1939. Studies in the biochemistry of microorganisms. LX. Griseofulvin, $C_{17}H_{17}O_6Cl$, a metabolic product of *Penicillium griseofulvum.* Biochem. J., *33*, 240.

Pagolotti, A.L., Ivanetich, K.M., Sommer, H., and Santi, D.V. 1976. Thymidylate synthetase: studies on the peptide containing covalently bound 5-fluoro-2-deoxyuridylate and 5,10-methylenetetrahydrofolate. Biochem. Biophys. Res. Commun., *70*, 972.

Peil, H.G. 1981. Open clinical study on the efficacy and tolerance of ciclopiroxolamine in vulvovaginal candidosis. Arzneimittelforschung, *31*, 1366.

Perfect, J.R., Savani, D.V., and Durack, D.T. 1986. Comparison of itraconazole and fluconazole in treatment of cryptococcal meningitis and candida pyelonephritis in rabbits. Antimicrob. Agents Chemother., *29*, 579.

Pierce, A.M., Pierce, H.D., Unrau, A.M., and Oehlschlager, A.C. 1978. Lipid composition and polyene resistance of *Candida albicans* mutants. Can. J. Biochem., *56*, 135.

Pine, L. 1986. Actinomyces and microaerophilic actinomycetes. In *Infectious Diseases and Medical Microbiology.* 2nd Edition. Edited by A.I. Braude, C.E. Davis, and J. Fierer. Philadelphia, W.B. Saunders, p. 391.

Polak, A. 1979. Pharmacokinetics of amphotericin B and flucytosine. Postgrad. Med. J., *55*, 667.

Polak, A., and Scholer, H.J. 1973a. Fungistatic activity, uptake and incorporation of 5-fluorocytosine in *Candida albicans* as influenced by pyrimidines and purines. I. Reversal experiments. Pathol. Microbiol., *39*, 148.

Polak, A., and Scholer, H.J. 1973b. Fungistatic activity, uptake and incorporation of 5-fluorocytosine in *Candida albicans* as influenced by pyrimidines and purines. II. Studies on distribution and incorporation. Pathol. Microbiol., *39*, 334.

Polak, A., and Scholer, H.J. 1975. Mode of action of 5-fluorocytosine and mechanisms of resistance. Chemotherapy, *21*, 113.

Pratt, W.B., and Fekety, R. 1986. *The Antimicrobial Drugs.* New York, Oxford University Press, p. 320.

Prince, H.N. 1959. Effect of pH on the antifungal activity of undecylenic acid and its calcium salt. J. Bacteriol., *78*, 788.

Qadripur, S.A., Horn, G., and Hohler, T. 1981. On the local efficacy of ciclopiroxolamine in onychomycoses. Arzneimittelforschung, *31*, 1369.

Readio, J.D., and Bittman, R. 1982. Equilibrium binding of amphotericin B and its methyl ester and borate complex to sterols. Biochim. Biophys. Acta, *685*, 219.

Restrepo, A., et al. 1988. Treatment of chromoblastomycosis with itraconazole. Ann. N.Y. Acad. Sci., *544*, 504.

Reynolds, E.S., Tomkiewicz, Z.M., and Dammin, G.T. 1963. The renal lesion related to amphotericin B treatment for coccidioidomycosis. Med. Clin. North Am., *47*, 1149.

Riley, C.M., and James, M.O. 1986. Determination of ketoconazole in the plasma, liver, lung, and adrenal of the rat by high-performance liquid chromatography. J. Chromatogr., *377*, 287.

Rippon, J.W. 1982. Pharmacology of antimycotic drugs. In *Medical Mycology.* 2nd Edition. Philadelphia, W.B. Saunders, p. 723.

Rippon, J.W. 1988a. Actinomycosis In *Medical Mycology.* 3rd Edition. Philadelphia, W.B. Saunders, p. 30.

Rippon, J.W. 1988b. Mycetoma. In *Medical Mycology.* 3rd Edition. Philadelphia, W.B. Saunders, p. 80.

Rippon, J.W. 1988c. Nocardiosis. In *Medical Mycology.* 3rd Edition. Philadelphia, W.B. Saunders, p. 53.

Robertson, D.B., and Maibach, H.I. 1987. Dermatologic pharmacology. In *Basic and Clinical Pharmacology.* 3rd Edition. Edited by B.G. Katzung. Norwalk, Connecticut, Appleton and Lange, p. 767.

Rothman, S., Smeljamic, A.M., and Shapiro, A.L. 1945. Fungistatic action of hair fat on *Microsporum audouini.* Proc. Soc. Exp. Biol. Med., *60*, 394.

Ruiz, A., Neilson, J.B., and Bulmer, G.S. 1982. Control of *Cryptococcus neoformans* in nature by biotic factors. Sabouraudia, *20*, 21.

Rustia, M., and Shubik, P. 1978. Thyroid tumors in rats and hepatomas in mice after griseofulvin treatment. Br. J. Cancer, *38*, 237.

Ryder, N.S., Frank, I., and Dupont, M.-C. 1986. Ergosterol biosynthesis inhibition by the thiocarbamate antifungal agents tolnaftate and tolciclate. Antimicrob. Agents Chemother., *29*, 858.

Saag, M.S., and Dismukes, W.E. 1988. Mini-review. Azole antifungal agents: Emphasis on new triazoles. Antimicrob. Agents Chemother., *32*, 1.

Sande, M.A., and Mandell, G.L. 1985. Antimicrobial agents: antifungal and antiviral agents. In *Goodman and Gilman's The Pharmacological Basis of Therapeutics*. Edited by A.G. Gilman, L.S. Goodman, T.W. Rall, and F. Murad. New York, Macmillan, p. 1219.

Santi, D.V., McHenry, C.S., and Sommer, H. 1974. Mechanism of interaction of thymidylate synthetase with 5-fluorodeoxyuridylate. Biochemistry, *13*, 471.

Sarosi, G.A., and Davies, S.F. 1986. Histoplasmosis. In *Infectious Diseases and Medical Microbiology*. 2nd Edition. Edited by A.I. Braude, C.E. Davis, and J. Fierer. Philadelphia, W.B. Saunders, p. 863.

Sarosi, G.A., et al. 1988. Chemotherapy of the pulmonary mycoses. Am. Rev. Respir. Dis., *138*, 1078.

Schacter, L.P., Owellen, R.J., Rathbun, H.K., and Buchanan, B. 1976. Antagonism between miconazole and amphotericin B. Lancet, *2*, 318.

Scholer, H.J. 1980. Flucytosine. In *Antifungal Chemotherapy*. Edited by D.C.E. Speller. New York, Wiley, p. 35.

Scott, F.W., et al. 1975. Teratogenesis in cats associated with griseofulvin therapy. Teratology, *11*, 79.

Seki, S., et al. 1963. Laboratory evaluation of M-1028 (2,4-5-Trichlorophenyl-gamma-iodopropargyl ether), a new antimicrobial agent. Antimicrob. Agents Chemother., *3*, 569.

Shadomy, S. 1969. In vitro studies with 5-fluorocytosine. Appl. Microbiol., *17*, 871.

Shadomy, S., et al. 1985. Treatment of systemic mycosis with ketoconazole: in vitro susceptibilities of clinical isolates of systemic and pathogenic fungi to ketoconazole. J. Infect. Dis., *152*, 1249.

Shah, V.P., Epstein, W.L., and Riegelman, S. 1974. Role of sweat in accumulation of orally administered griseofulvin in skin. J. Clin. Invest., *53*, 1673.

Shaw, M.A., Gumbleton, M., and Nicholls, P.J. 1987. Interaction of cyclosporin and itraconazole. (Letter.) Lancet, *2*, 637.

Sheets, J.J., and Mason, J.I. 1984. Ketoconazole: a potent inhibitor of cytochrome P-450-dependent drug metabolism in rat liver. Drug Metab. Dispos., *12*, 603.

Shepard, J.H., Canafax, D.M., Simmons, R.L., and Najarian, J.S. 1986. Cyclosporin-ketoconazole: a potentially dangerous drug-drug interaction. Clin. Pharm., *5*, 468.

Sloboda, R.D., et al. 1982. Griseofulvin: association with tubulin and inhibition of in vitro microtubule assembly. Biochem. Biophys. Res. Commun., *105*, 882.

Smith, A.G. 1984. Potentiation of oral anticoagulants by ketoconazole. Br. Med. J. (Clin. Res.), *228*, 188.

Smith, E.B. 1976. New topical agents for dermatophytosis. Cutis, *17*, 54.

Steer, P.L., Marks, I., Klite, P.D., and Eickhoff, T.C. 1972. 5-Fluorocytosine, an oral antifungal compound. Ann. Intern. Med., *76*, 15.

Stern, J.J., et al. 1988. Oral fluconazole therapy for patients with acquired immunodeficiency syndrome and cryptococcosis: experience with 22 patients. Am. J. Med., *85*, 477.

Stevens, D.A. 1988. The new generation of antifungal drugs. Eur. J. Clin. Microbiol., *7*, 732.

Stockley, R.J., et al. 1986. Ketoconazole pharmacokinetics during chronic dosing in adults with haematological malignancy. Eur. J. Clin. Microbiol., *5*, 513.

Sugar, A.M., and Saunders, C. 1988. Oral fluconazole as suppressive therapy of disseminated cryptococcosis in patients with acquired immunodeficiency syndrome. Am. J. Med., *85*, 481.

Sugar, A.M., et al. 1987. Pharmacology and toxicity of high-dose ketoconazole. Antimicrob. Agents Chemother., *31*, 1874.

Tanner, A.R. 1987. Hypothyroidism after treatment with ketoconazole. Br. Med. J. (Clin. Res.), *294*, 125.

Tapazoglou, E., et al. 1986. High-dose ketoconazole therapy in patients with metastatic prostate cancer. Am. J. Clin. Oncol., *9*, 369.

Thaler, M., et al. 1988. Hepatic candidiasis in immunocompromised patients: a new or evolving syndrome. Ann. Intern. Med., *108*, 88.

Torres, J., Savopaulos, C., and Dittmar, W. 1981. Open clinical trial in dermal mycoses of a 1% ciclopiroxolamine solution in polyethylene glycol 400 carried

out in FR Germany, study with shortened therapy. Arzneimittelforschung, *31*, 1373.

Tosh, F.E., Hammerman, K.J., Weeks, R.J., and Sarosi, G.A. 1974. A common source epidemic of North America blastomycosis. Am. Rev. Respir. Dis., *109*, 525.

Trachtenberg, J., and Zadra, J. 1988. Steroid synthesis inhibition by ketoconazole: sites of action. Clin. Invest. Med., *11*, 1.

Tucker, R.M., Williams, P.L., Arathoon, E.G., and Stevens, D.A. 1988. Treatment of mycoses and itraconazole. Ann. N.Y. Acad. Sci., *544*, 451.

Tucker, R.M., et al. 1988. Pharmacokinetics of fluconazole in cerebrospinal fluid and serum in human coccidioidal meningitis. Antimicrob. Agents Chemother., *32*, 369.

Umstead, G.S., Babiak, L.M., and Tejwani, S. 1987. Immune hemolytic anemia associated with ketoconazole therapy. Clin. Pharm., *6*, 499.

Utz, J.P., et al. 1968. 5-Fluorocytosine in human cryptococcosis. Antimicrob. Agents Chemother., *8*, 344.

Van Cauteren, H., Heykants, J., DeCoster, R., and Cauwenberg, G. 1987. Itraconazole: pharmacologic studies in animals and humans. Rev. Infect. Dis., *9*, 543.

Van Cutsem, J., Van Gerven, F., and Janssen, P.A.J. 1987. Activity of orally, topically, and parenterally administered itraconazole in the treatment of superficial and deep mycosis: animal models. Rev. Infect. Dis., *9*, 515.

Van den Bossche, H., et al. 1980. In vitro and in vivo effects of the antimycotic drug ketoconazole on sterol synthesis. Antimicrob. Agents Chemother., *17*, 922.

Vandevelde, A.G., Mauceri, A.A., and Johnson, J.E., III. 1972. 5-Fluorocytosine in the treatment of mycotic infections. Ann. Intern. Med., *77*, 43.

Van't Wout, J.W., Mattie, H., and Van Furth, R. 1988. A prospective study of the efficacy of fluconazole (UK-49, 858) against deep-seated fungal infections. J. Antimicrob. Chemother., *21*, 665.

Walsh, T.J., and Pizzo, P.A. 1988. Nosocomial fungal infections: a classification for hospital-acquired fungal infections and mycoses arising from endogenous flora or reactivation. Annu. Rev. Microbiol., *42*, 517.

Warnock, D.W., Turner, A., and Burke, J. 1988. Comparison of high performance liquid chromatographic and microbiological methods for determination of itraconazole. J. Antimicrob. Chemother., *21*, 93.

Weber, K., Wehland, J., and Herzog, W. 1976. Griseofulvin interacts with microtubules both *in vivo* and *in vitro*. J. Mol. Biol., *102*, 817.

Wehland, J., Herzog, W., and Weber, K. 1977. Interaction of griseofulvin with microtubules, microtubule protein, and tubulin. J. Mol. Biol., *111*, 329.

Wempen, I., Duschinsky, R., Kaplan, L., and Fox, J.J. 1961. Thiation of nucleosides. IV. The synthesis of 5-fluoro-2'-deoxycytidine and related compounds. J. Am. Chem. Soc., *83*, 4755.

Williams, D.J., Marten, R.H., and Sarkany, I. 1958. Oral treatment of ringworm with griseofulvin. Lancet, *2*, 1212.

Wilson, L. 1970. Properties of colchicine binding protein from chick embryo brain: interactions with vinca alkaloids and podophyllotoxin. Biochemistry, *9*, 4999.

Woestenborghs, R., Lorreyne, W., and Heykants, J. 1987. Determination of itraconazole in plasma and animal tissues by high performance liquid chromatography. J. Chromatogr., *413*, 332.

Wood, P.R., and Tarbit, M.H. 1986. Gas chromatographic method for the determination of fluconazole, a novel antifungal agent, in human plasma and urine. J. Chromatogr., *383*, 179.

Woods, R.A., Bard, M., Jackson, I.E., and Drutz, D.J. 1974. Resistance to polyene antibiotics and correlated sterol changes in two isolates of *Candida tropicalis* from a patient with an amphotericin B-resistant funguria. J. Infect. Dis., *129*, 53.

Woolley, D.W. 1944. Some biological effects produced by benzimidazole and their reversal by purines. J. Biol. Chem., *152*, 225.

Wright, D.G., Robichaud, K.J., Pizzo, P.A., and Deisseroth, A.B. 1981. Lethal pulmonary reactions associated with the combined use of amphotericin B and leukocyte transfusions. N. Engl. J. Med., *304*, 1185.

Yamaguchi, H., et al. 1986. In vitro activity of ME1401, a new antifungal agent. Antimicrob. Agents Chemother., *30*, 705.

Yu, R.J., and Blank, F. 1973. On the mechanism of action of griseofulvin in dermatophytosis. Sabouraudia, *11*, 274.

Zinsser, H. 1988. Systemic mycoses. In *Zinsser Microbiology*. 19th Edition. Edited by W.K. Joklik, H.P. Willett, D.B. Amos, and C.M. Wilfert. Norwalk, CT, Appleton and Lange, p. 895.

CHAPTER 25

PRINCIPLES OF VIRAL CONTROL
AND TRANSMISSION

Herbert N. Prince, Daniel L. Prince, and Richard N. Prince

INACTIVATION CURVES

The inactivation of bacteria and viruses is in general a first-order kinetic reaction. When plotted, the graph of the survivors versus time is a straight line (Hiatt, 1964). Killing curves of different shapes can be obtained by the use of heat, irradiation, or chemical germicides, depending upon either the homogenicity or the heterogenicity of the viral suspension. Few data are available, however, on samples of dried viruses as required in the hard-surface virucide method of the United States Environmental Protection Agency (EPA).

Early Data

The early data of Salk with formaldehyde inactivation of poliovirus (Salk and Gori, 1960) and Gerber et al. (1961) with simian virus 40 (SV-40) have led to the understanding of multiple component curves. The curve arises from a viral population with different sensitivities. Those that are more sensitive are inactivated first with a steep slope, whereas at the end only the most resistant ones survive, with a shallower slope for their survival curve. Thus, extrapolation of survivors from the shape of a killing curve cannot always be made without specific knowledge of the chemical nature of either the germicide or the surface of the virus particle. In the Salk experiments, dilute formaldehyde solution reacted with the protein coat of the virus gradually producing a slowdown in rate of inactivation. Gard (1957) explained this by postulating that it became increasingly difficult for the aldehyde to reach the nucleic acid core of the virus (the formaldehyde-fixed capsid having become impervious to further diffusion of aldehyde into the nucleoprotein core), leading to a decreased inactivation rate with time. A biphasic curve was produced when the infectivity of suspended virus was studied over several days. The curve described a dual population of sensitive as well as resistant viral particles. This curve was used by manufacturers of "killed" polio vaccine to estimate the length of time for complete inactivation of the virus subsequent to incubation of virus in *diluted* formaldehyde. It was a tragic underestimation and underscored the danger inherent to overdilution of aldehydes in the destruction of infectivity. Failure to properly understand the kinetics of the formaldehyde inactivation curve led to deaths from incompletely "killed" polio vaccine. Thus, attention was drawn for the first time to the relationship between the physicochemical nature (density, protein) of the viral particle and the chemical nature of the virucide. In this example, *injection* of a formaldehyde-treated virus introduced infectious nucleic acid within the host, even though the outer protein capsid had been fixed. Moreover, for the first time, although unappreciated by virologists at that time, a relationship between the surface chemistry of the virion and the chemistry of the inactivator was inferred.

Klein-DeForest Scheme

Almost a decade passed before the now-classic studies of Klein and DeForest (1963, 1965) on the chemical nature of viral inactivation explained the inferences of the Salk data and revealed that, in addition to the concentration and physical aggregation of the virions, the chemical nature of the viral surface had a remarkable bearing on the loss of infectivity. These data have now been embodied in a concept named the Klein-DeForest Scheme (Prince, 1983). According to this scheme, viruses can be divided into groups A, B, and C (Klein and DeForest, 1963 and 1983) with respect to inactivation of lipophilic (enveloped, lipid membrane) and hydrophilic (naked) viruses.

Specific physicochemical groups of viruses are now generally recognized to behave similarly with respect to sensitivity to chemical agents, and viruses can be putatively ranked in terms of their overall resistance to disinfectants such as phenolics (e.g., orthophenyl phenol), quaternary ammonium compounds (e.g., dual com-

Table 25–1. *Virucidal Effect of Aliphatic Alcohols Against Certain Viruses*

Virus	Methanol	Ethanol	Isopropanol	Butanol
Lipophilic		Increasing Activity		
Vaccinia	±	+	+ +	NT
Influenza A$_2$	+ +	+ +	+ +	+ + + +
Herpes simplex I	+	+ +	+ + +	+ + + +
Partial Lipophilic				
Adeno 2	+	+ +	+ +	NT
Adeno 7	NT	+ + +	+ + +	NT
Hydrophilic		Increasing Activity		
Polio 1	+ + +	+ + +	+	0
Coxsackie B$_1$	+ + +	+ + +	+	NT
ECHO 6	+ + +	+ + +	+	NT
Rhino 17	NT	+ + +	+	NT
Coxsackie B$_2$	NT	+ + + +	+	NT

		Concentration Required to Inactivate in 10 Minutes or Less
		(%)
Lipophilic	±	50
	+	40
	+ +	30
	+ + +	20
	+ + + +	10
Partial Lipophilic	+	60
	+ +	50
	+ + +	30
Hydrophilic	0 =	Inactive undiluted
	+	90–95
	+ + +	40–70
	+ + + +	30

NT = Not tested.

Adapted from Klein, M., and DeForest, A. 1983. Principles of viral inactivity. In *Disinfection, Sterilization, and Preservation*. 3rd Edition. Edited by S.S. Block. Philadelphia, Lea & Febiger.

pounds such as BTC-2125M, D-125), halogens (e.g., chlorine and iodine compounds such as hypochlorite, chlorine dioxide, iodine, and iodophors), basic aliphatic amines (e.g., chlorhexidine), aldehydes (e.g., formaldehyde, glutaraldehyde), lower aliphatic alcohols (e.g., ethanol, isopropanol), and other agents.

Tables 25–1 to 25–3 are a general summary of the work of Klein and DeForest with respect to the effect of various classes of chemical agents against a variety of viruses. Table 25–1 shows that virucidal activity of alcohols is related to both the chemical nature of the germicide and the chemical nature of the viral surface, as discussed later in this chapter. Table 25–2 extends this observation to phenolics and quaternary ammonium salts that are effective mainly against lipophilic viruses, but shows the broader spectrum of activity for oxidizing agents and aldehyde agents against both lipophilic and hydrophilic viruses. Table 25–3 further categorizes the three Klein-DeForest groups in terms of viral chemistry and general sensitivity to disinfectants. Table 25–4 ranks viruses in

more specific terms according to increasing resistance to chemical germicides, based upon the Klein-DeForest scheme and upon data from our laboratory.

In spite of the data in Table 25–4, however, the United States EPA does not allow the use of prototype testing for viruses, as is the case with bacteria (Fed. Reg. 1975). This position is supported by the exceptions that are known to exist to the dogma of the Klein-DeForest scheme (Klein and DeForest, 1983) (e.g., 10% benzalkonium chloride inactivated Coxsackie B$_5$ but not Coxsackie B$_1$ or B$_2$, or ECHO types 6 and 9). Many European countries, however, do allow prototype testing; the issue remains unresolved at the international level. It is generally thought that intertaxon predictions are more reliable than intrataxon predictions, e.g., inactivation of polio will predict inactivation of influenza but inactivation of Coxsackie B$_1$ may not predict for the inactivation of other Coxsackie A's, B's, or ECHO virions, all members of the picornaviridae.

The lipid nature of the viral envelope is a result of the unique budding process that occurs during replication and extrusion from the host cell. The membrane is "stripped" away, as it were, from the host cell and becomes the outer envelope of the emerging virus, either as a viral particle (HIV) or as a viral filament (influenza).

The presence of the lipid membrane enables the reverse process of viral entry to take place either by the process of dissolution-fusion upon the receptor sites of the host cell or by the process of endocytosis.

Referring again to the data in Table 25–1, a general pattern seems to obtain between the molecular weight of an alcohol and the susceptibility of various lipid-containing and lipid-free viruses, although a certain overlapping does exist. The effect of molecular weight is seen to the greatest extent when one observes the results with Coxsackie B$_1$ and B$_2$ viruses.

Although the early work of Klein and DeForest (1963) suggested the predictability of virucidal effects, later work of Klein and DeForest (1983) revealed that a wide range of alcohol concentrations was required to inactivate similar viruses. For example, these workers showed that ECHO 18 virus was inactivated in suspension in 10 min at room temperature by 30% ethanol, whereas ECHO 9 required 70%; similarly, 30% isopropanol inactivated ECHO 18, but ECHO 6 and ECHO 9, Coxsackie B$_1$, B$_2$, and B$_3$, and rhinovirus 17 required as high as 90 to 95%. Furthermore, according to the authors, 2% formalin inactivated poliovirus type 3, whereas 8% was required to inactivate type 1. Thus, the EPA requirement of *per species testing* instead of *prototype screening* seems to remain appropriate. In other words, Klein-DeForest predictions notwithstanding, there are no definitive published studies that would allow broad predictions on sensitivity or resistance for all members of a taxon, e.g., influenza A$_2$ (Japan 57/305) for all type A influenzas, Adeno 2 for all adenoviruses, rhino 14 for all rhinoviruses, etc.

Furthermore, caution must be exercised in using hy-

Table 25–2. *Chemical Guide to Viral Inactivation—Minimum Concentration of Virucide Inactivation in 10 Minutes*

Virus	Sodium Hypochlorite	Isopropanol	Ethanol	Benzalkonium Chloride and Derivatives	Iodophor as I_2	Ortho Phenylphenol G	Glutaraldehyde
Polio I	200 ppm[a]	95% active	70% active	10% inactive[b] D-125 inactivates in 30 min	150 ppm[a]	12% inactive[b]	2%[a]
Coxsackie B₁	200 ppm[a]	95% active	50% active	10% inactive[b]	150 ppm[a]	12% inactive	1%[a]
Adeno 2	200 ppm[a]	50% active	50% active	700–1000 ppm active (400 ppm partial)	150 ppm[a]	0.12%[c]	0.04%[a]
Vaccinia	200 ppm[a]	30% active	40% active	100 ppm[c]	75 ppm[a]	0.12%[c]	0.02%[a]
Herpes	200 ppm[a]	20% active	30% active	100 ppm[c]	75 ppm[a]	0.12%[c]	0.04%[a]
Influenza A	200 ppm[a]	30% active	30% active	1000 ppm[c]	75 ppm[a]	0.12%[c]	0.02%[a]
HIV-1 (AIDS)	50 ppm[e]	35% active[e]	50% active[e]	BTC 2125 dual[f] quat 70–100 ppm (formulation D-125 in 30 sec)	35–75 ppm[f]		0.12%[f]
Feline[d] parvovirus	2000 ppm ≥4 log reduction	50% inactive in 10 min	50% inactive in 10 min	5000 ppm inactive in 10 min	5000 ppm 1-log reduction	10% inactive in 10 min	1% (2-log reduction)
Hepatitis B	Limited data of Bond et al. (1983) and Prince, D.L. (unpublished) and Thraenhart, O. suggest the absence of marked resistance.						

[a]Shows the marked activity of halogens and glutaraldehyde.

[b]Shows the inactivity of lipophilic substances against hydrophilic viruses in 10 min.

[c]Shows the activity of lipophilic substances against lipophilic viruses, which generally mimics effects against vegetative bacteria.

[d]Some inactivations can occur with high-passage strains and a combination of agents and synergists in the formulation; contact times may have to be extended in presence of minimum protein load of 5% serum. Data from Scott (1980). Customary 10-min contact time ineffective (incomplete to partial inactivation). Similar results are seen with canine parvovirus.

[e]See Martin, et al., 1985.

[f]See Prince and Prince, 1989.

[g]Commercial disinfectant containing 2.8% o-phenyl phenol and 2.7% o-benzyl-p-phenol. Aryl substituted and halogenated phenols are poorly soluble substances and difficult to study as pure compounds at physiological pHs.

Data from Klein, M., and DeForest, A. 1963. The chemical inactivation of viruses. In Proceedings of the Chemical Specialty Manufacturing Association, 49th Midyear Meeting, pp. 116–118; Klein, M., and DeForest, A. 1983. Principles of viral inactivity. In *Disinfection, Sterilization, and Preservation*. 3rd Edition. Edited by S.S. Block. Philadelphia, Lea & Febiger; Scott, F.W. 1980. Virucidal disinfectants and feline viruses. Am. J. Vet. Res., 41, 410–414; Prince, H.N. 1983. Disinfectant activity against bacteria and viruses; a hospital guide. Partic. Microb. Control, 2, 55–62; and Martin, L.S., McDougal, J.S., and Loskoski, S.L. 1985. Disinfection and inactivation of the human T lymphotropic virus type III/LAV. J. Infect. Dis., 152, 400–403.

Table 25–3. *Sensitivity to Disinfectants*

Klein-DeForest Category	Solubility	Chemical Structure	Sensitivity
(A) Lipid*	Lipophilic (envelope)	Nucleic acid + capsid + envelope	*Marked* Myxoviruses Respiratory syncytial Herpes Human immunodeficiency
(B) Nonlipid	Hydrophilic (no envelope)	Nucleic acid + capsid	*Slight* Polio Coxsackie, ECHO Rhino
(C) Nonlipid	Intermediate (capsomeric lipophilicity)	Nucleic acid + capsid	*Moderate* Adeno Reo SV-40 Rota

*The lipophilicity of group A is based upon destruction by diethylether or adsorption of viruses by lipids such as cholesterol, palmitic acid, or hexadecylamine, as well as by inactivation by lipophilic germicides such as quaternary ammonium compounds and other polar or nonpolar detergents.

Table 25–4. *Ranking of Viruses by Susceptibility* to Chemical Germicides (10-Min Exposure at 20–25°C)*

Virus		Viral Susceptibility Group	Active Agents†
Myxoviruses, herpesviruses, retroviruses, vaccinia, toga, bunya, arena, corona, rhabdo, other lipophilic viruses		A	Halogens Aldehydes Quaternary ammonium compounds (quats) Phenolics Alcohols H_2O_2 Proteases Detergents
Vaccinia	B_1	B	Halogens
Adenoviruses	B_2		Aldehydes
Rotavirus	B_3		Quats
Papovaviruses	B_4		Phenolics
Hepatitis B virus (probable)			Alcohol
			H_2O_2
Picornaviruses			
Coxsackie A		C	Alcohol alone or in combination with quats; quat mixtures at *longer* contact times
Coxsackie B			
ECHO			Halogens
Rhino			Aldehydes
Polio			Phenolics
Hepatitis A virus			H_2O_2
Parvoviruses		D	Halogens Aldehydes (variable) Quat and phenolics (variable) with synergists and longer contact time (e.g., 30–60 min) H_2O_2
Viroids		E	Halogens/H_2O_2 Nucleic acid inactivators RNAase
Prions		F	2N NaOH effective. None of the common chemical agents; routine autoclaving ineffective

*Susceptibility is the ability of the agent to inactivate the surface apparatus while not necessarily destroying the replicating ability of the core nucleic acid. The susceptibility of hepatitis B virus (HBV) is probably within groups A to B.

†Disinfectant formulations are influenced by co-ingredients and "inerts," consequently in certain cases activity, solubility and stability can be "built" or synergized into a product.

Note: Bacteriophages generally display sensitivity similar to lipid-containing viruses. Quaternary ammonium compounds have been found to be more effective against T-1 and T-4 coliphages than phenolics or hypochlorites (Prince et al 1990) in experiments designed to mitigate the contamination of *Eschericha coli* pilot and production batches during the production of genetically engineered products (e.g., insulin).

drophilic surrogate viruses as predictive assays for lipophilic viruses, especially when studies with increased protein load (serum or mucin) are undertaken. All the studies to date that have shown how difficult it is to inactivate a hydrophilic virus and how easy it is to inactivate a lipophilic agent have been performed with relatively low protein load. It must be determined whether increased protein load is more protective for lipophilic viruses such as herpes and influenza, viruses with an affinity for mucous membranes and mucopolysaccharides. No data are available on the relative shielding effect of protein and mucin on these two chemical classes of virus. In fact, the possibility may exist that in the presence of high organic load, some myxoviruses may be more difficult to inactivate than their nonenveloped counterparts because of their special affinity for organic matter, which, in turn, may protectively encapsulate the virion from the germicide. These studies should be pursued.

CLASSIFICATION OF VIRUCIDAL DISINFECTANTS

Spaulding (1968), Favero (1983) and, more recently, Rutala (1989) have emphasized the concept of "high-level" and "low-level" disinfectants, designations based upon the critical, semicritical, or noncritical nature of the article treated. This approach, although useful and popular, tends to overemphasize the theoretic application of pure active ingredients and to overlook that surface fomites and devices are treated in practice with mixtures of substances. These mixtures or products are comprised basically of "actives," solvents, detergents, anticorrosives, metal chelators, buffers, and other so-called "inerts." Just as the United States Food and Drug Administration (FDA) does not recognize that three different pharmaceutical companies producing the same antibiotic or the same hypotensive agent are producing the same drug (a drug consists of *all* the ingredients *plus* the manufacturing process), the EPA does not recognize that three separate disinfectants produced with the same concentration of the same active ingredient are the same germicidal product. Accordingly, the EPA has chosen not to categorize disinfectants, as per the United States Centers for Disease Control (CDC), but has chosen to require statistically dependable antimicrobial tests for each product allowing the label claim to speak for itself. The "high-level/low-level" taxonomy leads to generalizations such as the statement that iodophors, phenolics, and isopropanol (70%) are "low level," whereas ethanol (70%) is "high level" (a conclusion based upon the resistance of poliovirus). In fact, poliovirus is a relatively unimportant target organism in either environmental or nosocomial disease transmission; furthermore, polio can be inactivated by isopropanol requiring a concentration of 95%. Finally, the relegation of such important disinfectants as quaternary ammonium compounds (for which, among other things, Domagk won the Nobel prize in 1939) and phenolics as "low level" does disservice to the fact that, when used properly, these agents kill the majority of important vegetative pathogens and all the lipophilic virus so far tested and that their rate of kill is exceeded only by halogens. Surely, they are inferior to other germicides, but a term other than "low level" should be used for such active materials.

In short, the Spaulding concept based upon the sterilization of contaminated medical instruments and upon key organisms such as polio, tuberculosis, and spores is sound, but the bifurcation into "high" and "low" and the elimination of the category of "intermediate" implies to the practitioner either "good" or "bad." Perhaps the terms broad spectrum, moderate spectrum, and narrow spectrum may be more descriptive of the usefulness of these agents. After all, penicillin, which inhibits essentially only cocci and *Treponema* and not the dozens of gram-negative rods, tuberculosis, yeasts, molds, and viruses, is certainly not a "low-level" antibiotic. Antimicrobial designations, whether for disinfectants or for chemotherapeutics, should be based upon common principles of nomenclature.

SCALE OF SUSCEPTIBILITY

Table 25–5 is an approximate disinfection scale for all the categories of microorganisms likely to be encountered in medical and veterinary environments. Reference to this chart can help one to make sensible decisions about which disinfectant to use in a particular situation. When fecal contamination is likely (possible rotavirus or Coxsackie virus), a disinfectant with a rhinovirus claim (common cold) would be superior to one with only a

Table 25–5. *Approximate Disinfection Scale for All Organisms in Order of Increasing Resistance (Response to Commercial Disinfectants)*

Microbial Susceptibility Group*	Microorganisms (Dried on Carriers)
A	Retroviruses (AIDS), ortho and paramyxoviruses, herpes viruses, vaccinia, corona, other enveloped viruses, gram-negative rods and some filamentous fungi; some gram-positive cocci
B	*Staphylococcus aureus*, some diphasic and filamentous fungi, yeasts and algae, some gram-negative rods, hepatitis B(?)
C	Adenoviruses
D	Mycobacterium tuberculosis (BCG strain)† rotaviruses, reoviruses, some mold ascospores
E	Picornaviruses (polio, rhino) Parvoviruses (SS DNA), Hepatitis A
F	Bacterial endospores (*Bacillus*, *Clostridium*); viroids
G	Prions (chronic infectious neuropathic agents, slow viruses)

*Exceptions will be found to exist among and between the various susceptibility groups listed in Table 25–5, but the broad outline of comparative susceptibility has become a basic principle in disinfectant biology.

†Unfortunately little information is available on human strains, such as H37Ra, H37Rv, the various scotochromogens, drug resistant forms, *Mycobacterium avium* intracellulare, and species of *M. fortuitum* and *M. chelonii* as well as pathogenic actinomycetes.

tuberculosis claim. This table makes it clear that a knowledge of the spectra and modes of action of chemical agents can aid in the rational selection of disinfectant agents. Thus, for example, if a hospital disinfectant kills *Staphylococcus aureus*, it is clearly capable of inactivating practically all agents in susceptibility group A, i.e., common (but not all) gram-negative rods, as well as lipophilic viruses such as influenza and herpes. If a disinfectant is capable of passing the EPA virucide test against poliovirus or a rhinovirus (the most difficult of the common infectious disease agents to inactivate by the EPA test within 10 mins), little doubt exists that it is truly a broad-spectrum disinfectant in terms of susceptibility groups A, B, C, and D.

Still, it can be difficult to predict the activity of a formulation (as opposed to a pure "active") because various ratios of excipients, sequestrants, solvents, detergents, and actives produce nonspecific and synergistic effects. For example, the presence of alcohol, detergents, and wetting agents will enhance all virucidal claims. Formulations containing quaternary ammonium compounds are generally less active against enteroviruses and adenoviruses (as compared to their antibacterial effect) than are formulations containing phenolics, aldehydes, or halogens. Most hospital disinfectants, whether they contain iodophors, phenolics, or quaternary ammonium compounds, are equally effective

Table 25–6. *Mechanism Categories of Agents Cited in Table 25–4*

Category	Agent
Denaturants (physically disrupt protein or lipid structures)	Quaternary ammonium compounds* Chlorhexidine Phenolics Acids Bases Alcohols
Reactants (form or break covalent bonds)	Aldehydes Enzymes
Oxidants (increase positive valence of C, S, or N)	Halogens H_2O_2 Ozone

*These agents combine virucidal properties with detergency.

against lipophilic viruses such as influenza, AIDS, and herpes. The benefits of quaternary ammonium compounds in hospitals are generally underestimated because they lack activity against tuberculosis in endoscopic procedures. Putting this aside, they are truly broad spectrum and biodegradable and are relatively non-toxic making them extremely important environmental germicides. Their rate of kill is exceptionally fast.

MECHANISM OF ACTION

All the agents listed in Table 25–4 can be classified into three groups based upon mechanism of action, as set forth in Table 25–6, which describes the denaturing, reacting, or oxidizing properties of most disinfectants.

The quaternary ammonium compounds and phenolics are highly effective against lipophilic viruses. Quaternary ammonium compounds as pure substances have the advantage of detergency, and at the use-dilution they possess little to no toxicity; in limited concentrations, they can be used for food contact surfaces.

The combination of glutaraldehyde and phenol (so-called glutaraldehyde-phenate) does not qualitatively broaden the virucidal spectrum of glutaraldehyde alone. The presence of "phenate" does not contribute to the activity of these agents because it is merely the salt of phenol; the microbicidal effect of this and all other organic acids is associated with the undissociated acid alone.

The mechanism of action of other virucidal agents is shown in Table 25–7. These agents, representing a variety of chemical and physical techniques, inactivate viruses for the most part by means of a covalent reactant pathway. It should be made clear that these agents, as well as all disinfectants, "inactivate" viruses by disrupting their surface structures. Antibacterial activity, on the other hand, is frequently associated with intracellular events. Disruption of the viral surface disturbs the es-

sential lock-and-key configuration of attachment and receptor sites on the virion and host cell surfaces. When associated with disinfectants, then, the term "viral inactivation" means that the viral particles are no longer capable of independent attachment to and absorption into the host cell. As long as the nucleic acid portion of the virion is intact, however, and if by some extraordinary means the naked nucleic acid should enter the cell, replication is theoretically possible. This possibility has been demonstrated with RNA from phenol-extracted poliovirus (Bitton, 1980).

CLASSIFICATION OF VIRUSES

At present, 18 families of animal viruses that are, in turn, subdivided into genera are recognized. Table 25–8 summarizes the salient physicochemical properties of these groups in terms of symmetry, size, envelope, capsomeres, and nucleic acid. The taxonomy depicted in Table 25–8 conforms to international nomenclature. The citations on sensitivity to disinfectants are based upon the presence or absence of lipid envelopes. Disinfectant chemists are interested in these lipid envelopes, as well as the protein capsid, as they hopefully develop wider-spectrum and less-toxic virucides. Medicinal chemists, on the other hand, are more interested in the nucleic acid content as a target for chemotherapeutic attack. The prions and viroids are discussed separately in the chapter because they are not true viruses.

Although AIDS captured the imagination of the world in 1982 (as did canine parvovirus in 1978), the Filoviridae (Marburg and Ebola agents) described in Table 25–8 are the most mysterious of all human viruses. They appeared suddenly in Germany and Yugoslavia in 1967 among laboratory workers working with African green monkey cell cultures (*Cercopithecus aethiops*). The virus was then nosocomially spread to hospital personnel. It was determined that the green monkeys came from Uganda, yet

Table 25–7. *Mode of Action of Miscellaneous Agents*

Agent	Mechanism
Ethylene oxide, β-propiolactone	Reactant; alkylating agent affecting protein and nucleic acid (radiomimetic agent)
Glycols	Denaturants
Ultraviolet light	Reactant; at 240 to 280 nM destroys nucleic acid
Ionizing irradiation*	Reactant; produces free radicals, especially in presence of air; can preserve anti- genicity.
Mercurials	Reactant; converts sulfhydryl groups to disulfide bonds

*Gamma irradiation of viruses produces first order reaction inactivation (Mahnel et al 1980) and is generally more effective than either UV light or β-propiolactone (Elliot LH, et al 1982). Viruses are in general more resistant to gamma irradiation than bacteria or fungi with the exception of *Streptococcus fecalis* (Stettmund and Mahnel 1980) and this resistance is more related to size than to nucleic acid content.

Table 25–8. *18 Families of Animal Viruses According to Host Range of Infection (General Outline of Sensitivity to Virucidal Disinfectants)*

Family	Human	Animal	Birds	Sensitivity to Disinfectants
Adenoviridae (naked, DNA)	Human adenoviruses	Equine adeno, infectious canine hepatitis, murine, bovine & others	Several	Moderate
Arenaviridae (enveloped, RNA)	Lymphocytic choriomeningitis (LCM); Lassa fever (highly infectious); Bolivian hemorrhagic fever; Argentine (Junin) hemorrhagic fever; Machudo virus	LCM of mice and hamsters	—	High (limited testing)
Bunyaviridae (enveloped, RNA)	Bunyamwera disease, California encephalitis; Sandfly fever; Napes virus; Sicilian virus; Rift Valley fever; Congo hemorrhagic fever	Rift Valley fever; Nairobi sheep disease	—	High (limited testing)
Caliciviridae (naked, RNA)	Possibly the Norwalk gastroenteritis agents* and others involved with gastroenteritis, such as Hawaii, Montgomery County, W, Taunton, Marin County, Snow Mountain Agents	Vesicular exanthema 1–12 of swine; San Miguel sea lion virus 1–8; feline and calf caliciviruses	—	Low (limited testing)
Coronaviridae (enveloped, RNA)	Human corona as common cold, urinary tract infections and possible pneumonia and possible gastroenteritis	Transmissible gastroenteritis of swine, hemagglutinating encephalomytis of swine, feline infectious peritonitis virus, mouse hepatitis virus	Infectious bronchitis virus of fowl; turkey bluecomb virus	High (limited studies)
Filoviridae (enveloped, RNA)	Marburg and Ebola diseases (hemorrhagic) (highly infectious)	Marburg and Ebola of A.G. monkeys, guinea pigs, hamsters and mice (all experimental)	—	High (limited testing)
Hepadnaviridae† (enveloped, DNA)	Hepatitis B virus (HBV)	Hepatitis B-like viruses of woodchuck, ground hog, and squirrel; these viruses are antigenically similar or identical to human HBV; HBV can infect chimpanzees as shown by serology and elevated liver aminotransferases	Peking duck; HBV-like	High to moderate (limited testing) (extensive testing in Germany by Thraenhart, MADT assay).
Herpesviridae (enveloped, DNA)	HSV-1 (HHV-1); HSV-2 (HHV-2); VZV (HHV-3); EB (HHV-4); CMV (HHV-5), HHV-6; HHV-7; B-virus	Bovine virus mammillitis; B-virus monkeys; pseudorabies (swine); equine rhinopneumonitis; murine CMV; chimp herpes virus; feline viral tracheitis; frogs, reptiles	Marek's disease of fowl, turkey herpes virus plus many others	High (limited testing)
Orthomyxoviridae (enveloped, RNA)	Influenza A, B, & C	Influenza A, B, & C	Avian influenza	High
Papovaviridae (naked, DNA)	At least 9 wart* viruses, BK, JC, polyoma agents of humans (not associated with neoplasms)	Shope papilloma of rabbits; SV-40 virus in monkey; others	—	Moderate (limited studies)
Paramyxoviridae (enveloped, RNA)	Paraflu 1, 2, 3, and 4; mumps; measles; respiratory syncytial virus (RSV); Newcastle disease (NDV); conjunctivitis	NDV, Paraflu (Sendai) of mice; paraflu 3 of cattle; rinderpest of cattle; canine distemper; bovine respiratory syncytial virus; pneumonia virus of mice	Paraflu of birds	High
Parvoviridae (naked, DNA)	No specific human disease; parvo-like agent (PVLA) is candidate virus; adeno-associated virus (AAV)	Feline panleukopenia, canine parvovirus,‡ mink enteritis virus; Aleutian mink disease; bovine parvovirus; porcine parvovirus; RVHD;§ H-1 virus of rats & hamsters, minute virus of mice (MVM)	Goose parvovirus	Low (limited testing)

Table 25–8. *18 Families of Animal Viruses According to Host Range of Infection (General Outline of Sensitivity to Virucidal Disinfectants)* (Continued)

Family	Human	Animal	Birds	Sensitivity to Disinfectants
Picornaviridae (naked, RNA)	Enteroviruses polio 1, 2, 3; Coxsackie virus A$_{1-22}$, B$_{1-6}$; ECHO virus 1–9; human enterovirus 68–71; hepatitis A virus (human enterovirus 72); rhino viruses 1–113.	Enterovirus swine vesicular disease; murine polio; porcine enterovirus 1–8; bovine enterovirus 1–7; bovine rhinovirus 1–2; equine rhinovirus 1–2; foot-and-mouth disease virus; EMC (Col-Sk, Mengo).	—	Low
Poxviridae (naked, DNA)	Vaccinia; molluscum contagiosum	Fowlpox; monkeypox; sheeppox; smallpox; swinepox; mousepox; lumpy skin disease; rabbit fibroma; goatpox	A variety	Moderate
Rhabdoviridae (enveloped, RNA)	Rabies; vesicular stomatitis (VSV); Mokola virus; piryvirus, and others	VSV; rabies; piryvirus; Mokola infection; necrosis of fish; (vast host range includes insects, fish, mammals, plants)	Lagos bat virus; rabies	High (limited testing)
Reoviridae RNA (naked RNA) (respiratory enteric orphans)	Reo 1, 2, 3, diarrhea, possibly Colorado tick fever, rotaviral gastroenteritis	Reo 1, 2, 3 of mice (steatorrhea); blue tongue disease; African horse sickness; hemorrhagic disease of deer; rotaviral diarrheas; simian rota SA-11; porcine rota SB-2; porcine osu; chicken rotavirus	—	Low
Retroviridae (enveloped, RNA)	Human T-lymphocyte viruses (Gallo): HTLV-I (T-cell leukemia); HTLV-II (hairy cell leukemia); HTLV III (LAV); (HIV-1) (AIDS); HIV-2 (AIDS) (Oleske, Denny)	Bovine leukosis; feline sarcoma; baboon, gibbon ape and woolly monkey leukemia; reptilian oncoviruses; mouse mammary tumor virus; Visna virus of sheep	Avian reticuloendotheliosis; sarcoma and leukosis viruses	High (limited testing)
Togaviridae (enveloped, RNA) (Flaviviridae)	(a) Eastern equine encephalitis; (EEE); West E.E., Semliki fever; yellow fever; Murray Valley fever, Dengue; Sindbis; Japanese encephalitis; Venz. *encephalitis*; (b) Rubella (German measles) (c) Hepatitis C	Same arbovirus as insect vectors of human encephalitides; hog cholera, lactic acid dehydrogenase virus of mice, border disease of sheep; bovine viral diarrhea	High (limited studies) Further taxonomy; Genus *Arbovirus* (yellow fever group of about 70 agents) (Dengue) Genus *Pestivirus* (hog cholera, bovine viral diarrhea) Genus *Hepatovirus* (hepatitis C) (HCV) portions of genome are similar to tobacco X virus	

*Virus not propagated in laboratories.

†Note: Does not include:

HAV.................................. picornavirus (RNA)
HCV (togaviridae) .... flavivirus (RNA) (enveloped)
Hepatitis Delta............................viroid (RNA)
Hepatitis E................enteric non-A, non-B (calicivirus)

‡Probable new mutant from feline agent first appearing in 1978.

§Rabbit viral hemorrhagic disease (RVHD) or necrotic hepatitis virus of rabbit appeared in 1984 in China and may be derived from porcine parvovirus (Gregg and House, 1989) or from the Caliciviridae (Kitching, 1989) (Xu and Chen, 1989).

As a general rule, although insufficient testing has been done, the enveloped virions (lipophilic DNA and RNA) are the easiest to inactivate within 10 min including HIV-1 and the naked viruses (hydrophilic DNA and RNA) the most difficult. For the 18 currently recognized families, the great majority (11) are enveloped, and within this group the majority are RNA (9 of 11). Of the 7 naked families, again the majority (4 of 7) are RNA. It is generally suspected that among the naked virions, the parvoviruses (Scott, 1980), reoviruses, picornaviruses, and caliciviruses are the most difficult to inactivate. However, no comparative side-by-side studies have appeared involving standardized test methods, for example, as set forth by EPA or ASTM. Such studies are required before this general guideline becomes a fixed concept.

follow-up tests on 200 wild animals yielded no antibody. Domesticated guinea pigs used for food in Zaire harbored Marburg antibodies, but it is believed that guinea pigs, just like humans, are infected via incidental horizontal or zigzag transmission from a yet-unknown reservoir. The last epidemic occurred in 1979 and was caused by Ebola virus, a serologic variant of Marburg in the Sudan where 24 of 34 cases were fatal. In 1976 simultaneous epidemics occurred in Zaire and the Sudan with 430 deaths in 500 cases. Like the virus of Lassa fever, Marburg virus is extremely dangerous to work with, and medical personnel treating these patients are at high risk. Use of disinfectants is obligatory, and limited evidence indicates that quaternary ammonium compounds, phenolics, aldehydes, and halogens are effective, but insufficient tests have been done. Universal CDC precautions should be taken including barrier procedures, protective clothing, and Biosafety Level Number 4 laboratory facilities.

The widest host range in nature is within the Rhabdoviridae (rabies group), with an animal reservoir descending into the insects and fish. The narrowest host range is possibly within the Parvoviridae or Caliciviridae, which are among the least infectious of all human viruses. The human and animal host ranges of these 18 families are summarized in Table 25–9. The nomenclature in Table 25–9 is further extended to include certain genera as well as families in accordance with a growing trend toward the Linnaean binomials characteristic of other branches of biology.

PROPAGATION OF VIRUSES AND HOST RESPONSES

Cell cultures (Tables 25–10 and 25–11), also called tissue cultures, are the most common host for replication of viruses. From the point of view of longevity, the cultures are of two types: immortal and limited (mortal). Immortal lines are capable of infinite serial transfers. Such cells are usually malignant polyploid, epithelial cells (e.g., H.Ep.2, HeLa) or CD-4-positive T lymphocyte cells (such as H-9). Mortal cell lines are typically diploid cells capable of only a limited number of transfers. From a cytologic point of view, cell cultures can be divided into two types: epithelial and fibroblastic; the epithelial cell cultures are polygonal and the fibroblastic are spindle shaped (connective tissue type). Table 25–10 outlines some of the preferred tissue culture systems for

Table 25–9. *The 18 Families of Animal Viruses According to Chemical and Physical Properties and Genetic Information*

Families & Genera	Symmetry	Number of Capsomers	Types	Presence of Envelope	Approx. Diameter of Virion (nM)	Nucleic Acid	Approx. Number of Genes
Adenoviridae Mastadenovirus (infects mammals) Aviadenovirus (infects birds)	Icosahedral	252	At least 37	No	70–90	ds DNA	30
Arenaviridae Arenavirus	Complex	N/A	Lassa Fever Machupo LCM	Yes	50–300	ss RNA, segmented	10
Bunyaviridae Bunyavirus (Bunyamwera)	Helical	N/A	Bunyamwera, Rift Valley fever	Yes	90–100	ss RNA, segmented	>3
Caliciviridae (tentative group)	Icosahedral	32	Possibly Norwalk agent (cannot be cultured); (doesn't infect animals); (several orphan viruses detected by EM in stools)	No	23–34	unknown	
Coronaviridae Coronavirus	Complex	N/A	Cornaviruses	Yes	80–130	ss RNA	30
Filoviridae	—	N/A	Marburg; Ebola	Yes		ss RNA	
Hepadnaviridae	Complex	N/A	Hepatitis B (similar to woodchuck hepatitis) and duck hepatitis	Complex coats; HBsAg	42	ds DNA, circular	4
Herpesviridae Herpesvirus (human herpes)	Icosahedral	162	(a) HHV-1 (oral mucocutaneous) (b) HHV-2 (genital) (c) HHV-3 (varicella/zoster) (d) HHV-4 (Epstein-Barr) (e) HHV-5 (cytomegalovirus-CMV) (f) HHV-6 (T-cell, 1986) (g) HHV-7 (T-cell, 1990) (h) Pseudorabies (veterinary)	Yes	150–200	ds DNA	160
Orthomyxoviridae Influenzaviruses Influenza	Helical; sialic acid receptors, neuraminidase hemagglutinin chick embryo sensitive, highly mutable		Influenza A, A₁, A₂ Influenza B Influenza C	Yes	80–120	ss RNA, segmented	10

Table 25–9. *The 18 Families of Animal Viruses According to Chemical and Physical Properties and Genetic Information* (Continued)

Families & Genera	Symmetry	Number of Capsomers	Types	Presence of Envelope	Approx. Diameter of Virion (nM)	Nucleic Acid	Approx. Number of Genes
Papovaviridae (a) Polyomavirus (rodents & primates) (b) Papillomavirus (produces papillomas)	Icosahedral	32	Papilloma; (warts); BK; JC; SV-40; Mouse polyoma	No	45–55	ds DNA	5–8
Paramyxoviridae (a) Paramyxoviruses: (Newcastle dis.) (b) Morbillivirus; measles (c) Pneumovirus; (respiratory syncytial RSV)	Helical	N/A	Parainfluenza 1, 2, 3 Measles (lacks neuraminidase); Mumps (lacks neuraminidase; no HA) RSV, NDV, Sendai, SV-5	Yes	150–300	ss RNA	>10
Parvoviridae Parvovirus (infects vertebrate hosts)	Icosahedral	32	Canine and Feline parvo virus of animals; PVLA of humans (not cultured); (possible viral hemorrhagic disease of rabbits)	No	18–26	ss DNA	3–4
Picornaviridae (a) Enterovirus (enteric) (b) Rhinovirus (respiratory)	Icosahedral	32	Polio 1, 2, 3; Coxsackie A_{22}; Coxsackie B_{16}; ECHO 31; FMV; HAV; (hepatitis A); Rhinol 113; EMC (rodents; possibly man)	No	20–30	ss RNA	4–6
Poxviridae Orthopoxvirus (vaccinia and smallpox)	Very complex brick-shaped	N/A	Vaccinia; smallpox; ectromelia; rabbitpox; monkeypox	Complex coats ether resistant	230–400	ds DNA	300
Reoviridae (a) Reovirus (b) Orbivirus (c) Rotavirus	Icosahedral	32	Reo 1, 2, 3; Rotavirus	No	60–80	ds RNA, segmented	10–12
Retroviridae (tumors)	Complex, possibly Icosahedron	N/A	HTLV-I HTLV-II HIV-1, 2 (HTLV-III, LAV); Rous sarcoma	Yes	90–120	ss RNA duplicate copies segmented; reverse transcriptase	4
Rhabdoviridae (a) rabies group (b) Vesiculovirus (vesicular stomatitis group)	Helical	N/A	Rabies VSV	Yes (least lipophilic of the RNA enveloped viruses)	70 × 175	ss RNA	5
Togaviridae (Flaviviridae) Alphavirus: (group A arboviruses) (group B arboviruses) Rubivirus = rubella	Icosahedral	32	Dengue fever; arboviruses; EEE, VEE Sindbis WEE; rubella; hepatitis C (HCV)	Yes	50–70	ss RNA	10

N/A = Not applicable, capsomers are found only in cubical (icosahedral) viruses.

Table 25–10. *Tissue Culture Hosts of Choice for Some Common Viruses*

Tissue Culture	Some Viruses that Will Replicate*
HeLa H.Ep. 2 (E)	Polio, vaccinia, Coxsackie, adeno, herpes, ECHO
WI-38 MRC-5 (F)	Polio, vaccinia, Coxsackie, herpes, rhino, CMV, measles, corona
Rabbit kidney (E)	Herpes
Monkey kidney (E)	Polio, ECHO, Coxsackie, influenza, measles, rubella
Human leukemic cells: PHA-stimulated human blasts (L); H-9; MT-2 cells	HIV-1, HIV-2

*Detection end points are cytopathic effect (CPE), plaques, giant cells, syncytial formation, human O, chick, or guinea pig red blood cells (hemadsorption) for influenza and other myxoviruses; reverse transcriptase (RT) or p24 Elisa Antigen Capture for HIV-1,2 or dye uptake-tetrazolium salt reduction in viable cells, as well as immunofluorescence (IF) or DNA-probes.

E = epithelial; F = fibroblastic; L = lymphoid.

some common viruses. The table indicates which viruses may be propagated in six of the most frequently used cell lines which are categorized as epithelial or fibroblastic. Table 25–11 is a comprehensive summary of the propagation techniques for a wide range of viruses. It is diagnostically oriented with respect to clinical source, host range, and pathognomonic signs.

Cell cultures are fed with complex mixtures of amino acids, carbohydrates, purines, and pyrimidines, plus trace elements and vitamins and various balanced salt solutions. These are often supplemented with high concentrations of blood serum (5 to 20%) during primary explantation to form a confluent cell sheet and with lower concentrations (0 to 2%) for maintenance of the culture. RPMI 1640 is an example of a completely synthetic medium that may or may not be supplemented with serum (Table 25–12). The composition of so-called minimal essential media and balanced salt solutions can be modified by systematically deleting components of a basic RPMI-type formulation. The pH and pCO_2 of the various cultures must be maintained and poised by the inclusion of buffer systems (usually $NaHCO_3$). Incubation is accomplished in the presence of 5 to 8% CO_2 or, in the absence of CO_2, in tightly screw-capped vessels. Defined refeeding schedules are mandatory for each cell line.

Chick embryos (Table 25–13) are common host systems, with the allantoic cavity, amniotic cavity, and surface of the chorioallantoic membrane (CAM) as the usual routes of inoculation. Detection end points are death, CAM pocks, and hemagglutination from the chorioallantoic fluid. Table 25–13 summarizes some of the common host-virus relationships with this method of propagation. The use of this system is of value when cytotoxicity in cell culture virucide assays is a problem. Low dilutions of virus and disinfectants are tolerated by chick embryos (9 to 10 days) and produce no "carryover" antiviral effect. Thus, the use of neutralizers and detoxification is not

necessary. Avian embryos have been used for many years in vaccine production.

Mice are not frequently used as host systems. Like chick embryos, however, they can be of value in virucide experiments because they respond with less toxicity to germicides than cell culture (Table 25–14). Albino mice, 9 to 12 g, can be injected intranasally with influenza and subcutaneously, intraperitoneally, and/or intracerebrally with encephalomyocarditis virus (EMC), vaccinia, and herpes virus. Coxsackie viruses are best inoculated into suckling mice. Human rhinovirus, ECHO viruses, and adenoviruses cannot infect mice or any other animal. Table 25–14 summarizes comparative virulence titrations from our laboratory in various hosts. The wide host range for cell cultures is apparent, and the limited usefulness of the chick embryo in virucide analysis is obvious, being limited basically to influenza.

Table 25–15 shows some of the variation encountered when trying to select the host of choice in tissue culture systems. Such preliminary range-finding tests are extremely important in virus inactivation assays because the greater the number of infectious viral particles, the less the possibility that cytotoxicity will invalidate the test, according to the strict requirements of the EPA (no virus detected at any log dilution, with at least a 3 log [99.9%] reduction). It is obvious from these data that the rhesus monkey kidney cell culture, chick embryo CAM, and mouse-brain models are all equally sensitive to vaccinia virus. If toxicity were not a problem and speed and expense were of paramount importance, the rhesus monkey kidneys would be the host of choice in this example of a vaccinia virus inactivation experiment. The chick embryo would give excellent results and less toxicity, but it would be more time consuming. The mouse is a reliable but expensive model.

BASIC TEST PROCEDURES

Virucide tests are basically of two types: suspension and carrier. Both are finite contact tests, as opposed to the antiviral chemotherapy experiments as conducted in the pharmaceutical industry. These tests are discussed in more detail elsewhere in this chapter. The original suspension test was published by Klein and DeForest (1963) and consisted of a 10-minute contact at room temperature followed by log-dilution titrations in cell cultures or chick embryos. A 1-hour suspension test to determine the mechanism of action of pharmaceutically active antivirals was later published by Grunberg and Prince (1970). The current EPA test requires that the disinfectant be tested against a dried film of the virus in the presence of 5% serum. Evidence with hepatitis B virus (HBV), rotavirus, picornaviruses, transmissible gastroenteritis virus of swine, and others indicates that dried virus is more resistant than suspended virus (Bond et al., 1983; Lloyd-Evans et al., 1986; Klein and DeForest, 1983; Nakao et al., 1978; Schurmann and Eggers, 1983).

The official EPA carrier method for viruses was first proposed in the Federal Register of June 25, 1975 and

Table 25–11. *Comprehensive Schedule of Host Systems in Isolation, Propagation, Identification, and Antiviral Testing of the Common Viruses of Man and Animals*

Virus	Clinical Material	Susceptible Host	Cell Culture Response	Type Blood for HA
Adeno	Eye, throat swab	H.Ep. 2, HEK, HeLa	CPE (rounded cells)	Rat or Rhesus
Arbo	Autopsy, serum CSF	S. mice (death), duck embryo BHK, vero cells	Plaques	Goose
Corona	Throat and nasal	HETOC, HEK, MRC-5 S. mice (death)	Cilia, inhibition, CPE	Chick
Coxsackie A	Feces and throat	S. mice (death) (flaccid paralysis) MkK, H.Ep. 2, WI-38	CPE	
Coxsackie B	Feces and throat	S. mice (death) (spastic paralysis) MkK, WI-38, H.Ep. 2	CPE	
Cytomegalo	Urine and throat	HEL, MRC-5	CPE (giant cells, focal lesions)	Sheep
ECHO	Feces	MkK, HEL	CPE	
Epstein-Barr	Throat and blood	Lymphoid cells	Experimental transformation	
Hepatitis B virus	Blood, semen, vaginal secretions, CSF	Chimpanzee	None; EM Dane particles in plasma, HBsAg and HB antibody markers in plasma; transfected cell cultures available	—
Herpes simplex	Throat and vesicles buccal, eye, genital	HEL, H.Ep. 2, CE, WI-38, MRC-5, rabbit kidney S. mice (death)	CAM (pocks) (death), CPE	Sheep
HIV (AIDS) (LAV)	Blood, semen	PHA-stimulated blasts, CD-4-positive T cells, MT-2 cells, CD-4 Hela cells, Molt cells, MT-4	Syncytia, p24, reverse transcriptase, antigen capture p24 (ELISA), viability, TTC reduction	—
Influenza	Nasal and throat	AMN, eggs, CE, PMK	Amniotic fluid (HA test), HAd on inoculated cell cultures	Guinea pig chick, human O
LCM	Blood and CSF	3-week mice	BHK cells	
Measles	Throat and urine	PMK, MRC-5	CPE	Vervet
Mumps	Throat	PMK	HAd on inoculated cell cultures, syncytial CPE on some cultures	Guinea pig
Parainfluenza	Throat	PMK, CE	HAd on inoculated Guinea pig cultures	
Polio	Feces and CSF	PMK, WI-38, H.Ep. 2, HeLa	CPE	
Rabies	Brain	3-week mice, WI-38, duck embryo	Death (IC inoc.) CPE	
Reo	Throat and feces	PMK, HEK	CPE	
Respiratory syncytial	Nasal and throat	H.Ep. 2, PMK	CPE	
Rhino	Nasal and throat	HEL, WI-38; MRC-5	CPE	
Rota	Feces	(V-1) (Vero)	CPE	
Rubella	Throat	PAGMK, RK-13	No CPE in PAGMK; use ECHO 11 interference test for ID	1-day-old chick
Vaccinia	Vesicles	CAM, PMK, CE, WI-38, H.Ep. 2	Pocks on CAM, CPE (rounding)	Human O, chick
Varicella-zoster	Vesicles	HEL, MRC-5	CPE	
Variola	Vesicles (smallpox)	CAM, cell culture	CPE, pocks on CAM	
Pseudorabies	Nasal swabs, CNS	Vero, BHK	CPE	
Canine distemper	Nasal, oral, conjunctival swabs, CSF	Dog kidney, Vero, alveolar macrophages	CPE	

ALL = allantoic cavity; AMN = amniotic cavity; BSS = balanced salt solution; BHK = baby hamster kidney cells; CC = cell culture; CAM = choriollantoic membrane; CE = chick embryo; CNS = central nervous system; CPE = cytopathic effect; CSF = cerebral spinal fluid; D. emb. = duck embryo; HA = hemagglutination test; HAd = hemadsorption; HEK = human embryonic kidney; HEL = human embryonic lung fibroblasts; HETOCH = human embryonic tracheal organ culture; H.Ep. 2 = human epithelioma number 2; IC = intracerebral; INT = interference test; LCM = lymphocytic choriomeningitis; MRC-5 = Medical Research Council; OC-43 = coronavirus strain; PAGMK = primary African green monkey (PrAFMkK); PMK = primary Rhesus monkey kidney (RhMkK) (LLC); RK = rabbit kidney cells; RSV = respiratory syncytial virus; S. mice = suckling mice

Table 25–12. *RPMI 1640*

Component	(mg/L)
Amino Acids	
L-Arginine (free base)	200.00
L-Asparagine	50.00
L-Aspartic acid	20.00
L-Cystine	50.00
L-Glutamic acid	20.00
L-Glutamine	300.00
Glycine	10.00
L-Histidine (free base)	15.00
Hydroxyproline	20.00
L-Isoleucine	50.00
L-Leucine	50.00
L-Lysine HCl	40.00
L-Methionine	15.00
L-Phenylalanine	15.00
L-Proline	20.00
L-Serine	30.00
L-Threonine	20.00
L-Tryptophan	5.00
L-Tyrosine	20.00
L-Valine	20.00
Vitamins	
p-Aminobenzoic acid	1.00
d-Biotin	0.20
Ca D pantothenate	0.25
Choline chloride	3.00
Folic acid	1.00
Inositol	35.00
Nicotinamide	1.00
Pyridoxine HCl	1.00
Thiamine HCl	0.20
Inorganic Salts	
Ca $(NO_3)_2 \cdot 4H_2O$	100.00
KCl	400.00
$MgSO_4 \cdot 7H_2O$	100.00
NaCl	6000.00
NaHCO	2000.00
$Na_2HPO_4 \cdot 7H_2O$	1512.00
Other Components	
Glucose	2000.00
Glutathione (reduced)	1.00
Phenol red	5.00

Table 25–13. *Common Viral Inoculations in the 9- to 10-Day Chick Embryo*

Virus	Route	Endpoint
Influenza	Intramniotic	Hemagglutination (HA)
Newcastle (NDV)	Intra-allantoic	of guinea pig or chick RBC or human O
Parainfluenza		
Herpes	Onto the chorioallantoic	Pocks on the CAM
Vaccinia	membrane (CAM)	

appears in the Pesticide Assessment Guidelines, Subdivision G, Product Performance, as well as in EPA proposed method DIS/TSS-7 (November 12, 1981). The assay, which is similar to the method required in Canada, requires that 2 batches of the disinfectant be tested against a recoverable virus titer of at least 10^4 (dried virus) from the test surface (petri dish, glass slide, steel cylinder, etc.) within 10 mins. European and U.K. tests in general employ a non-carrier suspension. The product must demonstrate complete inactivation of the virus at all dilutions. When cytotoxicity is evident, at least a 3-log reduction in titer must be obtained for any virus, including human immunodeficiency virus type 1 (HIV-1), for which restrictive claims are allowed. The American Society for Testing Materials (ASTM) has published both a suspension and a carrier test through Committee E-35 under the guidance of J. Chang, D. Fredell, and M. Mahl. McDuff and Gaustad (1976) described a carrier test that incorporated the use of Association of Official Analytical Chemists (AOAC) stainless steel cylinders in testing for virucidal activity against herpes virus and poliovirus type 1. The data from these assays were for the most part consistent, but the authors indicated that more collaborative work was needed.

Variations in results will occur, especially when too little attention is paid to areas of the test that have not been standardized, such as end-points, refeeding schedules, and incubation times. Klein and DeForest (1983) have also pointed out that viral aggregation is an important variable in the viral pool. Naked virions (picornaviruses, adenoviruses, papovaviruses) occur as aggregates or crystalline arrays within the infected cell, whereas herpes and influenza viruses bud individually from the cell membrane.

Problems of Neutralization/Detoxification

Effect of Serum on Virucidal Activity

Herpes Simplex Virus Type 2. In testing for the inactivation of viruses, conventional neutralizers such as polysorbate (Tween), azolectin, and reducing agents cannot be used because they are toxic to cell cultures. Thus, a nontoxic neutralizer such as serum is often used. Accordingly, we performed some experiments on serum with herpes virus and on HIV-1 in collaboration with T. Denny and J. Oleske of New Jersey Medical School. A series of suspension tests were performed in our laboratory in the presence of 5% serum wherein equal parts of phenol solution and undiluted tissue culture pools were incubated at room temperature for 10 mins. Dilutions of the disinfectant-virus reaction mixture were then inoculated into H.Ep.2 cells and were observed for cytopathic effects (CPE) for up to 8 days, along with saline-virus controls. Virucidal effects were determined by calculation of the median tissue culture infective dose ($TCID_{50}$). The results are shown in Table 25–16. Only the 2.5% concentration was active.

The experiment was repeated with increasing concentrations of serum up to 50% without any loss of activity.

Table 25–14. *Comparative Virulence of 7 Viruses in 3 Host Systems*

Virus	Cell Culture $TCID_{50}{}^a$	Mouse LD_{50} Mice[b]	Chick Embryo $EID_{50}{}^c$
Col Sk (EMC)	$10^{-4.7}$	$10^{-6.7}$	
(RNA ether-resistant)	$10^{-6.3}$	$10^{-6.8}$	No take
	$10^{-7.5d}$	$10^{-6.5}$	
Herpes simple type 1	$10^{-5.8}$	$10^{-6.5}$	$10^{-3.5}$
(DNA ether-sensitive)	$10^{-6.3}$	$10^{-6.0}$	$10^{-3.0}$
	$10^{-7.7}$	$10^{-6.7}$	$10^{-3.0}$
			Pocks on CAM
Cox B₁ RNA	$10^{-3.8}$	$10^{-4.4}$	
(ether-resistant)	$10^{-6.0}$	$10^{-4.5}$	No take
	$10^{-5.5}$	$10^{-4.7}$	
ECHO 9	$10^{-5.6}$		
(Cox A₂₃)	$10^{-5.5}$	No take	No take
(RNA ether-resistant)	$10^{-4.7}$		
Rhino	$10^{-4.7}$		
(RNA ether-resistant)	$10^{-4.0}$	No take	No take
	$10^{-5.5}$		
Influenza A₂	$10^{-4.3}$	$10^{-4.4}$	$10^{-7.0}$
(J-305-57)	$10^{-5.5}$	$10^{-2.8}$	$10^{-6.0}$
(RNA ether-resistant)	$10^{-4.0}$	$10^{-2.5}$	$10^{-7.5}$
		Intranasal infection	
Adeno	$10^{-5.5}$		
(DNA, ether var.	$10^{-6.0}$	No take	No take
or resistant)	$10^{-4.8}$		

$TCID_{50}$, LD_{50}, EID_{50} = Median tissue culture infected, median lethal, and median egg infectious dose, respectively.
[a]CPE in Rhesus monkey kidney cells at 4 to 10 days (or WI-38).
[b]9- to 12-g weaning albino mice, 0.1 ml IP at 10 days for paralysis and death.
[c]9- to 10-day chick embryos, 0.1 ml IA, 48 hours, 35°C, CAF harvest for HA 0.5%. GPRBC (1 hour at room temperature or overnight at 4°C).
[d]Blind passage (no CPE) of 5-day supernatant via intraperitoneal injection in mice (death in 7 days if virus present in cell culture).
From Gibraltar Biological Laboratories. 1977–1978. Unpublished data presented at ASTM E-35 Committee Meetings: Cleveland, 1977; Philadelphia, 1978.

*H.Ep. 2 cells in microtiter plates, 35°C, 5% CO_2, MEM with Earle's base, 8 days.
†General level of toxicity to be expected with most germicides.

Thus, even though phenol required relatively high concentrations to inactivate this lipophilic virus, it had the advantageous property of being refractive to the neutralizing effect of serum. These herpes studies were repeated with additional virucides, as well as with glutaraldehyde and a chlorine compound against HIV-1 (see later).

Phenol is less active against Klein's group A lipophilic viruses than less-soluble derivatives, ortho-phenylphenol and ortho-benzyl-p-chlorophenol; however, it is more active than these against Klein's group B hydro-

philic viruses but at higher concentrations (Klein and DeForest, 1983).

The data in Table 25–17 show the ability of serum to neutralize the virucidal activity of the dual quaternary ammonium compound BTC-2125M and sodium hypochlorite, but at relatively high concentrations. Raising the concentration of the germicide or increasing the exposure time would, of course, overcome this neutralizing effect. Normal household bleach (5.25% sodium hypochlorite) retained activity against a high protein load when diluted 1:10 (as recommended by CDC) or 1:20

Table 25–15. *Titration Data Obtained with Vaccinia (Wyeth Strain)**

Host	Result	Comment	Toxicity of Germicides†
1. Tissue culture (WI-38)	$TCID_{50} = 10^{-3.5}$	0	High
2. Tissue culture (Rhesus MkK)	$TCID_{50} = 10^{-6.0}$	+	High
3. Chick embryo (dropped CAM)	$EID_{50} = 10^{-6.0}$ or higher	+	Low
4. Mice (intracerebral)	$LD_{50} = 10^{-6.0}$ or higher	+	Practically none

0 = Viral concentration insufficient to obviate cytotoxicity in EPA assay; + = acceptable for EPA qualification, assuming no more than 3 logs of toxicity (viral concentration sufficient); tissue culture infection ($TCID_{50}$), median egg infectious disease (EID_{50}), and median lethal dose$_{50}$ (LD_{50}) respectively.

Table 25–16. *Effect of Various Concentrations of Phenol* on Herpes Simplex Virus Type 2†(HSV-2) with 5% Serum*

% Phenol Concentration Reagent (Reaction Mixture)	$TCID_{50}$ (CPE End Point) Phenol	$TCID_{50}$ (CPE End Point) Control	Effect
1.0 (0.5)	$10^{-7.0}$	$10^{-7.0}$	Inactive
2.0 (1.0)	$10^{-6.5}$	$10^{-6.5}$	Inactive
5.0 (2.5)	$<10^{-1.0}$	$10^{-6.5}$	5-log reduction

*Pure studies with phenolic derivatives are difficult to control because of poor solubility, which necessitates the addition of detergents or alcohol. Consequently, data with pure phenol or its sodium salt are easier to analyze and easier to perform, especially with viruses that are susceptible to detergents and/or alcohol.

†H.Ep. 2 cultures in MEM, 10 days at 37°C, microtiter-CO_2

$TCID_{50}$ = Median tissue culture infective dose; CPE = cytopathic effect.

when added in equal parts to the serum-virus contaminant; however, it was partially active in the presence of a final concentration of 2.5% serum when diluted 1:100 and it was essentially inactive at 1:100 when the serum level was raised to 10% (5.0% final concentration in the reaction mixture). Care must be taken with the indiscriminate use of hypochlorite in the presence of blood or other organic matter at dilutions greater than 1:10. Studies with bacteria and spores show similar effects. For large spills, it will always be safer to apply a volume of bleach or quaternary ammonium compound greater than the volume of contaminant. Both isopropanol and ethanol were refractive to blood serum in this herpes assay (i.e., possessed high serum activity); however, this would not necessarily be true with more resistant viruses. The quaternary ammonium compound was at least

as serum active as 1:20 bleach (but less serum active than 1:10 bleach) and had superior serum activity to 1:100 bleach. The nonspecific virucidal effect of serum was also evident; when virus was incubated with equal parts of 100% serum (to give 50% final serum concentration), a 100-fold decrease in the $TCID_{50}$ as compared to 5% serum was observed.

Human Immunodeficiency Virus Type 1 (HIV-1). Studies on the optimal yield of HIV-1 in T cells and on the effect of serum on the anti-HIV-1 activity of chlorine dioxide and glutaraldehyde were performed in a collaboration between our laboratory facility and T. Denny, H. Adieuh, and J. Oleske of the Department of Pediatrics and Immunology, New Jersey Medical School, Newark as part of a joint project on the laboratory inactivation of AIDS virus. A glass surface was contaminated with an HIV-1 pool propagated first in phytohemagglutinin-stimulated blasts and then H-9 cells (Popovic et al., 1984) maintained with RPMI 1640 supplemented with 20% fetal calf serum plus penicillin and streptomycin. One ml virus was dried to a film for 45 mins at 37°C and then treated with 1.0 ml disinfectant at the use-dilution (a 1:2 reaction mixture) for 10 mins at 20°C. A low-protein assay was also run using an HIV-1 pool containing 10% fetal calf serum with disinfectant added to the dry film at the ratio of 0.5 ml virus to 5.0 ml disinfectant (1:10 reaction mixture). These 2 conditions simulated low and high levels of blood or culture spills in the hospital or in the laboratory. After treatment for 10 mins the film was rapidly diluted in neutralizing/detoxifying broth from 10^{-1} to 10^{-6}, and 1.0-ml aliquots were inoculated into screw-capped flask cultures (37°C) containing 10 ml of H-9 cells at a concentration of 5×10^5 ml. Viability of the cells at

Table 25–17. *Effect of Increasing Serum Concentration Against Herpes Simplex Virus Type 2 (HSV-2) $TCID_{50}$—10-Min Contact in Suspensions at 20 to 25°C*

Concentration of Fetal Calf Serum (%) (R)	(R-M)	$TCID_{50}$ ($<10^{-1}$ or $<10^{-2}$ = Virus Not Detected Below Toxic Level of Germicide) D-125 1000 ppm Quat (BTC 2125M)	70% Isopropanol	70% Ethanol	Glut 0.12%	NaClO (5.25%) 1:10 0.5%	NaClO 1:20 0.25%	NaClO 1:100 0.05%	Saline 0.85%
5	(2.5)	$<10^{-2a}$	$<10^{-2a}$	$<10^{-2a}$	$<10^{-1a}$	$<10^{-2a}$	10^{-1a}	$10^{-3.5b}$	$10^{-6.5}$
10	(5.0)	$<10^{-2a}$	$<10^{-2a}$	$<10^{-2a}$	$<10^{-1a}$	$<10^{-2a}$	10^{-1a}	$10^{-5.5b}$	$10^{-6.5}$
20	(10.0)	$<10^{-2a}$	$<10^{-2a}$	$<10^{-2a}$	$<10^{-1a}$	$<10^{-2a}$	10^{-1a}	$10^{-6.5c}$ Inactive	$10^{-6.5}$
50	(25.0)	$10^{-2.5b}$	$<10^{-2a}$	$<10^{-2a}$	$10^{-1.5b}$	$<10^{-2a}$	$10^{-3.5b}$	$10^{-5.5c}$ Inactive	$10^{-5.5}$
75	(37.5)	$<10^{-5.5c}$ Inactive	$<10^{-2a}$	$<10^{-2a}$	$10^{-2.0b}$	$<10^{-2a}$	$10^{-5.5c}$ Inactive	$10^{-5.5c}$ Inactive	$10^{-5.5}$
100	(50.0)	$<10^{-4.5c}$ Inactive	$<10^{-2a}$	$<10^{-2a}$	$10^{-3.5b}$	$<10^{-2a}$	$10^{-5.5c}$ Inactive	$10^{-4.5c}$ Inactive	$10^{-4.5}$

The components were mixed in equal parts; glut = Alkaline glutaraldehyde; (R) = reagent concentration, (R-M) = final concentration of reagent in reaction mixture

$TCID_{50}$ = median tissue culture infectious dose, as calculated by the dose-response method of Reed and Muench (1938); a = complete inactivation (italicized); b = partial inactivation (>90%); c = no inactivation (no decrease in viral titer).

initiation was at least 85% as determined by trypan blue exclusion and cell photometry. Cultures were fed twice weekly and the supernatants were assayed after 7 to 14 days for HIV by enzyme-linked immunosorbent assay (ELISA) detection of p24 antigen using Abbott reagents. This procedure conformed to the requirements of the EPA disinfectant branch. The results are shown in Table 25–18. Additional data on the effects of serum on anti-herpes simplex virus (anti-HSV) and anti-HIV activity have been published elsewhere (Prince et al., 1990).

The data in Table 25–18 show clearly that, as with the serum experiments with herpes, lipophilic viruses such as HIV-1 that normally display great sensitivity to virucides become appreciably resistant (or the germicide becomes less active) in the presence of more elevated concentrations of organic load, such as can be found in blood, semen, feces, urine, and vaginal and buccal secretions. It is possible that viruses that are dissimilar with regard to chemical sensitivity (hydrophilic versus lipophilic) might demonstrate a more equivalent degree of resistance as the tolerance threshold of the enveloped virion is raised in the presence of protein or other organic matter. Studies like this should be pursued.

The ability of serum to inactivate or neutralize certain virucides also makes it a generally useful reagent for detoxifying virucides as they are brought over into the cell culture system, especially for cationics, alkalis, acids, oxidizing agents, and aldehydes. Detoxification is less of a problem in chick embryos and in animals. The problems of neutralization and detoxification are unique in virology and, as mentioned previously, cannot be solved by the simple addition of polysorbates, azolectin, or reducing agents, as with antibacterial and antifungal assays. Such neutralizers are frequently more toxic to the cell culture than the germicides themselves. Neutralization and detoxification, in the absence of gel filtration, are best accomplished by rapid dilution in nonspecific atoxic dilution blanks, such as trypticase soy broth supplemented to 20% with inactivated mammalian blood serum. When neutralization cannot be accomplished

chemically, procedures such as centrifugation and/or Sephadex filtration are helpful (see later).

Proof of neutralization can be accomplished by running a separate set of controls wherein disinfectant dilutions alone are added to the cell cultures, and virus at low multiplicity of infection is immediately back inoculated and then followed in the usual manner for rate and extent of replication. When contact times are short (30 s to 3 mins), virus-germicide reaction mixtures have to be rapidly removed from the suspension. For example, for a 30 s contact, recovery should commence by pipette removal at 20 s. Before the assay, however, a validation run should be performed to show that the rapid manipulations of removal, dilution, and inoculation are temporally possible.

Gel Filtration for Neutralization of Virucidal Agents

This method is applicable when toxicity cannot be eliminated by other means, such as dilution or serum.

Summary of Method. After exposure of virus to disinfectant, the virus-disinfectant suspension is applied to a column of Sephadex LH-60-120. The column is placed in a centrifuge and is centrifuged to separate virus from disinfectant (30 mins $600 \times g$) by gel filtration. The filtrate (column flow-through that contains the virus) is assayed in the appropriate host system. The untreated virus control suspension is similarly gel filtered, and the virus titer of the filtrate is determined by assay of infectivity. The residual cytotoxicity of the disinfectant is determined by gel filtration of the disinfectant control under the same conditions. The gel filtration procedures described in this standard are a modification of the EPA method of Blackwell and Chen (1970). The pioneer efforts of these men as well as G. Bass, G. Asbury, T. Czerkowicz, and A. Beloian at the former EPA laboratory in Beltsville, Maryland cannot be underestimated in respect to standardization of disinfectant methods. The performance and enforcement criteria as developed by other EPA personnel (R. Engler, J. Jenkins, D. Gusse, W. Campbell, J. Lee, E. Brown, V. Goncarovs, and J. Wills), as well as by W. Rutala and E. Cole of the Uni-

Table 25–18. *Effect of Serum on Anti-Human Immunodeficiency Virus (HIV) Activity* (Induction of Tolerance to Disinfectants)*

Virucide	High Soil — Virus in 20% Serum with Equal Ratio of Disinfectant (1:2)		▲ log	Low Soil — Virus in 10% Serum with Virus Disinfectant Ratio of (1:10)		▲ log	RPMI 1640 TC Control
Chlorine dioxide product	$10^{-4.5}$†	T O L E R A N T	1.0	$<10^{-1.0}$	S E N S I T I V E	<4.0	$10^{-5.5}$
1:16 Dilution of 2% glutaraldehyde product	$10^{-3.5}$		2.0	$<10^{-1.0}$		<4.0	

*H-9 assay system. Collaboration with T. Denny and H. Adieuh and Dr. J. Oleske, New Jersey Medical School, Newark, NJ.
†TCID$_{50}$ as measured by ELISA antigen capture for p24 core protein at 14 days in H-9 suspension cultures, 10^5 cells/10 ml RPMI flask culture.

versity of North Carolina, have all contributed to a growing consensus that these tests require the collaboration of government, academia, and industry, as has been stressed by Favero and Groeschel (ASM, 1987; ASM, 1990).

Operating Technique. Suspend Sephadex in a large excess of sterile distilled or deionized water in an Erlenmeyer flask. Use sufficient Sephadex for the number of columns to be prepared (approximately 0.5 g Sephadex/column). Close the flask with plastic film or closure and allow Sephadex to swell overnight at 4°C.

Remove the cap from the syringe tip, remove the plunger from the syringe, and place the syringe in an 18 × 150-mm test tube or in a suitable tube holder above a sink or liquid receptacle.

Place a small wad of glass wool in the syringe to cover the internal tip opening. Swirl the Sephadex slurry and pipette Sephadex into the syringe. Allow excess water to drain, and repeat until a desired bed size of Sephadex has formed. If the column is not used immediately, seal or plug the syringe tip, add a layer of distilled water above the column, cover with Parafilm, and store at 4°C.

To use the column allow the water to flow through, then equilibrate with phosphate buffered saline (PBS) by passing 10 ml PBS through the column.

Cover the column with Parafilm or other film and place the column in a sterile 15- or 50-ml conical centrifuge tube. Place the tube with the column in the centrifuge and centrifuge at approximately 600 × g for 3 mins to clear the void volume. Record the rpm used for this step.

Remove the column, discard the void volume, and replace the column in a new tube.

Gently pipette 0.6 or 1.2 ml the virus-disinfectant mixture (depending on column size) onto the Sephadex, place the column in the centrifuge, and centrifuge again for 3 mins at exactly the same rpm as in the previous step.

Remove the column from the centrifuge, collect the filtrate (column flow-through), and titrate for infectivity.

The virus and disinfectant control samples are handled in the same manner.

Spray Products. Prior to applying the virus-product mixture to a Sephadex column, the volume of the mixture is adjusted to 2.0 ml with an appropriate aqueous medium, such as water, PBS, tissue culture medium, or neutralizer solution.

Chemical Neutralizers. When used, the chemical neutralizer is added after the contact time, and the virus-disinfectant-neutralizer mixture is applied to the Sephadex column.

Carryover Antiviral Effect of Contact Virucides

Limited work has been done on the in vitro and in vivo antiviral effects of virucidal disinfectants such as quaternary ammonium compounds, phenolics, aldehydes, and halogens. In general, when such germicides are added to cell culture systems in noncytotoxic tolerated concentrations, carryover antiviral effects are not seen (Prince, unpublished data; Klein and DeForest,

1963). This is consistent with the finding that potential topical antiviral ointments and lotions containing quaternary ammonium compounds, phenolics, and/or aldehydes have not been found to be chemotherapeutically active for herpetic skin and/or eye infections.

Grunberg and Prince (1970) studied the antiviral effects of a series of isoquinolines in three models: (1) direct contact suspension test; (2) in vitro cell culture assay; and (3) mouse infections followed by intraperitoneal treatment with maximum tolerated doses. The results are summarized in Table 25–19.

The two compounds that were active in tissue culture (dehydroisoquinoline acetamide [DIQA] against Coxsackie B_1 and dehydroemetine against influenza A) were active neither by suspension contact nor by animal injections. Finally, none of the in vivo activities against Columbia-SK (Col SK), ECHO 9, Coxsackie B_1, influenza A, or herpes simplex type 1 could be predicted from either the suspension or cell culture in vitro systems. These data suggested that contact virucides, successful cell culture compounds, and compounds active in vivo may express their antiviral effect in each case by different mechanisms and that no correlation existed between in vitro and in vivo data. There are no published studies to show that a correlation exists between a contact virucidal effect from a germicide and a "carryover" antiviral or chemotherapeutic effect in time culture.

Additional experiments in our laboratory with quaternary ammonium and phenolic compounds against HIV-1 using an EPA-approved protocol have shown similar results, as shown in Table 25–20. These data show that use of rapid dilution and serum as described in this protocol is an effective neutralizing technique.

IMPROVEMENT AND STANDARDIZATION OF VIRUCIDE ASSAYS

The American Society of Microbiology, under the co-chairmanship of Drs. Martin Favero and Dieter Groeschel, convened a workshop in Arlington, Virginia on chemical germicides in the health-care field (ASM, 1987). The procedures are published (Favero and Groeschel, 1987). A portion of the recommendations of the virus working group are described here, especially with regard to standardization of the assay.

In 1971, the EPA established guidelines for the testing of virucides involving the use of viral films dried onto carriers, such as glass slides or petri dishes. There are no Association of Official Analytical Chemists (AOAC) methods for testing the virucidal properties of disinfectants. Numerous suspension tests are used in Europe and in the United Kingdom. During the period 1975 to 1985, the E-35 Committee of the American Society for Testing Materials developed and approved two virucidal methods, a carrier and a suspension test. The EPA/ASTM method has been the basis of virucide registration in the United States and has been used for the following groups of viruses: myxoviruses, paramyxoviruses, rhinoviruses, enteroviruses, adenoviruses, herpes viruses, reoviruses,

Table 25–19. *Lack of Correlation Within Suspension, Cell Culture, and in Vivo Systems*

	Activity Profile on Direct Contact (Suspension in Saline)				
Compound	A Col-SK	B ECHO 9	C Coxsackie B₁	D Influenza A	E Herpes
1. DIQA					
2. Dehydroemetine					
3. Papaverine	■■■■■				

	Activity Profile in Tissue Culture (Rh M.K)				
Compound	Col-SK	ECHO 9	Coxsackie B₁	Influenza A	Herpes
4. DIQA			■■■■		
5. Dehydroemetine				■■■■	
6. Papaverine					

	Activity Profile in Vivo (Mice)				
Compound	Col-SK	ECHO 9	Coxsackie B₁	Influenza A	Herpes
7. DIQA	■■■■	■■■■		■■■■	■■■■
8. Dehydroemetine	■■■■		■■■■		
9. Papaverine	■■■■		■■■■		■■■■

DIDA = Dehydroisoquinoline acetamide; ■■■■■ = antiviral effect detected.

As can be seen, the single-contact virucidal activity could not be confirmed in vitro (T.C.); i.e., papaverine inactivated Col SK virus in saline suspension (A-3), but had no effect against the virus in rhesus monkey kidney cells (A-6). DIQA (C-4) and dehydroemetine (D-5) were effective against Coxsackie B₁ and influenza A, respectively, but were inactive in vivo (C-7 and D-8). Furthermore, none of the 8 in vivo activities were predicted from any of the in vitro results.

rotaviruses, and pox viruses. Recently, the EPA TSS-7 guideline, which describes carrier tests only, has been the basis of approved protocols (Gibraltar Biological Laboratories, 1987) for testing against the AIDS virus as well as against hepatitis B virus (Gibraltar Biological Laboratories, 1990). Both the ASTM and EPA methods are extremely conservative. There is no evidence that they have overestimated the potency of chemical virucides, except the possibility exists that the moderate protein load requirement (5% blood serum) may be inadequate to gauge antiviral potency properly in the case of blood spills, as well as in fecal and tissue environments. This is especially true in light of the comprehensive rotavirus experiments of Springthorpe et al. (1986) and Lloyd-Evans et al. (1986).

At the workshop, a program of ongoing review and revision of methods was recommended, including testing against HBV. It was concluded that the current ASTM and EPA methods require further standardization, especially in regard to host systems, protein load, length of incubation, and uniformity of viral strains. A follow-up international meeting was held in 1990 (ASM, 1990) at which there was a consensus that quantitative carrier tests of dried organisms were more stringent than suspension tests, such as are used in Europe. In addition further validation of the MADT procedure for anti-HBV activity was presented (Thraenhart, 1990; Prince, 1990).

INACTIVATION OF VIRUSES IN MONOCLONAL PRODUCTS

Principles of viral inactivation can be incorporated into sound quality-assurance programs for monoclonal products. The FDA (Hoffmann, 1987; Code of Federal Regulations, 1985) has set limits concerning the viral and molecular contamination of MA products (derived from

Table 25–20. *Human Immunodeficiency Virus (HIV) Rechallenge Assay Using Trypticase Soy Broth with Serum to 20% as Dilution Blank*

Concentration of Phenolic or Quat* on Disinfecting Surface	Concentration in Cell Culture Recovery Medium	Presence of Cytotoxicity	Presence of HIV-1	Back Reinoculation Challenge for "Carryover" Presence of HIV-1
Undiluted	10^{-1} virus 70 ppm	+	n.t.	n.t.
(700 ppm aqueous)	10^{-2} virus 7.0 ppm	0	0	+ †
10 min at 20 to 25°C to dried	10^{-3} virus 0.7 ppm	0	0	+ †
film of HIV-1 in 10% serum	10^{-4} virus 0.07 ppm	0	0	+ †

*D-125 also active after 30-s contact.
†Elisa antigen capture for p24 core antigen in H-9 supernatant after 7 and 14 days of incubation at 37°C in RPMI 1640₈₀ FCS₂₀.
n.t. = not tested; + = virus detected, proving absence of nonneutralized "carryover" of antiviral effect; 0 = no virus detected

Table 25–21. *Agents Prohibited by FDA in MA Products*

Virus	Nucleic Acid	Size (nm)
Murine-derived hybridomas		
Reo type 3	ds RNA; N	75–80
Hantaan	ss RNA; E	90–100
Polyoma	ds DNA; N	45–55
Pneumonia virus of mice	ss RNA; E	150–300
Mouse adenovirus	ds DNA; N	65–80
Minute virus of mice	ds DNA; N	18–20
Mouse hepatitis	ss RNA; E	75–160
Ectromelia	ds DNA; E	230–400
Sendai	ss RNA; E	150–300
Mouse encephalomyelitis (Theiler's GD VII)	ss RNA; N	22–30
LCM	ss RNA; E	50–300
Mouse salivary gland (murine CMV)	ds DNA; E	100–200
EDIM	Unknown	Unknown
Thymic	Unknown	Unknown
LDH	ss RNA; E	150–300
Human-derived hybridomas		
Epstein-Barr virus (EBV)	ds DNA; E	100–200
Cytomegalovirus (CMV)	ds DNA; E	100–200
Retroviruses (HIV)	two RNA strands; E	80–120
Hepatitis B virus surface antigen	ds DNA; E	42

ds = double stranded; N = naked; ss = single stranded; E = enveloped; nm = nanometer.

Table 25–22. *Ranking of Hybridoma Adventitious Viruses Based on Their Resistance to Disinfection**

Agent	Family	
Pneumonia virus of mice	Paramyxoviridae	
Sendai	Paramyxoviridae	
Mouse salivary gland	Herpesviridae	
LCM	Arenaviridae	Increasing
LDH	Togaviridae	
Mouse hepatitis	Coronaviridae	resistance
Polyoma	Papovaviridae	
Ectromelia	Poxviridae	to
Reo type 3	Reoviridae	
Mouse adenovirus	Adenoviridae	virucides
Mouse encephalomyelitis (Theiler's GD VII)	Picornaviridae	
Minute virus of mice	Parvoviridae	

*In order of increasing resistance to chemical inactivation.
Adapted from Prince, HN 1983. Disinfectant activity against bacteria and viruses: a hospital guide. Partic. Microb. Control, 2, 55–62; and Klein M, and DeForest A. 1983. Principles of viral inactivity. In *Disinfection, Sterilization, and Preservation.* 3rd Edition. Edited by S.S. Block. Philadelphia, Lea & Febiger.

murine hybridomas) that are intended for human use. These adventitious viral agents are listed in Table 25–21. Because it is expensive and time consuming to assay MA products for all these viruses, Prince and Prince (1988), using the concept of the "scale of disinfection," proposed an inoculated product bioindicator scheme as a way to validate that the manufacturing process can yield a virus-free product. This is an assay system similar to the use of spore strips as biologic indicators in the validation of sterilization cycles.

Table 25–22 shows a resistance ranking of the hybridoma viruses mentioned in the FDA *Points to Consider* (Hoffmann, 1987). Clearly, viral inactivation of a murine hybridoma inoculated at the start of manufacture with nonenveloped (naked) virus such as mouse encephalomyelitis (Picornaviridae), minute virus of mice (Parvoviridae), or reotype 3 (Reoviridae) would suggest that all the other more sensitive viruses (e.g., enveloped) were also inactivated. Similarly, hepatitis B virus surface antigen inactivation in a "spiked" MA might serve as a bioindicator for inactivation of Epstein-Barr virus (EBV), cytomegalovirus (CMV), and human immunodeficiency virus type 1 (HIV-1). Table 25–23 shows the various steps during the MA process wherein inactivation of a "spiked" organism might indicate the absence of all the other possible adventitious agents. Results in our laboratory with Sindbis virus and infectious bovine rhinotracheitis are summarized in Table 25–24.

The data in Table 25–24 show that Sindbis virus, a lipophilic virion, was stable up to the point of lyophili-

zation, but the application of dry heat produced a steady decline in infectivity. Additional validation experiments are required, but these suggest that other lipophilic agents (enveloped), such as cited in Table 25–21, would show similar predictable degrees of inactivation. The physical factors producing inactivation in the manufacturing process are assumed to bear some mechanistic relationship to chemical inactivation with regard to the denaturation of surface appendages.

Table 25–24 shows a steady decline in viral titer with a dramatic break point after lyophilization and none detectable after the third heat cycle. These results suggest that "spiking" experiments that quantitatively demonstrate the removal/inactivation of resistant indicator virus,

Table 25–23. *Components of Process Validation; Inactivation of Viruses**

Basic biochemical procedures
　Salt fractionation of culture or ascites fluids
　Size exclusion chromatography
　Affinity chromatography
　Ion-exchange chromatography
　Ultracentrifugation
　Lyophilization
　Polyacrylamide gel electrophoresis
　Agarose gel electrophoresis
　Ultrafiltration

Physical or chemical procedures
　Elevated temperature
　pH variation
　Exposure to:
　　Organic solvents
　　Chelating agents
　　Nucleases

*The procedures listed can be used alone or in series to inactivate and/or remove polynucleotides and/or viruses from biologic products.

Table 25–24. *Spiking Experiment**

	Log 10 (pfu/ml)	
Component of Process	Sindbis	IBR
Viral inoculum	9.00	8.1
Inoculum after freeze-thawing	8.20	0
Factor 8 spiked then frozen	7.10	0
Lyophilization	6.87	0
24 h dry heat (68°C)	3.41	0
48 h dry heat (68°C)	2.02	0
72 h dry heat (68°C)	<0.04	0

*Factor 8 was spiked to 10^9 or 10^8 pfu/ml with Sindbis virus or infectious bovine rhinotracheitis (IBR) virus, respectively. The spiked factor 8 preparation was then exposed to the manufacturing process in the sequence: freezing, lyophilization, dry heat. Samples were removed at each process steps and plague assays were performed with chick embryo fibroblasts. The change in log is calculated from the difference in infectivity relative to the inoculum after freeze-thawing. Infectious bovine rhinotracheitis was completely inactivated by freeze-thawing.

can provide assurance that the final bulk lot is free of less-resistant viruses. Accordingly, the time-consuming and expensive murine antibody production (MAP) tests, as set forth in Table 25–21, can be reduced to one or two indicator tests. Furthermore, by the application of direct antigen-capture ELISA methods coupled to in vitro and in vivo enrichment procedures, one can rapidly detect the presence of indicator strains. Such techniques have been used in our laboratory for the screening of MA products derived from human hybridomas for HIV-1 p24 core antigen (Table 25–25).

The data in Table 25–25 represent the starting point for a series of validation experiments the purpose of which would be to show that negative detection of HIV-1 by the direct antigen-capture method would correlate with a high degree of assurance that agents of concern to the FDA such as HSV or CMV are absent. Thus, virologic research on the inactivation of viruses by chemical agents can extend useful extrapolations to quality-control techniques in biotechnology.

TRANSMISSION OF VIRUSES

One reason for the use of disinfectants is to prevent contamination or disease. Another reason is to prevent objectional overgrowth (e.g., mildew, putrefaction). Where do viruses and virucides fit? With regard to overgrowth there is no fit at all—viruses do not produce mildew and they do not produce odors. This uniqueness with respect to other environmental pests is placed into fuller perspective in Table 25–35, which summarizes the spectrum of dangers from bacteria, fungi, and viruses. With regard to their residence on or in inanimate habitats, therefore, can they produce disease? It is a question of transmission, viral concentration, host susceptibility, and portal of entry. For infectious diseases, viruses included, there are three routes of transmission: (1) *horizontal*; (2) *vertical*; and (3) *zigzag*. Disinfectants are involved with zigzag transmission.

Horizontal Transmission

Horizontal transmission (HT) is best exemplified by person-to-person droplet infection (influenza, rubella, scarlet fever) and person-to-person intimate contact (venereal diseases, transfusion of contaminated blood). HT is prevented by avoidance of contact, barriers, or by the use of antiseptics or other virucidal strategies.

Vertical Transmission

Vertical transmission (VT) occurs during birth either by transplacental (congenital) infection (rubella, AIDS) or by vaginal passage (herpes, gonorrhea). VT is prevented by the use of chemotherapeutic agents.

Zigzag Transmission

This common mode of transmission is either (1) *animate*, i.e., animal to insect to animal (arthropod-borne) such as Eastern equine or Colorado tick fever encephalitis or (2) *inanimate*, i.e., animal to fomite to animal.

There is invasive zigzag transmission (ZZT) and topical ZZT. Their role in viral infection control is shown in Table 25–26. Inanimate ZZT is discussed further because it can be prevented with disinfectants.

Table 25–25. *Direct Screening of Monoclonal Antibodies for Human Immunodeficiency Type 1 (HIV-1) p24 Antigen**

Specimen	Absorbance at 492 nm		Comment
1	0.078	0.082	Nonreactive
2	0.077	0.080	Nonreactive
3	0.140	0.077	Nonreactive
4	0.085	0.080	Nonreactive
5	0.075	0.065	Nonreactive
6	0.096	0.114	Nonreactive
7	0.091	0.119	Nonreactive
Controls			
negative	(1) 0.095		Nonreactive
	(2) 0.089		Nonreactive
	(3) 0.144		Nonreactive
	Mean = 0.109		
positive	(1) 1.387		Reactive
	(2) 1.357		Reactive
	Mean = 1.372		

*The presence or absence of HIV-1 p24 antigen was determined by relating the absorbance of the specimen to the cutoff value. The cutoff value is the absorbance of the negative control mean plus the factor 0.50. (Specimens with absorbance values less than the cutoff value are considered nonreactive by the criteria of the test.) For the run to be valid, the difference between the means of the positive and negative controls should be 0.400 or greater.

Cutoff value

Difference of positive and negative control means: 1.372–0.109 = 1.263

To confirm that the antigen detected in a positive reaction is associated with infectious virus, the MA is incubated in H-9 cells for 7 to 14 days. The supernatant is analyzed for p24 antigen or for reverse transcriptase enzymatic activity.

Table 25–26. *Routes of Infection: Zigzag Vectoring by Fomites*

INVASIVE TRANSMISSION *(Invasive ZZT)*		*(Patient-Care Equipment)*
	Critical*	*Semicritical†*
(Patient → Device → Patient)	Arthroscopy, angioscopy Laparoscopy Bronchoscopy Respiratory equipment Tracheoscopy Endoscopic accessories such as biopsy forceps and suction valves, implants, catheters, dialysis equipment, needles, syringes, IV tubing	Colonscopy Sigmoidoscopy Hydrotherapy tanks Breathing circuits Other extracorporeal devices

Potential Transmission Via Devices to:	*Viruses Transmitted*
(a) Lung	Myxoviruses, VZV, adeno, CMV, EB, RSV
(b) Trachea	Myxoviruses, VZV, adeno, CMV, EB, RSV, parainfluenza
(c) Intestine	Rota, Coxsackie, Hepatitis, HIV, ECHO, polio, reo, adeno, plus the Norwalk, Hawaii, W, and Montgomery County agent
(d) Oral cavity	Myxoviruses, adeno, herpes, EB
(e) Kidneys	CMV, vaccinia
(f) Venereal	Herpes, HIV, EB
(g) Cardiovascular	EMC, Coxsackie, HSV, HIV, hepatitis B, hepatitis C, EB, rubella
(h) Brain	CJD virus, measles, kuru, Alzheimer's disease, other encephalitides

TOPICAL TRANSMISSION *(Topical ZZT)*	
	(Non-critical Equipment or Surfaces)‡
(Patient → Surface → Patient)	(Bedpans, furniture, linens, bedrails, floors, kitchen utensils, etc.) lab equipment

Potential Transmission from Surfaces Via Hands to:	*Viruses Transmitted*
(a) Hands	Rhinoviruses (hand to mouth, hand to eye or nose)
(b) Nose	Rotaviruses, HSV-1, 2, HIV, RSV, Adeno, ECHO, HBV, Polio, HAV
(c) Eyes	Coxsackie, smallpox, possibly others
(d) Mouth	

*Equipment that normally enters sterile tissue.
†Equipment that comes in contact with mucous membranes or broken skin.
‡Articles with hard surfaces, environmental.

Invasive Transmission

Invasive ZZT is of most concern during endoscopic procedures; of less concern is getting influenza from a bathtub or AIDS from a doorknob.

AIDS virus (HIV-1) can be transmitted by all three routes as follows: horizontal (venereal), vertical (placental or congenital), zigzag (contaminated needles). This is another unique feature of this organism. Thus, the role of disinfectants should not be underestimated in the care of a disease that, although not contagious, can be spread by triple transmission.

Invasive transmission from incompletely disinfected devices can cause tuberculosis, hepatitis, and bacterial infections such as *Pseudomonas* and *Salmonella* (Greene et al., 1974; Hawkey et al., 1981; Webb and Vall-Spinosa, 1975; Dawson et al., 1982; Leers, 1980; Dwyer et al., 1987; Wheeler and Kaiser, 1987; Bond, 1987; Bond et al., 1979). Of course, there is always the fear of acquiring AIDS, herpes, and respiratory and enteric viruses during endoscopic procedures such as bronchoscopy and colonoscopy.

Topical Transmission (Viral Transmission from Fomites)

Topical ZZT is of constant concern but is more difficult to prove. Vectoring probably occurs via the hands and then back to the susceptible host (surface to mouth, surface to eye, surface to open wound, etc.). Assiduous treatment of surfaces is important in eradication of topical transmission, especially in hospitals or other environments where high viral levels can be expected from either normal shedding or spills or splashes in either the clinic or the laboratory.

The application of virucidal disinfectants is appropriate for the following viruses because evidence does exist for transfer *via the zigzag route*.

Rhinoviruses. Hendley et al. (1978) suggested that rhinoviruses could be shed to hands and then to inanimate objects, which are then touched by a susceptible person and inoculated into the conjunctival or nasal mucosa. Reagan et al. (1981) presented data on human rhinoviruses that showed that shedding to environmental surfaces might cause such surfaces to serve as fomites for susceptible individuals. Hendley et al. (1973) showed the ability of rhinoviruses to be transferred to hands by rubbing contaminated areas. Rhinoviruses are responsible for more than one-third of all common colds. The large quantities of viruses present in nasal secretions readily contaminate the hands of infected individuals. The virus can be transmitted via an inanimate object (clothing or hard surfaces) to the recipient's hands, which then can inoculate the mucous membranes of the eyes and nose. This transmission is thought to require as little as a single viral particle to initiate infection (Hendley et al., 1978).

Hepatitis B Virus (HBV). Favero et al. (1979) described mechanisms of transmission of HBV infection ranging from overt parenteral (direct percutaneous inoculation by contaminated needles) as a high probability to transfer of infective material via vectors or inanimate environmental surfaces (e.g., toothbrushes, drinking cups, and horizontal surfaces in hospitals) as a low probability. Transmission to dialysis personnel from hepatitis B surface antigen (HBsAg)-positive patients or from contaminated instruments and environmental surfaces has been reported (Snydman et al., 1976).

Although the subject of hepatitis virus is discussed elsewhere in this volume, a discussion on principles of inactivation should properly include data on a hepatitis B antigen destruction assay.

In our laboratory we have turned to an in vitro destruction test as a means of quickly and inexpensively evaluating anti-HBV agents. The suspension test described herein has been used to evaluate 21 substances (Table 25–27). The test is conservative in the sense that some efficacious agents may not be detected, but those that achieve a ≥80% reduction in reactivity of HBsAg with anti-HBsAg antibody may meet EPA criteria when an approved test becomes available.

The test system reported here is known as a "Qualitative third generation enzyme-linked immunosorbent assay for the detection of hepatitis B surface antigen subtypes ad and ay in human serum or plasma." It is an acceptable method for the evaluation of human vaccines for HBV (21 CFR).

The method used was as follows: 0.5 ml liquid disinfectant was added to 0.5 ml human serum that contained relatively high amounts of HBsAg for the period of time indicated. HBsAg-negative human serum was used to stop the reaction and to perform dilutions; 0.2-ml aliquots were added to microtiter wells coated with a highly purified antibody specific for HBsAg, subtypes ad and ay, prepared in guinea pigs.* The addition of a sample containing HBsAg binds to the solid-phase antibody during the initial incubation at 45°C. At the completion of the incubation period, the HBsAg-disinfectant sample was removed by aspiration and the well thoroughly washed five times with distilled water. In the second incubation at 45°C, chimpanzee anti-HBsAg-alkaline phosphatase conjugate bound to the solid-phase anti-

*NML ELISA Antibody to Hepatitis B Surface Antigen (Chimpanzee Alkaline Phosphatase Conjugate Organon Teknika Corporation, Box 15969, Durham, NC, 27704–0969)

body-antigen complex. After the incubation period, the contents of the well were aspirated and the well was washed as previously. The reaction was visualized by the addition of the substrate for alkaline phosphatase (p-nitrophenyl phosphate) for 45 mins at 45°C. 1N sodium hydroxide was used to terminate the enzyme-substrate reaction and to stabilize the yellow color. When the disinfectant successfully modified or destroyed HBsAg, antigen was not available for binding to the solid-phase antibody and therefore no color developed. Spectrophotometric measurements were made at 492 nm. Other steps were as described by the manufacturer.

The results indicate that the halogen compounds were among the most effective agents. The novel hypochlorite is among the fastest acting sporicides that we have evaluated, having a D_{10} value of approximately 25 s. The antiseptic iodophors tested ranged in activity from 29% (prediluted douche) to 96% (surgical scrub). Sodium hypochlorite (525 ppm) produced a 93% destruction in 20 mins.

The halogenated substituted alcohol-phenol (Chlorophenyl) was also highly effective and warrants further evaluation.

The dental impression materials were effective, albeit less so than most compounds tested. The experimental design had to be modified, however, to test these products because the formed impressions were tested adding HBsAg to a bored-out well 6 mm in diameter and 6 mm in depth.

An alcohol-quaternary ammonium compound was completely inactive, whereas a BTC 2125M one-step hospital detergent formulation was effective.

Our results may prove to correlate with the Morphological Alteration and Disintegration test (MADT) used in Europe (Thraenhart, 1987; Kuwert et al., 1982). A major advantage of the HBsAg test is that electron microscopy is not required. The MADT electron microscopic method is accepted by the EPA for the registration of certain anti-HBV claims in the United States.

Fixatives such as formaldehyde have been reported to be ineffective in this assay at sporicidal concentrations (Bond et al., 1983). Thus, although the test described herein may not be suitable for all types of disinfectants, it would appear to be useful for the evaluation of nonfixative-type disinfectants.

Parainfluenza. Transmission requires close contact. Direct large-particle transmission or hand-to-hand spread directly via fomites can occur.

Respiratory Syncytial Virus (RSV). RSV is the most important cause of lower respiratory disease in children under 2 years of age and is most frequently transmitted horizontally by close person-to-person contact. The virus can be recovered, however, from gowns and paper tissues and after 7 hours on counter tops (Hall, 1977). Infectious virus can be transferred from these environmental surfaces to hands or from hand to hand (Hall et al., 1980).

Creutzfeldt-Jakob Disease (CJD) Virus. There is evi-

Table 25–27. *In Vitro Destruction of Hepatitis B Surface Antigen (HBsAg) in Order of Increasing Effectiveness*

Final Concentration of Active Ingredient in Reaction Mixture	% Destruction		
	Average of Two Replicates	Exposure* in Minutes	Organic Load
1. n-alkyl (68% ^{12}C, 32% ^{14}C) dimethyl, ethyl benzyl, ammonium chlorides 0.05% n-alkyl (60% dimethyl, benzyl, ammonium chloride 0.07%, isopropyl alcohol 4%)	0	10	50
2. Alginate impression material containing a nonionic detergent	11	30	50
3. Silicone quaternary 3-(trimethoxysiyl) propyldimethyl octadecyl ammonium chloride 21%, methanol 24.5%	14	35	50
4. Polyvinyl siloxane impression material	29	30	50
5. 2% chlorhexidine	47	20	50
6. PVP I solution 2.5%	54	20	50
7. Novel alcohol containing 35% EtOH (triple A)	63	24	50
8. Virex II (696 ppm quaternary ammonium compound)	69	30	10
9. D-125 (352 ppm active quat) BTC 2125M formulation	77	21	50
10. Novel alcohol containing 50% EtOH (triple A)	79	24	50
11. 0.7% formaldehyde	81	30	50
12. Chlorophenyl (isopropyl alcohol 4.4% sodium salt of 2,2'-methylenebis (3,4,6 trichlorphenol) (Hexachlorophene 0.5%)	(a) 86 (b) 80	20 13	50
13. 0.525% Household bleach	93	20	50
14. 2% Formaldehyde	94	30	50
15. Public places (1200 ppm, quat) formulation	94	30	10
16. 1.1% glutaraldehyde (reused 28 days)	95	30	50
17. PVP I scrub, (2.5%)	96	20	50
18. Novel hypochlorite (25%)	98	30	50

*Purified HBsAg, in human serum, was mixed in a 1:1 ratio with the disinfectant.

dence of transmission of CJD from contaminated human growth hormone (HGH) derived from human pituitaries. Accidental transmission of CJD to humans appears to have occurred after corneal transplantations, contaminated EEG electrode implantation (Prusiner and McKinley, 1987), and from surgical operations using contaminated instruments or apparatus. EEG electrodes stored in ethanol-formalin for several years were still capable of producing CJD in a chimpanzee 18 months after experimental implantation. In the 4 fatal cases of cerebral dysfunction and dementia discussed by Prusiner and McKinley (1987), patients aged 20 to 34 years who were treated with HGH during the period of 1969 to 1979 displayed incubation periods of 5 to 22 years. Incubation periods of 2 to 3 decades have been reported for kuru amongst New Guinea cannibals. CJD is detected upon autopsy at a rate of 1 per 10,000. In the absence of suitable germicides, the precautions of the Centers for Disease Control (CDC) for hepatitis virus (with special attention to "sharps" during surgery or autopsy) would appear to be prudent.

Smallpox. In addition to the comments of Valenti et al. (1980) on the hospital environment (and fomites such as linen) as a potential problem for infection-control personnel, especially for respiratory diseases, direct evidence has long been available incriminating fomites in smallpox transmission. Taylor and Knowlden (1957) discussed the role of fabrics as fomites and reported the occurrence of secondary cases of smallpox among laundry sorters in England. In addition, smallpox infection was attributed to contaminated textile articles by Cram (1951) during a smallpox outbreak in England as well as a hospital outbreak (Downie et al., 1965).

It is true that smallpox (variola) has been eradicated from the world by vaccination, and because no animal reservoir exists (as there is with influenza and rabies), it is not likely to return. Because smallpox immunization is not always a routine pediatric practice, however, unvaccinated laboratory workers are at risk for mild vaccinal infections. In addition, person-to-person (horizontal) or fomite transfer (zigzag), must be considered in a transfer setting originating in the laboratory environment and extending to neonates in a hospital or at home. Indeed, the transfer of smallpox virus and poliovirus from experimentally contaminated swatches of fabric (after drying) to previously sterile fabric has been shown by Sidwell et al. (1970).

Herpes Simplex and Human Immunodeficiency Viruses (HSV and HIV). The ability of HSV and HIV to be experimentally transferred by contact to dental impressions has been reported by Hammesfahr et al. (1989). These investigators demonstrated that the incorporation of virucides into the impression material prevented transfer, thus severing the potential zigzag chain of transmission from patient to fomite to doctor. Infection of laboratory or hospital personnel via contaminated instruments or surfaces is remote, however, especially with the use of CDC universal precautions.

Polio and Coxsackie Viruses. An experiment performed in our laboratory has shown that poliovirus type 1 and Coxsackie B$_1$ virus can be transferred from a finger-contaminated toothbrush to a tube of toothpaste (outside and inside the threaded extrusion nozzle), from toothpaste to toothbrush, and from toothbrush to toothbrush for at least 6 hours after inoculation. The enteroviruses were propagated in rhesus monkey kidney fed with Morgan and Parker's medium 199 and were incubated in screw-capped tubes for up to 7 days at 35°C. Virus was detected by cytopathic effect at 3, 5, and 7 days, as compared to virus-free cytotoxicity toothpaste controls. Sterile gloves were worn and then inoculated with virus as a means to contaminate the fomites. Again, the problem of hands (in this case poorly washed fecal-contaminated hands of children) as vectors to fomite surfaces and then zigzag back to man is highlighted by these experimental data.

Rotavirus. A series of papers have reported on the inanimate transfer of rotavirus from feces to fomites with evidence on the role of improperly disinfected fomites in the nosocomial spread of rotaviral gastroenteritis (Halvorsrud and Orstavik, 1980; Ryder et al., 1977; Sattar et al., 1986).

Adenovirus. Dawson and Darrel (1973) reported an outbreak of epidemic keratoconjunctivitis caused by adenovirus type 8 in a physician's office where 21 of 98 persons who were subjected to ophthalmic procedures later developed infections. In these cases, the zigzag transmission started with the physician's own eye infection, then proceeded to his hand, and then to a tonometer; the horizontal spread was hand to eye. Prince (1984) quantitated the survival time of various viruses on a hard surface and calculated D$_{10}$ values for desiccation resistance, the D$_{10}$ value being defined as the length of drying time at 20 to 25°C to reduce the viral titer by 1-log. The data are shown in Table 25–28 and confirm the likelihood of viruses remaining viable on inanimate surfaces. These data confirm the work of Mahl and Sadler (1975) who showed that viruses can survive for at least 8 weeks on common environmental surfaces. The data also show that desiccation resistance correlates with disinfectant resistance with the highest D$_{10}$ value (13.5 h) obtained for polio. Similar data for HIV-1 have been reported by Resnick et al. (1985).

NOSOCOMIAL VIRAL INFECTIONS—ROUTES OF TRANSMISSION

Hospital-acquired infections are not limited to bacterial and mycotic infections, although nosocomial spread of these agents is more common and is better documented (CDC, 1981, 1986). There is evidence, either by horizontal (person-to-person) transmission or by zigzag transmission (fomites) that viral infections can be acquired in health-care settings. Infection-control programs, therefore, must incorporate the usual barrier and gowning precautions plus the use of disinfectants with known virucidal properties, in addition to vigorous implementation of handwashing procedures. Valenti et al. (1980) studied the incidence of a variety of viral infections and arrived at the following conclusions:

1. The majority of hospital-acquired viral infections occurred in the pediatric and psychiatric services and were due to close person-to-person contact (horizontal transmission).
2. Viruses produced 78%, 71%, 5%, and 2% of nosocomial respiratory, gastrointestinal, disseminated or blood, and skin/soft tissue viral nosocomial illness in their study.
3. Herpes virus infections were more frequent in patients 14 years and older.
4. Respiratory syncytial virus (RSV), influenza, adenoviruses, and parainfluenza infections were more common in patients <3 years.
5. Patients with nosocomial virus infections were on average hospitalized 9.3 days longer than uninfected controls.
6. Topical zigzag transmission is possible (fomite to hand).

The nosocomial characteristics of each disease studied were characterized according to viral agent. The fomite-transferred viruses, as previously mentioned (rhinovirus, hepatitis B virus, parainfluenza, respiratory syncytial and adenovirus), also produced nosocomial infections. In addition, nosocomial person-to-person incidents have been recorded for herpes viruses, influenza, varicella-zoster virus, cytomegalovirus, rubella, measles, mumps, Creutzfeldt-Jakob disease, rotavirus, parvovirus, Coxsackie A and B viruses, ECHO, Lassa fever virus, and the Marburg and Ebola agents. The nosocomial factors involved with the following viral diseases were reviewed by Valenti et al. (1980) and are summarized here. The letter E at the end of each paragraph indicates an enveloped virus (lipophilic). Information on hepatitis B virus (HBV) is presented elsewhere in this volume, but it is well documented that dialysis patients can become infected from contaminated blood and equipment.

Influenza Virus. Influenza A and B virus infections are among the most contagious diseases of man. Person-to-person spread is thought to take place mostly by small-particle aerosols because large concentrations of virus are present in respiratory tract secretions and are available for dispersion as small aerosol particles produced by coughing, sneezing, or talking. (E)

Respiratory Syncytial Virus (RSV). RSV is the most important cause of lower respiratory disease in children less than 2 years of age. The primary mode of transmission is close person-to-person contact, with occasional small-particle aerosol transmission. Virus can be shed to environmental surfaces and thence to hands. (E)

Parainfluenza Virus. Transmission requires close respiratory contact. Direct large-particle transmission or hand-to-hand spread directly or via fomites can occur. (E)

Table 25–28. *Drying of Viral Films with 5% Serum at Room Temperature*

Virus	Host	ID_{50}s per Device*			D_{10}†
		N_0 (0-Time)	N_1 (24 Hour)	N_1 (48 Hour)	
Influenza A$_2$ J-305/57 (Asian) GBL 505	Chick embryo	1.0×10^7	$<1.0 \times 10^1$	—	4 hours
HSV-1 (Sabin) GBL 504	H.Ep. 2	5.0×10^7	5.0×10^5	$<1.0 \times 10^1$	7 hours
Vaccinia (Wyeth) GBL 506	MRC-5	5.0×10^6	1.0×10^5	$<1.0 \times 10^1$	8.5 hours
Polio I GBL 507	MRC-5	1.0×10^6	8.0×10^4	5.0×10^1	13.5 hours
HIV type I‡ on glass	H-9 System (Gallo)	2.0×10^6	10 min 20°C 1.0×10^6	24 hours R.T. $2 \times 10^{3.0}$ 7 days R.T. 1.0×10	$D_{10} = 8$ hours

*ID_{50} = infectious dose 50% per device as calculated by the method of Reed and Muench from the data obtained in cell cultures or in chick embryos.

†D_{10} estimated from data of Prince, H.N. Medical Device and Diagnostic Industries, July 1984, Canon Communications, and current data for HIV; time to reduce infectivity by 1-log or 90%. (D_{10} values for viruses on high-density polyethylene hip cups after 24 hours at room temperature.)

‡At 37°C HIV is inactivated within 6 days; in T.C. liquid at room temperature it retains more infectivity then when dry; HIV data from GBL virology laboratory, unpublished.

Rhinovirus. These agents are responsible for one-third of all "common colds" and cause exacerbations of chronic bronchitis. The large concentration of viral particles from nasal secretions contaminates hands. Hand-to-hand and environmental hand-to-fomite-to mucous membrane transmission can occur (Gwaltney et al., 1978). Handwashing is important in breaking the chain of transmission.

Human Herpes Virus. Members of the family Herpesviridae include: (1) herpes simplex type 1 (oral); (2) HSV type (genital); (3) varicella-zoster virus (VZV); (4) Epstein-Barr virus (EBV); (5) cytomegalovirus (CMV); and (6) the newly described human herpes virus 6 (CDC, 1988) and human herpes virus 7 (Frenkel et al., 1990). The foregoing are designated respectively as HHV-1, HHV-2, HHV-3, HHV-4, HHV-5, HHV-6, and HHV-7. Of these, HHV-3 (VZV chicken pox, varicella shingles) is the most capable of nosocomial transmission by direct contact or by small-particle aerosols. Varicella pneumonia can be a serious consequence. For all other herpes viruses, close person-to-person contact is required. Transmission of herpes zoster (HHV-3) from shingles patients to produce chickenpox has occurred, but this is far less common than transmission from patients with chickenpox. This is because there is less oral shedding of VZV from older shingles patients than from chickenpox patients. Localized herpes zoster requires wound and skin precautions to prevent infection by direct contact with either wounds or with secreta-contaminated articles. As with chickenpox, zoster patients require strict isolation in a private room with negative air pressure.

HHV-1 transmission from symptomatic and asymptomatic hospital personnel to patients is well documented. Hospital personnel have become infected by direct inoculation of finger from an infected patient's mouth (herpetic whitlow). Genital herpes (HHV-2) in mothers at term produces infection in the newborn about 40 to 60% of the time, and half these infections are fatal or severe. Women with genital herpes may transmit virus either postnatally or upon close contact. Therefore, personnel should observe wound and skin precautions with gowns and gloves for direct contact with perineal pads, dressings, and linen, which should be double-bagged. Cytomegalovirus (HHV-5) requires close contact for transmission and is more likely to be acquired in the hospital from congenital transfer, blood transfusions, immunosuppression, and renal transplants. Care should be taken in the handling of secreta, excreta, soiled articles, and linens from these patients. (E)

Rubella (German Measles) Virus. As a respiratory pathogen, close person-to-person contact is required. Outbreaks in hospitals have been reported. Precautions are especially required for congenital rubella including handwashing, private room, mask, gown, gloves, and attention to excreta, soiled articles, blood, needles, secreta, and linens. (E)

Creutzfeldt-Jakob Disease (CJD) Virus. CJD is not contagious in the usual sense. Nosocomial transmission has been reported (corneal transplant) and zigzag transmission via contaminated stereotactic electrodes from previous neurosurgery is known. Precautions should be taken with brain biopsy material, blood, and CSF, similar to those recommended by the CDC for hepatitis B virus. Disinfection can only be accomplished with concentrated NaOH or sodium hypochlorite followed by autoclaving for at least 2 hours. Contaminated instruments, tables, floors, and countertops should be treated with strong alkali or hypochlorite (not conventional disinfectants), followed by routine washing with soap and water or detergent disinfectant, such as a quaternary ammonium compound in lower dilution than cited as a label claim.

Rotaviral Gastroenteritis. Human rotavirus (HRV) is

also called the human reovirus-like agent or infantile gastroenteritis virus. It is a major cause of gastroenteritis in infants and children during the winter in temperate climates. Transmission is by the fecal-oral route, and nosocomial infections have been documented. Articles or surfaces contaminated with feces should be decontaminated, especially with disinfectants tolerant to organic matter (Sattar et al., 1986).

Parvoviral-like Gastroenteritis. The Norwalk, Hawaii, W, and Montgomery County agents are a major cause of gastroenteritis in children and adults and are thought to be spread by fecal and oral transmission. Nosocomial infection is believed to be possible but has not been demonstrated. These agents are relatively resistant to many disinfectants. Hypochlorite is useful as well as iodophors and glutaraldehyde. Claims for activity of quaternary ammonium compounds and phenolics are not substantiated. These agents, if used, must be potentiated with other agents or left in contact for longer periods of time. There is controversy concerning the parvocidal effect of these latter agents.

Adenovirus. These agents can be isolated from the throat, feces, and eyes of infected individuals, and fecal shedding can persist for many months. The viruses cause a variety of clinical conditions including conjunctivitis, keratoconjunctivitis, adenopharyngoconjunctival fever (APC fever), pneumonia, and a pertussis-like syndrome. Transmission is by the respiratory route in all age groups; the eye is also a portal of entry. The fecal-oral route is more frequent in children than in adults. Adeno 8 is the only strain to cause epidemic keratoconjunctivitis because it satisfies receptor sites on the cornea. Nosocomial infections have been documented for both patient and personnel. Virus can be spread and may persist on linens and articles and surfaces contaminated with secreta or excreta.

Nonpolio Enterovirus (ECHO, Coxsackie). Most nosocomial outbreaks have been reported in neonatal units. Transmission is by the fecal-oral route, with a probability of hand-to-fomite spread. Droplet infection has been described, and virus can be recovered from the oropharynx and rectum. Enteroviruses have been isolated from houseflies and cockroaches, which animals may promote zigzag spread. Patients may be asymptomatic or may have fever, rash, upper respiratory or gastrointestinal symptoms, meningitis, encephalitis, myocarditis, or pleurodynia. Often, nursery outbreaks can be traced to a congenitally infected infant with secondary horizontal transmission from infant to infant or zigzag via the hands of personnel. Maternal transmission may occur before or during delivery (vertical) or after delivery (horizontal). Careful handling of feces, secretions, soiled objects, and instruments is advised. Enteroviruses are relatively resistant to disinfectants, but ethanol, glutaraldehyde, hypochlorite, and higher concentrations of isopropanol can be effective.

Lassa Fever Virus. An airborne outbreak was reported in 1972 in a hospital in Africa (Buckley and Casals, 1973;

Valenti et al., 1980). Person-to-person spread is believed to have occurred via contact with blood, urine, and respiratory secretions. Lassa fever, a fatal and highly contagious hemorrhagic illness, is for the most part confined to Africa. (E)

The following viruses are of less importance in nosocomial spread.

Epstein-Barr Virus (EBV) (HHV-4). Nosocomial infection is rare. Infection has occurred through blood transfusion and from contaminated dialysis equipment. (E)

Measles (Rubeola) Virus. Nosocomial infection is now rare because of continued use of measles vaccine; hospital outbreaks are large when they do occur. One of the most easily transmitted diseases of man, the virus spreads from the respiratory tract by small-particle aerosols as well as by close contact. Spread from nasal or respiratory secretions via hands to nasal mucosa has been suspected. Measles encephalitis can be a serious consequence. (E)

Mumps Virus. Less contagious than either measles or varicella (chickenpox), transmission occurs by large droplets spread from the respiratory tract and salivary glands. Nosocomial episodes are not common; outbreaks are common in schools, families, and in the military. (E)

Poliovirus. Nosocomial spread is no longer a problem. Virus shedding can persist for a brief period following the administration of oral polio vaccine. The incidence of vaccine-induced paralysis from the attenuated oral strain is 0.44/million vaccinated.

Rabies Virus. Nosocomial rabies is uncommon; however, cases of human-to-human or zigzag transmission from corneal transplantation have been reported (Centers for Disease Control, 1980). Laboratory personnel working with bats and other susceptible animals are at risk, especially in regard to aerosolization of cultures. Corneas from individuals who have died with a history of dementia, encephalopathy, undiagnosed neurologic disease, multiple sclerosis conjunctivitis, or other viral diseases including hepatitis B, rabies, or Creutzfeldt-Jakob disease should not be used for transplants. (E)

Table 25–29 outlines some of the precautions suggested from the studies of Valenti et al. (1980). As can be seen, the most extensive precautions are required for hepatitis B virus as well as smallpox and the Lassa, Marburg, and Ebola agents.

PRIONS AND VIROIDS—A DISINFECTANT DILEMMA

It was formerly thought that all infectious diseases of plants and animals were caused either by mitotic microorganisms (bacteria, fungi, yeasts, protozoa) or by viruses. Now it is known that smaller and less complex agents can be involved and they are called viroids and prions.

Viroids

Viroids were first discovered in 1971. These agents only infect higher plants. There are 12 viroid diseases of

Table 25–29. *Precautions to be Taken for Transmission by Aerosol and via Soiled Articles (As Relates to Shedding and Portal of Entry)*

Viral Illness	Mask	Gloves	Soiled Articles From			Blood Needles
			Excreta	Secreta	Linen	
Respiratory Viruses						
Influenza A, B (E)	X					
Rhinoviruses		X		X		
RSV (E)				X		
Varicella (E)	X	X	X	X	X	
Herpes Zoster (E)	X	X	X	X	X	
HSV-I, II (E)		X		X		
EBV (E)		X		X		
CMV (congenital) (E)		X	X		X	
Hepatitis						
A	X	X	X	X	X	X
B (E)	X	X	X	X	X	X
(non-A, non-B)	X	X	X	X	X	X
Exanthematous Virus						
Rubella (congenital)	X	X	X	X	X	X
(acquired) (E)	X	X		X		
Measles (E)	X			X		
Mumps (E)	X			X		
Gastrointestinal						
Rotavirus		X	X	X		
Parvo-like		X	X	X		
Other (non rota)		X	X	X		
Arenaviruses						
Lassa fever (E)	X	X	X	X	X	X
Smallpox	X	X	X	X	X	X
Adenovirus	X	X	X	X		
Slow virus (CJD)		X		X	X	
Rabies (E)	X	X		X	X	
Marburg virus (E)	X	X	X	X	X	X
Ebola virus (E)	X	X	X	X	X	X
Entero-picornaviruses						
Polio		X	X		X	
ECHO		X	X		X	
Coxsackie A, B		X	X		X	

E = enveloped.

Adapted from Valenti W.M., et al. 1980. Nosocomial virus infections. II. Guidelines for prevention and care of respiratory viruses, herpes virus and hepatitis virus. Infect. Control, *1*, 33–37; and Valenti WM, et al. 1980. Nosocomial viral infections. III. Guidelines for prevention and control of exanthemata, gastroenteritis, picornaviruses, and uncommonly seen viruses. Infect. Control, *1*, 38–49.

plants affecting primarily dicotyledons and at least one monocotyledon: potato spindle tuber virus (PSTV), citrus exocortis virus (CEV), chrysanthemum stunt virus (CSV), chrysanthemum chlorotic mottle virus (CCMV), cucumber pale fruit virus (CPFV), coconut cadang-cadang virus (CCCV), hop stunt virus (HSV), columnea latent virus (CV), avocado sunblotch virus (ASBV), tomato apical stunt virus (TASV), tomato plant macho virus (TPMV), burdock stunt virus (BSV). Our knowledge of viroid structure is far greater than that of prions. Viroids are not inactivated by detergents or phenol. The viroid is a small infectious agent composed of low-molecular-weight RNA found only in plants. Viroids introduce less RNA into their hosts than do viruses and they do not require the assistance of detectable "helper" viruses. The particle consists of simple, stunted, circular RNA molecules. Thus, it would seem that the true viruses, which contain nucleic acid and protein, have evolved from simpler viroids and prions, or that viroids and prions are degenerate viruses in a pattern of de-evolution. There are no known viroid diseases of animals; however, evidence indicates that the delta hepatitis virus of man is a parasitic viroid-like agent. (See the section on biologic considerations at the end of this chapter.) There are no known prion diseases of plants.

Prions

Six prion diseases are known, three of which are in man. Prion diseases of animals produce slow, wasting

Table 25–30. *Prion Diseases*

Agent	Disease
Scrapie (early 20th century)	Scrapie in goats, sheep, etc.
Transmissible mink encephalopathy (TME)	Mink
Chronic wasting disease (CWD)	Mule deer, elk
Creutzfeldt-Jacob Disease (CJD) (1920)	Man
Kuru (1957)	Man
	Ritualistic cannibals; 3–30 years incubation with death in 1–2 years; Eastern highlands of Papua, New Guinea
Gerstmann-Straussler syndrome (GSS) (1928)	Man
Questionable	Alzheimer's disease; amyotrophic lateral sclerosis (ALS); Parkinson's disease; multiple sclerosis; Huntingtons chorea

The most effective decontamination procedure for CJD clinical materials is 2N NaOH for 30 minutes at room temperture. Exposure to 1N NaOH is not completely effective.

neuropathic effects. Scrapie is the prototypic prion disease; others are listed in Table 25–30. These diseases were formerly categorized as chronic infection neuropathic agents (CHINA agents). Only kuru is under control since the advent of restriction in practices of eating the dead among New Guinea natives.

Prions are aggregates of protein rods and are believed to contain neither DNA nor RNA. There is not total agreement on the existence of prions or their chemical nature. They are small, proteinaceous, infectious particles that are resistant to nucleic-acid-modifying procedures. Whether or not nucleic acid is ever shown to be present, the protein is essential for infectivity.

Prusiner and McKinley (1987) and their colleagues have produced the greatest body of evidence on the infectious nature of prions. Prions are extremely resistant to inactivation by procedures that commonly destroy other microorganisms. Routine autoclaving is not completely effective. A rare clinical problem has been the decontamination of Creutzfeldt-Jakob disease (CJD)-infected materials, as discussed later.

Table 25–31 summarizes the inactivation data currently available for prions. Table 25–32 outlines the current recommended sterilization procedure for surgical instruments, as well as the ineffective techniques. Tables 25–31 and 25–32 clearly demonstrate the nature of the challenge that these most primitive infectious agents present to either the disinfectionist or the chemotherapist.

In summary, prion diseases are chronic, fatal diseases of the central nervous system. They are not common, but they may represent a larger problem in the future

Table 25–31. *Inactivation Data for Prions*

Treatment	Reduction of Infectivity
Triton X-100 (1%)	None
100°C for 3 min*	Slight reduction
pH 3.5	None
pH 10.0	Slight decrease
65°C plus (1%) Sodium dodecyl sulfate	None (partial SDS + phenol)
Protease digestion	Decrease

Temperature (C)	No. Minutes	
60	30	None
80	30	None
100	10	Partial
100	30	Partial
Autoclave 121°C 30 min		Marked reduction
Autoclave 121°C 4 hours		Marked reduction but still present, depending upon organic load and heat penetration.

*Resistance to heat is a general feature of prions

as current orphan diseases become etiologically untangled. Thus, no one knows the true extent to which current disinfectant agents (including cold sterilizing solutions and oxidizing agents) are ineffective or the extent to which there is a future pressing need. Because these may represent the most chemically resistant and most untreatable of all infectious diseases, we hope that the list does not grow.

CURRENT VIRUCIDES AND ANTIVIRAL AGENTS

Virucides

Besides the usual array of germicides and "inerts" that comprise the disinfectant market (Tables 25–33 and 25–34), including the amphoterics used in Europe but not in the United States, mention should be made of metals and the recent work on polio inactivation by aluminum in water supplies (Thurman and Gerb, 1988) and of studies conducted by Murray (1980). These studies have shown an inactivating effect against poliovirus. The activity of aluminum against bacteria is not fully explored, but the oligodynamic effects of metal are well known (i.e., mercury, copper, and silver). Metallic aluminum was studied for possible use in conjunction with

Table 25–32. *Sterilization Procedures for Prions (Especially Surgical Instruments)*

Recommended (all 3 steps in sequence)
1. Autoclave 4½ hours (121°C, 15 psi)
2. 1 N NaOH autoclave for 1½ hours
3. 1 N NaOH for 30 min at 25°C 3 times

Ineffective (or partially effective)
  Ethylene oxide, UV, EtOH, Formalin, β-propiolactone, bleach, boiling, detergents, acids, ionizing radiation, alcoholic iodine, acetone

Table 25–33. *Comprehensive List of Ingredients Used as Disinfectant Formulations and Includes Both "Active" and "Inactives"*

Acidic anionic detergents	Phosphoric acid*
Amphoterics	Polyethoxypolypropoxypolyethoxyethanol-iodine complex
o-benzyl-chlorophenol	Pine oil
2-bromo-2-nitropropane, 1-3 diol (bronopol)	Povidone-iodine complex
Butoxypolyopropoxpolyethoxyethanol-iodine complex	Propionic acid*
Cetrimide	Propylene glycol*
Chloramine-T/	Sodium para-tertiary amyl phenate
Chlorhexidine acetate or gluconate (biguanides)	Sodium O-benzyl-p-chlorophenate
Chlorine dioxide	Sodium carbonate*
4-chloro-3,5-xylenol	Sodium dodecylbenzenesulphonate
Citric acid*	Sodium hypochlorite
Dodecylbenzenesulphonic acid	Sodium hydroxide*
Ethyl alcohol	Sorbic acid
Formaldehyde	Sodium o-phenylphenate
Glutaraldehyde	Sodium pentachlorophenate plus related chlorophenates
Glycerin*	Sodium sulfite*
Hydrochloric acid	Sulfonated oleic acid*
Hexachlorophene	Sulfuric acid*
Isopropyl alcohol	Triethanolamine*
Potassium bromide*	p-tertiary amyl phenol
Lactic acid*	Triethylene glycol*
Sodium chlorite	Trisodium phosphate*
Sodium metasilicate*	Tetrosodium ethylenediamine-tetraacetate*
Nonoxynol*	Methyl alcohol
Nonylphenoxypolyethylene ethanol-iodine complex	Xylenols
Phenol	
o-phenylphenol	
Oxalic acid*	

*Inerts (by definition; but all are potential amplifiers or synergists)

All the active ingredients in this table can inactivate vegetative bacteria and lipophilic viruses in Klein's group A when tested either in suspension or on carriers in the presence of 5% serum; only some of them can inactivate the more resistant picornaviruses. Increased activity against adenoviruses, rotaviruses, and picornaviruses can be obtained for some by a combination with "inerts" or alcohols. Additional information from the EPA on active and inert ingredients can be obtained from Federal Register, May 4, 1988, Part II, Environmental Protection Agency, 40CFR, pp. 15952–15999, as well as from EPA Lists of Chemicals Used as Inert Ingredients In Pesticides, List 1–4, July, 1986, 20 June, 1986 and October 1987. Disinfectant chemists readily point out that the activity of a complete formulation at a certain dilution is often more than the contributory effect of the "active" alone. As a result, it is difficult to standardize disinfectant tests with a reference control, such as with pharmacologics or antibiotics, since a "pure" standard, whether a quaternary salt, substituted phenol or aldehyde has less activity than the so-called "builders," "synergists" or "inerts" listed above.

Table 25–34. *Common Quaternary Ammonium Compounds with Aryl- and/or Alkyl-substitutes on the Tetravalent Nitrogen Shown as R (1–4)*

C12 (%)	C14 (%)	C16 (%)	C18 (%)	R2	R3	R4
40	50	10	—	Methyl	Methyl	Benzyl
50	30	17	3	Methyl	Methyl	Ethylbenzyl
68	32	—	—	Methyl	Methyl	Ethylbenzyl
50	30	17	3	Methyl	Methyl	Benzyl
	100% C10			C10	Methyl	Methyl
5	60	30	5	Methyl	Methyl	Benzyl
	Octyl			Octyl	Methyl	Methyl
	Octyl			Decyl	Methyl	Methyl

*All the quaternary ammonium compounds listed have about the same activity against bacteria and viruses, but they differ in terms of their activity in hard water and in the presence of organic load. They can be especially enhanced by the addition of alcohol, metal chelators, and certain nonionics. Activity in aqueous solutions is poor against TB and hydrophilic viruses.

or as an alternative to chlorine in drinking water. Almost complete inactivation was shown, and the infectious viruses were absorbed onto the surface of powdered metallic aluminum and then released from the metal as noninfectious particles. Analysis by electron microscopy, cesium chloride gradient centrifugation, and polyacrylamide gel electrophoresis indicated that either dissociation or destruction of the viral capsid protein occurred. Murray (1980) had shown earlier that aluminum degrades the RNA of intact poliovirus. Putting the two sets of data together, it would seem that the aluminum, probably as aluminum oxide and aluminum hydroxide on the surface of the metal, first cleaved the capsid protein allowing entry into the RNA core. Thus, aluminum, like formaldehyde, inactivates the polio particle by both a disruptive surface event and an internal nucleoprotein event. It is not known whether a similar virucidal effect exists for enveloped lipophilic virus. These agents can possibly shield the metal from the outer protein shell via lipid envelope interference. Studies of this nature on novel virucides are extremely important, given the long-term survival of poliovirus, hepatitis A, and rotavirus in community water supplies, as well as in bottled water; these viruses frequently exhibit resistance to inactivation by conventional chemical or physical agents (Biziagos et al., 1988). The effects of metallic and ionic silver and organosilver compounds on microorganisms are well known and are discussed elsewhere in the volume. Silver has been used in drinking water for many years in Europe and its usefulness as an antiseptic as well documented.

Future Research

There is a spectrum of danger from microorganisms in the environment (Table 25–35). It is important for disinfectant research to develop new germicides that are less toxic to man, animals, and plants and that are more compatible with the environment and are not inactivated by protein. For years, disinfectant research has revolved around reformulating and/or mixing well-known chemicals and improving test methods to meet regulatory requirements. Not since the development of chlorhexidine in 1954 has anything really new appeared. Emerging organisms and a fragile environment demand a more serious effort.

Antiviral Agents (Chemotherapeutics)

A brief summary of the most widely studied antiviral agents is given in this section. The agents included in this review are active in vitro (cell culture), in vivo (rodent, rabbits), and clinically in man. None are active as disinfectants. Further, none of the disinfectant compounds are on this list, although iodine is known to be effective in herpes eye infections. Phosphonoacetic acid, an organic acid, is as close as any chemotherapeutic agent has come to even the vaguest similarity to standard disinfectants and antiseptics. This follows the general finding over the years that the standard active ingredients in disinfectant formulations are essentially inactive as chemotherapeutics, with the exception of the prophy-

lactic uses of iodine, iodophors, hexachlorophene, and chlorhexidine as antiseptics, surgical scrubs, and other preoperative skin-degerming applications. Klein and DeForest (1963) first reported that tolerated (noncytotoxic) levels of quaternary ammonium compounds, phenolics, halogens, alcohols, and aldehydes that are "carried over" without neutralization to all culture recovery tubes *did not* repress viral replication.

Acyclovir. This agent 9-[2-hydroxyethoxy) methylguanidine] (trade name Zovirax, Burroughs Wellcome) is a topical antiherpetic (ophthalmic); it is used orally and topically for recurrent genital herpetic attacks and is also effective against herpes encephalitis.

Iododeoxyuridine (IDU) (IUDR). This agent [2'-deoxy-5'-iodouridine] (trade name Stoxil, SKF) is used topically for herpes simplex keratitis (eye infections); it is not active systemically. IDU, the first successful antiviral (1962), is for DNA viruses only.

Trifluoridine (TFT). This agent [5'-trifluoromethyl-2'-deoxyuridine] (trade name Viroptic, Burroughs Wellcome) is used topically for herpes simplex keratitis. The drug is effective against DNA viruses only.

Vidarabine. This agent [9-B-D-arabinofuranosyladenine (Ara-A)] (trade name Vira-A, Parke-Davis) is used topically for herpes simplex keratitis; intravenously against herpes zoster and herpes encephalitis. This agent is for use against DNA viruses only; it is not effective in genital herpes.

Ribavirin. This agent [1-B-D ribofuranosyl-1H, 1, 2, 4-triazole-3-carboxamide] (trade name Virazole, ICN) was the first broad-spectrum antiviral, active in cell culture against most DNA and RNA viruses including human immunodeficiency virus (HIV). The aerosolized drug is used against respiratory syncytial virus (RSV), the intravenous formulation is used against Lassa fever, and aerosol and oral preparations are effective against influenza.

Phosphonoformate (PFA). This agent [derivative of phosphono acetic acid] (CNa_3O_5P) (trade name Foscarnet, ASTRA) inhibits herpes viruses and HIV in cell culture. It is used topically for male genital herpes and intravenously against cytomegalovirus (CMV) in allograft recipients.

Amantadine (1-adamantanamine) HCl. This agent [$C_{10}H_{17}$ N•HCl] (trade name, Symmetrel, Du Pont) is used primarily as an oral prophylactic for influenza A_2 infections; a derivative, rimantadine, is equally active plus shows a therapeutic effect orally against influenza A_2.

3' Azidothymidine (AZT). This agent [3'-azido-3'-deoxythymidine] (trade name, Retrovir, Burroughs Wellcome) has limited activity orally against HIV-1 (AIDS). Drug resistance is now known to develop.

Suramin. This drug (a naphthalene sulfonic acid $[C_{51}H_3 4N_6Na_6O_{23}S_6]$) is used for early African trypanosomiasis; it has also shown activity as a reverse transcriptase inhibitor in a few AIDS patients.

HPA 23. This agent (a tungstoantimony compound, $[(NH_4)_{17}$ Na/NaW$_{21}$ Sb$_9$O$_{86}$•14 H$_2$O]) is unique as an in-

Table 25–35. *Germicides are Applicable: Spectrum of Dangers from Disinfectant Targets*

Site	Odors	Mildew	Slime		Infections
Home/Office	(X)	(X)	0	X	Respiratory fungi (SBS) Home Care (AIDS) Feces Dermatophytes Legionella
Public Facilities (restrooms, gyms)	(X)	(X)	(X)	X	Herpes Fecal Contamination Dermatophytes
Restaurants	(X)	(X)	(X)	(X)	Salmonella Staph Campylobacter Enteroviruses Hepatitis
Food	(X)	(X)	(X)	(X)	Salmonella Staph Campy Enteroviruses Hepatitis Botulism

Pharmaceuticals,
  Devices
	(X)	(X)	(0)	(X)	Sterility
					  Contamination
					USP Limits
					GMP Limits
					Pyrogens
					Nosocomial Infections

Hospitals,
  Laboratories
  Sickrooms
	(X)	(X)	0	(X)	Nosocomial
					  (environmental)
					  devices and instruments
					  hands, etc.

Bacteria and Fungi

Viruses

(X) = Applicable, occurrence is highly probable
 X = Applicable, occurrence is probable but not high risk
 0 = Not applicable, occurrence is not probable
SBS = Sick building syndrome

organic substance against the reverse transcriptase of AIDS virus in limited clinical study.

The detection of the chemotherapeutic activity of antiviral agents is accomplished primarily in cell culture systems or chick embryos followed by in vivo studies in mice, guinea pigs, and rabbits. These tests are calibrated against 10 to 100 median tissue culture infective dose ($TCID_{50}$) of challenge virus and must be controlled wherever possible with standard antiviral agents such as AZT (HIV-1), IUDR (herpes and other DNA viruses), amantadine (influenza), and ribavirin. In vitro screening methods for HIV-1 or HIV-2 are available using, for example, a cytopathic effect (CPE)-viability assay with MT-2 cells or a p24 core antigen detection assay (ELISA) in an H-9 immortal cell system (Prince, Geering, and Freeman, 1990).

The use of virucides as antiseptics against target pathogens is not easily studied in a clinical setting because the viruses are not resident flora and volunteer inoculation studies are impractical because of the virulence and potential invasiveness of such agents as herpes simplex virus, HIV, ECHO, Coxsackie, rotaviruses, etc. Human and animal skin in vivo and in vitro methods are available, as well as classic infectious disease models such as topical HSV-2 vaginitis in mice (with accompanying central nervous system effects) or topical HSV-1 dendritic keratitis in the rabbit eye. Agents such as para-chloro-meta-xylenol (PCMX), chlorhexidine, polyvinyl-pyrolidone-Iodine (PVP-I), nonoxynols, and alcohols can be studied in this way.

BIOLOGIC CONSIDERATIONS

The principles of viral inactivation are entirely different from other antimicrobial activities. Indeed, even the principles of viral chemotherapy lack many similarities to the antimicrobial therapy of bacterial, fungal, and protozoan diseases. The effects of chemical germicides on a virion deal exclusively with surface events—the chemical or physical derangement of the protein and/or lipid structures essential to the attachment and penetration of the viral particle to specific receptor sites on the host cell. The effect of a cationic substance such as a quaternary ammonium salt on a bacterial cell is an event proximal to the virucidal germicide. In the case of the quaternary ammonium compound, subsurface organelles, such as the lipopolysaccharide cytoplasmic membrane, are disrupted causing leakage of essential cell components. For oxidizing agents (chlorine, iodine, bromine, peroxides), external (capsid) and internal (nucleoprotein) covalent changes are involved. Even these are not strictly surface phenomena, however. The antibacterial effects of phenolics and aldehydes require cell entry and deal primarily with internal cytoplasmic events related neither to the maintenance of cell constituents nor to the ability of a microbe to attach to the receptor. These, too, are not surface events. With regard to bacteria, however, the adhesion hypothesis (Mackowiak, 1982) does offer some similarities to the viral surface event. In this model, a difference is emphasized between the total killing of a bacterium and the destruction of its infectivity (i.e., the potential for associated flora to produce disease). The term "associated flora" replaces the term "normal flora."

Accordingly, because adhesions must be fully intact to attach to a host receptor (e.g., *Salmonella* within the small intestine; gonococci for the urethral mucosa), a sublethal dose of a germicide may allow outgrowth of exposed cells to an in vitro recovery broth, but in fact the recovered organisms may have lost all virulence in vivo or even the ability to become normal or associated flora. Indeed, this is *disinfection* in the true sense, as opposed to cell death, i.e., the ability to selectively strip from the cell the ability to attach and potentially invade while metabolism and reproductive functions remain intact. This phenomenon is selective. It has not been named but it can be called *depathogenization* or *sub-disinfection*. It is a subtle mechanism constantly operative in nature, and it is perhaps the reason that the myriad viable bacteria on and in our environment do not produce more infections than they do. Differences exist among dead bacteria (cannot grow), avirulent bacteria (can grow but cannot infect), and virulent bacteria (can grow and can infect). As a matter of fact, subdisinfection occurs simply on drying as well as during culture transfers. It is reversed upon animal passage. Most bacteria in the environment, especially if spilled from frequently transferred cultures, are avirulent and, with the exception of endoscopes and blood products, pose little threat. Bacteria may be "alive" but noninfectious. Viruses may be "dead" but still infectious (if somehow the nucleic acid enters the host's cytoplasm or nucleus).

Therefore, bacteria and viruses share a surface apparatus in common. For viruses it is essential for their continued replication, and for bacteria (those that are pathogenic) it is essential for infection but not for a free-living existence. Nonetheless, the term disinfectant remains fixed to the concept of killing viruses and vegetative cells. In the United States (but not all countries), it is meant strictly to define the chemical process by which microorganisms are killed on inanimate surfaces. Thus, for bactericides and fungicides we use the word "kill" and for viruses we use the word "inactivate." One cannot kill what is not alive, and viruses fulfill only one of the criteria for "life" (viruses do not *grow* and they do not exhibit *irritability*, they merely *replicate*). Viruses replicate in a quasisexual process that involves attachment of an appendage to a receptor followed by injection of genetic material into a single cell wherein it may reside as a latent virus or may replicate subsequently bursting out with lethal consequences for the host cell.* This extraordinary series of cellular and subcellular events speaks to the origin of viruses themselves. Surely, requiring living cells, viruses evolved after the bacteria and lower plants and animals. A genetic intrusion theory would allow that they entered the cells as degenerate mitochondria or plasmids from higher or similar organisms and then produced biochemical misbehavior; a genetic extrusion theory would suggest that they are bits of DNA or RNA somehow lost from the same cell, encapsidated elsewhere, and then able to re-enter with total commandeering of the biochemical machinery of the cell that once produced it. In any event, virucidal germicides (as incorrect as the term "virucide" may be) promote destruction of the entry mechanism, whereas current clinically useful antiviral agents (except for antibodies) for the most part promote cessation of intracellular biosynthetic events.

A fuller examination of the theory surrounding virucidal activity, whether for disinfectants or for antiseptics, which could possibly lead to newer generations of less-toxic, broad-spectrum germicidal agents, requires a probe into the biochemistry, cytology, and genetics of the animal and plant cell that is beyond the scope of this chapter. Such a probe would not exclude inquiry into bacterial and plant viruses as well the double-stranded RNA "killer" viruses of yeast (Williams and Leibowitz, 1987).

Viruses are especially dangerous because they are *highly infectious by the respiratory route* and because they are *especially resistant to drug therapy*. The most infectious and fatal are Lassa fever virus within the *Arenaviridae* and the Marburg-Ebola agent within the *Filoviridae*. These are relatively recent (last 20 years) and no one knows where they originated. The AIDS virus, although among the most fatal, is among the least contagious, requiring either venereal or intravenous contact and transmitted neither by aerosol nor by insects. So therefore, the air that we breathe is potentially the most disastrous source of lethal virus, and the only thing worse than the epidemics of rabies, yellow fever, plague,

---

*An exception occurs with the arboviruses, which are neither latent nor lytic in the insect; the virions are synthesized and secreted without any harmful effect on the arthropod vector.

influenza, and AIDS that have struck mankind from reservoirs in the animal kingdom would be a T-cell lymphotropic virus or a neurotropic virus with a respiratory portal of entry. If it came from the plant kingdom via pollen or dust, it would be disastrous, the ultimate irony. Take note, in the first place, that there are similarities between the wound-tumor virus of clover and the *Reoviridae* in animals and man and, in the second place, that structures have been found in plant viroids that are similar to the delta particle of hepatitis. How susceptible are these structures to a mutation toward human receptor compatibility? Are they examples of molecular conservation of fundamental genetic morphology, or are they suggestions of evolution from one kingdom to the next? Can plant viruses invade the animal kingdom? The plants gave rise to the animals and, ironically, if it is in the scheme of things, they may be able to do the reverse.

REFERENCES

American Society of Microbiology (ASM). 1987. Germicides in the health care field. ASM News, 53, 327.

American Society of Microbiology (ASM). 1990. International Symposium on Chemical Germicides, Atlanta, GA.

Biziagos, E., Passagot, J., Crance, J.M., and Deloince, R. 1988. Long-term survival of hepatitis A virus and polio virus type 1 in mineral water. Appl. Environ. Microbiol., 54, 2705–2710.

Blackwell, O.H., and Chen, J.H.S. 1970. Effects of various germicide chemicals on H. Ep 2 cell culture and herpes simplex virus. J. Assoc. Off. Anal. Chem., 53, 1229–1236.

Bitton, G. 1980. *Experimental Virology*. New York, John Wiley & Sons.

Bond, W.W. 1987. Virus transmission via fiberoptic endoscope: recommended disinfection. JAMA, 257, 843–844.

Bond, W.W., Favero, M.S., Mackel, D.C., and Mallison, G.F. 1979. Sterilization and disinfection of flexible fiberoptic endoscopes. AORN J., 30, 350–351.

Bond, W.W., Favero, M.S., Peterson, N.J., and Ebert, J.W. 1983. Inactivation of hepatitis B virus by intermediate-to-high level disinfectants. J. Clin. Microbiol., 18, 535–538.

Buckley, S.M., and Casals, J. 1973. Lassa fever, a new viral disease of man from West Africa. A.₂ M. J. Trop Med. Hyg., 223, 279–283.

Centers for Disease Control. 1980. Human-to-human transmission of rabies via a corneal transplant. MMWR, 29, 25–26.

Centers for Disease Control. 1981. *Guidelines for the Prevention and Control of Nosocomial Infections*. Atlanta, GA, Centers for Disease Control.

Centers for Disease Control. 1986. Guidelines for handwashing and hospital environmental control—1985. Garner, J.S., and Favero, M.S. Am. J. Infect. Control, 14, 110–126.

Centers for Disease Control. 1988. HHV-6 evidence suggests novel herpes virus does not potentiate AIDS. AIDS Weekly, Sept. 5, 1988, page 2.

Chandler, R.C. 1961. Experimental scrapie illness in mice. Lancet, 1, 1378–1879.

Code of Federal Regulations (CFR). 1985. General biological product standards part 610. In *Food and Drugs Code of Federal Regulations*. Title 21. Washington, D.C., Office of the Federal Register, National Archives and Records Administration, United States Government Printing Office, pp. 42–67.

Cram, B.R. 1951. Smallpox outbreak in Brighton, 1950–1951. Public Health, 64, 123–128.

Dawson, C.R., and Darrel, R. 1973. Infectivity due to adenovirus type 8 in the United States: an outbreak of epidemic keratoconjunctivitis originating in physician's office. N. Engl. J. Med., 268, 1031–1034.

Dawson, D.J., Armstrong, J.G., and Blackblock, Z.M. 1982. Mycobacterial cross-contamination of bronchoscopy specimens. Ann. Rev. Respir. Dis., 126, 1095–1097.

Downie, A.W., et al. 1965. The recovery of smallpox virus from patients and their environment in a smallpox hospital. Bull. WHO, 33, 615–622.

Dwyer, D.M., et al. 1987. *Salmonella newport* infections transmitted by fiberoptic colonoscopy. Gastrointest. Endosc., 33, 84–87.

Elliot, L.E., McCormick, J.B., and Johnson, K.M. 1982. Inactivation of Lassa Marburg and Ebola viruses by gamma irradiation. J. Clin. Microbiol., 16, 704–708.

Favero, M.S. 1983. Chemical disinfection of medical and surgical materials. In *Disinfection, Sterilization, and Preservation*. 3rd Edition. Edited by S.S. Block. Philadelphia, Lea & Febiger.

Favero, M.S., and Groeschel, D.H.M. (Eds.). 1987. *Chemical Germicides in the Health Care Field*. Washington, D.C., American Society of Microbiology.

Favero, M.S., Maynard, J.E., and Leger, R.I. 1979. Guidelines for the care of patients hospitalized with viral hepatitis. Ann. Intern. Med., 91, 872–876.

Federal Register, EPA Virucide Disinfectant Efficacy Testing, June 25, 1975, p. 11625.

Frenkel, N., et al. 1990. Isolation of a new herpesvirus from human CD4⁺ T cells. Proc. Natl. Acad. Sci. U.S.A., 87, 748–752.

Gard, S. 1957. Chemical inactivation of viruses. Ciba Found. Symp., 123–146; 1960. Theoretical considerations in the inactivation of viruses by chemical means. Ann. N.Y. Acad. Sci., 83, 638–648.

Gerber, P., Hottle, G.A., and Grubbs, R.E. 1961. Inactivation of vacuolating viruses (SV-40) by formaldehyde. Proc. Soc. Exp. Biol. Med., 108, 112.

Gibraltar Biological Laboratories. 1977–1978. Unpublished data, presented at American Society for Testing Materials E-35 Committee Meetings, Cleveland, 1977, and Philadelphia, 1978.

Gibraltar Biological Laboratories, 1987. Protocol for inactivation of human immunodeficiency viruses on inanimate surfaces. EPA, 9 September, 1987.

Gibraltar Biological Laboratories. 1990. Protocol for Morphologic Alteration and Destruction Test (MADT) for inactivation of hepatitis B virus. EPA, 12 July, 1990.

Greene, W.H., et al. 1974. Esophagoscopy as a source of *Pseudomonas aeruginosa* sepsis in patients with acute leukemia: the need for sterilization of endoscopes. Gastroenterology, 67, 912–919.

Gregg, D.A., and House, C. 1989. Necrotic hepatitis of rabbits in Mexico: a parvovirus. Vet. Rec., 125, 603–604.

Grunberg, E.M., and Prince, H. 1970. Experimental methodology and the search for effective antiviral agents. Ann. N.Y. Acad. Sci., 173, 122–130.

Gwaltney, J.M., Mosolski, P.B., and Hendley, J.O. 1978. Hand to hand transmission of rhinovirus. Ann. Intern. Med., 88, 453–467.

Hall, C.B. 1977. The shedding and spreading of respiratory syncytial virus. Pediatr. Res., 11, 236–239.

Hall, C.D., Douglas, R.G., and Geiman, J.M. 1980. Possible transmission by fomites of respiratory syncytial virus. J. Infect. Dis., 141, 98–102.

Halvorsrud, J., and Orstavik, I. 1980. An epidemic of rotavirus-associated gastroenteritis in a nursing home for the elderly. Scand. J. Infect. Dis., 12, 161–164.

Hammesfahr, P.D., Bennett, R.J., Jeffries, S.R., and Prince, R.N. 1989. Antiviral properties of self-disinfecting impression materials. Presented at the March 19, 1989 meeting of the American Association of Dental Research, San Francisco.

Hawkey, P.M., et al. 1981. Contamination of endoscopes by *Salmonella species*. J. Hosp. Infect., 2, 373–376.

Hendley, J.O., Mika, L.A., and Gwaltney, J.M. 1978. Evaluation of virucide compounds for rhinovirus on hands. Antimicrob. Agents Chemother., 14, 690–694.

Hendley, J.O., Wenzel, R.P., and Gwaltney, J.M. 1973. Transmission of rhinovirus colds by self-inoculation. N. Engl. J. Med., 288, 1361–1364.

Hiatt, C.W. 1964. Kinetics of the inactivation of viruses. Bacteriol. Rev., 28, 150–163.

Hoffmann, T. 1987. *Points to Consider in the Manufacture of Monoclonal Antibody Products for Human Use* (1987 CHFN 830). Bethesda, MD, Chairman Hybridoma Committee, Office of Biologics Research and Review, United States Food and Drug Administration. U.S. Govt. Printing Office, Washington, D.C.

Kitching, R.P. 1989. Cited in Vet. Res., July 15, 1989 (U.K.)

Klein, M., and DeForest, A. 1963. The chemical inactivation of viruses. In Proceedings of the Chemical Specialty Manufacturing Association, Chicago, 49th Midyear Meeting, pp. 116–118.

Klein, M., and DeForest, A. 1965. Chemical inactivation of viruses. Fed. Proc., 24, 319 (Abstr. 1052).

Klein, M., and DeForest, A. 1983. Principles of viral inactivity. In *Disinfection, Sterilization, and Preservation*. 3rd Edition. Edited by S.S. Block. Philadelphia, Lea & Febiger, pp. 422–434.

Kuwert, E., Thraenhart, O., Dermietzel, R., and Scheiermann, N. 1982. Zur Hepatitis B-Viruswirksamkeit und Hepato-viruzidie von Desinfektion sverfahren auf der Grundlage MADT, Medizin Hygiene, Prävention, Verlag, Maing, Germany.

Leers, W.D. 1980. Disinfecting endoscopes: how not to transmit *Mycobacterium tuberculosis* by bronchoscopy. Can. Med. Assoc. J., 123, 275–280.

Lloyd-Evans, N., Springthorpe, V.S., and Sattar, S.A. 1986. Chemical disinfection of human rotavirus-contaminated surfaces. J. Hyg. Camb., 97, 163–173.

McDuff, C.R., and Gaustad, J.W. 1976. Test method for determination of virucide efficacy of liquid surface disinfectants. J. AOAC, 59, 1151–1155.

Mackowiak, P.A. 1982. The normal flora. N. Engl. J. Med., 307, 83–85.

Mahl, M.C., and Sadler, C. 1975. Virus survival on inanimate surfaces. Canad. J. Microbiol., 1, 819–823.

Mahnel, H., Stettmund Von Brodorotti, H., and Ottis, K. 1980. Sensitiveness of viruses to gamma irradiation. Zbl. Bakt. I. Abt. Orig. B170, 57–70.

Martin, L.S., McDougal, J.S., and Loskoski, S.L. 1985. Disinfection and inactivation of the human T lymphotropic virus type III/LAV. J. Infect. Dis., *152*, 400–403.

Murray, J.D. 1980. *Physical Chemistry of Virus Adsorption and Degradation on Inorganic Surfaces. Its Relation to Waste Water Treatment.* EPA–600/ 2–80–134, United States Environmental Protection Agency.

Nakao, J., Hers, R.G., Bachman, P.A., and Mahnel, H. 1978. Inactivation of transmissible gastroenteritis (TGE) virus. Berl. Munch. Tierarztl. Wochenschr., *91*, 353–357.

Popovic, M., Sarngadharan, M.G., Read, E., and Gallo, R.C. 1984. Detection, isolation, and continuous production of cytopathic retroviruses (HTLV-III) from patients with AIDS and pre-AIDS.

Prince, D.L., and Prince, R.N. 1988. Quality assurance of monoclonal products: virologic and molecular biologic considerations. J. Indust. Microbiol., *3*, 157–165.

Prince, D.L., Prince, R.N., and Prince, H. 1990. Inactivation of human immunodeficiency virus type 1 and herpes simplex virus type 2 by commercial hospital disinfectants. Chem. Times Trends, February 1990: pp. 13–16.

Prince, D.L., Geering, G., and Freeman, L. 1990. ASM Intern Germicide Conference, Atlanta, GA, 1990 Proceedings. Publish. Amer. Soc. Microbiol. Washington, D.C.

Prince, H.N. 1983. Disinfectant activity against bacteria and viruses: a hospital guide. Partic. and Microb. Control, *2*, 55–62.

Prince, H.N., and Rubino, J. 1984a. Bioburden dynamics: the viability of microorganisms on devices before and after sterilization. Med. Device Diagn. Indust.

Prince, H.N. 1984b. Diagnostic medical microbiology. In *CRC Handbook of Microbiology.* 2nd Edition. Vol. VI: *Growth and Metabolism.* Edited by A.I. Laskin and H. Lechevalier. Boca Raton, FL, CRC Press, pp. 209–233.

Prince, H.N., and Grunberg, E., 1970. Experimental methodology and the search for effective antiviral agents. Ann. N.Y. Acad. Sci., *173*:122–130.

Prince, H.N. 1990. Problems in virus testing. American Society for Microbiology. Proceedings of International Conference on Chemical Germicides, Atlanta, GA. (ASM Publications, Washington, D.C.)

Prusiner, S.B., and McKinley, M.P. (Eds.). 1987. *Prions.* San Francisco, Academic Press.

Prusiner, S.D., Groth, D.F., and Martinez, H.M. 1980. Scrapie in hamsters. Biochemistry, *19*, 4883.

Reagan, K.J., McGrady, M.L., and Crowell, R.L. 1981. Persistence of human rhinovirus infectivity under diverse environmental conditions. Appl. Environ. Microbiol., *41*, 618–620.

Resnick, L., et al. 1985. Stability and inactivation of HTLV-III/LAV under clinical laboratory environments. JAMA, *255*, 1887–1891.

Rutala, W.A. 1989. Draft guideline for selection and use of disinfectants. Am. J. Infect. Control, *17*, 24A–38A.

Ryder, R.W., Mcgowan, J.E., Hatch, M.H., and Palmer, E.L. 1977. Reovirus-like agent as a cause of nosocomial diarrhea in infants. J. Pediatr., *90*, 698–702.

Salk, J.E., and Gori, J.B. 1960. A review of the theoretical experimental and practical considerations in the use of formaldehyde for the inactivation of polio virus. Ann. N.Y. Acad. Sci., *83*, 609–637.

Sattar, S.A., Lloyd-Evans, N., Springthorpe, V.S., and Nair, R.C. 1986. Institutional outbreaks of rotaviruses diarrhea: potential role of fomites and environmental surfaces as vehicles for virus transmission. J. Hyg., *96*, 277–289.

Schurmann, W., and Eggers, H.J. 1983. Antiviral activity of an alcoholic hand disinfectant: comparison of the in vitro suspension test with in vivo experiments on hands and on individual fingertips. Antiviral Res., *3*, 25–41.

Scott, F.W. 1980. Virucidal disinfectants and feline viruses. Am. J. Vet. Res., *41*, 410–414.

Sidwell, R.W., Dixon, G.J., Westbrook, L., and Forziati, F.H. 1970. Quantitative studies on fabrics as disseminators of viruses. IV. Virus transmission by dry contact on fabrics. Appl. Microbiol., *19*, 950–954.

Snydman, D.R., Bryan, J.A., Macon, E.J., and Gregg, M.D. 1976. Hemodialysis associated hepatitis. Am. J. Epidemiol., *104*, 563–570.

Spaulding, E.H. 1968. Chemical disinfection of medical and surgical materials. In *Disinfection, Sterilization, and Preservation.* 1st Edition. Edited by S.S. Block and C.A. Lawrence. Philadelphia, Lea & Febiger, pp. 517– 531.

Springthorpe, V.S., Grenier, J.L., Lloyd-Evans, N., and Sattar, S.A. 1986. Chemical Disinfection of Human Rotavirus: Efficacy of Commercially Available Products in Suspension Test. J. Hyg. Camb., *97*, 139–161.

Stettmund Von Brodorotti, H., and Mahnel, H. 1980. Inactivation of viruses and bacteria in sewage sludge by gamma radiation. Zbl. Bakt. I. Abt. Orig. B170, 71–81.

Taylor, J., and Knowlden, T. 1957. *Principles of Epidemiology.* London, J.A. Churchill, p. 108.

Thraenhart, O. 1987. Current status of virus disinfection in Germany and some notes on the morphological alteration and disintegration test (MADT). Presented at the American Society of Microbiology Symposium on Chemical Germicides in the Health Care Field, Arlington, VA, November 1987.

Thraenhart, O. 1990. Problems in virus testing. American Society for Microbiology. Proceedings of International Conference on Chemical Germicides, Atlanta, GA. (ASM Publications, Washington, D.C.)

Thurman, R.B., and Gerb, C.P. 1988. Characterization of the effect of aluminum metal on polio virus. J. Indust. Microbiol., *3*, 23–38.

Valenti, W.M., et al. 1980. Nosocomial viral infections. II. Guidelines for prevention and care of respiratory viruses, herpes virus and hepatitis virus. Infect. Control, *1*, 33–37.

Valenti, W.M., et al. 1980. Nosocomial viral infections. III. Guidelines for prevention and control of exanthemata, gastroenteritis, picornaviruses and uncommonly seen viruses. Infect. Control, *1*, 38–49.

Webb, S.F., and Vall-Spinosa, A. 1975. Outbreak of *Serratia marcescens* associated with flexible fiber bronchoscope. Chest, *68*, 708.

Wheeler, R.W., and Kaiser, A.B. 1987. Mycobacterial contamination of bronchoscopy specimens and possible pulmonary infection due to an inability to disinfect the suction valves of bronchoscopes. Abstract 27th Intersci. Conf. Antimicrob. Agents Chemother., *71*, 108.

Williams, T., and Leibowitz, M.J. 1987. Conservative mechanism of the in vitro transcription of killer virus of yeast. Virology, *158*, 231–237.

Xu, Z.J., and Chen, W.X. 1989. Viral haemorrhagic disease in rabbits: a review. Vet. Res. Commun., *13*, 205–212.

CHAPTER 26

MEASURES FOR DISINFECTION AND CONTROL OF VIRAL HEPATITIS

Olaf Thraenhart

Many viruses of various taxonomic virus groups can infect the liver of humans and cause hepatitis as a clinical entity, as shown in Table 26–1. Viruses that induce hepatitis as a cardinal symptom are the hepadnavirus group with the hepatitis B virus (HBV) and the hepatitis delta agent (HDV), the unclassified and not completely identified non-A, non-B (NANB) viruses with at least two virus groups of enterally (HEV) and parenterally (HCV) transmitted NANB viruses, and hepatitis A virus (HAV) of the picornavirus group.

Yellow fever (YF) of the flavivirus group, and cytomegalovirus (CMV) of the herpes virus group, also cause hepatitis as the cardinal symptom of these infections. In addition, other viruses such as other picornaviruses (Coxsackie and ECHO viruses), herpes viruses [herpes simplex (HSV), varicella zoster (VZV), and Epstein-Barr (EBV)] cause hepatitis as a secondary symptom.

In general, however, the term "viral hepatitis" refers to infections caused by at least five viruses, namely, HAV (previously called infectious or epidemic hepatitis), HBV (previously called serum hepatitis), HDV, which occurs only together with HBV, and NANB. Viral hepatitis is a major public-health problem occurring endemically in all parts of the world. Until now there seems to have been no decrease in the incidence of either enterally or parenterally transmitted viral hepatitis.

Table 26–1. *Viruses that Induce Hepatitis in Man*

Virus Group	Nucleic Acid	Virus Type	Cardinal Symptom	Secondary Symptom
Hepadna	DNA	HBV	+	−
(satellite)	RNA	HDV	+	−
Flavi	RNA	HCV	+	−
YF	RNA		+	−
(calici)	RNA	HEV ?	+	−
Picorna	RNA	HAV	+	−
		Coxsackie	−	+
		ECHO	−	+
Reo	RNA	Reo	−	+
Herpes	DNA	CMV	+	−
		HSV	−	+
		VZV	−	+
		EBV	−	+
Pox	DNA	Variola major	−	+

HBV = Hepatitis B virus; HDV = hepatitis D virus; HCV = hepatitis C virus, NANB = non-A, non-B; HEV = hepatitis E virus; HAV = hepatitis A virus; CMV = cytomegalovirus; HSV = herpes simplex virus; VZV = varicella zoster virus; EBV = Epstein-Barr virus; YF = yellow fever.

+ = hepatitis is the cardinal and/or secondary symptom

− = hepatitis is not the cardinal and/or secondary symptom

? = nucleic acid not yet known

In Table 26–2 the number of hepatitis cases reported by medical personnel to the German Federal Health Office, the Bundesgesundheitsamt, Berlin (Lange and Masihi, 1989), are shown as an example of the viral hepatitis situation in Germany. The table could lead one to the conclusion that in Germany the total number of viral hepatitis infections has diminished since 1981 because the absolute figures show a decrease from close to 20,000 cases in 1981 to under 10,000 cases in 1988. This reduction by 50% affected the numbers of HAV as well as HBV. The ratios between the numbers of HAV:HBV are stable, however, being 1:0.8 for the period 1981 to 1982, when the vaccination against HBV started, as well as 4 years later for the period 1986 to 1987. Constant ratios of 1:0.65 are estimated for the time periods 1981–1982:1986–1987 for HAV and HBV. Because it is unlikely that both groups of infections with completely different modes of transmission and possibility of prophylactic measurements decline at the same rate, Lange and Masihi (1989) concluded that the epidemiology of hepatitis did not change despite the introduction of a vaccination against HBV, but that the reporting of cases has decreased in recent years.

PATHOGENESIS

Acute viral hepatitis is a generalized infection, with emphasis on inflammation of the liver. The clinical picture of the infection varies in its presentation from asymptomatic or subclinical through mild gastrointestinal symptoms and the anicteric form of the disease to acute illness with jaundice, severe prolonged jaundice, and acute fulminant hepatitis.

Hepatitis B and coinfection with delta agent and NANB hepatitis may be associated with a persistent carrier state. These forms of infections may progress to chronic liver disease. Moreover, evidence indicates that hepatocellular carcinoma is associated with HBV.

HEPATITIS B VIRUS (HBV)

Characteristics

The HBV belongs to the virus family Hepadnaviridae (the hepatitis B-like viruses) (Gust et al., 1986).

Virions of HBV consist of a lipid-containing envelope (containing hepatitis B surface antigen [HBsAg]) surrounding a nucleocapsid (containing hepatitis B core antigen [HBcAg]). Virions are 42 nm in diameter (the Dane particle) and nucleocapsids are 18 nm; HBsAg particles are either 22 nm in diameter or filaments of different length. The genome consists of one molecule of DNA, which is circular, and mainly double-stranded, with a large, single-stranded gap; its size is 3.2 kilobase pair (kbp) when fully double-stranded. Virions have polypeptides making up the HBcAg and the hepatitis B e antigen (HBeAg).

DNA replication involves repair of the single-stranded gap, conversion to a supercoiled helix, and transcription to two classes of RNA, mRNA for protein synthesis and genomic DNA (Locarnini and Gust, 1988).

Pathology

Replication of HBV in hepatocytes takes place in the nucleus (with HBcAg accumulation); HBsAg production occurs in the cytoplasm in massive amounts. It is shed into the blood, producing antigenemia. Persistence is common and is associated with chronic disease and neoplasia.

The range of target cells of the human organism susceptible to HBV infection has been shown to be wider than initially predicted. In addition to hepatocytes, the viral genome is found in peripheral leukocytes of asymptomatic and sick chronic carriers either in free or integrated form (Pontisso et al., 1984; Shen et al., 1986; Yoffe et al., 1986). The frequency correlates to the presence of HBeAg in serum, representing replicative activity of the virus. The finding of HBV DNA in leukocytes is of importance because the peripheral blood mononuclear cells might transmit the infection even when virus production by hepatocytes has ceased (Locarnini and Gust, 1988).

Epidemiology, Transmission, and Control Measures

Although some other chains of infection in hepatitis B, such as horizontal and vertical transmission and intrafamiliar and sexual spread of the virus, have been established, the nosocomial cycle of the disease in the broader sense plays the major part in sustaining the virus within the populations of highly developed countries. According to Pantelick et al. (1981), 25% of the hepatitis cases within hospitals were acquired by contaminated instruments and/or human blood products, 21% after contact with infected patients, and 18% through needlestick accidents; in 36% of cases, the exact means of infection could not be determined.

Chronic or transient human virus carriers not suspected of carrying the virus are the basic reservoirs for transmission of HBV. As shown in Table 26–3, many body fluids of infected persons contain HBsAg, such as blood, ascites, liquor cerebrospinalis, and synovial fluid. HbsAg is also detected in many excretions such as urine, saliva, semen, breast milk, tears, and sweat, but not in feces. Infectious HBV, however, has been detected only in blood, semen, and saliva. The relative highest amount of infectious virus is present in the blood. Therefore, blood and blood products are acknowledged to be the main vehicle for HBV. Shikata, et al. (1977) showed that a serum positive for HBsAg and HBeAg could be diluted to 10^{-8} and still infect susceptible chimpanzees. Therefore, minimal blood spills may become sources of infection. Even when the blood has dried, it remains infective, as Bond et al. (1980) were able to show.

Saliva of some persons infected with HBV has been shown to contain HBV DNA at concentrations of 1:1000 to 1:10,000 of that found in the infected person's serum (Jenison et al., 1987). HBsAg-positive saliva was infectious when injected into experimental animals and after

Table 26–2. *Hepatitis Cases as Reported to the German Federal Health Office in Berlin*

Year	Total	Hepatitis A	(%)	Hepatitis B	(%)	Unclassified	(%)
1988	9,700	5500	56.7	3500	36.1	700	7.2
1987	11,312	5875	51.9	4444	39.3	993	8.8
1986	12,195	5897	48.4	5101	41.8	1197	9.8
1985	15,113	7276	48.1	6185	40.9	1652	10.9
1984	17,152	7886	46.0	7064	41.2	2202	12.8
1983	15,984	6496	40.0	7303	45.7	2185	13.7
1982	19,395	9065	46.7	7324	37.8	3006	15.5
1981	19,892	9181	46.2	7317	36.8	3393	17.0

From Lange, W., and Mahisi, K.N. 1989. Zur Morbidität der Hepatitis infectiosa. Bundesgesundheitsbl., *32*, 223–226.

Table 26–3. *Hepatitis B Surface Antigen (HBsAg) Contamination and Infectivity of Body Fluids and Human Secretions and Excretions Compared with Human Immunodeficiency Virus (HIV) Contamination*

Body Fluids	HBsAg	HBV	HIV
Blood, serum, plasma	+ + +	+ + +	+ + +
Ascites	+	?	?
Pleural fluid	+	?	?
Synovial fluid	+	?	?
Cerebrospinal fluid	+	?	+
Excretions			
Semen	+ + +	+ + +	+ + +
Vaginal fluid	+	+	+
Saliva	+	+	+
Urine	+	−	+
Nasopharyngeal washing	+	−	−
Feces	−	−	−
Breast milk	+	−	−
Tears	−	−	−
Sweat	±	−	−

+ + + = high concentration
+, ± = low concentration
− = not detected
? = not clear

human bite exposures (Cancio-Bello et al., 1982), although HBsAg-positive saliva has not been shown to be infectious when applied to oral mucous membranes in experimental primate studies.

There are great variations of the presence of HBV markers in different populations. Within an area differences exist in specific groups of the population. Szmuness et al. (1978) found a "north-south gradient" in so far as the carrier rate in the northern parts of Europe and in North America is estimated to be 0.1 to 0.5% of the population, whereas this rate is 1 to 3% in Mediterranean countries and in Central and South America. In northern Africa, the rate is 3 to 5%, but a rate of 6 to more than 10% is observed in Africa south of the equator and in Southeast Asia, especially in China, Taiwan, and the Philippines. The cumulative infection rates, which are calculated from the three HBV markers HBsAg, anti-HBs, and anti-HBc, vary between 7 and 12% in northern Europe and North America, but are as high as 60 to 90% in Africa, South America, and Southeast Asia. HBV in-

fections are acquired in the Northern Hemisphere mainly during the third to sixth decades of life, whereas in the Southern Hemisphere they are acquired particularly from birth to the second decade of life. It is not yet clear whether HBV infection is primarily a tropical illness introduced in the northern regions because of increasing travel and tourism.

In the Northern Hemisphere, transmission of HBV occurs mainly in situations where blood leaves the human body, as in the medical field and among drug addicts.

Moreover, emergency workers have an increased risk of hepatitis B infections. The degree of risk correlates with the frequency and extent of blood exposure when performing work-related activities.

In addition, HBV transmission in hospitals is related significantly to the extraordinary amounts of HBV-contaminated blood from patients who are staying in the hospital to be treated for hepatitis or other diseases. Unvaccinated personnel or patients without HBV anamnesis are especially at risk. These risks are highest in hemodialysis units, clinical and microbiologic laboratories, urologic clinics, surgeries, and psychiatric clinics (Kuwert, Scheiermann, and Thraenhart, 1982). A high positivity of HBV markers among the personnel of a central hospital kitchen and laundry unit may be due to the proportion of workers who are inhabitants of countries with endemic HBV.

In the United States, the total number of HBV infections was estimated in 1987 to be 300,000/yr, with approximately 57,000 (25%) infected persons developing acute hepatitis. Of these infected individuals, 18,000 to 30,000 (6 to 10%) will become HBV carriers, with the danger of developing chronic liver disease and infecting others. Moreover, 12,000 health-care workers whose jobs entail exposure to blood become infected with HBV each year; 500 to 600 of them are hospitalized, 700 to 1200 become HBV carriers, and approximately 250 die (Mullan et al., 1989).

Hepatitis B virus (HBV) transmission can occur inside and outside the medical field as follows:

1. Vertical transmission from the mother to the child by virus transfer via placenta or during the birth by oral aspiration of HBV-positive blood of the mother (direct contact).

2. Horizontal intrafamiliar transmission of HBV by intimate contact such as sexual intercourse, kissing (direct contact), or use of toothbrushes and toys (indirect contact).
3. Direct virus transfer by blood transfusion, organ transplantation, or blood products.
4. Direct percutaneous virus inoculation with a contaminated needle in connection with withdrawal of blood (needle-stick accident).
5. Percutaneous virus inoculation with sharp contaminated instruments from an infected to an uninfected person.
6. Percutaneous transfer of infective blood into minute cutaneous scratches, abrasions, burns, or other small lesions by skin-to-skin contact (direct contact) or by contaminated instruments or surfaces (indirect contact).
7. Contamination of mucosal surfaces by infective blood or infective fluids in connection with mouth pipetting, label licking, splashes, contact with instruments, or contact with contaminated environmental surfaces (indirect contact) or other means.

Mother-to-child transfer of HBV seems to be an important mode for HBV epidemiology and the induction of the chronic carrier status (Blumberg and Hesser, 1975). In comparison to areas with endemic HBV infections, such as Southeast Asia, because of the low carrier rate in adults, vertical transmission is of secondary importance in North America and Europe.

Risk factors for the transmission are hepatitis B surface and e antigens (HBsAg and HBeAg) in the serum of the mother. In contrast, detection of anti-HBeAg is an indicator of low probability of mother-to-child transfer of HBV. Vertical transmission was observed mainly when the mother acquired the HBV infection during the end of pregnancy, i.e., during the third trimester or shortly before birth (Schweitzer, 1975).

The infection rate is lower when the mother was a chronic HBsAg carrier before pregnancy or when she contracted the HBV infection in early pregnancy. Whether transplacental infection occurs by an active virus transfer through the placenta or by a passive transfer through an injury of the placenta is not known. Although HBsAg has been detected in breast milk, this mode of transfer is unlikely to occur (Beasley et al., 1975).

Prevention of vertical transmission of HBV is possible by screening of high-risk women (McQuillan et al., 1987), by active immunization of the population in endemic areas, or by passive immunization of newborns (Cossart and Cohen, 1976).

Within families, HBV transmission is of importance if a family member is an HBsAg chronic carrier also carrying HBeAg and DNA polymerase in the serum. The virus is predominantly transferred by the oral route, either directly by kissing or indirectly by several family members using the same toothbrush. Sexual intercourse may be another route of virus transfer. The mother seems to be the primary transmitter (Kashiwagi et al., 1984).

Active vaccination of the uninfected family members is the most appropriate control measure. If, however, vaccination is contraindicated because of some disease or a lack of response to the vaccine, hygienic measures and possibly the use of HBV-effective disinfectants should be considered.

Blood transfusion and organ transplantation had a high risk of direct HBV transmission in the medical environment before routine screening of blood. Now, donors of organs for transplantation are also screened for HBsAg as well as human immunodeficiency virus (HIV) and cytomegalovirus (CMV). Otherwise, approximately 10 to 15% of all viral hepatitis cases would be caused by blood transfusion by HBV (Aach and Kahn, 1980). Therefore, by far the most important task in preventing this kind of transmission is the reliable detection of HBV carriers among blood and organ donors and elimination of these persons from donation (Ranki et al., 1988). Semen donors should also be screened because Berry et al. (1987) observed transmission of HBV by artificial insemination.

Blood products such as factor VIII concentrates involve a considerable risk of transmission of HBV, as well as non-A, non-B (NANB) hepatitis. The risk has been reduced by heat treatment of these plasma derivatives (Hollinger et al., 1984; Mauler et al., 1987). Brackman and Egli (1988), however, found a residual HBV infectivity in heat-inactivated factor VIII concentrates. Another procedure for HBV inactivation is treatment with beta-propiolactone (Heinrich et al., 1987). Prince et al. (1983) were able to show that a combination of beta-propiolactone, Tween 20, and ultraviolet treatment was also effective in inactivation of HBV.

Testing for HBsAg is the favored method at present, but additional tests might be introduced for screening donated blood and organs in the future. For example, nucleic acid hybridization in serum gives a direct measure of the numbers of virions present and is thus a measure of the activity of the viral infection. Whereas the detection of HBsAg and DNA showed a 66 to 74% correlation, the figure for HBeAg and DNA was 83 to 100% (Liebermann et al., 1983; Scotto et al., 1983).

Recent studies have revealed that infectious HBV may be present in cases that would have been considered noninfectious by serologic criteria. Scotto et al. (1983) and Wu et al. (1986) found that 18 to 30% of anti-HBeAg-positive carriers were HBV-DNA positive. HBV DNA was also frequently present in patients suffering from HBsAg-negative chronic liver disease (Brechot et al., 1985).

The direct percutaneous needle stick is by far the most important mode of transmission. The probability of acquisition of HBV infection from an HBV-positive patient in connection with a needle-stick accident was estimated by Werner and Grady (1978) to be 19% and by Seef et al. (1978) to be 27%. Because today only disposable needles and syringes are used in the medical field in developed countries, this kind of transmission occurs mainly after the process of blood-taking from a patient by direct percutaneous inoculation into the body of medical personnel. Laboratory workers are also at risk, however, when blood samples are sent together with the contaminated needle to the laboratory.

In addition, blood contamination of a glass vial for a drug occurred, and 10 of 61 patients of a hemodialysis unit were infected when an HBsAg carrier prepared the drug for injection and pricked herself with a needle before drawing up the anesthetic (Alter et al., 1983).

Active and/or passive immunization of medical personnel is the method of preventing HBV transmission by needle sticks. In addition, in laboratories that receive samples with blood-contaminated needles, needles should be carefully discarded, and the probably contaminated tubes, etc., must be disinfected.

Percutaneous inoculation with sharp and HBV-contaminated instruments such as knives inside or outside the medical field, and tattooing instruments as well, may play a considerable part in the chain of HBV transmission (Kent et al., 1988; Slater et al., 1988). Decontamination of instruments by effective disinfection is a prerequisite for efficient protection against HBV transmission by this route.

No risk of iatrogenic transmission seems to exist through jet injectors or contact lenses, even if they are used on successive patients during initial testing for the correct size (Scheid et al., 1982).

It is difficult to evaluate the significance of percutaneous transfer of infective blood into minute cutaneous scratches, abrasions, burns, or other small lesions by skin-to-skin contact or contact with contaminated instruments or surfaces. The greatest risk may exist in clinical and microbiologic laboratories and in pathologic departments because of blood handling. Again, hygienic precautions and the use of HBV-effective disinfectants are mandatory.

The controversial dispute whether HBV can be transmitted by surfaces cannot be answered, but the regulation of the German Federal Health Office that makes disinfection mandatory in all clinical departments in which patients with immunosuppression are located or from which infections may be spread seems to be a useful precaution (Bundesgesundheitsamt Berlin, 1976).

As mentioned previously, in clinical and microbiologic laboratories, pathologic departments, and all other departments where floors may become contaminated by blood, even in the smallest amounts, disinfection of table tops as well as floors is a necessity for prevention of transmission of HBV as well as other infectious agents. In the past, when no hepatitis B vaccination was available, these procedures together with general hygienic precautions, of which wearing gloves seems to be the most important, led to the protection of personnel in a virologic laboratory. In contrast, clinical laboratories, in which personnel were not aware of the risk of contracting an HBV infection, had a high incidence of this disease. Contamination of mucosal surfaces such as nose, mouth, and eyes by infective blood or infective fluids

may occur in connection with mouth pipetting, label licking, and splashes, especially in laboratories. The mode of transmission by a splash into the eye has been demonstrated (Bond et al., 1980). Favero et al. (1986) stress that direct droplet contact may also occur by centrifuge accidents or on removal of rubber stoppers from tubes. Hygienic precautions and guidelines for prevention of infections in laboratories should be followed because virus disinfection cannot prevent this kind of transmission.

Mucosal surfaces, such as nose, mouth, and eye, but also internal mucosal surfaces, such as the gastrointestinal, urogenital, or respiratory tracts, come in contact with various instruments in the medical field, e.g., endoscopes, tonometers, etc. Bond and Moncada (1978), Morris et al. (1975), Massarrat and Schiff (1975), and Birnie et al. (1983) showed that transmission via endoscopes is possible. That only few cases have been observed by this route (Villa et al., 1984) may be due to the longstanding practice of intensive cleaning and disinfection of these instruments.

Airborne HBV transmission has been suggested, but does not seem to exist (Petersen et al., 1979).

There is no fecal-oral transmission of HBV because of an inhibitor in human feces and intestinal mucosa (Piazza et al., 1973). According to Favero et al. (1986), however, HBV-contaminated materials can initiate infection when they enter the mouth. In this case, the HBV must enter the host's vascular system via the mucosal surface of the mouth and not the intestine and could be grouped in the previously mentioned second mode of transmission, i.e., percutaneous transfer.

Indirect virus transfer by pharmaceutically processed blood or constituents of the human body that may contain HBV, such as plasma fractions or dura mater, are no longer observed because various procedures of HBV inactivation by physical and/or chemical means have been taken in the manufacture.

"Multimodal Network" of Control of HBV in Hospitals

To reduce nosocomial hepatitis B virus (HBV) infection, it is necessary to take different control precautions aimed at inanimate vectors, blood and organ donation, blood products, medical personnel, and patients.

Sterilization and disinfection of instruments, laundry, and environmental surfaces are aimed at the control of inanimate vectors. General hygiene precautions and disinfection of hands should be observed by medical personnel and patients. Screening of blood and organ donors for HBV markers has proved to be most efficient for the control of the otherwise uncontrollable chain of infection. Active and passive immunization of medical personnel has led to the reduction of the risk of HBV infection, especially by needle-stick accidents.

Recommendations for Inactivation of HBV in the Laboratory

Favero et al. (1986) stress the primary overall strategy of preventing viral hepatitis by consistent observance of

Table 26–4. *Multi-modal Network for the Control of Nosocomial HBV Infections*

	Environmental Vectors	Blood and Organ Donation	Blood Products	Personnel	Patients
General hygienic measure	+ +			+ +	+
Decontamination					
Thermal sterilization	+ +[1]		+ +		
Chemical disinfection	+ +[2]		+ +	+ +[3]	+
Screening for HBV-markers		+ + +	+ + +	+ +	+
Immunization				+ +	+

[1]Thermo resistant instruments

[2]Instruments

  Laundry

[3]Environmental surfaces

  Hands

blood precautions, which are necessary not only in microbiologic laboratories, but also in any laboratory that investigates blood samples from human beings. Such precautions involve the observance of the general hygienic guidelines practiced routinely in laboratories and the use of only high- and intermediate-level disinfectants. These guidelines, drawn up by Favero et al. (1986), are shown in Table 26–5.

Official Guidelines for Sterilization and Disinfection of HBV in Prehospital Health Care of the United States Centers for Disease Control

Table 26–6 summarizes the guidelines for reprocessing methods for the equipment used in prehospital health care, set up by the United States Department of Health and Human Services Public Health Service, Centers for Disease Control (Mullan et al., 1989). According to these guidelines, sterilization has the highest priority for decontaminating instruments or devices that penetrate skin or contact normally sterile areas of the body. High-level disinfectant should be used for any reusable instruments or devices that come in contact with mucous membranes, such as endoscopes. Intermediate-level disinfectant is recommended for surfaces that come in contact only with the skin and have been visibly contaminated with blood or bloody body fluids. In these cases, surfaces must be precleaned.

For handwashing, the CDC recommends washing with warm water and soap. Only when handwashing facilities are not available should a waterless antiseptic hand cleanser be used. Spills of blood should be promptly decontaminated using a United States Environmental Protection Agency (EPA)-approved germicide or a 1:100 solution of household bleach while one is wearing gloves.

Laundry should be washed normally according to washing machine and detergent manufacturers' recommendations.

With regard to the guideline concerning hand washing, the high resistance of HBV to different pH values should be considered. It is recommended to disinfect the hands with an HBV-effective germicide and then wash them with water and soap. Otherwise, hands can

be rubbed with a disinfectant prepared for this use. In every case, only an HBV-effective germicide should be used.

Official Recommendations for Sterilization and Disinfection of HBV of the German Federal Health Office

For the prevention and control of hospital infections, one must use the disinfectants and disinfection procedures that are active against viruses according to the list of tested and accepted disinfectants and disinfection procedures (Bundesgesundheitsamt Berlin, 1987).

Official recommendations for sterilization and disinfection for viral hepatitis have been revised by the German Federal Health Office (Bundesgesundheitsamt Berlin, 1988). This list includes thermal treatment, such as boiling in water with addition of 0.5% soda, incineration, and water steam disinfection. Further, chemical germicides that are listed as virucidal germicides include chlorine, aldehydes, and halogens. The combination of chemical and physical treatment consists of chemical treatment in conjunction with elevated temperatures. Various manufacturers have developed different procedures.

Special procedures have been developed for the disinfection of laundry in washing machines where the laundry is washed and decontaminated for 15 min at +85°C or 10 min at +90°C.

A combination of chemical-thermal treatment would consist of using aldehyde-containing germicides for 15 min at +50°C or chlorine-containing germicides for 10 min at +60°C. Disinfection procedures for instruments have been elaborated by the manufacturers of washing machines. The "System Miele" (Firma Miele, Gütersloh, Germany) consists of disinfection for 10 min at +93°C in the Miele washing machine with a disinfectant.

Importance of Disinfection in Controlling HBV Infections

Hepatitis B virus (HBV) is an important cause of nosocomial infections. The direct transmission of HBV, the primary source of HBV infections, cannot be combated

Table 26–5. *Some Physical and Chemical Methods for Inactivating Hepatitis B Virus (HBV)[a]*

Class	Concentration or Level	Activity
Sterilization		
Heat		
Moist heat (steam under pressure)	250°F (121°C), 15 min	
	Prevacuum cycle, 270°F (132°C), 5 min	
Dry heat	170°C, 1 hr	
	160°C, 2 hrs	
	121°C, 16 hrs or longer	
Gas		
Ethylene oxide	450–500 mg/L, 55–60°C	
Liquid[b]		
Glutaraldehyde, aqueous	2%	
Hydrogen peroxide, stabilized	6–10%	
Formaldehyde, aqueous	8–12%	
Disinfection		
Heat		
Moist heat	100°C	High
Liquid		
Glutaraldehyde, aqueous[c]	Variable	High
Hydrogen peroxide, stabilized	6–10%	High
Formaldehyde, aqueous[d]	3–8%	Intermediate to high
Iodophors[e]	30–50 mg/L free iodine;	Intermediate
	70–150 mg/L available iodine	
Chlorine compounds[f]	50–500 mg/L free available chlorine	Intermediate

[a]Comment. Adequate precleaning of surfaces is the first prerequisite for any disinfection or sterilization procedure. The longer the exposure to a physical or chemical agent, the more likely it is that all pertinent microorganisms will be eliminated. Ten minutes of exposure may not be adequate to disinfect many objects, especially those that are difficult to clean because of narrow channels or other areas that can harbor organic material as well as microorganisms; thus, longer exposure times, i.e., 20 to 30 min, may be necessary. This is especially true when high-level disinfection is to be achieved. Although alcohols (e.g., isopropanol) have been shown to be effective in killing HBV, we do not recommend that they be used generally for this purpose because of their rapid evaporation and the consequent difficulty in maintaining proper contact times.

[b]This list of chemical germicides contains generic formulations. Other commercially available formulations can also be considered for use. Users should ensure that the formulations are registered with the United States Environmental Protection Agency. Information in the scientific literature or presented at symposia or scientific meetings can also be considered in determining the suitability of certain formulations.

[c]Several glutaraldehyde-based proprietary formulations are on the market in the United States, i.e., low-, neutral-, or high-pH formulations recommended for use at normal or elevated temperatures with or without ultrasonic energy and also a formulation containing 2% glutaraldehyde and 7% phenol. The manufacturer's instructions regarding use as a sterilant or disinfectant or anticipated dilution use should be closely followed.

[d]Because of the continuing controversy over the role of formaldehyde as a potential occupational carcinogen, the use of formaldehyde is recommended only in limited circumstances under carefully controlled conditions, i.e., disinfection of certain hemodialysis equipment.

[e]Only those iodophors registered with the Environmental Protection Agency as hard-surface disinfectants should be used, and the manufacturer's instructions regarding proper use, dilution, and product stability should be closely followed. Iodophors formulated as antiseptics are not suitable for use as disinfectants.

[f]There currently is a chlorine dioxide formulation registered with the Environmental Protection Agency as a sterilant and disinfectant (depending on contact time). The manufacturer's instructions regarding its use as a sterilant or disinfectant or anticipated dilution during use should be closely followed. An inexpensive, broad-spectrum disinfectant for use on table tops and similar surfaces can be prepared by diluting common household bleach (5.25% sodium hypochlorite) to obtain at least 500 ppm free available chlorine (e.g., ¼ c bleach/gal tap water). This dilution should be freshly made each day, and caution should be taken because chlorine compounds may corrode metals, especially aluminum.

From Favero, M.S., Petersen, N.J. and Bond, W.W. 1986. Transmission and control of laboratory-acquired hepatitis infection. In *Laboratory Safety: Principles and Practices*. Edited by B.M. Miller, et al. Washington, D.C., American Society for Microbiology, pp. 49–58.

by disinfection procedures, but situations do exist in the medical field where disinfection procedures are able to break some chains of HBV transmission.

Moreover, the necessity of carrying out disinfection against HBV remains even after the introduction of active immunization against hepatitis B. Certainly, the risk of contracting a hepatitis B infection for medical personnel or patients undergoing long-term hemodialysis is minimized when they receive complete active immunization against HBV. All patients with a defective immune system or patients undergoing immunosuppressive therapy

still have a high infection risk, however, because they cannot be vaccinated or they would not be able to induce a sufficient immune response to a vaccination against HBV (Scheiermann and Kuwert, 1984).

Because more and more hospital patients in the Northern Hemisphere suffer from tumors, various immunologic diseases, including AIDS, or burns, or undergo severe operations, which in themselves suppress immunity, or are treated with immunosuppressive drugs, especially after bone marrow or organ transplantation, the problem of the care of immunocompromised patients

Table 26–6. *Reprocessing Methods for Equipment Used in the Prehospital* Health-Care Setting for Decontamination of HBV*

Sterilization:	Destroys:	All forms of microbial life including high numbers of bacterial spores
	Methods:	Steam under pressure (autoclave), gas (ethylene oxide), dry heat, or immersion in Environmental Protection Agency (EPA)-approved chemical "sterilant" for prolonged period of time, e.g., 6–10 hrs or according to manufacturers' instructions; note: liquid chemical "sterilants" should be used only on those instruments that are impossible to sterilize or disinfect with heat
	Use:	For those instruments or devices that penetrate skin or contact normally sterile areas of the body, e.g., scalpels, needles, etc.; disposable invasive equipment eliminates the need to reprocess these types of items; when indicated, however, arrangements should be made with a health-care facility for reprocessing of reusable invasive instruments
High-Level Disinfection:	Destroys:	All forms of microbial life except high numbers of bacterial spores
	Methods:	Hot-water pasteurization (80–100°C, 30 min) or exposure to an EPA-registered "sterilant" chemical as above, except for a short exposure time (10–45 min or as directed by the manufacturer)
	Use:	For reusable instruments or devices that come into contact with mucous membranes (e.g., laryngoscope blades, endotracheal tubes, etc.)
Intermediate-Level Disinfection:	Destroys:	*Mycobacterium tuberculosis*, vegetative bacteria, most viruses, and most fungi, but not bacterial spores
	Methods:	EPA-registered "hospital disinfectant" chemical germicides that have a label claim for tuberculocidal activity; commercially available hard-surface germicides or solutions containing at least 500 ppm free available chlorine (a 1:100 dilution of common household bleach, approximately ¼ c bleach/gal tap water)
	Use:	For those surfaces that come into contact only with intact skin, e.g., stethoscopes, blood pressure cuffs, splints, etc., and have been visibly contaminated with blood or bloody body fluids. Surfaces must be precleaned of visible material before the germicidal chemical is applied for disinfection
Low-Level Disinfection:	Destroys:	Most bacteria, some viruses, some fungi, but not *Mycobacterium tuberculosis* or bacterial spores
	Methods:	EPA-registered "hospital disinfectants" (no label claim for tuberculocidal activity)
	Use:	These agents are excellent cleaners and can be used for routine housekeeping or removal of soil in the absence of visible blood contamination
Environmental Disinfection:		Environmental surfaces that have become soiled should be cleaned and disinfected using any cleaner or disinfectant agent intended for environmental use. Such surfaces include floors, woodwork, ambulance seats, countertops, etc.
IMPORTANT:		To ensure the effectiveness of any sterilization or disinfection process, equipment and instruments must first be thoroughly cleaned of all visible soil

*Defined as setting where delivery of emergency health-care takes place prior to arrival at hospital or other health-care facility.
From Mullan, R.J., et al. 1989. Guidelines for prevention of transmission of human immunodeficiency virus and hepatitis B virus to health-care and public-safety workers. MMWR, *38*.

is difficult and growing. These patients can only be protected against infections, including HBV, by disinfection procedures.

According to the German guidelines for the prevention and control of nosocomial infection (Bundesgesundheitsamt Berlin, 1976), disinfection is mandatory in departments of hospitals in which immunosuppressed patients are staying or from which infectious agents can be spread to other departments. Instruments, hands, skin, bed linen, floors, and table surfaces have to be disinfected.

In connection with the aim of reducing nosocomial HBV infections, disinfectants should be judged by their ability to inactivate HBV (Kuwert and Thraenhart, 1977). Moreover, decontamination of HBV should include all the previously mentioned surfaces even if there is only a slight chance that they may be contaminated. Only the entirety of the disinfection procedure guarantees the full protection of the patient (Kuwert, Thraenhart, Dermietzel, and Scheiermann, 1982).

Since the occurrence of AIDS, the importance of disinfectants and disinfection procedures against HBV has increased because the human immunodeficiency virus (HIV) is excreted from nearly the same body fluids as HBV (see Table 26–3), and the World Health Organization (WHO) (1989) recommends the use of HBV-effective disinfectants.

In conclusion, the control of germicidal activity against HBV is of high priority. HBV infection is a significant nosocomial infection, and disinfection procedures recommended for the inactivation of HBV are approved for HIV disinfection.

Methods for the Control of HBV-Virucidal Activity of Disinfectants

The principles of tests for investigation of virucidal activity in Germany are the basis for the development of such tests and assessment of the results. The virucidal activity of a disinfectant as determined in Germany and some other European countries is carried out according to a guideline prepared by the German Federal Health Office (BGA) and the German Society Against Virus Diseases (DVV) (Kuwert et al., 1982). These guidelines contain some essentials that may be summarized here.

Virus disinfection is the inactivation of the infectivity of the complete virus particle by a disinfectant. The inactivation of the infectivity has to be measured quantitatively. The inactivation has to be followed kinetically; i.e., the infectivity of a virus suspension has to be tested with every concentration of a disinfectant for at least three exposure times. The choice of exposure time depends on the anticipated use of the germicide. Disinfectants for instruments or surfaces are tested for exposure times of 0, 15, 30, and 60 min; those for skin or hands are tested for 0, ½, 1, 2, and 5 min.

All tests are suspension tests; i.e., a virus suspension is mixed with the disinfectant. Carrier tests are not yet included because of difficulties in standardizing such tests and making them reproducible (Kuwert and Spicher, 1982).

The suspension tests are carried out with three protein concentrations in comparison to measure the influence of unspecific protein load on the activity of the germicide. The protein loads are 10% fetal calf serum (approximately 13 to 23 mg protein/ml suspension), 0.2% bovine serum albumin (approximately 8 to 15 mg protein/ml suspension). One test set is carried out without addition of protein solution (<0.1 mg protein/ml suspension). For the control of the test system, the inactivation kinetic of a 0.7% (w/v) formaldehyde solution is followed in parallel.

Virucidal activity of a disinfectant is assumed if, after a given exposure time, inactivation of at least 99.99% (reduction of median infective dose [ID_{50}] $\geq 10^4$) of the infectivity of the four test viruses with the three protein loads can be proved.

Virus inactivation by any disinfectant has to be tested against four test viruses, selected on the basis of representative structures and elevated resistance to chemical reagents. Moreover, test viruses were chosen to represent important agents in human medicine. Along this line, it was decided to favor poliovirus type 1, wild-type strain, adenovirus, papovavirus SV-40, and vaccinia virus. According to Kuwert et al. (1982), it seems to be unnecessary and impracticable to test the virucidal activity of all viruses for which a manufacturer claims the virucidal activity of a germicide. Thus, this joint BGA/DVV guideline constitutes the minimal requirements. This means that other tests can be performed in addition, but a certificate stating the virucidal activity of a disinfectant is issued by the DVV if the minimal requirements are fulfilled.

Because disinfection with proved hepatovirucidal disinfectants definitely plays a major role in the interruption of the chain of HBV infection, the HBV virucidal activity of disinfectants for use against HBV has to be tested. The HBV virucidal effect, however, i.e., the inactivation of the HBV by a disinfectant, can so far only be determined in vivo by the chimpanzee infection assay. However, animal protection prohibits the use of primates for routine tests on commercial products.

Attempts to Establish an Infectivity Test in Tissue Culture. The standardization of an infectivity assay for measuring the inactivation of the infectivity of HBV in a tissue culture system would be optimal for the HBV testing of germicides.

Conditions for a HBV infectivity assay can be defined as follows:

1. Use of infectious complete HBV particles for the reaction with the germicide;
2. Replication of HBV to high concentrations of infectious HBV to perform the virus testing;
3. Availability of a highly susceptible cell line to measure the residual infectivity;
4. Quantification of the infectivity;
5. Reproducibility of titrations; and
6. Practical assay for measuring the residual infectivity.

Many groups tried to multiplicate HBV in tissue culture cells. These studies are especially undertaken with human hepatomo cell line (HepG2) (Bchini et al., 1990; Roingeard et al., 1990; Loncarevic et al., 1990); or in a primate kidney cell line (Takeshima et al., 1989). The results, however, show that the attempts to infect tissue culture cells with the complete HBV failed up to now. The following conclusions can be drawn:

1. HepG2 cells cannot be infected with complete infectious Dane particles (DP);
2. Only a transfection of HepG2 cells with HBV-DNA is successful;
3. After HBV-DNA transfection of HepG2 cells a transient production of a low amount of complete HBV occurs. This virus is infectious in chimpanzees;
4. The main proportion of replicated material after HBV-DNA transfection, however, are HBV nucleocapsids.
5. The production of infectious HBV is so low that it is easier to screen patients for Dane particles in their blood than to prepare virus preparations from DNA transfected HepG2 cells.
6. Bchini et al. (1990) found only a marginal signal and no tests for demonstration of complete HBV were given;
7. Moreover, no quantitative data are presented in this publication.

According to these results, the prerequisites for a HBV infectivity assay in tissue cultures for testing of germicides are still not fulfilled:

1. No infectious complete HBV virus can infect HepG2 cells;
2. No high concentrations of virus can be produced;
3. No quantitative titrations are possible to perform;
4. No data on reproducibility are available;
5. Determination of antigens in the cells were shown. However, these antigens may be HBs-antigen which were taken into cells, when a large amount of HBs-antigen is inoculated onto tissue culture cells.

HBV-Virucidal Activity of Chemical Disinfectants or Physical Insults as Measured in the Chimpanzee. Chimpanzee experiments were performed to prove the resistance of HBV. Determination of the efficiency of thermal treatment (Shikata et al., 1978) and testing of the effect of formaldehyde on the infectivity of HBV have been carried out by several groups (Stephan and Prince, 1982; Hollinger et al., 1982; Tabor and Gerity, 1982; Thraenhart et al., 1982). The results are shown in Table 26–7, which shows that a considerable resistance of the HBV to chemical compounds and thermal treatment was demonstrated. Bond et al. (1981, 1983) were able to show that, even in dried human HBV-positive plasma, HBV was still infectious after resuspending the HBV suspension for chimpanzees.

This resistance may to some extent be due to the preparation of the different virus suspensions, i.e., purification and concentration of infectivity. However, that only 99.9% of the infectivity of a partly purified and concentrated HBV suspension without serum or other proteins was inactivated after 1 hr at +20°C indicates a resistance to formaldehyde equal to that of poliovirus in this experiment (Thraenhart et al., 1982).

In conclusion, HBV seems to be a relatively resistant virus. Favero et al. (1986) classified the resistance of HBV somewhat above tuberculosis bacteria but below bacterial spores.

Methods for Testing Other Than HBV Virucidal Effects of Chemical Disinfectants or Physical Insults.

Chimpanzee experiments are hardly suitable for elaboration of quantitative and kinetic aspects of hepatitis B virus (HBV) disinfection.

We had to overcome the dilemma that, on the one hand, a simple animal model or tissue-culture method was not and in 1991 is still not available for the investigation of HBV infectivity and, on the other hand, a test for the investigation of disinfectants for their HBV ac-

tivity was urgently needed. Stephan (1989) found that bacteriophages were inactivated during the process of preparation of plasma and plasma derivates with beta-propiolactone and ultraviolet irradiation. In earlier studies, inactivation of HBV infectivity was observed in the chimpanzee (Stephan et al., 1988). From these results the authors discuss the possibility of using bacteriophages for tests for HBV virucidal activity. According to Spicher (personal communication), however, no analogy of inactivation of animal and human viruses and bacteriophages appears to exist in light of his experiments (unpublished results). Therefore, the German Society for Hygiene and Microbiology and the German Society against Virus Diseases (DVV) does not recommend any tests with bacteriophages for determining the virucidal activity of a disinfectant. This decision is in accord with other European organizations. The Association Francaise de Normalisation (AFNOR) abolished the use of bacteriophages for virucidal label claim, and introduced standard tests on the basis of animal viruses (polio, adeno, orthopox), suspension test, and evaluation of the inactivation kinetic instead (AFNOR, 1989). These are very similar to the German BGA/DVV guidelines (Kuwert et al., 1982). Alternative methods using HBV have been developed. These methods do not measure the infectivity, but other markers that should be correlated with the infectivity as far as possible.

The following parameters that are under consideration (Deinhardt et al., 1983) are discussed in the inverse sequence of accumulated experience: (1) biologic integrity of the HBV DNA; (2) enzymatic activity of the HBV DNA polymerase; (3) antigenic reactivity of the virus particles or the structural antigens (HBsAg, HBcAg, HBeAg); and (4) physical integrity of the infectious HBV virus particle.

Table 26–7. *Inactivation of Hepatitis B Virus (HBV) Infectivity as Measured with the Chimpanzee Test*

Tested Procedure		Results and Remarks	Reference
10 hrs +60°C		Partial inactivation	Soulier et al., 1972
10 hrs +60°C		Complete inactivation* (>1000 ID$_{50}$/ml)	Tabor and Gerity, 1982
0.7% (w/v) Formaldehyde	1 hr +20°C	Partial inactivation (99.9%)	Thraenhart et al., 1982
5% (succinic dialdehyde) Gigasept	1 hr +20°C	Complete inactivation (>10^9 ID$_{50}$/ml)†	"
Beta-propiolactone/UV treatment for preparation of blood derivates		Complete inactivation	Stephan and Prince, 1982
Formalin 1:4000	72 hrs +37°C	Complete inactivation (10^5 ID$_{50}$/ml)	Tabor and Gerity, 1982
Sodium hypochlorite	10 min +20°C	Complete inactivation (10^6 ID$_{50}$/doses) of dried and resuspended HBV-positive plasma	Bond, et al. 1983
500 mg Free Cl$_2$	10 min +20°C	"	"
Glutardialdehyde 2% (w/v)	10 min +20°C	"	"
Glutardialdehyde + phenol	10 min +20°C	"	"
Isopropylalcohol 70%	10 min +20°C	"	"
Aldehyde mixture (Kohrsolin 3%)	60 min +20°C	Complete inactivation	Howard et al., 1983
Alcohol mixture (Sterillium 99%)	5 min +20°C	"	"

*No HBV infection of chimpanzee after inoculation of the material

†Estimation of HBV concentration is based on the regression of the dose-response relationship of ID$_{50}$ and first appearance of HBsAg in the blood of the inoculated chimpanzee.

Biologic Integrity of HBV DNA. HBV DNA can be detected by the spot hybridization test with 10 to 100 μl serum. The sensitivity of the technique allows the detection of 10^4 target DNA molecules (Krogsgaard et al., 1986). The destruction of the HBV genome should lead to the loss of infectivity, but no results have been published that prove that the method is not unspecifically influenced by the various compounds of a disinfectant.

Enzymatic Activity of HBV DNA Polymerase. A considerable reduction of HBV DNA polymerase was determined after reaction of HBV with pure chemicals such as sodium hypochlorite, 20% diethyl ether, and 70% ethyl alcohol. Thermal treatment of HBV at $+60°C$ also resulted in a significant decrease of the activity of DNA polymerase (Nath and Fang, 1982).

Sherertz et al. (1986), however, found that although DNA polymerase was negative after simulating electrodesiccation with reusable needle electrodes, complete HBV particles were still found in the electron microscope.

Moreover, the method of determination of the DNA polymerase seems to be extremely dependent on the conditions of the reaction and may therefore not be suitable for testing disinfectants (Siegert, 1982). It is also not yet clear whether the DNA polymerase is an essential marker for the infectivity, because Will et al. (1982) were able to infect chimpanzees with HBV DNA without DNA polymerase.

Antigenic Reactivity of Structural Antigens. Proteins of the HBV surface (HbsAg) or of the inner part (HBcAg, HBeAg) may influence the adsorption of the virus to susceptible cells or may take part in the infection process. Tests measuring the antigenicity of the structural antigens (HBsAg, HBcAg, HBeAg) therefore offer a simple procedure to follow the change of the antigen concentration during the reaction of these antigens and the germicide (Frösner et al., 1982).

Exposure of HBsAg particles under conditions generally effective for HBV inactivation, however, has little effect on the antigenicity of HBsAg (Skelly et al., 1981). There is also the question whether the decrease of the antigenicity is correlated with the inactivation of HBV infectivity. Moreover, it is uncertain whether test results obtained with noninfectious virion-free HBV proteins can be transferred to the condition of the complete infectious HBV, because physical and biochemical differences exist. Moreover, reduction of antigenicity of a virion-free and thereby noninfectious antigen suspension, e.g., HBV vaccines, with HBsAg or test kits containing any HB antigen, and possibly treated for HBV inactivation, are not consistent with the principles of testing the virucidal activity of disinfectants: inactivation of infectivity cannot be tested with separate virus proteins, antigens, or genomes, but only with complete virus particles.

In an HBV-containing suspension such as serum, however, the antigen is the quantitatively dominating particle. Even in an HBV suspension that is partly purified and concentrated by ultracentrifugation, HBsAg contaminates the fraction with HBV (Thraenhart et al., 1982). Therefore, it is impossible to associate an antigen loss of HBsAg solely with the HBV.

When such partly purified and concentrated HBV suspensions after reaction with a germicide are subjected to another rate zonal ultracentrifugation (see the method of the morphologic alteration and disintegration test [MADT] later in this chapter), HBsAg was detected in fractions of lower density than that of HBV. Table 26–8 shows that HBsAg in the mean virus-containing fraction was 121 and 91% after treatment with aldehydes in comparison to the untreated virus control. The infectivity of these suspensions was, however, $10^{6.5}$ chimpanzee infectious units (ID50) and $<10^{1.0}$ in the aldehyde-treated preparations in comparison to $10^{9.5}$ in the control (Thraenhart et al., 1982).

In another chimpanzee experiment, complete reduc-

Table 26–8. *Comparison of Infectivity, Hepatitis B Surface Antigen (HBsAg), and Physical Integrity of a Hepatitis B Virus (HBV) Suspension Partly Purified and Concentrated by Ultracentrifugation (Fraction with 38–42% Sucrose) in a Chimpanzee Experiment Treated with 0.7% (w/w) Formaldehyde (b), or 5% Succinic Dialdehyde Solution (c), in Comparison with the Untreated Virus Control (a)*

| | Infectivity (Chimpanzee) | | Physical Integrity (MADT) | | | | HBs Antigenicity (AUS-RIA) Sum of HBsAg in* | | | |
| | | | | | | | All Fractions † | | DP Containing ‡ Fractions | |
Reagent	ID_{50} ($-log_{10}$)§	% Inactivation	Alteration Phases	% Alteration	% Disintegration	% HBV-Destruction	CPM	%	CPM	%
a	9.5	0	0,1	<10	0	<10	13,900	100	4,740	100
b	6.5	99.9	1,2	20	50	60	18,200	131	5,731	121
c	<1.0	>99.99	2,3	>99	80	>99.98	19,190	138	4,319	91

*The partly purified and concentrated HBV suspensions used for the infectivity and morphologic alteration and disintegration test (MADT) control were subjected to another rate zonal ultracentrifugation.

†Sum of CPM in all fractions after rate zonal ultracentrifugation.

‡CPM of the fraction with maximal number of DP of the virus control.

§Estimation of HBV concentration is based on the regression of the dose-response relationship of ID_{50} and first appearance of HBsAg in the blood of the inoculated chimpanzee.

tion (17 ng/ml) of HBsAg without any loss of infectivity for four chimpanzees was demonstrated during the purification of factor VIII concentrates. Only after an additional step of inactivation was it impossible to demonstrate either HBsAg or infectivity (Hilfenhaus and Weidmann, 1986). It seems, therefore, that the test for HBs antigenicity reduction is not a reliable method.

Physical Integrity of the Infectious HBV Virus Particle. In analogy to Leuwenhook, who tested the change of the structure of bacteria after reaction with germicides under an optical microscope (Block, 1987), the morphologic alteration and disintegration of the HBV virion after reaction with a disinfectant can be determined under an electron microscope. This "morphologic alteration and disintegration test," the MADT, has been standardized after investigation of more than 100 different disinfectants, chemical compounds, and various physical inactivation procedures, such as heat or ultrasonic treatment (Thraenhart et al., 1978).

Furthermore, the hypothesis of the MADT, i.e., that the physical destruction of the virus particle is correlated with the inactivation of the infectivity, was proved in a chimpanzee experiment (Thraenhart et al., 1982; Kuwert, Thraenhart, Dermietzel, and Scheiermann, 1982).

Similar and stereotype alterations of the HBV virions were detected independently of the type of reagent or disinfection procedure reacting on the HBV, as presented in Figure 26–1. The intact Dane particle (DP) [alteration phase (AP) 0] is altered from a change in the outer membrane of the virion (AP 1) to the alteration of outer and inner structures of the virion, which are still visible (AP 2), however, with increasing concentration of a germicide or prolongation of the exposure time. Before the ultimate disintegration of the DP, the virion appears as a polygonal particle without any substructures and a diameter of less than 40 nm (AP 3). It was therefore possible to characterize three different alteration phases (AP) of the virions, as schematically represented in Figure 26–2.

By enumeration of the ratio of intact to altered DP as a function of the exposure time, kinetic curves show graphically the increase of alteration and disintegration of intact DP by germicides. These kinds of dose-response curves are similar to those for inactivation of infectivity.

In analogy to virus inactivation, the term "HBV-destroying activity," which can be calculated from the ratio of the remaining intact DP fraction (see the following method of the MADT), was introduced to make clear that the change of the physical appearance and disintegration of the DP under the electron microscope may not reflect the inactivation of infectivity in every case. Drees (1966) suggested, however, that those disinfectants that induce physical disintegration of the virus particles seem to be ideal germicides. Situations where inactivation of infectivity occurs without any morphologic alteration cannot be excluded. The reverse, however, conservation of infectivity after virion disintegration, seems to be highly improbable.

From the result of the chimpanzee experiment, it was possible to conclude that, by inoculation of an untreated HBV suspension with 100% intact DP, a more active HBV infection was induced than by inoculation of an HBV suspension containing only 40% intact DP with a partial inactivation of infectivity of >99.9%. With an HBV suspension in which no intact DP was detected after intense searching (<0.1% intact DP), no HBV infection was induced (inactivation of infectivity of >99.99%) (Table 26–8). The demonstration of intact DP is therefore an indicator of infectivity.

From the results of the infectivity experiment, the following minimal requirements were defined for assessing that a certain concentration of a disinfectant and a defined exposure time have an effective HBV-destroying activity. The mixture of disinfectant and HBV suspension may contain after the reaction:

1. No intact HBV particles after intense searching and 80% or more disintegration of HBV particles for germicides to be used in HBV-risk areas.
2. No intact HBV particles after intense searching and less than 80% disintegration of HBV particles for germicides to be used for HBV prophylaxis.

The method for the morphologic alteration and disintegration test (MADT) (Thraenhart et al., 1982; Kuwert, Thraenhart, Dermietzel, and Scheiermann, 1982) is as follows: For conducting the MADT, HBV rich fractions are concentrated and partly purified from serum or plasma of HBsAg, HBeAg, and Dane particle positive patients. This is done in 2 steps: 9 ml of the serum diluted 1:2 is layered onto a 2 ml gradient of sucrose (1 ml of 10 and 20% sucrose) in tubes of the rotor 50 Ti. HBV and HBsAg is "trapped" (McNaughton and Mathews, 1971) under the sucrose after ultracentrifugation at 40000 rpm at +10°C for 2 hrs in a H L8-70 centrifuge (Beckman Instruments, Palo Alto, California). The pellet is resuspended in a volume of 2 ml in phosphate buffered saline (PBS) and layered on top of a linear gradient of sucrose (5 to 60% w/w) of the SW 40 rotor.

After ultracentrifugation in a L8-70 centrifuge with 37000 rpm at +10°C for 4 hrs, fractions of 11 drops are collected from the bottom. The fractions of 38 to 42% sucrose, which contain the partly purified, concentrated, and infectious HBV virions (Thomssen et al., 1978) and some HBsAg, are pooled and used for the MADT without additional protein load.

For the MADT without additional protein load, electron microscopical formvar-coated copper grids are layered on top of a drop of this pool for 20 min at room temperature for adsorption of HBV. After washing off the sucrose from the grids with PBS, the grids are put on a drop of the disinfectant under test and, for control purposes, on a drop of bidistilled water and on a drop of 0.7% (w/w) formaldehyde for the respective exposure times as recommended in the German joint BGA/DVV guideline on testing chemical disinfectants for virucidal activity (Kuwert et al., 1982). After washing off the disinfectant and performing the negative or positive staining

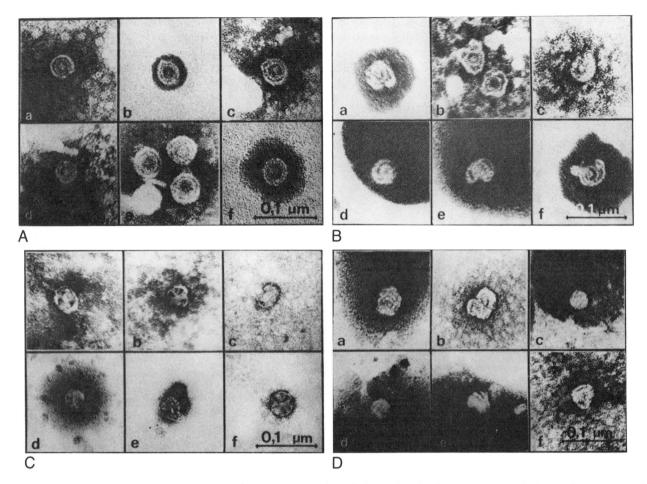

Fig. 26–1. Alteration phases (AP) of Dane particles (hepatitis B virions [HBV]) observed in the electron microscope before or after reaction with buffer, water, chemicals, or germicides at +20°C. *A,* AP 0, intact structure of the HBV, no morphologic alterations; representative virus particles were photographed after contact with double-distilled water for 15 min (a), phosphate-buffered saline (pH 7.2) for 15 min (b), 70% (v/v) ethyl alcohol for 15 min (c), tap water for 15 min (d), phosphate-buffered saline (pH 7.2) for 15 min (e), and 70% (v/v) ethyl alcohol for 15 min (f). *B,* AP 1, alteration of the outer membrane of the virion; representative particles were photographed after contact with 2% (v/v) formaldehyde for 15 min (a), 5% (v/v) succinic dialdehyde for 2 min (b), 70% (v/v) ethyl alcohol for 15 min (c), 1% of an oxide-releasing disinfectant (Dentavon) for 5 min (d), 0.1% of a sodium hydroxide-containing commercial disinfectant (Maranon H) for 5 min (e), and 2% of a disinfectant containing an aldehyde mixture (Lysoform 2000) for 5 min (f). *C,* AP 2, alteration of outer and inner structures of the virion, which are still visible, however; representative particles were photographed after reaction with 2% (v/v) formaldehyde for 1 hour (a), with 5% (v/v) succinic dialdehyde (Gigasept) for 2 min (b), 70% (v/v) ethyl alcohol for 15 min (c), 2% of an oxide-releasing disinfectant (Dentavon) for 5 min (d), 0.1% of a sodium hydroxide-containing commercial disinfectant (Maranon H) for 5 min (e), and 2% of a disinfectant containing an aldehyde mixture (Lysoform 2000) for 5 min (f). *D,* AP 3, alteration of all substructures resulting in virus particles that appear as polygonal particles without any substructure and a diameter of less than 40 nm; representative particles were photographed after reaction with 2% (v/v) formaldehyde for 1 hour (a), with 5% (v/v) succinic dialdehyde (Gigasept) for 15 min (b), 70% (v/v) ethyl alcohol for 15 min (c), 2% of an oxide-releasing disinfectant (Dentavon) for 5 min (d), 0.1% of a sodium hydroxide-containing commercial disinfectant (Maranon H) for 30 min (e), and 2% of a disinfectant containing an aldehyde mixture (Lysoform 2000) for 15 min (f).

with phosphotungstic acid or with potassium permanganate and uranyl acetate of the grids, the morphology of the HBV of the different tests is quantitatively examined under the electron microscope.

For the MADT with additional protein load, the pellet of the first ultracentrifugation is resuspended in PBS with 0.2% bovine serum albumin and mixed with equal volumes of the disinfectant, bidistilled water, or formaldehyde. After expiry of the exposure times, dilution with ice-cold buffered saline, trap and gradient ultracentrifugation, as mentioned above, is carried out, the fractions

of 38 to 42% sucrose are pooled and the number of the altered and unaltered HBV are counted.

For the estimation of alterative activity, the ratio of the unaltered HBV (AP 0 and 1) to the altered HBV (AP 2 and 3) is calculated. The degree of disintegration is the ratio of the total number of HBV virions in the test to the total number in the control with double-distilled water.

The HBV-destroying activity is the overall parameter of the alterative and disintegrative activity of a germicide. This activity depends on the concentration of the dis-

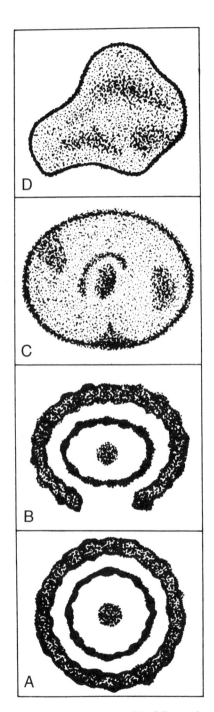

Fig. 26–2. Schematic representation of the different alteration phases (AP) of Dane particles (DP) as visualized after reaction with germicides or physical treatment. *A,* AP 0: morphologic integrity of the DP; *B,* AP 1: alteration of the outer membrane, but the core is still intact; *C,* AP 2: alteration of the outer membrane and inner core; substructures still visible; *D,* AP 3: round to polygonal particles with a diameter of 38 to 40 nm without any substructures.

infectant reacting for an exposure time on the HBV virions. The HBV-destroying activity is estimated according to the equation:

$$1 - a/b \cdot c/d$$

where a = number of Dane particles (DP) of alteration phase (AP) 0 and 1; b = number of all DP (AP 0 to 3) in the test, which was counted for the estimation of "a"; c = number of all DP per 125 μm^2 in the test; d = number of all DP per 125 μm^2 in the control assay with double-distilled water (Table 26–9).

As mentioned previously, the degree of morphologic damage was correlated with the loss of infectivity in an infection experiment in a chimpanzee. This experiment was conducted and the results were as follows:

For animal-protection reasons, only three animals were available for this experiment, one for each treated HBV suspension, a procedure also chosen by Bond et al. (1983). Although this procedure does not allow a statistical analysis, it is possible to draw conclusions concerning the inactivation of HBV infectivity from this experiment by taking earlier experiences with HBV titrations in chimpanzees into consideration. From such virus titrations, the inverse correlation of infectivity titer (ID_{50}) and the first appearance of hepatitis B surface antigen (HBsAg) were established by Murray et al. (1955). This correlation was also demonstrated by Barker et al. (1975) and Shikata et al. (1978). Moreover, we found that the results of the investigations of Barker et al. (1975) and Shikata et al. (1978), which were carried out in two different laboratories at different times, showed no significant differences concerning the dose response of the time of first HBsAg detection after inoculation and concentration of the inoculum. Therefore, it was possible to combine the results and determine a correlation coefficient of r = 0.85 for both data sets (n = 26) and a regression line of y = (13.636 − 1.262 · x) · 7 or approximately x = 11 − 1/9 · y, where x = $\log_{10}$ of HBV concentration (ID_{50}) and y = day p.i. of first HBsAg appearance in the serum of the chimpanzee. This kind of estimation of the virus concentration allowed the calculation of relative infectious chimpanzee units (ID_{50}) and spared animals that otherwise would have been necessary to sacrifice for titration purposes.

Each of the three chimpanzees, which were HBsAg negative more than half a year before the beginning of the inoculation, received one of the following intravenously: (a) an untreated partially purified and concentrated DP suspension; (b) the same preparation after reaction with 0.7% (w/v) formaldehyde; or (c) the same preparation after reaction with a 5% (v/v) succinic dialdehyde preparation (Gigasept, Fa. Schülke and Mayr, Hamburg) at +20°C for 1 hr.

The undiluted DP was derived from sera of 2 patients who were HBsAg positive and from whom contact cases with HBV infections were known. This HBV suspension had 10^{11} DP particles/ml, which were intact, an antigenicity of HBsAg of 101 times above the negative control, corresponding to a titer of 1:10,000, and an antigenicity

Table 26–9. *An Example of the Determination of the Hepatitis B Virus (HBV) Destroying Activity*

Result of Electron Microscopy

	Counted Virions	Alteration Phase 0 and 1	Alteration Phase 2 and 3	Alteration (%)	Disintegration (%)
Disinfectant	100	30	70	70	90
Double-distilled water	1000	950	50	5	0

Calculation of HBV-destroying activity by the disinfectant

According to the foregoing formula:

a = 30
b = 100
c = 100
d = 1000

$$\text{HBV-destroying activity} = 100 \cdot \left(1 - \frac{30}{100} \cdot \frac{100}{1000}\right) = 100\,(1 - 0.03) = 97\%$$

Alternative calculation:

Alteration   70%
Disintegration   90%

Ratio of not altered fraction $= (1 - 0.7) = 0.3$
Ratio of undisintegration fraction $= (1 - 0.9) = 0.1$

HBV-destroying activity $= 100 \cdot (1 - (0.3 \cdot 0.1)) = 97\%$

of HBeAg 6 times above the doubled counts per minute-value of the negative controls. After treatment, the HBV suspensions contained 100% (a), 40% (b), and <0.1% (c) physically intact DP.

The first appearance of HBsAg in the sera of the chimpanzees was detected at day 13 (a) and day 40 (b) after inoculation. The maximum titer was 1:51,000 at day 40 (a) and 1:15,000 at day 98 (b); the duration was 85 (a) and 79 (b) days. HBeAg appeared at day 19 (a) and day 49 (b), the maximal titers were 1:>1024 at day 70 (a) and 1:300 at day 70 (b), and the duration was 65 (a) and 35 (b) days. DP was found in concentrations of 10^8 DP/ml serum at day 40 (a), but not in b or c. Anti-HBc was detected first at day 40 (a) and day 70 (b); the maximum titer was 1:7800 at day 98 (a) and 1:4000 at day 193 (b). Anti-DP was detected first at day 49 (a) and day 70 (b); the maximum titers were 1:8000 at day 119 (a) and 1:1000 at day 193 (b). Anti-HBs was first determined at day 98 (a) and day 84 (b); the maximum titers were 1:20 from day 193 to 332 (a) and 1:300 at day 334 (b). Anti-HBe appeared first by day 193 (a and b); the maximum titer was 1:5 at day 245 (a) and 1:39 at day 332 (b). The duration of all antibodies was >100 days for a and b. The enzymes GGT, GOT, and GPT were elevated approximately 60 to 160 days p.i. for a and b. On day 98, acute (a) and at day 193, subacute (b) hepatitis was diagnosed patho-histologically. None of the foregoing HBV marker or enzymes became positive, and no histopathologic change of the liver occurred with c. This animal could be infected by the original untreated HBV suspension 332 days after the first inoculation, however, as shown by HBsAg antigenemia from day 77 to 100 with a maximum titer of 1:20,000, HBeAg determination of 1:17 at day 100, and induction of anti-HBc, anti-Hbs, and anti-HBe.

By applying the foregoing regression equation to our results, the infectious concentrations worked out to be approximately ID$_{50}$ $10^{9.5}$ (a), $10^{6.5}$ (b), and ID$_{50}$ <10^1 (c).

Thus, an alteration of 20% and disintegration of 50%, i.e., a HBV-destroying effect of 60%, resulted in a loss of infectivity of 99.9%, whereas a complete alteration (>99%) and 80% disintegration resulted in a complete loss of infectivity (>99.99%).

Comparison of the Alternative Methods for Testing of Virucidal Activity. Methodologic difficulties exist in testing complex mixtures of germicides for the biologic integrity of hepatitis B virus (HBV) DNA and DNA polymerase, and no infectivity experiments exist for correlation of these results. No correlation of infectivity and HBc or HBe antigenicity has been proved.

No correlation was found in comparative experiments with the morphologic alteration and disintegration test (MADT) and HBeAg using partly purified and concentrated HBV suspension (Thraenhart and Kuwert, 1984). Most experience so far has been gathered with the MADT and HBsAg test.

In some comparisons between the MADT and HBs antigenicity of partly purified and concentrated HBV suspensions (Table 26–10), a 77 to 93% reduction of the HBsAg in the case of >99% HBV activity in the MADT was shown, but the meaning of this result is not clear (Thraenhart and Kuwert, 1984).

Results of HBsAg and infectivity did not show that these two parameters correlate. In one chimpanzee experiment, the HBsAg value remained at 95%, but no infectivity was induced (Thraenhart et al., 1982). In another chimpanzee experiment, four of four chimpanzees contracted HBV infections despite complete reduction of HBsAg below the detection level (Hilfenhaus and Weidmann, 1986).

So far, definition of minimal criteria for the evaluation of a disinfection procedure has been possible for the MADT only on the basis of an infectivity experiment. For such disinfection procedures, the concentration of a germicide and the necessary exposure time for an efficient HBV-destroying activity are determined. In Eu-

Table 26–10. *Comparison of Physical Destruction of HBV (MADT), HBs and HBe Antigen Reduction*

Disinfectant	Concentration Vol (%)	Exposure Time (min)	HBV Physical Destruction (MADT) (%)	HBsAg Reduction* (%)	HBeAg Reduction* (%)	Chimpanzee Test Reduction of Infectivity	Reference
Double-distilled water	—	5	0	0	0	n.d.	Thraenhart and Kuwert (1984)
Formaldehyde	0.7 w/v	5	<20	0 (238)†	7	n.d.	
PVP-iodide in aqueous solution	25	5	20	0 (166)†	49	n.d.	
	50	2	20	0 (188)†	41	n.d.	
Aldehydic germicide for hands	50	2	>99.9	69	44	n.d.	
	75	2	>99.9	77	42	n.d.	
	90	1	>99	68	n.d.	n.d.	
Formaldehyde	0.7 w/v	30	<20	0 (154)†	0 (151)†	n.d.	
		60	20	10	0 (117)†	n.d.	
Two aldehydic germicides for hands	90	1	>99	n.d.	0	n.d.	
		1.5	>99.9	93	0 (117)†	n.d.	
		2	>99.9	93	0 (119)†	n.d.	
		5	>99.9	93	0	n.d.	
Sodium hypochlorite	2	30	>99	92	0 (127)†	n.d.	
		60	>99.9	94	0 (122)†	n.d.	
	3	30	>99.9	95	0 (159)†	n.d.	
PBS	—	60	<10	0	n.d.	0	Thraenhart et al. (1982)
Formaldehyde	0.7 w/v	60	60	0 (121)†	n.d.	99.9	
Succinic aldehyde	5	60	>99	9	n.d.	>99.99	
Cryoprecipitate	—	—	n.d.	0	n.d.	0 (4/4)‡	Hilfenhaus and Weidmann (1986)
Purified F VIII concentrate	—	—	n.d.	>94	n.d.	0 (4/4)‡	
Purified F VIII concentrate heat treated	—	—	n.d.	>94	n.d.	100 (0/7)‡	

n.d. = Not done

*HBsAg and HBeAg were determined by radioimmunoassay (RIA).

†Increase of antigenicity. (% values of HBsAg)

‡(4/4) = 4 infected 14 total inoculated animals

rope, the MADT is acknowledged by several national official authorities as the alternative method for testing HBV activity of germicides. The same is true for the United States. Only recently the Environmental Protection Agency (EPA) of the U.S. government approved a MADT protocol adapted to the U.S. regulations of virucidal testing (H. Prince, Gibraltar Lab., personal communication, 1990) as the single alternative method besides the chimpanzee test.

HBV-Destroying Activity as Determined by the MADT. CHEMICAL COMPOUNDS. Because of the lack of data on the virucidal activity of most disinfectant substances or physical procedures, results obtained with the MADT are presented.

Double-distilled water and tap water did not induce any alteration or disintegration of the structures of HBV. We found that even after an exposure time of 10 hrs with distilled water or tap water, no significant HBV-destroying activity was observed. Even after 50 hrs of exposure time, only 40% of the Dane particle (DP) was altered.

pH values of 4.0 to 10.0 were tolerated up to 60 min.

A pH value of 12.0 resulted in complete alteration and partial disintegration after 5 min. A mixture of KOH and ethyl alcohol with a pH of 13.4 induced an alteration and disintegration of more than 90% in each case after 15 min reaction time. Even in the range of pH 2.0, an alteration and disintegration of 50% in each case was determined, i.e., an HBV-destroying activity of 75%. According to these results, HBV seems to be more sensitive to an excess of OH⁻ ions than H⁺ ions.

More than 50 disinfectants containing different compounds were tested for HBV-destroying activity. These tests were undertaken with exposure times used under practicable conditions. "Long-time disinfection," i.e., exposure time of >15 to 60 min, is used for instruments, environmental surfaces, and laundry. "Short-time disinfection," with exposure times up to 5 min, is the practice for disinfection of hands and skin surface. Disinfectants for long-time disinfection contain mostly aldehydes, oxygen-releasing agents, halogen-containing compounds, and phenolic derivates. Germicides for short-time disinfection contain mostly alcohols and organic iodine compounds.

A direct correlation exists between the HBV-destroying activity of the different aldehydes at a constant concentration and the length of the exposure time. When, however, kinetics of several concentrations of one aldehyde are compared, differences are obvious between glutardialdehyde and the other aldehydes. The non-glutaraldehydes are characterized by a direct correlation between the aldehyde concentration and the degree of HBV destruction. The situation with glutardialdehyde, on the other hand, is complex due to its characteristics: this compound has a germicidal and a fixative activity by crosslinkage of proteins. At lower concentrations, the HBV-destroying activity seems to be more pronounced than the fixative activity, whereas the fixative activity is preponderant at higher concentrations (Thraenhart, 1990).

When germicides that contain glutardialdehyde have to be tested with the MADT, the disinfectant must pass the pass/fail criteria of the MADT at a concentration level for use or lower. However, for safety reasons, additional results of virucidal tests with resistant viruses should be considered when a concentration of a glutardialdehyde-containing compound shall be recommended.

Commercially available disinfectants that contain a mixture of mono- and dialdehydes and possibly tensides or other surface-active substances showed better HBV-destroying activity than single aldehydes. Differences among such germicides were considerable, however.

It may be concluded that aldehydes are able to destroy HBV, but there seems to be an inverse correlation of concentration and exposure time. Mixtures of aldehydes and ethyl alcohol that are dispersed on environmental surfaces have HBV-destroying activity, which may be attributed to the aldehyde because alcohol in usable concentrations in germicides had a low HBV-destroying activity.

Germicides based on sodium hypochlorite are used for the disinfection of machines for hemodialysis. This compound is active against HBV: an exposure time of only 5 min with a dilution of 1% caused alteration of DP of 60% and disintegration of 50%. The disintegration increased to 90% when a 2% solution was used. The activity of this preparation was inhibited by the protein load, however.

Oxygen-releasing disinfectants such as permanganate, peracetic acid, or other per-acids are receiving ever-increasing interest as compounds for disinfectants because of their environmental compatibility. These compounds with a wide pH range had a good and fast alterative and disintegrative HBV-destroying activity in relatively low concentrations of 0.5 to 2.0%. These germicides were found to be active in concentrations of 0.5 to 2.0% after an exposure time of 5 min. The HBV-destroying activity was between 85 and >99% using a 1% solution of persuccinic acid. According to these results, oxygen-releasing compounds can be used for short- and long-time disinfection.

Quaternary ammonium compounds were tested with the MADT, mainly in mixtures with other germicidal reagents. The HBV-destroying activity of single quaternary ammonium compounds may be quite different. Results of detailed studies will be available soon.

Short-time disinfection is of high priority especially for hand decontamination. Disinfectants for hand decontamination are mainly based on alcohols with a maximum content of 70% alcohol. We find differences of the HBV-destroying activity of such a concentration for exposure times for 1 to 15 min; however, ethyl alcohol in a concentration of 82% (w/v) led to a complete alteration of HBV after 5 min.

The addition of H_2O_2 increased the HBV activity considerably. Most probably, the active compound, i.e., H_2O_2, is intensified in its effect by the alcohol, which seemed to have a carrier function. This concept led to the development of a hand germicide on the basis of alcohol plus H_2O_2 (Spitaderm, Firma Henkel, Düsseldorf). After an exposure time of 2 min, all DP were significantly altered and disintegrated. In a practice-oriented experiment, this disinfectant fulfilled the minimal requirements set up for the MADT in risk areas when the undiluted disinfectant was applied three times for a minute. A disinfectant on the basis of an arylated phenolic compound (Primasept M, Firma Schülke & Mayr, Hamburg) was the first hand disinfectant against HBV that showed an HBV-destroying activity of >99% after 1 min.

Iodine is still the best disinfectant for skin disinfection. It is also used for long-time disinfection of hemodialysis instruments. Different preparations of high-molecular organic iodine (polyvinyl pyrollidone iodine) had quite different HBV-destroying activities, ranging from no effect to significant A&D. This variability of activity was also observed for enteroviruses (Wallis et al., 1963; Drulak, Wallbank, and Lebtag, 1978; Kappel, 1974; Sporkenbach, 1980). Drulak et al. (1978) therefore considered iodine a critical virucidal disinfectant. Recently, the phenomenon of variability of germicidal activity of organic iodine products has been attributed to the amount of free (≥ 10 ppm) iodine and its constant availability (G. Schwarzmann, Sempach, personal communication, 1989). Under this condition (12 ppm), we found HBV-destroying activity after an exposure time of 5 min, but no HBV-destroying activity was observed with germicides with 2 to 5 ppm free available iodine.

Only a slight effect on HBV was found when a germicide on the basis of mercury borate and isopropyl alcohol (Merfen) was used.

To simulate the conditions in practice, the MADT was carried out with and without additional protein load. In this "environmental MADT," the protein load was approximately 10 to 20 mg protein/ml. Under these conditions, the HBV-destroying activity was inhibited to some extent.

On the basis of the results of the MADT experiments, a gradient of the HBV-destroying activity of different germicides and reagents was formulated (Tables 26–11 and 26–12). According to this gradient, compounds with oxygen-releasing acids are followed in their HBV-destroying activity by aldehydes, halogens, arylated phenolic compounds, PVP iodine, and alcohols.

PHYSICAL PROCEDURES. Thermal treatment of plasma for 10 hrs at +60°C, which gave inconsistent results in the infectivity experiment, resulted in an insignificant alteration and disintegration (A&D) when stabilizers used for the preparation of factor VIII preparations were added. A temperature of 98°C, however, induced complete A&D after a 3-min reaction, i.e., >99% HBV-destroying activity. At +121°C for an exposure time of 15 min, only a few DP of alteration phase (AP) 2 and 3 were detected. No DP was observed at +134°C for 15 min.

Ultrasonic treatment at 35 KHz of 120 to 140 w up to 30 min had no effect on the physical structure of the HBV, although the temperature of the DP suspension increased from +17 to +35°C.

It may be concluded that the physical integrity of HBV has a high resistance against thermal and ultrasonic procedures.

COMBINED PHYSICAL AND CHEMICAL PROCEDURES. When chemical disinfectants, e.g., aldehyde, oxygen-releasing acids, and KOH, are combined with ultrasonic or thermal treatment, this combination has an additive effect on the destruction of the DP. Such HBV destruction was only noticed, however, when chemical germicides had an HBV-destroying activity on their own.

HEPATITIS D VIRUS (HDV)

Characteristics

The agent of delta virus (HDV) is a defective satellite of HBV requiring the presence of HBV for its replication and assembly. The virion is 35 to 37 nm in diameter and consists of an envelope made of hepatitis B surface antigen (HBsAg) surrounding a structure containing the delta antigen and an ssRNA genome with a size of 1.75 kb. HDV has not yet been classified, and its taxonomic position is far from clear.

Epidemiology and Transmission

Because HDV requires active help of functions from HBV for its replication, infection with HDV only occurs in patients with acute or chronic HBV infections. HDV is therefore endemic among the HBV carrier population and is identified in different parts of the world where HBV occurs.

High-risk groups include intravenous drug users and hemophiliacs. In hemodialysis units, HDV has been transmitted by the use of a dialysis machine contaminated by an HDV-positive patient.

Control and Disinfection

Because HDV is accompanied by HBV infection in every case, control measurements of HBV infections such as screening, disinfection, and vaccination against

HBV should also control the transmission of HDV (Lettau et al., 1986).

HEPATITIS A VIRUS (HAV)*

Characteristics

Hepatitis A virus (HAV) is an enterovirus of the family Picornaviridae (type: Enterovirus 72 = HAV). As a picornavirus, the naked virion of HAV (Zuckerman, 1988a) has icosahedral symmetry and is 30 nm in diameter. Other characteristics of HAV and picornaviruses are also identical (Deinhardt et al., 1984). The genome consists of one molecule of infectious ssRNA of 7.2 to 8.4 kilobase (kb) and have four major polypeptides. RNA replication involves the synthesis of a complementary RNA that serves as template for genome RNA synthesis. Genome RNA also serves as mRNA, being translated into a polyprotein that is cleaved into all the viral proteins, including those that serve as enzymes for specific cleavages. Replication involves translation of a large precursor polyprotein and post-translational cleavage into functional polypeptides. Replication and assembly take place in the cytoplasm, and virus is released via cell destruction. The virus has a narrow host range.

Only one serotype of HAV has been identified so far in natural and experimental infections as well as by cross-neutralization tests (Lemon and Binn, 1983).

Epidemiology and Transmission

HAV occurs endemically in all parts of the world, but the exact incidence is difficult to estimate because of the high proportion of asymptomatic and anicteric infections, differences in surveillance, and differing patterns of the disease. Serologic surveys have shown that although the prevalence of hepatitis A in industrialized countries, particularly in northern Europe, North America, and Australia, is decreasing, the infection is almost universal in most countries (Zuckerman, 1988a).

According to serologic studies, the infection rate is related to age and socioeconomic status. In northern Europe, North America, and Australia, 5 to 20% of the population has anti-HAV antibody by the age of 20 years and 40 to 50% by the age of 50 years, whereas in most other countries, up to 90% of the population is infected by the age of 10 years. With improvements in sanitation and socioeconomic status, the incidence of hepatitis declines rapidly. This epidemiologic pattern is an indication of the efficiency of hygienic precautions and water sanitation.

HAV infection is frequently contracted by travellers from areas with high sanitation standards to areas of low sanitation standards.

Occasional sexual transmission may occur among homosexual men, particularly those who practice oral-anal

*Dr. R. Scheid and Prof F. Deinhardt of Munich carried out most of the inactivation experiments of HAV. Unpublished data were kindly made available and are gratefully acknowledged.

Table 26–11. *Examples of Morphologic Alteration and Disintegration Test (MADT) Results Obtained with Germicides Containing Different Classes of Active Compounds*

Main Active Compound in Germicide and Concentration	Reaction Time (min)	MADT without Protein				MADT with Protein			
		Alteration Phases	Alteration[a] (%)	Disintegration (%)	HBV Destruction (%)	Alteration Phases	Alteration (%)	Disintegration (%)	HBV Destruction (%)
5% 100 g (v/v)[b]	2	0, 1, 2	50	<10	<55	n.d.	n.d.	n.d.	n.d.
0.34 g 6.8 g succinic dialdehyde	15	2, 3	>90	30	>93	n.d.	n.d.	n.d.	n.d.
0.225 g 4.5 g dimethoxytetra-	30	n.d.	n.d.	n.d.	n.d.	0, 1	10	10	20
hydrofuran	60	3	>90	>90	>99	1, 2	50	50	75
0.225 g 4.5 g formaldehyde	120	n.d.	n.d.	n.d.	n.d.	2, 3	>90	>80	>98
	240	3	>90	>90	>99	n.d.	n.d.	n.d.	n.d.
100% (v/v)[c]	5	1, 2, 3	80	50	90	1, 2, 3	80	80	96
0.13% formaldehyde	15	2, 3	>90	50	>95	2, 3	>90	>90	>99
0.065% glyoxal	30	3	>90	>90	>99	3	>90	>90	>99
0.019% glutaraldehyde	60	3	>90	>90	>99	3	>90	>90	>99
38.4% ethanol									
2% (w/v)[d]	5	3	>90	>90	>99	3	>90	>90	>99
0.3% tetra-acetylethylendiamine									
0.4% sodium perborate									
0.176% glyoxal[e] 2% (v/v)	60	3	>90	>90	>99	3	>90	>90	>99
0.090% glutaraldehyde									
0.088% glyoxal[e] 1% (v/v)	60	2, 3	>90	50	>95	n.d.	n.d.	n.d.	n.d.
0.045% glutaraldehyde	120	3	>90	>90	>99	2, 3	>90	>90	>99
	240	3	>90	>90	>99	2, 3	>90	>90	>99
100% (w/v)[f]	1	1, 2	80	20	84	n.d.	n.d.	n.d.	n.d.
70.0% 2-propanol	2	2, 3	>90	70	>97	n.d.	n.d.	n.d.	n.d.
0.5% chlorhexidine digluconate	5	3	>90	80	>98	n.d.	n.d.	n.d.	n.d.
0.45% hydrogen peroxide	15	3	>90	>90	>99	n.d.	n.d.	n.d.	n.d.
Formaldehyde	15	0, 1	<10	<10	<20	0, 1	<10	<10	<20
0.7% (w/v)	60	0, 1	<10	<10	<20	0, 1	<10	<10	<20
Tap water	60	0, 1	<10	—	<10	0, 1	<10	—	<10

HBV = hepatitis B virus; n.d. = not done.

[a] Alteration phases 2 and 3
[b] Gigasept
[c] Incidin Special Spray
[d] Sekusept Pulver
[e] Incidur
[f] Spitaderm

Table 26–12. *Activity Gradient of Hepatitis B Virus (HBV) Destruction by Different Chemical Compounds*

Compounds	Exposure Time Necessary for HBV Destruction	Effective Concentration Range	Inhibition by Proteins
Oxygen cleaving (per acids)	Short	Low	Rel. Low
Aldehydes	Long	Low	
	Short	High	Rel. Low
Chlorine cleaving	Short	Low	Rel. High
Organic iodine	Short	≥10 ppm*	(?)
Alcohols	Short	High (≥80%) (w/v)	(?)
Phenolic compounds	Long	Rel. High	(?)

(?) = Further investigations necessary.
*Only if ≥10 ppm free iodine available (G. Schwarzmann, personal communication, 1989).

contact (Zuckerman, 1988a), or lesbians (Walters and Rector, 1986).

In developed countries, the infection occurs mainly in crowded situations such as nursery schools, institutions for the mentally handicapped, or homes for old people. Nosocomial transmission of HAV from patients to staff members, though unusual, may happen, especially from infected children in whom an illness obscures the early diagnosis of HAV (Reed et al., 1984; Baptiste et al., 1987). Nosocomial transmission most often occurs via nurses, and the HAV infection may spread from one child to others in the hospital, to nurses, and even to family members (Klein et al., 1984).

Transmission is predominantly by the fecal-oral route, usually by person-to-person contact. Outbreaks result most frequently from fecal contamination of drinking water and food. The consumption of raw vegetables or inadequately cooked shellfish or food handled after preparation by HAV-infected persons presents a high risk of transmission in areas with endemic HAV (Deinhardt et al., 1984; Lowry, et al., 1986) because healthy persons excrete HAV in their stool in endemic regions (De Filippis et al., 1987). Biziagos et al. (1988) were able to show that HAV survives in water, even in mineral water at +4°C, for 1 year.

Virus Stability

Chemical Disinfectants

Hepatitis A virus (HAV) has the same resistance to chemical reagents as other picornaviruses, as demonstrated by Scheid et al. (1981b) by comparing several chemicals used for the decontamination of water, such as sodium hypochlorite iodine, potassium permanganate, chloramine T, peracetic acid, and quaternary ammonium compounds.

Only recently, Mbithi, Springthorpe, and Sattar (1990) published data on the resistance of HAV against 20 different formulations. The virus was artificially suspended in 10% feces of a 5-month-old healthy baby for testing. The suspension was centrifuged to remove gross particulate matter. Thereafter, the supernatant was passed through a 0.22 μm filter, dried on a steel disk under ambient conditions for 20 mins and brought in contact with the germicide for 1 min. Only 3 of the 20 tested formulations proved to be effective against HAV. These were: 2% glutaraldehyde; 0.4% quaternary ammonium (QAC) with 23% hydrochloric acid; sodium hypochlorite with at least 5,000 ppm of free chlorine (Table 26–13).

According to these authors the following can be concluded:

1. "Chlorine resistance of HAV is similar to that of other fecally-suspended enteroviruses dried on environmental surfaces.
2. The inability of formulations with pH of nearly 2 to inactivate the virus reflects the high acid resistance of HAV.
3. The results of this study are an additional proof of the poor virucidal properties of QAC; the efficacy of the single QAC-based formulation against HAV was most likely due to its high HCl content.
4. Presence of isopropyl or ethyl alcohol in QAC formulations or phenolics were not effective against HAV.
5. Even 6% hydrogen peroxide could not inactivate HAV on environmental surfaces."

HAV is ether-resistant and stable at pH 3.0. The virus is inactivated by ultraviolet irradiation and by treatment with a 1:4000 concentration of formaldehyde solution at +37°C for 72 hrs. There is also evidence that HAV is inactivated by chlorine at a concentration of 1 mg/L for 30 min (Grabow et al., 1983; Abb and Deinhardt, 1986) and by ozone (Botzenhart and Herbold, 1988).

In Table 26–14, the results of some of the inactivation experiments by Scheid and Deinhardt (personal communications, 1989) are presented.

Formaldehyde at a concentration of 1:4000 at +37°C for 72 hrs inactivated semipurified viral preparations; however, a formalin solution of 1:350, which is equal to 0.1% (w/v) formaldehyde, inactivated HAV incompletely after an exposure time of 1 hr at room temperature. 70% alcohol reduced the infectivity by $\log_{10}$ median infective dose $(ID_{50}) = 2.25$ at room temperature for 3 mins. Even after 12 hrs, however, alcohol was not able to inactivate HAV completely, although an inactivation of $\log_{10} ID_{50} = 4.75$ was observed (Scheid et al., 1981b).

Table 26–15 gives inactivation results of Scheid and Deinhardt (personal communication, 1989) with disinfectants that could be used for decontamination of drinking water and shows that sodium hypochlorite, iodine, and potassium permanganate would be effective disinfectants when one is traveling in endemic areas.

Thermal Treatment and Irradiation

The high resistance of HAV at room temperature was verified by McCaustland et al. (1982), who showed that fecal specimens containing HAV remain infective even after drying and storage at +25°C and 42% relative humidity for at least 30 days.

Also from results of Scheid et al. (1981b) and additional data (Zuckerman, 1988a), which are summarized in Table 26–16, it can be concluded that HAV is relatively stable against thermal treatment. HAV is stable for >1 yr of storage at −20 to −70°C for at least 1 hr at 50 to 60°C, and even after 6 to 12 hrs of exposure to +60°C, residual infectivity could be observed. At +100°C, HAV was inactivated within 5 mins.

Siegl (1984) points out significant differences between poliovirus and HAV concerning temperature resistance. When polio or hepatitis A virus particles were heated at pH 7 for 10 mins, 50% of the polio virions were disintegrated after heating at 43°C but hepatitis A virions needed a temperature of 61°C for 50% disintegration. In the presence of 1M $MgCl_2$, which stabilizes enteroviruses, the $T_{50,10}$ for poliovirus and HAV shifted to 61 and 81%, respectively.

Table 26–13. *Inactivation of HAV by Different Germicides*

Disinfectant		Dilutions Tested	pH	Recommended For	Log Reductions
Commercial Formulations					
(1)	2.0% Glutaraldehyde	Undiluted	7.5	Medical instruments	>4
(2)	6% Sodium hypochlorite	1:18 (to give 3000 ppm free chlorine)	10.9	General purpose disinfectant	<1
(2a)	6% Sodium hypochlorite	1:11 (to give 5000 ppm free chlorine)	11.2	"	>4
(3)	2.75% Sodium chlorite and 15.10% organic acid	1:12	2.9	Instruments and environmental surfaces	<1
(4)	15.5% Iodophor and 6.5% phosphoric acid	1:214 (to give 75 ppm titratable iodine)	2.8	Highly contaminated areas, isolation rooms and food contact surfaces	<1
(5)	17.84% Iodophor	1:173 (to give 75 ppm titratable iodine)	5.2	Surfaces and skin	<1
(6)	0.5% Sodium Q-benzyl-p chlorophenol and 0.6% Sodium lauryl sulphate	Undiluted	12.7	Environmental surfaces	<1 <1
(7)	0.1% Q-phenyl-phenol, 70% ethyl alcohol and 0.14% chlorhexidine gluconate	Undiluted	2.4	Surfaces and instruments in medical, dental, and veterinary clinics	<1
(8)	0.4% QAC 1 and 23% HCl	Undiluted	0.4	Surfaces, toilet bowls and urinals	>4
(9)	10.76% QAC 2, 10.76% QAC 3 & 16% isopropanol	1:500 (to give 430 ppm QAC)	6.3	General purpose surface and equipment cleaning	<1
(10)	0.3% QAC 4, 45% isopropyl alcohol, 3% triethylene glycol and 2% propylene glycol	Undiluted	7.6	Environmental surfaces	<1
(11)	2.7% QAC 5	Undiluted	9.2	Environmental surfaces	<1
(11a)	2.7% QAC 5	1:33	8.9	Environmental surfaces	<1
(12)	2.7% QAC 5 and 70% ethanol	Undiluted	10.1	Environmental surfaces	<1
Noncommercial Formulations					
(13)	10% Chloramine T	1:18 (to give 3000 ppm free chlorine)	7.7	Food equipment and environmental surfaces	<1
(13a)	10% Chloramine T	1:11 (to give 5000 ppm free chlorine)	8.0	"	<1
(14)	3.125% Iodophor	Undiluted	1.8	Instruments and environmental surfaces	<1
(15)	70% Ethanol	Undiluted	5.2	General surfaces	<1
(16)	Glacial acetic acid	1:33 (to give 3% acid)	2.6	Environmental surfaces	<1
(16a)	Glacial acetic acid	1:10 (to give 10% acid)	2.2	"	<1
(17)	35% Peracetic acid	1:33	2.4	Isolators, medical and surgical equipment and environmental surfaces	<1
(17a)	35% Peracetic acid	1:10	2.2	"	<1
(18)	85% Phosphoric acid	1:33	2.3	Environmental surfaces	<1
(18a)	85% Phosphoric acid	1:10	1.8	"	<1
(19)	10% Citric acid	1:3 (to give 3.3% acid)	2.9	Environmental surfaces	<1
(19a)	10% Citric acid	1:2 (to give 5% acid)	2.6	Environmental surfaces	<1
(20)	30% Hydrogen peroxide	1:10 (to give 3% hydrogen peroxide)	6.8	Surgical implants, ventilators, utensils, and thermoplastic equipment	<1
(20a)	30% Hydrogen peroxide	1:5 (to give 6% hydrogen peroxide)	6.6	"	<1

QAC = quaternary ammonium compound.
QAC 1 = n-alkyl (50% C14, 40% C12, 10% C16) dimethyl benzyl ammonium chloride.
QAC 2 = n-alkyl (60% C14, 30% C16, 5% C12, 5% C18) dimethyl benzyl ammonium chloride.
QAC 3 = n-alkyl (68% C12, 32% C14) dimethyl benzyl ammonium chloride.
QAC 4 = n-alkyl (C12 40%, C14 50%, C16 10%) dimethyl benzyl ammonium chloride.
QAC 5 = n-alkyl (50% C14, 40% C12, 10% C16) n-n-dimethyl n-benzyl ammonium chloride.
From Mbithi, J.N., Springthorpe, V.S. and Sattar, S.A. 1990. Chemical disinfection of hepatitis A virus on environmental surfaces. Appl. Environ. Microbiol., 56, in press.

Table 26–14. *Inactivation of Hepatitis A Virus (HAV) by Chemical Compounds*

Disinfectant	Concentration	Exposure Time	Temperature (°C)	Inactivation ($\log_{10} ID_{50}$)
pH = 3	—	3 hrs	+37	No complete inactivation
Formalin 1:350	(0.1 g/L)	60 min	Room	3.0 (incomplete inactivation)
Sodium hypochlorite	10 mg/L	15 min	Room	3.0
Iodine	3 mg/L	15 min	Room	3.0
Potassium permanganate	30 mg/L	15 min	Room	3.0
Chloramine T	1 g/L	15 min	Room	<3.0
Peracetic acid	300 mg/L	15 min	Room	<3.0
Alcohol	70%	3 min	Room	2.25
Alcohol	70%	12 hrs	Room	4.75 (incomplete inactivation)

From Scheid, R. and Deinhardt, F. 1989. Personal communication.

Moreover, Biziagos et al. (1988) found differences in the temperature sensibility of poliovirus and HAV; whereas poliovirus was not detected at room temperature after 300 days, HAV was still infectious.

Irradiation with ^{60}Co with a dose of 150 to 1200 krad led to only a slight reduction of HAV infectivity (Scheid et al., 1981a).

Ultraviolet radiation inactivates HAV (Zuckerman, 1988a).

Methods for Control of Virucidal Activity of Disinfectants

Hepatitis A virus (HAV) replicates in several types of cell culture of primate origin without cytopathic effect (Scheid et al., 1981a). HAV can also be titrated with a plaque assay on B-SC-1 cells (Anderson, 1987).

HAV remains predominantly cell associated in most infected cell cultures. Viruses adapted to growth in cell culture may become attenuated (Provost et al., 1988; Hu et al., 1988). Whether the rapid change of virulence in tissue-culture cells may cause difficulties for the standardization of test procedures for testing virucidal activity of germicides is not yet known. It is therefore advisable to test the virucidal activity with one stock virus of the same passage (Scheid, personal communication, 1989).

HAV virucidal activity of HAV-inactivation procedures can be investigated by using the human hepatocellular carcinoma cell line PLC/PRF/5, Hep3B2.17 or human embryo fibroblast cells. Virus multiplication must be

made visible by immunofluorescence because HAV does not induce cytopathogenic effects (Scheid et al., 1981a).

After proving that germicides inactivate HAV and poliovirus to the same extent (Scheid and Deinhardt, 1981), a test for the virucidal activity against poliovirus, which is much easier to perform, seems to be sufficient, at least for chemical disinfectants as recommended in the joint guidelines of the German Federal Health Office and the German Society against Virus Diseases (Kuwert et al., 1982).

Control and Disinfection

Because HAV is shed and transmitted by the fecal route and shedding of the virus occurs mainly during the late incubation period and the beginning of the prodromal period, strict cleanliness should be observed, and the use of disinfectants effective against picornaviruses is recommended in areas with high HAV incidence, such as in crowded situations and in tropical countries. Sterilization of water by chlorine (Abb and Deinhardt, 1986) or chemicals is recommended, as indicated in Table 26–15.

In case of short visits to tropical countries, normal

Table 26–15. *Inactivation of 99.9% of Hepatitis A Virus (HAV) Infectivity After an Exposure Time of 15 min at Room Temperature by Different Disinfectants for Decontamination of Drinking Water (Concentrations of Virucidal Activity Are Compared with the Upper Level of Palatability)*

Disinfectant	Concentration of the Disinfectant of	
	HAV Inactivation	Upper Level of Palatability
Sodium hypochlorite	≤10 mg/L	100 mg/L
Iodine	3 mg/L	30 mg/L
Potassium permanganate	30 mg/L	30 mg/L
Chloramine T	>1 g/L	10 mg/L
PS15 (15% peracetic acid)	>300 mg/L	300 mg/L

From Scheid, R., and Deinhardt, F. 1989. Personal communication.

Table 26–16. *Inactivation of Hepatitis A Virus (HAV) at Different Temperatures*

Temperature °C	Exposure Time	Inactivation ($\log_{10} ID_{50}$)
−70	6 months	0
−20	6 months	0
+4	16 weeks	0.5
Room	1 week	0
Room	4 weeks	2.0
Room	8 weeks	≥3.5†
+32	1 week	2.0
+32	14 days	≥4.0
+37	14 days	≥4.25
+37	4 weeks	≥4.25†
+56	6–12 hrs	≥5.25
+56	24 hrs	≥4.25
+60	6–12 hrs	<5.25*
+85	1 min	>5.25

*But residual infectivity in passage.
†Below level of detection.

From Scheid, R., and Deinhardt, F. 1989. Personal communication.

Table 26–17. *Characteristics and Resistance to Ether and Thermal Treatment of the "GB" Isolate*

Size	20–30 nm
Buoyant density (CsCl)	1.18–1.23
Ether	
20%, 12 hrs, +4°C	Stable
50%, 12 hrs, +4°C	Incomplete inactivation
Thermal treatment	
+50°C, 30 min	Stable
+56°C, 30 min	Stable or resistant*
+60°C, 30 min	Inactivated
+100°C, 5 min	Inactivated

*Results of different laboratories.
From Deinhardt, F. et al. 1975. Personal communication.

human immunoglobulin, containing at least 100 IU anti-HAV antibody/ml, should be administered intramuscularly before exposure to the virus (Zuckerman, 1988a).

Vaccines are under development and may be available shortly (e.g., Provost et al., 1988; Flehmig et al., 1988).

NON-A, NON-B (NANB) HEPATITIS VIRUSES

The agents of non-A, non-B (NANB) hepatitis fall into at least two categories, of which one or more than one virus is transmitted by the fecal-oral route (epidemic form), sometimes provisionally called HEV. The second category of NANB hepatitis viruses, which are parenterally transmitted and of which one provisionally named HCV, seems to have some characteristics of the virus group (HCV).

Until now, all attempts to characterize these viruses of HCV and HEV in detail and possible other NANB hepatitis viruses have failed, but antigens of one HEV have been identified and antibodies determined (Krawczynski and Bradley, 1989). No classification is possible so far, and hardly any information on the biologic behavior of these viruses is available.

ENTERALLY TRANSMITTED NANB HEPATITIS (ENANB OR HEPATITIS E VIRUS [HEV])

Isolates from the stool of patients show different appearances under the electron microscope.

An "HEV" was already isolated in 1975 (Deinhardt et al., 1975). This so-called "GB" isolate had some characteristics similar to picornaviruses, such as a size of 20 to 30 nm, a buoyant density of 1.18 to 1.23, and a high stability, as shown in Table 26–17.

With this kind of virus, it was possible to infect marmosets by the intramuscular (Peterson et al., 1978) or oral (Deinhardt et al., 1975) route. The incubation time was 14 to 21 days (IM route) or 12 to 47 days (12, 12, 19, 47 days) (oral route).

Purcell and Ticehurst (1988) also describe particles of a structure that are similar to HAV. These authors presume that ENANB may possibly be type 2 of HAV.

Particles of 27 to 30 nm were observed by Bradley et al. (1988b) in outbreaks of ENANB in different regions of the world. In addition, these authors found particles of 27 to 34 nm with a sedimentation coefficient of 180 S (Bradley et al., 1987, 1988a; Bradley and Balayan, 1988). The virus was unstable to freeze-thawing and storage at +4 to 8°C. It also disintegrated when pelleted from CsCl density-gradient fractions, which may be a Norwalk virus-like behavior. Krawczynski and Bradley (1989) have detected the HEV antigen of the 32- to 34-nm virus in hepatocytes of macaques.

Epidemiology and Transmission

A significant proportion of the acute hepatitis that occurs in young and middle-aged inhabitants in Asia, South America, and Africa appears to be caused by HEV. Both epidemic and sporadic forms of HEV have been observed. According to Purcell and Ticehurst (1988), the clinical attack rate in epidemics is highest in young adults and lower in the very young and very old. The mortality rate, which is normally low, is high in pregnant women.

Usually, contaminated drinking water is the source of infection and can cause fulminant epidemics. For example, in 1973, approximately 10,000 cases were reported in the Kathmandu valley (Kane et al., 1984). There is, however, a relatively low incidence of clinical disease observed in case contacts. For example, only 2.4% of household contacts of HEV patients developed clinical illness during the epidemic in the Kathmandu valley (Kane et al., 1984).

Control and Disinfection

Although a low resistance of HEV was observed by Bradley et al. (1988b), that another HEV may have a high resistance to environmental conditions cannot be excluded.

These infections can be prevented by improving water sanitation. Travellers to tropical and subtropical countries should boil drinking water or use disinfectants as approved by Scheid and Deinhardt for HAV during their stay (see Table 26–15).

PARENTERALLY TRANSMITTED NANB HEPATITIS

Characteristics

According to reported studies, the existence of at least two transmissible agents has been documented (Bradley and Maynard, 1983).

According to the first results, one virus seems to have some characteristics of retroviruses (Zuckerman, 1988b), such as positive reverse transcriptase, particles with a diameter of approximately 60 to 90 nm with a density of 1.13 g sucrose/ml and an antigenic cross-reactivity with glycoprotein of human immunodeficiency virus (HIV) (Seto and Gerety, 1985).

The virus was resistant to 20 or 83% chloroform in one case, but sensitive in another case (Feinstone et al., 1983). The chloroform-sensitive virus passed through an

80-nm filter, had a sedimentation coefficient of 200 to 280 S, and had a buoyant density in CsCl of 1.24 g/ml.

Hepatitis C virus (HCV) is not yet characterized. The morphology is unknown. According to filtration experiments, the diameter may be <80 nm; it should have an envelope and contain a ssRNA coding for 7300 bp (Beach and Bradley, 1990; Moeckli et al., 1990). Structural proteins and enzymes seem to have some relationship with flaviviruses, but classification in this group is uncertain (Beach and Bradley, 1990; Miller and Purcell, 1990).

Epidemiology and Transmission

Parenterally transmitted non-A, non-B (NANB) viruses have been found in every country and share a number of features with hepatitis B. This form of hepatitis has been most commonly recognized as a complication of blood transfusion. Hellings et al. (1985) detected transmission of NANB by mononuclear leukocytes of a chronic patient. In spite of screening of blood donations for HBsAg, hepatitis is still transmitted, and 90% may be accounted for NANB.

Transmission may also be possible by administration of blood-clotting factors VIII and IX. Moreover, other routes of transmission may be identical to those of hepatitis B virus (HBV) (Dienstag, 1983a, b).

In addition, significant numbers of cases are not associated with transfusion and may account for 10 to 25% of all adult patients, predominantly males, with recognized viral hepatitis. The route of infection has not been identified so far. Although the illness is mild and often subclinical or anicteric, severe hepatitis with jaundice and even fulminant hepatitis may occur. The virus has a high virulence with intensive intrafamilial spreading.

Clinical evidence based on observations of multiple attacks of hepatitis in individual patients led to the suggestion that probably more than one virus exists.

HCV is transmitted by transfusion, but transmission via inanimate vectors, such as hemodialysis machines, may be important (own unpublished results).

Because of the similarity of transmission of some of the NANB and HBV, the same multimodal network as proposed for HBV will probably be efficient for the control of NANB and HCV (see Table 26–4). In particular, screening of blood donations and possibly organ donation with newly developed tests will reduce transmission of this virus.

Few data are available concerning the inactivation of the viruses by chemical or physical means.

One of the agents was inactivated by formalin 1:2000 at +37°C for 72 to 76 hrs (Tabor, 1982), heating at 100°C for 5 min (Yoshizawa et al., 1981) and possibly at 60°C for 10 hrs (Gerety and Iwarson, 1986). Hollinger et al. (1984) demonstrated the efficiency of a thermal treatment of a human factor VIII concentrate at +60°C for 10 hrs.

According to Kernoff et al. (1987), however, no inactivation occurs by "wet heating." For the inactivation of the Hutchinson strain of NANB blood derivatives, Prince et al. (1985) successfully used beta-propiolactone and ultraviolet irradiation. Even beta-propiolactone alone

was able to inactivate this virus strain (Stephan et al., 1988). No data are available for the resistance of HCV to chemical agents (January 1991).

REFERENCES

Aach, R.D., and Kahn, R.A. 1980. Post-transfusion hepatitis: current perspectives. Ann. Intern. Med., 92, 539–546.

Abb, J., and Deinhardt, F. 1986. Hepatitis A. In Viral Hepatitis: Clinics in Tropical Medicine and Communicable Diseases. Edited by A.J. Zuckerman. London, W.B. Saunders, pp. 303–319.

AFNOR. 1989. Antiseptiques et desinfectants, 2nd Edition. AFNOR, Paris, France.

Alter, M.J., Ahtone, J., and Maynard, J.E. 1983. Hepatitis B virus transmission associated with a multiple dose vial in a hemodialysis unit. Ann. Intern. Med., 99, 330–333.

Anderson, D.A. 1987. Cytopathology, plaque assay, and heat inactivation of hepatitis A virus strain HM175. J. Med. Virol., 22, 35–44.

Baptiste, R., Koziol, D., and Henderson, D.K. 1987. Nosocomial transmission of hepatitis A in an adult population. Infect. Control, 8, 364–370.

Barker, L.F., et al. 1975. Hepatitis B virus infection in chimpanzees: titration of subtypes. J. Infect. Dis., 132, 451–458.

Bchini, R., et al. 1990. In vitro infection of human hepatoma (HepG2) cells with hepatitis B virus. J. Virol., 64(6), 3025–3032.

Beach, M., and Bradley, D.W. 1990. Analysis of the putative nonstructural gene region of hepatitis C virus. In The 1990 International Symposium on Viral Hepatitis and Liver Disease. Houston, April 4–8, p. 139.

Beasley, R.P., Stevens, C.E., Shiao, I.S., and Meng, H.C. 1975. Evidence against breast feeding as a mechanism for vertical transmission of hepatitis B. Lancet, 2, 740–741.

Berry, W.R., Gottesfeld, R.L., Alter, H.J., and Vierling, J.M. 1987. Transmission of hepatitis B virus by artificial insemination. JAMA, 257, 1079–1081.

Birnie, G.G., et al. 1983. Endoscopic transmission of hepatitis B virus recent advancements lower risk of hepatitis infections in health professionals (news). Georgetown Univ. Sch. Dent. Mirror, 47, 14–15.

Biziagos, E., Passagot, J., Crance, J.M., and Deloince, R. 1988. Long-term survival of hepatitis A virus and poliovirus type 1 in mineral water. Appl. Environ. Microbiol., 54, 2705–2710.

Block, S.S. 1987. Historical review. In American Society for Microbiology Symposium on Chemical Germicides in the Health Care Field. Arlington, VA, Nov. 2–4.

Blumberg, B.S., and Hesser, J.E. 1975. Viral hepatitis: modes of transmission and the role of the carrier. In Transmissible Disease and Blood Transfusion. Edited by T. Greenwalt and G.A. Jamieson. New York, Grune & Stratton, pp. 67–80.

Bond, W.W., and Moncada, R.E. 1978. Viral hepatitis B infection risk in flexible fiberoptic endoscopy. Gastrointest. Endosc., 24, 225–230.

Bond, W.W., et al. 1980. Transmission of type B viral hepatitis via eye inoculation of a chimpanzee. J. Clin. Microbiol., 15, 533–534.

Bond, W.W., et al. 1981. Survival of hepatitis B virus after drying and storage for one week. Lancet, 1, 550–551.

Bond, W.W., Favero, M.S., Petersen, N.J., and Ebert, J.W. 1983. Inactivation of hepatitis B virus by intermediate-to-high-level disinfectant chemicals. J. Clin. Microbiol., 18, 535–538.

Botzenhart, K., and Herbold, K. 1988. Abtötung von Hepatitis-A-Virus im Wasser durch Ozon (Inactivation of hepatitis A virus in water by ozone). Z. Gesamte Hyg., 34, 508–510.

Brackmann, H.H., and Egli, H. 1988. Acute hepatitis B infection after treatment with heat-inactivated factor VIII concentrate (letter) effect of dry-heating of coagulation factor concentrates at 80°C for 72 hours on transmission of non-A, non-B hepatitis. Study group of the UK Haemophilia Centre Directors on Surveillance of Virus Transmission by Concentrates. Lancet, 2, 814–816.

Bradley, D.W., et al. 1987. Enterically transmitted non-A, non-B hepatitis: serial passage of disease in cynomolgus macaques and tamarins and recovery of disease-associated 27- to 34-nm viruslike particles enterically transmitted non-A, non-B hepatitis—Mexico. MMWR, 36, 597–602.

Bradley, D., et al. 1988a. Aetiological agent of enterically transmitted non-A, non-B hepatitis. J. Gen. Virol., 69, 731–738.

Bradley, D.W., et al. 1988b. Enterically transmitted non-A, non-B hepatitis: etiology of disease and laboratory studies in nonhuman primates. In Viral Hepatitis and Liver Disease. Edited by A.J. Zuckerman. New York, Alan R. Liss, pp. 138–147.

Bradley, D.W., and Balayan, M.S. 1988. Virus of enterically transmitted non-A, non-B hepatitis. (Letter.) Lancet, 1, 819.

Bradley, D.W., and Maynard, J.E. 1983. Non-A, non-B hepatitis: research progress and current perspectives. Dev. Biol. Stand., 54, 463–473.

Brechot, C., et al. 1985. Hepatitis B virus DNA in patients with chronic liver disease and negative tests for hepatitis B surface antigen. N. Engl. J. Med., 312, 270–276.

Bundesgesundheitsamt Berlin. 1976. *Richtlinie für die Erkennung, Verhütung and Bekämpfung von Krankenhausinfektionen.* Stuttgart, Gustav Fischer-Verlag.

Bundesgesundheitsamt Berlin. 1987. Liste der vom Bundesgesundheitsamt geprüften und anerkannten Desinfektionsmittel und -Verfahren. Bundesgesundheitsbl., 30, 279–292.

Bundesgesundheitsamt Berlin. 1988. Merkblatt Nr. 21; Virushepatitis. Verhütung und Bekämpfung; Ratschläge an Ärzte und Zahnärzte. Ausgabe Juli 1987. Bundesgesundheitsbl., 31, 185–190.

Cancio-Bello, T.P., et al. 1982. An institutional outbreak of hepatitis B related human biting carrier. J. Infect. Dis., 146, 652–656.

Cossart, Y.E., and Cohen, B.J. 1976. Transmission of hepatitis B to fetus and infant. In *Liver Disease in Infancy and Childhood.* Edited by S.R. Berenberg. Baltimore, Williams & Wilkins, pp. 180–188.

De Filippis, P., et al. 1987. Detection of hepatitis A virus in the stools of healthy people from endemic areas. Eur. J. Epidemiol., 3, 172–175.

Deinhardt, F., Habermehl, O., Kuwert, E., and Spicher, G. 1983. Stellungnahme zur Prüfung von Desinfektionsmitteln auf Wirksamkeit gegenüber dem Hepatitis B-Virus. Bundesgesundheitsbl., 26, 222–222.

Deinhardt, F., et al. 1975. Hepatitis in marmosets. Am. J. Med. Sci., 270, 73–80.

Deinhardt, F., et al. 1984. Viral hepatitis A: virus, disease, and control. In *Applied Virology.* Edited by E. Kurstak. New York, Academic Press, pp. 365–376.

Dienstag, J.L. 1983a. Non-A, non-B hepatitis. I. Recognition, epidemiology, and clinical features. Gastroenterology, 85, 439–462.

Dienstag, L.L. 1983b. Non-A, non-B hepatitis. II. Experimental transmission, putative virus agents and markers, and prevention. Gastroenterology, 85, 743–768.

Drees, O. 1966. Über den Wirkmechanismus viruzider Desinfektionsmittel. Zentralbl. Bakteriol. Mikrobiol. Hyg., 201, 358–359.

Drulak, M., Wallbank, A.M., and Lebtag, I. 1978. The relative effectiveness of commonly used disinfectants in inactivation of echovirus 11. J. Hyg. Camb., 81, 77–87.

Drulak, M., et al. 1978. The relative effectiveness of commonly used disinfectants in inactivation of coxsackievirus B5. J. Hyg. Camb., 81, 389–397.

Favero, M.S., Petersen, N.J., and Bond, W.W. 1986. Transmission and control of laboratory-acquired hepatitis infection. In *Laboratory Safety: Principles and Practices.* Edited by B.M. Miller, et al. Washington, D.C., American Society for Microbiology, pp. 49–58.

Feinstone, S.M., et al. 1983. Inactivation of hepatitis B virus and non-A, non-B hepatitis by chloroform. Infect. Immun., 41, 816–821.

Flehmig, B., et al. 1988. Progress in the development of an attenuated, live hepatitis A vaccine. In *Viral Hepatitis and Liver Disease.* Edited by A.J. Zuckerman. New York, Alan R. Liss, pp. 87–90.

Frösner, G., Jentsch, G., and Uthemann, H. 1982. Zerstörung der Antigenität und Beeinflussung der immunchemischen Reaktivität von Antigenen des Hepatitis B-Virus (HBs-Ag, HBc-Ag und HBe-Ag) durch Desinfektionsmittel—ein Prüfungsmodell. Zentralbl. Bakteriol Mikrobiol. Hyg. (B), 176, 1–14.

Gerety, R.J., and Iwarson, S.A. 1986. Non-A, non-B hepatitis. In *Viral Hepatitis: Clinics in Tropical Medicine and Communicable Diseases.* Edited by A.J. Zuckerman. London, W.B. Saunders, pp. 441–458.

Grabow, W.O., Gauss-Müller, V., Prozesky, O.W., and Deinhardt, F. 1983. Inactivation of hepatitis A virus and indicator organisms in water by free chlorine residuals. Appl. Environ. Microbiol., 46, 619–624.

Gust, I.D., et al. 1986. Taxonomic classification of human hepatitis B virus. Intervirology, 25, 14–29.

Heinrich, D., et al. 1987. Virus safety of beta-propiolactone treated plasma preparations: clinical experiences. Dev. Biol. Stand., 67, 311–317.

Hellings, J.A., van der Veen-du Prie, J., Snelting-van Densen, R., and Stute, R. 1985. Preliminary results of transmission experiments of non-A, non-B hepatitis by mononuclear leucocytes from a chronic patient. J. Virol. Methods, 10, 321–326.

Hilfenhaus, J., and Weidmann, E. 1986. Pasteurization as an efficient method to inactivate blood borne viruses in factor VIII concentrates. Arzneimittelforschung, 36, 621–625.

Hollinger, F.B., Dolana, G., Thomas, W., and Gyorkey, F. 1984. Reduction in risk of hepatitis transmission by heat-treatment of a human factor VIII concentrate. J. Infect. Dis., 150, 250–261.

Hollinger, F.B., et al. 1982. Reduction of infectivity of hepatitis B-virus (HBV) and a non-A, non-B hepatitis agent by heat treatment of human antihemophilic factor (AHF) concentrates. In *Second International Max v. Pettenkofer Symposium on Viral Hepatitis,* Munich, Oct. 19 to 22.

Howard C.R., et al. 1983. Chemical inactivation on hepatitis B virus: the effect of disinfectants on virus-associated DNA.

Hu, M., et al. 1988. Attenuated hepatitis A virus for vaccine development: attenuation and virulence for marmosets. In *Viral Hepatitis and Liver Disease.* Edited by A.J. Zuckerman. New York, Alan R. Liss, pp. 81–82.

Jenison, S.A., Lemon, S.M., Baker, L.N., and Newbold, J.E. 1987. Quantitative

analyses of hepatitis B virus DNA in saliva and semen of chronically infected homosexual man. J. Infect. Dis., 156, 299–306.

Kane, M.A., et al. 1984. Epidemic non-A, non-B hepatitis in Nepal: recovery of a possible etiologic agent and transmission studies in marmosets. JAMA, 252, 3140–3145.

Kappel, E.E. 1974. Über den Einfluss chemischer Desinfektionsmittel auf die Struktur von Poliovirus-Teilchen. Hamburg, Medical inaugural dissertation, University of Hamburg.

Kashiwagi, S., et al. 1984. Transmission of hepatitis B virus among siblings. Am. J. Epidemiol., 120, 617–625.

Kent, G.P., et al. 1988. A large outbreak of acupuncture-associated hepatitis B. Am. J. Epidemiol., 127, 591–598.

Kernoff, P.B., et al. 1987. Reduced risk of non-A, non-B hepatitis after a first exposure to "wet heated" factor VIII concentrate. Br. J. Haematol., 67, 207–211.

Klein, B.S., et al. 1984. Nosocomial hepatitis A: a multinursery outbreak in Wisconsin. JAMA, 252, 2716–2721.

Krawczynski, K., and Bradley, D.W. 1989. Enterically transmitted non-A, non-B hepatitis: identification of virus-associated antigen in experimentally infected cynomolgus macaques. J. Infect. Dis., 159, 1042–1049.

Krogsgaard, K., et al. 1986. Hepatitis B virus DNA in hepatitis B surface antigen-positive blood donors: relation to the hepatitis B system and outcome in recipients. J. Infect. Dis., 153, 298–303.

Kuwert, E.K., and Spicher, G. 1982. Kommentar zur Richtlinie des Bundesgesundheitsamtes und der Deutschen Vereinigung zur Bekämpfung der Viruskrankheiten zur Prüfung von chemischen Desinfektionsmitteln auf Wirksamkeit gegen Viren. Bundesgesundheitsbl., 26, 413–417.

Kuwert, E., and Thraenhart, O. 1977. Theoretische, methodische und praktische Probleme der Virusdesinfektion in der Humanmedizin. Immun. Infekt., 4, 125–137.

Kuwert, E., Scheiermann, N., and Thraenhart, O. 1982. *"Transmission der Hepatitis-Viren, Hepatitis A, B sowie Non A/Non B. Infektionsquellen, Risikobereiche, Übertragungswege, Immunisierung."* Mainz, mhp-Verlag.

Kuwert, E., Thraenhart, O., Dermietzel, R., and Scheiermann, N. 1982. *Zur Hepatitis B-Viruswirksamkeit und Hepatoviruzidie von Desinfektionsverfahren auf der Grundlage des MADT.* Mainz, mhp-Verlag.

Kuwert, E., Thraenhart, O., Dermietzel, R., and Scheiermann, N. 1984. The morphological alteration and disintegration test (MADT) for quantitative and kinetic determination of hepato-virucidal effect of chemical disinfectants. Hyg. Med., 9, 1–6.

Kuwert, E., et al. 1982. Richtlinie des Bundesgesundheitsamtes und der Deutschen Vereinigung zur Bekämpfung der Viruskrankheiten zur Prüfung von chemischen Desinfektionsmitteln auf Wirksamkeit gegen Viren. Bundesgesundheitsbl., 25, 397–398.

1990. Guidelines of Bundesgesundheitsamt (BGA; German Federal Health Office) and Deutsche Vereinigung zur Bekämpfung der Viruskrankheiten e.V. (DVV; German Association for the Control of Virus Diseases) for Testing the Effectiveness of Chemical Disinfectants Against Viruses. Zbl. Hyg., 189, 554–562.

Lange, W., and Masihi, K.N. 1989. Zur Morbidität der Hepatitis infectiosa. Bundesgesundheitsbl., 32, 223–226.

Lemon, S.M., and Binn, L.N. 1983. Antigenic relatedness of two strains of hepatitis A virus determined by cross-neutralization. Infect. Immun., 42, 418–420.

Lettau, L.A., et al. 1986. Nosocomial transmission of delta hepatitis. Ann. Intern. Med., 104, 631–635.

Liebermann, H.M., et al. 1983. Detection of hepatitis B virus DNA directly in human serum by a simplified molecular hybridization test: comparison to HBeAg/anti-HBe status in HBsAg carriers. Hepatology, 3, 285–291.

Loncarevic, I.F., et al. 1990. Replication of hepatitis B virus in a hepatocellular carcinoma. Virology, 174(1), 158–168.

Locarnini, S.A., and Gust, I.D. 1988. Hepadnaviridae: hepatitis B virus and the delta virus. In *Laboratory Diagnosis of Infectious Diseases: Principle and Practice.* Vol. II. *Viral, Rickettsial, and Chlamydial Diseases.* Edited by E.H. Lennette, P. Halonen, and F.A. Murphy. New York, Springer-Verlag, pp. 750–796.

Lowry, P.W., et al. 1989. Hepatitis A outbreak on floating restaurant in Florida, 1986. Am. J. Epidemiol., 129, 155–164.

Madeley, C.R. 1988. Unclassified viruses and caliciviridae: other viruses associated with gastroenteritis. In *Laboratory Diagnosis of Infectious Diseases: Principle and Practice.* Vol II. *Viral, Rickettsial, and Chlamydial Diseases.* Edited by E.H. Lennette, P. Halonen, and F.A. Murphy. New York, Springer-Verlag, pp. 806–818.

McCaustland, K.A., et al. 1982. Survival of hepatitis A virus in feces after drying and storage for 1 month. J. Clin. Microbiol., 16, 957–958.

McNaughton, P., and Mathews, R.E.F. 1971. Sedimentation of small viruses at very low concentrations. Virology, 45, 1–9.

McQuillan, G.M., et al. 1987. Prevention of perinatal transmission of hepatitis B virus: the sensitivity, specificity, and predictive value of the recommended screening questions to detect high-risk women in an obstetric population. Am. J. Epidemiol., 126, 484–491.

Massarrat, S., and Schiff, W. 1975. Virusübertragung durch Endoskope. Med. Klin., 70, 392–392.

Mauler, R., Merkle, W., and Hilfenhaus, J. 1987. Inactivation of HTLV-III/LAV, hepatitis B and non-A, non-B viruses by pasteurization in human plasma protein preparations. Dev. Biol. Stand., 67, 337–351.

Mbithi, J.N., Springthorpe, V.S., and Sattar, S.A. 1990. Chemical disinfection of hepatitis A virus on environmental surfaces. Appl. Environ. Microbiol., 56, in press.

Miller, R.H., and Purcell, R.H. 1990. Hepatitis C virus shares protein sequence similarity with plant and animal viruses. In *The 1990 International Symposium on Viral Hepatitis and Liver Disease*. Houston, April 4–8, p. 140.

Moeckli, R.A., et al. 1990. Epitope mapping of the HCV nonstructural region. In *The 1990 International Symposium on Viral Hepatitis and Liver Disease*. Houston, April 4–8, p. 139.

Morris, I.M., Cattle, D.S., and Smith, B.J. 1975. Endoscopy and transmission of hepatitis B. Lancet, 2, 1152.

Mullan, R.J., et al. 1989. Guidelines for prevention of transmission of human immunodeficiency virus and hepatitis B virus to health-care and public-safety workers. MMWR, 38.

Murray, R., et al. 1955. Effect of ultraviolet radiation on the infectivity of iatrogenic plasma. JAMA, 157, 8–14.

Nath, N., and Fang, C. 1982. Effect of selected physicochemical agents on the stability of HBV specific DNA polymerase. In *Viral Hepatitis: 1981 International Symposium*. Edited by W. Szmuness, H. Alter, and J.E. Maynard. Philadelphia, Franklin Institute Press, p. 623–624.

Pantelick, E.L., Miller, D.J., and Steere, A.C. 1981. Nosocomial hepatitis B in personnel during an 8 year period: policies for screening and pregnancy in high risk areas. Hyg. Med., 6, 51 (abstract).

Petersen, N.J., Bond, W.W., and Favero, M.S. 1979. An air sampling for hepatitis B surface antigen in a dental operatory. J. Am. Dent. Assoc., 99, 465–467.

Peterson, D.A., et al. 1978. Virus excretion, antibody development and changes in rosette formation of lymphocytes during non-B hepatitis in marmosets. Prim. Med., 10, 280–287.

Piazza, M., Distasio, G., Maio, G., and Marzano, L.A. 1973. Hepatitis B antigen inhibitor in human feces and intestinal mucosa. Br. Med. J., 2, 334–337.

Pontisso, P., Poon, M.C., Tiollais, P., and Brechot, C. 1984. Detection of hepatitis B virus DNA in mononuclear blood cells. Br. Med. J., 288, 1563–1566.

Prince, A.M., et al. 1985. Inactivation of the Hutchinson strain of non-A, non-B hepatitis virus by combined use of beta-propiolactone and ultraviolet irradiation. J. Med. Virol., 16, 119–125.

Prince, A.M., Stephan, W., Kotitschke, R., and Brotman, B. 1983. Inactivation of hepatitis B and non-A, non-B viruses by combined uses of Tween 80, beta-propiolactone, and ultraviolet irradiation. Thromb. Haemost., 50, 534–536.

Provost, P.J., Emini, E.A., Lewis, J.A., and Gerety, R.J. 1988. Progress toward the development of a hepatitis A vaccine. In *Viral Hepatitis and Liver Disease*. Edited by A.J. Zuckerman. New York, Alan R. Liss, pp. 83–86.

Provost, P.J., et al. 1986. New findings in live, attenuated hepatitis A vaccine development. J. Med. Virol., 20, 165–175.

Purcell, R.H., and Ticehurst, J.R. 1988. Enterically transmitted non-A, non-B hepatitis: epidemiology and clinical characteristics. In *Viral Hepatitis and Liver Disease*. Edited by A.J. Zuckerman. New York, Alan R. Liss, pp. 132–137.

Ranki, M., Syvänen, A.-C., and Söderlund, H. 1988. Nucleic acids in viral diagnosis. In *Laboratory Diagnosis of Infectious Diseases: Principle and Practice*. Vol. II. *Viral, Rickettsial, and Chlamydial Diseases*. Edited by E.H. Lennette, P. Halonen, and F.A. Murphy. New York, Springer-Verlag, pp. 132–151.

Reed, C.M., Gustafson, T.L., Siegel, J., and Duer, P. 1984. Nosocomial transmission of hepatitis A from a hospital-acquired case. Pediatr. Infect. Dis., 3, 300–303.

Roingeard, P., et al. 1990. Immunocytochemical and electron microscopic study of hepatitis B virus antigen and complete particle production in hepatitis B virus DNA transfected HepG2 cells. Hepatology, 11(2), 277–285.

Scheid, R., and Deinhardt, F. 1981. Biochemische, physikalische und immunologische Charakterisierung von Hepatitisviren. In *Leberdurchblutung und Kreislauf*. Edited by W. Tittor and G. Schwalbach. Stuttgart, Georg Thieme Verlag, pp. 121–127.

Scheid, R., Deinhardt, F., Frösner, G., and Gauss-Müller, V. 1981a. Further characterization of hepatitis A virus. Med. Microbiol. Immunol., 169, 134–134.

Scheid, R., Deinhardt, F., Frösner, G., and Gauss-Müller, V. 1981b. Further studies on the inactivation of hepatitis A virus (HAV). In 38. *Tagung der DGHM*. Göttingen, Oct. 5 to 8.

Scheid, R., et al. 1982. Inactivation of hepatitis A and B viruses and risk of iatrogenic transmission. In *Viral Hepatitis: 1981 International Symposium*. Edited by W. Szmuness, H.J. Alter, and J.E. Maynard. Philadelphia, Franklin Institute Press, pp. 627–628.

Scheiermann, N., and Kuwert, E.K. 1984. Active hepatitis B immunization with an experimental German vaccine. I. Immunogenicity studies in healthy adults. II. The primary 19S and 7S responses to HBsAg in healthy adults.

III. Immunogenicity studies in hemodialysis patients. Zentralbl. Bakteriol. Mikrobiol. Hyg. (A), 257, 439–455.

Schweitzer, I.L. 1975. Infection in neonates and infants with the hepatitis B virus. Prog. Med. Virol., 20, 27–48.

Scotto, J., et al. 1983. Detection of hepatitis B virus DNA in serum by a simple spot hybridization technique: comparison with results for other viral markers. Hepatology, 3, 279–284.

Seef, L.B., and the Veterans Administration Cooperative Study Group. 1978. Type B hepatitis after needle-stick exposure: prevention with hepatitis B immune globulin. Final report of the Veterans Administration Cooperative Study. Ann. Intern. Med., 88, 285–293.

Seto, B., and Gerety, R.J. 1985. A glycoprotein associated with the non-A, non-B hepatitis agent(s): isolation and immunoreactivity. Proc. Natl. Acad. Sci. U.S.A., 82, 4934–4938.

Shen, H.-D., et al. 1986. Hepatitis B virus DNA in leukocytes of patients with hepatitis B virus-associated liver diseases. J. Med. Virol., 18, 201–211.

Sherertz, E.F., et al. 1986. Transfer of hepatitis B virus by contaminated reusable needle electrodes after electrodesiccation in simulated use. J. Am. Acad. Dermatol., 15, 1242–1246.

Shikata, T., et al. 1978. Incomplete inactivation of hepatitis B virus after heat treatment at +60°C for 10 hours. J. Infect. Dis., 138, 242–244.

Shikata, T., et al. 1977. Hepatitis B e antigen and infectivity of hepatitis B virus. J. Infect. Dis., 136, 571–576.

Siegert, W. 1982. Die Dane-Partikel assoziierte DNA-Polymerase: Biochemische Grundlagen und klinische Bedeutung der Hepatitis B. Lab. Med., 6, 77–81.

Siegl, G. 1984. The biochemistry of hepatitis A virus. In *Hepatitis A*. Edited by R.J. Gerety. New York, Academic Press, pp. 9–32.

Skelly, J., Howard, C.R., Zuckerman, A.J. 1981. Hepatitis B polypeptide vaccine preparation in micelle form. Nature, 290, 51–54.

Slater, P.E., et al. 1988. An acupuncture-associated outbreak of hepatitis B in Jerusalem. Eur. J. Epidemiol., 4, 322–325.

Soulier, J.-P., et al. 1972. Prevention of virus B hepatitis (SH hepatitis). Am. J. Dis. Child., 128, 429–434.

Sporkenbach, J. 1980. Über die fehlende inaktivierende Wirkung einiger PVP-Jod-Verbindungen gegenüber Poliomyelitis- und Adenovirus. Hyg. Med., 5, 357–362.

Stephan, W. 1989. Inactivation of hepatitis viruses and HIV in plasma and plasma derivatives by treatment with beta-propiolactone/UV irradiation. Curr. Stud. Hematol. Blood Transfus., 122–127.

Stephan, W., et al. 1988. Inactivation of the Hutchinson strain of hepatitis non-A, non-B virus in intravenous immunoglobulin by beta-propiolactone. J. Med. Virol., 26, 227–232.

Stephan, W., and Prince, A.M. 1982. Beta-propiolactone/ultraviolet treatment: quantitative studies on effectiveness for inactivation of hepatitis B virus. Zentralbl. Bakteriol. Mikrobiol. Hyg. (A), 251, 418–418.

Szmuness, W., Harley, E.J., Ikram, H., and Stevens, C.E. 1978. Sociodemographic aspects of the epidemiology of hepatitis B. In *Viral Hepatitis*. Edited by G.N. Vyas, S.N. Cohen, and R. Schmid. Philadelphia, Franklin Institute Press, pp. 297–320.

Tabor, E., and Gerety, R.J. 1982. A survey of formalin inactivation of hepatitis A virus, hepatitis B virus, and a non-A, non-B hepatitis agent. In *Second International Max v. Pettenkofer Symposium on Viral Hepatitis*. Munich, Oct. 19 to 22.

Takeshima, H., Namiki, M., Inokoshi, J., Lee, T., Abe, A., Suzuki, Y., and Omura, S. 1989. Stable expression of hepatitis B virus genome in a primary kidney cell. Arch. Virol., 109(2), 35–49.

Thomssen, R., Gerlich, W., and Stamm, B. 1978. Hepatitis B: Erreger und Infektionsverlauf unter Berücksichtigung vorläufiger Ergebnisse einer Gemeinshaftsstudie. Bundesgesundheitsbl., 21, 337–344.

Thraenhart, O., and Kuwert, E. 1984. Zur Wirksamkeitsprüfung von Desinfektionsmitteln gegenüber dem Hepatitis B-Virus unter besonderer Berücksichtigung des MADT. Hyg. Med., 9, 385–390.

Thraenhart, O., Gesemann, M., and v.Heinegg, E. 1989. Virologisches Infektionsrisiko im Rettungsdienst unter besonderer Berücksichtigung von AIDS und Hepatitis B. In *Duisburg Vortrag auf der 9. Tagung der Sektion Rettungswesen, 9. und 10. Juni*. Heidelberg, Springer-Verlag.

Thraenhart, O., et al. 1978. Influence of different disinfection conditions on the structure of the hepatitis B virus (Dane particle) as evaluated in the morphological alteration and disintegration test (MADT). Zentralbl. Bakteriol. Mikrobiol. Hyg. (A), 242, 299–314.

Thraenhart, O., et al. 1982. Comparison of the morphological alteration and disintegration test 1 (MADT) and the chimpanzee infectivity test for determination of hepatitis B virucidal activity of chemical disinfectants. Zentralbl. Bakteriol. Mikrobiol. Hyg. (B), 176, 472–484.

Thraenhart, O. 1990. Principles and problems of virus testing. Abstract. ASM International Symposium on Chemical Germicides, Atlanta, July 27–28, 1990.

Villa, E., et al. 1984. Gastrointestinal endoscopy and HBV infection: no evidence for a causal relationship. A prospective controlled study. Gastroint. Endosc., 30, 15–17.

Wallis, G., Behbehani, A.M., Lee, L.H., and Bianchi, M. 1963. The ineffectiveness of organic iodine (Wescodyne) as a viral disinfectant. Am. J. Hyg., 78, 325–329.

Walters, M.H., and Rector, W.G. 1986. Sexual transmission of hepatitis A in lesbians (letter) leads from the MMWR: non-A, non-B hepatitis associated with a factor IX complex infused during cardiovascular surgery—Arizona. JAMA, 256, 573–574.

Werner, B.G., and Grady, G.F. 1978. Accidental hepatitis-B-surface-antigen-positive inoculations. Ann. Intern. Med., 88, 285–293.

Will, H., et al. 1982. Cloned HBV DNA causes hepatitis in chimpanzees. Nature, 299, 740–742.

World Health Organization. 1989. *Guidelines on Sterilization and High-Level Disinfection Methods against Human Immunodeficiency Virus (HIV)*. Geneva, WHO AIDS Series 2.

Wu, J.-C., et al. 1986. Analysis of the DNA of hepatitis B virus in the sera of Chinese patients infected with hepatitis B. J. Infect. Dis., 153, 974–977.

Yoffe, B., Noonan, C.A., Melnick, J.L., and Hollinger, F.B. 1986. Hepatitis B virus DNA in mononuclear cells and analysis of cell subsets for the presence of replicative intermediates of viral DNA. J. Infect. Dis., 153, 471–477.

Yoshizawa, H., et al. 1981. Demonstration of two different types of non-A, non-B hepatitis by reinjection and cross-challenge studies in chimpanzees. Gastroenterology, 81, 107–113.

Zuckerman, A.J. 1988a. Picornaviridae: hepatitis A virus. Chapter 38. In *Laboratory Diagnosis of Infectious Diseases: Principle and Practice*. Vol. II. *Viral, Rickettsial, and Chlamydial Diseases*. Edited by E.H. Lennette, P. Halonen, and F.A. Murphy. New York, Springer-Verlag.

Zuckerman, A.J. 1988b. Unclassified: non-A, non-B hepatitis. Chapter 40. In *Laboratory Diagnosis of Infectious Diseases: Principle and Practice*. Vol. II. *Viral, Rickettsial, and Chlamydial Diseases*. Edited by E.H. Lennette, P. Halonen, and F.A. Murphy. New York, Springer-Verlag.

CHAPTER 27

HUMAN IMMUNODEFICIENCY VIRUS (HIV) DISINFECTION AND CONTROL

Jeffrey Rubin

In the summer of 1981, infectious disease specialists read with interest reports by the Centers for Disease Control of two clusters of otherwise healthy young and middle age men, one with a rare type of protozoan (pneumocystis carinii) pneumonia and the other with a rare form of cancer, Kaposi's sarcoma. It was understood at the time that these cases represented phenomena not previously seen, but no one could appreciate that these would be the first recognized cases of what was to become the greatest public health problem of the latter twentieth century, a devastating new epidemic. The Centers for Disease Control formed a task force to study these cases, and it soon became apparent that a common thread existed among the afflicted men: homosexuality. Shortly after, the syndrome was also noted in clusters of intravenous drug abusers (Centers for Disease Control, 1981a, 1981b). It became clear that affected individuals had an underlying basic immune defect rendering them susceptible to opportunistic infections and cancers; the disease became known as acquired immunodeficiency syndrome (AIDS), later found to be caused by a retrovirus.

As the epidemic spread and its morbidity, mortality, and profound social and economic implications became apparent, a major shift in health care priorities resulted. In the early 1980s it was generally felt that medical science had, at long last, a handle on the control and prevention of infectious disease with the costs of treating these illnesses representing less than 5% of all illness costs in the United States (Fox, 1987). AIDS was to change these perceptions drastically. The Centers for Disease Control estimates the cost of caring for such infected individuals to be 28 to 30 billion dollars in the year 1991 alone!

As knowledge increased, the causative retrovirus was identified as the human immunodeficiency virus (HIV), formerly called human T-cell lymphotropic virus type III (HTLV-III). The virus produced a severe immunodefi-

ciency mostly as a result of selective destruction of a lymphocyte, the T-4 helper lymphocyte, essential for identifying foreign antigen and maintenance of a competent immune system. Other cells in the brain and nervous system were later determined to be specifically targeted as well. The virus was first isolated from afflicted individuals in 1984 as described in a series of articles appearing in *Science* (Gallo et al., 1984; Popovic et al., 1984; Sargadharan et al., 1984). Two types of HIV are now recognized. HIV-I causes disease in the United States and throughout the world; HIV-II was discovered in West Africa (Clavel et al., 1986) and causes a similar disease there, with a few sporadic cases imported to the Americas (CDC, 1988a)

The virus is widely believed to have originated in Africa, with retrospective studies indicating seropositivity there extending back as far as two or more decades (Saxinger et al., 1985; Naharias et al., 1986).

As mentioned, HIV is cytopathic to the T-4 helper lymphocyte, a cell crucial to the body's immune response. Susceptibility to a spectrum of opportunistic infections and cancers results, pneumocystic carinii pneumonia (PCP) and Kaposi's sarcoma (KS) being by far the most common of these seen in affected persons. Less frequently seen are other viruses, bacteria, protozoans, fungi, and yeasts attacking the immunocompromised host. *Mycobacteria*, especially *M. tuberculosis* and *M. avium-intracellulare*, infect HIV-positive individuals at a greatly increased rate, causing an increased incidence of these infections especially in areas where HIV is prevalent (Rieder and Snider, 1986; McEuen, 1988; CDC, 1987e). Treating AIDS involves specifically managing the opportunistic infections and cancers. Additionally, new antiviral agents targeting HIV are being increasingly used. Azidothymidine, widely used to treat HIV-infected individuals, seems to prolong survival and decrease the frequency of opportunistic infections without significantly affecting or improving immune function (Fischel et al., 1987; Lane et al., 1989).

Treating HIV infection with its associated opportunistic diseases is complex and involves every body system. Goldsmith (1988) states, "Many physicians have modernized Osler's old rubric on syphilis. Now it's 'to know HIV disease is to know medicine!' " Harrington thinks that optimal management of AIDS patients requires highly specialized resources available in large medical centers (Florida Medical Assn., 1989). It is not, he says, a primary care disease.

It is estimated that 1½ million Americans may be infected with HIV, and that as many as 5 to 10 million individuals may be infected worldwide (Mann and Chin, 1988). The vast majority of these persons are asymptomatic, unaware of their infected status, and infectious to others (see *Transmission and Epidemiology*).

A few weeks after initial infection, individuals may develop an influenza-like illness that subsides (Cooper et al., 1985). Some patients may develop a persistent generalized lymph-node enlargement (PGL) as a single sign; this is believed to be an intermediate progression of disease. Others become symptomatic with anorexia, weight loss, diarrhea, chills, night sweats, and fevers, and are diagnosed as having AIDS-related complex (ARC). When specific opportunistic infections or cancers appear, the diagnosis of acquired immunodeficiency syndrome (AIDS) can be made (CDC, 1985b; CDC, 1987c). Diagnosed cases of AIDS are in essence "the clinical endpoint of the continuum of infection with HIV . . . " (CDC, 1989).

In July of 1989 the CDC reported 100,000 cases of AIDS in the U.S. It is estimated that by 1992 there will be 500,000 cases of AIDS in the Western Hemisphere (Quinn et al., 1989), with an incalculable implication for health care, economic, and social systems. Of the 1½ million people infected in the U.S—given the fact that 20 to 30% of these will develop AIDS in 5 years—it is estimated that 270,000 cases of AIDS will develop in the U.S. by 1991 (Fauci, 1988). In spite of these statistics, some progress has been made. Improved diagnostic techniques, new treatment methods and drugs, and general increased medical awareness and knowledge of HIV infection have all resulted in improvement of mean survival rates in the past few years (Florida Medical Assn., 1989).

VIROLOGY

The human immunodeficiency virus is thought to have crossed the species barrier, possibly first infecting humans from a primate species in Africa. A Simian T lymphotrophic virus (STLV-III) found in sick macaques and well African green monkeys has polynucleotide sequence homology and serologic reactivity very close to those of HIV (Kawti, 1985).

HIV is an RNA retrovirus similar to cytopathic lentiviruses causing related disease in animals. Examples include visna virus of sheep, equine infectious anemia virus, and feline immunodeficiency virus (Fauci, 1988).

The visna virus of sheep causes a lymphadenopathy, encephalitis, susceptibility to infections (especially a bacterial pneumonia), and generalized wasting symptoms analogous to HIV infection in humans. Other human retroviruses have been associated with oncogenic potential and found in patients with rare forms of leukemia.

The structure of HIV consists of a glycoprotein envelope and a core protein surrounding two strands of RNA. An enzyme, reverse transcriptase, transcribes viral RNA into DNA, allowing the virus to incorporate itself into the host genome. With HIV, the effect of this integration is cytopathic, producing premature death of the infected cell. As mentioned, HIV has a predilection for the helper T-4 lymphocyte, but also for neurons (Shaw et al., 1985; Ho et al., 1985a), producing severe immune dysfunction and neurologic disease respectively.

Clinical testing for HIV infection usually involves commercially available tests for antibody, which include the ELISA (enzyme-linked immunosorbent assay), performed in laboratories throughout the U.S. Some false positivity occurs, and a confirmatory Western Blot test is performed on ELISA-positive blood. Commercial testing to determine presence of HIV viral antigens in infected individuals is under development. Culturing for HIV is done in specialized laboratories, and is difficult and expensive.

TRANSMISSION AND EPIDEMIOLOGY

The brochure distributed by the Centers for Disease Control (CDC, 1988c) to every home in America in June of 1988 stressed that "who you are has nothing to do with whether you are in danger of being infected with the AIDS virus. What matters is what you do." High-risk behavior, such as sharing contaminated needles by intravenous drug abusers and male homosexual activity, together account for about 91% of AIDS cases in the U.S. Heterosexual contact, exposure to contaminated blood and blood products, and perinatal transmission from infected mother to newborn infant account for almost all the remaining cases. A small number of health-care workers have become infected with HIV from contaminated needles and other sharp instruments, and non-parenterally by exposure to blood of infected individuals.

Present cases of AIDS may not accurately reflect current HIV infection patterns because "the median interval between infection with HIV and onset of AIDS is nearly 10 years" (CDC, 1989b).

Procedures for control and the need for HIV disinfection must be considered in the light of an appreciation of the modes of transmission of the virus. Fortunately, HIV, unlike measles or influenza, is not easily transmitted. With education, preventive measures in terms of control of high-risk behavior can and has effectively controlled its spread.

HIV has been isolated from human blood, semen, tears, saliva, breast milk, urine, cerebrospinal fluid, lymph and brain tissue, bone marrow, and cervical and vaginal secretions (Lifson, 1988; Matlow and Fisher,

1989; Fujakawa et al., 1985a,b; Shaw et al., 1985; Groopman et al., 1984; Thiry et al., 1985; Vogt et al., 1986; Wofsy et al., 1986).

Again HIV is, in the vast majority of instances, transmitted through sexual contact or exposure to infected blood or blood components. In light of the large number of people infected with HIV and reported cases of health-care workers apparently becoming infected through exposure to infected patients' blood, the CDC recommends that "all patients be considered potentially infected with HIV and/or other blood-borne pathogens" and rigorous adherence to infection control procedures be followed in *all* patients (universal precautions) to minimize the risk of exposure to potentially infected blood and body fluids. Exposure to blood or body fluids containing visible blood is to be scrupulously avoided with barrier methods (CDC, 1988d).

HIV is spread similarly to hepatitis B virus. There are, however, over one hundred million viral particles per milliliter in hepatitis-B–infected blood, whereas in HIV there are only one hundred viral particles per milliliter of blood (CDC, 1985c). The practical implications of this are found in prospective studies of accidental needle-sticks containing HIV-contaminated blood. The rate of seroconversions was found to be 0.3% for HIV, compared to a 6 to 30% rate when exposed to hepatitis-B–contaminated needles (Loshen, 1988). A case reported of a health-care worker stuck with a needle from a patient infected with HIV and hepatitis B virus resulted in infection with hepatitis B, but tests for HIV antibody remained negative after 15 months (Gerberding et al., 1985).

It is important to stress that numerous studies indicate the risk to health-care workers to be extremely low (McEvoy et al., 1987). Gerberding et al. (1987) studied 270 health-care workers, 75% of whom worked closely with AIDS or ARC patients for a year or more, with 35% of these sustaining a total of 342 accidental parenteral exposures to HIV-infected body fluids. None of these subjects was positive on enrollment, and of 175 retested 10 months later, all were negative for antibody. He concluded that health-care workers are at minimal risk of HIV transmission from occupational exposure to patients with AIDS or ARC even when "intensively exposed for prolonged periods of time."

HIV has been isolated from saliva of infected individuals, but very infrequently (Lifson, 1988; Ho et al., 1985b). One case of suggested horizontal transmission of HIV between two siblings was attributed to a bite (Wahn, 1986). A number of other studies followed persons bitten by HIV-infected individuals, but did not identify any seroconversions (Drummond, 1986; Lifson, 1988). No evidence that HIV has been transmitted by kissing alone has been reported, although transmission through saliva is theoretically possible and "it is prudent to avoid extensive exposure to saliva from infected individuals" (CDC, 1987a).

HIV has been isolated from tears (Fujikawa et al.,

1985a) and contact lenses of infected individuals (Tervo et al., 1986). There is, however, no evidence that HIV has been transmitted from ophthalmic procedures or contact lens fitting (Conte, 1986). Nevertheless, because of theoretic possibilities, specific recommendations have been promulgated by the CDC for ophthalmic procedures (CDC, 1987a; CDC, 1985a).

HIV has rarely been isolated from the urine of infected individuals (Lifson, 1988), and several studies showed no seroconversions in persons exposed to urine of infected patients (Gerberding et al., 1987). Again CDC guidelines suggest precautions to avoid repeated exposure to possibly infected urine.

HIV has been isolated from cell-free breast milk (Thiry et al., 1985). Possible transmission to infants from infected breast milk has been reported (Ziegler et al., 1985; LePage et al., 1987). The CDC recommends that infected mothers avoid breast feeding. This is important because not all infants born to infected mothers will become infected through pregnancy, labor, or delivery (CDC, 1985d). Also, cases of infants breast-fed by infected mothers but *not* becoming infected have been reported (Senturia et al., 1987).

Extensive studies of households containing HIV-infected individuals indicate no evidence of transmission through kitchen utensils or shared bath and toilet facilities (Lifson, 1988). CDC guidelines do not restrict infected persons from sharing office equipment, telephones, toilets, showers, water fountains, or swimming pools. No transmission has been reported in school, office, or factory settings (CDC, 1985c)

Seventy-eight percent of children with AIDS acquired the disease perinatally from infected mothers, 19% from blood or blood products, and 4% from undetermined means of exposure (CDC, 1989b).

Very rare instances of transmission from skin grafts (Clarke, 1987), bone transplants (CDC, 1988f), and artificial insemination (Stewart et al., 1985) have been reported.

Since the development of antibody testing of blood and blood products in late Spring of 1985, the risk of transmission from this source is extremely low. Immune globulin preparations, recent therapeutic products for hemophilia patients, and hepatitis B vaccines prepared from pooled blood have been shown to be free of HIV (CDC, 1986a; CDC, 1988e; CDC, 1984).

No evidence exists that HIV is spread by arthropods. A study by the CDC in Belle Glade, Florida strongly suggested HIV was *not* transmitted by mosquitos in this area of very high HIV incidence (CDC, 1986e).

Physical and Chemical Agents and HIV Control

The truth is that at the present time studies on the activity of disinfectants against HIV are scant in the literature. Nevertheless, it is generally accepted that standard disinfection procedures used in hospitals and medical and dental facilities are adequate to disinfect instruments and items contaminated with body fluids from individuals infected with HIV (CDC, 1987a).

Two widely used methods to determine viability of HIV include determination of reverse transcriptase activity and the ability of virus to infect T-cell lines of tissue culture. Infectivity of HIV has been demonstrated when reverse transcriptase activity cannot be detected, and viral activity in cell culture appears to be the more sensitive method.

Physical Agents

The CDC found that drying HIV causes a rapid ("within several hours") 90 to 99% reduction in concentration of virus, but cell-free HIV could be detected "up to 15 days at room temperature and up to 11 days at 37°C" (CDC, 1987b).

Spire et al. (1985b) found that HIV was 100% inactivated by heating at 56°C for 30 minutes, but inactivation was 0% at 37°C, 40% at 42°C, and 63% at 48°C for this same period. The authors found that addition of 50% human serum to the solution did not affect inactivation at 56°C. Additionally, the authors reported that HIV was relatively resistant to gamma rays and ultraviolet light in doses much higher than those used for foodstuffs and in operating theaters and laboratories.

McDougal et al. (1985) also found HIV to be "heat labile with little difference in thermal decay when virus is present in culture media, serum, and liquid factor VIII." HIV was inactivated by exposure to both low and high extremes of pH (Martin et al., 1985).

Chemical Agents

Resnick et al. (1986) found that either 0.5% sodium hypochlorite (10% solution of household bleach), 70% alcohol, or a combination of quaternary ammonium chlorides (0.08%) completely inactivated very concentrated HIV within 10 minutes. The authors also found fixing infected cells with alcohol and acetone abolished ability to recover virus after 20 minutes of exposure. In view of the effectiveness of hypochlorite (bleach) in inactivation of HIV, it has been strongly recommended for distribution to intravenous drug abusers to disinfect their needles (Chaisson et al., 1987).

Martin et al. (1985) confirmed HIV to be inactivated by alcohols, hypochlorite, detergent NP-40 (but not Tween-20), hydrogen peroxide, phenolics, and paraformaldehyde at "concentrations well below those usually formulated for use as disinfectants or in the laboratory." Spire et al. (1984) studied reverse transcriptase activity of HIV after exposure to 1% glutaraldehyde and 25% ethanol, finding this viral activity to be very sensitive to these agents in these concentrations. Fresh solutions of the above were recommended to disinfect medical instruments. Hypochlorite (0.2%) was similarly tested and found to be effective, and was recommended for disinfecting potentially contaminated benches and floors.

Quinnan et al. (1986) found HIV to be "efficiently inactivated by formalin, beta-propiolactone, ethyl ether, detergent, and ultraviolet light plus psoralen."

The CDC feels the above studies suggest that no changes in basic currently recommended sterilization, disinfection, or housekeeping strategies are necessary to deal with HIV.

Practical Considerations

A number of studies using various physical and chemical agents applied to laboratory specimens from patients to render these specimens safer for handling by personnel have been reported. That such treatment does not significantly alter the results of analyses is of obvious importance. Physical and chemical agents have likewise been studied to treat biologic products to render them safe from infective transmission without significantly diminishing therapeutic efficacy.

Ball et al. (1987, 1985a, 1985b), noting previously reported studies describing effectiveness of 56°C heating against HIV, found that heat treatment of plasma "caused clinically insignificant alteration in the results of electrolyte, urea, creatinine, albumin, and glucose concentration but did specifically alter total protein and enzyme activity." Cell agglutination and hemolysis made blood specimens treated with heat unsuitable for hematologic analyses. The authors found that beta-propiolactone added to blood was effective against HIV and did not significantly alter most blood analyses for constituents including electrolyte, plasma protein, hemoglobin, white cell, and platelet counts.

Goldie et al. (1985) in an article in *Lancet* present a summary of analytic results on serum after heat treatment (56°C for 30 minutes), concluding that "most enzymes apart," heat treatment appeared to have little or no effect on analytic results. The authors suggest that heat treatment of serum before analysis "could allow AIDS patients to be offered a near-normal range of laboratory tests without great expense and without hazard to laboratory workers."

On the other hand, Ronalds et al. (1986), in a letter to the editor, offer a word of caution. They stress that, in their experience, heat treatment may alter antibody and other serum components. The authors present as example evidence the fact that heat treatment resulted in false-positive results in tests for antibody to HIV in two commercial procedures.

Eglin and Wilkinson (1987) pasteurized pooled breast milk infected with HIV in concentrations greatly exceeding "any potential natural HIV infectivity" at 56°C for 30 minutes. This completely eliminated reverse transcriptase activity. The authors concluded that pasteurization of pooled breast milk eliminated risk of HIV infection, making HIV antibody testing of donors unnecessary.

Studies of pasteurization of antithrombin III concentrate (Piszkiewicz et al., 1988) at 60°C for 7 minutes "caused infectivity of HIV to drop below the level of detectability." Prince et al. (1986) found tri(n-butyl) phosphate and sodium cholate effective in inactivating HIV diluted in factor VIII within 20 minutes at 24°C. Margolis (1986) described a process of heat sterilization of lyophilised factor VIII at 60°C for 3 days with amino acids as a stabilizer to inactivate HIV. Rouzioux et al. (1985) first reported that heat treatment of factor VIII used in a test group resulted in no seroconversions (development of antibody to HIV) among recipients, whereas use of untreated factor VIII was associated with a high rate of seroconversions. Unfortunately, significant percentages of hemophiliacs (CDC, 1987b) became HIV-antibody–positive before the testing of blood donors and before the rendering of this therapeutic blood product safe by heat treatment.

In studies with UV irradiation of blood products, Prodouz et al. (1987) found a dose-dependent reduction in virus titres (using attenuated poliovirus as a "model of a hardy RNA virus"). He did note, however, "moderate" platelet and plasma dysfunction with virucidal doses.

Since early 1985 all donated blood and plasma has been screened for HIV antibody, greatly reducing the possibility of transmission of HIV from blood and blood products. Donors are additionally screened for history of high-risk behavior and rejected as donors if such history is positive. Groopman et al. (1985) first reported two cases, one with AIDS and one with ARC, that were HIV-virus–positive but antibody-negative. Salahuddin et al. (1984) found HIV present in asymptomatic seronegative individuals. In June of 1986 the CDC reported a transfusion-associated HIV infection resulting from a seronegative donor (CDC, 1986d). Methods to destroy virus present in blood of donors in early stages of infection, when detectable antibody may be absent without destroying functional value of the blood elements, have been studied.

Mathews et al. (1988) used a "photodynamic method" (a hematoporphyrin photosensitizer) known to destroy viruses without significant changes in blood cell number, red cell lysis, plasma proteins, and other hematologic elements. The authors suggested that this approach showed promise in solving the problem of undetectable HIV and other infectious agents in blood and blood products.

HIV Disinfection and Control in Clinical Settings

As noted previously, transmission of HIV iatrogenically through blood and blood products, tissue transplants, artificial insemination, breast feeding, and accidents among health-care workers represent a small fraction of overall HIV infections.

Among health-care workers occupational risk of HIV infection is very small and most often associated with percutaneous inoculation from sharp instruments contaminated with infected blood (Gerberding et al., 1987). The risk of HIV infection following needle sticks contaminated with blood from known HIV-infected patients has been determined by various studies to be less than 1% (CDC, 1988b). The risk of exposure from infected blood on nonintact skin or mucous membranes is believed to be much lower than from percutaneous needlestick. That a small number of such cases have been reported (CDC, 1987d) underscores the need to strictly adhere to CDC recommendations for minimizing risk of exposure to blood and body fluids containing visible

blood in health-care settings. Health-care workers are urged to regard *all* patients as potentially infected with HIV and other blood-borne pathogens and adhere to recommendations in *all* patients ("universal precautions"). Recent specific detailed recommendations regarding HIV prevention have been prepared by the CDC in the major areas of medical practice, the workplace, and other settings (CDC, 1989a, 1988d, 1987a, 1986c,d, 1985a,c,d).

General Housekeeping and Management of Infectious Waste

Environmental surfaces visibly soiled with bloody or body fluids containing visible blood should be immediately cleaned. A 10% solution of household bleach is cheap, effective, and generally recommended. Other disinfectant-detergents registered with the EPA may be used (CDC, 1987a; Conte, 1986). Soiled linen should be bagged immediately and washed at temperatures of at least 71°C for 25 minutes (CDC, 1987a). The CDC (1987a) recommends that infectious waste be incinerated or autoclaved before disposal in landfills, but bulk blood and fluids may be carefully poured down drains connected to sanitary sewers.

Ophthalmology

Isolation of HIV from tears (Fujikawa et al., 1985a) conjunctival epithelium (Fujikawa et al., 1985b), the cornea (Salahuddin et al., 1986), and contact lenses in HIV-positive patients (Terro et al., 1986) along with the greatly increased incidence of HIV infection has caused concern about the potential for accidental transmission to eye physicians and associated health-care workers. The CDC published in 1985 precautions for health-care workers in preventing possible transmission in this setting (CDC, 1985a). A 5- to 10-minute exposure to a fresh solution of 3% hydrogen peroxide, or a 1/10 dilution of household bleach, or a 70% ethanol or a 70% isopropanol solution should be used on all instruments coming into direct contact with the eye. The devices should be thoroughly rinsed in tap water and dried before reuse. Hard lenses can be treated with heat of 78 to 80°C (172 to 176°F) for 10 minutes. Rigid gas-permeable trial-fitting lenses should be treated with hydrogen peroxide as described above (CDC, 1985a).

Tervo et al. (1987) detailed the effects of disinfection solutions on various ophthalmologic instruments and described methods of disinfection of specific instruments as tonometers and contact lenses. Vogt et al. (1986) tested various commercially available cleaning solutions and found them able to disinfect contact lenses exposed to HIV.

Donors of corneas should be tested prior to transplantation, although no reports of seroconversions from corneal transplants have been reported even among patients known to have received corneas from seropositive donors (Govig et al., 1988; Pepose et al., 1987a, 1987b).

"Universal precautions" do not apply to tears, because

the risk of transmission from this fluid is believed to be extremely low or nonexistent (CDC, 1988d).

Dentistry

The risk of occupationally acquired HIV infection in dentistry is believed to be very low (Klein et al., 1988). Of 1231 dentists and hygienists practicing in an area of high AIDS incidence and participating in the study, one dentist (0.1%) was found to be HIV-antibody positive. The infected dentist had no exposure to a known HIV-infected person and denied other risk factors. There was, however, a history of needlestick injuries, trauma to the hands, and failure to routinely use gloves when providing care (CDC, 1987a).

Cottone and Molinari (1987) show a photo of a dentist and dental assistant performing a simple operative procedure on a mannequin with dye used to simulate saliva. The dye is seen to splatter the faces, hair, hands, and chest, completely contaminating the operator and assistant. As previously noted, HIV has been isolated from saliva of infected individuals, but very infrequently (Ho et al., 1985b). If blood is present in the saliva, the risk of the presence of virus is greatly increased. Splashing of hepatitis B virus on the cornea of a chimpanzee resulted in infection of the animal (Bond et al., 1982).

In July, 1990 the Centers for Disease Control (CDC, 1990) reported a case of possible transmission of HIV to a young woman during an invasive dental procedure. A careful epidemiologic investigation could not establish an alternative source for her HIV infection. Two years prior to her diagnosis of AIDS the patient had two teeth extracted by a dentist who had AIDS. The above patient recalled that the dentist used gloves and a mask. Analysis of HIV isolated from the patient and dentist showed close similarities of the viral DNA sequences. CDC concluded that this case was "consistent with transmission of HIV to a patient during an invasive dental procedure although the possibility of another source of infection cannot be entirely excluded" and that "regardless of the interpretation of the findings in this investigation, adherence to universal precautions, including prevention of blood contact between health-care workers and patients and proper sterilization and disinfection of patient-care equipment, is important for prevention of transmission of bloodborne pathogens in health-care settings."

In January, 1991 the CDC updated the above case reporting four additional patients of the dentist who are infected with HIV. Two of these patients were infected with HIV strains closely related to those of the first patient and to the dentist as determined by viral DNA sequencing. One of these patients was an elderly female with no HIV risk factors and whose spouse of more than 25 years tested negative for HIV antibody. The other was a young man with multiple heterosexual partners. His wife and other female sexual partners who were tested were HIV seronegative. All three patients made numerous visits to the dentist between 1984 and 1989 for a variety of procedures. In 1989 two of the above patients

had prophylaxis performed on the same day but it is unknown if the dentist provided dental care on that day.

Investigation of the dental practice revealed no written policy or training course offered to the dentist's staff and there was no protocol for reporting injuries (as needlesticks). The dentist and an assistant recapped needles using a two-handed technique in which the exposed needle is held in one hand and the cap in the other. There was no information on any specific incidents that could have exposed the patients to the dentist's blood. Staff members stated that barrier precautions were introduced into the office in 1987 (latex gloves and masks). All surgical instruments were autoclaved and nonsurgical instruments were autoclaved or immersed in liquid chemical germicide for varying lengths of time. Other dental equipment, such as handpieces, were either wiped with alcohol or immersed in a liquid chemical germicide at irregular intervals. Germicides known to be available were isopropyl alcohol and 2% glutaraldehyde. CDC reports "the dental practice had no written protocol or consistent pattern for operatory cleanup and instrument reprocessing." The dentist "occasionally received prophylactic treatment from the hygienists; at least one hygienist topically treated an oral lesion of the dentist on one occasion in 1987."

CDC concluded that the precise mode of transmission to the three above mentioned patients is unknown. All three had invasive procedures at a time when the dentist was known to be infected. The dentist may have sustained needlestick injury during two-handed recapping or other sharp instrument injury. Barrier techniques were used but not consistently and not in compliance with recommendations. Barriers "do not prevent sharps injuries and puncture or cut wounds . . . this may have allowed dentist's blood to enter an open wound or contact mucous membranes of a patient directly." CDC also suggests that instruments contaminated with HIV infected blood may have been involved in transmission but felt this to be less likely than direct blood-blood transfer because HIV ". . . does not survive in the environment for extended periods, and has not demonstrated resistance to heat or to commonly used germicides." These cases represented the first time that HIV-possible transmission from a HCW to patients is reported. CDC again stressed "strict adherence to universal precautions including proper cleaning and sterilization or disinfection of instruments and other patient care equipment." (CDC, 1991).

In 1986 the CDC published its recommended infection-control practices for dentistry (CDC, 1986b). These include use of protective attire and other barrier techniques, handwashing, use and care of sharp instruments, and specific disinfection and sterilization procedures for instruments, surfaces, supplies, and materials, handling of biopsy material, and disposal of waste.

It is widely accepted that 2% alkalinized glutaraldehyde is the most effective immersion disinfectant. Cottone and Molinari (1987) noted that in 1978 the American

Dental Association's Council of Dental Therapeutics concluded that quaternary ammonium compounds were not acceptable for disinfection of instruments and surfaces, and yet a 1984 survey revealed that 47% of dentists responding used these compounds for these purposes.

Hemodialysis

In the 1970s the incidence of hepatitis B surface antigen positivity in hemodialysis units was very high: 16% among patients and 2.4% among staff working in the units (Szmuness et al., 1974). In 1982 the incidence decreased to 0.5% among patients and 0.4% among staff members (Favero, 1985a). These differences are believed due to adoption of strict infection-control practices. Because HIV is transmitted similarly to hepatitis B virus, the same sterilization and disinfection procedures should be protective against HIV transmission (CDC, 1986c).

There have been no reported cases of HIV transmitted at dialysis centers; a study of 520 patients in these centers concluded that HIV was not transmitted in this setting (Peterson et al., 1986). In fact, no spread of HIV from hemodialysis or any other type of medical equipment has been reported as a result of inadequate disinfection (Ayliffe, 1988).

The CDC recommends that dialysis fluid pathways be cleaned with 500 to 750 ppm sodium hypochlorite for 30 to 40 minutes or 1.5 to 2% formaldehyde overnight (CDC, 1987a). HIV patients need not be isolated from other patients in the dialysis unit (CDC, 1985c).

Endoscopy

Endoscopy brings health-care personnel into close contact with potentially infectious secretions and blood, and there has been special concern regarding the transmission of HIV in this setting. There have been, however, no documented cases of transmission of HIV by endoscopy.

Seventy-four percent of respondents to a study involving 196 adult gastroenterology training programs at university medical centers in the United States believed that endoscopy in patients with AIDS "entailed some potential risk of transmission to endoscopic personnel," although the majority (61%) believed the risk was minimal. Forty-six percent, however, used instruments specifically reserved for these patients (Raufman and Straus, 1988).

Nosocomial infections following endoscopy are rare but are reported in the literature (Webb and Vall-Spinosa, 1975; Pereira et al., 1974; O'Connor and Axon, 1983; Dean, 1977; Hawley et al., 1981; Tufnell, 1976; Beecham et al., 1979; CDC, 1977). The cause of these infections was believed to be due to inadequately disinfected endoscopes.

Birnie et al. (1983) reported a case of hepatitis B "almost certainly acquired at endoscopy from an instrument sterilized in the conventional manner (activated glutaraldehyde) but which had been used the previous day on a patient with bleeding esophageal varices who was incubating type B viral hepatitis." The source of the prob-

lem was believed to be an inadequately disinfected channel of the instrument.

In 1980, a survey of 52 large endoscopy units showed that less than half were using effective disinfecting schedules (Axon and Cotton, 1983). Katner et al. (1988) found in an American Academy of Family Physicians survey of 1585 randomly selected physicians responding that 67% of these physicians performing endoscopic examinations used disinfection procedures inadequate to inactivate HIV when compared to recommended procedures of the Centers for Disease Control.

Studies previously cited have shown HIV to be inactivated by many commonly used disinfecting agents. The CDC recommends (CDC, 1987a) that devices that come in contact with mucous membranes "be sterilized or receive high level disinfection . . . (such) medical devices or instruments should be thoroughly cleaned before being exposed to the germicide, and the manufacturer's instructions for the use of the germicide should be followed . . . it is important that the manufacturer's specifications for compatibility of the medical device with chemical germicides be closely followed."

Katner et al. (1988) stresses the importance of removal of all organic material prior to immersion in disinfectant. The Working Party of the British Society of Gastroenterology (1988) suggests that only properly trained individuals clean and disinfect endoscopes. This committee suggests that only fully immersible endoscopes be used and that "nonimmersible instruments be phased out in favor of newer immersible endoscopes."

Aliberti (1987) noted the difficulty in properly cleaning valves for forceps openings and suggested "inserting a pipe cleaner or cotton-tipped swab through the valve opening and immersing in disinfectant. Due to the spring-like configurations, accessories such as biopsy forceps are also extremely difficult to clean and disinfect. It is recommended that these accessories as well as the valves for forceps openings be purchased in sufficient quantity to allow for ethylene oxide sterilization or for prolonged disinfection by chemical agents."

Spector (1987), as editor of the *Laryngoscope*, responded to concern regarding "improper cleaning of endoscopes and the spread of infectious disease, specifically hepatitis B and AIDS" with the following procedure:

1. A 10-minute soak in sterilized soap and water
2. Thorough rinse in distilled water
3. Ten-minute soak in a 2% glutaraldehyde preparation buffered in an alkali pH 8.6 or a 1:16 dilution of a germicide containing 2% glutaraldehyde and 7% phenol
4. Air dry 10 minutes
5. Ten-minute soak in sterilized soap and distilled water
6. Thorough rinse with distilled/sterile water

Ayliffe et al. (1986) recommended 30-minute immersion of endoscopes in 2% gluaraldehyde for patients known to be positive for HIV antibody. Specter states, however, that the use of glutaraldehyde may "diminish the life expectancy of fiberoptic instruments, since the rubber and plastics become brittle and crack."

Others have expressed reservations and concerns about glutaraldehyde's irritant and sensitizing potential in persons exposed to this agent. Trigg (1984), noting in a survey she conducted that 55% of the hospitals replying reported reactions to glutaraldehyde among staff, nevertheless went on to state that "until a substitute that has the same properties as glutaraldehyde is found, there is no option but to continue using it for hospital equipment." Babb (1988) recommends that gloves be worn, immersion tanks be covered, and the agent be used and stored away from personnel. He stresses that all traces of glutaraldehyde be removed before an instrument or device be reused. Automated enclosed systems for washing and disinfecting instruments are available. They reduce staff exposure but are expensive.

Ayliffe et al. (1986), stressing the allergic and irritating qualities of glutaraldehyde, alone recommend two other aldehyde preparations as alternatives in disinfecting endoscopes. These are Sporicidin containing 2% glutaraldehyde and 7.05% phenol, and Gigasept containing succinic acid dialdehyde and formaldehyde. These combinations, according to the authors, are highly effective, nondamaging to instruments, and less irritating. The authors state, however, that Sporicidin is five times more expensive than 2% glutaraldehyde alone. Sporicidin is said by the manufacturer to kill HIV in 1 minute at room temperature (Hanson et al., 1988). Hanson feels aldehydes are the only disinfectants suitable for use with fiberoptic instruments, but quotes Spire et al. (1984) as the authors of the only real study testing the activity of glutaraldehyde against HIV: "The method used does not permit reliable extrapolation of the results to clinical practice."

Scheidt (1980) found that certain gram-negative organisms (*Pseudomonas, Klebsiella,* and *Serratia*) required 45-minute immersion in glutaraldehyde to destroy them, and recommended ethylene oxide sterilization as an alternative for endoscopes.

CONCLUSION

No proven infection with HIV has resulted from inadequately sterilized or disinfected instruments or equipment. Methods and procedures generally accepted for other pathogens appear to be adequate in preventing transmission of HIV by this route.

Health-care workers are at very low risk of becoming infected in the workplace. The few cases of transmission from accidental exposure to infected blood, however, underscore the importance of knowledge and strict adherence to CDC procedures and recommendations. Health-care workers must be carefully trained in these procedures as well as in the epidemiology, transmission, and prevention of HIV infection.

As important as it is, adequate sterilization, disinfection, and protective procedures in the health-care setting play a small role in the overall prevention of transmission of HIV. At a time when safe and effective drugs for curing, or vaccines for preventing, HIV infection may be years in the future, education of the public to reduce high risk behavior is by far the most critical aspect in bringing this new and devastating epidemic under control.

REFERENCES

Aliberti, L.C. 1987. The flexible sigmoidoscope as a potential vector of infectious disease, including suggestions for decontamination of the flexible sigmoidoscope. Yale J. Biol. Med., *60*, 19–26.

Axon, A.T.R., and Cotton, P.B. 1983. Endoscopy and infection. Gut, *24*, 1064–1066.

Ayliffe, G.A., Babb, J.R., and Bradley, C.R. 1986. Disinfection of endoscopes. J. Hosp. Inf., *7*, 296–299.

Ayliffe G.A. 1988. Equipment related infection risks. J. Hosp. Inf., *11*(Suppl. A), 279–284.

Babb, J.R. 1988. Methods of reprocessing complex medical equipment. J. Hosp. Inf., *11*(Suppl. A), 285–291.

Ball, M.J., and Griffiths, D. 1985a. Effect on chemical analyses of beta-propiolactone treatment of whole blood and plasma. Lancet, 1160.

Ball, M.J., and Griffiths, D. 1985b. Heat treatment of whole blood and serum before chemical analysis. Lancet, 1160–1161.

Ball, M.J. 1987. Effects of two disinfectant treatments on laboratory analyses. J. Roy. Soc. Med., *80*, 882–884.

Beecham, H.J., Cohen, M.L., and Parkin, W.E. 1979. Salmonella typhinurium transmission by fiberoptic upper gastrointestinal endoscopy. JAMA, *241*, 1013–1015.

Birnie, G.G., et al. 1983. Endoscopic transmission of hepatitis B virus. Gut, *24*, 171–174.

Bond, W.W., et al. 1982. Transmission of type B viral hepatitis via eye inoculation of a chimpanzee. J. Clin. Microbiol., *15*, 533.

Centers for Disease Control

1977. Salmonella gastroenteritis acquired from gastroduodenoscopy. M.M.W.R., *26*, 266.

1981a. Pneumocystis pneumonia—Los Angeles. M.M.W.R., *30*, 250–252.

1981b. Kaposi's sarcoma and pneumocystis pneumonia among homosexual men—New York City and California. M.M.W.R., *30*, 305–308.

1984. Hepatitis B vaccine: Evidence confirming lack of AIDS transmission. M.M.W.R., *33*, 685–687.

1985a. Recommendations for preventing transmission of human T-cell lymphotrophic virus type III/lymphadenopathy-associated virus from tears. M.M.W.R., *30*(34), 533–535.

1985b. Revision of the case definition of acquired immunodeficiency syndrome for national reporting—United States. M.M.W.R., *34*, 373.

1985c. Recommendations for preventing transmission of infection with human T-lymphotropic virus type III/lymphadenopathy-associated virus in the workplace—Summary. M.M.W.R., *34*, 681–686.

1985d. Recommendations for assisting in prevention of perinatal transmission of human T-lymphotropic virus type III/lymphadenopathy-associated virus and acquired immunodeficiency syndrome. M.M.W.R., *34*, 721–732.

1986a. Safety of therapeutic immune globulin preparations with respect to transmission of human T-lymphotropic virus type III/lymphadenopathy-associated virus infection. M.M.W.R., *35*, 231–233.

1986b. Recommended infection control practices for dentistry. M.M.W.R., *35*, 237–242.

1986c. Recommendation for providing dialysis treatment to patients infected with human T-lymphotropic virus type III/lymphadenopathy-associated virus. M.M.W.R., *35*(23), 376–383.

1986d. Transfusion-associated human T-lymphotropic virus type III/lymphadenopathy-associated virus infection from a seronegative donor—Colorado. M.M.W.R., *35*(24), 389–391.

1986e. Acquired immunodeficiency syndrome (AIDS) in western Palm Beach County, Florida. M.M.W.R., *35*(39), 609–612.

1987a. Recommendations for prevention of HIV transmission in health-care settings. M.M.W.R., *36*, 2S–17S.

1987b. Human immunodeficiency virus infection in the United States: A review of current knowledge. M.M.W.R., *36*, S6, 1–42.

1987c. Revision of the CDC surveillance case definition for acquired immunodeficiency syndrome. M.M.W.R., *36*(1), 155.

1987d. Update: Human immunodeficiency virus infections in health-care workers exposed to blood of infected patients. M.M.W.R., *36*(19), 285–289.

1987e. Tuberculosis and acquired immunodeficiency syndrome—New York City. M.M.W.R., *36*, 785.

1988a. AIDS due to HIV-2 infection—New Jersey. M.M.W.R., *37*, 33–35.

1988b. Acquired immunodeficiency syndrome and human immunodeficiency virus infection among health-care workers. M.M.W.R., *37*(15), 229–234.

1988c. Understanding AIDS: An information brochure being mailed to all U.S. households. M.M.W.R., 37(17), 262–269.

1988d. Update: Universal precautions for prevention of transmission of human immunodeficiency virus, hepatitis B virus, and other blood borne pathogens in health-care settings. M.M.W.R., 34(24), 377–388.

1988e. Safety of therapeutic products used for hemophilia patients. M.M.W.R., 37(29), 441–450.

1988f. Transmission of HIV through bone transplantation: Case report and public health recommendations. M.M.W.R., 37(39), 597–599.

1989a. Guideline for prevention of transmission of human immunodeficiency virus and hepatitis B virus to health care and public safety workers. M.M.W.R., 38, S–6, 1–37.

1989b. AIDS and human immunodeficiency virus infection in the United States: 1988 update. M.M.W.R., 38, S–4.

1990. Possible transmission of human immunodeficiency virus to a patient during an invasive dental procedure. M.M.W.R., 39(29), 489–493.

1990. Update: Transmission of HIV infection during an invasive dental procedure—Florida. M.M.W.R. 40(2), 21–27.

Chaisson, R.E., et al. 1987. HIV, bleach and needle sharing. Lancet, 1430.

Clarke, J.A. 1987. HIV transmission and skin grafts. Lancet, 983.

Clavel, F., et al. 1986. Isolation of a new human retrovirus from West African patients with AIDS. Science, 233, 343–346.

Conte, J.E. 1986. Infection with human immunodeficiency virus in the hospital. Ann. Int. Med., 105, 730–736.

Cooper, D.A., et al. 1985. Acute AIDS retrovirus infection. Lancet, 1, 537–540.

Cottone, J.A., and Molinari, J.A. 1987. Selection for dental practice of chemical disinfectants and sterilants for hepatitis and AIDS. Aust. Dent. J., 32(5), 368–374.

Dean, A.G. 1977. Transmission of salmonella typhii by fibreoptic endoscopy. Lancet, 2, 134.

Drummond, J.A. 1986. Seronegative 18 months after being bitten by a patient with AIDS. JAMA, 256, 2342–2343.

Eglin, R.P., and Wilkinson, A.R. 1987. HIV infection and pasteurization of breast milk. Lancet, 1093.

Fauci, A.S. 1988. The human immunodeficiency virus: infectivity and mechanisms of pathogenesis. Science, 239, 617–622.

Favero, M.S. 1985. Recommended precautions for patients undergoing hemodialysis who have AIDS or non-A, non-B hepatitis. Infect. Control, 6(8), 301–305.

Fischl, M.A., et al. 1987. The efficacy of azidothymidine (AZT) in the treatment of patients with AIDS and AIDS related complex: a double blind placebo controlled trial. N. Engl. J. Med., 317, 185–191.

Florida Medical Association. 1989. Clinical manual on HIV and AIDS. Florida Medical Assn. and Florida Department of Health and Rehabilitative Services, Jacksonville, FL.

Fox, D.M. 1987. AIDS and the American Health Polity: The history and prospects of a crisis of authority. In AIDS, The Burdens of History. Edited by E. Fee and D.M. Fox.

Fujikawa, L., et al. 1985a. Isolation of human T-lymphotrophic virus type III from the tears of a patient with AIDS. Lancet, 2, 529–530.

Fujikawa, L., et al. 1985b. Human T-cell leukemia/lymphotrophic virus type III in the conjunctival epithelium of a patient with AIDS. Am. J. Ophthalmol., 4, 507–509.

Gallo, R.C., et al. 1984. Frequent detection and isolation of a cytopathic retrovirus (HTLV-III) from patients with AIDS and at risk of AIDS. Science, 224, 500–503.

Gerberding, J.L., Hopewell, P.C., Kaminsky, L.S., and Sandie, M.A. 1985. Transmission of hepatitis B without transmission of AIDS by accidental needlestick. N. Engl. J. Med., 312, 56–57.

Gerberding, J.L., et al. 1987. Risk of transmitting the HIV, CMV, HBV to HCWs exposed to patients with AIDS and AIDS related conditions. J. Infect. Dis., 156(1), 1–8.

Goldie, D.J., McConnell, A.A., and Cooke, P.R. 1985. Heat treatment of whole blood and serum before chemical analysis. Lancet, 1160–1161.

Goldsmith, M. 1989. Seasoned AIDS warriors extend arms to rookies in the battle against HIV disease. JAMA, 262(3), 326–327.

Govig, B., Jackson, W.B., and Gilmore, N. 1988. Preventing transmission of human immunodeficiency virus in ophthalmologic practice. Can. J. Ophthalmol., 23(1), 5–7.

Groopman, J.E., et al. 1985. Antibody seronegative human T-lymphotropic virus type III infected patients with AIDS or related disorders. Blood, 66(3), 742–744.

Hanson, P.J.V., Jeffries, D.J., Batten, J.C., and Collins, J.V. 1988. Infection control revisited: dilemma facing today's bronchoscopists. B.M.J., 297, 185–187.

Hawley, P.M., et al. 1981. Contamination of endoscopes by salmonella species. J. Hosp. Infect., 2, 373–376.

Ho, D.D., et al. 1985a. Isolation of HTLV-III from cerebrospinal fluid and neural tissues of patients with neurologic symptoms related to AIDS. N. Engl. J. Med., 313, 1493–1497.

Ho, D.D., et al. 1985b. Infrequency of isolation of HTLV-III virus from saliva in AIDS. N. Engl. J. Med., 313, 1606.

Kanti, P.J., et al. 1985a. Serologic identification and characterization of a macaque T-lymphotrophic retrovirus closely related to HTLV-III. Science, 228, 1199–1201.

Kanti, P.J., et al. 1985b. Isolation of T-lymphotrophic retrovirus related to HTLV-III/LAV from wild-caught African green monkeys. Science, 230, 951–954.

Katner, H.P., Buckley, R.L., Smith, M., and Henderson, A.M. 1988. Endoscopic cleaning and disinfection procedures for preventing iatrogenic spread of human immunodeficiency virus. J. Fam. Pract., 27(3), 271–276.

Klein, R.S., et al. 1988. Low occupational risk of human immunodeficiency virus infection among dental professionals. N. Engl. J. Med., 318, 86–90.

Lane, H.C., Falloon, J., and Walker, R.E. 1989. Zidovudine in patients with human immunodeficiency virus (HIV) infection and Kaposi's sarcoma. Ann. Intern. Med., 111, 41–56.

Lepage, P., et al. 1987. Postnatal transmission of HIV from mother to child. Lancet, 2, 400.

Lifson, A.R. 1988. Do alternate modes for transmission of human immunodeficiency virus exist? JAMA, 259(9), 1353–1356.

Loschen, D.J. 1988. Protecting against HIV exposure in family practice. Am. Fam. Pract. Phys., Jan., 213–219.

Mann, J.M., and Chin, J. 1988. AIDS: A global perspective. N. Engl. J. Med., 319(5), 302–303.

Margolis, J. 1986. Heat sterilization to inactivate AIDS virus in lyophilised factor VIII. Aust. N. Z. J. Med., 16, 413.

Martin, L.S., McDougal, J.S., and Loskoski, S.L. 1985. Disinfection and inactivation of the HTLV-III/LAV. J. Infect. Dis., 152(2), 400–403.

Matlow, A.G., and Fisher, B.K. 1989. The acquired immunodeficiency syndrome. In Sexually Transmitted Diseases. Edited by L.C. Parish and F. Gschuait. Berlin, Springer-Verlag.

Matthews, J.L., et al. 1988. Photodynamic therapy of viral contaminants with potential blood banking applications. Transfusion, 28(1), 81–83.

McDougal, J.S., et al. 1985. Thermal inactivation of the acquired immunodeficiency syndrome virus, HTLV-III/LAV, with special reference to antihemophilic factor. J. Clin. Invest., 76, 875–877.

McEuen, M. 1988. Tuberculosis—threshold of an epidemic. J. Fla. Med. Assoc., 75, 355.

McEvoy, M., et al. 1987. Prospective study of clinical, laboratory, and ancillary staff with accidental exposures to blood or body fluids from patients infected with HIV. Br. J. Med., 294, 1595–1597.

Nahamias, A.J., et al. 1986. Evidence for human infection with HTLV-III/LAV like virus in central Africa. Lancet 1, 1279–1280.

O'Conner, H.J., and Axon, A.T.R. 1983. Gastrointestinal endoscopy, infection and disinfection. Gut, 24, 1067–1077.

Pepose, J.S., et al. 1987a. Serologic markers after the transplantation of corneas from donors infected with human immunodeficiency virus. Am. J. Ophthalmol., 103, 798–801.

Pepose, J.S., et al. 1987b. Screening cornea donors for antibodies against human immunodeficiency virus. Ophthalmology, 94, 95–99.

Pereira, W., et al. 1974. Complications of fiberoptic bronchoscopy. Am. Rev. Resp. Dis., 109, 67.

Peterson, T.A., et al. 1986. HTLV-III/LAV infection in hemodialysis patients. JAMA, 255(17), 2324–2326.

Piszkiewica, D., et al. 1988. Inactivation of HIV in antithrombin-III concentrate by pasteurization. Transfusion, 28(2), 198.

Popovic, M., Sargadharan, M.C., Read, E., and Gallo, R.C. 1984. Detection, isolation and continuous production of cytopathic retrovirus (HTLV-III) from patients with AIDS and pre-AIDS. Science, 224, 497–500.

Prince, A.M., Horowitz, B., and Brotman, B. 1986. Sterilization of hepatitis and HTLV-III viruses by exposure to tri (n-butyl) phosphate and sodium cholate. Lancet, 706–710.

Produoz, K., Fratantoni, J.C., Boone, E.J., and Bonner, R.F. 1987. Use of laser-UV for inactivation of virus in blood products. Blood, 70(2), 589–592.

Quinn, T.C., Zacarias, F.R.K., and St. John, R.K. 1989. AIDS in the Americas. N. Engl. J. Med., 320(5), 1005–1007.

Quinnan, G.V., et al. 1986. Inactivation of human T-cell lymphotropic virus, type III by heat, chemicals and irradiation. Transfusion, 26(5), 481–483.

Raufman, J.P., and Straus, E.W. 1988. Endoscopic procedures in the AIDS patient: risks, precautions, indications and obligations. Gastroenterol. Clin. North Am., 17(3), 495–505.

Resnick, L., et al. 1986. Stability and inactivation of HTLV-III/LAV under clinical and laboratory environments. JAMA, 255(14), 1887–1891.

Rieder, H.L., and Snider, D.E. 1986. Tuberculosis and acquired immunodeficiency syndrome. Chest, 90(4), 469.

Ronalds, C.J., Grint, P.C.A., and Kangro, H.D. 1986. Disinfection and inactivation of HTLV-III/LAV. J. Infect. Dis., 153(5), 996.

Rouzioux, C., et al. 1985. Absence of antibodies to AIDS virus in hemophiliacs treated with heat-treated factor VIII concentrate. Lancet, 271.

Salahuddin, S.Z., et al. 1984. HTLV-III in symptom-free seronegative persons. Lancet, 2, 1418.

Salahuddin, S.Z., et al. 1986. Isolation of human T-cell leukemia/lymphotrophic virus type III from the cornea. Am. J. Ophthalmol., *101*, 149–150.

Sargadharan, M.G., et al. 1984. Antibodies reactive with human T-cell lymphotrophic retroviruses (HTLV-III) in serum of patients with AIDS. Science, *224*, 506–508.

Saxinger, W.C., et al. 1985. Evidence for exposure to HTLV-III in Uganda before 1973. Science, *227*, 1036–1038.

Scheidt, A. 1980. Persistent contamination of the flexible fiberbronchoscope following disinfection in aqueous glutaraldehyde. Chest, *78*(2), 352–353.

Senturia, Y.D., Ades, A.E., Peckham, C.S., and Giaquinto, C. 1987. Breast feeding and HIV infection. Lancet, *2*, 400–401.

Shaw, G.M., et al. 1985. HLTV infection in brains of children and adults with AIDS encephalopathy. Science, *277*, 177–182.

Spector, G.J. 1987a. Letter. Laryngoscope, *97*(11), 1367.

Spector, G.J. 1987b. Cleaning of endoscopic instruments to prevent spread of infectious disease. Laryngoscope, *97*, 887.

Spire, B., Barré-Sinoussi, F., Montagnier, L., and Chermann, J.C. 1984. Inactivation of lymphadenopathy associated virus by chemical disinfectants. Lancet, 899–901.

Spire, B., et al. 1985. Inactivation of lymphadenopathy associated virus by heat, gamma ray, and ultraviolet light. Lancet, 188–189.

Stewart, G.J., et al. 1985. Transmission of human T-cell lymphotrophic virus type III (HTLV-III) by artificial insemination by donor. Lancet, 581.

Szmuness, W., et al. 1974. Hepatitis B infection. A point prevalence study in 15 U.S. hemodialysis centers. JAMA, *227*, 901–906.

Tervo, T., et al. 1986. Recovery of HTLV-III from contact lenses. Lancet, *1*, 379–380.

Tervo, T., et al. 1987. Updating of methods for prevention of HIV transmission during ophthalmological procedures. Acta. Ophthalmol (Copenhagen), *65*, 13–18.

Thiry, L., et al. 1985. Isolation of AIDS virus from cell-free breast milk of three healthy virus carriers. Lancet, *2*, 891–892.

Trigg, J.A. 1984. A sensitive issue. Nursing Mirror (N.A.T.N. Suppl.), 6–8.

Tufnell, P.G. 1976. Salmonella infections transmitted by a gastroscope. Can. J. Pub. Health, *67*, 141–142.

Vogt, M.W., et al. 1986a. Isolation of HTLV-III from cervical secretions of woman at risk of AIDS. Lancet, 525–527.

Vogt, M.W., et al. 1986b. Safe disinfection of contact lenses after contamination with HTLV-III. Ophthalmology, *93*, 771–774.

Wahn, V., et al. 1986. Horizontal transmission of HIV infection between two siblings. Lancet, 694.

Webb, S.F., and Vall-Spinosa, A. 1975. Outbreak of serratia marcescens associated with the flexible fiber bronchoscope. Chest, *68*(5), 703–708.

Wofsy, C.B., et al. 1986. Isolation of AIDS-related retrovirus from genital secretions of woman with antibodies to the virus. Lancet, 527–529.

Working Party of British Society of Gastroenterology. 1988. Cleaning and disinfection of equipment for gastrointestinal flexible endoscopy: interim recommendations of a working party of the British Society of Gastroenterology. Gut, *29*, 1134–1151.

Ziegler, J.B., Cooper, D.A., Johnson, R.O., and Gold, J. 1985. Postnatal transmission of AIDS associated retrovirus from a mother to an infant. Lancet, *1*, 896–897.

CHAPTER 28

ANTIPROTOZOAN, ANTHELMINTIC, AND OTHER PEST MANAGEMENT COMPOUNDS

S.E. Leland, Jr.

The importance of diseases caused by protozoan and helminth parasites is measured in human terms by the millions of individuals worldwide that die annually from malaria and schistosomiasis (blood flukes) and economically in the case of domestic animals, where the annual production loss due to internal parasites is estimated to be over $1.2 billion in the United States alone. An additional $3.0 billion loss in livestock production was also estimated to occur annually because of arthropod pests (Drummond et al., 1981), some of which serve as intermediate hosts or vectors for helminth or protozoan parasites.

The parasitic diseases caused by the protozoa and helminths are of a nature that sets them apart from most of the other disease-producing organisms. Special principles inevitably must be considered for each species of parasite and dictate the measures used in control. The use of chemical agents represents an important aid and component of most control programs but is not a substitute for other measures, such as sanitation or vector control, in an overall program. Nonetheless, the situation may be extremely subjective, such as one in which a heavily parasitized human, fancied pet, or otherwise valuable creature is concerned, and the more objective principles of the overall control program may be of less immediate demand. Here the practitioner may need to rely heavily on chemotherapy to buy time in order to get a control program in operation. However, if the host-parasite balance ultimately is to be shifted in favor of the host, inevitably an overall control program must be established, with prevention receiving emphasis.

Generally, a parasite is either biologically or economically more vulnerable to attack at one stage of its life cycle than at another, but measures exerted in favor of the host may be necessary on all fronts in the ideal control program. Thus, pressures may be exerted directly against the free-living stages outside the host or indirectly against the intermediate host where one is required in the completion of the life cycle, or directly against the adult parasite populations in the definitive host.

COMPOUNDS DIRECTED AGAINST THE FREE-LIVING STAGES OF THE PARASITE

The free-living stages include the encysted stages of some protozoa; the egg and/or larval stages of some of the cestodes (tapeworms) and nematodes (roundworms); and the egg, miracidial, cercarial, and metacercarial stages of some of the trematodes (flukes).

A comprehensive treatise concerning sanitary measures and the chemicals tested under laboratory conditions on the free-living stages of nematodes was set forth by Cameron (1941). The close association of these stages with feces, vegetation, soil, or large volumes of water has frustrated the use of some chemicals, whereas the application of others has resulted in the destruction of associated flora and fauna. In addition, nature has endowed the free-living stages of many parasites with qualities of resistance to chemical attack. For example, relatively high concentrations of formaldehyde, sulfuric acid, ammonium hydroxide, and cresol are necessary to prevent sporulation of coccidial oocysts. Ascaris eggs are also resistant to chemical disinfectants and temporary immersion in strong chemicals. Thus, a need exists for a safe effective compound that could, for example, be sprayed on pastures, ponds, the lawns of pet owners, or other areas suspected of harboring infective stages.

The practical application of chemical agents against free-living stages is limited to closely defined circumstances. Heavy applications of brine to the soil of dog runs, for example, prevent the development of hookworm larvae but destroy all plant life. The penetrability of colloidal iodine makes the suspensoid destructive to oocysts of *Eimeria tenella* and infective nematode larvae where the material can be brought in contact with exposed oocysts or larvae. Ammonia gas and strong ammonia solutions are lethal for oocysts (Horton-Smith et al., 1940) and have been recommended for scrubbing down infective premises and equipment. In the classic work of York and Adams (1926) the resistance of *Entamoeba histolytica* cysts to various drugs and chemicals was explored using in-vitro cultivation of the exposed cysts as a criterion for viability. Under these conditions the lethal concentrations of HCL, chlorine, mercuric chloride, potassium permanganate, formaldehyde, lysol, and carbolic acid were ascertained. Tetraglycine hypoperiodide compounded with the acidic excipient, disodium dihydrogen pyrophosphate, and talc is cysticidal for *E. histolytica* and cercaricidal for schistosomes. It has been applied as a disinfectant of water canteens by the United States Army. Jarroll et al. (1981) studied the dynamics of chlorine disinfection of water containing *Giardia lamblia* cysts and noted that pH, chlorine demand, and temperature of the water influence successful inactivation. Chlorination alone as a dependable means of water treatment in the absence of a cyst filtration component is in question. In recent years a new class of solid-phase disinfectants has emerged in which triiodide (Triocide) or pentaiodide (Pentacide) is complexed to the strong base, quaternary ammonium anion exchange resin. As demand-release disinfectants, they release the active agent to the microorganism or to organic molecules in solution but introduce little or no disinfectant residual in the aqueous environment. When water containing microorganisms is allowed to flow through these resins, collisions of the microorganisms with the iodinated beads results in release of iodine to the microorganism with subsequent devitalization. A broad-spectrum water disinfectant, based on this principle, with the pentaiodide-resin has been efficacious against a large number of bacterial genera, virus, and representative parasites such as *G. lamblia*, *G. muris*, and *Cryptosporidium parvum* (Marchin et al., 1983, 1985; Upton et al., 1988). Marchin et al. (1983, 1985) noted that in all trials and at all concentrations of *G. lamblia* or *G. muris* cysts that were tested, there was significant excystation when the cysts were passed through the triiodide-resin. This was in contrast to the results with the pentaiodine-resin, where essentially complete devitalization of the cysts was obtained. Noting that cysticidal activity of traditional chlorination is problematic, the authors point out that the Pentacide can be manufactured to yield an iodine residual of 8.0 to 0.5 ppm, whereas in the case of the Triocide a nearly undetectable residual can be achieved. The use of the two resins in series, therefore, results in the Triocide sequestering residual iodine released by the Pentacide. The authors suggest the iodinated resin-disinfectants merit consideration as alternate devices where safe, potable water is needed. The Environmental Protection Agency has ruled that iodine disinfection is acceptable for short-term, limited, or emergency use but that it is not recommended for longterm or routine community water supply application where the iodide-containing

species may remain in the drinking water (Schaub, 1986). Marchin and Fina (1989) have reviewed the commercial devices on the market that utilize iodinated resin disinfectants. The iodine resin devices have been used in camping equipment and embassies in countries abroad. The iodine resins have also found successful application in the manned U.S. Space Program. Upton et al. (1988) reported the oocysts of *C. parvum* were retained on a pentaiodide resin column in a one-hit manner and that, although killing of parasites may occur within the column, the greatest effect may have been electrostatic retention.

Methyl bromide is lethal for most parasite ova (Swanson, 1943) and coccidial oocysts (Clapham, 1950), but practical use of fumigation procedures is limited by cost, methods of application, and toxicity.

A more successful application of the chemical attack against the free-living stages in some cases has been accomplished indirectly through the oral administration of compounds to the parasitized host (feed-through). Thus, daily administration of small amounts of phenothiazine to sheep, cattle, or horses results in sufficient concentration in the excreted feces to prevent larval development of most gastrointestinal nematodes. Feed-through administration of diflubenzuron and tetrachlorvinphos is also used to control arthropod development in excreted feces. Several techniques have evolved that depend on the recovery of worm eggs from the feces, followed by incubation in serial concentrations of a compound in order to determine the influence on egg embryonation or ability to hatch. Thiabendazole at a concentration of less than 1 ppm in vitro was shown to completely inhibit embryonic development of *Ascaris suis* (Egerton, 1961). Leland and Bogue (1964) observed inhibition of larval development of *Strongyloides ransomi* from the egg when thiabendazole was mixed with the feces at concentrations down to 25 to 50 ppm (g of drug/g of feces). Likewise, Stone et al. (1964) reported that when thiabendazole was added to charcoal-feces cultures, the eggs of *Ancylostoma caninum* failed to develop into infective larvae. Le Jambre (1976) and Kirsch (1978) employed an egg-hatch technique to measure benzimidazole resistance in certain strains of gastrointestinal nematodes of sheep. Resistance to benzimidazole anthelmintics in vivo was detectable in vitro by reduction or loss in ovicidal activity.

COMPOUNDS DIRECTED AGAINST THE INTERMEDIATE HOSTS OF THE PARASITE OR THE PARASITE WITHIN THE INTERMEDIATE HOST

The intermediate host is biologically required for the completion of the life cycle of some parasites in that some development or maturation takes place and makes the parasite capable of infecting the definitive host. This is in contrast to mechanical vectors that are not required biologically to complete the life cycle but serve in a dissemination capacity. Designation as an intermediate host relates to the host that harbors larval stages of the helminth or asexual stages of a protozoan, whereas the definitive host harbors the adult plus, in some cases, larval stages of a helminth, or the sexually mature stages plus asexual stages in the case of a protozoan.

In the case of some parasites that require an intermediate host, the life cycle has been successfully interrupted through the use of chemical agents directed against these vectors. Intermediate hosts for protozoan or helminth parasites are represented in several of the major animal groupings, including vertebrates. However, chemical agents have been used most extensively against certain invertebrate intermediate hosts.

Insecticides

The discovery of longlasting synthetic organic compounds such as chlorophenothane (DDT) revolutionized the concept of vector control and, for a time, control and even eradication of many arthropod-borne diseases on a worldwide basis seemed within reach. However, the protective hand of nature was destined to intervene in defense of even these undesirable species that man seeks to render extinct. Thus, a case in point is insecticide resistance. Cooperative efforts among field observers, the research institutes in Europe, Asia, and America, and the World Health Organization (WHO, 1964) confirmed resistance in mosquitoes. Since house flies first developed resistance to DDT in 1946, more than 428 species of arthropods were reported to have developed strains resistant to one or more pesticides. Resistance to pesticides is generally regarded as one of the most serious obstacles to effective pest control (Georghiou and Mellon, 1983). The demise of DDT was further ensured with the advent of research that established its low order of biodegradation in the environment, its resistance to mammalian metabolism, and its solubility in fatty tissues. Thus, animals exposed to DDT in the environment (soil, water, plant tissue, etc.) accumulate the chemical in their fatty tissues and, as prey, cause further accumulation in their predators; this condition in the food chain is termed biomagnification.

However, lest we deal too glibly with the established negative aspects of DDT, we should allude to a consideration that has recently become part of the pesticide vernacular, the cost-benefit ratio. In the case of DDT, numerous deaths and immeasurable suffering from malaria and other insect-borne diseases were prevented during World War II. Because of its effectiveness and low cost (less than $.22 per lb), DDT was used extensively following the war against agricultural insect pests. Its overuse and abuse, along with the influence on the environment and human health, resulted in the EPA banning its use, effective January 1, 1973, except for products used: (1) to control vector diseases by U.S. Public Health and other Health Service Officials, (2) by USDA or military for health quarantine, (3) in formulations for controlling human body lice (dispensed by physicians only), and (4) other situations considered on a case basis.

The lesson to be learned from the rise and fall of DDT is well stated by Ware (1978): "There is an absolute need for an informed, cautious, and—according to available knowledge—correct way of employing a specific chemical for pest control; it is quite likely that new 'DDT cases' are in the making; and, consequently, there is necessity for basic research performed in autonomous institutions not subject to the need for competing in the economic market place. And, because this research is basic, as opposed to applied, it will of necessity be slow, expensive, long-term and not immediately applicable."

Among the compounds used for the destruction of larval or adult arthropods in their particular habitat (residual sprays) are the organophosphates dimpylate (Diazinon), dichlorovos (DDVP, Vapona), dimenthoate (Cygon), fenthion (Baytex, Tiguvon), tetrachlorvinphos (stirofos, Rabon), and the pyrethroids fenvalerate (Ectrin) and permethrin (Expar, Permectrin and many other brands). Synergists such as N-octy bicycloheptene dicarboximide (MGK 264) and peperonyl butoxide are used to stabilize and prolong the active life of rotenone, pyrethrins, allethrin, and other synthetic pyrethroids. A more comprehensive list of compounds with their physical and chemical characteristics has been compiled elsewhere (Sine, 1989). Mock (1987, 1988) lists current compounds used in beef cattle and swine.

Additional classes of chemical substances are emerging through accelerated basic and biologic research efforts. Insect growth regulators (IGRs) are agents that interfere with normal insect development. Because most IGRs interfere with the juvenile-hormone-regulated growth process, these compounds are also known as juvenile hormone mimics, juvenile hormones, juvenile hormone analogs and synthetic juvenile hormones. Other forms of IGRs include cyromazine (a triazine-type IGR), L-canavanine (an arginine analogue) and diflubenzuron (a chitin synthase inhibitor) (Mock and Greene, 1989). Most IGRs exert their influence by interfering with cuticle development, causing sterility or death of the insect. In some cases, death may occur at a stage beyond the one that was exposed to the IGR. Current information on a number of IGRs indicates a high degree of safety for man and animals. Methoprene (Altoside SR-10) is now marketed for mosquito control in cattle mineral (Altoside) or bolus (Inhibitor) formulations for horn fly control, and as a flea larvicide (Precor). Diflubenzuron is marketed in cattle bolus (Vigilante) for horn fly and face fly control. Cyromazine (Larvalex) is used as a feed additive to provide fly control in and around caged or slatted flooring in layer and breeder poultry (chickens only) operations.

Another group of chemical substances, called sex pheromones, are produced and released by insects and cause a sexual response or attraction to the opposite sex of the same species. Some substances attract or sexually excite both sexes and are known as aggregating pheromones. Pheromones find application in suppression of insect populations as attractants in bait traps and in conjunction with chemical sterilants or insecticides. The Z isomer of a synthetic pheromone (Z)-9-trecosene (Muscalure) is used in several commercially prepared house fly baits in combination with either the carbamate insecticide methomyl or the organophosphate bomyl. The significance of the isomerism was demonstrated in experiments by Carlson et al. (1971), where more flies were attracted with 50 μg of the Z isomer than with 200 μg of the E isomer.

A mixture of 10 chemicals, including butyl alcohols, dimethyl disulfide, phenol, p-cresol, indole, and acetic, benzoic, butyric, and valeric acids (swormlure-2), was used in detection and suppression systems for adult screw worms, *Cochliomyia hominivorax* (Snow et al., 1982).

In some host-parasite cycles, the intermediate host is an external parasite on the definitive host for varying periods of time. For example, the dog flea, *Ctenocephalides canis*, the cat flea, *C. felis*, the human flea, *Pulex irritans*, and the louse of the dog, *Trichodectes canis*, can harbor the cysticercoid larva of the tapeworm *Dipylidium caninum*. The cysticercoid develops into an adult tapeworm when dog, cat, or man ingests the infected intermediate host.

Chemical agents are directed against ectoparasites and in this manner apply pressure at this point in the life cycle of the internal parasite. The chemical agents are applied topically in the form of dusts, dips, sprays, pourons, spot-ons, and impregnated ear tags, and orally as systemics or feed-throughs to the host harboring the arthropod ectoparasites. Examples of these agents are found in several chemical groupings and include: the plant products rotenone and the pyrethrins; the chlorinated hydrocarbons methoxychlor, toxaphene, and the gamma isomer of benzene hexachloride (lindane); the organophosphates; dimpylate (Diazinon), dichlorvos, famphur, fenthion, malathion, coumaphos, and trichlorfon; the carbamate carbaryl (Sevin); the formamidine amitraz (Mitaban, Taktic); and the pyrethroids fenvalerate (Ectrin), permethrin (Expar, Permectrin, and others), flucythrinate (Guardian), and cypermethrin. A more extensive list of these agents and their physical and chemical characteristics was compiled by Theodorides (1985) and Moch (1987, 1988).

Repellents

By limiting exposure to ectoparasites, repellents likewise reduce contact between the arthropod intermediate host and definitive host. Such repellency is usually limited to a matter of hours; for continued protection frequent applications may be necessary. Some repellent are not used on the host; di-n-butylsuccinate (Tabatres), for example, is applied to premises but not to livestock. Dimethyl phthalate is used as a repellent for mosquitoes, flies, fleas, and chiggers. Di-n-propyl isocinchromeronate (MGK 326) is used as a spray on livestock and agricultural premises. The compound 2, 3:4, 5 bis (2-butyline) tetrahydro-2-furfural (MGK 11) has been used in combination with insecticidal compounds for fleas, lice, and ticks on dogs and cats. Sine (1989) lists various compounds used as repellents and provides their chemical and physical descriptions.

Molluscicides

Molluscicidal compounds are used in the chemical control of the intermediate hosts of disease-producing trematodes of man and domestic animals. The molluscan host in many instances is the weakest link in the life cycle of these parasites. The choice and use of compounds as molluscicides require consideration of diversity and extent of habitat, physiologic differences, habits, and ecology of the various snail species. The molluscicides currently used in control programs are: niclosamide as the ethanolamine salt (Bayluscid), pentachlorophenol (PCP), and methocarb (Mesurol).

Rodenticides

Some parasites utilize rodents as an intermediate host, as for example the rat in the case of the tapeworm *Taenia taeniaformis* of the cat, and the nematode *Trichinella spiralis* of swine. Rodenticides can therefore be utilized to control the intermediate host. Their use, however, must be conditioned since, as in completion of the life cycle of the parasite the definitive host comes in contact with the intermediate host, so may the definitive host come in contact with the rodenticide. Lethal quantities of the rodenticide may reach the definitive host by direct consumption of bait or by ingestion of the poisoned intermediate host.

Compounds with rodenticidal activity are found in the following groups:

Botanical
    The alkaloid, strychnine ($C_{21}H_{22}N_2O_2$)
    Red squill, from *Urginea martima*, the sea onion
Coumarins
    Dicumarol
    Warfarin
    Coumochlor (Tomorin)
    Coumatetralyl (Racumin)
    Coumafuryl (Fumarin)
    Diphacinone (Diphacin)
Indandiones
    Chlorophacinone
    Pindone (Pival)
Pyriminilureas
    Pyriminil (Vacor)
Others
    Alpha-Naphthylthiourea (Antu)
    Phosphorus
    Sodium fluoroacetate (1080)
    Thallium sulfate
    Zinc phosphide
    Sodium cyanide (fumigant)

Hone and Mulligan (1982) reviewed the literature on 38 vertebrate pesticides. Information was provided on physical and chemical properties, mode of action, known antidote, legal status, and chronic and acute toxicity. Sine

Table 28–1. *Compounds Directed Against Protozoans, Helminths, and Other Pests*

Group and/or Compound		*Formula*	*Sensitive Organisms*	*References*
Alkaloids	Emetine	 Emetine dihydrochloride	Amebae	Norris and Ravdin (1988)
	Quinine* Quinidine (d-enantiomer of Quinine)	 *6-methoxy-α-(5-vinyl-2-quinuclidinyl)-4-quinolinemethanol	Malaria	Desjardins and Trenholme (1984)
	Amprolium	 1-(4-amino-2-n-propyl-5-pyrimidinylmethyl) -2-picolinium chloride hydrochloride	Coccidia	Cuckler et al. (1960)
Antibiotics	Avermectin (eight major naturally occurring compounds) from *Streptomyces avermitilis*	 A_1 R_5 = CH_3 A_2 R_5 = CH_3 B_1 R_5 = H B_2 R_5 = H a series R_{25} = $CH(CH_3)C_2H_5$ b series R_{25} = $CH(CH_3)_2$	Nematode parasites of cattle, sheep, dogs, and chickens	Campbell (1985)
	Ivermectin (MK-933, abamectin, Ivomec, Eqvalan). 22,23-Dihydroavermectin B_1 is a synthetic derivative of avermectin B_1 and exists as a mixture containing not less than 80% of the B_{1a} and not more than 20% of the B_{1b} form of 22,23-Dihydroavermectin.		Broad-spectrum anthelmintic activity in sheep, cattle, dogs, poultry; activity against parasitic arthropods; horses	Campbell (1985)
	Hygromycin B	 Fermentation product of *Streptomyces hygroscopicus*	Intestinal nematodes of swine and poultry	Shumard and McCowen (1963)
	Monensin	 Fermentation product of *Streptomyces cinnamonensis* $C_{36}H_{62}O_{11}$	Avian coccidia	Shumard and Callender (1967)

Table 28–1. *Compounds Directed Against Protozoans, Helminths, and Other Pests* Continued

Group and/or Compound		Formula	Sensitive Organisms	References
Antimony Compounds	Lithium antimony thiomalate Stibophen Potassium antimony tartrate Sodium antimony tartrate Antimony dimercaptosuccinate Ethylstibamine (Neostibosan) Sodium antimony gluconate* Antimony-N-methyl-glutamine (Glucantime, Rhodis)	*(structure)* *Sodium antimony gluconate (Solustibosan, Pentostam)	*Leishmania donovani* *Leishmania tropica* *Leishmania braziliensis* Schistosomes in humans (Penta and Trivalent antimonials)	Marr (1984) Bennett and Depenbusch (1984)
Atabrine (quinacrine HCl, mepacrine 2HCl)		*(structure)* 6-chloro-9-(4-diethylamino-1-methyl-butyl-amino)-2-methoxyacridine dihydrochloride	Malaria *Leishmania tropica* *Giardia lamblia* Adult tapeworms in man	Desjardins and Trenholme (1984) Theodorides (1985)
Benzimidazole Carbamates	Albendazole Cambendazole Fenbendazole Mebendazole Oxibendazole Oxfendazole Thiabendazole*	*(structure)* *2-(4′thiazolyl)-benzimidazole	Gastrointestinal nematodes of horses, sheep, cattle, swine, poultry, and man	Drudge (1964) Drudge et al. (1964) Leland and Combs (1965) Theodorides (1985)
Bephenium/Thenium Compounds	Bephenium hydroxynaphthoate	*(structure)* $C_{11}H_7O_3{}^-$ Benzyldimethyl-2-phenoxy-ethylammonium-3-hydroxy-2-naphthoate	Mucosa-dwelling intestinal nematodes of cattle, sheep, dogs, and man	Csaky and Barnes (1984)
	Thenium closylate	*(structure)* $C_6H_4ClO_3S$ N,N-dimethyl-N-2-phenoxyethyl-N-2′-thenylammonium-p-chlorobenzenesulfonate	*Ancylostoma caninum* *Uncinaria stenocephala*	Rawes and Clapham (1961)
Bisphenols	Bithionol* Dichlorophen (di-phenthane-70) Hexachlorophene	*(structure)* *2,2′-thiobis(4,6-dichlorophenol)	Tapeworms Flukes	Kendall and Parfitt (1962) Theodorides (1985)
Chlorinated Hydrocarbons	Tetrachlorethylene	*(structure)* Tetrachlorethylene	Hookworms in humans Flukes in humans	Theodorides (1985)

Table 28–1. *Compounds Directed Against Protozoans, Helminths, and Other Pests* Continued

Group and/or Compound		Formula	Sensitive Organisms	References
Chloroquine (Aralen)		7-chloro-4-(4-diethylamino-1-methylbutylamino) quinoline diphosphate	Malaria Amebae Giardia Flukes	Norris and Ravdin (1988) Desjardins and Trenholme (1984)
Coumarins	Warfarin* Dicumarol	*3-(α-acetonylbenzyl)-4-hydroxycoumarin	Rodents	Hone and Mulligan (1982) Sine (1989) Csaky and Barnes (1984)
Cyanine Dyes	Pyrvinium pamoate* Dithiazanine iodide Quinazine toluene sulphonate Stilbazium iodide	*Bis-6-dimethylamino-2-[(2,5-dimethyl-α-phenyl-3-pyrrolyl vinyl]-1-methyl-quinolinium pamoate	Pinworms Strongyloides *Trichuris trichiura* Microfilaria	Csaky and Barnes (1984)
Diamidines	Stilbamidine Diaminazineaceturate Pentamidine* Propamidine	*4,4'-diamidino-1,5-diphenoxypentane	Leishmania Trypanosomes	Marr (1984) Meshnick (1984)
Diodoquin		Diiodohydroxyquinoline	Amebae Balantidium Giardia	Norris and Ravdin (1988)
Disophenol (DNP)		2,6-di-iodo-4-nitrophenol	*Ancylostoma caninum*	Theodorides (1985)

Table 28–1. *Compounds Directed Against Protozoans, Helminths, and Other Pests* Continued

Group and/or Compound		Formula	Sensitive Organisms	References
Insect Growth Regulators (IGRs)	Diflubenzuron		Mosquitoes Flies	Sparks and Hammock (1983)
	Methoprene		Face and horn flies	Mock (1987) Miller et al. (1978)
Imidazothiazoles	Levamisole	1-2,3,5,6-tetrahydro-6-phenyl-imidazo-[2,1-*b*]-thiazole HCl	Lungworm and gastrointestinal nematodes of swine and cattle	Lindquist et al. (1971) Leland et al. (1980)
	Tetrahydropyrimidine (imidazothiazole derivative) Pyrantel pamoate Pyrantel* tartrate Morantel tartrate	*trans-1,4,5,6-tetrahydro-1-methyl-2-[2-(-thienyl) vinyl] pyrimidine	Gastrointestinal nematodes of dogs, horses, and swine	Lyons et al. (1975) Roberson (1977)
Nitroimidazoles	Metronidazole (Flagyl)* Ornidazol (Tiberal) Tinidazole (Fasigyn)	*1(2'-hydroxyethyl)-2-methyl-5-nitroimidazole	Trichomonads in humans Amebiasis	Norris and Ravdin (1988)
Niclosamide	Ethanolamine salt form (Bayluscide) used as molluscicide	N-(2'-chloro-4-nitrophenyl)-5-chlorsalicylamide	Tapeworms Mollusks	Boisvenue and Hendrix (1965) Sine (1989)
Niridazole (Ambilhar)		1-(5-nitro-2-thiazolyl)-2-imidazolidinone	Schistosomes and *Dracunculus medinensis*	Bennett and Depenbusch (1984)
Organophosphates	Trichlorphon* Ruelene Coumaphos Dichlorvos	*0,0-dimethyl-1-hydroxy-2-trichloroethyl phosphonate	Gastrointestinal nematodes of cattle, sheep, and swine	Broome (1962) Theodorides (1985)

Table 28–1. *Compounds Directed Against Protozoans, Helminths, and Other Pests* Continued

Group and/or Compound		Formula	Sensitive Organisms	References
Phenothiazine		Thiodiphenylamine	Gastrointestinal nematodes of horses, sheep, and cattle	Broome (1962) Drudge et al. (1964) Leland et al. (1957)
Piperazines	Diethylcarbamazine* Piperazine citrate Piperazine adipate	*1-diethylcarbamyl-4-methylpiperazine	Ascarids in man and animals Filaria	Csaky and Barnes (1984)
Phermones	(z)-9-tricosene (muscalure)		House fly	Carlson et al. (1971)
Phthalates	Dimethylphthalate (DMP)	dimethyl-1,2-benzenedicarboxylate	Flies Fleas Chiggers	Sine (1989)
Pyrethroides	Cypermethrin Fenvalerate Flucythinate Permethrin Pyrethrin*	2,2,dimethyl-3-(2-methylpropenyl)cyclokpro-panecarboxylic acid ester with 4-hydroxy-3-methyl-2-(2,4-pentadienyl)-2 cyclopenten-1-one	Mites Lice Ticks	Mock (1987, 1988)
Sulfonamides	Sulfaguanidine* Sulfadimidine Sulfaquinoxaline Sulfamethoxine Sulfamethazine Sulfadoxine Sulfalene Sulfamethoxazole	*p-aminobenezenesulfonylguanidine	Coccidia Malaria	Desjardins and Trenholme (1984)
Suramin (Bayer 205)		Sodium salt of 8,8'-[3″,3″ '-ureylene-bis(3″ ″-benzamido-4″ ″ -methyl-benzamido) bis-1,3,5-naphthalenetrisulfonic acid	Trypanosome and filaria in humans	Meshnick (1984)

(1989) also provides a list of rodenticides with related characteristics.

Nondestructive Treatment

Some compounds are used in the nondestructive treatment of the intermediate hosts. In the case of some parasites, man or a domesticated animal is the intermediate host. The bladderworms of the *Taeniidae* are an example, and in such cases the immediate goal is to free the intermediate host of the larval stages. In general, chemical agents have not been successful against these stages. Control through chemotherapy has been achieved by treatment of the definitive host for the adult parasite, thereby reducing the opportunity for intermediate hosts to become infected.

Technically speaking, man is an intermediate host to the species of *Plasmodium* that cause human malaria, because the sexual cycle occurs in the mosquito. This host-parasite relationship is also true in avian malaria.

COMPOUNDS DIRECTED AGAINST THE PARASITIC STAGES IN THE DEFINITIVE HOST

The definitive host harbors the adult or sexually mature parasite and such larvae, or developmental stages that occur between the time of infection and patency. Although the use of chemical agents against these stages actually represents chemotherapy, which is not a major topic for consideration here, some mention is deemed appropriate to achieve greater perspective concerning the generally complex life cycle these organisms undergo. In addition, certain compounds administered to the host exert their influence against the preinfective stages in the excreted feces of the host (feed-through). Certain of the compounds used chemotherapeutically against the protozoans, helminths and other pests are also used as disinfectants for other organisms discussed in this volume and, thus, have overall interest.

Because the function of a successful chemotherapeutic agent is to exert maximum destructive influence on the parasite while exerting no influence or only minimal undesirable effect on the host, the resulting differential in essence defines the practical activity a particular compound may possess. Included in Table 28–1 are examples of chemotherapeutic agents with the general group of parasites against which they have been used or tested.

Thus, a wide variety of chemical substances have been employed for the control or treatment of diseases caused by protozoa or helminths. These substances have been directed at a variety of situations in the life cycle of the various parasites, including the free-living stages, the intermediate host or vector, and against specific points in the parasitic stages. Active compounds are represented in many of the major chemical groupings. These compounds have evolved almost entirely from empirical methods of screening, and only in retrospect has mode of action been studied. The complicated relationship existing between host and parasite has limited the infor-

mation available concerning basic physiology and biochemistry of the parasitic stages, so that a rational or guided approach to chemotherapy has not always been possible. As the fund of knowledge concerning the metabolic reactions of these parasites increases, possibly through improved in vitro cultivation or other means (Mansour, 1979), the differential metabolic processes between host and parasite may allow predictable selection of antiprotozoan and anthelmintic compounds. Since the last edition of this book, continued and somewhat increased interest in the mode of action of chemical agents used against parasites and pests has occurred, as exemplified by Campbell (1985) and recorded by Csaky and Barnes (1984).

REFERENCES

Bennett, J.L., and Depenbusch, J.W. 1984. The chemotherapy of schistosomiasis. In *Parasitic Diseases*. Volume 2, The chemotherapy. Edited by J.M. Mansfield. New York, Marcel Dekker, pp. 73–117.

Boisvenue, R.J., and Hendrix, J.C. 1965. Prophylactic treatment of experimental *Raillietina cesticillus* infection in chickens with Yomesan. J. Parasitol., *51*, 519–522.

Broome, A.W.J. 1962. Mechanisms of anthelmintic action with particular reference to drugs affecting neuromuscular activity. In *Drugs, Parasites, and Hosts*. Edited by L.G. Goodwin and R.H. Nimmo-Smith. Boston, Little, Brown, pp. 43–61.

Campbell, W.C. 1985. Ivermectin: An Update. Parasitol. Today, *1*, 10–16.

Cameron, T.W.M. 1941. Epidemiology and sanitary measures for the control of nemic parasites of domesticated animals. In *Introduction to Nematology*, Section II, Part II. Babylon, Edited by M.B. Chitwood, pp. 302–308.

Carlson, D.A., et al. 1971. Sex attractant pheromone of the house fly. Isolation, identification and synthesis. Science, *174*, 76–77.

Clapham, P.A. 1950. On sterilizing land against poultry parasites. J. Helminthol., *24*, 137–144.

Csaky, T.Z., and Barnes, B.A. 1984. *Cutting's Hand Book of Pharmacology—The Actions and Uses of Drugs*. 7th Edition. Norwalk, CT, Appleton-Century-Crofts.

Cuckler, A.C., Garzillo, M., Malanga, C., and McManus, E.C. 1960. Amprolium I. Efficacy for coccidia in chickens. Poult. Sci., *39*, 1241.

Desjardins, R.E., and Trenholme, G.M. 1984. Antimalarial chemotherapy. In *Parasitic Diseases*. Volume 2, The chemotherapy. Edited by J.M. Mansfield. New York, Marcel Dekker, pp. 1–71.

Drudge, J.H. 1964. Control of migrating *Strongylus vulgaris*. Mod. Vet. Pract., *45*, 29.

Drudge, J.H., Szanto, J., Wyant, Z.N., and Elam, G. 1964. Field studies on parasite control in sheep: comparison of thiabendazole, ruelene, and phenothiazine. Am. J. Vet. Res., *25*, 1512–1518.

Drummond, R.D., Lambert, G., Smalley, H.E., and Terrill, C.E. 1981. Estimated losses of livestock to pests. In *CRC Hand Book of Pest Management in Agriculture*. Volume 1. Edited by D. Pimentel. Boca Raton, FL, CRC Press, pp. 111–127.

Egerton, J.R. 1961. The effect of thiabendazole upon Ascaris and Stephanurus infections. Parasitol., *47*(Suppl.), 37.

Georghiou, G.P., and Mellon, R.B. 1983. Pesticide resistance in time and space. In *Pest Resistance to Pesticides*. Edited by G.P. Georghiou and T. Saito. New York, Plenum Press, pp. 1–46.

Hone, J., and Mulligan, H. 1982. Vertebrate Pesticides. Edited by John Pitt. Science Bulletin 87. Dept. Agri., New South Wales, Division of Res. & Advisory Services, Haymarket, Sydney, Australia.

Horton-Smith, C., Taylor, E.L., and Turtle, E.E. 1940. Ammonia fumigation for coccidial disinfection. Vet. Rec., *27*.

Jarroll, E.L., Bingham, A.K., and Meyer, E.A. 1981. Effect of chlorine on *Giardia lamblia* cyst viability. Appl. Environ. Microbiol., *41*, 483–487.

Kendall, S.B., and Parfitt, J.W. 1962. The chemotherapy of fascioliasis. Br. Vet. J., *118*, 1–10.

Kirsch, R. 1978. *In vitro* and *in vivo* studies on the ovicidal activity of fenbendazole. Res. Vet. Sci. 25, 263–265.

Le Jambre, L.F. 1976. Egg hatch as an in vitro assay of thiabendazole resistance in nematodes. Vet. Parasitol., *2*, 385–391.

Leland, S.E., Jr., and Bogue, J.H. 1964. Laboratory tests on the anthelmintic activity of thiabendazole against the free-living stages of *Strongyloides ransomi*. J. Parasitol., *50*(Suppl.), 61.

Leland, S.E., Jr., and Combs, G.E. 1965. Tests of anthelmintic activity (utilizing experimental challenge) against the migratory stages of *Strongyloides ransomi* in pigs. Am. J. Vet. Res., *26*, 932–938.

Leland, S.E., Jr., Drudge, J.H., and Wyant, Z.N. 1957. Strain variation in the response of sheep nematodes to action of phenothiazine III. Field observations. Am. J. Vet. Res., *18*, 851–860.

Leland, S.E., Jr., et al. 1980. Economic value and course of infection after treatment of cattle having a low level of nematode parasitism. Am. J. Vet. Res., *41*, 623–633.

Lindquist, W.D., Leland, S.E., Jr., and Ridley, R.K. 1971. Field experiment on Levamisole against certain helminths in pigs, with emphasis on tests of activity against lungworms. Am. J. Vet. Res., *32*, 1301–1304.

Lyons, E.T., Drudge, J.H., and Tolliver, S.C. 1975. Field tests of three salts of pyrantel against internal parasites of the horse. Am. J. Vet. Res., *36*, 161–166.

Mansour, T.E. 1979. Chemotherapy of parasitic worms: New biochemical strategies. Science, *205*, 462–469.

Marchin, G.L., and Fina, L.R. 1989. Contact and demand release disinfectants. In *Critical Reviews in Environmental Control*. Edited by C.P. Straub. Boca Raton, FL, CRC Press, *19*, 277–290.

Marchin, G.L., Fina, L.R., and Lambert, J.L. 1985. The biocidal properties of the pentacide/demand-type resin I$_5$. Proc. Am. Water Works Assoc., Water Qual. Tech. Conf., Dec 8–11, pp. 461–472.

Marchin, G.L., Fina, L.R., Lambert, J.L., and Fina, G.T. 1983. Effect of resin disinfectants -I$_3$ and -I$_5$ on *Giardia muris* and *Giardia lamblia*. Appl. Environ. Microbiol., *46*, 965–969.

Marr, J.J. 1984. The chemotherapy of Leishmaniasis. In *Parasitic Diseases*. Volume 2. The chemotherapy. Edited by J.M. Mansfield. New York, Marcel Dekker, pp. 201–227.

Meshnick, S.R. 1984. The chemotherapy of african trypanosomiasis. In *Parasitic Diseases*. Volume 2. The chemotherapy. Edited by J.M. Mansfield. New York, Marcel Dekker, pp. 165–199.

Miller, R.W., Picken, L.G., and Hunt, L.M. 1978. Methoprene: Field tested as a feed additive for control of face flies. J. Econ. Entomol., *71*, 274–278.

Mock, D.E. 1987. Managing insect problems on beef cattle. Publication C-671 (Revised). Cooperative Extension Service, Kansas State Univ., Manhattan, KS.

Mock, D.E. 1988. Lice, mange and other swine insect problems. Publication C-766 (Revised). Cooperative Extension Service, Kansas State Univ., Manhattan, KS.

Mock, D.E., and Greene, G.L. 1989. Current approaches in chemical control of stable flies. In *Symposium: Current Status of the Stable Fly in the United States*. Misc. Pub. Entomol. Soc. Am., *74*, 46–53.

Norris, S.M., and Ravdin, J.I. 1988. The pharmacology of antiamoebic drugs. In *Amebiasis—Human Infection by Entamoeba histolytica*. Edited by J.I. Ravdin. New York, Wiley & Sons, pp. 734–740.

Rawes, D.A., and Clapham, P.A. 1961. A new anthelmintic thenium (N:N-dimethyl-N-2-phenoxyethyl-N-2'-thenylammonium) p-chlorobenzene sulphonate: its activity against hookworms and roundworms in the dog. Vet. Rec., *73*, 1755–1758.

Roberson, E.L. 1977. Chemotherapy of parasitic diseases. In *Veterinary Pharmacology and Therapeutics*. 4th Edition. Edited by L.M. Jones, N.H. Booth, and L.E. McDonald. Ames, Iowa, The Iowa State University Press.

Schaub, S.A. 1986. Report of task force on guide standard and protocol for testing microbiological water purifiers. Washington, D.C., U.S. Environmental Protection Agency.

Shumard, R.F., and Callender, M.E. 1967. Monensin, a new biologically active compound VI. Anticoccidial activity. Antimicrob. Agents Chemother., 369–377.

Shumard, R.F., and McCowen, M.C. 1963. Antibiotics as anthelmintics. Antimicrob. Agents Chemother., 588–596.

Sine, C., Editor. 1989. Section C—Pesticide Dictionary Cl-C318. In *Farm Chemicals Hand Book*. Willoughby, OH, Meister Publishing.

Snow, J.W., et al. 1982. Swormlure: Development and use in detection and suppression systems for adult screwworm (Diptera: Calliphoridae). Bull. Entomol. Soc. Am., *28*, 277–284.

Sparks, T.C., and Hammock, B.D. 1983. Insect growth regulators: resistance and the future. In *Pest Resistance to Pesticides*. Edited by G.P. Georghiou and T. Saito. New York, Plenum Press, pp. 651–668.

Stone, O.J., Mullins, J.F., and Willis, C.J. 1964. Inhibition of nematode development with thiabendazole. J. Invest. Dermatol., *43*, 437.

Swanson, L. 1943. Control of cattle-parasitic and free-living nematodes by soil fumigation with methyl bromide. Proc. Helm. Soc. Wash., *10*, 1–3.

Theodorides, V.J. 1985. Antiparasitic drugs. In *Parasitology for Veterinarians*. 4th Edition. Edited by J.R. Georgi. Philadelphia, W.B. Saunders, pp. 187–226.

Upton, S.J., Tilley, M.E., Marchin, G.L., and Fina, L.R. 1988. Efficacy of a pentaiodide resin disinfectant on *Cryptosporidium parvum* (Apicomplex:Cryptosporidiidae) oocysts in vitro. J. Parasitol., *74*, 719–721.

Ware, G.W. 1978. *The Pesticide Book*. San Francisco, W.H. Freeman.

World Health Organization. 1964. The medical research program of the WHO—report of the Director General 1958–1963. Geneva.

York, W., and Adams, A.R.D. 1926. Observations on *Entamoeba histolytica*. II. Longevity of the cysts in vitro and their resistance to heat and to various drugs and chemicals. Ann. Trop. Med. Parasitol., *20*, 317–326.

PART IV

Chemical and Physical Sterilization

CHAPTER 29

STERILIZATION BY HEAT

L.J. Joslyn

Sterilization is an absolute term meaning the destruction of all life. A radical process, sterilization generally alters or damages the type of materials subjected to pasteurization,* disinfection, and other substerilizing or "inhibitory" treatments. Sterilizing agents are classified as "physical" or "chemical," and these in turn are either liquid, gaseous, or electromagnetic radiation. However, there are no sharp distinctions in nature. Physical agents may induce the formation of lethal chemicals; heat and osmotic pressure, produced by reacting chemical sterilizing agents, may be responsible in part for the destruction of microorganisms.

The oldest and most recognized agent of destruction is heat. From early recorded history, due consideration was given to dangers associated with the inception and transmission of disease. The use of fire and water as purifying agents was incorporated in the Mosaic Law. Moist and dry heat are classic sterilizing media. Moist heat includes either saturated steam or boiling water. Although boiling water at ambient pressures is not a good sterilizing agent because of its relatively low temperature, its principal advantage is its availability. Steam under pressure is inexpensive and sterilizes penetrable materials and exposed surfaces rapidly.

Dry heat, on the other hand, is relatively slow, requiring higher temperatures of application. However, dry heat will penetrate all kinds of materials, such as oils, petrolatum, and closed containers, that are not permeable to steam.

KINETICS OF THERMAL DESTRUCTION OR INACTIVATION

Thermal death of bacterial cells and spores is exponential. Chick (1908, 1910) indicted that a monomolecular chemical reaction is necessary for such a first-order relationship. Weiss (1921) and Esty and Meyer (1922) found that the destruction curves of *Clostridium botulinum* were essentially linear (Amaha and Sakaguchi,

*See Chapter 44 for definition of terms.

1957). Knaysi (1930), on the other hand, disagreed with the monomolecular theory because the majority of survivor curves are sigmoidal rather than linear exponential curves. Loeb and Northrup (1917) and Finney (1952) propounded what Charm (1958) called "the distribution of resistance theory." Charm (1958) used a kinetic approach to derive the equation describing the exponential survival curve, which is based on the kinetics of inactivation. Plotting the probit of the survival on logarithmic probability paper against the log of exposure time, Fernelius et al. (1958) were able to change the sigmoidal survival curve to a linear relationship. Reynolds and Lichtenstein (1952) and Kaplan et al. (1953) indicated that thermal death rate curves of the putrefactive anaerobe (PA 3679) were sigmoidal rather than linear, indicating thermal resistance distribution.

Lewis (1956) obtained different values for the destruction rate constant, k, for different times of heating based on the estimation of decimal reduction times (D values) by statistical analysis. The D value is the reciprocal of k and is the time necessary to reduce a microbial population by one log or 90% at a given temperature. Using Bigelow and Esty's (1920) thermal death time tube method, Anand (1961) found that four out of seven of the organisms he subjected to thermal analysis followed exponential destruction rates. Destruction rate curves, he found, were of two types, either of increasing or decreasing death rate of spores.

Edwards, Busta, and Speck (1965) found both nonlinear time-survivor and decimal reduction rate (survival) curves for the ultrahigh-temperature treatment of *Bacillus subtilis* spores. Williams (1929) indicated an increasing thermal death rate for *B. subtilis* spores. Kaplan et al. (1953) found an initial deviation or lag from linearity in the death rate of the putrefactive anaerobe. The increasing rate of thermal destruction could be caused by one or more of the following: (1) the presence of nonuniform heat-resistant spores (El-Bisi and Ordal, 1956a; Ball and Olson, 1957); (2) the inactivation of germination and growth inhibitors (Humphrey and Nickerson, 1961;

El-Bisi and Ordal, 1956*b*); (3) more than one event in the overall lethal reaction; or (4) the existence of a "heat stimulation" factor. Anand (1961*a*) further ascribes the decreasing order of death to two or more heat-resistant variants in the strain.

Although the controversy continues, there seems little reason to doubt that the order of death is a first-order reaction mechanism that can be designated mathematically in several ways. One such form is:

$$N_t = N_0 e^{-kt}$$

where N_0 is the starting number of a population, N_t is the number surviving at any time, t, and k is the death rate constant. The negative sign indicates that the exponential is regressing.

Activation, Inactivation, and Dormancy

It seems to be well understood that deviation from the linear logarithmic nature of the survival curve is generally due to two basic factors: (1) The presence of a hump or "lag" in the initial portion of the survival curve of a heat-resistant population of spores is due to Anand's "heat stimulation" or what is understood as "heat activation" (Evans and Curran, 1943; Curran and Evans, 1945, 1946, 1947; Shull and Ernst, 1962; Busta and Ordal, 1964). (2) The tailing of the final portion is due, no doubt, to more than one thermoresistant variant in the population.

An energy of *activation* is generally necessary to initiate a chemical or biologic process, in this case, the energy necessary to release spores from their *dormant* state to begin their germination process. An activation energy is also required to initiate *inactivation* (destruction) of microorganisms.

The activation portion of the survival curve of spores is not generally observed in the survival curves of vegetative cells. If such an anomaly exists, it could be explained on the basis of other factors, such as thermal lag or protective effects for vegetative cells that are not always as predominant as the activation principle for spores. Where such determinations are conducted carefully, thermal lags can be minimized. The activation energy required to indicate germination along portions of a survival curve of a population of spores becomes more or less pronounced under the following circumstances:

1. *The Innate Heat Resistance of the Strain.* The more heat resistant a strain, the more likely it is to have a pronounced activation requirement. Spores of *Clostridium thermosaccharolyticum* are a unique example of this, reported by Perkins (1965) to have a D value of 110 minutes at 121°C. On this basis, it would require over 11 hours to kill a population of a million spores. This is about 44 times the resistance of spores ordinarily used as sterility indicators. The spores of this species also require an abnormal activation to germinate at 121°C for 30 minutes. The survival curve of spores of the thermophile *Bacillus stearothermophilus* (Fig. 29–1)

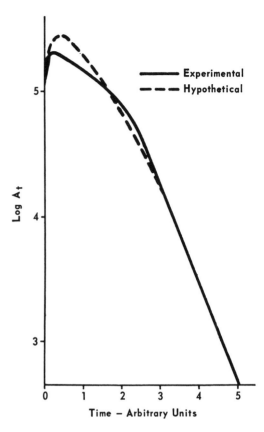

Fig. 29–1. A typical survival curve of *Bacillus stearothermophilus* spores on filter paper strips exposed to steam above 121°C. A_t represents the number of surviving spores forming visible colonies on agar. The hypothetic curve is from the formula of Shull, Cargo, and Ernst (1963).

shows not only an initial lag but also a pronounced hump.

2. *The Temperature of Treatment.* The lower the treatment temperature, the more pronounced the initial lag is apt to be because of a relatively slow activation rate. On the other hand, as the treatment temperatures are raised, the activation time is reduced, the hump becomes higher, and the lag time shorter, approaching extinction because of the inability to adequately observe the effect of short increments of time. This may explain in part some of the confusion that exists with respect to the initial portion of survival curves—whether they are indeed linear or curvilinear depends to a great degree on these factors.

3. *The Outgrowth Media.* The degree of spontaneous germination (Powell and Hunter, 1955) and the contribution to germination from constituents of the growth media (Hyatt and Levinson, 1961) will influence the shape of the initial phase of the survival curve determined by colony court.

4. *The Incubation Temperature.* The incubation temperature also may contribute to the activation of a fraction of the spores in the population (Busta and Ordal, 1964).

5. *The Past History of the Crop.* Drying or wetting, storage temperature, and freeze-thaw cycles all will contribute to the shape of the survival curve as it relates to inactivation required for germination and growth into visible colonies.

Other factors, such as clumping, diffusion, and thermal lags (Hansen and Riemann, 1963), some already alluded to and others to be mentioned, may influence the response to heat treatment and the ultimate determination of survival curves, but such factors do not affect the characteristic activation principle that is inherent in the heat-resistant spore.

It would be reasonable to assume that all the spores in a homogeneous population are "dormant" and that the growth media might contain small amounts of activation chemicals sufficient to activate only a low percentage of spores. In addition to this, the incubation temperature would activate a small percentage of spores, accounting for the small fraction of spores that always seem to germinate spontaneously and grow to visible colonies. Finley and Fields (1961) demonstrated a heat-induced dormancy for *B. stearothermophilus* spores at temperatures between 80° and 100°C, below what they termed the occurrence of true activation temperatures. This is difficult to prove, because the activation rate may be slow and may exactly match an inactivation rate. It is apparent that the shape of the survival curves of *B. stearothermophilus* spores and spores of other heat-resistant species indicates that activation must precede inactivation. In any case, the inactivation of dormant spores must proceed at an extremely slow rate compared to that of activated spores.

Shull et al. (1963) derived the equation that undoubtedly describes the interaction of activation and inactivation on the thermal treatment of heat-resistant dormant spores of *B. stearothermophilus*. Applying this equation to many survival curves that were determined under carefully controlled conditions, the equation was found to be reasonably accurate.

Other factors beside activation and inactivation that could influence the shape of a survival curve have been mentioned. If these are minimized, and if the germination and growth media, incubation temperature, and spore crops are kept essentially the same, whether or not chemical activators are incorporated in the growth media, much information can be gleaned from heat spore-destruction studies based on the determination of survival curves and the use of the survival equation. One can compare the effect of heat treatments at different temperatures for the activation and destruction rates of spores of the same species, compare those characteristics of different strains or species at the same temperature, or compare the effect of constituents of various growth media to alter the rate patterns of a species.

In making comparisons based on inactivation rates and heat resistance in the past, it was necessary to use either the linear portion of the curve or to assume that survival curves are always exponential. Nonetheless, it seems that both heat activation and inactivation obey first-order kinetics (Busta and Ordal, 1964), in combination and in that order, and that the moment a spore becomes activated it is subjected to the inactivation law. This makes the mathematic delineation somewhat complex, but a straight-forward mathematic analysis of the relationship yields the following equations from Shull et al. (1963):

$$(1) \quad A_t = A_0 e^{-kt} + \frac{\alpha N_0}{k - \alpha}(e^{-\alpha t} - e^{-kt})$$

$$(2) \quad L_t = N_t + A_t$$

where A_0 and A_t are the numbers of activated spores at times zero and t, respectively, as determined by colony count. N_0 and N_t are the numbers of spores not activated at times zero and t, respectively, and N_0 is determined from $N_0 = L_0 - A_0$; α is the activation rate constant. One can solve for α knowing other constants. k is the inactivation rate constant and can be determined from the linear portion of the curve, which occurs after all spores have been activated. L_0 and L_t are the total numbers of viable spores at times zero and t. L_0 can be determined from the relation $L_0 = k \int_0^\infty A_t \, dt$ by taking the products of k and the area under the survival curve of A_t.

The first term, $A_0 e^{-kt}$, of equation (1) describes the first-order death of the initial activated spore population, and the second term, $\frac{\alpha N_0}{k - \alpha}(e^{-\alpha t} - e^{-kt})$, describes the activation and subsequent death of the original nonactivated population. Figure 29–1 shows the fit of the calculated hypothetic curve to experimental results. By use of this equation, one can accurately determine the starting number of the viable population and the rate constants for comparative purposes. It is perhaps a wishful thought that such a model could be applied to compare various sterilizing agents wherever an activation principle would be operative—that is, to use minimal treatments of combinations of agents to best advantage. For example, to chemically activate harmful spore populations to reduce the heat requirement for total destruction would minimize adverse effects of heating. These effects could be quantitated by advantageous use of the mathematic relationship, comparing the rate constants under various conditions. For example, elevated temperatures make generally resistant bacterial spores more susceptible to destruction by inordinately low levels of gamma irradiation (Reynolds, 1969; Reynolds et al., 1970). Of course, the same could be said for treatment by low concentrations of ethylene oxide gas at elevated temperatures (Ernst and Doyle, 1968).

Busta and Ordal (1964) determined the thermodynamic properties of heat activation under carefully controlled conditions using thermodynamic relationships after determining Arrhenius activation energy by plotting the logarithm of reaction velocity against the reciprocal of absolute temperature (Fig. 29–2). Because E_0 and the

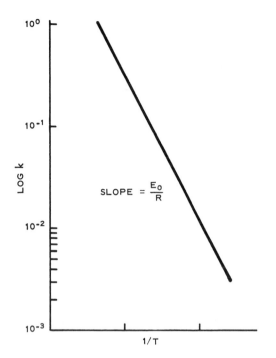

Fig. 29–2. A typical Arrhenius plot of the log of a rate constant, K_1, and the reciprocal of the absolute temperature.

standard enthalpy $\Delta H\ddagger$ were nearly the same for their system, they found $\Delta H\ddagger = 27,900$ calories per mole; $\Delta F\ddagger = 25,100$ to $26,400$ calories per mole; and $\Delta S\ddagger = 4.6$ to 8.1 calories per mole-degree. Interestingly, Grecz et al. (1972) found the formation energies for the presumed elements of heat resistance to be closely within this range of thermodynamic values for *Clostridium botulinum*.

If one assumes 20,000 calories per mole per strong chemical bond, the $\Delta H\ddagger$ value just given would indicate the breaking of a strong and a weak chemical bond, or several weak bonds. The Arrhenius equation is represented by $k = Ce^{(-E/RT)}$, where C is a constant, E is the activation energy, T, absolute temperature, and R, the gas constant.

Charm (1958) calculated the activation energies in several organic media and in distilled water for inactivation of spores of *C. botulinum* and PA 3679. These energies varied from 68,500 to 64,500 BTU per cell for *C. botulinum* and 58,250 to 55,500 BTU, per cell for PA 3679.

Amaha and Sakaguchi (1957) determined the thermodynamic relationships and the activation energies for the inactivation of spores of *Bacillus natto*, *B. megatherium* and *B. mycoides*, comparing these with similar data for the protein denaturation of hemoglobin, trypsin and pancreatic lipase. These are values for: $E_0 = 40,800$ to $77,314$ calories per mole; $\Delta H\ddagger = 40,160$ to $76,600$ calories per mole; $\Delta S\ddagger = 44.7$ to 152 calories per degree-mole; $\Delta F\ddagger = 25,000$ calories per mole in nearly every case. Trypsin and pancreatic lipase compared favorably with *B. megatherium* spores, and hemoglobin very favorably with the other two species of spores. Wang,

Scharer, and Humphrey (1964) determined the Arrhenius activation energy for the inactivation of *B. stearothermophilus* spores. These were 83.6 kcal per mole, and the enthalpy and entropy changes were 84.4 kcal per mole and 157 calories per mole-degree, respectively. It is concluded that the same order of magnitude exists for both reactions, inactivation of spores and denaturation of protein, and the large values of E_0 and ΔS are characteristic of protein denaturation. Urbakh (1961) also determined that the number of broken chemical bonds from the kinetics of protein denaturation is related to at least one labile site.

Thermal Death Point and Thermal Death Time

The thermal death point is the lowest temperature at which a suspension of bacteria is killed in 10 minutes. This standard has been almost completely abandoned because of the inherent variables associated with culturing and test methods.

Thermal death time, a standard used in the canning industry, is the shortest time necessary to kill all the microbes in or on a menstruum at a specific temperature. Thermal death times are subject to error for reasons discussed.

Death Rate Constants

Because death is a first-order exponential, or logarithmic, function, death rate constants have been used widely for comparative purposes. Based on the death rate function, data have been extrapolated over wide ranges to predict sterilization times. As has been stated, such extrapolations may be valid for vegetative cells, but not for heat-resistant spore populations, especially not if the spores require activation. Just as activation distorts a survival or thermal death curve in its initial stages, as has been stated, so the presence of heat-resistant variants in a strain causes tailing of the final portions of the survival curve.

The use of D values has been prominent as a tool for the extrapolations stated previously. Stumbo, Ball, Schmidt, and others have done a great deal of work in this field (Schmidt, 1957). This subject is covered in greater detail in another chapter. Notice is here directed to some obvious pitfalls in the use of D values. No matter how they are determined, the gravest possibility of error exists in those cases in which the survival curve is sigmoidal or partially sigmoidal in shape. D values are based on the assumption that such curves are linear; they are only so in special cases. D values are sometimes calculated on the basis of end-point determinations, assuming a straight-line logarithmic survivor curve drawn from the starting point of a number of viable organisms to the point of extinction or end point of such a population. A D value determined in this manner provides nothing, in fact, other than the largest possible value for the slope. It would seem from this that the end-point determination at least provides an adequate safety factor for subsequent extrapolations.

There was a case in our laboratory in which D values

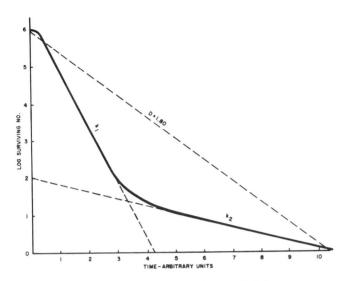

Fig. 29–3. A thermal treatment survival curve of a dichotomous population of spores having thermal death rate constants K_1 and K_2, showing the D value from end-point determinations.

were calculated for soil samples based on partial survival data (for end-point determinations) for spores subjected to dry heat. These D values were then extrapolated to provide time-temperature values for the complete destruction of hypothetic starting populations. No doubt in soil there is a great variety of heat-resistant strains. Figure 29–3 shows a simplified survival curve for a hypothetic situation for a dichotomous population heat-treated at some sterilizing temperature. From the figure, the solid line is the resultant of two death rate curves, the constants of which are k_1 for the less resistant and k_2 for the more resistant one. The value of D is indicated, based on the slope of the straight line connecting the starting number (10^6 spores) with the end point (one viable spore or less). In the actual case, a relatively few (represented by 100 in this case) heat-resistant spores were undoubtedly protected in some way in the soil menstruum, because isolates of the same spores were found to be not nearly as heat resistant as the soil treatments indicated.

These D-value data were extrapolated by others from the actual curves to provide sterilization times for the heat treatment of "planetary landers." For the reason stated, such end-point determinations should provide the highest D values, and therefore sterility would be adequately assured, especially if several more D values were added for safety. However, in the hypothetic case, the end-point determination is based on the destruction of only a few highly protected spores. One could add many thousands of the low or moderate heat-resistant spores without compromising sterility, but the addition of only a relatively few of the highly protected heat-resistant spores could discount the sterilization based on such a D-value extrapolation. It is highly probable that a degree of protection similar to that encountered in soil is attained by spores encased in solid materials. This

point will be discussed further in the section titled *Protective Effects.*

If the straight line portion of a sigmoidal thermal death curve is used for the determination of death rate D to determine sterilization times, a dangerous error would also accrue because D would have a low value, resulting in low estimates of the actual time required to kill a known population of spores. Use of any portion (Reynolds and Lichtenstein, 1952) of a survival curve to determine D values will result in error that will be compounded if D is used to compute other values that are extrapolations of it.

D values, therefore, are valid only in situations in which the treatment temperature is high enough to discount the effect of activation and the population is of uniform resistance.

The Temperature Coefficient

The thermodynamic temperature coefficient is usually expressed as Q_{10}. Chemical reactions generally proceed at a rate that increases as temperature increases. For every 10°C rise in temperature, reaction rates for chemical reactions usually double. From Rahn (1945):

$$Q_{10} = \frac{(\text{Rate at T} + 10)}{\text{Rate at T}} = \frac{K\,(T + 10)}{K_t}$$

$$= \exp\left(\frac{\mu}{2} \cdot \frac{10}{T\,(T + 10)}\right)$$

it can be seen that as absolute temperature T becomes larger, Q_{10} decreases with increasing temperature. Rahn (1945) indicated Q_{10} values of 2, 3, and 4 at 20 to 30°C for normal chemical reactions and 1.36, 1.62, and 1.84 at 170 to 180°C. For dry-heat sterilization, a Q_{10} of 3 could be expected at a room temperature range and 1.6 for the range 170 to 180°C. For steam denaturation of proteins, however, Q_{10} values go from 10, 20, and 100 at 50 to 60°C to 4.8, 7.7, and 23.0 at 120 to 130°C. To quote from Rahn (1945), "The low coefficient is the reason why the various laboratory manuals disagree widely on the times and temperatures necessary to sterilize dry glassware. There is no disagreement about the sterilization of media in the autoclave because the temperature coefficient in this case is so high that an increase of 2° to 3°C cuts the sterilizing time in half."

Using average Q_5 values determined in phosphate buffer for the temperature range 95 to 100°C, Amaha and Sakaguchi (1957) calculated Q_{10} values for spores of *B. natto, B. megatherium,* and *B. mycoides* to be 16.96, 6.25, and 13.17, respectively, which were in the range expected for the denaturation of protein.

THERMAL RESISTANCE OF SPORES

Heat resistance varies among proteins, among microbial species, and among bacterial spores. Many of the bacterial spores are the forms of life most resistant to most chemical and physical killing agents, and particularly to heat. There is a notable difference between thermal resistance to moist heat and to dry heat. A species of bacterial spore highly resistant to moist heat is not necessarily highly resistant to dry heat and vice versa. A case in point is the comparison of spores of the thermophile *B. stearothermophilus* with spores of the mesophile *B. subtilis* var. *niger*. These are the spores most often used to monitor sterilization processes for moist and dry heat, respectively. To inactivate 100,000 spores of *B. stearothermophilus* in saturated steam at 121°C requires 12 minutes of exposure, but 1,000,000 spores of *B. subtilis* are inactivated in less than 1 minute at the same temperature. However, *B. subtilis* var. *niger* is much more resistant to dry heat than *B. stearothermophilus* when both are subjected to the same high temperature.

Other factors can enhance or lower the heat resistance of spores. An innate thermoresistance appears to be associated with certain spores of bacteria that characterizes them as having a greater resistance to heat than other spores. Beyond this, however, environmental influences such as pH, ion concentrations, and constituents of growth and sporulating media enhance the thermoresistance of spores. Sommer (1930) demonstrated that spores of *Clostridium botulinum* grown in 4% peptone resisted 100°C for 1.5 to 2.5 hours, but the addition of phosphate increased the heat tolerance to 4 hours. Increasing the concentration of peptone or adding glucose did not increase this resistance, although more growth occurred. Attempts to find increased resistance by selection failed in the 15 strains tested.

Amaha and Ordal (1957) indicated that differences in degree and rate of thermal destruction might be associated with the loss of cations that enhance the thermoresistance of spores. To quote these authors, "The rate of loss of viability would be greater in the presence of increased phosphate concentration or in the presence of more powerful or more specific chelating agents."

Powell (1953) isolated dipicolinic acid, DPA (pyridine-2,6-dicarboxylic acid) from spores of *Bacillus megatherium*, and Perry and Foster (1955) studied its biosynthesis in *B. cereus*. DPA has been found in all bacterial endospores examined (Wooley and Collier, 1965), yet it seems to be absent from nonresistant vegetative cells (Church and Halvorson, 1959). DPA has been recognized as an agent in establishing thermoresistance (Collier and Murty, 1957; Church and Halvorson, 1959; Hashimoto et al., 1960; Byrne et al., 1960). Another agent of thermoresistance is calcium (Sugiyama, 1951; Slepecky and Foster, 1959). Refractility to heat of the spore and the amount of DPA synthesized were found to be proportional to the amount of calcium available where calcium was in limiting concentrations (Young and Fitz-James, 1962).

Both aerobic and anaerobic bacterial spores contain large quantities (5 to 15% dry weight) of DPA. Church and Halvorson (1959) found that phenylalanine present in the sporulation medium reduced DPA formation. Using this suppressing agent, these authors sought to find the relationship among DPA content, viability, and thermoresistance of spores. Viability was independent of DPA content above 1.2%; rate of inactivation decreased with increased DPA content; reducing DPA 60% or more made spores more heat sensitive and caused them to germinate spontaneously (Keynan et al., 1962). Day and Costilow (1964) indicated that heat resistance developed coincidentally with synthesis of DPA. Levinson et al. (1961) found no direct relationship between thermoresistance and DPA or calcium content, but a good agreement was found between calcium-to-DPA ratio and thermal resistance of spores.

Grecz et al. (1972) indicated a correlation between the thermodynamic stabilities of the Ca(II)-DPA chelate in model systems and the in vivo heat resistance of Ca(II)-DPA-containing spores of *Clostridium botulinum*.

Zytkovicz and Halvorson (1972) state that "It has been well documented that DPA is a major constituent of bacterial spores, and it is believed that its calcium salt is a major contributing factor to heat resistance," quoting many of the authors already mentioned in this chapter.

In view of the previous statement that activation precedes inactivation, it seems to be apparent that the activation principle is related to dissolution of the Ca(II)-DPA complex. Grecz et al. (1972) indicated that the rate of loss of DPA on heating seemed to be related to the thermal death of spores and that heat-resistant strains apparently lose DPA less quickly than heat-sensitive strains.

pH and Ion Exchange Effects

Additionally, dissolution of the Ca(II)-DPA complex or loss of DPA from the spores by any means, such as by ion exchange effects at different pH levels, will result in a related loss of heat resistance (Grecz et al., 1972). The kinetics of release of Ca(II)-DPA from *Bacillus stearothermophilus* spores is related to conditions of time, temperature, and pH (Brown and Melling, 1973).

Bacterial death rates are higher in acid or alkaline media than in neutral suspensions (Rahn, 1945). Walker (1964) stated that a higher recovery of survivors resulted in the neutral pH zone. Citrate, phthalate, or ammonium buffers reduced thermoresistance of spores compared to those in phosphate buffer. Spores are more readily inactivated at low pH, because the pH could influence the type of ions that would adsorb on the spore surface, which in turn would alter heat stability (Alderton and Snell, 1963). Alderton and Snell (1963) suggested that spores exhibit a base exchange behavior: "This function is pronounced, and compositional manipulation by this route can be used to reduce, restore, and enhance heat resistance of fully formed spores. Some properties of spores may be correlated with the behavior of ion exchange gels." The spore exchanger resembles a weak

Pyridine-2,6-dicarboxylic acid (dipicolinic acid, DPA)

cation exchange system; therefore, the hydrogen ion, possessing the greatest exchange potential, would displace other cations. This base exchange mechanism allows for the adsorption of calcium in excess of the DPA chelation equivalent reported by Levinson et al. (1961) and Lechowich and Ordal (1962).

The Process of Spore Biosynthesis of Heat-Resistant Components

Halvorson (1957) indicated that sporulation is a multiphase process. First, the refractile cell is formed, and then DPA is synthesized; the development of the thermoresistant spore is a final, separate process. Young and Fitz-James (1962) reported that the spore coat and exosporium of *B. cereus*, during formation peripheral to the outer cortical membrane, take up calcium and synthesize DPA. Wooley and Collier (1965) found that calcium accumulation occurred early in sporogenesis and preceded both biosynthesis of DPA and thermoresistance for *Clostridium roseum*.

Warth et al. (1962, 1963) concluded that the most heat-resistant spores contained the highest amounts of diaminopimelic acid (DAP) and hexosamine. They concluded further that these peptide constituents resided in the cortex and are "involved in the basic mechanism of heat stabilization of spores." Gerhardt and Ribi (1964) studied the structural details of the exosporium of spores of *Bacillus cereus* and *B. anthracis* by electron microscopy and x-ray diffraction analysis. They found two main layers, an outer layer of "hair-like projections" and an inner layer that "had a hexagonally perforate surface pattern of holes, and was made up of four lamellae."

In the outer coat or the exosporium, some basic structure similar to a honeycomb seems to exist, made up perhaps of the diaminopimelic acid-glucosamine complex. Filling the honeycomb would be the calcium-DPA chelate, and adsorbed to it, calcium in the base cation exchange fashion. Activation by heat would be similar to melting wax from a honeycomb, and chemical activation similar to dissolving the honey. Activation therefore would remove the heat-refractile and diffusion barrier for either subsequent germination and growth via the absorption and diffusion of water and nutrient materials or the penetration of heat for protein denaturation. Excellent reviews of the nature of spore biosynthesis have recently appeared (Halvorson et al., 1972).

Calcium is notably associated with both heat-refractile and relatively water-insoluble compounds. Such an exosporium depleted of calcium and DPA would be expected to act like a porous membrane, which swells under hydrostatic pressure on the absorption of water. Swelling is typical of the germinating spore.

The composition of spore coats suggested that polypeptides have the capability for extensive intra- and intermolecular bonding of the hydrophobic type (Tipper and Ganthier, 1972). Increased density is produced by increased binding of heavy atoms, which is presumed necessary for sporulation (Highton, 1972). Furthermore, Grecz et al. (1972) state that the binding of Ca(II)-DPA

results in a hydrophobic condition. The release of the chelate, however, increases hygroscopicity.

Protective Effects

Sobernheim and Mündel (1938) found that sterilization of spores contained in soil required 6 to 8 times longer by moist heat than sterilization of the same number of spores cultured from soil. Likewise, Doyle and Ernst (1967) have found that sterilization of spores contained in soil required 15 to 20 times longer by dry heat than sterilization of the same number of spores cultured from soils. The presence of organic matter can protect spores during heating. Peptone, albumin, nucleic acids, sugars, and starch all provided protection at certain concentrations (Sykes, 1963: Walker, 1964). Protection of spores by anhydrous materials such as oils and fats (Yesair et al., 1946; Rahn, 1945) against destruction by steam is equivalent to treatment with dry heat.

Although Sykes (1963) related "in-crystal" protection to chemical agents, spores occluded in crystal structures display a phenomenal resistance to destruction by heat. Ernst and Doyle (1965), attempting to simulate the same degree of protection afforded by soil, occluded spores of several bacteria in various crystals (Fig. 29–4). Spores of *B. subtilis* var. *niger* on paper strips are killed in steam at 121°C in less than 1 minute; however, the same number of spores occluded in insoluble calcium carbonate crystals survived for more than 2 hours. The crystals were of uniform microscopic size (*circa* 100 μm), and each crystal contained about 100 viable spores. Dry-heat resistance was also maximized by this protection. At 121°C, spores of *B. subtilis* var. *niger*, occluded in crystals of calcium carbonate as described, had a 900-fold increase in resistance to steam and a 9-fold increase in resistance to dry heat for the same total number of spores.

Koesterer (1964) noted a high degree of resistance to dry heat for destruction of natural flora in certain soils. Spores added back to certain materials, especially the soils mentioned, increased heat resistance by many times (Bruch et al., 1963; Bruch, 1964). Ernst and Doyle (1965) have produced phenomenal heat resistance by manipulating combinations of protective materials. The highest resistance seems to accrue from the use of the crystal occlusion of spores as the basic unit.

It is possible that the heat resistance of natural flora is much greater than is now imagined. It seems from these studies that the greatest protection is afforded to those spores occluded within highly water-insoluble crystals that are generally composed of those heat-refractile elements mentioned previously. Attempts to determine viability by usual procedures would leave such protected microbes intact within their crystals. Koesterer (1964) inferred, on the basis of recovery techniques that would not release microbes from their insoluble environment, that his data indicated that situations could exist in which the dry-heat treatment of 135°C for 24 hours, recommended at that time for the sterilization of "planetary landers," would not sterilize. Experience in this field suggests that occlusion of spores in and between

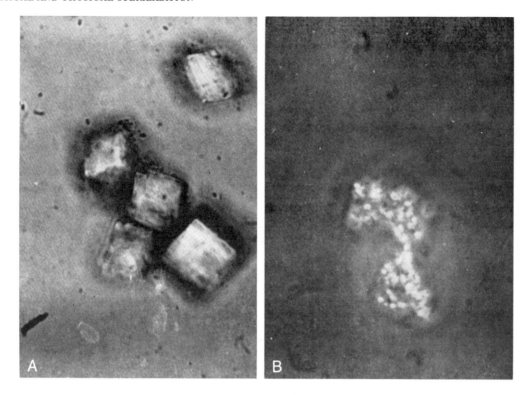

Fig. 29–4. Crystals of CaCo₃ occluding spores of *Bacillus subtilis* var. *niger. A*, Phase, showing individual spores. *B*, Phase, showing spores being released by dissolving crystals (× 2500).

materials of spacecraft construction would indeed fall into the category of great protection against dry-heat sterilization.

Because sterilization by dry heat is an oxidation process (Rahn, 1945), Ernst and Doyle (1965) feel that protection is afforded spores in highly heat-resistant soils in such a manner so as to inhibit the availability of oxygen to the oxidative site to reduce the oxidation rate extensively. Such protection could be afforded by the presence of antioxidants associated with spores. Experiments incorporating various antioxidants with spores of *B. subtilis* var. *niger* that are subjected to hot air treatments indicate that increased heating times are necessary to produce the same degree of destruction as that of unassociated spores.

Michener et al. (1959) also found that substances having antioxidant or reducing powers either did not enhance the killing rate of heat-resistant spores in moist heat or actually protected the spores to a great extent. The protective effect was due to reducing agents that may have been augmented by metallic ions, because these were mostly salts.

Thermodynamic Effects and Protection at the Molecular Level

Silverman et al. (1963) found phenomenal protection afforded to 43 isolates from Mohave desert soil that survived 170°C for 4 to 5 days under vacuum at a pressure of 6 × 10⁻⁹ torr. Of the same isolates exposed to 120°C for 3 hours at atmospheric pressure, only 5 survived.

Much needs to be done to determine the basic mechanisms involved in heat inactivation of spores in particular. Charm (1958) presented a hypothetic model depicting heat-sensitive volumes within the cell surrounded by heat transfer units, water molecules, having an energy distribution of which only a fraction possessed inactivation energy. There would be a certain energy transfer frequency between a vibrating water molecule possessing inactivation energy colliding with a sensitive volume. From these considerations, Charm derived the logarithmic survival curve.

Comparing heat destruction of spores of *B. subtilis* var. *niger* in air at various temperatures, using the data of Koesterer (1964), with their destruction at the same temperatures under conditions of ultrahigh vacuum (Silverman et al., 1963), we could not reasonably correlate by any means by kinetic theory (Present, 1958) the difference in destruction time for the same number of spores with the phenomenal difference in energy transfer capability, discounting the effect of radiant heat, or assuming radiant heat to be the same in each case. The difference in energy transfer for the two systems is nearly proportional to the number of available gas molecules (related to the number of collisions per unit area). This comes to many orders of magnitude (about eight, all assumptions being correct), whereas the actual difference between destruction time at atmospheric pressure and the ultrahigh vacuum of Silverman et al. is two to three times higher for ultrahigh vacuum. This indicates one of two things: (1) When energy transfer is considered at the molecular level, dry heat-resistant spores are much more susceptible to heat under vacuum; or (2) under vacuum, protective heat-refractile elements are "boiled off," leaving a naked spore more susceptible to killing by radiant heat. This latter point would tend to explain in part why the differential of heat resistance comparing spores in soil versus unprotected spores is much greater in ultrahigh vacuum than in air at atmospheric pressure. A greater degree of protection is afforded to the spore in soil from radiant heat than from heat by convection. On the other hand, delayed killing under vacuum may be due simply to a reduced oxidation rate (Rahn, 1945), and the apparent enhancement of the antioxidants removing the little available oxygen.

Davis et al. (1963) provide data that seem to refute these arguments, at least in the case of *Aspergillus niger* spores. They state that resistance patterns vary according to individual species. The spores of *A. niger* did not survive 1 day at 90°C under atmospheric pressure, but survived 4 to 5 days at 88°C under ultrahigh vacuum. The order was reversed at 60°C, however, such that ultrahigh vacuum was much more destructive than atmospheric pressure.

The problem is extremely complex. There is evidently a subtle interplay between the various elements, external and internal, relative to the spore and its gross composition. What effect does the "boiling off" of water molecules or the fusion of chemical constituents within, on, or in the immediate environment of the spore have on the absorption of heat, thus protecting the spore from a lethal effect?

Rough determinations using kinetic theory calculations were applied to the ultrahigh vacuum. Assuming reported inactivation energy values for the destruction of one or two strong chemical bonds, evaporation of "bound" water from spores of *Bacillus subtilis* var. *niger* to maintain thermal balance for the application of about 85 kcal per mole would require the loss of between 25 and 50 water molecules per spore within a prescribed period. A loss of water at a rate less than necessary to maintain thermal balance (which would be the case where available water molecules would decrease) would determine the time required for sufficient energy to accumulate at the lethal bond. One would expect such a mechanism to be much more critical under ultrahigh vacuum.

From heat transfer considerations, it seems that the amount of available heat, even if one assumes extremely low efficiencies, is far in excess, by many orders of magnitude, of that indicated as necessary for inactivation by the kinetic data reported in the literature. It seems also that supposed protective effects apparently go far beyond conceptual models. Somewhere between these extremes may be the answer. By most considerations, the reported kinetic energy data seem to be too low. This is augmented by the fact that such data are based upon questionable rate relationships and lead to the conclusion that present concepts need to be investigated more thoroughly.

THERMAL INACTIVATION OF VIRAL PARTICLES

It is generally agreed that virus particles are much less resistant to thermal inactivation than bacterial spores. However, in the case of serum hepatitis virus, because of the nature of its environment, the virus is afforded a great degree of protection by an organic menstruum. Ginoza et al. (1964) examined the inactivation by heat of single-stranded virus nucleic acids. They determined, from kinetics of inactivation, that the two classes of nucleic acids are inactivated by first-order processes that are distinctly different, in that a single phosphodiester bond is cleaved to inactivate the RNAs of TMV and R17, and a single depurination inactivates DNA of φX 174. The pH effects relating to the stability of the nucleic acid strands are evidently similar to those for protein denaturation, and interestingly, similar first-order reaction kinetics and energy values apply for the destruction of viral particles by heat.

MECHANICS OF STEAM STERILIZATION

Sterilization by steam under pressure is nearly universally applied except where penetration or heat and moisture damage is a problem. Steam sterilization equipment is found in a wide variety of shapes and sizes in hospitals, clinics, microbiologic laboratories, and industrial production facilities. Steam sterilization works better than some other forms of sterilization because steam destroys most resistant bacterial spores in a brief exposure and heats rapidly because of mass heat transfer as it condenses.

Construction

The construction of a steam autoclave is shown in the longitudinal cross section of Figure 29–5. The basic system consists of a steel shell equipped with a sealable door on one end and a permanent closure (backhead) on the other end. A thermostatically trapped steam jacket surrounds the autoclave on all sides (except the backhead and the door). Both the main shell and the jacket are fed with steam through control valves, and both are equipped with pressure gauges and safety relief valves. A chamber temperature indicator/controller probe is generally located in the chamber drain vent line. Additional necessary design elements of the sterilizer are the baffle, water separator, and splash pan.

Design Principles

Well designed steam sterilization equipment delivers steam to the bacterial sites throughout the load. The major problems during this process are air removal, superheat, load wetness, and material damage.

Air Removal

Chamber air is the factor most detrimental to efficient steam sterilization. If temperature varies in the chamber environment and cold spots occur in a load, air has not

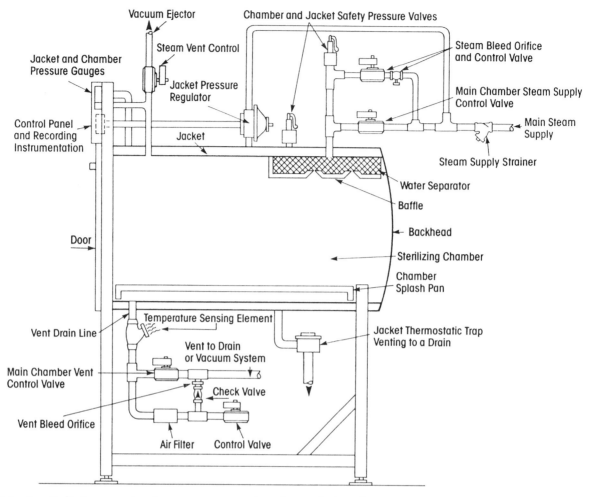

Fig. 29–5. Longitudinal cross section of a steam pressure sterilizer showing the basic features.

been adequately removed from the sterilizing environment. The basic techniques for removing air are (1) gravity displacement, (2) dilution by mass flow, (3) dilution by pressure pulsing, (4) high-vacuum sterilization, and (5) pressure pulsing with gravity displacement.

Gravity Displacement

This method is a standard air removal technique. It takes advantage of fluid displacement characteristics resulting from a large differential in specific gravity between air and steam, in addition to a mass flow displacement motivating force. As shown in Figure 29–6, steam is initially admitted to the top of the sterilizing chamber through a main steam control valve, a water separator, and a baffle. Because steam is lighter than air, it forms a stratified layer across the top of the sterilizer. Although air is diffusing into the steam layer, as a related rates function, the steam mass displaces the air downward faster than the air can diffuse into the constantly renewed supply of pure steam. In effect, the steam wavefront acts as a piston driving the air out of the bottom of the chamber through the drain vent. As air diffuses out of the load, a continuous steam and drain vent bleed sweep

this air out of the chamber throughout the sterilization process.

The water separator and the steam baffle play important roles. High-velocity steam, even when flowing through well trapped steam supply piping, carries a considerable amount of entrained water, which will result in poor steam quality. The gross water carryover is observable, but the atomized particulate water droplets are not. To minimize excessive wetting of materials, a water separator is used to remove the atomized water particles and the raw entrained water, providing steam with a quality of 98% or better. The water separator introduces tortuous paths for the steam molecules. Heavier atomized water particles and entrained water collide with the separator path walls, where they coalesce with other water particles and drain out of the bottom portion of the separator. Here the water is directed to the chamber drain, while the pure steam continues through the maze. Typical water separators are made from porous stones, metal, and plastics or fiber mesh of wire or plastic.

The steam separator, in conjunction with the baffle, also functions to reduce the velocity of steam entering

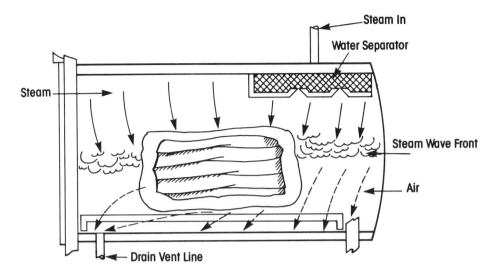

Fig. 29–6. Characteristics of a gravity displacement steam sterilizer.

the chamber. This reduction is necessary for efficient gravity displacement of air from the sterilizing chamber. If the steam enters the chamber at a high velocity, turbulence causes the steam to mix with air. Although this air can be removed by mass-flow dilution, this is considerably less efficient than gravity displacement. The effect of high-velocity steam can be observed in an unheated steam sterilizer by admitting steam into the chamber with the door open. A properly designed baffle will produce a visible smooth cloud layer at the top of the chamber when the steam contacts the cold air and condenses as shown in Figure 29–7. An inefficient baffle design will produce an obvious swirling mixing of the air and steam.

Data (Joslyn, 1976) indicate that for efficient gravity displacement, the steam velocity should be reduced to approximately 1 foot per second as it enters the chamber top. During testing, it was observed that, regardless of the flow rate, baffles on the side that do not extend to the chamber top are particularly prone to air-steam mixing as steam flows to the chamber top.

Proper sizing of the chamber drain vent also is a factor in efficient gravity displacement. Figure 29–6 shows a towel test pack being sterilized in a gravity displacement sterilization process. When steam is admitted to the chamber, if the drain vent line is sized properly, the chamber pressure will not exceed 1 to 2 psig. As the steam wavefront sweeps by the pack, the partial pressure of air in the pack is essentially at atmospheric pressure. An improperly sized chamber drain vent results in an immediate increase in chamber pressure when steam is admitted to the chamber. If, for example, the chamber pressure is increased to 20 psig, the partial pressure of air compressed into the pack is twice that at atmospheric pressure. Because air diffusion is slow and more than retards steam heating of porous loads, it is desirable to minimize the amount of air in the pack during the gravity

displacement process. This factor applies to other air removal techniques to be discussed.

In general, gravity displacement processes are adequate for sterilizing unwrapped or lightly wrapped materials. For denser, porous materials, gravity displacement is both less predictable and less efficient than other methods of removing air. Thus, particularly for dense porous loads, the primary disadvantage of the gravity displacement process is the inability to ensure that all parts of the load receive proper exposure time at temperatures adequate for sterilization.

Dilution by Mass Flow

Dilution of air from a sterilization environment using this method deserves little recognition in steam sterilization, except possibly for high-speed flash sterilization of unwrapped instruments. This is because mass-flow dilution requires considerably more energy and time to remove air from the sterilizing environment than does gravity displacement.

In dilution by mass flow, the concentration of air in the chamber is reduced by using steam as a diluent. As steam is admitted to the chamber, air and steam vent from the chamber at the same rate. Assuming the air and steam are totally mixed, the dynamic removal of air from the system can be predicted by the equation:

$$A = A_i e^{-\frac{Xt}{V}}$$

where A is the air concentration per unit volume at any time (t), A_i is the initial air concentration per unit volume, X is the input/output volumetric flow rate, and V is the chamber volume.

Dilution by Pressure Pulsing

In principle, pressure pulsing reduces the concentration of air in a sterilizing environment by pressurization with a diluent gas (steam) and evacuation or venting the resulting mixture of air and steam. This is repeated until

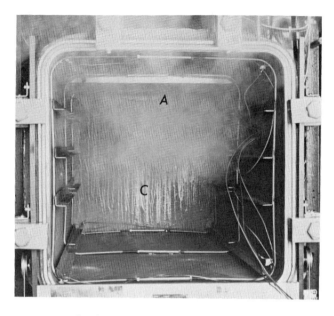 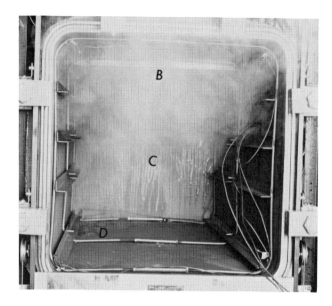

Fig. 29–7. Chamber water separator and baffle design for gravity displacement. *A*, Improper design results in mixing of air and steam. *B*, Proper design results in a smooth cloud layer that acts as a piston to displace air from the chamber. *C*, Entrained water from the steam supply is separated and runs down the backhead to the drain. *D*, Accumulation of water on the chamber floor. Photographs courtesy of Sybron Corporation, Medical Products Division, Rochester, NY.

the air concentration is reduced to below a pre-determined acceptable concentration. Assuming uniform mixing of air and steam, a mathematic model showing the approximate partial pressure of air after each pulse is given by:

$$A_n = \frac{P_2 (A_{n-1})}{P_1}$$

where A_n is the partial pressure of air in the sterilizing chamber following each pressure pulse (n), A_{n-1} is the partial pressure of air in the sterilizing chamber prior to each pressure pulse, P_2 is the final absolute chamber pressure on evacuation, and P_1 is the final absolute chamber pressure during pressurization. Analysis of this equation shows that an increased partial pressure of steam (P_1 increases) and lower vacuum levels (P_2 decreases) result in an increase in the rate of air removal. In practice, the calculated number of pulses required for removal of air to a partial pressure less than 5 mm Hg results in a load temperature that will generally follow the temperature and pressure of saturated steam in the chamber (no thermal lag). Figure 29–8 shows the heating character of a pressure-pulsing system versus a single high vacuum to remove sufficient air for uniform heating of a single towel pack. With deeper vacuum levels, air removal is efficient and fewer pulses are required to reduce the concentration of air to acceptable levels for efficient steam heating. When the vacuum is less than 250 mm Hg, the air removal characteristics are more like a high-vacuum system. This includes the potential of a small-load effect (see *High-Vacuum Sterilization*).

An interesting characteristic of pressure-pulsing systems is that air is removed more efficiently from dense porous loads than from the sterilizing chamber. This is because pressurization of the system compresses air into a spherical ball in the load. At the depth at which steam does penetrate, it condenses and heats the material. When the chamber pressure is reduced, the air expands into the heated region, and the steam revaporizes because of the lower pressure. This drives the air out of the load. Thus, the relative inefficiency of the pressure-pulsing system is the result of the remaining chamber air being re-entrained in the load during repressurization.

High-Vacuum Sterilization

High-vacuum sterilization was one of the methods developed early in the course of steam sterilization development. Steam penetration of dense porous loads was found to improve when deep vacuums were used to remove air initially from the sterilizing chamber prior to admitting steam. As the vacuum level approached 20 mm Hg, the heat-up of a fully loaded sterilizer followed the temperature profile of the sterilizing chamber environment. Bowie (1961) demonstrated how a small, dense, porous load placed in the same sterilizer exhibited a significant thermal lag unless a prevacuum level of 5 mm Hg or less was drawn. Even this vacuum level was found to be ineffective in preventing a "small-load effect" dependent upon the size of the sterilizing chamber. Rowe et al. (1961) indicated that "high speed" prevacuum sterilization required production of a sufficiently low partial pressure of air throughout a system such that, when distributed throughout the load, the amount of air available for any given pack would not interfere significantly with heating during the sterilization process. Joslyn (1978) demonstrated that the "small-load effect" is a pre-

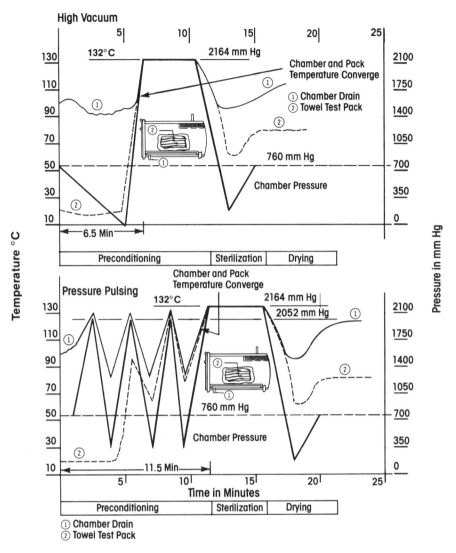

Fig. 29–8. High-vacuum air removal is a special case (one pulse) of a pressure-pulsing air removal system. When the partial pressure of air in the chamber is below 5 mm Hg, heating in the load generally follows the chamber steam temperature, as shown, with 42-towel double-muslin-wrapped test packs.

dictable cause-and-effect relationship based upon (a) the specific heat of the load; (b) the difference between the temperature of the load and the eventual exposure temperature; and (c) the total amount of chamber air.

In principle, the number of BTUs required to heat a load to a given temperature will result in condensation of a proportional number of cubic feet of steam (mixed with air). This leaves the noncondensable air within the load being heated. As a dynamic process, continued steam condensation concentrates chamber air within the load. This ultimately retards the rate at which steam can penetrate, resulting in a thermal lag in pack heating. To prevent this, the total amount of air in the system should exhibit a partial pressure less than 50 mm Hg when compressed to a volume of 1 cubic foot. Functionally, this is the mechanism behind air entrainment measured with the Bowie and Dick type test currently being used

to evaluate the efficiency of vacuum-type sterilizers in hospitals (AAMI, 1980). The typical effect of chamber air relative to various prevacuum levels and load heat lag is shown in Figure 29–9.

High prevacuum sterilizers generally are not desirable for sterilization processes. Ernst and Josyln (1967) found that high vacuums cause dehydration of many materials. Upon heating of linens, tremendous heat energy was released upon hydration, resulting in superheated steam in the pack. A second finding was that air in the system caused charring of the fabric. It was hypothesized that the superheated steam was acting as a catalyst for oxidation, and part of the heat energy observed was from the oxidation reaction.

The interesting part of the residual air phenomenon was that biologic indicators were inactivated in half the time when compared to an equivalent exposure time in

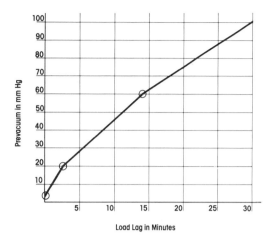

Fig. 29–9. The delay time for a 42-towel double-muslin-wrapped test pack to reach a chamber temperature of 132°C after prevacuums to various vacuum levels (small-load effect).

saturated steam. Pflug (1977) and Joslyn (see later section entitled *Chamber Air*) have found that naked spore strips are more resistant to sterilization in saturated steam than spore strips in glassine envelopes. Based upon heat transfer considerations, one would expect the reverse. This would suggest a synergistic effect of air in the glassine envelope and steam on biologic inactivation, as is hypothesized to occur in the charring of linens.

Additional problems with high prevacuum sterilizers relate to an inordinately high probability that porous loads will not be effectively sterilized owing to the extreme sensitivity to air leaks in the system and the expense of equipment required to attain the deep vacuum levels. In general, high-vacuum sterilization can be replaced by more effective methods.

Pressure Pulsing with Gravity Displacement

Proper application of pressure-pulsing and gravity displacement techniques provide the most effective method of removing air from a sterilizing chamber. In a typical cycle, shown in Figure 29–10, air is removed by evacuating the sterilizer chamber to a predetermined pressure. At this pressure, steam is admitted to the chamber at a rate equal to the vacuum pump capacity to maintain the given vacuum level. After a timed interval, the majority of chamber air is removed by gravity displacement. The partial pressure of the air in the load is at the chamber vacuum level, but the partial pressure of air in the chamber becomes almost negligible. As the system is pressurized with steam, the load air is compressed, and steam heats a larger portion of the pack. As the sterilizing chamber is evacuated a second time, air in the load expands. A portion of the steam that condensed in the load during heating revaporizes at the lower pressure, driving the air out of the load into the sterilizing environment. The air is again removed by gravity displacement. This procedure is repeated until air is removed from the system sufficiently such that no thermal lag is noted on heating of the load to the desired exposure temperature.

The key to an effective process is the use of gravity displacement to minimize re-entrainment of air during pressurization. The velocity of steam admitted to the chamber during gravity displacement is critical (see previous section entitled *Gravity Displacement*). A high-velocity steam flow results in mass-flow dilution, which still works but is considerably less efficient. Figures 29–10 and 29–11 show the proper heating characteristic of a towel pack versus the characteristics when the steam is admitted to the chamber at too high a velocity, with all other conditions the same.

Airtightness of the Sterilizer Chamber

Regardless of which technique of air removal is used, proper conditioning of the load prior to the exposure time at a given temperature is vital. Under normal conditions, the process should ensure that the entire load will be exposed for a sufficiently long time at a high enough temperature to be acceptably sterilized.

Common causes of air in the sterilizing chamber with vacuum sterilizers are air leaks through mechanical components such as valves and door gaskets. Even with diligent equipment check-out efforts, the sterilizer may develop an air leak between tests or exhibit intermittent leak problems that compromise proper sterilization.

In a test of ten prevacuum steam sterilizers, Darmady et al. (1964) showed that not one was able to produce and maintain the conditions advocated by authorities for effective sterilization. A good sterilization process design ensures air removal and airtightness of the sterilization chamber. Perkins (1969) suggested the maximum permissible leak rate should not exceed 1 mm Hg per minute at a chamber pressure of 12 mm Hg in the sterilizing chamber as measured by absolute pressure gauges or switch arrangements. AAMI (1980) and AORN (1980) recommended running a Bowie and Dick type test pack daily to ensure adequate sterilizing efficiency. This is not a test that can be performed during regular processing. Joslyn (1976) developed a method to directly quantitate air in the sterilizing chamber and thus to demonstrate that it has been adequately removed during preconditioning.

Henfrey (Medical Research Council, 1964) developed a load simulator that is actually an air accumulator positioned to collect residual air. It compares temperature in the chamber drain with temperatures achieved in the load sensor. An accumulation of air will not allow the cycle timing to proceed until the preset temperature has been attained in the load sensor. This technique, although good in theory, has suffered from poor design.

Above-Atmospheric Steam Sterilization

Joslyn (1988) discovered that air could be removed from the sterilizing chamber and the load in a process performed at above-atmospheric pressure with a short conditioning period comparable to that achieved with vacuum sterilization processes. Referring to Figure 29–12, the sterilization process consists of a sequence of pressure pulses and steam flushes performed at above

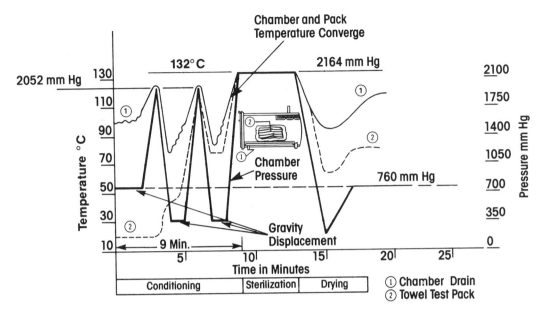

Fig. 29–10. Heating characteristic of a 42-towel double-muslin-wrapped test pack in a properly designed combination pressure-pulsing with air displacement process.

atmospheric pressure. The positive pressure prevents air from leaking into the sterilizing chamber. Short conditioning times and rapid heating were achieved while adding the dependability of sterilization, even when air leaks were created in the sterilizing chamber to simulate mechanical problems. No positive biologic indicators or negative chemical indicator results have been reported for the new process since the initial validation in a hospital application (Anonymous, 1988). In addition to typical health-care facility applications, it is projected that this technology will provide reliable sterilization in applications in which the sterilizing chamber would be more prone to leakage problems, as in military applications where equipment is frequently moved, such as in field hospitals.

Superheated Vapor

The departure of superheated steam from a liquid/vapor equilibrium saturation curve is commonly expressed in two ways. (1) The *degree of superheat*, often called simply superheat, is the temperature excess above the temperature of saturated steam at the same pressure. For example, if the pressure is 29.825 psia and the temperature is 132.2°C, we find that the temperature of

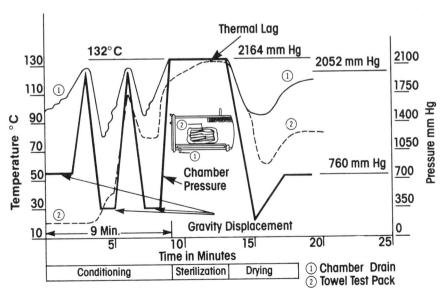

Fig. 29–11. Heating of a 42-towel double-muslin-wrapped test pack in a combination pressure-pulsing and air displacement process as in Figure 29–10, but with chamber turbulence due to improper baffle design.

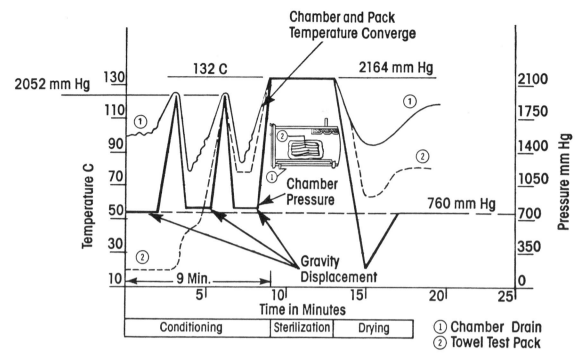

Fig. 29–12. Heating characteristic of a 42-towel double-muslin-wrapped test pack in the Joslyn above-atmospheric pressure steam sterilization process.

saturated steam at 29.825 psia is 121.1°C. The superheat is then 132.2° − 121.1° = 11.1°C. (2) The *relative humidity* (RH) is the ratio of the actual pressure of the vapor to the pressure of saturated steam at the same temperture. For the previous example, pressure equaling 29.825 psia and the temperature equaling 132.2°C, the pressure of saturated vapor at a temperature of 132.2°C is 41.856 psia. The relative humidity of the steam is then 29.825/41.856 = 0.713.

In a pure steam system, relative humidity or superheat can be measured with pressure and temperature instrumentation. In air-steam mixtures, various other techniques are required.

Saturated steam and superheated steam behave like any gas mixture. In the presence of water at thermal equilibrium with the saturated steam, the superheated steam will lose its additional heat energy when it contacts water or any surface below the saturation temperature. The rate of heat transfer is essentially equal for both saturated and superheated steam until the material being heated reaches the dew point temperature for the superheated steam. Then heating by mass heat transfer stops in a superheated steam environment. Superheated steam is metastable but will exist where a hot surface, a drop in pressure across an orifice, or other modifying factors provide the appropriate boundary conditions.

During steam sterilization, some degree of superheat can be tolerated, but higher degrees result in a loss of sterilizing efficiency (Walter, 1948). Savage (1937) found that as deviation from the saturation phase boundary increased, the rate of spore destruction decreased phe-

nomenally. These data would indicate that at temperatures above 132°C, superheat becomes inconsequential. However, this is an area that requires more investigation using appropriately designed test equipment. Rates of reaction are so fast at temperatures above 121°C that the accuracy of test results must be considered questionable for any of the test methods reported to date. In general, based upon the bacteriologic results obtained at lower temperatures, superheat below 5°C (approximately 85% RH) should not be objectionable.

Superheated steam can arise from several sources. Jacket heat that is above the sterilizing temperature produces heating of materials with high emissivity characteristics by radiant heat transfer to the surface of materials in the sterilizing chamber. As steam is admitted to the sterilizing environment and passes through the material, it picks up heat from both the chamber walls and the material, resulting in superheat in a surface layer of the material.

Superheating can also result from the characteristics of materials. Walter (1942), Henry (1959), Knox et al. (1960), and Bowie (1961) showed that superheating occurs in steam sterilizers because of the combined effects of heat transfer from steam to the fabric and an exothermic heat energy released on hydration of excessively dried materials that normally maintain a certain hydration level (e.g., cotton fabrics, paper products). This phenomenon is particularly noticeable in the center of a load. When the materials have a low specific heat and high insulative properties, the load retains the heat generated during hydration. Ernst and Joslyn (1967) also found that the presence of air can increase the temperature in towel packs tremendously, resulting in charring during high-vacuum sterilization (see *High-Vacuum Sterilization*).

Temperature measurements in an environment are often thought to be superheat when actually they represent radiant energy from the jacket being measured. The intensity of thermal radiation passing between surfaces is not affected appreciably by the presence of intervening media because, unless the temperature is high enough to cause ionization or dissociation, monatomic gases and most diatomic gases, as well as air, are transparent. Thus, unless temperature measurement sensors are properly shielded, radiant energy from the jacket can heat the sensor, producing a higher temperature indication than actually exists in the environment. Numerous factors contribute to radiant heat transfer, including material emissivity, the distance from the heat source, and shape factors (Kreith, 1973).

Load Wetness

In a wet state, sterilized materials are more susceptible to recontamination. Beck and Collette (1952) and Probst (1953) proved that bacteria readily pass through wet or damp wrapping materials. To lessen the problem of wetness, most steam sterilization processes provide a drying phase. In gravity sterilizers, the door is sometimes opened partially so that steam vents out of the chamber while radiant and convective heat from the sterilizing chamber provide the heat energy to dry the load. This is not a preferred method, because unsterile air contacts the load at a vulnerable time.

A second method uses an aspirator to pull steam out of the sterilizing chamber while admitting air through a bioretentive filter until the load is sufficiently dried. It is important to remove the steam through the top of the chamber while admitting air in the bottom (the reverse of gravity displacement) until the sterilizer door is opened. This is because steam would accumulate at the top of the chamber and would not be totally removed. Hospital autoclave operators frequently have reported burns from rising steam after opening the autoclave door and reaching for panel controls, which are often located above the door. Steam causes severe burns with only a moment's contact.

Drying in vacuum sterilizers generally produces acceptably dry loads under normal conditions. Following sterilization, the chamber is evacuated to between 100 and 40 mm Hg absolute. This revaporizes a percentage of the condensate and dries the load.

Chamber Water

Most modern sterilizers are rectangular vessels to minimize floor space and maximize loading volume. The flat bottoms generally are not adequately sloped for water to exit the drain vent; therefore, low spots retain condensate in the chamber (Fig. 29–7). Following sterilization, rapid venting of the sterilizing chamber results in violent ebullition of the water on the hot floor of the autoclave chamber. This ebullition propels water up onto materials being processed and causes spot wetting on the bottom of wrapped materials. Such gross wetting is not always dried during the drying process. To prevent this wetting, some manufacturers provide a splash pan (Fig. 29–5).

Steam Quality

The quality of steam is the weight of dry steam present in a mixture of dry saturated steam and entrained water. If the steam quality is 97%, the wet steam mixture consists of 3 parts by weight of saturated water and 97 parts by weight of saturated steam. Ideal steam for sterilization is 100% saturated steam. Factors such as boiler priming, poorly trapped steam supplies, and normal pipe wall condensation entrained by high-velocity steam flow all contribute to produce a steam quality that is less than 100%.

Steam quality for steam sterilization can be controlled, however, at the point of use (in the autoclave chamber) by using a steam separator and baffling. These design elements ensure that an autoclave will perform consistently regardless of the steam quality delivered to the autoclave.

Steam quality affects the degree of sterilization and dryness of processed materials. When materials such as dressings, linens, and outer wrappings are sterilized, the fabrics can become saturated with moisture. Excessive wetting of the materials hinders diffusion of air from the load. The phenomenon is similar to tying the pant legs of a pair of trousers for flotation in water. When the material is dry, air passes freely. When the material is wet, the diffusivity of air through the material decreases. This trapped air can reduce significantly the rate at which a dense porous load will heat.

Following sterilization, grossly wetted materials are not easily dried. Penikett et al. (1959) reported that materials are noticeably damp when containing 6% water by weight. Figure 29–13 shows the typical moisture gain of a 12-pound towel pack, with various percentages of initial pack moisture following sterilization in 99% saturated steam and one postvacuum to 100 mm Hg. It can be seen that a high initial pack moisture results in increased moisture gain. Figure 29–14 shows the increase in moisture gain relative to steam quality for a towel pack with an initial pack moisture level of 3%. The moisture gain increases as the steam quality decreases. It should be noted that steam quality is much more important in pressure-pulsing systems because more steam is used to eliminate air from the system.

Deleterious Effects in Sterilization by Heat

In the science of sterilization, one of the considerations is the rate of material degradation relative to the rate of biologic inactivation. Studies of steam corrosion and its inhibition (Holmlund, 1965), damage to fabrics and rubber (Medical Research Council, 1964; Henry, 1964; Fallon and Pyne, 1963) and nutritional degradation (Stumbo, 1973) have shown that short high-temperature sterilization processes have fewer deleterious effects for

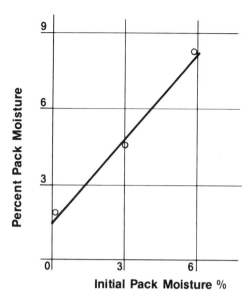

Fig. 29–13. Percentage of moisture in a 12-pound towel pack with various initial moisture contents following high-vacuum sterilization with 99 + % saturated steam at 132°C and one postvacuum to 100 mm Hg.

equivalent bacterial inactivation. Proteins generally suffer under heat treatments, and carbohydrates are sometimes caramelized. Caramelized products have been implicated as toxic agents. Such chemical degradation is a particularly important facet of sterilization process design for parenterals.

Figure 29–15 shows the degradation of thiamine at various sterilization temperatures. At elevated temperatures, degradation is significantly less and nearly independent of any selected process lethality (F_0). In the food industry, the concept of minimal degradation has stimulated activity revolving about the sterilization and aseptic packaging of food products such that they can be transported and stored without refrigeration (U.S. Department of Energy, 1979). Many heat-sensitive fluids have been sterilized using ultrahigh-temperature sterilization (above 132°C) without noticeable organoleptic or minimal catabolic degradation.

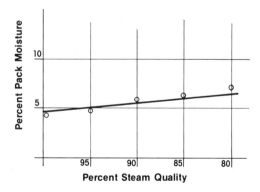

Fig. 29–14. The effect of steam quality on moisture gain for a 12-pound towel pack with 3% initial moisture content following high-vacuum sterilization at 132°C and one postvacuum to 100 mm Hg.

Sterilization of Liquids

Major technologic changes are occurring in the sterilization of liquids and semiliquid materials in the food and pharmaceutical industries. One of the major reasons is the growth of autoclavable flexible packaging. The materials developed for autoclavable pouches not only provide superior barrier properties for a long shelf life, seal integrity, toughness, and puncture resistance, but also enhance thermal processing. Flexible packaging (Fig. 29–16) can increase the ratio of heating surface to volume and reduce heat penetration depth such that materials can be heat-sterilized with significantly less thermal lag between the surface and the center. Likewise, materials can be cooled readily. Thus, less exposure time is required at a given temperature to achieve sterilization. To ensure a thin, high surface area, the pouch geometry should be constrained during processing as shown in Figure 29–17. This provides a more consistent heat character from one pouch to the next.

Industrial sterilization techniques are improving. The trend is toward continuous sterilization processes in which each individual item is processed sequentially rather than the classic bulk sterilization of large loads. In the sequential method, not only can equivalent loads be processed, but if the equipment fails, a smaller amount of the product is lost. This is important because of the high cost of preparation and packaging prior to sterilization. During continuous sterilization the item can be manipulated to improve heating and cooling. One method tumbles a liquid container end over end so that air in the container agitates the liquid to produce more uniform heating.

Utsumi et al. (1975) and Stenstrom (1974) have developed methods to rapidly heat fluids independent of the container material (except metal containers) using dielectric heating with microwaves. Anyone involved with the design of microwave equipment knows that field standing waves are generally uncontrollable, resulting in one object heating preferentially before the next. In a continuous sterilization process, however, in which one object is processed at a time, the thermal heating characteristics of each product can be controlled and measured by nonintrusive means.

Ultrahigh-temperature (UHT) sterilization of heat-sensitive fluids was promoted in early 1964 by Ellertson and Pearce. In these processes, fluids are heated rapidly to a given temperature for an appropriate exposure time and cooled in heat exchangers. More recently, the Department of Energy (1979) sponsored a grant to study direct sterilization of heat-sensitive fluids by a method whereby the fluid to be sterilized is pumped directly into a steam environment as shown in Figure 29–18. The liquid falls freely through the steam as a thin film, where it is "instantaneously" heated to the steam temperature. The positive pressure in the chamber forces the fluid out of the chamber, where it is rapidly cooled by the heat of vaporization at a lower pressure. Both methods require aseptic packaging techniques. Milk sterilized by this

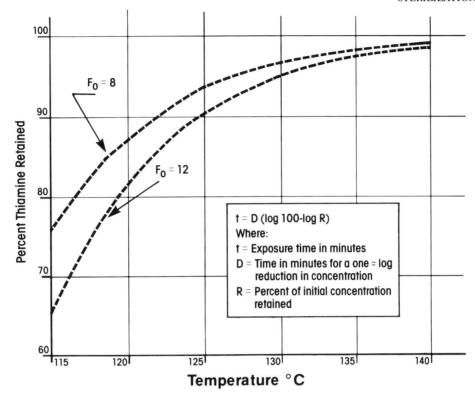

$$t = D (\log 100 - \log R)$$

Where:

t = Exposure time in minutes

D = Time in minutes for a one = log reduction in concentration

R = Percent of initial concentration retained

Fig. 29–15. Degradation of thiamine relative to steam sterilization effect at various temperatures, demonstrating that less degradation occurs at elevated temperatures for a given sterilization effect.

method underwent only trace amounts of organoleptic and catabolic degradation. Many foods that can be processed in this way do not require refrigeration during shipping or storage, resulting in tremendous energy savings.

STERILIZATION BY DRY HEAT

As Rahn (1945) pointed out, a great deal of confusion exists regarding the proper time-temperature relationships for sterilization by dry heat. As Rahn implied, this is due to many conflicting reports in the literature based upon the fact that the killing of spores by dry heat reflects

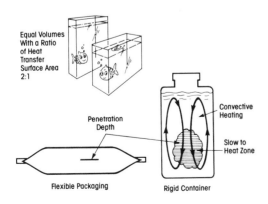

Fig. 29–16. Increased surface-to-volume relationship and reduced heat penetration depth achievable with autoclavable flexible packaging.

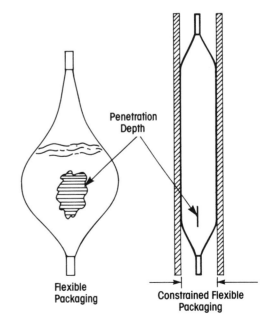

Fig. 29–17. More-consistent heat character of product being sterilized was maintained by constraining the flexible packaging into consistent dimensions.

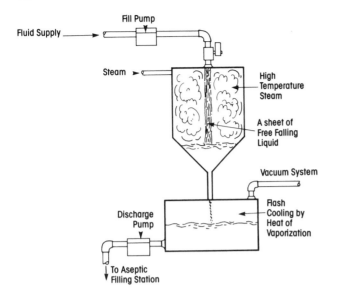

Fig. 29–18. Free-fall method of rapidly heating liquids in steam and rapid cooling after sterilization.

low Q_{10} ratios as compared to moist heat. There are also many complicating factors associated with destruction by dry heat. Whereas steam sterilization is usually accomplished with saturated moisture, the moisture involved in dry-heat sterilization may vary considerably. The death rate of spores might be expected to change with the continued application of heat, especially at lower heating temperatures, because of the loss of moisture. However, Oag (1940) found an abrupt change in resistance at 160°C, above which temperature spores were killed much more rapidly. Some reasonable areas of explanation may involve protective effects already discussed, relating to the diffusion of heat, amount of heat available from the heating medium, amount of available moisture and heat lost owing to change of state, and changes occurring at the spore surface and in its immediate surroundings.

Although the mechanism for destruction by dry heat is primarily an oxidation process, it may not be exclusively so in all cases, because dry heat must be a relative term. Lewith (1890) found different coagulation temperatures for protein containing different amounts of water. From Perkins (1960):

Egg albumin + 50% water coagulates at 56°C.
Egg albumin + 25% water coagulates at 74° to 80°C.
Egg albumin + 18% water coagulates at 80° to 90°C.
Egg albumin + 6% water coagulates at 145°C.
Egg albumin + 0% water coagulates at 160° to 170°C.

A great amount of interest is presently being generated relating the water activities of spores of bacteria with their thermal resistance (Pflug, 1965). The water activity, A_w, is related to the concentration and is expressed as a fraction of the pure component in the standard state, where $A_w = 1$. Waldham and Halvorson (1954) suggested that heat resistance of spores may be due to "bound protein," in that there is evidence that the polar groups

are masked, so that spores lose their affinity for water. Marshall et al. (1962) found the water activity of spores of *Bacilli* and *Clostridia* during storage after freeze drying affected their viability after storage at 25°C. At A_w values between 0.2 and 0.8, there was no loss of viability, but at A_w less than 0.2, losses were marked. Resistance to heating was greatest after storage at A_w values of 0.4 to 0.8. Oxidation may also play a small part in the death of bacterial spores by moist heat, as indicated by the reduced D values obtained when antioxidant materials were added to the spore suspensions exposed to heat (Michener et al., 1959).

Although great strides have been made in improving and developing other methods of sterilization, little has been accomplished where sterilization by dry heat is concerned. Sterilizers are still essentially the same as they were a decade ago. This neglected area has recently been given great impetus by those concerned with the sterilization of extraterrestrial "planetary landers" to prevent contamination of virgin preserves for the sake of future exobiologic experiments. Therefore, the sterilization of the interior of solids is of great concern in this program, whereas before the concern was primarily the sterilization of surfaces of such materials. One of the sterilizing agents with general penetrating properties for all kinds of materials is dry heat.

Other means of sterilizing by dry heat are infrared and incineration. Infrared will transmit only by direct rays to the surfaces exposed to the radiation. Penetration must be by conduction. Many instruments in a load, for example, would be shielded from the infrared by other instruments in the direct path. Heating of such shielded materials would require convection heat transfer from the previously heated materials, resulting in delays and tendencies toward unequal heating.

The most effective means for the sterilization of air is incineration (Cherry et al., 1963), which, however, is destructive. When destruction is of no concern, incineration is efficient and effective as a means of killing harmful microorganisms and disposing of contaminated materials.

The time-temperature relationships for sterilization with hot air suggested by Perkins (1960) are as follows:

170°C (340°F) .... 60 minutes
160°C (320°F) .... 120 minutes
150°C (300°F) .... 150 minutes
140°C (285°F) .... 180 minutes
121°C (250°F) .... Overnight

These temperatures relate to the time of exposure after attainment of the specific temperature and do not include heating lags.

Heat availability has much to do with the efficacy of the heat treatment as it relates to heat conductivity. The greatest amount of heat is available from steam, but the temperature necessary to effect sterilization would require steam pressures beyond the range of practicability. Thus, the agent of choice, air, is not the best heat transfer medium by any means, but it is the least expensive. Heat transfer can be accelerated by moving the air stream, because a grave limitation in dry-heat sterilization by static means is severe stratification and lack of diffusion in and around relatively cool materials.

Hot air sterilizers are usually heated electrically and can be designed to provide heaters underneath a perforated bottom plate to provide natural convection currents. Cool instruments, for example, will cool the air surrounding them. This air will move in a downward direction, and the air in contact with the heaters will move upward, setting up convection currents. This type of sterilizer is the *gravity convection* type. On the other hand, *mechanical convection sterilizers* are fitted with a motor-driven squirrel-cage fan, which assists in air circulation, increasing heat transfer by convection.

Dry heat should be used only for those materials that cannot be sterilized by steam, when the moisture would either damage the materials or they would be impermeable to it. Such materials are petrolatum, oils, powders, sharp instruments in particular, and glassware. It is necessary not to overload a dry-heat sterilizer with materials; overloading delays heat convection either by circulation or by heat absorption. Sufficient space should be left between materials for good circulation. Wrappings and other barriers should be kept to a minimum. A heavy load of instruments would require an abnormally long time to heat, and organic matter on the instruments would tend to char and bake on them.

The principal advantage of dry-heat sterilization is its penetrating power. It is not as corrosive as steam for metals and sharp instruments and it does not erode ground glass surfaces. Therefore, glass can be sterilized at much higher temperatures for shorter periods of time.

The disadvantages of dry-heat sterilization are as follows:

1. *Heating is slow.* Diffusion and penetration of heat are slow because the heat transfer medium is poor, and there is a distinct lack of available heat compared to steam particularly.
2. *It requires long sterilizing periods.* Long exposure times are required because the killing rate by dry heat is slow, as is heat absorption.
3. *It requires high temperatures.* These temperatures may be deleterious to materials.
4. *Materials are damaged.* Deterioration of materials occurs with oxidation. Killing by dry heat is an oxidation process, and the medium that facilitates this killing action also augments its deleterious effects.
5. *There is a tendency to stratify.* A severe tendency to stratify over a considerable range of temperature must be overcome.

MEASUREMENT OF THE EFFICIENCY OF STEAM STERILIZATION PROCESSES WITH BIOLOGIC AND PHYSICAL/CHEMICAL INDICATORS

Biologic Indicators

Biologic indicators (BIs) are standardized preparations of specific microorganisms resistant to a sterilization

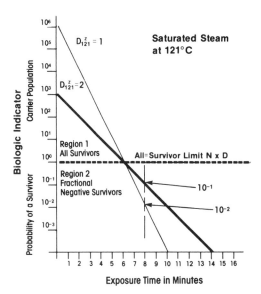

Fig. 29–19. Biologic indicator inactivation characteristics during steam sterilization at 121°C.

process. In the purest form, the microorganisms are added directly to the item being sterilized. When this approach is not practical, an alternative is to add the organisms to carrier materials that have compositions as similar as possible to the package or item being sterilized, such that the effects of the sterilization process are similar (USP, 1980). BIs that survive a sterilization process provide evidence of an ineffective process.

Historically, BIs have been the accepted referees for determining the adequacy of sterilization processes. This is logical in that sterilization-inactivation kinetics are derived from biologic testing. BIs have retained prominence as the preferred standard for monitoring the effectiveness of steam sterilization processes owing to an ability to sense and integrate not only time and temperature factors but also miscellaneous conditions, such as superheat, physical characteristics, or constituents in a medium being sterilized, that influence the rate of biologic inactivation. When properly applied, BIs can be used to evaluate process effectiveness without physically influencing the test results. The ability of the BIs to reflect the effects of various conditions on biologic inactivation without influencing microenvironmental conditions is the key element differentiating between BIs and physical/chemical indicators (P/CIs) or instrumentation for evaluating process effectiveness.

Under given sterilization conditions, the intrinsic inactivation characteristics of BIs are the D value and the initial carrier organism population. The exposure time transition point, or all-survivor limit, at which BIs all culture positive as opposed to producing fractional negative cultures, is a product of the logarithm of the number of organisms per carrier (N) times the D value, as shown in Figure 29–19.

Infinite combinations of D values and carrier populations result in inactivation curves that intersect at a given all-survivor limit. Mathematically, exposure periods equal to or less than this time result in positive cultures for all of these combinations. For exposure intervals greater than this, the different BI characteristics produce a significant difference in probability of a survivor. An example of this can be seen in Figure 29–19. Two BI curves are shown at an 8-minute exposure for the two curves shown passing through an all-survivor limit of 6 minutes. The BI curve with a D value of 1 minute has a 1-in-10^2 probability of a survivor, where the BIs with a D value of 2 minutes have a 1-in-10 probability of a survivor. BIs with lower D values have a greater differentiation between the all-survivor limit and the fractional negative region.

Lethality factors, such as F_0 and F_T^Z values, are the method of expressing effectiveness of steam sterilization processes by physical measurement that most professional organizations (PDA, 1978) and official compendia (USP XIX, 1975 and USP XX, 1980) have accepted. These factors are treated extensively in the literature (FDA, 1978; Phillips and Miller, 1973; Stumbo, 1973). Coexistence of lethality factors and BIs for specifying and measuring process effectiveness requires an understanding of the relationship between the two.

The all-survivor limit is the common denominator for equating BI resistance to sterilization with lethality factors. N times the D value at a given temperature should be equal to the desired process lethality factor. When the test organism Z value is the same as the Z value for calculating the process lethality, the BI's all-survivor limit (D_T^Z times N) correlates mathematically with the lethality factor (F_T^Z) calculated over the range of process temperatures. Obviously, validation of process lethality with BIs is limited to lethality factors that are obtainable relative to a practical BI D value and carrier population.

There is some controversy over methods for and accuracy of determining BI Z values and D values. Still, in practice, it is not unreasonable to expect BIs to exhibit variation in characteristics. Z values for *Bacillus stearothermophilus* NCA 1518 (BSTM), which is typically used to validate the effectiveness of steam sterilization, are typically reported to range from 8.9 to 11.1°C (16 to 20°F) or more. Such variations can alter significantly the correlation between results with BIs or any relationship to a standard lethality factor such as an F_0 value. Figure 29–20 shows an example of process lethality factors and BI all-survivor limit variations during a hypothetic sterilization process due to different Z values. In this cycle, a design minimum process $F_{121°C}^Z$ of 8 was selected. Three BIs, A, B, and C, with Z values of 8.9°, 10°, and 11.1°C (16°, 18°, and 20°F) respectively, and D values of 1.6 as determined at 121°C, are selected such that the all-survivor limits are equal:

$$N \times D_{121°C}^{8.9°C} = N \times D_{121°C}^{10°C} = N \times D_{121°C}^{121°C} = F_{121°C}^Z$$

Calculations show that a higher Z value provides a more conservative lethality factor and all-survivor limit for temperatures above the base temperature (T_B) relative to the generally accepted lethality factor (F_0).

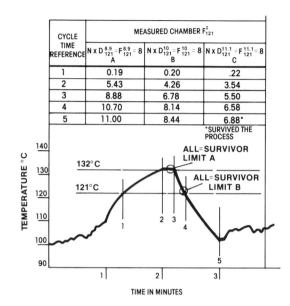

CYCLE TIME REFERENCE	MEASURED CHAMBER F_{121}^Z		
	$N \times D_{121}^{8.9} = F_{121}^{8.9} = 8$ A	$N \times D_{121}^{10} = F_{121}^{10} = 8$ B	$N \times D_{121}^{11.1} = F_{121}^{11.1} = 8$ C
1	0.19	0.20	.22
2	5.43	4.26	3.54
3	8.88	6.78	5.50
4	10.70	8.14	6.58
5	11.00	8.44	6.88*

*SURVIVED THE PROCESS

Fig. 29–20. Computer-simulated relationship between BIs all-survivor limits (D times N) and lethality factors (F) for various Z values in a steam sterilization process.

Below the reference temperature, a lower Z value results in a more conservative estimate relative to an F_0 value. Thus, the range of lethality factors and all-survivor limits obtained depends upon the shape of the sterilization process temperature profile. Computer simulation of various hypothetical sterilization temperature profiles, using a range of Z values from 8.9 to 11.1°C indicates the calculated lethality factors and all-survivor limits will range typically from an equivalent of 5.5 to 11 relative to an F_0 of 8 (USP XX minimum suggested article lethality, 1980) and from 8 to 17 relative to an F_0 of 12 (PDA suggested minimum article lethality for the overkill method, 1980).

Physical/Chemical Indicators (P/CIs)

P/CIs are devices designed to provide information relative to the achievement of one or several of the conditions necessary to destroy microorganisms resistant to sterilization. When used in a sterilization process, P/CIs are used to indicate that the sterilization process was performed and to ensure proper product packaging, sterilizer load configurations, and functioning of the processing equipment.

Potential use of P/CIs for measuring sterilization process effectiveness is of major interest to those responsible for process development and sterility assurance. The low cost and immediate indication that sterilizing conditions have been achieved without the necessity of support equipment and facilities (media, incubation areas, and transfer hoods) promote the liberal use of these devices. Many of these devices also provide a permanent record of the achievement of appropriate sterilizing conditions. These features could result in a higher assurance of proper sterilization.

Reports have indicated that P/CIs exhibit questionable

performance. Negative criticism can often be attributed to the failure of the authors to recognize appropriate design intent and application or to have accepted performance standards. BIs did not receive the same criticism in many reports even though historically they also have not demonstrated, and often still do not demonstrate, resistance to sterilization equivalent to acceptable minimum sterilization standards such as those proposed by Perkins (1978). Negative criticism can also be attributed to inadequate methods or equipment for evaluating the various devices. It was only in 1980, for instance, that standards were suggested for BI test apparatus (AAMI, 1980). This was in recognition that variation among test systems was the cause of inconsistent unacceptable biologic test results from one laboratory to the next or even in the same test apparatus. Nonetheless, a stigma (real or not) exists relative to the credibility of using P/CIs for validating effectiveness of a sterilization process.

Some difference of opinion exists about desirable performance characteristics for P/CIs for sterilization in industrial settings versus the health care institutions. Industrial sterilization is generally performed in well instrumented equipment with consistent load configurations. A professional staff of sterilization scientists work on industrial sterilization. Financial, regulatory, and professional interests promote both cost containment and product quality. Industrial scientists have demonstrated improved product quality and throughput with equivalent sterilization effectiveness by performing steam sterilization at selected temperatures for minimum exposure periods. Toward this end, professional organizations have effectively promoted lethality factors for simplicity in estimating process lethality in addition to consistency in the design and evaluation of sterilization processes over a range of sterilization temperatures. Additionally, calibrated BIs are used to validate the process in conjunction with the instrumentation. This trend toward consistency indicates a need for P/CIs to be used in industrial sterilization that correlates with BIs and lethality measured with instrumentation.

Sterilization in health care institutions is generally performed in poorly instrumented equipment that is used to sterilize a variety of load configurations. The staff is usually not trained in sterilization technology and does not generally perform in-house testing of sterilization processes. To ensure adequate sterilization, extended exposure times and P/CIs that require long exposure times before the achievement of sterilization conditions is indicated have been suggested (AORN, 1980).

Unfortunately, extending exposure periods and using P/CIs that require longer periods to indicate that conditions for sterilization have been achieved will not ensure proper sterilization. Figure 29–21 shows chemical indicator sheets, chemical indicators, and a BI placed in a towel pack and sterilized in saturated steam at 134°C for 10 minutes. The most difficult location for steam to penetrate was not the geometric center of the packs, as

one might assume. Furthermore, the slow-to-heat location shifts randomly from one pack to the next. It is only because the sheet-type P/CI provides information about the entire cross section of the towel pack that a cold spot might be detected consistently. The indicators requiring extended exposure times before indicating that sterilization conditions have been achieved may or may not detect a cold spot depending upon the position of the spot in the test pack. One should recognize, based upon the position shown, that BIs would not have indicated a deficiency. Indicating devices are instruments to measure the conditions at the point of use. They cannot compensate for the inefficiency of a sterilization process. Liberal use of the correct type of calibrated indicator for a given pack or load (the sheet type in this example) is the best way to ensure sterilization effectiveness.

At elevated temperatures, overprocessing defeats two of the primary advantages of high-temperature sterilization: reduced load degradation and increased sterilization throughput rate. Steam sterilization studies have shown that, as a related rate function, bacterial inactivation is generally faster than material degradation at elevated temperatures. In health care institutions, load degradation is often not addressed, because of the difficulty in identifying and quantifying the deleterious effects of sterilization upon the variety of items processed. Many central supply supervisors have indicated that with current materials being used, no general load degradation problems have been noted.

Biologically Based P/CIs

Indicators that are biologically based are considered different from P/CIs that might be used to evaluate sterilization process lethality. There are conditions under which indicators that are referred to as BIs are more appropriately classified as biologically based P/CIs. One of the most commonly used biologically based P/CIs consists of test organisms on a carrier strip enclosed in a bioretentive vented container with a crushable ampule of culturing medium. Owing to thermal lag, this type of indicator often exhibits Z values as high as 30°C as determined between test temperatures of 121 and 132°C. With such a high artificial Z value, correlation to accepted process lethality factors for most items being sterilized is impossible. The design of this type of indicator also prohibits evaluation of the influence of superheat upon biologic inactivation because the "carrier system" acts as a dew point apparatus. Steam or superheated steam contacting the ampule and container condenses and wets the carrier strip. Thus, the test organism on the carrier strip will not be subjected to superheat conditions as often reported in steam sterilization of dehydrated materials. By definition, this type of indicator should not be considered a true BI in most applications.

A second biologically based P/CI commonly used is a sealed ampule containing a culturing medium and microorganisms. In some applications, this system acts as a BI, but misapplication can result in meaningless correlation to sterilization process effectiveness. In an ap-

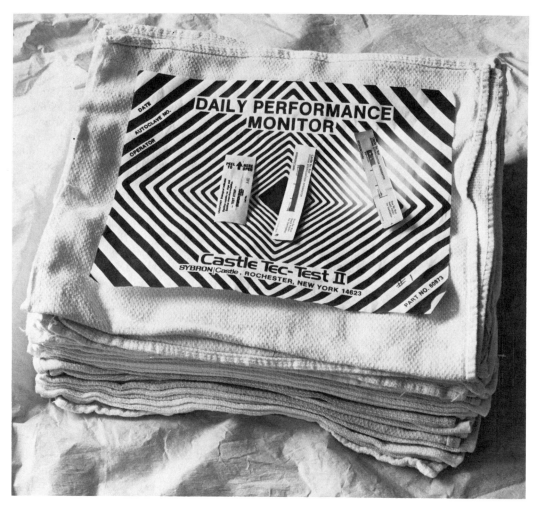

Fig. 29–21. BIs and P/CIs used in Bowie- and Dick-type towel packs to monitor steam sterilization effectiveness in high-vacuum sterilization with an air leak. Courtesy of Sybron Corporation, Medical Products Division, Rochester, NY.

propriate application of this type of indicator, the heat character of the ampule is the same as the heat character of the load. Thus, the biologic inactivation is related to the item being sterilized, assuming the test organism has the same Z value both in or on the item being sterilized and in the test BI ampule. In health care institutions, these ampules are frequently used inappropriately to monitor flash (high-temperature, short-duration) steam sterilization processes.

Figure 29–22 shows BI ampule heating and cooling characteristics during a flash cycle. The ampule is heated by mass heat transfer resulting from steam condensing on the ampule. This is a fast heating mechanism. Depending upon the rate of chamber heatup time, the ampule may exhibit a slight thermal lag. This lag results in less biologic inactivation or lethality than is actually achieved during this portion of the process. After reaching a given exposure temperature, the sterilizer is rapidly cooled by venting the steam. The ampule, however, does not cool rapidly because the only mechanisms for removing heat are convection and radiant heat transfer.

These are slow heat transfer mechanisms, resulting in a gross thermal lag and consequently significantly higher ampule biologic inactivation or lethality factors than were attained in the process.

Evaluation of these ampule thermal characteristics shows that an overall actual process lethality can be obtained that is significantly less than would be measured using the BI ampule. The difference between proper versus improper use of the BI ampule, in this case, is the thermal time constant of the ampule. The time constant is the time required for an object to reach 63% of a step change in temperature in a specific medium. At elevated temperatures, the thermal time constant is increasingly significant relative to the ability of a BI or a P/CI to represent the achievement of sterilization process lethality. To follow the kinetics of biologic inactivation for BSTM in saturated steam, BIs and P/CIs should have a time constant on heating and cooling that approaches those shown in Figure 29–23.

Unfortunately, performance differences for biologic indicators relative to application considerations are not ad-

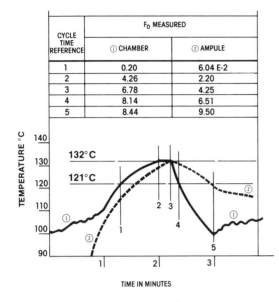

CYCLE TIME REFERENCE	F_0 MEASURED	
	① CHAMBER	② AMPULE
1	0.20	6.04 E-2
2	4.26	2.20
3	6.78	4.25
4	8.14	6.51
5	8.44	9.50

Fig. 29–22. BI ampule heating and cooling characteristics relative to chamber and ampule F_0 values.

equately recognized in practice, even though professional organizations, articles, and official compendia clearly point out the consideration of performance as similar as possible to the package or item being sterilized (Perkins, 1978) (HIMA, 1978; USP, 1975 and 1980). Considering the limitations of biologically based P/CIs, other nonbiologically based P/CIs would be as effective for process indicators while providing the following advantages: they are less expensive, provide immediate indication of conditions achieved, provide a permanent process record, do not require culturing media and incubation facilities, and do not require aseptic transfer techniques or sterility maintenance of the culturing system.

Performance Characteristics for BIs and P/CIs

The objective of sterilization process monitoring is to provide an indication that ensures that minimal acceptable sterilization conditions have been achieved. Approaches include biologic inoculated carriers, printed chemistry, specific melt temperature fusible pellets, and fusible pellets with a wicking member. There are four basic types of indicators: Single transition point indicators, single transition point integrating indicators, integrating P/CIs, and BIs.

Single Transition Point Indicators

Single transition point indicators are devices that provide an indication that a specific temperature has been attained. Some of these devices require the presence of moisture for an indication. In general, there is no correlation between the achievement of any minimal acceptable lethality except at temperatures above 140°C, where sterilization is considered instantaneous.

Single Transition Point Integrating Indicators

Single transition point integrating indicators are devices that require a given time after reaching a specific temperature before indicating that they have been exposed to the appropriate sterilizing conditions. Moisture may be required to produce an indication. These devices are applicable over a limited temperature range. Care must be exercised with indicators used to measure process lethality when the rate of physical/chemical reaction is greater than the rate of biologic inactivation for temperature excursions above the design trigger point of the indicator. In this situation, the achievement of sterilizing conditions can be indicated prematurely.

Integrating P/CIs

Integrating P/CIs, like BIs, have rates of physical/chemical reactions that change with temperature. When the change in rate of reaction corresponds with the biologic system, direct correlation to process lethality factors and biologic inactivation can be attained. This in-

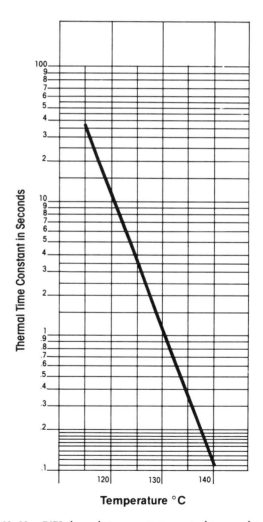

Fig. 29–23. P/CI thermal time constant required to correlate with the rate of inactivation for *Bacillus stearothermophilus* NCA 1518, assuming a Z value of 10°C and $D_{121°C}$ value of 1.5 minutes.

cludes lethality during heating and cooling. These devices may require the presence of moisture for operation. An analogue indicator of this type of device offers the advantage of providing correlation to various degrees of sterilization. This is useful for monitoring lower lethality processes required for heat-labile materials where initial bioburden (number and type of organisms) is known and controlled.

BIs

BIs differ from P/CIs in that they are influenced by known and unknown factors that influence biologic inactivation and do not influence microenvironmental conditions being measured. Owing to the probabilistic nature of survivors, BIs provide a rough yes/no indication of having been exposed to adequate sterilizing conditions. Sublethal process lethality measurement can be made using plate count enumeration methods, but this is not generally performed. Typical commercial BIs survive exposure to steam sterilization processes with F_0 values from 5 to 10. Some of the highly resistant BIs will survive a process with F_0 values of 12 and above. For measurement of process lethality factors above 12, it is generally more practical to use P/CIs and instrumentation.

Indicators that are used for monitoring sterilization of nonheat-labile or low-heat-labile materials should be similar for both industrial and hospital steam sterilization. Figure 29–24 shows the relationship between lethality factors and BI performance characteristics at 121°C that generally have been accepted as the challenge for ensuring the effectiveness of steam sterilization processes. Typical BIs for monitoring steam sterilization consists of 10^5 to 10^6 BSTM organisms per carrier. The D value, as determined at 121°C, generally ranges from 1 to 2 minutes. BIs with D values less than 1.5 were once acceptable; however, current literature (USP XX, 1980) suggests a minimum acceptable article lethality (F_0) of 8. This fact would require BIs with $D_{121°C}$ values above 1.5 minutes. BIs approach a maximum practical all-survivor limit of 12 minutes at 121°C. This corresponds to an F_0 of 12. BIs that can survive sterilization at 121°C for up to 12 minutes exhibit high D values and approach a limit relative to the number of organisms that can practically be inoculated or found naturally on a carrier material. Thus, the maximum process lethality (F_0) that can be practically measured using BIs is 12. This fact concurs with the PDA (1980) recommendation of an F_0 of 12 as the minimum article lethality, for steam sterilization processes where bioburden and organism resistance studies are not performed on nonheat-labile materials to be sterilized.

BIs do not generally survive an F_0 of 12, but the probabilistic nature of biologic systems can result in occasional survivors with process lethality factors above 12. When BIs are used in parallel with P/CIs, a positive BI culture results in uncertainty relative to the credibility of the performance of the P/CIs. Hospital professional organizations recommend reprocessing loads where BIs culture positive (AAMI, 1980; AORN, 1980; HIMA, 1978). To

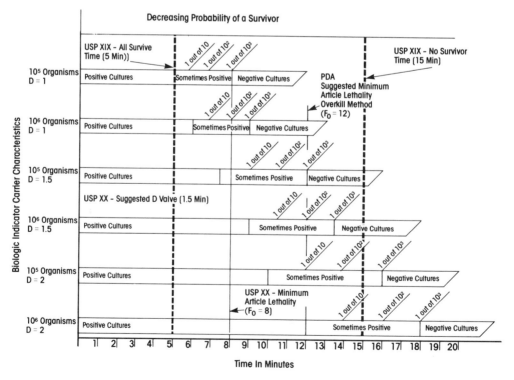

Fig. 29–24. Survival characteristics of BIs at 121°C relative to USP XIX suggested performance characteristics and minimum article lethality (F_0) recommended in literature.

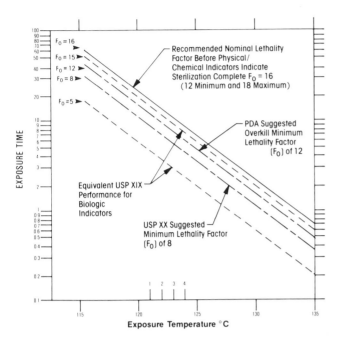

Fig. 29–25. The calculated equivalent performance characteristics of BIs relative to suggested process lethality factors and a recommended performance range for integrating P/CIs (assuming a Z value of 10°C).

minimize this type of result, P/CIs selected should require F_0 values greater than the all-survivor limit of the BI used with an F_0 of 12 as the minimum for the P/CI. Where the BI and P/CI rates of reaction correlate, the probability of a survivor is constant at various exposure temperatures. In general, P/CIs that require a nominal F_0 of 16 prior to indicating that conditions for sterilization are complete will be compatible with most commercial BIs used in health care institutions.

The use of lethality factors provides a common language for relating the performance characteristics of BIs and P/CIs. Figure 29–25 shows the calculated equivalent F_0 for BIs versus suggested minimum sterilization process lethalities and my recommended performance requirements for P/CIs. By superimposing actual P/CI exposure time, temperature, and indication performance characteristics on this figure, a user can readily select P/CIs that meet appropriate exposure time criteria before indicating that conditions have been met over the range of temperatures applicable to the sterilization process.

Moisture

Many steam sterilization indicators claim that the presence of moisture is required before the indicator will function. This capability can be misleading because, depending upon the sensitivity to moisture levels, the P/CI indication could be meaningless. Alderton and Snell (1970) and Murell and Scott (1966) demonstrated that water activity (A_w) or relative humidity (RH) can change the resistance of many bacterial spores, including *Bacillus stearothermophilus*. Although the results of the investigators do not agree precisely, there is a definite

trend in the information indicating that at approximately 85% RH (5°C superheat) and below, the resistance of most bacterial spores increases markedly. Based upon this information, it appears that a first approximation of moisture sensitivity for P/CI design should require exposure to steam environments greater than 85% RH if there is to be a direct relationship to biologic inactivation.

MEASURING THE PERFORMANCE CHARACTERISTICS OF BIOLOGIC INDICATORS FOR STEAM STERILIZATION PROCESSES

Failure to obtain repeatable measurement of biologic indicator performance characteristics has been a growing area of concern to manufacturers, professional organizations, and regulatory agencies. Macek (1972) and Mayernik (1972) conducted studies to evaluate the reproducibility of BI performance data obtained from industrial test apparatus. In these collaborative studies, *B. stearothermophilus* NCA 1518 (BSTM) from the same manufacturing lot were distributed to independent investigators for their evaluation. The results of these tests varied significantly, not only from one laboratory to the next, but also in repeated tests within the same test apparatus. These test results are a good indication that the test apparatus is a significant variable in BI performance evaluation.

Equipment Design

Joslyn (1979) evaluated equipment instrumentation and mechanical designs currently being used to measure the performance characteristics of BIs at several laboratories. The equipment examined exhibited greater variation than was recognized by the users with respect to control of known process variables such as exposure time and temperature. Typical temperature control accuracy varied from ± 1 to ± 4°C from the desired test temperature. Exposure time varied from ± 3 to ± 8 seconds from the desired exposure time.

To estimate the relative significance that exposure time and temperature could have for measurement of biologic inactivation characteristics (D and Z values), mathematic models were used to develop cause-and-effect relationships. Assuming exposure time and temperature variations of ± 3 seconds and ± 1°C, the log variation for a six log reduction in a biologic population was calculated to range from +1.83 to −1.41 at 121°C and +2.89 to −2.03 at 132°C as shown in Table 29–1. The calculated apparent D values due to exposure time and temperature variation ranged from 0.76 to 1.32 minutes relative to a hypothetic D value of 1 minute at 121°C, and from 0.04 to 0.09 minutes relative to a D value of 0.06 at 132°C. This represents a potential difference in D values measured at the respective temperatures of −72 and +125°C. A Z-value determination error was calculated using the log variation values. Under the worst case, Z-value variation could range from 7.3 to 11.9°C. This is an error

Table 29–1. *The Accumulative Log Variation and Apparent D Values Calculated at 121 and 132°C Relative to a Hypothetic 6-Log Reduction in a Biologic Population Based upon Low D and Z Values (i.e., $D_{121°C}^{8.9} = 1$ Minute) Where the Test System Temperature Control Accuracy Is ±1°C and Exposure Time Is ± 3 Seconds*

Hypothetic			Exposure Temperature			
			121°C		132°C	
$D_{121°C}^{8.9}$ Value	Z Value	Process Variable	(+)	(−)	(+)	(−)
1	8.9°C	Exposure Time ±3 seconds (at temperature limits)	.06	.04	1.12	.66
		Exposure Temperature ±1°C	1.77	1.37	1.77	1.37
		Total Log Variation	1.83	1.41	2.89	2.03
		Apparent $D_T^{8.9}$ Value ($D = t/N_o\text{-}N_u$)	.76	1.31	.04	.09

of from +3 to −1.6°C relative to a hypothetic Z value of 8.9°C.

It was concluded that if the test systems examined are representative examples of equipment being used to validate BI performance, then consistent results could not be expected. Consequently, the accuracy of most BI performance data reported to date would be questionable.

An extensive instrumentation and system design evaluation had been performed to determine design control limits for test equipment that could be reproduced (Joslyn, 1976). Equipment was developed that could accurately maintain steam test environments at 115 to 135°C to within ± 0.2°C. Injection and retrieval of test samples from the test environment was achieved to within ± 3 seconds. Referring to Table 29–2, the influence this test system's control accuracy would have upon biologic inactivation characteristics was estimated. At 121°C, the calculated log variation and apparent D value variation was negligible. At 132°C, however, the log variation ranged from +1.22 to −1.12, resulting in apparent D values of 0.05 to 0.07 minutes relative to a hypothetic D value of 0.06. The reason for the larger log variation at 132°C is that exposure time becomes a major process variable as the temperature increases. Although the exposure time control could be feasibly reduced to within ± 2 seconds, experience has indicated that it is unlikely that mechanical test equipment could be fabricated re-

peatedly to accurately control exposure time within this limit. Given these physical design limits for exposure time and temperature control accuracy, the calculated variation in the Z value could range from 8.2 to 9.8°C, as compared to a hypothetic Z value of 8.9°C.

Oxborrow et al. (1988) of the Food and Drug Administration coordinated a collaborative study for the Association for the Advancement of Medical Instrumentation (AAMI) to examine the variability of Joslyn versus non-Joslyn Biologic Indicator Evaluator Resistometers (BIER). The study showed that the overall variance of the Joslyn BIER test units was 50% of that attained with non-Joslyn test systems. Replicate tests were performed with different types of culturing media. As expected, the culturing media significantly influenced the recovery of stressed organisms, producing a wide range of variance in survivor characteristics. Because culturing media is a major variable in the measurement of survivor characteristics, this has to be taken into account when trying to attain repeatable results.

Chamber Air

Anomalies were noted in BI inactivation characteristics during testing. BIs consisting of filter paper strips inoculated with BSTM spores enclosed in a glassine bioretentive envelope were found to be less resistant than inoculated spore strips without the glassine envelope

Table 29–2. *The Accumulative Log Variation and Apparent D Values Calculated at 121 and 132°C Relative to a Hypothetic 6-Log Reduction in a Biologic Population Based upon Low D and Z Values. (i.e., $_{121°C}^{8.9} = 1$ Minute) Where the Test System Has Been Optimized to Accurately Control within ±.2°C with an Exposure Time within ±3 Seconds*

			Exposure Temperature			
			121°C		132°C	
D_{121}^Z Value	Z Value	Process Variable	(+)	(−)	(+)	(−)
1	8.9°C	Exposure Temperature ±.2°C	.3186	.3025	.3186	.3025
		Exposure Time ±3 Seconds (At Temperature Limit)	.0520	.0470	.9060	.8170
		Total Log Variation	.3706	.3495	1.2246	1.1195
		Apparent D Value	.9418	1.0618	.0482	.0714

under the same test conditions. Pflug (1977) has reported this phenomenon also. It was further observed that BIs (in glassine) sandwiched together produced results indicating that the center BIs were less resistant than the outer BIs. This is contrary to the expected results considering thermal lag. Based upon these observations and the results obtained in high vacuum sterilization processes, it was hypothesized that a synergistic effect of air and steam was increasing the rate of biologic inactivation. Preliminary testing conducted in air-steam mixtures has shown that for spore strips tested in saturated steam at 121°C with no air, a D value of 1.6 minutes was observed. A D value of 1.0 minute at 121°C was observed with spore strips from the same lot tested in an air-steam mixture where the partial pressure of air was 0.5–2 psi.

These results indicated that air in the test system is a major variable. Because the air concentration in a steam environment (concentration gradients) is difficult to control, it appears that repeatable test results require the removal of air from the test system.

Considerations for the Future

Much remains to be learned about the kinetics of moist-heat sterilization. Accurately controlled test apparatus designs are a key issue in developing an ability to identify and investigate the influence of process variables such as air and superheat on biologic inactivation. Such variables will have to be addressed relative to the use of BIs and P/CIs for validating the effectiveness of steam sterilization processes and establishing test procedures for measuring the characteristics of process indicators.

SYMBOLS, DEFINITIONS AND EQUATIONS

Symbols and Definitions

Unless otherwise indicated, the following terms are used as defined:

F_0 = A lethality factor equating the equivalent time in minutes at various temperatures required to produce a given sterilization effect in saturated steam at 121°C where the Z value is 10°C.

F_T^Z = A lethality factor equating the equivalent time in minutes at various temperatures required to produce a given sterilization effect relative to a given set of initial sterilizing conditions.

D_T^Z = The time in minutes, under any set of sterilizing conditions, required to reduce a biologic population by 90% as calculated from an initial D value, where T_B and Z have been determined.

Z = The number of degrees C necessary to change the F_0, F_T, or D values by a factor of 10.

t = Exposure time in minutes.

D = The time in minutes, under any given set of sterilizing conditions, required to reduce a biologic population by 90%.

D_R = The time in minutes, under any given set of conditions, required to reduce the quality or quantity of a substance by 90%.

N = Log of the number of organisms per BI carrier.

R = The percent quality or quantity of a substance retained.

T = Temperature in degrees C.

T_B = The base test reference temperature in degrees C.

L_T^Z = The logarithmic rate of reduction in a biologic population.

N_0 = The log of the initial number of organisms per carrier.

N_u = The log of the number of organisms per carrier after exposure to given sterilization conditions.

Equations

(1) $$F_0 = \int 10^{\frac{T - 121°C}{10}} dt$$

(2) $$F_T^Z = \int 10^{\frac{T - 121°C}{z}} dt$$

(3) $$t = D_R (\log 100 - \log R)$$

(4) $$D_T^Z = D \times 10^{\frac{T_B - T}{z}}$$

(5) $$L_T^Z = 1/D_T^Z$$

(6) $$D = t/(N_0 - N_u)$$

REFERENCES

AHA, 1979. Guidelines for the hospital central service department. American Hospital Association.

AAMI, 1980. Good hospital practice: Steam sterilization and sterility assurance. Association for the Advancement of Medical Instrumentation, ST. 1–1980.

Alder, V.G., and Alder, F.I. 1961. Preserving the sterility of surgical dressings wrapped in paper and other materials. J. Clin. Pathol., 14, 76–79.

Alder, V.G., and Gillespie, W.A. 1939. Automatic high pre-vacuum steam sterilisation for surgical dressings and gloves. Drayton Regulator & Instrument Co., Ltd., West Drayton, England.

Alderton, G., and Snell, N. 1970. Chemical states of bacterial spores: heat resistance and kinetics at intermediate water activity. Appl. Microbiol., 19, 565–572.

Alderton, G., and Snell, N. 1963. Base exchange and heat resistance in bacterial spores. Biochem. Biophys. Res. Commun., 10, 139–143.

Amaha, M., and Ordal, J.Z. 1957. Effect of divalent cations in the sporulation medium on the thermal death rate of Bacillus coagulans var. thermoacidurans. J. Bacteriol., 74, 596–604.

Anand, J.C. 1961a. Heat resistance and shape of destruction rate curves of sporulating organisms. J. Sci. Ind. Res., 20C, 295–298.

Anand, J.C. 1961b. Density of bacterial spores and their destruction rate by heat. J. Sci. Ind. Res., 20C, 353–355.

Anonymous. 1988. The Joslyn process: A new sterilizer technology. J. Health Care Mat. Manag., 6(3), 62–64.

Association of Registered Nurses Journal. 1980. Recommended practices for in-hospital sterilization. AORN J., 225–230.

Ball, C.O. 1943. Short-time pasteurization of milk. Ind. Eng. Chem., 35, 71–84.

Ball, C.O., and Olson, F.C.W. 1957. Sterilization in Food Technology. New York, McGraw-Hill, p. 159.

Barker, H.A. 1933–1934. The effect of water content upon the rate of heat denaturation of crystallizable egg albumin. J. Gen. Physiol., 17, 21–34.

Beck, C.E., Shay, D.E., and Purdum, W.A. 1953. An evaluation of paper used for wrapping articles to be sterilized. Bull. Am. Soc. Hosp. Pharm., 10, 421–427. (See also 12, 511, 1955.)

Beck, W.C. 1976. A new instrument for measuring and for monitoring the time and temperature of steam sterilizers. Guthrie Bulletin, Vol. 45.

Beck, W.C., and Collette, T.S. 1952. False faith in the surgeon's gown and surgical drape. Am. J. Surg., 83, 125.

Bigelow, W.D. 1921. The logarithmic order of thermal death time curves. J. Infect. Dis., 29, 528–536.

Bigelow, W.D., and Esty, J.R. 1920. Thermal death point in relation to time of typical thermophilic organisms. J. Infect. Dis., *27*, 602–617.

Black, S.H., and Gerhardt, P. 1962. Permeability of bacterial spores. IV. Water content, uptake and distribution. J. Bacteriol., *83*, 960–967.

Bowie, J.H. 1961. The control of heat sterilizers. Sterilization of surgical materials. Report of a symposium. London, Pharmaceutical Press, pp. 109–142.

Bowie, J.H. 1958*a*. Health Bulletin (Edinburgh, Scotland), *16*, 36.

Bowie, J.H. 1958*b*. Requirements for an automatically controlled, high prevacuum sterilizer, XVI, No. 2 Health Bulletin, Edinburgh.

Bowie, J.H. 1955. Pharm. J., *174*, 473.

Bowie, J.H., Kelsey, J.C., and Thompson, G.R. 1963. The Bowie and Dick autoclave tape test. Lancet, *1*, 586.

Brown, M.R.W., and Melling, J. 1973. Release of dipicolinic acid and calcium and activation of *Bacillus stearothermophilus* spores as a function of time, temperature, and pH. J. Pharm. Pharmacol., *25*, 478–483.

Bruch, C.W. 1964. Some biological and physical factors in dry heat sterilization; a general review. In *Life Sciences and Space Research*. Volume 2. (Edited by M. Florkin and A. Dollfus.) Amsterdam, North-Holland Publishing Company, pp. 357–374.

Bruch, C.W., Koesterer, M.G., and Bruch, M. 1963. Dry heat sterilization; its development and application to components of exobiological space probes. Dev. Ind. Microbiol., *4*, 334–342.

Bundeson, H.N., Danforth, T.F., Woolley, H., and Lehner, E.C. 1953. Thermal destruction of *Mycobacterium tuberculosis* var *bovis* in certain liquid dairy products. Am. J. Public Health, *43*, 185–188.

Busta, F.F., and Ordal, Z.J. 1964. Heat-activation kinetics of endospores of *Bacillus subtilis*. J. Food Sci., *29*, 345–353.

Byrne, A.F., Burton, T.H., and Koch, R.B. 1960. Relation of DPA content of anaerobic bacterial endospores to their heat resistance. J. Bacteriol., *80*, 139–140.

Charbeneau, G.T., and Berry, G.C. 1959. A simple and effective autoclave method of handpiece and instrument sterilization without corrosion. J. Am. Dent. Assoc., *59*, 732–737.

Charm, S.E. 1958. The kinetics of bacterial inactivation by heat. Food Technol., *12*, 4–9.

Cherry, G.C., Kemp, S.D., and Parker, A. 1963. The sterilization of air. Prog. Ind. Microbiol., *4*, 35–60.

Chick, H. 1910. Disinfection by chemical agencies and hot water. J. Hyg., *10*, 237–286.

Chick, H. 1908. An investigation of the laws of disinfection. J. Hyg., *8*, 92–158.

Chick, H., and Martin, C.J. 1910. On the "heat coagulation" of proteins. J. Physiol. (Lond.), *40*, 404–430.

Christie, J.E. 1957. Muslin vs. paper autoclave wrappers—a hospital study. Hosp. Top., Part I, *35*, 117–121; Part II, *35*, 111–116.

Church, B.D. 1963. Hospital laundry hazards leading to recontamination of washed bedding. Proc. Natl. Conf. on Institutionally Acquired Infections. Atlanta, Ga., U.S. Dept. HEW, Publ. No. 1188, p. 70.

Church, B.D., and Halvorson, H. 1959. Dependence of the heat resistance of bacterial endospores on their dipicolinic acid content. Nature, *183*, 114–125.

Collier, R.E., and Murty, G.G.K. 1957. The correlation of dipicolinic acid synthesis with the sporulation of *Clostridium roseum*. Bacteriol. Proc., *5*, 32.

Crowley, M.C., Charbeneau, G.T., and Aponte, A.J. 1959. Preliminary investigation of some basic problems of instrument sterilization. J. Am. Dent. Assoc., *58*, 45–49.

Curran, H.R. 1952. Symposium on the biology of bacterial spores. V. Resistance in bacterial spores. Bacteriol. Rev., *16*, 111–117.

Curran, H.R., and Evans, F.R. 1947. The viability of heat-activatable spores in nutrient and non-nutrient substrates as influenced by pre-storage and post-storage heating and other factors. J. Bacteriol., *53*, 103–113.

Curran, H.R., and Evans, F.R. 1946. The viability of heat-activatable spores in nutrient and non-nutrient substrates as influenced by pre-storage and post-storage heating. J. Bacteriol., *51*, 567–568.

Curran, H.R., and Evans, F.R. 1945. Heat activation inducing germination in the spores of thermotolerant and thermophilic aerobic bacteria. J. Bacteriol., *49*, 335–346.

Darmady, E.M., Drewett, S.E., and Hughes, K.E. 1964. Survey on pre-vacuum high-pressure steam sterilizers. J. Clin. Pathol., *17*, 126–129.

Darmady, E.M., Hughes, K.E.A., Jones, S.D., and Verdon, P.E. 1959. Failure of sterility in hospital ward practice. Lancet, *1*, 622–624.

Davis, N.S., Silverman, G.J., and Keller, W.H. 1963. Combined effects of ultrahigh vacuum and temperature on the viability of some spores and soil organisms. Appl. Microbiol., *11*, 202–210.

Day, L.E., and Costilow, R.N. 1964. Physiology of the sporulation process in *Clostridium botulinum*. I. Correlation of morphological changes with catabolic activities, synthesis of dipicolinic acid, and development of heat resistance. J. Bacteriol., *88*, 690–694.

Deindoerfer, F.H., and Humphrey, A.E. 1959*a*. Microbiological process discussion. Analytical method for calculating heat sterilization times. Appl. Microbiol., *1*, 256–264.

Deindoerfer, F.H., and Humphrey, A.E. 1959*b*. Microbiological process dis-

cussion. Principles in the design of continuous sterilizers. Appl. Microbiol., *1*, 264–270.

Doyle, J.E., and Ernst, R.R. 1967. Resistance of *Bacillus subtilis* var *niger* spores occluded in water-soluble crystals to three sterilizing agents. Appl. Microbiol. *15*, 726–730.

Ecker, E.E., and Smith, R. 1937. Sterilizing surgical instruments and utensils. Mod. Hosp., *48*, 92–98.

Eckert, E.R.G. 1959. *Heat and Mass Transfer*. New York, McGraw Hill, 339, 519–520.

Edwards, J.L., Jr., Busta, F.F., and Speck, M.L. 1965. Thermal inactivation characteristics of *Bacillus subtilis* spores at ultrahigh temperatures. Appl. Microbiol., *13*, 851–857.

El-Bisi, H.M., and Ordal, Z.J. 1956*a*. The effect of certain sporulating conditions on the thermal death rate of *Bacillus coagulans* var. *thermoacidurans*. J. Bacteriol., *71*, 1–9.

El-Bisi, H.M., and Ordal, Z.J. 1956*b*. The effect of sporulation temperature resistance of *Bacillus coagulans* var. *thermoacidurans*. J. Bacteriol., *71*, 10–16.

Ellertson, M.E., and Pearce, S.J. 1964. Some observations on the physical-chemical stability of sterile concentrated milks. J. Dairy Sci., *47*, 564–569.

Enright, J.B., Sadler, W.W., and Thomas, R.C. 1957. Pasteurization of milk containing the organism of Q fever. Am. J. Public Health, *47*, 695–700.

Enright, J.B., Sadler, W.W., and Thomas, R.C. 1956. Observations on the thermal inactivation of the organism of Q fever in milk, J. Milk Food Tech., *19*, 313–318.

Ernst, R.R. 1977. Sterilization by heat. In *Disinfection, Sterilization and Preservation*. 2nd Edition. Philadelphia, Lea & Febiger.

Ernst, R.R. 1963. Factors influencing retained air and air entrainment in steam sterilizers. A Castle Company Report.

Ernst, R.R. 1960. The kinetic energy barrier retains air in dressing packs in steam sterilizers. A Castle Company Report.

Ernst, R.R., and Doyle, J.E. 1968. Sterilization with gaseous ethylene oxide: a review of chemical and physical factors. Biotechnol. Bioeng., *10*, 1–32.

Ernst, R.R., and Doyle, J.E. 1965. The resistance of spores occluded in crystals to three sterilizing agents. Unpublished work.

Ernst, R.R., and Joslyn, L.J. 1967. High vacuum sterilization—The deleterious effect of air steam mixtures. Unpublished work (A Castle Company Research Project).

Ernst, R.R., and Kretz, A.P., Jr. 1964. Compatibility of sterilization and contamination control with application to spacecraft assembly. J. Am. Assoc. Contam. Control, *3*, 10–15.

Esty, J.R., and Meyer, K.F. 1922. The heat resistance of spores of *B. botulinus* and allied anaerobes. J. Infect. Dis., *31*, 650–663.

Evans, F.R., and Curran, H.R. 1943. The accelerating effect of sublethal heat on spore germination in mesophilic aerobic bacteria. J. Bacteriol., *46*, 513–523.

Fallon, R.J. 1963. Wrapping of sterilized articles. Lancet, *2*, 785.

Fallon, R.J., and Pyne, J.R. 1963. The sterilisation of surgeon's rubber gloves. Lancet, *1*, 1200–1202.

Felicotti, E., and Esselen, W.B. 1957. Thermal destruction rates of thiamine in pureed meats and vegetables. Food Technol., *11*, 77.

Fernelius, A.L., et al. 1958. A probit method to interpret thermal inactivation of bacterial spores. J. Bacteriol., *75*, 300–304.

Finley, N., and Fields, M.L. 1961. Heat activation and heat-induced dormancy of *Bacillus stearothermophilus* spores. Appl. Microbiol., *10*, 231–236.

Finney, D.J. 1952. *Statistical Method in Biological Assay*. New York, Hafner Publishing Co.

Gerhardt, P., and Ribi, E. 1964. Ultrastructure of the exosporium enveloping spores of *Bacillus cereus*. J. Bacteriol., *88*, 1774–1789.

Gifford, G.E. 1960. Occurrence of morpholine in steam and its solution during autoclaving. J. Bacteriol., *80*, 278–279.

Ginoza, W., Hoelle, C.J., Vessey, K.B., and Carmack, C. 1964. Mechanisms of inactivation of single-stranded virus nucleic acids by heat. Nature, *203*, 606–609.

Glassman, P. 1964. Proper care enables longer trouble-free use of stainless steel instruments. Hosp. Top., *42*, 107–109.

Grecz, N., Tang, T., and Rajan, K.S. 1972. In *Spores V*. Fifth International Spore Conference (H.O. Halvorson, R. Hanson and L.L. Campbell, Eds.). American Society for Microbiology, Washington, 53–60.

Halvorson, H.O. 1957. Rapid and simultaneous sporulation. J. Appl Bacteriol., *20*, 305–314.

Halvorson, H.O., Hanson, R., and Campbell, L.L. (Eds.) 1972. In *Spores V*. Fifth International Spore Conference, American Society for Microbiology, Washington.

Halvorson, H.O., and Zeigler, N.R. 1933. Application of statistics in bacteriology, a means of determining populations by the dilution method. J. Bacteriol., *25*, 101–121.

Hansen, N.H., and Reimann, H. 1963. Factors affecting the heat resistance of non-sporing organisms. J. Appl. Bacteriol., *26*, 314–333.

Harrington, R., Jr., and Karlson, A.G. 1965. Destruction of various kinds of mycobacteria in milk by pasteurization. Appl. Microbiol., *13*, 494–495.

Harvey, J.L. 1957. Use of octadecylamine in steam lines of food and drug establishments. Fed. Register, *22*, 9594.

Hashimoto, T., Black, S.H., and Gerhardt, P.V. 1960. Development of fine structure, thermostability, and dipicolinate during sporogenesis in a bacillus. Can. J. Microbiol., *6*, 203–212.

Hayakawa, K. 1978. A critical review of mathematical procedures for determining proper heat sterilization processes. Food Technol., *32*, 59–65.

Heiser, A.H. 1964. Hydrostatic sterilizers. Food Process, *25*, 86–91.

Henfrey, K.M. 1961. Personal communication (Ernst, R.R.)

Henfrey, K.M. 1970. Personal communication (Ernst, R.R.)

Henry, P.S.H. 1964. The effect on cotton of steam sterilization with pre-vacuum. J. Appl. Bacteriol., *27*, 413–421.

Henry, P.S.H. 1959. Physical aspects of sterilizing cotton articles by steam. J. Appl. Bacteriol., *22*, 159–173.

Henry, P.S.H, and Scott, E. 1963. Residual air in the steam sterilization of textiles with pre-vacuum. J. Appl. Microbiol., *26*, 234–245.

Highton, P.J. 1972. Changes in the structure of mesosomes and cell membrane of *Bacillus cereus* during sporulation. In *Spores V*, Fifth International Spore Conference (Edited by H.O. Halvorson, R. Hanson and L.L. Campbell). American Society for Microbiology, Washington, 13–18.

HIMA. 1978. Medical Device Sterilization Monograph: Biological and Chemical Indicators. Health Industry Manufacturers Association. Report. No. 78–4.4.

Holmlund, L.G. 1965. Steam corrosion and steam corrosion inhibition in autoclave sterilization of dental and surgical steel materials. Biotechnol. Bioeng., *7*, 177–198.

Hoyt, A., Chaney, A.L., and Cavell, K. 1938. Steam sterilization and effect of air in the autoclave. J. Bacteriol., *36*, 639–652.

Humphrey, A.E., and Nickerson, J.T.R. 1961. Testing thermal death data for significant non-logarithmic behavior. Appl. Microbiol., *9*, 282–286.

Hunter, C.L.F., Harbord, P.E., and Riddett, D.J. 1961. Packaging Papers as Bacterial Barriers. Symposium on Sterilisation of Surgical Materials. London, Pharmaceutical Press.

Hyatt, M.T., and Levinson, H.S. 1961. Interaction of heat, glucose, L-alanine, and potassium nitrate in spore germination of *Bacillus megaterium*. J. Bacteriol., *81*, 204–211.

Joslyn, L.J. 1980. The design and elevation of sterilization processes. Unpublished text from which Chapter 1 was contributed.

Joslyn, L.J. 1979–1981. Personal Consultations on Irradic Biological Indicator Inactivation Kinetics.

Joslyn, L.J. 1978. Air detecting device for steam or gas sterilizers. U.S. Patent 4,115,068.

Joslyn, L.J. 1976–1981. Investigation of temperature and exposure time control limits of apparatus for testing rates of reaction of chemicals and degradation of materials in saturated steam environments. Macedon, N.Y., Joslyn Valve Co., Process Development Project.

Joslyn, L.J. 1976. Methods and apparatus for detecting entrapped air in a steam sterilizer. U.S. Patent 3,967,494.

Joslyn, L.J. 1976. Empirical determination of steam flow rates for maximum gravity displacement efficiency. Macedon, N.Y., Joslyn Valve Co., Research Project.

Joslyn, L.J. 1988. Above atmospheric steam sterilization process. U.S. Patent No. 4,759,909.

Kaplan, A.M., Lichtenstein, H., and Reynolds, H. 1953. The initial deviation from linearity of the thermal death rate curve of a putrefactive anaerobe. J. Bacteriol., *66*, 245–256.

Karlson, K.E., Ruley, W., and Dennis, C. 1959. A quantitative evaluation of the permeability of wet surgical drapes to *Staphylococcus aureus*. Surg. Forum, *IX*, 568–571.

Katzin, L.I., Standholzer, L.A., and Strong, M.E. 1943. Application of the decimal reduction time principle to a study of the resistance of coliform bacteria to pasteurization. J. Bacteriol., *45*, 265–272.

Kells, H.R., and Lear, S.A. 1960. Thermal death time curve of *Mycobacterium tuberculosis* var. *bovis* in artificially infected milk. Appl. Microbiol., *8*, 234–236.

Kelsey, J.C. 1965. Sterilisation and disinfection technologies and equipment. J. Med. Lab. Technol., *22*, 209–215.

Keynan, A., and Halvorson, H. Transformation of a dormant spore into a vegetative cell. Spores III. Symposium, Ann Arbor, Michigan, American Society for Microbiology, October 1964, 176.

Keynan, A., Murrel, W.G., and Halvorson, H.O. 1962. Germination properties of spores with low dipicolinic acid content. J. Bacteriol., *83*, 395–399.

Keynan, A., et al. 1964. Activation of bacterial endospores. J. Bacteriol., *88*, 313–318.

Knaysi, G. 1930. Disinfection. IV. Do bacteria die logarithmically? J. Infect. Dis., *47*, 322–327.

Knox, R., and Penikett, E.J.K. 1958. Influence of initial vacuum on steam sterilization of dressings. Br. Med. J., *6*, 680–682.

Knox, R., and Pickerill, J.K. 1964. Efficient air removal from steam sterilizers without the use of high vacuum. Lancet, *1*, 1318–1321.

Knox, R., Penikett, E.J.K., and Duncan, M.E. 1960. The avoidance of excessive

superheating during steam sterilizing of dressings. J. Appl. Bacteriol., *23*, 21–27.

Koesterer, M.G. 1964. Thermal death studies on microbial spores and some considerations for the sterilization of spacecraft components. Dev. Ind. Microbiol., *6*, 268–276.

Krieth, T.J. 1973. Principles of heat transfer. In *Text Educational Publishers*. 3rd Edition. 219–243, 532.

Lechowich, R.V., and Ordal, Z.J. 1962. The influence of the sporulation temperature on the heat resistance and chemical composition of bacterial spores. Can. J. Microbiol., *8*, 287.

Levinson, H.S., Hyatt, M.T., and Moore, F.E. 1961. Dependence of the heat resistance of bacterial spores on the calcium:dipicolinic acid ratio. Biochem. Biophys. Res. Commun., *5*, 417–421.

Lewis, J.C. 1956. The estimation of decimal reduction times. Appl. Microbiol., *4*, 211–221.

Lewith, S. 1890. Ueber die ursache der widerstandsfahigkeit der sporen gegen hohe temperaturen. Ein beitrag zur theorie der desinfection. Arch. Expo. Pathol. Pharmakil., *26*, 341–354.

Licciardello, J.J., and Nickerson, J.T.R. 1963. Some observations on bacterial thermal death time curves. Appl. Microbiol., *11*, 476–480.

Loeb, J., and Northrup, J.H. 1917. On the influence of food and temperature upon the duration of life. J. Biol. Chem., *32*, 103–121.

Lund, D.B. 1978. Statistical analysis of thermal process calculations. Food Technol., *32*, 3, 76.

Macek, T.J. 1972. Biological indicators. A USP Review. Bull. Parent. Drug Assoc., *26*, 18–25.

Marshall, B.J., Murrell, W.G., and Scott, W.J. 1962. The effect of water activity, solutes and temperature on the viability and heat resistance of freeze-dried bacterial spores. J. Gen. Microbiol., *31*, 451–460.

Mayernik, J.J. 1972. Biological indicators for steam sterilization—A U.S.P. collaborative study. Bull. Parent. Drug Assoc., *26*, 205–211.

Medical Research Council Working Party. 1964. A third communication. Sterilization by steam under increased pressure. Lancet, *1*, 193–195.

Medical Research Council Working Party. 1959. A report. Sterilization by steam under increased pressure. Lancet, *1*, 425.

Michener, H.D., Thompson, P.A., and Lewis, J.C. 1959. Search for substances which reduce the heat resistance of bacterial spores. Appl. Microbiol., *7*, 166–172.

Murray, D.S., and Talbot, J.M. 1964. Sterile supplies for a hospital group. Hospitals, March, 3–11.

Murrell, W.G., and Scott, W.J. 1966. The heat resistance of bacterial spores at various water activities. J. Gen. Microbiol., *43*, 411–425.

Murrell, W.G., and Warth, A.D. 1965. Composition and heat resistance of bacterial spores III. American Society for Microbiology, 124.

Oag, R.K. 1940. The resistance of bacterial spores to dry heat. J. Pathol. Bacteriol., *51*, 137–141.

Oxborrow, G.S., Twohy, C.W., and Demetrius, C.A. 1968. Biological indicator evaluator resistometer (BIER) collaborative studies for ethylene oxide and steam: determination of variability.

PDA, 1978. Validation of steam sterilization cycles. Parenteral Drug Association. Technical Monograph, No. 1.

Penikett, E.J.K., Rowe, T.W.G., and Robinson, E. 1959. Vacuum drying of steam sterilized dressings. J. Appl. Bacteriol., *71*, 282–290.

Perkins, J.J. 1978. *Principles and Methods of Sterilization in Health Sciences*. 2nd Edition. Springfield, Ill., Charles C Thomas, 479–490.

Perkins, J.J. 1948. Preparation and sterilization of surgical instruments. The Surgical Supervisor, *8*, 15–22.

Perkins, J.J. Bacteriological and surgical sterilization by heat. In *Antiseptics, Disinfectants, Fungicides, Chemical and Physical Sterilization*. (Edited by G.F. Reddish.) Philadelphia, Lea & Febiger.

Perkins, W.E. 1965. Production of *Clostridial* spores. J. Appl. Bacteriol., *28*, 1–16.

Perkins, W.E., Ashton, D.H., and Evanco, G.M. 1975. Influence of value of *Clostridium botulinum* on the accuracy of process calculations. J. Food Sci., *40*, 1189.

Perry, J.J., and Foster, J.W. 1955. Studies on the biosynthesis of DPA in spores of *Bacillus cereus* var. *mycoides*. J. Bacteriol., *69*, 337–346.

Pflug, I.J. 1977. Microbiology and Engineering of Sterilization Processes. Parenteral Drug Association. Philadelphia, PA, 124–125.

Pflug, I.J. 1965. Personal communication to R. Ernst.

Pflug, I.J. 1960. Thermal resistance of microorganisms to dry heat: design of apparatus, operational problems and preliminary results. Food Tech., *14*, 483–487.

Pflug, I.J., and Smith, G.M. 1977. The use of biological indicators for monitoring wet heat sterilization process. In *Sterilization of Medical Products*. Gaushran and Kereluk, 222.

Phillips, G.B., and Miller, W.S. 1973. *Industrial Sterilization*. Duke University Press, 239–282.

Powell, J.F. 1957. Biochemical changes occurring during spore germination in *Bacillus* species. J. Appl. Bacteriol., *20*, 349–358.

Powell, J.F. 1953. Isolation of dipicolinic acid from spores of *Bacillus megatherium*. Biochem. J., *54*, 210–211.

Powell, J.F., and Hunter, J.R. 1955. Spore germination in the genus *Bacillus*: The modification of germination requirements as a result of pre-heating. J. Gen. Microbiol., *13*, 59–67.

Present, R.D. 1958. *Kinetic Theory of Gases*. New York, McGraw-Hill.

Prickett, E. 1953. Processing of surgical instruments. From a study of the operating room, School of Nursing, University of Pittsburgh and Methods Engineering Council.

Probst, H.D. 1953. The effect of bacterial agents on the sterility of surgical linen. Am. J. Surg., *86*, 301–308.

Rahn, O. 1945. Physical methods of sterilization of microorganisms. Bacteriol. Rev., *9*, 1–47.

Rahn, O. 1943. The problem of the logarithmic order of death in bacteria. Biodynamics, *4*, 81–130.

Rahn, O. 1932. *Physiology of Bacteria*. Philadelphia, Blakiston.

Rahn, O. 1929. The size of bacteria as the cause of the logarithmic order of death. J. Gen. Physiol., *13*, 179–205.

Reynolds, H., and Lichtenstein, H. 1952. Evaluation of heat resistance data for bacterial spores. Bacteriol. Rev., *16*, 126–135.

Reynolds, M.C. 1969. The feasibility of thermoradiation for sterilization of spacecraft—A preliminary report. Research Report SC-RR-70-423, Sandia Laboratory, Albuquerque.

Reynolds, M.C., Lindell, K.F., and Laible, N. 1970. A study of the effectiveness of thermoradiation sterilization. Research Report SC-RR-70-423, Sandia Laboratory, Albuquerque.

Rowe, T.W.G., Kusay, R., and Skeleton, E. 1961. The application of vacuum to steam sterilizers. Paper submitted to 2nd International Congress of I.O.V.S.T., Washington.

Savage, R.H.M. 1959. Principles underlying steam sterilization. Report of a Symposium. Pharmaceutical Press, London, pp. 1–11.

Savage, R.H.M. 1937. Experiments on the sterilizing effects of mixtures of air and steam, and of superheated steam. Q. J. Pharmacol., *10*, 451–462.

Schmidt, C.F. 1957. Thermal resistance of microorganisms. In *Antiseptics, Disinfectants, Fungicides, and Chemical and Physical Sterilization*. 2nd Edition. (Edited by C.F. Reddish.) Philadelphia, Lea & Febiger, pp. 831–884.

Shull, J.J., and Ernst, R.R. 1962. Graphical procedure for comparing thermal death of *Bacillus subtilis* spores in saturated and superheated steam. Appl. Microbiol., *10*, 452–457.

Shull, J.J., Cargo, G.T., and Ernst, R.R. 1963. Kinetics of heat activation and of thermal death of bacterial spores. Appl. Microbiol., *11*, 485–487.

Silverman, G.J., Davis, N.S., and Keller, W.H. 1963. Exposure of microorganisms to simulated extraterrestrial space ecology. In *Life Sciences and Space Research*. Volume II. (Edited by M. Florkin and A. Dolfus.) Amsterdam, North-Holland Publishing Company, pp. 372–384.

Slepecky, R., and Foster, J.W. 1959. Alterations in metal content of spores of *Bacillus megaterium* and the effect of some spore properties. J. Bacteriol., *78*, 117–123.

Sobernheim, G., and Mündel, O. 1938. Grundsatzliches zue technick der sterilisations prufung. II. Verhalten der erdsporen bei der dampfsterilisation. Ihre ignung als sporen test. Z. Hyg. Infectionskrankh., *121*, 90–112.

Sommer, E.W. 1930. Heat resistance of the spore of *Clostridium botulinum*. J. Infect. Dis., *46*, 85–114.

Spaulding, E.H. 1939. Chemical sterilization of surgical instruments. Surg. Gynecol. Obstet., *69*, 738–744.

Speck, M.L. 1961. Bactericidal aspects of high temperature pasteurization of ice cream mix. J. Milk Food Tech., *24*, 378–381.

Speers, R., Jr., and Shooter, R.A. 1966. Use of double-wrapped packs to reduce contamination of the sterile contents during extraction. Lancet, *2*, 469–470.

Stenstrom, L.A. 1974. Heating of products in electromagnetic field. U.S. Patent 3,809,845.

Struve, M., and Levine, E. 1961. Disposable and reusable surgeons' gloves. Nurs. Res., *10*, 79–86.

Stumbo, C.R. 1973. Thermobacteriology in food processing. New York, Academic Press, pp. 235–247.

Sugiyama, H. 1951. Studies on factors affecting the heat resistance of spores of *Clostridium botulinum*. J. Bacteriol., *62*, 81–96.

Sykes, G. 1963. The phenomenon of bacterial survival. J. Appl. Bacteriol., *26*, 287–294.

Townsend, C.T., Esty, J.R., and Baselt, F.C. 1938. Heat resistance studies on spores of putrefactive anaerobes in relation to determination of safe processes for canned foods. Food. Res., *3*, 323–346.

Tipper, D.J., and Ganthier, J.J. 1972. Structure of the bacterial endospore. In *Spores V*, Fifth International Spore Conference (Edited by H.O. Halvorson, R. Hanson and L.L. Campbell). American Society for Microbiology, Washington, 3–12.

Underwood, W.B. 1941. *A Textbook of Sterilization*. 2nd Edition. Chicago, Lakeside, Donnelley.

United States Department of Energy. 1979. Sterile acceptable milk (SAM). D.O.E. Final Report, Prepared under Grant No. EC77-S-07-1689 by University of Maryland, College Park.

United States Pharmacopeia (USP) XIX, 1975. 710–713.

United States Pharmacopeia (USP) XX, 1980. 1037–1039.

Urbakh, V.Y. 1961. Thermodynamics of protein denaturation. Biofizika., *6*, 748–750.

Utsumi, I., et al. 1975. Method and apparatus for the sterilization of ampoules with pharmaceutical liquid therein. U.S. Patent 3,885,915.

Waldham, D.G., and Halvorson, H.O. 1954. Studies on the relationship between equilibrium vapor pressure and moisture content of bacterial endospores. Appl. Microbiol., *2*, 333–338.

Walker, G.C., and Harmon, L.G. 1966. Thermal resistance of *Staphylococcus aureus* in milk, whey and phosphate buffer. Appl. Microbiol., *14*, 584–590.

Walker, H.W. 1964. Influence of buffers and pH on the thermal destruction of spores of *Bacillus megatherium* and *Bacillus polymyxa*. J. Food Sci., *29*, 360–365.

Walter, C.W. 1948. *The Aseptic Treatment of Wounds*. New York, Macmillan.

Walter, C.W. 1948. Sterilization. Surg. Clin. North Am., *28*, 350.

Walter, C.W. 1938. Technique for the rapid and absolute sterilization of instruments. Surg. Gynecol. Obstet., *67*, 244.

Wang, D.I.C., Scharer, J., and Humphrey, A.E. 1964. Kinetics of death of bacterial spores at elevated temperatures. Appl. Microbiol., *12*, 451–454.

Warth, A.D., Ohye, D.F., and Murrell, W.G. 1962. Spore cortex formation, composition and heat resistance. Congress for Microbiology, Abstract No. A2.2, Montreal, 16.

Warth, A.D., Ohye, D.F., and Murrell, W.G. 1963. The composition and structure of bacterial spores. J. Cell Biol., *16*, 569–592.

Weiss, H. 1921. The heat resistance of spores with especial reference to the spores of *B. botulinus*. J. Infect. Dis., *28*, 70–92.

Whittenberger, J.L. 1949. Steam sterilization of paper-wrapped packages. Framingham, Mass., Dennison Mfg. Co.

Wilkinson, G.R., Peacock, F.G., and Robins, E.L. 1960. A shorter sterilising cycle for solutions heated in an autoclave. J. Pharm. Pharmacol., *12*, 197T–202T.

Williams, O.B. 1929. The heat resistance of bacterial spores. J. Infect. Dis., *44*, 421–465.

Wooley, B.C., and Collier, R.E. 1965. Changes in thermoresistance of *Clostridium roseum* as related to the itracellular content of calcium and dipicolinic acid. Can. J. Microbiol., *11*, 279–285.

Yesair, J., Bohrer, C.W., and Cameron, E.J. 1946. Effect of certain environmental conditions on heat resistance of micrococci. J. Food Res., *11*, 327–331.

Young, I.E., and Fitz-James, P.C. 1962. Chemical and morphological studies of bacterial spore formation. IV. The development of spore refractility. J. Cell Biol., *12*, 115–133.

Zeller, H., Wedemann, W., Lance, L., and Gildemeister, E. 1942. In *The Pasteurization of Milk*. Edited by G.S. Wilson. London, Arnold, 148.

Zimmerman, D.R., and Wostmann, B.S. 1963. Vitamin stability in diets sterilized for germ free animals. J. Nutr., *79*, 318–322.

Zytkovicz, T.H., and Halvorson, H.O. 1972. In *Spores V*. Fifth International Spore Conference (Edited by H.O. Halvorson, R. Hanson and L.L. Campbell). American Society for Microbiology. Washington, 40–52.

CHAPTER 30

STERILIZATION FILTRATION

R.V. Levy and T.J. Leahy

The history of filtration dates so far back that details of its invention and initial use lie buried in the unrecorded past. An early example of filtration was the Egyptian practice of straining grape juice through fabrics. Carthage was famous for the clarity of its wines and must have used some method of filtration.

This chapter deals with a technology that goes a step beyond clarification—the technology related to the complete removal of microorganisms and particles to a specific size range from liquid or gas to produce a product that meets the current guidelines set by the Food and Drug Administration/Bureau of Drugs and the United States Pharmacopeia (USP XXII, 1990). Although filtration and filter media are used to effect a number of separations of various types, e.g., solid/liquid, electrophoretic, and molecular, the discussion here is limited to the removal of microorganisms and microscopic particles.

With varying success, filtration has been used for years as a means of stabilizing pharmaceutical and biologic solutions. Probably the first filters designed for the removal of bacteria from solution were constructed by Pasteur and Chamberlain in 1884 (Sykes, 1965). These were produced in the shape of hollow, unglazed candles by heating a mixture of quartz sand and kaolin to a temperature just below the sintering point. Later, fibrous asbestos pad filters, developed in Germany and known as Seitz filters, came into common use. Retention of bacteria by these media depends on absorption of bacteria to the porous inner structure and random entrapment throughout the filter matrix. In 1922, Zsigmondy and Buchmann introduced a true membrane filter for the removal of bacteria from solution. A screen-like filtration medium was produced by forming a thin microporous structure composed of inert cellulose esters. The filters were able to retain particles larger than the pore size at or near their surface. The Germans used this technology to determine bacterial contamination of potable water supplied during World War II. The technology was then used to develop a controlled manufac-

turing process in the United States after the war. Since then, membrane filter technology has advanced markedly, particularly in the last three decades.

Commercially available membranes were first manufactured in two pore sizes: 0.45 μm and 0.80 μm. Although the 0.45 μm-pore–sized membrane was quickly applied to the removal of bacteria, yeast, and molds from biologic and pharmaceutical fluids, it became apparent in the late 1960s that a pseudomonad-like organism associated with proteinaceous solution could pass through that membrane during the filtration process. A membrane with a pore size of 0.22 μm was then introduced for critical sterilizing filtration applications.

Today, in addition to its many other commercial and scientific applications, filtration is used extensively in the production of sterile and particle-free biologic pharmaceutical fluids that cannot be purified by any other means. Modern pharmaceutical manufacturers and the U.S. Food and Drug Administration have imposed rigid performance criteria on filtration media, particularly those used to produce small-volume parenteral drug products (FDA, 1985).

FILTER CLASSIFICATION

Literally hundreds of materials have been employed as filter media. Among the more familiar are porous fibrous materials such as paper and felt. Fabrics of woven yarns, monofilament plastics, or fine metal wire also serve as filter media, as do perforated or chemically etched metal sheets. Beds of fine granular materials, such as sand or charcoal, can also be used for filtration. Pores can be introduced either mechanically or physiochemically into sheets of polymeric material to form coarse or fine filter media. Sintered powders and unglazed ceramic materials have long been used for exceedingly fine filtration.

The filtration process consists of passing a mixture of fluid and solids through a porous medium that retains the solids on its surface, entraps them within its matrix, or both. Filters may be categorized as primarily depth, surface, or screen filters, depending on their composition and construction characteristics, particle/fluid/filter interactions, and mechanisms of filtration. The distinction between depth, surface, and screen filters is of considerable importance, particularly to pharmaceutical process filtration.

When used independently, no one type of filter will be cost-effective for most high-volume pharmaceutical filtration applications requiring complete removal of microorganisms and particles down to a specific size level. High-volume microfiltration usually calls for removing particles in a precise, definable way and at an optimal cost. The most effective way to accomplish this is to capitalize on the complementary properties of depth, surface, and screen filters. Depth and surface filtration is the most economical way to remove the great bulk of the particulate burden from a fluid. This is accomplished through filtration, which has been recently reviewed (Meltzer, 1989). Final, highly efficient filtration can be provided only by a screen filter placed downstream of depth or surface filters. The optimum choice of filters involves a careful weighing of two factors: filtration efficiency and dirt-handling capacity.

PREFILTRATION

Depth Filters

A depth filter consists of fibrous, granular, or sintered materials, pressed, wound, fired, or otherwise bonded into a tortuous maze of flow channels. Particles in a fluid that pass through the irregular channels defined by the tortuous orientation are retained by a combination of effects or mechanisms. The principal retention mechanisms, particularly for small particles, are mechanical entrapment and random adsorption, which occurs throughout the depth of the filter matrix. Figure 30–1 illustrates the combination of retention mechanisms inherent in depth filters. Materials that have been commonly used include fiberglass, cotton, wool, and resin-bonded laminates of paper, asbestos, and other inorganic fibers, porcelain, and diatomaceous earth.

Because of the types of materials and methods of fabrication, depth filters cannot be realistically assigned an absolute particle-retention rating. Instead, they are assigned a normal rating, i.e., some particle size above which a certain percentage of contaminants will be retained.

The nominal rating can be determined experimentally after fabrication by passing a test fluid through the depth filter. This fluid, having a known concentration of suspended particles and a known size distribution, is assayed with membrane filters (screen-type filters) before and after filtration. Particle size counts are made on both assay filters, and the percentage retained (in various size ranges) by the depth filter is calculated. It is important to note that the nominal rating of a depth filter is valid

only under a strictly defined set of conditions (flow, temperature, pressure, and viscosity).

Changes in any one of these parameters may affect the retention mechanisms and may have an important bearing on critical filtration. For instance, when a solid contaminant in a fluid winds its way through a depth filter, it follows the path of least resistance until it becomes trapped or is adsorbed. As the pressure differential increases, which often results from filter clogging or an increase in operating pressure, particles and microorganisms are driven deeper into the matrix. Eventually, these will move into the filtrate. In sterile filtration applications, the consequences are noteworthy, because sterility is lost.

Advantages of Depth Filters

The advantages of depth filters may be summarized as follows: (1) Because depth filters can collect contaminants throughout their thicknesses, and because they have relatively large spaces between the interstices as compared to surface or screen filters, they normally exhibit a highest "dirt-handling" capacity. (2) Depth filters will retain a large percentage of contaminants smaller than their normal size rating because of adsorption.

Disadvantages of Depth Filters

The following are considered disadvantages of depth filters: (1) Media migration, or the tendency of the filter media (filter fragments) to slough off during filtration, is a severe drawback peculiar to all depth filters (Fig. 30–2). Although continuous throughout the life of the filter, media migration becomes more pronounced when a hydraulic surge or continuous flexing of the filter matrix takes place. (2) Release of microorganisms initially trapped in the matrix downstream also presents a problem, particularly during long filtration runs. If adsorption has played a role in the removal of certain particles, even minute changes in the fluid/particle/filter matrix interactions may trigger a release of those particles. Under certain conditions, microorganisms may reproduce within the filter matrix, penetrate deeper into the matrix, and emerge on the downstream side to contaminate the filtrate (Dwyer, 1968). This phenomenon is often called growthrough. (3) Because they have no meaningful pore size, depth filters impose no definite limitation on the size of particles that may pass through. (4) The relatively large amounts of liquid product retained by depth filters (holdup volume) can be a serious shortcoming when filtering solutions that are valuable.

Surface Filters

A surface filter is composed of multiple layers of media, usually glass or polymeric microfibers. When a fluid is passed through a surface filter, particles larger than the spaces between the microfiber matrix are retained, primarily on the surface. In addition, smaller particles may be trapped within the matrix, giving a surface filter the advantages of both depth and membrane filters.

Surface filters are typically constructed of polypro-

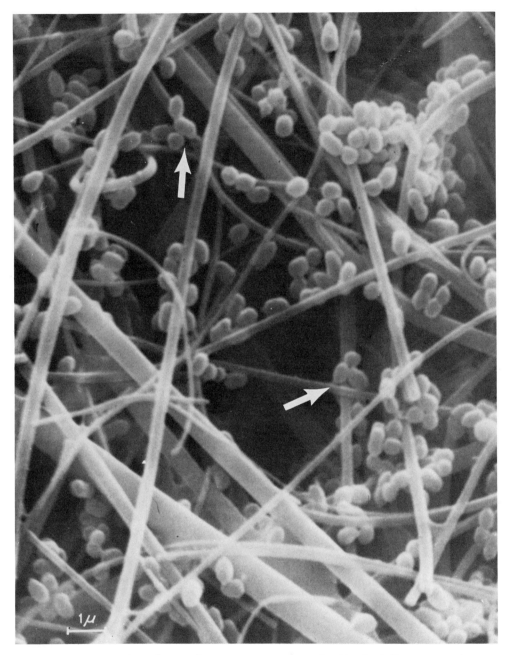

Fig. 30–1. Scanning electron micrograph of *Pseudomonas diminuta* ATCC 19146 on a glass fiber depth filter. Arrows indicate examples of bacterial cells adsorbed to fibers.

pylene, cellulose/resin–bonded paper, or fiberglass/paper. Unlike depth filters, surface filters can be pleated and supported by base materials for incorporation into a cartridge format. Recent advances in the fabrication of base support materials (usually polypropylene) have permitted the use of thinner support layers and permitted the addition of more filter material per cartridge. Cartridges that provide 6 to 9 square feet of effective filtration area are common.

The latest addition to the list of surface filters are ceramic filters. Ceramic filters are composed of high-purity alumina compounds. These filters can be used to clarify liquids, such as beers and juices, containing high solids, or can concentrate very fine solids whose diameters are less than 10 μm. Ceramic filters have many advantages over more traditional filter materials:

1. They can be cleaned and steam sterilized in place
2. Their filtration rates are higher and more stable in tough applications, e.g., high-viscosity fluids
3. They have the widest compatibility of any filters and can be used with solvents and hazardous materials

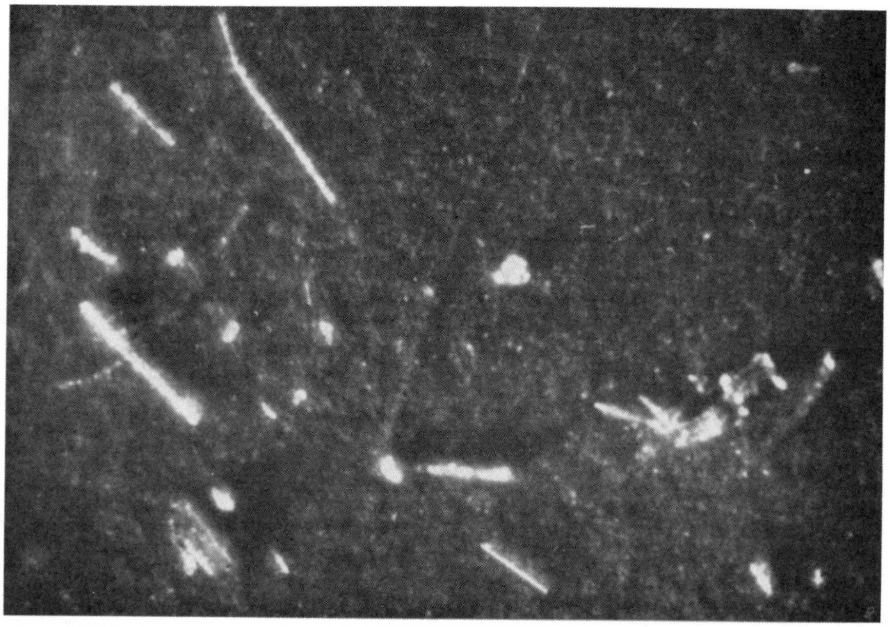

Fig. 30–2. Media migration debris (resin and glass particles, and asbestos fibers) was collected on a black membrane filter (screen filter) downstream from a resin-bonded depth filter (× 225).

4. They are long-lived and extremely durable
5. They can be backflushed
6. They can be used in both dead-ended and tangential flow modes

At this stage in development, no ceramic filters exhibit validated, sterilizing-grade performance.

STERILIZING FILTRATION

Screen or Membrane Filters

Screen or membrane filters are used to achieve controlled and predictable particle removal, particularly for final filtrations that produce a sterile effluent. A screen filter is a highly uniform, rigid, and continuous structure with regularly spaced uniform meshes, spaces, or holes. When a fluid is passed through the filter, all particles and microorganisms larger than the hole size will be retained entirely on its surface. Particles that penetrate the surface are caught within the matrix if they are large enough to be retained by the pores. Examples of screen filters are stainless steel, nylon or Dacron mesh, and—of particular interest here—microporous membrane filters.

Particle Retention Rating

The primary filtration mechanism of a membrane filter is physical sieving, whereby all particles larger than the hole or pore size are retained at or near its surface (Fig. 30–3). Uniformity of pore size permits well defined limits of particle retention to be determined by appropriate testing, i.e., high bacterial challenge levels at a defined number of microorganisms per square centimeter of effective filtration area equals no passage detected.

Advantages of Membrane Filters

The following may be considered advantages of using membrane filters: (1) Filter efficiency is independent of flowrate and pressure differential for particles larger than the pore size. (2) There is no media migration with membrane filters because of their homogeneous structure, nor do such filters permit passage of particles or organisms larger than the most open pore size, even at pressure differentials approaching 500 psi. (3) Large inflexible particles tend to form a coarse mat on the membrane filter surface. Though interfering little with flow, this porous mat acts as a depth filter by retaining particles smaller than the membrane pore size, thereby increasing the efficiency of the membrane filter. (4) Practically no product is retained within the membrane filter and its holder or housing. Membrane filters are thin (< 150 μm), and because there is little void volume between the filter surfaces and the inner walls of the holder or housing, fluid retention is further minimized.

Disadvantages of Membrane Filters

The following may be considered disadvantages to using membrane filters: (1) Because of their surface-retention mechanism, membrane filters have a relatively low dirt-handling capacity, particularly if the particles approximate the pore size of the filter surface. Such particles stop up the pores and prevent fluid flow. (2) Not all particles smaller than its pore size will pass through the membrane filter. Some of these particles will be collected on the membrane surface, and some will be trapped in the tortuous capillaries themselves. If there is a sufficient number of these smaller particles, a rapid buildup in pressure differential will result.

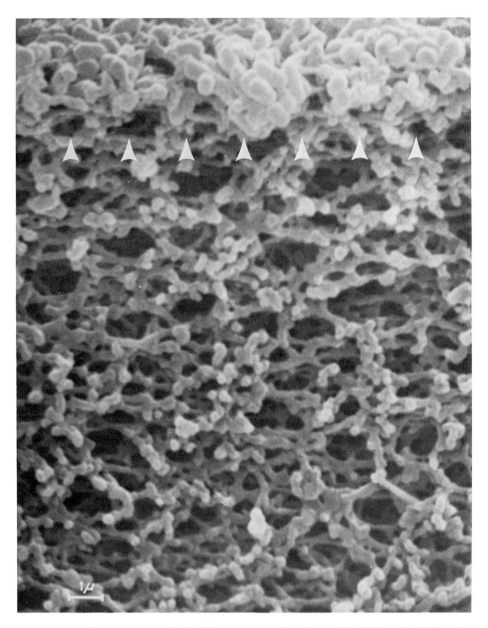

Fig. 30–3. Cross-sectional scanning electron micrograph of a 0.22-μm pore-sized membrane filter challenged with *Pseudomonas diminuta* ATCC 19146. Arrows indicate interface of membrane surface and internal polymer structure. A layer of bacterial cells is shown trapped at the surface.

Filter Combinations: An Economic Consideration

Because depth and surface filters retain large amounts of fine particulates, they find wide use as prefilters for membrane filters. Materials used as the prefilter medium are generally low in cost compared to membrane filters. It is important then that they remove the larger share of particulate contamination so that the life of the membrane filter is extended as far as possible, acting as an insurance policy by removing all particles and microorganisms to a high level of efficiency.

To maximize the effective life of a membrane filter of a particular pore size, a prefilter must have not only the proper retention efficiency, but also the optimum filtration area. The membrane-filter pore size determines the retention efficiency required of the prefilter, i.e., the prefilter must remove most of the particulates that approximate the absolute pore size rating of the membrane filter. For example, if product considerations dictate the use of a 0.45-μm-pore–sized membrane filter, the nominal rating of the prefilter must be at least 0.5 μm. This introduces a problem, however, because filtration systems that use prefilters with a nominal rating of 0.5 μm usually require high pressures to produce high-volume production flow rates, unless the prefilter filtration area is sufficiently large. With the proper filtration area, a prefilter that has the required retention efficiency will make the most efficient and economic use of the membrane filter. At the same time, the filtration capability of

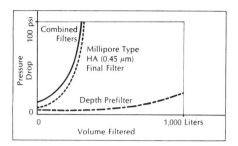

Fig. 30–4. Screen filter protected by relatively coarse prefilter. Inadequate prefiltration has resulted in premature clogging of screen filter.

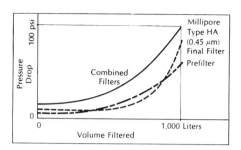

Fig. 30–6. Properly matched prefilters and screen filter, resulting in full use of both filter capacities and complete filtration of batch.

the prefilter will be utilized most fully. For the example just cited, the optimum filtration area ratio of prefilter to membrane filter is approximately 10:1. The ratio is optimal because it reduces the face velocity and pressure differential, thus increasing the retention efficiency of the prefilter.

Figures 30–4 through 30–6 show how the twin concepts of efficiency and dirt-handling capacity apply in a typical process. In this case, it is assumed that the fluid is being filtered at a constant flow-rate through a series of two filters, the first a depth prefilter and the second a screen filter (in this case a 0.45-μm-pore–sized membrane). It is also assumed, for this example, that the processor is handling a batch size of 1000 L and has a pump that can deliver a maximum pressure of 100 psi.

One fact is immediately apparent: as particles accumulate in and on the two filters, both flow resistance and pressure drop increase. The three figures illustrate the startling disparities, however, in the performance achieved with different prefilters.

Figure 30–4 shows what happens when the 0.45-μm screen filter is protected by a relatively coarse, or loose, prefilter. Pressure drop as a function of volume is shown for each filter by the broken lines. The combined pressure drop is represented by a solid line. Here, evidently, the prefilter is not providing enough retention efficiency to protect the final filter because there is little pressure buildup across the prefilter. As a result, the poorly protected final filter plugs rapidly, and maximum pressure is exceeded, with most of the batch still to be processed.

The situation is different in Figure 30–5. Here a much tighter prefilter has been used. In this case the prefilter

has more than adequate retention efficiency but insufficient dirt-handling capacity. This time it is the prefilter that clogs prematurely.

Figure 30–6 shows what happens when the prefilter has just the right retention efficiency and dirt-handling capacity. The properties of the two filters are perfectly matched, and the overall pressure drop has just reached the pressure limits of the system as the last of the batch has been processed. Note that at the end of the run, both filters have exhausted almost all their dirt-handling capacity.

For contrast, Figure 30–7 shows what would have happened if the final filter had been used alone, with no prefilter. It can be seen that the life of the filter is drastically shortened without prefiltration.

CONTAMINATION AND THE ROLE OF FILTRATION

Types of Contaminants

This section reviews the nature of contaminants, their harmful effects, and the usual methods for removing them. Three broad classes of contaminants are found in biologic and pharmaceutical solutions: (1) dissolved impurities, (2) microorganisms, and (3) suspended particulate matter.

Dissolved contaminants can be subdivided into inorganic (ionic) and organic impurities. Inorganic salts find their way into water supplies from soil, rocks, tanks, pipes, and other sources. Organic compounds include lignins, tannins, detergents, polysaccharides, proteins,

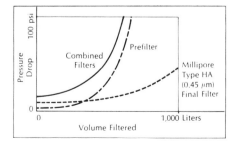

Fig. 30–5. Screen filter protected by prefilter with too little dirt-holding capacity, leading to premature clogging of prefilter.

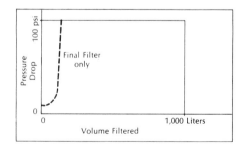

Fig. 30–7. Without prefiltration, the screen filter quickly clogs, resulting in a small throughput.

and other biodecomposition products. Water is the major source of dissolved impurities.

Microorganisms are a problem whether alive or dead. Alive, they can multiply at logarithmic rates. Dead, they are a source of pyrogens and can lead to sterile abscesses and particulate agglomeration. Because of the low absorption characteristics of membrane filters, pyrogens in solution are not removed. Marcus et al. (1959) reported that a high pyrogenic activity may be attributed to the presence of bacterial cells. Intact cells may be removed quantitatively, but no assurance can be given that cell lysis, and thus release of the soluble pyrogenic constituents into the solution, has not taken place. Particulate matter includes colloidal solids, metal, asbestos, cotton, dust, lint, and an endless variety of other solid contaminants, including microorganisms.

Harmful Effects of Particles

Microbiologic contamination of injectable drugs and solutions is obviously undesirable and should be avoided at all costs. The case against particulate matter is not as obvious, but there is growing clinical evidence that it can be a serious hazard.

A study at the Edinburgh Royal Infirmary in Scotland produced evidence that a patient might receive from 100,000 to 2,000,000 particles larger than 1 μm during extensive intravenous therapy (Myers, 1972) (Fig. 30–8). Studies made elsewhere indicate that this is not unusual. In one FDA survey of more than 300,000 bottles of intravenous solutions supplied by 6 manufacturers to 360 hospitals, visible particulate matter was found in some of the products of each manufacturer (Goddard, 1966). Garvan and Gunner (1971) showed that granulomas typical of those caused by a foreign body could be produced

experimentally in the lungs of rabbits by infusing intravenous solutions that appeared to be free of visible particles. For every half liter of intravenous fluid, they found 5000 granulomas scattered throughout both lungs.

Autopsies performed on children who had received intravenous fluids prior to death from various causes revealed pulmonary vascular granulomas containing cellulose fibers. The frequency varied with the volume of fluid received; however, when the patient had been given 40 L, vascular granulomas were found in one out of every ten serial sections (Garvan and Gunner, 1971). Granulomas were also found in the brain of a patient who received saline intra-arterially during cerebral angiography. Dr. Albert M. Jonas of the Yale University School of Medicine (1966) cited an instance in which a particle produced a partial occlusion of the central retinal artery, which could have resulted in blindness (Fig. 30–9).

The body's response to infused particles varies with the size, shape, and chemical nature of the particles, where they become occluded, and the host's response (Jonas, 1966). The major pathologic consequences appear to be (1) direct blockage of the blood vessels by foreign matter, (2) clot formation and emboli resulting from the tendency of red cells to adhere to particles (Jonas, 1966; Plumer, 1970), (3) local granulomas resulting from inflammatory reactions where a particle is embedded in tissue, and (4) antigenic reactions with allergenic consequences (Jonas, 1966).

Even where particles are relatively inert, as in glass, and may be absorbed in time, blockage may persist in the form of cell growth around the particle. Moreover, blockage may have done its damage by the time the

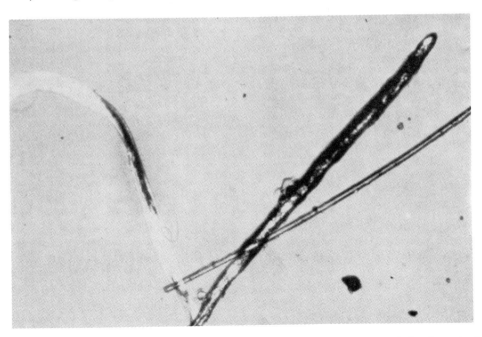

Fig. 30–8. Fibrous contamination isolated on a Millipore filter from I.V. solution (× 75). Courtesy of the Edinburgh Royal Infirmary, Edinburgh, Scotland.

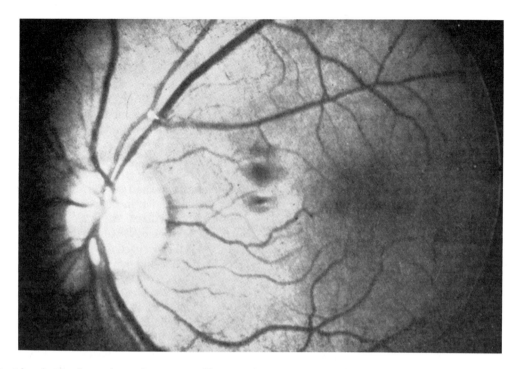

Fig. 30–9. Partial occlusion of central retinal artery caused by particulate contaminant in the vascular system.

particle is absorbed. Particles can cause harm in several other ways. Particles from an incompletely dissolved lyophilized drug may become lodged at some point, causing excessive localized drug concentration and tissue damage. Dead bacteria or mycotic spores may cause pyrogenic reactions or a sterile abscess. Inhaled asbestos has been strongly implicated in the formation of some pulmonary diseases, including cancer. Asbestos particles are found commonly in solutions in which asbestos is still used for prefiltration and clarification. Their presence in injectable solutions is highly undesirable (Turco and Davis, 1973).

Another form of particles not often considered in this context are the visible and subvisible precipitates that often form as a result of drug incompatibilities or interactions between packaging materials. After being filtered out and concentrated by the venous system, these small particles may become chemically active in unintended ways. Insoluble matter raises a potential danger of embolism, myocardial damage, and effects on other organs such as the liver and kidneys (Plumer, 1970).

Sources of Contamination

Some of the major contamination sources that need to be recognized and dealt with in the design of a work area and apparatus for handling critical drugs and solutions are listed as follows:

1. The manufacturing area, including its physical layout, location, traffic patterns, and use, influence the particulate burden in the air. Most airborne microscopic contaminants are found clinging to dust or lint that is churned up by the movement of people.

2. The original solution and ingredients are potential sources of contaminating debris, dissolved impurities, and microorganisms. Dead bacteria and mycotic spores left over from such sterilization processes as autoclaving or UV irradiation remain a threat as particles and as sources of pyrogens. "Purified" water may be laden with deionization beads, carbon granules, and other entrained particles from the purification process or transfer lines and vessels (Figs. 30–10 and 30–11). Chemical incompatibility is another common problem that may lead to insoluble precipitates, and lyophilized additives may fail to go entirely into solution.

3. Equipment, piping, vessels, and nearly every surface to which the fluid is exposed can contribute contaminants. Particles are inevitable wherever there are moving parts, valves, bungs, O-ring seals, threaded connectors, rubber tubing, or any surface subject to abrasion or wear, as in even the most well designed filling machines and apparatus. Researchers have found, too, that rubber disintegrates with age and repeated autoclavings (Garvan and Gunner, 1971).

4. Containers are another major source of particles. Both glass and rubber particles are shed when a rubber stopper is forced into a bottle. With additives purchased in glass ampules, the simple act of breaking open the ampule releases a shower of glass fragments. Turco and Davis (1972) made a study of glass particles produced by ampules during high-dosage treatment with furosemide. They found that thousands of glass particles, ranging from 5 to 100

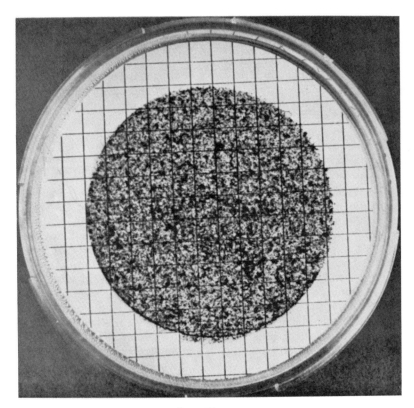

Fig. 30–10. Particulate contamination from tap water on a membrane filter.

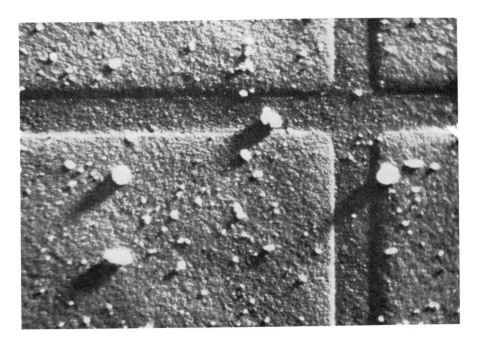

Fig. 30–11. Particles collected on a Millipore filter from a distilled water reservoir.

μm, were injected into the patient during treatment.

5. Depth filtration media slough off countless fibers, sintered glass, and sintered metal continually during filtration. All depth filtration media are prone to "media migration."
6. People shed dandruff, hair, clothing fibers, and bacteria in abundance.

General Methods of Removal

The method used to remove a particular class of contaminants depends not only on the nature of the contaminants, but also on the desired levels of purity. If the product must be sterile, just one viable organism represents a failure, because it could quickly reinfect and multiply within the fluid.

Dissolved organic impurities in water are removed most effectively by reverse osmosis or by charcoal or activated carbon. A well designed still will remove most organic impurities, but some impurities have boiling points near or even below that of water and may therefore pass over with the vapor phase. Dissolved inorganic impurities can be removed by reverse osmosis, distillation, ion exchange, or continuous deionization (CDI). For example, in a mixed-bed ion-exchange column, anion-exchange resins scavenge the negatively charged ions, and cation resins bind the positively charged ions. Deionization is inherently more efficient than distillation for removing ionic impurities.

Microorganisms may be dealt with in a number of ways; however, the most reliable methods of producing a sterile fluid with the highest assurance of sterility are heat or chemical sterilization and sterilizing filtration. There are many circumstances in which neither heat nor chemical sterilization is acceptable. Moreover, simply killing microorganisms does not eliminate them as a source of pyrogens or agglomerating particles. If a fluid is heat-labile, filter sterilization is the only practical alternative. Particulate matter is removed most effectively by filtration. Where a liquid needs to be substantially free of particles larger than a specific size—certainly true of all parenteral products—highly efficient filtration is essential.

DESIGNING A CLEANING SYSTEM

The major sources of contamination are listed above. In this section, we review some of the specific steps that can be taken to control contamination from each of those sources.

Mixing and Filling Areas

If at all feasible, "clean-room" conditions should prevail in all work areas used for the mixing, handling, or filling of injectable drugs and solutions. Ideally, such liquids should be exposed only in a laminar-air-flow hood or work area in which airborne contaminants are continually swept away by the forced flow of filtered air. Precautions, such as positive room pressure consisting of filtered air, will help prevent the flow of contaminated outside air into the work area. The proper use of laminar flow prevents turbulence that scatters and redistributes particles. All solid surfaces should be hard and smooth so they may be cleaned easily and do not provide places for dirt and bacteria to accumulate. Fabrics that release lint and surface finishes that flake or chip should be avoided. Clean-room technology is discussed only briefly here, because many excellent reference works are available.

Filtration Equipment Design

Because clean-room equipment design is beyond the scope of this chapter, the discussion here is confined to systems for sterilizing or ultraclean filtration.

No cleaning method can render a surface totally free of contaminating particles. Even the most well designed system will contribute some contamination. Therefore, placement of the membrane filter at the last possible point in the system is recommended.

Because of its uniformity, a membrane filter is quickly clogged by particles that are nearly the same size as its pore openings. The lifetime of a membrane filter can be prolonged considerably by introducing a depth prefilter (which is particularly efficient at removing particles in that size range) upstream.

Valve actuation is a major source of contamination. The more complicated its design and the larger its internal surfaces, the greater its contribution to particulate contamination. Of all available types, however, ball valves and diaphragm valves are easiest to flush and clean because of their simple flow path. They are therefore the most suitable valves for a critical filtration system. In any case, always place all valves upstream of the final membrane filter.

Vacuum filtration is not recommended for sterilizing or ultraclean filtration. Positive pressure is preferred for the following reasons: (1) It allows higher flow rates (vacuum limited to one atmosphere); (2) it prevents leakage into the system, which could admit contamination; (3) it dispenses sterile, particle-free filtrate directly into the final container; (4) it allows integrity testing; (5) it prevents vaporization of solvents, which could result in loss of product and formation of potentially explosive vapor; and (6) it minimizes foaming and denaturation of protein solutions.

For small volumes, pressure may be provided with a small hand syringe; however, use a Luer-Lok, not a Luer-Slip, fitting. For large volumes, use either a suitable sanitary pump (rotary gear, cradle-mounted tubular, or centrifugal pump), or use water-pumped, medical-grade nitrogen to pressurize the product. Nitrogen is an inert gas that will not change pH or oxidize the product. Compressed air is likely to contain water droplets, bacteria, particles, and oil vapor from the compressor seal.

The amount of contamination generated by a system is directly related to the number of valves, joints, junctions, and surface areas. Therefore, keep a system as simple as possible.

Use internally polished stainless steel piping, sanitary fillings, and stainless steel pressure vessels. Avoid threaded fittings when possible; if they must be used, wrap all threaded stainless steel connections with a single overlapping turn of nonadhesive Teflon tape to prevent seizing. Wrap so that tightening the fitting tightens the tape.

Use tubing made of polyethylene, polyvinylchloride, silicone rubber, gum rubber, or Teflon. Plastic tubing is preferable to rubber because rubber crumbles with age. Plastic tubing should be composed of FDA-approved materials. Avoid surgical latex and black rubber tubing, which contain extractables that will leach out during autoclaving. If tubing will be autoclaved, pretreat by coiling in a pan of water and autoclaving for one cycle.

Preparation of Equipment

Four important considerations apply to sterilizing filtration, regardless of the materials to be filtered.

1. The entire filter holder and its associated tubing, connections, reservoir vessel, and receiving vessel must be thoroughly cleaned and rinsed with distilled water (or equivalent) before each use. (Disposable units that are precleaned and sterilized by the manufacturer are exceptions to this rule.) Of special importance is the cleaning of the equipment when filtering protein solutions where residuals from previous runs may introduce pyrogens into the subsequently filtered solution. The filter holders must be constructed of high-grade stainless steel so that they do not add ionic species contamination to the solution being filtered.
2. In large-volume sterile filtration applications, the assembled filter holder and connecting hoses should be autoclaved together and an aseptic connection should be made to a sterile receiving tank, pump, or filter. For smaller applications, wherever practical, it is advisable to autoclave the filter holder assembly tubing and receiving flask.
3. In large-volume sterile filtration applications, the concept of cleaning "in place" (CIP) is frequently practiced. The CIP process involves a fluid delivery system that supplies the processing system with cleaning agent and rinses. Each system must be controlled for flow rates, cleaning agent parameters (e.g., concentration and temperature), and system parameters (e.g., surface finish). Each system must be evaluated for system efficiency and validated for performance. Adams and Agarwar recently reviewed CIP system design (1989).
4. Where particulate cleanliness as well as sterility is important, membrane filtration should always be the final step in the process and should be placed as close as possible to the sterile receiving container. Excessive downstream tubing or piping can easily contribute to bacterial and particulate contamination if improperly cleaned and sterilized and should be eliminated.

Container Preparation

Approach the washing of ampules, vials, and bottles with the same care used in preparing the liquid product. The best way to minimize clinging particles and residues is to follow the normal detergent washing and rinsing with high-velocity spray rinse using filtered distilled or filtered deionized water. One manufacturer washes intravenous solution bottles with an initial rinse of hot water and detergent, followed by six rinses of tap water and two final rinses of distilled water. Water used for the final rinses should be filtered through a membrane filter with a pore size of at least 1.2 μm.

Bottles that have been chipped or scratched should be thrown away, because they are likely to shed particles and abrade stoppers. Particulate contamination from rubber bungs can be reduced by lacquering and pretreating them by boiling or autoclaving. This opens their pores and flushes out trapped particles. Stoppers also should be rinsed with filtered water after they are washed.

People and Clothing

A person doing moderate exercise will generate about a million particles 0.5 μm in size and larger per minute. The outer dermal layer is constantly sloughing off. Minute particles of dandruff, dry skin, pieces of hair, bacteria, and dirt on the hands or under the nails are persistent sources of contamination wherever there is human activity. The normal clothes people wear are also contamination sources because both fibers and individual particles of dirt are retained by clothing. The sloughing off of contaminants from the body and clothing is aggravated by movement of the body and by contact with floors and furniture surfaces.

To minimize such contamination, keep traffic and human activity to a necessary minimum, and perform critical procedures in a laminar-air-flow hood. Avoid the use of abrasive cleaners during critical operations. The use of clean-room garments such as gloves, hoods, gowns, or coveralls is also highly recommended. In some instances, it may even be advisable to wear a surgical mask to prevent contamination from the breath. Clean-room garments are made of tightly woven monofilament synthetics to prevent the formation of lint and to serve as a filter that encloses the wearer. The tight weave minimizes the number of particles escaping from the wearer into the environment. Some fabrics are also designed to minimize static electricity.

PERFORMANCE CHARACTERISTICS OF MEMBRANE FILTERS

Flow Rate

The rate at which a clean liquid will flow through a membrane filter (volume filtered per unit of time) is a function of filtration area, differential pressure, and fluid viscosity. This relationship is shown in the following equation:

$$Q = C_1 \frac{A*P}{V}$$

where Q is flow rate, A is filtration area, P is differential pressure, V is viscosity of the liquid, and C_1 is the resistance to fluid flow of the filtration medium. From this, a number of things are apparent:

1. Flow rate is directly proportional to pressure differential. This applies only to a clean liquid. Clogging, of course, will increase resistance to flow.
2. Flow rate is directly proportional to the effective filtration area for a disk filter.
3. Decreasing fluid viscosity (by raising temperature, for instance) will yield a proportional increase in flow rate.
4. The resistance to flow offered by the filter medium (C_1) is, of course, related to open pore volume and pore size. The size and quantity of contaminants trapped on a filter surface affect the amount of open pore volume and therefore diminish flow. Particle size is a factor because a pore is blocked more effectively by a contaminant that closely approximates it in size.

Throughput

Throughput is the total volume of fluid that will pass through a filter before it clogs. Practically speaking, the filter is considered clogged when the pressure differential across the filter reaches the practical limits of the system, or when flow has decreased to the point at which it becomes impractical to continue.

In theory, one should choose the smallest, and therefore least expensive, filter that will provide enough throughput for the job, although a somewhat larger filter may be advisable so that filtration of the last few milliliters of liquid does not take an undue amount of time.

Serial Filtration

Serial filtration consists of filtering a liquid through a series of filters that have progressively finer pores. Often, the series consists of a stack of disks installed in a single filter holder.

When membrane filters are stacked on top of each other in the same filter holder, each is operated with mesh separators, so that little surface area is blocked by contact with the filter above. Placing a mesh separator directly on the filter support screen also facilitates removal of the final membrane filter.

The first disk may be a depth prefilter and the others membrane filters, each with a pore size smaller than the one preceding it. The same concept holds true when using filter elements with larger surface areas, such as pleated cartridges.

Serial filtration is often the most economical and, in some cases, the only means of filtering a liquid that is heavily burdened with colloidal material. Each membrane filter removes the bulk of the solids most likely to clog the filter that follows it, resulting in greater overall throughput.

FILTER INTEGRITY TESTING

Bubble Point

An important advantage of a membrane filter is its ability to be nondestructively tested for integrity before and after filtration. Commonly used integrity tests are the bubble point, diffusive air flow, and pressure hold tests. Each test was recently reviewed by Meltzer (1989b, 1989c).

Membrane filters are composed of a sponge-like matrix of a solid polymer with open pores of a narrow size distribution. When this structure is full of a wetting liquid (e.g., water in a hydrophilic membrane), a gas (e.g., air) will displace the liquid from the pores only if the gas pressure is high enough to overcome the local liquid-surface-tension–induced capillary forces. The critical pressure at which this occurs is controlled by the size of the pores and the surface tension of the wetting liquid (Fig. 30–12). The bubble point is determined experimentally by noting the pressure at which gas bubbles flow from the downstream side of the membrane or filter, hence the name "bubble point pressure" (Fig. 30–13). The relationship between the bubble point pressure and the pore size is an inverse one (i.e., the bubble point is higher for smaller pores), and thus a large opening defect is identified by a bubble point below the manufacturer's bubble point specification for the integral membrane.

Diffusion Testing

Another valid integrity test that is especially useful for large-area filters is the diffusion test. In this test, the rate for flow of a gas is measured as it diffuses through the water in a wetted integral filter or convectively flows through defects in a nonintegral filter.

Diffusive flow through an integral membrane consists of a three-step process: (1) solution of the test gas in the liquid on the high-pressure upstream side of the membrane, (2) migration of individual gas molecules through the liquid (described mathematically by Fick's law of diffusion), and (3) evaporation of the gas molecules on the low-pressure downstream side of the membrane. The overall rate at which this occurs depends on (1) the solubility of the gas in the liquid, (2) the diffusivity of the gas through the liquid, (3) the pressure difference between the upstream and downstream sides, (4) the temperature, (5) the membrane thickness and porosity, and (6) the total frontal area of the membrane in the filter.

If a diffusion-test pressure is selected appropriately by the filter manufacturer (typically near 80% of the normal bubble-point pressure), then defective filters can be identified as those for which measured gas flow rates are higher than the manufacturer's specification for acceptable flow rates (Fig. 30–14).

Because of the dependence of the overall diffusion rate

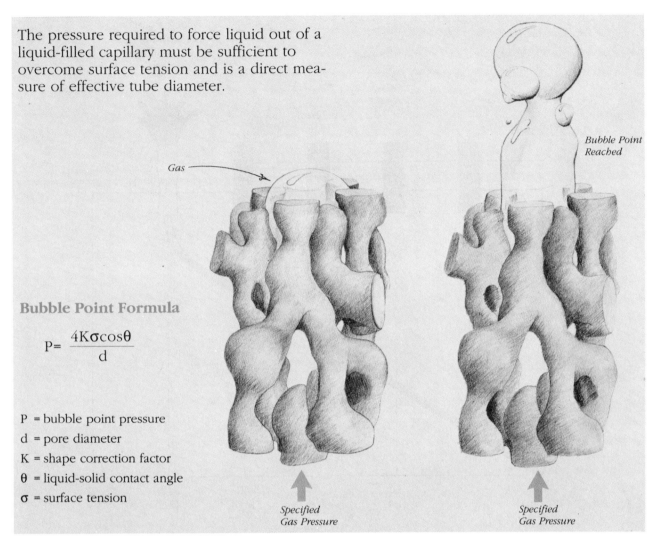

The pressure required to force liquid out of a liquid-filled capillary must be sufficient to overcome surface tension and is a direct measure of effective tube diameter.

Gas

Bubble Point Reached

Bubble Point Formula

$$P= \frac{4K\sigma\cos\theta}{d}$$

P = bubble point pressure

d = pore diameter

K = shape correction factor

θ = liquid-solid contact angle

σ = surface tension

Specified Gas Pressure

Specified Gas Pressure

Fig. 30–12. Bubble point pressure determination. Courtesy of Millipore Corporation.

on the membrane area, the amount of diffusion that is experienced by small-area filters (those with areas less than approximately 2000 cm², for example) is not enough to confuse the identification of the bubble point. Instead, the difference observed visually between the effluents at pressures below and above the bubble point is quite dramatic. (For small-area devices, little or no flow is observed below the bubble point, whereas very large flow rates are observed at pressures above the bubble point.) However, the larger diffusive flows experienced by large-area devices result in a much less dramatic difference in what is observed immediately below and above the bubble point, which in turn makes identification of bubble point much more difficult. Consequently, many manufacturers provide sensitive, automated equipment to perform both the diffusion and bubble-point tests (Fig. 30–15).

The reliability and accuracy achieved during the operation of each integrity test device should be qualified during installation and during operation. The instru-

ment's performance should be recorded and analyzed during use with the actual fluid(s) being tested (Lee, 1989). By following the manufacturer's recommendations for the appropriate test and test conditions for the filter in question, users can obtain quantitative results that, when compared to the manufacturer's specifications, determine the integrity of the filter.

Significance of Integrity Tests

A key feature of an integrity test is its ability to predict performance. In sterilization by filtration, the removal of microorganisms to high levels of efficiency is the most critical performance characteristic. Sterilizing filters must perform to total removal levels of 10^{10} to 10^{11} total microorganisms. Expressed in percentage of efficiency, the removal ability equates to greater than 99.999999999%, a high level indeed. This high efficiency is needed because even one organism emerging from a sterilizing filter can render the filtrate nonsterile.

The performance of other methods of sterilization,

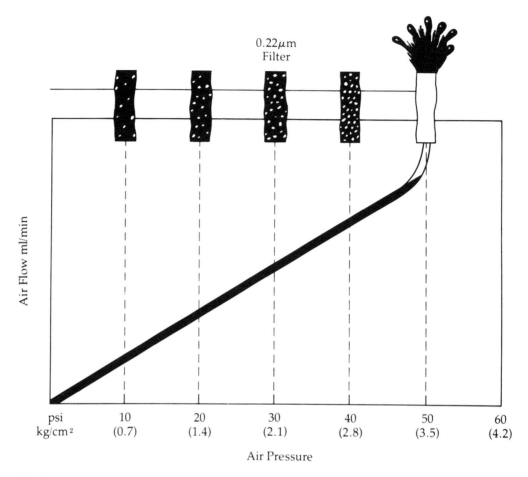

Fig. 30–13. Air flow through a wetted porous structure as a function of air pressure applied to a wetted membrane structure. Air flow is linear according to Fick's Law of Diffusion. A sharp departure from linearity is evident at the bubble point (approximately 50 psi applied air pressure).

such as autoclaving, are often characterized by two parameters: physical and biologic. For example, the physical measurements of an autoclave's performance includes the time/temperature profile of the sterilization cycle. Examples of physical measurement on sterilizing filters include bubble-point and diffusional air flow determinations. A biologic parameter would be a measure, expressed in quantitative terms, of the microbial kill by a sterilization system. Generally, the spores of *Bacillus stearothermophilus* are used for testing biologic performance in autoclaves. *Pseudomonas diminuta*, described in the next section, is the analogous biologic indicator (BI) for sterilizing filtration.

The fact that a relationship exists between the two parameter characterizations is an important feature. The physical measurement should predict the biologic performance of the sterilization system. In an analogous manner, the most useful integrity test of filtration is one that provides information on its ability to remove microorganisms.

MICROBIAL RETENTION TESTING

Microbe-Based Challenge Testing

The earliest report of a microbial (bacterial) retention test being used to predict the performance properties of membrane filters was presented by Elford (1931). Although his studies emphasized membrane formation, he investigated several biologic applications for his filters. Using three different genera of bacteria, he showed that retention of microorganisms by filters of various pore sizes depended on the size of microorganisms used in the test. These tests were performed on membranes composed of nitrocellulose. Studies were carried out at low-pressure drops across the filter, and little attention was given to the culturing of the test microorganisms.

Bowman et al. (1967) described a microbial retention test for membrane filters. They isolated an organism contaminating a protein solution and described it as a small pseudomonad that, when present in high concentrations,

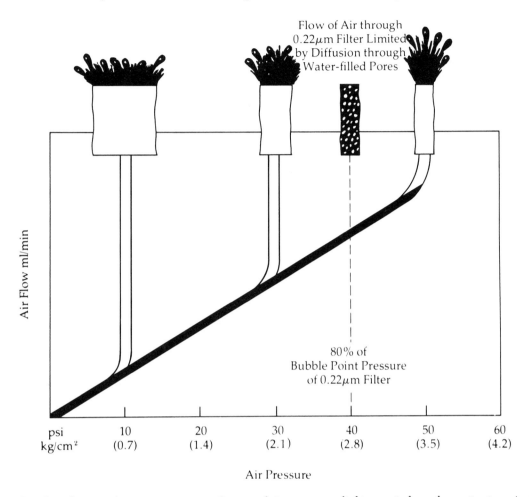

Bulk Flow of Air through 1.2μm Filter

Bulk Flow of Air through 0.45μm Filter

Bulk Flow of Air through 0.22μm Filter

Flow of Air through 0.22μm Filter Limited by Diffusion through Water-filled Pores

Air Flow ml/min

80% of Bubble Point Pressure of 0.22μm Filter

| psi | 10 | 20 | 30 | 40 | 50 | 60 |
| kg/cm² | (0.7) | (1.4) | (2.1) | (2.8) | (3.5) | (4.2) |

Air Pressure

Fig. 30–14. Air flow through a wetted porous structure as a function of air pressure applied to a wetted membrane structure. An integrity test pressure applied at 80% of the bubble point of a 0.22-μm membrane filter will discriminate between defective or large-pore-sized filters, because air flow will depart dramatically from the linear relationship predicted by Fick's Law.

consistently passed through a 0.45-μm membrane filter; they used this as their test microorganism. Realizing the need for a standardized test microorganism, they deposited it with the American Type Culture Collection (ATCC). Subsequently, the organism was identified as *Pseudomonas diminuta* and given the accession number of 19146.

Rogers and Rossmoore (1970) later proposed a procedure for determining the "biologic" pore size of membrane filters. Their intent was to develop a pore-size characterization of microporous membranes using biologic methods as a supplement to physical measurements. While also employing *P. diminuta* for sterilizing grade membranes, they were able to examine larger pore sizes by using microbes of greater dimensions.

P. diminuta is a small (0.2 μm to 1.5 μm), asporogenous, gram-negative rod. It possesses a single, polar flagellum that has a uniquely short wavelength (0.6 μm). *P. diminuta* forms small colonies 1 to 2 mm in diameter

on soybean casein digest agar after 48 hours of incubation at 30°C. The colonies exhibit a light tan pigment and are round and slightly convex, with entire edges. Morphologically, *P. diminuta* is difficult to differentiate from other pseudomonads.

In contrast to most pseudomonads, *P. diminuta* exhibits limited biochemical activity. The organism does not produce acid from glucose, and most carbohydrates are not used by the organism as carbon sources. It can be differentiated from other bacterials using the API NFT (Anytabs) test strip by its single positive CAP reaction. A member of the *diminuta* RNA homology group (Group IV), *P. diminuta* is characteristically cytochrome-oxidase and catalase positive. Ballard et al. (1968) provide a comprehensive review of the taxonomy and physiology of this organism.

Just as heat resistance of *Bacillus stearothermophilus* spores is an important factor in steam-sterilization testing, the size of the test microbe is critical for the deter-

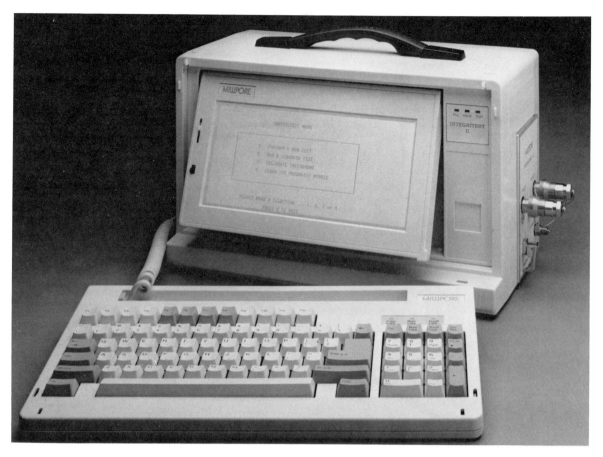

Fig. 30–15. Example of a portable, automated integrity test device for measuring diffusional air flow. Courtesy of Millipore Corporation, Bedford, MA.

mination of retention characteristics of membranes. In much the same way that D values (a measure of thermal resistance) can fluctuate for a particular strain of *B. stearothermophilus* spores, the size of bacteria, for instance, can vary with different physiologic states and with different cultivation media.

Microbial Size

Size is controlled by two factors: the organism's environment and its genetics. The environmental influences that affect size include changes in the growth phase of an organism, nutrient content of culture medium, and concentration of dissolved oxygen. The size of an microorganism changes as the organism goes through the various growth phases. Figure 30–16 shows typical bacterial growth curves obtained by plotting either log of bacterial mass (a measure of size) or log of bacterial numbers versus time of incubation.

In the late 1920s, Henrici (1928) observed that freshly inoculated cells show a size increase during the lag phase while the organism adjusts to a new environment. In so doing, the cell increases its intracellular components (ribosomes, mRNA, enzymes) and thus prepares for the increase in the cellular division rate that is to follow. After this preparation, the organism enters the expo-

nential growth phase, a time of rapid growth. During the transition from the exponential to the stationary phase, cells again become smaller because they divide faster than they grow. Although the extracellular concentration of nutrients is depleted, the organism is still capable of maintaining a growth rate (i.e., continuation of division) by using intracellular reserves. As the cell depletes the intracellular reserves its size decreases, and the population enters the stationary phase of growth.

The stationary phase is that period of growth during which the number of cells no longer increases, i.e., during which there is essentially a zero growth rate. Once into stationary phase, although there is no net increase in bacterial numbers, the population is still in a dynamic state. While some cells continue to divide at a basal rate, others die because of the severity of the environment (lack of nutrients and accumulation of waste products). Cultures from late stationary phases may have a level of viable cells equivalent to that of early stationary-phase cultures, but they may also contain many dead cells and much autolytic cellular debris. The entire surface of a membrane must be challenged with viable bacterial cells for the retention test to be severe. If significant portions of the membrane being tested become clogged with debris, the viable cells cannot effectively challenge that

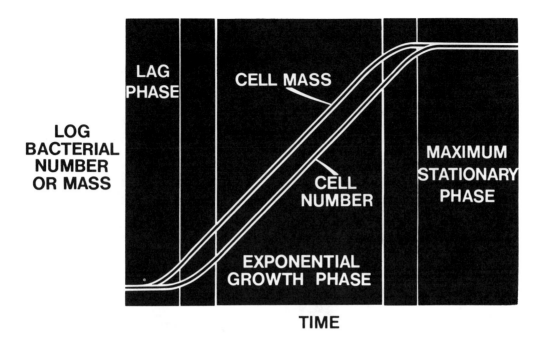

TIME

Fig. 30–16. Typical bacterial growth curves obtained by plotting either log of bacterial mass (a measure of size) or log of bacterial numbers versus time of incubation.

portion of the membrane. The particulate debris and viable cells in this case must compete for test sites on the membrane surface; thus, results of retention tests may be falsely negative.

Early stationary phase cultures are clearly the most appropriate for bacterial retention testing of membrane filters because they are small, are still capable of further division, and have few dead and dying cells in the population. Choice of the growth phase requires a thorough understanding of the population dynamics of the test organism under defined conditions and of cultivation.

The cultivation medium can also have a profound effect on both cell size and cell arrangement. Schaechter et al. (1958), working with another gram-negative bacterium, *Salmonella typhimurium*, observed profound effects, caused by different cultivation media, on cell size and composition (RNA and DNA). They concluded that size and composition depended on the growth rate afforded by the medium, an increase in growth rate resulting in an increase in cell size. Other workers have found substantial increases in cell size and mass under conditions of progressively faster growth rates (Herbert, 1958; Maaloe and Kjeldgaard, 1966).

A similar response has been observed with *Pseudomonas diminuta* cultivated under various conditions (Leahy and Sullivan, 1978). This response is illustrated in the two scanning electron micrographs seen in Figure 30–17. Figure 30–17 shows *P. diminuta* grown in saline lactose broth (SLB), a medium widely used in cultivations for retention testing. The organisms are coccobacillary and occur primarily as single cells. Comparatively little detrital material is seen with light microscopic viewing of wet-mount or stain preparations.

The formula for SLB is as follows: 7.6 g NaC1; 970.0 ml Reagent Grade H_2O; 30.0 ml Lactose Broth (1.3 g Dehydrated Lactose Broth per 100 ml Reagent Grade water). SLB is, in essence, a dilute solution of saline to which limiting sources of carbon and nitrogen are added. *P. diminuta* exhibits a generation time of 2.6 hours in this medium and reaches cell densities of 10^7 organisms/ml at 18 to 22 hours incubation at 30°C.

Figure 30–17 also shows *P. diminuta* cultivated in soybean casein digest broth. In contrast to SLB cultivation, here *P. diminuta* is larger, forming cells that are distinctly rod shaped (aspect ratios approximately 4:1). In addition, multiple cell clusters, or rosettes, are formed. These rosettes are commonly composed of 10 to 15 cells each. Wet-mount and stain preparations show extensive clumping. These clumps can result in particles whose effective filtration size is approximately five times that of a single cell in SLB. It has been shown that such clusters tend to artificially increase retention efficiencies of membrane filters (Rogers and Rossmoore, 1970). Leahy and Sullivan (1978) provide a more detailed description of *P. diminuta* cultivation for retention testing.

Validation of Membrane Filter Performance

P. diminuta has been widely used to validate bacterial retention in filtration. *P. diminuta* ATCC 19146 has emerged as the biologic indicator of choice in sterilizing filtration performance and is recognized as such by organizations by the Health Industry Manufacturers Association (HIMA, 1982) and the American Society of Testing Materials (ASTM, 1987). It is used by almost all manufacturers of membrane filters to qualify the retention properties of their sterilizing grade membranes. It has also been used extensively by the pharmaceutical in-

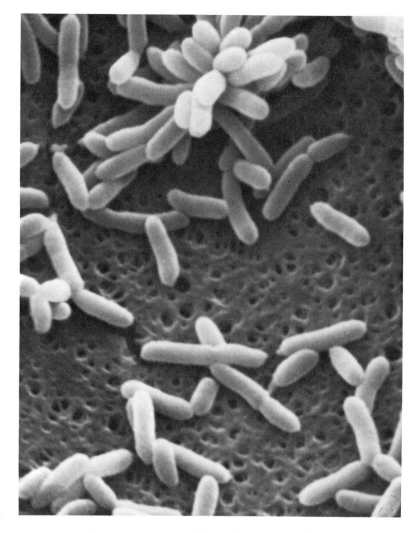

A

Fig. 30–17. Scanning electron micrograph showing the typical morphology of *Pseudomonas diminuta* ATCC 19146 when cultivated in trypticase soy broth (soybean casein digest broth) *(A)* and in saline lactose broth *(B)*.

dustry during development and qualification of sterilization processes that use filters as the sterilizing agent.

Choosing *P. diminuta* as a test organism to validate the performance of membrane filters follows the same logic used in the choosing *Bacillus stearothermophilus* for steam sterilization and *B. subtilis* var. *globigii* for ethylene oxide sterilization. When considering physical chemical agents such as steam and ethylene oxide, the most logical choice for a test organism is one that has been shown to be resistant to the agent to be applied, as have the two spore-forming organisms just mentioned. Similarly, small pseudomonads rigorously challenge the ability of a filtration system to physically exclude and therefore remove bacteria. *P. diminuta* is a natural candidate for a test organism for several reasons. It was originally isolated from contaminated solutions after filtration. Under properly controlled cultivation conditions, the cells are small (0.2 μm to 0.9 μm), nearly spherical (most cells have a length to width ratio of 2:1), and arranged singly (nonaggregated). In addition, the

organism is easily maintained and can be grown to high cell densities in a short time (18 to 24 hours).

P. diminuta is also widely used in studies on both the theoretical and practical aspects of bacterial retention. Reti (1976) used *P. diminuta* to show the relationship between integrity testing and bacterial retention. In a similar study, Pall and Kirnbauer (1978) also demonstrated a relationship between integrity test values and the retention of *P. diminuta*. Tanny et al. (1979) used *P. diminuta* to suggest a role for adsorption during the filtration process. Reti et al. (1979) examined the impact of multiple filter layers and chemical composition of suspending media on *P. diminuta* retention. Wallhausser (1979a and b) has published reports on the performance of filtration products for retention of *P. diminuta*. Most recently, Levy (1987a) used *P. diminuta* as a test microorganism to study the effects of solution chemistry (pH, viscosity), surfactant (Triton X-100), divalent ($MgCl_2$), and trivalent ($AlCl_3$) cations on the retention of these bacteria by polyvinylidene fluoride (PVDF) membranes.

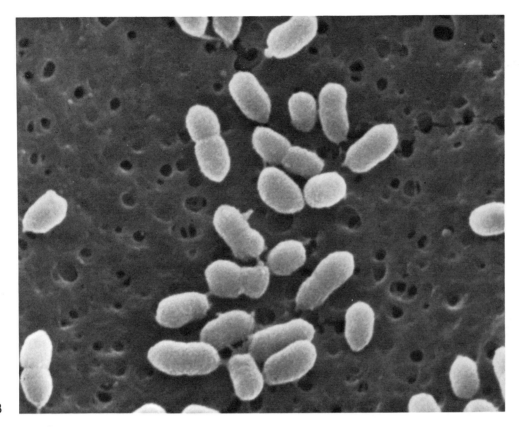

B

Fig. 30–17. *Continued.*

He demonstrated that retention was independent of solution attributes and pressure of filtration (30 to 50 psid). A summary of the literature to date regarding the role of adsorption in sterilizing filtration may be found in Levy (1987b) and Meltzer (1987).

Although the physical makeup of the hardware needed for microbial retention testing may vary according to the filtration system under study, there are several common procedural parameters that should be considered when performing such testing: (1) consistent and well documented cultivation of *P. diminuta*, (2) a minimum concentration of *P. diminuta* per unit area of the filter, (3) the use of sensitive recovery methods for *P. diminuta*, (4) simulated process conditions, e.g., transmembrane pressure drop and duration of filtration, and (5) the chemical attributes of the suspending vehicle.

The impact of cultivation on the suitability of *P. diminuta* for retention testing has been discussed previously.

Clearly, the number of organisms that challenge a filter per unit area of the filter is an important test variable. Elford (1933) observed that passage of microorganisms through membranes with even larger pore sizes (greater than 0.5 μm) depended on the number of organisms present. Wallhausser (1979a) obtained a similar result in his testing of filter cartridges. This phenomenon may be illustrated by the data shown in Table 30–1. Passage of *P. diminuta* through a 0.45-μm pore will not occur until some threshold value is exceeded. Below that threshold,

Table 30–1. *Effect of Bacterial Challenge Level On Passage of* Pseudomonas Diminuta *Through a 0.45-μm Pore-Size Membrane Filter*

	Total Number of Organisms Challenging Filter	*Total Number of Organisms Passing Through Filter*
Retention	10^2	0
	10^4	0
Threshold	10^6	10^0
	10^8	10^2
	10^{10}	10^4

the filtrate is sterile. Although bioburdens of liquids that are sterilized by filtrations are often known, reliable sterilization procedures should take into account an unexpected increase of bioburden and should also provide some margin of safety to obtain sterile filtrates. In this way, sterilizing filters are commonly challenged at relatively high concentrations of microorganisms to validate their performance. A suggested minimum concentration of 10^7 organisms/cm^2 of effective filtration area will adequately challenge a filtration element (FDA, 1987).

The sensitivity of any test for bacterial retention depends to a great extent on the efficient detection of any organism that may traverse the filter. Because the presence of even one organism in the filtrate is significant, recovery methods for the test organism should be as

Table 30–2. *Bacterial Retention Test Performed By Recirculation of Continually Inoculated Liquid Through a 0.22-μm Pore-Size Membrane Filter. Test Organism: Pseudomonas Diminuta; Test Duration 16 Hours*

Replicate	Microbial Challenge per cm² of Filter Area	Total Microbial Challenge	LRV*
1	1.6×10^7	7.6×10^9	>9.88
2	1.3×10^7	6.0×10^9	>9.78
3	1.9×10^7	8.9×10^9	>9.95
4	1.4×10^7	6.6×10^9	>9.82

* Log reduction value.

sensitive as possible. Maximum sensitivity may be achieved by examining the entire filtrate for sterility. Aliquot sampling of the filtrate (i.e., testing only a portion of the filtrate rather than all of it) will miss organisms when they are in low concentrations (less than one organism per 100 ml). The United States Pharmacopeia (USP XXII, 1990) describes sterility test methods that may be applied to sterility testing of large fluid volumes.

Leahy and Sullivan (1978) described a modification of the USP method that allows quantitation of bacterial passage instead of merely growth/no-growth results.

Time is another factor that may influence the performance of bacterial filtration. Although most sterilizing filtrations are limited to short run times (less than 8 hours), extended filtrations may allow the penetration of microorganisms and growth through a filter. Howard and Duberstain (1980) showed that filters that were constantly fed well water show passage of microorganisms as a function of time. Generally, passage did not occur until after 24 hours and increased with time.

Leahy et al. (1980) showed that sterilizing grade filters were completely retentive to daily challenges of 10^6 of a variety of microorganisms. Experiments were run for 28 days under simulated conditions of continuous ambulatory peritoneal dialysis. It appears that the impact of time includes a subset of variables that affect retention. Examples of these are (1) numbers and types of microorganisms in liquid stream, (2) physiochemical makeup of liquid stream (e.g., temperature, pH, ionic strength), and (3) nutritional makeup of liquid stream (i.e., stimulatory or inhibitory to microbial growth).

Table 30–2 contains data on *P. diminuta* retention using a test system that recirculates fluid containing a constant feed of organisms for 16 hours. The experimental conditions were designed to simulate pharmaceutical-type filtrations. Sterilizing filters (0.22-μm pore size) successfully retained all organisms throughout the test period. The factor of time must be considered, however, when determining the useful life of a filtration element.

Another important factor in bacterial retention is the pressure drop across the filter element. Leahy and Sullivan (1978), Reti et al. (1979), and Tanny et al. (1979) have shown the dependence of transmembrane pressure

on bacterial retention. These studies used filters having pore sizes larger than those recommended for sterilization. This effect is illustrated by the data in Table 30–3. At pressure drops that differ by an order of magnitude, there is a corresponding order-of-magnitude change in the rate of bacterial passage. The efficiency of retention decreases with increasing pressure drop. It is important to note that sterilizing filters (0.22 μm pore size) are independent of pressure, i.e., no passage is detected at any of the test pressures. Performance tests, however, should be run at relatively high transmembrane pressures (e.g., 30 psid) to maximize the likelihood of detecting bacterial passage if it is to occur.

Sterilizing filtration has been applied to a wide variety of liquids that differ in their physical and chemical attributes, including pH, ionic strength, polarity, surface tension, and viscosity. It is therefore impossible to design any one bacterial retention test procedure that considers all these variables. The general principles outlined in the preceding paragraphs, however, have been used in evaluating many of these conditions. Reti et al. (1979) examined the effect of divalent cations and surfactants on bacterial retention. Robertson and DeVisser (1980) studied *P. diminuta* retention using liquids that varied in surface tension, ionic strength, and viscosity. In both studies, bacterial retention was not affected, i.e., the sterilizing filters under study remained completely retentive. Leahy (1985) and Levy (1987a) have completed the most extensive examination of chemical attributes of the liquid vehicle on filter performance.

Quantification of Bacteria Retention and Relationship to Integrity Test

The quantification of microbial kill is an important element in the characterization of any sterilization system. For such sterilization methods as those using steam or ethylene oxide, the rate of kill is described as the D value. The D value, expressed in minutes, is the amount of exposure time to the conditions of sterilization that results in a 1-log reduction in bacterial numbers. It is the relationship between microbial kill and some physical measurement of the sterilization system that allows prediction of sterilization performance.

The quantification of bacterial retention by membrane filters may also be determined experimentally. Reti (1976) and Leahy and Sullivan (1978) have proposed the term *beta ratio* to express the microbial removal efficiency of filters. The beta ratio was defined as the number

Table 30–3. *Impact of Transmembrane Pressure (Δᴾ) on Retention of* Pseudomonas Diminuta

Pore Size of Membrane Filter (μm)	LRV*	
	5 psiΔᴾ	50 psiΔᴾ
0.22	>10^{10}	>10^{10}
0.45	8.653	7.602
0.65	4.613	3.146
0.80	2.000	1.322

* Log reduction value.

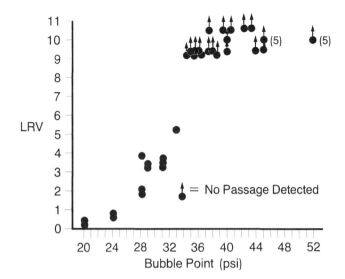

Fig. 30–18. Bacterial removal (LRV) as a function of membrane bubble point. Data points with an arrow indicate no passage (I.E., complete retention) of *Pseudomonas diminuta* ATCC 19146.

of organisms challenging the filter divided by the number that pass through the filter. In a later study, Pall and Kirnbauer (1978) proposed the term *titer reduction* (T_R), which is synonymous with the beta ratio. In an effort to standardize terminology, HIMA has adopted the log reduction value (LRV) as an expression of the microbial removal efficiency by filters. The LRV is the $\log_{10}$ of the beta ratio. An LRV is obtained by determining the total number of microorganisms that are used to challenge a filter. The filtrate is assayed to determine the total number of microorganisms that have passed through the filter. The base-ten logarithm of the ratio of these determinations is the LRV. Such terminology is useful for filters that exhibit high levels of retention efficiency. For example, a filter with an LRV of 8 is capable of reducing the number of test microorganisms by eight orders of magnitude. If this retention efficiency was expressed as a percentage, the value would be 99.999999%. Sterilizing filters do not commonly exhibit passage of test organisms; such filters, therefore, are assigned LRVs that are expressed as "greater than" the $\log_{10}$ of the total challenge level.

Studies continue to establish the relationship between LRV and integrity test values. Reti (1976) and Pall and Kirnbauer (1978) provided the original data demonstrating such a relationship. Many manufacturers of membrane filters have developed an extensive quality-control data base that contains the results of thousands of integrity-test values and corresponding bacterial retention tests for sterilizing grade filters. Figure 30–18 contains data showing the relationship between LRV and bubble point on membrane filters composed of polyvinyldine fluoride. As the bubble point increases and pore size decreases, the LRV increases in a linear fashion. It is interesting to note that as the bubble point approaches that of a sterilizing-grade filter (45 psi), no passage of

microorganisms is observed. In fact, complete retention is obtained at bubble points below the minimum established for sterilizing filters of this type. This allows for some margin of safety with respect to bacterial retention.

It is important to realize that the relationship between any integrity test method and bacterial retention (LRV) must be established for each type of filter. Currently, different types of membrane filters are composed of a variety of different polymers (e.g., cellulose esters, polyvinyldine fluoride [PVDF], polytetrafluorethylene [PTFE], polysulfones, and nylons). Polymers may differ in their wetting characteristics, which can affect the integrity test value of a filter. When interpreting the relationship between the integrity test and bacterial retention, close attention should be paid to the conditions of both physical (integrity) and biologic (retention) testing.

Manufacturers of membrane filters often will provide data on the comparison between their suggested integrity test and bacterial retention for their products. In addition, they can provide guidance on performing and interpreting integrity tests obtained from the wide variety of fluids that are sterilized by filtration.

STERILIZATION OF AIR AND OTHER GASES BY FILTRATION

Filters are by far the most commonly used devices for the sterilization of air and other gases. The relative ease of handling, the low cost per unit volume of air sterilized, and the efficiency in removing not only microorganisms but also other submicrometer particles as well, all account for their extensive use today. Filtration is the method used for the sterilization of both small and large volumes of air and gas. The mechanics are such that large volumes may be processed economically. For efficient and economic operation, however, the aerosol content of the gas to be filtered must be low. This is of particular importance with the high-efficiency filters in use today for the removal of bacteria, yeasts, and molds.

Microorganisms, particles, or droplets of liquid dispersed in a gas are referred to as aerosols. The behavior of aerosols is of concern in many scientific and industrial applications. Dwyer (1966) reports that particles suspended in a gaseous medium behave according to the classic law of mechanics. Complications are involved, however, because the mass of these particles is so small that they have an extremely small inertia but high viscous drag properties. Dwyer points out that this is not surprising when one considers that for a spherical particle, inertial effects are a function of the cube of the radius, whereas the viscous drag effects are a manifestation of surface area and are a function of the square of the radius. One would expect, then, that as particle size is decreased, the viscous effects would become more predominant.

Many viable microorganisms exist as aerosols. In fact, the air around us serves as the vehicle for many species of bacteria, molds, yeasts, and their spores. The fact that microorganisms are ever present is of particular concern to the food and beverage processing industries, the pharmaceutical industry, hospitals, and the many smaller laboratories requiring sterile environments. The fact that postoperative infections in hospitals are not uncommon points to the necessity of controlling the microbiologic aerosol population in the air-handling systems—certainly in the operating room.

Of particular importance to operating rooms in hospitals is a new trend in contamination control known as the laminar-flow principle. This concept has been highly developed in the aerospace and microelectronic industries, where work is of such a critical nature that the presence of particles in the micrometer and submicrometer range cannot be tolerated. The "white room" or "clean room" was designed for such critical manufacturing applications. A bank of HEPA filters comprises one complete wall of the room, whereas the opposite wall is a matrix of louvered exhaust ducts. When air or gas is flowing in a laminar fashion, there is essentially no mixing of fluid elements normal to the direction of flow. Gases tend to flow in a laminar configuration at low velocities. As the velocity of the gas increases, however, a critical point will be reached at which turbulence and eddy currents will be formed. It stands to reason, then, that the cleanest possible place in a clean room is directly in front of the air filter. Any contamination generated would be removed in laminar fashion to the exhaust ducts.

Many hospital operating facilities are now employing the laminar-flow principle. A bank of bacterial retentive filters is placed above the operating table connected to an air-handling system. Curtains or some other means of enclosing the immediate area are used. The immediate environment is then sanitized before the scheduled operation. Sterile laminar-flow air envelops the patient and operating team, and any microbial aerosol contamination generated during the operation is quickly carried away. Whitfield (1967), in a microbiologic study of laminar-flow rooms, proposed that the same kind of control possible for particulates would be possible for bacteria because bacteria are within the same size range as the particles and are nonmobile. Coriell and McGarrity (1967), in a microbiologic study of laminar-flow rooms, proposed the same thing. The feasibility of this seemed likely, because (as stated above) bacteria were within the same size range as the particles, and are nonmobile. Coriell and McGarrity (1967), using the vertical laminar-flow principle in a hospital operating room, demonstrated that the bacterial count dropped to zero 2 minutes after the filter unit was started. Bacterial counts promptly returned when the unit was turned off.

Mechanisms of Retention in Gas Filters

It is interesting to note that the actual passageways through the gas filter may be large compared with the size of the particles or microorganisms being trapped, but the mechanism of filtration is such that efficiency in removing small particles is high. Dwyer (1966) indicates that a filter having an effective diameter on the order of

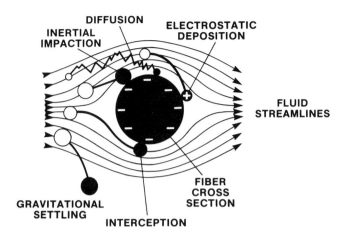

Fig. 30–19. Mechanisms of filtration in gas streams.

5 to 100 μm will remove more than 99% of submicrometer particles. One of the chief ways of increasing the efficiency of a filter is to reduce the spacing between the fibers. Filters constructed of fine rather than coarse fibers will tend to decrease the gap. Dwyer (1966) related that the removal of particles of microorganisms from air and other gases may be attributed to the following five basic mechanisms (Fig. 30–19):

Interception. Interception is simply the contacting of the surface of the microorganism to the surface of the filter. An assumption is made and can be readily demonstrated that particles will adhere to the filter surface once they make contact. Interception would be favored, then, by a small fiber diameter of the filter matrix.

Sedimentation. The mechanism is probably of secondary practical importance because the settling rate of microorganisms is low. If a stream of gas is flowing through a filter matrix, eventually the microorganisms will settle on the surfaces of the filter fibers.

Impaction. The momentum of microorganisms traveling in a gas stream will not allow them to make sharp changes of direction, and so they will impact on the fiber surface. The efficiency of impaction is favored by a higher gas velocity through the filter and again by small fiber diameter of the filter matrix, which would mean a more abrupt change in the flow path of the gas.

Diffusion. Low velocities of air or gas through the filter matrix favor diffusion. Bacteria will undergo Brownian movement to some extent and will diffuse to the surfaces of the fiber matrix.

Electrostatics Gas flowing through a filter matrix causes a triboelectric effect resulting in the charging of the filter fibers. The charge acquired depends on the nature of the fiber. Microorganisms carrying a charge become attracted to the surfaces of the filter. Rossano and Silverman (1954) showed that coating the fibers of a filter with a good electrical insulator increases the efficiency of the filter. In a sterile filtration application, the filters must not become moist or the retention effect caused by the electrostatic charge could be dissipated.

Thus, hydrophobicity is an important characteristic of air filters.

These particle-capture mechanisms lead to a most penetrating particle size and dictate that it is desirable to construct a filter with a surface area as large as is practical. Accomazzo and Grant (1986) reported that the most penetrating particles for fibrous filter media and for membrane filters have been measured to be 0.15 μm and 0.05 μm, respectively. Retention ratings for HEPA fiberglass filters have been determined to be ≥ 99.99%, and for typical membrane filters ≥ 99.9999999%.

These mechanisms dictate that it is desirable to construct a filter with a surface area as large as is practical. A large surface area will maintain a low pressure differential across the filter and will maintain filter efficiency by decreasing the translational velocity of the gas. Large surface areas of high-efficiency filters in use today are obtained by pleating the filter back and forth around fluted separator plates.

Depth-Type Fibrous Media

Of the two types of filter materials used in air sterilization, depth and membrane, the fibrous depth type is the most common when large volumes of air must be handled. Fiberglass is the material from which many depth-type filters are made. The gas passing through the matrix of such filters follows a tortuous path, and the microorganisms present will be trapped both on the surface and within the depth of the filter.

Membrane Filters

Membrane filters are becoming increasingly important in critical gas sterilizing applications. The collection mechanism of membrane filters is such that they will retain microorganisms smaller than the specified pore size directly on the immediate surface of the filter. Megaw and Wiffen (1963) have demonstrated that a filter having an average pore diameter of 0.8 μm will retain particulate material as small as 0.05 μm. The mechanism

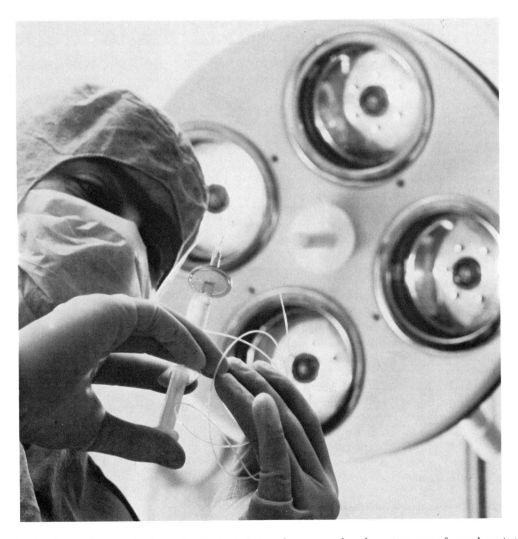

Fig. 30–20. Epidural analgesia administration is a pain-relieving technique for surgery when the maintenance of normal respiratory function is desirable. Here, a small Millex membrane filter unit is being used in line to help minimize the risk of infection.

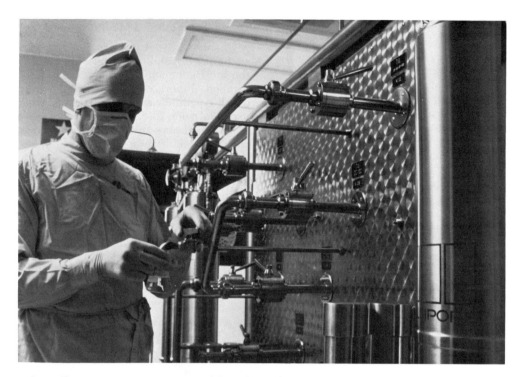

Fig. 30–21. A sterilizing filtration system, representative of those that perform to critical specifications, is shown here in use at Pharmacia AB in Uppsala, Sweden.

of electrostatic charge is probably more responsible than any other for this retention.

Of growing importance is the sterile filtration of medicinal gases such as oxygen delivered to a patient in an oxygen tent over a long period. The fact that the membrane filter is a homogeneous integral structure that will not allow parts of itself to be released downstream is extremely important. An added advantage of placing a membrane filter directly in the line coming from the oxygen tank is that any particulate contamination, such as metallic particles and fibers from the tank and valves, is quantitatively removed along with any microorganisms.

Membrane filters are ideally adaptable to the filtration of venting air for sterile tanks or containers from which sterile pharmaceuticals are being withdrawn. Sparging for fermentation applications is ideally suited to membrane filtration because an entire filtration element may be sterilized in place.

An in-line membrane filter must be of the hydrophobic type; otherwise, moisture droplets, often found in pressurized gas systems, could wet a nonhydrophobic membrane to the extent that a pressure above the bubble point (previously described in this chapter) of the membrane would be required to force air through. In addition, wetting of an air filter may decrease its retention efficiency.

Recently, large-area hydrophobic membrane filter systems have been used in conjunction with large-production fermentation systems requiring sterile air. Unlike the conventional depth-filter units, the membrane sys-

Table 30–4. *Some Typical Groups of Fluids Treated By Absolute Filtration*

Antibiotics
Ophthalmic solutions
Intravenous solutions
Intravenous additives
Hyperalimentation fluid
Diagnostic drugs
Radiopharmaceuticals
Allergenic extracts
Organ preservation fluids
Irrigation solutions for surgery
Peritoneal dialysis fluids
Pharmaceutical makeup water
Diagnostic growth media
Tissue culture medium
Serum and serum fractions
Vaccines
Narcotics
Steroids
Fermentation products
Oil-base pharmaceuticals
Veterinary products
Air and other gases

tem does not allow bacterial passage if challenged with large amounts of moisture from the pressure system.

Applications

The applications involving sterilizing filtration are many and varied. From laboratory applications to those in the pharmaceutical, medical, or fermentation industries, new uses are being found each year. New filtration products and procedures are under continuous development.

For more than 30 years, sterilization by membrane filtration has been an accepted standard procedure. In many cases, it is the only practical method for assuring that a variety of products reach the end user in sterile form. Figures 30–20 and 30–21 illustrate the broad range of applications for sterile filtration from processing large volumes of parenteral drugs to small volumes of fluids at the point of use. Table 30–4 lists a cross section of general categories with which sterilizing filtration is advantageous.

The specific apparatus to be used depends on the volume to be filtered and to some extent on the amount of contamination in the solution. For the filtration of parenteral solutions, two categories have been established: (1) Small- Volume Parenteral (SVP) sterilization, in which a single dose is less than 100 ml, and (2) Large-Volume Parenteral (LVP) sterilization, in which a single dose is 100 ml or greater.

As has been described in this chapter, sterilization by membrane filters is a significant and demanding application. To remove all bacteria, the membrane pore size must be smaller than the bacteria and must be uniform throughout. The filter element must be properly sealed to prevent bypass and to allow sterilization of the filter and housing before use. Finally, quality assurance requires that the entire system be tested for integrity before and after use. Regardless of the manufacturing process, variation in dosage form, type of container, and drug or vehicle chemistry, the product must be sterile in the final container.

REFERENCES

Accomazzo, M.A., and Grant, D.C. 1986. Mechanisms and devices for filtration of critical process gases. In *Fluid Filtration: Gas*. Volume 1. ASTM STP 975. Edited by R.R. Raber. Philadelphia, American Society of Testing Materials, pp. 402–420.

Adams, D.G., and Agarwal, D. 1989. Clean-in-place design. BioPharm, 2(6), 48–57.

American Society of Testing Materials (ASTM). 1986. Determining the bacterial retention of membrane filters utilized for liquid filtration. In *1986 Annual Book of Standards*. Volume 14.02. Designation F838–83, pp. 938–944.

Ballard, R.W., Doudoroff, M., and Stanier, R.Y. 1968. Taxonomy of the aerobic pseudomonads: Pseudomonas diminuta and P. vesiculare. J. Gen. Microbiol., 53, 349–361.

Bowman, F.W., Calhoun, M.P., and White, M. 1967. Microbiological methods for quality control of membrane filters. J. Pharm. Sci., 56, 453–459.

Coriell, L.L., and McGarrity, G.J. 1967. Elimination of airborne bacteria in the laboratory and operating room. Bull. Parent. Drug Assoc., 21, 46–51.

Dwyer, J.L. 1968. The technology of absolute microfiltration. Tech. Q. Master Brewers Assoc. Am., 5(4), 246G.

Dwyer, J.L. 1966. *Contamination Analysis and Control*. New York, Reinhold.

Einstein, A., and Muhsa, H. 1923. Experimentalle Bestimmung der Kanalweite von Filtern. Dtsch Med. Wochenschr., SLIX, 1012.

Elford, W.J. 1933. The principles of ultrafiltration as applied in biological studies. Proc. R. Soc., 112B, 384–406.

Elford, W.J. 1931. A new series of graded collodian membranes suitable for general bacteriological use, especially in filterable virus studies. J. Pathol. Bacteriol., 34, 505.

Food and Drug Administration (FDA). 1987. *Guideline on sterile drug products produced by aseptic processing*. Washington, D.C., Center of Drugs and Biologics and Office of Regulatory Affairs, June 1987.

Food and Drug Administration (FDA). 1985. *Compliance Program Guidance Manual, CP7356.002A, Small Volume Parenterals*. Washington, D.C., Center of Drugs and Biologics and Office of Regulatory Affairs, October 1985.

Garvan, J.M., and Gunner, B.W. 1971. Particulate contamination of intravenous fluids. Br. J. Clin. Pract., 25, 119–121.

Goddard, J.L. 1966. Address to the Parenteral Drug Association. Bull. Parent. Drug Assoc., 10, 183–188.

Health Industry Manufacturers Association (HIMA). 1982. Microbiological evaluation of filters for sterilizing liquids. HIMA Document No. 3, Volume 4, April 1982.

Henrici, A.T. 1928. *Morphologic Variation and the Rate of Growth of Bacteria*. London, Bailliere, Tindall and Cox.

Herbert, D. 1958. Some principles of continuous culture. In *Recent Progress in Microbiology*. Edited by G. Tunevall. Springfield, IL, Charles C Thomas, pp. 381–402.

Howard, G., Jr., and Duberstain, R. 1980. A case of penetration of 0.2-μm rated membrane filters by bacteria. J. Parent. Drug Assoc., 34, 95–102.

Jonas, A.M. 1966. Potentially hazardous effects of introducing particulate matter into the vascular system of man and animals. Proceedings FDA Symposium of Safety of Large Volume Parenteral Solutions, Washington, D.C., pp. 23–27.

Leahy, T.J., and Sullivan, M.J. 1978. Validation of bacterial retention capabilities of membrane filters. Pharm. Tech., 2, 65–75.

Leahy, T.J., Sullivan, M.J., Slingeneyer, A., and Mion, C. 1980. The efficiency of microbial retention by peritoneal dialysis filters. Trans. Am. Soc. Artif. Intern. Organs, 26, 225–230.

Lee, J.Y. 1989. Validating an automated filter integrity test instrument. Pharm. Tech., 13, 48–56.

Levy, R.V. 1987a. The effect of pH, viscosity and additives on the bacterial retention of membrane filters challenged with *Pseudomonas diminuta*. In *Fluid Filtration: Liquid. Volume II*. American Society for Testing Materials, Special Technical Publication 975, pp. 80–89.

Levy, R.V. 1987b. The mechanisms and reliability of sterilizing filtrations with microporous membranes. Paper presented at the Pharm Tech Conference '87, East Rutherford, New Jersey, 22–24 September, 1987.

Maaloe, O., and Kjeldgaard, N.O. 1966. *Control of Macromolecular Synthesis*. New York, W.A. Benjamin.

Marcus, S., Anselmo, C., and Luke, J. 1959. Studies on bacterial pyrogenicity. II. A bacteriological test for pyrogens in parenteral solutions. J. Am. Pharm. Assoc., 49, 616–619.

Megaw, W.J., and Wiffen, R.D. 1963. The efficiency of membrane filters. Int. J. Air. Water Pollut., 7, 501–509.

Meltzer, T.H. 1987. *Filtration in the Pharmaceutical Industry*. New York, Marcel Dekker, p. 1091.

Meltzer, T.H. 1989a. Filtration: the practice of prefiltration and its related considerations. Ultrapure Water, 6(3), 24–34.

Meltzer, T.H. 1989b. Filtration. A critical review of filter integrity testing. Part I—The bubble point method; assessing filter compatibility; initial and final testing. Ultrapure Water, 6(4), 40–51.

Meltzer, T.H. 1989c. Filtration. A critical review of filter integrity testing. Part II—The diffusive air flow and pressure-hold methods; assessing filter compatibility; initial and final testing. Ultrapure Water, 6(5), 44–56.

Myers, J.A. 1972. Interim report on a clinical trial of the Millipore infusion filter unit. Pharm. J., 208, 547–549.

Pall, D.B., and Kirnbauer, E.A. 1978. Bacteria removal production in membrane filters. Abstr. 52nd Colloid and Surface Science Symposium, ACS, Knoxville, Tennessee.

Plumer, A.L. 1970. *Principles and Practice of Intravenous Therapy*. Boston, Little, Brown.

Reti, A.R. 1976. An assessment of test criteria for evaluating the performance and integrity of sterilizing filters. Bull. Parent. Drug Assoc, 31, 187–194.

Reti, A.R., Leahy, T.T., and Meier, P.M. 1979. The retention mechanism of sterilizing and other submicron high efficiency filter structures. In *Proceedings of Second World Filtration Congress*. London, pp. 427–435.

Robertson, J.H., and DeVisser, A. 1980. Microbiological qualification and validation of sterilizing membrane filters. New York, Abstr. Interphex USA.

Rogers, B.G., and Rossmoore, H.W. 1970. Determination of membrane filter porosity of microbiological methods. In *Developments in Industrial Microbiology*. Volume II. Edited by C.J. Corum. Washington, D.C., American Institute of Biological Sciences, pp. 453–459.

Rossano, A.T., Jr., and Silverman, L. 1954. Electrostatic effects in fiber filters for aerosols. Heat. Ventil. Ref., 51, 102–108.

Schaechter, M., Maaloe, O., and Kjeldgaard, N.O. 1958. Dependency on medium and temperature of cell size and chemical composition during balanced growth of *Salmonella typhimurium*. J. Gen. Microbiol., 19, 595–605.

Sykes, G. 1965. *Disinfection and Sterilization*. 2nd Edition. Philadelphia, J.B. Lippincott.

Tanny, G.B., Strong, D.K., Presswood, W.G., and Meltzer, T.H. 1979. Adsorptive retention of *Pseudomonas diminuta*, by membrane filters. J. Parent. Drug Assoc., 33, 40–51.

Technical Staff. 1960. *Handbook of Filtration*. Mt. Holly Springs, Eaton-Dikeman Company.

Turco, S., and Davis, N.M. 1973. Clinical significance of particulate matter: a review of the literature. Hosp. Pharmaceut., 8(5), 137–319.

USP XXII. 1990. *The United States Pharmacopeia.* Easton, Mack Printing Co.

Wallhausser, K.H. 1979a. Is the removal of microorganisms by filtration really a sterilizing method? J. Parent. Drug Assoc., *33,* 156–191.

Wallhausser, K.H. 1979b. Recent studies on sterile filtration. Pharm. Ind., *41,* 475–481.

Whitfield, W.J. 1967. Microbiological studies of laminar flow rooms. Bull. Parent. Drug Assoc., *21,* 37–45.

Zsigmondy, R., and Buchmann, F. 1922. U.S. Patent No. 1,421,341.

ACKNOWLEDGMENTS

The authors gratefully acknowledge the technical assistance of Scott Emory and Perry Schwartz and the editorial assistance of Denise Boyd.

CHAPTER 31

STERILIZATION BY ULTRAVIOLET IRRADIATION

I.L. Shechmeister

The practical applications of ultraviolet irradiation (hereafter designated as UV) depend on the killing action of the radiation on agents such as yeasts, molds, bacteria, rickettsiae, mycoplasma, and viruses. Some of the other effects of UV include increases in the rate of mutation, chromosomal aberration, and changes in cellular viscosity. UV affects such vital processes as respiration, excitability, and growth. A number of reviews and books have been written about the mechanisms of UV action on microbial agents and photoreactivation (Wang, 1976; Harm, 1980; Hader and Tevini, 1987). The *Illuminating Engineering Society Lighting Handbook* (Kaufman, 1987) and *Germicidal Lamps and Applications* (Philips' Gloeilampenfabriken, 1985) contain concise discussion of applications of UV.

FUNDAMENTAL CONCEPTS OF UV

Basic Physics

Radiant energy can be studied when it is intercepted by matter and converted into thermal, chemical, or mechanical energy. Radiations are usually divided into two main groups: corpuscular and electromagnetic wave radiations. Corpuscular radiations are exemplified by streams of atoms, electrons, and protons. Electromagnetic wave radiations comprise the wide range of radiations from the longest radio waves without a detectable biologic effect, through infrared or heat rays, and visible light, to UV, roentgen rays (x rays), gamma rays, and secondary cosmic rays. Although the speeds of corpuscular radiations differ, electromagnetic rays travel at the same rate of 186,000 miles per second; however, they differ in length. The shorter radiation waves are measured in nanometers (nm). One nanometer is equivalent to 10^{-9} meters. Although radiation travels as a wave, it acts as if it were produced and delivered in discrete amounts of energy called quanta. Quanta of electromagnetic radiant energy, or photons, are emitted from radiation sources. The energy of these photons depends directly on the frequency of radiation. The speed trav-eled per second by the radiation waves, c, is determined by the number of oscillations per second, or f, also known as the frequency, and the wavelength, or λ; thus, $c = f\lambda$ or $f = \dfrac{c}{\lambda}$. The energy of a quantum E is given by the product of $h \times f$, that is to say $E = hf$ or $E = \dfrac{hc}{\lambda}$ where h is Planck's constant (6.62×10^{-27} erg-seconds). The energy of a photon, therefore, increases with increasing frequency or with decreasing wavelength. This equation clarifies the relatively inappreciable photochemical and photobiologic effects of infrared radiation in contrast to the marked effects of UV. The germicidal effect of UV could result from absorbed radiation and from an indirect effect of toxic compounds produced in the surrounding medium. However, the latter mode of action appears improbable. Therefore, availability of large-energy quanta that are poorly absorbed at a particular wavelength will lead to an inefficient reaction. The absorbed quanta must be of sufficient magnitude to initiate and maintain a given photoreaction.

Mechanism of Action

Although the UV spectrum includes a range from 15 nm to the rays bordering on the visible, the region of greatest interest to us is from 220 to 300 nm, often called the "abiotic" region. LD_{50} values of UV for some unicellular organisms have been assembled by Spector (1956). UV radiation is called "nonionizing," because most organic molecules require wavelengths below 180 nm to effect ionization. Because of this, for all practical purposes ionization may be excluded as one of the immediate consequences of UV irradiation in biologic materials. Only a few comments about the mechanism of the killing effect of UV are presented at this time. A more complete discussion is given by Hader and Tevini (1987).

As indicated previously, the chemical details of the lethal action have been studied intensively during the past 25 to 30 years. Nevertheless, exciting as it is, the available information should be viewed as initial steps in clarification of this process. The early observations by Gates (1928) pointed out the bactericidal action of different wavelengths of monochromatic UV. These so-called action spectra showed the similarity of, and hence the probable relation between, the germicidal wavelengths and those absorbed by nucleic acids or nucleic acid constituents. Studies of action spectra of mutagenic effects and retardation of cell division suggested that these conditions are caused by the effect of UV on nucleic acids (Ciese, 1968). Of the components of nucleic acids, sugar phosphates do not absorb UV significantly above 220 nm. Because pyrimidines are much more sensitive to UV than purine bases, the major effects of mutagenic and lethal UV on biologic systems are attributed to photochemical transformations of pyrimidine bases (Patrick and Rahn, 1976). It appears that the sterilizing UV acts on cellular DNA primarily by producing links between successive pyrimidines on a DNA strand to form dimers. It has been suggested that they are formed primarily of adjacent thymine residues in the same strand (Hanes, 1964). Thymine dimers have become specifically linked to loss of tranforming ability of bacterial DNA. Cytosine-thymine mixed dimers and cytosine-cytosine dimers have been also identified in DNA from normal and transforming bacterial strains exposed to UV, as well as in cellular DNA of irradiated bacteria, protozoa, and mammalian cells; although these dimers are identified less frequently than thymine- thymine dimers, they interfere with replication and also lead to death of the cells (Setlow and Carrier, 1966; Harm et al., 1971). According to Rahn (1973), UV irradiation of DNA results in the formation of various kinds of photoproducts that may have a disruptive influence on the local integrity of the DNA structure. The cross-linking of DNA and protein plays a significant role in the killing of UV-irradiated cells (Smith, 1976). The predominant photoproduct in UV-irradiated bacterial spores, 5-thyminyl-5,6-dihydrothymine, has been shown to cause lethal effects. It is not found in vegetative bacterial cells. Damage other than formation of pyrimidine dimers may also contribute to the denaturation of irradiated DNA. As yet, there is no clear indication of the other forms this damage takes.

Much fewer data are available on the photochemistry of RNA than on that of DNA. Hydrates and uracil dimers have been observed in irradiated RNA, and both products can cause UV inactivation of RNA. Other pyrimidine photoproducts have been detected; however, the nature of their possible inactivation of RNA is not established (Gordon et al., 1976).

Survival curves of viruses with single-stranded DNA or single-stranded RNA can be drawn on a semilogarithmic paper approximately as a straight line. Survival curves of cells with double-stranded DNA as the target for UV action, however, show minor shoulders followed by a straight-line relationship over a considerable range of values. Maximum bacterial effectiveness is manifested at about 265 nm, with a sharp decline at about 290 to 300 nm and with progressively lower effectiveness through the visible-light range.

Several factors influence bacterial sensitivity to UV. The more important are (1) pH, (2) sensitivity at different stages of bacterial growth cycle, the greatest activity being in the logarithmic growth phase, and (3) presence of spores, which are about twice as resistant as vegetative cells. There is no agreement regarding sensitivity to UV and cell moisture content. There are also inconsistent results in the attempted correlation of susceptibility of airborne bacteria to UV at different relative humidities. Genetic constitution, exemplified by *Escherichia coli* B/r, a strain resistant to radiation and isolated by Witkin (1946), and postirradiation treatment may account for great variation in survival of irradiated organisms. Estimation of survival can be influenced by the nature of the medium used for assay of bacterial growth and by various "reactivations."

Reactivation of Irradiated Microbial Agents

There is a delicate balance in living things between the deterioration of cellular components after exposure to UV and their biochemical repair. If the amount of damage exceeds the cell's capacity to repair this damage, the cell will die. The reversal of injurious effects of UV by visible light, i.e., photoreactivation, was recognized as a general phenomenon following its rediscovery by Kelner (1949) in bacteria and by Dulbecco (1955) in bacteriophage. Fungus spores, bacteria, animal and plant cells, viruses, and nucleic acids inactivated by UV are photoreactivated by treatment with visible light or near UV, in the vicinity of about 330 to 480 nm. Mutations and cytologic changes induced by UV are also reversed by such treatment (Giese, 1973; Wolff, 1972). Until the initial studies by Kelner, DNA exposed to UV was consideree to be permanently destroyed. A photoreversible irradiation product of thymine was isolated and identified as thymine dimers by Beukers and Berends (1960). It has been shown that different pyrimidine dimers formed after exposure of cells, such as *Escherichia coli*, to UV in the lethal range of about 220 to 290 nm were photoreactivated to a different extent, and never completely. This indicated that other photoproducts were formed in UV-treated cells. The operational concept of the "killed" state does not necessarily represent irreversible destruction of viability. If cellular injury is reversible, the damaged cells may recover to produce visibly discernible structures. At this time our understanding of recovery mechanism is based primarily on results of studies with bacteria and viruses. Although more than one mechanism can lead to photoreactivation, the most common and usually the most effective mechanism is photoenzymatic repair of damaged DNA and RNA (Harm, 1976). A photoreactivating light-dependent enzyme can split pyrimidine dimers in situ, restoring normal structure. This has been demonstrated in a wide variety of cellular systems. It can also bring about direct chemical conversion of thymine dimers to thymine. The UV-damaged free viral RNA and many RNA-containing plant viruses can be photoreactivated. It is suggested that a process similar to enzymatic photoreactivation of UV-damaged DNA is responsible for this phenomenon (Varghese, 1972).

Spontaneous reversion of photoproducts to the original undamaged state is another, and the simplest, mechanism of repair, primarily dependent upon the environmental conditions. For example, chemical composition and pH of postirradiation plating medium and incubation temperature greatly influence the survival of UV-irradiated *E. coli* B cells. The third mechanism of repairing damage produced by UV radiation utilizes two enzymes and takes place in the dark; it is known as dark recovery. One enzyme is hydrolytic in nature and excises the dimers produced by UV. The second enzyme is a polymerase and replaces the excised regions by copying the undamaged strand.

APPLICATION OF UV ENERGY

Viruses, mycoplasma, bacteria, and fungi may be destroyed by UV, whether they are suspended in air or in liquids or deposited on surfaces. Because UV will not penetrate most substances, foods and fabrics, for example, cannot be sterilized by this radiation. The more important applications of UV are directed at (1) destruction of airborne organisms, establishing by this action satisfactory air hygiene; (2) inactivation of microorganisms located on surfaces or suspended in liquids, but accessible to UV; and (3) protection and disinfection of many products of unstable composition that cannot be treated by conventional methods. Bacterial spores are more resistant than vegetative bacteria, and there is a wide difference between species (Baylin and Waites, 1979). A much higher degree of irradiation is required to sterilize microbes suspended in a liquid such as broth than for those suspended in water or buffer. When placed on a surface, the nature of the material on which droplets are deposited is important. For example, aluminum and glass surfaces were sterilized, but not wood, rubber, or paper exposed even for 4 hours at 120/μW/cm^2. The use of UV against microbial agents deposited on surfaces of different chemical nature is a subject of continued studies. UV pass-through chambers for disinfecting single sheets of paper contaminated with *Bacillus subtilis* spores and *Serratia marcescens* (Phillips and Novak, 1956), as well as paper contaminated with *Mycobacterium tuberculosis* (Haber et al., 1970), have been described. UV was used for sterilization of local anesthetic cartridges (Ciarlone and Fry, 1980) and disinfection of dental materials (Boylan et al., 1987); although microbes on surfaces were killed rapidly, shadowed areas were not readily affected. A number of microbial cultures were effectively eliminated from a tonometer using a special UV sterilizer (Sherman, 1974). However, it is misleading to generalize about the efficacy of UV, because a large number of microbial agents may be killed while the surface may not necessarily be sterilized (Morris, 1972).

Prior to application of UV to air sanitation, the effects of UV on bacterial and viral aerosols have been studied under a variety of conditions (Wells, 1955; Jensen, 1964; Smith et al., 1964). *Escherichia coli* has been adopted by many as the standard test organism in air sanitation, even though it is seldom found naturally in the airborne state. Reid et al. (1956) suggested the use of *Streptococcus viridans* as a more realistic index of air hygiene. The environmental conditions frequently suggest the use of different organisms for this purpose; for example, *Staphylococcus aureus* serves as a realistic indicator for air contamination in hospitals. Dust-borne organisms may be shielded from UV by solids in the dust particles.

Reports on the effect of relative humidity (RH) on the sensitivity of bacterial aerosols have been equivocal. Although some workers reported decreased killing of airborne organisms by UV at humidities in excess of 60 to 70%, other investigators did not agree with these results. Riley and Kaufman studied the effect of RH on the inactivation of *Serratia marcescens* by UV in a specially designed apparatus (1972). They concluded that at RH above 60 to 70%, there was a sharp decline in the number of killed organisms; that in the middle range of RH the sensitivity of their bacteria to UV was greater than that reported by other investigators; and that at low humidities, i.e., below 40%, again there was a decrease in the number of killed organisms. Some claimed that the aerosols were more sensitive than suspensions in liquids, whereas others stated that organisms on agar and in the air were equally sensitive to UV. Unfortunately, the inactivating effect of radiation was compared regardless of age or state of bacterial suspension. Exponential or sigmoidal survival curves were observed, depending on these and other experimental conditions.

Germicidal Lamps

The most practical method of generating UV radiation is by passage of electric discharge through low-pressure mercury vapor enclosed in special glass tubes, known commercially as germicidal lamps. The principle of all germicidal lamps is the same, that of electron flow between electrodes through ionized mercury vapor. The arc in a fluorescent lamp operates on the same basic principle and produces the same type of UV energy. The difference between the two is that the bulb of the fluorescent lamps is coated with a phosphor compound that converts UV to visible light. The glass used in ordinary fluorescent lamps filters out all germicidal UV. The germicidal lamp is not coated with phosphor and is made of special glass that transmits the UV generated by the mercury in addition to visible light. About 95% of the UV is in wavelengths of 253.7 nm. These lamps have germicidal efficiency of 5 to 10 times that of high-pressure quartz mercury arcs (400 to 60,000 mm Hg or 0.5 to 75 atm).

Killing, K, or inactivation of microorganisms as a result of exposure to UV light, is expressed as the product of the intensity, I, of germicidal energy and time, t. Consideration of this relation, $K = It$, leads to postulation that the same exposure can be obtained using either high intensity for a short time or low intensity for a proportionally longer period. Under practical conditions, the exposure time is dictated by the particular situation.

Operational efficiency of germicidal lamps depends on the surrounding temperature and movement of air. Commercial lamps are generally designed to operate most efficiently at an ambient temperature of 27°C. Cooling the lamp below 27°C by passing air currents over it or by submerging it in liquid lowers its output. Special lamps that operate efficiently under otherwise undesirable conditions are available commercially.

In addition to transmission of 253.7 nm, the glass used in low-pressure mercury lamps will transmit a certain amount of 184.9-nm energy. Energy of this wavelength forms ozone by breaking the bonds of the oxygen molecule. The amount of ozone produced is controlled entirely by the transmission of the glass tubes and decreases more rapidly than emission of 253.7-nm energy with the age of a lamp. The concentration of ozone in a given area is measured in parts of ozone per million parts of air. The amount of ozone will vary with temperature, humidity, and air movement. Special germicidal lamps are made with glass envelopes allowing transmission of high concentration of 184.9-nm energy along with the germicidal 253.7-nm energy. These are used in industry for preservation of food. Ozone has antimicrobial action, but not of practical significance when human beings are subjected to it. Ozone is also used in many situations to eliminate or suppress objectionable odors and to impart a clean, fresh smell to air.

Germicidal tubes depreciate rapidly during the first 100 hours of operation; consequently, commercial tubes are rated initially as though they had already operated for 100 hours. Meters are available to monitor the output of a particular lamp, as well as to measure the intensities of germicidal energy at various locations in the room and reflectance of germicidal energy by walls and ceilings (Jagger, 1961; Mpelkas, 1983).

Various germicidal tubes are available, operating at different current ratings. The maximum intensity of a tube is provided at its own surface. Absorption of UV by air is negligible. However, distance from the source of radiation imposes certain restrictions in calculation of intensity. An inverse relationship exists between distance from the source and intensity of radiation out to about one-half of the effective length of the source, and between the square of the distance at greater than this length from the source. Slim-line germicidal lamps start instantly and use a coil filament on each end that operates hot. Lamp life is governed by the electrode life and frequency of starts. These lamps are used when high ultraviolet intensity is desired, as in treatment of water or air or of products on conveyor belts. Cold cathode bactericidal lamps also start instantly but are not affected by number of starts. Their useful life is determined entirely by the transmission of the bulb. They have a longer life than other lamps and perform well at cold temperatures. Because of their long life and moderate intensity,

they are often used in occupied areas and when frequent starting is desirable. Most bactericidal lamps operate best in still air at room temperature, and thus UV output is measured at an ambient temperature of 77°F. Higher or lower temperatures decrease the output of the lamp.

The lamps should be cleaned periodically by wiping with a cloth dampened in alcohol or ammonia and water to maintain maximum output of UV. No oils or waxes should be used for moistening the wiping cloth. When a lamp drops to about 60% of its 100-hour rating, or after it has been used for three- fourths of its rating time, it should be replaced.

Installation of UV lamps in an enclosed space has become an exacting procedure that should be handled by a lighting engineer. Preliminary ideas regarding certain aspects of installation may be gathered from pamphlets and handbooks put out by the manufacturers of these lamps (Mpelkas, 1983; Philips' Gloeilampenfabriken, 1985).

ACTION OF UV ON MICROBIAL AGENTS IN AIR

Sampling Devices

Most of the reports dealing with air hygiene describe the effect of a particular antimicrobial agent either on a total number of airborne organisms or on the concentration of a chosen "indicator" organism. However, there is no agreement regarding the organism to be used for indication of microbial air pollution, the most appropriate instrument for air sampling, and the culture medium for reliable and reproducible results.

Mircoorganisms may be found in air as part of small "droplet nuclei" or as components of larger aggregates of microbes (Wells, 1955). Little movement of air is required to keep droplet nuclei suspended, and adventitious currents may result in their dispersal over wide areas. Large droplets will settle out eventually to become part of the dust. UV is more effective against droplet nuclei than against large airborne microbial aggregates.

To ascertain the number of airborne agents, numerous sampling devices have been described and evaluated. A review by Akers and Won (1969) discusses the quantitative methods for assay of living airborne microorganisms. To obtain reliable information regarding biologic properties of a given microbial aerosol, one may have to resort to a comparative evaluation of several different types of samplers. Sampling methods include deposition on agar, impingement on liquid and solid media, filtration, centrifugation, and thermal precipitation. Some of the instruments have also been used for sampling viral and rickettsial content of air. An adequate sampling device should be characterized by high efficiency, wide range of applicability, easy operation, quick sampling, simple construction, portability, low initial cost, and inexpensive maintenance. These instruments may collect airborne aggregates without breaking up the clumps of organisms, or the procedure may disperse an aggregate into the component agents. The older literature indicates that many investigators preferred the simple but inefficient method of enumerating smaller or larger sedimenting aggregates by counting colonies developing on nutrient medium in petri dishes exposed for a given period to the tested air. Also, certain factors affecting practical use of UV for disinfecting purposes should be kept in mind when using sampling devices in laboratory or field studies. The heterogeneity of biologic populations in a given environment and the presence of protecting substances influence the rate of microbial inactivation (Morris, 1972).

Lethe

The concentration of bacteria in a given enclosed environment varies directly with the supply of fresh air, which is measured in units of room-volume replacement, or so-called air change. One air change cannot completely replace all the air and the suspended organisms, for the incoming air is diluted by the outgoing air. The fraction remaining after one air change is 36.8% of the air and bacteria originally present. Increasing the number of turnovers of air, using fresh filtered air for this purpose, has as one of its limitations the creations of drafts. Similar removal of airborne organisms may be achieved by judicious use of UV energy. The amount of UV necessary to kill the bacteria in one turnover of air is known as lethe and is expressed in watt-minutes per square foot. It is possible to obtain conditions equivalent to 60 to 180 air changes per hour, or 1 to 3 changes of air per minute at the breathing level.

Standards for Exposure to UV

UV light is capable of damaging sensitive tissues and is ineffective if not properly directed in sufficient intensity. Although maximum erythemal effect is produced by 298.6 nm, the erythemal effect of commercially available sources of 253.7-nm energy is about half as great as that of the optimal wavelength. Consequently prolonged exposure to germicidal intensities of UV may lead to undesirable physiologic effects. These are manifested primarily by reddened skin and irritated eyes. Precautions should always be taken to shield the eyes, not only from direct radiation from a lamp or reflector but also from continued exposure to radiation reflected by room surfaces, clothing, and furnishings. The glass in conventional eyeglasses protects from direct radiation but not from UV entering from the side. Clear plastic shields are available to protect the face. Protection of hands and arms is desirable if there is prolonged exposure to high concentration of UV. Special fixtures have been designed to guard against this contingency. The extent of daily exposure by occupants of the room determines the type of UV lamp and fixture most suitable for the particular installation. The mean room intensity may be considerably higher if one irradiates intensively the air above normal eye level, using specially screened reflectors and UV-absorbing paint (Sylvania, 1983).

Methods for Irradiation of Air

Irradiation of upper air by germicidal lamps placed on walls slightly above eye level will effectively reduce bacterial concentration in the entire room, because there is continuous local interchange of upper and lower room air by convection, allowing irradiation of 1 to 3 room air changes per minute (Riley, 1977). It is estimated that irradiation of the upper part of the room with a given intensity of UV is equivalent to irradiation of the whole room with one-half to one-third this intensity.

Kethley and Branch (1972) pointed out that, in installing UV lamps to improve sanitary ventilation, the location of lamps should be matched to the air distribution system of the room. The type of air system that promotes mixing throughout an air space should be most suitable for this purpose. In their experiments using upper-air UV radiation against artificially produced *Serratia marcescens* aerosols, they reported that equivalent sanitary ventilation of 39 changes of air per hour was obtained using 2.7-μm aerosol particles, compared to 18 changes her hour when 5.2-μm aerosol particles were produced. In addition, they emphasized the importance of the location of sampling devices within the room used for their studies. Riley et al (1971a, b) investigated convective air change in rooms with UV-irradiated upper air. The efficiency with which airborne test organisms were removed from the lower part of the room was used to evaluate convective air mixing between the upper and lower parts of the room. Rates of disappearance of test organisms were more than twice as fast when the air entering the ceiling was 3°F or more cooler than the air in the lower part of the room. Upper-air treatment with UV for disinfection of air in the lower part of a room was a function of good mixing of air as well as the rapid disinfection of upper air. Riley et al. (1976) nebulized various mycobacteria into the air of a room equipped with upper-air irradiating UV fixtures and monitored the rate of microbial disappearance. *Mycobacterium tuberculosis* was approximately ten times as susceptible to UV as *M. phlei*. Their value for equivalent sanitary ventilation using *M. tuberculosis* as the test organism was 25 changes of air per hour, a somewhat lower number than that obtained by Kethley and Branch (1972) using *Serratia marcescens*.

Germicidal fixtures may be either recessed in the wall or surface-mounted on the wall and may be open or louvered (Mpelkas, 1983). Their installation should be influenced by the reflectance of UV from the walls and ceiling. Reflectance of aluminum metal and paints ranges from about 40 to 80%, compared to that of oil-based paint of 3 to 10% (Morris, 1972). The distribution of radiation from different UV fixtures has been determined. Properly designed fixtures have not been found to expose occupants of the room to dangerous levels of UV; however, improper use of UV lamps or fixtures can lead to injuries such as erythema and conjunctivitis (Stamp and Muth, 1978; Wulf, 1980).

Another method of reducing airborne organisms consists of placing germicidal tubes without reflectors in heating and air-conditioning ducts serving the room in question. The size and shape of the duct, the UV reflection characteristics of the walls, and the number of the lamps determine the efficiency of the method. Disinfection of air with this UV tube is affected by conditions such as temperature, humidity, and air velocity (Riley and Kaufman, 1972). Arrangement of lamps perpendicular to the flow of air in the duct is important in order to obtain full utilization of the emitted UV energy. The lamps are best installed after the filters, where air velocity is slowest, to allow for longer exposure to UV. It is desirable to have the walls of the ducts painted with highly reflective aluminum paint. This arrangement is not tenable with smaller window-fitted air-conditioning units. Here lamps are introduced parallel to airflow and still effectively reduce bacteria in the circulated air. In this situation, the UV room air conditioner recirculates relatively clean air at constant temperature and relative humidity and provides the room with bacteriologically purified air, comparable to a system that uses 100% fresh air.

The third method of irradiating the air in the enclosed space is by radiation from unshielded, naked lamps. This method of keeping out microorganisms has proved effective in protection of various products during their manufacture or storage and in handling pathogenic organisms in glove boxes and safety cabinets. In the latter, there should be at least 40 μW/cm^2 UV at the base of the cabinet (Morris, 1972). Similarly, barriers to microorganisms are set up by the use of narrow intensive curtains of UV across openings or in front of hospital cubicles. One should consider, however, that possibilities exist for interpersonal transmission of organisms in space enclosed by these barriers.

The use of UV in air disinfection is desirable in preventing the spread of airborne microbial agents. Indoor installation of UV is much more effective than mechanical ventilation in reducing the concentration of airborne microbes. The Center for Disease Control recommends that both procedures be used to reduce the airborne load (Center for Disease Control, 1971). Fresh air accomplishes the same effect outdoors. Because people move about in many indoor atmospheres, an individual protected by the UV environment may become infected in unprotected locations. Persons living in a special environment, such as a hospital or a convalescent home, may benefit significantly from the added protection offered by the UV installation.

Experiments in Hospitals

Numerous and extensive experiments were conducted to determine the efficacy of UV light for protection against infections in hospitals and for reduction of the incidence of respiratory infections in populations routinely sharing a common environment, as exemplified by wards, schools, and barracks. An excellent recent review of prevention of nosocomial infections by UV was published by Levenson et al. (1986).

The first successful application of UV air disinfection in the hospital was pioneered by Hart (1938), followed by Overholt and Betts (1940). Hart installed unshielded UV lamps a short distance above the operating team in a surgical amphitheater, allowing the intensity of radiation to be 18 to 30 μW/cm^2 at the level of the operating table. Prior to the use of UV, postoperative mortality from overwhelming infection after clean operations was 1.12% (19 deaths after 1782 operations). Twenty-nine years after the installation of UV lights (Hart, 1960), no such deaths occurred following 2600 operations, including thoracoplasties and neurosurgery. During the same period, wound infection rates dropped from 11.6% (207 of 1782 operations) to 0.25% (6 of 2460 operations) in clean primary incisions. According to Hart, contamination with staphylococci did not present a problem because continuous use of UV during and between operations controls the spread of bacteria by air. He considers the air route of spread to be the greatest factor in seeding of clean operative wounds and exposed sterile supplies with pathogenic bacteria. Hart emphasized the use of adequate precautions for the patient and the surgical team, as well as the necessity of installing the proper equipment.

In spite of these results, the use of direct UV did not achieve wide popularity and had only limited acceptance. In 1962, it was estimated that about 15 hospitals were using this procedure in the United States (Ad. Hoc. Committee of the Committee on Trauma, 1964). Although alarm over the epidemic of infections due to *Staphylococcus aureus* in supposedly clean wounds was evident from a number of publications (Koontz, 1958; Gaulin, 1957; Altemeier, 1958), the medical profession as a whole has not become convinced of the practicability of using UV. This attitude could be attributed primarily to the following factors. The intensity of UV was considered to be insufficient; there was a lack of control of relative humidity in the operating rooms; dirty tubes precluded penetration of UV; and the installation was expensive and difficult because the decrease in UV intensity is inversely proportional to the square of the distance from the source.

Smith et al. (1964) reported on their 2-year study using the Linde-Robbins UV aseptic air system installed in the entire operating suite, obstetric room, nursery, and emergency room of a new 60-bed hospital. Careful hospital design allowed this air system to counteract the negative factors just mentioned and to function at above 99% efficiency in killing airborne *Pseudomonas*, *Bacillus subtilis*, and *Staphylococcus aureus*. Of 3971 operations performed by 90 surgeons over 22 months, no bacteria were recovered in air sampled with petri dishes. The infection rate in this hospital was 0.002%. In another hospital using the same system only in surgery, a 0.0019% infection rate was recorded over 2 years. This is compared with a 1.3% rate in two hospitals without the Linde-Robbins UV system. The authors pointed out that surgical infection rates usually vary from 0.96 to 13.6%. It is interesting to note that the results of a survey carried out by the authors revealed that 20 U.S. and Canadian hospitals in the planning or building stages were incorporating the aseptic air units as a part of the design. Using a similar apparatus and Anderson's air sampler (1958), Jensen (1964) obtained an inactivation rate of greater than 99% for adenovirus type 2 and the Coxsackie B, influenza A, Sindbis, and vaccinia viruses.

In contrast to these data by Hart and by Smith et al. are the results reported by the National Academy of Sciences (1964) on a carefully controlled study carried out in five university medical centers that installed UV lamps in 16 operating rooms and recorded observations for 27 months. There was two- to four-fold reduction of airborne contamination. A total of 15,613 operative wounds in 14,854 patients were followed. There were 1157 definite infections within 28 days after operation. In the "refined-clean" wounds, radiation reduced postoperative infection rate from 3.8 to 2.9%, a statistically significant effect. A slight difference favoring irradiation (from 7.5 to 7.3%) occurs in "other" clean wounds. Infection was encountered more frequently, but not significantly so, in irradiated wounds than in nonirradiated wounds in three other categories of wounds. Although irradiation reduced the risk of postoperative infection by about 25% among patients with "refined-clean" wounds, 80% of all definite infections were in other wound classifications. The net effect of UV on the entire series was negligible. However, the overall infection rates varied from 3 to 11.7% in five institutions, indicating the importance of factors other than airborne organisms in wound infections.

Lewis and Burke (1969) concluded that UV used with an intensity of 35 μW/cm^2 at the level of the operating table was effective in reducing sepsis in prolonged clean neurosurgical procedures. Wright and Burke (1969) used UV only during actual surgical procedures, shielding the patient and staff with glasses and paper or cloth hoods. In their experience, the infection rate after craniotomies dropped from 5.3 to 0.7% and after laminectomies from 4.1 to 0.3%. Goldner et al. (1980) described a group of total hip arthroplasty operations carried out during 1974 and 1975 and found that UV significantly reduced airborne organisms. From 1969 to 1977 UV replaced routine use of antibiotics in 1322 total hip replacements. The wound infection rate was only 0.68% in refined clean cases. Lowell and Kundsin (1978) and Lowell et al. (1980) approved the use of UV in the operating room and concluded that with modest expense, risk, and inconvenience they improved the operating room environment and lowered the risks of surgery for their patients undergoing total joint replacement. Carlsson et al. (1986) believe that UV reduced the airborne organisms significantly in their study of total hip replacements. However, they suggest that "UV-irradiation alone in a conventionally ventilated operating room would probably not be sufficient to achieve ultra clean air." It is interesting to note that at present, even with these encouraging results,

there is no consensus regarding the use of UV light in the operating room.

Some investigators suggest that procedures of ventilation alone can reduce hospital sepsis rates. It has been suggested that ventilation removes many large as well as small airborne particles; UV acts primarily against bacteria in the small airborne particles, the microbial agents in the larger particles being shielded from irradiation. Some suspect that only large particles may contain enough organisms to initiate sepsis (Williams et al., 1966).

Infection is a major problem in dialysis treatment, and the dialyzing room should be as free of microbial agents as possible. Inamoto et al. (1979) suspended a 15-watt bare UV lamp from the ceiling and used it after working hours. Bacteria were killed even in the area of low UV intensity, possibly by reflected rays and ozone. Easy application and low cost would make this method more advantageous than other procedures used in room disinfection. Orange et al. (1985) indicate that UV can be used to sterilize the junction in equipment using a bag of dialysis fluid. This may be of considerable importance, inasmuch as peritonitis may occur because of contamination of the connector during bag changing. The authors suggest that "There are many other possible applications for a U.V. system in sterilizing extracorporeal fluid connections, especially for immunocompromised patients in whom infection of intravenous catheters is a serious problem."

The many hospital infections have been discussed extensively (Williams et al., 1966; APHA, 1970; Levenson et al., 1986). Nagasawa et al. (1970) described the use of UV in the operating rooms and other locations, as well as in procedures such as treatment of contaminated linen and bedmaking, in hospitals in Japan. Also, Greene (1970) pointed out in more general terms the use of UV in air and surface disinfection in American hospitals.

The first installation of UV barriers was employed to separate units that housed patients with different contagious diseases, or to separate wards that housed patients with contagious diseases from other wards in the hospital. It has been demonstrated that such barriers have been successful in reducing respiratory cross-infection in children's hospitals (Friederiszick, 1954; Laurell and Range, 1955). Barriers to microorganisms were created by curtains of UV light from tubes carefully arranged above open ends of cubicles so as not to harm the occupants. Of the several field trials, the one conducted at The Cradle from 1939 to 1946 showed that in the ward with UV curtains, the number of cross-infections per year was one-twentieth that of the control unit.

Reduction of bacterial contamination, as well as reduction in cross-infections, has also been reported when only the upper air of a ward was irradiated. Higgons and Hyde (1947), on the basis of the results of their 6-year study in an institution completely equipped with UV lamps, endorsed the expenditure necessary for their installation, and held the lights responsible for the prevention of spread of airborne infections. More recently, Botzenhart et al. (1976) concluded from their studies dealing with clinical uses of UV that, with the exception of the barrier technique, UV did not substantially reduce the number of microorganisms in the air. They suggested that it is important to establish the acceptable upper number of microorganisms in the air of hospital wards and operating theaters for evaluating the effectiveness of air disinfection by UV. Bagshawe et al. (1978), in presenting their design for construction of isolation wards, suggested the use of UV as a barrier at room doors. They also commented on the need for standards for establishing significant reduction of airborne microbes.

The potential value of irradiating air of a tuberculosis ward was demonstrated by Riley et al. (1962). None of the guinea pigs receiving irradiated air developed tuberculosis, whereas 63 infections occurred in guinea pigs subjected to untreated air from the ward. Burk et al. (1978) believe that maintenance of adequate ventilation systems and UV can minimize the frequency and intensity of future infant exposure to tuberculosis in nurseries. They suggest that the application of current knowledge of technology makes nosocomial neonatal tuberculosis a preventable disease. Riley (1977) suggested that there is epidemiologic evidence that the spread of influenza can be prevented in a hospital patient population that stays continuously in a building with upper-air irradiation throughout.

Air disinfection in corridors serves the dual purpose of protecting occupants of the corridor from airborne infection and of preventing transmission of airborne organisms from one part of the building to another. Corridor irradiation isolates rooms along the corridor from the rest of the building (Ayliffe et al., 1971). It may be desirable to have more reflected UV in corridors, because less time is usually spent in these areas than in the patients' rooms (Riley and Kaufman, 1971).

Experiments in Schools and Barracks

Although UV light will effectively reduce the number of airborne organisms, its usefulness as a measure for the control of infections in schools is equivocal. This is accentuated by the numerous out-of-school contacts, each contact acting as a potential biologic atomizer. Careful epidemiologic analysis presented by Wells (1955) and by the Air Hygiene Committee (Medical Research Council, 1954) should be studied in order to better evaluate the potential uses and limitations of UV irradiation of the air.

Another application of UV to reduce the incidence of infections of the upper respiratory tract has been to irradiate the upper, and occasionally also the lower, air of the sleeping quarters of a training school for boys and barracks of military personnel. In all field investigations, inhabitants of the irradiated environment had a certain degree of contact with individuals not living in treated quarters. This occurred in places such as dining halls, gymnasiums, recreation halls, and movie theaters.

Although it has been shown that practical intensities of UV light have a marked effect in lowering the bacterial contamination of the air equivalent to more than 100 air changes per hour, a need was indicated for a more thorough study of UV and of the factors that determine the occurrence and incidence of respiratory disease among the recruits (Miller et al., 1948; Langmuir et al., 1948).

UV in Laboratories for Infectious Diseases and in Other Locations

The potential health hazards in biologic research have been discussed in some detail by Hellman et al. (1973) and by Wedum and Barkley (1972). Over 2520 laboratory infections were attributed to nonviral agents by Lennette (1973), probably only a small fraction of the cases that have actually occurred (Wedum and Barkley, 1972). In tumor virus research, there are indications that laboratory accidents, procedures, or equipment have caused significant inoculation of personnel with research material, leading to detectable serologic conversion. Incorporation of microbiologic safety measures in the design of biomedical laboratories has been discussed by Phillips and Runkle (1967). These measures stress the importance of preventing the escape and possible spread of infectious agents. The use of UV is particularly important in establishing the so-called secondary barriers providing separation between infected areas in the building and the outside community and between the individual infectious areas. It has been suggested that UV be employed in personnel air locks and door barriers, equipment air locks and pass boxes, isolation cubicles, treatment of air from safety hoods, animal inoculation and autopsy cabinets, and shoe storage racks and clothing discard containers. Ceiling-mounted or wall-mounted UV lights are useful, as are the lights in the heating and ventilation systems. UV barriers have been used, together with certain special ventilating procedures, for separation of infectious animals from laboratory personnel and from other normal and infected animals. Direct UV irradiation of room air and room surfaces is useful in many situations in the laboratory, particularly because a common source of laboratory-acquired infection is the inhalation of accidentally or experimentally created microbial aerosols. A UV sterilizer has been designed and used successfully in eliminating high concentrations of vegetative cells and spores for small volumes of air. This instrument has been used to sterilize contaminated exhaust air obtained from experimental chambers housing forcibly aerated cultures or from chambers designed for study of bacterial aerosols (Miller et al., 1955).

The principles of air sanitation by UV also apply to places of public gathering, particularly in industry and in special situations such as physicians' waiting rooms, animal hospitals, kennels, dairy barns, stables, calf pens and maternity pens, the poultry business, and housing for small animals such as chinchilla, mink, and foxes.

ACTION OF UV ON MICROBIAL AGENTS SUSPENDED IN LIQUIDS

Purification of Water

Microorganisms withstand considerably more UV in water than in dry air. Commercially available sources of

UV at present offer limited but important application in industries practicing bacteriologic control that require or desire nonchlorinated water, as well as in areas where drinking water is or may be unsafe (Huff et al., 1965; Atlantic UV Corporation, 1972). Commercial UV units are available that allow flow-rates of water from 75 to 20,000 gallons per hour. Certain purification systems have been designed to deliver 253.7-nm energy in excess of 30,000 µW/sec/cm². These instruments are germicidal lamps enclosed in a quartz protection sleeve, allowing for higher lamp temperatures required for optimium output of UV. Although laboratory devices have been developed that may destroy 100% of water-borne bacteria under certain conditions, complete sterility is not necessary for production of potable water as long as water conforms with the Public Health Service Drinking Water Standards. When this is accomplished, the unique advantage of the UV treatment is that nothing is added to the water. UV water purification has been applied to water wells, cisterns, and swimming pools to avoid heavy chlorination, and where biologically pure water is desirable or required. Such situations include bacteria-free water for use in breweries, wineries, soft drink and water bottling facilities, and in the pharmaceutical, cosmetic, food, and electronic industries. The bactericidal treatment of liquids in general is defined by certain factors that control the amount of energy available to a suspended organism from a UV source, and by the resistance of water-borne microorganisms to the radiation. The degree of penetration of UV and the rate of flow of liquid through a particular purifying device are factors of primary importance. Transmission of UV through water is an inverse function of its mineral and organic content (Dohnalik, 1965). In practice, the variation of degree of absorption was shown to be due almost entirely to dissolved iron salts. In addition to these factors, the intensity of UV output of a lamp depends on the primary voltage, water temperatures, and burning hours of a lamp.

UV is a valuable tool for limited purification of water, particularly when used under special conditions. UV has been used successfullly to control microfouling communities responsible for slime formation on optical surfaces immersed in sea water (Di Solvo and Cobet, 1974). Box et al. (1982, 1984) believe that UV may be used to sterilize eye drops and other aqueous liquids. Herald et al. (1962) discussed the successful use of UV in treating closed and semiclosed aquarium systems. Huff et al. (1965) evaluated the use of a commercial UV disinfecting system for water designed primarily for shipboard use. *Escherichia coli*, the index organism of water pollution, has been tested in this system, as were *Aerobacter aerogenes* and a number of viruses. The viruses were inactivated, and over 99.9999% of the bacteria were killed, yielding good potable water. Other procedures have been used successfully aboard ships to treat drinking water with UV (Goethe et al., 1969; Mueller et al., 1970). Recently, Severin (1980) and Chang et al. (1985) stated

that UV is an effective and practical alternative to chlorine as a means of disinfecting municipal wastewater effluent. When UV-treated secondary effluent was given to trout, no adverse effects were observed, whereas chlorinated effluent produced fish kills. Myhrstad (1979) demonstrated that UV may be regarded as an alternative method to chlorination of sewage from an activated sludge process.

Hospital water distribution systems can be a source of nosocomial infections with *Legionella pneumophilia*. Comparative evaluation of different agents used with a hospital plumbing system (Muraca et al., 1987) suggested that UV may be a primary or supplemental method for disinfection. The Legionella Monitoring Committee (Helms et al., 1988) confirmed the efficacy of UV for disinfection of *L. pneumophilia* in water in the laboratory and cooling tower.

UV is valuable for treating sea water used in the shellfish industry, because chlorine has an adverse effect on feeding activity of oysters. The Kelly-Purdy UV generating unit (Kelly, 1961) effectively destroyed excessive numbers of coliform organisms, the three types of poliovirus, certain types of echoviruses, selected coxsackieviruses, and some reoviruses added to the tested water (Hill et al., 1969, 1970).

Purification of Liquids Other Than Water

The application of UV to liquids more absorptive, and possibly more viscous, than water resulted in the development of special equipment counteracting this condition by allowing adequate time for exposure of a moving thin film of liquid to the radiation (Buttolph et al., 1953). Even under these conditions, it has been difficult to produce commercially available instruments applicable to milk control, although it has been established that exposure to UV significantly lowers the visible count of thermophilic and thermoduric bacteria. These results suggest a possible use of UV radiation to supplement pasteurization. UV irradiation of products such as fruit juices, wine, and beer has not been achieved on a commercial scale, largely because of limitations imposed by the products, i.e., suspended solid particles or chemical instability. In clear water, over 50% of the radiation energy is lost at a depth of less than 5 cm, and in river water it may be lost within 1 cm. Irradiation of the dialysis fluid to prevent bacteremia during hemodialysis was found to be superior to the conventional filtration procedure (Tolon et al., 1977). Experimental use of UV lamps did not lead to flow rate and pressure problems encountered when conventional filtration was employed.

Preparation of Immunizing Antigens

Applications of UV to sterilization of bacterial and viral suspension for preparation of immunizing antigens was stimulated by the work of Hodes et al. (1940), who used a mercury resonance bulb to produce nonvirulent, but immunizing, rabies vaccine. Levinson and coworkers (1945) pioneered exposure of a continuously flowing thin film of fluid containing microbial agents for less than a second to a high-pressure mercury vapor lamp, having a large proportion of radiation of less than 200 nm. Many bacterial and viral suspensions were sterilized in this manner—*Salmonella enteritidis, Staphylococcus aureus, Streptomyces viridans, Diplococcus pneumoniae,* fixed rabies virus, virus of lymphocytic choriomeningitis, and St. Louis encephalitis virus. UV irradiation of viruses resulted in a higher degree of immunity in mice than was shown by phenolized preparations, and exhibited no loss of potency after 6 months at 5°C. Improvement in this procedure was made by exposing a thin film of antigenic material introduced by gravity or under pressure directly to a UV lamp emitting most radiation at 253.7 nm. In this manner, the immunizing property of rabies virus was not affected after exposure to five times the amount of radiation necessary to inactivate the virus (Habel and Sockrider, 1947). It was pointed out that the continuous flow technique could be adapted to commercial scale production. Purified rabies vaccine of suckling rat brain free from encephalitogenic activity was prepared after treatment with UV (Lavender, 1970). Application of UV radiation for production of antituberculosis vaccine from a highly virulent human strain, and comparison of this agent with the immunizing property and stability of BCG, resulted in controversial reports (Saber et al., 1950; Milzer et al., 1950; Seagle et al., 1953).

Exposure of a thin film of psittacosis (Francis et al., 1947), poliomyelitis (Milzer et al., 1945), St. Louis encephalitis, lymphocytic choriomeningitis, and vaccinia viruses, as well as of suspensions of certain bacteria and of toxins, to UV light showed the superiority of the resultant vaccines to those produced by heat or chemicals, in regard both to antigenicity and to keeping qualities of the product (Milzer and Levinson, 1949; Collier et al., 1955).

Although UV need not destroy the immunizing property of inactivated suspensions of microbial agents, as measured in animals by protection tests, the effect of radiation on reactivity of antigens must be kept in mind. Although UV-inactivated vaccinia virus produced neutralizing antibody and resistance to challenge in rabbits, it was active in only about half of human volunteers (Kaplan et al., 1962). That care should be used in application of UV for vaccine production can be surmised from reports by Kleczkowski (1962), Kleczkowski and Gold (1962), and Porter and Maurer (1962), which stated that exposure of human, horse, and bovine serum albumins, as well as of tobacco mosaic virus, to UV led to alteration or destruction of their antigenic properties, when measured in vitro.

Irradiation of Plasma

Lo Grippo and his associates have successfully sterilized human plasma by treating it with beta-propiolactone (BPL) and 253.7-nm UV light. In contrast to the 3 to 60% hepatitis attack rate of pooled plasma treated with UV alone, transfusion hepatitis did not develop in any of 581 patients receiving a total of 280 L of plasma sub-

jected to combined BPL-UV treatment. In all, 1410 transfusions were administered from 1956 to 1961 using 30 lots of plasma from 2065 donors (Lo Grippo et al., 1964a). No toxic or allergic reactions were encountered that could be attributed to the treated plasma. Of a number of procedures tried by the authors, the combined treatment just described proved to be the only one that was successful (Lo Grippo et al., 1964b). In addition, this procedure was used successfully in treatment of 268 homografts, 117 bone and 15 cartilage transplants, and 12 administrations of bovine platelet factor 3 (Lo Grippo, 1960). The procedure was monitored by adding *Escherichia coli* and T-3 bacteriophage. These agents were destroyed, as were the 19 animal viruses tested in plasma. Stephan (1971) reported that human serum exposed to 254-nm energy in a rotary flow apparatus was administered during 3 years to more than 200,000 patients without incidence of hepatitis. He also reported (Stephan, 1973) that cold sterilization using beta-propiolactone and subsequent UV irradiation of all human sera tested for hepatitis suppressed the risks to laboratory personnel using potentially infective reagents. The efficacy of this treatment has been demonstrated for HAV, HBV, NANBHV, and HIV (Stephan, 1989). This combined treatment does not interfere with purification procedures for the production of hepatitis B virus surface antigen or with the immunogenicity of this preparation (Stephan and May, 1976; Stephan et al., 1981). Kallenbach et al. (1989) believe that UV light may be used to disinfect human blood products and calf serum used in cell cultures, without loss of resulting material to support cell growth.

USE OF UV IN INDUSTRY AND IN SPECIAL SITUATIONS

Air is the important vehicle of microorganisms that may become responsible for deterioration and spoilage of many consumable products—bread, meat, beer, wine, soft drinks, dairy products, and others. Judicious applications of UV light can neutralize this possibility. Basic principles of protection by UV irradiation are those already discussed and include (1) reduction of airborne organisms in usually occupied locations, (2) irradiation of the product during processing, and (3) destruction of organisms that settle on surfaces and become part of the dust. Successful application of these principles that was claimed to raise the quality of apple cider and of wine (Avakian, 1971; Harrington et al., 1968) also reduced contamination of various other products, such as syrups and soft drinks, and reduced the growth of mold in equipment or on walls as well as on preserved products such as meat in cold storage. Special devices have been developed to expose surfaces of granular material such as sugar crystals to germicidal UV energy in order to destroy objectionable thermophilic contaminants causing trouble when the sugar is used in canning. A significant increase of the case life of beef was reported after exposure of muscle and fat surfaces to UV for 2 minutes (Reagan et al., 1973). Treatment with UV reduced by about 80% the bacterial count of spores in meat processing (Wolkowick et al., 1971).

Special UV lamps were used successfully to control microbial and insect population under different conditions. Thus, Riordan (1969) reduced the population of *Aeedes aegypti*, but warned that treatment with 253.7-nm energy should not be regarded as a practical alternative to irradiation or other means of sterile male technique of insect control. Species of *Trichophyton* and *Candida albicans* have been killed in shoes (Gemeinhardt, 1972). Thomson and Norn (1969) reported that an adequate degree of safety has been achieved by treating tonometer prisms with absolute alcohol and then irradiating the prisms with UV light.

Application of localized radiation over production lines is used by the pharmaceutical industry in sterile transfer rooms and hoods, in filling and capping rooms, in air-duct systems to provide sterile air to working areas, and in any locations or situations in which microbial contamination may be a problem. Although no claims are made for complete removal of microorganisms, it is indicated that better sanitation is brought about as a result of UV radiation. In addition, certain chemicals and plastics were sterilized by UV without producing untoward changes (Salalykin et al., 1963). Finally, one must not omit from this discussion the use of UV in many research procedures requiring the use of certain filter membranes, special plastic-coated instruments, and similar apparatuses that cannot be subjected to conventional microbial decontamination. A more complete discussion of application of UV in industry can be found in Philips' Gloeilampenfabriken (1985) and in the Sylvania bulletin (1983).

REFERENCES

Ad Hoc Committee of the Committee on Trauma, Division of Medical Sciences NAS-NRC. 1964. Post-operative wound infections: the influences of UV irradiation of the operating room and of various other factors. Ann. Surg. *160*, Supplement.

Akers, A.B., and Won W.D. 1969. Assay of living airborne microorganisms. In *An Introduction to Experimental Aerobiology.* Edited by R.L. Dimmick and Ann B. Akers. New York, Wiley-Interscience, pp. 55–99.

Altemeier, W.A. 1958. The problem of post-operative wound infections and its significance. Ann. Surg., *147*, 770–774.

American Public Health Association. 1970. *Infection Control in the Hospital.* Chicago, American Hospital Association.

Anderson, A.A. 1958. New sampler of collecting, sizing and enumeration of viable airborne particles. J. Bacteriol., *76*, 471–488.

Atlantic Ultraviolet Corporation, New York. 1972. Sanitation ultraviolet water purifiers. Pamphlet No. 200–201.

Avakian, B.B. 1971. Investigation of sterilizing doses of ultraviolet radiation and ultrasonic waves for the treatment of basic microflora in wine. Biol. Zh. Arm., *24*, 90–94.

Ayliffe, G.A.J., Collins, B.J., Lowbuty, E.J.L., and Wall, M. 1971. Protective isolation in single-bed rooms; studies in a modified hospital ward. J. Hyg., *69*, 511–527.

Bagshawe, K.K., Blowers, R., and Lidwell, O.M. 1978. Isolating patients in hospital to control infection. Part III—Design and construction of isolation accommodation. Br. Med. J., *6139*, 744–748.

Bayliss, C.E., and Waites, W.M. 1979. The combined effect of hydrogen peroxide and ultraviolet irradiation on bacterial spores. J. Appl. Bacteriol., *47*, 263–269.

Beukers, R., and Berends, W. 1960. Isolation and identification of the irradiation product of thymine. Biochim. Biophys. Acta, *41*, 550–551.

Botzenhart, K., Ruden, H., Tolon, M., and von K. Scharfenberg, M. 1976. Clinical uses of ultraviolet light radiation. Prakt. Anaesth., *76*, 320–327.

Boylen, R.J., Goldstein, G.R., and Schulman, A. 1987. Evaluation of ultraviolet disinfection unit. J. Prosthetic Dent., *58*, 650–654.

Box, J.A., Sugden, J.K., and Younis, N.M.T. 1982. The use of ultraviolet light to sterilize water. Pharm. Acta. Helv., *57*, 330–333.

Box, J.A., Sugden, J.K., and Younis, N.M.T. 1984. An examination of the sterilization of eye drops using ultraviolet light. J. Parent. Sci. Tech., *38*, 115–121.

Brewer, J.H., and Phillips, G.B. 1971. Environmental control in the pharmaceutical and biological industries. Crit. Rev. Environ. Control., *1*, 467–506.

Burk, J.R., et al. 1978. Nursery exposure of 528 newborns to a nurse with pulmonary tuberculosis. South Med. J., *71*, 7–10.

Buttolph, L.J., Haynes, H., and Matelsky, I. 1953. *Ultraviolet Product Sanitation.* Pamphlet LD–14. Cleveland, General Electric Co.

Carlsson, A.S., Nilsson, B., Walder, M.H., and Osterbertg, K. 1986. Ultraviolet radiation and air contamination during total hip replacement. J. Hosp. Infect., *7*:176–184.

Center for Disease Control, Health Services and Mental Health Administration, Atlanta, U.S. Department of Health, Education, and Welfare. 1971. Notes on air hygiene, summary of conference on air disinfection. Arch. Environ. Health, *23*, 473–474.

Chang, J.C.H., et al. 1985. UV inactivation of pathogenic and indicator microorganisms. Appl. Environ. Microbiol., *49*, 1361–1365.

Clarlone, A.E., and Fry, B.W. 1980. Decreased vasoconstrictor content in local anesthetic cartridges exposed to ultraviolet irradiation. J. Dent. Res., *59*, 724.

Collier, L.H., McClean, D., and Vallet, L. 1955. The antigenicity of ultraviolet irradiated vaccinia virus. J. Hyg., *53*, 513–534.

Di Solvo, L.H., and Cobet, A.B. 1974. Control of estuarine microfouling sequence on optical surfaces using low-intensity ultraviolet irradiation. Appl. Microbiol., *27*, 172–178.

Dohnalik, K. 1965. Efficiency of devices for the disinfection of water by ultraviolet radiation. Gaz. Voda. Tech. Sanit., *39*, 14–16.

DuBuy, H.G., et al. 1948. An evaluation of ultraviolet radiation of sleeping quarters as supplement of accepted methods of disease control. Am. J. Hyg., *48*, 207–226.

Dulbecco, R. 1955. Photoreactivation. In *Radiation Biology.* Volume II. Edited by A. Hollaender. New York, McGraw-Hill, pp. 455–486.

Francis, R.D., Milzer, A., and Gordon, F.B. 1947. Immunization of mice against viruses of the Psittacosis group with ultraviolet inactivated vaccines. Proc. Soc. Exp. Biol. Med., *66*, 184–186.

Friederiszick, F.K. 1954. New experiences with ultraviolet air disinfection in a children's hospital. Strahlentherapie, *95*, 491–495.

Gates, F.L. 1928. On nuclear derivatives and the lethal action of ultraviolet light. Science, *68*, 479–480.

Gaulin, R.P. 1957. Air conditioning the hospitals. Hospitals, *31*, 43–74.

Gemeinhardt, H. 1972. The question of killing foot fungi in shoes with ultraviolet rays. Z. Gesamte Hyg., *18*, 9–14.

Giese, A.C. 1973. *Cell Physiology.* Philadelphia, W.B. Saunders, pp. 228–231.

Giese, A.C. 1968. Ultraviolet action spectra in perspective: with special reference to mutation. Photochem. Photobiol., *8*, 527–546.

Giese, A.C. 1950. Action of ultraviolet radiations on protoplasm. Physiol. Rev., *30*, 431–458.

Goethe, H., Zorn, E., and Mueller, G. 1969. Hygienic problems of drinking water supply aboard marine vessels with special regard for vacuum evaporations and for water sterilization by ultraviolet rays. Staedtehygiene, *20*, 1–3.

Goldner, J.L., et al. 1980. Ultraviolet light for control of airborne bacteria in the operating room. In *Airborne Contagion.* Edited by R.B. Kundsin. Ann. N.Y. Acad. Sci., *353*, 27.

Gordon, M.P., Huang, C., and Hurter, J. 1976. Photochemistry and photobiology of ribonucleic acids, ribonucleoproteins, and RNA viruses. In *Photochemistry and Photobiology of Nucleic Acids.* Volume II. Edited by S.Y. Wang. New York, Academic Press, pp. 265–309.

Greene, V.W. 1970. Disinfection and sterilization practices in American hospitals. In *Disinfection.* Edited by M.A. Bernarde. New York, Marcel Dekker, pp. 702–756.

Greenlee, R.G., Terrill, R.J., and Sloan, J.W. 1951. Homologous serum hepatitis after transfusions of blood and ultraviolet irradiation plasma. Tex. State J. Med., *47*, 831–835.

Habel, K., and Sockrider, B.T. 1947. A continuous flow method of exposing antigens to ultraviolet radiation. J. Immunol., *56*, 273–279.

Hader, D.P., and Tevini, M. 1987. *General Photobiology.* New York, Pergamon Press.

Harm, W. 1980. *Biological Effects of Ultraviolet Radiation.* New York, Cambridge University Press.

Harm, W. 1976. Repair of UV-irradiated biological systems: Photoreactivation. In *Photochemistry and Photobiology of Nucleic Acids.* Volume II. Edited by S.Y. Wang. New York, Academic Press, pp. 219–263.

Harm, W., Rupert, C.S., and Harm, H. 1971. The study of photoenzymatic repair of ultraviolet lesions in DNA by flash photolysis. In *Photophysiology.* Volume VI. Edited by A.C. Giese. New York, Academic Press, pp. 279–324.

Harrington, W.O., and Hills, C.H. 1968. Reduction of the microbial population of apple cider by ultraviolet irradiation. Food Technol., *22,* 117–120.

Hart, D. 1960. Bactericidal ultraviolet radiation in the operating room. Twenty-nine-year study of control of infection. JAMA, *172,* 1019–1027.

Hart, D. 1938. Sterilization of the air in the operating room with bacterial radiation. J. Thorac. Surg., *7,* 525–535.

Haynes, R.H. 1964. Microbial inactivation and recovery. Photochem. Photobiol., *3,* 429–450.

Hellman, A., Oxman, M.N., and Pollack, R. (eds.) 1973. *Biohazards in Biological Research.* New York, Cold Spring Harbor Laboratory.

Helms, C.M., et al. 1988. Legionella Monitoring Committee. Legionaire's disease associated with hospital water system. JAMA, *259,* 2423–2428.

Herald, E.S., Dempster, R.P., Walters, C., and Hunt, M.L. 1962. Filtration and ultraviolet sterilization of sea water in large, closed and semi-closed aquarium system. Bull. Inst. Oceanog. Monaco Spec., *13,* 49–61.

Higgons, R.A., and Hyde, G.M. 1947. Effect of ultraviolet air sterilization upon incidence of respiratory infections in a children's institution. A six-year study. N.Y. State J. Med., *47,* 707–710.

Hill, W.F., Jr., Hamblet, F.E., and Benton, W.H. 1969. Inactivation of poliovirus type I by the Kelly-Purdy ultraviolet seawater treatment unit. Appl Microbiol., *17,* 1–16.

Hill, W.F., Jr., Hamblet, F.E., Benton, W.H., and Akin, E.W. 1970. Ultraviolet devitalization of eight selected enteric viruses in estuarine water. Appl. Microbiol., *19,* 805–812.

Hodes, M.L., Webster, L.T., and Lavin, G.I. 1940. The use of ultraviolet light in preparing a non-virulent antirabies vaccine. J. Exp. Med., *72,* 437–444.

Hosler, W.W. 1951. Germicidal ultraviolet tubes kept Strong-Cobb packing pure. Elec. Prod. Mag., *24,* 115.

Huber, T.W., Reddick, R.A., and Kubica, G.P. 1970. Germicidal effect of ultraviolet irradiation on paper contaminated with mycobacteria. Appl. Microbiol., *19,* 383–384.

Huff, C.B., Smith, M.F., Boring, W.D., and Clarke, N.A. 1965. Study of ultraviolet disinfection of water and factors in treatment efficiency. Public Health Rep., *80,* 695–705.

Inamoto, H., et al. 1979. Dialyzing room disinfection with ultraviolet irradiation. J. Dial., *3,* 191–205.

Jaggar, A. 1961. A small and inexpensive ultraviolet dose-rate meter useful in biological experiments. Radiol. Res., *14,* 394–403.

James, G., Korns, R.F., and Wright, A.W. 1950. Homologous serum jaundice associated with use of irradiated plasma. JAMA, *114,* 228–229.

Jensen, M.M. 1964. Inactivation of airborne viruses by ultraviolet irradiation. Appl. Microbiol., *12,* 418–420.

Kallenbach, N.R., et al. 1989. Inactivation of viruses by ultraviolet light. In *Virus Inactivation in Plasma Products.* Curr. Stud. Hematol. Blood Transfus. Morgenthaler, J.J. (Ed.) Basel, Karger, No. 56, pp. 70–82.

Kaplan, C., McClean, D., and Vallet, L. 1962. A note on the immunogenicity of ultraviolet irradiated vaccinia virus in man. J. Hyg., *60,* 79–83.

Kaufman J.E. (Ed.) 1987. Nonvisual effects of radiant energy. In *IES Lighting Handbook.* Application Volume. New York, Illuminating Engineering Society, pp. 1–20.

Kelly, C.B. 1961. Disinfection of sea water by ultraviolet radiation. Am. J. Public Health, *51,* 1670–1680.

Kelner, A. 1949. Effect of visible light on the recovery of *Streptomyces griseus* conidia from ultraviolet irradiation injury. Proc. Natl. Acad. Sci., *35,* 73–79.

Kethley, T.W., and Branch, K. 1972. Ultraviolet lamps for room air disinfection: Effect of sampling location and particle size of bacterial aerosol. Arch. Environ. Health, *25,* 205–214.

Kleczkowski, A. 1962. Destruction of antigenicity in vitro of human serum albumin and of tobacco mosaic virus by UV radiation. Photochem. Photobiol., *1,* 291–297.

Kleczkowski, A., and Gold, A.H. 1962. Effects of ultraviolet radiation on antigenicity of horse serum albumin: formation of new determinants. Photochem. Photobiol., *1,* 299–304.

Koontz, A. 1958. The operating room as a source of wound infections. Am. Surg., *34,* 358–361.

Langmuir, A.D., Jarrett, E.T., and Hollaender, A. 1948. Studies of the control of acute respiratory diseases among naval recruits; the epidemiological pattern and the effect of ultraviolet irradiation during the winter of 1946–1947. Am. J. Hyg., *48,* 240–251.

Laurell, G., and Range, H. 1955. Ultraviolet air disinfection in children's hospital. Acta Paediatr., *44,* 407–425.

Lavender, J.F. 1970. Purified rabies vaccine (suckling rat brain origin). Appl. Microbiol., *19,* 923–927.

Lennette, E. 1973. Potential hazards posed by nonviral agents. In *Biohazards in Biological Research.* Edited by A. Hellman, M.M. Oxman, and R. Pollock. New York, Cold Spring Harbor Laboratory, pp. 47–63.

Levenson, S.M., Trexler, P.C., and ven der Waaij, D. 1986. Nosocomial infection: prevention by special clean-air, ultraviolet light, and barrier (isolator) techniques. Curr. Probl. Surg., *23,* 452–558.

Levinson, S.O., et al. 1945. A new method for the production of potent inactivated vaccines with ultraviolet irradiation. II. Sterilization of bacteria and immunization with rabies and St. Louis encephalitis virus. J. Immunol., *50,* 317–329.

Lewis, W.R., and Burke, J.F. 1969. Effect of ultraviolet radiation on post-operative neurosurgical sepsis. J. Neurosurg., *31,* 533–537.

Lo Grippo, G.A. 1960. Investigation of use of beta-propiolactone in virus inactivation. Ann. N.Y. Acad. Sci., *83,* 578–594.

Lo Grippo, G.A., Wolfram, B.R., and Rupe, C.E. 1964a. Human plasma treated with ultraviolet and propiolactone. Six-year clinical evaluation. JAMA, *1987,* 722–726.

Lo Grippo, G.A., Wolfram, B.R., and Brock, E.B. 1964b. Propiolactone plus ultraviolet-treated plasma without hepatitis. Arch. Surg., *88,* 721–724.

Lowell, J.D., and Kundsin, R.B. 1978. The operating room and the ultraviolet environment. Med. Instrum., *12,* 161–164.

Lowell, J.D., Kundsin, R.B., and Schwatz, C.M. 1980. Ultraviolet light and reduction of deep wound infection following hip and knee arthroplasty. In *Airborne Contagion.* Edited by R.B. Kundsin. Ann. N.Y. Acad. Sci., *353,* 285.

McLaren, A.D., and Shugar, D. 1964. *Photochemistry of Proteins and Nucleic Acids.* New York, Macmillan.

Miller, O.T., Schmitt, R.F., and Phillips, G.B. 1955. Application of germicidal ultraviolet in infectious disease laboratories. I. Sterilization of volumes of air by ultraviolet irradiation. Am. J. Public Health, *45,* 1420–1423.

Miller, W.R. 1948. Evaluation of ultraviolet radiation and dust control measures in control of respiratory disease at a naval training center. J. Infect. Dis., *82,* 86–100.

Milzer, A., and Levinson, S.O. 1949. Active immunization of mice with ultraviolet inactivated lymphocytic choriomeningitis virus vaccine and results of immune serum therapy. J. Infect. Dis., *85,* 251–255.

Milzer, A., Levinson, S.O., and Lewis, M.D. 1950. Immunization of mice with ultraviolet killed tuberculosis vaccines. Proc. Soc. Exp. Biol. Med., *75,* 733–736.

Milzer, A., Oppenheimer, F., and Levinson, S.L. 1945. A new method for the production of potent inactivated vaccines with ultraviolet irradiation. III. A completely inactivated poliomyelitis vaccine with Lansing strain in mice. J. Immunol., *50,* 331–340.

Morris, E.J. 1972. The practical use of ultraviolet radiation for disinfection processes. Med. Lab. Technol., *29,* 41–47.

Morse, M.L., and Carter, C.E. 1949. The effects of ultraviolet irradiation on the synthesis of nucleic acid by E. coli. Bacteriol. Proc., *49,* 14.

Mpelkas, C.C. 1983. Germicidal and short-wave ultraviolet radiation. Engineering Bull. 0-342. Sylvania Lighting Center, Danvers.

Mueller, G., Goethe, H., and Herrmann, R. 1970. Bacteriological examinations for disinfecting drinking water of ships by means of ultraviolet irradiation. Zentralbl. Bakteriol. Mikrobiol. Hyg. (A), *215,* 555–562.

Muraca, P., Stout, J.E., and Yu, V.L. 1987. Killing of *Legionella pneumophilia* within a model plumbing system. Appl. Environ. Microbiol., *53,* 447–453.

Myhrstad, J.A. 1979. Disinfection of sewage by ultraviolet irradiation. NIPH Ann., *2,* 11–16.

Nagasawa, S., Tsuchiya, T., and Nishimura, H. 1970. Hospital infection. In *Disinfection.* Edited by M.A. Benarde. New York, Marcel Dekker, pp. 257–290.

National Academy of Sciences–National Research Council. Report on an Ad Hoc Committee. 1964. Post-operative wound infection: The influence of ultraviolet irradiation of the operating rooms and various other factors. Ann. Surg., *160*(Suppl.), 1–192.

Organe, G.V., Henderson, I.S., and Leung, A.C.T. 1985. Ultraviolet light as a sterilizing agent for extracorporeal fluid tubing connections. Intern. J. Artif. Org., *8,* 125–129.

Overholdt, R.H., and Betts, R.H. 1940. Comparative report on infection of thoracoplasty wounds: experiences with ultraviolet irradiation of operating room air. J. Thorac. Surg., *9,* 520–529.

Patrick, M.H., and Rahn, R.O. 1976. Photochemistry of DNA and polynucleotides: Photoproducts. In *Photochemistry and Photobiology of Nucleic Acids.* Volume II. Edited by S.Y. Wang. New York, Academic Press, pp. 35–95.

Philips' Gloeilampenfabriken. 1985. *Germicidal Lamps and Applications.* N.V. Eindhoven, the Netherlands.

Phillips, G.B., and Novak, F.E. 1956. Application of germicidal ultraviolet in infectious disease laboratories. II. An ultraviolet pass-through chamber for disinfecting single sheets of paper. Appl. Microbiol., *4,* 95–96.

Phillips, G.B., and Runkle, R.S. 1967. Laboratory design for microbiological safety. Appl. Microbiol., *15,* 378–389.

Porter, D.D., and Maurere, P.H. 1962. Modified bovine serum albumin. IX. The effect of ultraviolet irradiation on the immunological properties. Photochem. Photobiol., *1,* 91–96.

Qualls, R.G., and Johnson, J.O. 1983. Bioassay and dose measurement in UV disinfection. Appl. Environ. Microbiol., *45,* 872–877.

Rahn, R.A. 1973. Denaturation in ultraviolet-irradiated DNA. In *Photophysiology.* Volume VIII. Edited by A.C. Giese. New York, Academic Press.

Reagan, J.O., Smith, G.C., and Carpenter, Z.C.C. 1973. Use of ultraviolet light for extending the case life of beef. J. Food Sci., *38*, 929–931.

Reid, D.D., Lidwell, W.C., and Williams, R.E.O. 1956. Counts of air-borne bacteria as indices of air hygiene. J. Hyg., *54*, 524–528.

Riley, R.L. 1977. Ultraviolet air disinfection for protection against influenza. Johns Hopkins Med. J., *140*, 25–27.

Riley, R.L. 1974. Airborne infection. Am. J. Med., *57*, 466.

Riley, R.L., and Kaufman, J.E. 1972. Effect of relative humidity on the inactivation of *Serratia marcescens* by ultraviolet radiation. Appl. Microbiol., *23*, 1113–1120.

Riley, R.L., and Kaufman, J.E. 1971. Air disinfection in corridors by upper air irradiation with ultraviolet light. Arch. Environ. Health, *22*, 551–553.

Riley, R.L., Knight, M., and Middlebrook, G. 1976. Ultraviolet susceptibility of BCG and virulent tubercle bacilli. Am. Rev. Respir. Dis., *113*, 413–418.

Riley, R.L., Permutt, S., and Kaufman, J.E. 1971a. Convection, air mixing and ultraviolet air disinfection in rooms. Arch. Environ. Health, *22*, 200–207.

Riley, R.L., Permutt, S., and Kaufman, J.E. 1971b. Room air disinfection by ultraviolet irradiation of upper air: further analysis of convective air exchange. Arch. Environ. Health, *23*, 35–39.

Riley, R.L., et al. 1962. Infectiousness of air from a tuberculosis ward. Ultraviolet irradiation of infected air: comparative infectiousness of different patients. Am. Rev. Respir. Dis., *85*, 511–525.

Riordan, D.F. 1969. Effects of ultraviolet radiation on adults of *A. aegypti.* Mosq. News, *29*, 427–431.

Salalykin, V.I., Lebedeva, S.A., and Ostromogolskii, D.T. 1963. Sterilization of urea by means of ultraviolet rays. Vopr. Neirokhir., *1*, 10–11.

Sarber, R.W., Nungester, W.J., and Stimpert, F.D. 1950. Immunization studies with irradiated tuberculosis vaccines. Am. Rev. Tuberc., *62*, 418–427.

Seagle, J.B., Karlson, A.G., and Feldman, W.H. 1953. Irradiated antituberculosis vaccine, including comparison with BCG in experimentally infected guinea pigs. Am. Rev. Tuberc., *67*, 341–353.

Setlow, R.B., and Carrier, W.L. 1966. Pyrimidine dimers in ultraviolet-irradiated DNAs. J. Mol. Biol., *17*, 37–254.

Severin, B.F. 1980. Disinfection of municipal wastewater effluents with ultraviolet light. J. Water Pollut. Control, *52*, 2007–2018.

Sherman, S.E. 1974. Evaluation of an improved ultraviolet tonometer sterilizer. Am. J. Ophthalmol., *78*, 329–330.

Smith, K.C. 1976. The radiation-induced additions of proteins and other molecules to nucleic acids. In *Photochemistry and Photobiology of Nucleic Acids.* Volume II. Edited by S.Y. Wang. New York, Academic Press, pp. 187–218.

Smith, L.R., Garrett, C.M., and Woodhall, E.C. 1964. Improved ultraviolet irradiation: further studies in the control of infection in the operating room. J. Int. Coll. Surg., *42*, 38–43.

Spector, W.S. (ed.) 1956. *Handbook of Biological Data.* Philadelphia, W.B. Saunders, p. 474.

Stamps, J.T., and Muth, E.R. 1978. Reducing accidents and injuries in the dental environment. Dent. Clin. North Am., *22*, 389–402.

Stephan, W. 1973. Hepatitis-free reagents in tests for Australia antigen. Vox Sang., *24*(Suppl.), 78–79.

Stephan, W. 1971. Hepatitis-free and stable human serum for intravenous therapy. Vox Sang., *20*, 442–457.

Stephan, W., and May, G. 1976. Sterilized hepatitis B (surface) antigen for production of specific antisera. Vox Sang., *31*, 416–422.

Stephan, W., Berthold, H., and Prince, A.M. 1981. Effect of combined treatment of serum containing hepatitis B virus with beta-propiolactone and UV irradiation. Vox Sang., *41*, 134–138.

Stephan, W. 1989. Inactivation of hepatitis viruses and HIV in plasma and plasma derivatives by treatment with B-propiolactone/UV irradiation. In *Virus Inactivation in Plasma Products.* Curr. Stud. Hematol. Blood Transf. No. 56. Moreen Thaler J.J. (Ed). P122–127.

Sylvania. 1983. *Germicidal and Shortwave Ultraviolet Radiation.* Engineering Bulletin O-342.

Thomson, V.F., and Norn, M.S. 1969. Disinfection of Goldman's applanation tonometer prisms by means of ultraviolet light. Acta Ophthalmol., *47*, 1207–1218.

Tolon, M., Botzenhart, K., Wilbrandt, R., and Alsleben, J. 1977. Filtration and irradiation of the dialysis fluid to prevent bacteremia during hemodialysis. Med. Klin., *72*, 1451–1454.

Wang, S.Y. (ed.) 1976. *Photochemistry and Photobiology of Nucleic Acids.* Volume II. New York, Academic Press.

Wedum, A.G., and Barkley, W.E. 1972. Handling infectious agents. JAVMA, *161*, 1557–1567.

Wells, W.F. 1955. *Airborne Contagion and Air Hygiene.* Cambridge, Harvard.

Wells, W.F., Wells, M.W., and Wilder, T.S. 1942. The environmental control of epidemic contagion: I. An epidemiologic study of radiant disinfection of air in day schools. Am. J. Hyg., *35*, 97–121.

Widmer, W. 1951. Three new twists with ray lamps. Food Ind., *23*, 144.

Williams, R.E.O., Blowers, R., Garrod, L.P., and Shooter, R.A. 1966. *Hospital Infection.* London, Lloyd-Luke, pp. 197–230.

Witkin, E.M. 1946. Inherited differences in sensitivity to radiation in *Escherichia coli.* Proc. Natl. Acad. Sci., *32*, 59–68.

Wolff, S. 1972. Chromosome aberrations induced by ultraviolet radiation. In *Photophysiology.* Volume VII. Edited by A.C. Giese. New York, Academic Press, pp. 189–205.

Wolkowiak, E., Aleksandrovska, I., Witky, A., and Watyochowicz, I. 1971. Studies on sterilization in spices in meat processing by means of ultraviolet radiation. Med. Weter, *27*, 694.

Wright, R.L., and Burke, J. 1969. Effect of UV radiation on postoperative neurosurgical sepsis. J. Neurosurg., *31*, 533–537.

Wulf, H.C. 1980. Work in ultraviolet radiation. Contact Dermatitis, *6*, 72–76.

CHAPTER 32

STERILIZATION AND PRESERVATION BY IONIZING IRRADIATION

G.J. Silverman

The use of radiation for commercial applications requires a multidisciplinary approach. Playing an integral role in this effort is the microbiologist who is responsible for determining the inherent radiation resistance of microorganisms, and also for investigating the influences of a variety of environmental and physical factors on radiation resistance.

The two main commercial applications of ionizing radiation are for the preservation of foods and for the sterilization of medical products. The commercial applications of ionizing radiation for the preservation of foods has experienced only limited success in the past decade. The main deterrents to more widespread utilization has been the presence of radiation off-flavors and the requirement for sufficient toxicologic testing. In 1989, 36 countries, including the United States (Federal Register, 1981), have approved the marketing of a wide variety of irradiated foods (Council for Agricultural Science and Technology, 1989; Loaharanu, 1989).

In contrast, the use of radiation to sterilize medical products is widespread, and its applicability is increasing because it has proven to be an economic and reliable sterilizing agent (Masefield et al., 1978).

The primary intent of this section is to impart a sense of the applicability and the limitations in the use of ionizing radiation as a lethal agent against microorganisms. This chapter does not attempt to deal with the subject of technologic aspects of irradiation facilities (Gaughran and Goudie, 1978; Takehisa and Machi, 1987).

DESCRIPTION OF RADIATION ENERGY

In general, radiation may be classified into two groups: (1) electromagnetic and (2) particle radiation. The various types of ionizing radiation in the electromagnetic spectrum produce bactericidal effects by transferring the energy of a photon into characteristic ionizations in or near a biologic target. In addition to creating pairs of positive and negative electrons, ions can also produce free radicals and activated molecules. These effects, which are produced without any appreciable rise in temperature, have been termed "cold sterilization" when applied to the destruction of microorganisms.

Electromagnetic Radiation

Of the types of irradiation suggested or used for the destruction of microorganisms, microwave, ultraviolet, gamma (γ), x rays, and electrons, only the latter three will be dealt with in this chapter. Inactivation by ultraviolet radiations is discussed in Chapter 31. The question of whether the lethal action of microwave energy is due to a thermal effect is unresolved at present, although studies have indicated a possibility that electromagnetic and other nonthermal mechanisms may be operative (Chipley, 1980). X-radiation and gamma radiation, although identical in nature, have different origins. The emission of an x ray from an atom occurs when there is a transition of an electron from an outer shell to a vacancy further within an inner shell and is produced by bombarding a heavy metal target with fast electrons in a manmade accelerator. Gamma radiation is the result of a transition of an atomic nucleus from an excited state to a ground state, as in certain radioactive materials. The electromagnetic radiation differs only in frequency over a wavelength of 0.0001 to 10 Å. X rays and gamma rays have considerable penetrating power; intensity will generally be in accordance with the equation:

$$\frac{I}{I_0} = e^{-\mu_1 x}$$

where I/I_0 is the ratio of intensity, and μ_1 is the linear absorption coefficient, which depends upon the composition of the material and the wavelength of energy in passage through a sample of thickness x. It is usual to characterize the penetrating power of these rays by the half-thickness value based upon this equation or by the use of the mass absorption coefficient μm; $\mu m = \mu_1/\rho$, where ρ is the density.

The relationship between a quantum of energy of photon E, its wavelength λ, and its frequency v is:

$$E = hv = \frac{hc}{\lambda}$$

where c is the speed of light and h is Planck's constant. It follows that the higher the frequency, the more energy there is per quantum of radiation. Gamma rays emitted by ^{60}Co, to date the main isotopic source of radiation used for microbiologic inactivation studies, emit photons mainly at 1.17 and 1.33 MeV (million electron volts) and have a half-life of 5.2 years. ^{137}Ce emits photons at 0.661 MeV and has a half-life of 33 years. X rays can be produced over an extremely wide range of wavelengths. Soft x rays have wavelengths of approximately 0.1 Å; hard x rays have shorter wavelengths and are more penetrating.

Particle Radiation

The particles usually considered of importance in radiation biology are the α, β, neutron, meson, positron, and neutrino. The only particle that currently is applicable to sterilization is the β particle or electron. Alpha particles, although capable of causing dense ionizations, have limited penetrating ability; neutrons, which are uncharged, have great penetrating power into matter but are unacceptable because they induce radioactivity. Mesons and protons are produced only by expensive, high-energy machines.

Beta radiation, arising from radioactive disintegrations, consists of electrons with a single negative charge and a low mass. Beta radiation from an isotopic source cannot penetrate materials deeply, but electrons (cathode rays) produced in manmade machines can be accelerated to high energies with a subsequent improvement in penetrating ability. The penetration of electrons into matter is expressed by the Feather equation:

$$R_{max} = \frac{0.542E - 0.133}{\rho}$$

where R_{max} is the maximum range (g/cm³) for cathode rays in matter of density ρ, and E is the voltage (MeV) by which the electrons have been accelerated. The penetrating abilities of the various radiations are compared in Table 32–1 (Hannan and Thornley, 1957).

Radiation Units

The roentgen (r) is the unit of radiation dose of exposure. It can be related to the absorbed dose, the rad, or to the newly introduced SI unit, the gray (Gy), by appropriate factors (Table 32–2).

Linear Energy Transfer (LET)

The characteristic property of high-energy radiation is to cause ionization in the material in which the radiation is absorbed. In addition to ions, many molecules are also

Table 32–1. *Useful Penetrations Achieved with Different Ionizing Radiations Using Typical Irradiation Sources*

		Useful Penetration (cm)	
		Irradiating from One Side	*Irradiating from Both Sides*
γ rays	Co⁶⁰	10.2	40.6
X-rays	50 KeV	<0.1	~0.5
	10 MeV	12.7	61.0
Cathode rays	1 MeV	~0.3	~0.8
	5 MeV	1.8	4.3
	10 MeV	3.8	8.6
β rays	Sr⁹⁰	<0.1	~0.3

*The dose received at any one point will exceed 60% of that at points of maximum intensity.

From Hannan, R.S., and Thornley, M.J. 1957. Radiation processing of foods. Food Mfg., Oct.–Dec., 1.

converted to free radicals and excited molecules. Neither x-radiation nor gamma radiation, being uncharged, causes ionization directly. Electrons lose energy by inelastic scattering (at low energy) and by bremsstrahlung (at high energies). It is the interaction of the irradiation energy with matter that alters irradiation material. These interactions of energy with material are represented schematically in Figure 32–1.

At any given time, all portions of a material are not equally subjected to the energy of ionizing radiations. Ionizing radiations are by nature discrete, and in passage through a material, the photons or electrons produce a number of localized events along their passage or "track." Certain portions may not experience any alteration while an adjacent area is being subjected to intense energy. Along a track, photons of energy ionize the material and also produce free radicals and excited atoms. Secondary electrons, if they possess sufficient energy, ionize or excite an additional number of adjacent atoms, forming a spur of delta rays. The sequence of events along a track is therefore localized and intense, and the alterations in those molecules affected are severe, because many chemical bonds are altered by less than 100 eV. These reactions are also rapid. Obviously, the presence of a spur widens the effective range of the photon track.

The distance between primary ionization events that occur along the track depends on the photon energy and

Table 32–2. *Units and Conversion Factors in Radiation Chemistry*

1 roentgen (r) =	2.58 × 10⁻⁴ coulombs/kg (standard conditions)
1 rad =	100 erg/g
=	10⁻² joules/kg
=	6.29 × 10¹³ eV/g
=	2.4 × 10⁻⁶ cal/g
1 gray (Gy) =	100 rad
1 Megarad (Mrad) =	10⁶ rad
G value =	molecules of a product/100 eV absorbed

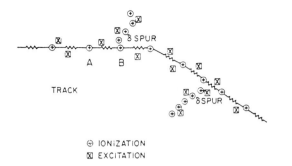

Fig. 32–1. Photon energy interaction with matter and a diagrammatic depiction of events along an ionizing track.

the absorbing material. A method of expressing this is by Linear Energy Transfer (LET), which is usually expressed as eV/Å or KeV/μ. The ionizations and excitations will have values ranging from zero to a maximum value, and in practice, either an average value is employed or the distribution is described. The LET increases with the square of the charge on the particle and decreases as its speed increases. For example, ^{60}Co γ rays have a mean LET of 0.42 in water; 200 KeV x-rays, 2.8; and x-rays from polonium, 150 (Swallow, 1977). The distance A to B of Figure 32–1 will be much greater for γ rays than for α particles.

Radiolysis Reactions

Upon being exposed to radiation energy, water and organic molecules are altered. Water is ionized and a hydrated electron (e_{aq}^-) is produced along or adjacent to the radiation track:

$$H_2O \leadsto H_2O^+ + e_{aq}^-$$

There are a number of theories as to the fate of the electron in further reactions (Vereshchinskii and Piakaev, 1964; Swallow, 1977; Chatterjee, 1987). Ignoring detailed mechanisms, the overall reactions for the positive water ion and the electron, and dependence upon the reaction conditions, the species produced are:

$$H_2O \leadsto H, e_{aq}^-, OH, H_3O^+, H_2O, H_2, H_2O_2,$$
$$OH^-, HO_2, O_2, O_2^-, HO_2^-.$$

(Magee and Chatterjee, 1987). The free radicals produced in the more densely ionized portion of the track will recombine, whereas in other portions of the track, where diffusion occurs, these radicals will react with solute. Therefore, the extent of the interactions between the solute and those produced by radiolysis depends upon concentration.

In the presence of oxygen, significant quantities of the hydroperoxyl radical ·HO$_2$ are formed which, in turn, produces H$_2$O$_2$:

$$2 \cdot HO_2 \rightarrow H_2O_2 + O_2$$

The longevity of the H$_2$O$_2$ molecule can be appreciable. Oxygen can also be formed by other reactions involving

the OH radical and H$_2$O$_2$. Hydrogen peroxide and the hydroperoxyl radical may act as oxidizing or reducing agents. In acid media, the HO$_2$ radical is undissociated and is a strong oxidant and a weak reducing agent, whereas the O$_2$ ion obtained from the dissociation of the HO$_2$ radical can act as a reducing agent.

These species, i.e., OH·, e_{aq}^-, and H·, etc., are capable of degrading and altering a variety of organic materials and biochemicals. These interactions are beyond the scope of this chapter and are reviewed in other sources (Swallow, 1977; Taub et al., 1979; Gaughran and Goudie, 1978; Mee, 1987).

LETHAL EFFECTS OF IRRADIATION ON MICROORGANISMS

Intracellular Effects

Lesions caused by the direct action of ionizing irradiation on a target molecule are the result of energy being transferred within the target molecule itself, in contrast to indirect action resulting from the diffusion of radicals produced in the adjacent volume (Lea, 1956). Indirect effects, in a sense, are still within an organism, but inactivate the organism by diffusion to, and by reacting with, a sensitive target site. The diffusion distance can be of the order of 40 Å, although larger values have been reported. This should not be confused with another type of effect—an environmental effect caused by radicals and other radiation-produced compounds formed extracellularly and that still can be lethal to a cell. Some of these compounds, hydrogen and organic peroxides and radicals, have appreciable longevity in menstruums and can be demonstrated as postirradiation effects.

Ionizing radiations can cause a wide variety of physical and biochemical effects in microorganisms. It is most likely, however, that the primary cellular target that governs the loss of viability is the DNA molecule of the cell (Ginoza, 1967). Sparrow et al. (1967) correlated the radiosensitivity of 79 organisms ranging from viruses to higher plants and animals with their chromosome volume. The larger the volume, the more sensitive the biologic unit was to ionizing radiation. It also appears that appreciable differences in radiosensitivity may be the result of an ability to repair DNA damage rather than an inherent radiation resistance of the DNA target (Davies and Sinskey, 1973; Davies et al., 1973; Town et al., 1971; Matsuyama, 1973).

In this presentation, microbial survival is defined as an ability of a microorganism to be able to either reproduce significantly in broth or to form a macrocolony on a nutrient agar, after being exposed to radiation.

Environmental Effects

One may consider those lethal effects that originate in the menstruum as a type of indirect effect. The influence of the menstruum can be altered by (1) using dried preparations in order to restrict the moisture content only to that closely associated with the cell; (2) freezing the menstruum and cells to minimize the migration of free radicals; (3) varying the LET and consequently radicals and molecular products produced by radiation; (4) varying the temperature during irradiation; and (5) varying the concentration of a solute or organic material under consideration. Although most of the lethal damage to a cell is considered to occur as a result of direct action, the radiation sensitivity that a microbial population displays can be altered experimentally. Representative factors that alter radiation resistivity and compounds that can sensitize or protect organisms from the lethal action of ionizing radiation are presented in Table 32–3. Many of the compounds listed must be present during the irradiation process to be effective. The modification of the

lethal effects of irradiation can vary from a relatively modest effect by freezing to orders of magnitude by sensitizers or protectors.

To decrease or eliminate the microbial population from a surface or within a material by ionizing radiation involves additional considerations. The microbial contaminants will consist of mixed flora, distributed in a manner characteristic of the material. Microorganisms growing as a dense mass in a restricted area, or diffuse when dispersed in a liquid, will be destroyed at different rates by an equivalent dose and dose distribution. The physiologic state of the organisms will vary, and the composition of the menstruum surrounding the microorganisms may also vary from that of an inert substance to a

Table 32–3. *Factors That Modify Radiation Resistivity*

Modifier	Examples	Effect on Resistivity	Conditions that Influence Modifier
Irradiation atmosphere	Oxygen	Decrease	Reducing agents Protectors Anaerobiosis by microbial metabolism or by dose, catalase
Protectors	Sulfhydryl-containing compounds Reducing agents Alcohols Glycerol Dimethyl sulfoxide Proteins Carbohydrates	Increase	Oxygen pH Temperature Sensitizers
Sensitizers	N-ethylmaleimide Quinones Iodoacetic acid p-Chloromercuribenzoic acid Nitrous oxide Dimethyl sulfoxide Halides Nitrites Nitrates Radiation products H_2O_2	Decrease	Oxygen pH Temperature Protectors Catalase Superoxide dismutase OH scavengers Spore or vegetative cell
Temperature	Freezing Elevated	Increase Decrease	
Water content of cell	Desiccation of cell	Can increase if vegetative; decrease if spore or yeast	Relative humidity Oxygen
Recovery techniques	Incubation temperature Composition of medium Salts Diluent Oxygen	Variable	
Age of microorganism		Variable depending upon stage of growth cycle	
Dose rate	Greater than 10^4 rad/μs	Decrease at high rates	Oxygen
Pulse		Decrease	
Type of energy	Co-60 vs. electron	Co-60 more lethal	
Composition of support surface		Variable	Relative humidity Oxygen

plant or animal tissue of high complexity. It would be fortuitous if the survival curve for this mixed microflora were to be exponential (see the following) in all cases. Instances in which the flora is not equally distributed may necessitate an additional dosage. Morever, there will be interactions involving the organism, the material in which it is embedded, and the LET of the ionizing track. For this reason, there may be differences of opinion, dependent on the experimental parameters, regarding the determination of effective dosages to be employed for either radiopasteurization or radiosterilization.

Radiation Resistivity

Although many factors influence the radiation resistivity of various microorganisms, they can generally be classified as to inherent resistivity (Table 32–4). Bacterial spores, with few exceptions, are the most resistant to radiation, gram-negative rods the most sensitive, and yeast and fungi of intermediate resistance.

A number of exceptions exist. *Deinococcus radiodurans, D. radiophilus, D. proteolyticus,* and *D. radiopugnans* are four gram-positive, heat-sensitive, desiccant-resistant, vegetative, red pigmented organisms that are extremely resistant to radiation (Brooks et al., 1980; Murray, 1986). Nonpigmented gram-negative vegetative cells may also be radioresistant. *Moraxella osloensis* (Moraxella-acinetobacter), *Arthrobacter radiotolerans,* *Pseudomonas radiora* and *Acinetobacter radioresistens,* which was isolated from irradiated tampons and also from soil, have all been shown to be highly radiation resistant (Welch and Maxcy, 1975; Sanders and Maxcy, 1979; Nishimura et al., 1988). The four *Deinococcus* species, *Moraxella osloensis,* and *Pseudomonas radiora* have also been shown to have complex, lipid and protein-containing thick cell walls (Sanders and Maxcy, 1979). Recently a red (pink) pigmented, gram-negative, rod, *Deinobacter grandis* was found to also be extremely radiation resistant (Oyaizu et al., 1987).

Osterberg (1974) also noted that 11 out of 12 of the most resistant microorganisms isolated from suture material were either pink or red. In fact, the most resistant organism was a pink pigmented micrococcus having a population frequency of 0.03% and a 10^{-6} inactivation dose of 2.5 Mrad. One white pigmented yeast (0.05% frequency) required 2.1 Mrad to attain a 10^{-6} inactivation dose.

The data presented in Tables 32–3 and 32–4 are useful for comparative purposes, but in actuality can serve only as a guide to the course of action to be taken in specific circumstances.

Survival Curves

The destruction of organisms during irradiation may be characterized by their survival curves. This relationship is obtained by graphing the logarithm of survival fraction (concentration of survivors, N/concentration of the original population, No.) versus dose. Some representative types of curves are shown in Figure 32–2. The Type 2 curve is called exponential (Lea, 1956); the Type 1 curve is usually termed sigmoidal, multihit, or multitarget and is a simpler representative of this type of curve. At low doses, a shoulder is observed, with an intercept obtained by extrapolation (extrapolation number, N) (Alper, 1961), the curve becoming exponential at the higher doses. For organisms such as *Deinococcus (Micrococcus) radiodurans* (Anderson et al., 1956), and radiation-resistant mutants of *Salmonella typhimurium* (Davies and Sinskey, 1973), the magnitude of the shoulder is appreciable before exponential death occurs and is probably due to a repair mechanism (Mosely and Laser, 1965; Davies et al., 1973). In examining Figure 32–2, one should note that for each of the three curves, a different dosage is required in order to inactivate 99% of the cells.

For the nonexponential curve of Type 1, Lea (1956) has used the following equation:

$$\text{Fraction surviving} = 1 - (1\text{-}e^{-x})^n; \quad X = KD$$

where K is the slope of the linear portion of the survival curve expressed as reciprocal of kiloroentgens (kr^{-1}), and D is the dose. K should be independent of n, and n should be greater than or equal to 1. Anellis et al. (1965) found that, for *Clostridium botulinum* 33A, X = -13.43D and n = 80 in buffer and -9.04D and 90, respectively in pea puree.

The third curve, Type 3, in Figure 32–2, has been interpreted as caused by microbial populations that are nonhomogeneous with regard to resistivity. A higher proportion of the less resistant cells are inactivated first, leaving the more resistant cells to tail out. One should not assume that a tailing effect occurs only in a Type 3 curve; it has been reported to occur in studies with *Clostridium botulinum* (Grecz et al., 1965), with yeast (Kuprianoff, 1963), and with salmonellae in dried foodstuffs (Mossel and DeGroat, 1965). Some of these effects are due to cultural problems and repair mechanisms, but some cannot be readily explained (Cerf, 1977).

APPLICATION OF IONIZING RADIATION FOR THE DESTRUCTION OF MICROORGANISMS

There are essentially two approaches to the use of radiation: partial and/or selective destruction of the microbial flora (radiation pasteurization) and the complete destruction of the microbial flora (radiation sterilization).

Radiation Sterilization of Food

If the intent is to produce a sterile food product, certain conditions must be met. For maximal shelf stability, not only microorganisms but tissue enzymes should also be inactivated. Even though chemical changes in the food constituents can still occur, the food should be capable of possessing a long storage life without needing refrigeration. Enzymes require a higher irradiation dosage for inactivation than microorganisms (Table 32–4); therefore, a substerilization thermal treatment may be required to supplement radiation.

Table 32–4. *Radiation Resistivities of Microorganisms and Other Biologic Units*

Species	D10* (Mrad)	Presence of a "Shoulder" (Mrad)	Irradiation Menstruum	References (see footnotes)
Anaerobic Spore Formers				
Clostridium botulinum Type A 36	0.33	0.4	Buffer	b
Type B	0.11–0.33	0.4–1.0	Buffer	a,b
Type D	0.22	0.25–0.35	Water	a
Type E Beluga	0.08	0.25–0.35	Water	a
Type F	0.25	0.25–0.35	Water	a
C. sporogenes	0.16–0.22	0.25–0.35	Water	a
C. perfringens	0.12–0.20	0.25–0.35	Water	a
C. tetani	0.24	0.25–0.35	Water	a
Aerobic Spore Formers				
Bacillus subtilis	0.06		Saline + 5% gelatin	c
B. pumilus E601	0.17	1.1	Water	n
	0.30		Dried	p
B. pumilis ATCC 27142	0.14–0.40		Dried, medical devices, drugs, natural substances	d
B. sphaericus C₁A	1.00		Dried, organic	p
Vegetative Bacteria and Fungi				
Salmonella typhimurium	0.02		PO₄ buffer	e
S. typhimurium R6008	0.13	0.4	PO₄ buffer	m
Pseudomonas spp.	0.006		PO₄ buffer	e
Lactobacillus brevis NCDO 110	0.12	0.02–0.05	PO₄ buffer	d
Staphylococcus aureus	0.02		PO₄ buffer	h
Streptococcus faecium	0.28		Dry state	i
Deinococcus radiodurans	0.22	1.2	PO₄ buffer	j
Moraxella osloensis	0.58		Ice	o
Acinetobacter radioresistens	0.13–0.22		PO₄ buffer	q
Aspergillus niger	0.05		Saline + 0.5% gelatin	c
Saccharomyces cerevisiae	0.05		Saline + 0.5% gelatin	c
Viruses				
Foot-and-mouth	1.3		Frozen at −60° C	k
Coxsackievirus	0.45		Eagle + 2% BSA	f
Process requirements‡				
Trichina inactivation	0.02–0.05			l
Enzyme inactivation	2.0–10.0			l
Insect deinfestation	0.1–0.5			l
Effect of Food Constituents on Radioresistance				
C. botulinum Types A, B	0.34–0.42		Beef	h
S. typhimurium	0.08		Egg yolk magma	g
S. seftenburg	0.09		Egg yolk magma	g

*Rads required to decrease the initial population by one logarithm.
†No shoulder-dose required for 10⁴ inactivation.
‡Complete destruction (megarad).

References

a. Roberts and Ingram (1965)
b. Grecz (1965)
c. Lawrence et al. (1953)
d. Prince and Rubino (1984)
e. Thornley (1963)
f. Sullivan et al. (1971)

g. Brogle et al. (1954)
h. Kreiger et al. (1983)
i. Christensen (1964)
j. Duggan et al. (1963)
k. McCrea and Horton (1962)
l. Bellamy (1959)

m. Davies and Sinskey (1973)
n. Van Winkle et al. (1967)
o. Welch and Maxcy (1975)
p. Gaughran and Goudie (1978)
q. Nishimura et al. (1988)

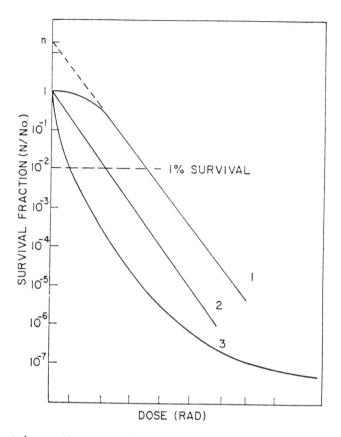

Fig. 32–2. Schematic diagram of survival curves. N = survivors of irradiation dose (arbitrary units in rad); N_0 = original number of microorganisms; n = extrapolation number.

In order to establish a sterilizing dose for a given material, one must be able to balance the radiation tolerance of a material against that dose of radiation considered necessary to establish sterility. For relatively inert materials such as hides and plastics, large doses can be used with relative impunity, but for materials more susceptible to radiation, such as foodstuffs, greater care must be taken in establishing a minimal dose so as to balance acceptance with safety. A material being irradiated will not require a "come-up" time as in thermal heating, but will be instantaneously penetrated by the ionizing track. Nevertheless, the material will act as a shield, which, although not usually serious for penetrating rays such as gamma rays, will deter the extent of the penetration of beta and alpha rays. Of a more indeterminate nature is the previously mentioned fact that many irradiated organisms are not inactivated logarithmically.

The most severe constraint required for the application of ionizing radiations to the sterilization of food materials is the equivalent 12D requirement for *C. botulinum*, a requirement also imposed on thermal processing. Although relatively heat sensitive, the spores of *C. botulinum* are among the most radiation-resistant organisms

and generally demonstrate a sigmoidal type of survival curve (Roberts and Ingram, 1965; Ross, 1974).

In essence, the 12D requirement means that if a given dose reduces a population of organisms by one logarithmic cycle (a D_{10} value), then the material should be exposed to the equivalent of 12D values for sterilization. It is not feasible to conduct inoculated-pack studies with 10^{12} organisms per can, so that studies are designed to determine D_{10} values and to calculate the equivalent 12D.

A practical difficulty lies in accurately estimating the D_{10} value. For the Type 2 curve (Fig. 32–2), the D_{10} value can be obtained from any portion of the straight line, but in other types of curves, its interpretation is more difficult.

Methods for obtaining D_{10} values are those of Stumbo et al. (1950), Stumbo (1973), and Schmidt and Nank (1960). Stumbo et al. (1950) adapted the most-probable-number (MPN) technique for obtaining the D_{10} value and derived an equation capable of treating either inoculated or indigenous organisms. From the Halvorson and Ziegler (1933) MPN equation:

$$\bar{x} = 2.303 \log \frac{n}{q}$$

where $\bar{x}$ is the MPN of surviving spores per unit, n the number of units irradiated, and q the number of units rendered sterile. The D_{10} value is derived by using the equation:

$$D_{10} = \frac{\text{dose}}{\log (\text{bioburden}) - \log \bar{x}}$$

This model assumes exponential inactivation.

Schmidt and Nank (1960) proposed the use of an equation for calculating a 12D sterilization dose:

$$D_{10} = \frac{\text{dose}}{\log m - \log S}$$

where m is the number of spores per can multiplied by the number of cans at each dose, and S is the number of spoiled cans per dose at partial spoilage. This equation involves inoculated-pack studies for deriving partial spoilage data. The use of this equation also requires that the influence of the menstruum be minimal and assumes that one spore survives per can. They suggested that a D_{10} value of 0.4 Mrep be used, giving a 12D value of 4.8 Mrep or the equivalent of 0.37 rad and 4.45 Mrad, respectively, and which should inactivate 10^{12} spores of *C. botulinum*.

Bridges (1964) states that it is unlikely that the population in any food containing *C. botulinum* will exceed 10^1 to 10^2 per g and that 4.8 Mrep should destroy a population of 10^{12} spores per g (having a radiation resistance equivalent to that of *C. botulinum*).

Other approaches to deriving a sterilization dose have not required the assumption that the bioburden has exponential inactivation kinetics. These include the use of the Spearman-Karber equation and the Weibull distribution (Anellis and Werkowski, 1968, 1971). Ross (1974) also indicated that for partial spoilage data for inoculated-pack studies on foods, the Weibull distribution was operative, but not the lognormal function, and that it is even doubtful that the inactivation kinetics of *C. botulinum* are exponential, although they are often assumed to be so. Ross (1976) subsequently included techniques for involving the shifted exponential (shoulder) function as well as a normal distribution for estimating 12D and also methods to determine whether simple exponential distribution of inactivation kinetics is applicable and what approaches to subsequently use.

In the U.S. Army radiation sterilization program, the experimental 12D sterilizing dose (ESD) on enzyme-inactivated foods inoculated with 10^7 spores of *C. botulinum* types A and B varies between 1.5 to 2.0 Mrad for cured foods such as bacon or pork sausages to 3.5 to 4.5 Mrad for pork or beef. Irradiation is conducted at −30°C (Josephson et al., 1973; Rowley et al., 1978). The experiments for ESD must include tests not only for viability but also for toxin (Greenberg et al., 1965).

The requirement for 2 to 5 Mrad has the capability of causing organoleptic and flavor deterioration in food materials. Quality deterioration will not be discussed in any detail, but in practice, two methods (see Table 32–3)

have been used to decrease off-flavors in foods: (1) the exclusion of oxygen during irradiation (nitrogen and anoxic packs) and (2) the use of low temperatures. The use of cysteine and free radical acceptors is of limited value in foods.

Radiation Pasteurization of Food

The doses employed are considerably lower for pasteurization than those used for sterilization, usually 1 Mrad or less, and consequently, the product undergoes less off-flavor development. In general, the gram-negative indigenous psychrophiles are much more radiation sensitive than the remaining flora and are considered the main spoilage agents. The net result therefore will be one of microbial selection; the more radiation-sensitive microorganisms will be rendered nonviable, the most numerous organisms decreased, and the spoilage pattern, it is expected, altered and inhibited. Radiation pasteurization has also been advocated for the destruction of the ubiquitous organism, salmonella, from egg, poultry, and meat products.

Radiopasteurization can extend the shelf life of a variety of fresh food products if certain factors are considered: (1) The initial numbers of microorganisms must be reasonably low. (2) The irradiated product should be maintained at a refrigeration temperature as low as possible. (3) The packaging must be of the proper type. (4) Recontamination after irradiation must be minimal. (5) The dosage should be low enough to preserve the characteristic odor and flavor of the fresh product. It must be realized, though, that not all foods, e.g., vegetables and dairy products, can tolerate radiation energy without undergoing significant changes in such aspects as flavor and texture.

Seafood, one of the most perishable of foods, and subject to dose-dependent radiation off-flavor, has been considered to be adaptable to radiopasteurization. The optimum dose depends upon the species of fish (Ronsivalli et al., 1965). The doses employed have usually been less than 1 Mrad and can be less than 0.5 Mrad (MacLean and Welander, 1960; Masurovsky et al., 1963; Miyauchi et al., 1964; Spinelli et al., 1965; IAEA, 1973). There is a definite selection of microorganisms by irradiation. Corlett et al. (1965) studied the microbial shifts occurring in Dover sole after irradiation and storage at 6°C. In the nonirradiated samples, spoilage was caused predominately by pseudomonads. *Achromobacter* and yeasts predominated in the sample irradiated at 0.4 Mrad and below. The micrococcus that survived irradiation did not grow at 6°C, and at 0.5 Mrad, the surviving yeasts were the main spoilage organisms. Packaging and the atmosphere have also been shown to select the subsequent growth of survivors (Sinskey et al., 1967).

Urbain (1966) reviewed those parameters required to make radiation of fresh meats and poultry a commercial reality. He found that the dose, the presence of phosphates, and the packaging materials had to be carefully selected before success could be achieved. A panel was able to detect off-flavors in cooked poultry irradiated with

0.46 Mrad and stored for up to three weeks at 1.1°C (MacLeod et al., 1969).

Other food materials have also been subjected to irradiation in order to extend their shelf lives, to decrease their bioburden, to deinfest, and to delay the onset of fungal growth. Shea (1965) has summarized the results with fruits. The radiation dosage employed has been in the range of 150 to 200 Krad, and although the shelf life has not been greatly extended, radiation is claimed to have reduced the incidence of premature spoilage. A tendency toward softening has been noted for fruits and vegetables (Etchells et al., 1961; Martin and Techenor, 1962; Truelsen, 1963) which, in some cases, has led to superior final products for specific purposes, such as canning or dehydration (Kadar, 1986).

Dehydrated onion powder irradiated with 0.9 Mrad did not undergo any deleterious changes in either aroma or taste (Silberstein et al., 1979), and the microbial population was reduced to below 25,000/g. Pruthi (1980) and Grecz et al. (1986) found radiation effective in decreasing the microbial flora of the normally heavily-contaminated spices and condiments.

The elimination of salmonellae from the food chain by irradiation has been attempted in poultry and eggs (Thornley, 1963; Comer et al., 1963; Idziak and Incze, 1968). A dose of 0.5 Mrad is recommended by Thornley (1963) for a $7D_{10}$ reduction in frozen egg, and a dose of 0.65 Mrad for a $0.2D_{10}$ reduction in *Salmonella typhimurium* in frozen horsemeat (Ley et al., 1963).

The elimination of the natural microflora in radiopasteurized foods may allow subsequent growth by the surviving spores. *C. botulinum* type E, which can grow at temperatures as low as 4°C (Schmidt et al., 1962) has been of concern. The incidence of these organisms has been low, and outgrowth and toxin production is inhibited at low refrigeration temperatures. *C. perfringens* does not appear to multiply below 20°C and should not be a problem if the food product is properly refrigerated (Barnes et al., 1963; Midura et al., 1965).

Viruses that are relatively heat sensitive are highly resistant to irradiation (Kaplan and Moses, 1964; Kenny et al., 1969), as are toxins (Wagenaar and Dack, 1960; Roberts et al., 1965; Patel et al., 1989), and their control depends mainly upon preventing the introduction of significant concentrations.

Radiation Sterilization of Medical Products

The sterilization by radiation of drugs, pharmaceuticals, and tissue for transplantation (Table 32–5) has met with a measure of success (Phillips, 1973; Gaughran and Goudie, 1978; Silverman, 1979; Masefield, 1981). Some radiation side effects such as a decrease in immunogenicity in bone graft material are beneficial, but radiation can also cause a decrease in mechanical strength. These disadvantages have not prevented the use of irradiated bone cartilage and skin for grafts. Radiosterilization has been advocated for the dry constituents used in tissue culture and in the manufacture of vaccines. It has also been suggested for the pasteurization of the vaccines

themselves, especially to remove radiation-sensitive bacteria.

In the sterilization of medical devices, a highly successful application of radiation, the initial approach was to require a standard dose in order to attain a safety factor equivalent to 10^{-6} (6D). Many countries employ a standard, minimal absorbed sterilization dose of 2.5 Mrad. If some other dose is used, then process effectiveness must be validated. Using a standard dose for sterilization penalizes those processors manufacturing products having a low bioburden, whereas products having a high bioburden may not be properly sterilized. The current approach (see the following) is to depend upon substerilization dosages to determine the bioburden and its distribution of resistances (White, 1973; Tallentire and Khan, 1978; Whitby and Gelda, 1979; Davis et al., 1981; Doolan et al., 1985; Fitch et al., 1985). This information is then applied to models to derive an estimation of the sterilization dose (AAMI, 1981).

Irradiation with 2.5 Mrad of the five drugs listed in Table 32–5 resulted in three of them, ampicillin, tetracycline, and pilocarpine, retaining sufficient qualities to meet official criteria, with atropine and chloramphenicol failing (Diding et al., 1979). It appears that radiation is no more damaging to many pharmaceuticals than heat or other methods of sterilization, especially if the product is in a dry state or in the presence of a protector. Irradiation might be used more, because feasibility studies have indicated its effectiveness, if, instead of employing a minimum dose of 2.5 Mrad, an effectively lower dose, based upon good manufacturing procedures and a low bioburden, can be used.

The use of gamma radiation to sterilize hospital supplies such as plastic hypodermic syringes, sutures, and containers is the main commercial application of ionizing radiation (Oliver and Tomlinson, 1960; Powell and Bridges, 1960; Darmady et al., 1961; Burt and Ley, 1963; Ley, 1971; IAEA, 1974; Gaughran and Goudie, 1974, 1978; Silverman, 1979; Masefield, 1981). Examples of contamination levels on medical items are shown in Table 32–6 (Silverman, 1978). Although the bioburden can be at high concentrations, it is generally low when proper manufacturing procedures are employed. Horakova et al. (1978) reported that the distribution of organisms on gauze swabs was not a Poisson distribution. Surveys of initial contamination levels indicate that most disposable syringes contain less than 100 aerobic or anaerobic organisms (Sztanyik, 1974). Artandi (1974) found a similar range of low contamination for sutures. The resistivities of various isolates from manufacturing environments or products differed by a factor of 2 to 9 (Table 32–7; Silverman, 1978). The differences in resistivities in these studies might have been due as much to experimental techniques as to inherent microbial resistivities. Burt and Ley (1963) were able to achieve a calculated inactivation factor of 10^{15} with 2.5 Mrad for *Bacillus pumilus* dried on various surfaces in air and of 10^7 in anoxia. They did note a protective effect for cells dried onto a surface

Table 32–5. *Examples of Products Sterilized by Radiation**

Graft†	Drugs‡	Other
Lyophilized bone	Chloramphenicol	Vaccines Ointments
Cartilage	Ampicillin trihydrate	Powder Talc
Tendons, fascia	Tetracycline hydrochloride	Syringes Sutures
Skin	Atropine sulfate	Containers
Heart valve	Pilocarpine hydrochloride	Sheets Sponges Surgical equipment

*Gaughran and Goudie (1979); Masefield (1981).
†Irradiated after lyophilization.
‡Irradiated as a powder.

Table 32–6. *Bioburden Concentrations Associated with Medical Items*

Reference	Material	Microorganisms/ Item
Horakova and Buriankova, 1975	Surgical gloves	0–100
Horakova et al., 1978	Gauze swabs	100–20,000
Miller and Berube, 1978	Syringes	0–46
Osterberg, 1973	Dry sutures	10–400
Cook and Berry, 1968	Syringes	0–150
Fitch et al., 1985*	Syringes	7.5–24

*Noted that some samples were too numerous to count.

Table 32–7. *Examples of D_{10} Values and the Inactivation Factor for 10^{-6} Reduction of Isolates Obtained Either from Medical Products or the Manufacturing Environment*

Reference	Organism	D_{10} (Krad)	Inactivation Factor for 10^{-6} (Mrad)
Christensen, 1978	Gram-positive rod		2.5–4.5
	Diplococcus		3.0–5.0
Bochkarev et al., 1978	Staphylococci	120 ± 45	
	Streptococci	160 ± 70	
	Sporeformer	205 ± 105	
	Gram-negative		
		105 ± 50	
	Nonsporeformer	110 ± 50	
	Fungi		
Whitby, 1978	Gram-positive rod	25–42	
	Gram-negative rod	25–35	
	Gram-positive coccus	25–42	
	Yeast	25–40	
Osterberg, 1974*	Yeast (white)		2.1
	Yeast (pink)		1.6
	Micrococcus (pink)		2.5
	Sporeforming rod (red)		0.9–1.6
	Non-sporeforming rod (red)		1.0–1.5
Czerniawski and Stolarczyk, 1974	Sporeformers and micrococci	25–56	3†–3.5‡

*Assuming 10 organisms per device
†100 organisms per device
‡1000 organisms per device

having some degree of solubility as compared to a surface that was insoluble.

The safety of a 2.5-Mrad dose and the use of *B. pumilus* as a test organism have been questioned (Christensen, 1964, 1978; Christensen and Holm, 1964; Christensen et al., 1967) and the substitution of *Streptococcus faecium*, an opportunistic pathogen found in manufacturing and assembly areas with a radioresistivity greater than many microbial spores (see Table 32–4), has been suggested. It has therefore been proposed that for ^{60}Co sterilization, 3.2 (3.5 Mrad for electrons), 4.5, and 5.0 Mrad be used for items containing an average count below 50, between 50 and 500, and between 500 and 5000 organisms per item, respectively (Christensen, 1973; Gaughran, 1982). This results in a probability of sterility of approximately 10^{-6} (White, 1973). While *S. faecium* (ATTC 19581), as well as *Bacillus sphaericus* C_1A, and *B. pumilus* E601, have been suggested for sterility controls (see Table 32–4), Czerniawski and Stolarczyk (1974) used actual isolates and corrected for the incidence of each class of resistant organisms in deriving a sterilization dose of 3.5 Mrad for an inactivation factor (sterility coefficient) of 10^{-6} for a contamination level of 1000 organisms per product, and of 3 Mrad if 100 organisms per product are present. Osterberg (1973, 1974), assuming a bioburden of 10 organisms per suture, and for an inactivation dose of 10^{-6}, derived sterilization dose requirements of 0.7 to 2.5 Mrad for vegetative cells and 0.9 to 1.9 Mrad for spores. These studies also indicated (Osterberg, 1974; Whitby and Gelda, 1979) that the most resistant organisms were present in low (0.03 to 0.05%) numbers.

Tallentire and Khan (1978) employed substerilization doses to characterize the distribution and size of the bioburden on medical devices. They indicated that extrapolations, which assume either a Poisson or an exponential bioburden distribution, may not be applicable and that information on bioburden distribution is necessary for modeling. White (1973) proposed the use of three doses, two substerilizing and one sterilizing, for characterizing the bioburden. None of these approaches will be valid if a resistant tail (Fig. 32–2) is present.

The subcommittee on radiation sterilization of the Association for the Advancement of Medical Instrumentation (AAMI, 1981; Davis et al., 1981) has suggested a number of approaches for deriving a sterilization dose, based upon the bioburden. A number of procedures are recommended, all depending upon obtaining accurate estimations of the initial numbers of organisms and their distribution of radiation resistivities by incremental (substerilization) dosing. The procedures allow the selection of sterility assurance levels (probability of being nonsterile) of from 10^{-3} to 10^{-6}. Moreover, the models incorporate the use of verification procedures for evaluation of the effectiveness of the processing procedures. An audit of the sterility dose is also provided to compensate for any factors that increase the sterilizing dose. A basic assumption is "that the bioburden is a mixture of homogeneous populations, each of which behaves in a 'D_{10}' fashion." These techniques will detect subpopulations containing significant numbers of highly resistant organisms.

The AAMI procedures also require that the processor, in addition to determining the proper sterilization dose, deliver the proper dose by effective good manufacturing procedures (FDA, 1979) and employ accurate dosimetry. Proper application can result in the use of a dosimetric release procedure, that is, the product can be released as sterile upon verification that the intended and correct radiation dose was used without the requirement for sterility testing. This is an advantage, because a sterilization dose required to obtain a safety factor of 10^{-6} cannot be verified by accepted sterility testing procedures because they generally suffer a contamination frequency of approximately 1 in 10^3 to 10^4.

Other Applications

Radiation has been used to treat sewage and industrial sludges in order to reduce the microflora. It has also been successfully employed for sterilizing feed for gnotobiotic animal studies and for hospital patients requiring sterile foods. Relatively low doses of radiation will deinfestate grain and destroy *B. anthracis* spores in goat hair (Horne et al., 1959).

STERILIZATION BY GAS PLASMA

A gas plasma, also called a glow discharge plasma or low-temperature gas plasma, is a gas that contains an essentially neutral cloud of electrons, ions, free radicals, and dissociated and/or excited atoms or molecules produced as a result of an electrical discharge, including the accompaniment of ionizing radiation—principally ultraviolet light (Bithell, 1982). This type of gas plasma has average electron energies of 1 to 10 eV and electron densities of 10^9 to 10^{12}/cm^3 (Gut Boucher, 1980). With the exception of electrons, all other charged or excited units in the gas plasma significantly contribute to microbial lethality (Bithell, 1982).

Menashi (1968) described an apparatus capable of producing a gas plasma at atmospheric pressure by generating a corona discharge and that was capable of destroying microorganisms on the surfaces of materials and devices. The original apparatus has been modified by others, and a current gas plasma sterilizing apparatus generally consists of a sterilization chamber able to withstand a vacuum of at least 200 μm, a radio-frequency generator, an impedance matching network, and gauges for admitting controlled amounts of gases for generating the gas plasma. Additional features may be ports or doors constructed so as to prevent the escape of ultraviolet light created during production of the gas plasma and a water jacket for cooling the gas plasma stream. Although gas plasma generators normally operate in the frequency range of 1 to 30 Megahertz, higher frequencies, in the microwave region of 100 to 300,000 Megahertz, can also be used. The gas plasma generated at microwave frequencies have a longer life and greater penetrability. One advantage of sterilization with a gas plasma is that unlike methods involving a sterilant agent such as ethylene oxide, sterilization by a gas plasma does not leave any agent residue on the sterilized material.

The carrier gases used to generate a gas plasma can be argon, helium, xenon, nitrogen, oxygen, or carbon dioxide. Although nonoxidative gases were initially considered more desirable for generating gas plasmas for sterilization, subsequent studies showed that equal, if not greater, microbial lethality was obtained under vacuum with a gas plasma derived from oxygen or a mixtures of gases made by the addition of aldehydes or nitrous oxide to the carrier gas (Fraser et al., 1976; Gut Boucher, 1980). A gas plasma, generated mainly from the germicide, hydrogen peroxide, has been reported to be an effective sterilant (Jacobs and Lin, 1988).

A gas plasma may be generated continuously or pulsed. When generated the particles in the gas plasma may reach 500°C or higher, but usually cool to less than 100°C when impacting the target molecule. When necessary, additional cooling of the gas plasma can be achieved with the use of a cooling jacket around the plasma-generating chamber or by pulsing (Fraser et al., 1976). The penetration of narrow cavities or apertures in articles normally difficult for plasmas to sterilize can be achieved by cyclically varying chamber pressure (Bithell, 1982).

Four studies have described microbiologic challenges to measure the sterilization efficacy of this technology, but only one included medical devices. Menashi (1968) stated that 4×10^6 microbial spores (not identified) can be inactivated in less than 0.1 second. Fraser et al. (1976), although noting that a reduction of 99% of a spore population (not identified) was achieved within 2 minutes, suggested that longer periods were necessary for sterility. More extensive studies, using 10^6 to 10^9 spores of *Bacillus subtilis* (ATCC 19659) and *Clostridium sporogenes* (ATCC 3584) in the sporicidal test of the Association of Official Analytical Chemists, found that exposure to various aldehyde gas plasmas for contact times of between 10 and 30 minutes was sufficient for achieving sterility. Jacobs and Lin (1988) sterilized paper discs and surgical blades inoculated with approximately 10^5 to 10^6 spores of *Bacillus subtilis* (var. *globigii*) enclosed in spun-bonded polyethylene envelopes. After a pretreatment consisting of a 10-minute exposure to a hydrogen-peroxide atmosphere under reduced pressure, they were subjected to a hydrogen-peroxide gas plasma. Sterility was achieved within 60 minutes, and usually in less than 30 minutes.

The initial gas plasma apparatus sterilized objects that were not packaged. Proposals for maintaining sterility of the processed items were to (1) package after sterilization, (2) sterilize the objects in a package with one open seam to allow the entry of plasma, and then seal the open seam after sterilization, or (3) to use packages with an orifice for plasma entry which, after sterilization, is

sealed by taping. Using these techniques it is difficult to ensure a high degree of product sterility. Recently Bithell (1982) proposed that items be sterilized in "porous" packaging materials, such as polyethylene, which allows the passage of the lethal plasma cloud into the package interior. Jacobs and Lin (1988) found that polyethylene or a composite of polyethylene with polyethylene terephthalate was satisfactory for sterilization by a hydrogen-peroxide gas plasma. It was also stated that although paper packaging can be used, longer sterilization times are necessary because of paper's reactivity with the gas plasma.

A wide variety of articles and devices such as catheters, surgical tubing, scissors and scalpels, prosthetic or body implant devices, pharmaceutical preparations, and fruits and vegetables, as well as the use of this technique for sterilizing articles during space travel, have been proposed as candidates for surface sterilization or decontamination by gas plasma. The technologic as well as the economic feasibility of this technique for application to such a wide variety of products remains to be demonstrated.

REFERENCES

AAMI, 1981. Process control guidelines for radiation sterilization of medical devices. Arlington, VA, Association for the Advancement of Medical Instrumentation.

Alper, T. 1961. Effects on subcellular units and free living cells. In *Mechanisms in Radiobiology.* Edited by M. Errera and A. Forssberg. New York, Academic Press.

Anderson, A.W., et al. 1956. Studies on a radio-resistant micrococcus. I. Isolation morphology, cultural characteristics and resistance to gamma radiation. Food Technol., 10, 575.

Anellis, A., and Werkowski, S. 1971. Estimation of an equivalent "12D" process by the normal distribution method. Can. J. Microbiol., 17, 1185.

Anellis, A., and Werkowski, S. 1968. Estimation of radiation resistance values of microorganisms in food products. Appl. Microbiol., 16, 1300.

Anellis, A., Grecz, N., and Berkowitz, D. 1965. Survival of *Clostridium botulinum* spores. Appl. Microbiol., 13, 397.

Artandi, C. 1974. Microbiological control before and after sterilization: Its effect on sterility assurance. In *Experiences in Radiation Sterilization of Medical Products.* Vienna, IAEA.

Barnes, E.M., Despaul, J.E., and Ingram, M. 1963. The behavior of a food poisoning strain of *Clostridium welchii* in beef. J. Appl. Bacteriol., 26, 415.

Bellamy, W.D. 1959. Preservation of foods and drugs by ionizing radiations. In *Advances in Applied Microbiology.* Edited by W.W. Umbreit. New York, Academic Press.

Bithell, R.M. 1982. Plasma pressure pulse sterilization. U.S. Patent No. 4,348, 357.

Bochkarev, V.V., et al. 1978. Ecological studies of radiation sensitivity in microorganisms at some enterprises of medical industry. In *Sterilization of Medical Products by Ionizing Radiation.* Montreal, Multiscience Publ., Ltd., p. 46.

Bridges, B.A. 1964. Microbiological aspects of radiation sterilization. Prog. Ind. Microbiol., 5, 283.

Brogle, R.C., et al. 1954. Use of high voltage cathode rays to destroy bacteria of the *Salmonella* group in whole egg solids, egg yolk solids, and frozen egg yolk. Food Res., 22, 572.

Brooks, B.W., et al. 1980. Red-pigmented micrococci: A basis for taxonomy. Int. J. System. Bacteriol., 30, 627.

Burt, M., and Ley, F.J. 1963. Studies on the dose requirement for the radiation sterilization of medical equipment. I. Influence of suspending media. J. Appl. Bacteriol., 26, 484.

Cerf, O. 1977. Tailing of survival curves of bacterial spores. J. Appl. Bacteriol., 42, 1.

Chatterjee, A. 1987. Interaction of ionizing radiation with matter. In *Radiation Chemistry, Principles and Application.* Edited by Farhataziz and M.A.J. Rogers. New York, VCH Publishers.

Chipley, J.R. 1980. Effects of microwave irradiation on microorganisms. Adv. App. Microbiol., 26, 129.

Christensen, E.A. 1978. The role of microbiology in commissioning a new facility and in routine control. In *Sterilization of Medical Products by Ionizing Radiation*. Edited by E.R.L. Gaughran and A.J. Goudie. Montreal, Multiscience Publ. Ltd., p. 50.

Christensen, E.A. 1973. Hygienic requirements, sterility criteria and quality and sterility control. In *Manual on Radiation Sterilization of Medical and Biological Materials*. Vienna, IAEA.

Christensen, E.A. 1964. Radiation resistance of enterococci dried in air. Acta Pathol. Microbiol. Scand., *61*, 483.

Christensen, E.A., and Holm, N.W. 1964. Inactivation of dried bacteria and bacterial spores by means of ionizing radiation. Acta Pathol. Microbiol. Scand., *60*, 253.

Christensen, E.A., Holm, N.W., and Juul, F.A. 1967. Radiosterilization of medical devices and supplies. In *Radiosterilization of Medical Products*. 265 (STL/PUB/157). Vienna, IAEA.

Comer, A.G., Anderson, G.W., and Garrard, E.H. 1963. Gamma irradiation of Salmonella species in frozen whole egg. Can. J. Microbiol., *9*, 321.

Cook, A.M., and Berry, R.J. 1968. Microbial contamination of disposable hypodermic syringes prior to sterilization by ionizing radiation. Appl. Microbiol., *16*, 1156.

Corlett, D.A., Lee, J.S., and Sinnhuber, R.O. 1965. Application of replica plating and computer analysis for rapid identification of bacteria in some foods. II. Analysis of microbial flora in irradiated dover sole *(Microstomus pacificus)*. Appl. Microbiol., *13*, 818.

Council for Agricultural Science and Technology. 1989. Ionizing energy in food processing and pest control. Task Force Report No. 115. Ames, Iowa.

Czerniawski, E., and Stolarczyk, L. 1974. Attempt to establish the ionizing radiation dose to be used in the sterilization of one-use medical equipment units. Acta Microbiol. Pol. Ser. B6, 177.

Darmady, E.M., et al. 1961. Radiation sterilization. J. Clin. Pathol., *14*, 55.

Davies, R., and Sinskey, A.J. 1973. Radiation-resistant mutants of *Salmonella typhimurium* LT2: Development and characterization. J. Bacteriol., *113*, 133.

Davies, R., Sinskey, A.J., and Botstein, D. 1973. Deoxyribonucleic acid repair in a highly radiation-resistant strain of *Salmonella typhimurium*. J. Bacteriol., *114*, 357.

Davis, K.W., Strawderman, W.E., Masefield, J., and Whitby, J.L. 1981. DS gamma radiation dose setting and auditing strategies for sterilizing medical devices. In *Sterilization of Medical Products*. Vol. II. Edited by E.R.L. Gaughran and R.F. Morrissey. Montreal, Multiscience Publ. Ltd.

Diding, N., et al. 1979. Irradiation of drugs with Co-60 and electrons. In *Sterilization by Ionizing Radiation*. Edited by E.R.L. Gaughran and A.J. Goudie. Montreal Multiscience Publ. Ltd.

Doolan, P.T., et al. 1985. Towards microbiological quality assurance in radiation sterilization processing: a limiting case model. J. Appl. Bacteriol., *58*, 303.

Duggan, D.E., Anderson, A.W., and Elliker, P.R. 1963. Inactivation of the radiation-resistant spoilage bacterium, *Micrococcus radiodurans*. I. Radiation inactivation roles in three meat substrates and in buffer. Appl. Microbiol., *11*, 398.

Etchells, J.L., Costilow, R.N., Bell, T.A., and Rutherford, H.A. 1961. Influences of gamma radiation on the microflora of cucumber fruit and blossoms. Appl. Microbiol., *9*, 145.

FDA, 1979. Good Device Manufacturing Practices. U.S. Government Printing Office.

Federal Register, 1981. Policy for irradiated foods: Advance notice of proposed procedures for the regulation of irradiated foods for human consumption. *46* (59), 18992.

Fitch, F.R., et al. 1985. Towards microbiological quality assurance in radiation sterilization processing: simulation of the radiation inactivation process. J. Appl. Bacteriol., *58*, 307.

Fraser, S.J., Gillette, R.B., and Olsen, R.L. 1976. Sterilizing process and apparatus utilizing gas plasma. U.S. Patent No. 3, 948, 601.

Gaughran, E.R.L. 1982. International aspects of radiation sterilization processing. Med. Dev. Diag. Ind., *4*, 33.

Gaughran, E.R.L., and Goudie, A.J. 1978. *Sterilization of Medical Products by Ionizing Radiation*. Montreal, Multiscience Publ. Ltd.

Ginoza, W. 1967. The effects of ionizing radiation on nucleic acids of bacteriophages and bacterial cells. Annu. Rev. Microbiol., *21*, 325.

Grecz, N. 1965. Biophysical aspects of Clostridia. J. Appl. Bacteriol., *28*, 17.

Grecz, N., Al-Harithy, R., and Jaw, R. 1986. Radiation sterilizing of spices for hospital food services and patient care. J. Food Safety, *7*, 241.

Grecz, N., Snyder, O.P., Walker, A.A., and Anellis, A. 1965. Effect of temperature of liquid nitrogen on radiation resistance of spores of *Clostridium botulinum*. Appl. Microbiol., *13*, 527.

Greenberg, A., Bladel, B.O., and Zingelmann, W.J. 1965. Radiation injury of *Clostridium botulinum* spores in cured meat. Appl. Microbiol., *13*, 743.

Gut Boucher, R.M. 1980. Seeded gas plasma sterilization system. U.S. Patent No. 4,207,286.

Halvorson, H.O., and Ziegler, N.R. 1933. Application of statistics to problems in bacteriology. I. A means of determining bacterial population by the dilution method. J. Bacteriol., *25*, 101.

Hannan, R.S., and Thornley, M.J. 1957. Radiation processing of foods. Food Mfg., Oct.-Dec., 1.

Horakova, V.C., Cerney, P., and Sladka, D. 1978. Experiences with radiation sterilization in Czechoslovakia. In *Sterilization of Medical Products by Ionizing Radiation*. Edited by E.R.L. Gaughran and A.J. Goudie. Montreal, Mutiscience Publ. Ltd., p. 119.

Horakova, V.C., and Buriankova, E. 1975. Presterilization contamination of disposable medical products and the choice of minimum sterilization dose. In *Radiosterilization of Medical Products*. Vienna, IAEA.

Horne, T., Turner, G.C., and Willis, A.T. 1959. Inactivation of spores of *Bacillus anthracis* by gamma-radiation. Nature, *183*, 475.

IAEA, 1974. *Experiences in Radiation Sterilization of Medical Products*. Vienna, International Atomic Energy Agency.

IAEA, 1973. *Radiation Preservation of Foods*. Vienna, International Atomic Energy Agency.

Idziak, E.S., and Incze, K. 1968. Radiation treatment of foods. I. Radurization of fresh eviscerated poultry. Appl. Microbiol., *16*, 1061.

Jacobs, P.T., and Lin, S. 1988. Hydrogen peroxide plasma sterilization. U.S. Patent No. 4,756,882.

Josephson, E.S., et al. 1973. Radappertization of meat products and poultry. In *Radiation Preservation of Foods*. Vienna, IAEA, p. 471.

Kadar, A.A. 1986. Potential applications of ionizing radiation in post harvest handling of fresh fruits and vegetables. Food Technol., *40*, 117.

Kaplan, H.S., and Moses, L.E. 1964. Biological complexity and radiosensitivity. Science, *145*, 21.

Kenny, M.T., Albright, K.L., Energy, J.B., and Bittle, J.L. 1969. Inactivation of rubella virus by gamma radiation. J. Virol., *4*, 807.

Krieger, R.A., Snyder, OP., and Pflug, I.J. 1983. *Clostridium botulinum* ionizing radiation D-value determination using a micro food sample system. J. Food Sci., *48*, 141.

Kuprianoff, J. 1963. Food irradiation research in Western Germany. In *Radiation Research, Proceedings of an International Conference*. Edited by F.R. Fisher. Natick, Army Natick Laboratories. NTIS PB-181506.

Kadar, A.A. 1986. Potential applications of ionizing radiation in post harvest. (sic)

Lawrence, C.A., Brownell, L.E., and Graikoski, J.T. 1953. Effect of cobalt-60 gamma radiation on microorganisms. Nucleonics, *11*, 9.

Lea, O.E. 1956. *Actions of Radiations on Living Cells*. London, Cambridge University Press.

Ley, F.J. 1971. Gamma radiation for product sterilization. J. Soc. Cosmet. Chem., *22*, 711.

Ley, F.J., and Tallentire, A. 1965. Radiation sterilization—the choice of dose. Pharm. J., Sept., 216.

Ley, F.J., Freeman, B.M., and Hobbs, B.C. 1963. The use of gamma radiation for the elimination of salmonella from various foods. J. Hyg. Camb., *61*, 515.

Ley, F.J., et al. 1972. Radiation sterilization: Microbiological findings from subprocess dose treatment of disposable plastic syringes. J. Appl. Bacteriol., *35*, 53.

Loaharanu, P. 1989. International trade in irradiated foods: Regional status and outlook. Food Technol., *43*, 77.

MacLean, D.P., and Welander, C. 1960. The preservation of fish with ionizing radiation: Bacterial studies. Food Technol., *14*, 261.

MacLeod, C.M., Farmer, F.A., and Nelson, H.R. 1969. Organic evaluation of low-dose irradiation chicken stored under refrigerated conditions. Food Technol., *23*, 104.

Magee, J.L., and Chatterjee, A. 1987. Theoretical aspects of radiation chemistry. In *Radiation Chemistry, Principles and Application*. Edited by Farhataziz and M.A.J. Rogers. New York, VCH Publishers, p. 138.

Martin, D.C., and Techenor, D.A. 1962. Effects of low-dose irradiation and storage on acceptability of broccoli, sweet corn, and strawberries. Food Technol., *16*, 96.

Masefield, J. 1981. Advances made in cobalt-60 gamma sterilization. In *Sterilization of Medical Products*. Vol. II. Edited by E.R.L. Gaughran and R.F. Morrissey. Montreal, Multiscience Publ. Ltd.

Masefield, J., Davis, K.W., Strawderman, W.E., and Whitby, J.L. 1978. A North American viewpoint on selection of radiation sterilization dose. In *Sterilization of Medical Products by Ionizing Radiation*. Edited by E.R.L. Gaughran and A.J. Goudie. Montreal, Multiscience Publ. Ltd., p. 332.

Masurovsky, E.B., Voss, J.S., and Goldblith, S.A. 1963. Changes in the microflora of haddock fillets and shucked soft-shelled clams after irradiation with Co^{60} gamma rays and storage at 0° C and 6° C. Appl. Microbiol., *11*, 229.

Matsuyama, A. 1973. Present status of food irradiation research in Japan with special reference to microbiological and entomological aspects. In *Radiation Preservation of Food*. Vienna, IAEA.

McCrea, J.F., and Horon, R.F. 1962. Literature survey of viruses and rickettsiae in foods. Q.M. Research and Engineering Center, Natick, MA, Contract DA19-129-QM-1810. Report No. 4 Final.

Mee, L.K. 1987. Radiation chemistry of biopolymers. In *Radiation Chemistry, Principles and Application*. Edited by Farhataziz and M.A.J. Rogers. New York, VCH Publishers.

Menashi, W.P. 1968. Treatment of surfaces. U.S. Patent No. 3,383,163.

Midura, T.F., Kempe, L.L., Graikoski, J.T., and Milone, N.A. 1965. Resistance of *Clostridium perfringens* Type A spores to γ-radiation. Appl. Microbiol. *13*, 244.

Miller, W.S., and Berube, R. 1978. Environmental control and bioburden in manufacturing processes. In *Sterilization of Medical Products by Ionizing Radiation*. Edited by E.R.L. Gaughran and A.J. Goudie. Montreal, Multiscience Publ. Ltd.

Miyauchi, D., Eklund, M., Spinelli, J., and Stoll, N. 1964. Irradiation preservation of Pacific coast shellfish. I. Storage life of king crab meats at 33° F. and 42° F. Food Technol., *18*, 928.

Moseley, B.E.B., and Laser, H. 1965. Repair of x-ray damage in *Micrococcus radiodurans*. Proc. R. Soc. London, *162*, 210.

Mossel, D.A.A., and DeGroat, A.P. 1965. The use of pasteurizing doses of gamma-radiation for the destruction of salmonellae and other enterobacteraceae in some foods of low water activity. In *Radiation Preservation of Foods*. NAS/NRC Publ. 1273.

Murray, R.G.E. 1986. Family II. Deinoccaceae. In *Bergey's Manual of Systematic Bacteriology*. Vol. 2. Baltimore, Williams & Wilkins, p. 356.

Nishimura, Y., Ino, T., and Iizuka, H. 1988. *Acinetobacter radioresistens* isolated from cotton and soil. Int. J. Syst. Bacteriol. *38*, 209.

Oliver, R., and Tomlinson, A.H. 1960. The sterilization of surgical rubber gloves and plastic tubing by means of ionizing radiation. J. Hyg. Camb., *58*, 465.

Osterberg, B. 1974. Radiation sensitivity of the microbial flora present on suture material prior to irradiation. Acta Pharm. Suecica, *11*, 53.

Osterberg, B. 1973. Microbiological evaluation of suture items before radiation sterilization. Appl. Microbiol., *26*, 354.

Oyaizu, H., et al. 1987. A radiation-resistant rod-shaped bacterium, *Deinobacter grandis* gen. nov., sp. nov., with peptidoglycan containing ornithine. Int. J. Syst. Bacteriol., *37*, 62.

Patel, U.D., Govindarajan, P., and Dave, P.J. 1989. Inactivation of aflotoxin B_1 by using the synergistic effect of hydrogen peroxide and gamma radiation. Appl. Environ. Microbiol., *55*, 465.

Phillips, G.O. 1973. Medicines and pharmaceutical base materials. In *Manual on Radiation Sterilization of Medical and Biological Materials*. Tech. Rept. Ser. No. 149. Vienna, IAEA, p. 207.

Powell, D.B., and Bridges, B.A. 1960. Processing by irradiation. I. Sterilization of medical and pharmaceutical products. Radiat. Res., *13*, 151.

Prince, H.N., and Rubino, J.R. 1984. Bioburden dynamics: the viability of microorganisms on devices before and after sterilization. Med. Dev. Diag. Ind., *6*, 47.

Pruthi, J.S. 1980. *Spices and Condiments: Chemistry, Microbiology, Technology*. New York, Academic Press.

Roberts, T.A., and Ingram, M. 1965. Radiation resistance of spores of Clostridium species in aqueous suspension. J. Food Sci., *30*, 879.

Roberts, T.A., Ingram, M., and Skulberg, A. 1965. The resistance of spores of *Clostridium botulinum* type E to heat and irradiation and the resistance of *Clostridium botulinum* type E toxin to radiation. J. Appl. Bacteriol., *28*, 125.

Ronsivalli, L.J., Steinberg, M.A., and Seagram, H.L. 1965. Radiation preservation of fish of the northwest Atlantic and the Great Lakes. In *Radiation Preservation of Foods*. NAS/NRC Publ. 1273.

Ross, E.W. 1976. On the statistical analysis of inoculated packs. J. Food Sci., *41*, 578.

Ross, E.W. 1974. Statistical estimation of 12D for radappertized foods. J. Food Sci., *39*, 800.

Sanders, S.W., and Maxcy, R.B. 1979. Patterns of cell division, DNA base compositions and fine structures of some radiation-resistant vegetative bacteria found in food. Appl. Environ. Microbiol., *37*, 159.

Schmidt, C.F., and Nank, W.K. 1960. Radiation sterilization of food. I. Procedures for the evaluation of the radiation resistance of spores of *Clostridium botulinum* in food products. Food Res., *25*, 321.

Schmidt, C.F., Nank, W.K., and Lechowich, R.V. 1962. Radiation sterilization of food. II. Some aspects of the growth, sporulation, and radiation resistance of spores of *Clostridium botulinum*, type E. J. Food Sci., *27*, 77.

Shea, K.G. 1965. The USAEC program on food irradiation. In *Radiation Preservation of Foods*. NAS/NRC Publ. 1273.

Silberstein, O., Kahan, J., Penniman, J., and Henzi, W. 1979. Irradiation of

onion powder: Effects on taste and aroma characteristics. J. Food Sci., *44*, 971.

Silverman, J. 1979. Advances in radiation processing. In *Trans. 2nd Internatl. Mtg. Radiation Processing*. Radiat. Phys. Chem., Vol. 14.

Silverman, G. 1978. Radiation sterilization-process development. In *Proc. of Educational Conference Sterile Products*. Detroit, Biomed. Div. Am. Soc. Qual. Control. p. 29.

Sinskey, J., Pablo, I.S., Silverman, G.J., and Ronsivalli, L. 1967. Effect of packaging on the major microbial flora of irradiated haddock. Nature, *213*, 425.

Sparrow, A.H., Underbrink, A.G., and Sparrow, R.C. 1967. Chromosomes and cellular radiosensitivity. I. The relationship of D_0 to chromosome volume and complexity in seventy-nine different organisms. Radiat. Res., *32*, 915.

Spinelli, J., Ecklund, M., Stoll, N., and Miyauchi, D. 1965. Irradiation preservation of Pacific coast fish and shellfish. Food Technol., *19*, 126–130.

Stumbo, C.R. 1973. *Thermobacteriology in Food Processing*. New York, Academic Press.

Stumbo, C.R., Murphy, J.R., and Cochran, J. 1950. Nature of thermal death time curves for PA 3679 and *Clostridium botulinum*. Food Technol., *4*, 321.

Sullivan, R., et al. 1971. Inactivation of thirty viruses by gamma radiation. Appl. Microbiol., *22*, 61.

Swallow, A.J. 1977. Chemical effects of irradiation. In *Radiation Chemistry of Major Food Components*. Edited by P.S. Elias and A.J. Cohen. New York, Elsevier Scientific Publ. Co., p. 5.

Sztanyik, L.B. 1974. Application of ionizing radiation to sterilization. In *Sterilization by Ionizing Radiation*. Edited by E.R.L. Gaughran and A.J. Goudie. Montreal, Multiscience Publ. Ltd.

Tallentire, A., and Khan, A.A. 1978. The sub-process dose in defining the degree of sterility assurance. In *Sterilization of Medical Products by Ionizing Radiation*. Edited by E.R.L. Gaughran and A.J. Goudie. Montreal, Multiscience Publ. Ltd.

Takehisa, M., and Machi, S. 1987. Radiation processing and sterilization. In *Radiation Chemistry, Principles and Application*. Edited by Farhataziz and M.A.J. Rogers. New York, VCH Publishers.

Taub, I.A., et al. 1979. Effect of irradiation on meat proteins. Food Technol., *33*, 184.

Thornley, M.J. 1963. Microbiological aspects of the use of irradiation for the elimination of salmonellae from foods and feeding stuffs. IAEA Tech. Rep. Ser. 22.

Town, C.D., Smith, K.C., and Kaplan, H.S. 1971. Production and repair of radiochemical damage in *Escherichia coli* deoxyribonucleic acid; its modification by culture conditions and relation to survival. J. Bacteriol., *105*, 127.

Truelsen, T.A. 1963. Radiation pasteurization of fresh fruits and vegetables. Food Technol., *17*, 336.

Urbain, W.M. 1966. Technical and economic considerations in the preservation of meats and poultry by ionizing radiation. In *Food Irradiation*. Vienna, IAEA.

Van Winkle, W., Borick, P.M., and Fogarty, M. 1967. Destruction of radiation-resistant microorganisms on surgical sutures by ^{60}Co-irradiation under manufacturing conditions. In *Radiosterilization of Medical Products*. Vienna, IAEA.

Vereshchinskii, I.V., and Pikaev, A.K. 1964. *Introduction to Radiation Chemistry*. New York, Daniel Davey & Company.

Wagenaar, R.O., and Dack, G.M. 1960. Studies on type A *Clostridium botulinum* toxin by irradiation with cobalt-60. Food Res., *25*, 279.

Webb, R.B. 1964. Physical components of radiation damage in cells. In *Physical Processes in Radiation Biology*. Edited by L. Augustein, R. Mason, and B. Rosenberg. New York, Academic Press.

Welch, A.B., and Maxcy, R.B. 1975. Characterization of radiation-resistant vegetative bacteria in beef. Appl. Microbiol., *30*, 242.

Whitby, J.L. 1978. Memorandum to AAMI Subcommittee on Radiation Sterilization.

Whitby, J.L., and Gelda, A.K. 1979. Use of incremental doses of Cobalt-60 radiation as a means to determine radiation sterilization dose. J. Parent. Drug Assoc., *33*, 144.

White, J.D.M. 1973. Biological control of industrial gamma radiation sterilization. In *Industrial Sterilization*. Durham, Duke University Press.

CHAPTER 33

STERILIZATION WITH ETHYLENE OXIDE AND OTHER GASES

Anthony N. Parisi and William E. Young

Little was it realized when ethylene oxide (ETO) was discovered, how important a role this chemical would play in the health care of the world populations (Wurtz, 1859). This chemical has made the medical device industry as it is known today possible by allowing manufacturers to use low cost, thermoplastic materials for sterile disposable medical devices. It took some 64 years after ETO's discovery, however, before its biocidal activity was first reported. These initial reports were of its activity as an insecticide (Cotton and Roark, 1928). Not long after that the first patents were applied for the use of ethylene oxide for the destruction of microorganisms in spices and gums. Griffith and Hall (1940, 1943) in these patents were the first to describe an industrial gaseous ethylene oxide sterilization process. The process they described employed vacuum chambers and pure (100%) ethylene oxide gas. Considerable experimentation took place in the 1940s and 1950s that demonstrated that laboratory plastics, medical and biologic preparations, hospital bedding, plastic bandages, medical instrumentation, surgical transplants, and many other items could be successfully sterilized using this chemical agent. ETO is the primary gas used in hospitals to sterilize items that cannot be sterilized by steam. In addition, those industries supplying the hospitals with medical devices use ETO sterilization for products that are sensitive to the heat of steam sterilization or that contain materials not compatible with radiation sterilization.

The sterilization of medical products by other gaseous agents such as propylene oxide, formaldehyde, methyl bromide, and beta-propiolactone has not been as extensive, but these agents have been used in disinfection applications (Russell, 1976; Bruch, 1961; Bruch and Bruch, 1970). In particular, propylene oxide has been used for the sterilization of food products. New technologies emerging in the late 1980s and early 1990s are discussed; the reader is referred to Bruch and Bruch (1970) and Phillips (1977), who have reviewed earlier work with ETO and other gaseous agents for disinfection and sterilization, and to the Health Industries Manufacturers Association for a look into the near future (HIMA, 1989).

This chapter includes information on microbial activity of ETO, biologic indicators, worker safety, toxicity, sterilization equipment, cycle development, process validation, routine process control, emission control, and sterilant residues.

ETHYLENE OXIDE

Ethylene oxide, also known as epoxyethane or dimethylene oxide, is a colorless gas. It reacts with many chemicals such as alcohols, amines, organic acids, and amides, and is used in the manufacture of many surface-active agents. The physical properties of ETO are listed in Table 33–1. Ethylene oxide is soluble in water at 10°C and will form polyglycols in the presence of a base, water, or both. The vapors of this gas are flammable and explosive; however, the fire hazards can be reduced by using ETO diluted with carbon dioxide (Coward and Jones, 1952) or fluorocarbon (Kaye, 1959; Haenni et al., 1959). Based on information developed in the 1980s, this gas has now been classified as both a mutagen and carcinogen, resulting in stricter regulations on its use. The physical properties of some ETO mixtures currently available are listed in Table 33–2. The use of fluorocarbon mixtures over carbon dioxide mixtures for sterilization offers many advantages; however, because of recent implications of halocarbons and their effect on the ozone layer, restrictions on its use are rapidly emerging (EPA, 1988, 1989). A more detailed list of the properties of ethylene oxide is given by Cawse et al. (1980).

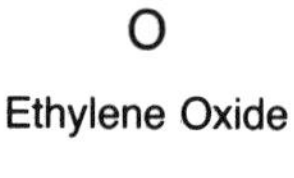

$$H_2C - CH_2$$
$$\diagdown \diagup$$
$$O$$

Ethylene Oxide

Table 33–1. *Physical Properties of Ethylene Oxide**

LIQUID

Molecular weight	44.05
Apparent specific gravity at 20/20°C (68/68°F)	0.8711
Δ Sp. gr./Δt at 20° to 30°C (68° to 86°F)	0.00140
Coefficient of expansion at 20°C (68°F)	0.00161
Water solubility	Complete
Heat of vaporization at 1 atm	6.1 kcal/g-mole
Surface tension	28.0 dynes per cm
Viscosity at 10°C (50°F)	0.28 cps
Vapor pressure at 20°C (68°F)	1095 mm Hg
Boiling point at 760 mm.	10.4°C (50.7°F)
at 300 mm.	−11.0°C (−12.2°F)
at 10 mm.	−66°C (−86.8°F)
Δ BP/ΔP at 740 to 760 mm Hg.	0.033°C per mm
Freezing point	−112.6°C (−170.7°F)
Refractive index, n_o at 7°C (44.6°F)	1.3597
Heat of fusion	1.236 kcal/g-mole
Specific heat at 20°C (68°F)	0.44 cal per g per °C
Explosive limits in air at 760 mm Hg..upper	100% by volume
lower	3% by volume
Flash point, Tag open cup (ASTM Method D 1310)	< −18°C (<0°F)

VAPOR

Critical temperature	196.0°C (384.8°F)
Critical pressure	1043 psia
Autoignition temperature in air at 1 atm	429°C (804°F)
Decomposition temperature of pure vapor at 1 atm	560°C (1040°F)
Heat of combustion of gas, gross	312.15 kcal/g-mole
Heat of formation	12.2 kcal/g-mole

*Data from Union Carbide Corp., New York

Table 33–2. *Properties of Ethylene Oxide Mixtures*

	Carbon Dioxide Mixtures			Fluorocarbon Mixture
Ethylene Oxide				
% by Weight	10	20	30	12
% Gas Volume	10	20	30	27
Carbon Dioxide				
% by Weight	90	80	70	—
% Gas Volume	90	80	70	—
Fluorocarbon 12				
% by Weight	—	—	—	88
% Gas Volume	—	—	—	73
Vapor Pressure (full cylinder) at 21°C (70°F), psig	750	675	600	60
Ethylene Oxide, mg/L at 54°C (130°F)	470 (29.4 psig)	1020 (33.0 psig)	1167 (22.0 psig)	600 (7.3 psig)
Flammability	Nonflammable	16.5 to 43.5% in air with spark ignition at atmospheric pressure.	Approximately the same flammability range as the 80/20 mixture.	Nonflammable in storage and shipment and in concentration used in practice in ordinary rooms or vaults or in suitable vacuum fumigation vaults.

(Mixtures available from Union Carbide Corp., Linde Division, South Plainfield, N.J.)

The microbiologic activity of gaseous agents has been the subject of many articles that review the sporicidal and bactericidal activity of gaseous agents (Phillips, 1952, 1968, 1977; Bruch, 1961; Kereluk and Lloyd, 1969; Bruch and Bruch, 1970; Kereluk, 1971; Russell, 1976). The objective of this section is to expand the database on the activity of ETO and other gaseous agents.

Phillips (1977) suggested that the microbiologic activity of ETO was due to alkylation of sulfhydryl, amino, carboxyl, phenolic, and hydroxyl groups in the spore or vegetative cell. Alkylation is the replacement of a hydrogen atom with an alkyl group. In a bacterial cell or spore, this type of substitution can cause injury or death.

Experimental evidence indicates that the reaction of ETO with nucleic acids is the primary cause of bactericidal and sporicidal activity. Alkylation of the guanosine triphosphate of DNA in *Salmonella senftenberg* was shown by Michael and Stumbo (1970) to cause the cells to lose the power of reproduction. In addition, Winaro and Stumbo (1971) showed that the lethal effect of ETO on spores of *Clostridium botulinum* Type A was due to alkylation of guanine and adenine components of DNA.

ETO is used as a sterilant because of its ability to inactivate all microorganisms. Phillips was one of the first investigators to quantitate the ETO resistance of bacterial cells and spores (Bruch, 1961). The earlier literature showed that bacterial spores are more resistant to ETO than bacterial cells, yeasts, and molds are (Bruch, 1961). Phillips (1977) has indicated that bacterial spores are five to ten times more resistant to ETO than bacterial vegetative cells are.

A summary of published reports on microbial resistance to ETO is shown in Table 33–3. Only general statements can be made about these data because the experimental methods and exposure conditions vary from study to study. Kereluk et al. (1970) found that the spores of *Bacillus subtilis* var. niger exhibited higher resistance to ETO exposure than the spores of *Clostridium sporogenes*, *Bacillus stearothermophilus*, or *B. pumilus* did. The vegetative cells tested in this study had similar resistance to ETO when compared to the spore form, except for *B. subtilis* var. niger spores, which exhibited greater resistance to ETO than the vegetative form did. Other microorganisms that have been tested, such as spores of *B. coagulans*, conidiospores of *Aspergillus niger*, vegetative cells of *Lactobacillus brevis*, *Leuconostoc mesenteroides*, *Hansenula anomala*, and *Saccharomyces cerevisiae*, have been shown to have a lower resistance than the spores of *Bacillus subtilis* do (Blake and Stumbo, 1970; Liu et al., 1968; Dadd and Daley, 1980).

In addition to being effective against bacteria, molds, and yeasts, ETO has also been shown to inactivate viruses. Studies have been conducted on the use of ETO as a sterilizing agent for blood and plasma, insect viruses, animal viruses, and human viruses (Klarenbeek and Van Tongeren, 1954; Tompkins and Cantwell, 1975; Savan, 1955; Matthews and Hofstad, 1953; Sidwell et al., 1969;

Hartman et al., 1955). A summary of some of the studies on virus inactivation is shown in Table 33–4.

The consistent ETO resistance pattern of *Bacillus subtilis* var. niger (*globigii*) spores is the basis for the USP XXI recommendation that this organism be used as the biologic indicator of choice in monitoring of ETO sterilization cycles (USP, 1985).

PROPYLENE OXIDE

Propylene oxide is also known as epoxy propane. For its chemical and physical properties the reader is referred to the Merck Index (1983).

$$H_3C—CH——CH_2$$
$$\diagdown\ \diagup$$
$$O$$

Propylene Oxide

Propylene oxide hydrolyzes in the presence of moisture to form propylene glycol, which is nontoxic.

Gaseous propylene oxide (PO) is used to sterilize food products (Alguire, 1963). Liquid propylene oxide has also been used as a sterilizing agent for disinfectants (Hart and Brown, 1974; Hart and Ng, 1975). Blanchard and Hanlin (1973) showed that PO was effective in inactivating microorganisms on pecans. Bruch and Koesterer (1961) showed that PO was effective as a decontaminant for flaked and powdered foods, but not for dried foods, as is ethylene oxide. They also showed that PO was more active at lower relative humidity (RH) for *B. subtilis* var. niger spores. Himmelfarb et al. (1962), however, found the opposite for *B. subtilis* spores and gram-positive cocci. Additional information on *B. subtilis* var. niger inactivation by PO is contained in a more recent report by Tawaratani et al. (1981).

A summary of some data on the microbiologic activity of propylene oxide is presented in Table 33–5. Similar to that of ETO, the mode of action of PO has been shown to be due to the alkylation of guanine of DNA that results in single-strand breaks of DNA (Tawaratani et al., 1980; Tawaratani and Shibasaki, 1973).

FORMALDEHYDE

$$H_2C = O$$

Formaldehyde

Formaldehyde is more widely known as a fumigant for buildings and rooms, especially in poultry husbandry (Russell, 1976). It has also been used in low-temperature steam-formaldehyde sterilization in Europe.

Formaldehyde has been shown to be effective against bacteria and bacterial spores (Acklund et al., 1980; Braswell et al., 1970) and vegetative bacterial cells (Williams, 1980). Acklund et al. (1980) showed that at 20°C and a relative humidity of approximately 100%, a 6-log reduction of *B. subtilis* spores was obtained after 1.5 hours exposure to 300 µg/L whereas at 250 µg/L, only a 4-log

Table 33–3. *Ethylene Oxide Resistance of Vegetative Cells and Bacterial Spores*

Organism	Carrier Material	Test Temperature (°F)	Relative Humidity (%)	Ethylene Oxide Conc. (mg/L)	D value (min)	Reference
Bacillus subtilis var. niger	Paper	130	30–50	500	3.5	Kereluk and Gammon, 1973
	Plastic	130	30–50	500	6.7	Kereluk et al., 1970
	Paper	130	60 ± 10	600	2.1–2.4	Reich, 1980
	Paper	130	65 ± 15	600	2.2–5.8	Gillis et al., 1976
	Paper	130/140	40–60	540–580	2	Jones and Adams, 1981
	Paper	130	60 ± 10	600 ± 20	3.0–3.4	Caputo et al., 1980
	Paper	130	50 ± 10	1200	1.8	Reich, 1980
	Paper	118	40	300/900	7.6/3.5	Caputo and Mascoli, 1980
	Paper	90/150	40	500	13.0/1.6	Caputo and Mascoli, 1980
B. subtilis (ATCC 9524)	Paper	104	30–35	700	14.5–15.3	Marletta and Stumbo, 1970
	Paper	104/176	30–35	700	14.7/0.7	Liu et al., 1968
B. coagulans	Paper	86/140	30–35	700	10.4/3.07	Blake and Stumbo, 1970
B. stearothermophilus	Paper	130	30–50	500	2.6	Kereluk et al., 1970
B. pumilus	Paper	130	30–50	500	2.2	Kereluk et al., 1970
Clostridium botulinum	Paper	104	47	700	11.0/11.5	Savage and Stumbo, 1971
Type A (strain 62)		104	11–33	700 ± 20	6.0/11.8	Winaro and Stumbo, 1971
	Paper	122	33	700	5.75	Kuzminski et al., 1969
		122	73	700	5.10	
		158	33	700	1.74	
		158	73	700	1.95	
C. sporogenes	Paper	130	30–50	500	2.8–3.3	Kereluk and Lloyd, 1969
Salmonella senftenberg	—	104	11–33	700 ± 20	3.3–5.9	Michael and Stumbo, 1970
Escherichia coli	—	104	11	700 ± 20	2.9	Michael and Stumbo, 1970
Streptococcus faecalis	Plastic	130	30–50	500	2.0–3.75	Kereluk et al., 1970
Leuconostoc mesenteroides	Paper	86	30–35	700	3.45	Blake and Stumbo, 1970
Lactobacillus brevis	Paper	86	30–35	700	5.88	Blake and Stumbo, 1970
Micrococcus radiodurans	Plastic	130	30–35	500	3.0	Kereluk et al., 1970
Aspergillus niger conidiospores	Paper	86	30–35	700	11*	Blake and Stumbo, 1970
Hansenula anomala	Paper	86	30–35	700	6*	Blake and Stumbo, 1970
Saccharomyces cerevisiae	Paper	86	30–35	700	5.5*	Blake and Stumbo, 1970

*Time for 99.9% reduction in population.

reduction was obtained after 6 hours of exposure. As with ETO, propylene oxide (PO), and beta-propiolactone (BPL), relative humidity of the environment is critical for the optimum bactericidal activity of formaldehyde (Hoffman and Spiner, 1970). The mechanism of action of formaldehyde is assumed to be due to the reaction with cell protein and DNA or RNA (Russell, 1976).

BETA-PROPIOLACTONE

$$H_2C — CH_2$$
$$O — C = O$$

Beta-Propiolactone

Beta-propiolactone (BPL) has been recommended as a substitute for formaldehyde in the disinfection of chamber rooms and buildings (Hoffman and Warshowsky, 1958). Hoffman and Warshowsky indicated that beta-propiolactone was approximately 4000 times more active than ETO and 25 times more effective than formalde-

hyde. BPL is not recommended as a substitute for ETO because of its lack of "penetrating power." Also, it has been shown to be carcinogenic in mice, and therefore a probable safety hazard (Searle, 1961).

The microbiologic activity of BPL is due primarily to alkylation of DNA (Kubinski and Kubinski, 1978). The resistance of *Bacillus subtilis* spores exposed to beta-propiolactone (Table 33–5) has been shown to be greater than that of *B. stearothermophilus* and *Clostridium botulinum* (Curran and Evans, 1956). As in ethylene oxide sterilization, the control of relative humidity is critical in sterilization using beta-propiolactone (Hoffman, 1968). Also, this gas has been shown to be effective against viruses (Dawson et al., 1959; Yabrov et al., 1978; Dawson et al., 1960; Garlick and Avery, 1976; Parker, 1975).

EMERGING TECHNOLOGIES

Chlorine Dioxide

Chlorine dioxide (ClO_2) has long been used for disinfecting drinking water and bleaching paper pulp. The

Table 33–4. *Resistance of Viruses to Ethylene Oxide*

Virus	Carrier Material	Test Condition	Relative Humidity (%)	Ethylene Oxide Conc.	Reduction in Infectivity Titer	Reference
Influenza B	Horse serum	60 minutes at 39°F then 95°F for 24 hours	—	10,000 mg/L	$\geq 10^{4.7}$	Ginsberg and Wilson, 1950
Influenza A	Horse serum	60 minutes at 39°F then 95°F for 24 hours	—	10,000 mg/L	$\geq 10^3$	Ginsberg and Wilson, 1950
Newcastle	Horse serum	60 minutes at 39°F then 95°F for 24 hours	—	10,000 mg/L	$\geq 10^6$	Ginsberg and Wilson, 1950
Mouse encephalomyelitis	Horse serum	60 minutes at 39°F then 95°F for 24 hours	—	10,000 mg/L	$\geq 10^{2.6}$	Ginsberg and Wilson, 1950
Foot-and-mouth	Tissue suspension	Room temperature	—	540 mg/L	$\geq 10^{5.8}$	Fellowes, 1960
Vaccinia	10% Rabbit	—	—	1% v/v	$\geq 10^5$	Wilson and Bruno, 1950
Vaccinia	dried	6 hr at 77°F		1500 mg/L	$\geq 10^3$	Jorgensen and Lund, 1972
Equine encephalomyelitis	water	1 hr at 64° to 68°F		10%	$\geq 10^4$	Bucca, 1956
Coxsackie B3	dried	6 hr at 77°F	—	1500 mg/L	$\geq 10^3$	Jorgensen and Lund, 1972
Echo II	dried	6 hr at 77°F	—	1500 mg/L	$\geq 10^3$	
Coliphage	water and serum	98°F	50	500 mg/L	3.4–6.4 min for 90%	Gammon et al., 1971

lethal effect of chlorine dioxide in aqueous solutions is well documented (Benarde et al., 1965; Roller, 1978; Olivieri et al., 1985).

More recently, the Scopas Technology Company has investigated the use of chlorine dioxide gas to sterilize medical devices. Their studies have shown that even at low concentrations (20 mg/L), chlorine dioxide is an effective sterilant (Table 33–5). Additionally, Rosenblatt and Knapp (1988) have reported on the importance of relative humidity for microbial inactivation and conclude that 50% or higher is optimal for sterilization.

Chlorine dioxide is, however, a powerful oxidizer (Sax,

Table 33–5. *Resistance of Bacteria and Virus To Other Chemical Sterilant Gases*

Gaseous Agent	Bacteria/Virus	Carrier Material	Test Temp. (°C)	Gas Conc.	Relative Humidity (%)	D-value (min.)	Reference
Propylene oxide	B. subtilis var. niger	Paper	36–38	410 mg/L	80/90	144/216	Bruch and Koesterer, 1961
	B. subtilis var. niger	Paper	36–38	830 mg/L	80/90	96/120	Bruch and Koesterer, 1961
	B. subtilis	Wool patches	35	1 cm³/L	1/98	974/54	Himmelfarb et al., 1962
	B. stearothermophilus	Wool patches	35	1 cm³/L	1/98	112/15	Himmelfarb et al., 1962
	E. coli	Wool patches	35	1 cm³/L	1/65	24/6	Himmelfarb et al., 1962
	S. aureus	Wool patches	35	1 cm³/L	1/98	155/8	Himmelfarb et al., 1962
Beta propiolactone	B. subtilis var. niger	Cloth patches	27 ± 2	0.1 mg/L	80 ± 5	42	Hoffman and Warshowsky, 1958
	Encephalomyelitis virus	Cotton patches	26	2.4 mg/L	90	0.5*	Dawson et al., 1959
Chlorine dioxide	B. subtilis	Porcelain	27–30	20 mg/L	80/90	23.6	Rosenblatt and Knapp, 1988
	C. sporogenes	Porcelain	27–30	20 mg/L	80/90	22.1	Rosenblatt and Knapp, 1988
	S. aureus	Porcelain	27–30	20 mg/L	80/90	2.6	Rosenblatt and Knapp, 1988
	Ps. aeruginosa	Porcelain	27–30	20 mg/L	80/90	2.3	Rosenblatt and Knapp, 1988
Ozone	B. subtilis var. niger	Stainless steel	25 ± 2	8%†	85 ± 5	4.01	Karlson, 1988
	E. coli	Stainless steel	25 ± 2	8%	85 ± 5	0.97	Karlson, 1988
	S. aureus	Stainless steel	25 ± 2	8%	85 ± 5	<0.5	Karlson, 1988
	Ps. aeruginosa	Stainless steel	25 ± 2	8%	85 ± 5	1.74	Karlson, 1988

*LD_{50}.
†Percentage by weight.

1979), which must be taken into consideration when choosing the product and packaging materials. Because the reactivity is selective, some materials, such as titanium, stainless steel, silicone rubber, ceramics, polyvinyl chloride, and polyethylene are unaffected by exposure to the gas.

Ozone

Like chlorine dioxide, ozone (O_3) has also been used to treat drinking water and to bleach paper pulp. In addition, it is used to sterilize sewage water and treat waste gas.

Ozone is not a new sterilant. Studies performed on the water supply of Lille, France in 1899 (Celmette and Roux) demonstrated that ozone was an effective sterilant. What makes ozone interesting today is its potential for sterilizing medical devices. Karlson (1988) has reported the effects on a wide variety of microorganisms at concentrations ranging from 2 to 10% by weight. D-values for some of these microorganisms exposed to 8% ozone concentrations are provided in Table 33–5.

Because of the highly oxidative properties of ozone, the use of this sterilant appears to be well directed for resterilizing hospital instruments composed of materials such as noble metals, titanium, stainless steel, silicone rubber, ceramics, polyvinyl chloride, and polyurethane.

Vapor Phase Hydrogen Peroxide

Liquid phase hydrogen peroxide has been a widely used surface disinfectant for aseptic food and dairy packaging. It is also used for processing systems, spacecraft hardware, hemodialyzers, and sewage effluent, as well as for numerous other living and nonliving surfaces (Toledo et al., 1973; Wardle and Renninger, 1975; Spaulding et al., 1977). One of the earliest recorded uses of liquid hydrogen peroxide as a bactericide was published in 1883 for the preservation of milk (Schrodt, 1883). Since then, there have been numerous publications on liquid hydrogen peroxide sterilization and disinfection (King et al., 1969; Greene and Urban, 1985; Ito, 1973). For a comprehensive early literature review on liquid hydrogen peroxide antimicrobial activity, we refer the reader to von Bockelman and von Bockelman (1972).

A new patented sterilization system based on a vapor phase of hydrogen peroxide has been approved by the United States Environmental Protection Agency (HIMA, 1989). This system provides a rapid, low-temperature technique which, because of its low toxicity, eliminates much of the potential public health hazard associated with sterilants such as formaldehyde and ethylene oxide. The A.O.A.C. sporicidal results have revealed that the vapor phase of hydrogen peroxide is as highly sporicidal, as indicated in the patents that recently discovered this technology. Because of the low dose needed to sterilize surfaces, this sterilization technique opens the door to in situ and in vivo sterilization. A number of prominent biotechnology, pharmaceutical, food, and scientific laboratory companies have begun to explore this new sterilant, because contamination is a severe problem in their industries.

Gas Plasma Sterilization

A new sterilization process based on gas plasma technology was patented in 1987 by Surgikos, Inc., a Johnson and Johnson Company (Jacobs and Lin, 1987; HIMA, 1989). The process utilizes radio frequency energy and hydrogen peroxide vapor to create a low-temperature hydrogen peroxide gas plasma and achieve relatively rapid sterilization. The sterilization cycle consists of the following steps: Articles to be sterilized are placed in the chamber, the door is closed, and a vacuum is drawn within the chamber. A solution of hydrogen peroxide is injected into the chamber and vaporized. The vapor diffuses throughout the chamber and surrounds the items to be sterilized. At the end of the diffusion phase, radio frequency is applied to the chamber. The radio waves break apart the hydrogen peroxide vapor into reactive species (free radicals), which form a gas plasma. The gas plasma is maintained long enough to interact with and kill microorganisms. During this gas plasma phase, the hydrogen peroxide is continuously depleted as the active (free radical) components recombine into oxygen and water. At the completion of the plasma phase, the source of the radio waves is turned off, the vacuum is released, and the chamber is returned to atmospheric pressure by introducing filtered air. Because the process temperature does not exceed 40°C, the technology is particularly well suited to materials that cannot be steam sterilized.

FACTORS AFFECTING MICROBIOLOGIC ACTIVITY

The major factors that affect the inactivation of microorganisms by ETO are gas concentration, temperature, relative humidity, and exposure time. The substrate or "carrier" material that contains the microorganisms may also affect the inactivation rate.

Gas Concentration

Survivor curves for the inactivation of *Bacillus subtilis* var. niger (*globigii*) spores at different ETO concentrations are shown in Figure 33–1 (Caputo and Rohn, 1982). As the gas concentration increases from 50 to 500 mg/L, the inactivation rate increases significantly. At gas concentrations greater than 500 mg/L, there is no significant increase in the rate of spore inactivation. Kereluk et al. (1970) showed that, for *B. subtilis* var. niger spores, for gas concentrations of 200 to 1200 mg/L, the most dramatic decrease in resistance occurs when the given concentration is increased from 200 to 400 mg/L at 54.4°C. At specific temperatures and above a certain concentration of ETO, Ernst and Shull (1962) showed that increasing concentrations no longer increased inactivation (zero order). They indicated that for each concentration of ETO there is a minimum Q_{10} value (factor by which, for every 10°C change in the temperature, the inactivation rate changes). A Q_{10} of 1.8 was reported in their

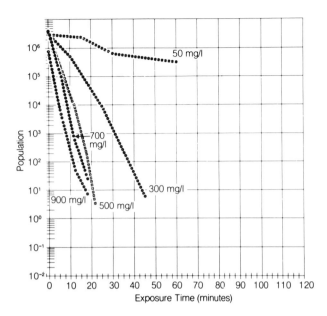

Fig. 33–1. Inactivation of *Bacillus subtilis* var. niger (globigii) spores at different ethylene concentrations at 117.5°F and 40% relative humidity.

study, in which the concentration was greater than the minimum concentration needed for zero order. Larger Q_{10} values (2.3 to 3.2) were found for temperatures at which the concentration was limiting to the reaction rate.

Temperature

Inactivation of *B. subtilis* var. niger spores at various temperatures are shown in Figure 33–2 (Caputo and Rohn, 1982). The Q_{10} value for this data is approximately 1.9. This corresponds to the value reported by Ernst and

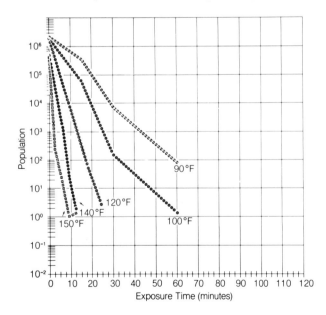

Fig. 33–2. Inactivation of *Bacillus subtilis* var. niger (globigii) spores at different temperatures at 500 mg/L ethylene oxide and 40% relative humidity.

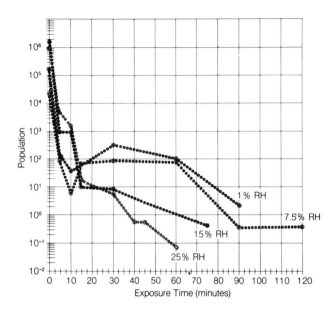

Fig. 33–3. Inactivation of *Bacillus subtilis* var. niger (globigii) spores at relative humidities of 1 to 25% at 500 mg/L ethylene oxide and 117.5°F.

Shull (1962) of 1.8 for *B. subtilis* var. niger and 2.18 reported for *B. subtilis* (ATCC 9524) by Liu et al. (1968). A Q_{10} value of 1.55 to 1.64 has been reported for spores of *B. coagulans* (Blake and Stumbo, 1970), and a Q_{10} of 1.7 to 2.2 for spores of *Clostridium botulinum* (Kuzminski et al., 1969). These data indicate that, in general, for every 10°C change in temperature, the inactivation rate for spores to ETO will double when the concentration is not limiting.

Relative Humidity

Relative humidity (RH) has long been recognized as a critical factor in ETO sterilization. Tawaratani et al. (1980b) concluded that the difference in sensitivity of spores to gaseous sterilants at various relative humidities was due mainly to the difference of the spore water content, and that the amount of gas absorbed by the spores was secondary. They found that a maximum value of lethality for RH was 33%. This confirmed the work of Gilbert et al. (1964), who found that *Bacillus subtilis* spores, preconditioned and exposed at the same relative humidity (range 1 to 98%), were inactivated more readily at 33% RH. At humidities of 1 to 22%, the survivor curves were concave upward (nonlinear). Spores preconditioned at low relative humidities or exposed to a vacuum prior to exposure at 33% RH had increased resistance, and the survivor curves were also concave upward. It was found that the effect could be reversed by excessive wetting of the spores. Studies by Caputo and Rohn (1982) demonstrated that at humidities between 30 and 75%, the inactivation curves were linear, whereas below 30%, nonlinearity exists (Figs. 33–3 and 33–4).

Kaye and Phillips (1949) have demonstrated the need for relative humidities of at least 30% for effective ETO sterilization. Kereluk et al. (1970) concluded that the

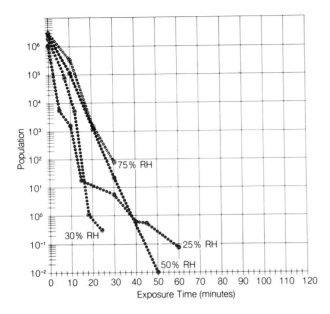

Fig. 33–4. Inactivation of *Bacillus subtilis* var. niger (globigii) spores at relative humidities of 25 to 75% at 500 mg/L ethylene oxide and 117.5°F.

Table 33–6. *Resistance (D Values) of* Bacillus subtilis *(globigii) Spores on Various Carrier Materials*

Carrier	Test Conditions*			
	300 mg/L ETO		600 mg/L ETO	
	41°C	52°C	41°C	52°C
Paper	17.0	10.6	7.1	3.7
Dialysis Membrane	53.5	12.4	19.4	6.8
Sheet PVC	10.9	4.6	6.3	2.6
Silicon Rubber	5.6	7.6	4.1	4.3
PVC Tubing	14.5	4.1	4.8	4.4
Nylon Sutures	15.3	3.8	4.3	2.6
Aluminum	26.0	8.8	7.0	4.6
Polyester	10.0	5.0	5.5	5.5
Natural Rubber	10.5	5.2	3.9	1.9
Siliconized Rubber	9.4	5.7	3.9	2.5

*RH = 50%, D values in minutes.

water content of the microenvironment of the spores had a greater influence on ETO spore resistance than the relative humidity in the sterilizing atmosphere. The requirement for the presence of water for ETO sterilization is not surprising, because water will react with ETO to open the epoxide ring (Politzer et al., 1978) and allow it to react with the cell. Another benefit of humidifying with steam is to help bring the materials being sterilized to process temperature.

Carrier Material

The ETO resistance of spores has been shown to be affected by carrier material for the spores (Bruch and Bruch, 1970). The effect of the type of carrier or spore substrate material on spore D values is shown in Table 33–6 from data by Rohn et al. (1981). It was reported that a possible cause of the differences in substrate results is related to the differences in absorbency among the test substrate materials. Therefore, the ratio of reactants (i.e., ETO and water) delivered to the spores during exposure is affected by the absorbing characteristics of the carrier material. The difference in resistance does not appear to be due to occluded spores, because no evidence of this was found on scanning electron micrographs of spores on plastic, paper, or aluminum (Figs. 33–5, 33–6, 33–7).

Microorganism

The water content of the spore is critical in ETO sterilization, as mentioned earlier in the discussion of relative humidity. In addition, the cleanliness of the cell suspension has been shown to significantly influence the inactivation rate of spores or vegetative cells (Bruch and Bruch, 1970). A number of factors in the preparation of

microorganisms have been shown to affect the response of microorganisms to heat (e.g., growth medium, incubation time and temperature, and storage conditions), and it should not be unexpected that the same factors can influence the response of microorganisms to ETO. Some of these factors have yet to be investigated and

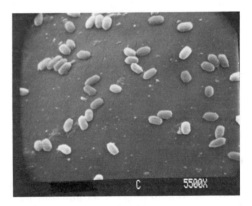

Fig. 33–5. Scanning electron micrograph of *Bacillus subtilis* var. niger (globigii) spores on dialysis membrane material.

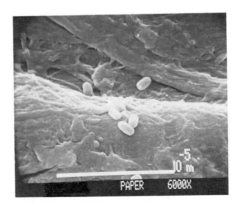

Fig. 33–6. Scanning electron micrograph of *Bacillus subtilis* var. niger (globigii) spores on a paper carrier.

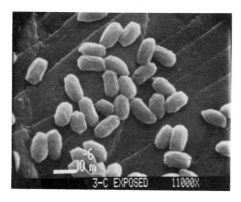

Fig. 33–7. Scanning electron micrograph of *Bacillus subtilis* var. niger (globigii) spores on an aluminum carrier.

may be found to be as critical in affecting ETO resistance as they are in affecting heat resistance.

An issue that should be carefully addressed relates to the poststerilization holding conditions for biological indicators (BIs). It has been demonstrated that microbial inactivation continues after the completion of the cycle because of residual ETO. Therefore the most rigid test of cycle effectiveness is shown when BIs are tested soon after the completion of the cycle. The possible microbiocidal effect of the test (BI) substrate outgassing should be known.

Because gas concentration, temperature, humidity, and the condition of the microorganisms can significantly affect a microorganism's response to ETO, any microorganism used to evaluate the lethal effect of an ETO sterilization cycle should be standardized (Bruch and Bruch, 1970). The USP XXI (1985) suggests testing parameters and the limits of response for spores used as ETO biological indicators.

Equipment

A variety of equipment has evolved over the years for ethylene oxide treatments. The equipment has ranged from the chamber of Griffith and Hall (1940, 1943) to the sample atmospheric pressure metal fumigation chambers and gas-tight plastic bags reported by Phillips (1977).

The basic scheme for a gas sterilizer is represented in Figure 33–8. The vessels range in size from only a few cubic feet as commonly found in laboratories and hospitals to large medical device and food processing (primarily spice decontamination) vessels up to 2000 or more cubic feet of product capacity. Regardless of the size of the vessel, the elements of the process that must be controlled are identical. An ETO sterilizer is basically a pressure vessel with the capacity to evacuate air, warm and moisturize the product uniformly, add the sterilant gas at a specific temperature, and finally, remove the gas after a specified interval.

Ethylene oxide gas sterilization vessels have changed little over the past 10 to 15 years. The major design changes that have occurred have primarily been to en-

sure the homogenicity of the sterilizer internal environment by the use of recirculation devices such as fans and external recirculation loops. An added benefit of these modifications is that temperature variability and low-sterilization-rate cold spots are reduced or eliminated.

Because of the need to minimize the potential for sterilizer operators' exposure to ETO when unloading freshly sterilized material, some sterilizers have been equipped with automatic opening doors that operate from the control panel and large exhaust systems at the distal end of the vessel. The door is opened, the evacuation begins, and fresh air uncontaminated by ETO flows past the operator doing the unloading.

When product configurations tolerate vacuums in the range of 20 to 30 mm Hg (absolute), it is most economical to use 100% ethylene oxide. It must be recognized that because the gas is highly flammable, extreme caution must be employed in process and control equipment. All parameter and control devices must be certified as safe for use in such environmental conditions.

Typical cycle profiles are shown in Figures 33–9 and 33–10.

Sterilant Mixtures

Although a number of mixtures of ethylene oxide and CO_2 have been used in the past, most have been replaced by a nonflammable mixture of 12% ethylene oxide and 88% chlorofluorocarbon (Freon). These cycles typically employ a mild initial vacuum step to remove as much air as possible, and are used to sterilize products whose componentry or packaging cannot withstand the severe vacuums associated with 100% ETO cycles.

Recent research has lead to the development of environmentally compatible cycles using nitrogen and ETO. Nitrogen-based cycles have been developed as alternatives to the ETO/Freon mixtures. The cycle employs a series of mild vacuum steps with each vacuum being replaced by nitrogen. The number of evacuation plus nitrogen backfill steps must be sufficient to ensure that the oxygen level remaining is insufficient to support combustion when the sterilant is added in the pure or 100% form.

Most cycles used today employ multiple air-wash steps after the conclusion of sterilizing gas exposure. This is to ensure that upon opening the sterilizer door, the worker is exposed to a minimal amount of ETO. Also, it has been found that the air washes help reduce product sterilant residuals.

Because most early sterilization equipment was of a simple design, the sterilization process and its control was also believed to be simple and uncomplicated. As the use of this chemical sterilant grew in popularity, scientific studies demonstrated that effective reproducible sterilization was not as uncomplicated as it was believed, and that it required the controlled interaction of the parameters of heat, moisture, and gas concentration.

As the complexities of ethylene oxide sterilization become understood, it was soon recognized that more sophisticated control of the parameters would be necessary.

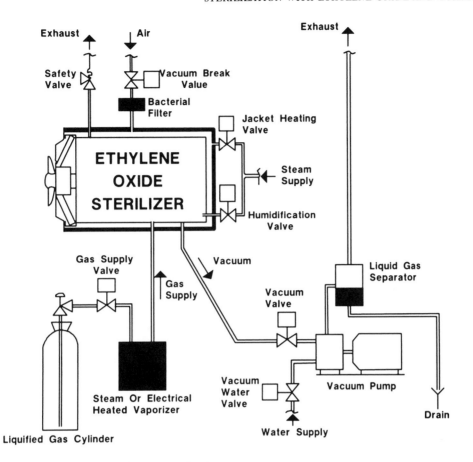

Fig. 33–8. Illustration of an ethylene oxide sterilization vessel and supportive system.

These typical sterilization control monitoring systems, although increasing in sophistication, were similar in principle and composed of several sequenced electro-mechanical devices, such as pressure switches, timers, and temperature controllers.

In sterilization processing there must be consistent assurance that multiple sterilization parameters (pressures, temperatures, times, rates, and sterilant concentrations) are adequately controlled, monitored, and doc-

umented. Table 33–7 from Burrell et al. (1979) shows that a simple ethylene oxide sterilization cycle typically requires at least 12 different hardware components. As multiplicity of cycles and additional process constraints are placed upon the various parameters, the need for increased individual components increases accordingly in both hardware components and the control system.

Some of the most noted changes and improvements in recent years have occurred in the area of sterilizer

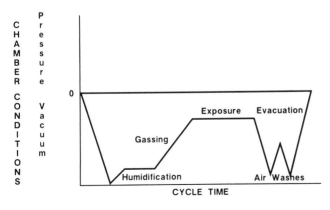

Fig. 33–9. Typical cycle dynamics for a 100% ethylene oxide sterilization cycle.

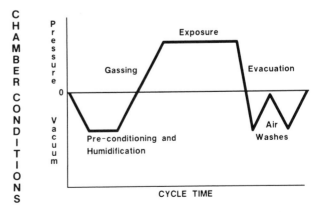

Fig. 33–10. Typical cycle dynamics for a 12/88 ethylene oxide sterilization cycle.

Table 33–7. *Electromechanical Components Required for a Simplified Ethylene Oxide Process: Minimal Controller Constraints for Sterilization Control*

Cycle Step	Pressure	Time	Temperature
Initial vacuum	PS1		
Vacuum dwell	PS2	TM1	
Steam injection	PS3		
Steam dwell		TM2	
Gas charge	PS4		TC1
Exposure period	PS5	TM3	TC2
Final vacuum	PS6		
Air inbleed	PS7		

From Burrell, R.L., Wein, R.Z., and Parisi, A.N. 1979. Scot (Sterilization Computer Operating Terminal) for sterilization control and monitoring. J. Parent. Drug Assoc., 33, 363–371.

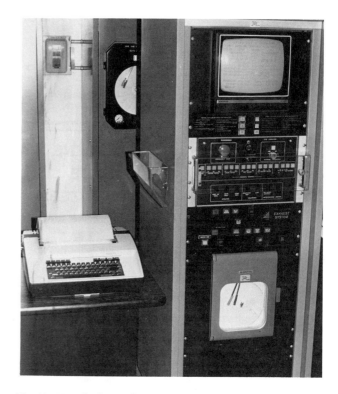

Fig. 33–11. The "SCOT" system.

control systems. With the advent of microprocessor technology, the availability of low-cost hardware, and the application of these to process control systems, it was not long before this technology was applied to sterilizer control systems. The microprocessor approach dramatically minimizes the number of individual hardware components required in electromechanical systems. Microprocessor systems operate from set points and control algorithms incorporated into the system's software. The result is that the multiple pressure switches of the electromechanical-type systems can be replaced with a single pressure transducer, several timers, and an electronic clock.

The main elements of a computer-based control system are described by Burrell et al. (1979) and Parisi (1981) for the "SCOT" system (Sterilizer Computer Operating Terminal), the first of a series in operation at various Baxter/Pharmaseal facilities (Fig. 33–11). In other systems, such as the Vacudyne and AMSCO systems, a magnetic coded card contains cycle-specific data to direct the computer.

A manual backup system is a common component of computer-based systems and is completely independent. It is used primarily for troubleshooting. It can, however, be used for cycle operation in the event of computer problems. A keyed lock is commonly provided to limit access to this system.

ETHYLENE OXIDE STERILIZATION OF MEDICAL PRODUCTS

The three major elements in ethylene oxide sterilization of medical products are (1) preparation of the product, (2) delivery of sterilization parameters, and (3) the removal of the residual sterilizing agent.

The manufacture of a medical product for sterilization must follow Good Manufacturing Practice (GMP) guidelines. The product must be produced in such a manner as to control microbial contamination (bioburden). Other influencing factors to be considered are usually related to complexity of the product in packaging and loading configuration, which are directly controlled by the man-

ufacturer and, as such, need to be optimized for a given product or vessel size.

The product complexity is usually determined by the product engineers, who should be aware of requirements of the sterilization process. The objective in preparation of the product for sterilization is to provide uniform temperature and relative humidity by using either specified rooms or the sterilizing chamber itself. Advantages and disadvantages exist with both systems and need to be evaluated by each manufacturer.

The second major element is the one most manufacturers consider when validating an ethylene oxide cycle. This element—delivery of sterilization parameters to the product—is critical. The fact that a sterilization chamber operates at a specific temperature, pressure, or gas concentration does not guarantee sterility.

The factors important in delivery of sterilization parameters that influence sterility are:

1. Product and product bioburden
2. Packaging, loading, and mass
3. Precycle conditioning (heat and humidity)
4. Gassing time
5. Gas concentration
6. Exposure time
7. Exposure temperature
8. Exposure relative humidity
9. Evacuation time
10. Uniformity of conditions in the load

The last major element in ethylene oxide sterilization is the removal of residual sterilizing agent. This is usually accomplished through sterilizer chamber evacuation with multiple air washes, with dedicated aeration chambers at elevated temperatures, or with both. As discussed earlier, this has two effects: the reduction of worker exposure to the gas and the reduction of product sterilant residuals (Santello, 1989). A portion of the gas that is contained within the product at the conclusion of a sterilization cycle rapidly degasses from packaging components and thus is of concern to sterilizer worker safety, whereas it is the slower product desorption that poses concern to the patient.

In 1978 the U.S. Food and Drug Administration published proposed limits for the ethylene oxide sterilant residuals in product for both medical devices and drugs (FDA, 1978). Although these proposals were never finalized, they have become generally accepted. The validity of the claim that these 1978 proposed levels provide patient safety was supported in the Environ Report (HIMA, 1988). It therefore can be expected that a new proposed regulation will be developed.

A number of analytic methods are available to determine ETO residual agents as well as other byproducts of ETO sterilization (Warren, 1971; Romano and Renner, 1975; AAMI, 1986). It has become common industry practice to use methods to extract the ETO residues from a product under evaluation that stimulate actual product use. For example, a product that contacts aqueous media, such as blood, is extracted in water. An implant, however, because it would probably expose the body to its complete complement of residue over time, would be extracted through a solvent process that totally dissolved the component (HIMA, 1980; AAMI, 1986). Factors that have an impact on the removal of residual agents are:

1. Product, materials, and configuration
2. Packaging, loading, and mass
3. Exposure gas concentration
4. Temperature during exposure and aeration
5. Air washes
6. Time and environment of aeration

Significant changes in any of these elements should be evaluated in terms of the influence on microbial lethality as well as influence on toxicity and safety to the worker and the user.

Cycle Development

Cycle development is the process of defining the sterilization cycle parameters such that the product maintains its intended function and has a predetermined probability of nonsterility or sterility assurance level (SAL).

Preliminary studies should be performed at various sterilization cycle parameters to understand their effects on the product and its packaging. Acceptable values can then be established for temperature, humidity, gas concentration, and pressure differential prior to cycle development. The desired SAL must also be defined prior to cycle development. Typically, the SAL will be based on the intended use of the product and may range from

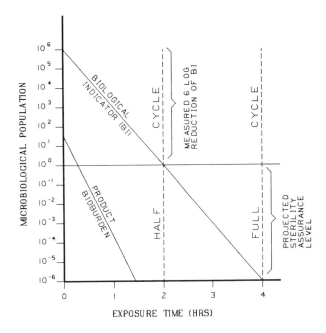

Fig. 33–12. Overkill (120) approach to cycle development.

10^{-3} to 10^{-6}. A SAL of 10^{-3} may be appropriate for a topically applied product, whereas as an SAL of 10^{-6} would be required for a product that was invasive and would contact blood.

Unlike moist heat sterilization, there is no mathematical model that will integrate the synergistic effects of the ETO cycle parameters. Therefore, after selecting the cycle temperature, humidity, and gas concentration, a biological indicator or the product bioburden can be used to establish the exposure time.

The "overkill" or "12D" approach is the most common method of cycle development (AAMI, 1988). This method assumes that the product bioburden or initial contamination level consists of less than or equal to 10^6 organisms that have a resistance that is less than or at least equal to that of the biological indicator. It also assumes that the challenge can be reduced to 10^0 at one-half the normal exposure time (Fig. 33–12). Although little information regarding product bioburden is required, the assumptions must be confirmed. The inactivation of the biological indicator on which the exposure time will be based, must occur at the most difficult-to-sterilize location within or on the product. Figure 33–13 shows how fractional exposure evaluations can be used to determine the most difficult-to-sterilize product location. From this, the minimum exposure time can be determined.

Because few products manufactured today in a GMP environment actually contain such bioburden levels or resistance, alternative methods of cycle development can be considered. The combined biological indicator/bioburden approach sets the initial contamination level at the maximum observed value of product bioburden (but not less than 10^3) and assumes that the resistance of the

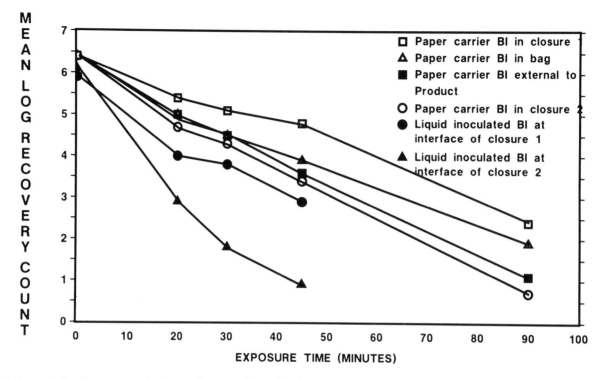

Fig. 33-13. Fractional exposure evaluations to determine the product location that is most difficult to sterilize.

bioburden is less than or equal to that of the biological indicator. This method requires that bioburden enumeration be routinely performed and that the assumption regarding resistance be confirmed (Fig. 33-14.)

If the assumption of relative resistance in the "overkill" or "combined biological indicator/bioburden" approach is not correct, then cycle development must be performed using the actual product with its normally occurring bioburden to determine exposure time.

Validation

Process validation is a documented program that provides a high degree of assurance that a specific process will consistently produce a product meeting its predetermined specifications and quality attributes. Process validation is a requirement of the current Good Manufacturing Practice regulations, 21 CFR, parts 210-211 (Vogel, 1989), and a draft guideline on the general principles of process validation has been developed by the FDA (1983).

Process validation is an essential part of ethylene oxide sterilization and has been the subject of a number of documents published by trade associations and other groups (MEDISPA, 1975; HIMA, 1978; AAMI/ANSI, 1988). There are three major elements of the validation program: installation qualification, performance qualification, and certification.

The installation qualification element requires that the sterilization equipment, including the preconditioning and aeration facilities, be reviewed and tested to verify that they operate within specified parameters. The

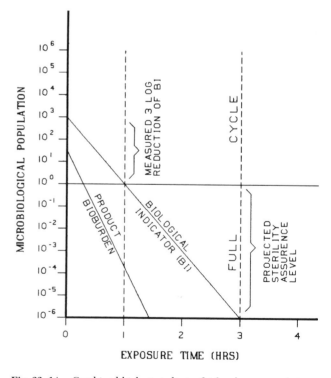

Fig. 33-14. Combined biologic indicator/bioburden approach to cycle development.

equipment configuration and operation should be documented through drawings and text that describe the sequence of operation and safety systems. In addition, calibration and maintenance procedures must be developed as part of this element. Finally, the acceptable results of the equipment operation, calibration, process control, temperature distribution, and safety systems must be documented. Product is not required for this element of validation.

The performance qualification element requires that the established process can be delivered in a reproducible way. Typically, three studies are performed here which include the most difficult-to-sterilize load configuration(s). The product should contain a sufficient number of biological indicators and thermocouples to evaluate the efficacy and uniformity of the process throughout the load. The placement of biological indicators should be at the most difficult-to-sterilize location within the product (as determined in cycle development), and the thermocouples should accompany the biological indicator in a nearby location. A successful performance qualification should include, from consecutive studies, the appropriate spore log reduction of the biological indicator at half cycle, a temperature distribution within specified limits, and a successful product/package evaluation. The acceptable results of this element must also be documented.

The certification element requires that all of the above documentation be reviewed by a designated person(s). If the documentation confirms that all requirements have been met, then the validation program will be approved and the sterilization system released for routine use.

It has become generally accepted practice that once a process has completed its initial validation program, the process efficacy should be requalified on an annual basis (AAMI, 1986).

Environment and Safety

A comprehensive industry study of the safety of medical devices after sterilization by ETO concluded that if an ETO-sterilized product is released for sale in accordance with the FDA proposed maximum residue limits (FDA, 1978), exposure to the ETO residue is unlikely to cause significant risks to human health. Recently, the FDA's center for Devices and Radiological Health (CDRH) presented its internal risk assessment, which supports the safety of the 1978 proposed limits (Cyr et al., 1989). Although at the time of this writing no formal FDA regulation exists, a new FDA proposal is anticipated.

The achievement of acceptable ethylene oxide residue levels is most commonly accomplished by simply holding the products in a quarantine area for the time deemed necessary by outgassing studies. If it is desired to accelerate the outgassing period, heated aeration rooms or chambers are usually employed (Santello, 1989). It should be noted that this is effective only for ethylene oxide and not practical for the less volatile residues ECH and EG. For information regarding residue testing,

product sampling, and laboratory analytical procedures, the reader is referred to the AAMI Recommended Practice for the Determination of ETO Residuals (AAMI, 1986). A guideline for the determination of ECH and EG is currently being finalized by the same AAMI Task Force.

In 1986 the state of California enacted the Safe Drinking Water and Toxic Enforcement Act, commonly known as "Proposition 65," which requires that a business may not "expose any individual to a chemical known to the state to cause cancer or reproductive toxicity without giving clear and reasonable warning" (Allen, 1989). Ethylene oxide is among the chemicals cited as both a carcinogen and a reproductive hazard. Therefore, if a manufacturer has ethylene oxide residues from the sterilization process present on a product at the time of sale in amounts greater than 20 μg, it must currently warn as follows: "This product contains a chemical known to the State of California to be a reproductive hazard." At the time of this writing a number of other states are considering similar legislation.

Toxicity

Since the last edition of this book was published there has been considerable activity involving the toxicity, mutagenicity, and carcinogenicity of ethylene oxide. This has had a significant impact on those who use ethylene oxide as a sterilizing agent. Restrictions on its use have included the amount permitted to exit the sterilizers to the atmosphere. These restrictions have been imposed by individual states, air pollution control boards, and districts. The Environmental Protection Agency (EPA) is currently considering a federal ETO emissions standard. Specific regulations, however, are not expected until 1991 (EPA, 1985). At least ten states now place limitations on these gaseous emissions. As a result, about one-half of the medical device manufacturers were reported as controlling ETO emissions from chamber vents (Jorkasky, 1988). Scrubbers that convert ethylene oxide to less toxic ethylene glycol have been employed successfully to control ETO emissions (Santello, 1989). Gas reclamation and recycling systems are also employed that trap, condense, and reconstitute the chamber emissions. Incinerators can be used only on pure ethylene oxide or non-Freon mixtures to convert the ETO to the harmless compounds of CO_2 and H_2O.

The Occupational Safety and Health Administration (OSHA), which has authority over workplace safety, published a final ruling on ETO in 1984 that reduced the permissible worker 8-hour time-weighed exposure (TWA) level from 50 parts of ETO per million parts of air (50 ppm) to 1 part of ETO per million parts of air (1 ppm) (OSHA 1984). In 1988 OSHA amended its existing standard by adopting an Excursion Limit (EL) for ETO of 5 parts of ETO per million parts of air (5 ppm) averaged over a 15-minute sampling period (OSHA, 1988).

Not only has the sterilizing gas come under considerable scrutiny and tightened regulations as just discussed, but also the most common safety diluent gas,

Freon. Freon, the diluent gas used in the common mild vacuum cycles, is a chlorofluorocarbon (CFC); this class of chemicals is implicated in depletion of the protective ozone layer of the stratosphere. An international treaty to reduce CFC emissions, known as the Montreal Protocol, was signed in 1987 and is now in the ratification stage in 45 nations. The U.S. EPA has already approved restrictions on both production and consumption (EPA, 1988). With the restrictions and significant anticipated cost increases for CFCs, a switch from the CFC/ETO cycles to alternative mild vacuum low-explosive hazard cycles is rapidly taking place. Nitrogen/ETO cycles, as discussed earlier, already are being employed, and an increase in the use of CO_2/ETO mixtures such as 10% ETO/90% CO_2 can also be expected.

REFERENCES

AAMI. 1986. *Recommended practice for determining residual ethylene oxide in medical devices*. Arlington, VA, Association for the Advancement of Medical Instrumentation.

AAMI/ANSI. 1988. *Guideline for industrial ethylene oxide sterilization of medical devices*. Arlington, VA, Association for the Advancement of Medical Instrumentation.

Acklund, N.R., Hinton, M.R., and Denmeade, K.R. 1980. Controlled formaldehyde fumigation system. Appl. Environ. Microbiol., 39, 480–487.

Alguire, D.E. 1963. Effective sterilization with 100% ethylene oxide. Bull. Parent. Drug Assoc., 17, 1–8.

Allen, E.H. 1989. California Proposition 65. In *Sterilization in the 1990's*. Report 89-1. Washington, D.C., Health Industry Manufacturers Association.

Benarde, M.A., Israel, B.M., Olivieri, V.P., and Granstrom, M.L. 1965. Efficiency of chlorine dioxide as a bactericide. Appl. Microbiol., 13(5), 776–780.

Blake, D.F., and Stumbo, C.R. 1970. Ethylene oxide resistance of microorganisms important in spoilage of acid and high-acid foods. J. Food Science, 35, 26–29.

Blanchard, R.O., and Hanlin, R.T. 1973. Effect of propylene oxide treatment on the microflora of pecans. Appl. Microbiol., 26, 768–772.

Braswell, J.R., Spiner, D.R., and Hoffman, R.K. 1970. Absorption of formaldehyde by various surfaces during gaseous decontamination. Appl. Microbiol., 20, 765–769.

Bruch, C.W. 1961. Gaseous sterilization. Ann. Rev. Microbiol., 15, 245–262.

Bruch, C.W., and Bruch, M.K. 1970. Gaseous disinfection. In *Disinfection*. Edited by M.A. Benarde. New York, Marcel Dekker.

Bruch, C.W., and Koesterer, M.G. 1961. The microbicidal activity of gaseous propylene oxide and its application to powdered or flaked foods. J. Food Science, 26, 428–435.

Bucca, M.A. 1956. Effect of various chemical agents on eastern equine encephalomyelitis virus. J. Bacteriol., 71, 491–492.

Burrell, R.L., Wein, R.Z., and Parisi, A.N. 1979. Scot (Sterilization Computer Operating Terminal) for sterilization control and monitoring. J. Parent. Drug Assoc., 33, 363–371.

Caputo, R.A., and Mascoli, C.C. 1980. The design and use of biological indicators for sterilization cycle validation. Med. Device Diagn. Ind., August.

Caputo, R.A., Rohn, K.J., and Mascoli, C.C. 1980. Biological validation of an ethylene oxide sterilization process. In *Developments in Industrial Microbiology*. Volume 22. Society for Industrial Microbiology.

Caputo, R.A., and Rohn, K.J. 1982. The effects of ETO sterilization variables on BI performance. Med. Device Diagn. Ind., 4, 37–41.

Cawse, J.N., Henry, J.P., Swartzlander, M.W., and Wadia, P.H. 1980. Ethylene oxide. In *Encyclopedia of Chemical Technology*. Volume 9. 3rd Edition. Edited by Kirk and Othmer. New York, Wiley.

Celmette, A., Roux, W. 1899. Ann. Inst. Pasteur, 13, 344.

Cotton, R.T., and Roark, R.C. 1928. Ethylene oxide as a fumigant. Eng. Chem., 20, 805.

Coward, H.F., and Jones, G.W. 1952. Limits of flammability of gases and vapor. Bureau of Mines Bulletin No. 503.

Curran, H.R., and Evans, F.R. 1956. The effects of β-propiolactone on bacterial spores. J. Infect. Dis., 99, 212–218.

Cyr, H.W., Glaser, Z., and Jacobs, M.E. 1989. A CDRH risk assessment of ethylene oxide residues on medical devices. In *Sterilization in the 1990's*. Report 89-1. Washington, D.C., Health Industry Manufacturers Association.

Dadd, A.H., and Daley, G.M. 1980. Resistance of micro-organisms to inactivation by gaseous ethylene oxide. J. Appl. Bacteriol., 49, 89–101.

Dawson, F.W., Hearn, H.J., and Hoffman, R.K. 1959. Virucidal activity of β-propiolactone vapor. I. Effect of β-propiolactone on Venezuelan equine encephalomyelitis virus. Appl. Microbiol., 7, 199–201.

Dawson, F.W., Janssen, R.J., and Hoffman, R.K. 1960. Virucidal activity of β-propiolactone vapor. II. Effect on the etiological agents of smallpox, yellow fever, psittacosis and Q fever. Appl. Microbiol., 8, 39–41.

E.P.A. 1985. U.S. EPA assessment of ethylene oxide as a potentially toxic air pollutant. Federal Register, 50, 40286, October 2, 1985.

E.P.A. 1988. U.S. Environmental Protection Agency Protection of Stratospheric Ozone. Federal Register, 53, 30566, August 12, 1988.

E.P.A. 1989. Protection of stratospheric ozone. Federal Register, 54, 13502, April 3, 1989.

Ernst, R.R., and Shull, J.J. 1962. Ethylene oxide gaseous sterilization. I. Concentration and temperature effects. Appl. Microbiol., 10, 337–341.

Fellows, O.N. 1960. Chemical inactivation of foot and mouth disease virus. Ann. NY Acad. Sci., 83, 595–608.

Food and Drug Administration. 1978. Ethylene oxide, ethylene chlorohydrin, and ethylene glycol: Proposed maximum residue limits and maximum levels of exposure. Federal Register, 43(122), 27474–27483, June 23, 1978.

Food and Drug Administration, 1983. Guideline on the General Principles of Process Validation. Division of Drug Quality Compliance (HFN-320) Office of Drugs, National Center for Drugs and Biologics. Rockville, MD, Food and Drug Administration.

Gammon, R.A., Kereluk, K., and Lloyd, R.S. 1971. Ethylene oxide inactivation of coliphage. Dev. Ind. Microbiol., 12, 273–277.

Garlick, B., and Avery, R.J. 1976. Inactivation of New Castle disease virus by β-propiolactone. Arch. Virol., 52, 175–179.

Gilbert, G.L., et al. 1964. Effect of moisture on ethylene oxide sterilization. Appl. Microbiol., 12, 496–503.

Ginsberg, H.S., and Wilson, A.T. 1950. Inactivation of several viruses by liquid ethylene oxide. Proc. Soc. Exp. Biol. Med., 73, 614–616.

Greene, D.F., and Urban, V.L. 1985. U.S. Patent 4,518,585, "Hydrogen Peroxide Disinfecting and Sterilizing Compositions."

Griffith, C.L., and Hall, L.A. 1940. Sterilization process. U.S. Patent No. 2,189,947.

Griffith, C.L., and Hall, L.A. 1943. Sterilization process. U.S. Patent re 22,284.

Haenni, E.O., et al. 1959. New non-flammable process for sterilizing sensitive materials. Ind. Eng. Chem., 51, 685–688.

Hart, A., and Brown, M.W. 1974. Propylene oxide as sterilizing agent. Appl. Microbiol., 28, 1069–1070.

Hart, A., and Ng, S.N. 1975. Effect of temperature on the sterilization of isopropyl alcohol by liquid propylene oxide. Appl. Microbiol., 30, 483–484.

Hartman, F.W., Kelly, A.R., and LoGrippo, G.A. 1955. Four-year study concerning the inactivation of viruses in blood plasma. Gastroenterology, 28, 244–256.

HIMA. 1978. Validation of sterilization systems. Report 78-4-1. Washington, D.C., Health Industry Manufacturers Association.

HIMA. 1980. Guidelines for the analysis of ethylene oxide residues in medical devices (Document No. 1, Vol. 1). Washington, D.C., Health Industries Manufacturers Association.

HIMA. 1988. Ethylene oxide residues on sterilized medical devices. Report 88-6. Washington, D.C., Health Industry Manufacturers Association.

HIMA. 1989. *Sterilization in the 1990's*. Report 89-1. Washington, D.C., Health Industry Manufacturers Association.

Himmelfarb, P., El-Bisi, H.M., Read, R.B., and Litsky, W. 1962. Effect of relative humidity on the bactericidal activity of propylene oxide vapor. Appl. Microbiol., 10, 431–435.

Hoffman, R.K., and Spiner, D.R. 1970. Effect of relative humidity on the penetrability and sporicidal activity of formaldehyde. Appl. Microbiol., 20, 616–619.

Hoffman, R.K. 1968. Effect of bacterial cell moisture on the sporicidal activity of β-propiolactone vapor. Appl. Microbiol., 16, 641–644.

Hoffman, R.K., and Warshowsky, B. 1958. Beta-propiolactone vapor as a disinfectant. Appl. Microbiol., 6, 358–362.

Ito, K.A. 1973. "Resistance of Bacterial Spores to Hydrogen Peroxide." Food Technology, 11:59–66.

Jacobs, P.T., and Lin, S.M. 1987. Hydrogen peroxide plasma sterilization system. U.S. Patent No. 4,643,876.

Johnston, Apple, Baker, 1948. Determination of olefins and gasoline—application of infrared spectroscopy. Ind. Eng. Chem., 20, 805.

Jorgensen, R.H., and Lund, E.L. 1972. Studies on the inactivation of viruses by ethylene oxide. Acta Vet. Scand., 13, 520–527.

Jorkasky, J.F. 1988. Health Industry Manufacturers Association, before the U.S. GPA National Air Pollution Control Technique Advisory Committee meeting on ethylene oxide emissions from commercial sterilization sources.

Karlson, E.L. 1988. A revolutionary sterilization system employing ozone: the Karlson sterilizer. Washington, D.C., Health Industries Manufacturers Association. HIMA Conference Proceedings, pp. 66–74.

Kaye, S., and Phillips, C.R. 1949. The sterilizing action of gaseous ethylene oxide. IV. The effect of moisture. Am. J. Hyg., 50, 296–300.

Kaye, S. 1959. Non-inflammable ethylene oxide sterilant. U.S. Patent No. 2,891,838.

Kereluk, K. 1971. Gaseous sterilization: methyl bromide, propylene oxide and ozone. In *Progress in Industrial Microbiology*. Volume 10. Edited by D. Hockenhull. New York, Churchill Livingstone.

Kereluk, K., and Gammon, R.A. 1973. The microbiocidal activity of ethylene oxide. In *Developments in Industrial Microbiology*. Volume 14. Washington, DC, AIBS.

Kereluk, K., Gammon, P.A., and Lloyd, R.S. 1970. Microbiological aspects of ethylene sterilization. II. Microbial resistance to ethylene oxide. Appl. Microbiol., *19*, 152–156.

Kereluk, K., and Lloyd, R.S. 1969. Ethylene oxide sterilization. A current review of principles and practices. J. Hosp. Res., *7*, 7–75.

King, W.L., and Gould, G.W. 1969. "Lysis of Bacterial Spores with Hydrogen Peroxide." J. Appl. Bact., *32*, 481–490.

Klarenbeek, A., and van Tongeren, H.A.E. 1954. Virucidal action of ethylene oxide gas. J. Hyg., *52*, 525–528.

Kubinski, Z.O., and Kubinski, H. 1978. Alterations in *Bacillus subtilis* transforming DNA induced by β-propiolactone and 1,3-propane sulfone, two mutagenic and carcinogenic alkylating agents. J. Bacteriol., *136*, 854–866.

Kuzminski, L.N., Howard, G.L., and Stumbo, C.R. 1969. Thermochemical factors influencing the death kinetics of spores of Clostridium botulinum 62A. J. Food Sci., *34*, 561–567.

Liu, T.S., Howard, G.L., and Stumbo, C.R. 1968. Dichlorodifluoromethane-ethylene oxide mixture as a sterilant at elevated temperatures. Food Technol., *22*, 86–89.

Marletta, J., and Stumbo, C.R. 1970. Some effects of ethylene oxide on *Bacillus subtilis*. J. Food Sci., *35*, 627–631.

Matthews, J., and Hofstad, M.S. 1953. The inactivation of certain animal viruses by ethylene oxide (Carboxide). Cornell Vet., *43*, 452–461.

Medispa 1975. Process guide for the ethylene oxide sterilization of single use medical products made primarily from plastics and rubber. London, Medical Sterile Products Association.

Merck Index. 1983. 10th edition. Rahway, NJ, Merck & Company. 7757.

Michael, G.T., and Stumbo, C.R. 1970. Ethylene oxide sterilization of *Salmonella senftenberg* and *Escherichia coli*: Death kinetics and mode of action. J. Food Sci., *35*, 631.

Olivieri, V.P., Hauchman, F.S., Noss, C.I., and Vasl, R. 1985. Mode of action of chlorine dioxide on selected viruses. Chem. Environ. Impact Health Eff. Proc. Conf. 5th, pp. 619–634.

OSHA. 1984. U.S. Department of Labor, Occupational Safety and Health Administration. 29 CFR Part 1910. Occupational exposure to ethylene oxide, final standard. Federal Register, *49*, 25733, June 22, 1984.

OSHA. 1988. U.S. DOL, OSHA, 29 CFR Part 1910, Occupational exposure to ethylene oxide. Final Standard. Federal Register, *53*, 11413, April 6, 1988.

Parisi, A.N. 1981. Advances in ethylene oxide sterilization. In *Sterilization of Medical Products*. Edited by E.R.L. Gaughran and R.F. Morrissey. Montreal, Multiscience Publications.

Parker, J. 1975. Inactivation of African horse-sickness virus by betapropiolactone and by pH. Arch. Virol., *47*, 357–365.

Phillips, C.R. 1952. Relative resistance of bacterial spores and vegetative bacteria to disinfectants. Bacteriol. Rev., *16*, 135–138.

Phillips, C.R. 1968. Gaseous sterilization. In *Disinfection, Sterilization, and Preservation*. 1st Edition. Edited by C.A. Lawrence and S.S. Block. Philadelphia, Lea & Febiger.

Phillips, C.R. 1977. Gaseous sterilization. In *Disinfection, Sterilization, and Preservation*. 2nd Edition. Edited by S.S. Block. Philadelphia, Lea & Febiger.

Politzer, P., Daiker, K.C., Estes, V.M., and Baughman, M. 1978. Epoxide-nucleophile interactions: Acid catalyzed reaction of ethylene oxide with water. Int. J. Quantum Chem. Quantum Biol. Symposium, *5*, 291–299.

Reich, R.R. 1980. Effect of sublethal ethylene oxide exposure on *Bacillus subtilis* spores and biological indicator performance. J. Parent. Drug Assoc., *34*, 200–211.

Reich, R.R. 1980. Storage stability of *Bacillus subtilis* ethylene oxide biological indicators. Appl. Environ. Microbiol., *39*, 277–279.

Rohn, K., Caputa, R., and Stryker, D., 1981. Ethylene oxide resistance and population stability of *Bacillus subtilis* var. niger (globigii) spores on various

carrier materials. Presented at the American Society for Microbiology annual meeting, March 1–6.

Roller, S.D. 1978. Some aspects of the mode of action of chlorine dioxide on bacteria. Master's Thesis. The Johns Hopkins University, Baltimore, MD.

Romano, S.J., and Renner, J.A. 1975. Comparison of analytical methods for residual ethylene oxide analysis. J. Pharm. Sci., *64*, 1412–1417.

Rosenblatt, A.A., and Knapp, J.E. 1988. Chlorine dioxide gas sterilization. HIMA Conference Proceedings, pp. 47–50.

Russell, A.D. 1976. Inactivation of non-sporing bacteria by gases. Soc. Appl. Bacteriol., *5*, 61–68.

Santello, L. 1989. Controlling ethylene oxide and chlorofluorocarbon emissions at sterilization factilities. In *Sterilization in the 1990's*. Report 89-1. Washington, D.C., Health Industry Manufacturers Association.

Savage, R.A., and Stumbo, C.R. 1971. Characteristics of progeny of ethylene oxide treated *Clostridium botulinum* type 62A spores. J. Food Sci., *36*, 182–184.

Savan, M. 1955. The sterilizing action of gaseous ethylene oxide on foot-and-mouth disease virus. Am. J. Vet. Res., *16*, 158–159.

Sax, N.I. 1979. Dangerous properties of industrial materials. 5th Edition, 486.

Schusky. 1958. Testimony by James F. Jorkasky, Health Industry Manufacturers Association, before the U.S. EPA National Air Pollution Control Technique Advisory Committee Meeting on Ethylene Oxide Emissions from Commercial Sterilization Sources, May, 1988.

Schrodt, M. 1883. "Ein neues Konservierungsnaittel fur Milch und Butter." Milch-Zig 13, 785.

Searle, C.E. 1961. Experiments on the carcinogenicity and reactivity of β-propiolactone. Br. J. Cancer, 15, 804–811.

Sidwell, R.W., Dixon, G.J., Westbrook, L., and Dulmadge, E.A. 1969. Procedure for the evaluation of an ethylene oxide gas sterilizer. Appl. Microbiol., *17*, 790–796.

Spaulding, E.H., Cundy, K.R., and Turner, F.J. 1977. "Chemical Disinfection of Medical and Surgical Materials." In Disinfection, Sterilization and Preservation. ed. Block, S.S. pp. 654–684.

Tawaratani, T., and Shibasaki, I. 1973. Change in the chemical resistance of heat sensitive and heat resistant bacterial spores against propylene oxide. Hakko Kogaku Zasshi, *51*, 819–814.

Tawaratani, T., Hirano, Y., and Shibasaki, I. 1981. Selection of conditions in gaseous propylene oxide sterilization. Hakko Kogaku Kaishi, *59*, 111–118.

Tawaratani, T., Sawada, T.H., Yuichiro, I., and Shibasaki, I. 1980. Mechanism of the bacterial action of propylene oxide. Hakko Kogaku Kaishi, *58*, 331–337.

Tawaratani, T., Inui, Y., and Shibasaki, I. 1980. Effect of moisture on the sporicidal activity of sterilants against bacterial spores. Hakko Kogaku Kaishi, *58*(2), 85–93.

Toledo, R.T., Escher, F.E., and Ayres, J.C. 1973. Sporicidal properties of hydrogen peroxide against food spoilage organisms. Appl. Microbiol., *26*, 592–597.

Tompkins, G.J., and Cantwell, G.E. 1975. The use of ethylene oxide to inactivate insect viruses in insectaries. J. Invertebr. Pathol., *25*, 139–140.

United States Pharmacopeia. 1980. USP XX. Rockville, MD, United States Pharm. Conv.

Vogel, P. 1989. In *The Gold Sheet*. Vol. 23(5) P. 5 F-D-C Reports, Inc. Chevy Chase, MD.

von Bockelman, I., and von Bockelman, B. 1972. "The Sporicidal Action of Hydrogen Peroxide. A Literature Review." Lebensmittel-Wissenschott Technologie 5, p. 22.

Wardle, M.D., and Renninger, G.M. 1975. Bactericidal effect of hydrogen peroxide on spacecraft isolates. Appl. Microbiol., *30*, 710–711.

Warren, B. 1971. The determination of residual ethylene oxide and halogenated hydrocarbon propellants in sterilized plastics. J. Pharm. Pharmacol., *23*, 1705–1755.

Williams, J.E. 1980. Formalin destruction of salmonellae in poultry litter. Poult. Sci., *59*, 2717–2724.

Wilson, A.T., and Bruno, P. 1950. The sterilization of bacteriological media and other fluids with ethylene oxide. J. Exp. Med., *91*, 449–458.

Winaro, F.G., and Stumbo, C.R. 1971. Mode of action of ethylene oxide on spores of Clostridium botulinum 62A. J. Food Sci., *36*, 892–895.

Wurtz, V.A. 1859. Ueber das aethylenoxyd. Annalender Chemi *110*, 125.

Yabrov, A., Artsob, H., and Spence, L. 1978. A simple method for the inactivation of St. Louis encephalitis virus preparations for immunofluorescent microscopy. Can. J. Microbiol., *24*, 72–74.

CHAPTER 34

GLUTARALDEHYDE

E.M. Scott and S.P. Gorman

Glutaraldehyde is a powerful biocidal agent having the advantage of continued activity in the presence of organic material. It has an established reputation for the chemosterilization of equipment that cannot be sterilized by traditional physical methods. The first indications of its antimicrobial potential came from a survey of saturated dialdehydes by Pepper and Lieberman in 1962 in their search for an efficient substitute for formaldehyde. In the following year Stonehill et al. (1963) advocated that a suitably alkalinated solution of glutaraldehyde was rapidly sporicidal, and toward the end of 1963, a glutaraldehyde formulation was marketed for use as a chemosteriliser.

The continuing interest in the compound is reflected in the numerous publications, even in recent years, on such basic aspects as its structure, activity, and mechanism of action. Particular emphasis is currently being applied to the toxicology of glutaraldehyde while much attention continues to be focused on increasing the range of applications and improvements in formulation of the compound. These various areas are discussed within this chapter in relation to the antimicrobial properties of glutaraldehyde.

CHEMICAL PROPERTIES

Structure

Glutaraldehyde (1,5-pentanedial) appears in the official monographs of the United States and British pharmacopoeias as Glutaral Concentrate and Strong Glutaraldehyde Solution, respectively. Other synonyms used are Glutaric Dialdehyde and Glutardialdehyde. It is usually supplied as an amber-colored liquid of acidic pH. The saturated 5-carbon dialdehyde was first synthetized by Harries and Tank (1908). As with other aldehydes, the two aldehyde groups react readily under suitable conditions, particularly with proteins (Bowes and Cater, 1966; Hopwood et al., 1970).

A single absorption maximum at 280 nm is exhibited by pure glutaraldehyde, though a second maximum at 235 nm is normally observed in commercial solutions because of the presence of impurities of polymers (Anderson, 1967; Hardy et al., 1969). The impurity may be removed by several methods (Pease, 1964; Fahimi and Drochmans, 1965; Anderson, 1967; Hopwood, 1972; Dijk et al., 1985). Appearance of the 235-nm absorbing polymer in pure solutions depends on storage temperature (Gillett and Gull, 1972; Stibenz, 1973) and the rate of the polymerization depends on temperature and pH (Rasmussen and Albrechtsen, 1974; Gorman and Scott, 1979a).

The ratio of monomer to polymer and type of polymer present have been the subjects of numerous publications (Gorman et al., 1980). Essentially it is considered that the presence of free aldehyde groups is a prerequisite for good biocidal activity. Schemes depicting glutaraldehyde polymerization in both acid and alkaline aqueous solution are outlined in Figures 34–1 and 34–2 (Gorman and Scott, 1980). At acid pH glutaraldehyde is in equilibrium with its cyclic hemiacetal and polymers of the cyclic hemiacetal, as proposed by Hardy et al. (1969, 1976a). Increase in temperature produces more free aldehyde in acid solution, whereas in alkaline solution loss of reactive aldehyde groups is possible. When pH is raised to the neutral or basic range the dialdehyde undergoes an aldol condensation with itself followed by dehydration to generate α,β unsaturated aldehyde polymers. Progression to the higher polymeric form (Figure 34–2b) can also occur with increased time and pH. As the pH is raised, n increases in value until the polymer precipitates from solution. Loss of reactive aldehyde groups could therefore be responsible for the rapid loss of biocidal activity of alkaline solutions on storage. A study by Margel and Rembaum (1980) into the structure of the solid aldol condensation product showed that polymerization of glutaraldehyde under basic conditions results in the formation of water-soluble and insoluble polymers, and that these polymers contain unconjugated aldehyde, conjugated aldehyde, hydroxyl, and carboxyl groups. A number of other studies, under the direction

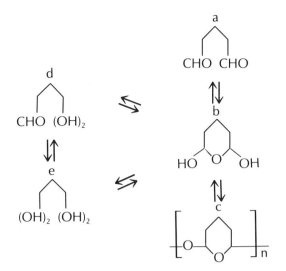

Fig. 34–1. Glutaraldehyde polymerization in aqueous acid media: (a) Monomer, (b) cyclic hemiacetal, (c) acetal-like polymer, (d) monohydrate, (e) dihydrate.

of Tashima in Japan, investigated the several products formed in the aldol condensation of glutaraldehyde and concluded that these new oligomers were glutaraldehyde trimer, pentamer, and heptamer having a 1,3,5-trioxane skeleton (Hashimoto et al., 1983; Tashima et al., 1987a,b, 1988, 1989). In particular, glutaraldehyde trimer, 2,4,6-tris(4-oxobutyl)-1,3,5-trioxane, was named "paraglutaraldehyde," and this was proposed as being responsible for the precipitation observed occasionally during chemosterilization with alkaline glutaraldehyde.

Increased activity in acid solution through application of heat or ultrasonics (Boucher, 1975) can be explained by displacement of equilibrium towards the monomer (Figure 34–1a). A scheme relating these various factors to biocidal activity is described in Figure 34–3.

Analysis

Various methods have been used to determine glutaraldehyde concentration. Measurement of the complex absorbances resulting from glutaraldehyde reaction with 2,4-dinitrophenylhydrazine (Jones and Hancock, 1960) or 3-methyl-2-benzothiazolone hydrazone (Paz et al., 1965) were early reported methods. A relationship be-

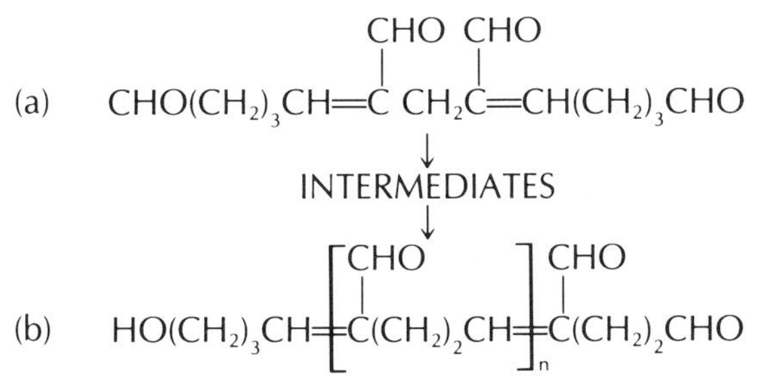

tween concentration and osmolality of glutaraldehyde solutions has also been employed (Fahimi and Drochmans, 1965; Smith and Farquhar, 1966).

A number of methods involving measurement of the 235-nm and 280-nm absorption maxima have also been reported. The purification index (P.I.), defined as A_{235}/A_{280}, where A_{280} is the UV absorbance of monomeric glutaraldehyde at its λ_{max} 280 nm, and A_{235} is that of polymeric glutaraldehyde at its λ_{max} 235 nm, has been widely employed to grade glutaraldehyde products. Lower P.I. values represent higher purity. However, care must be taken in the application of this index in the light of recent findings by Tashima et al. (1987a,b). These authors discovered a commercial glutaraldehyde product to contain an impurity that exhibits absorption at 280 nm but not at 235 nm, indicating the unreliability of the P.I. value. Munton and Russell (1970a) used a 235-nm absorbance to concentration relationship. The 280-nm absorbance maximum was employed by Anderson (1967) and Stibenz (1973), though Stibenz suggested that for routine laboratory use a chemical titration method would be most suitable. Titration methods have been described by Anderson (1967) and Frigerio and Shaw (1968).

Hajdu and Friedrich (1975), while studying the reaction of glutaraldehyde with hydroxylamine, hydrazine, and methylamine, found that a characteristic change in absorbance occurred. From this they developed a spectrophotometric method for the determination of low concentrations of the aldehyde in the presence of substrates absorbing in the same wave-length region.

Other methods of analysis have been developed for specific reasons such as the determination of glutaraldehyde at low levels in hospital air (Wliszczak et al., 1977). A number of chromatographic methods have also been described. These gas chromatographic (Lyman et al., 1978; Harke and Pust, 1978) and high-performance liquid chromatographic (HPLC) methods (Tashima et al., 1987a) have compared favourably with UV methods. It is advised that the chromatographic methods should be used in preference to the UV-absorption (235/280 nm) or UV spectrophotometric method (hydroxylamine) according to Millership (1987) and Tashima et al. (1988).

Reaction with Proteins

The chemistry of the reaction of glutaraldehyde with proteins continues to be investigated; it is likely that several reactions occur, giving rise to a number of products. Several studies of glutaraldehyde interaction with proteins in vitro have been published (Habeeb and Hiramoto, 1968; Blass et al., 1976; Kirkeby and Moe, 1986), shedding some light on this subject. The composition/purity of the glutaraldehyde solution is known to dictate the type of reaction products formed with amino acids (Kirkeby et al., 1987). The rate of reaction with protein is pH-dependent and increases considerably over the pH 4 to 9 range (Hopwood et al., 1970), and it is known that the reaction gives rise to a product (or products) that is stable to acid hydrolysis and a chromophore with an absorbtion maximum at 265 nm. The stability of the

(a) $CHO(CH_2)_3CH=\underset{\underset{CHO}{|}}{C}\ CH_2\underset{\underset{CHO}{|}}{C}=CH(CH_2)_3CHO$

$\downarrow$

INTERMEDIATES

$\downarrow$

(b) $HO(CH_2)_3CH=\underset{\underset{CHO}{|}}{\left[C(CH_2)_2CH=\right.}\underset{\underset{CHO}{|}}{\left.C\right]_n(CH_2)_2CHO}$

Fig. 34–2. Glutaraldehyde polymerization in aqueous alkaline media. Aldol-type polymer (a) progresses to higher polymeric form (b) with time and increased pH.

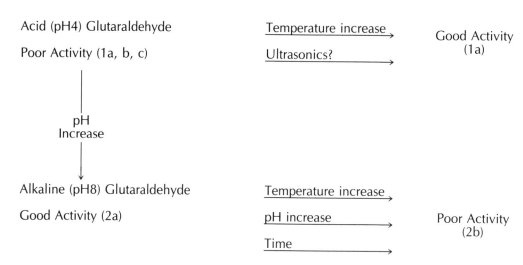

Acid (pH4) Glutaraldehyde

Poor Activity (1a, b, c)

Temperature increase →

Ultrasonics? →

Good Activity
(1a)

pH
Increase

Alkaline (pH8) Glutaraldehyde

Good Activity (2a)

Temperature increase →

pH increase →

Time →

Poor Activity
(2b)

Fig. 34–3. Influence of time, temperature, and pH on the biocidal activity of acid and alkaline glutaraldehyde solutions: 1a,b,c and 2a,b relate to state of the molecule as described in Figs. 34–1 and 34–2.

cross-linkages to acid hydrolysis rules out Schiff base formation (Reichlin, 1980).

Monsan et al. (1975) stated that the aldol-type polymers formed in alkaline solution react with amino groups to give an imino bond stabilized by resonance with the ethylenic double bond (Fig. 34–4), and proposed that glutaraldehyde does not react with proteins in its free form but as an unsaturated polymer. On the other hand, the tanning actions of aqeuous solutions of purified and unpurified glutaraldehyde are almost identical (Hardy et al., 1976a,b, 1977, 1979), indicating that a possible cross-linking reaction does not depend on the initial presence of unsaturated compounds. In a study of the mechanism of cross-linking of proteins, Cheung et al. (1985), employing bovine pericardium, suggested that glutaraldehyde fixes primarily the surface of the fibers and creates a polymeric network that hinders the further cross-linking of the interstitium of the fiber.

Proteins are composed of amino acids, some of which contain free amino groups that readily react with glutaraldehyde. In particular, lysine possesses an ξ-amino group that is the principal side chain of the molecule and

therefore accessible to glutaraldehyde (Korn et al., 1972). Hardy and colleagues (1979) have proposed a further mechanism to explain the nature of glutaraldehyde-protein cross-links. The reaction of free aldehyde with a primary amine of the protein is followed by condensation of additional free glutaraldehyde and leads to the formation of a 1, 3, 4, 5 substituted pyridinium salt analogous to the amino acid desmosine (Fig. 34–5). This mechanism ties in with the observation of a new absorption peak at 265 nm as proteins are cross-linked, and the lability of pyridinium type cross-link to alkaline hydrolysis is similar to protein-glutaraldehyde cross-links treated in the same manner (Woodroof, 1978). The pyridinium linkage is not the only type of cross-link in glutaraldehyde-treated proteins, but it most likely represents a significant portion of these, with other possibilities existing.

The reaction of glutaraldehyde with adenosine, cytidine, and guanosine and with the equivalent deoxyribonucleosides has been investigated by Hemminki and Suni (1984). Multiple products were seen in HPLC for adenine and guanine nucleosides. In each nucleoside the

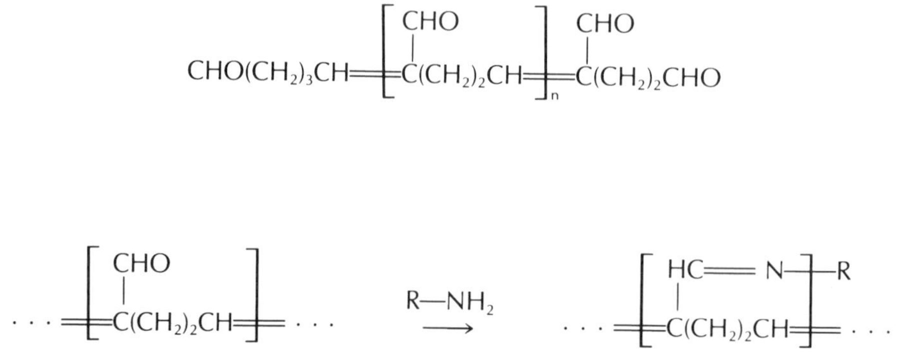

Fig. 34–4. Reaction of aldol-type polymers of glutaraldehyde with amino groups.

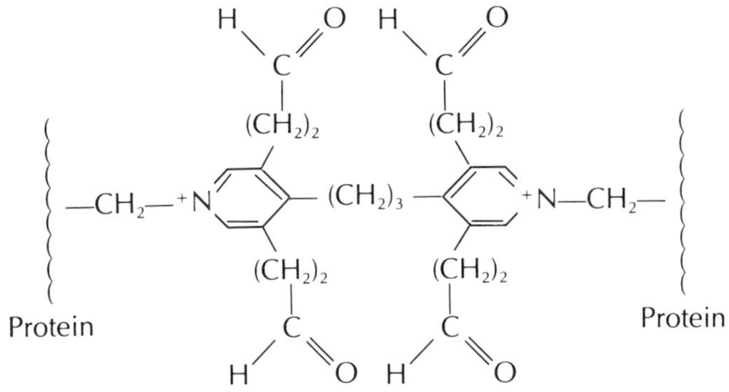

Fig. 34–5. A protein pyridinium crosslink resulting from glutaraldehyde reaction with protein.

site of reaction was shown to be the exocyclic amino group. Chemically the bonds were thought to be Schiff bases.

ANTIMICROBIAL PROPERTIES

Glutaraldehyde displays a broad spectrum of activity and rapid rate of kill against the majority of microorganisms (Table 34–1). Borick (1968) classed glutaraldehyde as a chemosterilizer capable of destroying all forms of microbial life including bacterial and fungal spores, tubercle bacilli, and viruses. Spaulding et al. (1977) also classified glutaraldehyde as a high-level germicide capable of producing sterility if the exposure was long enough.

Effect on Spores

The ability of glutaraldehyde to kill bacterial spores is, perhaps, its most important property. Useful sporicidal activity is a relatively rare property of chemical disinfectants, which are generally bactericidal only. Glutaraldehyde is the only aldehyde to exhibit excellent sporicidal activity (Table 34–2), an activated 2% solution having a greater effect than 8% formaldehyde against a range of spores (Table 34–3).

The time required for sterilization by a chemical agent is based upon the killing time achieved by the agent against a reasonable challenge of resistant spores. At the common use-dilution of 2%, glutaraldehyde was capable of killing spores of *Bacillus* and *Clostridium* spp. in 3 hours (Stonehill et al., 1963; Borick et al., 1964). Rubbo et al. (1967) reported a 99.99% kill of spores of *Bacillus anthracis* and *Clostridium tetani* in 15 and 30 min, respectively. It was apparent from their results that not all species were equally susceptible, and of those organisms tested *Bacillus pumilis* was the most resistant. Dyas and Das (1985) compared the sporicidal activity of 2% glutaraldehyde against *B. subtilis* var. *globigii*, *B. stearothermophilus*, and *Clostridium difficile*. The aerobic species, normally chosen for test purposes, survived for 2 hours, but *Cl. difficile* was killed in under 10 min.

Boucher (1974) found that *B. subtilis* spores were the most resistant to treatment with glutaraldehyde. Using the Association of Official Analytical Chemist (AOAC) sporicidal test and vacuum-dried spores, he found that 10 hours was necessary for complete kill. Babb et al. (1980), in an investigation including nine glutaraldehyde formulations, reported that all were effective against a spore suspension of *B. subtilis* var. *globigii* in 3 hours or less. A similar result was obtained with a challenge of 10^6 spores dried onto aluminum foil. These authors commented that a 3-hour exposure should be sufficient for practical purposes, particularly as spores are infrequent on clean medical equipment. Other work, using similar time-survivor measurements and aqueous suspensions of *B. subtilis* spores, indicated that a 3-hour period gave approximately a 6-log drop in viable count (Sierra and Boucher, 1971; Kelsey et al., 1974; Forsyth, 1975; Miner et al., 1977).

Glutaraldehyde appears to have a significant advantage over other compounds for which claims of sporicidal activity have been made, although some newer combinations, such as mixtures of hypochlorite and alcohol (Coates and Death, 1978; Gorman et al., 1983a, 1984a) and buffered hypochlorite solutions (Babb et al., 1980) are more powerful.

Antibacterial Activity

Vegetative bacteria are readily susceptible to the action of glutaraldehyde. As shown in Table 34–4, a 0.02% aqueous alkaline solution is rapidly effective against gram-positive and gram-negative species, and a 2% so-

Table 34–1. *Lethal Effects of Aqueous 2% Alkaline Glutaraldehyde Solutions*

Type of Microorganism	Specific Organism(s)	Killing Time
Vegetative bacteria	Staphylococcus aureus Streptococcus pyogenes S. pneumoniae Escherichia coli Pseudomonas aeruginosa Serratia marcescens Proteus vulgaris Klebsiella pneumoniae Micrococcus lysodeikitcus	< 1 min
Tubercle bacillus	Mycobacterium tuberculosis H37Rv	< 10 min
Bacterial spores	Bacillus subtilis B. megaterium B. globigii Clostridium tetani C. perfringens	< 3 h
Viruses	Polio types I and II Echo type 6 Coxsackie B-1 Herpes simplex Vaccinia Influenza A-2 (Asian) Adeno type 2 Mouse hepatitis (MHV3)	< 10 min

Based on Borick, P.M. 1968. Chemical sterilizers (chemosterilizers). Adv. Appl. Microbiol., *10*, 291–312.

Table 34–2. *Comparative Sporicidal Activities of Some Aldehydes*

Aldehyde	Chemical Structure	Sporicidal Activity
Formaldehyde (methanal)	HCHO	Good
Glyoxal (ethanedial)	CHO·CHO	Good
Malonaldehyde (propanedial)	CHO·CH$_2$·CHO	Slightly Active
Succinaldehyde (butanedial)	CHO·(CH$_2$)$_2$·CHO	Slightly Active
Glutaraldehyde (pentanedial)	CHO·(CH$_2$)$_1$·CHO*	Excellent
Adipaldehyde (hexanedial)	CHO·(CH$_2$)$_4$·CHO	Slightly Active

*In simplest form: see text also.

Table 34–3. *Comparison of the Sporicidal Activity of Formaldehyde and Glutaraldehyde*

	Time (hr) Required to Kill	
Spores	2% Activated Glutaraldehyde*	8% Formaldehyde*
Bacillus globigii	2–3	>3
B. subtilis	2	>3
Clostridium tetani	<2	>3
C. perfringens	2–3	>3

*Age of Solutions: 18 hr.

From Stonehill, A.A., Krop, S., and Borick, P.M. 1963. Buffered glutaraldehyde, a new chemical sterilizing solution. Am. J. Hosp. Pharm., 20, 458–465.

lution is capable of killing any vegetative species, including *Staphylococcus aureus, Proteus vulgaris, Escherichia coli,* and *Pseudomonas aeruginosa* within 2 min (Stonehill et al., 1963). McGucken and Woodside (1973) reported a complete kill in 10 min of *E. coli* (2 × 10^8 cells/ml) by 100 μg/ml alkaline glutaraldehyde, compared with a 45% kill produced by acid solution.

Glutaraldehyde preparations passed the Kelsey-Sykes capacity test with and without yeast, using *Ps. aeruginosa* as the test organism, compared with hypochlorite, which failed the test when yeast was added (Babb et al., 1980). Using stainless steel penicylinders, neoprene "O" rings, and polyvinyl tubing as carriers for a range of organisms including *Ps. aeruginosa* and *Mycobacterium smegmatis* to simulate in-use conditions for the sterilization of instruments, catheter tubing, and anaesthetic equipment, Leers et al. (1974) found a glutaraldehyde preparation more effective on all three carriers than Savlon, which was only partially effective.

Table 34–4. *Susceptibilities of Nonsporing Bacteria to 0.02% Aqueous Alkaline Glutaraldehyde*

	Inactivation Factor After Exposure (Min)			
Organism	5	10	15	20
Staphylococcus aureus	10^1	10^2	10^4	10^4
Escherichia coli	10^1	10^1	>10^6	>10^6
Pseudomonas aeruginosa	<10^1	10^1	10^1	10^4

From Rubbo, S.D., Gardner, J.F., and Webb, R.L. 1967. Biocidal activities of glutaraldehyde and related compounds. J. Appl. Bacteriol., 30, 78–87.

Effect on Mycobacteria

The tubercle bacillus is more resistant to chemical disinfectants than other nonsporing bacteria. Because glutaraldehyde is widely used for the cold sterilization of respiratory equipment that may be contaminated with tubercle bacilli, it must have good activity against these organisms. Earlier reports of glutaraldehyde activity against mycobacteria have been conflicting, with some claiming good mycobactericidal activity (Stonehill et al., 1963; Borick et al., 1964; Snyder and Cheatle, 1965; Miner et al., 1977). Others have shown a slow action against *Mycobacterium tuberculosis* (Rubbo et al., 1967), being less effective than formaldehyde or iodine (Bergan and Lystad, 1971) or hypochlorite (Relyveld, 1977). A report by Leers (1980) recommended 2% glutaraldehyde treatment for 10 to 30 min for the chemical disinfection of fiberoptic endoscopes, where iodophore disinfection had not destroyed the tubercle bacillus. The use of glutaraldehyde as an alternative to other disinfectants in tuberculosis laboratory discard jars was recently investigated by J. Collins (1986). A 5-log reduction in viability of clinical isolates of *M. tuberculosis* was obtained within 10 to 30 min at 25°C using alkaline glutaraldehyde, even in the presence of neutralizing materials such as swab sticks and sputum.

A possible explanation for these varying conclusions has been provided by a recent report by Asczenzi et al. (1986), which found the official AOAC test procedure to be nonquantitative and to lack precision and accuracy. They concluded that use of carriers increased variability of results. The importance of accurate temperature control was also highlighted (F. Collins, 1986a). A significant change in rate of kill of *M. bovis* BCG by glutaraldehyde was observed as temperature was increased from 20° to 25°C. Clumping of bacilli was proposed as another cause of erroneous results.

The choice of organism for use in mycobactericidal tests is also controversial. Best et al. (1988) used *M. smegmatis* in suspension and a variety of carriers in the presence of sputum to assess mycobactericidal activity of disinfectants. In these tests glutaraldehyde produced in excess of a 6-log reduction in viable count after 1 min of contact. However, van Klingeren and Pullen (1987) have suggested that *M. smegmatis* is more susceptible to disinfectants than *M. tuberculosis,* and therefore its use as a test organism is not appropriate. These authors suggested using *M. terrae,* which produced results more

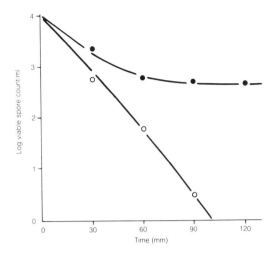

Fig. 34–6. Effect of 0.5% glutaraldehyde on spores of *Aspergillus niger*. ●, Acid glutaraldehyde; ○, alkaline glutaraldehyde. From Gorman, S.P., and Scott, E.M. 1977a. A quantitative evaluation of the antifungal properties of glutaraldehyde. J. Appl. Bacteriol., *47*, 463–468.

closely related to *M. tuberculosis* in the suspension test employed. Once again a glutaraldehyde formulation was found to be rapidly cidal. Variation in resistance to glutaraldehyde was shown by different strains of mycobacteria, with strains of *M. avium* and *M. intracellulare* requiring over 20 and 40 min, respectively, to achieve a 99% kill (F. Collins, 1986b). Differences in sensitivity to glutaraldehyde between laboratory strains and clinical isolates had been observed previously (Carson et al., 1978).

In conclusion, claims of glutaraldehyde activity against mycobacteria must be regarded with caution, taking into account the method and temperature used in the assessment and the criteria employed to measure success or failure of disinfection. All reports indicate activity of glutaraldehyde against these organisms; it is the rate of kill that is affected by method and conditions used. The practical implications of these reports are that adequate time for decontamination of equipment must be allowed.

Antifungal Activity

Glutaraldehyde has been shown to exhibit potent activity against a range of fungi, including the dermatophytes *Trichophyton interdigitale* and *Microsporium gypseum*, the yeasts *Candida albicans* and *Saccharomyces cerevisiae*, the common spoilage molds *Mucor hiemalis*, *Rhizopus stolonifer*, and *Penicillium chrysogenum*, and the resistant fruit spoilage mold *Byssochlamys fulva* (Dabrowa et al., 1972; Gorman and Scott, 1976a; Tadeusiak, 1976; Gorman and Scott, 1977a).

Fungicidal activity of a 0.5% glutaraldehyde solution is illustrated in Figure 34–6 against spores of *Aspergillus niger*. This fungus was found to be more resistant than other fungi to glutaraldehyde (Rubbo et al., 1967; Gorman and Scott, 1977a). However, in common with a range of other fungal species both mycelial growth and

sporulation are inhibited by 0.5% alkaline glutaraldehyde, whereas spore swelling is entirely halted by a 0.5% solution. *A. niger* and *A. fumigatus* were found to be the most resistant fungi encountered in a comparative study of fungicidal activity of disinfectants (Terleckyj and Axler, 1987). Sonacide (an acid-based glutaraldehyde formulation) was effective against both fungi; however, a glutaraldehyde-phenate mixture (sporicidin) was not effective, even after 90 min of contact.

Antiviral Activity

Reliable scientific evidence of virucidal activity of disinfectants has become increasingly necessary as more information becomes available implicating direct contact with infected material as a significant means of transmission of infection. Two recent publications, while developing a test method to determine virucidal activity of disinfectants, have confirmed the excellent antiviral activity of glutaraldehyde. Boudouma et al. (1984), using an ultrafiltration dilution technique to separate disinfectant from virus, demonstrated that 2% glutaraldehyde was rapidly cidal to poliovirus type 1. Tyler and Ayliffe (1987) described a surface test in which a standard challenge of 3×10^7 plaque-forming units of herpes simplex was allowed to dry onto coverslips before exposure to a range of disinfectants. No virus was recovered after 1 min of contact with 2% alkaline glutaraldehyde, and overall glutaraldehyde and ethanol or isopropanol were the most active of all the agents tested.

A number of earlier reports showed that glutaraldehyde was effective against a range of viruses (Blough, 1966; Graham and Jaeger, 1968; Schumann and Grossgebauer, 1977; Shen et al., 1977), even in the presence of high levels of organic matter (Saitanu and Lund, 1975; Evans et al., 1977). Enveloped lipophilic viruses usually show significantly less resistance than the nonlipid viruses. This was found to be the case in the report by Klein and Deforest (1963), in which the nonlipid enteroviruses—polio, echo, and coxsackie—showed greater resistance to disinfection with glutaraldehyde than other virus groups. A potentiated acid glutaraldehyde formulation was also shown to have weak activity against coxsackievirus B5 and echovirus 11 in studies by Drulak et al. (1978a,b) and to be less effective than ethanol or a chlorine based disinfectant against reovirus 3 (Drulak et al., 1984).

Many recent reports have concentrated on hepatitis and human immunodeficiency virus (HIV). A summary of activity of glutaraldehyde against these viruses is given in Table 34–5. Viral hepatitis B continues to be a major health hazard, especially among health-care professionals. Because of the definite risks to personnel and the lack of data relating to disinfectant activity toward hepatitis B virus (HBV), infection-control bodies have tended to recommend only strong disinfectants such as glutaraldehyde for treatment of HBV-contaminated material. These recommendations are now supported by evidence that glutaraldehyde is capable of inactivating HBV antigen (Adler-Storthz et al., 1983) and destroying

Table 34–5. *Evidence of Antiviral Activity of Glutaraldehyde Against Human Immunodeficiency Virus (HIV) and Hepatitis A (HAV) and Hepatitis B Virus (HBV)*

Virus	Assay Method	Treatment Conditions*	Result	Reference
HIV	Reverse transcriptase	0.125% glutaraldehyde (Room temperature)	Enzyme inactivation	Spire et al. (1984)
HAV	Infective titre and antigenicity	0.5% glutaraldehyde, 3 min (23°C)	>3 log reduction >80% reduction	Passagot et al. (1987)
HBV	Antigenicity	2% alk glutaraldehyde, 10 min (25°C)	>90% reduction	Alder-Storthz et al. (1983)
	Infectivity (Direct chimpanzee inoculation) (as above)	2% alk glutaraldehyde, 10 min (20°C, pH 8.4)	No infection developed	Bond et al. (1983)
		0.1% alk glutaraldehyde, 5 min (24°C)	No infection developed	Kobayashi et al. (1984)

*The pH of glutaraldehyde employed is not mentioned in some references.

HBV infectivity (Bond et al., 1983; Kobayashi et al., 1984). Loss of HBV infectivity was determined by direct inoculation of chimpanzees with HBV that had been dried in human plasma and then exposed to disinfectant. The animals did not develop infection, from which it was concluded that infectivity was destroyed. However, because HBV infectivity was also inactivated by other "weaker" disinfectants, Bond et al. (1983) concluded that it did not present a special problem for disinfectants. Hepatitis A is also a major public health problem, especially in developing countries where the disease is endemic. Passagot et al. (1987) proposed that an effective disinfectant that was not inactivated by organic matter would help reduce the risks of epidemics. They demonstrated that glutaraldehyde produced a time-and-concentration–dependent reduction in HAV titer and a decrease in antigenicity.

The risk of catching acquired immunodeficiency syndrome (AIDS) particularly from articles contaminated with blood, has been a major concern of the past few years. Spire et al. (1984) concluded that the causative virus, HIV, displayed sensitivity to chemical disinfection similar to that of other enveloped viruses, and recommended that 1% glutaraldehyde should be suitable for disinfection of medical instruments. Reverse transcriptase was used as an indicator of viral inactivation, and although this assay was demonstrated by Resnick et al. (1986) to be less sensitive than measurement of infectious virus titer, these authors also concluded that HIV behaved similarly to other enveloped viruses.

Rotaviruses are responsible for numerous outbreaks of acute gastroenteritis in young children. The possible risk of transmission of these viruses by contaminated hand or fomite contact could be reduced by good disinfection practice. In an evaluation of disinfectant activity against human rotaviruses, 2% alkaline glutaraldehyde solution in the presence of an organic load produced at least a 3-log reduction in virus plaque titer within 1 min in a suspension test (Springthorpe et al., 1986) and using virus-contaminated inanimate surfaces (Lloyd-Evans et al., 1986).

Resistance

Reports in the literature of resistance of microorganisms to glutaraldehyde resulting in contamination and occasionally infection may be attributed to two factors. Firstly, where reference is made to outbreak of infection or spread of contamination through use of glutaraldehyde (Ringrose et al., 1968; Bassett, 1971; Ayliffe and Deverill, 1979), the agent was invariably employed as a disinfectant rather than as a sterilizing agent. The short time available between patients on, for example, endoscopy lists, has necessitated a reduction in contact time for decontamination in many instances, and this has inevitably led to the reported cases. Indeed, Scheidt (1980) found that 45 min of glutaraldehyde contact was necessary to achieve sterilization of heavily contaminated flexible-fiber bronchoscopes.

A second factor, however, that must also be considered is intrinsic organism resistance. Carson et al. (1978) have shown that TM strains of *Mycobacterium chelonei* survived 60 min of exposure to 2% alkaline glutaraldehyde, although no survivors of ATCC strains of *M. chelonei* or *M. fortuitum* were detected in fluids assayed at 2 min of contact time. With 0.2% glutaraldehyde both TM and ATCC strains showed survivors at 96 hours of exposure time. *M. chelonei* organisms have been reported as intrinsic contaminants of porcine prosthetic heart-valve tissues treated and stored, respectively, in 1% and 0.2% glutaraldehyde solutions (Laskowski et al., 1977; Anon, 1977). Disinfectant solutions used to treat materials and equipment for patient use must therefore be carefully evaluated in terms of their potential for harboring rather than eliminating contaminants.

There are, however, dangers inherent in these evaluations. Glutaraldehyde (0.05%) was shown in vitro to rapidly inactivate *Pseudomonas aeruginosa* (Rubbo et al., 1967), but glutaraldehyde (2%) failed to disinfect ultrasonic nebulizers heavily contaminated with *Pseudomonas* species (Pierce et al., 1970). In a study by Carson et al. (1972) comparing the resistances of naturally occurring and subcultured cells of a strain of *Ps. aeruginosa* to glutaraldehyde, results showed that the resistance of the

Table 34–6. *Revival of Alkaline Glutaraldehyde-Treated* Bacillus subtilis *Spores Following Coat Removal and Resuscitation*

Treatment Sequence	% Survivors Following Dilution and Incubation in:		
	25%v/v Ringer's	GM	GM + Lysozyme
a **Glutaraldehyde 2% (3h)**	0.0006	0.0006	0.0004
b UDS	0	0	0.038
c Sonication 10 min	0	0	0.046
d Sonication 10 min	0	0	0.032
a **Glutaraldehyde 2% (10h)**	0	0	0
b UDS	0	0	0.004
c Sonication 10 min	0	0	0.006
d Sonication 10 min	0	0	0.0015
a **Glutaraldehyde 1% (10h)**	0.27	0.26	0.26
b UDS	0.035	0.075	0.75
c Sonication 10 min	0.016	0.013	2.20
d Sonication 10 min	0.018	0.031	1.05

NB: Initial viable spore count: 2×10^7 cfu/ml

GM, germination medium; UDS, urea/dithiothreitol/sodium dodecyl sulphate

Based on Gorman, S.P., Hutchinson, E.P., Scott, E.M., and McDermott, L.M. 1983b. Death, injury and revival of chemically treated *Bacillus subtilis* spores. J. Appl. Bacteriol., *54*, 91–99.

subcultured cells did not begin to approach the degree of resistance of the naturally occurring organism. These authors concluded that when results obtained solely with laboratory-adapted cells are extrapolated to naturally occurring populations in the hospital environment, significant error may be introduced in evaluating the efficiency and use of disinfectants.

Sporicidal results from our laboratory (Gorman et al., 1983b) have recently shown that a spore population of *Bacillus subtilis* treated with alkaline glutaraldehyde, and presumed dead, can be revived in defined germination medium following removal of the outer coat layers of the spore with selective agents and by application of ultrasonic energy (Table 34–6). A small proportion may be recovered after 3 to 10 hours of contact with 2% glutaraldehyde solutions by application of ultrasonic energy, lysozyme, and protein denaturing agents such as dithiothreitol and urea-mercaptoethanol. This revival may be academic in nature but it has implications in practice, especially in view of the differences in resistance exhibited by natural and subcultured populations as suggested above. Furthermore, there is a risk attached to the use of sublethal concentrations of glutaraldehyde (i.e., less than 2%) for sterilizing purposes. Such concentration levels may arise not only from in-use dilution but also from polymerization of alkaline solutions of glutaraldehyde and presence of organic matter (Gorman and Scott, 1977b).

The presence of various types and amounts of organic and inorganic materials, as well as changes in pH, may lead to adsorbtion, alteration, or inactivation of the disinfectant, significantly reducing recommended effective concentrations. Also, substandard preparation of the "activated" disinfectant, contamination of solutions, failure to replace solutions that have deteriorated on standing, or even dilution of residual glutaraldehyde solution may all modify the outcome of disinfection. Due attention should therefore be exercised in the use of glutaraldehyde, as with any disinfectant, to avoid such an occurrence.

Exceptional resistance to sterilization and disinfection is exhibited by the causitive agent of scrapie. Scrapie agent was shown to be more resistant than other organisms to glutaraldehyde and was not fully inactivated by 12.5% glutaraldehyde in 16 hours at 4°C (Dickinson and Taylor, 1978).

MECHANISM OF ACTION

Interactions with Bacterial Cell Constituents

Glutaraldehyde-protein interactions, as described earlier, indicate an effect of the dialdehyde on the surface of bacterial cells. Conclusions from a range of mode-of-action studies indicate a powerful binding of the aldehyde to the outer cell layers. Hughes and Thurman (1970) found that the dialdehyde reacted with 30 to 50% of the ε-amino groups in isolated peptidoglycan, and it was proposed that two tripeptide side-chains could be joined when free ε-amino groups are available. Treatment of *E. coli* cells and walls with alkaline glutaraldehyde greatly reduces, or completely prevents, lysis by 2% sodium lauryl sulphate at 35 to 40°C (McGucken and Woodside, 1973), and pretreatment of *Staphylococcus aureus* and *Pseudomonas aeruginosa* cells with glutaraldehyde reduces subsequent lysis by lysostaphin and EDTA-lysozyme (Russell and Haque, 1975; Russell and Vernon, 1975). Strengthening of the outer layers of spheroplasts and protoplasts by glutaraldehyde has also been reported (Munton and Russell, 1970b, 1973a).

Cell agglutination, shown to occur on addition of glutaraldehyde to various microorganisms, was considered by Navarro and Monsan (1976) to be due to the formation of intercellular bonds, thus confirming the hypothesis of a preferential action of glutaraldehyde on the outer layers of the cells. However, the biocidal effect of glutaraldehyde is unlikely to be due to a sealing of the cell envelope alone, according to studies by Gorman and Scott (1977c,d). Transport of a low-molecular-weight amino acid, α-amino-isobutyric-acid-1-^{14}C(14 C-AIB), was compared in glutaraldehyde-treated and untreated cells of *E. coli* and found to be reduced by only 50% in treated cells.

The reaction of glutaraldehyde with cytoplasmic constituents has received less attention. The inhibitory effect of the aldehyde on RNA, DNA, and protein syntheses in *E. coli* is practically complete within 10 min of adding the disinfectant and is due to inhibition of precursor uptake as a consequence of a glutaraldehyde-protein reaction in the outer structures of the cell (McGucken and Woodside, 1973). The reaction of the aldehyde with nucleic acids follows pseudo–first-order kinetics at high temperatures, but there is little evidence for the formation of intermolecular cross-links, even at the higher temperatures (Hopwood, 1975).

Comparatively few studies have examined the effects of glutaraldehyde on cell enzyme activity. Dehydrogenase activity is inhibited by concentrations that have little effect on cell viability (Munton and Russell, 1973a). This is possibly because the compound strengthens the outer cell surface and prevents ready access of substrate to enzyme. Ellar et al. (1971) found that glutaraldehyde prevented the selective release of certain enzymes from the cytoplasmic membrane of *Micrococcus lysodeikticus*. Various concentrations of glutaraldehyde inactivate several periplasmic enzymes (Done et al., 1965; Wang and Tu, 1969), including ATPase (Wetzel et al., 1970; Gorman and Scott, 1977c). Cheng et al. (1970) have shown that glutaraldehyde fixation causes a shift of ATPase from the periplasmic space to the cell surface. Thus, in addition to a sealing effect on the outer layer, glutaraldehyde also inactivates cell enzymes to achieve its rapid bactericidal effect (Gorman and Scott, 1977c).

Interaction with Bacterial Spores

The importance attached to the interaction of glutaraldehyde with bacterial spores is observed in the continuing interest shown by researchers in this area. Thomas and Russell (1974) have shown that low concentrations of glutaraldehyde (0.1% w/v) inhibit germination of spores of *Bacillus subtilis* and *B. pumilus*, whereas much higher concentrations (2% w/v) are sporicidal. The aldehyde, at acid and alkaline pH, appears to interact to a considerable extent with the outer layers of bacterial spores. This interaction reduces the release of dipicolinic acid (DPA) from *B. pumilus* and peroxide-induced lysis of spores subsequently treated with thioglycollic acid. However, the small differences in results obtained with acid and alkaline glutaraldehyde in respect of interaction with the spore coat did not correlate with the much greater sporicidal effect of the aldehyde at alkaline pH. The data indicated that acid glutaraldehyde could interact at the spore surface and remain there, whereas alkaline glutaraldehyde penetrates the spore.

A study by Gould and Dring (1975) found that spores of *B. cereus* became heat-sensitive in the presence of high concentrations of salts. The authors postulated that the cations interact with the loosely cross-linked and electronegative spore peptidoglycan to cause collapse of the cortex. Replacement of mobile counterions and a consequent fall in the osmotic dehydration of the spore core leads to a reduction in resistance. In this respect, replacement of the alkalinating agent or "activator salt" (e.g., $NaHCO_3$) in glutaraldehyde by, especially, divalent metal chlorides, retains a marked sporicidal effect in the absence of alkaline pH (Gorman and Scott, 1979a). This may indicate a role for the alkalinating agent or other cation addition in facilitating penetration and interaction of glutaraldehyde with components of the spore cortex or core.

An investigation in our laboratories by McErlean et al. (1980) into the resistance of ion-exchange and coat

Table 34–7. *Effect of Acid and Alkaline Glutaraldehyde on Ion-Exchange and Coat Defective Spore Forms of* Bacillus subtilis *at 20°C*

2% Glutaraldehyde	Time (min) to Kill 90% of Initial Spore Population*				
	Normal	H-form	Ca-form	UME	UDS
pH 7.9	85 (123)	95 (126)	30 (61)	47	<1
pH 4.0	190	220	97	85	16

*Initial spore count: 1.5×10^7 cfu/ml. H-form, hydrogen form; Ca-form, calcium form (ion-exchange spore forms); UME, urea/mercaptoethanol; UDS, urea/dithiothreitol/sodium dodecyl sulphate (spore coatless forms).

Figures in parentheses are for spores produced in defined liquid medium, otherwise spores were produced on solid medium.

Based on Gorman, S.P., Scott, E.M., and Hutchinson, E.P. 1984b. Interaction of the *Bacillus subtilis* spore protoplast, cortex, ion-exchange and coatless forms with glutaraldehyde. J. Appl. Bacteriol., 56, 95–102.

defective spores of *B. subtilis* to glutaraldehyde has also indicated the importance of the protective role of the spore coat. Gorman et al. (1984b) further examined the interaction of glutaraldehyde with normal and chemically altered spores of *B. subtilis* (Table 34–7). The Ca-form was more sensitive to glutaraldehyde (pH 4.0 and 7.9) than the normal or H-form, whereas removal of the spore coat, or coat protein, dramatically increased sensitivity of the spore to glutaraldehyde. Spore protoplasts offered no resistance to the action of glutaraldehyde. Pretreatment of coat-defective spores with glutaraldehyde (pH 7.9) reduced the rate of lysis by lysozyme and by sodium nitrite, thereby protecting the cortex. Glutaraldehyde at pH 4.0 had little effect.

Further observations inform us that uptake of acid glutaraldehyde by isolated spore coats follows a similar pattern to the uptake by intact spores. However, isolated spore coats take up alkaline glutaraldehyde at a faster rate than intact spores. These uptake patterns suggest that alkaline glutaraldehyde may penetrate beyond the coats in the intact spore, whereas acid glutaraldehyde may be confined to the spore coat layers. These results coupled with the possibility of revival of glutaraldehyde-treated spores (Gorman et al., 1983b), as discussed under *Resistance*, serve as strong evidence for a strictly glutaraldehyde–spore surface layer(s) reaction.

The emergence and development of resistance to glutaraldehyde (alkaline) in sporulating cells of *B. subtilis* has been investigated in our laboratories (Gorman et al., 1984b). Growth and sporulation were followed by electron microscopy and resistance assigned to specific stages in relation to phase brightness, ^{45}Ca, and DPA accumulation in the maturing spore (Fig. 34–7). A sequential development of resistance was observed with thermal resistance appearing first at early stage V of sporulation, corresponding to maturation of cortex and deposition of rudimentary spore coat material. Resistance to glutaraldehyde developed within the range t_5 to t_6 (i.e., 5 to 6 hours after exponential development), coinciding with

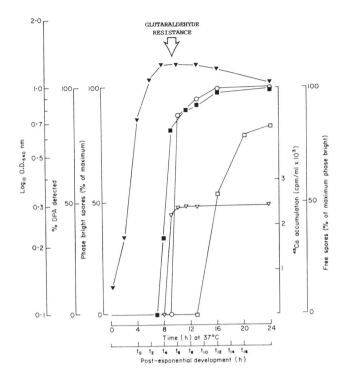

Fig. 34-7. Sporulation in *Bacillus subtilis* at 37°C from time of inoculation of nutrient medium to release of mature spore. Subscript t represents postexponential development. Resistance to glutaraldehyde (indicated by arrow) coincides with late stage V of sporulation at t5–t6. ▼, Optical Density (O.D.); ○, Dipicolinic acid (DPA) content; ■, phase bright spores; ▽, ^{45}Ca accumulation; □, free spores. Based on Gorman, S.P., Scott, E.M., and Hutchinson, E.P. 1984c. Emergence and development of resistance to antimicrobial chemicals and heat in spores of *Bacillus subtilis*. J. Appl. Bacteriol., 57, 153–163.

late stage V. Similar findings have recently been reported by Power et al. (1988). This development of resistance is in agreement with the observations stated above (Gorman et al., 1983b, 1984b) in respect of spore coat protection.

Interaction with Fungi and Viruses

Inhibition of germination, spore swelling, mycelial growth, and sporulation in fungal species at varying concentrations has been demonstrated by Gorman and Scott (1977a). The principal structural wall component of many moulds and yeasts in chitin, which resembles the peptidoglycan of bacteria and is thus a potentially reactive site for glutaraldehyde action. Other active sites could include the polysaccharide-protein complexes, found in yeast cells, and in which cystine residues, -S-S-bonds, are abundant. The formation of intercellular bonds in yeast causing agglutination of the cells as reported by Navarro and Monsan (1976) could also be a causative factor in death.

Few studies relate to mechanism of viral inactivation by glutaraldehyde. Sangar et al. (1973), working with foot-and-mouth-disease virus, found that glutaraldehyde-treated virus particles had a smaller sedimentation coefficient than normal particles. This, however, was in contrast to the effect observed on treated poliovirus when

no change occurred (Baltimore and Huang, 1968). Sangar et al. (1973) showed that considerable alterations in the arrangement of the RNA and protein subunits occurred. The overall structural integrity of the virus particle was not maintained. Wouters et al. (1973) have shown that prolonged exposure of poliovirus to the aldehyde increases its buoyant density and permeability to phosphotungstic acid.

It was suggested by Passagot et al. (1987) that interaction between glutaraldehyde and lysine residues on the surface of hepatitis A virus may occur, because this amino acid was present on the most exposed structural protein of the virus. Work with hepatitis B virus indicated that glutaraldehyde did not cause virus disruption, but results indicated that a "fixing" reaction occurred in a manner analogous to that seen for bacteria (Adler-Storthz et al., 1983).

Effect of Alkalination

Because the degree of biocidal activity observed in glutaraldehyde solutions is so markedly dependent on the pH of the solution, it seems appropriate to deal with this effect from a mechanistic viewpoint. The enhanced biocidal activity of glutaraldehyde in alkaline solution is thought to be due to an effect on the glutaraldehyde molecule in relation to polymerization, the outer layers of the microbial cell, or a combination of both. Effect of pH on the glutaraldehyde molecule has been discussed in detail previously (*Chemical properties*). The requirement that free aldehyde groups be present for optimum activity is well established (Rubbo et al., 1967; Boucher et al., 1973). Navarro and Monsan (1976) stated that the presence of free aldehyde groups in glutaraldehyde allows formation of an aldol-type polymer at alkaline pH. A similar biocidal effect may be obtained with substantially higher glutaraldehyde concentrations at acid pH.

A further interesting point developed from a study by Munton and Russell (1973b), who found that acid glutaraldehyde does not react immediately with the outer cell layers or to the same overall extent as an alkaline solution. This feature was considered by Navarro and Monsan (1976) to be compatible with the structure of the aldehyde at acid and alkaline pH. Subsequent data obtained on bacterial uptake of glutaraldehyde have supported these views (Gorman and Scott, 1977a). Uptake isotherms obtained from both acid and alkaline solutions are of the basic Langmuir (L) type, the acid solution having the further classification of L subgroup 2 and the alkaline, L subgroup 4, as illustrated in Figure 34-8. The second rise observed in the alkaline glutaraldehyde L-curve can be attributed to the development of fresh sites due to further penetration of the aldehyde and bicarbonate. The long plateau obtained for the acid solution indicates that a high-energy barrier has to be overcome before additional absorption can occur on new sites. This observation correlates with the increased biocidal activity obtained on heating acid glutaraldehyde solutions.

The effect of sodium bicarbonate and other alkalinating salts is likely to be on the bacterial cell rather than on

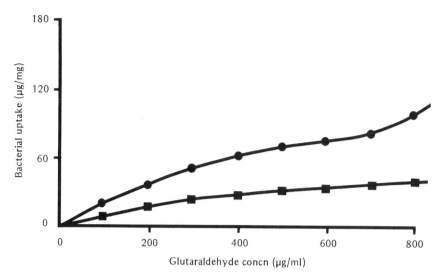

Fig. 34–8. Effect of concentration on uptake by *Escherichia coli* of added glutaraldehyde. ●, Alkaline glutaraldehyde; ■, acid glutaraldehyde. From Gorman, S.P., and Scott, E.M. 1977b. Uptake and media reactivity of glutaraldehyde solutions related to structure and biocidal activity. Microbios. Lett., *1*, 197–204.

the aldehyde molecule (Munton and Russell, 1970a). Support for this hypothesis of bicarbonate was obtained from cell leakage data (Gorman and Scott, 1977e) and proton magnetic resonance (PMR) studies by King et al. (1974). The loosely bound outer layer of the gram-negative cell can be removed by washing with 0.5 M sodium chloride or sodium bicarbonate (Gorman and Scott, 1977c). The alkalinating agent appears also to aid penetration of the glutaraldehyde molecule, as shown by its effect on the periplasmic-located enzyme, alkaline phosphatase (Gorman and Scott, 1977c). This enzyme is equally inhibited by acid and alkaline glutaraldehyde in NaCl-washed cells of *E. coli*, in contrast with the greater inhibitory action of alkaline glutaraldehyde on enzyme activity in whole cells.

Gorman and Scott (1977e) also examined the possibility of a bicarbonate effect on the glutaraldehyde molecule by estimating the degree of polymerization in acid and alkaline solutions. The degree of polymerization is extensive at alkaline pH but negligible in acid solution. This polymerization, leading to an extensive loss of aldehyde groups, is, however, measured in weeks rather than in the short periods (minutes or hours) in which biocidal activity of alkaline glutaraldehyde is observed. An immediate effect is not, therefore, apparent on the glutaraldehyde molecule, and consequently the primary effect of sodium bicarbonate must be on the bacterial cell.

Factors Influencing Efficacy and Evaluation of Activity

The antimicrobial activity of any compound cannot be looked at in isolation but must be described with reference to, for example, pH, temperature, organic challenge, and in-use dilution. Such factors significantly in-

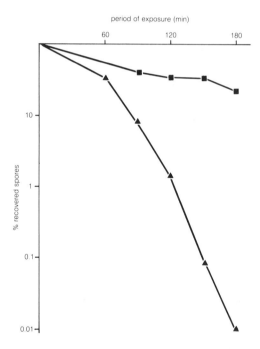

Fig. 34–9. Effect of glutaraldehyde (2%) on washed suspension of *Bacillus subtilis* spores (3 × 10^7 ml^{-1}). ▼, alkaline solution (sodium bicarbonate 0.3% activator) pH 7.9; ■, acid solution pH 4.0.

fluence the usefulness of the preparation and how it is used.

Reference has previously been made to the dramatic increase in biocidal activity of glutaraldehyde at alkaline pH. The difference in sporicidal activity of acid and alkaline solutions is illustrated in Figure 34–9. As temperature is increased, this difference in activity is reduced until at 70°C both are equally effective producing a complete kill of *Bacillus subtilis* spores (10⁷/ml) within 5 min (Sierra and Boucher, 1971).

Unfortunately alkaline solutions have poor stability, and a loss of antimicrobial activity is observed in such solutions on storage (Table 34–8). This is related to a drop in concentration of free aldehyde, which appears to be essential for biocidal activity. One estimate of the decrease in glutaraldehyde that can occur comes from a study by Borick (1968). This measured a fall from 2.1% (pH 8.5) to 1.3% (pH 7.4) over a period of 28 days at ambient temperatures. These values have been confirmed by Miner et al. (1977), who also showed that glutaraldehyde concentrations in solutions of pH 7.3 and lower were not affected by storage. As outlined in the section on *Novel Formulations*, several successful formulation exercises have resulted in much improved stability of alkaline glutaraldehyde solutions. Other preparations are formulated at a lower pH, some with other potentiators included to increase the otherwise low level of activity observed.

In practice, glutaraldehyde is generally available as a 2% solution to which an "activator" is added to bring the solution to alkaline pH. This activated solution has a limited shelf-life, on the order of 14 days. The problem of in-use dilution of glutaraldehyde solutions is of concern especially with regard to stabilized formulations designed for longer use. A long period of use would inevitably result in dilution of the sterilizing solution, which may be accompanied by pH changes and contamination by organic matter and contribute to loss of activity. Ayliffe et al. (1979) considered that repeated use of a solution, however stable, for more than 7 to 14 days was undesirable.

In-use conditions for disinfection and sterilization inevitably imply the presence of organic matter such as blood and pus. Ideally, therefore, a chemical agent should remain unaffected by organic matter. Many reports indicate a high resistance of glutaraldehyde to neutralization by organic matter, a surprising fact considering the reactivity of glutaraldehyde with protein. The presence of 20% blood serum (Borick et al., 1964) or 1% whole blood (Snyder and Cheatle, 1965) did not appear to adversely affect activity of glutaraldehyde. Using a specially devised test method, Miner et al. (1975) measured the concentration (% w/v) of sterile baker's yeast

(called the soil neutralization number) that a disinfectant could tolerate and still be able to kill bacteria in 10 min at 25°C. These authors found that 2% alkaline glutaraldehyde had a maximum neutralization number of 50% against *Staphylococcus aureus* and *Pseudomonas aeruginosa*. This was explained on the basis of the uptake pattern exhibited by glutaraldehyde, which is of the L (Langmuir) type. It was proposed that alkaline glutaraldehyde would react with a limited number of adsorption sites, either cell surfaces or other proteinaceous material, and would therefore remain relatively unaffected by a high content of organic matter.

One of the problems associated with determinations of the minimum inhibitory concentration (MIC) has been the reactivity of glutaraldehyde with constituents of the growth medium. Rubbo et al. (1967) noted a darkening of nutrient broth in the presence of glutaraldehyde, which was thought to explain the poor bacteriostatic results obtained. Furthermore, a 60% decrease in free aldehyde concentration occurs when alkaline glutaraldehyde is added to malt extract broth (Gorman and Scott, 1977b), although this is a fairly slow reaction over a 6-hour period at 37°C.

Neutralization of glutaraldehyde during in-vitro testing has been approached in a number of ways. In some reports no inactivator has been used; however, in such cases the results are only valid if dilutions were performed to subinhibitory levels. In a search for a suitable inactivator for glutaraldehyde, we found 1% glycine to be effective and nontoxic to the organism employed, *E. coli* (Gorman and Scott, 1976b). In a report on bactericidal activity of 40 potential disinfectant inactivators, Reybrouck (1978) also found glycine to be nontoxic to *Staphylococcus aureus* and *Pseudomonas aeruginosa*. Cheung and Brown (1982) similarly recommended glycine for neutralization of glutaraldehyde, though at a concentration of 2%. The higher concentration was recommended when high concentrations of glutaraldehyde are to be neutralized. Most of the other chemical inactivators used for glutaraldehyde inactivation have proven unsatisfactory (Munton and Russell, 1970a; Bergan and Lystad, 1971). Some methods of glutaraldehyde neutralization do not require the presence of an additional chemical inactivator; these include centrifuging the glutaraldehyde/cell mixture, followed by washing (Forsyth,

Table 34–8. *Effect of Storage on the Sporicidal Activity* of 2% Acid and Alkaline Glutaraldehyde (Based on Gorman and Scott, 1979a and b)*

Storage Time (weeks)	Acid		Alkaline	
	Time (min) for 99.9% Kill	Glutaraldehyde Concentration (%)	Time (min) for 99.9% Kill	Glutaraldehyde Concentration (%)
0	>300	2.0	40	2.0
2	>300	1.9	120–180	1.6
6	>300	1.5	>300	0.7
12	>300	1.5	>300	0.6
24	>300	1.5	>300	0.3

*Activity determined at 18°C against *Bacillus subtilis* (spore count: 10⁸/ml).

1975; Relyveld, 1977) and filtering with washing (Miner et al., 1977).

The methods and problems of biocidal testing require consideration, because they may influence claims for glutaraldehyde activity (see section on mycobacteria). The AOAC sporicidal test is well controlled and established as a standard procedure, although in the past this method has given variable results (Starke et al., 1975). Survival curves of treated spore suspensions provide more information on the kinetics of sporicidal action, but are also subject to wide variation. Many of the variables in such tests with glutaraldehyde were investigated by Forsyth (1975), who suggested improvements in the basic method. The problems of spore resistance as affected by method of preparation and recovery of spores after treatment would appear to warrant more attention. This aspect was illustrated by Hodges et al. (1980) using chemically defined and complex media for the production of *Bacillus subtilis* spores. The spore crops thus obtained differed in their resistance to glutaraldehyde. Reference to Table 34–7 allows comparison of glutaraldehyde (pH 7.9) sporicidal activity against spores and spore forms produced on solid medium and defined liquid medium in our laboratories. Significant differences in activity are observed (Gorman et al., 1984b). We have also shown that a progressive development of resistance to glutaraldehyde occurs on prolonged incubation of sporulating *B. subtilis* in sporulation medium (Gorman et al., 1984c). A time of 72 min was required for 2% glutaraldehyde to effect a 90% kill of 1-day *B. subtilis* spores, compared to 94 min required for 14-day spores.

Novel Formulations

Since the expiration of the original patent on the sterilizing action of alkalinated glutaraldehyde, many new products have been introduced, having equivalent activity and stability to the original patented product. In addition, in an attempt to improve the stability of activated glutaraldehyde, some preparations were formulated at lower alkaline pH values or at acid pH. This has the effect of reducing the rate of polymerization of glutaraldehyde and thus prolonging shelf-life. Microbiologic activity was maintained usually by the inclusion of a surfactant in the formulation. Jacobs (1986) described a glutaraldehyde composition containing an activator system that does not precipitate salts when diluted with hard water. This makes it possible to formulate solutions with an increased concentration of active glutaraldehyde to be diluted at the point of use without the attendant possibility of precipitate being deposited on sterilized surgical instruments. In a report by Babb et al. (1980), nine glutaraldehyde products were compared. All were effective against spores in suspension in 3 hours or less, but the acid glutaraldehyde preparations tested were less effective than alkaline ones, particularly against dried spores, and they also tended to be more corrosive.

Numerous attempts have been made to potentiate the antimicrobial activity of glutaraldehyde solutions. These have frequently involved addition of surface active agents: cationic (Stonehill, 1966), nonionic (Sidwell et al., 1970; Wilkoff et al., 1971), nonionic ethoxylates of isomeric linear alcohols (Boucher, 1971), amphoteric (Dick and Rombi, 1977), and anionic (Gorman and Scott, 1979a). Addition of inorganic cations will further increase activity (Gorman and Scott, 1979b), as does the use of ultrasonic energy (Sierra and Boucher, 1971). Addition of a second antimicrobial agent to provide a synergistic effect has also been reported. In this respect, addition of phenol to glutaraldehyde has proved to be beneficial (Schattner, 1978; Leach, 1981). Reports on other novel glutaraldehyde formulations have been reviewed by Gorman et al. (1980).

Toxicology

The use of glutaraldehyde for the chemical sterilization of heat-sensitive equipment is now widespread. This type of specialized use brings with it possible risks of toxic reactions occurring (1) to the individual handling the equipment during the disinfecting or sterilizing process and (2) to the patient exposed to equipment treated with glutaraldehyde—in some cases this may involve contact with the blood stream.

With regard to individuals being exposed to glutaraldehyde during handling of equipment, Axon et al. (1981), using results of a questionnaire, reported that 37% of endoscopy units using glutaraldehyde for disinfection reported health problems among their staff that were attributed to glutaraldehyde use. Other reports of occupational toxicity refer to small numbers of individuals (Sanderson and Cronin, 1968; Lyon, 1971; Hansen et al., 1983; Benson, 1984). Corrado et al. (1986) used provocation testing to determine allergic reactions in nurses who reported respiratory symptoms that they attributed to exposure to glutaraldehyde. Two of the four patients investigated had a confirmed reaction to glutaraldehyde. Estimates of percutaneous penetration of topically applied glutaraldehyde (10% aqueous solution) indicated that although no penetration of thick stratum corneum could be detected, approximately 3% penetrated epidermis and 3 to 13.8% penetration of thin stratum corneum occurred (Reifenrath et al., 1985). Irritation and one case of sensitization also resulted from application of glutaraldehyde to areas of thin stratum corneum. Evidence for a dose-dependent contact hypersensitivity response to glutaraldehyde was demonstrated in guinea pigs and mice (Stern et al., 1989). Inhalation is severely toxic when high-aldehyde concentrations are allowed to evaporate in a closed system. Meltzer and Henkin (1977) stated that single inhalations of concentrated vapors (25 and 50% glutaraldehyde) by rats for 6 to 8 hours did not kill any of the exposed animals.

It is important to reduce the risks of glutaraldehyde toxicity to staff by the use of clearly defined handling procedures such as wearing of rubber gloves (provided they are resistant to organic chemicals) and safety goggles. Siting of equipment in hoods or cabinets with exhaust is also necessary to prevent vapor inhalation. These and other safety measures were recommended by the Working Party of the British Society of Gastroenterology for cleaning and disinfection of endoscopes (Weller et al., 1988).

A number of publications have considered the risk to the patient from using glutaraldehyde-treated equipment. Varpela et al. (1971) showed that approximately 10% of glutaraldehyde absorbed by rubber or plastic parts was liberated in 24 hours. A useful and comprehensive report by Osterberg (1978) has studied the residual glutaraldehyde in plastics and rubbers after exposure to alkaline glutaraldehyde solution. The degree of absorption of glutaraldehyde into various materials correlated with time of contact between material and solution. The absorbed glutaraldehyde was confined to the surface of the exposed material, and a single 2-min rinse procedure significantly reduced glutaraldehyde levels. Further rinsing had little effect, although an extended immersion in rinsing solution did cause considerable desorption. On repeated exposure to glutaraldehyde, as would occur in practice, a build-up in glutaraldehyde levels was apparent only in latex rubber. Therefore, for this material, extended soaking and rinsing procedures were recommended. In a report on the use of glutaraldehyde to process tissue heart valves, Woodroff (1978) quoted a glutaraldehyde concentration of greater than 10 to 25 ppm as causing toxic effects on cells of any type. A protocol of three separate rinses in 500 ml of sterile normal saline for 2 min each with gentle agitation was recommended. This gave glutaraldehyde concentrations in the final rinse of less than 1 ppm. Glutaraldehyde release from bioprostheses can induce cytotoxic reactions (Woodroof, 1978; Gendler et al., 1984; Weibe et al., 1988). Various rinsing procedures have been recommended to reduce aldehyde levels, including rinsing followed by storage in glutaraldehyde-free solutions (Gendler et al., 1984).

The LD_{50} value of glutaraldehyde was estimated by Stonehill et al. (1963) to be 15 mg/kg in mice and 9.8 mg/kg in rats. According to Osterberg (1978) these values correlated with his own findings that damage to leucocytes was apparent only above a 100 μg/ml glutaraldehyde level. In addition, no erythrocyte damage occurred at the glutaraldehyde concentrations used. From his observations Osterberg concluded that even in extremely adverse circumstances, there was little risk of damage to blood cells due to the use of glutaraldehyde-treated apparatus. A potentiated acid glutaraldehyde was judged not to be teratogenic to mice in spite of using relatively high doses (Marks et al., 1980). Glutaraldehyde was not found to be mutagenic in the Ames test (Sasaki and Endo, 1978) and in four in-vitro systems involving microbial and mammalian-cell indicator tests (Slesinski et al., 1983).

APPLICATIONS

An increasing number of applications for glutaraldehyde continue to be found. Glutaraldehyde is used extensively in several major nonmicrobiologic areas, including the leather tanning industry and tissue fixation for electron microscopy. In a microbiologic context, glutaraldehyde has mainly been employed for the liquid chemical sterilization of medical and surgical material that cannot be sterilized by heat or irradiation.

Several advantages provide the basis for glutaraldehyde's use as a chemosterilizer:

1. Broad spectrum of activity, including sporicidal activity and rapidity of action
2. Activity in the presence of organic matter
3. Noncorrosive action toward metals, rubber, lenses, and most materials (although some formulations may not fulfill these criteria) (Ayliffe et al., 1979)
4. Lack of deleterious effects on cement and lenses of endoscopes

However, the increase in number of reports of occupational sensitivity reactions has resulted in growing concern about glutaraldehyde use, and adequate safety precautions are required to minimize risk of toxicity among operators (see toxicology section).

Disinfection of endoscopy equipment has become one of the main uses of glutaraldehyde. These instruments must be free of pathogens such as hepatitis B, HIV, and *Mycobacterium tuberculosis* to prevent transmission of infection between patients. The traditional heating methods of sterilization are unsuitable because they damage the instruments, and although ethylene oxide is recommended, it is not always available and is a time-consuming process. The requirement for a rapid turnover of equipment has necessitated rapid high-level liquid disinfection, and glutaraldehyde is regarded as the agent of choice (O'Connor and Axon, 1983; Ayliffe et al., 1986). A 30-min immersion was recommended following use of an endoscope on a patient or carrier of hepatitis B or AIDS, and a 1-hour immersion following use in a tuberculosis patient (Ayliffe et al., 1986). More recently, the interim report of the Working Party of the British Society of Gastroenterology recommended glutaraldehyde as a firstline disinfectant and proposed a 4-min soak as sufficient for inactivation of vegetative bacteria and viruses, including HIV and HBV (Weller et al., 1988). Many additional references have been made to the use of glutaraldehyde for rapid and safe disinfection of gastrointestinal endoscopy equipment (Axon et al., 1974; Tolon et al., 1976; Carr-Locke and Clayton, 1978; Noy et al., 1980).

Rittenbury and Hench (1965) were among the first workers to recommend glutaraldehyde for cold sterilization of hemostats, cystoscopes, food containers, and anaesthetic equipment. The success of this practice was confirmed by several authors (George, 1975; Lin et al., 1979). It has also proved useful for disinfection of urologic instruments (Mitchell and Alder, 1975) and gynecologic laparoscopy equipment (Loffer, 1980). Occasionally adverse effects of glutaraldehyde on medical equipment are observed (Mostafa, 1980).

Glutaraldehyde has been recommended for the decontamination of dental surgical instruments and working surfaces where the hepatitis B surface antigen (HBsAg) may be present (Anonymous, 1978). Glutaraldehyde-moistened sponges were shown by Christensen (1977) to be suitable for sterilizing dental equipment that could not be heat sterilized or immersed in a fluid bath because of large size, fixed position, or destructible parts. Also in the dental field, a low-concentration, stable glutaraldehyde disinfectant/cleaner was shown to be effective for aspirator care (Gorman and Scott, 1985).

The effectiveness of vapor-phase glutaraldehyde for surface disinfection against vegetative bacteria and spores was shown by Bovallius and Anas (1977) when in spite of its low volatility it was more effective than formaldehyde on an added amount basis. Nicklas and Bohm (1981) also found glutaraldehyde to have good disinfectant activity in the aerosol state and recommended it for disinfection of surfaces. In a related study, the effectiveness of glutaraldehyde in reducing surface contamination of packaged medical devices was investigated (Eskenazi et al., 1982). Glutaraldehyde was able to penetrate several types of packaging material, though not polyethylene film.

The treatment of viral warts with glutaraldehyde has been reported on several occasions (London, 1971; Bunney et al., 1976; Bunney, 1977). A 73.5% cure rate with 227 patients with viral warts treated with aqueous ethanol and collodion-based preparations of glutaraldehyde was demonstrated by Allenby (1977). A 10% solution (pH 4.2) in aqueous ethanol was found to be most convenient. Similar results are claimed for a recent presentation of glutaraldehyde (10%) as a semisolid aqueous-based gel for the treatment of plantar warts (Scott, 1982). Aqueous solutions of glutaraldehyde have been used to treat hyperhydrosis (Juhlin and Hansson, 1968), and topically applied glutaraldehyde has been effective in the treatment of onychomycosis (Suringa, 1970). Several dental applications have been described, including anti-caries formulations (Eigen, 1970; Litchfield and Vely, 1972). Hannah (1972) showed a glutaraldehyde-calcium hydroxide combination to be an effective pulp dressing for dental work.

Frequently in immunochemical work the need arises to link proteins to particles, to polymerize proteins, or to form covalent conjugates of proteins and smaller peptides (Reichlin, 1980). Glutaraldehyde is one of the few reagents that have been successfully used for all the above applications while also preserving the native antigenicity of the material under study. In the immunologic field glutaraldehyde has been used in the preparation of vaccines such as tetanus (Relyveld, 1973, 1975; Relyveld et al., 1973) and pertussis (Gupta et al., 1988). In a study of detoxification of tetanus toxin, glutaraldehyde proved to be most favorable compared to the activity of formaldehyde or β-propiolactone (Kunsel and Meissner, 1978). Kao et al. (1977) have described the use of the agent in radioimmune assays for a specific antigen. An interesting paper on the production of Type

I interferon has also appeared (Levon et al., 1980). This was induced by culturing human lymphocytes with cells infected with herpes virus and treated with glutaraldehyde. An excellent review by Relyveld and Ben-Efraim (1983) describes the preparation of vaccines by the action of glutaraldehyde on toxins, bacteria, viruses, allergens, and cells.

The antimicrobial properties of glutaraldehyde have also been applied in other areas. In the poultry industry, glutaraldehyde has been employed as a disinfectant in the immersion chilling of poultry (Mast and MacNeill, 1978). Thomson et al. (1977) showed that a 10-min pre-chill in 0.5% glutaraldehyde (pH 8.6) extended shelf-life of boiler carcasses at 2°C approximately 6 days beyond controls; salmonella transfer was also prevented. In the cosmetic industry glutaraldehyde has been recommended for disinfection of production equipment (Janik et al., 1977) and as a preservative (Meltzer and Henkin, 1970, 1977). The sterilization of fermentation media has been reported in the patent literature (Union Carbide, 1979). Glutaraldehyde also has certain advantages over formaldehyde as the preservative employed in the ancient art of embalming (Anonymous, 1962). In the veterinary field (Meaney, 1981), the introduction of glutaraldehyde as a teat-skin disinfectant for control of mastitis has been successful. Glutaraldehyde was shown to be more effective than iodine in preventing new intramammary infection, and no evidence of teat skin irritation was observed.

It appears that glutaraldehyde will continue to find new areas of useful application. A further example of this is its increasing role in combating microbial contamination, particularly sulphate-reducing bacteria, in oil-field water injection systems (Stott and Herbert, 1986).

REFERENCES

Adler-Storthz, K., Sehulster, L.M., Dreesman, G.R., and Hollinger, F.B. 1983. Effect of alkaline glutaraldehyde on Hepatitis B virus antigen. Eur. J. Clin. Microbiol., *2*, 316–320.

Allenby, C.F. 1977. The treatment of viral warts with glutaraldehyde. Br. J. Clin. Pract., *31*, 12–13.

Anderson, P.J. 1967. Purification and quantitation of glutaraldehyde and its effect on several enzyme activities in skeletal muscle. J. Histochem. Cytochem., *15*, 652–661.

Anonymous. 1962. Dialdehyde based fluids improve embalming procedures. Chemical Progress (Union Carbide Chemicals Co.), February.

Anonymous, U.S. Department of Health, Education and Welfare. 1977. Isolation of mycobacteria species from porcine heart valve prosthesis. Morbid. Mortal. Week. Rep., *26*, 42–43.

Anonymous. 1978. Expert group on hepatitis in dentistry. Report to the chief medical and dental officers of the Health Department of Great Britain. H.M.S.O. Publication.

Ascenzi, J.M., Ezzell, R.J., and Wendt, T.M. 1986. Evaluation of carriers used in the test methods of the Association of Official Analytical Chemists. Appl. Environ. Microbiol., *51*, 91–94.

Axon, A.T.R., Phillips, I., Cotton, P.B., and Avery, S.A. 1974. Disinfection of gastrointestinal fibre endoscopes. Lancet, *1*, 656–658.

Axon, A.T.R., et al. 1981. Lancet, *1*, 1093–1094.

Ayliffe, G.A., and Deverill, C.E.A. 1979. Decontamination of gastroscopes. Health Soc. Serv. J., May, 538–540.

Ayliffe, G.A., Collins, B.J., and Babb, J.R. 1979. Disinfection with glutaraldehyde. Br. Med. J., *1*, 1019.

Ayliffe, G.A., Babb, J.R., and Bradley, C.R. 1986. Disinfection of endoscopes. J. Hosp. Infect., *7*, 295–309.

Babb, J.R., Bradley, C.R., and Ayliffe, G.A. 1980. Sporicidal activity of glutaraldehydes and hypochlorites and other factors influencing their selection for the treatment of medical equipment. J. Hosp. Infect., 1, 63–75.

Baltimore, D., and Huang, A.S. 1968. Isopyonic separation of subcellular components from poliovirus-infected and normal HeLa cells. Science, 162, 572–574.

Bassett, D.J.C. 1971. Common-source outbreaks. Proc. R. Soc. Med., 64, 18–24.

Benson, W.G. 1984. Case report of exposure to glutaraldehyde. J. Soc. Occup. Med., 34, 63–64.

Bergan, T., and Lystad, A. 1971. Antitubercular action of disinfectants. J. App. Bacteriol., 34, 751–756.

Best, M., Sattar, S.A., Springthorpe, V.S., and Kennedy, M.E. 1988. Comparative mycobactericidal efficacy of chemical disinfectants in suspension and carrier tests. Appl. Environ. Microbiol., 54, 2856–2858.

Blass, J., Verriest, C., Leau, A., and Weis, M. 1976. Monomeric glutaraldehyde as an effective cross-linking reagent for proteins. J. Am. Leather Chem. Assoc., 74, 121–131.

Blough, H.A. 1966. Selective inactivation of biological activity of myxoviruses by glutaraldehyde. J. Bacteriol., 92, 266–268.

Bond, W.W., Favero, M.S., Petersen, N.J., and Ebert, J.W. 1983. Inactivation of Hepatitis B virus by intermediate-to-high-level disinfectant chemicals. J. Clin Microbiol., 18, 535–538.

Borick, P.M. 1968. Chemical sterilizers (chemosterilizers). Adv. Appl. Microbiol., 10, 291–312.

Borick, P.M., Dondershine, F.H., and Chandler, J.L. 1964. Alkalinised glutaraldehyde, a new antimicrobial agent. J. Pharm. Sci., 53, 1273–1275.

Boucher, R.M.G. 1971. Method and sporicidal compositions for synergistic disinfection or sterilisation. U.S. Patent Application No. 155, 233.

Boucher, R.M.G. 1974. Potentiated 1,5 pentanedial, a breakthrough in chemical sterilizing and disinfecting technology. Am. J. Hosp. Pharm., 31, 546–557.

Boucher, R.M.G. 1975. On biocidal mechanisms in the aldehyde series. Can. J. Pharm. Sci., 10, 1–7.

Boucher, R.M.G., Last, A.J., and Smith, G.K. 1973. Biochemical mechanisms of saturated dialdehydes and their potentiation by ultrasound. Proc. West. Pharmacol. Soc., 16, 282–288.

Boudouma, M., Enjalbert, L., and Didier, J. 1984. A simple method for the evaluation of antiseptic and disinfectant virucidal activity. J. Virol. Methods, 9, 271–276.

Bovallius, A., and Anas, P. 1977. Surface-decontaminating action of glutaraldehyde in the gas-aerosol phase. Appl. Environ. Microbiol., 34, 129–134.

Bowes, J.H., and Cater, C.W. 1966. The reaction of glutaraldehyde with proteins and other biological materials. J. R. Microsc. Soc., 85, 193–200.

Bunney, M.H. 1977. The treatment of viral warts. Drugs, 13, 445–451.

Bunney, M.H., Nolan, M.W., and Williams, D.A. 1976. An assessment of methods of treating viral warts by comparative treatment of trials based on a standard design. Br. J. Dermatol., 94, 667–679.

Carr-Locke, D.L., and Clayton, P. 1978. Disinfection of upper gastrointestinal fibreoptic endoscopy equipment: an evaluation of a cetrimide, chlorhexidine solution and glutaraldehyde. Gut, 19, 916–922.

Carson, L.A., Favero, M.S., Bond, W.W., and Petersen, N.J. 1972. Factors affecting comparative resistance of naturally-occurring and subcultured Pseudomonas aeruginosa to disinfectants. Appl. Microbiol., 23, 863–869.

Carson, L.A., Petersen, N.J., Favero, M.S., and Aguero, S.M. 1978. Growth characteristics of atypical mycobacteria in water and their comparative resistance to disinfectants. Appl. Environ. Microbiol., 36, 839–846.

Cheng, K.J., Ingram, J.M., and Costerton, J.W. 1970. Alkaline phosphatase localisation and spheroplast formation of Pseudomonas aeruginosa. Can. J. Microbiol., 16, 1319–1324.

Cheung, D.T., Perelman, N., Ko, E.C., and Nimni, M.E. 1985. Mechanism of crosslinking of proteins by glutaraldehyde 111. Reaction with collagen in tissues. Conn. Tiss. Res., 13, 109–115.

Cheung, H.Y., and Brown, M.R.W. 1982. Evaluation of glycine as an inactivator of glutaraldehyde. J. Pharm. Pharmacol., 34, 211–214.

Christensen, R.P. 1977. Effectiveness of glutaraldehyde as a chemosterilizer used in a wrapping technique on stimulated metal instruments. J. Dent. Res., 56, 822–826.

Coates, D., and Death, J.E. 1978. Sporicidal activity of mixtures of alcohol and hypochlorite. J. Clin. Pathol., 31, 148–152.

Collins, F.M. 1986a. Kinetics of the tuberculocidal response by alkaline glutaraldehyde in solution and on an inert surface. J. Appl. Bacteriol., 61, 87–93.

Collins, F.M. 1986b. Bactericidal activity of alkaline glutaraldehyde solution against a number of atypical mycobacterial species. J. Appl. Bacteriol., 61, 247–251.

Collins, J. 1986. The use of glutaraldehyde in tuberculosis laboratory discard jars. Lett. Appl. Microbiol., 2, 103–105.

Corrado, O.J., Osman, J., and Davies, R.J. 1986. Asthma and rhinitis after exposure to glutaraldehyde in endoscopy units. Hum. Toxicol., 5, 325–327.

Dabrowa, N., Landau, J.W., and Newcomer, V.D. 1972. Antifungal activity of glutaraldehyde in vitro. Arch. Dermatol., 105, 555–557.

Dick, P.R.G., and Rombi, M.A. 1977. New sterilizing compositions. French Patent No. 2,313,081.

Dickinson, A.G., and Taylor, D.M. 1978. Resistance of Scrapie agent to decontamination. N. Engl. J. Med., 229, 1413–1414.

Dijk, F., Oosterbaan, J.A., and Hulstaert, C.E. 1985. A rapid method for obtaining monomeric glutaraldehyde. Histochemistry, 83, 573–574.

Done, J., Shorey, C.D., Locke, J.P., and Pollak, J.K. 1965. The cytochemical localization of alkaline phosphatase in Escherichia coli at the electron microscope level. Biochem. J., 96, 27c–28c.

Drulak, M.W., et al. 1978a. The relative effectiveness of commonly used disinfectants in inactivation of coxsackievirus B5. J. Hyg. Camb., 81, 389–397.

Drulak, M.W., Wallbank, A.M., and Lebtag, I. 1978b. The relative effectiveness of commonly used disinfectants in inactivation of echovirus 11. J. Hyg. Camb., 81, 77–87.

Drulak, M.W., Wallbank, A.M., and Lebtag, I. 1984. The effectiveness of six disinfectants in inactivation of reovirus 3. Microbios, 41, 31–38.

Dyas, A., and Das, B.C. 1985. The activity of glutaraldehyde against Clostridium difficile. J. Hosp. Infect., 6, 41–45.

Eigen, E. 1970. Oral compositions containing non-toxic non-volatile aliphatic aldehydes. U.S. Patent No. 3,497,590.

Ellar, D.J., Munoz, E., and Salton, M.R.J. 1971. The effect of low concentrations of glutaraldehyde on Micrococcus lysodeikticus membranes. Biochem. Biophys. Acta, 225, 140–150.

Eskenazi, S., Bychkowski, O.E., Smith, M., and Macmillan, J.D. 1982. Evaluation of glutaraldehyde and hydrogen peroxide for sanitizing packaging materials of medical devices in sterility testing. J. Assoc. Off. Anal. Chem., 65, 1155–1161.

Evans, D.H., Stuart, P., and Roberts, D.H. 1977. Disinfection of animal viruses. Br. Vet. J., 133, 356–359.

Fahimi, H.D., and Drochmans, P. 1965. Essais de standardisation de la fixation au glutaraldehyde. J. Microsc., 4, 725–736.

Forsyth, M.P. 1975. A rate of kill test for measuring sporicidal properties of liquid sterilisers. Dev. Indust. Microbiol., 16, 37–47.

Frigerio, N.A., and Shaw, M.J. 1968. A simple method for determination of glutaraldehyde. J. Histochem. Cytochem., 17, 176–181.

Gendler, E., Gendler, S., and Nimni, M.E. 1984. Toxic reactions evoked by glutaraldehyde-fixed pericardium and cardiac valve bioprosthesis. J. Biomed. Mater. Res., 18, 727–736.

George, R.H. 1975. A critical look at chemical disinfection of anaesthetic apparatus. Br. J. Anaesth., 47, 719–722.

Gillett, R., and Gull, K. 1972. Glutaraldehyde—its purity and stability. Histochemistry, 30, 162–167.

Gorman, S.P., and Scott, E.M. 1976a. An assessment of the antifungal activity of glutaraldehyde. J. Pharm. Pharmacol., 28, 48.

Gorman, S.P., and Scott, E.M. 1976b. An evaluation of potential inactivators of glutaraldehyde in disinfection studies with Escherichia coli. Microbios Lett., 1, 197–204.

Gorman, S.P., and Scott, E.M. 1977a. A quantitative evaluation of the antifungal properties of glutaraldehyde. J. Appl. Bacteriol., 43, 83–89.

Gorman, S.P., and Scott, E.M. 1977b. Uptake and media reactivity of glutaraldehyde solutions related to structure and biocidal activity. Microbios Lett., 5, 163–169.

Gorman, S.P., and Scott, E.M. 1977c. Transport capacity, alkaline phosphatase activity and protein content of glutaraldehyde-treated cell forms of Escherichia coli. Microbios, 19, 205–212.

Gorman, S.P., and Scott, E.M. 1977d. Preparation and stability of mureinoplasts of Escherichia coli. Microbios, 18, 123–130.

Gorman, S.P., and Scott, E.M. 1977e. Effect of alkalination on the bacterial cell and glutaraldehyde molecule. Microbios Lett., 6, 39–44.

Gorman, S.P., and Scott, E.M. 1979a. Potentiation and stabilization of glutaraldehyde biocidal activity utilising surfactant-divalent cation combinations. Int. J. Pharm., 4, 57–65.

Gorman, S.P., and Scott, E.M. 1979b. Effect of inorganic cations on the biocidal and cellular activity of glutaraldehyde. J. Appl. Bacteriol., 47, 463–468.

Gorman, S.P., and Scott, E.M. 1980. The state of glutaraldehyde molecule in relation to its biocidal activity. J. Pharm. Pharmacol., 32, 131–132.

Gorman, S.P., Scott, E.M., and Russell, A.D. 1980. A review. Antimicrobial activity, uses and mechanism of action of glutaraldehyde. J. Appl. Bacteriol., 48, 161–190.

Gorman, S.P., Scott, E.M., and Hutchinson, E.P. 1983a. The effect of sodium hypochlorite-ethanol combinations on spores and spore forms of Bacillus subtilis. Int. J. Pharm., 17, 291–298.

Gorman, S.P., Hutchinson, E.P., Scott, E.M., and McDermott, L.M. 1983b. Death, injury and revival of chemically treated Bacillus subtilis spores. J. Appl. Bacteriol., 54, 91–99.

Gorman, S.P., Scott, E.M., and Hutchinson, E.P. 1984a. Hypochlorite effects on spores and spore forms of Bacillus subtilis and on a spore lytic enzyme. J. Appl. Bacteriol., 56, 295–303.

Gorman, S.P., Scott, E.M., and Hutchinson, E.P. 1984b. Interaction of the Bacillus subtilis spore protoplast, cortex, ion-exchange and coatless forms with glutaraldehyde. J. Appl. Bacteriol., 56, 95–102.

Gorman, S.P., Scott, E.M., and Hutchinson, E.P. 1984c. Emergence and development of resistance to antimicrobial chemicals and heat in spores of *Bacillus subtilis*. J. Appl. Bacteriol., 57, 153–163.

Gorman, S.P., and Scott, E.M. 1985. A comparative evaluation of dental aspirator cleansing and disinfectant solutions. Br. Dent. J., 158, 13–16.

Gould, G.W., and Dring, G.L. 1975. Heat resistance of bacterial endospores and concept of an expanded osmoregulatory cortex. Nature, 258, 402–405.

Graham, J.L., and Jaeger, R.F. 1968. Inactivation of yellow fever virus by glutaraldehyde. Appl. Microbiol., 16, 177.

Gupta, R.K., Saxena, S.N., Sharma, S.B., and Ahuja, S. 1988. Studies on the optimal conditions for inactivation of Bordetella pertussis organisms with glutaraldehyde for preparation of a safe and potent pertussis vaccine. Vaccine, 6, 491–496.

Habeeb, A.F.S.A., and Hiramoto, R. 1968. Reactions of proteins with glutaraldehyde. Arch. Biochem. Biophys., 126, 16–26.

Hajdu, J., and Friedrich, P. 1975. Reaction of glutaraldehyde with NH_2 compounds. A spectrophotometric method for the determination of glutaraldehyde concentration. Anal. Biochem., 65, 273–280.

Hannah, D.R. 1972. Glutaraldehyde and calcium hydroxide, a pulp dressing material. Br. Dent. J., 132, 227–231.

Hansen, K.S. 1983. Glutaraldehyde occupational dermatitis. Contact Dermatitis, 9, 81–82.

Hardy, P.M., Nicholls, A.C., and Rydon, H.N. 1969. The nature of glutaraldehyde in aqueous solution. J. Chem. Soc., (D), 565–566.

Hardy, P.M., Hughes, G.J., and Rydon, H.N. 1976a. Formation of quaternary pyridinium compounds by the action of glutaraldehyde on proteins. Chem. Soc. Chem. Comm., 5, 157–158.

Hardy, P.M., Nicholls, A.C., and Rydon, H.N. 1976b. The nature of the cross-linking of proteins by glutaraldehyde. Part I. Interaction of glutaraldehyde with the amino groups of 6-amino-hexanoic acid and of α-N-acetyl-lysine. J. Chem. Soc. Perkin., 1, 958–962.

Hardy, P.M., Hughes, G.J., and Rydon, H.N. 1977. Identification of a 3-(2-piperidyl)-pyridinium derivative (anabilysine) as a cross-linking entity in a glutaraldehyde-treated protein. J. Chem. Soc. Chem. Comm., 21, 759–760.

Hardy, P.M., Hughes, G.J., and Rydon, H.N. 1979. The nature of the cross-linking of proteins by glutaraldehyde. Part 2. The formation of quaternary pyridinium compounds by the action of glutaraldehyde on proteins and the identification of a 3-(2-piperidyl)-pyridinium derivative, anabilysine, as a cross-linking entity. J. Chem. Soc. Perkin. 1, 2282–2288.

Harke, H.P., and Pust, U. 1978. Quantitative determination of glutaraldehyde in disinfectants. Zentrabl. Bakteriol. Mikrobiol. Hyg. [B], 167, 87–89.

Harries, C.D., and Tank, L. 1908. Conversion of cyclopentene into the mono- and di-aldehyde of glutaric acid. Berichte., 41, 1701–1711.

Hashimoto, K., et al. 1983. Studies of aqueous solutions of glutaraldehyde by gas chromatography-mass spectrometry. Int. J. Mass Spect. Ion Phys., 48, 125–128.

Hemminki, K., and Suni, R. 1984. Sites of reaction of glutaraldehyde and acetaldehyde with nucleosides. Arch. Toxicol., 55, 186–190.

Hodges, N.A., Melling, J., and Parker, S.J. 1980. A comparison of chemically defined and complex media for the production of *Bacillus subtilis* spores having reproducible resistance and germination characteristics. J. Pharm. Pharmacol., 32, 126–130.

Hopwood, D. 1972. Theoretical and practical aspects of glutaraldehyde fixation. Histochem. J., 4, 267–303.

Hopwood, D. 1975. Reactions of glutaraldehyde with nucleic acids. Histochem. J., 7, 267–276.

Hopwood, D., Allen, C.R., and McCabe, C. 1970. The reaction between glutaraldehyde and various proteins: an investigation of their kinetics. Histochem. J., 2, 137–150.

Hughes, R.C., and Thurman, P.F. 1970. Cross-linking of bacterial cell walls with glutaraldehyde. Biochem. J., 119, 925–926.

Jacobs, P.T. 1986. Buffered glutaraldehyde sterilizing and disinfecting compositions. European Patent Application. Publication No. 0184297.

Janik, D., Hall, C.S., and De Navarre, M.G. 1977. Glutaraldehyde—a sanitizing agent for the equipment used in the manufacture of cosmetics. Cosmet. Toil., 92, 99–100.

Jones, L.A., and Hancock, C.K. 1960. Spectrophotometric studies of some 2,4-dinitrophyenyl-hydrazones. II. J. Am. Chem. Soc., 82, 105–107.

Juhlin, H., and Hansson, H. 1968. Topical glutaraldehyde for plantar hyperhidrosis. Arch. Dermatol., 97, 327–330.

Kao, W.W.-Y., Guzman, N.A., and Prockop, D.J. 1977. Use of glutaraldehyde-fixed *Escherichia coli* cells as a convenient solid support for radioimmune assays. Anal. Biochem., 81, 209–219.

Kedzia, W., et al. 1973. Antiseptic soaps. Anestezja Reanimacja Intensywna Terapia, 5, 309–319.

Kelsey, J.C., Mackinnon, I.H., and Maurer, I.M. 1974. Sporicidal activity of hospital disinfectants. J. Clin. Pathol., 27, 632–638.

King, J.A., Woodside, W., and McGucken, P.V. 1974. Relationship between pH and antibacterial activity of glutaraldehyde. J. Pharm. Sci., 63, 804–805.

Kirkeby, S., and Moe, D. 1986. Studies on the actions of glutaraldehyde, formaldehyde, and mixtures of glutaraldehyde and formaldehyde on tissue protein. Acta Histochem., 79, 115–121.

Kirkeby, S., Jacobsen, P., and Moe, D. 1987. Glutaraldehyde—"pure and impure." A spectroscopic investigation of two commercial glutaraldehyde solutions and their reaction products with amino acids. Anal. Lett., 20, 303–315.

Klein, M., and Deforest, A. 1963. The inactivation of viruses by germicides. Chem. Spec. Manuf. Assoc. Proc., 49, 116–118.

Kobayashi, H., et al. 1984. Susceptibility of Hepatitis B virus to disinfectants or heat. J. Clin. Microbiol., 20, 214–216.

Korn, A.H., Feairheller, S.H., and Filachione, E.M. 1972. Glutaraldehyde, nature of the reagent. J. Mol. Biol., 65, 525–529.

Kunsel, W., and Meissner, C. 1978. Studies into detoxification of tetanus toxin. Arch. Exp. Veterinarmed., 32, 823–830.

Laskowski, L.F., et al. 1980. Fastidious mycobacteria grown from porcine prosthetic-heart valve cultures. N. Engl. J. Med., 297, 101–102.

Leach, E.D. 1981. A new synergized glutaraldehyde-phenate sterilizing solution and concentrated disinfectant. Infect. Control., 2, 26–30.

Lebon, P., et al. 1980. Type I interferon induced by culturing human lymphocytes with cells infected with herpes virus and treated with glutaraldehyde. C. R. HEBD Seances Acad. ci. Ser. D. Sci. Nat., 290, 37–40.

Leers, W.D. 1980. Disinfecting fibreoptic endoscopes: how not to transmit *Mycobacterium tuberculosis* by bronchoscopy. J. Can. Med. Assoc., 123, 275–283.

Leers, W.D., McAllister, J.S., and MacPherson, L.W. 1974. A comparative study of Cidex and Savlon. Can. J. Hosp. Pharm., Jan.-Feb., 17–18.

Lin, K.S., Park, M.K., Baker, H.A., and Sidorowicz, A. 1979. Disinfection of anaesthesia and respiratory therapy equipment with acid glutaraldehyde solution. Resp. Care, 24, 321–327.

Litchfield, J.H., and Vely, V.G. 1972. Dialdehyde-containing anti-caries chewing gum compositions. U.S. Patent No. 3,679,792.

Lloyd-Evans, N., Springthorpe, V.S., and Sattar, S.A. 1986. Chemical disinfection of human rotavirus-contaminated inanimate surfaces. J. Hyg. Camb., 97, 163–173.

Loffer, F.D. 1980. Disinfection versus sterilisation of gynaecological laparoscopy equipment. Reprod. Med., 25, 263–266.

London, I.D. 1971. Buffered glutaraldehyde solutions for warts. Arch. Dermatol., 104, 440.

Lyman, G.W., Johnson, R.N., and Kho, B.T. 1978. Gas chromatographic determination of glutaraldehyde. J. Chromatogr., 156, 285–292.

Lyon, T.C. 1971. Allergic contact dermatitis due to Cidax. Oral Surg., 32, 895–898.

Marks, T.A., Worthy, W.C., and Staples, R.E. 1980. Influence of formaldehyde and sonacide (potentiated acid glutaraldehyde) on embryo and fetal development in mice. Teratology, 22, 51–58.

Margel, S., and Rembaum, A. 1980. Synthesis and characterization of poly(glutaraldehyde). A potential reagent for protein immobilization and cell separation. Macromolecules, 13, 19–24.

Mast, M.G., and MacNeil, J.H. 1978. Use of glutaraldehyde as a disinfectant in immersion chilling of poultry. Poult. Sci., 57, 681–684.

McErlean, E.P., Gorman, S.P., and Scott, E.M. 1980. Physical and chemical resistance of ion-exchange and coat defective spores of *Bacillus subtilis*. J. Pharm. Pharmacol., 32, 32P.

McGucken, P.V., and Woodside, W. 1973. Studies on the mode of action of glutaraldehyde on *Escherichia coli*. J. Appl. Bacteriol., 36, 419–426.

Meaney, W.J. 1981. Effective new teat disinfectant for dairy cows. Farm Food Res., 12, 13–15.

Meltzer, N., and Henkin, H. 1970. Glutaraldehyde—a new preservative for cosmetics. 6th Cong. Int. Fed. Soc. Cos. Chem. Preprints, Barcelona, 2, pp. 833–850.

Meltzer, N., and Henkin, H. 1977. Glutaraldehyde—a preservative for cosmetics. Cosmet. Toil., 92, 95–98.

Millership, J.S. 1987. A report on an initial comparative study of two methods for the determination of glutaraldehyde. J. Clin. Pharm. Ther., 12, 33–38.

Miner, N.A., Whitmore, E., and McBee, M.L. 1975. A quantitative organic soil neutralization test for disinfectants. In *Developments in Industrial Microbiology*. Vol. 16, Edited by Lubrecht and Cramer. Monticello, NY, pp. 23–30.

Miner, N.A., et al. 1977. Antimicrobial and other properties of a new stabilized alkaline glutaraldehyde disinfectant sterilizer. Am. J. Hosp. Pharm., 34, 376–382.

Mitchell, J.P., and Alder, V.G. 1975. The disinfection of urological endoscopes. Br. J. Urol., 47, 571–576.

Monsan, P., Puzo, G., and Mazarguil, H. 1975. Etude du mechanisme d'establissement des liaisons glutaraldehyde-proteines. Biochimie, 57, 1281–1292.

Mostafa, S.M. 1980. Adverse effects of buffered glutaraldehyde on the Heidbrink expiratory valve. Br. J. Anaesth., 52, 223–227.

Munton, T.J., and Russell, A.D. 1970a. Aspects of the action of glutaraldehyde on *Escherichia coli*. J. Appl. Bacteriol., 33, 410–419.

Munton, T.J., and Russell, A.D. 1970b. Effects of glutaraldehyde on protoplasts of *Bacillus megaterium*. J. Gen. Microbiol., 63, 367–370.

Munton, T.J., and Russell, A.D. 1973a. Effect of glutaraldehyde on cell viability, triphenyl tetrazolium reduction, oxygen uptake and β-galactosidase activity in *Escherichia coli*. Appl. Microbiol., *26*, 508–511.

Munton, T.J., and Russell, A.D. 1973b. Interaction of glutaraldehyde with spheroplasts of *Escherichia coli*. J. Appl. Bacteriol., *36*, 211–217.

Navarro, J.M., and Monsan, P. 1976. Etude du mechanisme d'interaction du glutaraldehyde avec les micro-organismes. Ann. Microbiol. (Paris)., *127B*, 295–307.

Nicklas, W., and Bohm, K.H. 1981. Studies on the usefulness of different disinfectants for the aerosol disinfection of surfaces. Zentrabl. Backteriol. Mikrobiol. Hyg. [B], *173*, 365–373.

Noy, M.F., Harrison, L., Holmes, G.K.T., and Cockel, R. 1980. The significance of bacterial contamination of fibreoptic endoscopes. J. Hosp. Infect., *1*, 53–61.

O'Connor, H.J., and Axon, A.T.R. 1983. Gastrointestinal endoscopy: infection and disinfection. Gut, *24*, 1067–1077.

Osterberg, B. 1978. Residual glutaraldehyde in plastics and rubbers after exposure to alkalinized glutaraldehyde solution and its importance on blood cell toxicity. Arch. Pharm. Chemi. Sci. Ed., *6*, 241–248.

Passagot, J., et al. 1987. Effect of glutaraldehyde on the antigenicity and infectivity of hepatitis A virus. J. Virol. Methods, *16*, 21–28.

Paz, M.A., et al. 1965. Detection of carbonyl compounds with N-methyl-benzothiazolone hydrazone. Arch. Biochem. Biophys., *109*, 548–559.

Pease, D.C. 1964. *Histological Techniques for Electron Microscopy*. 2nd Edition. New York, Academic Press, p. 58.

Pepper, R.E., and Lieberman, E.R. 1962. Dialdehyde alcoholic sporicidal compositions. U.S. Patent No. 3,016,328.

Pierce, A.K., Sanford, J.P., Thomas, G.D., and Leonard, J.S. 1970. Long term evaluation of decontamination of inhalation-therapy equipment and the occurrence of necrotizing pneumonia. N. Engl. J. Med., *282*, 528–531.

Power, E.G.M., Dancer, B.N., and Russell, A.D. 1988. Emergence of resistance to glutaraldehyde in spores of *Bacillus subtilis* 168. FEMS Microbiol. Letts., *50*, 223–226.

Rasmussen, K.E., and Albrechtsen, J. 1974. Glutaraldehyde. Influence of pH, temperature and buffering on the polymerisation rate. Histochemistry, *38*, 19–26.

Reichlin, M. 1980. Use of glutaraldehyde as a coupling agent for proteins and peptides. Methods Enzymol., *70*, 159–165.

Reifenrath, W.G., Prystowsky, S.D., Nonomura, J.H., and Robinson, P.B. 1985. Topical glutaraldehyde-percutaneous penetration and skin irritation. Arch. Dermatol. Res., *277*, 242–244.

Relyveld, E.H. 1973. Preparation de vaccins antitoxique et antimicrobiens a l'aide de glutaraldehyde. C.R. Acad. Sci. (Paris), *227*, 613–616.

Relyveld, E.H. 1975. Preparation de vaccins tetanique a l'aide du glutaraldehyde. Proceedings on the 4th International Conference on Tetanus, pp. 727–733.

Relyveld, E.H. 1977. Etude du pouvoir bactericide du glutaraldehyde. Ann. Microbiol. (Paris), *128B*, 495–505.

Relyveld, E.H., Girard, O., and Desormeau-Bedut, J.P. 1973. Procede de fabrication de vaccins a l'aide du glutaraldehyde. Ann. Immunol. Hung., *17*, 22–31.

Relyveld, E.H., and Ben-Efraim, S. 1983. Preparation of vaccines by the action of glutaraldehyde on toxins, bacteria, viruses, allergens and cells. In *Methods in Enzymology*. Volume 93. Edited by J.J. Langone and H. van Vunakis. London, New York, Academic Press, pp. 24–60.

Resnick, L., et al. 1986. Stability and inactivation of HTLV-III/LAV under clinical and laboratory environments. JAMA, *255*, 1887–1891.

Reybrouk, G. 1978. Bactericidal activity of 40 potential disinfectant inactivators. Zentrabl. Bakterior. Mikrobiol. Hyg. [B], *167*, 528–534.

Ringrose, R.E., et al. 1968. A hospital outbreak of *Serratia marcescens* associated with ultrasonic nebulizers. Ann. Intern. Med., *69*, 719–729.

Rittenbury, M., and Hench, M. 1965. Preliminary examination of an activated glutaraldehyde solution for cold disinfection. Ann. Surg., *161*, 127–130.

Rubbo, S.D., Gardner, J.F., and Webb, R.L. 1967. Biocidal activities of glutaraldehyde and related compounds. J. Appl. Bacteriol., *30*, 78–87.

Russell, A.D., and Haque, H. 1975. Inhibition of EDTA-lysozyme lysis of *Pseudomonas aeruginosa* by glutaraldehyde. Microbios, *13*, 151–153.

Russell, A.D., and Vernon, G.N. 1975. Inhibition of glutaraldehyde of lysostaphin-induced lysis of *Staphylococcus aureus*. Microbios, *13*, 147–149.

Saitanu, K., and Lund, E. 1975. Inactivation of entero virus by glutaraldehyde. Appl. Microbiol., *29*, 571–574.

Sanderson, K.V., and Cronin, E. 1968. Glutaraldehyde and contact dermatitis. Br. Med. J., *3*, 802–805.

Sangar, D.V., Rowlands, D.J., Smale, C.J., and Brown, F. 1973. Reaction of glutaraldehyde with foot and mouth disease virus. J. Gen. Virol., *21*, 399–406.

Sasaki, Y., and Endo, R. 1978. Mutagenicity of aldehydes in Salmonella. Mut. Res., *54*, 251–252.

Schattner, R.I. 1978. Buffered glutaraldehyde-phenol sterilizing compositions. U.S. Patent No. 4,103,001.

Scheit, A. 1980. Persistent contamination of the flexible fiber-bronchoscope following disinfection in aqueous glutaraldehyde. Chest, *78*, 352–353.

Schumann, K.O., and Grossgebauer, K. 1977. Experiments on disinfection of vaccinia virus embedded in scabs and/or at the hand. Zentralbl. Bakteriol. Mikrobiol. Hyg. [B], *164*, 45–63.

Scott, K.W. 1982. Glutaraldehyde gel for warts. Practitioner, *226*, 1342–1343.

Shen, D.T., Crawford, T.B., Gorham, J.R., and McGuire, T.C. 1977. Inactivation of equine infectious anaemia virus by chemical disinfectants. Am. J. Vet. Res., *38*, 1217–1219.

Sidwell, R.W., Westbrook, L., Dixon, G.J., and Happich, W.F. 1970. Potentially infectious agents associated with shearling bedpads. I. Effect of laundering with detergent-disinfectant combinations on polio and vaccinia viruses. Appl. Microbiol., *19*, 53–59.

Sierra, G., and Boucher, R.M.G. 1971. Ultrasonic synergistic effects in liquid-phase chemical sterilization. Appl. Microbiol., *22*, 160–164.

Slesinski, R.S., Hengler, W.C., Guzzie, P.J., and Wagner, K.J. 1983. Mutagenicity evaluation of glutaraldehyde in a battery of *in vitro* bacterial and mammalian test systems. Fd. Chem. Toxic., *21*, 621–629.

Smith, R.E., and Farquhar, M.G. 1966. Lysosome function in the regulation of the secretory process in cells of the anterior pituitary gland. J. Cell Biol., *31*, 319–348.

Snyder, R.W., and Cheatle, E.L. 1965. Alkaline glutaraldehyde—an effective disinfectant. Am. J. Hosp. Pharm., *22*, 321–327.

Spaulding, E.H., Cundy, K.R., and Turner, F.J. 1977. Chemical disinfection of medical and surgical materials. In *Disinfection, Sterilization and Preservation*. 2nd Edition. Edited by S.S. Block. Philadelphia, Lea & Febiger, pp. 654–684.

Spire, B., Barre-Sinoussi, F, Montagnier, L., and Chermann, J.C. 1984. Inactivation of lymphadenopathy associated virus by chemical disinfectants. Lancet, ii, 899–901.

Springthorpe, V.S., Grenier, J.L., Lloyd-Evans, N., and Sattar, S.A. 1986. Chemical disinfection of human rotaviruses: efficacy of commercially available products in suspension tests. J. Hyg., *97*, 139–161.

Starke, R.L., Ferguson, D., Garza, P., and Miner, N.A. 1975. An evaluation of the Association of Official Analytical Chemists sporicidal test methods. Dev. Indust. Microbiol., *16*, 31–36.

Stern, M.L., Holsapple, M.P., McCay, J.A., and Munson, A.E. 1989. Contact hypersensitivity response to glutaraldehyde in guinea pigs and mice. Toxicol. Ind. Health, *5*, 31–43.

Stibenz, V.D. 1973. About the spectrophotometric analysis and the index of purification E_{235}/E_{280} of glutaraldehyde. Acta Histochem., *47*, 83–88.

Stonehill, A.A. 1966. Sporicidal compositions comprising a saturated dialdehyde and a cationic surfactant. U.S. Patent No. 3,282,775.

Stonehill, A.A., Krop, S., and Borick, P.M. 1963. Buffered glutaraldehyde, a new chemical sterilizing solution. Am. J. Hosp. Pharm., *20*, 458–465.

Stott, J.F.D., and Herbert, B.N. 1986. The effect of pressure and temperature on sulphate-reducing bacteria and the action of biocides in oilfield water injection systems. J. Appl. Bacteriol., *60*, 57–66.

Suringa, D.W.R. 1970. Treatment of superficial onychomycosis with topically applied glutaraldehyde. Arch. Dermatol., *102*, 163–167.

Tadeusiak, B. 1976. Fungicidal activity of glutaraldehyde. Roc. Panstw. Zakl. Hig. (Poland), *27*, 689–695.

Tashima, T., et al. 1987a. Detection of impurities in aqueous solutions of glutaraldehyde by high performance liquid chromatography with a multichannel diode array UV detector. J. Electron Microsc., *36*, 136–138.

Tashima, T., et al. 1987b. Isolation and identification of new oligomers in aqueous solution of glutaraldehyde. Chem. Pharm. Bull., *35*, 4169–4180.

Tashima, T., et al. 1988. Relationship between precipitation in aqeuous solution of glutaraldehyde for chemosterilization and impurities detected by gas chromatography. Int. J. Pharm., *42*, 61–67.

Tashima, T., et al. 1989. Polymerization reaction in aqueous solution of glutaraldehyde containing trioxane-type oligomers under sterilizing conditions. Chem. Pharm. Bull., *37*, 377–382.

Terleckyj, B., and Axler, D.A. 1987. Quantitative neutralization assay of fungicidal activity of disinfectants. Antimicrob. Agents Chemother., *31*, 794–798.

Thomas, S., and Russell, A.D. 1974. Studies on the mechanism of the sporicidal action of glutaraldehyde. J. Appl. Bacteriol., *37*, 83–92.

Thomson, J.E., Cox, N.A., and Bailey, J.S. 1977. Control of salmonella and extension of shelf-life of broiler carcasses with a glutaraldehyde product. J. Food Sci., *42*, 1353–1355.

Tolon, M., Thofern, E., and Miederer, S.E. 1976. Disinfection procedures for fiberscopes in endoscopy departments. Endoscopy, *8*, 24–29.

Tyler, R., and Ayliffe, G.A.J. 1987. A surface test for virucidal activity of disinfectants: preliminary study with herpes virus. J. Hosp. Infect., *9*, 22–29.

Union Carbide Corp. 1979. Sterilization of fermentation media. Great Britain Patent No. 1,553,662,

Van Klingeren, B., and Pullen, W. 1987. Comparative testing of disinfectants against *Mycobacterium tuberculosis* and *Mycobacterium terrae* in a quantitative suspension test. J. Hosp. Infect., *9*, 292–298.

Varpela, E., Otterstrom, S., and Hackman, R. 1971. Liberation of alkalinized glutaraldehyde by respirators after cold sterilization. Acta Anaesthesiol. Scand., *15*, 291–298.

Wang, H.J., and Tu, J. 1969. Modification of glycogen phosphorylase by glutaraldehyde. Preparation and isolation of enzyme derivatives with enhanced stability. Biochemistry, *8*, 4403–4410.

Weller, I.V.D., et al. 1988. Cleaning and disinfection of equipment for gastro-intestinal flexible endoscopy: interim recommendations of a Working Party of the British Society of Gastroenterology. Gut, *29*, 1134–1151.

Wetzel, B.K., Spicer, S.S., Dvorak, H.F., and Heppel, L.A. 1970. Cytochemical localization of certain phosphatases in *Escherichia coli.* J. Bacteriol., *104*, 529–542.

Wiebe, D., Megerman, J., L'Italien, G.J., and Abbott, W.M. 1988. Glutaral-dehyde release from vascular prostheses of biologic origin. Surgery, *104*, 26–33.

Wikoff, L.J., Dixon, G.J., Westbrook, L., and Happich, W.F. 1971. Potentially infectious agents associated with shearling bedpads: effect of laundering with detergent-disinfectant combinations on *Staphylococcus aureus* and *Pseudomonas aeruginosa.* App. Microbiol., *21*, 647–652.

Wliszczak, W., Meisinger, F., and Kainz, G. 1977. Gaschromatographische bes-timmung de disinfektionsmittels glutaraldehyd in der luft von Krankenhau-sern. Mikrochim. Acta (Wien), II, 139–148.

Woodroof, E.A. 1978. Use of glutaraldehyde and formaldehyde to process tissue heart valves. J. Bioeng., *2*, 1–9.

Wouters, M., Miller, A.O.A., and Fenwick, M.L. 1973. Distortion of poliovirus particles by fixation with formaldehyde. J. Gen. Virol., *18*, 211–214.

PART V

Medical and Health-Related Applications

CHEMICAL DISINFECTION OF MEDICAL AND SURGICAL MATERIALS

M.S. Favero and W.W. Bond

The effective use of proper disinfection and sterilization procedures constitutes a significant factor in preventing nosocomial infections. Physical agents such as moist or dry heat play the dominant role in sterilization procedures in hospitals, and chemical germicides are used primarily for disinfection and antisepsis. In recent years there has been a virtual explosion in the numbers and types of chemical germicides available to health professionals in the United States. Almost 20 years ago, the American Society for Microbiology Ad Hoc Committee on Microbiologic Standards of Disinfection in Hospitals surveyed 16 hospitals in various parts of the United States (with a combined bed capacity of more than 9000) and found that the average number of different formulations used per hospital was 14.5, with a range of 8 to 22. A total of 224 products were used in the 16 hospitals, and 120 of them were proprietary products.

Chemical germicides used in the health-care setting are regulated by two government agencies: the U.S. Environmental Protection Agency (EPA) and the Food and Drug Administration (FDA). Chemical germicides formulated as disinfectants or sterilants are initially regulated and registered by the Disinfectants Branch, Office of Pesticides, EPA. The authority for this responsibility comes under the Federal Insecticide, Fungicide, and Rodenticide Act (FIFRA). The EPA requires manufacturers of chemical germicides formulated as sanitizers, general disinfectants, or disinfecting/sterilizing (sporocide) products to test formulations by using specific protocols for microbicidal activity, stability, and toxicity to humans. Also, if a germicidal chemical is advertised and marketed for use on a specific medical device, e.g., a hemodialysis machine or a flexible fiberoptic endoscope, then the germicide falls under the additional regulatory control of the FDA, Center for Devices and Radiological Health, which is the federal agency that regulates medical devices. Under the authority of the 1976 Medical Device Amendment to the Food, Drug and Cosmetic Act, a germicide that is marketed for use on a specific medical device is itself considered a medical device in a regulatory sense, and the manufacturer must, in addition to EPA registration, contact FDA and submit a premarket notification—510(k)—before the product can be legally marketed. Specific microbiologic activity data or other data such as device/chemical compatibility may be requested from the manufacturer before completion of the premarket notification process. Also, the FDA regulatory authority over a particular instrument or medical device dictates that the manufacturer is obligated to provide the user with adequate instructions for the "safe and effective" use of that instrument or device. These instructions must include methods to clean and disinfect or sterilize the item if it is marketed as a reusable medical device. Manufacturers must provide the users of these germicides with specific direction for use on the product label.

Currently, approximately 14,000 products have been registered with the EPA, and on the labels of these products, approximately 300 active ingredients have been listed. Of these 300 active ingredients, only 14 of them are in 92% of the registered products. Consequently, health-care professionals who are in charge of obtaining germicides should keep in mind that this field is highly competitive and that exaggerated claims are often made about the germicidal efficacy of specific formulations that may be very similar in composition and activity to other products. New formulations of chemical germicides that become commercially available should be scrutinized by health-care professionals, and it may also be necessary to consult with the Disinfectants Branch of the EPA or the Center for Devices and Radiological Health, FDA when questions regarding specific claims or patterns for use arise. Studies published in the scientific literature or presented at scientific meetings also provide important information on the capabilities or limitations of these formulations.

Chemical germicides that are formulated as antiseptics, preservatives, or drugs that are used on or in the human body or as preparations to be used to inhibit or kill microorganisms on the skin are regulated by the FDA. However, the FDA method of regulating these formulations is significantly different from the EPA method for regulating disinfectants. The FDA has an advisory panel that reviews nonprescription antimicrobial drug products. Manufacturers of such formulations voluntarily submit data to the panel, which in turn categorizes the products for their intended use, e.g., antimicrobial soaps, health-care personnel hand washes, patient preoperative preparations, skin antiseptics, skin wound cleansers, skin wound protectants, and surgical hand scrubs. Generic chemical germicides for each use are further divided into the following categories: I, safe and efficacious; II, not safe or efficacious; or III, insufficient data to categorize. Consequently, chemical germicides formulated as antiseptics and regulated by the FDA are categorized basically by use pattern and level of antimicrobial activity and are not regulated or registered in the same fashion that the EPA regulates and registers a disinfectant chemical for use on an inanimate surface. For more extensive discussions of these subjects the reader is referred to Chapter 58.

The Centers for Disease Control (CDC) is not a regulatory agency and does not test, evaluate, or otherwise recommend specific brand-name products of chemical germicides formulated either as disinfectants or sterilants, or as antiseptics, or as soaps for skin preparations. However, the Hospital Infections Program of CDC has published a guideline containing general considerations for methods and indications for handwashing, as well as strategies for disinfecting or sterilizing medical instruments and environmental surfaces (Garner and Favero, 1985). This guideline, which is updated periodically, is provided to all hospitals in the United States and should be consulted for current information and CDC recommendations for disinfection and sterilization strategies, environmental microbiologic control, and handwashing strategies.

The choice of specific disinfectants in association with protocols for cleaning is a decision that is made broadly and at various levels of hospital and other health-care facilities. No single chemical germicide procedure is adequate for all disinfection or sterilization purposes, and the realistic use of chemical germicides depends on a number of factors, which should be considered in selecting among the available procedures. These include the degree of microbial killing required; the nature and composition of the surface item or device to be treated; and the cost, safety, and ease of use of the available agents. In this chapter, we consider each of these factors and discuss practical methods for estimating the effectiveness of the various agents and procedures.

CATEGORIES OF MATERIALS

As used in this chapter, the term "medical and surgical materials" includes instruments and other medical devices or equipment, the use of which involve significant risk of transmitting infection to patients or hospital personnel. These items should be cleaned and then either sterilized or disinfected to prevent cross-contamination and possible transmission of infection.

The nature of instrument/medical-device/equipment disinfection or sterilization can be understood more readily if these items are divided into general categories, based on the risk of infection involved in their use, as first suggested by Dr. E. H. Spaulding (1972). Although one runs the risk of oversimplification in dividing medical devices into such categories, we have chosen to retain Dr. Spaulding's general classification system because it is fairly straightforward, logical, and has been used by epidemiologists and microbiologists for years when discussing or planning strategies for disinfection and sterilization. The CDC also uses this same basic system in its guidelines (Garner and Favero, 1985).

Spaulding believed that strategies for sterilization and disinfection could be better understood and implemented if instruments, equipment, and other medically related surfaces for patient treatment and care were categorized by the degree of risk of infection involved in their use. He described three categories of such items: critical, semicritical, and noncritical. In the present revision of this chapter, however, we have slightly modified and expanded Dr. Spaulding's classification scheme to more clearly differentiate the infection risks associated with medical instruments versus other medically related devices or environmental surfaces.

Critical instruments or devices, the first category, are so called because the risk of acquiring infection if the item is contaminated is substantial. These are instruments or objects that are introduced directly into the human body, either into or in contact with the bloodstream or normally sterile areas of the body. Examples include needles, scalpels, transfer forceps, cardiac catheters, implants, and also the inner surface components of extracorporeal blood flow devices such as of the heart-lung oxygenator and the blood-side of artificial kidneys (hemodialyzers). These items must be sterile before they can be used, and one of several accepted sterilization procedures should be chosen.

Instruments or devices in the second category are classified as *semicritical* in terms of the degree of risk of infection, and examples are flexible fiberoptic endoscopes, endotracheal and aspirator tubes, bronchoscopes, respiratory therapy equipment, cystoscopes, vaginal specula, and urinary catheters. Although these items come in contact with mucous membranes, they do not ordinarily penetrate body surfaces. Sterilization of many of these items, although desirable and often cost-effective if steam autoclaves can be used, is not absolutely essential. Semicritical instruments or devices should, at a minimum, be subjected to a powerful, broad-spectrum procedure that can be expected to destroy a few bacterial spores, most fungal spores, all ordinary vegetative bacteria, tubercle bacilli, and small or nonlipid viruses, and medium-sized or lipid viruses. In most cases, meticulous physical cleaning followed by an appropriate high-level disinfection treatment gives the user a reasonable degree of assurance that the items are free of pathogenic microorganisms.

The third category in order of relative risk of disease transmission is *noncritical instruments or devices*. These items usually come into direct contact with the patient but, in most instances, only with unbroken skin. Such items include face masks, blood pressure cuffs, most neurologic or cardiac diagnostic electrodes, or certain surfaces of x-ray machines. Use of these items carries relatively little risk of transmitting infection directly to patients. Consequently, depending on the particular item and the nature and degree of contamination during use, simple washing or scrubbing with a detergent and warm water may be sufficient for an adequate level of safety; however, in some instances, the added assurance of chemical disinfection with an intermediate- to low-level chemical germicide may be considered appropriate.

As mentioned previously, we have chosen to expand Dr. Spaulding's original classification of medically related surfaces to define more clearly the relative risks of disease transmission by these surfaces. An added category, and the one that carries the least risk of disease transmission, is *environmental surfaces*. This general category consists of a wide variety of surfaces that do not ordinarily come into direct contact with the patient, but if they occasionally do, it is only with intact skin. Although not directly implicated in transmission of disease within the hospital, these environmental surfaces may potentially contribute to secondary cross-contamination by hands of health-care workers or by contract with medical instruments that will subsequently come into contact with patients. In terms of relative potential for cross-contamination, the category of environmental surfaces may be further divided into at least two major subdivisions: (1) *medical equipment surfaces* such as frequently touched adjustment knobs or handles on hemodialysis machines, x-ray machines, instrument carts, or dental units, and (2) *housekeeping surfaces* such as floors, walls, tabletops, window sills, and so forth. Similar to noncritical medical instruments, adequate levels of safety for surfaces of medical equipment may be achieved by simple cleaning with a detergent and warm water or, depending on the equipment surface and the nature and degree of contamination, cleaning followed by application of an intermediate- to low-level chemical germicide. Housekeeping surfaces are those surfaces that, for the most part, have the least potential for cross-contamination among health-care personnel, patients, or medical equipment and instruments. Adequate safety levels can be achieved by maintaining these surfaces in a state of visible cleanliness by using water and a detergent or a hospital grade disinfectant/detergent designed for general housekeeping purposes (as indicated on the product label). Only in those instances in which there has been a *significant* spill of blood or other potentially infectious body fluid should

the added use of an intermediate-level chemical disinfectant be considered to ensure that such a surface is "safe."

The remainder of this chapter will consider disinfection or sterilization only in the context of "medical and surgical materials"; but it is clear that the choice of disinfecting methods rests largely with the judgment of the health-care professional. This is particularly true in the instance of many semicritical and most noncritical instruments or devices, and involved in this decision-making process are several factors, including the manufacturer's instructions, how the item will contact the next patient, the physical configuration (cleanability) of the item, the type and degree of contamination after use, the physical or chemical stability of the item, and the ease or difficulty in removing (rinsing, aerating) the chemical agent after the necessary exposure time. Ideally, the manufacturer's instructions for use of the item should include detailed instructions for all aspects of reprocessing, but in reality, this is not uniformly the case. Therefore, consistent and effective procedures for chemical disinfecting or sterilizing of medical and surgical materials often depend highly on the knowledge and judgment of the responsible health-care practitioner.

If all medical and surgical materials could be sterilized by steam autoclaving, there would be no need to establish these categories. In practice, however, many such medical devices and articles in everyday use cannot be sterilized by steam autoclaving, and chemical germicides must be used. In this context, one then must consider the differences between chemical sterilization and chemical disinfection.

ANTIMICROBIAL EFFECTIVENESS OF CHEMICAL GERMICIDES: DEFINITION OF TERMS

Although the definitions of sterilization, disinfection, and antisepsis (Block, 1983; Spaulding, 1972) have been accepted generally, it is common to see all three terms misused. The exact distinction among the three terms and the basic knowledge of how to achieve and monitor each state are important if the effective application of long-known principles is to be realized.

Sterilization

Sterilization is the use of a physical or chemical procedure to destroy all microbial life, including large numbers of highly resistant bacterial endospores. In the hospital, this specifically pertains to those microorganisms that may exist on inanimate objects. Moist heat by steam autoclaving, ethylene oxide gas, and dry heat are the major sterilizing agents used in hospitals. However, as will be discussed, a variety of chemical germicides have been used for purposes of sterilization and appear to be effective when used appropriately. These germicides used in a different manner may actually be part of a disinfection process. Unfortunately, some health-care professionals refer to disinfection as "sterilization," which leads to a degree of confusion that often becomes magnified with routine use. A good example of this is the use of glutaraldehyde-based germicides for the disinfection of certain flexible fiberoptic endoscopes. Some practitioners refer to this as "sterilization" of endoscopes. For instance, a 2% glutaraldehyde solution is capable of sterilization, but only after extended contact time in the absence of extraneous organic material. Unfortunately, flexible fiberoptic endoscopes of recent "totally immersible" design are not physically capable of withstanding repeated immersion in fluid for 6 to 10 hours—in fact, most manufacturers state that repeated prolonged immersion will damage the instruments, and recommend that routine immersion times not exceed 20 to 30 minutes. Thus, the procedure used for most flexible endoscopes is disinfection and not sterilization, in spite of the fact that colloquially this procedure is often referred to in the hospital as "sterilization."

Disinfection

Disinfection is generally a less lethal process than sterilization. It eliminates nearly all recognized pathogenic microorganisms but not necessarily all microbial forms (e.g., bacterial endospores) on inanimate objects. As can be seen by this definition, disinfection does not ensure an "overkill" and, therefore, disinfection processes lack the margin of safety achieved by sterilization procedures. The effectiveness of a disinfection procedure is controlled significantly by a number of factors, each of which may have a pronounced effect on the end result. Among these are the nature and number of contaminating microorganisms (especially the presence of bacterial endospores); the amount of organic matter (e.g., soil, feces, blood) present; the type and condition of the medical and surgical materials to be disinfected; and the temperature. Accordingly, disinfection is a procedure that reduces the level of microbial contamination, but there is a broad range of activity that extends from sterility at one extreme to a minimal reduction in the number of microbial contaminants at the other. Note that the acceptance of such distinction is consistent with the abilities of certain nonsporicidal disinfectant solutions to *completely destroy* microbial contamination on medical and surgical materials. Indeed, this probably happens often when spores are absent prior to the disinfection procedure. Nevertheless, these procedures should not be referred to as "sterilization" and, as will be discussed, not even as "high-level disinfection."

Decontamination

Decontamination is a term used to describe a process of treatment that renders a medical device, instrument, or environmental surface safe to handle; in the case of medical instruments or devices, a decontamination process or treatment does not necessarily mean that the item is safe for patient reuse. A decontamination procedure can range from sterilization or disinfection to simple cleaning with soap and water.

By definition, chemical disinfection differs from sterilization by its lack of sporicidal power. This is an oversimplification of the actual situation, because a few chemical germicides used as disinfectants do, in fact, kill large numbers of spores, even though high concentrations and several hours of exposure time may be required.

Nonsporicidal disinfectants may differ in their capacity to accomplish disinfection or decontamination. Some germicides rapidly kill only the ordinary vegetative forms of bacteria such as staphylococci and streptococci, some forms of fungi, and lipid-containing viruses, whereas others are effective against such relatively resistant organisms as *Mycobacterium tuberculosis* var. *bovis*, nonlipid viruses, and most forms of fungi. The latter group represents, therefore, a level of activity that is intermediate between that of sporicides and many commonly used germicides.

Absolute sterility is difficult to prove, and as a result it is common to define sterility in terms of the probability that a contaminating organism will survive treatment. For example, sterilizing processes are designed and often monitored using a high number (10^6 to 10^7) of dried bacterial endospores, and sterilization is defined as that state in which the probability of any one spore surviving is 10^{-6} or lower. As pointed out in other chapters in this book, this rationale has been used to establish cycles for steam autoclaves, dry air ovens, and ethylene oxide gas sterilizers, and it produces a great degree of overkill as well as a quantitative assurance of sterilization. It is nearly impossible to evaluate liquid chemical sterilization or disinfection processes by using these criteria. These procedures using chemical germicides do not have the same reliability as sterilization procedures such as steam autoclaving.

Antisepsis

An antiseptic is defined as a germicide that is used on skin or living tissue for the purpose of inhibiting or destroying microorganisms. Antiseptics will not be discussed in this chapter because they are treated elsewhere in this book, but it should be realized that the distinction between an antiseptic and a disinfectant often is not made. A disinfectant is a germicide that is used solely for destroying microorganisms on inanimate objects such as medical devices or environmental surfaces. An antiseptic germicide, however, is one that is used on or in living tissue. Although some germicides contain active chemicals that are used for both purposes (i.e., iodophors, alcohols), adequacy for one purpose does not ensure adequacy for the other. Consequently, it is not good practice to use an antiseptic for the purpose of disinfection and vice versa, because manufacturers specifically formulate these germicides for their intended use.

LEVELS OF DISINFECTANT ACTIVITY

Along with his categorization of medical and surgical materials, E. H. Spaulding proposed that three levels of germicidal action be recognized in order to properly carry out strategies for disinfection in hospitals. The pro-

Table 35–1. *Descending Order of Resistance to Germicidal Chemicals*

BACTERIAL SPORES

Bacillus subtilis
Clostridium sporogenes
↓
MYCOBACTERIA

Mycobacterium tuberculosis var. *bovis*
↓
NONLIPID OR SMALL VIRUSES

poliovirus
Coxsackie virus
rhinovirus
↓
FUNGI

Trichophyton spp.
Cryptococcus spp.
Candida spp.
↓
VEGETATIVE BACTERIA

Pseudomonas aeruginosa
Staphylococcus aureus
Salmonella choleraesuis
↓
LIPID OR MEDIUM-SIZED VIRUSES

herpes simplex virus
cytomegalovirus
respiratory syncytial virus
hepatitis B virus
human immunodeficiency virus

posed levels of activity ("high," "intermediate," and "low") are based on the fact that microorganisms can be categorized into several general groups according to their innate resistance levels to a spectrum of physical or chemical germicidal agents. These groups are listed in broad descending order of resistance in Table 35–1, and the examples of microorganisms represent some of the test organisms used to qualify germicides for a particular EPA registration category. The relationship of these general levels of microbial resistance to the levels of germicidal activity is shown in Table 35–2.

High-Level Disinfection

Most critical instruments and devices are heat-stable and are not adversely affected by repeated sterilizing cycles in a steam autoclave or dry-air oven. But other items in this category are not heat-stable (e.g., certain plastic or plastic-coated items) and must be sterilized by "cold" methods such as ethylene gas or powerful, broad-spectrum liquid chemical germicides. Relatively few critical instruments or devices in use today are routinely processed between patients by methods less rigorous than a sterilizing treatment. One notable exception to this is the "telescope" (optic-containing) portion of cer-

tain rigid endoscopic sets such as laparoscopes or arthroscopes. Although these instruments penetrate during use into normally sterile areas of the body, the widely-accepted between-patient processing method of high-level disinfection has been successful with no apparent adverse effect on patients (Ad Hoc Committee on Infection Control in the Handling of Endoscopic Equipment, 1980; Johnson et al., 1983). CDC guidelines recommend that sterilization of laparoscopes and arthroscopes is preferable but, if not feasible, then the minimum treatment should be high-level disinfection (Garner and Favero, 1985). It should be emphasized, however, that the optic portions of these types of endoscopes are relatively fragile, but they are constructed of smooth, easily cleanable surfaces with no internal channels and few surface irregularities. As a result, efficient precleaning of such items will ensure that little (if any) residual organic material and only low numbers of microorganisms will challenge the liquid chemical germicide in the subsequent disinfecting procedure.

High-level disinfection is the minimum treatment recommended by the CDC in guidelines for the reprocessing of semicritical instruments or devices (Garner and Favero, 1985), and as can be seen in Table 35–2, an essential property of a high-level disinfectant is a demonstrated level of activity against bacterial endospores. The capability of killing bacterial spores is an assurance of the relative power and activity spectrum of a germicide. Thus, if the contact time is long enough, this type of germicide can be used as a sterilant; it is important to recognize that contact time is the single important variable between sterilization or high-level disinfection with a specific chemical germicide.

High-level disinfectants are used often to treat certain medical and surgical materials and, in the absence of bacterial spores, are rapidly effective. The absence of spores normally cannot be ensured, although it has been shown that the number of spores on items subjected to such treatments are generally low (Spaulding, 1939). The sporicidal activity of the high-level disinfectant depends both on the specific chemical agent and the manner in which it is used. Table 35–3 shows several disinfectants that are categorized as having high-level activity. These include a number of glutaraldehyde-, chlorine dioxide-, hydrogen peroxide-, and peracetic acid-based formulations; these are commercially available germicides that have been approved by the EPA as sterilants/disinfectants. As will be pointed out later, the Association of Official Analytical Chemists' (AOAC) sporicidal test is highly stringent, so that chemical germicides designated as sterilants using AOAC test method are most likely to be effective in killing all groups of microorganisms, including high numbers of bacterial spores. Some of these products combine various chemicals such as glutaraldehyde with formaldehyde and glutaraldehyde with phenol or phenolic compounds. Peracetic acid in liquid and vapor states has been described in the past as a sterilant or disinfectant, but its application in high concentrations

Table 35–2. *Levels of Disinfectant Action According to Type of Microorganism*

| | Bacteria | | | | Virus | |
Level of Action	Spores	Tubercle Bacillus	Vegetative Cells	Fungi[1]	Nonlipid and Small	Lipid and Medium-Sized
High	+ [2,3]	+	+	+	+	+
Intermediate	− [4]	+	+	+	± [5]	+
Low	−	−	+	±	±	+

[1]Includes asexual spores but not necessarily chlamydospores or sexual spores.

[2]Plus sign indicates that a killing effect can be expected; a minus sign indicates little or no killing effect.

[3]Only with extended exposure times are high-level disinfectants capable of killing high numbers of bacterial spores in laboratory tests; they are however, *capable* of sporicidal activity (see text and Table 35–4).

[4]Some intermediate-level disinfectants (e.g., hypochlorites may exhibit some sporicidal activity; others (e.g., alcohols or phenolics) have no demonstrated sporicidal activity.

[5]Some intermediate-level disinfectants, although tuberculocidal, may have limited virucidal activity (see text).

presents major difficulties (Portner and Hoffman, 1968; Warshowsky et al., 1978), especially with medical and surgical items. However, germicidal products based on low-concentration mixtures of hydrogen peroxide and peracetic acid have recently been approved by the EPA as sterilant/disinfectants.

Germicides classified as sporicides have been shown to kill large numbers of resistant bacterial endospores under stringent test conditions, but may require as long as 24 hours of contact time to do so (Ortenzio, 1966). Although this type of germicide may qualify technically as a cold sterilant, it may receive little use as such because of the exposure time necessary. In addition, most medical devices in actual practice are not contaminated with extraordinarily high levels of bacterial endospores, so that if a small number of spores made up the initial population, sterilization may occur much more quickly than in 24 hours. In other words, given the circumstances of relatively few bacterial spores present, sterilization could theoretically be achieved by a weaker germicide. However, because medical devices and items are not routinely monitored microbiologically, one cannot consistently ensure the absence of bacterial spores, so that with certain critical types of medical devices and items, it may be good practice to rely on those germicides that have either been documented in the scientific literature to produce a sporicidal effect in a given amount of time or have been approved by the EPA as sterilant/disinfectants. In any event, these germicides can be expected to produce sterility if the exposure conditions in terms of contact time, temperature, pH, and other factors are met. The assurance of a sterilization process accomplished by a chemical germicide is significantly less than one accomplished by a physical process such as steam autoclaving or dry heat. The latter procedures are much less prone to be affected by human error than those associated with chemical germicides.

One question that is worthy of consideration is whether high-level germicides (sporicidal chemicals) should be promoted as sterilizing agents. For example, a variety of glutaraldehyde-based products registered by the EPA as sterilant-disinfectants have been marketed

for many years throughout the world. In recent years, however, the glutaraldehyde-based products in this EPA category have been joined by several other broad-spectrum germicide formulations containing active ingredients such as hydrogen peroxide, chlorine dioxide, and peracetic acid (Table 35–3). Although these formulations have been shown in laboratory tests to be capable of killing equivalent numbers and types of bacterial spores, as, for instance, a steam autoclave cycle, their use in the medical professions is almost exclusively limited to disinfection rather than sterilization.

The question of how many of these products should be classified as sterilizing agents is academic, because all of them require longer cycle times than a steam autoclave. Although the AOAC sporicidal test is stringent and is a major criterion used by the EPA for designating a germicide as a sterilant, actual procedures associated with the use of chemical germicides demand much more in the way of microbiologic verification because the potency of the chemicals is affected by the organic load of the device being processed, contact time, temperature, and the use history of the liquid product (age, dilution during use). The manufacturer's time and effort in designing and verifying the effectiveness of a sterilization process, as discussed in other parts of this book, are extensive and technically sophisticated. The same approach cannot be used in a modern hospital; in this setting, the use of biologic indicators with steam and ethylene oxide sterilizers is about the only direct procedure that can be done.

There is no direct way to microbiologically verify the sterility or the level of disinfection of medical devices and items without sampling the item itself. With heat or gaseous chemical sterilization procedures, each process cycle can be monitored to verify that the exposure parameters are capable of inactivating 10^6 to 10^7 bacterial endospores by using commercial biologic indicators. Liquid chemical sterilization or disinfection procedures cannot be monitored biologically; therefore, the existence of an established set of controls associated with the procedure as well as the liquid germicide itself takes on critical importance. A good example of this is the use of

Table 35–3. *Activity Levels of Selected Liquid Germicides[a]*

Procedure/Product	Aqueous Concentration[b]	Activity Level
STERILIZATION		
Glutaraldehyde	Variable[c]	
Hydrogen peroxide	6–30%	
Formaldehyde	6–8%[d]	
Chlorine dioxide	Variable[e]	
Peracetic acid	Variable[f]	
DISINFECTION[g]		
Glutaraldehyde	Variable	High to intermediate
Hydrogen peroxide	3–6%	High to intermediate
Formaldehyde	1–8%	High to low
Chlorine dioxide	Variable	High
Peracetic acid	Variable	High
Chlorine compounds[h]	500 to 5000 mg/L Free/available chlorine	Intermediate
Alcohols (ethyl, isopropyl)[i]	70%	Intermediate
Phenolic compounds	0.5 to 3%	Intermediate to low
Iodophor compounds[j]	40–50 mg/L free iodine; up to 10,000 mg/L available iodine	Intermediate to low
Quaternary ammonium compounds	0.1–0.2%	Low

[a]This list of chemical germicides centers on generic formulations. A large number of commercial products based on these generic components can be considered for use. Users should ensure that commercial formulations are registered with the EPA and, if used on medical instruments or devices, listed with the FDA. Information in the scientific literature or presented at symposia or scientific meetings can also be considered in determining the suitability of certain formulations; particular attention should be given to the manufacturer's instructions for use printed on the label of all EPA-registered products. Adequate precleaning of surfaces is the first prerequisite for any sterilizing or disinfecting procedure. The longer the exposure to a liquid chemical agent, the more likely it is that all pertinent microorganisms will be eliminated. Manufacturers' generally recommended exposure times may not be adequate to disinfect certain instruments or devices, especially those that are difficult to clean because of narrow channels or other areas that may harbor organic material as well as microorganisms; this is of particular importance when high-level disinfection is to be achieved.

[b]For sterilization or disinfection, refer to the manufacturers' instructions for exposure times and conditions as well as recommendations for rinsing and subsequent handling of processed items.

[c]There are several glutaraldehyde-based proprietary formulations on the U.S. market, e.g., low-, neutral-, or high-pH products recommended for use at normal or elevated temperatures with or without ultrasonic energy. Some of the products are supplied as ready-to-use preparations, and others are sold in concentrated forms, which require various dilutions to be made prior to a specific use; others may also require mixing of two or more components such as buffers or active ingredients (e.g., phenol and phenolic compounds). Therefore, it is imperative that the user of those products closely follow instructions of the manufacturer regarding use as a sterilant or disinfectant; some manufacturers supply test kits to aid in monitoring glutaraldehyde concentrations during the use-life of the product.

[d]Because of the ongoing controversy of the role of formaldehyde as a potential occupational carcinogen, the use of formaldehyde is limited to certain specific circumstances under carefully controlled conditions, e.g., for the disinfection of certain hemodialysis equipment. There are no EPA-registered products designed for liquid chemical sterilizing or disinfectant that contain formaldehyde.

[e]Chlorine dioxide is claimed to be the active chemical resulting from mixing water, sodium chlorite, and lactic acid in varying proportions depending on whether its intended use is as a sterilant or a disinfectant. Similar to that of other chlorine compounds, the spectrum of germicidal action is broad, but oxidative effects on metal or plastic surfaces may limit effective use.

[f]In recent years, a limited number of trade-name products containing low concentrations ($<0.1\%$) of peracetic (peroxyacetic) acid, combined with low concentrations ($<1.0\%$) of hydrogen peroxide at the in-use dilution, have been registered with the EPA as sterilants or sterilant/disinfectants. This combination of two powerful oxidizing chemicals at low concentration has made possible a rapid, broad spectrum of germicidal activity while minimizing negative affects such as corrosiveness, which occurs at higher concentrations of peracetic acid.

[g]As of December, 1988, there were approximately 85 proprietary formulations registered with EPA as "hospital disinfectants" that are also tuberculocidal, virucidal, and fungicidal. Among this registration listing are formulations composed of a single category of active ingredient (e.g., glutaraldehyde, phenolic, or iodophor), but others may contain such an array of "active" chemical agents that the user may have difficulty in attempting to define a generic classification. For this reason among others, the user is urged to pay particular attention to the information on the product label and accompanying package literature (spectrum of activity, approved use patterns, directions for use, safety precautions, etc.). At the present time, product information and claims in written or verbal advertising are not as closely regulated as information and claims on the product container label.

[h]Generic disinfectants containing chlorine are available in liquid or solid form, e.g., sodium or calcium hypochlorite. Although the indicated concentrations are rapid-acting and broad-spectrum (tuberculocidal, bactericidal, fungicidal, and virucidal), no proprietary hypochlorite formulations are formally registered with the EPA as such (common household bleach is an excellent and inexpensive source of sodium hypochlorite). Concentrations between 500 and 1000 mg/L chlorine are appropriate for the vast majority of uses requiring an intermediate level of germicidal activity; higher concentrations are extremely corrosive as well as irritating to personnel, and their use should be limited to situations in which organic material is difficult to clean (e.g., porous surfaces) or contains unusually high concentrations of microorganisms (e.g., spills of cultured material in the laboratory).

[i]The effectiveness of alcohols as intermediate-level germicides is limited, because they evaporate rapidly, resulting in very short contact times, and because they lack the ability to penetrate residual organic material. They are rapidly tuberculocidal, bactericidal, and fungicidal, but may vary in spectrum of virucidal activity (see text). Items to be disinfected with alcohols should be carefully precleaned and then totally submerged for an appropriate exposure time (e.g., 10 min).

[j]Only those iodophors registered with EPA as hard-surface disinfectants should be used, and the instructions of the manufacturer regarding proper dilution and product stability should be closely followed. Antiseptic iodophors are not suitable for disinfecting medical instruments or devices or environmental surfaces.

glutaraldehyde-based germicides, which are capable of sterilization, but only after extended contact time and in the absence of extraneous organic material. Unfortunately, some materials are not physically able to withstand immersion in these fluids for 6 to 10 hours. Even if prolonged contact time were possible, the treated materials would have to be retrieved from the germicide and handled with sterile implements, rinsed thoroughly with sterile water, dried with sterile towels (or in a special cabinet with sterile air) and, if not used immediately, stored in a sterile container to ensure that the materials remain sterile. However, it is common to observe staff members in hospitals and other settings soaking items in 2% glutaraldehyde germicides for 10 to 30 minutes, rinsing them in nonsterile water, and referring to the items as "sterile." This particular situation indicates a misunderstanding of the terms "sterile" and "disinfected" as well as overconfidence in a particular germicide and overestimation of the safety of the processed item.

Intermediate-Level Disinfection

Intermediate-level disinfectants are not necessarily capable of killing bacterial spores, but do inactivate *Mycobacterium tuberculosis* var. *bovis*, which is significantly more resistant to aqueous germicides than are ordinary vegetative bacteria (Table 35–2). These disinfectants are also effective against fungi (including asexual spores but not necessarily dried chlamydospores or sexual spores) as well as lipid and nonlipid medium-sized and small viruses. Examples of intermediate-level disinfectants include alcohols (70 to 90% ethanol or isopropanol), chlorine compounds (free chlorine, i.e., hypochlorus acids derived from sodium or calcium hypochlorite, gaseous chlorine, or chlorine dioxide, 500 mg/L), and certain phenolic or iodophor preparations, depending on formulation.

Although viruses and vegetative bacteria generally have similar susceptibilities to heat and other physical agents, Klein and Deforest (1983) observed that viruses may differ significantly in their susceptibilities to disinfectant chemicals. Further, they suggested that the presence or absence of lipid in the viral protein coat as well as the relative size of a virus may be useful guides in predicting viral susceptibility to a particular disinfectant. For instance, their data showed that small, nonlipid viruses were significantly more resistant to a spectrum of germicides than were medium-sized viruses or those with a lipid component in their protein coats. Some of the most widely used germicides (certain phenolics and quaternary ammonium compounds) failed to inactivate several small, nonlipid viruses tested (e.g., picornaviruses such as enteroviruses and rhinoviruses). Conversely, the presence of lipid component in viral composition was associated with a general susceptibility to all classes of germicides tested. Also, nonlipid viruses larger than picornaviruses (e.g., adenoviruses and reovirus) showed a sensitivity to the germicides similar to that of the lipid-containing viruses. Even though inter-

mediate-level (tuberculocidal) disinfectants are generally considered effective against a wide range of viruses, it is not necessarily true that they are capable of destroying all viruses. When choosing a chemical agent for a particular situation, it would be prudent for the user to thoroughly examine the EPA-registered label claims for specific activity of brand-name disinfectants and also to consult other chapters of this book as well as the scientific literature for information on the virucidal spectra of generic chemicals such as alcohols or halogens. For example, the human hepatitis viruses (hepatitis B virus and the non-A, non-B hepatitis viruses) are of current importance and concern in hospital infection control strategies. These viruses have not been cultured in the laboratory, and this difficulty has prevented EPA in certain instances from allowing activity claims on the labels or in advertising of commercial products. However, there is no evidence that any of these viruses are unusually resistant to disinfectants (Miner, 1978; Bond et al., 1977a).

In 1977, we proposed that the resistance level of the hepatitis B virus be considered to be between that of the tubercle bacillus and bacterial spores, but nearer the tubercle bacillus (Bond et al., 1977a). At that time, this type of rationale appeared reasonable, and it was thought that the most conservative approach would be to recommend at least high-level disinfecting procedures for all types of medical devices known or suspected of being contaminated with hepatitis B virus. When considering sterilization or disinfecting strategies for other hepatitis viruses that have not been studied extensively (hepatitis A virus and non-A, non-B hepatitis viruses), a similar rationale has been proposed (Favero et al., 1986). Subsequently, two studies employing direct inoculation of chimpanzees with disinfectant-treated human serum with high titers of hepatitis B virus have shown that a variety of intermediate to high-level disinfectant chemicals (two commercial glutaraldehyde-based products, 500 mg/L free chlorine from sodium hypochlorite, an iodophor product, 70% isopropanol, 80% ethanol and dilutions of glutaraldehyde as low as 0.1%) were shown to effectively inactivate the virus in relatively short exposure times and at low temperatures (Bond et al., 1983a; Kobayashi et al., 1984).

Another virus of current importance and concern in health-care settings is human immunodeficiency virus (HIV). Studies have shown that HIV is relatively unstable in the environment (Resnik et al., 1986) and rapidly inactivated after being exposed to commonly used chemical germicides at concentrations much lower than are used in practice (Spire et al., 1984, 1985; McDougal et al., 1985; Martin et al., 1985). When considered in the context of environmental conditions in health-care facilities, the demonstrated sensitivity of HIV in addition to low viral titers in blood of infected patients (circa 100 HIV/ml) has resulted in no changes of currently recommended strategies for sterilization, disinfection, or housekeeping (Centers for Disease Control, 1987). Even though the

EPA has recently approved specific HIV label claims for a large number of proprietary germicidal formulations (mostly those germicides used for housekeeping purposes), the presence or absence of such a claim should not be a major criterion in the selection of germicidal products.

Some chemical germicides with good tuberculocidal activity can destroy small nonlipid viruses. Klein and Deforest (1963) showed that both 70% ethanol and 70% isopropanol are rapidly virucidal; alcohols are also known to be rapidly tuberculocidal (Spaulding, 1964; Heister et al., 1968). Only ethanol, however, was found by Klein and Deforest to consistently destroy the small nonlipid viruses they studied, but Wright (1970a) reported that ethanol failed to kill a test virus that, on the basis of Klein and Deforest's study, would be expected to be susceptible. At best, an intermediate-level (tuberculocidal) disinfectant may not necessarily be an effective broad-spectrum virucide.

The major exception to the rule in the previous discussion of viral inactivation is the causative agent of Creutzfeldt-Jacob disease (CJD) or other related infectious agents responsible for certain fatal degenerative diseases of the central nervous system in humans or animals. These diseases, collectively referred to as "slow viral infections" (e.g., CJD or kuru in humans or scrapie in sheep or goats) are caused by agents that are commonly referred to as "unconventional viruses" (Anderson et al., 1988). As with the human hepatitis viruses, determination of specific virucidal activity of disinfectants is complicated by the fact that precise assays require large numbers of experimental animals and extended periods of postinoculation observation. Results of the limited studies to date on the physical and chemical inactivation kinetics of the scrapie agent have been inconsistent, but have suggested that "slow viruses" as a group have rather unusual levels of resistance (Asher et al., 1986). These controversial data have led to rather unconventional recommendations for disinfection and sterilization (Committee on Health Care Issues, ANA, 1986), and the existing guidelines for terminal processing of CJD agent-contaminated medical devices and surfaces far exceed the levels of treatment with conventional sterilization cycles. However, until the CJD and other related agents are studied further, it would be prudent for health-care workers to follow published guidelines, within reason, to maintain a rational balance among infection transmission risk, personal safety from toxic chemicals, and physical integrity of medical devices and environmental surfaces (Jarvis, 1982; Committee on Health Care Issues, ANA, 1986; Anderson et al., 1988).

The germicidal resistance of fungi is probably about the same as that of gram-positive vegetative bacteria (Petrocci, 1983; Prindle, 1983). However, experimental recognition of bacteriostasis may have been overlooked in many of these reports, and there is now a reason to believe that some forms of pathogenic fungi may be considerably more resistant than most vegetative bacteria.

Because it is likely that germicidal chemicals that are tuberculocidal and virucidal may not be capable of killing the more resistant fungi, intermediate-level germicides should be carefully examined with regard to demonstrated activity against specific groups or types of microorganisms (EPA-approved label claims or data in scientific literature).

Low-Level Disinfection

Low-level disinfectants are those that cannot be relied on to destroy, within a practical period, bacterial endospores, mycobacteria, all fungi, or all small or nonlipid viruses. These disinfectants may be useful in actual practice because they can rapidly kill vegetative forms of bacteria and most fungi as well as medium-sized or lipid-containing viruses. Examples of low-level disinfectants are quaternary ammonium compounds and certain iodophors or phenolics. In addition, the germicidal activity is flexible, depending on the concentration of the active ingredient. Disinfection levels of iodophors and phenolics may be classified as intermediate or low depending on the concentrations of the active ingredients. All germicidal chemicals do not have this capacity. For example, even a 5 to 10% concentration of a quaternary ammonium compound may fail to meet the tuberculocidal or virucidal criterion of intermediate-level disinfection (Klein and Deforest, 1963).

SELECTION OF DISINFECTION LEVEL

Patient-care instruments and devices have been categorized as critical, semicritical, and noncritical, and environmental surfaces have been categorized as medical equipment surfaces and housekeeping surfaces. The level of disinfection that should be used depends in part on the particular category and nature of the item and the manner in which it is to be used.

Critical Instruments or Devices

It would serve no useful purpose to attempt to name all of the critical instruments and devices and the large number of related medical and surgical materials in use in today's modern hospitals. The concept of a critical instrument is clear; the user must make his or her own list. All but a few articles in this category are either presterilized commercially or steam autoclaved by the user. A few important critical devices, however, are reused repeatedly and not steam autoclaved for one reason or another—for example, transfer forceps and container, an increasing number of plastic parts on medical devices, hemodialyzers, and certain rigid endoscopic devices or accessories to flexible fiberoptic endoscopes. To sterilize or disinfect these items, one must rely on proper use of certain chemical germicides formulated as sterilant/disinfectants and classified in this chapter as high-level disinfectants. Thorough cleansing must always precede chemical disinfection of such items, because the mechanical action alone can remove a large proportion of contaminating microorganisms and a good deal of organic material, which may tend to inactivate the germicide.

The number of bacterial spores is usually small, and they would not be expected to occur in relatively high numbers except when contaminated objects have not been well cleansed; this fact should not be interpreted as a rationale to substitute chemical sterilization for autoclaving when autoclaving is a feasible procedure. To do so would lower safety standards; also, using sterilant/disinfectant (high-level) chemical germicides is inconvenient because several hours must be allowed to ensure sterilization, and the exposed materials must be rinsed and dried or aired aseptically and kept in a sterile state before use.

One may debate the importance of an occasional bacterial endospore that remains viable after a critical device has been disinfected. There have been no epidemiologic studies that can settle this matter, but there are two points that deserve mention. First, critical instruments should, at a minimum, receive high-level disinfection; if feasible, these items should be sterilized. The second point pertains to the statement that most bacterial spores are nonpathogenic and thus may be ignored without incurring significant risk of infection. The distinction between pathogenic and nonpathogenic species is vague and relative rather than absolute, and in today's modern hospital environment, the host's level of resistance is the decisive factor in determining whether infection will develop. Classic nonpathogens such as *Bacillus subtilis* can produce serious and even fatal infections in immunosuppressed and immunocompromised hosts (Farrer, 1963; Conrad et al., 1971; Tuazon et al., 1979). But overriding the arguments regarding the possible consequences of infection with a sporeformer is the fact that sterilizing or high-level disinfecting (sporocidal) procedures have the *capability* of killing all other groups of microorganisms that may cause infection. Thus, application of a germicide with such broad-spectrum capability will increase levels of assurance that no infection will be transmitted from patient to patient.

Certain critical items deserve special attention. Sterility is essential for hypodermic needles because they enter deep tissues. Use of liquid germicides cannot guarantee sterility because of restricted access of the agent into the narrow lumen. Fortunately, the widespread use of presterilized disposable needles has almost eliminated the risky practice of reusing chemically sterilized needles. Even though disposable sterile items are now available, however, there is an increasing practice to keep costs down by reusing these items. A good example is the artificial kidney. Hemodialyzers are manufacturered and delivered to the user in a sterile state. Assurance that the item is sterile depends on the manufacturer's quality assurance and sterilization cycle verification programs.

Seventy percent of the chronic dialysis centers of the United States reuse hemodialyzers (Alter et al., 1989). This practice that has been performed for many years (Deane et al., 1978), and it appears that if cleaning and disinfection procedures are performed correctly (using good protocols), no infectious disease problems occur among patients who undergo dialysis with reused dialyzers. However, because these devices are not subjected to the same stringent sterilization cycles and controls that are performed by the manufacturer with new sterile dialyzers, the margin of safety, although it does exist, is not as great as it would be with the manufacturer's processing. Consequently, human error has occasionally caused a significant increase in side reactions or infections associated with the reuse of dialyzers (Favero, 1985; Gordon et al., 1989).

Semicritical Instruments or Devices

Instruments or devices in this category are likewise diverse, and the health-care worker should make his or her own listing unique to a particular medical practice. Basically, these are the items that make contact with mucous membranes during use but do not ordinarily penetrate the blood barrier or enter other normally sterile areas of the body. Examples in this category include flexible fiberoptic endoscopes, laryngoscopes, vaginal specula, anesthesia breathing circuits, a variety of dental equipment such as amalgam condensers, and a number of ophthalmic devices such as direct contact tonometers. Local host defense mechanisms can be expected to protect against challenges from small numbers of exogenous microorganisms, but these types of instruments should not be contaminated with a variety of vegetative bacteria, fungi, and viruses. Although sterilization is desirable and often the most economical procedure available (e.g., autoclaving), it is not absolutely essential, as is the case with critical items. For semicritical items that do not tolerate heat or cannot withstand repeated prolonged immersion in liquid chemical germicides or repeated exposures to ethylene oxide gas cycles, it is reasonable to use a high-level disinfection process. This is a procedure that is designed to destroy mycobacteria (e.g., *M. tuberculosis* var. *bovis*), small or nonlipid viruses, fungi, vegetative bacteria, and medium-sized or lipid viruses, and is accomplished with a high degree of assurance by using a germicide that is *capable* of killing large numbers of bacterial spores. It is important to note that the only difference between sterilization and high-level disinfection with a liquid germicide is length of contact time (Table 35–4). In this context, the reader should be aware of a potentially confusing situation in today's germicide marketplace. Several products currently registered with EPA as sterilant/disinfectant products give instructions for sterilization with a concentrated or slightly diluted product, and for disinfection with higher dilutions that exceed the capacity of the product's ability to inactivate bacterial spores. In these instances, if a sterilant/disinfectant chemical is diluted beyond its ability to kill bacterial spores (either prior to use or during use), then it no longer qualifies for Spaulding's or our designation of "high-level disinfectant." It is the responsibility of the user to read and interpret the EPA-approved product label to ensure this distinction of chemical potency as related to dilution, shelf life, and

Table 35–4. *Comparison of Environmental Protection Agency (EPA) Product Table Terminology and Centers for Disease Control (CDC) Germicidal Process Terminology*

EPA Product Classification	CDC Process Classification
"Sterilant/Disinfectant" (e.g., glutaraldehyde-, chlorine dioxide-, hydrogen peroxide-, or peracetic acid-based products)	"Sterilization"[a] (sporicidal chemical, prolonged contact time) "High-Level Disinfection"[b] (sporicidal chemical, short contact time)
"Hospital Disinfectant" with label claim for tuberculocidal activity (e.g., phenolics, iodophors, or chlorine compounds)[c]	"Intermediate-Level Disinfection"[d]
"Hospital Disinfectant" with *no* label claim for tuberculocidal activity; includes "Sanitizers" (e.g., quaternary ammonium compounds, some iodophors, and some phenolics)	"Low-Level Disinfection"[e]

[a]This type of sterilization procedure should be used *only* with those instruments (critical or semicritical) that are not heat-stable. As indicated in the text, sterilization with liquid chemical germicides is not capable of being monitored biologically and requires many cumbersome postexposure manipulations such as rinsing with sterile water and drying with sterile towels prior to use on a patient.

[b]High-level disinfection, as defined above and in the text, is appropriate for those semicritical instruments that are not heat-stable and therefore cannot be sterilized by steam autoclaving between uses. As with liquid chemical sterilization, thorough rinsing with sterile water after the required exposure time is appropriate.

[c]This class of germicide includes a number of generic hypochlorite formulations that are EPA-registered but do not have specific label designations of "Hospital Disinfectant" or "Tuberculocidal."

[d]Intermediate-level disinfection is appropriate for between-patient processing of certain noncritical instruments or devices or for environmental surfaces, particularly after significant spills of blood in any area or spills of microbial cultures in the laboratory.

[e]Low-level disinfection is appropriate for between-patient processing of certain noncritical instruments or devices or for routine cleaning and housekeeping. Manufacturer's label information, particularly for EPA-approved patterns of use, should be closely examined and followed.

use patterns. Some products in this category of germicide often provide test kits designed to aid the user in monitoring levels of active ingredients during the use life of the product.

Noncritical Instruments or Devices

This category of instruments or devices includes those instruments such as electrocardiogram electrodes, physical measurement devices, blood pressure cuffs, and stethoscopes that ordinarily touch only intact skin of the patient during routine use and seldom, if ever, become contaminated with patient material, in particular, blood. These items generally offer little risk of transmitting infectious agents; consequently, many individuals rely on detergent and water cleaning or the use of low-level disinfectants used either alone or in addition to the cleaning. Chemical disinfection is also widely practiced with low-level disinfectants used either alone or in addition to the cleansing, depending on the nature and degree of contamination during use. Examples of these types of disinfectants are shown in Tables 35–3 and 35–4.

Environmental Surfaces

As mentioned previously, we have chosen to slightly modify and expand Dr. Spaulding's classification of the inanimate environment in health care facilities in order to present a more rational perception of infection transmission risk. Recent reviews of environmental issues and the role of inanimate surfaces in transmission of nosocomial infection (Rutala and Weber, 1987; Rhame, 1986) suggest that direct patient contact with inadequately disinfected critical or semicritical medical instruments has been directly implicated in a wide variety of nosocomial infections, but that environmental surfaces (such as instrument knobs or handles, instrument carts, sinks, table tops, floors, or walls) may play theoretical but certainly less significant roles in disease transmission than medical instruments. With recent increases in levels of concern about transmission risks of a number of microbial agents, in particular, blood-borne viruses, it is not uncommon to observe a variety of health-care professionals decontaminating environmental surfaces in manners appropriate for medical instruments. Certainly, microbiologic assays of samples taken from many environmental sources have shown the presence of potentially pathogenic bacteria or fungi, but the direct relationship between the presence of these agents and the incidence of infection transmission has not been demonstrated. Other evidence, however, has suggested that innate microbial characteristics such as the ability of extremely high numbers of a particular pathogen to survive for extended periods in or on environmental surfaces may be related to an increased potential for environmentally mediated disease transmission. Several microorganisms having either one or both of these qualities are influenza or other upper respiratory tract viruses, *Clostridium difficile,* and hepatitis B virus (HBV).

Since the early 1970s, it has been recognized that many instances of hepatitis B infection among hemodialysis patients or clinical laboratory workers have not been accompanied by overt or recognized parenteral or mucous membrane contact. Subsequent studies have shown that a variety of environmental surfaces in areas such as hemodialysis units, clinical laboratories, and dental operatories where there is frequent contamination with blood may show the presence of hepatitis B surface antigen (HB$_s$AG), even in the absence of visible or even chemically detectable blood. Other studies have shown that hepatitis B virus occurs in extremely high numbers (between 10^8 and 10^9 HBV/ml) in the blood and blood components of infected persons (Shikata et al., 1977), that high numbers of HBV will survive for at least 1 week after drying and storage under typical ambient conditions (Bond et al., 1981), and that very small amounts of HBV-positive material placed or splashed into the eyes (and presumably on broken skin) will result in infection (Bond et al., 1982; Kew, 1973). For these reasons, HBV has come to be regarded by many infection control practitioners as a model "worst-case" scenario with respect to the potential for blood-borne cross-contamination and disease transmission among patients and health-care workers. With the observations that HBV does not appear to be unusually resistant to germicidal chemicals (Bond et al., 1983a; Kobayashi et al., 1984), a number of recent recommendations and strategies for employment of protective barriers (e.g., gloves, face protection), environmental controls or barriers (e.g., impervious coverings for frequently contaminated surfaces that are difficult to clean and disinfect), and general methods for cleaning and disinfecting have been based on this model (Favero, 1983; Centers for Disease Control, 1987).

Medical Equipment Surfaces

Examples of these types of surfaces are adjustment knobs, handles, buttons, or levers on a variety of medical equipment such as hemodialysis machines, x-ray machines, instrument trays and carts, and dental units. These surfaces almost never come into direct contact with the patient, but because of the nature of the treatment or the equipment design, may frequently become contaminated with patient material, particularly blood, and are repeatedly touched by health-care personnel during procedures involving parenteral or mucous membrane contact. These surfaces have a distinct potential for secondary transmission of microorganisms from patient to patient or from patient to health-care worker. A good example of this potential would be a dentist performing a surgical procedure and intermittently adjusting the dental unit light during progressive stages of the procedure; the light handle almost invariably becomes contaminated with blood and oral secretions and, if it is not adequately cleaned and disinfected after the procedure, may allow cross-contamination in subsequent procedures. Such equipment surfaces, at a minimum, should be cleaned of visible material using soap and water. It may also be prudent to disinfect with an intermediate-level germicide (Table 35–3).

Housekeeping Surfaces

Environmental surfaces such as floors, walls, sinks, table tops, and related objects are not associated with transmission of infections to patients or health-care workers, and, therefore, extraordinary attempts to disinfect these surfaces are not necessary. However, general cleaning and removal of visible soil should be done routinely. The chemicals appropriate for this routine clean-

ing are low-level disinfectants (e.g., EPA-registered, nontuberculocidal "hospital disinfectants"), but the actual removal of soil and microorganisms by scrubbing is probably at least as important as any germicidal activity of the cleaning agent used.

Special protocols to augment routine cleaning may be applicable if, in the judgment of responsible workers, specific sites within a health-care facility have become *significantly* contaminated with blood or other patient material. Such a strategy is relatively conservative and requires common sense judgment to determine the relative levels of disease transmission risk involved (e.g., the nature, size, and location of the spill). In the instance of a significant spill, the visible material should be cleaned from the surface and the immediate vicinity then disinfected with an intermediate-level germicide (Table 35–3); this can be done by moderately wetting the surface with germicide (wiping or spraying) and then allowing the surface to air dry.

Spills in certain clinical laboratory areas, however, may involve higher risks of disease transmission than in other areas of the health-care facility. Serology areas usually process large volumes of blood, and microbiology procedures involve the culturing or concentrating of pathogenic microorganisms. Because of the volume of human source material and high numbers of microorganisms associated with diagnostic cultures or concentrates, the use of an intermediate-level germicide for routine decontamination in the laboratory would be prudent. Significant spills of human source material should be cleaned and disinfected in the usual manner, but spills of cultured material should first be confined (if necessary) with absorbent material, then flooded with a germicide of at least intermediate level: the germicide should then be given time to exert its effect (i.e., 10 min or as directed on the product label) followed by cleaning of the surface and the reapplication of fresh germicide, as described above.

FACTORS INFLUENCING GERMICIDAL PROCEDURES

Microorganisms vary widely in their responses to physical and chemical stresses. The most resistant to such stresses are bacterial endospores, and few if any other microorganisms approach the broad resistance of endospores (Table 35–1). There are a number of factors, some of which are associated with the microorganisms themselves, and others with the surrounding physical and chemical environment, that influence the overall effectiveness of chemical germicides. Some factors are more important than others, but all of them should be considered when planning a strategy for the chemical disinfection of medical and surgical materials.

Nature of the Item To Be Disinfected or Sterilized

The easiest surface to disinfect or even sterilize chemically is one that is smooth, nonporous, and cleanable, such as a variety of unjointed retractors or probes. Crevices, joints, and pores in surfaces constitute barriers to the cleaning and subsequent penetration of liquid germicides, and can require prolonged contact times to accomplish disinfection; a disinfection procedure is highly likely to fail under these circumstances. If microorganisms are entrapped in occluded spaces or within organic materials, even an ethylene oxide sterilization procedure may fail, especially when the level of contaminating microorganisms is high and composed, even in part, of bacterial spores. In the past 25 years there have been a number of instruments or devices made of heat-sensitive materials that require that chemical germicides be used to accomplish sterilization or high-level disinfection. If sterilization is the objective of a treatment, contact times of 6 to 10 hours are required, and this is often detrimental to material in the devices. For example, flexible fiberoptic endoscopes cannot be subjected routinely to long contact times in liquid germicides without risking the eventual degrading of lenses or other components. For this reason, if sterilization is to be accomplished, ethylene oxide gas sterilization may be the only feasible treatment; even this treatment will rapidly degrade certain components of the endoscopes, and it also has the added negative factor of keeping the instrument out of service for the often lengthy period necessary for gas processing and aeration. Because these instruments are expensive and are used frequently, some practitioners have chosen to practice high-level disinfection rather than sterilization. Any alternative approach to reprocessing this category of instrument will be difficult until the manufacturers of the instruments alter the designs and materials to allow more efficient cleaning as well as physical stability.

The size of a medical device also limits the types of germicides that can be used and whether sterilization or high-level disinfection will be the intended treatment. If an instrument is too large to be conveniently and adequately immersed in solutions or placed in an ethylene oxide chamber, then disinfection may be accomplished only by cleaning and then wiping with liquid. This would include primarily noncritical devices.

Thus, the nature and use of a medical device or item may dictate the type and use of a chemical germicide. Practitioners should be aware of this, and when purchasing medical devices, at least one criterion to be considered should be the ease with which the device can be efficiently cleaned and sterilized or disinfected.

Number of Microorganisms Present

In general, the higher the level of microbial contamination, the longer must be the exposure to the chemical germicide before the entire microbial population is killed. This factor does not stand alone, because the amount of time necessary to inactivate 1000 bacterial spores would be significantly longer than the time required to inactivate 1,000,000 cells of *Staphylococcus aureus* or most other vegetative bacteria. When considering a natural microbial population composed of various types of microorganisms that have different degrees of

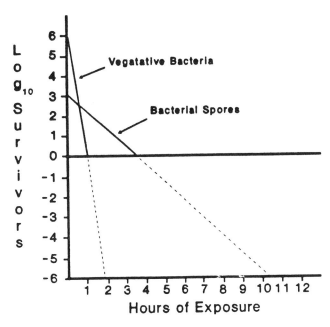

Fig. 35–1. Inactivation kinetics of a mixed microbial population.

resistance to physical or chemical stress, the survival curve with all factors controlled would be parabolic and not straight as it might be if a pure culture of a particular microorganism were used (Fig. 35–1). Furthermore, the most resistant microbial subpopulation, even through it may be present in a relatively lower concentration than the entire microbial population, tends to control sterilization or disinfection time (Bond et al., 1971).

Innate Resistance of Microorganisms

As mentioned above, microorganisms vary widely in their resistance to chemical germicides; thus, the types that are present on medical items or surgical materials may have a significant effect on the time as well as the concentration of germicides necessary for sterilization or disinfection. The most resistant types of microorganisms are bacterial spores, some of which are significantly more resistant to both chemical and physical stresses than a wide variety of other microorganisms (Bond et al., 1970, 1977b). In a broad descending order of relative resistance, considerably below that of bacterial endospores are the tubercle bacilli, small or nonlipid viruses, and vegetative fungi, as well as asexual fungal spores, vegetative bacteria, and medium-sized or lipid-containing viruses (Table 35–1). Obviously, the biggest difference in resistance is between bacterial spores and lipid viruses such as herpes viruses, hepatitis B virus, or human immunodeficiency virus. Smaller, but important, differences exist between the tubercle bacillus and non-acid-fast bacteria and among fungi and certain groups of viruses.

The differences in resistance exhibited by various vegetative bacteria to chemical germicides bacteria are relatively minor, except for the tubercle bacilli and other nontuberculous but acid-fast mycobacteria (Carson et al., 1978), which, presumably because of their hydrophobic cell surfaces, are comparatively resistant to a variety of disinfectants, especially those in the low-level category. Among the ordinary vegetative bacteria, staphylococci and enterococci are somewhat more resistant than most other gram-positive bacteria. It is interesting to note that antibiotic-resistant "hospital" strains of staphylococci do not appear to be more resistant to chemical germicides than are ordinary isolates. A number of gram-negative bacteria such as *Pseudomonas, Klebsiella, Enterobacter,* and *Serratia* also may show somewhat greater resistance to some disinfectants than other gram-negative bacteria. This may be significant because many of these gram-negative bacteria are frequently known to be responsible for outbreaks of hospital infections, especially in compromised hosts.

Gram-negative water bacteria, which have the ability to grow well and achieve levels of 10^3 to 10^7 cells per milliliter in distilled, deionized, or reverse-osmosis water, have been shown to be significantly more resistant to a variety of disinfectants in their "naturally occurring" state (i.e., isolated and grown in pure culture in water without subculturing on laboratory media) as compared with bacterial cells subcultured in the normal fashion (Favero et al., 1975; Carson et al., 1972). Figure 35–2 illustrates this phenomenon, which also has been shown to occur with nontuberculous mycobacteria (Carson et al., 1978). These differences in resistance become im-

portant when low-level disinfectants are used, particularly at marginal or dilute concentrations, or when disinfectants having greater germicidal properties are used inappropriately (e.g., surfaces are not adequately pre-cleaned prior to application of the germicide or significant organic loads are allowed to accumulate in the germicide container). The resistance of naturally occurring microorganisms also extends to bacterial spores, and it has been shown that naturally occurring bacterial spores in soil are significantly more resistant to dry heat than are subcultured spores (Bond et al., 1970).

Amount of Organic Soil Present

Blood, mucus, or feces, when present on items to be processed for reuse, may contribute to the failure of a given disinfection or sterilization procedure in three ways. The organic soil may contain large or diverse microbial populations, may occlude microorganisms and prevent penetration of chemical germicides, or the soil may directly and rapidly inactive certain germicidal chemicals such as chlorine and iodine-based disinfectants or quaternary ammonium compounds. The effect is correspondingly greater with weak concentrations and with low-level germicides than with strong concentrations and high-level germicides. In addition, this factor underscores the necessity and importance of thoroughly cleaning a medical device prior to chemical disinfection. Fail-

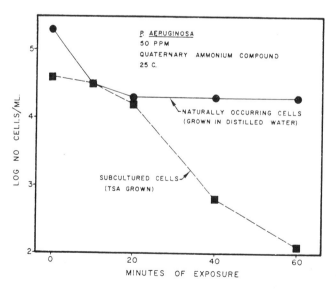

Fig. 35–2. Comparative survival of naturally occurring and subcultured cells of *Pseudomonas aeruginosa* exposed to a quaternary ammonium compound.

Table 35–5. *Tuberculocidal Activity of Alcohol, Phenolics, and Iodophor*

Compound	Disinfection Times
Phenolic I, 3%	2–3 hr
Phenolic II, 3%	45–60 min
Iodophor, 450 ppm	2–3 hr
Isopropanol, 70%	5 min

Simultaneous mucin-loop test. Number of *Mycobacterium tuberculosis* per loop was approximately 10^4.

From Spaulding, E.H. 1971. Role of chemical disinfection in the prevention of nosocomial infections. In *Proceedings of the International Conference on Nosocomial Infections, 1970.* Edited by P.S. Brachman and T.C. Eickhoff. Chicago, American Hospital Association, pp 247–254.

ure to do this may cause a disinfection or sterilization procedure to fail. In fact, physical cleaning is often the most important step in a disinfection process that by definition does not include the "overkill" factor of a sterilization process. Indeed, a report implicated a flexible fiberoptic endoscope in an outbreak of septicemia caused by *Serratia* (Webb and Vall-Spinosa, 1975). This instrument had been "sterilized" with ethylene oxide gas but had not been properly cleaned before the gassing cycle. Consequently, even a rigorous cycle capable of killing exposed bacterial spores may not kill even relatively delicate vegetative bacterial cells if these cells are protected by extraneous organic material. This factor also is intimately associated with the number of microorganisms present, so that effective cleaning procedures that remove organic soil simultaneously tend to substantially lower the general level of microbial contamination associated with the soil. More recent reports in the field of endoscopy have indicated that physically complex accessories to the endoscopic set, such as suction valves or biopsy forceps, may be extremely difficult or even impossible to clean and therefore have been responsible for transmission of a variety of organisms such as *Mycobacterium* spp. (Wheeler et al., 1989) and *Salmonella newport* (Dwyer et al., 1987). After investigating and reporting episodes of disease transmission, some workers have suggested the redesign of endoscopic equipment (Birnie et al., 1983).

Type and Concentration of Germicide Used

Generally, with all other variables constant, the higher the concentration of a chemical agent, the greater its effectiveness and the shorter the length of time required to disinfect or sterilize an item. What is not generally recognized, however, are the wide differences in potency that exist among chemical germicides used for the same purpose. For example, Spaulding (1971) compared the tuberculocidal activity between several proprietary phenolic and iodophor-based compounds to isopropanol and determined that there were significant differences in the amount of time to accomplish disinfection (Table 35–5).

Usually the disinfection time can be shortened substantially by increasing the use concentration. Some chemical germicides are appropriately used only at strong concentrations. This is true for many of the high-level chemical germicides such as glutaraldehyde-, hydrogen peroxide-, or chlorine dioxide-based products, which are sporicides. It is also true of ethanol and isopropanol because a dilution with water beyond 50 to 60% would reduce microbicidal activity. Some intermediate-level disinfectants may become useful sporicides when the concentration is increased significantly. This is probably true for hydrogen peroxide or chlorine-based products but is not true for all intermediate-level disinfectants, in particular, phenolics. In addition, complexed iodine solutions represent an instance in which there has been confusion with chemistry and strategies of use. As discussed below and elsewhere in this book, iodophor disinfectants are significantly affected by the amount of potassium iodide and water used in their formulation. Consequently, the label instructions describing a particular use dilution are much more critical than with other chemical germicides, because in the case of iodophors, use dilution is designed to yield the maximum amount of free iodine possible. Underdiluting or overdiluting the disinfectant may significantly reduce the germicidal potency. In other words, if an iodophor disinfectant is meant to be diluted 1:213, an undiluted or 1:10 aqueous dilution may have less microbicidal activity than the recommended use-dilution. Furthermore, it is not clear which iodine species should be used to gauge germicidal potency. Most iodophor disinfectants or antiseptics are formulated to contain a specific amount of complexed iodine, yielding a certain percentage of available iodine with an unspecified amount of free iodine contained in the use-dilution. Available iodine, which is simply the amount of iodine in solution that titrates with sodium thiosulfate, does not imply microbicidal effectiveness. Certainly, the amount of available iodine present is important because it can be converted to free iodine, depending on a number of other factors, including the amount of water present. Consequently, care should be taken to follow the manufacturer's instruction for proprietary disinfectant iodophor preparations so that the proper use-dilutions of the germicides are made.

Duration and Temperature of Exposures

As expected, with all other variables constant, the longer the germicidal process is continued, the greater its effectiveness. One possible exception would be with some low-level disinfectants with which there might be a minimum threshold concentration of the chemical that may have absolutely no killing effect on a microbial population no matter how long the contact time. For example, some quaternary ammonium disinfectants, either used in insufficient concentrations or in solutions that have deteriorated by age or by the presence of organic soil, might not only fail to kill some microbial populations (especially gram-negative bacteria) but may actually support their growth.

An increase in the temperature of a germicidal solution during the exposure time can significantly increase the efficacy of chemical germicides. However, temperature may be increased to such a point that the germicide itself degrades, reducing its potency or creating a health hazard by producing toxic fumes. This is especially true with germicidal disinfectants whose active components are halogens or aldehydes.

Other Factors

Depending upon the product, the pH of the solution, hardness of the water used for dilution, or presence of other chemicals such as soaps may have negative effects on germicidal potency. The label instructions on each proprietary formulation should be carefully examined and followed closely.

COMMONLY USED INSTRUMENT-EQUIPMENT GERMICIDES

As discussed previously, chemical germicides classified as disinfectants are by definition liquid formulations specifically used to inactivate microorganisms on inanimate objects. In health-care settings, they are commonly classified according to their spectrum of germicidal activities as high-, intermediate-, or low-level disinfectants, and this classification scheme corresponds with terminology found on the labels of all proprietory formulations registered by EPA (Table 35–4). The type of disinfectant that is chosen to accomplish a particular level of disinfection is related primarily to the item being disinfected, and whether that item is critical, semicritical, or noncritical in terms of the risk of transmitting infection, i.e., the degree of patient contact. Variables discussed previously, such as the nature of the contaminating material, the level of microbial contamination, and the temperature and concentration of disinfectant, are also important in the overall disinfection process. Further, one of the most important factors affecting the successful outcome of the disinfection process is the efficiency of the procedure that is used to physically clean an instrument prior to disinfection. Without proper cleaning, all disinfection processes are subject to failure, and even a sterilizing process may be compromised.

The chemical germicides discussed below are those that are commonly used in hospitals in the United States. Other workers have recently reviewed various classes and use patterns of chemical germicides used as disinfectants (Rutala and Weber, 1987; Rhame, 1986; Rutala, 1990).

Phenol Compounds

Phenol or carbolic acid is one of the oldest germicidal agents used in the hospital environment. The parent chemical has been replaced by hundreds of derivative compounds. These are referred to as phenol derivatives or phenolics. They are considered to be intermediate-to low-level disinfectants and are used primarily for disinfection purposes for a variety of environmental surfaces and for noncritical instruments or devices. The mechanism of action of phenol in high concentrations on the microbial cell appears to be a gross protoplasmic poison, penetrating and destroying the cell wall and precipitating cellular protein (Prindle, 1983). In lower concentrations, the eventual death of the bacterial cell appears to be due to inactivation of essential enzyme systems. Phenolics are considered fair-to-good bactericides, because they are stable and remain active after mild heating and prolonged drying. Subsequent application of moisture to a dry surface previously treated with a phenolic can redissolve the residual chemical so that it again becomes bactericidal. Concentrations of phenolics in the order of 1 to 2% remain active when in contact with organic soil, and for this reason phenolics are often one of the disinfectants of choice when dealing with gross organic contamination in general hospital housekeeping or for environmental disinfection in laboratory areas.

Their usefulness for the disinfection of semicritical instruments or devices is limited, however, because phenolics are generally difficult to rinse from most materials, and the residue may irritate patient tissue. Even when porous articles that are disinfected with phenolics can be rinsed thoroughly before use, there is still a possibility of residual disinfectant causing tissue irritation. Kahn (1970) reported that equipment and devices so treated caused depigmentation of skin and injury to mucous membranes. Brayman and Songer (1971) pointed out another aspect of phenol toxicity when they found hazardous concentrations in laboratory air near solutions that had been heated to 45°C (Wysowski et al., 1978). For these reasons and also because they are not sporicides, phenolics are not appropriate for disinfection of critical and semicritical instruments and devices. Phenolics have been shown to be effective but rather slow tuberculocides (Spaulding, 1971) (Table 35–5). Klein and Deforest (1983) reported that 5% phenol killed picornaviruses (nonlipid viruses), but as much as 12% o-phenylphenol did not. On the other hand, Wright (1970b) found several substituted phenolics to be effective against vesicular stomatitis virus. With the various formulations that are commercially available in the United States and the lack of consistent data about the germicidal spectrum of these products, it is somewhat difficult to suggest uses for phenolics beyond the disinfection of noncritical and very few semicritical instruments or devices. They are used primarily as environmental disinfectants in general housekeeping or in laboratory areas.

Quaternary Ammonium Compounds

A variety of quaternary ammonium compounds, including benzalkonium chloride and cetylpyridinium chloride, have been widely used since their introduction as germicides in 1935. As mentioned in Chapter 13, the mode of action of quaternary ammonium compounds appears to be associated with the agent's effect on the cytoplasmic membrane, which controls cell permeability. The "quats" were, for many years, the most popular of all classes of disinfectants primarily because of their blandness and low cost. In the laboratory, they appeared to be rapidly acting germicides against test bacteria in vitro, particularly the staphylococci, but under ordinary conditions of use, their germicidal action is somewhat questionable. They are classed as low-level disinfectants with relatively poor activity against gram-negative bacteria. In fact, commercial "preparations" have been shown to support the growth of *Pseudomonas* spp. (Adair et al., 1969). Dixon et al. (1976) have discussed the problems associated with the use of quaternary ammonium-based antiseptics and disinfectants in the hospital environment and have described several outbreaks of disease associated with gram-negative bacterial contamination of quaternary ammonium solutions.

When mixed with other chemical agents such as low concentrations of alcohol, certain proprietary formulations may be advertised as "tuberculocidal." However, quaternary ammonium compounds alone have no tuberculocidal activity, and because of this, they have a role in laboratory procedures for the isolation of tubercle bacilli from clinical materials (Wayne et al., 1962; Smithwick et al., 1975). Indeed, the general ineffectiveness of quaternary ammonium compounds against various gram-negative bacteria including *Pseudomonas* spp. (especially *P. aeruginosa*) was taken advantage of by laboratory workers in developing culture media that use quaternary ammonium compounds as an inhibitory factor against gram-positive organisms, allowing pseudomonads and some other gram-negative bacteria to be selectively isolated from mixed microbial populations. Also, Klein and Deforest (1963) found that benzalkonium chloride lacks activity against picornaviruses, even in 10% concentration. Because most quaternary ammonium compounds do not acquire even an intermediate-level activity at any usable concentration, they should not be used for disinfecting critical or semicritical medical instruments or devices.

These compounds are rapidly inactivated by contact with protein, cotton fibers, and other organic materials, and gram-negative bacteria such as *Pseudomonas, Enterobacter*, and *Serratia* spp. have frequently been noted to grow in certain formulations. However, most quaternary ammonium-based products are excellent cleansing agents that can be used effectively for housekeeping purposes in the hospital and other health-care settings.

Chlorine

Inorganic chlorine solutions in concentrations of 0.05 to 0.5% free chlorine are generally considered to be intermediate-level disinfectants and are among the most effective, most convenient, and least expensive germicides for specific site disinfection. The mode of action of free chlorine, unlike that of free iodine, is considered to be the inactivation of sulfhydryl enzymes and protein denaturation as well as the inactivation of nucleic acids. Solutions of 0.5% (household bleach contains approximately 5% sodium hypochlorite) have broad-spectrum germicidal activity. They exhibit sporicidal activity, are tuberculocidal, inactivate vegetative bacteria, and are fungicidal and virucidal. Klein and Deforest (1965) reported that all of 25 viruses, including the picornaviruses,

were inactivated in 10 minutes by as little as 0.02% available chlorine.

Free chlorine as derived from sodium hypochlorite or calcium hypochlorite has limited use on medical devices because of its corrosiveness. However, it can be used effectively in moderate concentrations for specific site decontamination of blood or body fluid spills, or for decontaminating spills of laboratory culture material. It has been used as a disinfectant for hydrotherapy baths and in hemodialysis systems but has the disadvantage of being corrosive to certain components of these devices. Hypochlorite solutions cannot be left for long periods in a dialysis machine, and the fact that it must be rinsed from the hemodialysis machine negates its overall efficacy; this is because gram-negative bacteria in the rinsing water tend to grow in these systems in the absence of a disinfectant (Favero et al., 1975; Favero and Petersen, 1977).

Iodophors

Tinctures of iodine and iodophors have been used for many years by health-care professionals for antisepsis and disinfection. Iodine (I_2) in its pure form is not very soluble in water and is saturated at 0.03%, which is 300 ppm free iodine (free iodine being the reactive chemical specie, I_2). Tinctures of iodine have been used primarily as antiseptic solutions, whereas iodophors are used as both antiseptics and disinfectants. Iodophors are the combination of iodine and a solublizing agent or carrier in which the resulting complex or combination in water acts as a reservoir of iodine and continuously liberates small amounts of free iodine. The number of carriers include polyvinylpyrrolidone ("PVP" or "povidone") and ethoxylated nonionic detergents (poloxamers). Iodine is believed to function as a general cellular poison and to affect both nucleic acids and proteins. Some iodophors have been marketed as disinfectants, and have the disadvantage of being unstable in the presence of very hard water, heat, and organic soil, but they appear to be reliable, general-purpose disinfectants if used in concentrations recommended by the manufacturer. Some metallic instruments can be corroded if they are routinely disinfected with iodophors for long periods; nonmetallic items are seldom physically damaged but may be stained or discolored. Iodophor disinfectants traditionally are classified as low- to intermediate-level disinfectants, depending on the concentration. However, as will be discussed, one cannot determine the concentration of the actual microbicidal agent (free iodine) from information on the label.

Formulations of iodophors usually list certain percentages of available iodine that have been used to indicate germicidal potency. This does not appear to be correct. There are many aspects related to the physical and organic chemistry of iodine complexes that are not understood fully. For example, a povidone-iodine germicide formulated as an antiseptic usually contains 10% providone-iodine and is said to yield 1% available iodine. The amount of free iodine present in these solutions has been reported to be approximately 1 ppm (Berkelman et al., 1981; Rodeheaver et al., 1976) and is controlled significantly by the amount of potassium iodide present as well as by the amount of water (see Chapter 8). Concentrated solutions of iodophor contain less free iodine in undiluted solutions than those that are diluted to a certain extent (Berkelman et al., 1982). It is almost impossible to chemically assay free iodine in the presence of complexed iodine without resorting to an extraction technique using solvents. Thus, it is clear that the manufacturer's direction for an iodophor disinfectant, which calls for a certain aqueous dilution of a concentrated product, is designed to give the maximum degree of microbicidal efficiency, which probably correlates with the amount of free iodine present. There is less free iodine in solution and, accordingly, less microbicidal activity when the product is diluted more or less than the prescribed amount. Available iodine does not appear to be a sufficient indicator of potency for iodophor germicides. Berkelman and colleagues (1981), for example, reported the recovery of *Pseudomonas cepacia* from blood cultures of 52 patients in four hospitals in New York City over a 7-month period from April through October 1980. Epidemiologic investigations revealed that the positive blood cultures indicated pseudobacteremias, and that the source of contamination was a commercially available 10% povidone-iodine antiseptic solution, which was used (incorrectly) both as an antiseptic and disinfectant. It was shown that *P. cepacia* gained entrance to blood culture tubes from povidone-iodine left on the skin prior to venipuncture or from povidone-iodine that was applied to blood culture bottle tops through which blood was inoculated by syringe into culture media. In addition, *P. cepacia* was isolated directly from the povidone-iodine solutions. There have been several other epidemiologic and microbiologic investigations that have documented intrinsic microbial contamination of iodophor antiseptic solutions. *Pseudomonas cepacia* has been associated both with pseudobacteremias (false-positive blood cultures) and peritoneal infections among patients undergoing peritoneal dialysis (Berkelman et al., 1981; Craven et al., 1981; Centers for Disease Control, 1989). *Pseudomonas aeruginosa* was associated with peritoneal infections, and the same organism was shown to be an intrinsic contaminant of poloxamer-iodine antiseptic solutions (Parrott et al., 1982; Berkelman et al., 1984). Laboratory investigations have shown that a probable mechanism of pseudomonad survival in a variety of chemically adverse environments is the development of extracellular matrices of polysaccharide materials (glycocalyx or biofilms) by the organisms during colonization of surfaces such as pipes in water treatment or distribution systems. Water passing through colonized pipes can sporadically carry the organisms embedded in masses of biofilm, and if the water is used to prepare an iodophor antiseptic solution, for instance, the biofilm can protect the embedded organisms from the germicidal effects of low free-iodine

levels. Similarly, if pipe systems colonized with biofilms containing pseudomonads are used to distribute or store the iodophor solution during the manufacturing process, portions of the biofilm can be stripped from the pipe surface and carried along with the germicide during fluid distribution. The organisms being protected by the biofilm matrix can survive for significant periods (e.g., for months) and exhibit an apparent level of resistance that would be expected of bacterial spores (Anderson et al., 1983, 1984; Berkelman et al., 1984; Bond et al., 1983b; Favero et al., 1983). Recently, Anderson and coworkers (1989a) demonstrated that gram-negative water bacteria can colonize polyvinyl chloride (PVC) water pipes, develop a biofilm matrix, and exhibit extreme resistance to a variety of chemical germicides. These reports are not the first to describe intrinsic microbial contamination of commercially available germicide solutions, but one would have thought that these solutions containing 1% available iodine would prevent the survival of vegetative bacteria (or perhaps even bacterial spores). Unfortunately, most investigators have tended to equate available iodine with free iodine. A review of the literature (see Chapter 8; Favero, 1982; Anderson, 1989b) concerning microbicidal capabilities of iodophor solutions reveals that prior to 1982, almost no one actually reported the amount of free iodine but rather expressed concentration either as a dilution of a particular formulation or, more often, as amounts of available iodine as mg per liter. This confusion may be due to equating the term "available iodine" with the term "available chlorine." The latter is defined as the amount of free (Cl_2 and $HOCl$) and combined chlorine (i.e., chloramines), both of which are microbicidal, although free chlorine is more active than combined chlorine. The term "available" when used with iodine means the amount that is titratable with sodium thiosulfate; available iodine, as such, is not microbicidal. Available iodine can be thought of as an expression of the reservoir of the complexed iodine, which slowly releases free iodine in a given solution. As the free iodine is depleted, more free iodine instantaneously takes its place. For example, with an iodophor disinfectant that has 1% (10,000 ppm) available iodine and 35 ppm free iodine, the free iodine, which is inactivated by reacting with organic materials or bacteria, is immediately replaced from the available reservoir. Likewise, when it is titrated with sodium thiosulfate, the free iodine concentration is instantaneously replaced from the reservoir of available iodine (even though it is the free iodine that is being titrated); the end result is 1% or 10,000 ppm available iodine. The amount of *free* iodine, however, is much less, i.e., 35 ppm free iodine.

This does not alter the rationale for classifying certain iodophor disinfectants as intermediate-level disinfectants, but it does present a problem in defining use-concentration. Because it is complicated to assay for free iodine in iodophor solutions, and because it is current practice for manufacturers to include the amount of available iodine (whether the amount is accurate or not) on product labels as an implication of potency, we have chosen to retain using available iodine as an indicator of potency for denoting strength in Table 35–3, but free iodine levels also are listed. It should be noted that with iodophors the manufacturer's directions are most critical with respect to actual use-dilutions with water, and care should be taken to follow label instructions closely.

Alcohols

The value of alcohol as a surgical germicide has been reviewed by Spaulding (1964). Ethyl and isopropyl alcohol are rapidly bactericidal intermediate-level disinfectants and are remarkably active against the tubercle bacillus (Table 35–5). Neither ethanol nor isopropanol are sporicidal and, indeed, both alcohols are sometimes used to store clean spore crops of *Bacillus* spp. and *Clostridium* spp. They are effective against all types of vegetative bacteria and fungi, but reports on the virucidal properties of alcohol indicate that the spectrum of activity may vary with the type of alcohol (Klein and Deforest, 1963; Wright, 1970a). Ethyl alcohol is broadly virucidal, but isopropyl alcohol activity is limited primarily to lipid-containing viruses.

Alcohols characteristically evaporate quickly and leave no residue on treated surfaces, which may or may not be an advantage, depending on the item being disinfected. In some instances, they have been known to dissolve the lens mountings of certain types of optical instruments, and when used for long exposures, they tend to harden and swell plastic tubing, including polyethylene. Further, rubber articles absorb alcohol, and irritation of the skin or mucous membranes may follow. Alcohols in a concentration of 70% by volume may be a reasonable choice for intermediate-level disinfection for noncritical and certain types of semicritical instruments, provided the items can be submerged to effect adequate contact contact time (e.g., 10 min). Because alcohols coagulate protein, they are poor cleaners, and rapid evaporation makes adequate contact times impossible on open surfaces; therefore, they are inappropriate for use on environmental surfaces.

Formaldehyde

Forty percent formaldehyde gas dissolved in water constitutes a 100% solution of formalin; 8% formaldehyde in water is 20% formalin. Depending on its concentration, formaldehyde is classified as a high-level (8% formaldehyde plus 70% alcohol) or intermediate to high-level (4 to 8% formaldehyde in water) disinfectant. Aqueous formaldehyde in concentrations less than 4% may have limited activity against *Mycobacterium* spp., particularly the atypical nontuberculous mycobacteria indigenous to certain potable water supplies. Formaldehyde has a broad spectrum of action on microorganisms, and its mode of action is by alkylation with amino and sulfhydryl groups of proteins and ring nitrogen atoms of purine bases such as guanine (Habeeb and Hiramoto, 1968). Sporicidal activity suggests that alkylation of nucleic acids may be more important in microbicidal action

than changes in protein constituents. The action of formaldehyde on a protein coat of poliovirus progressively slows down the killing rate by obstructing penetration of the nucleic acid core (Gard, 1959). As mentioned above, 8% formaldehyde in water is considered an intermediate- to high-level disinfectant; combining 8% formaldehyde in 65 to 70% isopropanol yields a compound that is rapidly bactericidal, tuberculocidal, and sporicidal, but the time required for achieving sterility using high numbers of spores as a challenge may be up to 18 hours or longer, depending on the test conditions (Spaulding, 1966, unpublished data). Although these solutions of formaldehyde are considered to be intermediate- to high-level germicides, the irritating fumes and potential carcinogenicity of formaldehyde limit its usefulness in the hospital environment, and its toxicity for tissue requires that disinfected materials be thoroughly rinsed before use. Because it is not corrosive to equipment associated with hemodialysis systems, formaldehyde is used in a concentration of 4% to disinfect dialysis systems and disposable hemodialyzers that are reused. In both instances, however, the problem of residual formaldehyde constitutes a potential health hazard to dialysis patients, and hemodialysis systems and hemodialyzers must be thoroughly rinsed free of formaldehyde prior to use.

Glutaraldehyde

Glutaraldehyde is a saturated dialdehyde that is chemically related to formaldehyde and has been shown to be two to eight times more sporicidal than formaldehyde (Borick, 1968). Like formaldehyde, the mode of action of glutaraldehyde on microorganisms is by alkylation, reactions with amino and sulfhydryl groups of proteins and ring nitrogen atoms of purine bases. Glutaraldehyde-based germicides have been used as disinfectants for many years since alkaline formulations were shown to be sporicidal (Boucher, 1972; Pepper and Chandler, 1963; Borick, 1968). The microbicidal activity of aqueous glutaraldehyde appears to increase when the pH is alkaline but declines after storage or use of the disinfectant (Borick, 1968). Neutral to acidic formulations are also sporicidal and this germicidal activity is increased by addition of heat or in the presence of ultrasonic energy (Sierra and Boucher, 1971; Boucher, 1974). In recent years, a large number of glutaraldehyde-based germicides with a variety of buffer systems, surfactants, and other additives have been approved by EPA as sterilant/disinfectants. A number of these products as they reach the user have concentrations of glutaraldehyde higher or lower than the earlier products with 2% "active" ingredient; some of these formulations are designed to be used undiluted as a sterilant or disinfectant (the only variable being contact time), and others may require or suggest dilution prior to use. In this latter instance, the user should be aware that dilution of any germicidal product results in a less powerful solution and perhaps one with a more narrow spectrum of microbicidal activity, e.g., it may no longer be capable of killing bacterial spores. For this reason, the user should carefully examine the EPA-approved product label to determine whether dilutions of a product, if recommended, remain capable of sterilization at extended contact times; if so, shorter contact times recommended for disinfection with the diluted product would be classed as "high-level" processes; otherwise, they would be "intermediate" at best. In practice, however, any product that is used more than once for sterilization or disinfection will lose potency for a variety of reasons, including dilution due to repeated exposures to moist or wet instruments, dilution due to use of certain automated disinfecting machines, accumulation of organic material from inadequately cleaned instruments, or innate chemical degradation within the germicide mixture. In other words, a chemical germicide invariably will lose potency if reused, and the rate of loss depends more on patterns and intensity of use than on the age of the solution (Bageant et al., 1981; Holmberg et al., 1984; Robison et al., 1988; Isenberg et al., 1988).

The exposure time recommended for disinfection with glutaraldehyde-based sterilant/disinfectants (and other like classes of germicides) is based on EPA-required test data for tuberculocidal activity and may vary from formulation to formulation, e.g., 10 to 90 minutes, depending on exposure temperature. Those products that contain only glutaraldehyde as the active ingredient have efficient bactericidal, fungicidal, and virucidal activity but are slowly tuberculocidal; the apparent reason for this is that the waxy cell-coating material common to all species of *Mycobacteria* retards the penetration of glutaraldehyde into the cells. Times necessary for efficient tuberculocidal activity may be shortened by additives such as other more rapidly tuberculocidal chemicals (e.g., phenol, phenolics, or alcohols) and/or surfactants to enhance penetration of glutaraldehyde.

Glutaraldehyde-based germicides are the most widely used sterilant/disinfectant products, especially for endoscopic and respiratory therapy/anesthesia instruments. They are noxious and irritating and may result in a variety of toxic reactions in health-care workers if proper ventilation and personal barriers (e.g., gloves, face protection), as recommended in product literature, are not consistently employed.

Hydrogen Peroxide

Hydrogen peroxide has been recognized as a germicide for more than a century (see Chapter 9). Application of low concentrations of unstable preparations to tissues containing inactivating levels of catalase led to unfavorable results; this agent has generally been abandoned as an antiseptic. However, it has recently been used in stabilized form. Currently, there is one EPA-registered sterilant/disinfectant formulation containing 6% hydrogen peroxide and several similarly registered products that contain low concentrations of both hydrogen peroxide and peracetic acid. Hydrogen peroxide has been shown to be bactericidal and virucidal (Mentel and Schmidt, 1973) and, in high concentration, sporicidal (Toledo et al., 1973). The latter investigators obtained

D-values of 0.8 to 7.3 minutes at 24°C with both aerobic and anaerobic spore suspensions by using 10 to 25% hydrogen peroxide. Wardle and Renninger (1975) showed that 10^8 aerobic spores were inactivated at 25°C in 60 minutes with a 10% concentration of hydrogen peroxide. Hydrogen peroxide in concentrations of 3 to 6% or in mixtures with peracetic acid constitutes a useful class of agents for sterilization or disinfection of a variety of materials, including medical and surgical devices.

Two recently developed methods under commercial investigation use low-temperature hydrogen peroxide vapor or hydrogen peroxide treated by glow-discharge plasma to disinfect or sterilize medical devices. Because the residual after such treatments is water and oxygen, there may be much interest in the near future in these approaches in replacing ethylene oxide sterilization where there is concern for airborne or residual germicide.

LABORATORY AND IN-USE TESTING OF CHEMICAL GERMICIDES

Two basic types of evaluation procedures can be used to compare the spectrum of microbicidal activity of various chemical germicides. First, laboratory in-vitro tests, using known numbers and types of microorganisms, can be performed to determine (1) the time (and temperature) needed to achieve disinfection for given concentrations of a chemical germicide in a particular procedure, or (2) the concentration of a germicide needed to produce a desired disinfection time under a given set of circumstances. The second type of test involves evaluation of a chemical germicide by an actual or simulated in-use test, along with an appropriate microbiologic assay. Depending on the test organisms used, the results can indicate the level of capabilities or activity spectrum of a disinfection procedure. Such tests may be performed with or without added organic loads.

In the United States, the basic laboratory tests for the evaluation of chemical germicides used by the EPA as well as many scientific investigators have been described by the AOAC (1984). The AOAC use-dilution method involves testing pure cultures of microorganisms either on surgical threads or small porcelain cylinders against a specific chemical germicide at a controlled contact time and temperature—usually 10 min at 20°C. It is designed as a dry test (i.e., the inoculum is placed in a receptacle and dried prior to exposure to the germicide). When 10^6 to 10^8 bacterial spores per test vehicle are used, such a test constitutes a fairly stringent challenge. With the dried inoculum, it is difficult for chemical germicides to penetrate to such an extent that the entire population is killed. The assay procedure is based on growth or no growth of surviving microorganisms after exposure of a specific number of carriers. If the test is designed as a sporicidal test, by definition it involves complete kill of 10^6 to 10^8 dried bacterial spores of *Bacillus subtilis* or *Clostridium sporogenes*. As mentioned previously, this constitutes a severe challenge that could be exceeded only by the use of naturally occurring spores, for example, those in the soil (Bond et al., 1970) or those embedded in dried organic material. Consequently, one can usually be assured that a chemical germicide that has been tested and approved by the EPA for use as a sporicide is an effective chemical sterilant if it is stored and used properly. Obviously, problems associated with misuse or improper preparation (e.g., excessive dilution of the product before use or during reuse or improper cleaning of an instrument) can contribute to the failure of a sterilization or high-level disinfection procedure.

The AOAC use-dilution test applied to vegetative bacteria is a somewhat less reliable indicator of germicide potency. The complete test set enables the EPA and manufacturers to provide a minimum set of guidelines for comparing and judging the activity level and spectum of germicidal products. However, this test does not constitute as severe a challenge when vegetative bacteria are tested as it does when germicides are challenged with bacterial spores. First, the factors influencing microbial resistance to germicides as discussed above in this chapter are greatly magnified when vegetative bacteria are involved; recent controversy, as discussed elsewhere (Rutala and Cole, 1987; Rutala, 1990), has centered around intra- and inter-laboratory inconsistencies and interpretation of laboratory data when testing vegetative bacteria, including *Mycobacterium tuberculosis* var. *bovis*. Furthermore, the number and type of species of bacteria used in these tests are limited. More importantly, they are pure cultures that have been subcultured for years and maintained in laboratories. That difference in itself will give a false sense of security because microorganisms in their naturally occurring state tend to be significantly more resistant to physical and chemical stresses than when they are subcultured (Carson et al., 1972 and 1978; Favero et al., 1975). Therefore, even though this type of test may provide the EPA, manufacturers, and investigators with a somewhat standardized basis for maintaining minimum criteria for comparing germicides, it cannot be used as the sole criterion for selecting chemical germicides to accomplish specific degrees of disinfection, whether it be sterilization or high to low levels of disinfection. This is especially true in a hospital setting.

Of great importance in the hospital environment is the manner in which the intended instrument or item is used, as well as the anticipated risk of disease transmission. In most instances, it is not necessary for hospital laboratories to test the antimicrobial effectiveness of commercial products unless such testing is part of a well designed and carefully controlled research or evaluation project. As mentioned previously, there are currently certain questions about the reproducibility or reliability of specific laboratory test methods, but basically one must rely on the testing methods and data required by the EPA for registration of disinfectant agents. It is a fairly good assumption that any chemical germicide registered with the EPA meets a general set of minimum

test criteria. There are times, however, when the use of a particular device or item is new or unique, the intended germicide has not been used previously in a specific manner, or it is a new germicide. In these cases, one may wish to do an in-use test. These tests should be well designed and can be conducted in one of two general ways.

The first type of in-use test is one in which the item is microbiologically assayed after it has been contaminated in actual use and after an appropriate germicidal treatment has been done. The type of microbiologic assay would depend on the intended outcome, i.e., sterilization or disinfection. For example, if the intended disinfectant level for a medical device is high, the microbiological criterion would be the absence of fungi and vegetative bacteria, but not necessarily of bacterial spores. Although this type of testing can be valuable, it is rather cumbersome, and few hospital laboratories have the resources to do it on a routine or even intermittent basis. This type of microbiologic testing is designed as part of a carefully designed research project and should not be incorporated into a program of routine microbiologic monitoring (Favero, 1985).

Another type of in-use test is to operate the medical device or instrument (for example, a hemodialysis machine) in the laboratory and provide a microbiologic challenge, either by inoculation of naturally occurring microorganisms or with pure cultures, and then perform the disinfection procedure, followed by a microbiologic assay. The microbiologic criterion would not change with respect to culture assay methods, but certain critical variables such as temperature, exposure time, and exact verified germicide concentrations can be controlled.

Some of the major reasons for inconsistencies between contact times derived from AOAC tests and from in-use tests are device-dependent and include design (texture, materials, and configuration of surfaces), the usual nature and amount of contamination, accessibility for cleaning, and the ease or difficulty of applying the germicide to all pertinent surfaces. Several studies (House and Henderson, 1965; Pierce et al., 1970) underscore the possible need for in-use testing of naturally contaminated equipment to establish more reliable contact times than those achieved with AOAC tests.

It is clear, then, that the actual effectiveness of a chemical germicide is influenced only in part by the nature of the active agent. Of equal and perhaps greater importance is the way in which it is used in the hospital settings. Many disinfectants, especially the low- and intermediate-level disinfectants, have little margin of safety, and their misuse may lead to failure of the intended process. Consequently, there is always a tendency for a hospital's infection control personnel to decide to use microbiologic cultures in a limited program to monitor the effectiveness of disinfection and sterilization procedures. We strongly discourage routine widespread environmental culturing, because it offers little usable data to infection-control personnel. Moreover, any environmental monitoring program must be well designed with a specific objective in mind (Favero and Bond, 1991). It would be difficult to justify, for example, evaluation of items or areas that are unlikely to play a role in disease transmission. Although floors or furniture and other noncritical items are routinely cleaned and, in certain instances, disinfected, they should *not* be tested, even to monitor the effectiveness of hospital housekeeping personnel; it has been said that a clean white glove is a more effective testing tool than is a culture plate in these areas. To the extent that it is used (and only when there is evidence that the devices are involved in infection transmission), microbiologic sampling should be limited to high-risk (critical or semicritical) items. Even then, microbiologic assays should not take the place of scrupulous attention to the actual performance of the cleaning and disinfection or sterilization procedures.

STRATEGIES FOR MONITORING CHEMICAL DISINFECTION OF SELECTED PATIENT CARE EQUIPMENT

Respiratory Therapy and Anesthesia Breathing Circuits

The most important part of an environmental control program to reduce infections transmitted directly or indirectly by respiratory therapy and anesthesia equipment breathing circuits is the use of proper cleaning and reprocessing procedures for reusable components (Favero and Bond, 1991). The most efficient and cost-effective way to accomplish these goals is to sterilize these devices with steam under pressure or with ethylene oxide. If this is not possible, the *minimal* procedure that should be used is one that achieves high-level disinfection. In this case these items may be spot-checked every few months or when disinfection or use procedures change. Routine or scheduled bacteriologic testing is not required. Although there is no adequate, well supported microbiologic guideline for this strategy, the most widely used criterion of acceptability is the absence of vegetative bacteria on components of the breathing circuits after the disinfection process (APHA, 1978; Favero, 1989).

Hemodialysis Systems

Gram-negative water bacteria can multiply rapidly in fluids associated with hemodialysis systems such as distilled, softened, deionized, and reverse-osmosis water, as well as in the dialysis fluid itself. Although these fluids do not need to be sterile, excessive levels of gram-negative bacteria pose a risk of pyrogenic reactions and septicemia. A quantitative microbiologic guideline for levels of contamination has been proposed (AAMI 1982, 1986; Favero and Petersen, 1977; Favero, 1985).

Dialysis fluids and water used to prepare dialysis fluids should be checked microbiologically at least once a month. Microbiologic guidelines for these procedures include sampling the water used to prepare dialysis fluid at the point at which it is mixed with concentrated di-

alysis fluid, and the level of bacterial contamination should not exceed 200 colony-forming units (CFU) per milliliter. Dialysis fluid should be sampled at the end of a dialysis treatment, and the level of bacterial contamination should not exceed 2000 CFU per milliliter. In both instances, routine standard plate count or membrane filter assay procedures using appropriate culture media such as tryptic soy agar can be used. Hemodialysis systems are among the few medical devices for which periodic microbiologic assays are recommended and for which one of the few microbiologic quantitative guidelines are actually based on epidemiologic studies (Favero and Petersen, 1977; Favero, 1985).

Arterial Pressure Transducers

Arterial pressure transducers have been incriminated in disease transmission, and the best means of control are adequate cleaning and sterilization as well as proper placement. Scheduled microbiologic sampling is not required, but these items should then be assayed occasionally to determine whether they are being sterilized properly. The criterion of acceptability is sterility (Beck-Sague and Jarvis, 1989).

Endoscopic Equipment

In recent years, flexible and rigid endoscopic devices for use on patients have increased in number and in complexity of design. These devices have the advantage in many cases of eliminating surgical procedures for clinical or diagnostic purposes, but because they touch mucous membranes or are placed into normally sterile areas of the body, they are in the category of semicritical-to-critical instruments. Ideally, all endoscopes including flexible fiberoptics should be appropriately cleaned and then sterilized between uses. In practice, however, the vast majority of all flexible or rigid endoscopic procedures performed worldwide are done with disinfected rather than sterilized optic portions of the endoscopic set. The reasons for this are that almost all optic portions of endoscopic devices are delicate and are, in varying degrees, degraded or destroyed by steam autoclaving; some endoscopes are damaged even by repeated ethylene oxide cycles, and this type of processing will remove the instruments from service for hours, sometimes even days, because of process and aeration times. In these instances, the absolute minimal strategy should be the use of meticulous cleaning and high-level disinfection (Bond et al., 1979; Garner and Favero, 1985; Ridgway, 1985; Bond, 1987a, 1987b; American Society for Gastrointestinal Endoscopy, 1988; British Society for Gastroenterology, 1988). A variety of chemical germicides that are classified as high-level disinfectants have already been discussed. When one selects a germicide for use with lensed instruments, not only the activity of the germicide must be considered but also the chemical compatibility after extended use with the instrument. Currently, the most widely used high-level disinfectants with endoscopic equipment are glutaraldehyde-based or hydrogen-peroxide–based germicides. As with other critical and semicritical items, the best method for ensuring the actual success of a disinfection procedure is strict adherence to established cleaning and disinfection protocols. Because of the physical variety and complexity of endoscopic devices, particularly flexible endoscopes, the user should pay particular attention to the device manufacturer's instructions for physical access and cleaning of all device surfaces; if patient material remains in or on instrument surfaces, practically all germicidal procedures short of a steam autoclave cycle may fail in their intended purpose (Dwyer et al., 1987; Wheeler et al., 1989). Scheduled microbiologic sampling is not required, but if it is done periodically the criterion of acceptability is the absence of vegetative bacteria.

Miscellaneous Procedures and Equipment

There are numerous items and patient-care equipment that pose varying degrees of infection risk associated with their use. They may make direct contact with skin and mucous membranes of body orifices or with the peritoneal cavity, but usually not with deep tissue. Items in this category, in addition to flexible fiberoptic and other endoscopic equipment, include hydrotherapy equipment, and peritoneal dialysis equipment, and certain dental handpieces or tooth scalers. With these items, as with others mentioned above, the most important element in environmental control is not microbiologic sampling but rather adherence to established protocols associated with the items' cleaning, preparation, disinfection or sterilization, length of use, and maintenance. Even spot-checking these items and procedures is not recommended in most cases because of the lack of meaningful microbiologic guidelines supported by epidemiologic criteria. One arbitrary guideline that can be used is the absence of recognized pathogens after a particular cleaning and disinfection procedure, which can be interpreted, from a realistic standpoint, as the absence of vegetative bacteria.

Unnecessary Microbiologic Assays

For a number of items and procedures in the hospital and other health-care environments, microbiological sampling on either a scheduled or periodic basis is not cost-effective or rational. These include sterile intravenous solutions, injectables, disposable syringes, disposable blood lines, artificial kidneys (even those that are reused), and all other items that are received in a sterile state. Equipment and solutions sterilized within the hospitals need not be sampled microbiologically. Instead, quality assurance testing associated with serilization procedures, such as appropriate biologic indicator spores (Favero and Bond, 1991), should be used to ensure that the sterilization process per se is performing to specifications and that the associated practices are being performed correctly.

It is recognized that inanimate surfaces and air associated with critical areas such as surgical suites and intensive care areas may contain, to varying degrees, reservoirs of microorganisms. However, the chance for disease transmission in environments that are routinely cleaned and maintained is remote. Environmental control procedures associated with housekeeping and engineering services should adhere to established cleaning, disinfection, and maintenance protocols. Microbiologic sampling on either a scheduled or periodic basis should not be done on floors, walls, intramural air, or other inanimate environmental surfaces. Conversely, appropriate sampling should be done when a disease outbreak appears to be associated with a certain part of the environment, such as the air ventilation system (Favero and Bond, 1991; Garner and Favero, 1985).

Environmental Microbiologic Sampling During Outbreaks of Disease

The strategy that should be used during an outbreak of disease with respect to environmental microbiologic sampling depends on several factors. First, the infection control practitioner/epidemiologist must determine whether certain procedures, equipment, instruments, or other parts of the environment have a direct or indirect role in the outbreak. An outbreak of nosocomial disease does not necessarily mean that environmental microbiologic sampling at any level is required. Second, if environmental microbiologic sampling is believed to be necessary, the microbiologist and infection control practitioner/epidemiologist should coordinate the sampling scheme and determine the assay procedures as well as the items or parts of the environment that require microbiologic assay.

The application of a microbiologic guideline in this context differs from one that is associated with scheduled or periodic sampling. During the investigation of an outbreak of nosocomial infection, environmental testing is usually directed toward the specific pathogenic microorganism. Consequently, if the outbreak is due to *Pseudomonas aeruginosa*, this organism is sought in or on the various environmental items sampled. In this respect, the guideline tends to be more qualitative than quantitative, although in some instances one must rely on established guidelines. For example, if there is an outbreak of pyrogenic reactions in a hemodialysis center, one would rely on established guidelines (AAMI, 1982; Favero and Petersen, 1977). If water or ice in a hospital is implicated in an outbreak of nosocomial salmonellosis, assays should be used for determining fecal coliform bacteria and the total number of microorganisms, as well as to identify salmonellae. Thus, the microbiologic guideline here is flexible and basically determined by the nature of the disease outbreak.

REFERENCES

AAMI. 1982. *American Standard for Hemodialysis Systems*. Arlington, VA, Association for the Advancement of Medical Instrumentation.

AAMI. 1986. *Reuse of Hemodialyzers*. Arlington, VA, Association for the Advancement of Medical Instrumentation.

AOAC. 1984. *Official Methods of Analysis*. 14th Edition. Arlington, VA, Association of Official Analytical Chemists.

APHA Committee on Microbial Contamination of Surfaces. 1978. A proposed microbiologic guideline for respiratory therapy equipment and materials. Health Lab. Sci., 15, 177–179.

Ad Hoc Committee on Infection Control in the Handling of Endoscopic Equipment (Association for Practitioners in Infection Control). 1980. Guidelines for preparation of laparoscopic instrumentation. A.O.R.N. J., 32, 65–76.

Adair, F.W., Geftic, S.G., and Gelzer, J. 1969. Resistance of Pseudomonas to quaternary ammonium compounds: I. Growth in benzalkonium chloride solution. Appl. Microbiol., 18, 299–302.

Alter, M.J., et al. 1990. National surveillance of dialysis-associated diseases in the United States, 1988. Trans. Am. Soc. Artif. Intern. Organs, 36, 107–118.

American Society for Gastrointestinal Endoscopy. 1988. Infection control during gastrointestinal endoscopy: guidelines for clinical application. Gastrointest. Endosc., 34(Suppl.), 37–40.

Anderson, L.J., et al. 1988. Nosocomial viral infections. In Laboratory Diagnosis of Infectious Diseases. Volume II: Viral, Rickettsial and Chlamydial Diseases. Edited by E.H. Lennette, F.A. Murphy, and P. Halonen. New York, Springer-Verlag, pp. 12–38.

Anderson, R.L., Berkelman, R.L., and Holland, B.W. 1983. Microbiologic investigations with iodophor solutions. In Proceedings of the International Symposium on Povidone. Edited by G.A. Digenis and J. Ansell. Lexington, KY, Univ. of Kentucky Press, pp. 146–157.

Anderson, R.L., et al. 1984. Investigations into the survival of Pseudomonas aeruginosa in poloxamer-iodine. Appl. Environ. Microbiol., 47, 757–769.

Anderson, R.L. 1989. Iodophor antiseptics: instrinsic microbial contamination with resistant bacteria. Infect. Control Hosp. Epidemiol., 10, 443–446.

Anderson, R.L., et al. 1990. Effect of disinfectants on pseudomonads colonized on the interior surface of PVC pipes. Am. J. Public Health, 80, 17–21.

Asher, D.M., Gibbs, C.J., and Gajdusek, D.C. 1986. Slow viral infections: safe handling of the agents of subacute spongiform encephalopathies. In Laboratory Safety: Principles and Practices. Edited by B.M. Miller, et al. Washington, D.C., American Society for Microbiology, pp. 59–71.

Bageant, R.A., et al. 1981. In-use testing of four glutaraldehyde disinfectants in the Cidematic washer. Respir. Care, 26, 1255–1261.

Beck-Sague, C., and Jarvis, W.R. 1989. Epidemic bloodstream infections associated with pressure transducers: a persistent problem. Infect. Control Hosp. Epidemiol., 10, 54–59.

Berkelman, R.L., et al. 1981. Pseudobacteremia attributed to contamination of povidone-iodine with Pseudomonas cepacia. Ann. Intern. Med., 95, 32–36.

Berkelman, R.L., Holland, B.W., and Anderson, R.L. 1982. Increased bactericidal activity of dilute preparations of povidone-iodine solutions. J. Clin. Microbiol., 15, 635–639.

Berkelman, R.L., et al. 1984. Intrinsic bacterial contamination of a commercial iodophor preparation: investigation of the implicated manufacturing plant. Appl. Environ. Microbiol., 47, 752–756.

Birnie, G.G., et al. 1983. Endoscopic transmission of hepatitis B virus. Gut, 24, 171–174.

Block, S.S. (ed.) 1983. Disinfection, Sterilization and Preservation. 3rd Edition. Philadelphia, Lea & Febiger.

Bond, W.W., Favero, M.S., Petersen, N.J., and Marshall, J.H. 1970. Dry-heat inactivation kinetics of naturally occurring spore populations. Appl. Microbiol., 20, 573–578.

Bond, W.W., Favero, M.S., Petersen, N.J., and Marshall, J.H. 1971. Relative frequency distribution of D125C values for spore isolates from the Mariner-Mars 1969 spacecraft. Appl. Microbiol., 21, 832–836.

Bond, W.W., Petersen, N.J., and Favero, M.S. 1977a. Viral hepatitis B: aspects of environmental control. Health Lab. Sci., 14, 235–252.

Bond, W.W., and Favero, M.S. 1977b. Bacillus xerothermodurans, sp. nov., a species forming endospores extremely resistant to dry heat. Intl. J. Syst. Bacteriol., 27, 157–160.

Bond, W.W., Favero, M.S., Mackel, D.C., and Mallison, G.F. 1979. Sterilization or disinfection of flexible fiberoptic endoscopes. A.O.R.N. J., 30, 350–352.

Bond, W.W., et al. 1981. Survival of hepatitis B virus after drying and storage for one week. Lancet, i, 550–551.

Bond, W.W., Petersen, N.J., and Favero, M.S. 1982. Transmission of type B viral hepatitis via eye inoculation of a chimpanzee. J. Clin. Microbiol., 15, 533–534.

Bond, W.W., Favero, M.S., Petersen, N.J., and Ebert, J.W. 1983a. Inactivation of hepatitis B virus by intermediate- to high-level disinfectant chemicals. J. Clin. Microbiol., 18, 535–538.

Bond, W.W., et al. 1983b. Observations on the sporicidal, bactericidal and virucidal activity of iodophors. In Proceedings of the International Symposium on Povidone. Edited by G.A. Digenis and J. Ansell. Lexington, KY, Univ. of Kentucky Press, pp. 167–177.

Bond, W.W. 1987a. Virus transmission via fiberoptic endoscope: recommended disinfeciton. JAMA, 257, 843–844.

Bond, W.W. 1987b. Disinfecting and sterilizing of flexible fiberoptic endoscopes (FEE) and accessories. Endosc. Rev., 5, 55–58.

Borick, P.M. 1968. Chemical sterilizers (chemo sterilizers). Adv. Appl. Microbiol., 10, 291–312.

Boucher, R.M.G. 1972. Advances in sterilization techniques: state of the art and recent breakthroughs. Am. J. Hosp. Pharm., 29, 661–672.

Boucher, R.M.G. 1974. Potentiated acid 1,5 pentanedial solution: a new chemical sterilizing and disinfecting agent. Am. J. Hosp. Pharm., 31, 546–557.

Brayman, D.T., and Songer, J.R. 1971. Phenol concentration in the air from disinfectant solutions. Appl. Microbiol., 22, 1166–1167.

British Society of Gastroenterology. 1988. Cleaning and disinfection of equipment for gastrointestinal flexible endoscopy: interim recommendations of a working party. Gut, 29, 1134–1151.

Carson, L.A., Favero, M.S., Bond, W.W., and Petersen, N.J. 1972. Factors affecting comparative resistance of naturally occurring and subcultured Pseudomonas aeruginosa to disinfectants. Appl. Microbiol., 23, 863–869.

Carson, L.A., Petersen, N.J., Favero, M.S., and Aguero, S.M. 1978. Growth characteristics of atypical mycobacteria in water and their comparative resistance to disinfectants. Appl. Environ. Microbiol., 36, 839–846.

Centers for Disease Control. 1987. Recommendations for prevention of HIV transmission in health-care settings. Morbid. Mortal. Weekly Rep., 36(No. 2s), 1–18.

Centers for Disease Control. 1989. Contaminated povidone-iodine solution: Texas. Morbid. Mortal. Weekly Rep., 38, 133–134.

Committee on Health Care Issues, American Neurological Association. 1986. Precautions in handling tissues, fluids, and other contaminated materials from patients with documented or suspected Creutzfeldt-Jacob disease. Ann. Neurol., 19, 75–77.

Conrad, J.E., Leadley, P.J., and Eickhoff, T.C. 1971. Bacillus cereus pneumonia and bacteremias. Am. Rev. Respir. Dis. 103, 711–714.

Craven, D.E., et al. 1981. Pseudobacteremia caused by povidone-iodine solution contaminated with Pseudomonas cepacia. N. Engl. J. Med., 305, 621–623.

Deane, N., et al. 1978. A survey of dialyzer reuse practice in the United States. Dialysis Transplant., 7, 1128–1130.

Dixon, R.E., et al. 1976. Aqueous quaternary ammonium antiseptics and disinfectants. JAMA, 236, 2415–2417.

Dwyer, D.M., et al. 1987. Salmonella newport infections transmitted by fiberoptic colonscopy. Gastrointest. Endosc., 33, 84–87.

Farrer, W.E. 1963. Serious infections due to "non-pathogenic" organisms of the genus Bacillus. Am. J. Med., 34, 134–141.

Favero, M.S., et al. 1975. Gram-negative water bacteria in hemodialysis systems. Health Lab. Sci., 12, 321–334.

Favero, M.S., and Petersen, N.J. 1977. Microbiologic guidelines for hemodialysis systems. Dialysis Transplant., 6, 34–36.

Favero, M.S. 1982. Iodine: champagne in a tin cup. Infect. Control, 3, 30–32.

Favero, M.S., Bond, W.W., Petersen, N.J., and Cook, E.H. 1983. Scanning electron microscopic observations on bacterial resistance to iodophor solutions. In Proceedings of the International Symposium on Povidone. Edited by G.A. Digenis and J. Ansell. Lexington, KY, Univ. of Kentucky Press, pp. 158–166.

Favero, M.S. 1985. Dialysis-associated diseases and their control. In Hospital Infections. 2nd Edition. Edited by J.V. Bennett and P.S. Brachman. Boston, Little, Brown, pp. 267–284.

Favero, M.S., Petersen, N.J., and Bond, W.W. 1986. Transmission and control of laboratory-acquired hepatitis infection. In Laboratory Safety: Principles and Practices. Edited by B.M. Miller, et al. Washington, D.C., American Society for Microbiology, pp. 49–58.

Favero, M.S. 1989. Principles of sterilization and disinfection. In Infections in Anaesthesia: Anaesthesiology Clinics of North America, 941–949.

Favero, M.S., and Bond, W.W. 1991. Sterilization, disinfection, and antisepsis in the hospital. In Manual of Clinical Microbiology. 5th Edition. Edited by A. Balows, et al. Washington, D.C., American Society for Microbiology, in press.

Gard, S. 1959. Theoretical considerations in the inactivation of viruses by chemical means. Ann. N.Y. Acad. Sci., 83, 638.

Garner, J.S., and Favero, M.S. 1985. Guidelines for handwashing and hospital environmental control. Atlanta, Centers for Disease Control, HHS publication No. 99-1117.

Gordon, S.M., Tipple, M.A., Bland, L.A., and Jarvis, W.R. 1988. Pyrogenic reactions associated with the reuse of hollow-fiber hemodialyzers. JAMA, 260, 2077–2081.

Habeeb, A.F.S.A., and Hiramoto, R. 1968. Reaction of proteins with glutaraldehyde. Arch. Biochem., 126, 16.

Heister, D., Shaffer, C.H., Jr., Hill, M., and Ortenzio, L.F. 1986. Studies on the A.O.A.C. Tuberculocidal Test. J. Assoc. Off. Anal. Chem., 51, 3–6.

Hoffman, R.K., and Warshowsky, B. 1958. Beta-propiolactone vapor as disinfectant. Appl. Microbiol., 6, 358–362.

Holmberg, S.D., Osterholm, M.T., Senger, K.A., and Cohen, M.L. 1984. Drug resistant salmonella from animals fed antimicrobials. N. Engl. J. Med., 331, 617–622.

House, R.J., and Henderson, R.J. 1965. Disinfecting the clinical thermometer. Br. Med. J., 2, 1404.

Isenberg, H.D., Giugliano, E.R., France, K., and Alperstein, P. 1988. Evaluation of three disinfectants after in-use stress. J. Hosp. Infect., 11, 278–285.

Jarvis, W.R. 1982. Precautions for Creutzfeldt-Jacob disease. Infect. Control, 3, 238–239.

Johnson, L.L., et al. 1982. Two percent glutaraldehyde: a disinfectant in arthroscopy and arthroscopic surgery. J. Bone Joint Surg., 64A, 237–239.

Kahn, G. 1970. Depigmentation caused by phenolic detergent germicides. Arch. Dermatol., 102, 177–187.

Kew, M.C. 1973. Possible transmission of serum (Australia-antigen-positive) hepatitis via the conjunctiva. Infect. Immun., 7, 823–824.

Klein, M., and Deforest, A. 1963. Antiviral action of germicides. Soap Chem. Spec., 39, 70–72, 95–97.

Klein, M., and Deforest, A. 1965. The chemical inactivation of viruses. Fed. Proc., 24, 319.

Klein, M., and Deforest, A. 1983. Principles of viral inactivation. In Disinfection, Sterilization and Preservation. 3rd Edition. Edited by S.S. Block. Philadelphia, Lea & Febiger, pp. 422–434.

Kobayashi, H., et al. 1984. Susceptibility of hepatitis B virus to disinfectants and heat. J. Clin. Microbiol., 20, 214–216.

McDougal, J.S., et al. 1985. Immunoassay for the detection and quantitation of infectious human retrovirus, lymphadenopathy-associated virus (LAV). J. Immunol. Methods, 76, 171–183.

Martin, L.S., McDougal, J.S., and Loskoski, S.L. 1985. Disinfection and inactivation of the human T lymphotropic virus type III/lymphadenopathy-associated virus. J. Infect. Dis., 152, 400–403.

Mentel, R., and Schmidt, J. 1973. Investigations on rhinovirus inactivation by hydrogen peroxide. Acta Virol., 17, 351–354.

Miner, N.A. 1978. Viral hepatitis: prevention and control. Postgrad. Med., 60, 19–22.

Ortenzio, L.F. 1966. Collaborative study of improved sporicidal test. J. Assoc. Off. Anal. Chem., 49, 721–726.

Parrott, P.L., et al. 1982. Pseudomonas aeruginosa peritonitis associated with contaminated poloxamer-iodine solution. Lancet, ii, 683–685.

Pepper, R.E., and Chandler, V.L. 1963. Sporicidal activity of alkaline alcoholic saturated dialdehyde solutions. Appl. Microbiol., 11, 384–388.

Petrocci, A.N. 1983. Surface-active agents: quaternary ammonium compounds. In Sterilization, Disinfection and Preservation. 3rd Edition. Edited by S.S. Block. Philadelphia, Lea & Febiger, pp. 309–329.

Pierce, A.K., Sanford, J.P., Thomas, G.D., and Leonard, J.S. 1970. Long-term evaluation of decontamination of inhalation therapy equipment and the occurrence of necrotizing pneumonia. N. Engl. J. Med., 282, 528–531.

Portner, D.W., and Hoffman, R.K. 1968. Sporicidal effect of peracetic acid vapor. Appl. Microbiol., 16, 1782–1785.

Prindle, R.F. 1983. Phenol compounds. In Sterilization, Disinfection and Preservation. 3rd Edition. Edited by S.S. Block. Philadelphia, Lea & Febiger, pp. 197–224.

Resnik, L., et al. 1986. Stability and inactivation of HTLV-III/LAV under clinical and laboratory environments. JAMA, 255, 1887–1891.

Rhame, F.S. 1986. The inanimate environment. In Hospital Infections. 2nd Edition. Edited by J.V. Bennett and P.S. Brachmann. Boston, Little, Brown, pp. 223–249.

Ridgway, G.L. 1985. Decontamination of fiberoptic endoscopes. J. Hosp. Infect., 6, 363–368.

Robison, R.A., Bodily, H.L., Robinson, D.F., and Christensen, R.P. 1988. A suspension method to determine reuse life of chemical disinfectants during clinical use. Appl. Environ. Microbiol., 54, 158–164.

Rodeheaver, G., et al. 1976. Pharmacokinetics of a new skin wound cleanser. Am. J. Surg., 132, 67–74.

Rutala, W.A., and Cole, E.C. 1987. Ineffectiveness of hospital disinfectants against bacteria: a collaborative study. Infect. Control, 8, 501–506.

Rutala, W.A., and Weber, D.J. 1987. Environmental issues and nosocomial infections. In Clinics and Critical Care Medicine: Infection Control in Intensive Care. Edited by B.F. Farber. New York, Churchill Livingstone, pp. 131–171.

Rutala, W.A. 1990. Guideline for selection and use of disinfectants. Am. J. Infect. Control, 18, 99–117.

Shikata, T., et al. 1977. Hepatitis B "E" antigen and infectivity of hepatitis B virus. J. Infect. Dis., 136, 571–576.

Sierra, G., and Boucher, R.M.G. 1971. Ultrasonic synergistic effects in liquid-phase chemical sterilization. Appl. Microbiol., 22, 160–164.

Smithwick, D.W., Stratigos, C.B., and David, H.L. 1975. Use of cetylpyridinium chloride and sodium chloride for the decontamination of sputum specimens that are transported to the laboratory for the isolation of Mycobacterium tuberculosis. J. Clin. Microbiol., 1, 411–413.

Spaulding, E.H. 1939. Chemical sterilization of surgical instruments. Surg. Gynecol. Obstet., 69, 738–744.

Spaulding, E.H. 1964. Alcohol as a surgical disinfectant. A.O.R.N. J., 2, 67–71.

Spaulding, E.H. 1971. Role of chemical disinfection in the prevention of nosocomial infections. In Proceedings of the International Conference on Nosocomial Infections, 1970. Edited by P.S. Brachman and T.C. Eickhoff. Chicago, American Hospital Association, pp. 247–254.

Spaulding, E.H. 1972. Chemical disinfection and antisepsis in the hospital. J. Hosp. Res., 9, 5–31.

Spire, B., Barre-Sinoussi, F., Montagnier, L., and Chermann, J.C. 1984. Inactivation of lymphadenopathy associated virus by chemical disinfectants. Lancet, ii, 899–901.

Spire, B., et al. 1985. Inactivation of lymphadenopathy-associated virus by heat, gamma rays, and ultraviolet light. Lancet, i, 188–189.

Toledo, R.T., Escher, F.E., and Ayers, J.C. 1973. Sporicidal properties of hydrogen peroxide against food spoilage organisms. Appl. Microbiol., 26, 592–597.

Tuazon, C., et al. 1979. Serious infections from Bacillus sp. JAMA, 241, 1137–1140.

Wardle, M.D., and Renninger, G.M. 1975. Biocidal effect of hydrogen peroxide in spacecraft bacterial isolates. Appl. Microbiol., 30, 710–711.

Wayne, L.G., Krasnow, I., and Kidd, G. 1962. Finding the "hidden positive" in tuberculosis eradication programs; the role of sensitive trisodium phosphate benzalkonium (Zephiran) culture technique. Am. Rev. Resp. Dis., 86, 537–541.

Webb, S.F., and Vall-Spinosa, A. 1975. Outbreak of Serratia marcescens associated with the flexible fiberbronchoscope. Chest, 68, 703–708.

Wheeler, P.W., Lancaster, D., and Kaiser, A.B. 1989. Bronchopulmonary cross-colonization and infection related to mycobacterial contamination of suction valves of bronchoscopes. J. Infect. Dis., 159, 954–958.

Wright, H.S. 1970a. Test method for determining the virucidal activity of disinfectants against vesicular stomatitis virus. Appl. Microbiol., 19, 92–95.

Wright, H.S. 1970b. Inactivation of vesicular stomatitis virus by disinfectants. Appl. Microbiol., 19, 96–98.

Wysowski, D.K., et al. 1978. Epidemic neonatal hyperbilirubinemia and use of a phenolic disinfectant detergent. Pediatrics, 61, 160–165.

CHAPTER 36

SURGICAL ANTISEPSIS

Dieter H.M. Gröschel and Timothy L. Pruett

Surgical antisepsis is the application of microbicidal or microbistatic antimicrobial chemicals to skin, mucosa, and wounds in order to reduce the risk of infection. Antimicrobials have been used at least since Pharaonic times in the form of natural products or chemicals to care for wounds and to prevent miasmata or contagia causing putrefaction and death (Craig, 1986; Dittrich, 1981). Semmelweis and Lister are the fathers of modern antisepsis, and their concept found support from the new science of bacteriology. The early bacteriologists, beginning with Robert Koch, studied the bacteria of the skin, suggested the possible contribution of these bacteria to the infection of wounds, and studied their reduction or elimination with antimicrobial agents. Price, in his classic study of 1938, showed that "skin bacteria are of two sorts, transients and residents." He demonstrated the effect of handwashing and of surgical scrubbing on the removal of skin flora and first showed that skin cannot be sterilized. Skin flora was studied by many investigators using various techniques (Larson, 1985), and many of these studies were summarized in the monographs of Aly and Maibach (1978), Maibach and Aly (1981), Noble (1981a), Noble and Somerville (1974), and Rosebury (1962)

AIMS OF ANTISEPSIS IN SURGERY

The major use of surgical antisepsis is the removal or reduction of normal flora by the topical application of antimicrobial substances to the skin before a surgical procedure. With preoperative scrubbing and patient skin preparation, one hopes to reduce both transient and resident flora to the fullest extent and to maintain this state for the duration of the surgical procedure. Despite confident statements that skin sterility can be achieved, considerable numbers of resident bacteria are found to survive antiseptic treatment in the deeper layers of the skin (Selwyn and Ellis, 1972). Lilly et al. (1979) tested alcoholic chlorhexidine in comparison with detergent preparations of chlorhexidine and hexachlorophene and

showed that the number of skin bacteria cannot be lowered below a certain level.

SKIN AND SKIN FLORA

Because an important function of the skin is to serve as a barrier against infection, antiseptic treatment should neither be toxic (Kramer et al., 1987) nor cause skin reactions (Mitchell and Rawluk, 1984; Roberts et al., 1981), nor should it interfere with the normal protective function of the skin. Removal of skin lipids, interference with the "acid mantle," and excessive drying may result in damage to skin, especially in frequent users of antiseptics such as surgeons and nurses (Larson, 1985). Frequent handwashing does some damage to the stratum corneum, as assessed with objective physiologic parameters by Larson et al. (1986). Such physiologic studies are needed for all antiseptics in addition to assessing efficacy, toxicity, absorption, and inactivation (Lowbury, 1981).

The skin is a multilayered surface with irregular pits, ridges, and creases covered by cornified epithelial cells that are loosely attached to the deeper cell layers and thus provide a nesting place for the bacterial flora as well as a potential source of airborne particles carrying microorganisms (Meers and Yeo, 1978). The surfaces are interrupted by the opening of sweat glands and pilosebaceous units. Because sweat is sterile, slightly acid, and flows continually, it keeps the sweat ducts clean of bacteria. In contrast, the ducts of sebaceous glands contain fatty and proteinaceous materials as well as cells, cell detritus, and salts that can serve as nutrients for a number of organisms of the resident flora. The fat covers the epidermal surface and makes it water repellent. Its composition changes with age and thereby affects the type and quantity of normal flora. Normal flora also differs on various parts of the body surface depending on the distribution of the skin secretory glands and their activity, the type, size, and density of hair, bacterial adherence, and antimicrobial antagonism (Aly and Maibach, 1981;

Larson, 1985; Noble, 1981b). Vorherr et al. (1980) have shown that certain regions of the body, such as the groin and the paragenital area of women, have high bacterial counts (up to 10^7 CFU/ml stripping solution). Price (1938) had already mentioned the studies of Preindlberger of 1891 regarding the bacteriology of the subungual space. Hann, confirming the studies of Price in 1973, showed that the resident flora is concentrated mainly around and under fingernails. Gross et al. reported in 1979 that the routine surgical scrub is not effective to reduce the subungual counts to acceptable levels, and McGinley et al. (1988) pointed out that this space is a significant reservoir of bacteria. Mahl (1989), recognizing the subungual space as a good indicator of the efficacy of personnel handwashes and surgical scrubs, developed a new method for testing of antiseptics by assessing the fluid obtained from artificially contaminated hands after scrubbing the subungal space with an automatic toothbrush.

The differentiation between transient and resident flora usually is considered to be important in deciding the role of each in nosocomial infections. The simple notion that transient bacteria are bad and the resident flora is harmless can no longer be supported. It was shown by Lowbury and his group during the height of the *Staphylococcus aureus* epidemic in the 1950s and 1960s (Lowbury, 1981) that this pathogen may become part of the resident flora and may even be disbursed in large quantities by "shedders." Gram-negative bacteria may also lodge persistently (Larson, 1981), especially in damaged or waterlogged skin. Guenthner et al. (1987) recovered gram-negative bacteria from nurses' hands after five consecutive handwashings with nonmedicated bar soap and tap water and proposed that these organisms, found independently of patient contact, should be considered nontransient (or transitional) flora. Noble (1981b) discussed the skin carriage of gram-negative bacteria, especially in axilla, groin, and toe webs, and reminded the reader that the patient may carry his own "environment" with him.

MUCOSA AND WOUNDS

Whereas antisepsis is more or less successful on unbroken skin, its use on exposed or visceral mucosa, open wounds, and burns is more problematic. Side effects due to the increased absorption of the antimicrobial chemical by the tissue and by the reduction of its activity by blood, exudates, and tissue result in less efficacious antiseptic regimens. Prevention of surgical infection as well as therapy of local infection is more effectively achieved with systemic antibiotics.

SURGEONS AND ANTISEPSIS

Surgeons have been aware since Lister that wound infections can be prevented by the topical use of antimicrobial chemicals. Handwashing and preoperative surgical scrubbing became part of the post-Listerian system of aseptic surgery introduced since 1882 by Trendelen-

Table 36–1. *European Hand Disinfection and Corresponding United States Terminology*

Europe	United States
Hygienic hand disinfection	Healthcare personnel handwash
Hygienic hand disinfection with residual action	Healthcare personnel handwash, residual (persistent) action (substantivity) desired
Surgical hand disinfection	Surgical hand scrub
Basic hand disinfection (Hände-Dekontamination)	Antimicrobial soap

From Deutsche Gesellschaft für Hygiene und Mikrobiologie. 1982. Richtlinie für Prüfung und Bewertung von Häude-Dekontaminationspräparaten. Zentralbl. Bakteriol. Hyg. B *182*, 562–570.

Food and Drug Administration. 1974. OTC topical antimicrobial products and drug and cosmetic products: establishment of a monograph and use of certain halogenated salicylanilides as active or inactive ingredients. Fed. Reg., *39*, 1210–1249; and Reybrouck, G. 1986. Handwashing and hand disinfection. J. Hosp. Infect., *8*, 5–23.

burg, von Bergmann, and Schimmelbusch in Germany and by Halsted in the United States, because bacteriologists could demonstrate that bacteria present on skin of surgeon or patient could cause wound infection. Antisepsis and asepsis contributed to the rapid development of surgery, and the advent of antibiotics promised further expansion of the surgical horizons. Infection remains a limiting factor of surgical success in certain patients, however, and cannot be controlled at all times by antibiotics alone. Fortunately, the surgical community has retained antisepsis as an important component of surgical technique (Altemeier, 1983; Hunt, 1981; Walter, 1978). Guidelines for the prevention of surgical wound infections by the American College of Surgeons (Altemeier et al., 1976) and by the United States Centers for Disease Control (CDC) (Garner, 1986) address the need for surgical antisepsis. The role of the skin flora in wound infection is clearly established (Maibach and Aly, 1981; Maki, 1986; Noble, 1986). A recent study by Horn et al. (1988) showed that the skin flora of personnel from different hospital services (dermatology and oncology) can differ in both its composition and its antimicrobial susceptibility. Dermatology personnel showed *Staphylococcus aureus* more frequently, whereas oncology personnel had a significantly higher carriage of gram-negative bacteria, yeasts, and multiple antibiotic-resistant corynebacteria. The isolates from nurses were resistant to many antibiotics, and two-thirds of the oncology nurses had methicillin-resistant staphylococci.

Surgeons throughout the world believe in the advantages of antisepsis, but the chemicals, their preparations, their testing and regulation are different in various countries. This starts with nomenclature (Table 36–1). Europeans often include degerming of skin in disinfection, whereas in the United States, disinfection and antisepsis are clearly separated (Gröschel and Spaulding, 1973; Reybrouck, 1986; Gröschel et al., 1989). Alcohol preparations have been widely used in Europe for all aspects of surgical antisepsis, but in the United States they have not been readily accepted, and aqueous chemical preparations with detergents are usually used (Larson, 1988; Stratton, 1986). Test methods for antiseptics are quite different (Ayliffe et al., 1975 and 1988; Bruch, 1983; DGHM, 1981; Dineen, 1978; FDA, 1974 and 1978; Hartmann, 1985; Lowbury, 1982; Mittermayer and Rotter, 1975; Reybrouck, 1986; Rotter, 1988), and the recommendations for the use of different preparations are not uniform. In the United States, antiseptics are classified by use and product categories (FDA, 1974 and 1978), and many of the products included in the United States Food and Drug Administration (FDA) listings have been used in surgical antiseptics over many years (Altemeier, 1983; Larson, 1988; Sebben, 1983).

The surgeon selecting an antiseptic must be familiar with the scope of activity, potential side effects, occasional failures, even potential contamination (such as reported for an iodophor by Berkelman et al., 1981, and Favero, 1982), cost effectiveness (Daschner, 1988), and last, not least, the art to motivate people to use these agents (Kaplan and McGuckin, 1986). The CDC recommendation (Garner and Favero, 1986) that handwashing with plain soap suffices for routine use in hospitals has been accepted with some reservations. Maki and Hecht (1982) showed that during the use of antiseptic handwashing in a surgical intensive care unit, the incidence of nosocomial infection was reduced by 50% when compared to the time when only nonmedicated soap was used. Massanari and Hierholzer (1984), in a similar study, found a reduction of nosocomial infections only in the medical, but not the surgical, intensive care units. Concerns abut the spread of methicillin-resistant *Staphylococcus aureus* (MRSA) and the introduction of universal precautions has led to renewed interest in the use of antiseptic handwashes, rather than using nonmedicated liquid soap. Tyzack (1985) reported that the use of povidone-iodine for handwashing, bathing, wound care, and prophylaxis was an effective component of controlling MRSA infections in his institution. Haley et al. (1985) tested different antiseptics for their killing effect within 15 s for three strains of MRSA and other nosocomial isolates and found that povidone-iodine was more rapidly bactericidal than 4% chlorhexidine gluconate, 1% p-chloro-m-xylenol, and 3% hexachlorophene. In a 2-year study, Onesko and Wienke (1987) showed that changing from a nonmedicated liquid hand soap to a 0.05% complexed iodine soap resulted in the reduction of overall nosocomial infection rates in high-risk areas by 21.5%, with the MRSA infection rate decreasing 80% per year. It is suggested that on surgical nursing units, especially intensive care units, antimicrobial-containing handwashing agents be used.

ANTISEPTICS USED IN SURGERY

In this chapter we use the definitions proposed by the FDA Over-the-Counter (OTC) Antimicrobial Panel II (FDA, 1978) for the use classification of antimicrobial products, as follows:

Health-care personnel handwash. A nonirritating antimicrobial-containing preparation designed for frequent use; it reduces the number of transient microorganisms on intact skin to an initial baseline level after adequate washing, rinsing, and drying, and it is broad spectrum, fast acting, and if possible, persistent.

Surgical hand scrub. A nonirritating, antimicrobial-containing preparation that significantly reduces the number of microorganisms on intact skin. A surgical hand scrub should be broad spectrum, fast acting, and persistent.

Patient preoperative skin preparation. A fast-acting, broad-spectrum, antimicrobial-containing preparation that significantly reduces the number of microorganisms on intact skin.

Skin wound cleanser. A nonirritating, liquid preparation (or product to be used with water) that assists in the removal of foreign material from small superficial wounds, does not delay wound healing, and may contain an antimicrobial ingredient.

The antimicrobial ingredients of such preparations were placed by the FDA OTC Antimicrobial Panel I (FDA, 1974) in three categories: category I, generally recognized as safe and effective and not misbranded; category II, not generally recognized as safe and effective or misbranded; and category III, available data insufficient to permit final classification at this time. Only antimicrobial ingredients placed in category I or III are currently marketed, as well as those approved through the FDA New Drug Application process such as chlorhexidine gluconate. Alcohols were not included in the OTC antimicrobial panel considerations, but were classified for first-aid use and preparation of the skin prior to an injection by another FDA panel (FDA, 1982). Because hexachlorophene is no longer generally available in the hospital and can be dispensed by prescription only, it is not included in this discussion.

For detailed information on the chemical, antimicrobial, and toxic properties of each active component, the reader is referred to the respective chapter of this book.

Alcohols

Alcohols are effective antiseptic agents with a broad spectrum of activity. The most widely used alcohol, isopropyl alcohol, kills bacteria, mycobacteria, fungi, and large and lipid-containing but not hydrophilic viruses in the use dilutions of 60 to 95%. Ethyl alcohol, on the other hand, does inactivate the hydrophilic viruses (Klein and Deforest, 1963). Alcohols offer the most rapid and greatest reduction of microbial counts on skin for personnel handwashing, surgical scrub, and patient preoperative skin preparation (Altemeier, 1983; Ayliffe, 1984; Lilly et al., 1979; Lowbury et al., 1974; Reybrouck, 1986; Rotter, 1984).

Alcohol preparations with emollient and refatting additives that also retard evaporation, and with other antimicrobial chemicals, have been used for several decades by European surgeons, but have not found wide acceptance in the United States, despite the statement of Price in the 1950s that "by and large ethyl alcohol is the most satisfactory and popular of all skin antiseptics" (quoted by Spaulding, 1964) and its promotion by Altemeier (1983), Beck (1980), Morton (1983), and Spaulding (1964). The call for more effective and rapidly acting antiseptics has increased the interest of health-care workers in alcohol antiseptics and has stimulated the industry to offer such preparations with and without the addition of an antimicrobially active chemical such as chlorhexidine gluconate.

Chlorhexidine

Chlorhexidine gluconate replaced hexachlorophene as an active ingredient for surgical antiseptics in the 1970s. In the 4% detergent preparation, it has a broad antimicrobial spectrum, but is less active against gram-negative than gram-positive bacteria, is not active against mycobacteria (Russell, 1982), is moderately active against fungi, and is generally active against viruses. Although not as rapidly acting as alcohol, chlorhexidine gluconate is a well-accepted surgical antiseptic with residual activity caused by its strong affinity for the skin and little interference by blood. It is also marketed now as a 0.5% tincture with alcohol, thereby combining the rapid effect of alcohol with the residual effect of chlorhexidine.

Iodine

Tincture of iodine has been used in surgery since its introduction by Grossich in Fiume in 1908 (Müller, 1950) for preoperative skin preparation. The old-fashioned tincture (7% iodine and 5% potassium iodide in 85% ethyl alcohol) was much too strong and caused considerable skin burns (Altemeier, 1983). The FDA OTC Antimicrobial Panel (1978) defined "iodine tincture" as a solution or tincture containing 2 ± 0.2 g iodine and 2.1 to 2.6 g sodium iodide in 100 ml purified water USP or in 44 to 50% ethyl alcohol.

Both preparations are reasonably safe and rapidly acting with a broad antimicrobial spectrum, but Altemeier (1983) found the solution to be inferior to the tincture in clinical use. He advocated the use of 1 or 2% iodine with an equal amount of potassium iodide in 70% ethyl alcohol as most effective in reducing skin flora. Iodine should be removed from the operative site immediately upon drying with 70% alcohol to prevent skin burns (FDA, 1978, p. 1247). This applies also to the use of tincture of iodine before punctures to obtain blood, body fluids, or tissue specimens. The problem of local toxicity has limited the use of tincture of iodine or aqueous iodine in recent years, mainly because of the arrival of the "tamed iodines" in the form of iodophor preparations.

Iodophors are complexes of iodine with carriers such as the nonsurfactant compound polyvinylpyrrolidone (povidone or PVP) or the surfactant compound poloxamer that slowly release free iodine and thereby reduce staining and local toxicity while retaining the broad antimicrobial activity of iodine.

Initially, iodophors were used widely on skin, mucosa, wounds, burns, and even in body cavities. Elevation of blood iodine levels were noted (FDA, 1978). Experimental data by Rodeheaver et al. (1982) showed that PVP iodine does not reduce the incidence of wound infection, and the addition of detergents even increased the wound infection rate. Van den Broek et al. (1982) showed that PVP iodine was toxic to phagocytes and was also inactivated by them. Iodophors, most commonly povidone or poloxamer-iodine, are used in concentrations of 0.75 to 2.0% available iodine (0.75 to 2 mg free iodine/L). Their activity is relatively slow, and the presence of organic materials neutralizes the free iodine. Studies following the surprising finding of Berkelman et al. (1981) of contamination of povidone-iodine with *Pseudomonas cepacia* showed that the ratio of free to bound iodine increases with dilution (Berkelman et al., 1982). Recently, a low-iodine hand soap (0.05% complexed iodine) was shown to be effective as a personnel handwashing agent (Onesko and Wienke, 1987).

Phenol Derivatives

Substituted phenols were discussed extensively by the FDA OTC Antimicrobial Panels (FDA, 1974 and 1978). One of the compounds widely used in the health-care field is *para*-chloro-*meta*-xylenol (PCMX) used in concentrations of 0.5 to 4%. It has a low level of germicidal activity (Favero, 1985), and its antimicrobial effectiveness is dependent on the formulation. PCMX as an active component of handwashing agents was reviewed by Larson and Talbot (1986).

PERSONNEL HANDWASHING WITH ANTISEPTIC PREPARATIONS

For over 140 years (Hebra, 1848), it has been known that infectious agents can be carried on hands. Whether acquired from corpses, patients, unclean dressings, or contaminated instruments and surfaces, they may survive as transient flora on the skin for some time, and some may become part of the "nontransient" flora (Gontijo et al., 1985; Guenthner et al., 1987; Larson, 1981 and 1984a; Lowbury, 1981). Handwashing has been accepted for many decades as the most effective way to interrupt the chain of transmission of infection from one person to another. The CDC *Guidelines for Handwashing and Hospital Environment Control* of 1985 recommend routine handwashing for at least 10 s, followed by a thorough rinsing under a stream of water (Garner and Favero, 1986). Plain soap is recommended unless otherwise indicated. According to CDC, the use of antimicrobial handwash preparations is indicated before the care of newborns, between patients in high-risk units, and before taking care of severely immunocompromised patients. CDC bases the recommendation for routine handwashing with plain soap on the statement that well-designed and controlled studies and the majority of expert advisors support the use of plain soap, whereas the use of antimicrobial handwashing agents has been proposed but lacked appropriate supporting data at the time of guideline formulation. Unfortunately, this guideline was interpreted in many hospitals to mean that antiseptic handwash agents were to be replaced in all hospital areas with nonmedicated soap. Routine handwashing practices in hospitals already were often less than optimal in frequency, length and technique of washing, and quantity of soap used (Albert and Condie, 1981; Donowitz, 1987; Larson, 1984b; Larson et al., 1987; Larson and Killien, 1982; Larson and Lusk, 1985). Thus, the removal of antimicrobial soaps with residual activity may have had a negative effect on infection control in some institutions.

Several studies demonstrated that handwashing with antiseptic soaps can reduce nosocomial infections (Maki and Hecht, 1982; Massanari and Hierholzer, 1984; Onesko and Wienke, 1987; Tyzack, 1985). Therefore, we believe that in surgical wards and clinics handwashing should be performed with antiseptic soaps or the more rapidly acting alcohol preparations, in order to eliminate the transient flora acquired from infected patients and to reduce the resident flora, which may include gram-positive and gram-negative bacteria of nosocomial significance (Beck, 1980; Lowbury, 1981; Guenthner et al., 1987; Morrison et al., 1986; Rotter, 1984). Handwashing frequency and technique are dependent on the motivation of personnel (Donowitz, 1987; Mayer et al., 1986), the selection of an acceptable handwashing agent, and the availability of either sinks for handwashing (Kaplan and McGuckin, 1986) or dispensers for waterless preparations (Beck, 1980). Senior clinicians and nurses play an important role both as decision makers and as role models for their associates.

When selecting an antimicrobial preparation for personnel handwashing, one should consider the following points: efficacy of removing and killing microorganisms; rapidity of antimicrobial action; persistent (residual) activity or substantivity; ease of use; and lack of skin irritation.

Using a standardized 15-s handwashing technique, Larson and Laughon (1987) tested chlorhexidine gluconate preparations in comparison with nonantiseptic soap and found that a single application of chlorhexidine-containing products did not reduce the transient skin flora any more than plain soap. After repeated washes (15) for 5 days, however, because of the persistent activity of the chemical, a significantly higher reduction of skin flora was noted with chlorhexidine, with 4% preparations being more effective than 2% preparations. Ulrich (1982) compared the effect of 0.5% chlorhexidine gluconate in 70% isopropyl alcohol with that of 7.5% povidone-iodine surgical scrub in a 15-s personnel handwash after artificial contamination. The alcoholic preparation produced significant lower counts with substantive (residual) effect after 24 washes over 8 hrs. A similar study comparing alcohol-based hand rinses with 4% chlorhexidine gluconate and plain soap (Larson, Eke, and Laughon, 1986) showed that alcohol rinses caused the most rapid, immediate reduction of skin flora, but that chlorhexidine resulted in more persistent reduction. Based on subjective measures of product acceptability, chlorhexidine

gluconate was the mildest and most preferred preparation.

Most earlier studies with antimicrobial detergent preparations were performed using 1- to 2-min exposure to the active agent. Rotter, Koller, and Wewalka (1980), using the Vienna test method (Rotter, 1984 and 1988), showed about a 3-log reduction of bacteria from artificially contaminated fingertips after a 2-min wash with povidone-iodine and after a 1-min wash with chlorhexidine gluconate. In comparison, a 1-min rubbing with 60% isopropanol resulted in a more than 4-log reduction. Ayliffe et al. (1988), using the same test method, compared 14 handwashing preparations. Again, alcoholic preparations showed the highest log reduction, followed by chlorhexidine and povidone-iodine, with chlorhexidine showing the best residual activity after 10 applications.

From these studies it is evident that alcohol preparations are the fastest acting and most effective, that chlorhexidine soap is the most acceptable for frequent washes because of mildness and persistent activity, that chlorhexidine-alcohol combines the rapidity of alcohol with the persistence of chlorhexidine, and that povidone-iodine requires at least a 2-min wash to fully develop its activity. Soaps containing PCMX (Davies et al., 1978; Sheena and Stiles, 1982) or triclosan (Ayliffe et al., 1988) are less effective than chlorhexidine and iodophor detergents, and the rapidity of their antimicrobial action is intermediate (Larson, 1988).

Because of universal precautions, health-care workers are supposed to wear gloves during patient contact if contamination with blood or body fluids could occur. The present recommendation is removal of gloves and handwashing after each contact. Gobetti et al. (1986) studied the use of different soaps in removing of bacteria from gloved hands and concluded that the gloved hand can be freed from bacteria by washing. A controlled, experimental trial by Doebbeling et al. (1988) showed that artificially contaminated gloves, after treatment with a 10-s wash with nonmedicated soap, a 60% isopropanol commercial preparation, or 4% chlorhexidine gluconate, were not consistently cleaned, and the hands of the study persons were contaminated with the test organisms after removal of the gloves after the use of nonmedicated soap. These authors concluded that it may not be prudent to wash and reuse gloves between patients.

SURGICAL SCRUB

The preoperative antiseptic preparation of the surgeon's hands and forearms has been accepted as an effective infection control measure since the late 1800s. Price (1938) performed the first scientifically sound study to show the effect of surgical scrubbing on the skin flora. Despite his and numerous subsequent studies, the technique and length of time required for the most effective surgical scrub is still being discussed, and no single procedure is accepted by all surgeons. In 1976, the American College of Surgeons listed four procedures in use at that time (Altemeier et al., 1976). In general, the surgical scrub requires that surgeons and nurses brush hands, fingernails, and forearms thoroughly with soap or an accepted antimicrobial compound such as a surgical hand scrub (FDA, 1978). After the scrub, the prepared areas are covered with a sterile gown and sterile gloves, adhering to the concept of asepsis by establishing an effective barrier between personnel and the patient's surgical wound.

In the past 20 years, numerous alterations of the "classic" scrub procedures were proposed and accepted. Bristle brushes were replaced by disposable plastic brushes and sponges impregnated with an antiseptic, antiseptic agents were changed, and the time of scrubbing was shortened (Sebben, 1983). Galle et al. (1978) addressed the question of using brushes for the surgical scrub. They compared the "classic" 10-min two-brush scrub using an iodophor surgical scrub preparation with a 5-min no-brush scrub using another iodophor and a 3-min no-brush with plain soap, drying with a sterile towel, and subsequent application of an ethanol-hexachlorophene foam. The shorter no-brush scrubs were as effective as the two-brush technique. Disposable sponge/brushes impregnated with the antimicrobial agents, chlorhexidine gluconate or povidone-iodine, were tested by Aly and Maibach (1983).

Decker et al. described in 1978 a mechanical device developed at the Walter Reed Army Medical Center, performing a 90-s jet washing that was more effective than the standard 10-min scrub used at Walter Reed at that time. Despite its announced advantages, this device has not made a major impact on the surgical scrub technique in other institutions.

Antimicrobially active scrubbing compounds other than alcohols have been shown to be more effective than soap and water, and many also have persistent and accumulative effects (Ayliffe, 1984; Lilly and Lowbury, 1971; Lowbury, 1982). Hexachlorophene, used widely as a 3% antiseptic soap, was replaced as a surgical scrub in the early 1970s when it was found to cause changes in the brain of infants because of absorption (FDA, 1972). Iodophors and, later on, chlorhexidine gluconate became the antiseptics of choice for surgical scrubbing. Peterson et al. showed in 1978 that a 6-min scrub with the newly introduced 4% chlorhexidine gluconate detergent preparation Hibiclens was effective to remove transient flora from the artificially infected hand and showed good activity and long-term (residual) activity against the resident flora. Generally, this new preparation was more effective than 0.75% povidone-iodine and 3% hexachlorophene soaps. This report confirmed earlier findings by Lowbury and Lilly (1973) in England where 4% chlorhexidine had been introduced several years before it was available in the United States. In the study by Aly and Maibach (1983) mentioned earlier, chlorhexidine gluconate reduced bacterial skin counts faster, to a greater degree, and more persistently. Like Lowbury and Lilly

(1974), these authors found chlorhexidine gluconate to be less affected by blood than povidone-iodine.

The time required for scrubbing with nonalcoholic agents is variously listed as being between 5 and 10 min for the classic scrubbing procedure (Price, 1938; Laufman, 1986) and with the use of modern antimicrobial agents (AORN, 1983; Garner, 1986; Larson, 1987 and 1988). When brushing with plain or antiseptic soap for 5 min and the use of 70% ethanol or an alcohol-hexachlorophene foam were combined, the time required for the first morning scrub was shortened (Altemeier et al., 1976). Significant reduction of skin bacteria both after the scrub and at the end of a surgical procedure was observed (Eitzen et al., 1979).

In Europe, alcohol preparations with or without the addition of other antimicrobially active chemicals have been used for a long time for the surgical scrub or "surgical hand disinfection," as it is commonly called in Europe and especially in German-speaking countries. A list of disinfectants approved for "surgical hand disinfection" by the German Society for Hygiene and Microbiology (DGHM, 1987) contains 50 different preparations; 23 alcohols, 23 alcohols combined with another antimicrobial agent such as chlorhexidine, a heavy metal, an iodophor, a phenol derivative or a quaternary ammonium compound, and 4 iodophors. These preparations are rubbed into the skin of the hands and forearms in 2 (or 3)-5 ml aliquots over a 5-min period. They are effective, because the tests required for approval (DHGM, 1981) are based on the Vienna Model proposed by Rotter et al. in 1974 (Rotter, 1984). Each compound must be compared with 60% n-propanol, the reference antiseptic. A 5-log reduction of the normal skin flora is achieved as compared to 2- to 3-log reductions seen with the antiseptic detergent agents commonly used in the United States. This approval (regulatory) requirement may, in part, explain the preference for alcohol over aqueous detergent preparations in Europe; however, the use of alcohol preparations for preoperative degerming of surgeon's hands was prevalent in Germany already in the mid 1950s when Gröschel was a medical student. Lowbury and collaborators had shown in 1964 that a 2-min standard handwash using 0.5% chlorhexidine in 70% ethanol reduced more of the resident skin flora than a 2-min wash with an antiseptic detergent. In 1974, Lowbury and his colleagues again studied alcohol and alcohol preparations and commented on the greater effect of alcohols in comparison with detergent washes, as well as the excellent residual effect and lower price of an alcohol preparation with 0.5% chlorhexidine (Lowbury, Lilly, and Ayliffe, 1974). Murie and Macpherson (1980) performed a clinical trial comparing preoperative "hand disinfection" with 0.5% chlorhexidine in 95% methanol after a "social" handwash with plain soap and water for 1 min, with a routine surgical scrub using 4.0% chlorhexidine gluconate detergent. They analyzed the wound infection rate after each scrubbing method and found no difference. They commented on the lower price of and the shorter scrub time with methanol-chlorhexidine and on the favorable acceptance by surgeons and nurses.

In the United States, iodophors and chlorhexidine gluconate soaps are still the preferred agents for surgical scrubbing, but it is anticipated that alcohol preparations such as those with 0.5% chlorhexidine will be used more frequently, not only in emergency medicine but also in operating rooms, especially by people with skin irritation due to detergent antiseptics. Generally, alcohol preparations are well accepted by the user (Larson et al., 1986), but their acceptance depends greatly on the emollients added to alcohol and their refatting capability.

PREOPERATIVE PREPARATION OF PATIENTS' SKIN

Antiseptic principles for the conduct of surgical procedures have been recognized since the time of Lister. Although much appears to be ritualistic, closer examination of the practice of surgery has led to recognized ways to increase and decrease the risk of infection in the surgical wound. Virtually all surgical procedures begin with the preparation of the skin at the site of incision as a first step in establishing a sterile surgical field. The bacteria of the skin that remain after a surgical scrub may colonize the incision and effect a postoperative wound infection.

There is no one way to prepare the keratinized skin surface for an operation. Lister's carbolic acid was the first of many agents used to reduce the risk of infection for the patient. The usual recommendation has been a 5-min scrub with an antimicrobial detergent (or 1-min alcohol wash) to remove skin debris as well as to defat the skin, exposing the bacteria within hair follicles. Application of an antiseptic solution (usually povidone-iodine or chlorhexidine) is then undertaken as the final preparation of the skin before draping (Gruendemann and Meeker, 1983). This approach has led to *excellent* clinical results of wound infections of 1 to 2% in clean cases (Cruse, 1975).

The duration of preparation, type of materials used, and use of barrier drapes have all been discussed for efficacy and cost. Geelhoed et al. (1983) and Alexander et al. (1985) compared wound infection rates after standard skin preparation (5- to 10-min iodophor scrub followed by painting of the skin surface) with a 1-min alcohol rinse of the operative site followed by the application of an incise drape with iodophor incorporated into the adhesive. These two methods proved to be equivalent in the prevention of wound infections. In an editorial comment to Alexander's report, Condon (1985) cautioned that for barrier drapes to work, they *must stick* to the skin; otherwise, such a preparation runs the risk of increasing wound infections. Brown et al. (1984) compared a standard povidone-iodine scrub to the operative site (6 min) followed by painting with aqueous povidone-iodine solution to a technique of dry gauze removal of obvious foreign material in umbilicus and skin folds followed by a spray application of 0.5% chlorhexidine gluconate in

Table 36–2. *Toxicity of Antimicrobial Agents to Fibroblasts in Comparison with Antibacterial Activity*

Agent	% Fibroblast Survival (24 hrs)	% Bacterial Survival (24 hrs)
Povidone-iodine		
0.01%	0	0
0.001%	105 ± 6	0
Sodium hypochlorite		
0.05%	0	0
0.005%	97 ± 6	0
0.0005%	107 ± 12	71 ± 5
Hydrogen peroxide		
3.0%	0	0
0.3%	0	103 ± 5
0.03%	41 ± 7	105 ± 8
Acetic acid		
0.25	0	78 ± 3
0.025	74 ± 7	97 ± 2

From Lineaweaver, W., et al. 1985. Topical antimicrobial toxicity. Arch. Surg., *120*, 267–270.

70% isopropyl alcohol. Although there was no significant difference in wound infection rates between the groups, the infection rate of 8.1% in the control group and 6.0% in the spray group was high and not stratified by classification of the surgical procedure (clean, contaminated, etc.). The optimal skin preparation for the conduct of a surgical procedure has not yet evolved. The general theme remains to eliminate (if possible) organisms residing on the skin of the patient with the expectation that there will be no bacteria to contaminate the wound and to produce postoperative infections. To the extent that a procedure is clean of endogenous contaminating organisms, this is a laudable, although not quite achievable, goal.

Surgical wound infections are often the result of many diverse factors. Even with similar skin preparations, different procedures have varied infection rates (Table 36–2). Some of the variables are manipulable by the surgeon, whereas others are not. Cruse (1988) had extensive experience studying factors in clinical wound infections.

Preoperative Hair Removal

Aesthetics often were the reason for preoperative removal of hair from the operative site. Seropian and Reynolds (1971) initially challenged this procedure by demonstrating that the infection rate after razor hair removal was almost 10 times higher than when a depilatory was used (5.6% vs. 0.6%). Later, Cruse, in an analysis of 18,090 clean cases, found an infection rate of 2.3% in shaved patients, of 1.7% in those with clipped hair, and of 0.9% in patients with no hair removed. It is important not to produce irregularities of the patient's skin before a surgical procedure. This leads to increased numbers of bacteria residing in the small crypts and cuts because of the trauma of shaving. Decreasing the resident population of bacteria with preoperative antiseptic showers the night prior to surgery reduces the risk of wound infection (2 to 3% vs. 1 to 3%).

Environmental Factors

Multiple factors have been associated with wound infections. Preoperative hospitalization increases the resultant risks of wound infection; 1-day, 1-wk, and more than 2-wk preoperative stays result in an infection rate of 1.2%, 2.1%, and 3.4%, respectively (Cruse and Foord, 1973).

A direct relation exists between length of operating time and infection rate, with the clean rate roughly doubling for every hour of operating time. This phenomenon is probably the consequence of proliferating bacteria within the wound and on the skin surface and increased injury to wound cells (desiccation, electrocautery, and retraction pressure) associated with long procedures.

It has been difficult to prove that contamination from dust and environment is implicated when the operating theater conforms to standard association regulations. As a general rule, less traffic, movement, chatter, and shorter hair decrease risks thought to be associated with surgical wound infections.

Patient-Related Factors

Increasing age, malnutrition, diabetes, and extreme obesity have all been associated with an increased risk of wound infections. It is important to recognize these factors in an attempt to minimize risk and to maximize effort to prevent surgical wound infections in these groups.

Surgeon-Related Factors

Cruse (1975) noted a decrease in the risk of wound infections over the period of time in which dissemination of information occurred. A host of surgical technical procedures can be used to minimize the risk of infection. Most surgeons are fully aware of these factors, and the publication of infection rates helps to reinforce their implementation. The Surgical Infection Society recently recommended the following:

In hospitals conducting 2000 or more operations per year involving surgical incisions through skin with subsequent primary closure, prospective wound surveillance will be conducted by the hospital epidemiologist (or other qualified person) of every such wound on a sufficiently frequent basis to determine if the wound heals primarily or if an infectious complication develops. Direct observation of surgical wounds by the surveyor is necessary to fulfill the requirements of this standard.

The surveyor will be responsible to and will report directly to the chief or director of surgery. Patients discharged from the hospital without apparent infectious wound complications will be followed up on or about the 30th day after surgery to determine if the wound has continued to heal without apparent complication. Such follow-up may be conducted by any method that will yield reliable data. The percentage of successful follow-up will be recorded.

Surgeon-specific and speciality service-specific wound infection rates will be determined by infection risk class and will be reported confidentially and in timely fashion to the chief or director of surgery. Personal surgeon-specific infection rates will also be reported confidentially and in timely fashion to each member of the surgical staff. It is recommended that data be appropriately coded to maintain confidentiality. Each hospital will determine the infection risk

Table 36–3. *Summary of Infections Following 100 or More Operations*

	National Research Council			Foothills Hospital		
		Infections			Infections	
Operative Procedure	No. of Wounds	No.	%	No. of Wounds	No.	%
General Surgery						
Radical mastectomy	227	43	18.9	—	—	—
Modified radical mastectomy	—	—	—	383	16	4.2
Appendectomy	551	63	11.4	1148	73	6.4
Cholecystectomy	756	52	6.9	1330	26	2.0
Inguinal hernia	1312	25	1.9	1857	9	0.5
Thyroidectomy	406	9	2.2	254	3	1.2
Nephrectomy	127	22	17.3	130	8	6.1
Orthopedics						
Bone biopsy and excision of bone lesion	109	6	5.5	372	10	2.7
Gynecology						
Abdominal hysterectomy with or without salpingo-oophorectomy	628	38	6.1	1823	77	4.2
Cardiovascular-Thoracic						
Exploratory thoracotomy (with or without biopsy)	137	8	5.8	54	3	5.6
Lobectomy segmental resection	131	9	6.9	145	8	5.5

From Cruse, P.J.E. 1975. Incidence of wound infection on the surgical services. Surg. Clin. North Am., 55, 1269–1275; and Cruse, P.J.E. 1988. Wound infections: epidemiology and clinical characteristics. In *Surgical Infectious Diseases.* 2nd Edition. Edited by R.J. Howard and R.L. Simmons. East Norwalk, CT, Appleton and Lange, pp. 319–329.

classification to be used in recording its data. (Condon et al., 1988)

The prevention of infection in the surgical wound is an important goal. No single factor may be isolated and given sole credit or blame for the result. Certainly, spontaneous generation of bacteria in wounds does not occur, and it is incumbent upon the operating team to keep the inoculum in the wound to an absolute minimum, to minimize the trauma inflicted upon the wound, and to promote the speedy repair of necessarily produced injuries.

ROLE OF ANTISEPTICS IN SURGICAL WOUNDS

The aim of treatment of injured tissue (whether by trauma or surgical procedure) is to provide optimal conditions for healing. It has long been recognized that infection or high tissue burden of bacteria will interfere with the biologic process of healing. To this end, "wound disinfectants" of a variety of types have been widely used by physicians and surgeons with the purpose of counteracting the detrimental effect of wound contamination and infection. As noted previously, the commonly used antiseptics are potent agents and have the capacity to injure not only the infectious organisms, but also viable human tissue. This double edge, whether the antiseptics produce more harm than good to the healing wound, is the problem confronting the practicing clinician.

Historical Perspective

The complication of wound infection was disastrous, with much morbidity and mortality, in the preantibiotic era. After Lister and Semmelweis had demonstrated the beneficial effect of disinfectants, much clinical attention was given to the careful and judicious application of antiseptics to the surgical wound. During the First World War, two schools of wound treatment arose: the "psychological school," which concentrated on aiding the body to clear infection, and the "antiseptic school," which attempted to kill microbes in a wound with a chemical agent.

The 1919, Hunterian Lecture before the Royal College of Surgeons was "The action of chemical and physiological antiseptics in a septic wound" by Alexander Fleming. During this discourse, the point was repetitively made that when wounds were analyzed, antiseptics of that era (carbolic acid, mercuric chloride, iodine, sodium hypochlorite, lysol, flavine, chloramine-T, hydrogen peroxide) did not effect a reduction in microbial burden. Conversely, wounds were often made more susceptible to microbial proliferation. It was hypothesized to be the consequence of the nonspecific effect of toxic chemicals on biologic tissues (antiseptics are unable to discriminate bacteria from viable or dead tissue), and the physical properties of a wound prevented contact between antiseptics and bacteria.

The debate is not over because industry has been responsive to developing newer antiseptics with different delivery systems. Advocates urge the practitioner to use these agents not only for disinfection of keratinized surfaces (skin, oropharynx, vagina), but also in epithelial or serosal surfaces (bladder, bowel, peritoneum) and directly in wounds (surgical wounds, pressure ulcers). Some of the information on this subject is reviewed and recommendations for practice are made.

Experimental Studies

The use of in vitro experiments to draw conclusions about the clinical environment is fraught with assumptions. The usual experiment to demonstrate bactericidal activity consists of placing bacteria, broth, and antiseptic in a single chamber and quantitating the number of viable organisms after a defined period of time (Lineaweaver et al., 1985; Gocke et al., 1985; Greenberg and Ingalls, 1958; van den Broek et al., 1982; Berkelman et al., 1982). These demonstrate that many agents (povidone-iodine, Dakin's solution, hydrogen peroxide) are effective at clinically relevant concentrations in effecting bacterial killing; however, missing from these studies are the usual controls for what is present in clinical wounds: large amounts of amorphous tissue. Fleming added tissue to antiseptics and bacteria under in vitro conditions and found that bacterial killing capacity was abrogated (Fleming, 1919). The effectiveness of antiseptic solutions on bacteria in the open healing wound is uncertain from the literature. One can surmise that efficacy is drastically reduced by inactivation of the antiseptic by the wound material.

Antiseptics are nonspecific in their interaction with living organisms, and normal mammalian cells are injured by antiseptic application. In 1958, Greenberg and Ingalls proposed a bactericide/leukocide ratio to evaluate disinfectants. Of 15 compounds analyzed, only 3 had less toxicity to phagocytes than to bacteria. Lineaweaver et al. (1985) have demonstrated that although fibroblasts survive in antibiotics, antiseptics (1% povidone-iodine, 0.25% acetic acid, 0.5% sodium hypochlorite, and 3% hydrogen peroxide) produce 100% cell death after 24 hours of in vitro exposure (Table 36–2). Impaired function of polymorphonuclear leukocytes (Lineawaver et al., 1985; van den Broek et al., 1982; Connolly and Gilmore, 1979), cytotoxicity to neoplastic tumor lines (Blenkharn, 1987), and injury to endothelial cells (Lineaweaver et al., 1985) have been reported with antiseptic use.

In vitro assays of cytotoxicity should draw criticism similar to that expressed for bacterial efficacy testing in vitro. Rarely, a control for tissue toxicity can be found in the wound. Antiseptics applied to wounds with large amounts of necrotic debris (fresh) would in all likelihood leave less of an injurious effect upon viable host cells than antiseptics placed in a fresh surgical wound. In vivo studies using experimental animal wounds have proved valuable in delineating the effect of antiseptics upon the healing process. Branemark and Ekholm (1967) demonstrated the effect of a quaternary ammonium compound (cetylpyridinium) upon an acute surgically created (no pus) wound. They demonstrated intravascular hemolysis, intravascular disruption of granulocytes, fibrin deposition on vascular endothelium, and tissue edema. Although other agents produced variable results, there was an overall deleterious effect by antiseptics upon the host cells of the *acute* surgical wound.

To evaluate the healing wound, Brennan and Leaper (1985) used an ear chamber in rabbits and tested Eusol, a calcium hypochlorite antiseptic with 0.3% available chlorine, povidone-iodine (5 and 1%), hydrogen peroxide, chloramine T (1% = 0.24% available chlorine), and chlorhexidine gluconate (0.05%). After approximately 4 weeks, all the agents tested caused adverse effects, but the hypochlorite antiseptics caused blood flow in the capillary of the granulation tissue to cease. Moreover, a delay in production of collagen was demonstrated when chloramine-T was applied to an experimental wound (Brennan et al., 1986). It has been suggested that a physician not put anything into a wound that could not safely be put in one's eye. MacRae et al. (1984) studied the corneal toxicity of some commonly used skin antiseptics comparing tincture of iodine, Hibiclens (4% chlorhexidine and detergent), pHisoHex (3% hexachlorophene and detergent), Lavacol (70% ethanol), 7.5% povidone-iodine scrub (with detergent), and 10% povidone-iodine solution in rabbits. With all products except 10% povidone-iodine solution, marked corneal epithelialization, conjunctival chemosis, and edema occurred (these effects were reversible within a week).

These studies suggest that the application of antiseptic solutions to open wounds is a risky procedure. In a study of experimental peritonitis, Ahrenholz and Simmons (1979) demonstrated that lethality was *increased* after the instillation of povidone-iodine. The balance between reducing bacterial numbers and injuring host mammalian cells is tenuous. On theoretic grounds, antiseptic solutions have little advantage over topical high-dose antibiotics, which have minimal toxicity to mammalian cells.

Clinical Studies

Since the time of Lister, physicians have put antiseptics onto wounds with the putative intent of "sterilizing" the wound and improving healing. Both the clinician and the patient invest much energy in the process. Clinical studies that demonstrate efficacy have been slow in coming, and consequently, one is left with multiple conflicting reports regarding the use of topical antiseptic agents in surgical wounds.

Morgan (1975) reviewed the English literature on topical therapy of pressure ulcers from 1900 to 1974. Although improved healing was often asserted, rarely was the claim supported by results that were controlled. The concluding paragraph noted that "no specific topical agent has been shown to be useful for pressure ulcers." More recently, Kucan et al. (1981) reported that as treatment for chronic pressure ulcers, povidone-iodine was no more effective in reducing wound bacterial numbers than physiologic saline. Topical silver sulfadiazine (1%) was effective in the reduction of pressure-ulcer bacteria, as it has been in the prevention of burn-wound infection.

The role of antiseptics in the contaminated wound has been open to much discussion. Because the contaminating inoculum is often polymicrobial and consists of unknown types and resistant bacteria, antiseptics have been used to decrease their numbers and, by analogy, the risk of wound infection.

Some studies show benefit from instillation of antiseptics into surgical wounds. Browne et al. (1978) reported that intraperitoneal taurolin (an agent that degrades to formaldehyde) both was nontoxic and improved survival rates. Gilmore and Sanderson (1975) used intraparietal povidone-iodine in patients with abdominal surgery and demonstrated a reduction of wound infections from 24% to 9%. A study to compare topical antiseptic (5% available iodine), aerosol (12% povidone-iodine) and topical polyantibiotic aerosolized powder (neomycin, bacitracin, and polymyxin B) during appendectomy was done by Gilmore and Martin (1974). The beneficial effect in the reduction of wound infections for povidone-iodine treatment to 8% (p<0.025) and polyantibiotic to 9.3% (p<0.06) was found when compared to controls with an infection rate of 16%. Sindelar et al. (1985) reported that intraperitoneal application of low-molecular-weight povidone-iodine solution reduced wound infections and intra-abdominal infectious complications when compared to saline lavage in 75 patients.

Becker (1966) reported that full-strength povidone-iodine does not reduce the incidence of wound infection in patients undergoing head and neck surgery and in fact may increase the risk. Viljanto (1980) found, in a series of 294 pediatric surgery patients, that treatment of an appendectomy wound with 5% povidone-iodine aerosol *increased* the wound infection rate (19% vs. 8% in controls). When the concentration of povidone-iodine was reduced to 1%, the increased wound infection rate diminished.

These studies strongly support the notion that the cytotoxicity demonstrated in the laboratory carries over to the clinic. If one applies an agent to a wound that is more toxic to host-reparative processes than bacteria, then the outcome will favor nonhealing and infection.

Other studies give equivocal results. In a small study by Vallance and Waldron (1985), saline lavage was compared to chlorhexidine gluconate and povidone-iodine. The incidence of postoperative fever, wound infection, and duration of hospital stay were unaffected by lavage grouping, and all deaths were due to either coexistent disease or severity of presenting disease. Parker and Mathams (1985) demonstrated no difference in wound infection rates in acute appendicitis when comparing metronidazole with either povidone-iodine or ampicillin.

The clinical experience serves many functions. It leaves enough vagaries and uncertainties to allow for individual opinion to persist with literature to support essentially any position on the use of antiseptics in wounds.

When examined in the light of in vitro studies and in vivo animal experiments, however, it must be concluded that the application of antiseptic solutions to surgical wounds is a risky procedure. There is a high likelihood that injury to the host cells (phagocytes, fibroblasts, endothelial cells) will be more prevalent than eradication of bacteria or fungi. The geography of wounds and the contact with biologic material resulting in inactivation of antiseptics makes this probable. The consequence of this series of events is the *increased* likelihood that a deleterious effect (i.e., delayed healing or wound infection) will occur. The maxim, "never put anything in a wound which you wouldn't place in your eye" is sound. Agents that redden the eye have a tendency to increase the chance of surgical wound infections (Bryant et al., 1984).

Use of Antiseptics to Prepare Contaminated Surgical Sites

Antiseptic solutions have proved utility in the preparation of thick keratinized surfaces for operative manipulation and have serious drawbacks when applied to injured wounds, no matter how contaminated with bacteria. It is often desirable to diminish the bacterial numbers in either mucosal-lined viscera or squamous cell-lined oropharynx and vagina/perineum (Byatt and Henderson, 1973). The "instant bowel prep," as popularized by Condon (Jones et al., 1976), was performed with the instillation of povidone-iodine into an isolated bowel segment (Rotstein et al., 1985). Experimentally, this proved to dramatically decrease the numbers of luminal bacteria; however, experimental models demonstrated that bowel-wall-associated organisms were minimally affected. Although used clinically with good results (Hay et al., 1985), there has been little information to suggest that intracolonic antiseptic is superior to the administration of systemic antibiotics. There is a worry that large amounts of iodine could lead to toxicity, although this is controversial (Globel et al., 1985). The use of oral hydrogen peroxide or povidone-iodine has been tried to decrease oral colonization of pathogens and to improve hygiene (Brun-Buisson et al., 1989). Its efficacy is not known, but the toxic potential is probably minimal if the agent used in small quantities.

Antiseptic solutions play an important role in surgery in preparation of patient and surgeon. The benefits are numerous and microbial killing is rapid and covers many types of microorganisms. Rarely are organisms "resistant" to antiseptics; even after multiple exposures, susceptibility remains (Gilmore, 1977). All this comes with a cost, however, and that typically resides in the toxicity to mammalian cells. Loss of cellular integrity and increased susceptibility to wound nonhealing are the detrimental side effects (Oberg and Lindsey, 1987). It is fortunate that good antibiotic agents are available to aid in the care of the contaminated wound.

REFERENCES

Ahrenholz, D.Z., and Simmons, R.L. 1979. Povidone-iodine in peritonitis. I. Adverse effects of local instillation in experimental *E. coli* peritonitis. J. Surg. Res., *26*, 458–463.

Albert, R.K., and Coudie, F. 1981. Hand-washing patterns in medical intensive care units. N. Engl. J. Med., *304*, 1465–1466.

Alexander, J.W., Aerni, S., and Plettner, J.P. 1985. Development of a safe and effective one-minute preoperative skin preparation. Arch. Surg., *120*, 1357–1361.

Altemeier, W.A. 1983. Surgical antiseptics. In *Disinfection, Sterilization, and Preservation*. 3rd Edition. Edited by S.S. Block. Philadelphia, Lea & Febiger, pp. 493–504.

Altemeier, W.A., Burke, J.F., Pruitt, B.A., and Sandusky, W.R. 1976. *Manual on Control of Infection in Surgical Patients*. Philadelphia, J.B. Lippincott.

Aly, R., and Maibach, H.I. 1978. *Clinical Skin Microbiology*, Springfield, IL, CC Thomas.

Aly, R., and Maibach, H. 1981. Factors controlling skin bacterial flora. In *Skin Microbiology: Relevance to Clinical Infection*. Edited by H.I. Maibach and R. Aly. New York, Springer, pp. 29–39.

Aly, R., and Maibach, H.I. 1983. Comparative evaluation of chlorhexidine gluconate (Hibiclens) and povidone-iodine (E-Z Scrub) sponge/brushes for presurgical hand scrubbing. Curr. Ther. Res., *34*, 740–745.

AORN Recommended Practice Subcommittee 1983. Proposed recommended practices for surgical scrubs. AORN J., *37*, 82–85.

Ayliffe, G.A.J. 1984. Surgical scrub and skin disinfection. Infect. Control, *5*, 23–27.

Ayliffe, G.A.J., Babb, J.R., Davies, J.G., and Lilly, H.A. 1988. Hand disinfection: a comparison of various agents in laboratory and ward studies. J. Hosp. Infect., *11*, 226–243.

Ayliffe, G.A.J., et al. 1975. Comparison of two methods for assessing the removal of total organisms and pathogens from the skin. J. Hyg. Camb., *75*, 259–274.

Beck, W.C. 1980. Alcohol foam for hand disinfection. ARON J., *32*, 1087–1088.

Becker, G.D. 1986. Identification and management of the patient at high risk for wound infection. Head Neck Surg., *8*, 205–210.

Berkelman, R.L., Holland, B.W., and Anderson, R.L. 1982. Increased bactericidal activity of dilute preparations of povidone-iodine solutions. J. Clin. Microbiol., *15*, 635–639.

Berkelman, R.L., et al. 1981. Pseudobacteremia attributed to contamination of povidone-iodine with *Pseudomonas cepacia*. Ann. Intern. Med., *95*, 32–36.

Blenkharn, J.I. 1987. The differential cytotoxicity of antiseptic agents. J. Pharm. Pharmacol., *39*, 377–479.

Branemark, P.I., and Ekholm, R. 1967. Tissue injury caused by wound disinfectants. J. Bone Joint Surg., *49*, 48–62.

Brennan, S.S., and Leaper, D.J. 1985. The effect of antiseptics on the healing wound: a study using the rabbit ear chamber. Br. J. Surg., *72*, 780–782.

Brennan, S.S., Foster, M.E., and Leaper, D.J. 1986. Antiseptic toxicity in wounds healing by secondary intention. J. Hosp. Infect., *8*, 263–267.

Brown, T.R., et al. 1984. A clinical evaluation of chlorhexidine gluconate spray as compared with iodophor scrub for preoperative skin preparation. Surg. Gynecol. Obstet., *158*, 363–366.

Browne, M.K., MacKenzie, M., and Doyle, P.J. 1978. A controlled trial of taurolin in established bacterial peritonitis. Surg. Gynecol. Obstet., *146*, 721–724.

Bruch, M.K. 1983. Methods of testing antiseptics: anti-microbials used topically in humans. In *Disinfection, Sterilization, and Preservation*. 3rd Edition. Edited by S.S. Block. Philadelphia, Lea & Febiger, pp. 946–963.

Brun-Buisson, C., et al. 1989. Intestinal decontamination for control of nosocomial multiresistant gram-negative bacilli: study of an outbreak in an intensive care unit. Ann. Intern. Med., *110*, 873–881.

Bryant, C.A., et al. 1984. Search for a nontoxic surgical scrub solution for periorbital lacerations. Ann. Emerg. Med., *13*, 317–321.

Byatt, M.E., and Henderson, A. 1973. Preoperative sterilization of the perineum: a comparison of six antiseptics. J. Clin. Pathol., *26*, 921–924.

Condon, R.E. 1985. Editorial comment. Arch Surg., *120*, 1361.

Condon, R.E., Haley, R.W., Lee, J.T., and Meakins, J.L. 1988. Does infection control control infection? (Panel Discussion, Surgical Infection Society, 1987), Arch. Surg., *123*, 250–256.

Connolly, J.C., and Gilmore, O.J.A. 1979. A study of the effect of povidone-iodine on polymorphonuclear leucocyte chemotaxis. Br. J. Exp. Pathol., *60*, 662–666.

Craig, C.P. 1986. Preparation of the skin for surgery. Infect. Control, *7*, 257–258.

Cruse, P.J.E. 1975. Incidence of wound infection on the surgical services. Surg. Clin. North Am., *55*, 1269–1275.

Cruse, P.J.E. 1988. Wound infections: epidemiology and clinical characteristics. In *Surgical Infectious Diseases*. 2nd Edition. Edited by R.J. Howard and R.L. Simmons. East Norwalk, CT, Appleton and Lange, pp. 319–329.

Cruse, P.J.E., and Foord, R. 1973. A five-year prospective study of 23,649 surgical wounds. Arch. Surg., *107*, 206–210.

Daschner, F.D. 1988. How cost-effective is the present use of antiseptics? J. Hosp. Infect., *11*(Suppl. A), 227–235.

Davies, J., Babb, J.R., Ayliffe, G.A.J., and Wilkins, M.D. 1978. Disinfection of the skin of the abdomen. Br. J. Surg., *65*, 855–858.

Decker, L.A., et al. 1978. A rapid method for the presurgical cleaning of hands. Obstet. Gynecol. *51*, 115–117.

Deutsche Gesellschaft für Hygiene und Mikrobiologie (DGHM). 1981. *Richtli-*

nien für die Prüfung and Bewertung chemischer Desinfektionsverfahren. Part 1. Stuttgart, Fischer.

Deutsche Gesellschaft für Hygiene und Mikrobiologie (DGHM). 1982. Richtlinie für die Prüfung and Bewertung von Hände-Dekontaminationspräparaten. Zentralbl. Bakteriol. Hyg. I. Abt. Orig. (B), *182*, 562–570.

Deutsche Gesellschaft für Hygiene und Mikrobiologie (DGHM). 1987. VII. Liste der nach den *Richtlinien für die Prüfung chemischer Desinfectionsmittel* geprüften und von der Deutschen Gesellschaft für Hygiene und Mikrobiologie als wirksam befundenen Desinfektionsverfahren. Wiesbaden, MHP Verlag.

Dineen, P. 1978. Hand-washing degerming: a comparison of povidone-iodine and chlorhexidine. Clin. Pharmacol. Ther., *23*, 63–67.

Dittrich, M. 1981. Geschichte de Antiseptik. In *Handbuch der Antiseptik.* Vol. I/2. Edited by W. Weuffen, et al. Berlin, VEB Verlag Volk und Gesundheit, pp. 13–38.

Doebbeling, B.N., Pfaller, M.A., Houston, A.K., and Wenzel, R.P. 1988. Removal of nosocomial pathogens from the contaminated glove. Ann. Intern. Med., *109*, 394–398.

Donowitz, L.G. 1987. Handwashing technique in a pediatric intensive care unit. Am. J. Dis. Child., *141*, 683–685.

Eitzen, H.E., Ritter, M.A., French, M.L.V., and Gioe, T.J. 1979. A microbiological in-use comparison of surgical hand-washing agents. J. Bone Joint Surg., *61*, 403–406.

Favero, M.S. 1982. Iodine-champagne in a tin cup. Infect. Control, *3*, 30–32.

Favero, M.S. 1985. Sterilization, disinfection and antisepsis in the hospital. In *Manual of Clinical Microbiology.* 4th Edition. Edited by E.H. Lennette, A. Balows, W.J. Hausler, and H.J. Shadomy. Washington, D.C., American Society for Microbiology, pp. 129–137.

Fleming, A. 1919. The action of chemical and physiological antiseptics in a septic wound. Br. J. Surg., *7*, 99–129.

Food and Drug Administration (FDA). 1972. Hexachlorophene as a component in drug and cosmetic products for human use. Fed. Reg., *37*, 20,160–20,164.

Food and Drug Administration (FDA). 1974. OTC topical antimicrobial products and drug and cosmetic products: establishment of a monograph and use of certain halogenated salicylanilides as active or inactive ingredients. Fed. Reg., *39*, 33,102–33,141.

Food and Drug Administration (FDA). 1978. OTC topical antimicrobial products: over-the-counter drugs generally recognized as safe, effective and not misbranded. Fed. Reg., *43*, 1210–1249.

Food and Drug Administration (FDA). 1982. Alcohol drug products for topical over-the-counter human use: establishment of a monograph and reopening of administrative record. Fed. Reg., *47*, 22,324–22,333.

Galle, P.C., Homesley, H.D., and Rhyne, A.L. 1978. Reassessment of the surgical scrub. Surg. Gynecol. Obstet., *147*, 214–218.

Garner, J.S. 1986. CDC Guideline for prevention of surgical wound infections, 1985. Infect. Control, *7*, 193–200.

Garner, J.S. and Favero, M.S. 1986. CDC Guidelines for handwashing and hospital environmental control, 1985. Infect. Control, *7*, 231–243.

Geelhoed, G.W., Sharp, K., and Simon, G.L., 1983. A comparative study of surgical skin preparation methods. Surg. Gynecol. Obstet., *157*, 265–268.

Gilmore, O.J.A. 1977. A reappraisal of the use of antiseptics in surgical practice. Ann. R. Coll. Surg. Engl., *59*, 93–103.

Gilmore, O.J.A., and Martin, T.D.M. 1974. Aetiology and prevention of wound infection in appendicectomy. Br. J. Surg., *61*, 281–287.

Gilmore, O.J.A., and Sanderson, P.J. 1975. Prophylactic interparietal povidone-iodine in abdominal surgery. Br. J. Surg., *62*, 792–799.

Globel, B., Globel, H., and Andres, C. 1985. The risk of hyperthyroidism following an increase in the supply of iodine. J. Hosp. Infect., *6*, 201–204.

Gobetti, J.P., Cerminaro, M., and Shipman, C. 1986. Hand asepsis: the efficacy of different soaps in the removal of bacteria from sterile, gloved hands. J. Am. Dent. Assoc., *113*, 291–292.

Gocke, D.J., Ponticas, S., and Pollack, W. 1985. *In vitro* studies of the killing of clinical isolates by povidone-iodine solutions. J. Hosp. Infect., *6(Suppl.)*, 59–66.

Gontijo, P.P., Jr., Stumpf, M., and Cardoso, C.L. 1985. Survival of gram-negative and gram-positive bacteria artificially applied to the hands. J. Clin. Microbiol., *21*, 652–653.

Greenberg, L., and Ingalls, J.W. 1958. Bactericide/leukocide ratio: a technique for the evaluation of disinfectants. J. Am. Pharm. Assoc., *47*, 531–533.

Gröschel, D.H.M., et al. 1989. Antisepsis and disinfection: need to clarify the terms. Zbl. Hyg., *188*, 526–532.

Gröschel, D., and Spaulding, E.H. 1973. Antisepsis or hand disinfection: an American contribution to the definition. Zentralbl. Bakteriol. Hyg. (B), *157*, 406–409.

Gross, A., Cutright, D.E., and D'Alessandro, S.M. 1979. Effect of surgical scrub on microbial population under the finger-nails. Am. J. Surg., *138*, 463–467.

Gruendemann, B.J., and Meeker, M.H. 1983. *Alexander's Care of the Patient in Surgery.* 7th ed., St. Louis, MO, C.V. Mosby, pp. 38–90.

Guenthner, S.H., Hendley, J.O., and Wenzel, R.P. 1987. Gram-negative bacilli as nontransient flora on the hand of hospital personnel. J. Clin. Microbiol., *25*, 488–490.

Haley, C.E., et al. 1985. Bactericidal activity of antiseptics against methicillin-resistant *Staphylococcus aureus.* J. Clin. Microbiol., *21*, 991–992.

Hann, J.B. 1973. The source of the "resident" flora. Hand, *5*, 247–252.

Hartmann, A.A. 1985. A comparison of the effect of povidone-iodine and 60% propanol on the resident flora using a new test method. J. Hosp. Infect., *6(Suppl. A)*, 73–80.

Hay, J.M., et al. 1985. The use of povidone-iodine enema as a pre-operative preparation for colorectal surgery: bacteriological study. J. Hosp. Infect., *6*, 115–116.

Hebra, F. 1848. Most important experiences about the etiology of puerperal fevers epidemic in birth institutions. Z. Gesellschaft K.K. Ärzte Wien, *2*, 242–244 (Transl. 1982. Infect. Control, *3*, 478–479).

Horn, W.A., Larson, E.L., McGinley, K.J., and Leyden, J.J. 1988. Microbial flora on the hands of health care personnel: differences in composition and antibacterial resistance. Infect. Control Hosp. Epidemiol., *9*, 189–193.

Hunt, T.K. 1981. Surgical wound infections: an overview. Am. J. Med., *70*, 712–718.

Jones, F.E., DeCosse, J.J., and Condon, R.E. 1976. Evaluation of "instant" preparation of the colon with povidone-iodine. Ann. Surg., *184*, 74–79.

Kaplan, L.M., and McGuckin, M. 1986. Increasing handwashing compliance with more accessible sinks. Infect. Control, *7*, 408–410.

Klein, M., and Deforest, A. 1963. Antiviral action of germicides. Soap Chem. Spec., *39*, 70–72, 95–97.

Kramer, A., Weuffen, W., and Adrian, V. 1987. Toxic risks by the use of disinfectants on skin. Hyg. und Med., *12*, 134–142.

Kucan, J.O., Robson, M.C., Heggers, J.P., and Ko, F. 1981. Comparison of silver sulfadiazine, povidone-iodine and physiologic saline in the treatment of chronic pressure ulcers. J. Am. Geriatr. Soc., *29*, 232–235.

Larson, E.L. 1981. Persistent carriage of gram-negative bacteria on hands. Am. J. Infect. Control, *9*, 117–119.

Larson, E. 1984a. Current handwashing issues. Infect. Control, *5*, 15–17.

Larson, E. 1984b. Effects of handwashing agent, handwashing frequency, and clinical area on hand flora. Am. J. Infect. Control, *12*, 76–82.

Larson, E. 1985. Handwashing and skin physiologic and bacteriologic aspects. Infect. Control, *6*, 14–23.

Larson, E. 1987. Skin cleansing. In *Prevention and Control of Nosocomial Infections.* Edited by R.P. Wenzel. Baltimore, Williams & Wilkins, pp. 250–256.

Larson, E. 1988. Guideline for use of topical antimicrobial agents. Am. J. Infect. Control, *16*, 253–266.

Larson, E., and Killien, M. 1982. Factors influencing handwashing behavior of patient care personnel. Am. J. Infect. Control, *10*, 93–99.

Larson, E., and Laughon, B.E. 1987. Comparison of four antiseptic products containing chlorhexidine gluconate. Antimicrob. Agents Chemother., *31*, 1572–1574.

Larson, E., and Lusk, E. 1985. Evaluating handwashing technique. J. Adv. Nurs., *10*, 547–552.

Larson, E., and Talbot, G.H. 1986. An approach for selection of health care personnel handwashing agents. Infect. Control, *7*, 419–424.

Larson, E, Eke, P.I., and Laughon, B.E. 1986. Efficacy of alcohol-based hand rinses under frequent-use conditions. Antimicrob. Agents Chemother., *30*, 542–544.

Larson, E., Eke, P.I., Wilder, M.D., and Laughon, B.E. 1987. Quantity of soap as a variable in handwashing. Infect. Control, *8*, 371–375.

Larson, E., et al. 1986. Physiologic and microbiologic changes in skin related to frequent handwashing. Infect. Control, *7*, 59–63.

Laufman, H. 1986. The operating room. In *Hospital Infections*, 2nd Edition. Edited by J.V. Bennett and P.S. Brachman. Boston, Little, Brown, pp. 315–324.

Lilly, H.A., and Lowbury, E.J.L. 1971. Disinfection of skin: an assessment of new preparations. Br. Med. J., *3*, 674–676.

Lilly, H.A., Lowbury, E.J.L., and Wilkins, M.D. 1979. Limits to progressive reduction of resident skin bacteria by disinfection. J. Clin. Pathol., *32*, 382–385.

Lineaweaver, W., et al. 1985. Topical antimicrobial toxicity. Arch. Surg., *120*, 267–270.

Lowbury, E.J.L. 1981. Topical antimicrobials: perspectives and issues. In *Skin Microbiology: Relevance to Clinical Infection.* Edited by H.I. Maibach and R. Aly. New York, Springer, pp. 158–168.

Lowbury, E.J.L. 1982. Special problems in hospital antisepsis. In *Principles and Practice of Disinfection, Preservation and Sterilization.* Edited by A.D. Russel, W.B. Hugo, and G.A.J. Ayliffe. Oxford, Blackwell Scientific, pp. 262–284.

Lowbury, E.J.L., and Lilly H.A. 1973. Use of 4% chlorhexidine detergent solution (Hibiscrub) and other methods of skin disinfection. Br. Med. J., *1*, 510–515.

Lowbury, E.J.L., and Lilly, H.A. 1974. The effect of blood on disinfection of surgeons' hands. Br. J. Surg., *61*, 19–21.

Lowbury, E.J.L., Lilly, H.A., and Ayliffe, G.A.J. 1974. Preoperative disinfection of surgeons' hands: use of alcoholic solutions and effects of gloves on skin flora. Br. Med. J., *4*, 369–372.

McCluskey, B. 1974. A prospective trial of povidone iodine solution in the prevention of wound sepsis. Aust. N.Z. J. Surg., *46*, 254–256.

McGinley, K.J., Larson, E.L., and Leyden, J.J. 1988. Composition and density of microflora in the subungual space of the hand. J Clin. Microbiol., *26*, 950–953.

MacRae, S.M., Brown, B., and Edelhauser, H.F. 1984. The corneal toxicity of presurgical skin antiseptics. Am. J. Ophthalmol., *97*, 221–232.

Mahl, M.C. 1989. A new method for determination of efficacy of health care personnel handwash. J. Clin. Microbiol., *27*, 2295–2299.

Maibach, H., and Aly, R. 1981. *Skin Microbiology: Relevance to Clinical Infection.* New York, Springer.

Maki, D.G. 1986. Skin as a source of nosocomial infection: directions for future research. Infect. Control, *7(Suppl.)*, 113–116.

Maki, D.G., and Hecht, J. 1982. Antiseptic-containing handwashing agents reduce nosocomial infections: a prospective study. In 28th Intersociety Conference on Antimicrobial Agents and Chemotherapy, Miami Beach, Am. Soc. Microbiol., Washington DC.

Massanari, R.M., and Hierholzer, W.J. 1984. A crossover comparison of antiseptic soaps on nosocomial infection rates in intensive care units. Am. J. Infect. Control, *12*, 247–248.

Mayer, J.A., et al. 1986. Increasing handwashing in an intensive care unit. Infect. Control, *7*, 259–262.

Meers, P.D., and Yeo, G.A. 1978. Shedding of bacteria and skin squames after handwashing. J. Hyg. Camb., *81*, 99–105.

Mitchell, K.G., and Rawluk, D.J.R. 1984. Skin reactions related to surgical scrub-up: results of a Scottish survey. Br. J. Surg., *71*, 223–224.

Mittermayer, H., and Rotter, M. 1975. Comparative investigations on the efficacy of tap water, some detergents and ethanol on the transient flora of the hands. Zentralbl. Bakteriol Mikrobiol. Hyg. (B), *160*, 163–172.

Morgan, J.E. 1975. Topical therapy of pressure ulcers. Surg. Gynecol. Obstet., *141*, 945–947.

Morrison, A.J., Gratz, J., Cabezudo, I., and Wenzel, R.P. 1986. The efficacy of several new handwashing agents for removing nontransient bacterial flora from hands. Infect. Control, *7*, 268–272.

Morton, H.E. 1988. Alcohols. In *Disinfection, Sterilization, and Antisepsis.* 3rd edition. Edited by S.S. Block. Philadelphia, Lea & Febiger, pp. 225–239.

Müller, R. 1950. *Medizinische Mikrobiologie.* 4th Edition. Munich, Urban and Schwarzenberg, p. 155.

Murie, J.A., and Macpherson, S.G. 1980. Chlorhexidine in methanol for the preoperative cleansing of surgeons' hands: a clinical trial. Scott. Med. J., *25*, 309–311.

Noble, W.C. 1981a. *Microbiology of Human Skin.* London, Lloyd Luke Medical Books.

Noble, W.C. 1981b. Microbiology of special sites in relation to infection. In *Skin Microbiology: Relevance to Clinical Infection.* Edited by H.I. Maibach and R. Aly. New York, Springer, pp. 40–44.

Noble, W. 1986. Skin as a source for hospital infection. Infect. Control, *7(Suppl.)*, 111–112.

Noble, W., and Somerville, D.A. 1974. *Microbiology of Human Skin.* Philadelphia, W.B. Saunders.

Oberg, M.S., and Lindsey, D. 1987. Do not put hydrogen peroxide or povidone iodine into wounds. Am. J. Dis. Child., *141*, 27–28.

Onesko, K.M., and Wienke, E.C. 1987. The analysis of the impact of a mild, low-iodine, lotion soap on the reduction of nosocomial methicillin-resistant *Staphylococcus aureus*: a new opportunity for surveillance by objectives. Infect. Control, *8*, 284–288.

Parker, M.C.O., and Mathams, A. 1985. Systemic metronidazole combined with either topical povidone-iodine or ampicillin in acute appendicitis. J. Hosp. Infect., *6*, 97–101.

Peterson, A.F., Rosenberg, A., and Alatary, D. 1978. Comparative evaluation of surgical scrub preparations. Surg. Gynecol. Obstet., *146*, 63–65.

Price, P.B. 1938. The bacteriology of normal skin: a new quantitative test applied to a study of the bacterial flora and the disinfectant action of mechanical cleansing. J. Infect. Dis., *63*, 301–318.

Reybrouck, G. 1986. Handwashing and hand disinfection. J. Hosp. Infect., *8*, 5–23.

Roberts, D.L., Summerly, R., and Bynre, J.P.H. 1981. Contact dermatitis due to the constituents of Hibiscrub. Contact Dermatitis, *7*, 326–328.

Rodeheaver, J., et al. 1982. The bactericidal activity and toxicity of iodine containing solutions in wounds. Arch. Surg., *117*, 181–186.

Rosebury T. 1962. *Micoorganisms Indigenous to Man.* New York, McGraw-Hill.

Rotstein, O.D., Wells, C.L., Pruett, T.L., Simmons, R.L. 1985. Reevaluation of the "instant" colon preparation with povidone-iodine. Surg. Forum, *36*, 70–71.

Rotter, M. 1984. Hygienic hand disinfection. Infect. Control, *5*, 18–22.

Rotter, M. 1988. Are models useful for testing hand antiseptics? J. Hosp. Infect., *11(Suppl.)*, 236–243.

Rotter, M., Koller, W., and Wewalka, G. 1980. Povidone-iodine and chlorhexidine gluconate-containing detergents for disinfection of hands. J. Hosp. Infect., *1*, 149–158.

Russell, A.D. 1982. Factors influencing the efficacy of antimicrobial agents. In *Principles and Practice of Disinfection, Preservation and Sterilization.* Edited by A.D. Russell, W.B. Hugo, and G.A.J. Ayliffe. Oxford, Blackwell Scientific, pp. 107–133.

Sebben, J.E. 1983. Surgical antiseptics. J. Am. Acad. Dermatol., *9*, 759–765.

Selwyn, S., and Ellis, H. 1972. Skin bacteria and skin disinfection reconsidered. Br. Med. J., *1*, 136–140.

Seropian, R., and Reynolds, B.M. 1971. Wound infections after preoperative depilatory versus razor preparation. Am. J. Surg., *121*, 251–254.

Sheena, A.Z., and Stiles, M.E. 1982. Efficacy of germicidal handwashing agents in hygienic hand disinfection. J. Food Protect., *45*, 713–720.

Sindelar, W.F., Brower, S.T., Merkel, A.B., and Takesue, E.I. 1985. Randomised trial of intraperitoneal irrigation with low molecular weight povidone-iodine solution to reduce intra-abdominal infectious complications. J. Hosp. Infect., *6*, 103–114.

Spaulding, E.H. 1964. Alcohol as a surgical disinfectant. AORN J., *2*, 67–71.

Stratton, C.W. 1986. Waterless agents for decontaminating the hands. Infect. Control, *7*, 186–187.

Tyzack, R. 1985. The management of methicillin-resistant *Staphylococcus aureus* in a major hospital. J. Hosp. Infect., *6(Suppl.)*, 195–199.

Ulrich, J.A. 1982. Clinical study comparing Hibistat (0.5% chlorhexidine gluconate in 70% isopropyl alcohol) and Betadine Surgical Scrub (7.5% povidone-iodine) for efficacy against experimental contamination of human skin. Curr. Ther. Res., *31*, 27–30.

Vallance, S., and Waldron, R. 1985. Antiseptic vs. saline lavage in purulent faecal peritonitis. J. Hosp. Infect., *6*, 87–91.

van den Broek, P.J., Buys, L.F.M., and van Furth, R. 1982. Interaction of povidone-iodine compounds, phagocytic cells, and microorganisms. Antimicrob. Agents Chemother., *22*, 593–597.

Viljanto, J. 1980. Disinfection of surgical wounds without inhibition of normal wound healing. Arch. Surg., *115*, 253–256.

Vorherr, H., Ulrich, J.A., Messer, R.H., and Hurwitz, E.B. 1980. Antimicrobial effect of chlorhexidine on bacteria of groin, perineum and vagina. J. Reprod. Med., *24*, 153–157.

Walter, C.W. 1978. The surgeon's responsibility for asepsis. Med. Instrum., *12*, 149–157.

CHAPTER 37

INFECTION CONTROL: APPLYING THEORY TO CLINICAL PRACTICE

Inge Gurevich

Florence Nightingale's admonition to do the patient no harm is as valid today as it was in the mid-1800s. She was well aware that the number of hospital-associated (nosocomial) infections that killed so many soldiers in military hospitals could be reduced by providing safe food and water, a clean environment, and aseptic technique. She thus predated the concept of infection control by over a hundred years (Cook, 1913). Miss Nightingale had to fight for her beliefs, but in time the concept of aseptic technique became well established and, indeed, resulted in drastic reductions of infection-related deaths until the discovery of antibiotics.

When it became obvious that antibiotics could cure many infections, the more tedious and costly aspects of aseptic technique fell by the wayside, and before long hospitals were plagued by outbreaks of staphylococcal and other infections once again. New technologies brought with them new pathogens. Patients were now kept alive by the use of respirators that provided the respiratory support they needed, but these lifesaving machines became reservoirs for the gram-negative rods, mainly the pseudomonads, that caused necrotizing pneumonias that killed as many patients as were saved by the respirators. In answer to these devastating new outbreaks, the 1960s saw the emergence of the English infection control sister, who was shortly joined by an American counterpart.

The new discipline we now call infection control was born in the early 1970s when the United States Centers for Disease Control (CDC) developed and taught its course on "Surveillance, Prevention and Control of Nosocomial Infections." Infection control practitioners were few and far between in the early 1970s and acceptance came slowly. Nosocomial infections continued to take a heavy toll among the 35 to 40 million patients who were hospitalized annually in the United States, however. As many of 5% of these patients, 2 to 2.5 million, developed

such infections, and about 50,000 to 80,000 still die of them.

In the mid-1970s, the cost of nosocomial infections was in excess of $1 billion (Dixon, 1978). Naturally, this figure has continued to rise along with the cost of health care in general. Thanks to efforts of the ever-growing number of infection control teams, however, the rate of some nosocomial infections began to decline in some hospitals. This was confirmed by the CDC's 3-year extensive and well-designed SENIC study (Study of the Efficacy on Nosocomial Infection Control). This study corroborated the belief that surveillance and control programs were able to decrease the risk of nosocomial infections in hospitals with an active infection control program with at least one infection control practitioner for each 250 hospital beds (Haley et al., 1980). The final stamp of approval was put on the concept of infection control in 1976 when the then Joint Commission of Accreditation of Hospitals (JCAH) made these programs mandatory. Infection control has now become a science with its own data base, an 9000-member National Association of Infection Control Practitioners (APIC), and a 300+-member Society of Hospital Epidemiologists (SHEA), with an ever-growing list of research and several journals devoted entirely to hospital infections and hospital epidemiology. Even with all the infection control measures at our disposal, however, the rate of nosocomial infections is slowly rising. There are several reasons for this increase. The acuity level of hospitalized patients is increasing, and we are able to do more for and to our patients. Surgery is more extensive, medications are more potent and more immunosuppressive, and patients are older and are kept alive longer. There are more invasive procedures: indwelling catheters, implanted pacemakers, joints, valves, and transplanted organs. The more critically ill the patient is, the more immunosuppressed he becomes, and the greater the risk is for developing an iatrogenic infection.

655

Table 37–1. *The Role(s) and Responsibilities of the Infection Control Practitioner*

   I. Prevention of nosocomial infection by:
      1. a. Monitoring clinical patient care practices
           invasive
           noninvasive
        b. Developing appropriate policies and procedures to improve practices, i.e., aseptic technique
      2. Providing input into policies related to a safe hospital environment for patients in all hospital departments and services, i.e., surgery, radiology, housekeeping, pharmacy, cardiac catheterization laboratory
      3. Guiding employee health services related to:
        a. Employees with potentially transmissible infections
        b. Protecting employees from patients' infections, i.e., vaccinations and postexposure prophylaxis
      4. Controlling transmissible infections by establishing appropriate categories of isolation and precautions
  II. Input into selection of patient-care products including sterilants, clinical disinfectants, and antiseptics
 III. Quality-assurance monitoring: hospital-wide, pertaining to infection control
 IV. Surveillance of nosocomial infections and patient-care outcomes by review of:
      1. Microbiology and other laboratory results
      2. Patients with temperature elevations
      3. Radiology reports
      4. Autopsy findings
      5. Antibiotics
  V. Outbreak (and pseudo-outbreak) investigation and epidemiologic studies
 VI. Education: hospital-wide for all services and departments
 VII. Research related to infection control practices
VIII. Review of antibiotic usage related to development of resistance patterns
 IX. Liaison and consultant to pertinent hospital committees
  X. Interface with regulatory agencies

How does the practical, if not the philosophic aspect of infection control relate to a book such as this? Table 37–1 lists some of the responsibilities and roles of an infection control practitioner, but the whole of an infection control program is vastly greater than the sum of its parts and beyond the scope of one chapter. Further information on other aspects of the discipline is available in books specifically written on the subject of infection control (Bennett and Brachman, 1987; Gurevich et al., 1984; Wenzel, 1987).

By mandate of the Joint Commission of Associations of Health Care Organizations (JCAHO) and of many individual states, infection control practitioners must have input into the policies and procedures that can affect the development of infection in every hospital service and department (JCAHO, 1989). All departments use products in one form or another for sanitation of the environment or for disinfection or sterilization of medical instruments. Therefore, another JCAHO standard states that infection control must have input into the selection of products used for sterilization, disinfection, and decontamination. Both these standards involve extensive knowledge of the activities throughout an institution.

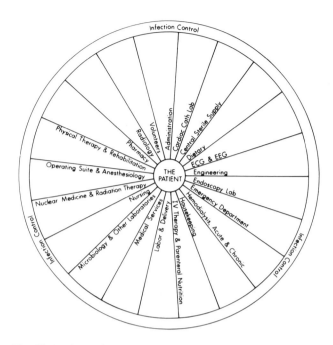

Fig. 37–1. Some departments requiring input and involvement by infection control.

This involvement is represented in Figure 37–1 in which the institution is depicted as a wheel with the patient at its hub. The spokes giving the wheel its form and support are the departments that serve the patient's needs. The infection control practitioner circulates along the wheel's periphery to ensure that each spoke's procedures and techniques ensure safe practices, including aseptic and sterile techniques, that will help in the prevention of nosocomial infection.

PREREQUISITES FOR THE DEVELOPMENT OF INFECTION

In order to assist clinicians in the prevention of nosocomial infections, infection control practitioners must be familiar with sequences and elements involved in the development of infection. The definition of a nosocomial infection is "an infection that was not present or incubating at the time of admission." There is no statement or implication that the infection was preventable, although 25 to 50% probably could be prevented, nor does the definition designate any particular origin or source for the pathogen because nosocomial infections can originate from the patient's own or endogenous flora or from exogenous sources. The development of any infection, including nosocomial infections, requires the existence of several prerequisites: (1) a source or reservoir for the pathogen; (2) a mode of transmission; (3) a portal of entry; and (4) a susceptible host who then in turn can become the source or reservoir, thus completing the circle or cycle.

Reservoir or Source

The reservoir for a nosocomial pathogen can be animate or inanimate. Among the most common animate sources is the patient with his own endogenous micro-flora. When the other prerequisites for the development of an infection are present, a normally nonpathogenic skin resident, *Staphylococcus epidermidis* or *Corynbacterium* species, can develop into a serious pathogen. The correct use of appropriate antiseptics can reduce this risk to some extent. The normal or transient microorganisms carried by physicians and nurses can also be a source of pathogens for their patients, as can contaminated invasive medical devices that were not adequately sterilized or disinfected. Hospital air (other than in an operating suite), floors, walls, and furniture are rarely involved in the process of infection and are not considered in this chapter in any detail.

Transmission

The second requirement for development of a nosocomial infection is that the organism must be transmitted or transported to an entry point into the body. Most nosocomial organisms are believed to be "transmitted" from their normal site of existence, on or within a patient, to an area of skin or mucous membrane whose integrity has been disrupted. Such is often the case in a wound infection or when a normally present skin inhabitant migrates into the patient's own blood along an intravascular catheter, or when a mucosal organism moves along a urinary catheter into the bladder. Other modes of transmission are via the hands of hospital personnel and by contaminated invasive devices. Recently, improperly sterilized equipment was responsible for infections in several patients undergoing urodynamic studies (Hamil et al., 1989). Contaminated antiseptic solutions such as benzalkonium chloride, iodophors, and chlorhexidine have caused a number of outbreaks (CDC, 1982; Sobel et al., 1982). Intravenous solutions can cause bacteremias if highly contaminated, and porcine heart valves preserved in contaminated glutaraldehyde have caused endocarditis (Lombardo et al., 1980).

Portals of Entry

Any disruption of the integrity of the skin or mucous membranes can provide a portal of entry for potentially pathogenic microorganisms. In the health-care setting, such portals of entry are constant, numerous, and unavoidable in most patients.

Susceptible Host

The last criterion for development of infection is that the person be susceptible to the particular infection that is threatening him. Vaccinations or naturally acquired infections are protective against some viral infections such as hepatitis B and the childhood exanthems. In general, however, there is increased susceptibility to bacterial and fungal infections in persons who are ill or immune suppressed or who have certain underlying conditions such as diabetes.

Hospital personnel can prevent the development of some nosocomial infections by limiting the sources of pathogens, i.e., by providing sterile or adequately disinfected instruments. They can protect the portals of entry in a limited way by using aseptic techniques and antisepsis for insertion of urinary and vascular catheters, for wound care, and for care of the patient on assisted ventilation. They cannot do much to influence the susceptibility of their patients. Health-care workers can have the greatest impact on prevention by limiting the transmission of organisms between personnel and patients, by perfecting aseptic or sterile technique, and by providing properly sterilized and disinfected instruments. This aspect is discussed in greater detail in the context of the material in this book.

GUIDELINES FOR INFECTION PREVENTION

Infection control measures can be divided into three categories, which closely parallel the categoric ranking schemes in the CDC's recommendations for prevention of infection in a variety of applications (CDC, 1983b). Category I consists of measures that are proved to be effective:

Measures in Category I are strongly supported by well-designed and controlled clinical studies that show their effectiveness in reducing the risk of nosocomial infections or are viewed as effective by a majority of expert reviewers. Measures in this category are viewed as applicable for most hospitals—regardless of size, patient population, or endemic nosocomial infection rates.

Category II pertains to presumably effective measures:

Measures in Category II are supported by highly suggestive clinical studies in general hospitals or by definitive studies in specialty hospitals that might not be representative of general hospitals. Measures that have not been adequately studied but have a logical or strong theoretical rationale indicating probable effectiveness are included in this category. Category II recommendations are viewed as practical to implement in most hospitals.

Category III often includes measures that are ritualistic, but not necessarily proved to be effective, i.e., preoperative shaving:

Measures in Category III have been proposed by some investigators, authorities, or organizations, but, to date, lack supporting data, a strong theoretical rationale, or an indication that the benefits expected from them are cost effective. Thus, they are considered important issues to be studied. They might be considered by some hospitals for implementation, especially if the hospitals have specific nosocomial infection problems, but they are *not* generally recommended for widespread adoption.

The choice and application of antiseptics usually falls into categories I and II and will be described first.

Clinical Considerations: Antiseptics

The word antisepsis implies that bacteria and other microorganisms are known to be present, and that the intent is to remove and kill as many of these as possible to prevent development of sepsis. One of the most important clinical applications of antiseptics is their use prior to performing an invasive procedure, be it surgery or insertion of an intravascular catheter. Each surgeon has a favorite preoperative regimen. As long as the post-operative wound infection rate in a hospital is within normal limits for that institution, and is not consistently higher than the so-called national norm, infection control will rarely be involved in the selection of these preoperatively used products, but will leave the choice to the individual surgeon.

It is different with antiseptics that are used for the preparation of the skin prior to insertion of intravascular lines, chest tubes, temporary pacemakers, and other such procedures. About 80% of hospitalized patients undergo insertion of an intravascular catheter (Teeger et al., 1983). It is thus one of the most frequently performed procedures in hospitals. Although the site of insertion (a mere puncture wound) is much smaller than a surgical incision, these lines stay in place for many days, they are inserted by members of many disciplines, not all of whom necessarily possess the skills necessary for success on a first attempt, and line-related sepsis is a major cause of morbidity and mortality in hospitalized patients. Therefore, infection control should be involved in all aspects of vascular cannulation and especially in the choice of products suitable for all levels of skill, keeping in mind the duration of intravenous access lines.

In recognition of the risk of sepsis accompanying intravascular cannulation, the CDC have issued guidelines for the prevention of this type of infection. They list four products that are suitable for skin preparation prior to intravascular catheter insertion. The products are tincture of iodine (1 to 2%), alcohol (70%), iodophor, and chlorhexidine (CDC, 1983c). Although all four products are equally effective, additional considerations can enter into the selection of one antiseptic over another. For example, tincture of iodine may be irritating, and if it is allowed to contact clothing or bedding, the stain is difficult to remove.

Alcohol readily and rapidly destroys organisms on the skin, and yet it may not be the ideal product for vascular access. For example, insertion of a central catheter into the subclavian vein can take 5 min or more, depending on the skill of the physician and the anatomic features of the patient. Alcohol has a slightly defatting action that can permit organisms present below the surface of the skin to contact the gloved fingers used to palpate for anatomic guideposts during insertion of the cannula. Because alcohol evaporates so rapidly, the gloved finger becomes contaminated from the skin of the patient, and the contaminating organisms can be introduced into the vascular system along with the catheter.

A wiser choice may be a longer-acting antiseptic such as povidone iodine, which leaves a clearly visible line of demarcation where it has been applied, both on the patient's skin and on the gloved fingers.

Making a choice among these four products listed as efficacious by the CDC is comparatively simple and carries no risk of making an erroneous decision. It is quite

another matter when choices of methods and products for sterilization or disinfection of medical devices and other patient-care products are involved.

Clinical Considerations: Sterilization

Ranked high among the proved (or Category I) measures for reducing the risk of infection is sterilization of invasive medical devices. Infection control practitioners must verify consistently that sterilization and quality-control procedures are strictly observed. Steam autoclaves as well as gas sterilizers should be challenged with live spore preparations at least once a week. Any load that includes an implantable item should also include a spore test, and the items should not be used until the spore test has been negative for 48 hrs (CDC, 1983a). Problems arise when standard 30-min steam autoclave and the longer and variable ethylene oxide sterilization procedures are not followed. For example, spore tests are rarely, if ever, used when items are flash sterilized in the operating suite. The purpose of a 3- to 5-min flash sterilization cycle is to quickly make available items that may have become contaminated inadvertently during a surgical procedure and that will be needed again shortly, if not at once. There is no time to wait 24 to 48 hours to check whether the simultaneously processed spores were killed, thus ensuring an effective sterilization cycle. In an emergency this risk is acceptable, but infection control practitioners must ensure that this flashing process is not abused for the sake of economics and convenience. Instead of investing in two or three additional pieces of an expensive item, only one may be available, and that one may simply be flashed three or four times a day between cases. This shortcut should not be permitted unless and until the scientific community can develop a rapid, fail-safe test for ensuring that an autoclave failure did not occur during the flashing process. Such misuse can be discouraged by requiring that a log book be kept of every item processed by flash sterilization. If an item is flashed too frequently in our institution, we strongly urge that more of these items be purchased. Although the initial expense may be high, the rotation of these instruments will prolong their life and will thus recoup the initial outlay.

Customized, implantable materials are often similarly flash sterilized, as a recent survey demonstrated, even though the CDC recommends against flash sterilization of implantable objects (Gurevich et al., 1989). This practice has been discouraged in our institution, but if an implantable item is flashed, a spore test must accompany it. If the spore test should read positive 24 and 48 hrs after the item has been implanted into a patient, the surgeon is notified.

CHEMICAL DISINFECTION AND STERILIZATION

Medical instruments can present further problems because they are becoming increasingly complicated and, therefore, more expensive. Some lensed instruments cannot tolerate even the lesser temperatures of ethylene oxide sterilization. Others are so expensive (an endoscope can cost more than $30,000) that seven or eight of them might be needed by a busy hospital service on any given day because of the prolonged aeration cycle. The cost would make purchase of so great a number impossible. An acceptable alternative for such devices is soaking in a chemical sterilizing-disinfecting solution.

This, however, entails extremely difficult decisions. The CDC has made recommendations for *antiseptics* and provided a choice of four acceptable products. No agency has provided such clear-cut choices for solutions used for sterilization or disinfection of medical instruments. Theoretically, the properties of the available generic products are well established, but the choice is made difficult by contradictory claims by the manufacturers regarding the potency of each individual formulation, effective concentrations, and ambient temperatures. The use of chemicals for disinfection and sterilization is becoming more widespread and therefore more lucrative. The ratio of dilution and the ability to reuse a solution for up to 6 weeks in some cases thus become important selling points. How these matters complicate the selection of a chemical sterilant/disinfectant will now be discussed.

Sterilization by Chemicals

Sterilization requires prolonged contact of the instrument with the sterilant, usually from 6 to 10 hrs. Some products may be heated, which can shorten the exposure time, but infection control practitioners must be sure that heating a product does not produce unacceptable fumes and the potential for increased toxicity. Labels on the chemical products must be read carefully because some manufacturers claim that products can be used for up to 30 days for disinfection, but that may not apply to sterilization. One manufacturer's label tells users that the product requires a 6 ¾-hr soak for the first 14 days of the product's use, but a 10-hr soak for the remainder of the product's total 30 days' use life. Such instructions are difficult to enforce and monitor, but if they are not followed, instruments may not be adequately sterilized. There is consensus, however, that if instruments can be submerged for 6 to 10 hrs, sterilization can be accomplished by a properly used chemical. A problem arises again if seven or more procedures, such as sigmoidoscopies or bronchoscopies, are performed on a daily basis. In order to sterilize the endoscopes between patients, seven or more would be required, and they can cost between $30,000 and $50,000 each: few hospitals or clinics will consider such an expenditure. Once again, a compromise has been developed, and medical devices can be divided into three types, each requiring a different "level" of disinfection (Spaulding, 1968):

Type 1 are critical devices that enter sterile tissue or the vascular system or through which blood will flow. These must still be sterilized.

Type 2 are semicritical devices. They come in contact with nonintact skin and mucous membranes; they must undergo high-level disinfection.

Type 3, noncritical items, are those that come in contact with intact skin, and they require low-level disinfection.

Sterilization for type 1 items has been discussed. Type 3 items simply require cleaning or sanitization and are not included in the discussion. The remainder of this chapter is devoted to a description of the difficulties infection control practitioners encounter when they follow the mandate of the JCAHO "to have input into the selection and use of products used for antisepsis, sterilization and disinfection" (JCAHO, 1989).

High-Level Disinfection

In order to ensure adequate disinfection of semicritical (type 2) instruments, high-level disinfection is recommended. Gastroscopes, sigmoidoscopes, and bronchoscopes fall into that category. A gray area is encountered with hysteroscopes and uroscopic instruments. Although they ultimately enter sterile tissue, they are introduced through highly contaminated body sites, the vagina and the urethra, respectively. Is high-level disinfection acceptable for these items? High-level disinfectants are capable of destroying all organisms except the most highly resistant spores. Are spores of concern in these instruments? Each individual infection control committee must make its own decision because no official guidelines exist. The most frequently used high-level disinfectants are the 2% glutaraldehydes. A combination glutaraldehyde-phenolic is also available. Although hydrogen peroxide is an acceptable alternative, according to textbook descriptions, CDC listings, and United States Environmental Protection Agency (EPA) approval, one such disinfectant label does not list the hydrophilic viruses as being killed during the 10-min exposure time recommended on the label (Table 37–2). A chlorine dioxide product has also been approved by the EPA as a clinical disinfectant/sterilant, but the label instructions suggest a temperature of 25°C, which is not ambient temperature, requires an external heat source, and may, therefore, produce fumes that are toxic to users.

Again, according to textbook descriptions and CDC recommendations, 2% glutaraldehyde is considered tuberculocidal. The in vitro test results apparently did not take ambient operating room temperatures into consideration (Favero, 1983; Scott and Gorman, 1983). In 1984, the manufacturer of a glutaraldehyde-based disinfectant distributed information that, upon retesting the product with the standard Association of Analytical Chemists test, the product was not found to be tuberculocidal. The manufacturer further labeled the product as requiring a longer contact time than the 10 min previously stated and a higher temperature for the disinfection of instruments contaminated with tubercle bacilli (Surgikos, 1984). The new temperature of 25°C is not achievable without the addition of a heating device, and glutaraldehydes may produce unpleasant and possibly toxic fumes at higher-than-ambient temperatures. This state-

Table 37–2. *Examples of Inter- and Intraproduct Differences in Instructions Regarding Reuse Life, Shelf Life, Dilution, and Spectrum of Activity*

Type of Product	Glutaraldehyde				Glutaralde- hyde/ Phenolic	Chlorine Dioxide	Hydrogen Peroxide
	I	II	III	IV	V	VI	VII
STERILIZATION	10 hrs reuse 14 days or 28 days*	10 hrs unused	8 hrs reuse 14 days* or 28 days	10 hrs 21°C† reuse 30 days	diluted –8 hrs first 14 days –10 hrs next 16 days undiluted –6 ¾ hrs	6 hrs 25°C† discard daily	6 hrs 6 wks reuse
DISINFECTION	10 min 20°C *reuse 14–28 days	10 min 20°C reuse 28 days	10 min 28 days *reuse 14–28 days	10 min 20°C dilute 1:4 not virucidal	10 min 20°C diluted 1:16	3 min 25°C† discard daily	10 min 20°C 6 wks reuse not for polio and other resistant viruses
TUBERCULOSIS	20 min 25°C† *reuse 14–28 days	10 min 20°C unused solu- tion	20 min 20°C *reuse 14–28 days 15 min 20°C freshly mixed solution	30 min 20°C –dilute 1:4 –reuse 21 days full strength reuse 42 days	10 min 20°C fresh solution 1:32 2 min full strength	3 min 25°C† discard daily	10 min 20°C 6 wks reuse

*Depends on which of 2 product formulations are used.

†See text about possible fumes or toxicity when solution is heated to this temperature.

ment brought the question about disinfectant efficacy to the attention of the infection control community. This manufacturer's statements were disputed by other manufacturers, but they clearly demonstrated that the results of disinfectant efficacy tests currently in use were not considered universally reliable. The statement and the subsequent publicity were the catalyst for certain actions by the EPA, which registers chemical sterilant/disinfectants. (The total process of registration is described elsewhere in this book.) Issuance of an EPA registration number does not include testing of the data submitted by those seeking registration because the EPA's test laboratories were closed by government action in 1982. Thus, the EPA simply reviews the data, which manufacturers submit in support of their claims, that the product kills certain bacteria, fungi, and viruses in a given time at a given temperature. If they meet test requirements, those data are accepted a face value. Right or wrong, those who use these products believe that an EPA registration number for approval of a product means that the product works as stated.

Because of the doubts brought into the open by this manufacturer's statement, in 1986 the EPA required that manufacturers of antimicrobial pesticides with existing tuberculocidal claims for reusable or "discarded daily" products resubmit their claims. The EPA did not approve or disapprove the new quantitative test method, but the agency required that resubmitted claims be based on any one of three now available and published tests, as follows (EPA, 1986):

1. The standard (old) AOAC tuberculocidal activity method. This requires the temperature of the germicidal solution to be 20°C or more, and the product must be tuberculocidal in 10 min. If this test were chosen, *one* additional sample of the disinfectant had to be tested by a laboratory of the registrant's (not the EPA's) choice using the same test criteria.

2. The AOAC tuberculocidal activity method, but with substantial modifications (of the time and temperature requirement).

3. The new quantitative method submitted by the Association of Analytical Chemists, but not yet verified by that organization's referee. It is this test on which the original manufacturer based his new claims, after he found that the old AOAC test methods did not kill 100% of the tubercle test bacilli.

As a result of this resubmission of claim data requirement, many products were denied reregistration, and some manufacturers voluntarily withdrew their claims for tuberculocidal activity (EPA, 1986).

The problem of tuberculocidal activity is important for the medical community. Tuberculosis is making a comeback in patients with the acquired immunodeficiency syndrome, many of whom require bronchoscopy as a means of diagnosing a variety of pulmonary infections. If the disinfectant is not effective at ambient temperatures and stated times, there is serious risk of cross-contamination among patients.

Infection control practitioners are concerned about the

lack of a universally accepted, collaboratively evaluated test that has been accepted unequivocally as reliable in the testing of chemical disinfectants. That manufacturers can use one of three tests, none of which meets those requirements, is disquieting.

The choice of a disinfectant is further complicated by the differences in claims made on disinfectant labels regarding shelf life, reusability, time and temperature, and which organisms are effectively destroyed. Table 37–2 shows a comparison of instructions among five glutaraldehyde-based products, a hydrogen peroxide product, and a chlorine dioxide disinfectant.

Label Instructions

There is unanimity on two directions found on all labels: (1) that the instruments to be disinfected must be thoroughly cleaned before immersion; and (2) that it is illegal to use the product other than as described.

Several products list a shelf life and an in-use or reuse period. In many instances, however, a product label states that the disinfectant can be reused for 14 to 30 days (depending on the product and whether it is diluted or not) for regular disinfection, but exceptions to this are found in other parts of the label. Instead of listing the variable times, dilutions and reuse instructions in one place, busy nurses must read the whole label to find out that, for tuberculocidal action of one product or sterilization with another, an unused solution must be used (Table 37–2).

For example, one label states that the product has a use and reuse life of 30 days. In different places on the label it states: (1) the product can be diluted (the ratio is given), but *if* diluted it can be used only for 21 days; (2) for disinfection of *Mycobacterium tuberculosis*, it is usable at full strength for 42 days; and (3) for sterilization at full strength, it can be used for 30 days. For sterilization, when diluted, only an 8-hr soak is required during the first 14 days of its use life, but for the next 16 days a 10-hr soak is required. Because diluting a product makes it less expensive, this is a selling point, but the variety of in-use instructions makes correct usage difficult.

The variable temperature requirements are most disturbing. As shown in Table 37–2, they vary from 20 to 21°C, 23°C, and 25°C. Only 20°C or less is ambient temperature; few if any users know this because many do not use the centigrade scale for room temperature. Being clinically oriented and unfamiliar with chemistry, they probably do not realize that temperature can affect a variety of functions in laboratory tests of solutions and therefore attach little importance to the temperature statements. Because at least three disinfectants require temperatures higher than room temperature (or longer contact) some instruments may not be adequately disinfected.

In a recently published *Guideline for Selection and Use of Disinfectants* sponsored by the Association of Practitioners in Infection Control (Rutala, 1990), the temperature requirements are for "room temperature."

The higher temperature requirement by some manufacturers of 25°C is not addressed.

One product label raises another problem. It states that the disinfectant is bactericidal, tuberculocidal, fungicidal, and virucidal. It lists only two lipophilic viruses, however. Few, if any, users will realize that the more resistant hydrophilic viruses may not be inactivated. As clinicians, nurses or doctors would simply believe that all viruses are killed by the product, and instruments may not be safe to use if disinfected with that product.

SUMMARY

Infection control practitioners clearly have a broad range of responsibilities within health-care settings. The clinical orientation and expertise of most infection control practitioners are invaluable in helping to reduce the risk of nosocomial infections in all patient-care activities; however, most have a limited understanding of the chemical and physical concepts involved in the evaluation of disinfectants. Few, if any, hospitals have the means or the knowledge to do it for them. Only two or three states test disinfectant claims, and the results have contained many discrepancies.

One hopes that the experts, whoever they may be, will develop, corroborate, and verify a uniformly reproducible and reliable test to evaluate disinfectant claims. It is further hoped that uniform recommendations can be developed for the reuse period of disinfectants, their dilution if any, their contact time, and realistic temperature requirements. When those data are available, infection control practitioners will be able to fulfill the least understood of their mandates, namely, to provide input into the selection of products used for sterilization, disinfection, and antisepsis.

REFERENCES

Bennett, J.V., and Brachman, P.S. (Eds.) 1987. *Hospital Infections*. 2nd Edition. Boston, Little, Brown.

Centers for Disease Control. 1982. *Pseudomonas aeruginosa* peritonitis attributed to a contaminated iodophor solution—Georgia. MMWR, *31*, 197–198.

Centers for Disease Control. 1983a. Guidelines for hospital environmental control. Am. J. Infect. Control, *11*, 97–115.

Centers for Disease Control. 1983b. Guidelines for prevention of surgical wound infections. Am. J. Infect. Control, *11*, 133–141.

Centers for Disease Control. 1983c. Guidelines for the prevention of intravascular infections. Am. J. Infect. Control, *11*, 183–193.

Cook, E. 1913. *Life of Florence Nightingale*. London, Macmillan.

Dixon, R.E. 1978. Effect of infections on hospital care. Ann. Intern. Med., *89*, 749–753.

Environmental Protection Agency (EPA). 1986. Summary of responses to tuberculocidal effectiveness data: call in notice. June, 1986.

Favero, M.S. 1983. Chemical disinfection of medical and surgical materials. In *Disinfection, Sterilization, and Preservation*. 3rd Edition. Edited by S.S. Block. Philadelphia, Lea & Febiger, pp. 463–492.

Gurevich, I., Tafuro, P., and Cunha, B.A. (Eds.) 1984. *The Theory and Practice of Infection Control*. New York, Praeger Scientific.

Gurevich I., Yannelli, B., and Cunha, B.A. 1989. Survey of techniques used for sterilization of facial implants. Am. J. Infect. Control, *17*, 35–38.

Haley, R.W., Quade, D., Freeman, H.E., and Bennett, J.V. 1980. CDC SENIC Planning Committee: the SENIC Project—Summary of Study Design. Am. J. Epidemiol., *111*, 472–485.

Hamil, R.J., Wright, C.E., Andres, N., and Koza, M.A. 1989. Urinary tract infection following instrumentation for urodynamic testing. Infect. Control and Hosp. Epidemiol., *10*, 26–32.

Joint Commission on Accreditation of Health Care Organizations (JCAHO). 1989. *Infection Control.* Chicago.

Lombardo, J.A., et al. 1980. Endocarditis due to an atypical mycobacteria following porcine heart valve replacement. Aust. N.Z. Med. J., *10*, 432–435.

Rutala, W.A. 1990. APIC guideline for selection and use of disinfectants. Am. J. Infect. Control, *18*, 100–117.

Scott, E.M., and Gorman, S.P. 1983. Sterilization with glutaraldehyde. In *Disinfection, Sterilization, and Preservation.* 3rd Edition. Edited by S.S. Block. Philadelphia, Lea & Febiger, pp. 85–88.

Sobel, J.D., Hashman, N., Reinherz, G., and Merzbach, D. 1982. Nosocomial *Pseudomonas cepacia* infection associated with chlorhexidine contamination. Am. J. Med., *73*, 183–225.

Spaulding, E.H. 1968. Chemical disinfection of medical and surgical materials. In *Disinfection, Sterilization, and Preservation.* 1st Edition. Edited by C.A. Lawrence and S.S. Block. Philadelphia, Lea & Febiger. pp. 517– 531.

Surgikos. 1984. *Letter to Health Care Professionals.* Arlington, TX.

Teeger, I.B., et al. 1983. An epidemiologic study of the risks associated with peripheral intravenous catheters. Am. J. Epidemiol., *118*, 839–851.

Wenzel, R.P. (Ed.) 1987. *Prevention and Control of Nosocomial Infections.* Baltimore, Williams & Wilkins, 1987.

CHAPTER 38

THE EPIDEMIOLOGY AND PREVENTION OF NOSOCOMIAL INFECTIONS

Consuelo M. Beck-Sague and William R. Jarvis

Nosocomial infections are those infections that develop during hospitalization and are neither present nor incubating at the time of the patient's admission. Most nosocomial infections become clinically apparent during hospitalization; however, infections with prolonged incubation periods, those with long latency periods, including many surgical wound infections (SWIs), those occurring in patients with short hospital admissions (nursery and obstetric patients), or those resulting from exposures in the outpatient department (day surgery) may become apparent after hospital discharge. Infections in newborns that are the result of passage through the birth canal and are not transplacentally acquired (such as herpes simplex or rubella) are also considered nosocomial (Garner et al., 1988). Agreement on a uniform set of nosocomial infection definitions, such as those published by the United States Centers for Disease Control (CDC), is a first step towards intra- and interinstitutional comparisons and eliminates subjective assessment of source of the infection (Garner et al., 1988). The current CDC definitions combine clinical findings and results of laboratory and diagnostic tests to determine the presence and anatomic site of nosocomial infections (Garner et al., 1988).

Nosocomial infections can be characterized as sporadic, endemic, or epidemic, on the basis of past occurrence of that disease in relation to time, place, and person (Brachman, 1986). The source of nosocomial infection can be either endogenous (from the patient's own flora) or exogenous (from a source other than the patient). Sporadic nosocomial infections occur occasionally and irregularly, without any specific pattern. Endemic nosocomial infections are often endogenous in origin and occur with ongoing and predictable frequency in a specific geographic area, population, and time period. An epidemic implies a significant increase in incidence of disease above the expected. The majority of nosocomial infections are endemic; that is, they occur with predict-

able frequency and are unrelated to other nosocomial infections occurring in a health-care setting (Wenzel et al., 1983). Such infections are often endogenous in origin and occur among immunocompromised, severely ill, or elderly patients.

Epidemic infections, which are temporally or geographically clustered, are less common and imply a common source (exogenous) or suggest increased person-to-person transmission. They are often associated with specific procedures or devices. Although epidemic nosocomial infections generally occur infrequently, in certain settings, such as intensive care units (ICUs), a substantial percentage of infections may occur in clusters (Wenzel et al., 1983). Moreover, increases in specific infections, such as group A streptococcal SWI or bloodstream infections (BSIs) due to unusual gram-negative organisms, such as *Ewingella* spp., are likely to represent epidemics. Goldmann suggests that even one such infection should be investigated as a possible epidemic because these infections are rarely sporadic (Goldmann, 1986).

SURVEILLANCE

Objectives

The purpose of surveillance of nosocomial infections should be to prevent infections by monitoring trends in infection rates, detecting outbreaks, and collecting data that will assist in identifying areas where prevention efforts should be instituted and enable evaluation of the effectiveness of introduced preventive measures. Periodically, surveillance objectives should be reviewed and a specific surveillance plan created to reach these goals. Although originally most infection control practitioners practiced hospital-wide surveillance, many now conduct focused or targeted surveillance. In focused surveillance, only high-risk populations, services, or sites of infection associated with the greatest morbidity and/or mortality are surveyed. Regardless of the type of surveillance, infection control practitioners should be aware that the methods used to detect infections, the frequency of performance of medical tests (e.g., blood culture, quantitative urine culture), and the intensity of surveillance activities all influence the likelihood of detecting infections (Haley and Schachtman, 1980).

Commonly, the introduction of new antimicrobial agents has been followed by a rapid tendency for organisms to develop resistance (McGowan, 1983). Monitoring resistance to antimicrobials, with the hope of delaying the emergence of highly resistant strains and preventing their predominance, has been a major goal of surveillance and prevention strategies. Despite intensive control measures, there has been a trend towards increasing percentage of nosocomial infections caused by multiply resistant pathogens (Allen et al., 1981; CDC, 1986). Moreover, the trend towards prolonged survival of immunocompromised patients who have prolonged exposures to multiple antimicrobials has created a population at high risk of nosocomial infection with pathogens that are difficult to diagnose and treat, particularly fungi and viruses (Winston et al., 1979). Although it is tempting to relate the changing causes of nosocomial infection and incidence of resistance to the introduction of new anti-

microbials, this obviously fails to take into consideration many other factors related to origins and mechanisms of resistance.

National Nosocomial Infections Surveillance

The National Nosocomial Infections Surveillance (NNIS) System is the only national surveillance system for nosocomial infections in the United States. Hospitals participating in NNIS are a nonrepresentative sample of United States hospitals. Between the system's inception in 1970 and 1986, all reporting hospitals conducted hospital-wide surveillance. In October 1986, a component system was introduced; hospitals could continue hospital-wide surveillance or choose to conduct focused surveillance, targeting ICUs, surgical, or high-risk nursery patients.

During the period from October 1986 through April 1989, 68,649 nosocomial infections caused by 81,325 pathogens were reported from the NNIS hospitals conducting hospital-wide surveillance. Urinary tract infections (UTIs), pneumonias, SWIs, and BSIs combined accounted for about 80% of reported nosocomial infections. UTIs, pneumonias, SWIs, and BSIs comprised 36%, 17%, 16%, and 12%, respectively. Infection rates (per 100 discharges) varied by site and service (Fig. 38–1). The overall nosocomial infection rate averaged 3.5 infections/100 admissions and ranged from a low of 0.1 in the ophthalmology service to a high of 14.6 in the

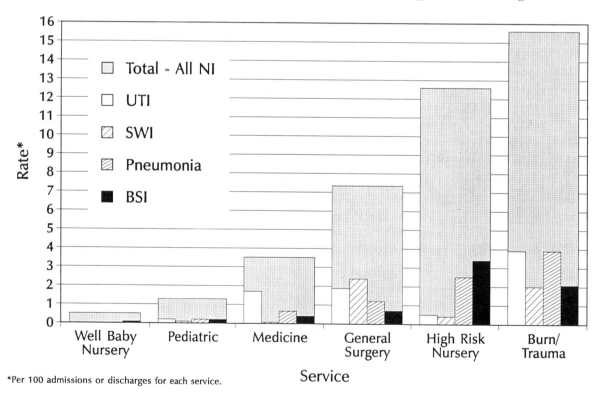

*Per 100 admissions or discharges for each service.

Fig. 38–1. Nosocomial infection (NI) rates by selected site and service, preliminary analysis National Nosocomial Infections Surveillance System. UTI = Urinary tract infection; SWI = surgical wound infection; BSI = bloodstream infection.

Table 38–1. *Preliminary Report of Hospital-Wide Surveillance Nosocomial Infection Rates,* by Service, and Intensive Care Unit (ICU) Nosocomial Infection Rates,† by Type of ICU, National Nosocomial Infections Surveillance System, October 1986 to April 1989*

HOSPITAL-WIDE SURVEILLANCE		ICU	
Service	Infection Rates	Type of ICU	Infection Rates
Medical			
Medicine	3.45	Coronary	12.1
Oncology	4.8	Respiratory	19.4
		Medical	22.3
Surgical			
Burn/trauma	14.64	Med/Surg	20.4
Cardiac surgery	10.10	Neurosurgical	18.5
Gynecology	2.61	Surgical	27.9
Dental	0.54	Burn	33.5
Ear, nose, throat	1.35	Trauma	34.2
General surgery	7.03		
Genitourinary	1.75		
Neurosurgery	6.42		
Ophthalmology	0.11		
Orthopedics	3.42		
Plastic surgery	1.97		
Obstetric	1.35		
Pediatrics			
Pediatric Service	1.27	Pediatric ICU	14.0
Newborn			
High-risk	13.86		
Well-baby	0.52		
All services	3.54	All ICUs	21.2

*Per 100 discharges.
†Per 1000 patient days.

burn/trauma (Table 38–1). Among different services, the infection rates varied by site. In the medicine service, the urinary tract was the most frequent site of infection, followed by the lower respiratory tract, bloodstream, and surgical wounds. In the pediatric and high-risk nursery services, BSI was first, followed by pneumonia, UTI, and SWI. Burn/trauma units had the highest rates of UTI and pneumonia. High-risk nurseries had the highest rates of BSI, and general surgery had the highest rates of SWI (Fig. 38–1).

The most frequently isolated pathogens reported in hospital-wide surveillance were *Escherichia coli* (15%), *Pseudomonas aeruginosa* (11%), and staphylococci (11%). The most frequently reported pathogens by site include *E. coli* for UTI, *Staphylococcus aureus* for SWI, *P. aeruginosa* for pneumonia, and coagulase-negative staphylococci for BSI (Fig. 38–2).

Hospitals conducting ICU surveillance reported 6595 nosocomial infections caused by 7546 pathogens during this period. The overall ICU nosocomial infection rate was 21.2/1000 patients days; rates ranged from 12.1/1000 patient days in coronary ICUs to 34.2 in trauma units (Table 38–1). In all ICUs combined, pneumonia was the most frequently diagnosed, accounting for 31.3% of

nosocomial infections, followed by UTI, BSI, and SWI. The most frequently isolated pathogens reported in ICU surveillance were *Pseudomonas* spp. (15%), coagulase-negative staphylococci (10%), and *Candida* spp. (9%). The site-specific distribution of pathogens reported from ICU patients differs from site distributions reported in hospital-wide surveillance (Fig. 38–3). *Candida* spp. was the most frequent pathogen causing UTI and the fourth most common cause of BSI; coagulase-negative staphylococci were the most common cause of BSI. Enterococci, coagulase-negative staphylococci, and *Candida* spp. accounted for a much greater proportion of infections in ICUs than in the hospital-wide component.

Hospitals conducting surgical patient surveillance reported a SWI rate of 2.3 infections/100 procedures (Horan et al., 1988).

RISK FACTORS

Factors that predispose patients to nosocomial infections can be classified as intrinsic or extrinsic. Intrinsic factors include characteristics of the patient, such as age, sex, underlying disease, and immune status. Extrinsic risk factors include those associated with the patient's

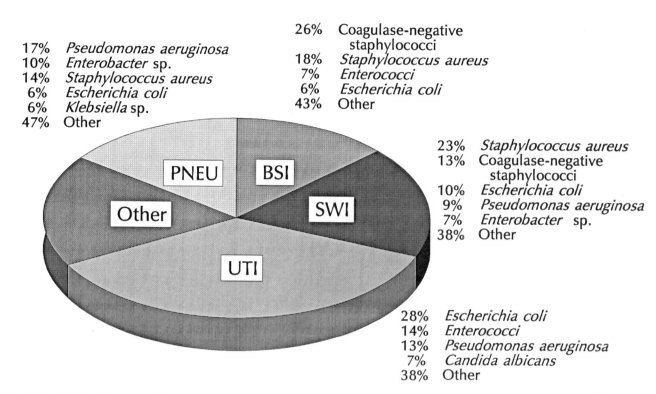

17% *Pseudomonas aeruginosa*
10% *Enterobacter* sp.
14% *Staphylococcus aureus*
6% *Escherichia coli*
6% *Klebsiella* sp.
47% Other

26% Coagulase-negative
staphylococci
18% *Staphylococcus aureus*
7% *Enterococci*
6% *Escherichia coli*
43% Other

23% *Staphylococcus aureus*
13% Coagulase-negative
staphylococci
10% *Escherichia coli*
9% *Pseudomonas aeruginosa*
7% *Enterobacter* sp.
38% Other

28% *Escherichia coli*
14% *Enterococci*
13% *Pseudomonas aeruginosa*
7% *Candida albicans*
38% Other

Fig. 38–2. Relative frequency of 8 common pathogens causing urinary tract infection (UTI), surgical wound infection (SWI), pneumonia (PNEU), and bloodstream infection (BSI) in hospital-wide surveillance, preliminary analysis National Nosocomial Infections Surveillance System (n = 81,325).

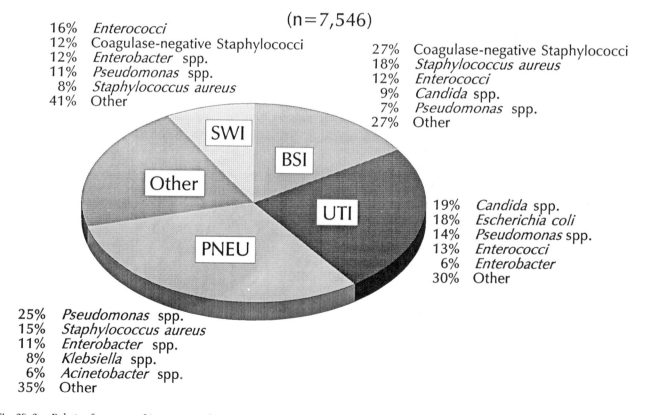

(n=7,546)

16% *Enterococci*
12% Coagulase-negative Staphylococci
12% *Enterobacter* spp.
11% *Pseudomonas* spp.
8% *Staphylococcus aureus*
41% Other

27% Coagulase-negative Staphylococci
18% *Staphylococcus aureus*
12% *Enterococci*
9% *Candida* spp.
7% *Pseudomonas* spp.
27% Other

19% *Candida* spp.
18% *Escherichia coli*
14% *Pseudomonas* spp.
13% *Enterococci*
6% *Enterobacter*
30% Other

25% *Pseudomonas* spp.
15% *Staphylococcus aureus*
11% *Enterobacter* spp.
8% *Klebsiella* spp.
6% *Acinetobacter* spp.
35% Other

Fig. 38–3. Relative frequency of 9 common pathogens causing urinary tract infection (UTI), surgical wound infection (SWI), pneumonia (PNEU), and bloodstream infection (BSI) in intensive care unit surveillance, preliminary analysis National Nosocomial Infections Surveillance System (n = 7546).

Table 38–2. *Risk Factors for Nosocomial Infections at Major Sites*

Site	Risk Factors
Urinary tract	Advanced age
	Female sex
	Breaks in closed system
	Failure of personnel handwashing
	Urinary tract or catheterization instrumentation
	Severity of illness
Pneumonia	Underlying disease
	Altered mental status
	Diabetes
	Alcoholism
	Intubation
	Mechanical ventilation
	Respiratory therapy equipment
	Tracheostomy
	Malnutrition
	Thoracoabdominal surgery
	Histamine II blockers, antacids
	Severity of illness
Bloodstream (primary)	Extremes of age
	Underlying disease
	Immunosuppression
	Burns
	Intravascular devices
	Severity of illness
Surgical wound	Advanced age
	Malnutrition
	Wound classification
	Prosthesis
	Type of prcedure
	Preoperative shaving
	Severity of illness

current hospitalization, including surgical procedures, diagnostic or therapeutic interventions, and personnel exposures. Although many factors increase the risk of virtually all nosocomial infections, such as severity of underlying illness, immunosuppression, advanced age, malnutrition, and surgical procedures, others affect the risk of a specific infection. Among these latter, mechanical ventilation specifically increases the risk of nosocomial pneumonia, for example (Table 38–2). In ICU patients, severity of underlying illness plays an important role in the risk and outcome of nosocomial infection. Site-specific risk factors are discussed later in this chapter.

The reduction of nosocomial infections by the identification of risk factors and the development, institution, and evaluation of efficacy of prevention measures is the principal objective of hospital epidemiology. Risk factors such as severity of illness are difficult to modify immediately. In contrast, extrinsic risk factors are more easily affected. Thus, the identification of extrinsic risk factors through analysis of surveillance data, controlled studies, and epidemic investigations is useful in modifying practices to reduce nosocomial infection.

PREVENTION

During the nineteenth century, as the awareness of how infectious diseases were transmitted grew, use of quarantine, or segregation of infected patients, was widely adopted. The promotion of disease reporting, quarantines, isolation and immunization of contacts, and disinfection of fomites as control measures, which flourished in the late nineteenth century, culminated in the publication of *Control of Communicable Diseases in Man* (APHA, 1980). At about the same time, a system of isolation precautions for specific categories of communicable diseases was introduced for hospitals in Paris (Richardson, 1915) and became widely used in United States hospitals.

In the 1970s, infection control activities in hospitals in the United States increased dramatically. In 1977, over 97% of hospitals reported the use of infection control practitioners (Emori et al., 1980). Most hospitals have an infection control committee. In the United States, the recommendation by the Joint Commission for Accreditation of Health-Care Organizations (JCAHO) that hospitals should have an infection control committee and infection control practitioners for accreditation has been a strong stimulus for hospitals to develop an infection control program, because accreditation is needed for a facility to qualify for Medicare funding.

At present, prevention of nosocomial infection is considered to rely primarily on patient-care practices. Many of these practices are described in the CDC *Guidelines for the Prevention and Control of Nosocomial Infections*. In the past decade, the percentage of hospitals with programs shown to be effective in preventing urinary tract infections (UTI), bloodstream infections (BSI), and pneumonia has increased. Classification of an infection as nosocomial does not imply preventability and is not synonymous with iatrogenic (Garner et al., 1988). Nevertheless, only approximately 9% of nosocomial infections are being prevented, whereas 32% could be prevented if all hospitals adopted the most effective programs (Haley et al., 1985c). In addition to patient-care practices, surveillance, isolation precautions, employee health, limited environmental control, and design of patient-care equipment all play important roles in the prevention and control of nosocomial infection.

Isolation Precautions

Isolation precautions are implemented when patients are suspected of having particular infections. These precautions have traditionally involved separating infected patients with other patients and from health-care workers using various types of barriers, such as gloves, gowns, masks, and isolation rooms (Garner and Simmons, 1983; CDC, 1987; Lynch et al., 1987). Isolation precautions for specific infections or categories of infection evolved from the concept of quarantines, and guidelines exist for instituting, maintaining, and discontinuing isolation precautions once a diagnosis is made or suspected (Garner and Simmons, 1983). Because most infections in hospitals may be transmissible before they are suspected, precautions that are universally applied are necessary to reduce the risk of transmission of pathogens to other patients and health-care workers. This is particularly true for community-acquired infections with prolonged asymptomatic periods, such as human immunodeficiency virus (HIV) or hepatitis B virus (HBV) (CDC, 1987). For this reason, precautions instituted for all patients are recommended to prevent transmission of bloodborne pathogens including HIV and HBV. Health-care workers should consider *all* patients as potentially infected with bloodborne pathogens and adhere rigorously to infection control precautions for minimizing the risk of exposure to blood and certain body fluids of all patients. These precautions eliminate the need for use of the isolation category of "blood and body fluid precautions" previously recommended for patients suspected or known to be infected with bloodborne pathogens. Other specific isolation precautions (i.e., enteric secretion, contact, strict), however, are still recommended for pathogens transmitted by nonbloodborne routes (CDC, 1988a; Garner and Simmons, 1983).

Employee Health

Almost 7 million persons, representing 5.6% of the United States labor force, are employed in health services. These persons may become infected outside the hospital or through exposure to infected patients. Subsequently, they may transmit infections to susceptible patients. The prevention of infectious disease transmission to and from health-care personnel depends on placement evaluations, including personnel health and safety education, immunizations, and work restrictions (Williams, 1983).

Placement evaluations should be limited to determining the worker's immunization status and obtaining a history of conditions that may predispose the health-care worker to acquiring or transmitting infectious diseases, such as tuberculosis, hepatitis, varicella zoster, and measles. Screening for serosusceptibility before immunization against measles, mumps, rubella, hepatitis, and influenza is not necessary for medical indications alone because previous infection is not a contraindication to immunization (Williams, 1983). No data suggest that routine physical examinations or laboratory tests are cost-beneficial; the placement medical history should indicate whether any laboratory studies are needed. Culture surveys of personnel are rarely, if ever, indicated either before or during employment. Unless a certain employee is epidemiologically linked to a cluster of cases, the results of such cultures are difficult to interpret and are seldom helpful in decision-making. The placement medical history can guide one to determine whether workers should have permanent restrictions to protect them from illnesses such as chicken pox, if they have not had the illness.

A number of disease processes, including hepatitis A, diarrhea, scabies, conjunctivitis, and group A strepto-coccal infections are indications for temporary exclusion of employees from patient care (Williams, 1983).

Because of the risk of occupational acquisition and perinatal transmission of certain viral infections, research has been directed at determining the risk to pregnant personnel of cytomegalovirus (CMV) or HIV infection. Data suggest that this risk of acquisition outside the hospital setting is greater than in the hospital, where the risk is low (Brady et al., 1987; Ahlfors et al., 1981).

Percutaneous exposure to blood of infected persons by needle sticks or sharp instruments appears to be the most efficient means of occupational transmission of bloodborne pathogens to health-care workers (Marcus et al., 1988). For this reason, universal precautions for the prevention of transmission of HIV, HBV, and other bloodborne pathogens focus on the prevention of needle sticks and other percutaneous exposures and provision of hepatitis B immunization for workers at high risk of occupational exposure (CDC, 1988a). An estimated 37% of such exposures reported in one study were judged to be preventable and occurred during high-risk procedures, including recapping, which are not recommended (Marcus et al., 1988). The prevention of percutaneous injuries should be a high priority for employee health and infection control departments and depends on several factors, including employee education on optimal disposal of sharp instruments and the availability of rigid, puncture-proof containers in patient-care areas to dispose of needles.

Environmental Control

Regularly scheduled culturing of the air, floor, walls, and table tops was widely practiced in hospitals in the United States before 1970 (Garner and Favero, 1985). In response to data suggesting that routine environmental culturing is wasteful and ineffective, many hospitals have gradually abandoned these procedures. In 1970, the Centers for Disease Control (CDC) and the American Hospital Association recommended the discontinuance of routine environmental culturing. Existing data showed that rates of nosocomial infection did not appear to relate to levels of microbial contamination of air or surfaces, and no meaningful standards existed for permissible levels of microbial contamination (Garner and Favero, 1985). The trend for hospitals to reduce the extent of environmental culturing has continued since the recommendation was made (Haley et al., 1980).

Two circumstances in which environmental culturing is recommended are: (1) monitoring the quality of water used to prepare dialysate; and (2) culturing epidemiologically identified sources during epidemic investigations. In hemodialysis units, routine microbiologic quantitative sampling is recommended of the water and dialysis fluids used with hemodialysis machines and for manual or automated disinfection of artificial kidneys (Favero, 1985). Gram-negative bacteria are able to reproduce rapidly in water and other fluids used in dialysis, and high microbial counts have been associated with pyrogenic reactions and bacteremia (Gordon et al.,

1988). Water used to prepare dialysis fluid and to disinfect artificial kidneys should not contain a total viable microbial count greater than 200 colony-forming units (CFU)/ml. The dialysis fluid at the end of dialysis treatments should contain less than 2000 CFU/ml (AAMI, 1986).

Often, during the course of epidemics, environmental culturing is undertaken to identify reservoirs or common sources of patient infections. Because no standards exist for the number or species of organisms acceptable for many environmental sources, the identification of even pathogenic organisms in such areas as walls, counters, floors, or air, may be, under most circumstances, impossible to interpret. It is essential that inanimate objects for culturing be selected carefully on the basis of epidemiologic evidence that they are linked to patients' infections. When intrinsic contamination of substances packaged as sterile is considered possible, local, state, and federal (Food and Drug Administration [FDA], CDC) officials should be contacted. The suspected items should be cultured by personnel familiar with appropriate techniques (Garner and Favero, 1985; CDC, 1986).

NOSOCOMIAL URINARY TRACT INFECTION (UTI)

Of the approximately 2 million patients who acquire nosocomial infections in acute-care hospitals annually, almost 40% have urinary tract infections (UTI), the most frequently diagnosed nosocomial infection (Garibaldi, 1981). In National Nosocomial Infections Surveillance (NNIS) hospital-wide surveillance, the UTI rate was 1.19 and ranged from 0.2/100 discharges in well-baby nurseries to 3.50 in burn/trauma units (Fig. 38–1). Overall, in NNIS ICUs, the UTI rate was 1.9/100 admissions (Jarvis et al., 1988). The major risk factors for nosocomial UTI include urinary tract catheterization and/or instrumentation; catheter-associated UTI rates ranged from 0 to 12/1000 catheter days (mean 8.0), whereas noncatheter-associated UTI rates ranged from 0 to 1.2/1000 patient days (Jarvis et al., 1988).

Pathogens

Among NNIS hospital-wide surveillance patients, *Escherichia coli* (28%), *Pseudomonas aeruginosa* (13%), and enterococci (14%) are the pathogens most frequently associated with UTI (Fig. 38–2). Among NNIS ICU patients, *Candida* spp. (19%) are more frequently isolated than *E. coli* (18%) and *Pseudomonas* spp. (14%) (Fig. 38–3).

Although mortality has been reported to be high following nosocomial UTI (Platt et al., 1982), in NNIS, UTIs are seldom reported to cause or contribute to death (CDC, 1986). The clinical severity of infection appears to be related to the severity of the patient's underlying illness and the ability to remove the invasive device (i.e., catheter) rather than to the species of infecting organisms or its antimicrobial susceptibility.

The majority of UTIs are endemic infections with strains of gram-negative organisms colonizing the gastrointestinal tract of catheterized patients. These organisms are generally not resistant to multiple antimicrobials and colonize the colon of patients as normal commensals. Epidemics of UTI are probably often missed because the background rate of UTI is high, and in most institutions, unusual, highly resistant organisms are infrequently associated with infection.

Patients' fecal contamination is an important reservoir of *E. coli*, whereas *P. aeruginosa* and *Serratia* spp. rarely colonize the intestinal tract, and reservoirs for these are usually contaminated inanimate objects, other common sources, or other infected patients (Garibaldi, 1981) (Table 38–3).

Risk Factors

The initial step in the pathogenesis of UTI is bacterial colonization of the lower urinary tract. Although this colonization most often follows catheterization, some host factors such as stones, caliceal and ureteral diverticula, hydronephrotic kidney, vesicoureteral reflux, bladder neck obstruction with urine residuals, and prostatic infection lead to the persistence of colonization and invasive symptomatic disease (Roberts, 1988). Virtually all these interfere with normal rapid urinary flow and bladder emptying, which appear to reduce colonization and the potential for progression from colonization to infection. Some diseases, such as diabetes mellitus, greatly increase the risk of UTI through multiple metabolic and neurogenic factors (Cox, 1988). Although cancer, immunosuppression, and advanced age increase the risk of all nosocomial infections, they seem to be associated with increased risk specifically of UTI.

Among intrinsic risk factors, female sex appears to be important in increasing the incidence of UTI (Table 38–2). The shorter length of the female urethra appears to provide ready access for bacterial invasion; however, hormonal factors may be associated with the increased risk because pregnancy appears to increase the incidence of bacteriuria in some populations. Although female sex appears to predispose patients to UTI, male patients with nosocomial UTI have significantly higher morbidity and mortality; this may be related to the finding that men who develop UTIs are generally older than women who develop nosocomial UTI (Carson, 1988).

Urethral catheterization is the single most important predisposing extrinsic factor in the development of UTI. Surgical manipulation of the urinary tract also increases the risk of bacterial colonization and subsequent infection. Antimicrobial prophylaxis in urologic surgery patients appears to reduce the incidence of postoperative UTI and may also reduce the development of sepsis after this type of surgery (Larsen et al., 1986). Because urethral catheterization, particularly prolonged catheterization, is the most important risk factor, however, and antimicrobials rarely affect the progression of UTI when the catheter remains in place, the limiting of this procedure is the most important strategy in reduction of UTI risk.

Table 38–3. *Reservoirs and Common Epidemiologic Patterns of Selected Pathogens Causing Nosocomial Urinary Tract Infection*

Pathogen	Reservoir	Epidemiologic Pattern
Escherichia coli	Fecal colonization	Endemic
Pseudomonas spp.	Common source	Epidemic (product contamination)
Enterococci	Fecal colonization	Endemic
Klebsiella spp.	Fecal colonization	Epidemic (autoinfection)
Proteus spp.	Other patients	Epidemic (autoinfection, cross-infection)
Serratia spp.	Other patients	Endemic
		Epidemic (cross infection)
Candida spp.	Skin colonization	Endemic

Prevention

Prevention of UTI depends on: (1) restriction of urinary tract catheterization to those for whom it is essential; (2) appropriate preparation of the insertion site and aseptic catheter insertion; and (3) maintenance of a closed urinary drainage system. Guidelines have been developed for the prevention of nosocomial UTI (Wong and Hooton, 1981). Some investigators suggest that intermittent catheterization with bladder emptying reduces the incidence of bacteriuria and subsequent UTI (Carson, 1988). When an indwelling catheter is essential, antiseptic cleaning of the meatus and aseptic insertion and the maintenance of a closed system with prompt removal of the catheter as soon as possible reduce the risk of UTI (Wong and Hooton, 1981). UTI inevitably occurs in patients with open systems after several days. Some studies suggest that antimicrobial prophylaxis and the use of sealed junction catheters may reduce the risk of UTI associated with certain urinary tract surgical procedures and instrumentation (Larsen et al., 1986; Platt et al., 1989).

NOSOCOMIAL PNEUMONIA

The lower respiratory tract is a frequent site of nosocomial infection; 16% of nosocomial infections in National Nosocomial Infections Surveillance (NNIS) hospital-wide surveillance are nosocomial pneumonia. Pneumonia rates per 100 discharges range from 0.03 in the obstetric and well-baby services to 2.5 in high-risk nurseries and 3.9 in burn/trauma units (Fig. 38–1). In high-risk nurseries, nosocomial pneumonia is more common than urinary tract infection (UTI), and in the burn/trauma unit, the rate is almost identical to that of UTI. Pneumonia is the most common nosocomial infection in all NNIS ICUs combined (Fig. 38–3).

Studies have shown that many nosocomial pneumonias are associated with upper respiratory tract, including oropharyngeal, colonization with hospital pathogens (Pennington, 1985). Most nosocomial pneumonias result from respiratory tract interventions, including endotracheal intubation, tracheostomy, and/or mechanical ventilation. In ICUs, ventilator-associated pneumonia rates range from 7 to 23.4/1000 ventilator days, whereas non-ventilator-associated rates ranged from 0.2.5/1000 patient days (Jarvis et al., 1988).

Pathogens

Among NNIS hospital-wide surveillance patients, *Pseudomonas aeruginosa* (17%), *Enterobacter* spp. (10%), and *Staphylococcus aureus* (14%) are the pathogens most frequently associated with nosocomial pneumonia (Fig. 38–2). In over 10% of pneumonias reported, no specific pathogen is identified. This suggests that microbiologic diagnosis of nosocomial pneumonia is more difficult than microbiologic diagnosis of infection at other sites. Indeed, the differentiation of incidentally colonizing pathogens from those truly responsible for infection may be difficult. The clinical picture itself is often confusing, particularly among critically ill patients: other factors, such as atelectasis, congestive heart failure, adult respiratory distress syndrome, and interstitial lung diseases may obscure the onset of pneumonia (Hessen and Kaye, 1988). A number of studies suggest that sputum cultures are frequently not useful in identifying the etiologic agents of pneumonia (Bamberger, 1988). Often, when routine diagnostic methods fail, sheathed fiberoptic bronchoscopy with quantitative culture and biopsy can provide a diagnosis. Occasionally, open lung biopsy is necessary.

Although most nosocomial pneumonias are caused by gram-negative organisms, *S. aureus*, and anaerobes, in immunocompromised hosts, fungi, mycobacteria, viruses, *Nocardia*, and *Pneumocystis carinii* are also often seen. Of all nosocomial infections, pneumonia is the leading cause of morbidity and mortality. Mortality due to nosocomial pneumonia varies by type of organism as well as underlying risk factors. Gram-negative pneumonias in hospitalized patients are associated with mortality rates that approach 70% (Wollschlager et al., 1988). Nosocomial pneumonias are the nosocomial infection most frequently associated with death (Gross and Van Antwerpen, 1983).

Risk Factors

The initial step in the pathogenesis of nosocomial pneumonia is colonization of the oropharynx (Pennington, 1985). Colonization rates vary with underlying disease; oropharyngeal colonization with gram-negative organisms is estimated to occur in approximately 18% of normal persons, 35% of moderately ill alcoholic and diabetic hospitalized patients, and 73% of moribund patients (Mackoviak et al., 1978).

Intrinsic risk factors related to motility of the airway and competence of the gag reflex may affect the risk of colonization and subsequent progression to pneumonia. Important host factors, such as immunosuppression, altered mental status, neurologic processes, and chronic obstructive pulmonary disease all increase the risk of developing pneumonia (Bamberger, 1988; Fels, 1988).

The most important risk factors for pneumonia are related to mechanical ventilation (see Table 38–2). Intubation bypasses the natural mechanical barrier and allows exposure of the lower respiratory tract to oropharyngeal flora. Intubation and tracheostomy increase the incidence of infection by approximately 20 and 25%, respectively (Wollschlager et al., 1988). Respiratory therapy and bronchoscopy equipment can serve as reservoirs for gram-negative organisms associated with nosocomial pneumonia and require appropriate disinfection or sterilization (Simmons and Wong, 1982).

Other important extrinsic risk factors for nosocomial pneumonia include thoracic and upper abdominal surgery and the use of antacids or histamine type 2 blockers (Bamberger, 1988). Virtually all surgical procedures performed under general anesthesia increase the risk of nosocomial pneumonia. Impairment of swallowing and respiratory clearance from instrumentation of the respiratory tract during surgery, anesthesia, operative pain, narcotics, and sedatives, all of which can result in aspiration or atelectasis, increase the risk of pneumonia. In one study, 3 out of 4 definite or probable cases of nosocomial pneumonia occurred in patients who had had surgical procedures; the risk of pneumonia was 38, 14, and 3.4 times greater for thoracoabdominal, thoracic, and abdominal surgical patients, respectively, than for patients without surgical procedures (Wollschlager et al., 1988). Multiple trauma patients also have an increased risk of nosocomial pneumonia, because of involuntary splinting and other factors.

Some epidemics of nosocomial pneumonia have been related to the use of contaminated respiratory therapy equipment (Table 38–2). The majority of these reported outbreaks have been associated with the use of contaminated humidification equipment, specifically reservoir nebulizers, including "room air humidifiers," which aerosolize water (Simmons and Wong, 1982). Water reservoirs of these nebulizers can easily become contaminated. Nebulizers that aerosolize water create particles of a size (1 to 2 μm) that can be deposited deep into the respiratory tract, where bacteria can more easily cause infection (Simmons and Wong, 1982).

Prevention

The prevention of nosocomial pneumonia largely depends on: (1) restricting the use of certain techniques (such as intubation and mechanical ventilation) to specific therapeutic indications; and (2) avoiding certain devices that are associated with a high risk of infection, such as nebulizers that create droplets to humidify air (Simmons and Wong, 1982). For patients undergoing surgical procedures for which the risk of nosocomial pneumonia is great, preoperative preparations should include therapy and instruction designed to prevent pulmonary complications (Simmons and Wong, 1982). These include treatment and resolution of preoperative pulmonary infections and discontinuance of smoking, and education and instruction on the use of respiratory therapy equipment to prevent atelectasis and pneumonia. Moreover, during the immediate postoperative period, deep breathing and coughing should be encouraged by early ambulation, incentive spirometry, and optimal pain control.

NOSOCOMIAL BLOODSTREAM INFECTION (BSI)

Nosocomial bloodstream infection (BSI) occurs in approximately 12.8% of patients diagnosed with nosocomial infection in National Nosocomial Infections Surveillance (NNIS) hospital-wide surveillance patients. ICUs have emerged as the highest risk area for all nosocomial infections, particularly BSI. In ICUs, approximately 1.3% of the patients develop a BSI, and BSIs comprise 15.8% of nosocomial infections (Jarvis et al., 1988) (Fig. 38–3). In a state surveillance system, 41% of all nosocomial BSI occurred among ICU patients; 8 of 11 outbreaks identified in this system involved BSI (Wenzel et al., 1983).

The major risk factor for nosocomial BSI is intravascular catheterization. Over 80% of BSI occurs among patients with intravascular lines. In NNIS ICU patients, the intravascular-line-associated BSI rate was 8.6/1000 line days, versus 0.02/1000 patient days among patients without vascular lines (Jarvis et al., 1988).

Pathogens

Among NNIS hospital-wide surveillance patients, Staphylococcus aureus (18%) and other staphylococcal species (26%) are the organisms most frequently associated with BSI (Fig. 38–2). Among NNIS ICU patients, 27% of BSIs are caused by coagulase-negative staphylococci, 18% by S. aureus, and 12% by enterococci; nearly 10% of ICU BSIs are caused by Candida species (see Fig. 38–3).

Surveillance of BSI in the United States suggests that in the 1980s, contamination of infusates became a relatively rare cause of BSI: gram-negative organisms, implicated in many of the outbreaks in the 1970s, became of only secondary importance. Enterobacter sp., Pseudomonas aeruginosa, and Serratia marcescens combined comprise only 13% of line-associated BSIs in ICUs. In contrast, over 50% are caused by gram-positive cocci, which are rarely infusate contaminants (Fig. 38–3).

The majority of nosocomial BSIs are endemic and are related to infection of the cannula wound by common skin contaminants. They develop as a complication of an identifiable local infection, often among immunocompromised or severely ill patients. Several studies have suggested that extrinsic contamination of infusates during conventional peripheral intravenous (IV) therapy is infrequent, unlikely to result in BSI, and completely eradicated, if low level, by replacement of the administration set (Maki et al., 1987a).

Contamination of infusates, the most common cause of recognized epidemic BSI, can be classified as intrinsic or extrinsic. Intrinsic contamination is caused by inadvertent introduction of microorganisms into substances intended for infusion at manufacture (Maki et al., 1976). This includes contamination of caps of containers of IV fluids and of blood components caused by unsuspected infections in donors. Since the nationwide outbreak of intrinsically contaminated IV fluids in the United States in 1971, no evidence of intrinsic IV fluid contamination causing BSI has been reported.

Extrinsic contamination of infusates, introduction of pathogens during use in a health-care setting, is more common and continues to be the most common cause of recognized epidemic BSI (Maki, 1977). Certain microorganisms are so prevalent in infusion-related sepsis— *Enterobacter cloacae* and *E. agglomerans, Pseudomonas cepacia,* and *Candida parapsilosis* in total parenteral nutrition—that their recovery from blood cultures in even one patient with the clinical picture of sepsis should prompt an immediate search for an infusion-related cause (Hamory, 1987). Contamination of stopcocks and hubs with gram-positive cocci, however, can also result in epidemic as well as endemic BSI and vascular infection (Sitges-Serra et al., 1983).

Risk Factors

The increasing incidence of BSI appears to be related to the use of prolonged central and peripheral IV cannulation. The initial step in the pathogenesis of catheter-related infections is the formation of a fibrin sheath around a cannula inserted into a vessel (Maki, 1981). This fibrin sheath is colonized, bacterial replication occurs, and bacteria are released into the blood. Most catheter-related infections are caused by skin microorganisms that invade the cutaneous tract during catheter insertion or during the course of intravascular therapy (Snydman et al., 1982). Loosening of the connection between intravascular access site and extension tubing, as well as stopcocks and hub contamination by skin organisms, has been recognized as an important cause of infections, however (Pemberton et al., 1984).

Intrinsic risk factors for BSI include extremes in age, which greatly affect immune response; rates are highest among low-birth-weight infants and elderly patients (Table 38–2). Patients with fatal underlying diseases are at greatest risk. In these patients, infections in other areas are not adequately contained and pathogens gain access to the blood, or small numbers of microorganisms can establish secondary BSI. Often these infections are not clearly related to intravascular therapeutic or monitoring interventions. In contrast, most primary BSI are related to some aspect of intravascular therapy, and multiple risk factors related to the use of intravascular devices have been identified (Table 38–2).

The majority of epidemic BSIs are primary, and in most, some aspect of infusion therapy or intravascular

monitoring is incriminated (Mermel and Maki, 1989). Except for epidemics involving neonates, severity of illness and immunocompetence do not appear to increase the risk of epidemic BSI: infection risk appears to be related almost exclusively to therapeutic and monitoring interventions (Maki, 1981; Wenzel et al., 1983).

Use of unreliable disinfectants for preparation of injection caps, cannula sites, and decontamination of transducer components has been the cause of numerous outbreaks (Maki, 1981). Extrinsic contamination of the fluid column in invasive pressure-monitoring systems, particularly because of inadequate disinfection of reusable pressure transducers, is among the most common causes of epidemic BSI (Mermel and Maki, 1989; Beck-Sague and Jarvis, 1989). The practice of warming or cooling infusates in contaminated water baths has also led to outbreaks of BSI (Rhame and McCollough, 1979). Similarly, cooling syringes by immersing them in ice and then connecting them to stopcocks to obtain blood specimens can readily contaminate both the stopcock and the fluid column (Stamm et al., 1975; Pien and Bruce, 1986).

Although extrinsic contamination of infusates is a frequent cause of epidemic BSI, it is a relatively rare cause of endemic nosocomial bacteremia (Maki et al., 1987a). Colonization of skin access site, contamination of hub, moisture, or blood beneath dressings, and duration of catheter placement have been demonstrated in several studies to be associated with local catheter-related infections: some studies have found significantly higher rates of local catheter-related infections with transparent dressings left on indefinitely; others have not (Maki et al., 1987b). The risk of transparent dressings, even when they are changed every 48 hrs, appears to be highest with central catheters (Conly et al., 1989).

Prevention

Guidelines are available for the prevention of nosocomial BSI associated with intravascular therapy and pressure monitoring (Simmons et al., 1981). Prevention of intravascular therapy-associated BSI depends on: (1) restricting the use of intravascular therapy/monitoring to those patients in whom it is essential; and (2) reducing catheter and infusate colonization; these are the most important preventable risk factors affecting the risk of BSI (Maki et al., 1987b). Several studies have estimated that 25 to 37% of BSIs are potentially preventable with an active and effective infection control program (Haley et al., 1985; Wenzel et al., 1983). Most studies have suggested the importance of skin disinfection prior to placement of the catheter because organisms contaminating the skin of the patient and/or personnel have been implicated (Salzman et al., 1967). Data suggest that the following infection control practices are appropriate for peripheral IV infusions under most circumstances: Administration sets and catheters may be changed together every 72 hrs, and dressings need to be applied only once, at the time of insertion, and do not need to be changed during the 72-hr period (Decker and Schaffner, 1987). Fluid containers should be changed every 24 hrs (Maki et al., 1987a). The use of the line for a number of procedures, such as hyperalimentation and blood transfusions, and their use in certain circumstances, such as in diaphoretic patients, may increase the risk of infection, and this has to be considered when determining adequate intervals for changes.

Invasive pressure monitoring, hyperalimentation, and multiple-lumen catheters entail greater risk to the patient of infectious morbidity and mortality; therefore, indications for their use should be carefully and frequently re-evaluated. Moreover, knowledge of and strict compliance with guidelines regarding their use should be a condition to their use (Williams, 1985; Mermel and Maki, 1989).

Close adherence to uniform protocols in insertion and maintenance of catheters appears to be a significant factor in reducing infectious complications. The use of IV therapy teams, which may be related to compliance with such protocols, appears to reduce the risk of catheter-related infection (Tomford et al., 1984).

SURGICAL WOUND INFECTION (SWI)

In National Nosocomial Infections Surveillance (NNIS) hospital-wide surveillance, 18.5% of nosocomial infections were surgical wound infections (SWI) (Fig. 38–2). In ICUs, SWIs comprise 8.4% of nosocomial infections (Fig. 38–3). Traditionally, SWIs have been categorized by the level of contamination experienced during the procedure. Contamination is categorized according to an algorithm that classifies the level of contamination from clean (class I) to dirty (class IV) procedures (Cruse and Ford, 1980). In the NNIS surgical patient component, SWI rates were 1.6 SWI/100 class I procedures, 2.7/100 clean-contaminated (class II) procedures, 3.1/100 contaminated (class III) procedures, and 6.7/100 dirty (class IV) procedures (Horan et al., 1988). Rates also varied by type of procedure: colorectal surgery (7.6%) had the highest SWI rate by operative procedure category (Horan et al., 1988). Lowest rates were observed in spinal fusions/laminectomies (1.9%) and cholecystectomies (2.2%) (Horan et al., 1988).

Pathogens

Among NNIS hospital-wide surveillance patients, *Staphylococcus aureus* (23%), coagulase-negative staphylococci (13%), *Escherichia coli* (10%), *Pseudomonas aeruginosa* (9%), and *Enterobacter* spp. (7%) are the pathogens most frequently isolated from SWI (Fig. 38–2). Among NNIS ICU patients, pathogens most frequently isolated from SWI include enterococci (16%), coagulase-negative staphylococci (12%), and *Enterobacter* spp. (12%) (see Fig. 38–3).

Risk Factors

The initial step in the pathogenesis of SWI is microbial contamination of the wound. The amount and type of microbial contamination of the wound, together with the condition of the wound at the end of the operation and the patient's ability to contain infection, determine whether an infection will be established and the outcome of the infection. Numerous factors, both intrinsic and extrinsic, affect SWI risk (Table 38–3).

Intrinsic factors relate to the resistance of the patient and include systemic and local factors. The importance of an adequate immune response and nutritional factors related to wound healing are great and can override even such vital factors as asepsis and contamination (Cruse and Ford, 1980). Organ transplantation has among the highest SWI rates largely because of the need to suppress the patient's immune response to prevent rejection of the transplant, making the patient, and particularly the incision, susceptible to infection.

Pathogens that cause SWI can be acquired from the patient (endogenous) or from hospital environment or personnel (exogenous). Endogenous sources appear to be responsible for the majority of infections, particularly when SWIs occurring in "clean" wounds are excluded. SWIs caused by gram-negative organisms are often endogenous and have as their source the gastrointestinal and genitourinary tracts and infections remote from the wound, such as urinary tract infections (UTIs). In contrast, certain organisms, such as group A streptococci, suggest personnel carriers and exogenous contamination.

Risk, severity, and outcome of infection are strongly influenced by the type of pathogen causing the infection, as well as the site of infection and multiple factors relative to the host and the procedure. For example, *Streptococcus viridans* rarely causes severe SWI outside the cardiovascular system, whereas group A streptococci are likely to cause severe infections regardless of site (Simmons, 1982).

A number of strategies have been developed to estimate the risk of SWI after a surgical procedure. Among the most widely used is the categorization of surgical procedures by wound class. Clean operations are those in which the gastrointestinal or respiratory tract was not entered, no apparent inflammation was encountered, and no break in aseptic technique was observed (Cruse and Ford, 1980). Clean-contaminated operations are procedures in which the gastrointestinal or respiratory tract was entered but no significant spillage was encountered. Contaminated operations are those in which acute inflammation without pus formation was encountered or in which gross spillage from a hollow viscus occurred. Fresh traumatic wounds and procedures in which major breaks in technique occurred are among these. Dirty operations are those in which pus was encountered or in which a perforated viscus was found.

Unfortunately, wound class alone does not incorporate the numerous additional factors that influence the risk for SWI such as age, sex, type of procedure, duration of the procedure, and underlying diseases. When these factors are incorporated into a surgical patient risk index, the risk of SWI varies widely among the traditional wound classes, from 1.1 to 15.8 among clean procedures and from 6.0 to 18.8 among contaminated procedures

(Haley et al., 1985a). When a patient risk index was developed by Haley et al. using number of discharge diagnoses >3, duration of procedure >2 hrs, thoracoabdominal procedures, and wound class, little variation in SWI rate was seen within the patient or site categories (Haley et al., 1985a).

Extrinsic risk factors predisposing patients to SWI are multiple and affect every aspect of the procedures, from preoperative hair removal and skin preparation to suturing and stapling of the wound. A number of factors associated with preoperative skin preparation have been associated with a marked increase in infection risk. Shaving of the patient's skin before surgery raises the risk of SWI, possibly by causing multiple microscopic nicks where bacterial growth can occur inaccessible to skin disinfection. The hands of surgical staff serve as reservoirs for organisms that can readily cause SWI. Likewise, the skin of the patient, particularly patients who have had prolonged preoperative stays before surgery, can be heavily colonized with a wide variety of potential pathogens.

Prevention

Prevention of SWI depends on: (1) reducing the amount and type of microbial contamination of the wound; (2) using techniques that protect the condition of the wound during the operation; and (3) enhancing the patient's ability to withstand microbial contamination. Guidelines for the prevention of SWI that outline prevention measures pre-, intra-, and postoperatively are available (Garner, 1985). Preoperative measures include treating known infections, keeping the preoperative stay short, bathing with a registered antiseptic, avoiding shaving, and correcting nutritional deficiencies. Intraoperative measures include appropriate preparation of the operative site with an FDA-registered antiseptic, adequate scrubbing of personnel's hands and use of sterile gloves, good operative technique, with gentle, expeditious, and careful handling of tissues, and appropriate use of prophylactic antimicrobials (Simmons, 1982).

Previous studies show that one of several important measures for reduction of SWI is to perform active SWI surveillance, which includes calculation of procedure-specific and surgeon-specific infection rates and the reporting of those rates back to surgeons (Haley et al., 1985b). In 1976, 19% of hospitals reported surgeon-specific infection rates to their surgeons; unfortunately, in 1983, only 13% of hospitals reported such rates to their surgeons (Haley et al., 1985c). If SWI rates are to be reduced, pre- and postoperative risk factors must be modified or controlled, but most important, the role of the surgeon in the origin of SWIs must be understood and comparative rates calculated, so surgical practices that result in infections can be investigated and modified.

REFERENCES

Ahlfors, K., Ivarrson, S.A., Johnsson, T., and Renmarker, K. 1981. Risk of cytomegalovirus infection in nurses and congenital infection in their offspring. Acta Pediatr. Scand., 70, 819–823.

Allen, J.R., Hightower, A.N., Martin, S.M., and Dixon, R.E. 1981. Secular trends in nosocomial infections 1970–1979. Am. J. Med., 70, 389.

American Public Health Association (APHA). 1980. Preface. In Control of Communicable Diseases in Man. 13th Edition. Edited by A.S. Benenson. Washington, D.C., American Public Health Association, pp. xix–xxvi.

Association for the Advancement of Medical Instrumentation (AAMI). 1986. Recommended Practice: Reuse of Hemodialyzers. Arlington, VA, Association for the Advancement of Medical Instrumentation.

Bamberger, D.M. 1988. Diagnosis of nosocomial pneumonia. Semin. Respir. Infect., 3, 140–147.

Beck-Sague, C.M., and Jarvis, W.R. 1989. Epidemic bloodstream infections associated with pressure transducers: a persistent problem. Infect. Control, 10, 54–60.

Brachman, P.S. 1986. Epidemiology of nosocomial infections. In Hospital Infections. Edited by J.V. Bennett and P.S. Brachman. Boston, Little, Brown, pp. 3–16.

Brady, M.T., Demmler, G.J., and Anderson, D.C. 1987. Brief report. Cytomegalovirus infection in pediatric house officers: susceptibility to and rate of primary infection. Infect. Control, 8, 329–332.

Carson, C.C. 1988. Nosocomial urinary tract infections. Surg. Clin. North Am., 68, 1147–1155.

Centers for Disease Control (CDC). 1986a. Guidelines for the Prevention and Control of Nosocomial Infections. Atlanta, CDC.

Centers for Disease Control (CDC). 1986b. National Nosocomial Infection Surveillance, 1984. CDC Surveillance Summaries, 35, 17SS–29SS.

Centers for Disease Control (CDC). 1987. Recommendations for prevention of HIV transmission in health care settings. MMWR, 36, 3s–17s.

Centers for Disease Control (CDC). 1988a. Update: Universal precautions for prevention of transmission of human immunodeficiency virus, hepatitis B virus and other bloodborne pathogens in health-care settings. MMWR, 37, 377–388 (a).

Centers for Disease Control (CDC). 1988b. Management of patients with suspected viral hemorrhagic fever. MMWR, 37 (Suppl. 3), 7–12 (c).

Conly, J.M., Grieves, K., and Peters, B. 1989. A prospective randomized study comparing transparent and dry gauze dressings for central venous catheters. J. Infect. Dis., 159, 310–319.

Cox, C.E. 1988. Nosocomial urinary tract infections. Urology., 32, 210–215.

Cruse, P.J.E., and Ford, R. 1980. The epidemiology of wound infections: a ten-year prospective study of 62,939 wounds. Surg. Clin. North Am., 60, 27–40.

Decker, M.D., and Schaffner, W. 1987. Intravenous therapy: expanding the bounds of safety. (Editorial). JAMA, 258, 2418–2419.

Elson, C.O., Halloi, K., and Balckstone, M.O. 1975. Polymicrobial sepsis following endoscopic retrograde cholangiopancreatography. Gastroenterology, 69, 507–510.

Emori, T.G., Haley, R.W., and Stanley, R.C. 1980. The infection control nurse in U.S. hospitals, 1976–1977: characteristics of the position and its occupant. Am. J. Epidemiol., 111, 592–607.

Favero, M. 1985. Dialysis-associated diseases and their control. In Hospital Infections. 2nd Edition. Edited by J.V. Bennett and P.S. Brachman. Boston, Little Brown, pp. 267–284.

Fels, A.O. 1988. Bacterial and fungal pneumonias. Clin. Chest Med., 9:449–451.

Garibaldi, R.A. 1981. Hospital acquired urinary tract infection. In CRC Handbook of Hospital Acquired Infections. Edited by R.P. Wenzel. Boca Raton, FL, CRC Press, pp. 371–412.

Garner, J.S., and Favero, M.S. 1985. Guideline for handwashing and hospital environmental control, 1985. In Guidelines for the Prevention and Control of Nosocomial Infections. Atlanta, Centers for Disease Control, pp. 4–18.

Garner, J.S. 1985. Guideline for prevention of surgical wound infections, 1985. In Guidelines for the Prevention and Control of Nosocomial Infections. Atlanta, Centers for Disease Control, pp. 1–9.

Garner, J.S., et al. 1988. CDC Definitions for nosocomial infections, 1988. Am. J. Infect. Control, 16, 128–140.

Garner, J.S., and Simmons, B.P. 1983. Guideline for isolation precautions in hospitals. In Guidelines for the Prevention and Control of Nosocomial Infections. Atlanta, Centers for Disease Control, pp. 1–81.

Goldmann, D.A. 1986. Epidemiology of Staphylococcus aureus and group-A streptococci. In Hospital Infections. Edited by J.V. Bennett and P.S. Brachman. Boston, Little, Brown, pp. 483–494.

Gordon, S.M., Tipple, M., Bland, L.A., and Jarvis, W.R. 1988. Pyrogenic reactions associated with the reuse of disposable hollow-fiber dialyzers. JAMA, 260, 2077–2081.

Gross, P.A., and Van Antwerpen, C. 1983. Nosocomial infections and hospital deaths. Am. J. Med., 75, 658–662.

Haley, R.W., and Schachtman, R.H. 1980. The emergence of infection surveillance and control programs in U.S. hospitals: an assessment, 1976. Am. J. Epidemiol., 111, 579–591.

Haley, R.W., et al. 1985a. The efficacy of infection surveillance and control programs in preventing nosocomial infections in U.S. hospitals. Am. J. Epidemiol., 121, 182–205.

Haley, R.W., et al. 1985b. Identifying patients at high risk of SWI: a simple multivariate index of patient susceptibility and wound contamination. Am. J. Epidemiol., *121*, 206–215.

Haley, R.W., et al. 1985c. Update from the SENIC project. Hospital infection control: recent progress and opportunities under prospective payment. Am. J. Infect. Control, *13*, 97–108.

Hamory, B.H. 1987. Nosocomial bloodstream and intravascular device-related infections. In *Prevention and Control of Nosocomial Infections*. Edited by R.P. Wenzel. Baltimore, Williams & Wilkins, pp. 283–319.

Hessen, M.T., and Kaye, D. 1988. Nosocomial pneumonia. Crit. Care Clin., *4*, 245–257.

Horan, T., et al. 1988. Surgical patient surveillance: preliminary NNIS experience with surgical wound infections. Association for Practitioners in Infection Control Annual Conference, Dallas, May 1–6, 1988 (abstr.).

Jarvis, W.R., et al. 1988. Intensive care unit surveillance for nosocomial infections: a national perspective. Association for Practitioners in Infection Control Annual Conference, Dallas, May 1–6, 1988 (abstr.)

Larsen, E.H., Gasser, T.C., and Madsen, P.O. 1986. Antimicrobial prophylaxis in urologic surgery. Urol. Clin. North Am., *13*, 591–604.

Lynch, P., Jackson, M.M., Cummings, M.J., and Stamm, W.E. 1987. Rethinking the role of isolation practices in the prevention of nosocomial infections. Ann. Intern. Med., *107*, 243–246.

Mackoviak, P.A., Martin, R.M., Jones, S.R., and Smith, J.W. 1978. Pharyngeal colonization by gram-negative bacteria in aspiration-prone persons. Arch. Intern. Med., *138*, 1224–1226.

Maki, D.G. 1977. Sepsis arising from extrinsic contamination of the infusion and measures for control. In *Microbiological Hazards of Infusion Therapy*. Edited by I. Phillips. Lancaster, England, MTP Press, pp. 99–141.

Maki, D.G. 1981. Epidemic nosocomial bacteremias. In *CRC Handbook of Hospital Acquired Infections*. Edited by R.P. Wenzel. Boca Raton, FL, CRC Press, pp. 371–512.

Maki, D.G., and Ringer, M. 1987b. Evaluation of dressing regimens for prevention of infection with peripheral intravenous catheters. JAMA, *258*, 2396–2403.

Maki, D.G., Botticelli, J.T., LeRoy, M.L., and Thielke, T.S. 1987a. Prospective study of replacing administration sets for intravenous therapy at 48- vs 72-hour intervals: 72 hours is safe and cost-effective. JAMA, *258*, 1777–1781.

Maki, D.G., et al. 1976. Nationwide epidemics of septicemia caused by contaminated intravenous products: I. Epidemiologic and clinical features. Am. J. Med., *60*, 471–485.

Marcus, R.A. 1988. Surveillance of health care workers exposed to blood from patients infected with the human immunodeficiency virus. N. Engl. J. Med., *319*, 1118–1124.

McGowan, J.E. 1983. Antimicrobial resistance in hospital organisms and its relation to antibiotic use. Rev. Infect. Dis., *5*, 1033.

Mermel, L.A., and Maki, D.G. 1989. Epidemic bloodstream infections from hemodynamic pressure monitoring: signs of the times. Infect. Control Hosp. Epidemiol., *10*, 47–53.

Pemberton, L.B., Lyman, B., Mandal, J., and Covinsky, J. 1984. Outbreak of *Staphylococcus epidermidis* nosocomial infections in patients receiving total parenteral nutrition. JPEN, *8*, 325–326.

Pennington, J.E. 1985. Nosocomial respiratory infection. In *Principles and Practice of Infectious Diseases*. Edited by G.L. Mandell, R.G. Douglas, and J.E. Bennett. New York, John Wiley & Sons.

Pien, F.D., and Bruce, A.E. 1986. Nosocomial *Ewingella americana* bacteremia in an intensive care unit. Arch. Intern. Med., *64*, 403–406.

Platt, R., Polk, B.F., and Murdock, B. 1982. Mortality associated with nosocomial urinary tract infection. N. Engl. J. Med., *307*, 637–641.

Platt, R., Polk, B.F., Murdock, B., and Rosner, B. 1989. Prevention of urinary tract infection: a cost-benefit analysis. Infect. Control Hosp. Epidemiol., *10*, 60–64.

Rhame, F.S., and McCollough, J. 1979. Nosocomial *Pseudomonas cepacia* infection. MMWR, *28*, 289.

Richardson, D.L. 1915. Aseptic fever nursing. Am. J. Nurs., *15*, 1082–1093.

Roberts, J.A. 1988. Role of aztreonam in urinary tract infections. Urology, *31*, 39–44.

Rose, H.D., and Schreier, J. 1968. The effect of hospitalization and antibiotic therapy on the gram-negative fecal flora. Am. J. Med. Sci., *255*, 228–232.

Salzman, T.C., Clark, J.J., and Klemm, L. 1967. Hand contamination of personnel as a mechanism of cross-infection in nosocomial infections. Antimicrob. Agents Chemother., 97–100.

Simmons, B.P. 1982. Guideline for prevention of surgical wound infections. In *Guidelines for the Prevention and Control of Nosocomial Infections*. Atlanta, Centers for Disease Control, pp. 1–9.

Simmons, B.P., and Wong, E.S. 1982. Guideline for prevention of nosocomial pneumonia. In *Guidelines for the Prevention and Control of Nosocomial Infections*. Atlanta, Centers for Disease Control, pp. 1–9.

Simmons, B.P., Hooton, T.M., Wong, E.S., and Allen, J.R. 1981. Guideline for prevention of intravascular infections. In *Guidelines for the Prevention and Control of Nosocomial Infections*. Atlanta, Centers for Disease Control, pp. 1–6.

Sitges-Serra, A., et al. 1983. Hub colonization as the initial step in an outbreak of catheter-related sepsis due to coagulase-negative staphylococci during parenteral nutrition. JPEN, *7*, 569–572.

Snydman, D.R., et al. 1982. Predictive value of surveillance skin cultures in total-parenteral nutrition-related infection. Lancet, *2*, 1385–1388.

Stamm, W.E., Colella, J.J., Anderson, R.L., and Dixon, R.E. 1975. Indwelling arterial catheters as a source of nosocomial bacteremia: an outbreak caused by *Flavobacterium* species. N. Engl. J. Med., *292*, 1099.

Tomford, J.W., et al. 1984. Intravenous therapy team and peripheral venous catheter catheter-associated complications: a prospective controlled study. Arch. Intern. Med., *144*, 1191–1194.

Wenzel, R.P., et al. 1983. Hospital acquired infections in intensive care unit patients: an overview with emphasis on epidemics. Infect. Control, *4*, 371–375.

Williams, W. 1983. CDC guideline for infections control in hospital personnel. In *Guidelines for the Prevention and Control of Nosocomial Infections*. Atlanta, Centers for Disease Control, pp. 1–25.

Williams, W. 1985. Infection control during parenteral nutrition therapy. J. Parenter. Enter. Nutr., *9*, 735–746.

Winston, D.J., Gale, R.P., Mayer, D.V., and Young, L.S. 1979. Infectious complications of human bone marrow transplantation. Medicine, *58*, 1.

Wollschlager, C.M., Conrad, A.R., and Khan, F.A. 1988. Common complications in critically ill patients. DM, *34*, 221–293.

Wong, E.S., and Hooton, T.M. 1981. Guideline for prevention of catheter-associated urinary tract infections. In *Guidelines for the Prevention and Control of Nosocomial Infections*. Atlanta, Centers for Disease Control, pp. 1–5.

CHAPTER 39

STERILIZATION, DISINFECTION, AND ASEPSIS IN DENTISTRY

Chris H. Miller and Charles John Palenik

The practice of dentistry spans a wide variety of oral treatments ranging from the simple polishing of a restoration to complex and extensive surgery of the osseous and soft oral-facial tissues. Standard procedures of sterilization, disinfection, and asepsis must be applied to all types of dental care to reduce the chances of cross-contamination that may lead to serious infectious diseases. Three major pathways for cross-contamination are: (1) patient to dental personnel; (2) dental personnel to patient; and (3) patient to patient. These pathways involve one or more of the three major routes by which microorganisms may be shared between individuals: (1) *direct contact* (touching oral surfaces and fluids); (2) *droplet infection* (airborne contamination with aerosols or splatter of oral and respiratory fluids); and (3) *indirect contact* (contact with contaminated instruments, environmental surfaces or hands). Depending upon the route of microorganism spread, microbes can enter the body through: (1) needlesticks and instrument punctures and cuts; (2) small breaks or cuts in the skin; (3) mucous membranes of the mouth, nose, eyes; (4) through open lesions; (5) inhalation; and (6) ingestion. Thus, the pathways for cross-contamination in dentistry involve numerous possible combinations of routes of microbe spread and entrance into the body, all of which must be addressed in a dental infection control program.

Cross-contamination from patient to the dental team mainly involves microorganisms present in the patient's mouth in saliva, blood, gingival crevice fluid, plaque, subgingival debris, or open lesions. The dental team may be exposed to these microbes through all three routes of spread by directly touching any oral surface, through dental aerosols and body fluid splatter, and by contact with previously contaminated instruments, surfaces, and supplies. In the absence of adequate protective measures, the dental team is exposed to the risk of infection by oral bacteria and bloodborne pathogens present in the patient's mouth. For example, the incidence of hep-

atitis B among dentists is about two to six times greater than that of the general population (Cottone, 1985). Similar increases occur among other health-care professionals who also have frequent exposures to human blood and body fluids that may harbor the virus of hepatitis B.

The risk of exposure to bloodborne pathogens such as hepatitis B and the human immunodeficiency virus for all health-care workers and the need for prevention have been recognized by the United States Centers for Disease Control (CDC, 1986; CDC, 1988b), by professional health-care organizations, including the American Dental Association (ADA, 1978; ADA, 1988a), and most recently by the Occupational Safety and Health Administration (OSHA) of the United States Department of Labor (OSHA, 1987; OSHA, 1989). Guidelines and specific local, state, and federal regulations now exist requiring all health-care facilities to practice specific sterilization, disinfection, and aseptic techniques.

Cross-contamination from a member of the dental team to the patient is a relatively rare event in dentistry that might involve the hands and respiratory fluids of dental personnel. This pathway of disease spread has been documented with case reports of dentist-to-patient transmission of hepatitis B (Cottone, 1985). Because these carrier dentists did not routinely wear gloves during care of the patient, it is assumed that the bloodborne virus periodically contaminated their hands as a result of blood or serum leaking through small cuts or abrasions. The virus was then apparently transferred to patients through a break in their oral mucosa during intraoral care. One instance of possible occupational spread of the human immunodeficiency virus from an infected dentist to a patient recently has been reported by the Centers for Disease Control (CDC, 1990)

Cross-contamination from one patient to another patient may occur by indirect routes through contaminated instruments, surfaces, equipment, or the hands of dental personnel. This pathway, involving improperly washed

Table 39-1. *Dental Instrument Recirculation Process*

1.	Presoak and Rinse	Submerge in detergent-disinfectant until time is available for full cleaning.
2.	Clean, Rinse, and Dry	Use ultrasonic cleaner and detergent. If instruments were used on a known infectious patient, you may heat sterilize first and then clean and proceed with subsequent steps. Clean and sterilize or disinfect nondisposable instrument trays used at chairside.
3.	Package	Add rust inhibitor to nonstainless steel instruments for steam sterilization. Package in proper wrap, bags, pouches, trays, or cassettes. Add spore tests and chemical indicators.
4.	Sterilize	Heat sterilize and process spore tests and check chemical indicators. Record results of monitoring.
5.	Store or Distribute	Sterilized trays, cassettes, or cloth-wrapped packs are ready for storage or use at chairside. Instruments in bags or pouches are properly stored or distributed at chairside on disposable trays, sterile trays, or at least on covered disinfected trays.

hands of a dental hygienist, has been documented in the spread of herpes simplex virus from a herpes labialis lesion of one patient to the mouths of several other patients resulting in herpes gingivostomatitis (Manzella et al., 1984).

The two main approaches to control cross-contamination involve reducing the dose of microorganisms that might be shared between patients and the dental team and increasing the resistance of the dental team through immunization against specific diseases. The infection control procedures in these approaches can be categorized into the seven major areas discussed in this chapter. These are: (1) proper instrument processing; (2) surface and equipment disinfection; (3) barrier techniques; (4) other aseptic techniques; (5) waste disposal; (6) immunization; and (7) laboratory asepsis.

INSTRUMENT PROCESSING

The goal of instrument recirculation is to prevent transfer of infectious agents to patients from contaminated instruments and at the same time to protect the staff who must handle these instruments. The steps in this process involve presoaking, cleaning, packaging, sterilization, monitoring, storage, and distribution, as summarized in Table 39-1.

Instrument Presoaking

If saliva and blood on instruments are allowed to dry, the cleaning process becomes more difficult. This occurrence is not uncommon, for seldom is it possible in a busy practice to clean instruments immediately after use. Thus, contaminated instruments should be presoaked in a detergent-disinfectant until time is available for full cleaning (Runnells, 1987a; Miller, 1989). This

process also is referred to as instrument "holding" and is most effective when it begins right at chairside. Alternatively, the used instruments can be placed in the presoak (holding) solution immediately after the patient is dismissed. This step in instrument recirculation prevents drying of blood and saliva, actually begins the cleaning process, and reduces the level of contamination, which is important when subsequent handling of the instruments occurs. Phenolic detergent-disinfectants work well as a presoak, but other types may be used. Do not hold the instruments in a presoak for more than a few hours, for the longer the instruments remain wet, the greater the chances for corrosion of nonstainless steel metals.

Be sure to wear heavy, puncture-resistant gloves when handling contaminated instruments. Wear heavy gloves and protective eyewear when mixing the presoak solution and when placing instruments into the solution.

If ultrasonic cleaning is used, place the contaminated instruments in the cleaning basket and then place the basket in the presoak solution. This will reduce the direct handling of the contaminated instruments. If one uses "plastic-type" instrument cassettes that retain the instruments during use at chairside and during ultrasonic cleaning, check with the manufacturer of the cassettes on which type of presoak solution to use that will not damage the cassette. After the presoak period, rinse the instruments under running tap water. Even though the presoak solution contains a disinfectant, it should be considered contaminated and should be changed at least once a day and discarded at the end of the day by someone wearing gloves, protective eyewear, and clinic attire.

Instrument Cleaning

The two approaches to instrument cleaning are hand scrubbing and ultrasonic cleaning. Hand scrubbing is directly contrary to one of the dogmas of infection control—reduce direct contact with contaminated surfaces as much as possible. Hand scrubbing increases such contact and involves the added danger of handling sharp and pointed objects (Palenik and Miller, 1980). If an item must be manually scrubbed, then heavy-duty utility gloves and protective eyewear and clinic attire MUST be worn. Splatter or aerosols generated during hand scrubbing must be held to a minimum. Scrubbing should be done in an area away from sterilized instruments, food, or beverages. Scrubbed instruments should be dried before being wrapped or packaged. This is especially valid for items to be sterilized in an unsaturated, chemical vapor sterilizer or dry-heat oven.

Ultrasonic cleaning is effective and is much more safe than hand scrubbing. Cleaners are available in a variety of sizes from several manufacturers and are reasonably priced. Each cleaner should be supplied with a metal cleaning basket, a lid that should be used at all times during operation, and clear instructions for use and care. An ultrasonic cleaning solution that is recommended for use in sonic cleaners should be used. Disinfectants should not be used in place of the cleaning solution. They are not designed for this use, and the heat generated during the cleaning process may inactivate them. The manufacturer's directions must be followed for optimal results.

For ultrasonic cleaning, the rinsed instruments contained in the cleaning basket are submerged into the cleaning solution. The basket suspends the instrument in the tank. Do not place loose instruments on the bottom of the tank, for this usually results in less effective cleaning. Place the lid on the cleaner and operate the unit for 6 to 10 min or until no visible debris remains. If the instruments are to be in cassettes, increase cleaning time to 15 min (Miller and Hardwick, 1988). Cleaning time is not time lost, for other tasks can be performed during this process. After cleaning, thoroughly rinse the instruments while they are still in the cleaning basket to remove dislodged debris, microorganisms, and residual cleaning solution.

If the instruments are to be sterilized in dry heat or in the chemical vapor sterilizer, or if they are to be disinfected in a chemical solution, they should first be dried to reduce chances of corrosion or diluting the disinfecting solution with residual water. Alternatively, for chemical vapor sterilization, the instruments may be dipped into alcohol or the special solution used in the sterilizer. If nonstainless steel instruments are to be sterilized in a steam autoclave, a rust inhibitor (dip or spray) such as sodium nitrite should be applied to the instruments after cleaning.

Ultrasonic cleaners are excellent for cleaning, and some cleaning solutions used may exhibit antimicrobial activity. Nevertheless, ultrasonic cleaners cannot be considered sterilizers. Thus, the cleaned and rinsed instruments must still be considered contaminated, and the used cleaning solution may be contaminated with live microorganisms. Use of the cleaning basket with handles avoids excessive contact with this solution, and rinsing after cleaning reduces this contamination on the instruments. The solution should be changed periodically, at least once a day, by someone wearing gloves and protective eyewear. At the end of the day, disinfect, rinse, and dry the cleaner chamber.

Instrument Packaging

Wrapped Instruments

This approach involves packaging cleaned instruments in an appropriate wrapping material before sterilization. The advantage is protection of the processed instruments from environmental contamination. The instruments may be packaged in functional sets and then opened at chairside, or they may be packaged in smaller groups or individually and distributed on sterile or disposable, or at least cleaned, disinfected trays for use at chairside.

Use a wrapping material that is designed as a sterilization wrap for the type of sterilizer to be used. Avoid thin paper bags. If these are used, sharp and pointed instrument tips will have to be covered to prevent bag puncture. "See-through" bags and pouches facilitate in-strument identification. One type is provided as a clear tubing on a roll that is cut and heat sealed. These are available for steam or dry-heat sterilization. Self-sealing "plastic"/paper pouches are also available for use in the steam autoclave or the chemical vapor sterilizer. A single-layer cloth wrap also may be used for steam sterilization. Sterilization paper wrap may be used for dry-heat sterilization as long as protrusion of sharp instruments is prevented.

Instruments in Trays or Cassettes

One option in this approach involves using a cassette that retains the instruments at chairside and during ultrasonic cleaning, rinsing, and subsequent sterilization (Miller and Hardwick, 1988). This maintains the instruments in functional sets and eliminates potentially dangerous handling of the contaminated instruments during the cleaning or distribution process. Following ultrasonic cleaning and rinsing, sterilizable supply items may be added to the cassette, and the cassette is wrapped, steam sterilized, and stored or used immediately.

The other option in this approach involves placing the cleaned instruments in one of several types of sterilizable trays. Solid-metal trays with lids that need no additional wrapping can be used in standard dry-heat sterilization. "Plastic-type" or metal trays for steam or chemical vapor sterilization must have no lids or be perforated to permit penetration of the steam or chemical vapors. These, like cassettes, must be wrapped before sterilization.

This approach of using sterilizable trays requires sterilizers with adequate chamber size to accommodate the trays. Larger-size office sterilizers are available.

Unwrapped Instruments

This approach involves sterilizing previously cleaned, unpackaged instruments in pans and then distributing them on trays or packaging them in functional sets before use. This approach also is used if instruments are merely disinfected in a solution rather than heat sterilized. *Processing unwrapped instruments is the least satisfactory approach.* It best lends itself to use if the instruments are going to be used immediately after sterilization and if they do not become contaminated with blood or saliva from hands, surfaces, or aerosols before use. Even if the instruments are to be used immediately after sterilization, they should be covered during the "trip" from sterilizer to chairside. In most instances, the sterilized instruments will be arranged on trays in specific setups. During this process, the instruments should be handled aseptically (e.g., with sterilized tongs) and, preferably, be placed on sterilized or disposable or disinfected trays and then covered. Placing the instruments in drawers at chairside is not recommended because the drawers are likely to be contaminated from previous instrument retrieval with saliva-coated fingers. A drawer distribution system of unwrapped instruments at chairside is plagued with great potential for cross-contamination.

Sterilization Versus Disinfection

Sterilization is defined as a process that kills all microorganisms, as verified by demonstrating the kill of bacterial spores (the most resistant of all microorganisms). Sterilization is the highest level of microbial kill. If a process can be routinely shown to kill bacterial spores, then it is correctly assumed that the process can kill all other microorganisms yielding sterilization. Disinfection is considered as a less lethal form of microbial killing usually involving use of a liquid germicide at room temperature. This process is directed at pathogenic microorganisms and is less lethal than sterilization because bacterial spores are not killed. Unfortunately, the level of killing that does occur on instruments submerged in a liquid germicide cannot be easily verified as the solution is used.

On the other hand, the level of killing that occurs in a heat sterilizer can be monitored by routine use of spore tests. Thus, the safest approach to preventing disease transmission by contaminated instruments is to sterilize them (with spore test monitoring) rather than to disinfect them.

The recommendations of the Centers for Disease Control (CDC) for infection control in dentistry state that:

> Surgical and other instruments that normally penetrate soft tissue and/or bone (e.g., forceps, scalpels, bone chisels, scalers, and surgical burs) should be sterilized after each use. Instruments that are not intended to penetrate oral soft tissues or bone (e.g., amalgam condensers, plastic instruments, and burs) but that may come into contact with oral tissues should also be sterilized after each use, if possible; however, if sterilization is not feasible, the latter instruments should receive high-level disinfection (CDC, 1986).

Sterilization Process

In dentistry, the three most commonly used forms of heat sterilization of instruments are: (1) the steam autoclave; (2) the chemical vapor sterilizer; and (3) dry heat. A fourth form of sterilization involves submerging instruments in a properly prepared glutaraldehyde solution for about 6 to 10 hrs; however, this method cannot be verified by spore testing and should be reserved for plastic and other items that melt in the three previously mentioned heat systems. Use of ethylene oxide gas is another method of sterilization that can be verified with spore testing. This method is primarily used in hospitals, some schools, and industry, however, with only minimal use in dental offices.

Microorganisms are killed within a few minutes after they come in direct contact with a heat-sterilizing agent (steam, chemical vapor, air) that is at the proper temperature. Thus, time, temperature, and exposure are the three key factors. The actual surfaces of the instruments must be exposed to the agent for the appropriate time, and the sterilizing agent must be at an appropriate temperature. Anything that interferes with exposure or temperature will prevent the sterilization or will extend the time required for sterilization.

A comparison of the three heat-sterilization methods appears in Table 39–2. Each of the three methods, when performed properly, will yield sterilization. Special care must be taken to follow the sterilizer manufacturer's directions for use and care. Moreover, follow the manufacturer's recommendation for the type of wrapping material to use, and routinely monitor the sterilizing process, as described later.

Steam Autoclave

Steam autoclaves are popular sterilizers in dental offices. A variety of models are available. Minimal features to look for are a temperature gauge independent of the pressure and an automatic timer that begins once the sterilizing temperature has been reached.

Chemiclave

The unsaturated chemical vapor sterilizer is gaining popularity in dental offices because of its noncorrosive form of sterilization. The sterilizing agent is mainly alcohol-formaldehyde vapor that is generated from the special solution added to the sterilizer for each run. Be sure instruments are dry or dipped in the special solution before sterilizing. This keeps the presence of water at a minimum, so the noncorrosive environment can be maintained.

Dry-Heat Ovens

More and more dry-heat ovens are being used in dental offices to sterilize items that may corrode in the steam autoclave. Smaller models are available through dental and scientific supply companies. Be sure the instruments are dry before sterilizing. Care should be taken during use of the dry-heat sterilizer not to open the door until the entire cycle is completed. Opening the door reduces the chamber temperature and requires that the sterilizing cycle be started again.

The newest type of dry-heat sterilizer is called a rapid heat-transfer unit, with claims of sterilization after 6 min at a chamber temperature of 375°F. This short sterilization time is reported to occur only with unwrapped instruments, however.

Sterilization Monitoring

Monitoring the sterilization process is one of the few standard quality-assessment procedures available in infection control. The three forms of monitoring are:

1. Physical monitoring: observation of sterilizer functioning (e.g., time, temperature, pressure).
2. Biologic monitoring: spore testing, the main guarantee of sterilization.
3. Chemical monitoring: color or physical change indicators that monitor exposure to sterilizing agents or conditions.

Proper monitoring involves all three forms and includes keeping records of the results. Physical monitoring consists of observing the gauges on the sterilizer and checking the timer to make sure the unit appears to be working properly. Weekly biologic monitoring (spore

Table 39–2. *Comparison of Heat–Sterilization Methods with Small Office Sterilizers*

Method	Standard Sterilizing Conditions*	Advantages	Precautions	Spore Testing
Steam autoclave	20 min at 250°F (15 psi)	Time efficient Good penetration Sterilization of water-based liquids	Do not use closed containers May damage plastic and rubber items Nonstainless steel metal items corrode Use of hard water may leave deposits	*Bacillus stearothermophilus* strips or vented vials
Unsaturated chemical vapor	20 min at 270°F (20–40 psi)	Time efficient No corrosion Quick drying of items after cycle	Do not use closed containers May damage plastic and rubber items Must use special solution Predry instruments or dip in special solution Ventilation must be adequate Cannot sterilize liquids	*Bacillus stearothermophilus* strips
Standard dry heat	60 min at 320°F	No corrosion Use of closed containers possible Large capacity per cost Items dry after cycle	Longer sterilization time Cannot sterilize liquids May damage plastic and rubber items Do not open door before end of cycle Predry instruments	*Bacillus subtilis* strips

* These conditions do not include warm-up time and may vary depending upon the nature and volume of the load. Sterilizing conditions in your office should be defined by results of routine spore testing.

testing) of dental office sterilizers is recommended by the CDC and American Dental Association (ADA) and is required for all hospital sterilizers (AAMI, 1988; ADA, 1988a). Spore testing should also be performed when changes in sterilizing procedures occur, with use of a new wrapping material or new types of instrument trays, with use of a new sterilizer, with use of a recently repaired sterilizer, and after training of new sterilization personnel (Table 39–3). Spore strips or vials should always be placed inside packages, bags, or trays next to

Table 39–3. *Spore Testing of Small Office Sterilizers*

When	Why
Once per week, PLUS	To verify proper use and functioning
Whenever a new type of packaging material or tray is used	To ensure that the sterilizing agent is getting inside to the surface of the instruments
After training of new sterilization personnel	To verify proper use of the sterilizer
During initial uses of a new sterilizer	To make sure unfamiliar operating instructions are being followed
First run after repair of a sterilizer	To make sure that the sterilizer is functioning properly
With every implantable device and hold device until results of test are known	Extra precaution for sterilization of item to be implanted into tissues
After any other change in the sterilizing procedure	To make sure change does not prevent sterilization

the instruments themselves just before placing the items into the sterilizer. Sterilization-monitoring services that function through the mail are available at a few dental schools and from some companies (ADA, 1988b). Most of these services can test steam autoclaves, chemiclaves, and dry-heat and ethylene oxide sterilizers. Some also provide infection control newsletters, certificates of participation, and an available contact to answer questions about infection control. The necessary supplies and instructions are sent, and the processed spore strips or vials are mailed back for culturing, analysis, and return of a testing report. Alternatively, steam autoclaves can be tested in the office with purchase of spore vials and an appropriate 56°C incubator for culturing. In-office testing of other types of sterilizers is more difficult (Miller, 1987).

Chemical monitoring of dental office sterilizers involves use of color change or other indicators (e.g., autoclave tape, special markings on bags, strips, packets) on the outside and inside of packs, bags, or trays. These indicators are available for all types of sterilizers and give immediate indication that the items have at least been exposed to the sterilizing agent or to sterilizing conditions.

Complete monitoring includes physical monitoring of every load, weekly spore testing, chemical monitoring on the outside of every pack and on the inside of at least one pack of each load, and keeping records of all monitoring.

Instrument Storage

Because of the need for rapid instrument recirculation in most offices, storage of instruments is usually not a problem. Some items that are used less frequently must be stored, however, and this relates to the question, "What is the shelf life of sterilized instruments?"

Unwrapped instruments have no shelf life. They are susceptible to contamination immediately after being removed from the sterilizer or disinfecting solution. The shelf life of sterile, wrapped instruments or instruments in completely closed containers depends upon the integrity of the wrap or container. If the wrap or container is not opened, punctured, or torn and remains sealed and dry, then internal sterility should be maintained indefinitely. Nevertheless, for safety's sake, paper- or cloth-wrapped instruments should be resterilized after 1 mo and plastic-wrapped items after 6 mo.

Care should be taken when handling sterilized packs so the wrapping material is not torn. If packs or trays are stored, the storage area should be dry, out of direct sunlight, away from heat sources, and free of dust (AAMI, 1988). Sterile instruments must be kept completely separated from nonsterilized instruments so there is no chance of intermingling. This is one of the advantages of using an external chemical indicator to identify packages or trays that have been processed through the sterilizer.

SURFACE AND EQUIPMENT DISINFECTION

Surface Contamination

Although epidemiologic evidence for transmission of diseases involving contaminated dental operatory surfaces is weak, such surfaces can become heavily contaminated during care of patients. Use of handpieces, ultrasonic scalers, and air-water syringes generates salivary aerosols and splatter containing microorganisms (Miller et al., 1971; Cochran et al., 1989). The smaller aerosol particles may remain airborne for some time, enhancing the possibility of inhaling microorganisms. The larger splatter droplets hit the skin, lips, and mucous membranes of the nose and eyes or settle rapidly and contaminate nearby operatory surfaces. These surfaces are also contaminated by touching with saliva/blood-coated fingers during care of patients. Although no evidence indicates dental aerosol spread of hepatitis B surface antigen (HBsAg) from HBsAg-positive patients (Petersen et al., 1979), other studies have shown that a variety of inanimate environmental surfaces can become contaminated with hepatitis B virus (HBV) particles (Lauer et al., 1979; Bond et al., 1977). Investigators have theorized that HBV contamination of surfaces may explain instances of disease transmission in the absence of overt percutaneous or mucous membrane exposures (Bond et al., 1977; Francis and Maynard, 1979). This hypothesis is strengthened by the finding that HBV in human plasma can remain infective for at least 1 wk in the dry state at a room temperature of 25°C (Bond et al., 1981).

Thus, operatory surfaces and equipment that are contaminated by touching or by salivary droplets may serve as a potential source of indirect spread of disease agents.

Approaches to Surface Care and Protection

Reducing the spread of disease agents involving contaminated operatory surfaces and equipment involves the

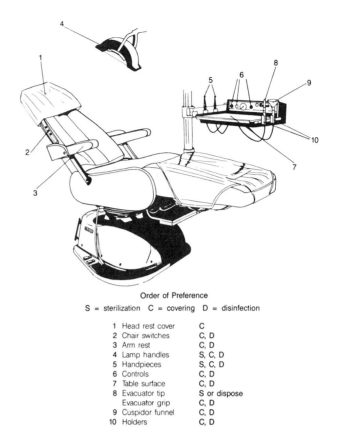

Order of Preference

S = sterilization C = covering D = disinfection

1	Head rest cover	C
2	Chair switches	C, D
3	Arm rest	C, D
4	Lamp handles	S, C, D
5	Handpieces	S, C, D
6	Controls	C, D
7	Table surface	C, D
8	Evacuator tip	S or dispose
	Evacuator grip	C, D
9	Cuspidor funnel	C, D
10	Holders	C, D

Fig. 39–1. Surface components of an operatory and their aseptic care. From Crawford, J.J. 1987, *Clinical Asepsis in Dentistry*, Mesquite, TX, Oral Med Press, p. 33.

following general approaches (Fig. 39–1; Crawford, 1987):

1. Determine which surfaces will be handled or contaminated with salivary droplets during an appointment and which will not.
2. Cover surfaces that may become contaminated, especially those that are difficult to disinfect (chair buttons, control switches, air/water syringe buttons, hoses, light handles).
3. Disinfect uncovered surfaces that become contaminated.

Surface Covers

The most effective and efficient way to prevent cross-contamination via operatory surfaces is to cover them with disposable plastic wrap, plastic sheets or tubing, plastic-backed paper, aluminum foil, or other material impervious to water (Crawford, 1987; Miller and Palenik, 1988b). Replace with fresh covers between each patient. It takes less time to replace the covers than it does to properly clean and disinfect a contaminated surface. It is not necessary to disinfect a properly covered surface between patients unless the cover fails or the surface is accidentally contaminated during cover removal.

Surface Cleaning

Uncovered contaminated surfaces must be precleaned and then disinfected. Because the presence of blood on uncleaned surfaces can reduce or impair germicide activity (Molinari et al., 1988), it is important to follow the CDC guideline to perform thorough cleaning before final disinfection (CDC, 1986). It is best to use a disinfectant cleaner, and this, along with the wearing of heavy-duty gloves, provides protection during cleaning and reduces the chances of spreading contamination to adjacent surfaces during the process (Miller, 1988a). It is also prudent to wear protective eyewear during the mixing and handling of cleaners and disinfectants. Water-based disinfectant solutions that solubilize organic matter (bleach) or those that contain detergents (complex phenolic agents and iodophors) can be used as cleaning agents for removing blood and organic films (Palenik et al., 1983).

Spray the surface with the disinfectant cleaner so the agent contacts the entire surface. If the item being cleaned has an irregular surface (i.e., handpiece), clean with a brush, preferably in the sink. Otherwise, vigorously wipe the sprayed surface with a paper towel or cleaning cloth saturated with the agent. Do not store the paper towel or cleaning cloth in the disinfectant cleaner. Wet it immediately before use. After brushing a handpiece in the sink, rinse with tap water and blot dry with paper toweling. Items with smooth surfaces should be wiped with toweling. These cleaned items are now ready for disinfection.

Surface Disinfection

The chemical nature and properties of liquid disinfectants and sterilants are described elsewhere in this book. Chemicals used for surface disinfection in the dental operatory should be specific for use on surfaces and should be registered with the United States Environmental Protection Agency (EPA) and be tuberculocidal. Such agents that have been accepted by the American Dental Association (ADA, 1988a) are considered to be effective against the relatively low levels of microbes left on dental equipment and surfaces after cleaning (Bond et al., 1983; Martin et al., 1985; Molinari et al., 1988; Rutala, 1989). These germicides that also possess cleaning properties include bleach (diluted 1:10 to 1:100 with water), complex phenols, and iodophors. Follow the manufacturer's directions on product labels, and use at least the minimum disinfection exposure time required for tuberculosis kill (OSAP, 1988).

For disinfection following the precleaning as described previously, reapply the disinfectant cleaner. If the item is to be used in the patient's mouth (e.g., handpiece), let the item remain moist for the appropriate tuberculocidal contact time specified on the label, and remove residual chemical with a water rinse. Other surfaces may be allowed to stand until the disinfectant evaporates or may be wiped dry after the specified contact time.

PROTECTIVE BARRIERS

Prevention of Contamination

The three basic steps in the development of an infectious disease are: (1) contamination (a portion of the body is exposed to microorganisms); (2) infection (the microorganisms survive and grow on or in the body); and (3) disease (growth of the microorganisms cause damage to our body).

Exposure to an infectious disease agent does not always lead to disease. In fact, disease is a rare event because our bodies are continuously bombarded by microorganisms from our environment. Three things determine whether disease develops after exposure: (1) the virulence of the disease agent (how strong are its disease-producing properties?); (2) the dose of the disease agent (how much of the disease agent enters our body?); and (3) the resistance of our body (how efficiently can our body fight off the disease agent?).

In preventing the transmission of infectious diseases in dentistry, little can be done to reduce the virulence of a disease agent that may be brought into the dental office. Increasing the resistance of our bodies to specific disease agents is possible, but only in a few instances through vaccination (e.g., hepatitis B vaccine). Thus, efforts must concentrate on reducing the dose or level of disease agents that might be transmitted to dental patients or to the dental staff.

Preventing or reducing contamination interferes with the initial step in the development of an infectious disease. It is always best to prevent contamination (when possible) than to rely totally upon our body's resistance to a given disease agent. One of the important approaches in attempts to accomplish this is the use of protective barriers such as gloves, eyewear, masks, face shields, and clinic attire to prevent or reduce exposure to potentially infectious materials.

Gloves

Gloves not only protect the hands of dental personnel from direct or indirect contamination by the patient's saliva and blood, but also protect the patient from contamination with microorganisms on the hands of dental personnel.

Gloves must be worn by the dental team where there is the potential to have direct skin contact with blood, other potentially infectious body fluids, mucous membranes, and nonintact skin and when handling items or surfaces soiled with blood or other potentially infectious materials (OSHA, 1989). Disposable gloves must be replaced when torn or punctured or when their ability to function as a barrier is compromised. They must not be washed or disinfected for reuse on another patient. Utility gloves may be cleaned and disinfected for reuse if the integrity of the glove is not compromised, but they should be discarded if they are cracked, peeling, discolored, torn, punctured, or exhibit other signs of deterioration.

Table 39–4 lists the several types of gloves used in

Table 39–4. *Types of Gloves*

Sterile:	Latex surgeon's
	Vinyl
	Latex examination
Nonsterile:	Latex
	Vinyl
	Copolymer
	Plastic (food handler)
	Heavy utility
	Dermal

dentistry (Palenik and Miller, 1988b). The sterile latex surgeon's gloves offer the best fit, with half-sizes and right and left thumb orientation. Nonsterile latex and vinyl examination gloves are adequate for nonsurgical intraoral procedures. Copolymer and the less expensive plastic ("food handlers") gloves have a poor fit, but can serve as an overglove for minor intraoral exams or for preventing the environmental spread of contamination from underlying saliva-coated latex or vinyl gloves. Heavy utility gloves should be worn during operatory cleanup when disinfecting surfaces, handling other chemicals, and handling contaminated instruments. Dermal gloves are made of thin cotton and are used as an underglove to reduce skin irritation from latex or vinyl gloves. Variations on the basic types of gloves include those that are hypoallergenic (powderless), colored, and even flavored.

Wide ranges (0–41%) in the prevalence of perforations (pinholes) in latex examination gloves have been reported with lot-to-lot and intralot variations (Paulssen et al., 1987; Miller, 1988b; Katz et al., 1989; CRA, 1989). The prevalence of perforations increases with intraoral use of both surgeon's and examination gloves, especially after 2 hrs (Otis and Cottone, 1989). Both sterile surgeon's and nonsterile patient-examination gloves are now regulated by the United States Food and Drug Administration (FDA) and are categorized as class I medical devices requiring general controls to ensure their safety and effectiveness (FDA, 1988; FDA, 1989). These recently increased regulations for patient-examination gloves are anticipated to enhance general quality (FDA, 1989). Accepted quality levels in respect to inherent perforations are 4.0 and 2.5% (maximum percentage of gloves with defects) for examination and sterile surgeon's gloves, respectively.

Gloving and Personal Protection

Small cuts and abrasions on the hands and fingers may serve as a route through which pathogenic microorganisms enter the body (Miller and Palenik, 1983; Miller, 1985). A study of 26 second-semester senior dental students who did not routinely wear gloves at chairside revealed a total of 101 areas of trauma (cuts and abrasions) on their hands (Allen and Organ, 1982). Twelve percent of these areas became painful upon swabbing with alcohol, suggesting an open epidermis. Of particular interest was that a few additional alcohol-induced painful responses were detected in visually intact areas between the fingernail and peripheral epidermis, including the subungual area. This indicates that even a close visual inspection of the hands may not detect areas that could serve as a portal of entry for microorganisms into the body.

Wearing gloves provides a physical barrier over such portals of entry for pathogenic organisms from the saliva or blood of dental patients. The lack of routine gloving is likely a major contributing factor to the alarmingly high occurrence of hepatitis B among dental personnel (Cottone, 1985). Like hepatitis B, herpetic whitlow (herpes simplex infection around the fingernails) is also an occupational disease of dental personnel (Rowe et al., 1982; Merchant, 1982; Palenik and Miller, 1982). Gloving prevents the occurrence of herpes simplex infections on the fingers acquired through direct contact with lesions or contaminated saliva.

Another personal-protection aspect of wearing gloves involves providing a barrier against contact with contaminated inanimate objects or with irritating chemicals used in the office. For example, office staff responsible for post-treatment operatory cleanup or use of disinfecting or sterilizing solutions should wear heavy rubber gloves. This reduces chances of accidental instrument puncture or direct contact with agents that may cause skin irritations or allergic reactions.

Handwashing and Gloving for Protection of Patients

Besides offering personal protection to members of the dental team, gloves also provide an important measure of protection to patients. Hands have long been known to be one of the most important sources of nosocomial infection, and handwashing is generally considered the single most important procedure for preventing such infections (Steere and Mallison, 1975; Palenik and Miller, 1981; Simmons, 1983). Surgical hand scrubbing is a standard procedure, but handwashing should also be performed before routine nonsterile gloving to reduce the number of skin microbes that multiply under the gloves and cause skin irritation. Recognized antiseptic handwashing agents that have residual activity on the skin (long-lasting effect) contain chlorhexidine gluconate or parachlorometaxylenol (Larson, 1988).

Although proper handwashing can remove the transient skin flora that usually contains potential pathogens, no handwashing procedure sterilizes the skin, not even properly performed surgical scrubs with antiseptic agents (Crawford et al., 1974; Gross et al., 1979). Thus, sterile gloving is used to prevent transmission of organisms not removed by handwashing.

Ungloved hands of dental personnel become contaminated with potentially infectious materials from patients' mouths. Blood impaction under the fingernails does occur, and this material may be retained for several days after treating a patient (Allen and Organ, 1982). This occult blood could serve as a source of infection for subsequent patients through a leaching process. Routine gloving would prevent blood or saliva impaction in those parts of the hands that are difficult to clean, such as under the fingernail or areas of dermatitis.

Microorganisms that might be present in the blood periodically contaminate the hands and fingers as a result of blood or serum leaking through small cuts or abrasions. This process may be enhanced if the site of the cut or abrasion is kept moist, as when performing bare-handed dentistry. This seems to be a likely route of hepatitis B virus transmission from carrier dentists to their patients.

The eight reported instances of hepatitis B virus transmission from dental personnel to patients has resulted in numerous cases of the disease (Cottone, 1985; Kane and Lettau, 1985; CDC, 1985a). Most of the implicated dental personnel acquired subclinical infections and became chronic carriers of the virus, none had worn gloves, and some had skin lesions or dermatitis on their hands. Although intact gloves would protect patients from this route of disease transmission, other routes of disease transmission from carrier dental personnel to patients clearly do exist.

The report of an outbreak of herpes simplex virus type I gingivostomatitis in a dental hygiene practice also offers a vivid line of evidence for the role of contaminated hands in disease transmission (Manzella et al., 1984). A hygienist with dermatitis on her ungloved hands contracted a herpes infection after treating a patient with active herpes labialis. Before vesicles developed in the areas of chronic dermatitis on her hands, she unknowingly transmitted the virus to other patients, resulting in gingivostomatosis in 20 of 46 patients treated over the next few days with ungloved hands.

Masks

Masks covering the mouth and nose were originally developed for the protection of the patient from respiratory organisms of health-care personnel. This is an important reason to use masks in dentistry, but equally important in dentistry is that masks protect the dental staff from the patient's microorganisms. They reduce the number of infectious particles that may enter the mouth or nose while one performs techniques that generate dental aerosols or splatter. Masks made of glass fiber or synthetic fiber mats appear to be more efficient in filtering bacteria than gauze or paper masks (Micik et al., 1971).

Surgical masks are available that claim at least a 98% bacterial filtration efficiency against particles that are 3 to 5 μm in diameter as determined by the modified Greene and Vesley method (Greene and Vesley, 1961). The filterability of any mask is destroyed if the mask does not fit well, however; this permits excessive contaminated air to leak around the edges of the mask (Pippin et al., 1987). A key feature of a mask is that it must be comfortable to wear, and for those who wear glasses, the mask should fit snugly over the bridge of the nose to reduce fogging of the glasses from exhaled air.

Masks are single-use disposable items and should not be reused with another patient and should be changed when wet.

Protective Glasses

Protective eyewear can reduce the chance of physical and microbial injury to the eyes (Palenik, 1981). Microorganisms may contact the eye by aerosol spray or droplet deposition. Tooth or restorative material expelled from the mouth also may be contaminated with potentially pathogenic microorganisms.

Usually, the eye eliminates transient infections, but if the contamination is heavy, if a highly virulent organism is involved, or if physical damage accompanies the contamination, serious disease may result. Of particular concern would be a herpes virus infection of the eye that may recur and produce more and more ocular damage. Hepatitis B may also develop after initial contamination of the eye with the virus (Kew, 1973; Bond et al., 1982).

Review of a report of 10 cases of ocular injuries sustained in dental offices demonstrates a compelling need for protective eyewear for both patients and dental personnel (Hales, 1970). The cases included impalement of a patient's eye by an excavator; corneal abrasions in patients from an exploding anesthetic carpule or a piece of acrylic denture tooth; subconjunctival hemorrhage after a dentist hit a patient's eye with his thumb; corneal abrasions and hemorrhage in dental assistants' eyes by projectiles emitted from patients' mouths during operative procedures; and damage to an assistant after splashing varnish into her eyes while working in the laboratory.

Protective eyewear should be worn at chairside, in the laboratory, in darkrooms, and in the sterilization area when mixing chemicals.

Face Shields

Plastic face shields have recently become more popular for use at chairside during procedures that generate salivary droplets. Face shields protect the skin, eyes, and mucous membranes of the mouth and nose from potentially infectious droplets, but offer little protection from inhalation of aerosols.

Clinic Attire

Dental procedures that generate salivary splatter contaminate clothing worn at chairside. Street clothes can be protected by fluid-resistant gowns. Clinic attire worn at work should be changed before leaving for home. Long-sleeve, disposable tops or short-sleeve, reusable tops appear to be the most appropriate. Those who wear long-sleeve garments at chairside must remember that aerosols and splatter contaminate the sleeves, which will come into close proximity to subsequent patients. Moreover, handwashing procedures between patients are hindered by long sleeves. Short-sleeve clinic attire permits washing of the forearms.

If a laundry service is not used and clinic attire is laundered at home, use bleach, detergent, and hot wash water whenever possible.

As a related precaution, keep your workshoes at work or at least out of reach of small children at home, because at work your shoes are constantly in contact with salivary splatter that rapidly settles to the floor.

ASEPTIC TECHNIQUES

Disposable Items

More and more disposable items are becoming available for use in dental care. From the point of view of infection control, a disposable item (defined as an item to be used once or only on one patient and then discarded) has major advantages in preventing disease transmission. Disposal of the item after use on one patient prevents transfer of microbes to another patient. The best-known example is the sterile disposable needle. Others include saliva ejector and high-volume evacuation tips, impression trays, prophy cups, brushes, surgical and examination gloves, and more recently, dental instruments, prophy angles, and light handle attachments.

Always use disposable needles and discard them properly after use on a single patient. Use other disposable items whenever possible, but compare their cost to that of using the nondisposable item. Take into consideration the frequency of item use and the labor dollars and any supplies required to properly prepare the reusable item for the next patient. This would include time needed to properly clean, package, and sterilize the item before reuse. Once you decide upon a disposable item versus a reusable item, do not try to save money and reuse the disposable item. Disposable items for patient care are not designed for reuse. In fact, the FDA states that you are liable for any problem that may develop from reuse of an item manufactured as disposable. Disposable patient-care items are always difficult or impossible to clean properly and are frequently damaged by cleaning agents and/or sterilization procedures.

Packaging and Dispensing

Aseptic storage and dispensing of supplies and instruments are difficult areas to control. The goal is to protect these items from contamination. Packaging of instruments in covered trays or sterilization bags or wraps after cleaning, but before sterilization, prevents their subsequent contamination, as described earlier. Packaging or dispensing instruments on trays or in drawers after sterilization permits contamination before use on the next patient. Storing previously sterilized or disinfected, unprotected instruments in a drawer at chairside results in contamination every time the drawer is opened and saliva-coated fingers are used to retrieve an instrument. Instruments should be cleaned, arranged in functional sets for use on a single patient, then packaged and sterilized.

Some manufacturers of dental supply-type items are beginning to package these items in unit doses for use on a single patient; however, many items are still bulk packaged, a method that increases the chances of contaminating many items in the package when one attempts to retrieve just one with saliva-coated fingers. The solution is to repackage in unit doses or devise an aseptic technique using forceps to retrieve a unit dose from the bulk package. If supplies must be stored near chairside, prevent their contamination from dental aerosols and splatter by storing them behind the patient or in drawers. Supply containers or drawer handles that are touched during care of patients must be covered or cleaned and disinfected between patients.

Limiting Surface Contamination

If an operatory surface is not contaminated during care of patients, then that surface need not be disinfected between patients. The fewer surfaces that must be disinfected between patients, the less time required for operatory cleanup. Contamination may occur by dental aerosols or splatter and by touching with saliva/blood-coated fingers or contact with contaminated items. Gloves used for care of patients are contaminated, and that contamination will be transferred to any surface touched by those gloves (e.g., switches, pens, charts, doorknobs, telephones, drawer knobs, cabinet handles, supply containers, unit surfaces, chairbacks).

Make every effort to dispense *all* items needed at chairside before the patient is seated. This includes placement of disposable surface covers as described earlier. Touch as few surfaces as possible with saliva/blood-coated fingers during care of patients. If possible, have an uninvolved person retrieve items needed unexpectedly. Have disposable plastic sheets or inexpensive plastic overlay (food handlers) gloves available to protect an uncovered surface that must be touched.

Preprocedure Mouthrinse

The application of Food and Drug Administration (FDA)-approved antiseptic agents to skin or mucous membranes before surgery or needle injection has been practiced for many years. The objective of this procedure is to reduce the number of microbes at the surgical site or needle injection site and to prevent entry of our body microbes into underlying tissues that may cause bacteremias, septicemias, or surgical site infections. These procedures reduce the chances of an autogenous infection (caused by our own microbes). The principle of these procedures is applied to reducing the spread of oral microbes to others. Use of a preprocedure, antiseptic mouthrinse approved for use in the mouth by the FDA reduces the number of oral microbes available for spread through aerosols, splatter, or direct contact (Litsky et al., 1970; Muir et al., 1978). Unfortunately, unless the antimicrobial agent has substantivity (residual or long-lasting activity), the microbes usually return to their original levels shortly after mouthrinsing long before most dental procedures are completed.

One agent appropriate for use as a preprocedure mouthrinse or subgingival irrigant is the bisbiguanide chlorhexidine. It has a broad spectrum of oral antimicrobial activity including activity against viruses and yeasts (Hennessey, 1973; Briner et al., 1986; Bernstein et al., 1988; Oosterwaal et al., 1989). It has been referred to as a "second-generation" antimicrobial agent because it has the property of substantivity that allows the agent to bind to and be slowly released from oral surfaces to provide an extended microbial kill (Kornman, 1986).

Reduction of Contaminated Dental Aerosols

Use of the rubber dam during dental procedures that generate salivary aerosols and splatter reduces the number of oral bacteria that are sprayed into the environment (Stevens, 1963; Cochran et al., 1989). The percentage of reduction in bacterial counts with use of the rubber dam can approach 100%, depending upon the type and site of the intraoral procedure and the environmental site of microbial sampling. The use of high-volume evacuation during operative procedures also reduces the production of both splatter and aerosols, but without simultaneous use of the rubber dam, this still permits the generation of considerable contamination (Cochran et al., 1989).

Handpiece Asepsis

Handpieces and dental-unit water lines can be microbially contaminated. This occurs through aspiration of oral fluids into the water-line by the action of a retraction valve in the line and by contamination from the unit water source (Gross et al., 1976; Bogga et al., 1984). Unless properly decontaminated, handpieces can serve as a source of cross-contamination, even if the outer surfaces have been properly disinfected. Handpieces should be sterilized between use on patients. Antiretraction valves should be added to the lines to reduce aspiration of oral fluids, and the handpiece and air/water syringe lines should be flushed into the sink before each use (Palenik and Miller, 1983; Scheid et al., 1982).

IMMUNIZATIONS FOR DENTAL PERSONNEL

Dental personnel are exposed daily in their offices, clinics, and laboratories to a variety of communicable diseases. Personal physical barriers, such as gowns, gloves, masks, and protective eyewear, help to prevent many cross-infections. Immunizations when available are the best methods for the prevention of disease, however. Maintenance of immunity is an essential part of any effective infection control program.

Topics reviewed in depth include immunization against hepatitis B, tetanus, influenza, and tuberculosis.

Hepatitis B

The Centers for Disease Control (CDC), (1989a) estimate that over 12,000 health-care workers occupationally acquire hepatitis B virus (HBV) annually. Of this group, 500 to 600 require hospitalization, whereas 700 to 1200 become chronic carriers. Chronicity increases dramatically the chances for transmission of HBV over extended intervals, for cirrhosis, for delta virus hepatitis, and for the development of primary hepatocellular carcinoma (Beasley and Hwang, 1984; Beasley et al., 1981). Out of the 12,000 health-care workers infected, about 250 will die (12 to 15 immediately of fulminant hepatitis and later 170 to 200 of cirrhosis and 40 to 50 of liver cancer).

Hepatitis B is a major occupational hazard for dental personnel, with attack rates among unvaccinated indi-

Table 39–5. *Prevalence of Hepatitis B Surface Antigen (HBsAg) Markers* in Selected Populations of American Dental Personnel*

Classification	Percent Positive (%)
Oral surgeon	18–30
Endodontist	9
Surgical specialist†	14
General practitioner	7–16
Periodontist	9.1
Dental hygienist	13–16.9
Dental assistant	12.9
Dental technologist	14.2
Office clerical worker	8.9
General population	3–5

* HBsAg and/or anti-HBsAg.

† Group included endodontists, oral surgeons, and periodontists.

Modified from Palenik, C.J., and Miller, C.H. 1987. Gloves and the practice of dentistry. Part I. A statement of need. J. Indiana Dent. Assoc., 66, 7–11.

viduals 3 to 10 times the 4% rate present in the general population (see Table 39–5). Hepatitis B is an especially difficult problem because many dental workers have repeated intimate contact with patient's body fluids and with items soiled with such fluids. HBV infection appears to be related more to the extent of exposure to blood than to the number or type of patients treated (CDC, 1987). The CDC (1989b) recommend that any health-care worker who is exposed to blood or blood-contaminated fluids on at least a monthly basis should be vaccinated.

The best protection against HBV acquisition is active immunization. Currently, three hepatitis B vaccines, Heptavax-B (plasma derived) or Recombivax-HB and Energix-B (yeast recombinant products) are commercially available in the United States. The most common vaccine regimen consists of doses given at 0-, 1-, and 6-month intervals. Current information indicates that the yeast-derived particles are immunologically equivalent to the plasma-derived hepatitis B surface antigen (HBsAg) (CDC, 1987; Zajac et al., 1986).

Injections administered intramuscularly in the deltoid muscle have produced seroconversion rates up to 95% in immunocompetent, seronegative individuals. Lower rates of protective antibody formation have been noted in persons over 40 yrs of age and among individuals who received their injections in the buttocks (as low as 70% seroconversion). Recent studies, however, indicate that genetic factors may significantly influence seroconversion rates (Williams, 1989; Keys, 1989). Complete protection against HBV includes postscreening for antibody levels (Palenik and Miller, 1988c). This procedure should be conducted 1 to 3 mos after the final injection. If seroconversion occurs after vaccination, protective levels of antibodies have been shown to persist for 7 yrs (CDC, 1989a).

Compliance with HBV vaccination among health-care workers has to be considered modest at best. Concerns expressed have included vaccine safety, cost, efficacy, pregnancy-related issues, lack of information on the vaccine, and perception of oneself to be at low risk. Hospital studies indicate vaccination levels improve when the series is paid for by the employer (Anderson and Hodges, 1983; DiAngelis et al., 1989). National studies show that dentists (about 60%) have the highest rate of vaccination among health-care workers (Verrusio et al., 1989). A recent survey of Indiana dental hygienists reported a vaccination level of 59.6% (Palenik et al., 1989).

In spite of the presence of proved occupational risk and the availability of safe and effective vaccines, only an estimated 30% of at-risk health-care workers have been vaccinated (CDC, 1987; Williams, 1989; Keys, 1989).

Tetanus

Tetanus (lockjaw) is a severe disease with a high case-fatality ratio. It can be an infectious complication of cuts and/or puncture wounds and is caused by the toxins of *Clostridium tetani*. Because tetanus endospores are continually present in the environment and because they are resistant to disinfection procedures, dental personnel must make an overt effort to control their spread. Also essential in the preventive process is the meticulous handling of all skin wounds and the monitoring of one's immune status (Palenik and Miller, 1988d).

Innate immunity to tetanus does not seem to exist in humans, nor does infection produce immunity to future attack; however, tetanus is a totally preventable disease. Absorbed tetanus toxoid (inactivated, but immunogenic) is the BEST prevention measure. Primary immunization usually begins as a neonate and consists of 3 injections given over a 1-yr period. Additional injections are given at 2 and 6 yrs of age. Commonly, tetanus toxoid is administered with diphtheria toxoid and the pertussis vaccine (DPT) to children. The CDC (1984, 1985b) currently recommend a tetanus booster every 10 yrs if there have not been any significant or suspicious wounds. A booster is appropriate for most minor (promptly cleaned, non-tetanus-prone) wounds if the last injection was over 5 yrs ago. Severe, neglected, or tetanus-prone wounds (those unclean defects contaminated with dead tissues and foreign materials that can support anaerobic growth) require immunization if the last booster was given more than 1 yr previously. It is wise to have all major wounds and any suspicious minor wounds professionally cleaned and treated and to have your immune status reviewed by a physician.

Influenza

Options for the control of influenza include chemoprophylaxis and/or therapy and vaccination. Antiviral drugs available are effective only against influenza A and are 70 to 90% effective in preventing illness. They also reduce the severity of symptoms when given after the onset of the disease. The use of drugs is not a substitute for vaccination. Vaccination of high-risk persons (being 65 yrs and older or having a chronic pulmonary, cardiovascular, or metabolic disease) each year before the influenza season is the single most important measure for reducing the impact of influenza (CDC, 1988a). Influenza vaccines are formulated of formaldehyde-inactivated influenza A and B viruses. The composition changes each year, to contain the viruses thought to be the "flu" season's predominant pathogens.

The CDC's Division of Immunization (1989b) has indicated that medical/dental staff illnesses (and absenteeism) during the influenza season could be reduced if all parties were immunized each fall. Vaccination would not only diminish spread within a dental work environment, but also would decrease the chances of transmission to patients and within employees' homes.

Tuberculosis

The risk for occupational acquisition of tuberculosis (TB) infection is low; however, transmission to practitioners in a primary-care medical clinic has been recently demonstrated (CDC, 1989c). The clinic offered extensive respiratory therapy to TB, AIDS, and TB/AIDS patients. Moreover, the clinic's ventilation system and separation of treatment areas were found to be inadequate.

The chances of transmission can be reduced by regular personal surveillance (and if positive, then promptly treated), the use of proper sterilization/disinfection methods, and the implementation of personal barrier precautions. At-risk dental personnel can be monitored for exposure by periodic tuberculin skin tests. The two-step Mantoux test appears to be the method of choice. Current guidelines recommend that health-care workers be tested at the start of their employment. The frequency of retesting is influenced by local TB levels and the number of exposures to known cases. Formulation of a skin-testing program should be made in consultation with a physician (Williams, 1989; Keys, 1989).

Immunization of health-care workers with the bacille Calmette-Guérin (BCG) vaccine is NO longer recommended. The effectiveness of the vaccine has long been a point of debate. In addition, confusion of Mantoux test results can occur when a vaccinated individual is investigated after a known exposure to TB.

Risk of Missed Opportunities

Immunization programs have been extremely successful in the prevention of diseases among children. Most of us are not aware of the continuing need for vaccinations during adulthood, however. An important percentage of vaccine-preventable disease occurs today in the adult population. Anyone who passes through childhood without immunization or infection is at risk. Many diseases are considerably more severe when contracted as an adult. The occupation and/or social behavior of adults also increase the chances of disease acquisition (Williams et al., 1988).

In addition to immunization against influenza, tetanus, and hepatitis B, dental personnel should discuss with their primary health-care provider their immune status to other vaccine-preventable diseases. These include pneumococcal pneumonia, measles, rubella, mumps, and poliomyelitis (CDC, 1989b).

LABORATORY ASEPSIS

Dental impressions and orally worn appliances can easily become contaminated with a patient's blood and saliva. Such fluids can contain overt pathogens, including the viral agents associated with hepatitis B, herpes simplex, and AIDS. Some of the microbes present can exist for extended periods outside their human hosts. Improper handling of such items offers the definite opportunity for cross-infection. Likewise, fabricated or repaired prostheses can become soiled with microorganisms of environmental or operator origin (ADA, 1988a; Merchant and Molinari, 1987; Palenik and Miller, 1988b).

As in the case of clinical dental asepsis, the zealous use of sterilization, disinfection, personal barrier techniques, and immunizations will dramatically reduce the chances of disease transmission.

Infection control procedures initially affect productivity; however, the potential risk to individuals working in the laboratory far exceeds the modest expense in time and materials associated with the process. It is expected that after a short acclimation period, efficiency will rise.

Pathways for Infection in the Dental Laboratory

Any item that has been used in the oral cavity or any item used on appliances or impressions is a potential source of infection. It is impossible to determine all highly infectious patients from medical histories and from conversations. Therefore, the only valid posture is to assume (and to act as if) all patients are highly infectious (ADA, 1985, 1988; CDC, 1989). The same sets of criteria and techniques must be used for all patients.

All items coming from the oral cavity must be sterilized or disinfected before being worked upon in the laboratory (ADA, 1985, 1988a; Miller and Palenik, 1988a). Procedures for each type of material vary, but they must be zealously used for each case. Laboratory infection control also involves the routine wearing of gloves and protective eyewear and, when necessary, masks.

If a contaminated item were to enter the laboratory, the chance exists that infectious materials could be spread to the prostheses or appliances of other patients. Unsuspecting laboratory personnel would also be at risk. In addition, a worker with an undetected disease could also serve as a source of infection. One way to minimize the effect of "internal contamination" is to isolate each case as best as possible. Selected amounts of necessary materials, such as pumice, must be segregated from large, common-source containers. This prevents the contamination of centrally stored materials. Small pieces of equipment (i.e., burs and stones and materials used to finish a case such as rouge and pumice) must either be sterilized or considered to be single-use, disposable items. Larger mechanical pieces of equipment, such as a lathe, must be disinfected routinely. Use of gloves,

masks, protective eyewear, and ventilation systems will enhance personnel protection.

Items that have been repaired or made in the laboratory must not be placed back into the patient's oral cavity without first being sterilized or disinfected. Such materials can easily become soiled during processing and thus could cause infection.

Infectious Disease Warnings Policy

Identifying Highly Infectious Patients

An integral part of an effective infection control program is the identification of highly infectious patients. Such categorizations are not intended to deny service, but rather to bring to the attention of the practitioner special medical concerns associated with such individuals. However, the variety of appliances or prostheses offered to such patients may be restricted or deferred (Palenik and Miller, 1985; Runnells, 1988; Verrusio et al., 1989).

Special Procedures for Highly Infectious Patients

All orally soiled sterilizable instruments and pieces of equipment must be placed in biohazard bags before being returned for processing. Disposable items are to be placed in separate bags and sealed before disposal. Disinfection procedures for environmental surfaces should be extremely thorough. Impressions and/or removed appliances must be disinfected before leaving the operatory area. As with all patients, appliances or prostheses must be disinfected before being returned to the patient. Reusable personal barriers, such as protective eyewear, should also be disinfected (ADA, 1988a; CDC, 1989a).

Personal Protection Policies

Personal Barriers

Gloves must be worn when handling all impressions and orally soiled appliances until they have been properly disinfected. Masks must be worn whenever rotary equipment (handpieces, lathes, etc.) or blast-cleaning machines are used. Protective eyewear must be worn whenever laboratory work is performed. Safety glasses with side shields afford the greatest protection.

The risks of eye injury in the dental laboratory are disturbingly high. Projectiles and aerosols generated by rotary equipment, blast-cleaning machines, high temperatures, heated waxes, molten metals, and strong acids and bases are all potentially hazardous. Fortunately, most eye injuries are minor, but a career-ending episode cannot be discounted. The chances of eye injury decrease dramatically with the routine use of protective eyewear (ADA, 1988a; Reis, 1986; Palenik, 1981).

Handwashing and Personal Hygiene

Hands must be washed whenever handling clinical case materials. Even though laboratory items are to be sterilized when possible or disinfected, the value of routine proper handwashing cannot be discounted (Guest and Cottone, 1987; ADA, 1988a). Clothing worn into the laboratory can become soiled with a variety of liquids and solid materials (Francis et al., 1981; Crawford, 1985). As with clothes worn in the clinic, special care should be extended to their cleaning. Laboratory clothing should be professionally laundered. When this is not possible, use high-temperature wash water and bleach. Shoes are underappreciated sources of cross-infection. It is best to have "work shoes." This would be a pair of comfortable shoes used only in clinics and laboratories. Hair, especially facial hair, is a proved mode of viral transmission. Rotary equipment can produce copious amounts of aerosols and particulate matter that can settle on hair. Although headcovers are not routinely advocated, daily shampooing is strongly encouraged, especially when returning home (ADA, 1988a; CDC, 1989a; Miller and Palenik, 1988a).

Work-Station Policy

All orally soiled items must be either sterilized or disinfected before they enter the laboratory. The process must be repeated when returning the items to the patient. Zealous use of this "double-disinfection" procedure greatly reduces the chances of cross-infection for both operator and patient. Because of their communal-use nature, all users of a dental laboratory must respect the rights and safety of other users (Miller and Palenik, 1988a).

Infection Control Procedures for the Fabrication and Repair of Prostheses and Appliances

Dental Impressions

Impressions easily become soiled with patients' blood, saliva, and plaque. Such contaminants contain the infectious agents of a variety of overt viral, bacterial, and fungal pathogens. Such microorganisms can be easily transferred to the skin or hair of the operator, to the instruments and pieces of equipment used, and to the general physical environment. Passage to the resultant stone casts has been demonstrated (Leung and Schonfeld, 1983). Obviously, without some special handling precautions and treatments, the chances of cross-infection are higher (ADA, 1985, 1988a; Palenik, 1981).

Gloves must be worn when handling orally soiled impressions until they have been properly disinfected. Masks and protective eyewear minimize exposure to chemical disinfecting agents and protect against aerosols and projectiles produced by rotary equipment (handpieces, lathes, etc.). Clinical or laboratory gowns/uniforms shield the operator, but they should be either professionally laundered or disposable.

The best way to deal with the problem of impression decontamination is chairside disinfection (ADA, 1985, 1988a; Runnells, 1988). Impressions are rinsed with tap water upon removal and then are placed into covered glass beakers or plastic jars or into zip-lock plastic bags that contain an appropriate disinfecting solution. After

10 to 15 min, the impression is removed and rinsed with tap water. The impression is ready for pouring. The disinfectant solution can be used only once. An alternative (and probably a less effective method) is to completely spray the impression after the initial water rinse. The impression is then wrapped in a paper towel moistened with disinfectant and is sealed in a zip-lock plastic bag. Exposure after spraying is also 10 to 15 min. It is important that the paper towel be kept moist. After treatment, the impression is rinsed well and is then ready to be poured (Miller and Palenik, 1988a).

Impression disinfection is an area of current research. Some impression materials are difficult to disinfect without physical damage, thus compromising their replication value. Moreover, the same type of impression material from different manufacturers reacts individually to the same disinfectant. Therefore, it is extremely important to select liquid agents that are compatible with a given impression material. A list of disinfectant-impression combinations appears in Table 39–6.

Some sources indicate that stone casts should also be treated (Palenik and Miller, 1988b; Merchant and Molinari, 1987). One possibility is to spray the casts with a disinfectant solution. Other suggestions are to expose the casts to ultraviolet light or autoclaving. Adding a disinfectant to the mixing fluid has also been advocated. One commercially available stone product has incorporated a disinfectant into the powder. The antimicrobial benefit (and lack of adverse reactions) of such processes has not been established. Therefore, no recommendation currently can be made.

Handling Orally Soiled Prostheses and Appliances

Most prostheses and appliances cannot withstand standard heat-sterilization procedures. The alternative is disinfection by immersion (ADA, 1988a; Runnells, 1987b, 1988).

After an item is removed from the oral cavity and is ready to be taken to the laboratory, it is rinsed well with tap water and is placed in a zip-lock plastic bag or glass beaker that contains an appropriate disinfecting solution (Table 39–7). After 10 to 15 min of immersion, the item is removed and rinsed well with tap water.

Some items may require cleaning prior to disinfection. WARNING: such debridement must be accomplished as best as possible chairside with the use of hand instruments and/or an ultrasonic cleaner. This is done by placing the item into a disinfectant-filled zip-lock bag or glass beaker and ultrasonically cleaning for 3 to 10 min. In some cases the disinfectant may have to be replaced by a special type of ultrasonic cleaning solution. Ultrasonic solutions, like disinfectants, may be used only once. Mechanical shell blasters may be used only on disinfected items (Miller and Palenik, 1988a; Palenik, 1981).

Grinding and Polishing

Laboratory work on impressions, appliances, and prostheses should only be performed on disinfected items. Bringing untreated materials into the laboratory estab-

Table 39–6. *Disinfecting Dental Impression Materials*

Impression Material†	Disinfectants*		
	Glutaraldehydes	Iodophors	Sodium Hypochlorite
Alginates‡	NO	YES	YES
Polysulfides	YES	YES	YES
Silicones	YES	YES	YES
Polyethers§	NO	NO	YES
Hydrocolloid‖	NO	YES	YES
Compound‖	NO	?	YES

*Solutions prepared according to manufacturers' recommendations for surface or immersion disinfection; WARNING: compatibilities of a disinfectant type with a given type of impression material vary per manufacturer.

†WARNING: Similar products from different manufacturers vary in their response to a given type of disinfectant.

‡If adverse response occurs, use a shorter immersion interval or spray impression well and place into a sealed plastic bag; combination synthetic phenolic compounds are acceptable for spraying of most types of impressions.

§Polyethers are unusually sensitive to immersion; if adverse response occurs, use a disinfectant with a shorter immersion interval (2–3 min), such as chlorine dioxide, or spray impression well with an acidic or alkaline glutaraldehyde and place into a sealed plastic bag.

‖Insufficient data currently available to make a recommendation.

Data from ADA. 1985. Guidelines for infection control in the office and the commercial dental laboratory. J. Am. Dent. Assoc., *110*, 969–972; ADA. 1988a. Johnson, G.H., Drennon, D.G., and Powell, G.L. 1988. Accuracy of elastomeric impressions disinfected by immersion. J. Am. Dent. Assoc., *166*, 525–530; Minagi, S., Fukushima, K., and Maeda, N. 1986. Disinfection method for impression materials. J. Prosthodont. Dent., *56*, 451; Miller, C.H., and Palenik, D.J. 1988. *Indiana University School of Dentistry Infection Control Manual*. Indianapolis, Indiana University, pp. II–19–26; Palenik, C.J., and Miller, C.H. 1989. Laboratory asepsis: disinfection of impression materials. Dent. Asepsis Rev., *10*, 1–2.

lishes the potential for cross-infection (ADA, 1988a; Miller and Palenik, 1988a; Runnells, 1988).

Burs and Stones. All burs and stones used in the laboratory must be sterilized prior to use and may be used only on a single patient before being sterilized again.

Dental Lathes and Ventilation. Operating a dental lathe provides an opportunity for both the spread of infection and for injury. The rotary action of the wheels, stones, and bands generates aerosols, splatter, and projectiles. Whenever the lathe is used, protective eyewear must be in place, the front Plexiglas shield must be down, and the ventilation system must be operating. The use of a mask is highly recommended. The air-suction motor should be capable of producing an air velocity of at least 200 ft/min. Maximum containment of aerosols and splat-

ter can be achieved when a metal enclosure (with hand holes) is adapted to the front of the lathe's hood. ALL attachments, such as the stones, rag wheels, and bands, must be sterilized between uses or be thrown away. The lathe unit must be disinfected twice a day (Miller and Palenik, 1988a).

Pumice. Fresh pumice and pan liners should be used for each individual case. The modest cost of pumice and the proved significant microbial contamination present in reused pumice prohibits multiple use (Craig, 1987; Miller and Palenik, 1988a).

Polishing Procedures. Polishing appliances and prostheses prior to delivery is necessary; however, polishing exposes the operator to potential cross-infection and physical injury. If the item being polished has been asep-

Table 39–7. *Disinfecting Prosthetic Devices and Appliances*

Prosthetic Device†	Disinfectants*		
	Glutaraldehydes	Iodophors	Sodium Hypochlorite
Complete Denture (plastic/porcelain)‡	NO	YES	YES
Removable Partial (metal/plastic)‡	NO	YES	YES/NO
Fixed (metal/plastic/ porcelain)‡	YES	YES	NO

*Solutions prepared according to manufacturers' recommendations for surface or immersion disinfection; routine immersion time is 30 min; WARNING: compatibilities of a disinfectant type with a given type of prosthetic material vary per manufacturer.

†Thorough rinsing of disinfected devices before laboratory processing or returning to patient is ESSENTIAL.

‡WARNING: Similar products from different manufacturers vary in their response to a given type of disinfectant.

Data from ADA. 1985. Guidelines for infection control in dental office and the commercial dental laboratory. J. Am. Dent. Assoc., *110*, 969–972; ADA. 1988. Infection control recommendations for the dental office and the dental laboratory. J. Am. Dent. Assoc., *116*, 241–248; Miller, C.H., and Palenik, C.J. 1988. *Indiana University School of Dentistry Infection Control Manual*. Indianapolis, Indiana University, pp. II–19–26.

tically prepared, the risks of infection are taken to a minimum. To avoid the potential spread of microorganisms, however, all polishing agents (i.e., rouge) should be obtained in small quantities from the large reservoirs. Unused agents should not be returned to the central stock, but rather should be thrown away. Most polishing attachments (i.e., brushes, wheels, cups) are single-use, disposable items. Reusable items should, if possible, be sterilized between uses or otherwise disinfected.

Intermediate Cases

Both complete and partial dentures undergo an intermediate wax try-in stage. Crowns, splinted bridges, and partial denture frameworks are often "test seated" prior to cementation or soldering. These devices, like wax try-in dentures, can become soiled with oral fluids. Before returning the items to the laboratory for further processing, they must be disinfected. The procedures in most cases are the same described for completed projects.

Returning Completed Cases

Appliances and prostheses returned to the patient are not free of microbial contamination. These organisms could come from other cases if aseptic procedures are not rigorously followed and from the operator's body. Many patients have open oral lesions or are sufficiently traumatized during treatment to facilitate easier microbial penetration. In addition, a growing number of patients have impaired immune defense systems or are in chemotherapy programs that render them more susceptible to infectious diseases. Disinfection procedures for such activities are best located at chairside.

DENTAL WASTE

Types of Waste

For many individuals, the terms "contaminated waste," "infectious waste," and "medical waste" are synonymous. Although the terms can apply to similar materials and are interrelated, they are by definition distinct (Table 39–8). Infectious waste is capable of causing an infectious disease. In order to be infectious, such waste must contain human pathogens with sufficient virulence and in ample quantity that exposure to the waste by a susceptible host could result in infection. Items soiled with blood or body secretions are contaminated waste. All infectious waste must be considered contaminated, but little contaminated waste is actually infectious. The presence of blood on a piece of cotton does not guarantee infectivity. The blood may be pathogen free or when dried may no longer have sufficient quantities of disease-causing microorganisms.

Much medical waste is contaminated, but only a small portion is potentially infectious. The general public, however, tends to believe anything soiled during the treatment of humans, by research animals, or in the laboratory to be a major threat to public safety. What is not common knowledge is that infectious waste, contam-

Table 39–8. *Definitions of Waste*

Term	Definition
Infectious waste	Waste capable of causing an infectious disease
Contaminated waste	Items that have had contact with blood or other body secretions
Hazardous waste	Waste posing a risk or peril to humans or the environment
Toxic waste	Waste capable of having a poisonous effect
Medical waste	Any solid waste* that is generated in the diagnosis, treatment, or immunization of human beings or animals in research pertaining thereto, or in the production or testing of biologicals. The term does not include any hazardous waste or household waste

*"Solid waste" includes discarded solid, liquid, semisolid, or contained gaseous materials.

Data from EPA. 1989. 40 CFR Parts 22 and 259: Standard for the tracking and management of medical waste. Fed. Reg., 54, 12,326–12,395; OSAP Research Foundation. 1988. Surface disinfection: procedures for disinfecting surfaces and equipment. *OSAP Position Statement No. 7–002*; Reis-Schmidt, T. 1989. Waste handling and processing standards developing for dentistry. Dent. Products Rep., 32, 46, 53, 58, 63.

inated waste, or medical waste does not contribute to the development of public health problems (Keene, 1988; Rutala, 1987). Such materials do pose a potential occupationally related threat to health-care workers. Good examples include human blood and sharps. With the proper use of universal barriers, sterilization, disinfection, sanitation methods, and immunizations, however, the risk to health-care providers can be held to an absolute minimum.

Background

During the summers of 1987 and 1988, a number of debris washups occurred in the United States. In some cases beaches were closed and local economies suffered. Intermixed with the arriving materials was a small amount of medical waste. Concerned citizens complained vehemently to their elected representatives. Most of the medical waste was found to be illegally dumped by waste handlers and the United States Navy. In response to the public outcry for remediation, however, Congress passed and President Reagan signed the Medical Waste Tracking Act (MWTA) of 1988, Public Law 100-582, (EPA, 1989). The Environmental Protection Agency (EPA) has historically regulated medical waste as general refuse under the Resource Conservation and Recovery Act, Subtitle D, and had issued guidelines for infectious waste management in 1986.

MWTA is a 2-yr demonstration program to develop a tracking system for regulated medical wastes (RMW). EPA has listed: (1) cultures and stocks; (2) pathologic wastes; (3) human blood and blood products; (4) sharps;

and (5) contaminated animal wastes as substantial threats to human health and wishes to regulate their disposal. Other types of wastes will be evaluated and added or dropped from the program. As of June 22, 1989, dental offices and other health-care facilities in five states, the District of Columbia, and Puerto Rico were obligated to participate. Seven Great Lake states initially included chose to opt out of the program. Dentists are required to segregate, package, label, and dispose of RMW as described in MWTA. Although the EPA has reduced the number of covered categories, MWTA has not been met with enthusiasm in all quarters. Some believe that the government overreacted to the washups and selected medical waste because of health-care's high visibility in the community and eagerness to maintain its reputation. Moreover, there is an increased possibility that viable tracking programs could be established among compliant (and regulated) health-care facilities. In addition to the federal government, a number of states, counties, and even cities have installed infectious waste laws of their own. Whether necessary or not, such actions have invariably had a negative impact on health-care costs.

Methods and Materials

Unfortunately, infectious waste disposal laws vary greatly throughout the United States. A lingering debate exists regarding which items or materials should be considered infectious and which are the proper methods for neutralization and disposal. With the mood set for increasing legislation, however, all health-care facilities, if not already affected, including dental offices, will probably soon be regulated to some extent. The most prudent action is to contact local (city and/or county) and state boards of health to determine what specific guidelines and laws are currently in place. Facilities not currently enrolled in MWTA may wish to review the mandates of the program and to estimate the costs associated if implemented on a national scale.

The Occupational Safety and Health Administration (OSHA, 1989) has recently issued some generic recommendations concerning infectious waste. The agency indicated that all infectious waste destined for disposal should be placed in closable, leakproof containers or bags that are color coded (in red) or labeled (with a fluorescent orange or orange-red biohazard symbol). If outside contamination of the container or bag is likely to occur, then a second container of approved design is to be placed over the original. Both OSHA (1989) and the Centers for Disease Control (CDC, 1989a) advocate *where local regulations allow* that infectious waste be incinerated or decontaminated (i.e., autoclaving) before disposal in a sanitary landfill. Where permitted, bulk blood, suctioned fluids, excretions, and secretions may be carefully poured down a drain connected to a sanitary sewer. In addition, sanitary sewers may be used to dispose of other infectious wastes capable of being ground and flushed into the sewer, where permitted.

Needle and Sharps Disposal

About Sharps

One important item that has not been a point of debate concerning medically generated waste is the handling of contaminated sharps. Sharps are items that can penetrate skin and include, but are not limited to, injection needles, scalpel blades, sutures, instruments, and broken glass. Proposed OSHA regulations indicate that, immediately after use, sharps are to be placed in closable, leakproof (at least the sides and bottom), puncture-resistant containers, "sharps boxes" (OSHA, 1989). These containers must be labeled or color coded with the distinctive biohazard legend for easy identification. The CDC (1989a) indicate that sharps containers should be located as close as practical to the work area. This means ideally that each dental operatory should be so equipped. There may be a need for multiple units in a dental laboratory. To prevent potential accidents, sharps such as needles should not be sheared, bent, broken, recapped, or resheathed by hand. Used needles are not to be removed from disposable syringes (OSHA, 1989).

Proper handling of sharps is essential because common personal protective barriers, such as gloves, do not totally prevent needlestick accidents. Of the 25 cases of occupationally acquired human immunodeficiency type 1 virus (HIV-1) infections noted to date, 19 involved sticks or cuts with contaminated sharps (CDC, 1989a). Fortunately, the efficiency of viral transfer has proved to be low. Studies relating number of needlesticks with known HIV-positive sharps to number of seroconversions appears to be about 1:250. With the ever-increasing number of AIDS and HIV-positive individuals, however, the risk of infection after an occupational accident must also increase (CDC, 1988b, 1989a).

Sharps and the MWTA

As described previously, the EPA's pilot Medical Waste Tracking Act (MWTA) became law in 1988 and was implemented in July of 1989 (EPA, 1989). Used and certain types of unused, discarded sharps and laboratory-generated waste items capable of puncturing skin are listed as specific types of regulated medical wastes (RMW) in the MWTA. Such items must be segregated from fluids and other forms of RMW. They must be packaged in rigid, leak-resistant, sealed containers, as previously described for RMW, but in addition the containers must be puncture resistant.

Although MWTA is currently applicable in a limited number of states and territories, many other states, counties, and cities have also passed RMW laws for sharps. In some areas, RMW generators cannot process any sharps containers in house, nor can they transport them off site. They must rely on local EPA-approved waste handlers for removal. MWTA does, however, allow generators of less than 50 lb/mo to ship sharps containers by registered mail, return-receipt requested. Several mail-in services currently exist. Usually, the company offers not only disposal services, but also the sharps containers themselves and mailing boxes. The MWTA and many local jurisdictions allow generators to treat and destroy RMW on site. If treatment and destruction are by means other than incineration, the generator must record quantities and percentages of RMW by weight processed.

On-Site Treatment

Because waste haulers charge a premium price for the removal of infectious materials, many dental offices elect to treat their sharps containers on site where legally permissible. Unfortunately, little information has appeared in the scientific literature to help practitioners; however, all sharps containers should be commercially available sealable units made for the sole purpose of collecting sharps. Such units should be made of leakproof, puncture-resistant plastic that is autoclavable. Containers should be filled no more than three-quarters full. The contents of some containers can be steam sterilized only while positioned on their sides with their vents left open. Containers left upright usually require additional exposure time to ensure sterility. Disposal of treated containers is then usually dictated by local or state code. In some areas, processed containers can be added to the regular ("household") waste. A call to one's state board of health should identify acceptable disposal procedures/methods (OSHA, 1989; Palenik and Miller, 1989a).

Dental Operatory Procedures

Because a patient can require multiple injections of anesthetic from a single syringe, dental practitioners have opposed the restriction on the recapping of needles (ADA, 1988a). They prefer to recap the needle and then to leave it on the bracket table. The remainder of the carpule can then be used if further anesthesia is needed; however, the CDC (1989a) and OSHA (1989) prohibit recapping by an unprotected two-hand method or the placement of used needles outside of sharps containers. Alternative and safe techniques include a mechanical cap-holding device that does not require hand contact with the needle or recapping with the use of forceps (ADA, 1988a). In addition, double-ended capped needles are more easily removed by the sharps containers than are uncapped needles.

Another potential use of a sharps container is for the disposal of extracted teeth. In most areas, extracted teeth are considered "human pathologic waste" and thus cannot be returned to patients. This does cause some consternation among pediatric patients. Resourceful dentists are now issuing "tooth fairy" vouchers to their young patients. Some problems exist with this method of disposal, however. Extracted teeth can be divided into two categories, namely, teeth *without* amalgam restorations and teeth *with* amalgam restorations. Teeth without amalgam can be placed into the sharps containers and steam sterilized along with the other contents. Teeth containing amalgam cannot be steam autoclaved (mercury would be released upon heating, thus creating a chemical hazard); rather, they should be treated in a 2 to 3.2% (full-strength) glutaraldehyde solution for 6 to 10 hrs, rinsed with tap water, wrapped in a gauze square, placed in a small plastic bag, and labeled with the office's address and the words "treated with glutaraldehyde." These materials are then disposed of in accordance with local rules (ADA, 1988a; Miller and Palenik, 1988a).

REFERENCES

Allen, A.L., and Organ, R.J. 1982. Occult blood accumulation under the fingernails: a mechanism for the spread of blood-borne infections. J. Am. Dent. Assoc., *105*, 455–459.

American Dental Association (ADA). 1978. Infection control in the dental office. J. Am. Dent. Assoc., *97*, 673–677.

American Dental Association (ADA). 1985. Guidelines for infection control in the dental office and the commercial dental laboratory. J. Am. Dent. Assoc., *110*, 969–972.

American Dental Association (ADA). 1988a. Infection control recommendations for the dental office and the dental laboratory. J. Am. Dent. Assoc., *116*, 241–248.

American Dental Association (ADA). 1988b. Biological indicators for verifying sterilization. J. Am. Dent. Assoc., *117*, 653–654.

Anderson, A.C., and Hodges, G.R. 1983. Acceptance of hepatitis B vaccine among high-risk health care workers. Am. J. Infect Control, *11*, 207–211.

Association for the Advancement of Medical Instrumentation (AAMI). 1988. *Good Hospital Practice: Steam Sterilization and Sterility Assurance.* Association for the Advancement of Medical Instrumentation. Arlington, VA.

Beasley, R.P., and Hwang, L.-Y. 1984. Epidemiology of hepatocellular carcinoma. In *Viral Hepatitis and Liver Disease.* Edited by G. N. Vyas, J.L. Dienstag, and J.H. Hoofnagle. Orlando, FL, Grune & Stratton, pp. 209–224.

Beasley R.P., Hwang, L.-Y., and Lin, C.C. 1981. Hepatocellular carcinoma and HBV: a prospective study of 22,707 men in Taiwan. Lancet, *2*, 1129–1133.

Bernstein, D., Schiff, G., Prince, A., and Briner, W. 1988. In vitro virucidal effectiveness of a 0.12% chlorhexidine (CH) mouthrinse. J. Dent. Res., *67* (special issue), 404, (abstr. no. 2329).

Bogga, B.S., Murphy, R.A., Anderson, A.W., and Punwami, I. 1984. Contamination of dental units cooling water with oral microorganisms and its prevention. J. Am. Dent. Assoc., *109*, 712–716.

Bond, W.W., Petersen, N.J., and Favero, M.S. 1977. Viral hepatitis B: aspects of environmental control. Health Lab. Sci., *14*, 235–252.

Bond, W.W., Favero, M.S., Petersen, N.J., and Ebert, J.W. 1983. Inactivation of hepatitis B virus by intermediate-to-high level disinfectant chemicals. J. Clin. Microbiol., *18*, 535–538.

Bond, W.W., et al. 1981. Survival of hepatitis B virus after drying and storage for one week. Lancet, *1*, 550–551.

Bond, W.W., et al. 1982. Transmission of a type B viral hepatitis via eye inoculation of a chimpanzee. J. Clin. Microbiol., *15*, 533–534.

Briner, W., et al. 1986. Effect of chlorhexidine gluconate mouthrinse on plaque bacteria. J. Periodont. Res., *21 (Suppl. 16)*, 44–52.

Centers for Disease Control (CDC). 1984. Adult immunization, recommendations of the immunization practices advisory committee (ACIP). MMWR, *33 (Suppl.)*, 10–11.

Centers for Disease Control (CDC). 1985a. Hepatitis B among dental patients—Indiana. MMWR, *34*, 73–74.

Centers for Disease Control (CDC). 1985b. Diphtheria, tetanus, and pertussis: Guidelines for vaccine prophylaxis and other preventive measures. MMWR, *34*, 405–414, 419–426.

Centers for Disease Control (CDC). 1986. Recommended infection control practices for dentistry. MMWR, *35*, 237–242.

Centers for Disease Control (CDC). Immunization Practices Advisory Committee. 1987. Update on hepatitis B prevention. Ann. Intern. Med., *107*, 353–357.

Centers for Disease Control (CDC). Immunization Practices Advisory Committee. 1988a. Prevention and control of influenza. MMWR, *37*, 361–364, 369–373.

Centers for Disease Control (CDC). 1988b. Update: Universal precautions for prevention of transmission of human immunodeficiency virus, hepatitis B virus and other blood-borne pathogens in health-care settings. MMWR, *37*, 377–382, 387–388.

Centers for Disease Control (CDC). 1989a. *Guidelines for Prevention of Transmission of Human Immunodeficiency Virus and Hepatitis B Virus to Healthcare and Public-safety Workers.* Atlanta, U.S. Department of Health and Human Services.

Centers for Disease Control (CDC). 1989b. *Immunization Recommendations for Health-Care Workers.* Atlanta, U.S. Department of Health and Human Services.

Centers for Disease Control (CDC). 1989c. *Mycobacterium tuberculosis* transmission in a health clinic—Florida, 1988. MMWR, *38*, 256–258, 263–264.

Centers for Disease Control (CDC). 1990. Possible transmission of human immunodeficiency virus to a patient during an invasive dental procedure. MMWR, *39*, 489–493.

Clinical Research Associates (CRA). 1989. Operating gloves, update. CRA Newslett., *13*, (Provo, UT).

Cochran, M.A., Miller, C.H., and Sheldrake, M.A. 1989. The efficacy of the dental dam as a barrier to the spread of microorganisms during dental treatment. J. Am. Dent. Assoc., *119*, 141–144.

Cottone, J.A. 1985. Hepatitis B virus infection in the dental profession. J. Am. Dent. Assoc., *110*, 617–621.

Craig, R.M. 1987. Infection control for the dental laboratory. Texas Dent. J. *104*, 6–11.

Crawford, J.J. 1985. State-of-the-art practical infection control in dentistry. J. Am. Dent. Assoc., *110*, 629–633.

Crawford, J.J. 1987. *Clinical Asepsis in Dentistry*. Mesquite, TX, Oral Med. Press, pp. 27–35.

Crawford, J.J., Parker, W.D., and Parker, N.H. 1974. Asepsis in periodontal surgery. J. Dent. Res., *53 (special issue)*, 99.

DiAngelis, A.J., Martens, L.V., Little, J.W., and Hastreiter, R.J. 1989. Infection control practices of Minnesota dentists: changes during 1 year. J. Am. Dent. Assoc., *11*, 299–303.

Environmental Protection Agency (EPA). 1989. 40 CFR Parts 22 and 259: Standard for the tracking and management of medical waste. Fed. Reg., *54*, 12,326–12,395.

Food and Drug Administration (FDA). 1988. 21 CFR Part 878: General and plastic surgery devices; general provisions and classifications of 51 devices; final rule. Fed. Reg., *53*, 23,856–23,877.

Food and Drug Administration (FDA). 1989. 21 CFR Part 880: Medical devices; patient examination glove; revocation of exemptions from the premarket notification procedures and the current good manufacturing practice regulations. Fed. Reg., *54*, 1602–1604.

Francis, D.P., and Maynard, J.E. 1979. The transmission and outcome of hepatitis A, B, and non-A, non-B: a review. Epidemiol. Rev., *1*, 17–31.

Francis, D.P., Favero, M.S., and Maynard, J.E. 1981. Transmission of hepatitis B virus. Semin. Liver Dis., *1*, 27–32.

Greene, V.W., and Vesley D. 1961. Method for evaluating surgical masks. J. Bacteriol., *83*, 663–667.

Gross, A., Cutright, D., and D'Allesandro, S. 1979. The effect of surgical scrub on microbial population under the fingernails. Am. J Surg., *138*, 463–467.

Gross, A., Devine, M.J., and Cutright, D.E. 1976. Microbial contamination of dental units and ultrasonic scalers. J. Periodontol., *47*, 670–673.

Guest, G.F., and Cottone, J.A. 1987. Personal protection: the first line of defense. Texas Dent. J., *104*, 16–18.

Hales, R.H. 1970. Ocular injuries sustained in the dental office. Am. J. Ophthalmol., *70*, 221–223.

Hennessey, T.D. 1973. Some antibacterial properties of chlorhexidine. J. Periodont. Res., *8 (Suppl. 12)*, 61–67.

Johnson, G.H., Drennon, D.G., and Powell, G.L. 1988. Accuracy of elastomeric impressions disinfected by immersion. J. Am. Dent. Assoc., *166*, 525–530.

Kane, M.A., and Lettau, L.A. 1985. Transmission of HBV from dental personnel to patients. J. Am. Dent. Assoc., *110*, 634–636.

Katz, J.N., Gobetti, J.P., and Shipman, C., Jr. 1989. Fluorescein dye evaluation of glove integrity. J. Am. Dent. Assoc., *118*, 327–331.

Keene, J.H. 1988. Infectious waste: a non-problem problem. APIC News, 7, 18.

Kew, M.C. 1973. Possible transmission of serum (Australia-antigen-positive) hepatitis via the conjunctiva. Infect. Immun., *7*, 823–824.

Keys, T.F. 1989. Immunization of health care workers: new concepts. Asepsis Infect. Control Forum, *11*, 14–15.

Kornman, K.S. 1986. The role of supragingival plaque in the prevention and treatment of periodontal disease: a review of current concepts. J. Periodont. Res., *21 (Suppl. 16)*, 5–22.

Larson, E. 1988. Guideline for use of topical antimicrobial agents. Am. J. Infect. Control, *16*, 253–266.

Lauer, J.L., VanDrunen, N.A., Washburn, J.W., and Balfour, H.H. 1979. Transmission of hepatitis B virus in clinical laboratory areas. J. Infect. Dis., *140*, 513–516.

Leung, R.L., and Schonfeld, S.E. 1983. Gypsum casts as a potential source of microbial cross-contamination. J. Prosthodont. Dent., *49*, 210–211.

Litsky, B.Y., Mascio, J.D., and Litsky, W. 1970. Use of an antimicrobial mouthwash to minimize the bacterial aerosol contaminations generated by the high-speed drill. Oral Surg., *29*, 25–30.

Manzella, J.P., et al. 1984. An outbreak of herpes simplex virus type I gingivostomatitis in a dental hygiene practice. JAMA, *252*, 2019–2022.

Martin, L.S., McDougal, J.S., and Loskoski, S.L. 1985. Disinfection and inactivation of the human T lymphotrophic virus III/lymphadenopathy-associated virus. J. Infect. Dis., *152*, 400–403.

Merchant, V. 1982. Herpes simplex virus infection: an occupational hazard in dental practice. J. Mich. Dent. Assoc., *64*, 199–203.

Merchant, V.A., and Molinari, J.A. 1987. Infection control in prosthodontics. Monitor, *9*, 3–4.

Micik, R.E., Miller, R.L., and Leong, A.C. 1971. Studies on aerobiology. III. Efficacy of surgical masks in protecting dental personnel from airborne bacterial particles. J. Dent. Res., *50*, 626–630.

Miller, C.H. 1985. Barrier techniques for infection control. J. Calif. Dent. Assoc., *13*, 54–59.

Miller, C.H. 1987. Heat sterilization assures microbe-free instruments. Dentist, *65*, 26–29.

Miller, C.H. 1988a. Surface disinfection. Dent. Assist., *8*, 21–22.

Miller, C.H. 1988b. Guidelines for gloving. Infect. Control Notes (Indiana University School of Dentistry), *1*, 1–2.

Miller, C.H. 1989. Instrument recirculation prevents infection transfer. Reg. Dent. Hyg., *9*, 18–21.

Miller, C.H., and Hardwick, L.M. 1988. Ultrasonic cleaning of dental instruments in cassettes. Gen. Dent., *36*, 31–36.

Miller, C.H., and Palenik, C.J. 1983. The case for gloves. Dent. Asepsis Rev., *4*, 1–2.

Miller, C.H., and Palenik, C.J. 1988a. *Indiana University School of Dentistry Infection Control Manual*. Indianapolis, Indiana University, pp. II–19–26.

Miller, C.H., and Palenik, C.J. 1988b. Surface disinfection. Dent. Asepsis Rev., *9*, 1–2.

Miller, R.L., Burton, W.E., and Spore, R.W. 1963. Aerosols produced by dental instrumentation. In *Proceedings of the First International Symposium on Aerobiology*. London. pp. 97–120.

Miller, R.L., Micik, R.E., Abel, C., and Ryge, G. 1971. Studies on dental aerobiology. II. Microbial splatter discharged from the oral cavity of dental patients. J. Dent. Res., *50*, 621–625.

Minagi, S., Fukushima, K., and Maeda, N. 1986. Disinfection method for impression materials: freedom from fear of hepatitis B and acquired immunodeficiency syndrome. J. Prosthodont. Dent., *56*, 451.

Molinari, J.A., Gleason, M.J., Cottone, J.A., and Barrett, E.D. 1988. Cleaning and disinfectant properties of dental surface disinfectants. J. Am. Dent. Assoc., *117*, 179–182.

Muir, K.F., Ross, P.W., and MacPhee, I.T. 1978. Reduction of microbial contamination from ultrasonic scalers. Br. Dent. J., *145*, 76–78.

Occupational Safety and Health Administration (OSHA) (U.S. Department of Labor). 1987. Joint advisory notice: Department of Labor/Department of Health and Human Services: HBV/HIV. Fed. Reg., *52*, 41,818–41,823.

Occupational Safety and Health Administration (OSHA) (Department of Labor). 1989. OSHA, 29 CFR Part 1910: Occupational exposure to blood-borne pathogens; proposed rule and notice of hearing. Fed. Reg., *54*, 23,042–23,139.

Office Sterilization and Asepsis Procedures (OSAP) Research Foundation. 1988. Surface disinfection: procedures for disinfecting surfaces and equipment. In *OSAP Position Statement No. 7-002*. Denver, OSAP.

Oosterwaal, P.J.M., Mikx, F.H.M., Vanden Brink, M.E., and Renggli, H.H. 1989. Bacteriocidal concentrations of chlorhexidine digluconate, amine fluoride gel and stannous fluoride gel for subgingival bacteria tested in serum at short contact times. J. Periodont. Res., *24*, 155–160.

Otis, L.L., and Cottone, J.A. 1989. Prevalence of perforations in disposable latex gloves during routine dental treatment. J. Am. Dent. Assoc., *118*, 321–324.

Palenik, C.J. 1981. Eye protection for the entire dental office. J. Indiana Dent. Assoc., *60*, 23–25.

Palenik, C.J., and Miller, C.H. 1980. Use of the ultrasonic cleaner in the dental office. J. Indiana Dent. Assoc., *59*, 11–12.

Palenik, C.J., and Miller, C.H. 1981. Handwashing. Dent. Asepsis Rev., *2*, 1–2.

Palenik, C.J., and Miller, C.H. 1982. Occupational herpetic whitlow. J. Indiana Dent. Assoc., *61*, 25–27.

Palenik, C.J., and Miller, C.H. 1983. Handpiece hygiene. Dent. Asepsis Rev., *4*, 1–2.

Palenik, C.J., and Miller, C.H. 1985. Treating highly infectious patients in the dental office. J. Indiana Dent. Assoc., *64*, 11–15.

Palenik, C.J., and Miller, C.H. 1987. Gloves and the practice of dentistry. Part I. A statement of need. J. Indiana Dent. Assoc., *66*, 7–11.

Palenik, C.J., and Miller, C.H. 1988a. Gloves and the practice of dentistry. Part 2. Selection and use. J. Indiana Dent. Assoc., *67*, 11–14.

Palenik, C.J., and Miller, C.H. 1988b. Disinfecting impression material. Dent. Asepsis Rev., *9*, 1–2.

Palenik, C.J., and Miller, C.H. 1988c. Hepatitis B vaccination. Dent. Asepsis Rev., *9*, 1–2.

Palenik, C.J., and Miller, C.H. 1988d. Tetanus—reviewing a persistent problem. Trends Techniques Contemp. Dent. Lab., *10*, 5, 18, 20, 22.

Palenik, C.J., and Miller, C.H. 1989a. Needle and sharps disposal. Dent. Asepsis Rev., *10*, 1–2.

Palenik, C.J., and Miller, C.H. 1989b. Laboratory asepsis: disinfection of impression materials. Dent. Asepsis Rev., *10*, 1–2.

Palenik, C.J., Singer, S.M., and Miller, C.H. 1983. Cleaning and sporicidal activities of common surface disinfectants. Int. Assoc. Dent. Res., *62*, 230 (abstr. no. 549).

Palenik, C.J., et al. 1989. Survey of infection control practices among Indiana dental hygienists. J. Dent. Res., 68, 958 (abstr.)

Paulssen, J., Eidem, T., and Kristiansen, R. 1987. Perforations in surgeon's gloves. J. Hosp. Infect., 11, 82–85.

Petersen, N.J., Bond, W.W., and Favero, M.S. 1979. Air sampling for hepatitis B surface antigen in a dental operatory. J. Am. Dent. Assoc., 99, 465–467.

Pippin, D.J., Verderome, R.A., and Weber, K.K. 1987. Efficacy of face masks in preventing inhalation of airborne contaminants. J. Oral Maxillofac. Surg., 45, 319–323.

Reis, T. 1986. Surveys indicate doctors donning gloves with increasing frequency. Dent. Products Rep., 20, 9–11, 78–79, 85–87.

Reis-Schmidt, T. 1989. Waste handling and processing standards developing for dentistry. Dent. Products Rep., 32, 46, 53, 58, 63.

Rowe, N.H., Heine, C.S., and Kowalski, C.J. 1982. Herpetic whitlow: an occupational disease of practicing dentists. J. Am. Dent. Assoc., 105, 471–473.

Runnells, R.R. 1987a. *Practical How To's of Dental Infection Control.* Fruit Heights, UT, I.C. Publications, pp. 39–55.

Runnells, R.R. 1987b. *Infection Control in the Former Wet Finger Environment.* Fruit Heights, UT. I.C. Publications, pp. 71–83.

Runnells, R.R. 1988. *Infection Control in the Dental Laboratory.* Fruit Heights, UT. I.C. Publications, pp. 41–49.

Rutala, W.A. 1987. Infectious waste—a growing problem for infection control. Asepsis Infect. Control Forum, 9, 2–5.

Rutala, W.A. 1989. Draft guideline for selection and use of disinfectants. Am. J. Infect. Control., 17, 24A–38A.

Scheid, R.C., et al. 1982. Reduction of microbes in handpieces by flushing before use. J. Am. Dent. Assoc., 105, 658–660.

Simmons, B.P. 1983. CDC guidelines for the prevention and control of nosocomial infections: guidelines for hospital environmental control. Am. J. Infect. Control, 11, 97–120.

Steere, A.C., and Mallison, G.F. 1975. Handwashing practices for the prevention of nosocomial infections. Ann. Intern. Med., 83, 683–690.

Stevens, R.E., Jr. 1963. Preliminary study—air contamination with microorganisms during use of the air turbine handpiece. J. Am. Dent. Assoc., 100, 237–239.

Verrusio, A.C., et al. 1989. The dentist and infectious diseases: a national survey of attitudes and behavior. J. Am. Dent. Assoc., 118, 553–562.

Williams, W.W. 1989. Immunization of health care workers: new concepts. Asepsis Infect. Control Forum, 11, 16–18.

Williams, W.W., et al. 1988. Immunization policies and vaccine coverage among adults, the risk for missed opportunities. Ann. Intern. Med., 108, 616–625.

Zajac, B.A., West, D.J., McAleer, W.J., and Scolnick, E.M. 1986. Overview of clinical studies with hepatitis B vaccine made by recombinant DNA. J. Infect., 13 (Suppl. A), 39–45.

CHAPTER 40

GERM-FREE TECHNOLOGY

Nobuhiko Ohnishi and Shogo Sasaki

The breeding of germ-free animals using strictly sterile procedure greatly facilitates the designing of experiments tailored to specific purposes, yielding straightforward results. From this standpoint, the apparatus are introduced together with some results obtained from their use. The latter half of this chapter on applications deals with bone marrow transplantations in mice and man, isolator systems for autopsy of infection cases, and instructions for producing germ-free animals by hysterectomy—all aspects of creating and maintaining germ-free environments, in the belief that such environments aid the development of medical science.

FUNDAMENTALS OF GERM-FREE TECHNOLOGY

Germ-Free Animals and Experimental Apparatus

The components required for setting up a germ-free experimental system are as follows (components are illustrated schematically in Figures 40–1 and 40–2):

Flexible Film Isolator Chamber

The chamber, 600 × 500 × 1200 mm for housing rats and mice, made of 0.5-mm–thick clear polyvinyl chloride (PVC) film, is placed on a trolley extending 50 mm beyond the dimensions of the chamber with screw holes for securing the sterile lock, V-shaped trap, and air inlet and outlet filters to the tabletop. We use 600 × 500 × 1200 mm isolators for housing rats and mice, but these dimensions can be altered freely. Openings are made in the chamber walls to accommodate one spray-gun port for decontamination, and 2 ports for air intake and exhaust made of 50-mm segments of 25-mm diameter clear PVC tubing. All ports used in the isolator are of these dimensions and material, and are made to fit No. 9 silicone rubber stoppers, selected for their resistance to acid corrosion. The chamber walls and ports, made of the same material, with differences only in thickness, are heat-sealed, whereas connections between the cham-

ber and objects such as the sterile lock made of different material are secured and sealed by tape.

Sterile Lock

The sterile lock is made of a 150-mm length of acrylic resin cylinder, 4 to 5 mm thick with an outer diameter of 320 mm. On one side of the chamber, two 150-mm diameter openings are made for gloves, and on the side opposite, a 200-mm diameter opening is created for the sterile lock, about 50 mm off the floor of the chamber. The sterile lock is inserted into the opening halfway, secured with 2 or 3 layers of filament tape, and another 3 or 4 layers of PVC (electrician's) tape. The taped lock is then rested on a stainless steel supporting structure, which is a stainless steel belt surrounding the bottom half of the lock with two legs for support bolted onto the table. A stainless steel belt to hold down the top half of the lock is then put in place and screwed onto the lower half, securing the lock to the table.

Air Filtration Units

Two air filtration units are prepared for the air inlet and outlet. The disc-shaped units are made of a pair of caps, coil springs, and clasps. Four No. 50 FG Filter Down (American Air Filter Co., USA) glassfiber mat air filters, 1000 × 30,000 × 12.5 mm, 1.25 μm diameter, are inserted between the two caps, protected by the springs and secured tightly by the clasps to prevent leakage of air. The opening on the side of the chamber is covered with polyester membrane, 50 × 50 mm, held in place by a rubber band, and the edges are trimmed. The membrane is secured by polyester tape, which should be done with care because the tape has little elasticity and can easily become creased or too thick, making it difficult to attach to the 25-mm diameter ports on the chamber. The tape should not be wound around more than 4 or 5 times.

The filtration unit is autoclaved with the polyester membrane side up and protected by cloth. After sterilization, the door should be left slightly ajar overnight to

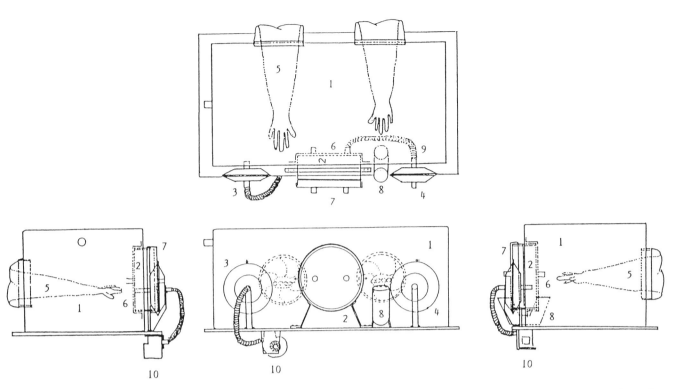

Fig. 40–1. PVC film isolator. 1, PVC chamber. 2, Sterile lock. 3, Air-intake filtration unit. 4, Exhaust air-filtration unit. 5, Neoprene gloves. 6, Inner cap. 7, Outer cap. 8, V-shaped trap. 9, Flexible pipe. 10, Motorized blower.

dry out the filter. Alternatively, it can be dried in a 37°C incubator. Care should be taken because use before the filter is completely dry will lead to contamination by airborne bacteria carried through the filter together with the moisture. Likewise, sterilizing cans and transfer containers must be kept dry.

After sterilization, the filter is connected to the chamber's air-inlet port and sealed tightly with PVC tape, making sure there is plenty of overlap. Insufficient overlap can lead to this connection being pulled apart when working inside the isolator, because the unit itself is stationary, being screwed onto legs that are bolted onto the table top.

When working with the gloves inside, it should be kept in mind that any movements that pull the opposite wall toward you are unsuitable. PVC isolators are easy to work with, being very flexible, but for the same reason their joints are vulnerable to excessive pressure.

Neoprene Gloves

Radio-isotope gloves, 0.8-mm thick, are attached to the two 150-mm diameter openings in the chamber using rings made of 20-mm segments of 250-mm diameter PVC cylinder. The ring is set inside the glove, forced through the opening halfway, and secured with three layers of filament tape. Further wrapping of 3 or 4 layers of PVC tape over the filament tape will prevent the glove from coming loose except under the most inordinate tension.

For the surgery isolator, the neoprene gloves are cut off at the wrist and surgical gloves are attached, using the same rings used for securing the neoprene gloves to the chamber. A surgery isolator set up in this manner permits experimentation that reproduces conditions similar to conventional surgery, making possible delicate procedures such as inserting a needle into the caudate veins of animals.

Inner Cap

Two ports made of 25-mm diameter PVC tubes to hold two No. 9 silicone rubber stoppers are attached to the inner cap in the same manner as the ports on the chamber. The inner cap, made of the same material as the chamber, is constructed in the shape of a brimmed hat, 2 to 3 mm smaller than the diameter of the sterile lock. The brim is provided to make it easier to slide the inner cap over the sterile lock with gloved hands. One end of a piece of flexible tubing is connected to one of the ports, and the other end of the tube is fitted to the air-outlet port. The other port on the inner cap is plugged with a rubber stopper, the removal of which will guide sterile air through the port, sterile lock, and sleeve, driving peracetic acid used for decontamination outside the isolator via the flexible pipe without having it come into contact with the animals inside. The inner cap is secured to the sterile lock with two rubber bands only, but sterility is maintained by the slight positive pressure inside the chamber, which keeps air from entering into the system.

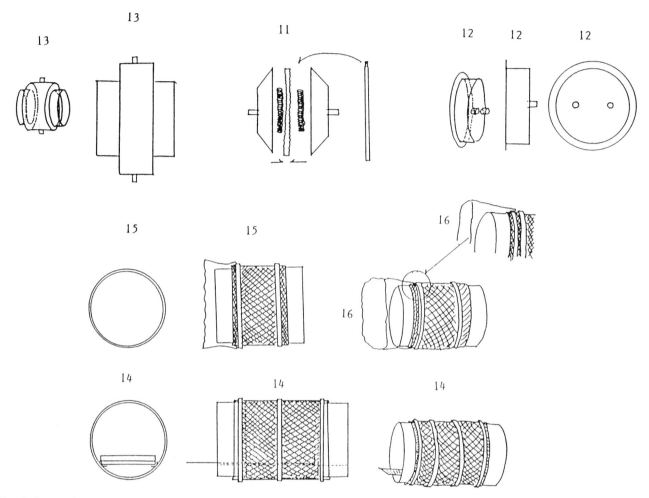

Fig. 40–2. Auxiliary apparatus. 11, Air-filtration unit. 12, Inner cap. 13, Sleeve. 14, Sterilizing can. 15, Mouse transport container. 16, Sleeve for transport container.

Uses for the sterile lock include the following:

Taking in heat-resistant materials that have been autoclaved in sterilizing cans into the chamber

Transferring animals from animal transport containers inside

Small amounts of acid-resistant instruments can be moved inside by placing in the sterile lock, closing the outer cap, introducing peracetic acid into the lock with a spray gun, and ventilating after 30 minutes

Similarly, use of peracetic acid in the sterile lock can be used for decontaminating materials on their way out of the isolator, such as animals, feces, and soiled bedding.

Rubber Bands

For securing the inner cap, synthetic rubber bands made of a compound of natural rubber and neoprene, 1 mm thick, 15 mm wide, and 200 mm in diameter, of superior acid-resistant quality should be used. They should not be too strong to be easily handled with gloved hands, but should have enough strength to prevent the inner cap from popping off under pressure of the peracetic acid sprayed into the sterile lock.

Outer Cap

The diameter of the outer cap, which is in the shape of a brimless hat, is of about the same as or slightly smaller than that of the sterile lock. The outer cap has ports to fit two No. 9 rubber stoppers, as on the inner cap. The cap is 50 mm in depth, and is slid over the sterile lock halfway and taped with PVC tape when airtightness is required.

V-Shaped Trap

For frequent removal of specimens from the isolator, it is preferable to use the V-shaped trap instead of the sterile lock, the use of which is not only time-consuming, but complex, raising the risk of contamination.

The V-shaped trap is installed between the sterile lock and air-outlet filter unit, and is belted down by a stainless steel belt, which is screwed onto the table. The trap is constructed of a bent piece of PVC pipe such as that used for drainage, 70 mm in diameter. A 10 to 20%

solution of hyamine (quaternary ammonium compound) (Domagk, 1935) is placed in the trap, forming a barrier between the interior and exterior of the chamber.

Small test tubes and butyl rubber stoppers stocked inside the chamber are used to pack specimens for removal. Butyl rubber stoppers are employed in this case because silicone rubber stoppers of this size are expensive. The test tube is propelled tail-end first through the trap with a tap of the finger. Forceps should be used to push the test tube through, should it get lodged in between. The test tube is then recovered from the outside and thoroughly rinsed with water before opening. Hyamine entering the test tube at this point will yield falsely negative results, whereas failure to complete this procedure under strictly germ-free conditions will make it impossible to distinguish whether a contaminant is from the animal or is the result of faulty technique (see under *Monitoring for Contamination*).

Sleeve

A sleeve made of cylindrical PVC film, the same material the chamber itself is made of, is used for connecting an isolator and a sterilizing can or for hooking up two isolators. The sleeve is 350 mm in length, and both ends are 320 mm in diameter but the midsection is a slightly larger 400 mm in diameter. Two ports are situated on opposing sides in the slightly larger midsection for accommodating a peracetic acid spray gun and an air-outlet pipe. The larger diameter of the midsection is to reduce the possibility of tearing the sleeve in pulling out the stainless steel rack from inside the sterilizing can, and for preventing spillage of peracetic acid used for decontamination into the chamber.

Sterilizing Cans

These are cylindrical containers 320 mm in diameter (the same as the sterile lock) and about 600 mm in length for sterilizing heat-resistant materials such as feed, water, and bedding (wood chips). The cylindrical portion and one end serving as the bottom of the can, which is bolted on, should be made of either stainless steel with perforations made with a drill, or stainless steel mesh. A stainless steel rack is placed inside, also perforated, for effective heat transfer; supports on which to place this rack are fixed inside the can. The rack is designed to make it easy to slide materials such as water bottles or packets of feed resting on the rack into the sterile lock. Folding up about 50 mm of the rear end of the rack will prevent materials from being left behind inside the can. The can is covered with four layers of filter paper and a layer of stainless steel mesh, and belted in four places by bands of stainless steel. The opening of the can is sealed with polyester membrane and PVC tape, which serves as a lid, before sterilization.

Waste Sterilizing Cans

These are of basically the same structure as the sterilizing cans above, but with an inner diameter easily fitting over the sterile lock. The inside rack is replaced by a pan the shape of a tube split in half with handles. It is designed to keep the materials in the can out of contact before autoclaving for containment purposes in infection experiments. Contamination from the isolator after use can be prevented completely by inserting rubber stoppers in the air inlet and outlet ports, securing the outer cap, and treating with peracetic acid.

Mouse Transport Containers and Special Sleeve

The following system has been adopted in our laboratory as an inexpensive and easily handled way for transferring germ-free mice from the breeders to the end-user:

One hundred millimeters of a 250-mm cardboard cylinder is joined to another 50-mm segment by a supporting structure made of metal insect screen in cylindrical shape 300-mm long, leaving a midsection of 150 mm of exposed screen cylinder. The inside of this structure is thus protected by the metal insect screen, which is secured to the cardboard cylinders by adhesive, and the outside of the insect screen is wrapped twice with glassfiber filter mats and a layer of cotton cloth for protection. This produces a semicollapsible structure that is convenient for transport. Both ends are fitted with tin lids, and the lid on the side of the 50-mm cardboard segment that forms the bottom of the container is sealed tightly with polyester tape.

The lid for the other end, polyester tape, and scissors are placed together with the container inside a sterilizing can, which is autoclaved, and introduced inside the isolator originally housing the animals.

This container is sufficient for holding 10 mice together with some bedding and feed up to 24 hours; after these are placed inside, the lid is put on and sealed with two layers of polyester tape. More than two layers will make it difficult to remove with forceps later on while working inside the isolator. Knives and scalpels should not be used for this or any other purpose inside breeding isolators because of the increased possibility of puncture they present. Procedures requiring their use should be performed inside surgery isolators equipped with surgical gloves hooked up to the breeding isolators via the sterile lock, so that contamination in the event of a puncture can be kept to a minimum.

For transferring the animals from the containers to the end-user isolator, a disposable sleeve designed specifically for this purpose to interface between the different diameters of the sterile lock and transfer containers is used. The sleeve, 320 mm in diameter on one end and 250 mm diameter on the other, is equipped with two ports on opposing sides in its midsection. One port is for the spray gun, and the other for ventilation and exhaust, relieving excess pressure build-up inside that would cause the sleeve to slip off at the ends.

The 250-mm diameter end of the sleeve is slid over the top end (100-mm segment side of the cardboard cylinder) about 50 mm beyond the tin lid, and sealed with four or five layers of PVC tape. This allows for about a 30-mm margin between the end of the tin lid and the

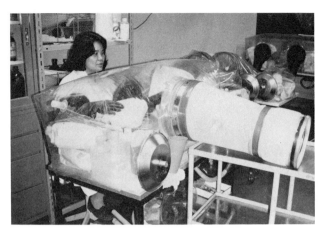

Fig. 40–3. Transfer of mice from a mouse transport container into an isolator.

position of the tape. This margin is sprayed with peracetic acid from inside the sleeve before it is secured to the sterile lock because it is difficult to reach by just spraying from the port. Care should be taken not to inhale the acid at this time.

The other end of the sleeve is then connected over the sterile lock; peracetic acid is introduced into the lock and evacuated three times over 30 min, and ventilated through the flexible pipe for another 30 min. The container is then slid partway through the sterile lock into the chamber, a procedure assisted by one person pushing from the rear end. Removal of the tape sealing the tin lid is best done with the container resting on the sterile lock. Utmost care should be taken to protect the sleeve from perforation by the sharp edges of the stainless steel rack in pulling it out from the container. The top of the tin lid is bent inside and the animals are removed (Fig. 40–3). Any peracetic acid remaining in the sleeve is caught by the inner cap and poured into the emptied container, where it will be absorbed by the bedding and removed from the chamber promptly to minimize its effect on the animals.

Polyester Membrane

Polyester film membranes are used for capping the sterilizing cans and the opening on the air-filtration units on the side connecting to the ports on the chamber. For example, the membrane is used to cover the opening on the side of the air-filtration units facing the chamber and is held in place with rubber bands; the edges are trimmed and secured with three or four layers of polyester tape before hooking up to the ports on the chamber.

Padding

Placing a soft PVC foam mat, about 3 mm thick, inside the chamber is useful for protecting the chamber floor.

Germ-Free Animal Feed

Purina is a well known source for this. See Gustafsson (1948) and Wostmann (1959).

Autoclave

The autoclave is one of the most important pieces of equipment required for dealing with germ-free animals. An important consideration is the capacity for complete exchange of air in the chamber with steam. Incomplete exchange will result in contamination coming from insufficiently sterilized feed with the core of solid feed not reaching sterilizing temperatures even under sufficient pressure. To avoid this, the chamber should be lowered to 60 cm/Hg pressure over 10 to 15 min, drawing air out of the feed before going into high-pressure steam sterilization for 20 min at $123 \pm 1°C$. This protocol will also keep heat destruction of the fortified vitamins contained in the feed at a minimum.

In recent years, slow virus infections by unconventional virus causing Creutzfeldt-Jakob disease, kuru disease, Gerstmann-Strausster disease in man, scrapie in sheep, and transmissible encephalopathy in mink have come to receive much attention (Brown et al., 1982; Gibbs et al., 1985; Traub et al., 1974). These diseases are all considered to be infections by the same virus, which can only be killed by decontamination at 130°C for over 60 min. It is projected that studies regarding such pathogens will increase in number, calling for increasingly efficient autoclaves. Hence, taking such tendencies into account, steam autoclaves—which are equipped to provide negative pressure as well, and which can operate at temperatures above 130°C—become a necessity. The ability for the system to be changed over to gas sterilization by a valve is also convenient, but is not as important as large capacity, considering the amount of materials needing sterilization for maintenance of germ-free animals. The autoclave in use at our laboratory is a square type capable of holding up to four sterilizing cans.

For more on germ-free animals and experimental apparatus, the reader is referred to Trexler and Reynolds (1957) and to Trexler (1959, 1964).

Peracetic Acid

Decontaminating the isolator chamber for rearing and experimenting with germ-free animals is done best by peracetic acid at present. Great care must be taken with its use, for although it is an effective sterilizing agent, it also causes acid burns on contact and difficulty in breathing and bronchitis upon inhalation. Immediate washing to dilute the acid can avert acid burns, and gargling is helpful in relieving shortness of breath. Inhalation can be circumvented by extending the exhaust pipe outdoors.

A 40% solution of peracetic acid diluted 1:20 with tap or distilled water (final concentration 2%), is used for decontamination. About 700 ml of this 2% solution is required for decontaminating a 500 × 600 × 1200 mm isolator.

After carefully sealing the outer cap with PVC tape, the connections between the chamber and the sterile lock, V-shaped trap, air intake and exhaust air filtration units, and neoprene gloves are carefully sprayed with peracetic acid. This process properly requires two people.

The acid is sprayed with a stainless steel spray gun fitted with a 25-mm gunhead to fit snugly into the 25-mm spraying port on the side of the chamber provided for this purpose. Compression is raised to 5 to 6 kg/cm² by a compressor equipped with a 50-L tank.

Items previously deposited in the chamber, e.g., cages, lids, flexible pipe, water containers, rags, forceps, and a wide-necked lidded polycarbonate jar for collecting peracetic acid from the initial decontamination, are also sprayed. The inner cap, two No. 9 silicone rubber stoppers, and PVC foam mat should be brought close to the spraying port by one person and gone over carefully by the other.

Ventilation is started in about 2 hours. For this, a flexible pipe is connected to the exhaust port of the air-outlet filtration unit, and the other end is extended outdoors. One arm is gently inserted into the glove, taking care not to suddenly increase the pressure inside the chamber, which would cause overflow of the hyamine solution in the V-shaped trap. First, the polyester membrane between the chamber and the exhaust filtration unit is broken with forceps. Next, the membrane sealing the air-inlet filtration unit is similarly broken, and the motorized blower switched on. To speed up ventilation, excess acid is mopped up with rags, wrung out into the stoppered inner cap, and transferred to the polycarbonate jar, which is promptly capped. When this jar is full, excess acid can be poured off into the V-shaped trap or empty water containers. The inside of the chamber should be dry in 24 hours, and the motorized blower should be of such capacity to handle this, for preventing undue acid corrosion resulting from longer exposure, although speeding up this process will adversely affect the animals. The appropriate capacity of a blower is that capable of exchanging air in the chamber 6 times/hour.

Under these conditions, it is possible to reuse the isolator over several years; only the gloves will need replacement from time to time, rendering the system cost-effective.

Introduction of feed, water, bedding, and animals through the sterile lock is effected by connecting the sterilizing cans and transport containers with the appropriate sleeve and decontaminating the inside of the sterile lock and sleeve with peracetic acid. The amount of acid solution involved in this procedure is 100 ml at most, but failure to ventilate properly will lead to denaturing of feed and animal suffocation, so that the process must be repeated each time. Decontamination of the sterile lock is carried out for 30 min, and ventilation is effected through the ventilation port on the inner cap drawing in sterile air, which is exhausted through the flexible pipe attached to the other port on the inner cap. It is unpragmatic to expect to ventilate to dryness in this case, so ventilation is carried out for about 30 min basically to remove the fumes and odor.

Following ventilation, the rubber stoppers are replaced on the inner cap, and the rubber band is removed. Excess peracetic acid collected in the inner cap is promptly removed so it does not come into direct contact with the animals or feed.

Peracetic acid should be kept refrigerated and used within 2 months from manufacture. Even then, deterioration is marked toward the end of that time, making it necessary to employ solutions stronger than the usual 2% for effective decontamination. Hence, because peracetic acid is an inexpensive agent, it is advisable to keep a fresh stock on hand at all times.

An alternative agent is Alcide ABQ (chlorine dioxide) (Alcide, U.S.A.), which is odorless and easy to handle, but which requires 6 hours at a constant concentration for decontaminating sporeforms. Furthermore, because this agent contains soap, it increases the danger of the inner cap popping off even when secured with a rubber band when sending the solution in under compression, making it an impractical choice for this isolator system.

For more on peracetic acid, see Greenspan and Mackellar (1951) and Greenspan (1946).

Gas Sterilization with Ethylene Oxide (EO)

This is used for sterilizing items such as weight scales for mice placed in sterilizing cans, and heat-labile antigens, which are also difficult to filter with Millipore filters. A good choice in selecting an autoclave is one that can be changed over to gas sterilization by a valve.

The gas sterilizer should be left to operate for over 4 hours at 40°C. However, this method of sterilization is the least desirable form of decontamination for materials having to do with germ-free animals.

For more on gas sterilization, see Foster (1959) and Phillips and Kaye (1949).

Millipore Filters

For transferring antigen-free feed synthesized from amino acids of less than 10,000 in particle weight into the isolator chamber, the synthetic feed is first passed through a 0.22-μm Millipore filter. The spray-gun port plugged with a No. 9 stopper on the side of the chamber is carefully wiped with 70% alcohol or povidone-iodine. Using a G21 needle, the feed is sent through to a container inside using a setup similar to that used for effecting blood transfusions. The feed is passed through another 0.22-μm Millipore filter in the process. Dealing with large quantities is easy with a large filter and pressurizing tank. Disposable Millipore filters are frequently used to introduce small amounts of agents or other fluids in this manner.

For more on Millipore filters, see Greenstein (1957), Greenstein et al. (1960), and Pleasants et al. (1970).

Sterilization of Feed

Apart from autoclaving, x-ray irradiation can also be used (Luckey et al., 1955). For sterilizing a 1.5-kg laminated bag of feed, 3000 Gy should be adequate. However, most of the solid feed for germ-free animal maintenance available today is formulated for autoclaving—i.e., fortified with surplus vitamins and nutrients, taking the loss from autoclaving into account. Hence, circumventing this loss by using x-ray irradiation will lead to an excess of nutrients, which can result in above-average growth of animals, creating difficulties in some experiments.

Items To Be Placed in the Isolator

Bedding is packed loosely in $60 \times 250 \times 300$ mm sterilizing bags, sealed, and perforated in 20 to 30 places with a pin. Water is placed in heat-resistant plastic containers (1-L polycarbonate containers are convenient), and together with bedding, should be sterilized and kept on stock.

Items to be sterilized in sterilizing cans include presterilized water; bedding; solid feed in $70 \times 100 \times 200$ mm stainless steel baskets; paper bags for packing animals or wastes for removal; rags; small test tubes (10×100 mm) and butyl rubber stoppers for sampling; syringes (1-ml and 2-ml tuberculin syringes); G27, G21, and 1 or 2 stomach probe needles (lumbar puncture needles with the end enlarged in a tear drop shape); and butyl rubber stoppers fitted with stainless steel tubes for the water feeding bottles.

Items to be placed inside before decontaminating the chamber are the inner cap with its two rubber stoppers; two acid-resistant rubber bands for securing the inner cap; forceps; a 600- to 700-mm length of 25-mm diameter flexible PVC tube with a connection on one end made to fit the ventilation port on the inner cap, and on the other end fashioned to connect to the air outlet of the chamber leading to the air filtration unit; polycarbonate cages and stainless steel lids doubling as a feed box that are small enough to be passed through the sterile lock; 250-ml polycarbonate water feeding bottles; 1-L polycarbonate water supply containers; a 1-L wide-necked polycarbonate jar with a lid for holding excess peracetic acid collecting after decontamination; and at least two rags.

Monitoring for Contamination

Needless to say, the animals must be maintained under germ-free conditions at all times, but it is difficult to prove that an animal is truly germ-free with the technology available today. Therefore, we must settle with proving the absence of bacteria that are detectable by the culturing techniques known, and even for this, a totally reliable analysis would entail enormous man-hours and expense, making it impractical. Also, the effort required for simply confirming that an animal is germ-free this way would amount to an end in itself, leaving no time for the original purpose of the study.

From the standpoint of the researcher, we would like to be able to start with the understanding that the animals guaranteed by the breeders to be germ-free are really so. We hope we can expect considerably strict control and testing on the part of the breeders, requiring only a minimal battery of basic testing for the researcher, to

which he could then add any other tests deemed necessary for the specific study, such as tests for virus, fungi, or mycoplasma.

The experimenter uses the three materials of fresh feces, drinking water, and swabs passed over the surface of apparatus as samples for monitoring. Feces are used because they are the easiest source for detecting contamination. Swabs are for detecting fungi. Monitoring is carried out as follows:

1. Cotton swabs are made and sterilized in a steam autoclave (dry-oven sterilization is unsuitable).
2. The sterilized swabs are moistened with drinking water inside the chamber.
3. The mouths of water-feeding bottles, interior surfaces of cages, backs of animals, vicinity of the air-outlet port, glove fingers, and other such sampling sites are swabbed.
4. A fresh piece of feces is diluted 20 times with water, because placing it directly in thioglycollate (TGC) medium would make it difficult to determine whether the clouding is due to feces or to contamination.
5. The $\times 20$ dilution is placed in two medium-sized test tubes containing TGC medium, two test tubes with cooked meat (CM) medium, and one test tube with potato dextrose (PD).
6. The swabs are also applied to this last PD medium test tube already containing the feces specimen.
7. The TGC and CM cultures at 20°C (or room temperature), and the PD culture at 20°C, are observed over 14 days.
8. Air-dried specimens are also made for the purpose of detecting bacteria that cannot be cultured.
9. When the results from the above cultures are equivocal, the medium is changed to solid media, and air-dried specimens are again made for microscopical analyses.

The above procedure is performed at the start of an experiment, and repeated upon completion of the study.

An alternative method is to set up a large supply isolator stocking large quantities of sterilized supplies such as feed, water, bedding, and apparatus required for animal maintenance and experimentation, together with a few monitor mice. The feces are collected from the monitor mice for testing on a regular basis; dissection of the mice and culturing of a whole-body homogenate promotes familiarization with and adept use of germ-free techniques, which is essential for obtaining stable results in any germ-free experiment.

The incidence of isolator contamination has not exceeded a few percentage points in our experience. At present, tests for contamination have been reduced to culturing feces in TGC at 37 and 20°C for 1 week followed by determination with gram staining.

Testing for Virus

Comparing C3H-strain GF and SPF mice reared in isolators following 10-Gy cobalt-60 irradiation through the PVC film of the chamber revealed survival to be 5 to 6 days for SPF mice, and 10 to 11 days for GF mice.

This is interpreted as an absence of the often-cited latent virus (Bernhard, 1963; Pollard, 1966; Jahuna and Pollard, 1967). In other words, the fact that the GF mice survived twice as long as their SPF counterparts after inducing viral proliferation by x-ray irradiation is believed to indicate that they were both germ-free and virus-free, although none of the GF animals were tested for virus after death.

APPLICATIONS OF GERM-FREE TECHNOLOGY

Bone Marrow Transplantations (BMT) in Mice

Reports on bone marrow transplantation in mice include those of Bealmear et al. (1983), Eastcott et al. (1981), Jones et al. (1971), Mauch and Hellman (1989), Onoe et al. (1980), Pollard and Truitt (1973, 1974), Truitt et al. (1974), Vallera et al. (1982), and Wade et al. (1987).

The accident at the Chernobyl nuclear plant was a turning point for BMT as therapy for acute leukemia and immunologic deficiencies in man, because since the accident rapid development has been seen on a global scale. However, there is a marked lack of animal experimentation in this area to provide fundamental data, and the feeling that the human therapy trials are surging ahead without sufficient backing cannot be denied.

The method of BMT in mice will now be described, citing the procedure employed in our laboratory, together with some data.

GF and SPF C3H/HeN mice are used as recipients, and C57BL/6N mice are used as donors. Thirty SPF C3H/HeN mice between 5 and 6 weeks of age are introduced into an isolator by first placing the mice in a paper bag decontaminated by alcohol without direct handling, putting the bag in the sterile lock, closing the lock, and retrieving the bag through the inner cap and transferring the mice to cages, 5 per cage. Arrangements are made with the breeders to have 30 GF mice also between 5 and 6 weeks of age delivered in transfer containers in batches of 15. The containers are connected in turn to one isolator using the specially designed sleeve, and the sterile lock is decontaminated with peracetic acid for 30 min and ventilated for another 30 min with the flexible pipe before the mice are transferred to the cages inside. This procedure is repeated for the second batch.

Ten-gray x-ray irradiation (Wilson, 1963; Wilson et al., 1964) is carried out after rearing the mice for 2 to 3 weeks, at which time the mice are 7 to 8 weeks old. Bone marrow is transplanted 24 hours later.

The following items are prepared for collecting and adjusting marrow to 3 to 4 × 10^7 cells/ml in the clean bench the following day: a wooden board on which to pin down mice, pins for holding down legs (syringe needles are convenient), scissors, five sets of one small and one large forceps, capillary pipettes and suction caps, gauze, a test tube rack, and a stocking or stainless steel

mesh for filtering marrow cells. The above materials are packed in sterilizing bags, autoclaved, and taken into the clean bench using sterilized surgical gloves and spraying with alcohol in the process.

Disposable 50-ml, 20-ml, and 5-ml syringes and G21 needles are used. Ten plastic petri dishes and 20 15-ml tissue-culture centrifuge tubes are sterilized by gas.

Two spraying bottles with 70% alcohol, a 500-ml bottle of RPMI–1640, tincture of iodine, and disinfecting cotton (immersed in 70% alcohol) are also taken into the clean bench after thoroughly spraying the containers with alcohol.

Forty-five donor mice are sacrificed in batches of 7 or 8 and are totally immersed in tincture of iodine for 3 to 5 min, making sure the iodine reaches all parts of the body including the armpits before moving the mice inside the clean bench with forceps. The technician working the clean bench must take care not to withdraw his hands from the work bench at any time.

The mice are successively pinned down to the board, and the femurs are removed. The abdominal muscles must not be disturbed in this process. Separate forceps and scissors are used for cutting into tissue and bone, and the instruments are cleaned with disinfecting cotton between each maneuver. The femur is severed at the joints and pooled in a petri dish filled with RPMI–1640. About 60 min should be sufficient for removing the femurs from all 45 mice.

Next, forceps and scissors are used to cut off both ends of the femur, and the marrow is pushed out carefully with RPMI–1640 in a 10-ml syringe fitted with a G21 needle, pooling the cells from the entire lot. Removing marrow in this manner from 90 femurs should be completed in about 40 min. The cells are separated into single cells by taking up into the above syringe and pushing out again several times. The suspension is passed through the mesh filter, collected in centrifuge tubes, centrifuged for 5 min at 1250 rpm, washed once, and resuspended in 17 to 18 ml RPMI. All procedures except for the centrifugation are carried out in the clean bench, so that care must be taken to carefully decontaminate the tubes with alcohol before they are returned to the clean bench. This process should yield a suspension of 3 to 4 × 10^7 cells/ml, which is passed into the isolator with a 20-ml syringe fitted with a G21 needle pushed through the rubber stopper, sealing the spraying port on the side of the chamber after disinfecting the surface of the stopper with tincture of iodine or 70% alcohol. The suspension is collected in a test tube inside the chamber, and 0.5 ml of the suspension is introduced slowly into each recipient mouse, directly into the heart, using a tuberculin syringe with a 28G needle.

To inject into the heart, the mice are held in a supine position with the left hand, and the position of the heart is approximated as being 2 mm below the line connecting the lowest point of the armpits, and 2 mm off-center to the right. The needle will come in contact with the heart when inserted about 3 mm at this point. A wrong move

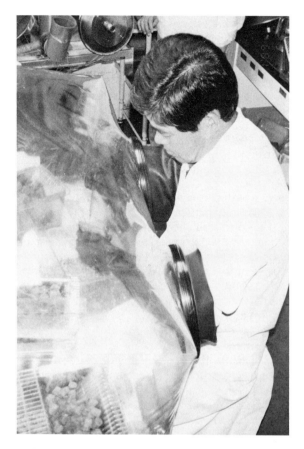

Fig. 40–4. BMT directly into the heart of mice carried out inside an isolator.

will release the cells into the lungs, resulting in its coming up through the nasal cavity and the suffocation of the animal. We have achieved a greater than 90% success rate with this technique. The established method of introduction into the caudate vein is not practical because of the difficulty it presents when working without changing to surgical gloves, and more important, because the brown coloring of C3H-strain mice makes it difficult to locate the vein. On the other hand, injecting the cells directly into the heart will ensure introduction of all 0.5 ml into the animal (Fig. 40–4).

After withdrawing the needle, astriction to the heart is applied for a while with the right hand.

The SPF recipients are also handled using the same germ-free techniques, because this will prevent contamination by such organisms as *Pseudomonas* and *Candida*, which are contacted through man, circumventing the need to introduce antibiotics into drinking water during the ensuing experiment.

This method has yielded a 100-day survival rate in GF mice of over 90%, whereas this rate was 18% in SPF animals when mismatched marrow was used (Van Bekkum et al., 1967). Treating the cells with monoclonal antibody raised the survival rate in SPF mice to 50% (Aizawa et al., 1981; Norin and Emerson, 1978).

BMT in Man

BMT is currently the most effective form of therapy for types of leukemia such as acute nonlymphocytic leukemia (ANLL), acute lymphoblastic leukemia (ALL), and chronic myelocytic leukemia (CML) that do not respond to chemotherapy (Bortin et al., 1988). Methods and therapeutic guidelines currently employed follow.

There are three systems for maintaining protective isolation: germ-free room systems, clean bench systems, and the isolator system (Trexler, 1974).

The isolator system is inexpensive and can be set up on short notice in an ordinary room, but the need to carry out all maneuvers through gloves places severe restrictions on the size of the chamber, making it an uncomfortable environment for the patient. In addition, the structure is such that it is easy for microorganisms to be retained in the event of faulty handling of patient excreta. The system has been largely overlooked as it now stands, and no recent modifications have been made, although the potential it holds is great.

We have adopted the germ-free room system in our hospital, where six high-efficiency particulate air (HEPA) filters (150 × 600 × 1500 mm) are positioned on the wall above the head of the patient in a 6000 × 4000 × 2500 mm room (Fig. 40–5). Sterile air flows horizontally over the patient and exits toward the anteroom located beyond the foot of the bed. The capacity of the HEPA filter is 0.5 m/sec, providing laminar air flow in an essentially horizontal direction. No fallout of bacteria to the floor was seen upon spraying 2 ml of a 10^8 cells/ml suspension of *E. coli* from a height of 1.5 m. Furthermore, dust-particle tests showed the room to be less than class 100 1 hour after operating the HEPA filters. A passbox for taking in food is provided for each room.

Methods for decontaminating a room prior to patient entry include fumigation by such gases as ethylene oxide, formaldehyde, and ozone, or vaporization of such agents as peracetic acid and chlorhexidine. Formalin gas sterilization (Glimstedt, 1932) is the form adopted in our hospital for creating a germ-free environment, and is effected as follows.

Six grams of formalin and 40 ml of water are placed in a vaporizer for every cubic meter of air, and the vaporizer is positioned in the center of the room. The room, including the HEPA filters, is sealed. The air-conditioning is turned off, and the vaporizer is turned on. Seven hours later, air-conditioning is resumed with the restart of laminar flow, and the room is ready for use in 2 days. Linen, supplies, medication, personal articles, and other items to be taken into the room are sterilized by using dry ovens or steam autoclaves, EO gas, irradiation, or filtration. Food can be sterilized by placing them in oven-proof glass dishes covered by three separate layers of aluminum foil, and baking them in an oven for 20 to 25 min at 250°C, which will kill even the spores.

To supply the sterilized meal to the patient, the outermost layer of foil is removed by the catering staff when placing the meal into the passbox of the catering room

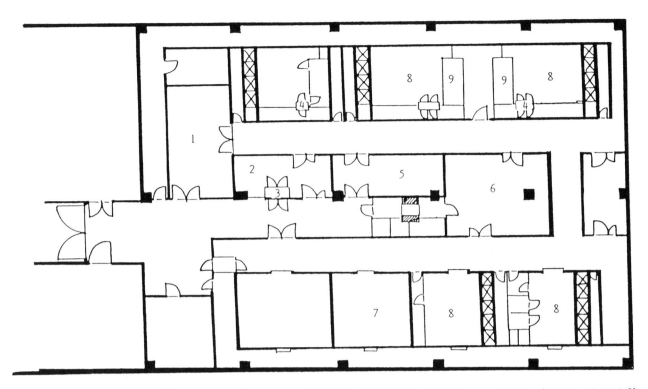

Fig. 40–5. Germ-free ward. 1, Sterilizing room. 2, Catering room. 3, Passbox A. 4, Passbox B. 5, Pharmacy. 6, Nurse's station. 7, PVC film isolator room. 8, Germ-free room. 9, HEPA filters.

for the germ-free ward without touching the second layer of foil; a nurse transfers it to the germ-free room passbox, removing the second layer with forceps and other instruments so as not to touch the third layer, which is removed by the patient.

Use of the oven is the primary mode of food sterilization, but it is important to provide a wider variety of germ-free foods by using other apparatus such as the autoclave and microwave oven. Fruit is given after decontaminating the outer surface with hibitane alcohol.

Feces are handled by a potty system holding plastic bags which are changed with each use. Because faulty handling here will lead to contamination of the entire room, alcohol and hibitane sprays are provided; instructing the patient on their use is one method. A washing basin with hibitane solution is also provided in each room.

The patient is prepared for entry into the germ-free room by first being primed with 2 g/m²/dose × 6 or 3 g/m²/dose × 10 cytosine arabinoside (Ara-C) from day −9 to day −5 before entry. A cardiovascular catheter is introduced into the patient prior to moving to the germ-free ward to facilitate treatment and testing over long periods. The catheter is inserted through an incision made in the external jugular vein to the middle cardiac vein, through which marrow cells, blood products, water, electrolytes, nutrients, and drug solutions are introduced. A 0.22-μm membrane filter is attached to the catheter for infusion of nutrients, and a three-way stop cock is positioned between the filter and the patient for

transfusion of blood components and other such materials needing no filtration.

Surface decontamination is effected by a 0.1% hyamine bath given in the anteroom; respiratory tract, vaginal, epidermal, and oral hygiene are maintained in the germ-free room itself.

From days −10 to −7 before BMT, the patient is placed on an oral regimen of vancomycin, polymyxin B, and nystatin (VPN) (Nagao et al., 1981); total-body irradiation (TBI) is given when decontamination of the intestinal tract is well underway. The moving couch method is used for the irradiation using KI gel 201 (Kurarey Co. Ltd., Japan) for bolus and 10 megavolt linear accelerator rays. The total dose of 12 Gy is fractionated into six installments over 3 days. The time for each session of TBI is just short of 30 min. This is achieved by using a dose rate of 16 cGy/min, which has been justified in our experience, because only 2 of 48 cases have been suspected of interstitial pneumonitis using this regimen. However, many aspects regarding total dose, dose fractionation, dose rate, and dosimetry have room for improvement in the future.

Twenty-four hours following TBI, bone marrow is transplanted. The largest number of cases involve transplantation of HLA-matched marrow from siblings. More recently, BMT has come to be carried out with HLA-mismatched marrow, and from donors who are not blood relatives. Agents such as cyclosporin (Gonwa et al., 1985) and cyclophosphamide (Collis and Steel, 1983) are used for immunosuppression, antibiotics for prevention of in-

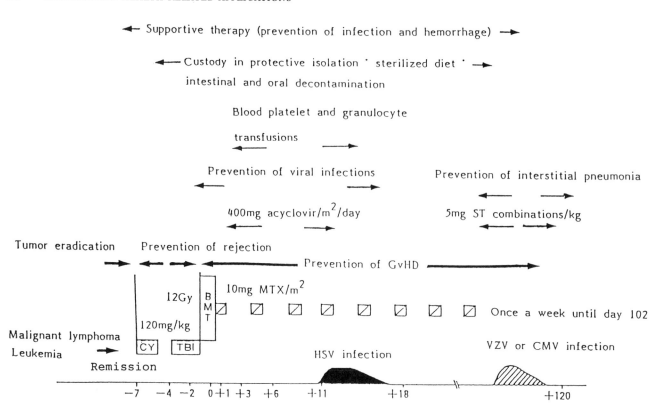

Fig. 40–6. Protocol for BMT in children and incidence of infectious disease.

fections, acyclovir for prevention of viral infection, and methotrexate for prevention of GvHD; these agents are employed as needed (Figs. 40–6, 40–7; Table 40–1).

The best results are obtained in using marrow from HLA-matched, MLC-negative siblings, but most patients do not have donors fitting this description. Recently, it has been revealed that there is no difference in the incidence of GvHD between matched and mismatched transplants, as long as HLA expression is the same, and we are coming to see greater numbers of possibilities in terms of donors.

On the other hand, there was a 15-year-old male with ALL treated by BMT from an identical twin, which presented no problems theoretically, but which ended in failure from recurrence when the grafted cells did not take even though there was no evidence of GvHD. Such cases illustrate the immaturity of this procedure, and the questions we have yet to answer.

However, we now know from experience that when *Candida* is detected during VPN decontamination, TBI should not be carried out until decontamination is complete, as unfavorable prognoses are seen in a markedly high percentage of cases in which the organism is again detected in the observation period after BMT. The presence of *Pseudomonas* should be regarded likewise.

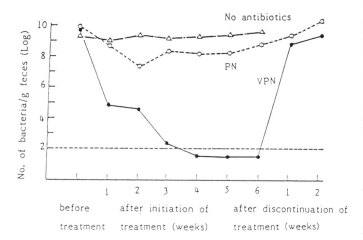

Fig. 40–7. Fluctuations in intestinal bacteria following administration of antibiotics.

Table 40–1. *Protocol for Human Decontamination*

Oral administration	
Vancomycin	30 mg/kg/day
Polymyxin B	12 mg/kg/day
Nystatin	6×10^4 units/kg/day (in 3 doses)
Inhalation	
Polymyxin B	5 mg
Amphotericin B	5 mg (every 6 hours)
Hibitane cream (1%)	2 applications/day (nasal, anal, and vaginal cavities)
Povidone-iodine (0.1%)	As gargle 4 times/day

Viral infections have long been the uncontrollable factor, but reports now indicate acyclovir to be effective against the herpes virus group (Gluckman et al., 1983).

Many problems remain to be solved in relation to BMT, apart from the obvious problems of GvHD and control of infections by virus and other microorganisms. They include pneumocystis carinii; psychological management; nutritional management; preparation of meals; nursing; generation, differentiation, culturing techniques, and genetic manipulation of marrow cells; development of a system for cryopreservation of an individual's cells (e.g., marrow and phagocytic cells including lymphocytes) taken in health; and a system for HLA registration.

PVC Isolators for Autopsy of Infection Patients (Fig. 40–8)

The number of autopsies involving Creutzfeldt-Jakob disease (CJD) (Koch et al.,1985), human immunodeficiency virus (HIV) and hepatitis B are on the rise. And with autopsies being an inescapable part of any medical institution, the incidence of infection of postmortem staff is also on the rise (Bernoulli, 1977; Elias, 1977; Gajdusek et al., 1977; Miller, 1988).

There are two systems for protection in use. One involves covering the entire body of staff by a completely watertight suit and helmet developed as a spin-off from NASA technology. The other involves the construction of a completely watertight room, decontaminated by a 5% solution of hypochlorous acid or, where it involves metals, 2% glutaraldehyde or 5% formaldehyde solution. Neither system is very practical considering the costs of maintenance, the restriction placed on movement in use, and the time reported for decontamination, which amounts to more than 24 hours using hypochlorous acid as the sterilant after handling cases of CJD.

We have developed a germ-free autopsy setup based on the isolator system, which is described below in detail as an easily adoptable system for preventing secondary infections among hospital personnel (Fig. 40–9).

Specifications

1. A stainless steel table built specifically for this purpose should be 600 × 2500 mm. The height should be adjustable by a mechanism for providing 100 to 200 mm of vertical slide, with hip level being the median height, allowing the table to be positioned at an optimal height for working. The tabletop is slanted so that it is 200 mm lower on the side of the sterile lock, and two hooks are provided at each end of the longitudinal side for tying down the chamber.

2. The chamber is basically the same as the PVC cham-

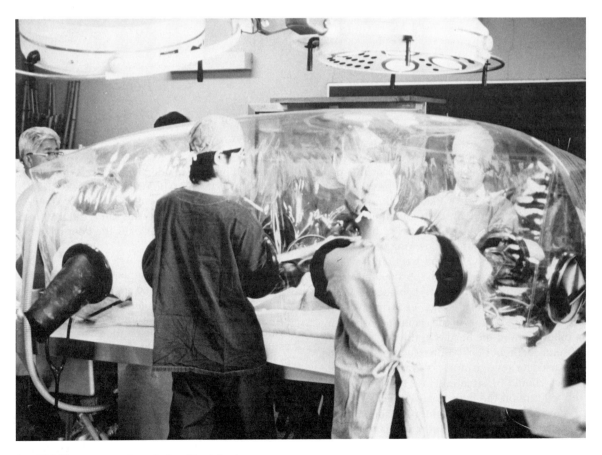

Fig. 40–8. PVC film autopsy isolator for handling infection cases.

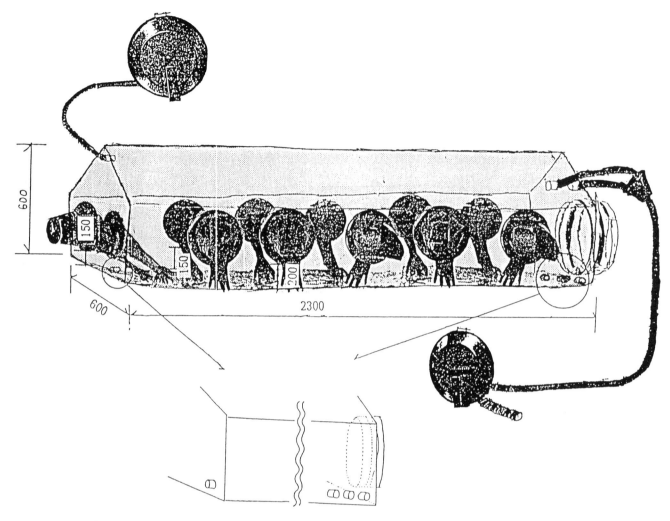

Fig. 40–9. PVC film autopsy isolator.

ber for germ-free animals, only larger (600 × 600 × 2300 mm), and is able to accommodate four or five persons working at the same time. Ten neoprene gloves designed to fit either hand are situated 200 mm off the floor of the chamber, five along each longitudinal side, enabling delicate procedures to be carried out by inserting the hands at any position. Covering these gloves with cotton gloves will provide good traction as well as protect them from puncture. On one short 600-mm side, a pair of regular neoprene gloves are provided 150 mm off the floor, enabling the blade of an electric saw to be worked on the occipital region of the cadaver, positioning a wooden pillow behind the head. On the other 600-mm side, a 300-mm segment of 550-mm diameter PVC pipe (such as that used for sewage pipes) is attached as a sterile lock. The lock should be situated close to the floor (approximately 30 mm off the floor at lowest point) to prevent the cadaver from getting caught in passing through the lock. The sterile lock is fitted into the chamber wall, secured with filament and PVC tape and, for added stability, rested on a block of wood formed to the contour

of the sterile lock (also about 30 mm at lowest point) positioned on the outside. Then the sterile lock is belted down tightly to the table with a stainless steel belt at a point 50 mm from the outer edge of the sterile lock.

3. A PVC foam mat, of the same quality used in the animal isolator, is used to cover the floor of the chamber for protection.

4. Air-filtration units are also the same as those used in the animal isolators. Air intake and exhaust ports made of PVC tubing are provided near the top of each end of the chamber, to which relatively long segments of flexible pipe are attached leading to the airfilters. The filtration units should be suspended with string from the ceiling so that their weight does not affect the inflation of the chamber and to protect them from the water used inside. The air-intake filters and motorized blower are also connected by a flexible pipe, long enough to avoid any tension.

5. Seven pieces of 25-mm diameter soft PVC tubing, 50-mm long each, are attached—one to the end opposite the sterile lock, and three along each longitudinal side close to the sterile lock and to the floor—as ports.

Two ports along the left side of the body in the chamber are used to pass through air hoses for supplying compressed air to the spray guns inside for peracetic acid atomization. Each hose is threaded through an opening made with a cork borer in a No. 9 silicone rubber stopper, fashioned to provide a watertight seal when inserted into the PVC port from outside the chamber, so it will remain intact even when the spray gun is pulled on from the inside. The length of the air hose from the rubber stopper to one spray gun should be adequate to reach the pair of gloves on the short 600-mm end, which are used to operate the spray gun. The air hose for the second spray gun should be long enough to permit insertion of the gunhead into the port on the inner cap for decontaminating the sterile lock. Two spray guns are used so that they can spray each other, because the grip of the guns are contaminated from handling with soiled gloves.

The third port on this side, used for draining the chamber, is left stoppered until use after decontamination.

The ports along the right side of the body in the chamber are used for drainage, for drawing in tap water, and for setting an aspirator in the same manner used to position the air hose. The aspirator is used for drawing off ascitic fluid, chest fluid, and water. The aspirated wastes are collected in a roll-away 200-L polyethylene tank, which is treated with sterilant after the autopsy. For example, for sterilizing CJD, the waste is used to adjust hypochlorite to a 5% hypochlorous solution and left for 24 hours before disposal.

On the 600-mm side opposite the sterile lock, the seventh port accommodates the cord of the electric saw. The saw should be equipped with a compact plug that can be passed through the port, with the cord fitted through a rubber stopper plugging into the port from inside the chamber, so the saw can be removed via the sterile lock with the electric cord, plug, and stopper attached. This means that care should be taken in using the saw not to pull strongly on the cord inside the chamber, because this will dislocate the stopper.

6. After depositing the cadaver in the isolator, a two-tiered stainless steel table is placed above the lower legs. This is used for holding instruments, sutures, and needles, as well as wide-necked lidded jars containing 10% formalin for collecting specimens. However, animals inoculated with specimens from CJD patients after soaking in 10% formalin for 1 year develop the disease without exception, showing formalin to be ineffective for disinfection. Therefore, CJD specimens should be fixed with 2% glutaraldehyde, although it is best to avoid collecting samples as much as possible.

Cotton used to stuff the chest and abdomen before closing up is packed in plastic bags to prevent water leakage. The board for cutting organs, the wooden pillow, linen string, and other such items are sterilized in the course of chamber decontamination by peracetic acid after use. Thick plastic bags able to withstand temperatures up to 130°C and impervious to peracetic acid are also among the supplies to be placed inside the isolator before use; these protect objects that are heat-resistant but susceptible to acid corrosion. Apparatus such as the electric saw, instruments, and scale for weighing organs are placed in the bags, which are tied securely with linen string to prevent entry of peracetic acid. When the necessary equipment is inside, the inner cap is put in place and the chamber is inflated by turning on the motorized blower.

7. To remove the cadaver from the isolator, first, a trolley the same height as the autopsy table is placed next to the sterile lock. A linear low-density polyethylene body bag (0.1 × 870 × 3000–3500 mm) is secured over the sterile lock with PVC tape. The cadaver is transferred to the bag, and the inner lid of the sterile lock is replaced after excess air in the body bag is evacuated by pressing down from the outside (Fig. 40–10). After tying off the bag tightly above the cadaver's head with a clipband, the sterile lock is decontaminated by peracetic acid left to react for 30 min. The tape securing the bag to the sterile lock is then removed, detaching the bag from the isolator.

8. The air-inlet and outlet ports are stoppered with No. 9 silicone rubber stoppers. Splattered blood (from using the electric saw to open the cranium) and tap water (used to rinse off the body surface after closing the abdomen) are aspirated, but the chamber is thoroughly gone over with 3 to 4% peracetic acid using the two spray guns, thus taking liquids that could not be aspirated into account. Because the chamber is large, it is advisable to always keep extra peracetic acid on hand inside the isolator.

9. After use, the chamber is decontaminated with peracetic acid for 2 hours after packing the acid-susceptible items in plastic bags. The chamber is then ventilated for several hours to evacuate the fumes and odor.

When the sterile lock is opened for cleaning up, the scale, electric saw, and other items packed in the plastic bags are placed inside an autoclave, where the bags are perforated with scissors for easy access of steam or gas. Together with the scissors used for perforation, the bags are autoclaved or treated with EO gas.

The principal features of this autopsy isolator are its simplicity, its ability to be set up anywhere, and, more than anything else, its inexpensive construction and maintenance costs, because once the apparatus is made, it can be reused over a long period. Because all work is done under containment, this isolator is capable of completely eliminating the possibility of secondary infections among postmortem staff. Sufficient training in using the completed isolator will serve to alleviate both the anxiety involved with using the apparatus and fear of secondary infections.

Establishment of a Germ-Free Line of Animals by Hysterectomy

The interested reader is referred to the protocol set forth by Prof. J.A. Reyniers of Notre Dame University for the production of germ-free animals, which is still widely used today (Reyniers and Sacksteder, 1957; Reyniers, 1959).

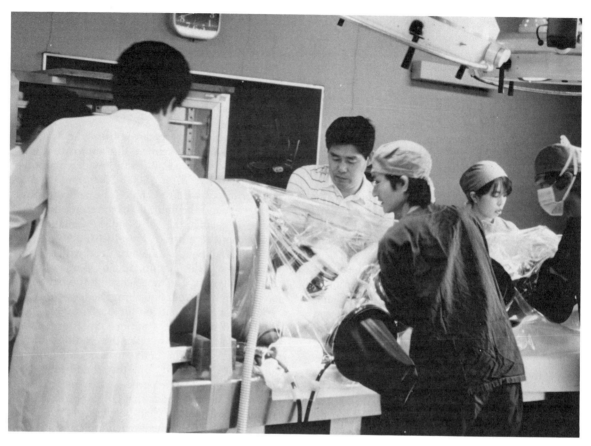

Fig. 40–10. Transfer of a body following autopsy through the sterile lock into a body bag.

The establishment of a germ-free line starts with the controlled breeding of animals for several generations; if this initial stage can be performed successfully, the rest of the procedure is not difficult. The procedure for establishing a germ-free line is now described, using mice as an example.

First of all, 10 males and 20 to 30 females of the strain to be made germ-free are reared on the same diet given to germ-free animals, which is autoclaved at $123 \pm 1°C$ for 20 min, from the time that begins immediately after weaning. Drinking water, likewise, is given sterilized. Mice and rats are mated at week 8 in combinations of 1:2–3 females, or 10 groups.

A total of 2 or 3 mice will become pregnant out of the 10 groups, and will yield about 10 mice/litter, which will average out to about 3 to 5 males per litter, although some litters will be composed only of females.

These F_1 mice are reared on a sterilized diet without mixing mice from different groups, and mated for F_2s. The procedure is repeated for producing F_3s, but while using only those groups of mice showing an increased birth-rate/litter. The F_3s thus produced should be about the same number and composition as the original set of animals, i.e., 10 males and 20 to 30 females, or slightly more.

Next, the F_3s are used to produce the germ-free an-

imals by hysterectomy. But before that, foster GF parents are prepared. Three groups of GF mice, each group consisting of 2 males and 5 females who have given birth 2 or 3 times, are housed separately, with 1 group/isolator. Seventy-two hours is allowed for mating time for the GF mice. Two days after mating GF mice, the F_3s of the mice from which germ-free animals are to be obtained are mated for 24 hours.

Preparations for the delivery of these animals are made as follows: Gauze, water, six or seven pieces of linen string, scissors, and five pairs of large and small forceps are wrapped in parchment paper or a sterilizing bag, sterilized, and placed in the isolators containing the GF foster parents.

Hysterectomies are performed on mice to be delivered germ-free 16 to 24 hours before they are due. Materials to be prepared for this are a board for holding down the mice, strings with which to hold down the hands and legs (strong enough to hold down a kicking animal), surgical gloves, operating cloth, autoclaved scissors, forceps, Kocher clamps, tincture of iodine and 70% alcohol spray for sterilization, and ether for lightly anesthetizing the animals to quiet them down. The hyamine solution in the V-shaped trap of the isolators containing the foster parents are warmed to 37°C with a heater, and the outer surface of the trap should be carefully decontaminated with tincture of iodine.

The hysterectomies are performed when the above setup is ready. Three people are required for this procedure, with the person working the isolator on standby, laying out gauze and scissors inside the chamber, spreading the parchment paper or sterilizing bags they came in, and passing one end of a piece of linen string through the V-shaped trap outside.

Approximately 16 to 24 hours before the mice are due, the pregnant mothers are lightly anesthetized, tied down to the board, and the entire body decontaminated with tincture of iodine. The animal is covered with an operating cloth leaving only the operative field in view. The epidermis and muscle layers are cut open, and the bicornuate uterus is laid bare. A Kocher clamp is positioned around the opening of the uterus, and the uterus is removed by an incision right below the clamp with scissors. The finger hole of the clamp is promptly tied to the end of the linen string trailing through the V-shaped trap, and the clamp and uterus are pulled through the hyamine solution into the chamber.

The uterus is laid out on the parchment paper, rinsed with drinking water, dried with gauze, and cut open with scissors. The fetuses are removed, wiped with gauze, and revived, protecting them from drops in body temperature.

The sequence from tying the uterus with the clamp to reviving the fetus should take no more than 60 seconds. The procedure should be simulated beforehand by the team of three, and carried out only when each person is thoroughly familiar with the sequence, because a year's effort will end in vain by failure at this point.

Further points that should be considered are the following:

1. No more than two litters should be contained in one isolator.
2. Animals less than 12 hours away from labor should not be used because of the likely possibility of contamination through the uterine opening, whereas fetuses removed 2 to 3 days before they are due are too small to be reared successfully.
3. Pregnant SPF mice whose abdomens do not protrude very much to the sides should not be considered for the hysterectomies, because such mice are carrying only a few fetuses. It is better to pick up 4 to 6 mice who appear to be pregnant with many fetuses for the procedure.
4. Within the isolator, the GF foster parents should already have given birth to more than 3 mice at the time of the hysterectomies. The original litter is replaced by the revived mice, and this exchange is effected easily by smearing the body surface of the newborns with feces of the foster parent. Primipara animals are not used as foster parents, because they will not nurse the foreign litter. Para II and Para III mice should accept and nurse the replacements without fuss.
5. If, upon reviving the fetuses, it becomes apparent that there are no males among the litter, or they are markedly underdeveloped, they should promptly be wrapped in the parchment paper together with the instruments used, and set aside, keeping the work area as clean as possible, to start work on the next uterus.
6. The offspring of the foster parents should be reared to be used later as GF monitor mice.
7. Only when the germ-free status of the X.GF mice reared by the foster parents is confirmed by tests for contamination using organ homogenate cultures and viral induction tests by 6 to 10 Gy irradiation using the GF monitor mice, can the previous generations of SPF animals be set aside. The monitoring needs to be continued until the X.GF animals produce their F_1s.
8. The physiologic properties of first-generation X.GF mice are almost unchanged from their SPF counterparts, so they should not be used for germ-free experiments. It is considered that GF characteristics are not fully exhibited until the F_3 generation at the earliest.

We have established lines of GF mice and nude rats as needed, and are currently in possession of a line of rnuGF nude rats produced in this manner.

REFERENCES

Aizawa, S., Sado, T., Muto, M., and Kubo, E. 1981. Immunology of fully H-2 incompatible bone marrow chimeras induced in specific-pathogen-free mice: Evidence for generation of donor- and host-H-2 restricted helper and cytotoxic T cells. J. Immunol., 127, 2426–2431.

Bealmear, P.M., Mirand, E.A., and Holterman, O.A. 1983. Modification of graft-vs-host disease following bone marrow transplantation in germfree mice. Biol. Cancer, 2, 409–421.

Bernhardt, W. 1963. Some problems of fine structure in tumor cells. Prog. Exp. Tumor Res., 3, 1–34.

Bernoulli, C., et al. 1977. Danger of accidental person-to-person transmission of Creutzfeld-Jakob disease by surgery. Lancet, 26, 478–479.

Bortin, M.M., Horowitz, M.M., and Gale, R.P. 1988. Current status of bone marrow transplantation in humans: report from the International Bone Marrow Transplant Registry. Nat. Immun. Cell Growth Regul., 7(5–6), 334–350.

Brown, P., Rohwer, R.G., Green, E.M., and Gajdusek, D.C. 1982. Effect of chemicals, heat, and histopathologic processing on high-infectivity hamster-adapted scrapie virus. J. Infect. Dis., 145(5), 683–687.

Collis, C.H., and Steel, G.G. 1983. Lung damage in mice from cyclophosphamide and thoracic irradiation. Int. J. Radiat. Oncol. Biol. Phys., 9, 685–689.

Domagk, G. 1935. Eine neue klasse von disinfektionsmitteln. Dtsch. Med. Wochenschr., 61, 829–832.

Eastcott, J.W., Broitman, S.A., and Bennett, M. 1981. Graft-versus-host reactions by NZB lymphoid cells exposed to major or minor histocompatibility antigens in irradiated adult mice. Cell. Immunol., 58, 124–133.

Elias, R., et al. 1977. Transmission of Creutzfeldt-Jakob disease to syrian hamster. Lancet, 26, 479.

Foster, H.L. 1959. Housing of disease-free vertebrates. Ann. N.Y. Acad. Sci., 78, 80–88.

Gajdusek, D.C., et al. 1977. Precautions in medical care of, and in handling materials from, patients with transmissible virus dementia (Creutzfeldt-Jacob disease). N. Engl. J. Med., 297(23), 1253–1258.

Gibbs, C.J., et al. 1985. Clinical and pathological features and laboratory confimation of Creutzfeldt-Jakob disease in a recipient of pituitary-derived human growth hormone. N. Engl. J. Med., 313(12), 734–738.

Glimstedt, G. 1932. Das leben ohne bakterien. Sterile aufziehung von meerschweinchen. Verh. Dtsch. Ges. Anat., 41, 79–89.

Gluckman, E., et al. 1983. Oral acyclovir prophylactic treatment of herpes simplex infection after bone marrow transplantation. J. Antimicrob. Chemother., 12(Suppl. B), 161–167.

Gonwa, T.A., et al. 1985. Failure of cyclosporine to prevent in vivo T cell priming in man. Transplantation, 40(3), 299–304.

Greenspan, F.P., and Mackellar, D.G. 1951. The application of peracetic acid germicidal washes to mold control of tomatoes. Food Technol., 5, 95–97.

Greenspan, F.P. 1946. The convenient preparation of peracids. J. Am. Chem. Soc., 68, 907.

Greenstein, J.P., Birnbaum, S.M., Winitz, M., and Otey, M.C. 1957. Quantitative nutritional studies with water-soluble, chemically defined diets. I. Growth, reproduction and lactation in rats. Arch. Biochem. Biophys., 72, 396–416.

Greenstein, J.P., Otey, M.C., Birnbaum, S.M., and Winitz, M. 1960. Quantitative nutritional studies with water-soluble, chemically defined diets. J. Natl. Cancer Inst., 24, 211–219.

Gustafsson, B.E. 1948. Germ-free rearing of rats. Acta Pathol. Microbiol. Scand., 73(Suppl.), 1–130.

Jahuna, M., and Pollard, M. 1967. Virus-like particles in 3-methylcholanthrene-induced primary and transplanted sarcoma of germfree rodents. Cancer Res., 27, 980–993.

Jones, J.M., Wilson, R., and Bealmear, P.M. 1971. Mortality and gross pathology of secondary disease in germfree mouse radiation chimeras. Radiat. Res., 45, 577–588.

Koch, T.K., Berg, B.O., Armond, S.J.De, and Gravina, R.F. 1985. Creutzfeldt-Jakob disease in a young adult with idiopathic hypopituitarism. Possible relation to the administration of cadaveric human growth hormone. N. Engl. J. Med., 313(12), 731–733.

Luckey, R.D., Wagner, M., Reyniers, J.A., and Foster, F.L. 1955. Nutritional adequacy of a semi-synthetic diet, sterilized by steam or by cathode rays. Food Res., 20, 180–185.

Mauch, P., and Hellman, S. 1989. Loss of hematopoietic stem cell self-renewal after bone marrow transplantation. Blood, 74(2), 872–875.

Miller, D.C. 1988. Creutzfeldt-Jakob disease in histopathology technicians. N. Engl. J. Med., 318(13), 853–854.

Nagao, T., Sawamura, S., Ozawa, A., and Sasaki, S. 1984. Clinical significance of gastrointestinal decontamination in leukemic patients. Appl. Gnotobiol. Infect. Prevent. Immunocomp. Host, (eds. Günther, I., Fink, W., Brigmohan-Günther, R.) 125–130.

Norin, A.J., and Emerson, E.E. 1978. Effects of restoring lethally irradiated mice with anti-Thy 1.2-treated bone marrow: graft-vs-host, host-vs-graft, and mitogen reactivity. J. Immunol., 120(3), 754–758.

Onoe, K., Fernandes, G., and Good, R.A. 1980. Humoral and cell-mediated immune responses in fully allogeneic bone marrow chimera in mice. J. Exp. Med., 151, 115–132.

Phillips, C.R., and Kaye, S. 1949. The sterilizing action of gaseous ethylene oxide. Am. J. Hyg., 50, 280–288.

Pleasants, J.R., Reddy, B.S., and Wostmann, B.S. 1970. Qualitative adequacy of a chemically defined liquid diet for reproducing germfree mice. J. Nutr., 100, 498–508.

Pollard, M., and Matsuzawa, T. 1966. Chemical prevention of radiation induced leukemia in mice. Proc. Soc. Exp. Biol. Med., 122, 539–542.

Pollard, M., and Truitt, R.L. 1973. Allogeneic bone marrow chimerism in germfree mice. I. Prevention of spontaneous leukemia in AKR Mice (37657). P.S.E.B.M., 144, 659–665.

Pollard, M., and Truitt, R.L. 1974. Allogeneic bone marrow chimerism in germfree mice. II. Prevention of reticulum cell sarcomas in SJL/J Mice (37837). Soc. Exp. Biol. Med., 145, 488–492.

Reyniers, J.A., and Sacksteder, M. 1957. Observation on the survival of germfree C3H mice and their resistance to a contaminated environment. Presented at the Eighth Annual Meeting of the Animal Care Panel, November 7–9.

Reyniers, J.A. 1959. Design and operation of apparatus for rearing germfree animals. Ann. N.Y. Acad. Sci., 78, 47–79.

Traub, R.D., Gadjusek, D.C., and Gibbs, C.J. 1974. Precautions in conducting biopsies and autopsies on patients with presenile dementia. J. Neurosurg., 41, 394–395.

Trexler, P.C., and Reynolds, L.I. 1957. Flexible film apparatus for the rearing and use of germfree animals. Appl. Microbiol., 5, 406–412.

Trexler, P.C. 1959. The use of plastics in the design of isolator systems. Ann. N.Y. Acad. Sci., 78, 29–36.

Trexler, P.C. 1964. Germfree isolators. Scientific American, 211, 78–88.

Trexler, P.C. 1974. Germ-free animal techniques and some clinical applications. Reprinted from The Glaxo, 39, 21–31.

Truitt, R.L., Pollard, M., and Srivastava, K.K. 1974. Allogeneic bone marrow chimerism in germfree mice. III. Therapy of leukemic AKR mice (38061). Soc. Exp. Biol. Med., 146, 153–158.

Vallera, D.A., Soderling, C.C.B., Carlson, G.J., and Kersey, J.H. 1982. Bone marrow transplantation across major histocompatibility barriers in mice. II. T cell requirements for engraftment in total lymphoid irradiation-conditioned recipients. Transplantation, 33(3), 243–248.

Van Bekkum, D.W., de Vries, M.J., and van der Waaij, D. 1967. Lesions characteristic of secondary disease in germfree heterologous radiation chimeras. J. Natl. Cancer Inst., 38, 223–228.

Wade, A.C., Luckert, P.H., Tazume, S., and Niedbalski, J.L. 1987. Characterization of xenogeneic mouse-to-rat bone marrow chimeras. I. Examination of hematologic and immunologic function. Transplantation, 44(1), 88–92.

Wilson, R. 1963. Survival studies of whole body X-irradiated germfree mice. Radiat. Res., 20, 477–483.

Wilson, R., Matsuzawa, T., and Connell, S.S.J. 1964. Hematological changes in germfree mice following whole body X-irradiation. Radiat. Res., 22, 249–250.

Wostmann, B.S. 1959. Nutrition of the germfree mammal. Ann. N.Y. Acad. Sci., 78, 175–182.

CHAPTER 41

DISINFECTION OF DRINKING WATER, SWIMMING POOL WATER, AND TREATED SEWAGE EFFLUENTS

Christon J. Hurst

The basic philosophy in the disinfection of drinking water, swimming-pool water, and treated sewage effluents is to destroy or remove infectious microorganisms so that the water or waste cannot transmit disease-producing biologic agents. Microbiologic agents found in water or waste can be removed in part by treatments such as storage and settling, biologic or chemical flocculation, and filtration. To prevent disease transmission by water or wastes, the final treatment should be disinfection. Proper and careful application of any of the numerous water or waste disinfection procedures will result in water that contains no demonstrable pathogenic microorganisms.

No matter which disinfectant is used to treat water or sewage effluents, reliable techniques for measuring the adequacy of treatment, and also for measuring the presence or absence of residual disinfectant, are desirable. A disinfectant residual protects the treated water from recontamination with pathogens and also inhibits the growth of nuisance organisms. Residuals are readily measured for the halogens, but measurement of residuals following ozone, silver, ultraviolet light, or heat disinfection may be impossible or at best difficult.

The generally accepted biologic measurement to determine the adequacy of water and waste disinfection is the test for organisms of the coliform group. A discussion of the principles involved in use and interpretation of coliform data obtained by the "most probable number" (MPN) technique was reported by Woodward (1957). Clark et al. (1957) summarized the principles involved in interpretation of the membrane filter (MF) results for detection of coliform organisms in water. The philosophy of the concept of indicator organisms of pollution, in this case the coliform group, was discussed in the National Interim Primary Drinking Water Regulations, Appendix A (1975) and summarized by Allen and Geldreich (1978).

In actual practice, because of the widespread use of chlorine, many water treatment plants base the adequacy of disinfection on the amounts of disinfectant applied and the residual disinfectant concentration. The amounts of disinfectant required to treat various waters adequately are defined in terms of reducing the coliform organisms to acceptable levels.

Whether the true biologic safety of water can be adequately measured by coliform counts has been questioned in view of data on the resistance of viruses and cysts to disinfection (Clarke et al., 1964; Scarpino et al., 1972; Liu, 1973; Chang, 1944). Marzouk et al. (1980), Gerba et al. (1979), Nestor (1980), and Sekla et al. (1980) reported that they found viruses in water samples that were considered acceptable as judged by coliform standards. Craun et al. (1976), Lippy (1978), Kirner et al. (1978) and Shaw et al. (1977) reported that coliform removal during the disinfection process was not an effective measure of the inactivation of *Giardia* cysts. Logsdon et al. (1981), however, reported that cysts were removed by proper filtration procedures. Cold water increases the life span of *Giardia* cysts, with temperatures less than 5°C allowing survival for about 2 months (Hibler et al., 1987). Furthermore, the cyst wall effectively protects the organism from many other adverse environmental factors, even postponing the biocidal activity of some disinfectants. The fact that lower temperatures decrease the rate at which cysts are inactivated by chlorine, coupled with the fact that lower temperatures naturally prolong cyst survival, may increase the risk of Giardiasis during colder seasons (Hibler et al., 1987). Walton (1961) has reviewed the effectiveness of water treatment processes as measured by coliform reduction.

Boardman and coworkers (1989) have reviewed the detection and occurrence of waterborne bacterial and viral pathogens. Sobsey (1989) has reviewed the inactivation of health-related microorganisms in water by disinfection processes. The review by Sobsey includes bacteria, viruses, and protozoan pathogens such as *Giardia lamblia*, *Cryptosporidium*, and free-living amoebae (e.g., *Acanthamoeba* species and *Naegleria* species). Free-living protozoa such as *Acanthamoeba* and *Tetrahymena* can be of particular concern during chlorine disinfection as they, themselves, can be more resistant than are bacteria (King et al., 1988). Bacterial pathogens that can remain viable following ingestion by the protozoa will likewise have an increased resistance to chlorine when inside the protozoa, and this way lead to persistence of bacteria in chlorine-treated water (King et al., 1988).

Factors affecting the efficiency of disinfection are dosage, contact time, temperature, turbidity, color, organic and inorganic material in the water, and pH. The effect of these factors varies with the disinfectant employed and will be discussed subsequently. Other important factors involved with water disinfection are the toxic byproducts that can result from the use of chlorine (Dugan, 1978) and alternative disinfectants (Bull, 1982). These will receive further mention in subsequent sections of this chapter.

DISINFECTION OF DRINKING WATER

The Safe Drinking Water Act (1974) included requirements for the promulgation of Primary Drinking Water Regulations that would apply to all public water supplies. These regulations were to contain a list of contaminants that have adverse effects on human health, maximum contaminant limit, and procedures and criteria to ensure that drinking water complied with the maximum contaminant levels. Such regulations were enacted by the U.S. Environmental Protection Agency with publication of the National Interim Primary Drinking Water Regulations (1975) and replaced the United States Public Health Service Drinking Water Standards (1962) and later the Final Rule for National Primary Drinking Water Regulations (U.S. EPA, 1989). Maximum contaminant limits were now applied for the first time for microorganisms and selected chemicals for all public water supplies serving 25 or more persons. It is axiomatic that the residual concentration of any water disinfectant must not be toxic to humans consuming the water. The role of adequate disinfection in the prevention of waterborne disease outbreaks has been summarized by Akin et al. (1982). A good general discussion of disinfection, including the chemistry of disinfectants, has been prepared by Bossart and McCreary (1983). One of the important aspects of drinking water disinfection is the frequent inability of laboratory-based models to accurately predict field results. This issue has been addressed by Wolfe and Olson (1985). Potassium permanganate has been used as a strong oxidant for the removal of iron and manganese from water supplies. This oxidant has been investigated by Yahya and coworkers (1989b) for its potential ability to help reduce the load of microorganisms in water. There

is not much additional information available on this subject.

Chlorine and Chlorine Compounds

Chlorine and its compounds are the most widely used drinking-water disinfectants. Morris (1971) estimated that over 95% of the existing water treatment facilities in the United States were disinfected with chlorine.

Chlorine and chlorine compounds are strong oxidizing agents, and their reactivity can be easily dissipated in reactions with organic and inorganic materials in water before efficient disinfection can occur. Chlorine is less reactive as pH increases, and reaction rates increase with increasing temperatures. Scarpino et al. (1972) reported, however, that this may not always be true, at least in the case of poliovirus 1. The nature and kinetics of reactions of chlorine with nitrogen-containing compounds (ammonia, amino acids, and proteins) have been studied by Griffin (1939), Fair et al. (1948), Palin (1945, 1950), and Wolfe et al. (1984).

Addition of chlorine gas to pure water results in the formation of a mixture of hypochlorous and hydrochloric acids.

$$Cl_2 + H_2O \rightleftharpoons HOCl + H^+ + Cl^-$$

The reaction is complete within seconds at ordinary water temperatures and at pH levels above 4. In dilute solutions, little Cl_2 exists in solution. The disinfecting action is associated with the HOCl formed. Hypochlorous acid dissociates as follows:

$$HOCl \rightleftharpoons H^+ + OCl^-$$

The degree of dissociation depends on pH and (much less) on temperature. Dissociation is poor at pH levels below 6. At pH levels of 6.0 to 8.5, a change occurs from undissociated HOCl to nearly complete dissociation. The same reactions occur regardless of whether chlorine gas or hypochlorite forms of chlorine are used in water disinfection, a point that not all investigators appreciate. To achieve good disinfection of water with chlorine, control of pH is critical. Chlorine has relatively little killing power in waters of pH 8.5 or above. Most potable waters, when chlorinated, have pH levels at which chlorine exists both as hypochlorous acid and hypochlorite ion. In water, hypochlorous acid and hypochlorite ion are defined as free available chlorine.

The reactions of chlorine with ammonia and nitrogen-containing organic substances are of great importance in water disinfection. Such nitrogen-containing substances react with hypochlorous acid to form chloramines of many sorts, known as *N*-chlor compounds (monochloramine, dichloramine, trichloramine, etc.). Such additional products retain some of the disinfecting power of hypochlorous acid, but are much less effective at a given level. These *N*-chlor compounds or chlorine-organic nitrogen compounds are defined as combined available chlorine. Shull (1981) reported on the experiences of a water treatment plant that had used chloramines as a primary disinfectant for over 50 years. He concluded that chloramines can be an effective primary disinfectant for coliforms and other bacteria in waters having a pH less than 8, provided that sufficient concentration and contact time are employed. No virus data were presented in the report.

The relative disinfecting effectiveness of free available chlorine and combined available chlorine on bacteria has been studied extensively by Butterfield and his associates (1943, 1946, 1948) and by Wattie and Butterfield (1944). Figure 41–1, constructed from their data, shows the superiority of free available chlorine (hypochlorous acid) versus combined available chlorine (monochloramine) against *Escherichia coli*. On the basis of these studies, Butterfield (1948) proposed minimum safe residual levels of free and combined available chlorine for the destruction of vegetative bacteria in water.

The relative resistance of bacteria and viruses, which may be very numerous in environmental waters (Walter et al., 1989), and cysts to chlorine is of obvious practical importance. Studies on the virucidal efficiency of chlorine have been reported by Clarke and Chang (1959), Clarke et al. (1964), Liu (1973), Engelbrecht et al. (1980), Sharp and Leong (1980), Jensen et al. (1980), Sharp et al. (1980), and others. The inactivation of heterotrophic bacterial populations in finished drinking water by chlorine and chloramines has been examined by Wolfe et al. (1985). Bacterial viruses have become of interest for their potential usefulness as indicators of disinfection effectiveness in substitution for human viruses (Sobsey et al., 1988). The advantages of using bacterial viruses include the fact that they do not present a pathogenic hazard to researchers. This interest has resulted in a number of studies addressing the disinfection of bacterial viruses, and in comparisons of the relative sensitivity of bacterial viruses and human viruses (Taylor and Butler, 1982). Grabow et al. (1983) have compared the sensitivity of bacteria and bacterial viruses to free chlorine residuals.

Other particularly notable factors with regard to the chlorine sensitivity of viruses are the possible role of dissolved salts as potentiators of virucidal effectiveness (Berg et al., 1989), the fact that viruses can vary greatly in their sensitivity to the disinfectant (Payment et al., 1985a), and the knowledge that ability of viruses to resist disinfection can depend upon such factors as the conformational form of the virus capsid proteins that surround and protect the viral nucleic acid genome (Young and Sharp, 1985). Detailed studies on the inactivation of cysts in water have been published by Chang (1944), Stringer and Kruse (1970), Stringer et al. (1975), Jarroll et al. (1981), DeJonckheere and Van De Voorde (1976), and Clark et al. (1989). Figure 41–2 was constructed from data of Butterfield et al. (1943), Clarke and Kabler (1954), Clarke et al. (1956), Weidenkopf (1958), and Engelbrecht et al. (1974) and indicates the relative resistance to hypochlorous acid of four viruses as compared to *E. coli*, *Mycobacterium fortuitum*, *M. phlei*, and the yeast *Candida parapsilosis*. With the exception of adenovirus type 3, all of the organisms tested are more resistant to hypochlorous acid than *E. coli*.

In practice, drinking water can be disinfected with either free residual chlorine or combined residual chlorine. Free residual chlorination involves addition of sufficient chlorine to water to produce a free available chlorine residual and to maintain it through all or part of the plant or distribution system. This procedure provides the most efficient disinfection. Although combined residual chlorination is less efficient in terms of rapidity of disinfection, it may be useful in maintaining a stable residual in the entire distribution system. Goshko et al. (1983) have found statistical associations between coliform density and chlorine residuals for some drinking water systems. Often both systems are used together; free residual chlorination is used before the water enters the distribution system, and combined residual chlori-

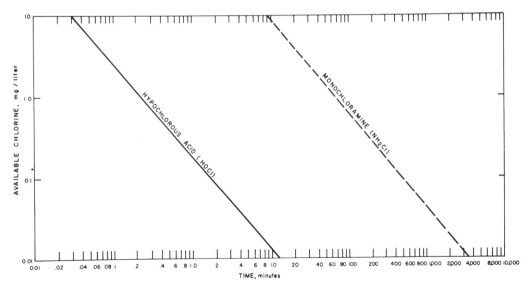

Fig. 41–1. Relationship between concentration and time for 99% destruction of *Escherichia coli* by two forms of chlorine at 2 to 6°C.

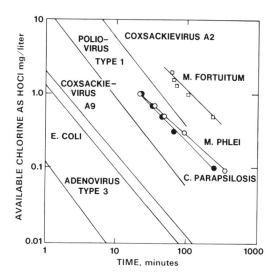

Fig. 41–2. Relationship between concentration and time for 99% inactivation for selected viruses and bacteria.

nation is used to maintain a residual in the system. In keeping with this approach, a study by Hubbs et al. (1981) recommended the application of free chlorine, followed 10 minutes later by ammoniation.

Turbidity in processed water can affect the efficiency of disinfection of the water. Culp (1974) and Cookson (1974) stated that turbidity levels of 0.1 to 1 Jackson Turbidity Unit were needed for good viral disinfection of water. Boardman and Sproul (1977) and Hoff (1978) found that viruses associated with inorganic particles having a turbidity level as high as 7 NTU were not protected during the disinfection process with chlorine. This is important, because Moore et al. (1975) and Schaub and Sagik (1975) found that viruses associated with clay particles are infective for cell cultures and animals. Hejkal et al. (1979) and Hoff (1978) reported that poliovirus associated with organic particles (fecal material or cell-associated virus) was inactivated at a slower rate than free virus. Hoff (1978) also reported that coliform bacteria associated with primary effluent solids and diluted to turbidity of 1 or 5 NTU were inactivated by chlorine at a much slower rate than was a laboratory culture of *E. coli*. These microorganisms are inactivated beyond detection limits when the chlorine concentration is high or the contact time prolonged. The results of this type of research confirm the need for a chlorine residual in a water distribution system.

Although the chlorination of drinking water is important for the inactivation of pathogenic microorganisms, the chlorination process can also lead to the formation of chloroform and other trihalomethane (THM) compounds, particularly when the water source is surface water (Rook, 1974; Bellar et al., 1974; Symons et al., 1975). Trihalomethane compounds are important because they are toxic chemicals and are possibly carcinogenic. Chloroform is a known carcinogen in test animals. The THM compounds apparently are formed from the reaction of chlorine with humic or fulvic acid. Reck-

how and Singer (1990) have published a detailed study on the formation of chlorination byproducts in drinking waters. Approaches for controlling the production of trihalomethanes have been summarized by Vogt and Regli (1981).

Chlorine Dioxide

The studies of Ridenour and Armbruster (1949), Ridenour et al. (1949), and Benarde et al. (1965) indicate that chlorine dioxide is an effective water disinfectant for achieving the destruction of bacteria. Chlorine dioxide is also a potent virucide (Scarpino et al., 1979; Hauchman et al., 1986; Noss et al., 1986) and is potentially effective against a recently recognized public health hazard, waterborne *Cryptosporidium* oocytes (Peeters et al., 1989). Their data show that its effectiveness is not lessened by increases in the pH of water; in fact, with increasing pH, lesser residuals are required because the biocidal efficiency of chlorine dioxide increases with increases in pH. Chlorine dioxide does not react as readily as chlorine with humic acid and other organic compounds found in water; therefore, lesser amounts of trihalomethanes are produced during chlorine dioxide disinfection of drinking water (Symons et al., 1976). The findings from a pilot study of chlorine dioxide use for reducing production of total trihalomethanes during the water treatment process have been published by Monscvitz and Rexing (1981).

Economic considerations have limited the wide use of chlorine dioxide as a water disinfectant. Miller et al. (1978) surveyed 105 water treatment plants in the United States and found that 84 plants use chlorine dioxide. Although multiple reasons were given for using chlorine dioxide, most plants used it to control taste and odor problems. Other reasons given were disinfection, iron and manganese control, control of organic substances, and color. The survey was expanded to include water treatment plants in other countries and showed that chlorine dioxide is used in at least 522 water treatment plants worldwide.

Formation of the organic byproducts chlorite ion and chlorate ion can be a problem in drinking water treatment processes that use chlorine dioxide as a disinfectant (Gordon et al., 1990). Myhrstad and Samdal (1969) have reported on a combination of methods for determining chlorine dioxide, chlorite, and chlorine in solution; additionally, they point out that the reduction of chlorine dioxide to chlorite has many practical consequences in general water treatment, including the toxicity of chlorite and its lower bactericidal effect. An update on this information has been published by the U.S. Environmental Protection Agency (1977). Calabrese et al. (1978) and Bull (1980) have also reported on the health effects of chlorine dioxide in water. The books *Chlorine Dioxide: Chemistry and Environmental Impact of Oxychlorine Compounds* by W.J. Masschelein (1979) and *Ozone/Chlorine Dioxide Oxidation Products of Organic Materials* (Rice and Cotruvo, 1978) are good reference sources for additional information about chlorine dioxide. Hoehn et al. (1990) have published a study that addresses odors reportedly associated with the use of chlorine dioxide as a drinking water disinfectant.

Bromine

Bromine has no known applications as a drinking water disinfectant; its use apparently has been limited to disinfection of swimming-pool waters and certain industrial wastes. The virucidal properties of bromine and related compounds have been reported by Floyd and Sharp (1978) and Olivieri et al. (1975); their bactericidal and cysticidal properties have been studied by Solo et al. (1975) and Stringer et al. (1975).

Iodine

Iodine, like bromine, has not been employed as a disinfectant for large public water supplies. Black et al. (1965), however, have reported a comprehensive study on its use to disinfect the water supplies of three Florida correctional institutions serving approximately 700 persons. The study continued for a period of 19 months under carefully planned chemical, bacteriologic, and medical controls. Their data show that iodine was an effective disinfectant of the two water supplies under investigation. Additionally, there was no evidence that iodine, under their experimental conditions, had any detrimental effect on general health or thyroid function. Iodine has been studied extensively as an emergency drinking water disinfectant or as a disinfectant for small individual supplies, primarily military.

Chambers et al. (1952) and Chang and Morris (1953) have studied the factors affecting the bactericidal, cysticidal, and virucidal efficiency of iodine in water. Their results show that iodine is an efficient water disinfectant. Its disinfecting ability is not affected by high pH (Alvarez and O'Brien, 1982) or the presence of organic or other nitrogen-containing substances as much as is chlorine. On a comparative mg/L basis, more iodine than chlorine is required for a comparable bacterial kill. Berg et al. (1964) reported extensive studies on the inactivation of certain enteroviruses by elemental iodine. Poynter et al. (1973), in their review of water disinfectants, devoted a section to the disinfectant activity of iodine. Chang (1958) reviewed in detail the chemistry of aqueous solutions of elemental iodine. Pyle and McFeters (1989) have published studies on the iodine sensitivity of bacterial isolates from the United States space shuttle's potable water system and from a prototype urine/wastewater recycling shower system, both disinfected with a demand-type iodinated anion exchange resin.

Ozone

Ozone is an unstable gas formed by the corona discharge of high-voltage electricity in dry air. Three atoms of oxygen are thus combined to form an O_3 molecule. It is a strong oxidizing substance, but it is unstable and therefore is usually generated at its point of application.

In Europe, particularly in France, ozone has been used as a water disinfectant in a number of water treatment plants. Miller et al. (1978) reported that over 1000 such installations are now in operation, mainly in Europe, but also including 23 in Canada. One of the largest drinking water treatment plants in the world using ozone is located in the city of Montreal; another is in Moscow. The United States has a few drinking water treatment plants that use ozone. It has been suggested that ozone may well be the most potent biocide among all of the current alternatives to free residual chlorine for use in drinking water disinfection (Hoff and Geldreich, 1981). A good history of the applications of ozone for disinfection purposes has been prepared by Rice et al. (1981).

Morris (1970) reported that in spite of the high efficiency of ozone, its use as a germicide has been limited because of major deficiencies in technology and unfavorable economics. The instability, low solubility, and difficulty of producing high partial pressures of O_3 have always made it hard to obtain a dosage of ozone high enough to satisfy demand and leave a measurable residue. This situation is changing, however, as ozone technology is improved (Miller et al., 1978; Opatken, 1978). As a way of surmounting some of these difficulties, Joret et al. (1986) suggested the employment of a progressive ozonation unit that employed preozonation, followed by coagulation-sedimentation, sand filtration, second-stage ozonation, carbon filtration, post-ozonation, and the addition of chlorine dioxide to provide a residual disinfection capacity.

Laboratory studies on the action of ozone on bacteria have been reported by Smith and Bodkin (1944), Dickerman et al. (1954), and Katzenelson et al. (1974). Its virucidal effect has been studied by Kessel et al. (1943), Evison (1978), Katzenelson et al. (1979), Roy et al. (1981, 1982), and Vaughn et al. (1987). Its effectiveness against cysts and oocysts has been examined by Newton and Jones (1949) and Peeters et al. (1989), respectively. The effect of particles on ozone disinfection was studied by Sproul et al. (1978), who reported that poliovirus 1 attached to cell fragments required a higher ozone residual for inactivation than virions attached to aluminum oxide or bentonite. These and other studies show that ozone is a highly effective disinfectant that kills bacteria, viruses, and cysts more rapidly than does chlorine. White (1972) ranks ozone and other disinfectants in the following order of decreasing efficiency: Ozone > chlorine dioxide > hypochlorous acid > hypochlorite ion > dichloramine > monochloramine.

The disinfecting capacity of ozone appears to be less affected by pH and temperature than that of chlorine. Some of the applications of ozone for water other than the disinfection of bacteria, viruses, and cysts are algae removal (oxidation); taste, odor, and color removal; and oxidation of soluble iron, manganese, organics, and suspended solids.

Ingols et al. (1959), Layton (1972), and Schecter (1973) have discussed methods for determining ozone in water. O'Donovan (1965), Evans (1972), and Miller et al. (1978) have published comprehensive and detailed reports on the use of ozone in water treatment. A discussion of ozonation and oxidation competition values, and their relationshlip to disinfection and microbial regrowth, has been published by Bancroft et al. (1984). The effect of suspended solids, in the form of kaolin and activated sludge, upon the disinfection effectiveness of ozone has been examined by Kaneko (1989). Two studies have reported on the use of peroxone treatment, the joint employ of hydrogen peroxide and ozone for achieving disinfection (Wolfe et al., 1989; Ferguson et al., 1990). These studies concluded that ratios of hydrogen peroxide to ozone of less than or equal to 0.3 to 1 would be optimal for disinfection.

Silver

The use of silver as a drinking water disinfectant has been much more popular in Europe than in the United States, and a voluminous literature is available on its application to water disinfection. A comprehensive review of the subject has been published in papers by Zimmermann (1952) and Woodward (1963). Additional information on its oligodynamic action, chemistry, and types of products available can be found in Chapter 18 of the third edition of this book. Generally, the literature on the effectiveness of silver in water disinfection is confusing and rather contradictory. This confusion reflects in part the variations in test procedures and, in some cases, is the result of failure to use a neutralizing agent in the reported tests. Inability to recognize or appreciate some of the unique properties of silver has also contributed to discrepancy.

The tendency of silver to adsorb onto surfaces can seriously interfere with bacteriologic tests of its effectiveness. This property of silver has been carefully studied by Chambers and Proctor (1960).

The low concentrations of silver used or suggested for use in water disinfection necessitate the use of a sensitive and accurate analytic procedure for measuring silver concentrations. A number of procedures have been employed (Feigl, 1928; Chambers et al., 1962; Uman, 1963; Lombardi, 1964), but a truly satisfactory technique has not yet been developed.

Wuhrmann and Zobrist (1958) published a comprehensive study on the efficacy of silver in water for inactivating *E. coli*. They evaluated the effects on inactivation times of silver concentration, exposure time, temperature, pH, phosphates, chlorides, and calcium. Their results demonstrate that the inactivation curves follow first-order reaction kinetics (Chick's law) under specific test conditions. Their data agree reasonably well with those of Chambers and Proctor (1960), but the results of Renn and Chesney (1953–1956) show inactivation curves that usually do not follow Chick's law.

Most investigators report that phosphates interfere with the bactericidal action of silver, but the levels of phosphates found in most natural waters probably would not be detrimental to silver disinfection. Calcium also interferes with the bactericidal effectiveness of silver; Wuhrmann and Zobrist (1958), for example, suggested that the time for 99.9% kill will be increased by 3 minutes for each 10 ppm of hardness at 20°C and pH 7.0. They

also reported that chlorides have a slowing effect on the disinfection action of silver.

Sulfides interfere seriously with the germicidal action of silver. Renn and Chesney (1953–1956) suggest that water containing more than 1 mg/L of sulfide is unsuitable for disinfection with the silver process they studied. Organic material, particulate or colloidal, also interferes with silver disinfection, but apparently not to the degree that it does with other water disinfectants, particularly chlorine.

The National Interim Primary Drinking Water Regulations (1975) has established a maximum contaminant limit of 0.05 mg/L for silver in drinking water. This limit is the same as that which was part of the United States Public Health Service Drinking Water Standards (1962), which was based on the observation that prolonged exposure to silver may give rise to the cosmetically objectionable argyria.

Ultraviolet Radiation

The disinfection of water by ultraviolet radiation (UV) from high-pressure mercury arc lamps has been used since 1909 (Ellis et al., 1941). During these early years, a number of cities in the United States and Europe had UV facilities capable of disinfecting as much as three million gallons of water per day. In fact, UV was used to disinfect city water supplies in England and Germany as late as 1935 (Phillips and Hanel, 1960). The cost of disinfecting public water supplies by UV in past years has greatly exceeded that of chlorination or ozone treatment, and consequently, the use of UV has become limited to special applications.

The germicidal effectiveness of UV varies with the wavelength of the radiation; wavelengths in the range of 250 to 260 nm are the most effective for killing microorganisms. Wavelengths in this region, sometimes called the abiotic region, are absorbed by the nucleic acid portions of the nucleoproteins, causing chemical alterations in the genetic material, with consequently lethal effects on the microorganism.

Over the years, a multitude of published reports have appeared in the literature documenting the bactericidal, virucidal, and fungicidal efficiency of UV. These studies resulted primarily from the availability of better types of artificial UV sources, e.g., the low-pressure mercury vapor lamp. This lamp emits nearly all of its UV energy at a wavelength of 253.7 nm, a wavelength with a high germicidal efficiency.

Phillips and Hanel (1960) have published a comprehensive report on the action and uses of UV, including an extensive listing of the susceptibility of various types of microorganisms, e.g., viruses, bacteria, bacterial spores, and fungi. Huff et al. (1965), Jepson (1972), and Yip and Konasewich (1972) have reported on UV disinfection of water and the factors influencing treatment efficiency. In spite of the fact that various types of microorganisms differ somewhat in susceptibility to UV, there is little question of the germicidal efficiency of UV if sufficient doses reach the organism.

A problem associated with UV inactivation of microorganisms is the phenomena of reactivation, which can occur when UV-inactivated microorganisms are exposed to light (photoreactivation) or remain unexposed to a light source (dark-repair mechanism). Photoreactivation of *E. coli* was demonstrated by Kelner (1949a and b). Carson and Peterson (1975) reported that *Pseudomonas cepacia* was photoreactivated by as much as one to four logs after exposure to UV. This organism could be a potential source of contamination in UV-treated waters. Photoreactivation is temperature dependent. The problem that reactivation poses when attempting to achieve effective bacterial inactivation by UV irradiation (Harris et al., 1987) does not exist when examining viruses, which are unable to directly repair the damage caused to them by UV irradiation. The effectiveness of UV treatment for inactivating a wide variety of animal virus groups has been assessed by von Brodorotti and Mahnel (1982). Kamiko and Ohgaki (1989) and Tartera et al. (1988) have published studies on UV inactivation of bacterial viruses, which have been proposed to serve as indicators of disinfection by this treatment technique.

Factors of importance in disinfecting water with UV are the presence of substances that prevent the penetration of the UV or absorb the UV energy. These include turbidity-causing particulate matter, organic compounds, iron salts, and colored compounds. Consequently, for UV to be most effective, the water must be pretreated to remove such contaminating constituents if they are present. This, of course, limits the application of UV to relatively small water supplies or to specialized uses unique to the food industry. For example, the bactericidal (Presnell and Cummins, 1972; Kelly, 1961) and the virucidal (Hill et al., 1971) efficiency of UV for treating estuarine water for use in shellfish purification systems has been studied and is presently considered the treatment of choice for disinfecting seawater. UV-treated water is also used in the dairy, beverage, and pharmaceutical industries, in which chemical treatment would adversely affect the marketable product.

UV meters are available that measure the UV dose during the exposure period. It should be recognized, however, that with UV, no residual disinfecting capacity exists as it does with chlorine, and treatment efficiency therefore is not measurable beyond the initial treatment. This, of course, limits the type of control desirable for adequate water quality management. Nevertheless, a number of UV water "sterilizers" are commercially available in which high-intensity lamps are used. These units do have value in customized applications and are advertised as being capable of treating up to 3000 gallons of water per hour. A study of methods for testing the efficacy of ultraviolet light disinfection devices for drinking water has been published by Tobin and coworkers (1983).

Ionizing Radiations

Ionizing radiations have been suggested as a potential means of water disinfection; however, little information is available on this application. Ridenour and Armbruster (1956) published data on the bactericidal effect of gamma radiation from ^{60}Co on normally contaminated surface water and laboratory-contaminated waters. Dosages of 100,000 rads were sufficient to kill 99% or more of the various test organisms in water. Lowe et al. (1956) also used ^{60}Co as a source of gamma rays and reported that dosages of 150,000 rads were required for 99% kill of various bacteria suspended in water. Ginoza (1968) reported that disinfection of water containing enteroviruses required a dose two to three times that required to disinfect the same concentration of bacteria in water. Sullivan et al. (1971) studied the inactivation of 30 viruses by gamma radiation and determined their D values (dose required for a 90% reduction in survivors). The radiation dose had to be increased more than threefold for inactivation of viruses that were suspended in culture medium instead of distilled water. The destruction rate curves were those of a first-order reaction.

Coagulation-Flocculation

The treatment methods of chemical coagulation, flocculation, sedimentation, and filtration in the drinking water plant serve to clarify the water, reduce the organic load, and greatly reduce the microbial count so that the post-treatment disinfectant can be more effective. These processes are a valuable and important means for reducing the microbial load of the water and appreciably reducing the amount of disinfectant that must be used.

Coagulation is achieved by the addition of soluble aluminum or iron salts or cationic organic polyelectrolytes. The microorganisms and the clay particles in the water are negatively charged. The trivalent metals and polyelectrolytes are positively charged and neutralize the charge on the microorganisms and clay particles, causing destabilization of the colloidal suspension with coagulation and agglomeration of the particles into microflocs. Metal salts with a valence charge of +1 or +2 are not as effective as those with the higher charge. Further, the aluminum and iron salts hydrolyze to produce a gelatinous polymer that, like the cationic polymers, mechanically entraps and adsorbs the microorganisms and clay particles. The salts can also react chemically with the free organic acid and thiol groups of proteins of the microorganisms and the soluble proteins, causing precipitation. Aluminum sulfate (alum) is used at a rate of 5 to 50 mg/L at an optimum pH range of 7 to 9, and ferric sulfate is used at the same rate with a pH range of 6 to 10 (Lorch, 1987).

The process of flocculation is the slow agitation of the agglomerated particles, aided by Brownian motion, to assist Van der Waal's forces and crystallization in increasing the size of the floc to effect more rapid sedimentation. Settling that could take decades in still water for tiny particles can be accomplished in hours as a result of flocculation. The settled matter is then separated by gravitational sedimentation and the finer particles are subsequently removed from the water by filtration of the supernatant.

There is considerable literature on the subject of the

removal of microorganisms (algae, bacteria, and viruses) by coagulation treatment, flocculation, sedimentation, and filtration, but one paper will serve to illustrate the effect of these operations in the purification of drinking water (Payment et al., 1985b). Seven drinking water plants were sampled twice a month for 12 months to evaluate the removal of indicator bacteria and cytopathogenic enteric viruses. The raw water was treated in all cases by prechlorination, coagulation, flocculation-sedimentation, filtration, ozonization, and final chlorination. Sampling was performed on the raw and finished waters and following each step of the treatment. The raw water in most plants was of poor quality, badly polluted with human and industrial wastes. The results varied, although the finished water in all cases was essentially free of indicator bacteria. The performance in eliminating viruses was less than perfect, but the water was still considered safe.

The authors concluded that the prechlorination-coagulation-sedimentation process appeared to be the most efficient step in reducing the number of microorganisms in the water. In the total treatment the coliform population was reduced by 6 $\log_{10}$, and viruses by 4 $\log_{10}$. In one plant the bacterial population was reduced by 1 $\log_{10}$ after prechlorination but was entirely eliminated following filtration, indicating that the processes of coagulation to filtration were responsible for the greatest removal of microorganisms. In the studies with viruses it was shown that disinfectant treatments following filtration did little to eliminate the surviving viruses. The average cumulative virus reduction was 95.15% after sedimentation and 99.97% after filtration, and did not significantly decrease after ozonation or final chlorination.

In an interesting case not related to drinking water but involving coagulation-flocculation removal of bacteria, a eutrophic recreational lake received two alum treatments for removal of phosphorus. During the treatment 95% of the bacterial population was removed from the water and deposited in the sediment at the bottom of the lake with the alum floc (Bulson et al., 1984). In another application, coagulation-flocculation is important in biologic waste treatment, even though there are no chemical additives to initiate the process. Here the microorganisms in the sludge themselves discharge natural polyelectrolytes such as proteins, protamines, nucleic acid, and pectic acid, which function as do the synthetic organic polyelectrolytes used in drinking water processes (Tenney and Stumm, 1965).

Heat

The disinfection of drinking water by boiling is probably the oldest method used by man and is still used in individual or emergency situations. Most water can be freed of infectious agents by simply boiling for 15 to 20 minutes.

Goldstein et al. (1960) have described a continuous-flow pasteurizer for disinfecting water. The unit may have applicability in treating farm pond, cistern, or other small water supplies. Stack (1973) indicates that microwave energy can be used to "sterilize" water by individuals or in emergency situations. If so employed, an energy saving of approximately 38% is obtained.

DISINFECTION OF SWIMMING-POOL WATER

As with drinking water disinfection, a basic philosophy in swimming-pool water disinfection is the destruction of pathogenic and other microorganisms of sanitary significance. The organisms in water entering the pool must be destroyed and, of even greater importance, the microorganisms contributed to the water by the bathers also must be destroyed. Because of this latter factor, pool water disinfection processes should be as rapid as possible. It is well documented that body secretions and excretions contribute large numbers of bacteria to pool waters and that these substances additionally impart a significant "disinfectant demand" to the water. The potential health hazards of swimming-pool waters are different from those of drinking water, since most swimmers try to avoid swallowing pool water. Thus, enteric organisms would appear to play a minor role in pool sanitation, with organisms of the nose, mouth, and throat playing the significant role. Although epidemiologic data do not indicate that pool water is important in the transmission of the more common enteric diseases, evidence suggests that there is an increased risk of respiratory or skin diseases to persons swimming in pools (Gallagher, 1948; Greenberg and Kupka, 1957; Schaefer, 1961). A potential hazard exists, and pool water therefore should be adequately disinfected at all times.

The ideal bacteriologic indicator organism of pool water sanitation has not been determined. Geldreich (1981), however, stated that the standard plate count is preferred to the total coliform count as the primary indicator organism and that supporting bacterial indicators should include *Streptococcus mitis*, *Streptococcus salivarius*, *Staphylococcus aureus*, and *Pseudomonas aeruginosa*. Warren and Ridgway (1978) found that staphylococci were more resistant to chlorine than *Streptococcus salivarius*, *E. coli*, or *Pseudomonas aeruginosa*. They also found staphylococci in swimming pools that were otherwise satisfactory. Crone and Tee (1974), Keirn and Putnam (1968), and Favero et al. (1964) suggested the use of staphylococci as indicators of pollution in swimming pools. They pointed out that these potential pathogens are valid indicators of pollution from the nose, mouth, and skin and also that they are more resistant to chlorine than are coliform bacteria.

A standard test for germicidal efficacy and acceptability of residual disinfecting activity in pool waters has been described by Ortenzio and Stuart (1964). Using this test procedure, Koski et al. (1966) have compared the disinfecting ability of chlorine, bromine, and iodine for swimming-pool water. Mallman (1962) discussed the use of cocci as indicators of pollution in pool water and also pointed out the pitfalls in collecting pool samples for bacteriologic analysis. He indicated that pools are "pockets of contamination," the contamination resulting largely from the secretions of the mouth and nose, and stressed the importance of collecting more than a single "grab" sample.

It is difficult to assess the relative importance of pool water per se in transmitting infections and the role of personal contact in and out of the pool in transmitting disease. For example, Ormsby (1955) reported on ocular diseases due to adenoviruses and presented data to indicate that swimming in pools is an important factor in transmission of these viruses. Other reports of disease due to adenoviruses associated with swimming in pools were described by Cockburn (1953) and Bell et al. (1955).

Caldwell et al. (1974) reported an epidemic of acute conjunctivitis in members of a swimming team. The team used a pool in which the pool filter and chlorinator had failed. The responsible organism was adenovirus 7. In contrast, Clarke et al. (1956) found that type 3 adenovirus was readily inactivated by chlorine and suggested that conjunctival irritation produced by swimming, coupled with the intimate contact among children at swimming pools, results in a rapid direct transmission of virus from person to person. Martone and coworkers (1980) have reported on an outbreak of adenovirus type 3 disease at a private recreation center's swimming pool. Keswick et al. (1981) examined the occurrence of enteroviruses in community swimming pools, finding 10 of 14 samples to contain infectious viruses. Three of those water samples were positive for virus in the presence of free chlorine, and two of the pools that contained viruses did exceed a 0.4 ppm free residual chlorine standard. All seven wading pools examined contained virus. Based upon the results of their study, it was concluded that total coliform bacteria were not adequate indicators of the presence of virus, because six of the samples were positive for virus but negative for coliforms, and that total bacterial plate counts appeared to provide a better indication of the sanitary quality of pool water (Keswick et al., 1981). Clearly, additional laboratory and epidemiologic studies are needed to assess the health hazards of swimming pools.

The three basic types of swimming pools used in the United States present different problems of disinfection. The fill-and-draw pool is the most difficult to disinfect. These pools are usually filled early in the day and are not drained until night. Under such conditions, problems of waste accumulation are obvious, and satisfactory disinfection is difficult. Flow-through pools are somewhat more satisfactory, since fresh water continuously replaces a portion of the pool water that is discharged to waste. Disinfection in these pools is also difficult and expensive.

Recirculating pools are the easiest to disinfect properly. Such pools usually have rapid, continuous recirculation of water that may be filtered in addition to being continually disinfected. Warren and Ridgway (1978), however, reported that a slime layer can build up on the surface of the filter medium when chlorination is stopped during the night, thus posing a potential risk to the first bathers in the morning. Adequate backwashing of the filters and a free chlorine level of 1.5 to 2.0 mg/L would alleviate this problem.

Chlorine and Chlorine Compounds

Chlorine or chlorine compounds are the most widely used disinfectants for swimming pools. Gaseous chlorine, calcium hypochlorite (in solution or as a solid), and sodium hypochlorite are all applied. As with drinking water disinfection, all forms are equally effective when residuals are measured as free available chlorine. In some pools, ammonia has been added along with chlorine to form a more stable or persistent chloramine. This does not appear to be a good practice, however, since chloramines are relatively slow disinfectants, and pool water should be disinfected rapidly. Mood (1950) studied the effect of free and combined chlorine on bacteria in swimming pools. He concluded that 0.4 to 0.6 mg/L of free chlorine in swimming pools is superior to 0.7 mg/L of combined chlorine.

Considerable interest has arisen in recent years on the use of high free residual chlorination (residuals above 1.0 mg/L) for swimming-pool disinfection. Robinton et al. (1957) have presented results on pool water converted from marginal to high free residual chlorine. The clarity and color of the pool water were improved and the bacterial densities drastically reduced. Swimmers no longer complained of eye irritation or chlorine odors. The authors stated that continuous maintenance of a sufficiently high free chlorine residual afforded complete protection against survival of any normal body bacteria in pool waters. They also suggested that bacteriologic tests on pools operated with high free residuals are unnecessary; a chemical test for chlorine residual would offer enough evidence for a safe or unsafe pool.

The use of chlorine stabilizers in pool disinfection, the chlorinated cyanurates (chlorinated cyanuric acid derivatives), has received some study during the past few years. They are complex nitrogen compounds that react with HOCl to form N-chloro derivatives. Their use in pool disinfection is primarily to provide a chlorine residual in outdoor pool water that is less subject to loss from the action of sunlight, aeration, and other factors. The disinfecting efficacy of these compounds as compared to HOCl is not clear. Stuart and Ortenzio (1964) stated that usual chemical tests for available chlorine in pools where chlorine stabilizers are present may provide results that must be interpreted entirely differently from those obtained on waters treated with gaseous chlorine and hypochlorites.

Andersen (1964) reported that significantly higher chlorine concentrations may be required in the presence of cyanuric acid, when compared with similar conditions in its absence, to achieve 99% bacterial death in 1 minute, even though the orthotolidine-arsenite (OTA) method indicated the chlorine residual as free available chlorine. Ditzel et al. (1961) and Warren and Ridgway (1978), however, reported that under swimming-pool conditions, the chlorinated cyanuric acids are as effective in killing bacteria as is sodium hypochlorite. Additionally, Kowalski and Hilton (1966) have evaluated data collected from the practical operation of swimming pools in St. Louis County, Missouri. They reported that pools treated with the chlorinated cyanurates had a better disinfection record than pools treated with other chlorine sources; they also point out that good disinfection was obtained with any chlorine source investigated, provided that an adequate available chlorine residual was continuously maintained in the pool. Chloramine-T has been examined as a possible alternative to free chlorine for water disinfection, particularly in slightly acidic waters (Gowda et al., 1986), and was found to be effective for adenovirus 3.

Chlorine Dioxide

Malpas (1973), in a brief review of disinfection of water with chlorine dioxide, cited several references on the favorable use of this disinfectant in swimming pools in Germany. Because of the success in Germany, the disinfectant was tested in a pool in England. The benefits of using chlorine dioxide were limited. Advantages were that chlorine dioxide did not cause eye irritation and the water was free from chlorinous odor, even though there was an excess of free chlorine in the pool water. The excess free chlorine was needed to reduce the formation of chlorite. Bacteriologic results were equivocal because of the free chlorine present. Disadvantages of chlorine dioxide were that the pool water became yellowish or greenish according to the concentration of the disinfectant. The measurement of the chlorine dioxide residual was more difficult than the measurement of the chlorine residual.

Iodine

In recent years, several studies have been conducted dealing with the use of iodine as a swimming-pool disinfectant. From the studies of Black et al. (1959), Marshall et al. (1960, 1962), Black (1961), and others, it appears that iodine residuals of 0.2 mg/L may be adequate to maintain pool water in good bacteriologic condition. In pools with high bathing loads, it is easier to maintain a desired residual with iodine than with chlorine, since iodine does not form additional products with ammonia, as does chlorine. Because of this, investigators reported that much less eye irritation occurs in iodinated pools than in chlorinated pools, and that most swimmers apparently prefer an iodinated pool. Some investigators reported that color control of iodinated pools requires close attention. A report on the safety of iodine as a pool disinfectant has been published by Byrd et al. (1963).

Favero and Drake (1964, 1966) have compared the microbial flora of swimming pools disinfected with chlorine and iodine. Their data show that although iodinated pools are usually free of coliform bacteria and enterococci, the total counts frequently became quite high. *Pseudomonas alcaligenes* and *Alcaligenes faecalis* were shown to be responsible for most (92 to 99%) of these high counts. The accumulation of high numbers of these organisms was shown to be due to their iodine resistance

and their ability to grow rapidly in pool water in the absence of free iodine. Although these organisms generally are not considered true pathogens, their presence in swimming-pool water appears undesirable, primarily because total counts are often used to evaluate the quality of swimming-pool water, and high total counts of these organisms in iodinated pools would interfere with the interpretation of tests used to determine the sanitary quality of swimming-pool water.

Bromine

Bromine has been used on a limited scale as a swimming-pool disinfectant. The Illinois Department of Health has conducted several studies with bromine and reports that less eye irritation and odor occur in brominated pools than in chlorinated pools and that the bactericidal efficacy of bromamines, as formed under pool conditions, is superior to that of chloramines. Johannesson (1960) presented data on the bactericidal effects, analytic chemistry, and reactions of free and combined bromine in swimming pools. Brown et al. (1964) reported on the disinfecting ability of a bromine-chlorine compound used in a large swimming pool.

Silver

Although silver has been used in Europe for swimming-pool disinfection, it has not been recommended for pool disinfection in the United States. Shapiro and Hale (1937), in studies of the Katadyn (silver treatment) process, reported that the 2-hour time requirement for effective results makes the process undesirable for pool water disinfection. Chlorides, ammonia, and organic matter were reported to interfere with treatment efficiency. There has been some resurgence of interest in the use of silver ions, in conjunction with simultaneously generated copper ions, for reducing the amount of free chlorine required to achieve effective disinfection of swimming pool waters (Landeen et al., 1989; Yahya et al., 1989a). The molecular mechanisms by which copper and silver ions act in bacterial and viral disinfection have been discussed by Thurman and Gerba (1989).

Algae Control

Swimming pools that have large numbers of bathers, and in which water is not periodically replaced, frequently develop serious algae infestations. In such pools, the objective should be to prevent the algae from multiplying to a point at which they are visible. In pools with obvious algae growth, applications of an algicide may result in cellular components being released into the water, with possible development of obnoxious tastes, odors, and water appearance. In such pools, the water should be drained and the walls scrubbed free of attached algae and then treated with an appropriate algicide. After the pool is refilled, careful and continuous use of algicides should be initiated to control further growth.

Chlorination plus copper sulfate at a concentration of 0.5 to 3.0 mg/L can be used to control algae in swimming pools. Taft (1965) recommended a residual copper concentration of 1 ppm in the pool water; however, Maloney and Palmer (1956) observed that copper sulfate appeared to be selective rather than general in its algicidal effects when used at concentrations of 2 mg/L or less.

Chlorine and iodine for the control of algae in swimming pools have been studied by Lackey et al. (1964). They concluded that effective algae control in pool water was readily achieved with 0.2 mg/L or less of free iodine (or its equivalent of free chlorine), provided the halogen demand of the water was first met. A paper by Black et al. (1970), however, indicates that iodine, although useful in pool water disinfection, cannot be recommended for general pool use because it does not control algae, particularly "black algae." These authors state that maintenance of a free chlorine residual will prevent the growth of algae in pools, but they have "not as yet identified an effective algicide that is compatible with iodine."

A number of chemical compounds that show promise as algicides have appeared on the market. These are listed by Palmer (1956) as quaternary ammonium compounds, rosin amines, quinones, "activated" silver, urea compounds, chlorophenates, organic zinc, modified copper compounds, and modified chlorine compounds. Many products, containing one or more of these chemicals, are commercially available and are advertised for algae control in swimming pools. Fitzgerald (1959) presented data on the bactericidal and algicidal properties of several commercial swimming-pool algicides and compared the results with those obtained with 1 mg/L of chlorine or 5 mg/L of copper. These compounds were tested against the bacteria present in raw sewage, using the manufacturers' recommended initial and weekly dosages. On the basis of the results obtained, he reported that the chemicals could be ranked as to their bactericidal properties in the following order (from most to least effective): Algimycin, chlorine, Algae-Nox, Exalgae, copper, Algae-Kill, Hyamine-2389, and Berkite No. 4. These same compounds (except chlorine and copper), when tested against three algae species, were ranked as to their algicidal properties in the following order: Algimycin, Algae-Nox, Exalgae, Hyamine-2389, Algae-Kill, and Berkite No. 4. Thus, the relative algicidal properties of these compounds were essentially the same as their bactericidal properties.

In a subsequent paper, Fitzgerald (1960) reported the factors in pool operation that contributed to the loss of activity of algicides. The factors considered were the adsorptive properties of diatomaceous filter media and the precipitation of copper compounds under different conditions in the water. The results of the adsorption studies demonstrated a loss of from 50% to greater than 67% of the algicidal property of four quaternary ammonium compounds, two amines, and a pyrimidine after treatment by a diatomaceous filter aid. There was apparently no loss of algicidal activity of the quinones tested, provided that the particular quinone examined was soluble in water and did not form an insoluble pre-

cipitate at the recommended use-dose. The removal from suspension of four copper compounds was also demonstrated to be affected by the hardness or alkalinity of water at pH 7. The ability of the four sources of copper tested to keep their copper in solution at pH 7 was ranked in increasing order: copper sulfate, Omazene, Algee-clear, and Cuprose. Thus, a decrease in the effectiveness of algicidal chemicals may be due to adsorption of the chemical on the pool filter medium or to a physical filtration of an insoluble form of the chemical. Fitzgerald suggests that algicides be added to swimming pools at frequent intervals to make up for these losses.

DISINFECTION OF TREATED SEWAGE EFFLUENTS

The primary objectives of sewage effluent disinfection are the killing of microbial pathogens, odor control, and microbial aftergrowth control. The killing of pathogenic microorganisms in sewage has obvious public health importance, since disease-causing organisms, if not destroyed, could be transmitted to man through sewage contamination of water used for drinking, food processing, irrigation, shellfish culture, or recreation. Control of odors from the microbial degradation of sewage components is not associated with public health, but is important from an aesthetic standpoint. Many types of microorganisms in sewage that can cause odor problems can be killed by the use of disinfectants. A sudden and sharp increase in bacterial populations in treated sewage or in water receiving treated sewage can be defined as "aftergrowth." Such increases in bacterial growth are usually of short duration and can be prevented by the effective use of disinfectants. Disinfection of treated sewage effluents has been studied for many years, and a great number of reports have been published.

Chlorine and its compounds are the chemicals most widely used in sewage disinfection. Chlorine is usually added ahead of the primary settling tank for odor control and terminally for disinfection. It should be stressed, however, that there is no consistently reliable disinfection control with standard sewage treatment practice (Kruse et al., 1973). Many of the disinfecting characteristics of chlorine have been established in highly purified water under highly controlled conditions. Under such conditions, it has been possible to evaluate precisely the effects of variations in pH, temperature, time, and disinfectant concentration on the relative efficiencies of free chlorine and monochloramine in killing organisms significant in wastewater treatment (Chambers, 1971). From an operational standpoint, however, the chlorination of wastewater effluents is complex, since it is difficult to maintain predictable levels of disinfecting efficiency.

The variable and unpredictable results observed in field studies derive largely from the complex and constantly changing compositions of sewage, which contains many kinds of organic and inorganic compounds, minerals, and gases. These materials react with chlorine to exert a demand that must be satisfied before adequate disinfection can occur. The demand can be roughly measured for a specific waste by determining the amount of chlorine that must be added to achieve a required amount of disinfectant activity (killing power) after a given interval of time. Even under the most desirable steady-flow conditions, however, changes in reactive materials, pH, temperature, suspended solids, and many other as yet ill-defined and unknown factors frequently make the resulting disinfection variable and rarely complete.

The use of breakpoint chlorination, as in water supply chlorination, is rarely practiced in sewage chlorination. The breakpoint is the point at which, theoretically, the chlorine demand has been satisfied. However, 10 mg/L of chlorine per 1 mg/L ammonia is required to reach the chlorine breakpoint (Collins et al., 1970). Sewage effluents may contain ammonia levels as high as 50 mg/L. Thus, 500 mg/L of chlorine theoretically would be required to reach breakpoint. This much chlorine added to sewage effluents not only would be economically prohibitive, but would also destroy the ecologic balance in the receiving waters. Brungs (1973) has reviewed the toxic effects of chlorine on aquatic life and reported on residual chlorine levels that can be tolerated by aquatic organisms, including fish. Haas et al. (1988) have published a study on the effect of disinfection upon receiving-water quality downstream of the discharge site.

Operational procedures compensating for the high chlorine dosages needed in sewage effluents containing high levels of ammonia have been described in full-scale sewage treatment plant studies oriented toward improving disinfection of sewage effluents (Kruse et al., 1973). In these studies, it was shown that dosages of chlorine far below the breakpoint effectively improved viral inactivation and coliform reduction. This was done by improving the sewage-chlorine mixing (flash mixing) and by lowering the chlorine-sewage pH. The combination of flash mixing and an acid feed for a reaction pH of 5.0 provided the equivalent disinfection observed when using four times the chlorine dosage in the absence of this combination. This reduced the total residual chlorine of more than 20 mg/L in the effluent to 3 mg/L residual, an acceptable chlorine level.

Many factors influence the efficiency of chlorination in controlling bacteria and viruses in wastewater effluents. Basically, maximum levels of oxidation are desirable because a completely oxidized and highly clarified effluent is disinfected with greater efficiency (Chambers, 1971). The chlorine requirement of sewage must be established for each individual treatment plant by correlating chlorine dosage, residual, and holding time, however, because of the differences in the composition of various wastes. If this is done, the probability of obtaining predictable and desired reduction in coliform content is enhanced. For example, septic sewage is high in ammonia and sulfides and therefore is a high consumer of chlorine. Industrial and commercial wastes containing high levels of reduced materials such as sulfur compounds, cyanides, phenols, and dyes will react with chlorine and reduce the oxidative efficiency desired for effective disinfection. Therefore, chlorine demand schedules must be developed so that chlorine feed rates may be adjusted to the varying requirements necessary to yield the desired results on a plant-by-plant basis. Other factors involved with the use of free chlorine and chloramines for wastewater disinfection include the fact that association of coliforms with wastewater particulates, especially those particles greater than seven micrometers in diameter (Berman et al., 1988), can afford the microbes with a significant protective effect. Den Blanken (1985) has attempted to model the effect of nitrification in the comparative disinfection of treated sewage with chlorine.

Some disinfectants other than chlorine suggested for sewage disinfection are chlorine dioxide, bromine, iodine, radiation, heat, UV, and ozone. Of these, ultraviolet light and ozone hold the most promise. Several new UV units for sewage disinfection have been developed and currently are being evaluated. Meckes (1982) has published a good study on the effectiveness of UV light disinfection in reducing the levels of specific bacterial strains. One major factor involved with the effectiveness of UV disinfection is the effect of particulates that, depending upon their physical nature, may absorb or scatter the radiation (Qualls et al., 1983). A general discussion on the disinfection of municipal wastewater effluents with UV has been published by Severin (1980). Ozone technology has also been improved. Ozone is a powerful oxidizing agent, approximately twice as powerful as chlorine. The oxidizing reaction occurs quickly and is effective in destroying organic odors and tastes as well as in killing bacteria and inactivating viruses. Ozone has been used for odor control in sewage treatment plants in New York, Florida, and Michigan (Evans, 1972). Full-scale ozone disinfection of wastewater has been studied by Rakness and Hegg (1980). Meckes et al. (1983) have examined the application of an ozone disinfection model for municipal wastewater effluents. Warriner and co-workers (1985) have suggested that fecal coliform organisms show promise as indicators for ozone disinfection. The major reason for this suggestion was the knowledge that fecal coliforms are more resistant to ozone than are certain viruses. Venosa et al. (1984) have suggested that for large treatment plants, treatment with ultraviolet light and ozone in a sequential arrangement was more cost-effective than either treatment alone. Bromine chloride may also provide a usable substitute for chlorine in wastewater disinfection applications, and the effectiveness of bromine chloride may be less affected by organic matter (Hajenian and Butler, 1980) than is chlorine. Additional information on treated sewage effluent disinfection can be found in the California Institute of Technology (1957) report, which contains 499 references, the Federation of Sewage and Industrial Wastes Association Manual of Practice No. 4 (1951), Progress in Wastewater

Technology (1979), and many of the standard textbooks of sanitary engineering.

Wastewater Renovation

Increasing populations, urbanization, and industrialization have placed severe demands on the water supplies of many areas of the United States and other countries. Thus, although the treatment of wastewater for reuse is not new, there has been great interest in recent years in water renovation by "advanced" waste treatment processes. Although the primary emphasis of advanced wastewater treatment has been other than disinfection, the final product water from advanced waste treatment processes must be readily disinfected to prevent the transmission of microbial pathogens.

Current "advanced" waste treatments that show most promise involve a series of processes that begin with conventional sewage treatment (Dean, 1965). The conventional treatment of choice is the activated sludge process carried to complete nitrification in order to eliminate ammonia from the product. Such treatment, if properly carried out, will also eliminate most sugars, amino acids, and other substances that cannot be removed by subsequent processes and can seriously interfere with disinfection of the final product. The activated sludge treatment effluent is clarified with lime, raising the pH to roughly 11. After filtration through a dual-media filter (coal and sand), the now clarified water is brought back to approximately pH 7 and chlorinated to help prevent bacterial growth in the carbon column that follows. Berg et al. (1968) reported that 98.6% to greater than 99.997% of seeded poliovirus in secondary effluent was removed by lime flocculation and sand filtration. The carbon column removes the remaining organic substances by adsorption and also rapidly removes the chlorine. It has been observed that large numbers of pseudomonads frequently develop in the bottom portions of the carbon column and cause gross contamination of the carbon filter effluent. Methods of preventing this growth require study.

The product water from the carbon column is completely colorless and free from odors and organic contamination and has a turbidity of less than 1 Jackson unit. If ammonia was removed by the activated sludge treatment, the water is easy to disinfect with chlorine and, in fact, will retain a chlorine residual for days. In some areas, the natural salt content of the water, coupled with that contributed by the municipality, will raise the level of total dissolved solids to about 500 mg/L, but usually below 1000 mg/L. Obviously, such water is too good to discard and could be used industrially. Careful post-disinfection of such water is necessary to protect against breakdowns in the treatment plant and to reduce the potential dangers of cross-contamination in industrial plants.

When it becomes necessary to reduce the salinity of water recovered by "advanced" treatments, a number of desalinization techniques are available, including electrodialysis, reverse osmosis, distillation, and freeze sep-

aration. All these processes are adversely affected by organic matter, and an organic-free feed probably will be required. Certain desalinization techniques inherently disinfect the product water, for example, high-temperature distillation, but not low-temperature vapor compression. Reverse osmosis, or hyperfiltration, generally disinfects as well as desalinizes water. An interesting observation is that it has been found necessary to chlorinate water before it comes in contact with reverse-osmosis membranes to prevent microbiologic growths from plugging the system. An additional benefit is that the chlorine is able to pass through the membrane and disinfect the effluent.

Electrodialysis, currently the most promising technique for removing a portion of the salts in renovated water, has little or no disinfecting capacity. The freeze-separation method produces crystals of ice that inevitably are contaminated with appreciable quantities of suspended solids, including bacteria. Water from this treatment process must be disinfected.

REFERENCES

Akin, E.W., Hoff, J.C., and Lippy, E.C. 1982. Waterborne outbreak control: which disinfectant? Environ. Health Perspect., *46*, 7–12.

Allen, M.J., and Geldreich, E.E., Jr. 1978. Evaluation of the microbiological standards for drinking water. Edited by C.W. Hendricks. EPA-570/9-78-00C. Washington, D.C., U.S. Environmental Protection Agency.

Alvarez, M.E., and O'Brien, R.T. 1982. Mechanisms of inactivation of poliovirus by chlorine dioxide and iodine. Appl. Environ. Microbiol., *44*, 1064–1071.

Andersen, J.R. 1964. A study of the influence of cyanuric acid on the bactericidal effectiveness of chlorine. Chicago, National Swimming Pool Institute Meeting.

Bancroft, K., et al. 1984. Ozonation and oxidation competition values relationship to disinfection and microorganisms regrowth. Water Res., *18*, 473–478.

Bell, J.A., et al. 1955. Pharyngo-conjunctival fever: Epidemiological studies of a recently recognized disease entity. JAMA, *157*, 1083–1092.

Bellar, T.A., Lichtenberg, J.J., and Kroner, R.C. 1974. The occurrence of organohalides in chlorinated drinking waters. J. Am. Water Works Assoc., *66*, 703–706.

Benarde, M.A., Israel, B.M., Olivieri, V.P., and Granstrom, M.L. 1965. Efficiency of chlorine dioxide as a bactericide. Appl. Microbiol., *13*, 776–780.

Berg, G., Chang, S.L., and Harris, E.K. 1964. Devitalization of microorganisms by iodine. I. Dynamics of the devitalization of enteroviruses by elemental iodine. Virology, *22*, 469–481.

Berg, G., Dean, R.B., and Dahling, D.R. 1968. Removal of poliovirus from secondary effluent by lime flocculation and rapid sand filtration. J. Am. Water Works Assoc., *60*, 193–198.

Berg, G., Sanjaghsaz, H., and Wangwongwatana, S. 1989. Potentiation of the poliocidal effectiveness of free chlorine by a buffer. J. Virol. Methods., *23*, 179–186.

Berman, D., Rice, E.W., and Hoff, J.C. 1988. Inactivation of particle-associated coliforms by chlorine and monochloramine. Appl. Environ. Microbiol., *54*, 507–512.

Black, A.P. 1961. Swimming pool disinfection with iodine. Water Sewage Works, *108*, 286–289.

Black, A.P., Lackey, J.B., and Lackey, E.W. 1959. Effectiveness of iodine for the disinfection of swimming pool water. Am. J. Public Health, *49*, 1060–1068.

Black, A.P., et al. 1970. The disinfection of swimming pool waters. Part 1. Comparison of iodine and chlorine as swimming pool disinfectants. Am. J. Public Health, *60*, 535–545.

Black, A.P., et al. 1965. Use of iodine for disinfection. J. Am. Water Works Assoc., *57*, 1401-1421.

Boardman, G.D., McBrayer, T.R., and Kohlhepp, P. 1989. Detection and occurrence of waterborne bacterial and viral pathogens. J. Water Pollut. Control Fed., *61*, 1097–1109.

Boardman, G.D., and Sproul, O.J. 1977. Protection of viruses during disinfection by adsorption to particulate matter. J. Water Pollut. Control Fed., *49*, 1857–1861.

Bossart, J.M., and McCreary, J.J. 1983. Disinfection. J. Water Pollut. Control Fed., *55*, 650–657.

Brown, J.R., McLean, D.M., and Nixon, M.C. 1964. Bromine disinfection of a large swimming pool. Can. J. Public Health, 55, 251–256.

Brungs, W.A. 1973. Effects of residual chlorine on aquatic life. J. Water Pollut. Control Fed., 45, 2180–2193.

Bull, R.J. 1980. Health effects of alternate disinfectants and their reaction products. J. Am. Water Works Assoc., 72, 299–303.

Bull, R.J. 1982. Toxicological problems associated with alternative methods of disinfection. J. Am. Water Works Assoc., 74, 642–648.

Bulson, P.C., Johnstone, D.L., Gibbons, H.L., and Funk, W.H. 1984. Removal and inactivation of bacteria during alum treatment of a lake. Appl. Env. Microbiol., 48, 425–430.

Butterfield, C.T. 1948. Bactericidal properties of chloramines and free chlorine in water. Public Health Rep., 63, 934–940.

Butterfield, C.T., and Wattie, E. 1946. Influence of pH and temperature on the survival of coliforms and enteric pathogens when exposed to chloramine. Public Health Rep., 61, 157–192.

Butterfield, C.T., Wattie, E., Megregian, S., and Chambers, C.W. 1943. Influence of pH and temperature on the survival of coliforms and enteric pathogens when exposed to free chlorine. Public Health Rep. 58, 1837–1866.

Byrd, O.E., Malkin, H.M., Reed, G.B., and Wilson, H.W. 1963. Safety of iodine as a disinfectant in swimming pools. Public Health Rep., 78, 393–397.

Calabrese, E.J., Moore, G.S., and Tuthill, R.W. 1978. Health effects of chlorine dioxide as a disinfectant in potable water. A literature survey. J. Environ. Health, 41, 26–31.

Caldwell, G.G., et al. 1974. Epidemic of adenovirus 7 acute conjunctivitis in swimmers. Am. J. Epidemiol., 99, 230–234.

California Institute of Technology, 1957. Report on the disinfection of settled sewage. Division of Engineering, Sanitary Engineering Research.

Carson, L.A., and Peterson, N.J. 1975. Photoreactivation of *Pseudomonas cepacia* after ultraviolet exposure: a potential source of contamination in ultraviolet-treated waters. J. Clin. Microbiol., 1, 462–464.

Chambers, C.W. 1971. Chlorination for control of bacteria and viruses in treatment plant effluents. J. Water Pollut. Control Fed., 43, 228–241.

Chambers, C.W., and Proctor, C.M. 1960. The bacteriological and chemical behavior of silver in low concentrations. Cincinnati, Tech. Rep., W60-4, R.A. Taft Sanitary Engineering Center.

Chambers, C.W., Proctor, C.M., and Kabler, P.W. 1962. Bactericidal effect of low concentrations of silver. J. Am. Water Works Assoc., 54, 208–216.

Chambers, C.W., Kabler, P.W., Malaney, G., and Bryant, A. 1952. Iodine as a bactericide. Soap Sanit. Chem., 28, 149–165.

Chang, S.L. 1958. The use of active iodine as a water disinfectant. J. Am. Pharm. Assoc., 47, 417–423.

Chang, S.L. 1944. Studies on *E. histolytica*. III. Destruction of cysts of *E. histolytica* by a hypochlorite solution, chloramines in tap water, and gaseous chlorine in tap water of varying degrees of pollution. War Med., 5, 46–55.

Chang, S.L., and Morris, J.C. 1953. Elemental iodine as a disinfectant for drinking water. Ind. Eng. Chem., 45, 1009–1012.

Clark, H.F., Kabler, P.W., and Geldreich, E.E. 1957. Advantages and limitations of the membrane filter procedure. Water Sewage Works, 104, 385–387.

Clark, R.M., Read, E.J., and Hoff, J.C. 1989. Analysis of inactivation of *Giardia lamblia* by chlorine. J. Environ. Engr., 115, 80–90.

Clarke, N.A., and Chang, S.L. 1959. Enteric viruses in water. J. Am. Water Works Assoc., 51, 1299–1317.

Clarke, N.A., and Kabler, P.W. 1954. The inactivation of purified Coxsackie virus in water by chlorine. Am. J. Hyg., 59, 119–127.

Clarke, N.A., Stevenson, R.E., and Kabler, P.W. 1956. The inactivation of purified type 3 adenovirus in water by chlorine. Am. J. Hyg., 64, 314–319.

Clarke, N.A., Berg, G., Kabler, P.W., and Chang, S.L. 1964. Human enteric viruses in water: Source, survival and removability. 1st International Conference on Water Pollution Research, September 1962, Volume 2. London, Pergamon Press, pp. 528–542.

Cockburn, T.A. 1953. An epidemic of conjunctivitis in Colorado associated with pharyngitis, muscle pain and pyrexia. Am. J. Ophthalmol., 36, 1534–1539.

Collins, H.F., Selleck, R.E., and White, G.C. 1970. Problems in obtaining adequate sewage disinfection. Proc. Natl. Spec. Conf. Disinfect., Amherst, Mass.

Cookson, J.T., Jr. 1974. Virus and water supply. J. Am. Water Works Assoc., 66, 707–711.

Craun, G.F., McCabe, L.J., and Huges, J.M. 1976. Waterborne disease outbreaks in the U.S. (1971–1974). J. Am. Water Works Assoc., 68, 420–424.

Crone, P.B., and Tee, G.H. 1974. Staphylococci in swimming pool water. J. Hyg. Cambridge, 73, 213–220.

Culp, R.L. 1974. Breakpoint chlorination for virus inactivation. J. Am. Water Works Assoc., 66, 699–703.

Dean, R.B. 1965. Personal communication.

DeJonckheere, J., and Van De Voorde, H. 1976. Differences in destruction of cysts of pathogenic and nonpathogenic *Naegleria* and *Acanthamoeba* by chlorine. Appl. Environ. Microbiol., 31, 294–297.

den Blanken, J.G. 1985. Comparative disinfection of treated sewage with chlorine and ozone effect of nitrification. Water Res., 19, 1129–1140.

Dickerman, J.M., Castraberte, A.O., and Fuller, J.E. 1954. Action of ozone on water-borne bacteria. J. N. Engl. Water Works Assoc., 68, 11–15.

Ditzel, R.G., Matzer, E.A., and Symes, W.F. 1961. New data on the chlorinated cyanurates. Swimming Pool Age, 35, 26–30.

Dugan, P.R. 1978. Use and misuse of chlorination for the protection of public water supplies and the treatment of wastewater. Am. Soc. Microbiol. News, 44, 97–102.

Ellis, C., Wells, A.A., and Heyroth, F.F. 1941. *The Chemical Action of Ultraviolet Rays*. 2nd Edition. New York, Reinhold Publishing Corp.

Engelbrecht, R.S., Foster, D.H., Greening, E.O., and Lee, S.H. 1974. New microbial indicators of wastewater chlorination efficiency. Environmental Protection Technology Series, EPA-670/2-73-082.

Engelbrecht, R.S., Weber, M.J., Salter, B.L., and Schmidt, C.A. 1980. Comparative inactivation of viruses by chlorine. Appl. Environ. Microbiol., 40, 249–256.

Evans, F.L. III (Ed.) 1972. *Ozone in Water and Wastewater Treatment*. Ann Arbor, Ann Arbor Science Publishers.

Evison, L.M. 1978. Inactivation of enteroviruses and coliphages with ozone in waters and waste waters. Prog. Water Technol., 10, 365–374.

Fair, G.M., et al. 1948. The behavior of chlorine as a water disinfectant. J. Am. Water Works Assoc., 40, 1051–1061.

Favero, M.S., and Drake, C.H. 1966. Factors influencing the occurrence of high numbers of iodine-resistant bacteria in iodinated swimming pools. Appl. Microbiol., 14, 627–635.

Favero, M.S., and Drake, C.H. 1964. Comparative study of microbial flora of iodinated and chlorinated pools. Public Health Rep., 79, 251–257.

Favero, M.S., Drake, C.H., and Randall, G.B. 1964. Use of staphylococci as indicators of swimming pool pollution. Public Health Rep., 79, 61–70.

Federation of Sewage and Industrial Waste Associations, 1951. Manual of Practice No. 4. Chlorination of sewage and industrial wastes.

Feigl, F. 1928. On silver-specific reagents and on a new sensitive silver indicator. Z. Anal Chem., 74, 380–386.

Ferguson, D.W., et al. 1990. Comparing peroxone and ozone for controlling taste and odor compounds, disinfection by-products, and microorganisms. J. Am. Water Works Assoc., 82, 181–191.

Fitzgerald, G.P. 1960. Loss of algicidal chemicals in swimming pools. Appl. Microbiol., 8, 269–274.

Fitzgerald, G.P. 1959. Bactericidal and algicidal properties of some algicides for swimming pools. Appl. Microbiol., 7, 205–211.

Floyd, R., and Sharp, D.G. 1978. Inactivation of single poliovirus particles by hypobromite ion, molecular bromine, dibromamine and tribromamine. Environ. Sci. Technol., 12, 1031–1035.

Gallagher, J.R. 1948. Swimming pools. N. Engl. J. Med., 238, 899–903.

Geldreich, E.E. 1981. Current status of microbiological water quality criteria. ASM News, 47, 23–27.

Gerba, C.P., et al., 1979. Failure of indicator bacteria to reflect the occurrence of enteroviruses in marine waters. Am. J. Public Health, 69, 1116–1119.

Ginoza, W. 1968. Inactivation of viruses by ionizing radiation and by heat. In *Methods in Virology*. Edited by K. Maramorosch and H. Koprowski. London, Academic Press.

Goldstein, M., McCabe, L.J., and Woodward, R.L. 1960. Continuous-flow water pasteurizer for small supplies. J. Am. Water Works Assoc., 52, 247–254.

Gordon, G., et al. 1990. Minimizing chlorite ion and chlorate ion in water treated with chlorine dioxide. J. Am. Water Works Assoc., 82, 160–165.

Goshko, M.A., Pipes, W.O., and Christian, R.R. 1983. Coliform occurrence and chlorine residual in small water distribution systems. J. Am. Water Works Assoc., 75, 371–374.

Gowda, N.M.M., Trieff, N.M., and Stanton, G.J. 1986. Kinetics of inactivation of adenovirus in water by chloramine-T. Water Res., 20, 817–823.

Grabow, W.O.K., et al. 1983. Inactivation of hepatitis A virus and indicator organisms in water by free chlorine residuals. Appl. Environ. Microbiol., 46, 619–624.

Greenberg, A.E., and Kupka, E. 1957. Swimming pool injuries, mycobacteria, and tuberculosis-like disease. Public Health Rep., 10, 902–904.

Griffin, A.E. 1939. Reaction to heavy doses of chlorine in various waters. J. Am. Water Works Assoc., 31, 2121–2129.

Haas, C.N., et al. 1988. Effects of discontinuing disinfection on a receiving water. J. Water Pollut. Control Fed., 60, 667–673.

Hajenian, H., and Butler, M. 1980. Inactivation of f2 coliphage in municipal effluent by the use of various disinfectants. J. Hygiene, 84, 247–255.

Harris, G.D., et al. 1987. Ultraviolet inactivation of selected bacteria and viruses with photoreactivation of the bacteria. Water Res., 21, 687–692.

Hauchman, F.S., Noss, C.I., and Olivieri, V.P. 1986. Chlorine dioxide reactivity with nucleic acids. Water Res., 20, 357–361.

Hejkal, T.W., Wellings, F.M., LaRock, P.A., and Lewis, A.L. 1979. Survival of poliovirus within organic solids during chlorination. Appl. Environ. Microbiol., 38, 114–118.

Hibler, C.P., et al. 1987. Inactivation of *Giardia* cysts with chlorine at 0.5°C to 5.0°C. Denver, American Water Works Association Research Foundation.

Hill, W.F., Jr., Akin, E.W., Benton, W.H., and Hamblet, F.E. 1971. Viral disinfection of estuarine water by UV. J. San. Eng. Div. ASCE, 87, 601–615.

Hoehn, R.C., et al. 1990. Household odors associated with the use of chlorine dioxide. J. Am. Water Works Assoc., 82, 166–172.

Hoff, J.C. 1978. The relationship of turbidity to disinfection of potable water. In *Evaluation of the Microbiology Standards for Drinking Water*. Edited by C.W. Hendricks. EPA-570/9–78–00C. Washington, D.C., U.S. Environmental Protection Agency.

Hoff, J.C., and Geldreich, E.E. 1981. Comparison of the biocidal efficiency of alternative disinfectants. J. Am. Water Works Assoc., 73, 40–44.

Hubbs, S.A., Amundsen, D., and Olthius, P. 1981. Use of chlorine dioxide, chloramines, and short-term free chlorination as alternative disinfectants. J. Am. Water Works Assoc., 73, 97–101.

Huff, C.B., Smith, H.F., Boring, W.D., and Clarke, N.A. 1965. Study of ultraviolet disinfection of water and factors in treatment efficiency. Public Health Rep., 80, 695–705.

Ingols, R.S., Fetner, R.H., and Eberhardt, W.H. 1959. Determining ozone in solution. Am. Chem. Soc. Adv. Chem. Ser., 21, 102–107.

Jarrol, E.L., Bingham, A.K., and Meyer, E.A. 1981. Effect of chlorine on *Giardia lamblia* cyst viability. Appl. Environ. Microbiol., 41, 483–487.

Jenson, H., Thomas, K., and Sharp, D.G. 1980. Inactivation of coxsackieviruses B3 and B5 in water by chlorine. Appl. Environ. Microbiol., 40, 633–640.

Jepson, J.D. 1972. Disinfection of water supplies by ultraviolet radiation. Water Treat. Exam., 64, 175–191.

Johannesson, J.K. 1960. The bromination of swimming pools. Am. J. Public Health, 50, 1731–1736.

Joret, J.C., et al. 1986. Virus inactivation during water treatment by a progressive ozonation unit. Water Res., 20, 871–876.

Kamiko, N., and Ohgaki, S. 1989. RNA coliphage QB as a bioindicator of the ultraviolet disinfection efficiency. Water Sci. Technol., 3, 227–231.

Kaneko, M. 1989. Effect of suspended solids on inactivation of poliovirus and T2 phage by ozone. Water Sci. Technol., 21, 215–219.

Katzenelson, E., Klether, B., and Shuval, H.I. 1974. Inactivation kinetics of viruses and bacteria in water by use of ozone. J. Am. Water Works Assoc., 66, 725–729.

Katzenelson, E., et al. 1979. Measurement of the inactivation kinetics of poliovirus by ozone in a fast-flow mixer. Appl. Environ. Microbiol., 37, 715–718.

Keirn, M.A., and Putnam, H.D. 1968. Resistance of staphylococci to halogens as related to a swimming pool environment. Health Lab. Sci., 5, 180–193.

Kelly, C.B. 1961. Disinfection of seawater by ultraviolet radiation. Am. J. Public Health, 51, 1670–1680.

Kelner, A. 1949a. Effects of visible light on the recovery of *Streptomyces griseus* conidia from ultraviolet irradiation injury. Proc. Natl. Acad. Sci. U.S., 35, 73–79.

Kelner, A. 1949b. Photoreactivation of ultraviolet-irradiated *E. coli*. J. Bacteriol., 58, 511–522.

Kessel, J.F., Allison, D.K., Moore, F.J., and Kaine, M. 1943. Comparison of chlorine and ozone as virucidal agents of poliomyelitis virus. Proc. Soc. Exp. Biol. Med., 53, 71–73.

Keswick, B.H., Gerba, C.P., and Goyal, S.M. 1981. Occurrence of enteroviruses in community swimming pools. Am. J. Public Health, 71, 1026–1030.

King, C.H., et al. 1988. Survival of coliforms and bacterial pathogens within protozoa during chlorination. Appl. Environ. Microbiol., 54, 3023–3033.

Kirner, J.C., Littler, J.D., and Angelo, L.A. 1978. A waterborne outbreak of giardiasis in Camas, Wash. J. Am. Water Works Assoc., 70, 35–40.

Koski, T.A., Stuart, L.S., and Ortenzio, L.F. 1966. Comparison of chlorine, bromine and iodine as disinfectants for swimming pool water. Appl. Microbiol., 14, 276–279.

Kowalski, X., and Hilton, T.B. 1966. Comparison of chlorinated cyanurates with other chlorine disinfectants. Public Health Rep., 81, 282–288.

Kruse, C.W., Kawata, K., Olivieri, V.P., and Longley, K.E. 1973. Improvements in terminal disinfection of sewage effluents. Water Sewage Works, 120, 57–64.

Lackey, J.B., Lackey, E.W., and Morgan, G.B. 1964. Iodine as an algicide for swimming pools. Eng. Prog. Univ. Fla., XVIII 1, Leaflet 171.

Landeen, L.K., et al. 1989. Microbiological evaluation of copper:silver disinfection units for use in swimming pools. Water Sci. Technol., 21, 267–270.

Layton, R.F. 1972. Analytical methods for ozone in water and wastewater applications. In *Ozone in Water and Wastewater Treatment*. Edited by F.L. Evans. Ann Arbor, Ann Arbor Science Publishers.

Lippy, E.C. 1978. Tracing a giardiasis outbreak at Berlin, New Hampshire. J. Am. Water Works Assoc., 70, 512–520.

Liu, O.C. 1973. Northeastern United States Water Supply Study. Potomac Estuary Water Supply: The Consideration of Viruses. Study Report: Environmental Protection Agency, United States Army Engineering Division, North Atlantic.

Logsdon, G.S., Symons, J.M., Hoye, R.L., Jr., and Arozarena. M.M. 1981. Alternative filtration methods for removal of Giardia cysts and cyst models. J. Am. Water Works Assoc., 73, 111–118.

Lombardi, O.W. 1964. Di-β-naphthylthiocarbazone (dinaphthizone) compared with dithizone as an analytical reagent for the determination of trace metals in natural waters. A preliminary investigation. Anal. Chem., 36, 415–418.

Lorch, W. 1987. *Handbook of Water Purification*. New York, Ellis Harwood Limited.

Lowe, H.N., Jr., Lacy, W.J., Surkiewicz, B.F., and Jaeger, R.F. 1956. Destruction of microorganisms in water, sewage and sewage sludge by ionizing radiations. J. Am. Water Works Assoc., 48, 1363–1372.

Mallmann, W.L. 1962. Cocci test for detecting mouth and nose pollution of swimming pool water. Am. J. Public Health, 52, 2001–2008.

Maloney, T.E., and Palmer, C.M. 1956. Toxicity of six chemical compounds to thirty cultures of algae. Water Sewage Works, 103, 501–503.

Malpas, J.F. 1973. Disinfection of water using chlorine dioxide. Water Treat. Exam., 22, 209–217.

Marshall, J.D., Jr., McLaughlin, J.D., and Carscallen, E.W. 1960. Iodine disinfection of a cooperative pool. Sanitarian, 22, 201–203.

Marshall, J.D., Faber, J.E., and Campbell, W.R. 1962. Advantages and limitations of iodine disinfection of an indoor swimming pool. I. Bacteriological analysis. Am. J. Public Health, 52, 1179–1185.

Martone, W.J., et al. 1980. An outbreak of adenovirus type 3 disease at a private recreation center swimming pool. Am. J. Epidemiol., 111, 229–237.

Marzouk, Y., Goyal, S.M., and Gerba, C.P. 1980. Relationship of viruses and indicator bacteria in water and wastewater of Israel. Water Res., 14, 1585–1590.

Masschelein, W.J. 1979. *Chlorine dioxide: Chemistry and Environmental Impact of Oxychlorine Compounds*. Edited by R.G. Rice. Ann Arbor, Ann Arbor Science Publishers.

Meckes, M.C. 1982. Effect of UV light disinfection on antibiotic-resistant coliforms in wastewater effluents. Appl. Environ. Microbiol., 43, 371–377.

Meckes, M.C., Venosa, A.D., and Evans, J.W. 1983. Application of an ozone disinfection model for municipal wastewater effluents. J. Water Pollut. Control Fed., 55, 1158–1162.

Miller, G.W., et al. 1978. An assessment of ozone and chlorine dioxide technologies for treatment of municipal water supplies. Environmental Protection Technology Series, EPA-600/2–78–147.

Monscvitz, J.T., and Rexing, D.J. 1981. A pilot study of chlorine dioxide use to reduce total trihalomethanes. J. Am. Water Works Assoc., 73, 94–96.

Mood, E.W. 1950. Effect of free chlorine and combined available residual chlorine upon bacteria in swimming pools. Am. J. Public Health, 40, 459–466.

Moore, B.E., Sagik, B.P., and Malina, J.F., Jr. 1975. Viral association with suspended solids. Water Res., 9, 197–203.

Morris, J.C. 1971. Chlorination and disinfection—state of the art. J. Am. Water Works Assoc. 63, 769–774.

Morris, J.C. 1970. Disinfection of water supplies. Soc. Water Treat. Exam. W.R.A. Symposium, "Water Treatment in the Seventies," pp. 160–176.

Myhrstad, J.A., and Samdal, J.E. 1969. Behavior and determination of chlorine dioxide. J. Am. Water Works Assoc., 61, 205–208.

National Interim Primary Drinking Water Regulations, 1975. U.S. Environmental Protection Agency, Federal Register, 40, 59566–59574.

Nestor, I. 1980. Enteroviruses in drinking water correlated with the physical-chemical and bacteriological indicators of water quality. Zentralbl. Bakteriol. Hyg. I. Abt. [Orig. B], 171, 218–223.

Newton, W.L., and Jones, M.F. 1949. The effect of ozone in water on cysts of *Endamoeba histolytica*. Am. J. Trop. Med., 29, 669–681.

Noss, C.I, Hauchman, F.S., and Olivieri, V.P. 1986. Chlorine dioxide reactivity with proteins. Water Res., 20, 351–356.

O'Donovan, D.C. 1965. Treatment with ozone. J. Am. Water Works Assoc., 57, 1167–1194.

Olivieri, V.P. et al. 1975. In *Disinfection—Water and Wastewater*. Edited by J.D. Johnson. Ann Arbor, Ann Arbor Science Publishers, pp. 145–162.

Opatken, E.J. 1978. Progress in wastewater disinfection technology. EPA-600/9–79–018. Cincinnati, Ohio, U.S. Environmental Protection Agency.

Ormsby, H.L. 1955. An interim report on ocular diseases due to APC viruses in Ontario. Can. J. Public Health, 46, 500–505.

Ortenzio, L.F., and Stuart, L.S. 1964. A standard test for efficacy of germicides and acceptability of residual disinfecting activity in swimming pool water. J. Assoc. Off. Agric. Chem., 47, 540–547.

Palin, A.T. 1950. A study of chloro derivatives of ammonia and related compounds, with special reference to their formation in the chlorination of natural and polluted waters. Water Water Eng., 50, 151–159, 189–200, 248–256.

Palin, A.T. 1945. The break point chlorination of water. J. Inst. Sanit. Eng., XLIV, 98–121.

Palmer, C.M. 1956. Evaluation of new algicides for water supply purposes. J. Am. Water Works Assoc., 48, 1133–1137.

Payment, P., Tremblay, M., and Trudel, M. 1985a. Relative resistance to chlorine of poliovirus and coxsackievirus isolates from environmental sources and drinking water. Appl. Environ. Microbiol., 49, 981–983.

Payment, P., Trudel, M., and Plante, R. 1985b. Elimination of viruses and indicator bacteria at each step of treatment during preparation of drinking water at seven water treatment plants. Appl. Environ. Microbiol., 49, 1418–1428.

Peeters, J.E., et al. 1989. Effect of disinfection of drinking water with ozone or chlorine dioxide on survival of *Cryptosporidium parvum* oocysts. Appl. Environ. Microbiol., 55, 1519–1522.

Phillips, G.B., and Hanel, E., Jr. 1960. Use of ultraviolet radiation in microbiological laboratories. Tech. Rept. No. BL 28. U.S. Army Chemical Corps Biological Laboratories, Fort Detrick.

Poynter, S.F.B., Slade, J.S., and Jones, H.H. 1973. The disinfection of water with special reference to viruses. Water Treat. Exam., 22, 194–206.

Presnell, N.W., and Cummins, J.M. 1972. Effectiveness of ultraviolet radiation units in the bactericidal treatment of seawater. Water Res., 6, 1203–1212.

Progress in Wastewater Technology, 1979. Edited by A.D. Venosa. EPA-600/9-79-018. Cincinnati, Ohio, U.S. Environmental Protection Agency, Municipal Environmental Research Laboratory.

Pyle, B.H., and McFeters, G.A. 1989. Iodine sensitivity of bacteria isolated from iodinated water systems. Can. J. Microbiol., 35, 520–523.

Qualls, R.G., Flynn, M.P., and Johnson, J.D. 1983. The role of suspended particles in ultraviolet disinfection. J. Water Pollut. Control. Fed., 55, 1280–1285.

Rakness, K.L., and Hegg, B.A. 1980. Full-scale ozone disinfection of wastewater. J. Water Pollut. Control. Fed., 52, 502–511.

Reckhow, D.A., and Singer, P.C. 1990. Chlorination by-products in drinking waters: from formation potentials to finished water concentrations. J. Am. Water Works Assoc., 82, 173–180.

Renn, C.E., and Chesney, W.E. 1953–1956. Reports to Salem-Brosius, Inc. on research on the Hyla system of water disinfection.

Rice, R.G., and Cotruvo, J.A. (Eds.) 1978. *Ozone/Chlorine Dioxide Oxidation Products of Organic Materials.* Cleveland, Ohio, Int. Ozone Inst.

Rice, R.G., et al. 1981. Uses of ozone in drinking water treatment. J. Am. Water Works Assoc., 73, 44–57.

Ridenour, G.M., and Armbruster, E.H. 1956. Effect of high-level gamma radiation on disinfection of water and sewage. J. Am. Water Works Assoc., 48, 671–676.

Ridenour, G.M., and Armbruster, E.H. 1949. Bactericidal effect of chlorine dioxide. J. Am. Water Works Assoc., 41, 537–550.

Ridenour, G.M., Ingols, R.S., and Armbruster, E.H. 1949. Sporicidal properties of chlorine dioxide. Water Sewage Works, 96, 279–283.

Robinton, E.D., Mood, E.W., and Elliot, L.R. 1957. A study of bacterial flora in swimming pool water treated with high free residual chlorine. Am. J. Public Health, 47, 1101–1109.

Rook, J.J. 1974. Formation of haloforms during chlorination of natural waters. Water Treat. Exam., 23(2), 234–243.

Roy, D., Englebrecht, R.S., and Chian, E.S.K. 1982. Comparative inactivation of six enteroviruses by ozone. J. Am. Water Works Assoc., 74, 660–664.

Roy, D., et al. 1981. Mechanism of enteroviral inactivation by ozone. Appl. Environ. Microbiol., 41, 718–723.

Safe Drinking Water Act, Public Law 93–523, December 16, 1974, 88 Stat. 1660. 42 United States Code (USC) 300f.

Scarpino, P.V., Brigano, F.A.O., Cronier, S., and Zink, M.L. 1979. Effect of particulates on disinfection of enteroviruses in water by chlorine dioxide. Environmental Protection Technology Series. EPA-600/2-79-054.

Scarpino, P.V., et al. 1972. A comparative study of the inactivation of viruses in water by chlorine. Water Res., 6, 959–965.

Schaefer, W.B. 1961. Swimming pool granuloma. Public Health Lab., 19, 65–66.

Schaub, S.A., and Sagik, B.P. 1975. Association of enteroviruses with natural and artificially introduced colloidal solids in water and infectivity of solids-associated virions. Appl. Microbiol., 30, 212–222.

Schecter, H. 1973. Spectrophotometric method for determination of ozone in aqueous solutions. Water Res., 7, 729–739.

Sekla, L., Stackiw, W., Kay, C., and Van Buckenhout, L. 1980. Enteric viruses in renovated water in Manitoba. Can. J. Microbiol., 26, 518–523.

Severin, B.F. 1980. Disinfection of municipal wastewater effluents with ultraviolet light. J. Water Pollut. Control Fed., 52, 2007–2018.

Shapiro, R., and Hale, F.E. 1937. An investigation of the Katadyn treatment of water with particular reference to swimming pools. J. N. Engl. Water Works Assoc., 51, 113–124.

Sharp, D.G., and Leong, J. 1980. Inactivation of poliovirus 1 (Brunhilde) single particles by chlorine in water. Appl. Environ. Microbiol., 40, 381–385.

Sharp, D.G., Young, D., Floyd, R., and Johnson, J.D. 1980. Effect of ionic environment on the inactivation of poliovirus in water by chlorine. Appl. Environ. Microbiol., 39, 530–534.

Shaw, P.K., et al. 1977. A communitywide outbreak of giardiasis with evidence of transmission by a municipal water supply. Ann. Intern. Med., 87, 426–432.

Shull, K.E. 1981. Experience with chloramines as primary disinfectants. J. Am. Water Works Assoc., 73, 101–104.

Smith, W.W., and Bodkin, R.E. 1944. Influence of hydrogen ion concentration on the bactericidal action of ozone and chlorine. J. Bacteriol., 47, 445.

Sobsey, M.D. 1989. Inactivation of health-related microorganisms in water by disinfection processes. Water Sci. Technol., 21, 179–195.

Sobsey, M.D., Fuji, T., and Shields, P.A. 1988. Inactivation of hepatitis A virus and model viruses in water by free chlorine and monochloramine. Water Sci. Technol., 20, 385–391.

Solo, F.W., Mueller, H.F., Larson, T.E., and Johnson, J.D. 1975. In *Disinfection Water and Wastewater.* Edited by J.D. Johnson. Ann Arbor, Ann Arbor Science Publishers, pp. 163–177.

Sproul, O.J., et al., 1978. Effects of particulate matter on virus inactivation by ozone. Proc. AWWA 1978 Annual Conference. Part II, Atlantic City, N.J., pp. 1–8.

Stack, D.B. 1973. Personal communication.

Stringer, R, and Kruse, C.W. 1970. Amoebic cysticidal properties. Proc. Natl. Spec. Conf. Disinfect., Amherst, Mass., pp. 319–338.

Stringer, R.P., Cramer, W.N., and Kruse, C.W. 1975. Comparison of bromine, chlorine and iodine as disinfectants for amoebic cysts. In *Disinfection Water and Wastewater.* Edited by J.D. Johnson. Ann Arbor, Ann Arbor Science Publishers, pp. 193–209.

Stuart, L.S., and Ortenzio, L.F. 1964. Swimming pool chlorine stabilizers. Soap Chem. Spec. 20, 79–82, 112–113.

Sullivan, R. et al. 1971. Inactivation of thirty viruses by gamma radiation. Appl. Microbiol., 22, 61–65.

Symons, J.M., et al., 1976. Interim treatment guide for the control of chloroform and other trihalomethanes. Cincinnati, Ohio, Water Supply Research Division, Municipal Environmental Research Laboratory, U.S. Environmental Protection Agency.

Symons, J.M., et al., 1975. National organics reconnaissance survey for halogenated organics. J. Am. Water Works Assoc., 67, 634–647.

Taft, C.E. 1965. Application of methods and materials for the control of algae. In *Water and Algae World Problems.* Edited by C.E. Taft. Chicago, Educational Publishers, Inc., p. 175.

Tartera, C., Bosch, A., and Jofre, J. 1988. The inactivation of bacteriophages infecting *Bacteroides fragilis* by chlorine treatment and UV-irradiation. FEMS Microbiol. Letters, 56, 313–316.

Taylor, G.R., and Butler, M. 1982. A comparison of the virucidal properties of chlorine, chlorine dioxide, bromine chloride, and iodine. J. Hygiene, 89, 321–328.

Tenney, M.W., and Stumm, W. 1965. Chemical flocculation of microorganisms in biological waste treatment. Water Poll. Control Fed. J., 37, 1370–1388.

Thurman, R.B., and Gerba, C.P. 1989. The molecular mechanisms of copper and silver ion disinfection of bacteria and viruses. CRC Crit. Rev. Environ. Control. 18, 295–315.

Tobin, R.S., et al. 1983. Methods for testing the efficacy of ultraviolet light disinfection devices for drinking water. J. Am. Water Works Assoc., 75, 481–484.

Uman, G.A. 1963. Spectrochemical method for silver. J. Am. Water Works Assoc., 55, 205–208.

U.S. Environmental Protection Agency, 1977. Ozone, chlorine dioxide, and chloramines as alternates to chlorine for disinfection of drinking water. State of the art. Cincinnati, Ohio, Water Supply Research, Office of Research and Development, U.S. Environmental Protection Agency.

U.S. Environmental Protection Agency. 1989. Final rule for national primary drinking water regulations. Federal Register, 54(124), 27486–27541.

U.S. Public Health Service, 1962. Drinking water standards. Public Health Service Publication No. 956. Washington, D.C., Government Printing Office.

Vaughn, J.M., et al. 1987. Inactivation of human and simian rotaviruses by ozone. Appl. Environ. Microbiol., 53, 2218–2221.

Venosa, A.D., et al. 1984. Disinfection of secondary effluent with ozone/UV. J. Water Pollut. Control Fed., 56, 137–142.

Vogt, C., and Regli, S. 1981. Controlling trihalomethanes while attaining disinfection. J. Am. Water Works Assoc., 73, 33–40.

von Brodorotti, H.S., and Mahnel, H. 1982. Comparative studies on the susceptibility of viruses to ultraviolet rays. Zentralbl. Veterinarmed., 29, 129–136.

Walter, R., et al. 1989. Viruses in river water and health risk assessment. Water Sci. Technol., 21, 21–26.

Walton, G. 1961. Effectiveness of water treatment processes as measured by coliform reduction. U.S. Department of Health, Education, and Welfare, Public Health Service Publication No. 898. Washington, D.C., Government Printing Office.

Warren, I.C., and Ridgway, J. 1978. Swimming pool disinfection. Technical Report TR90, Water Research Centre, Medmenham, England.

Warriner, R., et al. 1985. Disinfection of advanced wastewater treatment effluent by chlorine, chlorine dioxide, and ozone experiments using seeded poliovirus. Water Res., 19, 1515–1526.

Wattie, E., and Butterfield, C.T. 1944. Relative resistance of *Escherichia coli* and *Eberthella typhosa* to chlorine and chloramines. Public Health Rep., 59, 1661–1671.

Weidenkopf, S.J. 1958. Inactivation of type 1 poliomyelitis virus by chlorine. Virology, 5, 56–67.

White, G.C. 1972. *Handbook of Chlorination.* New York, Van Nostrand Reinhold.

Wolfe, R.L., and Olson, B.H. 1985. Inability of laboratory models to accurately predict field performance of disinfectants. In *Water Chlorination Chemistry,*

Environmental Impact and Health Effects. Volume 5. Edited by R.L. Jolley, et al. Chelsea, Lewis Publishers, pp. 555–573.

Wolfe, R.L., et al. 1989. Inactivation of *Giardia muris* and indicator organisms seeded in surface water supplies by peroxone and ozone. Environ. Sci. Technol., *23*, 744–745.

Wolfe, R.L., Ward, N.R., and Olson, B.H. 1984. Inorganic chloramines as drinking water disinfectants: a review. J. Am. Water Works Assoc., *56*, 74–88.

Wolfe, R.L., Ward, N.R., and Olson, B.H. 1985. Inactivation of heterotrophic bacterial populations in finished drinking water by chlorine and chloramines. Water Res., *19*, 1393–1403.

Woodward, R.L. 1963. Review of the bactericidal effectiveness of silver. J. Am. Water Works Assoc., *55*, 881–886.

Woodward, R.L. 1957. How probable is the most probable number? J. Am. Water Works Assoc., *49*, 1060–1068.

Wuhrmann, K., and Zobrist, F. 1958. Bactericidal effect of silver in water. Schweiz. Z. Hydrol., *20*, 218–254.

Yahya, M.T., et al. 1989. Swimming pool disinfection an evaluation of the efficacy of copper:silver ions. J. Environ. Health, *51*, 282–285.

Yahya, M.T., et al. 1989. Evaluation of potassium permanganate for inactivation of bacteriophage MS-2 in water systems. Form 261. Carus Chemical Company, Ottawa, Illinois.

Yip, R.W., and Konasewich, D.E. 1972. Ultraviolet sterilization of water—its potential and limitations. Water Pollut. Control (Can.), *110*, 14–18.

Young, D.C., and Sharp, D.G. 1985. Virion conformatinal forms and the complex inactivation kinetics of echovirus by chlorine in water. Appl. Environ. Microbiol., *49*, 359–364.

Zimmermann, W. 1952. Oligodynamische silberwerkung. I. Uber den werkungsmechanismus. II. Erfahrungen bei langerdauernder anwendung zur entseuchung dorflicher wassergewinnungsanlagen. Z. Hyg., *135*, 403–420.

CHAPTER 42

INFECTIOUS MEDICAL WASTES: TREATMENT AND SANITARY DISPOSAL

Seymour S. Block

When this chapter was introduced in the second edition of this book, in 1977, the problems associated with the proper treatment and disposal of medical wastes were recognized by professionals as important and deserving attention. In recent years, however, with the AIDS scare, the subject has ballooned, with the public and the U.S. Congress getting into the act. This change was precipitated during the summers of 1987 and 1988 when, according to *Time* magazine, "Medical debris, drug paraphenalia, and other waste washed up on beaches in New York, New Jersey, Rhode Island, Massachusetts and Connecticut. The medical debris included needles and syringes, prescription bottles, stained bandages, and containers of surgical sutures. There were dozens of vials of blood, three of which stained positive for hepatitis B virus, and at least six were positive for antibodies to the acquired immune deficiency syndrome (AIDS)." In addition, in Indiana and elsewhere newspapers reported improper dumping of medical wastes and children playing with infected hypodermic needles. The shocked public demanded action and Congress responded with hearings and legislation, requiring the Environmental Protection Agency (EPA) to track and report on the disposition of medical wastes in several eastern states as a pilot program. The states also reacted to the screaming headlines with stricter regulations on the treatment and disposal of medical wastes. In an early study for the EPA by myself (Block, 1974) most medical wastes were simply taken untreated to the city dump. Now treated wastes may be taken to a sanitary landfill, but not all landfills will accept medical wastes even though they are treated to meet regulations. The scene has definitely changed.

One change is reflected in the title of this chapter from "Infectious Hospital Wastes" to "Infectious Wastes." Although hospitals are still the major generator of potentially infectious wastes, many additional generators have appeared. According to 1985 data there were 13,200 freestanding laboratories, 180,000 private physicians' offices, and 100,000 dentists' offices. By 1986 estimates there were 3000 outpatient clinics and 20,000 nursing homes.

And in 1987 there were 650 ambulatory surgery centers and 860 freestanding dialysis centers. And these do not include all the 2000 home health agencies and other outpatient health-care facilities that generate medical waste. These health-care facilities are the major sources of infectious waste, but they are not the only ones. There are also academic and industrial research laboratories, the biotechnology industry, veterinary facilities, and the food, drug, and cosmetic industries.

In 1987 there were 7000 hospitals with a total of 1.267 million beds. Considering an occupancy rate of 68.9% (Rutala, 1989), a median hospital waste generation rate of 15 to 25 lbs. per patient per day (Torchia, 1988), and a total of 2.914 million pounds of infectious waste per day (3.3 pounds per patient) generated by hospitals in the United States, gives a total of about a billion pounds per year. The cost for medical waste disposal was $3.7 billion in 1988 and was predicted to grow to $10.7 billion in 1991. The Greater New York Hospital Association stated that a 500-bed hospital spends $600,000 a year to dispose of infectious waste. A single hospital in 1988 spent over $1 million on waste disposal (Goode, 1989). The Office of Technology Assessment (1988) reports that the cost of waste treatment can vary a hundredfold depending on the waste and the method used: from as little as a penny a pound for noninfectious general waste (landfilled) to as much as a dollar a pound for commercial offsite incineration.

What is infectious waste? The EPA defines infectious waste simply as "waste capable of producing an infectious disease." However, because there is no acceptable test of infectiousness, regulatory agencies identify waste depending on where it came from and what it contains. Under the definition employed, as little as 3% or as much as 90% of hospital waste could be classified as infectious. To help clarify the matter, the Medical Waste Tracking Act of 1989 (Federal Register, 1989), which was passed by Congress following the uproar over the beach pollution, dictates that the EPA must, at a minimum, include as infectious waste the following: cultures and stocks of infectious agents, pathologic wastes, blood and blood byproducts, used sharps, and contaminated animal parts and bedding. The EPA was also directed to list surgery wastes, laboratory wastes for research on infectious agents, dialysis wastes, isolation wastes, and discarded medical equipment that was in contact with infectious agents, unless the EPA found that potential mismanagement of such waste did not pose a substantial threat to health. If warranted, the EPA could add items to the list. Liberman (1988) has listed 12 types of infectious wastes.

TYPES OF INFECTIOUS WASTES

1. *Isolation wastes:* Wastes from hospital patients in isolation, to protect them from diseases of others, are not infectious unless the patient is also isolated because of illness with a communicable disease. However, under the Centers for Disease Control (CDC) Guidelines (Bond, 1988), blood and body fluids of all hospitalized patients are included in the infectious category under the doctrine of "universal precautions" because of the possibility that these fluids might contain human immunodeficiency virus (HIV), hepatitis B virus (HBV), or other blood-borne pathogens.

2. *Cultures and stocks of infectious agents:* This waste is generated in medical, pathologic, microbiologic, and research laboratories. It includes cultured specimens from patients, stocks maintained for research, and wastes from production of certain pharmaceuticals. This should be handled as infectious because it usually contains large quantities of microorganisms.

3. *Human blood and blood products:* These wastes are generated by blood banks, medical laboratories, dialysis centers, and pharmaceutical companies. They are potentially infectious because of the possible presence of pathogens, which may or may not have been demonstrated. These include, in addition to HIV and HBV, blood-borne diseases such as malaria, dengue, and congenital rubella.

4. *Pathologic wastes:* The body tissues, organs, and body parts that are removed during biopsy, surgery, and autopsy are termed pathologic wastes. These wastes have the potential of causing disease because of the possible presence of pathogens in the tissue. Therefore it is considered prudent to manage all pathologic wastes as infectious waste.

5. *Contaminated wastes from surgery and autopsy:* Waste generated during the surgery and autopsy of septic cases, or of patients with infectious diseases, may be contaminated with pathogens and should be managed as infectious waste. Under the doctrine of universal precautions all waste that has been in contact with patient blood and body fluids could be treated as infectious. This would include suction cannisters, tubing, sponges, lavage tubes, drainage sets, underpads, surgical gloves, soiled dressings, drapes, and gowns.

6. *Contaminated laboratory waste:* In this category are found culture dishes, devices used to inoculate, transfer, and mix cultures, and paper and cloth materials that were in contact with specimens or cultures. Laboratory waste includes all wastes that were in contact with pathogens that are not included in another category, such as cultures and sharps. These wastes may be especially hazardous because they may contain cultures of patient specimens that are antibiotic-resistant pathogens.

7. *Contaminated sharps:* Sharps include used hypodermic needles, syringes, Pasteur pipettes, broken glass, and scalpel blades. Sharps are a double hazard. They may inflict injury by cutting or puncture wounds and may cause infection by injecting pathogens into the flesh. Special precautions require sharps to be placed into thick plastic boxes so that they are separated from the other infectious waste and cannot cause injury.

8. *Dialysis unit wastes:* These are wastes that were in contact with the blood of patients undergoing hemodialysis. Because these patients receive frequent blood transfusions they are regarded as having a high incidence of hepatitis, taken as a group, even though previous tests for individuals may have been negative. Wastes in this category include disposable dialysis tubing and filters, sheets, towels, gloves, aprons, and lab coats. The major hazard is to the workers who are present at the point of use of these materials.

9. *Contaminated animal carcasses, body parts, and bedding:* The animals that contribute to these wastes were intentionally exposed to pathogens during research, production of biologicals, and testing of pharmaceuticals and must be treated as infectious waste.

10. *Discarded biologicals:* These consist of waste vaccines and other discarded biologicals produced by pharmaceutical companies for human or veterinary use. They are discarded because they are outdated, they failed to pass quality control, or the product is being removed from the market. They are managed as infectious waste because pathogens may be present although in most cases this would not be so.

11. *Contaminated food and other products:* In this category are foods, food additives, drugs, and cosmetics that are not safe for consumption because they are contaminated. These wastes should be treated so they are rendered unrecognizable and unusable.

12. *Contaminated equipment:* Equipment that became contaminated through inpatient care in medical and microbiologic laboratories, in research with infectious agents, and in the production and testing of some pharmaceuticals would be classified in this category. If equipment so contaminated is to be reused, it is necessary to see that it is properly decontaminated.

Under the doctrine of universal precautions hospitals may include a large amount of noninfectious waste with the infectious waste, depending on the hospital's interpretation of the doctrine. Some hospitals, for example, include all waste that has been in contact with patients to be sure that no infectious waste is missed. For safety, hospitals in the United States are required by the EPA to put all infectious waste in a red bag, whereas noninfectious waste is put into a clear colorless bag. (In Canada different types of wastes are separated into different colored bags.) Marrack (1988) reported on a study of the contents of 1022 pounds of red bag waste from two hospitals in the Houston area. "Disposable gowns and surgical drapes formed the bulk of the red bag contents. A scattering of paper plates, brown paper bags, cigarette packets, food wrappings and rubber gloves were observed." Total plastics made up 14.2% by weight of the red bag waste, with polyvinylchloride plastic making 9.4%. To examine the infectious potential, cultures were made of soiled swabs and other articles. *E. coli* and coagulase-negative streptococci were found. The articles cultured came mostly from the operating room, and the fact that few organisms were recovered was attributed to the general sterility and use of antibiotics in surgery. One thing that can be said about red bag waste is that it is anything but uniform, coming from so many different sources, making it difficult to generalize on its nature. In recent years the quantity of disposables has greatly increased, which has added to the volume of waste. Disposables have increased safety and convenience in hospital use. Table 42–1 lists disposable items employed in medical facilities, most of which are included in the red bag waste.

HOW HAZARDOUS IS RED BAG WASTE?

Hospitals and medical facilities are known sources of infectious organisms. It would be reasonable therefore to expect red bag waste to be infectious or even highly infectious. Government and hospital regulations require its collection and treatment as infectious material. The public regards it as highly dangerous. But is it really hazardous? Interestingly enough, a CDC guideline on infectious waste states, "There is no epidemiological evidence to suggest that most hospital waste is any more infectious than residential waste" (Garner and Favero, 1985).

Research at the University of West Virginia Medical Center (Burchinal and Wallace, 1971; Smith, 1970; Trigg, 1971; Wallace et al., 1972) revealed that pathogenic organisms can be present in hospital solid waste in significantly high concentrations, and especially so if an organic substrate is present. Coliform counts ranged from less than 1/g of refuse at some stations to as high as 8.6/g. Fecal streptococci ranged from less than 1/g to as high as 8.0/g, staphylococci from less than 2/g to 7.1/g, *Candida albicans* from less than 2/g to 3.8/g, *Pseudomonas* species from less than 2/g to 8.4/g, and spores from less than 1.5/g to 3.9/g (Trigg, 1971).

Substantial numbers of organisms of human origin were found, which suggests the presence of virulent pathogenic bacteria and viruses living in the solid waste in undetected numbers. *Bacillus* species made up 80 to 90% of all microbes observed, with staphylococci and streptococci each composing between 5 and 10% of the population. *Staphylococcus aureus* was by far the most prominent pathogen detected in the waste. Spore-forming organisms are not present in sufficient numbers to constitute a potential hazard if accepted methods of sterilization are followed. Nursing stations, such as in the operating rooms where pathologic waste is separated from other waste, show much lower microbial concentrations in general refuse than other stations. The stations

Table 42–1. *Disposable Items Available to the Hospital*

Alcohol swabs	Cartridge deionizers	Feeding tubes	Scalpels
Apparel and garments	Catheter adapters	Flask closures	Scalpels, blades, razors
Aprons	Catheter sets	Floor sweepers	Serving trays
Arm boards	Cloth cleaners	Gloves	Sheets
Bags	Collection units	Gowns	Shower caps
Bags and tubes	Conductive strips	Hypodermic needles	Specimen bags
Barium cups	Coverslips	Hypodermic syringes	Surgical gloves
Bassinets	Debubbling units	Infant formulas	Surgical masks
Beakers	Diapers	Infusion tubing	Surgical packs
Bedpan liners	Diaper liners	Kits	Syringes
Bed linens	Dinnerware	Limb holders	Tape measures
Bibs	Dishes: Food service	Masks	Trays and kits
Blankets	Douche bags	Obstetric packs	Trays and tubes
Blood clotting supplies	Drainage bags	Paper towels	Tumbler covers
Blood collection units	Drape packs	Petri dishes	Underpads
Blood lancets	Drawsheets	Pillows	Uniforms
Blood filters	Dressing trays	Pillow cases	Urinals
Blood transfusion sets	Enema administration	Pillow protector	Urinal covers
Boots	Units: Barium	Pipettes	Urine measurement device
Bottles	Enema bags	Pitchers	Utensils
Bottle caps	Enema solutions	Plastic containers	Utility bags
Carafes	Enema tubes	Prep sets	Washcloths
Capes	Examination gloves	Razors	

From "Medical Disposables" Marketing Guide and Company Directory. Technomic Publishing.

generating the refuse most highly contaminated with co-liform bacteria are those in the intensive care unit and pediatrics.

Virus survival studies indicate that almost all materials found in the hospital solid waste could be vehicles for transmission of viruses (Burchinal and Wallace, 1971; Wallace et al., 1972). Various types of waste were artificially contaminated with viruses to establish recovery times and rates. Vaccinia, polio 1, Coxsackie A-9, and influenza PR-8 were the viral strains used for inoculation. Paper and cotton fabric both held active viruses for long periods of time—from 5 to 8 days in most cases. Virus titer decreased in most cases at a steady rate with increasing time, implying that the agent loses its viability upon incubation.

Kalinowski et al. (1983) reported that the bacterial concentration of different types of hospital waste has 10 to 100,000 times less microbial contamination than household waste. Mose and Reinthaler (1985) showed a wider range of bacteria in hospital waste, but that, quantitatively, household refuse was more contaminated, especially with fecal bacteria. Almost one-third of all hospital waste showed no bacterial growth. In blood-drenched waste and serum samples 2% of all samples examined were anti-HBc and anti-HBe positive. Trost and Filip (1985) found that refuse from medical consulting rooms had generally lower microbial counts than municipal refuse. Fecal indicators and facultative pathogenic bacteria, however, were found more frequently and usually at higher concentrations in consulting room refuse. Salmonella was not found. The authors concluded that refuse from medical consulting rooms should be handled with caution, but that these kinds of refuse were not considered a source of acute risk. Jager et al. (1989) examined red bag waste from normal and high risk areas of large and small hospitals and found that the germ concentration of hospital waste was similar to or less than that of household refuse. The count of gram-negative rods in household refuse was 4 logs greater than that in operating room ward waste. These workers concluded that hospital wastes should be disposed of with special hygienic measures inside the hospital, but that outside the hospital they can be disposed of together with household refuse.

Considering the severity of the diseases that might be transmitted with infectious waste, HIV and HBV (AIDS and hepatitis) would potentially be the most dangerous. Studies of these diseases show that the risk for workers handling infected waste is no greater than that for the general population (Keene, 1988). In the case of HIV it is less than 1%, and for HBV it is 5 to 6%. The most hazardous component of the medical waste is the sharps, particularly the used hypodermic needles, because of their ability to puncture the skin and cause infection. This problem has received considerable attention. Jagger et al. (1988) studied the effect of 326 needlesticks of health-care workers during a 10-month period. None of the incidents resulted in a documented case of infectious disease. Kransinski et al. (1987) reported on 315 needlestick punctures in a 27-month period and found that two of the exposed workers developed hepatitis B. Rich-

ardson (1989) studied waste-handling personnel who handled biochemical waste. There were 210 needlesticks among 3000 hospital employees during the study but no documented cases of occupationally transmitted HBV. The City of New York sanitation department (1989) was concerned about needle puncture injuries of its garbage, refuse, and litter collectors on their city routes and in collecting noninfectious hospital waste, as well as some workers walking through landfill areas. In 39 months there were 224 needle puncture injuries reported, but none of the workers reported health problems resulting from the injuries.

It should not be surprising that there is a low incidence of disease. Despite popular opinion, diseases are not so easy to catch. Exposure is not synonymous with infection; although many are exposed, few become infected. There are four criteria for infection: (1) Presence of a pathogen with sufficient virulence. (2) An infectious dose. One or a few microorganisms are seldom enough to cause infection. The infectious dose varies by many orders of magnitude for different pathogens. (3) A necessary route of entry. Some pathogens infect through the respiratory tract, others through the alimentary canal, the blood, skin, etc. (4) And finally, there must be a susceptible host. Some people are resistant or immune to some diseases through genetics, race, sex, age, or vaccination. Many experts feel that the hazard of infectious waste is overblown: that it has been grossly overstated, that it exists largely in the public mind, and that we are dealing with perceived rather than real hazards. If this is so, where does it leave us? The course of action as recommended by the CDC (Bond, 1988) is one of caution with reason, as follows:

1. Establishing an Infective Waste Disposal Plan
   a. An infective waste management plan at a hospital, other health-care facility, or clinical/research laboratory should include strategies for identification (i.e., defining which wastes are considered infective), collection, handling, predisposal treatment, and terminal disposal of infective waste.
   b. An integral part of an effective infective waste disposal plan is the designation of the person or persons responsible for establishing, monitoring, periodically reviewing, and administering the plan.
2. Identification of Potentially Infective Waste
   a. Microbiology laboratory wastes, blood and blood products, pathology waste, and sharp items (especially needles) should be considered as potentially infective and handled and disposed of with special precautions as discussed below.
   b. Other items may be considered infective depending upon local and state regulations.
3. Handling, Transport, and Storage of Potentially Infective Waste
   a. Personnel involved in the handling and disposal of infective waste should be informed of the potential health and safety hazards and trained

in the appropriate handling and disposal methods.

b. If processing and/or disposal facilities are not available at the site of infective waste generation (i.e., laboratory, etc.) the waste may be safely transported in sealed impervious containers to another hospital area or other facility for appropriate treatment.

c. To minimize the potential risk for accidental transmission of disease or injury, infective waste awaiting terminal processing should be stored in an area accessible only to personnel involved in the disposal process.

4. Processing and Disposal of Potentially Infective Waste

a. Waste that has been designated as infective should either be incinerated or should be decontaminated prior to disposal in a sanitary landfill. Bulk blood, suctioned fluids, excretions, and secretions may be carefully poured down a drain connected to a sanitary sewer. Sanitary sewers may also be used for the disposal of other infectious wastes capable of being ground and flushed into the sewer.

b. Disposable syringes with needles, scalpel blades, and other sharp items capable of causing injury should be placed intact into puncture-resistant containers located as close as is practical to the area in which they were used. If predisposal autoclaving is performed, the container should maintain its puncture resistance after autoclaving to avoid subsequent physical injuries.

5. Special Precautions

Special waste-handling methods may be necessary for certain rare diseases or conditions such as Lassa fever. Concerns about blood-borne viruses such as HIV and subsequent implementation of "universal precautions" for infection control within the health-care environment necessitate no special alteration in current standards of waste management.

REGULATION OF INFECTIOUS WASTES

Federal Government Regulation

The EPA has the authority from Congress to regulate infectious waste under the Resource Conservation and Recovery Act of 1976 (RCRA) and the Medical Waste Tracking Act of 1988 (MWTA). The RCRA, which regulates hazardous waste, allows the EPA to regulate the management and disposal of infectious waste as hazardous waste. The EPA has not decided to issue final regulations because it has not perceived the problem of infectious waste to be severe enough to warrant regulation as hazardous waste. Instead the EPA issued a guidance manual on waste management in 1982, revised in 1986, which gave recommendations rather than specified legal requirements. The MWTA was passed by Congress in 1988 as a result of the reaction to the beach washups of medical waste along the Atlantic coast and the Great

Lakes. This act provided for the EPA to conduct a 2-year demonstration of the medical waste tracking program to determine the effectiveness of tracking regulations in reducing the threat of medical wastes to health and the environment. These regulations specified details as to the nature of the wastes considered for tracking, the documentation form required for waste shipped off-site from a medical facility, as well as information reports and records on the generation, handling, transportation, treatment, and disposal of the waste. When this program has been completed it is anticipated that the EPA will then issue regulations concerning measures such as off-site shipment of medical wastes.

The Occupational Safety and Health Administration (OSHA) is another federal agency that has regulatory power in the area of infectious waste. Under its jurisdiction an employer is required to present an employee with a workplace free from hazards that are likely to cause death or serious harm. The OSHA right-to-know regulations supply the employee with information on possible hazards to which he might be subjected. Although these regulations were originally written to pertain to chemical hazards, they apply as well to hazards resulting from infectious microorganisms. Although the OSHA has not yet issued regulations concerning infectious wastes, it did in 1987 recommend safety precautions for health-care workers with reference to HIV. As of 1989, the OSHA was considering converting these recommendations into regulatory requirements (OSHA, 1989).

State Controls

Whereas the federal regulations set the stage for control of infectious waste, individual states are more important in carrying out these programs. In 1987 the EPA conducted a survey that indicated that all but six of the states in the United States had enacted laws to regulate infectious waste as part of their hazardous waste program. These laws have been stiffened since that time, and it is doubtful that any state now remains that does not have some legislation on this subject. By and large these laws follow the EPA and CDC guidelines, but may be even more stringent. For example, the states may require that certain treatment be employed. Florida in its new regulations requires incineration of infectious waste. It will, however, permit other treatment processes, but evidence must be submitted demonstrating effectiveness of such treatments before they are approved by the Florida Department of Environmental Regulation. This department works closely with Florida's Department of Health and Human Services in these matters. Other states have similar agencies that provide such control.

Local Controls

Cities and counties have ordinances and codes that apply to waste collection, treatment, and disposal. These may determine what types of waste may be deposited in the local landfill, what materials may be discharged into the sanitary sewer, and whether a medical incinerator may be constructed in that city or county.

JCAHO Standards

The Joint Commission on Accreditation of Healthcare Organizations (JCAHO) exerts significant influence over hospitals in the United States through establishment of standards that hospitals must meet in order to become accredited (JCAHO, 1987). Under the JCAHO's 1988 accreditation standard, a hospital's infectious waste program must (1) control waste from its point of origin to its final disposal; (2) protect patients, personnel, visitors, and the environment; (3) include policies and procedures for identifying and managing hazardous materials and waste, including the substitution of less hazardous agents, process changes, isolation, and ventilation; (4) review operational policies and procedures at least annually by the respective safety or control committees, with recommendations, conclusions, and actions referred to those persons responsible for the hospital's quality assurance program; (5) provide job training to its waste handlers; (6) provide for the handling and disposal of hazardous gaseous, liquid and solid materials or waste, including packing, transport within the facility, and adequate and safe disposal facilities both on-site and off-site; (7) be established and operated in accordance with applicable law and regulation; and (8) observe safe and sanitary practices throughout the facility, including food preparation and serving, and patient care.

In 1987 and 1988 Rutala (1989) made a survey of 441 randomly selected hospitals in the United States to determine their waste-handling practices. The results of this survey indicated that the management of infectious waste is generally consistent with CDC guidelines and that, if anything, hospitals are overcautious by employing overly inclusive definitions of infectious waste.

TREATMENT OF INFECTIOUS WASTE

Doucet (1988) lists three major on-site treatment options available for infectious waste to render it noninfectious. These are incineration, steam sterilization (autoclaving), and shredding-milling coupled with chemical disinfection. These methods will now be described.

Incineration

Incineration is an ancient method for destroying wastes. It has long been used for the cremation of human and animal remains. Until 1957 most homeowners in southern California had backyard incinerators to dispose of their combustible refuse, and today many municipalities around the world use incineration to destroy wastes that will burn. Incineration has many desirable features. It destroys the structure and appearance of the waste; it reduces the volume by up to 95%; it permits energy in the waste to be recovered as heat; and the heat can destroy all microorganisms it reaches. These features have made it an appealing waste-treatment method for hospitals. But it also has disadvantages that are giving hospital managers second thoughts. Incinerators are expensive machines and are becoming increasingly more expensive. They require supervision by an engineer, and technical training is necessary for the operators. They require expensive maintenance and repair. The ash residue may contain toxic metals. And most disturbing is the problem of air pollution caused by incinerator effluent. Usually hospitals are located in densely inhabited

neighborhoods, and the smoke and gases from the incinerator can cause complaints and protest. The recent national attention to air pollution as well as to medical wastes has caused many regulatory bodies to require air pollution abatement equipment on incinerators to be installed within the near future. The cost of this equipment and its operation may significantly increase the cost of the incinerator. As a result, hospitals have considered getting out of the business, using the space for other hospital needs, and shipping the waste to off-site incinerators. James McLarney, an official of the American Hospitals Association, said, "There is only one hospital in California that still has a license to incinerate. The rest of them cannot meet the clean air rules" (*New York Times*, Nov. 20, 1990). Instead hospitals usually hire a hauler equipped to handle infectious wastes, who ships them to a single large incinerator that has high-technology antipollution equipment.

This procedure has been adopted by many hospitals. Larger operation permits more-efficient incineration and the use of air pollution abatement equipment. However, this too has problems. The cost for this service is high. The waste must be carefully packaged for off-site shipment. The hospital remains responsible if the shipper improperly handles the waste or fails to deliver it or treat it properly. And the waste-treatment company has problems in finding a site that is acceptable to the locality and the regulatory agencies. In the north-central part of Florida, for example, there have been six attempts to site medical waste incinerators within the past 2 years, with no success. In each case there was angry protest by the local citizens expressing the N.I.M.B.Y. syndrome ("not in my back yard"). The argument of whether to go off-site or stay on-site is one that hospital managers are seriously weighing at this time. Especially concerned are those hospitals with old, inefficient incinerators, where a decision must be made.

Types of Incinerators and Operation

Incineration is a process of combustion. It requires (1) air and fuel in proper proportions, (2) that the air, fuel, and combustible gases be adequately mixed, (3) that temperatures be sufficient for ignition of both solid fuel and the gaseous components, (4) that furnace volumes be large enough to provide the retention time needed for complete combustion, and (5) that furnace proportions be such that ignition temperatures are maintained and fly ash is minimized. All of these criteria must be met for proper combustion to occur.

The typical hospital incinerator, pathologic or biomedical incinerator, is a retort modular unit as shown in Figure 42–1. A pathologic incinerator is different from a refuse incinerator, which burns mainly paper. The pathologic incinerator has a large heater that will dry out animal bodies, surgery wastes, isolation wastes, agar media, blood bags, and other wet materials so they can be burned. The incinerator is usually cubical in shape with the secondary combustion chamber following the primary chamber. The chambers provide (1) for the volatilization of the water and combustible gaseous components of the waste, (2) for the mixture of air with these combustible components, and (3) for the burning of both

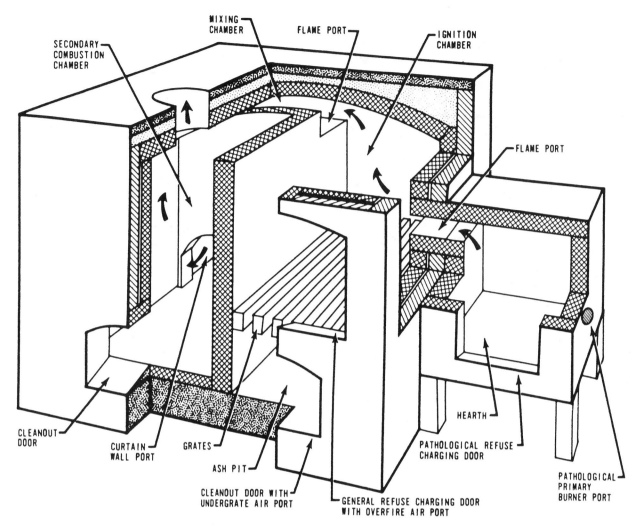

Fig. 42–1. Multiple-chamber incinerator with a pathologic-waste retort. (From Danielson, J.A., ed. 1973. Air Pollution Engineering Manual. Research Triangle Park, North Carolina, EPA Office of Air Quality Planning and Standards.)

the nonvolatile and volatile products that are combustible. Auxiliary fuel is provided to achieve the necessary temperature in each chamber. The gaseous combustion products and excess air are removed through the stack. The modular incinerator may be either an excess air or a controlled air (starved air) incinerator (Brunner and Brown, 1988). In the excess air incinerator waste is fired in the primary chamber. The secondary combustion chamber provides the residence time, temperature, and supplemental fuel for combustion of the unburned organics that are carried over from the primary chamber. The baffles inside the incinerator guide the combustion gases through 90° turns in both horizontal and vertical directions. These turns allow the soot to drop out of the flue gas stream so it does not escape through the stack with the effluent gas. The charge of waste is burned out over a period of hours. A typical operation might include charging during the day, then firing and burning toward evening, with burnout by the next morning, and ash removal before recharging. Air is injected into the primary and secondary combustion chambers through the

supplementary fuel burners. Each chamber has one or two burners to provide the heat necessary to raise the temperature to operating conditions. The primary combustion chamber should operate in the range of 1400°F (760°C) to 1800°F (982°C), and the secondary chamber at over 2000°F (1093°C), to make sure that all of the combustibles are consumed. Temperatures higher than 1800°F should be avoided in the primary chamber because the ash will begin to soften and melt with increasing temperature, and when it cools it will harden into a slag that may clog air ports, disable burners, and corrode the refractory. The retention time in the secondary chamber may be 0.5 to 2 seconds.

Efficient burning in an incinerator produces no unburned carbon or fly ash in the effluent, or uncombusted waste in the ash on the floor of the incinerator. A measure of the completeness of the latter is known as burnout. Poor burnout is indicated by large pieces of unburned or partially burned recognizable material. An EPA official told me of seeing, in incinerator residue, boxes of paper with the outside carton charred but the contents only scorched around the edges and otherwise unchanged. Poor burnout may result from overcrowding of materials in the incinerator, packing the contents too densely, not enough time for burnout, too low a temperature, insufficient air, too early shutdown, or improper incinerator design or operation. To determine whether infectious waste has been effectively destroyed or disinfected, biologic indicators, such as the spores of *Bacillus subtilis* var. *niger* or *globigii*, which are resistant to heat, may be added to the waste. The survival of the spores can be tested for in the ash and the stack emissions.

Some 5000 (about 90%) of the incinerators installed during the past 20 years are called controlled air or starved air incinerators. A controlled air incinerator differs from an excess air incinerator in that the former operates with only 40 to 80% of the stoichiometric air requirement in the primary chamber to provide the necessary temperature. Rather than oxidize the waste in the primary chamber, it is heated, dried, and volatilized, passing as combustible gases into the secondary chamber where the main burner provides combustion, and 100 to 140% of the stoichiometric air requirement is injected. The control of air in the primary chamber allows for control of the temperature and rate of throughput. This system has been popular because the reduced airflow in the primary chamber causes less carryover of entrained particles in the effluent, thus producing less smoke and fewer complaints of pollution. Brunner and Brown (1988), however, do not favor this type of incinerator for hospitals because of the extreme variation in hospital waste. The controlled air incinerator is designed to burn dry organic matter such as a paper waste, but the hospital waste is largely wet, and waste with a moisture content over 60% will not burn on its own at 1600°F. As shown in Table 42–2, much of the hospital or biomedical waste exceeds 60% moisture. Table 42–3 shows the variation in BTU and amount of air required for the different wastes. These workers (Brunner and Brown, 1988) state that this makes it virtually impossible for the controlled air process to be maintained when the stoichiometric ratio of air demand to pound of waste ranges from 1 to 16. They prefer instead the excess air system, which might be either the modular or the rotary kiln type.

The rotary kiln is a furnace that has been used in industry for many years to roast such things as cement. It is a horizontal cylinder lined with refractory that rotates about its horizontal axis as pictured in Figure 42–2. The waste is charged into the kiln and is constantly turned over at 1 to 3 rpm and moved through the kiln as regulated by the speed of rotation and angle of the kiln to the horizontal. The ash exits at the lower end while the off-gas and volatiles pass into the secondary combustion chamber directly above the kiln where the volatile organics are burned out. Excess air is supplied to both the kiln and secondary chamber. The turbulence of the kiln increases the particulate load of the flue off-gas; therefore this system requires more air emissions control than the modular units. The rotary kiln is run as a continuous system with a charging ram to feed the waste and with continuous discharge of ash. The rotary kiln is a relatively recent innovation for infectious waste incineration, only having been introduced by 1988 (Doucet, 1988). Although small units have been made, the rotary kiln is usually a large, expensive machine which is used in large off-site installations where its future appears to lie.

Incinerator Emissions

Just as it is jokingly said that a housewife dusting the house is just relocating the dirt, so it has been said that incinerating infectious waste just converts a hazard of one kind to a hazard of another kind. The hazardous products that might be present in incinerator emissions include hydrogen chloride (HCl), carbon monoxide (CO), nitrogen oxides (NO_x), sulfur dioxide (SO_2), polychlorinated biphenyls (PCBs), dioxins, furans, and particulates including compounds of mercury, arsenic, cadmium, and chromium. Because hospital incinerators are much smaller than municipal incinerators, in the past regulating agencies in most states didn't pay strict attention to the effluents of hospital incinerators. Now, however, that condition is being turned around and within a few years it is likely that all incinerators will require pollution abatement equipment. The PVC plastic used in the hospital represents about 9.4% of red bag waste and contributes to the formation of the chlorine-containing pollutants, HCl, PCBs, dioxins, and furans (Marrack, 1988). In a study of the effluent of Ontario waste incinerators, McClymont and Urbanski (1987) reported that, because of the PVC composition of the waste, the chlorine averaged 8.7 g/kg of waste and HCl emissions averaged 18.7 g HCl/kg of waste burned, based on the maximum half-hour average. HCl is not only toxic, it is highly corrosive in the environment and to the incinerator, its refractory lining, and the stack (EPA, 1986). It is clear from this that unless PVC is not incinerated, pollution abatement equipment is necessary. Pollution abatement equipment includes wet air scrubbers, dry collection systems, and electrostatic precipitators. Brunner and Brown (1988) feel that dry scrubbing systems are the most effective because most of the particulate discharge from a hospital incinerator is unburned organic matter, which is not easily wetted by water. Baghouse filters, electrostatic precipitators, and dry scrubbers will remove this particulate matter and the acid gases, which include carbon, the organics, the metals, HCl, SO_2, and NO_x. However the cost of this equipment in capital outlay and operation is high and no doubt will cause a large number of hospitals to choose off-site incineration or treatment systems other than incineration. According to Marrack (1988), options for reducing effluent pollution from incineration of red bag waste include (1) equipping all hospital incinerators with the best available control technology (BACT), (2) requiring red bag waste to be sent to an incinerator with BACT, (3) reducing the mass of red bag waste by in-house sterilization of some items, or (4) ceasing to use chlorine-containing materials.

The Incinerator as a Sterilizer

A question that has been the subject of a number of investigations is whether it is possible for pathogenic

Table 42–2. *Composition and Heat Value of Biomedical (Infectious, "Red Bag") Wastes*

Canadian Waste Class and Bag Color	Category Components	Weight % (as fired)	Moisture (% weight)	BTU/lb. (dry basis)	Heat Value BTU/lb. (as fired)
A1. Red Bag	Human anatomic	95–100	70–90	8,000–12,000	1,200
	Plastics	0–5	0–1	14,000–20,000	180
	Swabs, absorbents	0–5	0–30	8,000–12,000	80
	Disinfectants	0–0.2	0–0.2	11,000–14,000	20
A2. Orange Bag	Animal infected				
	Anatomic	80–100	60–90	9,000–16,000	1,500
	Plastics	0–15	0–1	14,000–20,000	420
	Glass	0–5	0	0	0
	Bedding, shavings, paper, fecal matter	0–10	10–50	8,000–9,000	600
A3a. Yellow Bag (lab waste)	Gauze pads, swabs, garments, paper, cellulose	60–90	0–30	8,000–12,000	6,400
	Plastics, PVC, syringes	15–30	0–1	9,700–20,000	3,250
	Sharps, needles	4–8	0–1	60	5
	Fluids, residuals	2–5	80–100	0–10,000	30
	Disinfectants	0–0.2	0–50	7,000–14,000	15
A3b. Yellow Bag (diagnostic waste)	Plastics	50–60	0–1	14,000–20,000	9,000
	Sharps	0–5	0–1	60	0
	Cellulosics	5–10	0–15	8,000–12,000	650
	Fluids, residual	1–20	95–100	0–10,000	30
	Disinfectants	0–0.2	0–50	11,000–14,000	20
	Glass	15–25	0	0	0
A3c. Yellow Bag (research and development)	Gauze, pads, swabs	5–0	0–30	8,000–12,000	1,000
	Plastics, petri dishes	50–60	0–1	14,000–20,000	9,000
	Sharps, glass	0–10	0–1	60	0
	Fluids	1–10	80–100	0–10,000	100
B1. Blue Bag	Noninfected animal				
	Anatomic	90–100	60–90	9,000–16,000	1,400
	Plastics	0–10	0–1	14,000–20,000	1,000
	Glass	0–3	0	0	0
	Beddings, shavings, fecal matter	0–10	10–50	8,000–9,000	600

Ontario Ministry of the Environment, 1986. Incinerator design and operating criteria. Vol. 2, Biomedical waste incinerators, October.

bacteria in red bag waste to pass through the incineration process without being killed and escape through the stack into the environment. In its Guide for Infectious Waste Management, the EPA noted that if incinerators are not operated properly viable pathogenic organisms can be released to the environment in stack emissions, residue ash, or wastewater (EPA, 1986). Certainly the temperatures in the combustion chambers are sufficient to destroy all living things, but any one or a combination of the following factors might interfere with the necessary time-temperature exposure of airborne microorganisms for sterilization: temperature gradients caused by intermittent incinerator use; linear velocities that exceed the incinerator design capacity and reduce retention time; internal conveyors; automatic vibrating grates; charging beyond capacity; excessive moisture content of refuse; short height of stack; and type of refractory lining.

Peterson and Stutzenberger (1969) studied the survival of bacteria in the incinerator residue. Four incinerators of different types, each with operating temperatures between 1200°F (649°C) and 2000°F (1093°C), were found to produce residues of remarkably different microbiologic quality (Table 42–4). Incinerator I produced a poor-quality residue, with no significant difference in the heat-resistant population (organisms viable after 30 minutes at 80°C) in the residue as compared to the initial waste. Physically, the residue contained unburned vegetables, animal wastes, and even newspapers with readable print. This was most evident when the incinerator was operating over its designed capacity owing to normal main-

Table 42–3. *Waste Combustion Characteristics*

Waste	BTU/lb.	lb. air/lb. waste
Pathologic	1,000	1
Paper	5,000	4
PVC	9,754	8
Polyurethane	11,203	9
Polystyrene	16,419	13
Polyethylene	19,687	16

Brunner, C.R., and Brown, C.H. 1988. Hospital waste disposal by incineration. JAPCA, 39, 164–168.

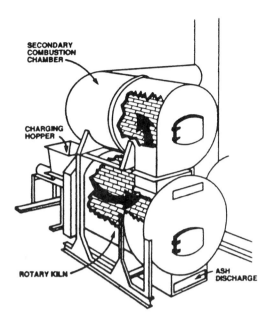

Fig. 42–2. Rotary kiln system. (Brunner, C.R., and Brown, C.H. 1988. Hospital waste disposal by incineration. JAPCA, *39*, 164–168.)

perature of 385°F (196°C) was necessary to prevent a sporadic release of the test organisms to the atmosphere. Overall it was found that a proper combination of three variables—air temperature, firebrick temperature, and retention time—is necessary to ensure a complete sterilizing effect. To this end, the exhaust stack played an important role by increasing the retention time and the effectiveness of the incinerator as a sterilizer.

Barbeito et al. (1968) challenged aerosols of *Bacillus subtilis* spores and vegetative cells of *Serratia marcescens* in two large air incinerators. Firebox temperature of 525°F (274°C) and retention time of 8.6 to 19.2 seconds sterilized dry Serratia cells. Wet spores of *Bacillus subtilis* were sterilized with firebox temperatures of 525 to 700°F (274 to 371°C). Barbeito and Shapiro (1977), using a semiportable pathologic incinerator and *B. subtilis* spores, found the temperatures required to sterilize the emissions from this incinerator were 1400°F (760°C) in the primary chamber, 1600°F (871°C) in the secondary chamber, and 1050°F (566°C) at the top of the stack. The retention time was 12.5 seconds at 1050°F (566°C). In another study (EPA, 1970), it was reported that 2 gram-positive bacilli per cubic foot of air were passing through the stack. Allen et al. (1989) questioned all the earlier studies as to the identity of the bacteria released in the stack gas and their source—namely, where did they come from? In their study, waste inoculated with *B. subtilis* spores was burned in a hospital incinerator and, although 1157 bacterial colonies per cubic meter were obtained from the stack gas, no *B. subtilis* were recovered. Identification of the bacteria indicated that they came neither from the waste nor the outside air but from the combustion air, which came from incinerator room air.

Steam Sterilization

Materials may be sterilized in several ways. Heat sterilization (other than incineration) may be accomplished by the use of steam (autoclaving) or dry heat. Both methods are used in microbiologic laboratories. Then there is chemical sterilization, with ethylene oxide and formaldehyde being examples of chemicals in use in hospitals. X-ray, gamma ray, and electron beam radiation are also used for sterilizing materials, but the method used primarily for sterilizing wastes in hospitals is steam sterilization. It is practical, effective, and cheap. The EPA and the National Research Council recommend

tenance shutdowns of one or more of the furnace units. Incinerator IV, in contrast, yielded a residue with a predominantly heat-resistant population of microorganisms, showing that most of the less hardy flora had been destroyed. The air temperatures (1200° to 2000°F or 649° to 1093°C) in all four of these incinerators were easily sufficient to kill all organisms. The presence of viable organisms in the refuse indicates that the residue never achieved these temperatures, and this is further supported by the presence of unburned materials.

Barbeito and Gremillion (1968) investigated the conditions necessary to ensure sterilization in an incinerator. Using an industrial refuse incinerator and *Bacillus subtilis* var. *niger* spores, they found that a combination of a top-of-the-stack temperature of 575°F (302°C) and a 41-second retention time inside the firebox of the incinerator were required to kill spores disseminated from a liquid suspension at a concentration of 5.3×10^9 spores per cubic foot of air flowing through the incinerator. In addition to the air temperature, a refractory lining tem-

Table 42–4. *Efficiency of Incinerator Operations in the Destruction of the Microflora Associated with Municipal Solid Wastes*

Material	Bacterial population*	I	II	III	IV
Solid Waste	Total cells	7.6×10^7	4.1×10^8	5.6×10^7	3.8×10^8
	Heat resistant†	4.2×10^4	6.8×10^4	2.7×10^4	1.7×10^4
	Total coliforms	6.2×10^5	4.8×10^6	5.4×10^5	1.2×10^5
	Fecal coliforms	9.1×10^4	4.0×10^5	1.2×10^5	2.3×10^4
Residue	Total cells	4.4×10^7	1.7×10^6	1.2×10^6	7.1×10^3
	Heat resistant†	1.0×10^5	2.0×10^4	3.9×10^3	4.4×10^3
	Total coliforms	1.5×10^4	2.3×10^2	4.1×10^1	5
	Fecal coliforms	2.4×10^3	9	5	<1

*Expressed as counts per gram
†Expressed as spores per gram
From Peterson, M.L., and Stutzenberger, F.J. 1969. Microbiological evaluation of incinerator operations. Appl. Microbiol., *18*, 8–13.

steam sterilization as the method of choice for treating waste cultures, stocks of infectious agents, biologicals, and contaminated labware. Further recommended for sterilization are isolation wastes, blood and blood products, and contaminated sharps. It can be seen from Table 42–5 that steam heat sterilizes at lower temperature than hot air heating and is much faster for the same temperature. For dry heat sterilization of solid, infectious wastes, the EPA recommends 160 to 170°C (320 to 338°F) for 2 to 4 hours (EPA, 1986). It is stated that these extensive time and energy requirements preclude common use of this treatment. To be most effective as a sterilizing agent, steam must be saturated with water vapor; thus it is referred to as moist heat, whereas hot air heating is referred to as dry heat. Superheated steam, or steam not saturated with water vapor, acts more like dry heat and is to be avoided. (For more detailed information on sterilization with steam refer to Chapters 6 and 29.) Wastes composed of cultures, tissues, and other materials with known pathogenic organisms may be routinely sterilized in small steam sterilizers within the laboratory or clinic where they are generated, whereas other cultures, such as blood samples, that might or might not contain infectious organisms may be sterilized with the red bag ("infectious") waste from the hospital or medical facility in large on-site sterilizers, or off-site in industrial-size retort units at regional waste facilities (Fig. 42–3).

Special problems pertain to the sterilization of waste. The first results from the fact that the waste is so variable in composition. Some materials require more time and temperature than other materials. This is because some wastes have greater heat capacity or lower heat conductivity than others. Some are wet and some are dry, some are acid and some are alkaline. This makes it difficult to know how to operate the sterilizer. It is best to try to standardize the load if that is possible. This may take planning and cooperation within the hospital. It may also require storage space, preferably refrigerated space, where different materials may be held prior to loading with a standard load. Another problem is that the waste is containerized, which is not the case in laboratory sterilization. The container may be sealed, as in the case of bottles of liquids that would spill if left open in the waste bin, or the red bags that would leak while being transferred through the hospital if not tied closed. Air is then entrapped within the container and steam is impeded from penetrating the containers; thus the contents, in effect, undergo dry heat sterilization rather than steam sterilization, requiring greatly increased time or higher temperature. Raising the temperature and doubling or tripling the usual time required for sterilization may overcome this problem. One manufacturer advises using 132°C (270°F), 28 to 30 psi steam pressure, for waste rather than 121°C (250°F), which is the temperature and pressure (15 psi) normally used in laboratory sterilizers (Cooney, 1988). One method for contending with the problem is to add water to the contents of the containers so that steam is produced inside the container as it is heated by the steam. Another is to open the container prior to sterilization or to puncture the plastic container bags so as to allow steam to penetrate and displace the air inside. This method was practiced by Rutala and colleagues (1982) in their experiments with laboratory microbiologic wastes. They employed 15-lb batches of contaminated petri plates infected with different bacteria, which they put into open or punctured polyethylene autoclave bags; these, in turn, were placed in steel or rigid polypropylene containers for autoclaving at 121°C. In the stainless steel container the bacteria were destroyed in 45 minutes whether or not 0.5 L of water was added to the plastic bags before autoclaving, but with the polypropylene containers bacterial destruction occurred only when water was added. In the absence of the added water sterilization required 60 minutes. With the steel container it took 90 minutes to destroy the spores of the biologic indicator, *Bacillus stearothermophilus*.

Table 42–6, which shows the work of Lauer and associates (1982) with autoclaved laboratory waste, indicates the problems in heat transfer with containers and moisture, such as found by Rutala et al. They showed that slower heat transfer occurred with polypropylene than with stainless steel and that further retardation was caused by the internal plastic bag, which they did not open. The beneficial effect of adding water to improve heat conduction and generate steam in the waste was also demonstrated. Water has a thermal conductivity 20 to 30 times greater than that of air, and for steel it is 100 to 500 times greater than for polypropylene. Many materials in wastes such as plastics, cloth, paper, and animal bedding are very poor thermal conductors, and heat transmission is therefore improved by adding water.

Table 42–5. *Temperature and Time* for Sterilization with Steam and Hot Air*

Steam			Hot Air		
°F	°C	Time (min.)	°F	°C	Time (min.)
240	116	30	250	121	Overnight
245	118	18	284	140	180
250	121	12	302	150	150
257	125	8	320	160	120
270	132	2	340	171	60

*Time counted only at maximum temperature, not when heating-up or cooling-down.

From Perkins, J.J., 1957. Bacteriological and surgical sterilization by heat. *Antiseptics, Disinfectants, Fungicides, and Chemical and Physical Sterilization.* Edited by G.F. Reddish. Philadelphia, Lea & Febiger.

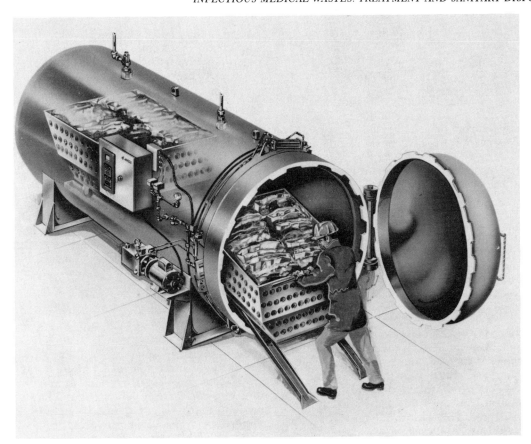

Fig. 42–3. Large steam sterilizer for biomedical wastes. (Courtesy of AMSCO.)

Air trapped inside the autoclave lowers the temperature because the air pressure prevents steam from filling the autoclave. This problem is handled with autoclaves either by displacing the air with steam by withdrawing the heavier air by gravity displacement, or by first drawing a vacuum on the autoclave chamber and contents prior to introduction of the steam. Even so, the nature of the items in the load may make it difficult to displace all the air, thus making certain parts of the autoclaved load cooler than other parts and keeping them from receiving the required heating for sterilization. To monitor this occurrence, various devices are employed. Thermocouples may be placed in various parts of the waste load to determine the temperature profile. Chemical and biologic indicators are also placed within the waste to determine whether the sterilization process is complete and effective. Chemical indicators give quick results but biologic indicators, which require days of incubation, are preferable because they take account of factors other than temperature. Improper sterilization may result from various factors. These include (1) overloading the unit (the larger the load, the longer it takes to heat), (2) poor-quality steam, (3) defective equipment, (4) improper load arrangement, (5) waste carriers that do not allow steam to circulate around and within the load, and (6) improper attention of the operators. Proper engineering supervision, operating standards, operator training, regular recordkeeping, and concerned hospital policy are all necessary to cope with these problems.

Table 42–6. *The Effect of Container and Added Water on the Temperature of Laboratory Waste in Steam Autoclave*

Container	Water Added?	Internal Plastic Bag	Temperature (°C) Reached (Minutes)		
			12	30	50
Steel	Yes	No	108	120	122
Steel	No	No	60	110	120
Steel	Yes	Yes	36	71	105
Polypropylene	Yes	No	—	—	108
Polypropylene	No	No	—	—	108
Polypropylene	Yes	Yes	—	—	99
Polypropylene	No	Yes	—	—	92

From Lauer, J.L., Battles, D.R., and Vesley, D. 1982. Decontaminating infectious laboratory waste by autoclaving. Appl. Environ. Microbiol., *44*, 690–694.

Special high-risk, infectious, biomedical wastes must be carefully sterilized under the supervision of a biosafety officer using sterilization monitoring and biohazard labeling. After sterilization, these wastes should be disposed of by incineration. Steam sterilization, although effective and low in cost, has limitations. It is not suitable for all biomedical wastes, such as chemotherapy wastes, which it may not destroy, or volatile chemical wastes, which would be vaporized and disseminated by the heat of the autoclave. It is not suitable for large quantities of body fluids and other liquids, which take too long to heat up. The same is true of carcasses of large animals, which heat up only slowly. Finally, autoclaving does not reduce the volume of the waste or change the external appearance of the items that are sterilized, as occurs in other treatments such as incineration, and the public is not prone to accept medical wastes as safe when they still look the same. In some hospitals the volume of the steam-sterilized waste is reduced by compression with the use of a waste compactor.

Mechanical-Disinfection Treatment (Hydro-Pulping)

The newest of the treatment systems and one of the three mentioned by Doucet (1988) is the shredding-milling and disinfectant system (Figs. 42–4 and 42–5) developed by Medical SafeTEC of Cincinnati. Also known as the mechanical-chemical system, this new system, according to Doucet, has demonstrated its utility for processing large quantities of wastes. He describes the process as follows: This system uses a two-stage shredding process, where the waste is first shredded, then reduced in a hammermill into small pieces. During the shredding process, sodium hypochlorite, bleach solution, is fed into the material. This provides contact with the free chlorine, which disinfects small pieces of waste material. The grinding operation certainly changes the appearance and the shape of the material, rendering it more suitable for off-site disposal in a general-waste landfill because it is unrecognizable as medical waste. The system comprises a conveyor system with two stages of shredding, a high-torque shredder, and a high-speed hammermill. The waste is sprayed with the chlorine solution during the shredding process and the entire system is kept under negative pressure. The air is drawn through a type of filtration system. At the discharge you can see the wet granulated material coming out on a conveyor belt. Nothing in the processed waste is recognizable. The conveyor belt is perforated for the residual liquids to drain underneath and be separated. Wastes are then collected in a cart.

The drained liquids are run into the sanitary sewer and the solid wastes from the cart are disposed of as noninfectious wastes in an ordinary landfill. As a result of the mechanical reduction and drainage of liquids the waste loses as much as 85% of its volume. This compares to up to 95% volume loss when waste is incinerated, and 30% volume reduction by autoclaving. Volume reduction is important when considering that the cost of tipping at most landfills is based on the volume of the waste, and that volume also increases the cost of transportation to the landfill. In the hammermilling operation glass bottles and tubes are reduced to sand and hypodermic needles

are cut up into small blunted pieces, which do not present a puncture hazard. The unit operates under reduced pressure with high-efficiency particulate air (HEPA) filtered air to prevent aerosols escaping into the room air, and automatic controls turn off the machine if this safety system fails. The machine is available in a hospital-sized unit that can handle 700 to 1500 pounds of waste per hour, and laboratory-sized units that will take 100 to 400 pounds per hour. Unlike the incinerator and steam sterilizer, this system has no difficulty with large volumes of water, but it will not handle large body parts. It does not produce air pollution but care must be taken with the quality of water it discharges to the sewer. The cost of a hospital-sized unit is about half that of an equal-sized incinerator, but more than an autoclave processing the same amount of waste. Reinhardt and Gordon (1991) have prepared a useful table comparing the three systems—steam sterilization, incineration, and the hammermill-disinfectant treatment. This is reproduced in Table 42–7.

Byer and Pickering (1989) reported on their experience with the hammermill-disinfection system in a large hospital in New Jersey. They listed 12 advantages of this system over their former system of autoclaving the waste. Among these are cost savings; 10:1 compaction of wastes; destruction of sharps; freedom from public relations problems due to waste appearance or effluent; and meeting EPA standards in producing a material that does not require special handling or tracking. Eitzen and French (1985) give eight advantages. Among these are low cost of operation; using only 100 KWH per ton of waste; elimination of need to store waste; use of any type of nonmetal waste collection container; and the fact that it is odorless and acceptable in regard to the noise level for hospital installation.

The microbiologic effectiveness of the hammermill-chemical treatment has been examined by Eitzen and French (1984), Denys (1989), and Denys (in press). Their findings showed that (1) with 0.15% free available chlorine as sodium hypochlorite, vegetative bacteria were quickly destroyed and never found in samples taken after 5 minutes following start of the process; (2) with 0.2%, spore formers were largely destroyed within 2 hours, and only low levels were detected; (3) indicator bacteria added to the waste prior to milling could not be detected in the room atmosphere, showing no microbial aerosol hazard to the system operator from operation of the equipment.

A variation of this mechanical-disinfection treatment has recently been developed in Germany, which employs heat by microwave instead of a chemical to produce disinfection. This is the Vetco Sanitec system offered in the United States by ABB Sanitec. It employs a shredder to granulate the waste and an auger to compact it. Then it is sprayed with water, which is heated to 203°F with the microwave generator to achieve disinfection. It is manufactured as a large unit that will handle 550 pounds per hour and a smaller one that will handle 220 pounds per hour. Both of these units are available for fixed or mobile operation. According to Cusak and Leinski (1988), a prototype had been in successful operation in

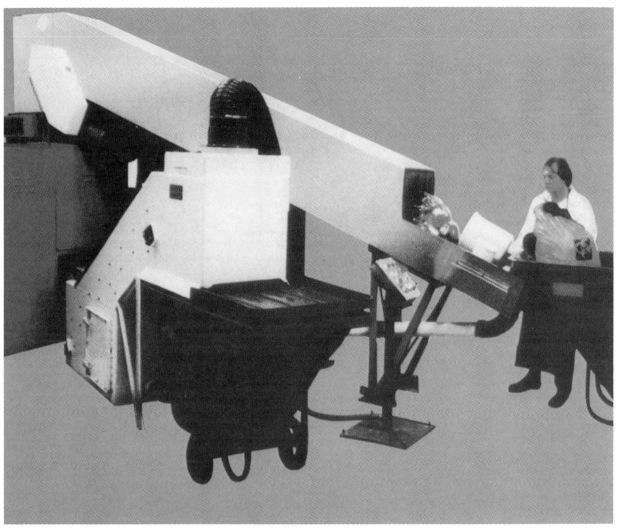

Fig. 42–4. Shredding-milling disinfectant system for infectious hospital wastes. (Courtesy of Medical SafeTEC.)

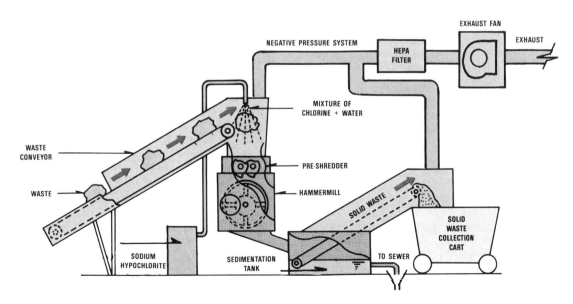

Fig. 42–5. Process diagram for the shredding-milling disinfectant system. (Courtesy of Medical SafeTEC.)

Table 42–7. *Comparison of Treatment Technologies*

	Type of Treatment Technology		
Factor	Steam Sterilization	Incineration	Hammermill/ Chemical Treatment
Operations			
Applicability	Most infectious wastes	Almost all infectious wastes	Most infectious wastes
Equipment operation	Easy	Complex	Moderately complex
Operator requirements	Trained	Highly skilled	Well trained
Need for waste separation	To eliminate nontreatable wastes	None	To eliminate nontreatables; for proper feeding
Need for load standardization	Yes	No	When feeding by type of waste
Effect of treatment	Appearance of waste unchanged	Waste burned	Waste shredded and ground
Volume reduction	30%	85–95%	Up to 85%
Occupational hazards	Low	Moderate	Moderate
Testing	Easy, inexpensive	Complex, expensive	Procotol under development
Potential side benefits	None	Energy recovery	Use of effluent in laundry
Onsite/offsite location	Both	Both	Both
Regulatory Requirements			
Medical waste tracking regulations	Applicable	Recordkeeping	Not applicable
Applicable environmental regulations	Wastewater	Air emissions, ash disposal, wastewater	Wastewater
Releases to air	Low risk via vent	High risk via emissions	Low risk via vent
Releases to water	Low risk via drain	Low risk via scrubber water	Moderate risk via wastewater
Disposal of residue	To sanitary landfill; potential problem with *red* bags	Ash may be a hazardous waste; if so, to RCRA-permitted landfill	Effluent to sanitary sewer, residue to sanitary landfill
Permitting requirements	None	For siting, air emissions	None
Costs			
Capital costs	Low	High	Moderate
Labor costs	Low	High	Moderate
Operating costs	Low	High	Moderate
Maintenance costs	Low	High	Moderate
Downtime	Low	High	Moderate to high

From Reinhardt, P.A., and Gordon, J.G. 1991. Treatment considerations and options. In *Infectious and Medical Waste Management.* Boca Raton, FL, Lewis Publishing, Inc., pp. 67–68.

Germany for 2 years, and several other units were being assembled in Germany and Holland.

SANITARY LANDFILL

Land disposal of waste is the time-honored method, recorded in the Bible: "Designate a place outside the camp where you can go to relieve yourself. As part of your equipment have something to dig with, and when you relieve yourself, dig a hole and cover up your excrement" (Deuteronomy 23:12–14). As of 1971, Iglar and Bond, reporting on waste disposal by 80 hospitals, noted that 73 of the 80 employed landfills. Of the 73, only 24 used sanitary landfills. Since that time uncontrolled dumping has been outlawed and sanitary landfill, while cheaper than other methods, has become more costly and harder to find. Furthermore, many sanitary landfills will not accept infectious waste, and those that do accept it require it to be sterilized first. Even when it is sterilized, it is still recognizable and landfill workers may

object to it. Landfill is off-site disposal, which requires manifests and packaging of the waste for highway transport, direct or via transfer stations to the landfill site. As in all highway transport, the community like the landfill workers may be concerned about exposure to hospital wastes even if they are sterilized. There is the option of contract disposal, where the hauler takes the waste to a landfill or incinerator. This removes the responsibility and burden from the hospital but it may cost from 30 cents to over a dollar a pound for that service.

Although there is ample evidence of pathogenic bacteria in the landfill, these pathogens are derived mainly from household wastes (which contain such things as diapers), which make up the major waste in the landfill. In any case, there is no evidence of a link between microorganisms in the landfill and human disease, such as exists between contaminated water and disease. One could question, therefore, whether untreated hospital waste would be a potential health hazard in the landfill. If the landfill is properly operated in an aerobic manner, the peak landfill temperature of 148°F (60°C) is sufficient for the inactivation of organisms. Kaplan and Melnick (1952) showed that poliovirus and Theiler's virus were rendered noninfective after heating to 131°F (55°C) for 30 minutes, and Gotaas (1956) showed that all bacterial pathogens (possibly excepting the tubercle bacillus) would be killed at 140°F (60°C) for 1 hour.

The potential for landfill workers to contact disease through exposure to fresh waste would seem to be great but their injuries tend to be sprains, cuts, and bruises rather than infectious diseases. A legitimate concern, however, is the presence of pathogens in landfill leachate. Studies by Cook et al. (1967) indicate that the leachate may contain various species of such entities as bacilli, brevibacteria, pseudomonas, clostridia, and humicola. The EPA (1973) found fecal streptococci in the upper part of the landfill but no bacterial or viral pathogens in the leachate. Zanoni (1972), in reviewing the literature on groundwater pollution by sanitary landfills, found few cases of serious or even troublesome contamination of groundwater directly attributable to sanitary landfills. With more-modern controls on landfills and leachates in recent years, this problem should be well under control.

Landfills are the final resting place for incinerator ash. If it contains toxic products it should be diverted to a special hazardous waste landfill. Sharps that have not been incinerated could cause puncture wounds, cuts, and scratches and should be treated by grinding them, imbedding them in plastic, or otherwise converting them to render them harmless. Pathologic wastes include body parts, which would cause aesthetic repulsion; these should be rendered unrecognizable by incineration or grinding prior to disposal in a landfill.

DISPOSAL TO SEWER

Infectious liquid wastes have been approved for disposal to the sewer by the CDC, and the grinding and flushing of solid waste out-of-sight by this available, handy mechanism has been most appealing. Wet grinding and drain removal of food wastes with the sink Dispos-All has suggested that this method could be adapted to hospital wastes as well.

Wet grinding is a means of reducing the waste for discharging it to the municipal sewage system. It has been frequently used for food wastes but is also being considered a means of handling the total waste (Anon., 1970; Weintraub and Kern, 1969; DeRoos, 1974). The Health Facilities Service Division, County of Los Angeles Health Department, was awarded a grant from the U.S. Public Health Service to study the use of grinders in hospitals, and test systems were installed at Children's Hospital of Los Angeles, a 330-bed pediatrics facility, and at Memorial Hospital in Panorama City, a 96-bed general hospital. The unit was a fixed-impeller type of grinder with a rotating 8-inch flywheel and stationary cutter blocks. Stainless steel knives were mounted below the cutter blocks to ensure an adequate fineness of grind, particularly when fibrous materials pass through the grinder.

The most serious problem encountered was the inability to grind soft materials such as tubing, rubber gloves, and the rubber plungers within syringes. Hard plastic, nylon, needles, and other solid objects were ground easily. Blockage of the traps serving the grinder was a problem, but once the materials passed into the hospital sewer, they traveled into the street sewer with no noticeable difficulty. Waste line blockage could be eliminated by using larger lines and an improved larger grinder. Other plumbing problems were blockage of the flywheel when solid objects such as surgical tools were dropped into the system, blockage of sump pumps used for elevating sewage from below ground, frequent maintenance chores because of dulling of the shear ring and cutter blocks, breaking of cutter knives, vibration, and noise from solenoid valves.

The major concern of municipal agencies is the effect of the ground waste on the sewage treatment facility. Tests in the municipal sewage transportation system for chloride, BOD, COD, and settleable solids revealed no significant changes in the sewage as a result of solid waste grinding. Consideration of the possibilities of disposal of ground plastics to the sewers on a citywide basis led to an estimate of a maximum of 500 lb/day of disposable plastics from medical and dental facilities. The total waste was anticipated to be about 50% plastic and 50% paper, with about 20 to 50% floatable. The bulk of ground plastic and related materials sent to a treatment plant should settle out as grit or should be removed during primary treatment. The other components of the waste should have little effect on the public health characteristics of the sewage since the city permits the disposal of garbage, blood clots, placentas, small vertebrate animals, and sterilized cultures from bioscience laboratories via grinders.

An air sampling program was conducted to determine if aerosol formation during grinding presented a hazard. The particle count in the room during grinding of the material was about the same as when the grinder was on but no material was being ground. No increase in aerosol concentration was observed during grinding of normally soiled syringes, and tracer organisms placed in the syringes were found in the air in only small concentrations.

Weintraub and Kern (1969, 1971) conclude that, given adequate facilities (including sufficient available water sources, adequately sized sewer connections, sufficient electrical power, and a large grinding unit), the disposal of hospital wastes into a sanitary sewer is feasible and desirable from the point of view of eliminating handling, storage, transportation, air pollution, and other problems of handling solid waste.

Objections to this method of treating waste include the difficulty in grinding all materials and the possibility of creating hazardous aerosols. Also, the form of the pathogenic wastes is changed, but the pathogens themselves are not affected. Thus, hazardous materials are introduced into city pipes, the volume of municipal effluents is increased (present systems have a limited capacity), and the costs of municipal sewage treatment are increased (Litsky et al., 1972).

For all its appeal this method for treating solid wastes has not caught on. Problems of piping and plugging in moving the solids through the sewage system, and re-

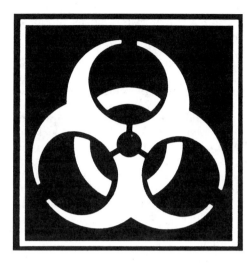

Fig. 42–6. The universal biohazard symbol, which warns of the presence of infectious materials.

luctance on the part of local sewage authorities to take on extra loads, including nondigestible solids, at a time when they have been unable to keep up with normal growth, has no doubt retarded development in this area. Another problem is that in times of heavy rain some sewers overflow into streams and rivers. Thus untreated, pathogen-laden sewage makes its way into bodies of water that may be used to supply water for drinking.

HANDLING, TRANSPORT AND STORAGE

The EPA (1986) has prescribed that closed bags of infectious waste should be placed in tied plastic bags, colored red for identification. Sharps and liquids should be put in suitable puncture-proof and leak-proof boxes or other containers with secured lids. These should be transported through the hospital or medical facility in wheeled, and preferably covered, carts. Chutes or dumbwaiters should not be used. Care must be taken not to tear open the bags during handling and transport. For off-site disposal, the bags should be packed in rigid containers such as wooden boxes or heavy cartons. If used again, the carts and boxes should be disinfected and not used for any other purpose. Dumpsters and trucks containing this waste should be kept closed and should be leak-proof. The univeral biohazard symbol (Fig. 42–6) should be displayed on all containers of infectious waste. If the waste is to be stored, assurance of its integrity must be maintained. Rodents and vermin must be eliminated or excluded by suitable packaging. The storage rooms should be properly designed for easy access and handling with mechanical devices. Temperature control with refrigeration should be provided to prevent putrefaction and odor. Wastes may be stored for one day at 64 to 77°F or 3 days at 34 to 45°F. Mixed wastes, that is, wastes containing hazardous chemicals as well as infectious wastes, should be separated and directed to a special landfill or incinerator that handles hazardous materials.

EMERGENCY PLANNING

In handling, transport, and storage there is always a chance for spillage to occur. Harvey W. Rogers of the National Institutes of Health (1988) gives some steps to be taken in such an event:

As more and more infectious waste is transported off-site for treatment or disposal, the likelihood for accidental spillage of the waste increases. Haulers of infectious waste must be prepared to take appropriate action in the event of a vehicular accident that results in a release of this cargo. There are several steps to take in such an event:

1. In the event of a major spill of material an appropriate emergency response agency (police, fire department or hazmat) should be notified.
2. Clean-up personnel should wear appropriate protective clothing such as boots, disposable coveralls and gloves.
3. To the maximum extent possible, clean-up personnel should use shovels, forks, tongs or other implements to retrieve and recontain spilled material.
4. The spill area should be decontaminated with the appropriate disinfecting solution. Hypochlorite solution works well for this purpose. A double application is sometimes recommended.
5. Cleanup gear appropriately should be decontaminated or discarded as infectious waste.
6. Incident reports should be completed as required.

The above steps would apply to most infectious waste spills and therefore should be a part of a spill plan. All haulers should be familiar with the details of how to carry out the above steps in an actual emergency.

Periodic drills should be staged to assure familiarity with the plan. Also, all actual spill episodes should be reviewed to see if the detailed response plan needs to be modified or refined.

SUPPLEMENT

After this chapter was in print, the U.S. Public Health Service made a report to Congress as required under The Medical Waste Tracking Act of 1988. This report is entitled The Public Health Implications of Medical Waste. A summary of this report with references is given here as a supplement to this chapter.

The Medical Waste Tracking Act of 1988 requires the administrator of the Agency for Toxic Substances and Disease Registry (ATSDR) to prepare a report on the health effects of medical waste. To comply with the act, ATSDR obtained data from professional associations, unions, and environmental, academic, and industrial groups.[1] The information and comments were collected during an extensive review process that involved an internal ATSDR panel; a federal advisory panel comprising representatives from Public Health Service (PHS) agencies, the Environmental Protection Agency, and the Health Care Financing Administration; an external peer review panel; public comments; and review by PHS and the Department of Health and Human Services. The findings were presented to Congress in *The Public Health Implications of Medical Waste: A Report to Congress.*[2] This report summarizes the conclusions and recommendations in the ATSDR report.

The report presented estimates of the number of persons injured by sharps in medical waste, the number

Estimated annual range of injuries, theoretical estimated annual number of hepatitis B virus (HBV) and HIV infections, and theoretical estimate of annual number of hepatitis B (HB) and AIDS cases in nonhospital and hospital employees as a result of medical waste-related injuries from sharps—United States, 1990

Employee group	Sharps injury range	HBV infections	HB cases	HIV infections	AIDS cases
Nonhospital					
Physicians	500–1,700	1–3	<1–2	<1	<1
Registered nurses	17,800–32,500	36–65	18–33	<1	<1
Licensed practical nurses	10,200–15,400	20–31	10–15	<1	<1
Emergency medical personnel	12,000	24	12	<1	<1
Dentists	100–300	<1	<1	<1	<1
Dental assistants	2,600–3,900	5–8	3–4	<1	<1
Refuse workers	500–7,300	1–15	<1–7	<1	<1
Hospital					
Physicians/Dentists/Interns	100–400	<1	<1	<1	<1
Registered nurses	9,800–17,900	20–36	10–18	<1–1	<1–1
Licensed practical nurses	2,800–4,300	6–9	3–4	<1	<1
Laboratory workers	800–7,500	2–15	1–8	<1	<1
Janitorial/Laundry workers	11,700–45,300	23–91	12–45	<1–3	<1–3
Hospital engineers	12,200	24	12	<1	<1

who may become infected with hepatitis B virus (HBV) and human immunodeficiency virus (HIV) as the result of medical waste-related sharp injuries, and the number who may develop hepatitis B and acquired immunodeficiency syndrome (AIDS) as the result of those injuries. (The number of other infections or infectious diseases related to medical waste could not be estimated because relevant data were not available.) These estimates are upper-limit theoretical estimates because the probability of infection is based on case studies of persons who came in contact with freshly drawn blood or other body fluids—an event more likely to occur during patient care than during medical-waste handling. In addition, some persons may be immune to HBV infection because of prior exposure or immunization.[3] The estimates did not take into account the rapid decline of viable HIV outside a living host. Because data were not available to determine how many janitorial and laundry workers, laboratory workers, and building engineers are employed at nonhospital facilities that generate medical waste, estimates could not be derived for these workers in these settings.

Based on available estimates, a maximum of <1-4 AIDS cases per year (<0.003%–0.01% of 33,173 AIDS cases in the United States reported to CDC in 1989)[4] occur in health-care workers as a result of contact with medical waste sharps (Table above). An estimated 80 to 160 hepatitis B cases per year may occur as a result of contact with medical waste sharps (0.05%–0.1% of 150,000 hepatitis B cases annually in the United States).[5]

Other findings included:
- Persons without occupational exposure are not likely to be adversely affected by medical waste generated in the traditional health-care setting.
- Outside the health-care setting, the potential for HBV or HIV infection in the general population following medical waste-related injuries is not likely to be a public health concern; however, needlestick injuries may cause local or systemic secondary infections.

- Increased in-home health care and other sources of nonregulated medical waste increase the likelihood that the general public may come in contact with medical waste.
- The estimated numbers of medical waste-related HIV and HBV infections and cases are of public health concern for selected occupations involved with medical waste (e.g., janitorial and laundry workers, nurses, emergency medical personnel, and refuse workers).
- The approximately 1.2 million U.S. intravenous-drug users (IVDUs)[6]—who have high rates of HIV and HBV infection—are a major source of discarded sharps. Although the general public may be at risk for injury and infection following contact with these discarded sharps, the potential risk for HIV and HBV infection from IVDU-related waste cannot be estimated.
- The potential for infection resulting from contact with nonsharp medical waste is likely to be substantially less than that related to contact with medical waste sharps, since a portal of entry must exist before contact with nonsharp medical waste for infection or disease to occur.
- Medical waste can be effectively treated by chemical, physical, or biological means (e.g., chemical decontamination, autoclaving, incineration, irradiation, and sanitary sewage treatment). Medical waste does not contain any greater quantity or different type of microbiologic agents than residential waste. In addition, properly operated sanitary landfills provide microbiologic environments hostile to most pathogenic agents. Therefore, untreated medical waste can be disposed of in sanitary landfills if procedures to prevent worker contact with this waste during handling and disposal operations are strictly followed.

References

1. Rodenbeck, S.E., and Lichtveld, M.Y. 1990. Report to Congress: the public health implication of medical waste. J Environ Health, 53:30–13.

2. ATSDR. The public health implications of medical waste: a report to Congress. Atlanta: US Department of Health and Human Services. Public Health Service, Agency for Toxic Substances and Disease Registry, Sept., 1990; document no. PB91-100271.
3. CDC. 1989. Racial differences in rates of hepatitis B virus infection—United States. 1976–1980. MMWR, 38:818–821.
4. CDC. 1990. HIV/AIDS surveillance report: year-end edition. Atlanta: US Department of Health and Human Services, Public Health Service, Jan.
5. CDC. 1989. Hepatitis surveillance report no. 52. Atlanta: US Department of Health and Human Services, Public Health Service.
6. Public Health Service. 1988. Report of the workgroup on intravenous drug abuse. Public Health Rep, 103(suppl 1):66–71.

REFERENCES

Allen, R.J., Brenniman, G.R., Logue, R.R., and Strand, V.A. 1989. Emission of airborne bacteria from a hospital incinerator. JAPCA, 39, 164–168.

Anonymous. 1969. Disposables are dangerous. Pa. Med., 71, 49.

Barbeito, M.S., and Gremillion, G.G. 1968. Microbiological safety evaluation of an industrial incinerator. Appl. Microbiol., 16, 291–295.

Barbeito, M.S., and Shapiro, M. 1977. Microbiological safety evaluation of a solid and liquid pathological incinerator. J. Med. Primatol., 6, 264–273.

Barbeito, M.S., Taylor, L.A., and Seiders, R.W. 1968. Microbiological evaluation of a large-volume air incinerator. Appl. Microbiol., 16, 490–495.

Block, S.S. 1974. Final Report EPA research grant 800189–02. Cincinnati, OH.

Bond, W.W. 1988. Universal precautions—impact on infectious waste categorization. Conference on Management of Medical and Infectious Waste—Practical Considerations. Washington, D.C., NIH, pp. 45–46.

Brunner, C.R., and Brown, C.H. 1988. Hospital waste disposal by incineration. JAPCA, 38, 1297–1308.

Burchinal, J.C., and Wallace, L.P. 1971. A study of institutional solid wastes. Department of Civil Engineering, West Virginia University, Morgantown.

Byer, H.G., Jr., and Pickering, J.E. 1989. A case study: A cost-effective approach to hospital infectious waste management. Conference on the Regulation and Management of Medical and Infectious Waste—II. Washington, D.C., Nov. 27–29, pp. 47–53.

City of New York, Dept. of Sanitation. 1989. Report on needle-puncture injuries. Through A. Lynn Harding, Conference on the Regulations and Management of Medical and Infectious Waste—II. Washington, D.C., Nov. 27–29, pp. 7–9.

Cook, H.A., Cromwell, L., and Wilson, H.A. 1967. Microorganisms in household refuse and seepage water from sanitary landfills. Proc. W. Va. Acad. Sci., 39, 107.

Cooney, T.E. 1988. Techniques for steam sterilizing laboratory waste. AMSCO Waste Processing Technical Report.

Cusak, J.L., and Leinski, H. 1988. Innovative new technology for disinfection of infectious wastes. 2nd Natl. Symp. Infectious Waste Management. San Francisco, Sept. 19–20; Boston, Oct. 3–4.

Danielson, J.A., ed. 1973. *Air Pollution Engineering Manual.* Research Triangle Park, Environmental Protection Agency, Office of Air Quality Planning and Standards, pp. 484–496.

Denys, G.A. 1989. Microbiological evaluation of the Medical SafeTEC mechanical/chemical infectious waste disposal system. 89 Ann. Mtg. A.S.M., New Orleans, LA, May 16.

Denys, G.A. In Press. Microbiological evaluation of the Medical SafeTEC Z-12,500 disposal system for chemical disinfection and grinding of infectious wastes. Appl. Environ. Microbiol., in press.

DeRoos, R.L. 1974. Environmental concerns in hospital waste disposal. Part II. Hospitals, 48, 120–123.

Doucet, L. 1988. A comparison of infectious waste treatment options. Conference on Management of Medical and Infectious Waste—Practical Considerations. Washington, D.C., pp. 51–53.

Eitzen, H.E., and French, M.L.V. 1984. Report on the microbiologic effectiveness of the Medical SafeTEC waste management system. Dept. Hospital Infection Control, Indiana University, April 3.

Eitzen, H.E., and French, M.L.V. 1985. Disposal of hospital waste. J. Hosp. Supply, Processing, and Distribution, July–Aug., pp. 64–65.

Environmental Protection Agency. 1970. Pathogens associated with solid waste processing. EPA Pub. No. EPA-SW-49r.

Environmental Protection Agency. 1973. Interim report 1, test cell 1, Boone County field site. Disposal Technology Branch, Solid Waste Research Laboratory, Cincinnati, OH.

Environmental Protection Agency. 1982. Draft manual for infectious waste management. SW-957. Washington, D.C., September.

Environmental Protection Agency. 1986. EPA guide for infectious waste management. U.S. EPA Office of Solid Waste and Emergency Response. NTIS PB86-199130, May.

Federal Register. U.S. Congress. 1989. March 24, p. 12325.

Garner, J.S., and Favero, M.S. 1985. Guideline for handwashing and environmental control—infectious waste. U.S. Dept. Health and Human Services, P.H.S., CDC, Atlanta, 99–117.

Goode, L.D. 1989. Flowing by the waste-side: The emerging national policy on medical waste. Acad. Med., 64, 514–515.

Gotaas, H.B. 1956. Composting-sanitary disposal and reclamation of organic wastes. WHO monograph Ser. No. 31.

Iglar, A.F., and Bond, R.G. 1971. Waste handling. Hospital solid waste disposal in community facilities. School of Public Health, University of Minnesota, Minneapolis.

Jager, E., Xander, L., and Ruden, H. 1989. Microbiological studies of wastes of various specialties at a large and small hospital in comparison to housekeeping waste. Zentralbl. Hyg. Umweltmed., 188, 343–364.

Jagger, J., Hunt, E.H., Brand-Elnaggar, B.A., and Pearson, R.D. 1988. Rates of needle-stick injury caused by various devices in a university hospital. N. Engl. J. Med., 319, 284–288.

Joint Commission of Accreditation of Healthcare Organizations (JCAHO). 1987. AMH/88: Accreditation manual for hospitals.

Kalnowski, G., Wiegand, H., and Ruden, H. 1983. Microbial contamination of hospital waste. Zentralbl. Bakteriol. Microbiol. Hyg., 178, 364–379.

Kaplan, A.S., and Melnick, J.L. 1952. Effect of milk and cream on the thermal inactivation of human poliomyelitis virus. Am. J. Public Health, 42, 525.

Keene, J.H. 1988. Hepatitis and AIDS—The risk of transmission from refuse. Conference on Management of Medical and Infectious Waste—Practical Considerations. Washington, D.C., pp. 19–21.

Kransinski, K., LaCouture, R., and Holzman, R. 1987. Effect of changing needle disposal systems on needle puncture injuries. Infect. Control, 8, 59–62.

Lauer, J.L., Battles, D.R., and Vesley, D. 1982. Decontaminating infectious laboratory waste by autoclaving. Appl. Environ. Microbiol., 44, 690–694.

Liberman, D.F. 1988. Occupational infections among waste handlers, transporters, and disposal facility operators. Conference on Management of Medical and Infectious Waste—Practical Considerations. Washington, D.C., pp. 27–31.

Litsky, W., Martin, J.W., and Litsky, B.Y. 1972. Solid waste: A hospital dilemma. Am. J. Nurs., 72, 10, 1841–1847.

Marrack, D. 1988. Hospital red bag waste. JAPCA, 38, 1309–1312.

McClymont, I.C., and Urbanski, R.J. 1987. Hydrogen chloride emissions from hospital waste incinerators. APCA Specialty Conference on Thermal Treatment of Municipal, Industrial, and Hospital Wastes. Pittsburgh, PA, November.

Medical Waste Tracking Act. 1988. Congress of the U.S. House of Representatives 351, Senate 2680.

Mose, J.R., and Reinthaler, F. 1985. Microbial contamination of hospital waste and household refuse. Zentralbl. Bakteriol. Mikrobiol. Hyg. (B), 181, 98–110.

Occupational Safety and Health Administration, U.S. Department of Labor. 1989. Occupational exposure to bloodborne pathogens; proposed rule and notice of hearing. Fed. Register, 54, 23,042–23,139, May 30.

Office of Technology Assessment. 1988. Testimony of Dr. Kathryn D. Wagner. Washington, D.C., Aug. 9.

Ontario Ministry of the Environment. 1986. Incinerator design and operating criteria. Vol. 2, Biomedical waste incinerators, October.

Perkins, J.J. 1957. Bacteriological and surgical sterilization by heat. In *Antiseptics, Disinfectants, Fungicides, and Chemical and Physical Sterilization.* Edited by G.F. Reddish. Philadelphia, Lea & Febiger.

Peterson, M.L., and Stutzenberger, F.J. 1969. Microbiological evaluation of incinerator operations. Appl. Microbiol., 18, 8–13.

Reinhardt, P.A., and Gordon, J.G. 1991. *Infectious and Medical Waste Management.* Chelsea, MI, Lewis Publishers, pp. 67–68.

Resource Conservation and Recovery Act. 1976. Congress of the U.S. Public Law 94-580, Oct. 21.

Richardson, J.H. 1989. Hepatitis B virus as an indicator of occupational infection risk in handlers and transporters of biomedical waste. Through A. Lynn Harding, Conference on the Regulation and Management of Medical and Infectious Waste—II. Washington, D.C., pp. 7–9.

Rogers, H.W. 1988. Infectious waste transport. Conference on Management of Medical and Infectious Waste—Practical Considerations. Washington, D.C., pp. 47–49.

Rutala, W.A. 1989. Management of infectious waste by U.S. hospitals. JAMA, 262, 1635–1640.

Rutala, W.A., Stiegel, M.M., and Sarubbi, F.A., Jr. 1982. Decontamination of laboratory microbiological waste by steam sterilization. Appl. Environ. Microbiol., 43, 1311–1316.

Smith, R.J. 1970. Bacteriological examination of institutional solid wastes. M.S. Thesis, West Virginia University, Morgantown.

Torchia, M. 1988. Hospitals and the medical waste disposal crisis. Conference on Management of Medical and Infectious Waste—Practical Considerations. Dec. 1,2, Washington, D.C., pp. 9–12.

Trigg, J.A. 1971. Microbial examination of hospital solid wastes. M.S. Thesis, West Virginia University, Morgantown.

Trost, M., and Filip, Z. 1985. Microbiological investigations on refuse from medical consulting rooms and municipal refuse. Zentralbl. Bakteriol. Hyg. (B), 181, 159–172.

Wallace, L.P., Zaltman, R., and Burchinal, J.C. 1972. Where solid waste comes from; where it should go. Mod. Hosp., 118, 92–95.

Weintraub, B.S., and Kern, H.D. 1971. Wet grinding units tested for disposal of hospital solid waste. J. Environ. Health, 33, 338.

Weintraub, B.S., and Kern, H.D. 1969. Use of wet grinding units for disposal of hospital solid wastes. Los Angeles Health Department, Los Angeles.

Zanoni, A.E. 1972. Ground-water pollution and sanitary landfills—A critical review. Ground Water, 10, 3.

CHAPTER 43

THE HAZARD OF INFECTIOUS AGENTS IN MICROBIOLOGIC LABORATORIES

R.W. McKinney, W.E. Barkley, and A.G. Wedum*

Control of hazard in the microbiologic laboratory has two objectives: first, to protect the diagnostic procedure or the experiment; and second, to protect the worker.

PROTECTION OF THE WORK

Historically and currently, the primary concern is to ensure sterile media for microbial growth, sterile glassware, instruments, and apparatus, and adequate subsequent decontamination by methods described in other chapters. The increasing use of tissue cultures demands strict adherence to aseptic techniques on the part of the worker and has necessitated reducing the microbial contaminants in such laboratories.

Man is a major contributor of contaminants, which he must control to protect his work. The soles of footwear can harbor more microorganisms per unit area than the floors on which the worker stands (Braymen et al., 1974). Careless work practices can establish and maintain numerous sources of contamination in the laboratory (Herman, 1968). The number of microbe-bearing particles shed from the skin of one person can easily be 200 to 1200 per minute (May and Pomeroy, 1973). Tremendous variations are possible from this source, even without the airborne microorganisms contributed by the ventilation system, supplies or specimen containers unpacked in the laboratory, cleaning and polishing procedures, motorized equipment, dirty clothing, and, worst of all, the practice of bringing animals or their cages into a room where cultures are inoculated or examined. The more detailed description of these sources of contamination, as described by Herman (1968), and the resultant airborne contamination that can be expected in the laboratory should be kept in mind: (1) large animal rooms and cage cleaning rooms—100 to 300 viable organisms per cubic foot of air; (2) small animal rooms and crowded work rooms—20 to 100; (3) large or active laboratories, crowded operating rooms, and patient care areas—4 to 20; and (4) clean rooms, sterile rooms, laminar flow units—0.01 to 4 organisms per cubic foot.

Air in rooms housing laboratory animals must also be controlled to avoid nonspecific deaths or invalidation of experiments caused by spread of indigenous infective agents or spread of experimental disease from cage to cage or room to room (Griesemer and Manning, 1973).

PROTECTION OF THE WORKER

In a well-constructed, well-run laboratory not handling highly infectious agents, conspicuous attention to protection of the worker legitimately may be a secondary matter, for the reason that with most microorganisms, the measures that adequately protect the experiment also protect the diagnostician or experimenter. Fortunately for the practice of microbiology, most microorganisms must be absorbed in large numbers to cause disease in a healthy person, and many human laboratory infections produce symptoms so mild that their true origin is neither suspected nor determined. The exceptions are relatively few, and well known. In establishing the precautions to take, the guidelines published by the Centers for Disease Control and the National Institutes of Health (DHHS, 1988a) serve as a valuable resource. This document describes the practices, procedures, and facility requirements for a broad variety of agents that have been involved in reported occupationally acquired infections. Guidelines for conduct of work involving recombinant DNA molecules are provided by the National Institutes of Health (DHHS, 1986).

Individual agents become less or more important as a cause of laboratory illness with changing trends in research and advances in medical practice. For instance: (1) Typhoid fever in laboratory technicians now is rare because the disease has declined in the general popu-

---

*Deceased

lation, and awareness of the dangers of mouth pipetting has increased; (2) effective vaccines have practically eliminated laboratory-acquired Rocky Mountain spotted fever, tularemia, typhus, Venezuelan encephalitis, and yellow fever; (3) Q fever and psittacosis probably are less often diagnosed as such since the advent of antibiotics, because the common use of antibiotics early in the development of respiratory symptoms and fever prevents a more serious illness.

On the other hand, laboratory-acquired hepatitis continues to be a significant concern despite the availability of a safe and effective vaccine for hepatitis B. Persons handling human blood and body fluids are at particular risk. Concern for the presence of the human immunodeficiency virus (HIV) is warranted when handling human specimens. Although the risk of infection with HIV for laboratory workers is low, the consequences of infection may be fatal. The mechanisms of hepatitis B and HIV infection in the laboratory are essentially the same; exposure through nonintact skin and mucous membranes and by direct inoculation. Recommendations for curbing transmission of hepatitis B and HIV are provided in a series of articles published in the Morbidity and Mortality Weekly Reports (MMWR, 1985b, 1987a, 1988b). Another potential source of serious human illness is the subhuman primate. Laboratory personnel handling Old World monkeys run the risk of acquiring B virus from a bite or contamination of broken skin or mucous membranes by an infected monkey (Hull, 1973; MMWR, 1987b).

ASSESSMENT OF RISK

The first step in selecting work practices to control an infectious agent is assessment of the risk involved. Some of the major guidelines in making this assessment include number and severity of laboratory infections; infectious dose for man; infection from procedure or equipment; infection of cagemate by inoculated animal; excretion of the infectious agent in urine, feces, or saliva, hazards peculiar to the animal species; increased susceptibility by sex or race; and availability of specific therapy or effective vaccine.

Reported Laboratory Infections

The first guideline in determining risk is the number of reported laboratory infections. Pike (1976, 1979) has provided comprehensive summaries and evaluations of 3921 laboratory-acquired infections. Fewer than 20% of all cases were associated with a known accident. Exposure to infectious aerosols was considered to be a plausible but unconfirmed source of infection for the more than 80% of the reported cases in which the infected person had "worked with the agent"—*Brucellosis*, typhoid, tularemia, tuberculosis, hepatitis, and Venezuelan encephalitis are the most commonly met serious bacterial and virus infections. Diarrheas acquired in the laboratory or animal room are common but less likely to be reported. The persons most often infected are the

Table 43–1. *Infective Dose for 25 to 50% of Volunteers*

Disease or Agent	Inoculation Route	Dose*
Scrub typhus	Intradermal	3†
Q fever	Inhalation	10
Tularemia	Inhalation	10
Malaria	Intravenous	10
Syphilis	Intradermal	57
Shigella flexneri	Ingestion	180
Anthrax	Inhalation	$\geq 1,300$
Typhoid fever	Ingestion	10^5
Tularemia	Ingestion	10^8
Cholera	Ingestion	10^8
Escherichia coli	Ingestion	10^8
Shigellosis	Ingestion	10^9

*Dose is in number of organisms.
†Mouse ID_{50} in this one instance.

workers at the bench, then the animal caretakers, then craftsmen serving the laboratories, dishwashers, and clerical personnel, then visitors and, rarely, janitors (Wedum, 1964).

A survey conducted by Skinhoj (1974) showed that personnel in Danish clinical chemistry laboratories had a reported incidence of hepatitis (2.3 cases per year per 1000 employees) seven times higher than that of the general population. Similarly, a survey by Harrington and Shannon (1976) indicated that medical laboratory workers in England had "a five times increased risk of acquiring tuberculosis compared with the general population." Hepatitis and shigellosis were also shown to be continuing occupational risks and, along with tuberculosis, were the three most commonly reported occupationally associated infections in Britain.

Changing trends in laboratory-acquired infections must not be interpreted as altering risk potential. Reports of laboratory-associated typhoid fever (USPHS, 1979a) and Q fever (USPHS, 1979b) indicate that the hazard of infection remains present and emphasize the need to maintain awareness of risk potential and to use good laboratory practices at all times.

Infective Human Dose

The variation in the minimum human infective dose can be tremendous, depending upon the organism, route of administration, and individual susceptibility. Data reported by several investigators, compiled and referenced elsewhere (Wedum et al., 1972), are summarized in Table 43–1.

A rule useful until proved otherwise is that the minimal animal and human infective doses are equal. There is experimental evidence for a significant correspondence among 15 or more human diseases of known cause. For instance, with *Mycobacterium tuberculosis*, 10 infective doses for the guinea pig were equal to one infective dose for man. With poliomyelitis virus TN strain type 2, the alimentary tract of the chimpanzee or cynomolgus monkey proved to be less susceptible to infection than the alimentary tract of man (Table 43–2) (Hellman et al.,

Table 43–2. *Microorganisms Required To Infect*

Tuberculosis or BCG	10 guinea pig ID equals 1 ID for man
Cholera	10^{11} vibrios for dog; 10^4 for man
Poliomyelitis type 2	Monkey gut is less susceptible than human gut
Q fever	One organism for guinea pig or man
Rubella	Monkey and man are about equal
Scrub typhus	1 mouse ID equals 1 human ID
Tularemia	10 organisms for mice, monkey, or man
Typhoid fever	10^{11} bacilli for chimpanzee; 10^8 or 10^9 for man
Venezuelan encephalitis	Monkey and man are about equal
West Nile virus	More virus to infect mice than man
Yaba pox virus	Monkey and man are about equal
Yellow fever	Monkey and man are about equal
Rhinovirus	Chimpanzee and man are about equal

1974–1975). Conversely, many animal disease agents rarely or never infect man.

Infection from Procedure or Equipment

The potential for aerosol release from procedures and equipment is an important guide in risk assessment. The route of infection of most laboratory illnesses has been attributed to the inhalation of aerosols (Sulkin, 1961). Experiments have confirmed that aerosols are produced during most common laboratory techniques or accidents. These show that each of us practices self-inoculation. Tables 43–3 and 43–4 present examples selected from comprehensive studies by Reitman and Wedum (1956) and Kenny and Sabel (1968).

Any laboratory procedure or operating equipment that imparts energy into a microbial suspension can be considered a potential source of aerosol (Chatigny et al., 1974). Dimmick et al. (1973) have developed an approach for estimating the rate of aerosol output from these sources for suspensions of varied microbial concentration. The measured aerosol output from a single procedure (Tables 43–3 and 43–4) is used to compute a characteristic ratio termed a "spray factor" for that procedure. The ratio is expressed as

Particles released per minute into the surrounding air

Concentration of viable units in the suspension

The rate of aerosol output for any procedure for which

Table 43–3. *Range of Viable Particles Recovered by Air Sampling During the Procedure or Accident Specified*

Pipette 30 ml culture into 50 ml test tube	0–5.5
Remove cotton plug from centrifuging tube	0.8–5
Remove cotton plug wet from flask after shaking	0–35
Remove 1 ml from vaccine vial by syringe	0.6–19
Streaking of petri plate	0–20
Insert inoculating loop (hot) into 100 ml culture	6–24
Decant centrifuge culture into flask	0–115
Mix culture in blender with worn bearing	12–126
Mix culture in blender with loose cover	77–1246
50 ml tube shatters and splashes in centrifuge	80–1800

Table 43–4. *Viable Particles Recovered Per Cubic Foot of Air Sampled During Procedures and Accidents*

Procedure or Accident	Number of Particles
Using sonic oscillator (minimal aeration)	6
Mixing culture with pipette	7
Overflow from mechanical mixer	9
Opening lyophilized cultures	135
Blending completed, top removed	1500
Dropping flask of culture	1551
Dropping lyophilized culture	4839

a spray factor has been determined can be calculated by multiplying the characteristic spray factor by the concentration of the suspension. Table 43–5 presents rates for selected procedures and accidents based on a concentration of 10^{10} viable organisms per milliliter. The computed output of aerosolized particles can be used to estimate corresponding inhalation dosages.

Infection of Cagemate by an Inoculated Animal

A fourth guide to risk, recognized as being unreliable at times, is available from experiments designed to determine whether an infected animal will transmit its disease to a normal cagemate. Such cross-infection is affected by many variables such as the microorganism, the animal and its age, method and volume of inoculation, feeding and watering, caging, urine and feces remaining in the cage, and cannibalism. A few illustrations, taken from a lengthy review by Wedum and Kruse (1969) of transmission and nontransmission, are provided in Table 43–6. Instances of cagemate transmission have been omitted when the challenge inoculum was an aerosol that incidentally was deposited on the fur of the challenged animal. In such a case, the transmission is by cross-contamination from the fur rather than by true transmission of infection. In this guide, the assumption is that if a normal cagemate can be infected, there is also a risk to the animal handler. The causative agents of tularemia, Q fever, coccidioidomycosis, and psittacosis are notorious causes of laboratory infections, yet they rarely infect cagemates. Four of the other five agents also are the cause of many laboratory infections and do infect cagemates. Our conclusion is that when infection of cagemates occurs, and especially if disease is transmited from one cage to another, it is a danger sign for the animal handler, unless there is a modifying factor such as the species specificity in avian disease.

Excretion of Microorganisms in Urine and Feces of Animals

The fifth guide lies in an evaluation of the infectious potential of the microorganism when it is excreted in the urine and feces of an experimentally inoculated animal.

It is surprising that so few human laboratory infections can definitely be attributed to this source. These have been reviewed elsewhere by Wedum (1974). Of the nearly 200 zoonotic diseases, at least 30 have significant

Table 43–5. *Aerosol Output for Select Procedures and Accidents Involving Suspension with Concentration of 10^{10} Viable Organisms Per ML*

Procedure or Accident	Spray Factor*	Aerosol Output
Blending completed, top removed	1.2×10^{-4}	1.2×10^6 particles/min
Mix culture in blender, loose cover	4×10^{-7}	4×10^3 particles/min
Using Sonic Oscillator		
Minimal aeration	5×10^{-7}	5×10^3 particles/min
Maximal aeration	1×10^{-4}	1×10^6 particles/min
Overflow from mechanical mixer	8×10^{-8}	8×10^2 particles/min
Streaking petri plate	4×10^{-8}	4×10^2 particles†
Dropping flask of culture	3×10^{-5}	3×10^5 particles†
Remove cotton plug from centrifuge tube	3×10^{-8}	3×10^2 particles†
Insert inoculating loop	3×10^{-8}	3×10^2 particles†
Opening lyophilized cultures	2×10^{-9}	2×10^1 particles†

transmissibility to man (Griesemer and Manning, 1973). Fifty or more disease agents, other than those causing intestinal disease in man, were found to be excreted in urine and feces of experimentally infected animals (Wedum and Kruse, 1969). Nevertheless, in reviewing infections among animal handlers, after eliminating cases due to recognized bites, cuts, and scratches, it is difficult to assess the importance of inhalation of microbe-bearing dust from cages or of manual contamination as a source of human infection. One reason is that it is common for animal caretakers to assist in inoculation and autopsy or in other procedures that may cause infection in the absence of a definite accident.

There have been some dramatic instances of laboratory infections from accidentally aerosolized urine and feces during research on the hemorrhagic fever viruses, in psittacosis-ornithosis, and in Q fever. There are also some surprises in the reported absence of the microorganisms in the urine and feces of animal inoculated with etiologic agents of Rift Valley fever, yellow fever, and some of the rickettsial diseases, all of which easily affect man in the laboratory in the absence of immunization (Table 43–7). It is apparent that the only safe policy is to take precautions appropriate to the disease based on an assumption that the inoculated microorganism will be excreted and made airborne.

Increased Human Susceptibility to Disease: Pregnancy, Immunodeficiency

A sixth factor begins with knowledge that viruses, bacteria, and at least one protozoan are known to have caused human malformations, abortion, or other undesirable effects (Blattner et al., 1973; Paranson et al., 1981). As a result, it is not uncommon for virologic laboratories to encourage or require removal of a woman during her pregnancy to a position that does not carry the risk of accidental viral inoculation. The National Institutes of Health Biohazard Safety Guide (1974) states that: "Women working with viruses should discontinue work with these agents as soon as pregnancy seems reasonably certain." Support for precautionary transfer from the virologic laboratory can be found in the increasing medical reluctance to immunize with live virus during pregnancy (Levine et al., 1974). For instance, the military medical services consider administration of any live virus vaccine during pregnancy to be medically contraindicated.

The effect of immunosuppression or immunodeficiency on human susceptibility to disease is too complicated to be summarized briefly, beyond stating that it is generally unfavorable. In cancer virology, immunosuppression usually facilitates tumor induction in an otherwise resistant animal (Dent, 1972).

Table 43–6. *Infection of Control Cagemate by Inoculated Animal*

Causative Agent Of	Animal Species Tested	Number of Species Showing Infection of Cagemate
Tularemia	Guinea pig, mice, rat, monkey	0
Q fever	Guinea pig, cat, hamster, monkey	2
Coccidioidomycosis	Guinea pig, dog, monkey	0
Psittacosis	Mice, chicken, monkey	0
Tuberculosis	Guinea pig, mice, rabbit, monkey	4
Brucellosis	Guinea pig, mice, chicken, swine, monkey	2
Venezuelan encephalitis	Guinea pig, mice, dog, horse, pigeon, monkey	3
Influenza	Mice, dog, ferret	2
Hemorrhagic fever-viral*	Guinea pig, hamster, mice, voles	4

*Junin, Machupo, hemorrhagic fever with renal syndrome.

Table 43–7. *Recovery of Infectious Agent From Urine or Feces*

Disease	No. of Animal Species	Recovery
Anthrax	16	16
Brucellosis	10	10
Q fever	11	8
Psittacosis	8	6
Melioidosis	7	7
Venezuelan encephalitis	6	3
Russian S-S encephalitis	5	4
Coccidioidomycosis	4	3
Rift Valley fever	5	0
Yellow fever	4	0

In this situation, it is recommended that laboratories handling hazardous infectious agents adopt a policy corresponding to that of the National Cancer Institute (1974): "Persons with reduced immunological competency, pregnant women, and patients under treatment with steroids or cytotoxic drugs, shall receive a medical evaluation before work in areas where (oncogenic) viruses are used."

Control Measures

The selection of appropriate control measures requires knowledgeable judgment of the risks by the laboratory director. Recommendations for control measures have been published by the Centers for Disease Control/National Institutes of Health (1988a), the National Cancer Institute (1974), and the National Institutes of Health (1986, 1978). The latter was published as a Laboratory Safety Monograph Supplement to the NIH Guidelines for Research Involving Recombinant DNA Molecules (NIH, 1986). The use of graded control measures is reflected in the guidelines and recommendations. The levels are identified by the numbers 1 through 4, which reflect in ascending order the practices and techniques, safety equipment and facility design required for the conduct of work of increasing hazard.

Control measures for biologic safety involve work practices, safety equipment and facilities. Maximization of these requires proper training and supervision of workers.

Work Practices

Rowe (1973) stated at the 1973 Asilomar Conference on Biohazards in Biological Research that " . . . much of microbiological safety consists of having good habits . . . Lab workers should have the operating room mentality, that there are clean and dirty areas with clearly defined but constantly changing boundaries. There is no reason why this mental approach should be restricted to microbiology, but it should be part of the training and lifelong habits of every lab worker; it is just as easy to work using good sterile technique as it is to use bad technique." We agree. To achieve a safe level of performance, however,

it is necessary that all laboratory workers understand the risks and become expert in procedures that provide protection. This is a responsibility shared by the laboratory director and the worker.

The laboratory director should establish the standards for activities that involve hazardous agents. These standards should describe requirements for protective clothing, mechanical pipetting devices, personal hygiene, and access control; identification and storage of materials; procedures for decontamination and disposal; and guidelines to ensure proper use of safety equipment. In addition, emergency procedures to be followed in the event of an exposure should be described.

Safety Equipment

The use of a safety equipment is the most common approach to controlling aerosols incidentally created by microbiologic procedures and accidents. This equipment is considered a primary barrier because it is applied at the source of the hazard, usually within a few inches of the person conducting the experiment. The most important items are the biologic safety cabinets and animal caging that minimizes escape of microbial aerosols.

There are three basic types of biologic safety cabinets. The types differ from one another in the degree of containment provided and the extent to which they provide protection against contamination of research materials.

The open-front (open-face) cabinet, or Class I cabinet, with an inward airflow from the room of 50 to 100 linear feet per minute (lfpm) serves primarily to protect the operator. Many interesting designs have been described by Chatigny and Clinger (1969), Evans et al. (1972), and Phillips (1961). Operator protection can be increased by insertion of a panel with portholes for hands. This will at least double the inward air velocity. A minimum of 75 lfpm is desirable in the absence of panel. This cabinet is suitable for most microbiologic diagnostic and research procedures. Because of potential and nonspecific contamination from the room, it is not recommended when protection of the experimental material is critical. However, the simplicity of the Class I cabinet has the advantages of easy measurement and control of airflow and no recirculation of exhaust air.

It is recommended that the exhaust air from Class I cabinets be treated with high-efficiency particulate air filters (HEPA). This filter has a particle collection efficiency of 99.97% or greater for particles in the respirable size range. The HEPA filter has been shown to retain coliphage and actinophage particles with diameters of 0.12 and 0.05 mμ, according to tests by Harstad and Filler (1969) and Roelants et al. (1968).

It is essential that regular periodic checks of the inward air velocity be performed, because a decline in airflow will occur with gradual loading of the filter. Malfunction of the exhaust system serving the cabinet can also contribute to loss of airflow. When filter replacement is indicated, the used filter either should be decontaminated in place or removed in a manner that prevents exposure of maintenance personnel. Gaseous decontamination

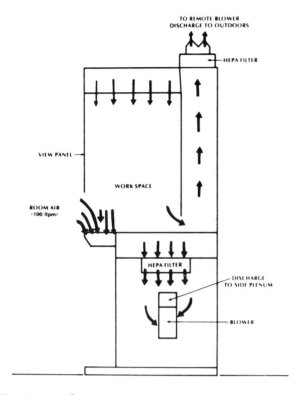

Fig. 43–1. Airflow pattern of the biologic safety cabinet.

with formaldehyde released by heated paraformaldehyde is effective (Taylor et al., 1969).

The downflow biologic safety cabinet (Class II) provides a rapid piston-action sweep of sterile air through the inside of the cabinet and a protective air curtain across the opening (Barkley, 1973). It protects experimental or diagnostic materials from contamination or cross-contamination while still protecting the worker (Fig. 43–1). These cabinets have been commonly referred to as laminar-flow biologic safety cabinets because the interior of the cabinet is basically a miniaturized clean room; i.e., HEPA-filtered air is supplied in a uniform manner to the cabinet interior at the top of the enclosure (ceiling) and is removed through grilles free from particulates. This air provides an environment for tissue culture and other systems that are susceptible to airborne contamination. The flow of air also contributes to personnel safety by entraining hazardous aerosols and transporting them to HEPA filters, where they are removed from the airstream before it is recirculated to or exhausted from the cabinet enclosure. Personnel safety is achieved primarily by maintaining an average inward air flow velocity across the front access opening of 75 to 100 lfpm. Class II cabinets offer several advantages over the Class I cabinet. These are (1) the greater dilution that occurs within the cabinet enclosure, (2) the uniform internal airflow, and (3) the rapid removal of entrained particles.

Class II cabinets should be tested on completion of new and relocated installation to establish proper performance. Annual testing is recommended. The proce-

dures to be used for the testing of Class II cabinets are described in Standard Number 49 published by the National Sanitation Foundation (NSF, 1987). Slide cassette programs describing the selection and effective use of laminar-flow biologic safety cabinets are available. Information regarding these programs is available from the Division of Safety, National Institutes of Health, Bethesda, MD 20892.

Class III cabinets are designed to completely isolate a hazardous operation by providing a physical barrier between the research worker and the research environment. These cabinets are fabricated with stainless steel or other impervious materials. All work within the cabinet enclosure is performed through impervious gloves that are attached to the walls of the cabinet. The interior space of the cabinet is maintained under negative pressure with respect to the pressure of the room where the cabinet is located. Exhaust air from Class III cabinets is filtered and incinerated or refiltered with HEPA filters before being discharged to the atmosphere. These cabinets can achieve a containment capability 10,000 times greater than Class I cabinets.

The housing of infected laboratory animals must be accomplished in accordance with proper animal husbandry (USPHS, 1986) and microbiologic practices (DHHS, 1988a). Collectively, these practices serve to minimize the risk of infection for the personnel and to prevent infection of the animals by the personnel or other infected animals.

A variety of caging units are available for the housing of the several species of animals used in infectious disease studies. They range from the simple open unit to the closed ventilated unit (Chatigny and Clinger, 1969) for work with high-risk agents such as Marburg and Lassa viruses. In the majority of cases, however, relatively simple and inexpensive methods are available for housing infected animals. The filter bonnet on mouse cages (Schneider and Collins, 1966) will prevent cross-infection between cages of mice, rats, and hamsters. Filter bonnets do contribute to an increase in temperature, humidity, and ammonia concentration (Simmons et al., 1968) but these effects can be offset by proper facility design and good animal husbandry. Giovanella and Stehlin (1973) reported excellent results using cages fitted with filter bonnets for the housing of "nude" (athymic) mice.

Several racks or shelving units that use directional outward airflow have been developed for the housing of normal and other animals where protection of the animal is required. Similar units using inward airflow have been developed. Most of these units, however, operate with low velocity, and their use with infected animals must be complemented with proper practices and procedures. A nonmobile rack with fixed air ducts and remote blower and filter, but with the convenience of an open-front inward-airflow containment system, has been used with infectious agents without intercage infection or infection of personnel (Chatigny and Clinger, 1969).

The advantage of designs that include airflow as a barrier to intercage and personnel infection is that they provide easier handling and servicing of the cages. These units have the inherent disadvantage of airflow barriers in that they provide only partial protection, and their use therefore must be controlled.

Secondary Barriers

Secondary protective barriers (Runkle and Phillips, 1969) such as air locks, clothing change rooms and shower rooms, ultraviolet lights, differential air pressures, and treatment of sewage, trash, and exhaust air are discussed at length in referenced sources. These barriers are used for isolating the laboratory environment to prevent spread of accidentally released microbial material. Secondary barriers traditionally have been installed to contain areas supporting activities that involved highly infectious agents. The basis for these control measures was to reduce the theoretical possibility that persons outside the laboratory might accidentally become infected. Actually, it has not been possible to find reports of laboratory-attributed infection in persons who never were in the laboratory building or who were not associated in some way with the laboratory (Wedum, 1974).

Close attention to provision and use of primary barriers will reduce the need for secondary barriers. Unfortunately there often is a tendency to install more secondary barriers than primary ones. We are inclined to believe this is caused by the willingness of the scientist to agree to almost any engineering safety design as long as it does not interfere with his customary practices of working on an open bench top.

The control of supply and exhaust air to provide for directional flow of air is an important protective measure that is recommended for all laboratories. Differential air pressures are selected so that clean air moves toward areas of highest potential hazard. This reduces the potential of an accidentally released aerosol being disseminated to adjacent areas. We recommend that the ventilation system be designed to supply clean air to the laboratory corridor for infiltration, under all operating conditions, of a minimum 50 cubic feet per minute (cfm) per doorway leading to the research space.

Exhaust air is a frequent cause for concern. If adequate primary barriers are used, treatment of the laboratory room air becomes less necessary, except in special cases, as in production processes. In some situations, the location of an exhaust discharge relative to a supply air intake may require treatment of the exhaust air. In these cases, it is advisable to consider alternative primary barriers or other actions that may eliminate the requirement for treating large volumes of exhaust air. It is to be noted that replacement of filters requires that the used filter be either decontaminated in place or removed in a manner that prevents exposure of personnel.

Recirculation of Air

The high cost of air conditioning justifies consideration of recirculation. There is no good microbiologic reason for not recirculating air from most biologic laboratories and animal rooms (Chatigny and Clinger, 1969; Runkle and Phillips, 1969). The exceptions are problems in control of odor; presence of toxic or flammable gas; excessive loading of filters with animal hair or other debris; laboratories studying dry micronized infectious particles or experimentally created infectious microbial aerosols; pilot plants growing pathogenic microorganisms in aerated tanks with agitators; facilities housing animals inoculated or infected with highly contagious animal diseases; and laboratories studying infectious agents that require Class III gas-tight cabinetry. In all other usual research and diagnostic laboratories, HEPA filtration before recirculation can remove the few infectious microorganisms that elude the primary barriers and remain viable. If there are no primary barriers, the laboratory personnel themselves serve as signal indicators; if they remain uninfected, the filtered recirculation of air that has not infected them will do no damage elsewhere.

However, there is a serious maintenance problem. Few institutions provide the engineering staff with the funds, equipment, personnel, time, and opportunity for specialized training necessary to service the HEPA filters and other elements of the recirculation system in a manner that guarantees continued effective filtration. Therefore, the expensive but foolproof system of 100% outside air often is chosen. A study of comparative costs would be interesting. For the same reason, it is recommended that the exhaust air from the laminar-flow biologic safety cabinet be exhausted to the outside rather than returned to the room through a HEPA filter. Laminar flow animal rooms that use recirculated air also have this maintenance problem if the room houses infectious agents.

REFERENCES

Barkley, W.E. 1973. Facilities and equipment available for virus containment. In *Biohazards in Biological Research*. Edited by A. Hellman, M.N. Oxman, and R. Pollack. New York, Cold Spring Harbor Laboratories, pp. 327–398.

Blattner, R.J., Williamson, A.P., and Heys, F.M. 1973. Role of viruses in the etiology of congenital malformations. In *Progress in Medical Virology*. Volume 15. Edited by J.L. Melnick. New York, Karger Basel, pp. 1–41.

Braymen, D.T., Songer, J.R., and Sullivan, J.F. 1974. Effectiveness of footwear and decontamination methods for preventing the spread of infectious agents. Lab. Anim. Sci., *24*, 888–894.

Chatigny, M.A., Barkley, W.E., and Vogl, W.A. 1974. Aerosol biohazard in microbiological laboratories and how it is affected by air conditioning systems. ASHRAE Trans., *80*, 463–469.

Chatigny, M.A., and Clinger, D.I. 1969. Contamination control in aerobiology. In *Introduction to Experimental Aerobiology*. Edited by R.L. Dimmick and A.B. Akers. New York, Wiley.

Dent, P.B. 1972. Immunosuppression by oncogenic viruses. In *Process in Medical Virology*. Volume 14. Edited by J.L. Melnick. New York, Karger Basel, pp. 1–35.

Department of Transportation, Code of Federal Regulation, 49 CRF 172.5, 173.386, 173.387, 173.388. Office of Hazardous Materials, DOT, Washington, 20590. Also published in the Federal Register, 30 September 1972 and 29 March 1973.

Dimmick, R.L., Vogl, W.F., and Chatigny, M.A. 1973. Potential for accidental microbial aerosol transmission in the biological laboratory. In *Biohazards in Biological Research*. Edited by A. Hellman, M.N. Oxman, and R. Pollack. New York, Cold Spring Harbor Laboratories, pp. 246–266.

Evans, C.G.T., Harris-Smith, R., and Stratton, J.E.D. 1972. The use of safety cabinets for the prevention of laboratory-acquired infections. In *Safety in Microbiology*. Edited by D.A. Shapton and R.G. Board. New York, Academic Press, pp. 21–36.

Giovanella, B.C., and Stehlin, J.S. 1973. Heterotransplantation of human malignant tumors in "nude" thymusless mice. I. Breeding and maintenance of "nude" mice. J. Natl. Cancer Inst., *51*, 615–619.

Griesemer, R.A., and Manning, J.S. 1973. Animal facilities. In *Biohazards in Biological Research*. Edited by A. Hellman, M.N. Oxman, and R. Pollack. New York, Cold Spring Harbor Laboratories, pp. 316–326.

Harrington, J.M., and Shannon, H.S. 1976. Incidence of tuberculosis, hepatitis, brucellosis and shigellosis in British medical laboratory workers. Br. Med. J., *1*, 759–762.

Harstad, J.B., and Filler, M.E. 1969. Evaluation of air filters with submicron viral aerosols and bacterial aerosols. Am. Ind. Hyg. Assoc. J., *30*, 280–290.

Hellman, A., Wedum, A.G., and Barkley, W.E. 1974–1975. Assessment of risk in the cancer virus laboratory (Preprint). Office of Research Safety, National Cancer Institute, Bethesda, MD.

Herman, L.G. 1968. Control of biological agents as contaminants in microbiological laboratories. In *Disinfection, Sterilization, and Preservation*. 1st Edition. Edited by C.A. Lawrence and S.S. Block. Philadelphia, Lea & Febiger, pp. 543–552.

Hull, R.N. 1973. Biohazards associated with simian viruses. In *Biohazards in Biological Research*. Edited by A. Hellman, M.N. Oxman, and R. Pollack. New York, Cold Spring Harbor Laboratories, pp. 3–40.

Kenny, M.T., and Sabel, F.L. 1968. Particle size distribution of *Serratia marcescens* aerosols created during common laboratory procedures and simulated laboratory accidents. Appl. Microbiol., *16*, 1146–1150.

Kruse, R.H., and Wedum, A.G. 1970. Cross-infection with eighteen pathogens among caged laboratory animals. Lab. Anim. Care, *20*, 541–560.

Levine, M.M., Edsall, G., and Bruce-Chwatt, L.J. 1974. Live-virus vaccines in pregnancy. Risks and recommendations. Lancet, *7871*, 34–37.

May, K.R., and Pomeroy, N.P. 1973. Bacterial dispersion from the body surface. In *Airborne Transmission and Airborne Infection*. Edited by J.F. Ph. Hers and K.C. Winkler. New York, John Wiley & Sons, pp. 426–432.

McGarrity, G.J., et al. 1969. Medical applications of dust-free rooms. III. Use in an animal care laboratory. Appl. Microbiol., *18*, 142–146.

National Sanitation Foundation Standard 49. Class II (Laminar Flow) Biohazard Cabinetry, 1987. NSF Building, Ann Arbor, MI 48105.

Paranson, I.M., Della-Porta, A.J., and Snowdon, W.A. 1981. Developmental disorders of the fetus in some anthropod-borne virus infections. Am. J. Trop. Med. Hyg., *30*, 660–673.

Phillips, G.B. 1961. Microbiological safety in U.S. and foreign laboratories. Tech. Study 35, AD–268635, National Technical Information Service, 5285 Port Royal Road, Springfield, VA.

Pike, R.M. 1979. Laboratory-associated infections: Incidence, fatalities, causes and prevention. Annu. Rev. Microbiol., *33*, 41–66.

Pike, R.M. 1976. Laboratory-associated infections: Summary and analysis of 3921 cases. Health Lab. Sci., *13*, No. 2, 105–113.

Reitman, M., and Wedum, A.G. 1956. Microbiological safety. Public Health Rep., *71*, 659–665.

Roelants, P., Boon, B., and Lhoest, W. 1968. Evaluation of a commercial air filter for removal of viruses from the air. Appl. Microbiol., *16*, 1465–1467.

Rowe, W. 1973. In *Biohazards in Biological Research*. Edited by A. Hellman, M.N. Oxman, and R. Pollack. New York, Cold Spring Harbor Laboratory, p. 352.

Runkle, R.S., and Phillips, G.B. 1969. *Microbial Contamination Control Facilities*. New York, Van Nostrand Reinhold.

Schneider, H.A., and Collins, G.R. 1966. Successful prevention of infantile diarrhea of mice during an epizootic by means of a new filter cage unopened from birth to weaning. Lab. Anim. Care, *16*, pp. 60–71.

Simmons, M.L., Robie, D.M., Jones, J.B., and Serrano, L.J. 1968. Effect of a filter cover on temperature and humidity in a mouse cage. Lab. Anim. Care, *2*, 113–120.

Skinhoj, P. 1974. Occupational risks in Danish clinical laboratories. II. Infections. Scand. J. Clin. Lab Invest., *33*, 27–29.

Sulkin, S.E. 1961. Laboratory-acquired infections. Bacteriol. Rev., *25*, 203–211.

Taylor, L.A., Barbeito, M.S., and Gremillion, G.G. 1969. Paraformaldehyde for surface sterilization and detoxification. Appl. Microbiol., *17*, 614–618.

U.S. Department of Health, Education and Welfare, Public Health Service. 1978. Laboratory Safety Monograph. A Supplement to the NIH Guidelines for Recombinant DNA Research. National Institutes of Health, Bethesda, MD 20892.

U.S. Department of Health, Education and Welfare, Public Health Service. 1979a. Morbidity and Mortality Weekly Report, *28*, 521–522; 593–594.

U.S. Department of Health, Education and Welfare, Public Health Service. 1979b. Morbidity and Mortality Weekly Report, *28*, 333–334.

U.S. Department of Health, Education and Welfare, Public Health Service. 1974. National Cancer Institute Safety Standards for Research Involving Oncogenic Viruses. National Cancer Institute, NIH 75–790, Bethesda, MD.

U.S. Department of Health, Education and Welfare, Public Health Service. 1974. *Biohazards Safety Guide*. Environmental Services Branch, NIH, Bethesda, MD.

U.S. Department of Health, Education and Welfare, Public Health Service. 1980. Code of Federal Regulations, 42 CFR 72.225. Centers for Disease Control, Atlanta.

U.S. Department of Health and Human Services, Public Health Service. 1985a. Guide for the Care and Use of Laboratory Animals. No. NIH 86–23, National Institutes of Health, Bethesda, MD.

U.S. Department of Health and Human Services, Public Health Service. 1985b. Morbidity and Mortality Weekly Report, Volume 34, No. 45. Centers for Disease Control, Atlanta.

U.S. Department of Health and Human Services, Public Health Service. 1986. National Institutes of Health Guidelines for Research Involving Recombinant DNA Molecules. Federal Register *51* (88), Part III, May 7, 1986, U.S. Government Printing Office, Washington, D.C.

U.S. Department of Health and Human Services, Public Health Service. 1987a. Morbidity and Mortality Weekly Report, Volume 36, No. 25, Centers for Disease Control, Atlanta.

U.S. Department of Health and Human Services, Public Health Service. 1987b. Morbidity and Mortality Weekly Report, Volume 36, No. 41, Centers for Disease Control, Atlanta.

U.S. Department of Health and Human Services, Public Health Service. 1988a. Biosafety in Microbiological and Biomedical Laboratories. Centers for Disease Control/National Institutes of Health. HHS Publication No. (CDC) 88–8395. U.S. Government Printing Office (Stock No. 17–40–508–3), Washington, D.C.

U.S. Department of Health and Human Services, Public Health Service. 1988b. Morbidity and Mortality Weekly Report, Volume 37, No. 24, Centers for Disease Control, Atlanta.

U.S. Department of Transportation. 1980. Code of Federal Regulations, 49 CFR 173, 886–173, 388. U.S. Government Printing Office, Washington, D.C.

Wedum, A.G. 1974. Biohazard control. In *CRC Handbook of Laboratory Animal Science*. Volume I. Edited by C. Melby and N.H. Altman. Cleveland, CRC Press, pp. 191–210.

Wedum, A.G. 1964. Laboratory safety in research with infectious aerosols. Public Health Rep., *79*, 619–633.

Wedum, A.G., and Kruse, R.H. 1969. Assessment of risk of human infection in the microbiological laboratory. Misc. Publication 30, AD–693258. Frederick Cancer Research Center, Frederick, MD.

Wedum, A.G., Barkley, W.E., and Hellman, A. 1972. Handling of infectious agents. Am. Vet. Med. Assoc. J., *161*, 1557–1567.

PART VI

Antimicrobials in Food Sanitation and Preservation

CHAPTER 44

ANTIMICROBIAL AGENTS USED IN AGRICULTURE

R.J. Lukens

Plant diseases take their toll in losses of crop production. Losses of feed, fiber, and ornamentals are held to about 14% in world production (Metcalf, 1971) with fungicides used on at least one half of the crops (Ordish and Mitchell, 1967). In 1969, over 4 million acres of crops in the United States were treated with fungicides at a cost of $55 million (Fowler and Mahan, 1973). Fungicides make up about 13% of pesticide production and sales, the largest portion of which is formulated into foliar protectants.

USES

Most fungicides used on crops protect the surface of the plants. Foliage and fruit are sprayed for protection against spotting and blighting diseases. Soil in seed beds or in planting rows is treated to protect young emerging seedlings from fungal attacks. With systemic fungicides, soil, seed, or leaf is treated for subsequent movement of fungicide to the site of infection.

The fungitoxicant is prepared in a safe, convenient way for application to crops by proper formulation. The active ingredients are stabilized to facilitate storage. All risks to humans and plants as well as to the equipment used for dispersion are minimized. Proper dilution, dispersion, and deposition of the toxic agents also are determined. Important factors of formulation and their role in the performance of a fungicide will be discussed briefly. These factors have been treated in greater detail elsewhere (Horsfall, 1945; Duyfjes, 1958; Martin, 1964).

Fungicides are diluted to workable quantities for application to plants. Clays, i.e., talc and kaolinite, are commonly used as diluents in dust, wettable powders, slurries, and sperill formulations, whereas water-immiscible solvents are used in emulsifiable concentrates, and water-miscible solvents are used in water-soluble formulations. Water added at the time of application of sprays further dilutes the fungicide to correct amounts for deposition on plant surfaces. The amount of water

added at this stage varies with the type of spraying equipment and speed of application.

Clay diluents have been selected for desired characteristics. Clays with high adsorbent capacity can be mixed with water-soluble and liquid toxicants to ensure a gradual release of toxicants in residues. Clays with high base exchange capacity or with humectant characteristics may hydrolyze certain fungicides to nonfungitoxic or phytotoxic products, as in the case of attapulgite and kaolinite with captan (Daines et al., 1957). Certain talcs, lacking these detrimental characteristics, are used as diluents with captan.

A wetting agent or spreader is incorporated into a formulation to cause the spray droplets to spread as films over the waxy surfaces of leaves and to seep into porous solids or obstacles on leaves, i.e., necrotic lesions, and masses of mycelia and spores. Martin (1964) described the wetting properties as the ability of a water film to persist rather than form a sphere and run off the leaf. The spreading property is the ability of water to spread in a film over a leaf surface. Once deposited and dried, the residue must resist wash-off by subsequent wetting from dew or rain.

Nonionic wetting agents are preferred to anionic types because the latter, being soluble in cool water, cause the dry residue to wash off plant surfaces when the surfaces become wet from dew or rain. Nonionic wetting agents, such as casein, gelatin, and oils, increase tenacity (ability to adhere to a surface) over deposits on drying.

Various accessory agents may be incorporated into the formulated product. Urea is frequently used to stabilize certain toxicants in storage. Sodium carbonate is used to buffer acidic decomposition products of toxicants that may form in residues and burn foliage. Dyes are incorporated into liquid formulations for identification purposes. Formulations for use on turf contain dyes to make the residues inconspicuous and to disguise diseased turf.

The size of particles in dry fungicide formulations affect many aspects of chemical control of plant diseases. As particle size decreases, deposition becomes more uniform because of an increase in the number of particles per unit area. Penetration of porous obstacles on leaf surfaces also improves. When a large particle is broken into smaller ones, the total exposed surface area of the material increases. Because adherence of residues to leaf surfaces depends on the contact of particle with leaf, the greater the exposed surface, the greater the tenacity. Similarly, fungitoxicity of a chemical deposit on a leaf surface, which depends upon exposed surface area, increases as particle size of the toxicant is reduced. However, loss in activity from decomposition and sublimation of the toxicant may increase as the particle size is decreased. Particles of 1 to 5 μm in diameter are commonly employed in fungicide formulations for attacking fungus spores ranging in size from 5 to 20 μm in dimension.

The effective concentration of fungicide in residues varies with the inoculum potential of the pathogen. In theory, as the number of spores settling on a leaf increases, the chance of a few spores alighting on unprotected areas also increases, as does the amount of fungicide required to minimize the chance for the fungus to find unprotected areas. Though ample fungicide is deposited on a leaf surface from a normal application of spray to withstand a high inoculum potential, wet weather, which favors buildup of inoculum potential, can deteriorate the protective residue. The protective coating is maintained during wet weather by more frequent applications of fungicide.

Although deterioration of spray residues is minimized in formulation, expanding surfaces of rapidly growing plant organs will crumble the protective covering. Thus, for protection against apple scab disease, frequent applications (every 5 to 7 days) are required during early growing season when buds are opening and young leaves are expanding. Later, when leaves and fruit have completed their growth, an occasional spray of fungicide will suffice to maintain a protective covering on plant surfaces.

Protective sprays applied to ripening fruit during late season may fail. The pathogens can bypass the protective barrier through the superficial injuries to which ripening fruit are prone. Fruit becomes more susceptible to some diseases on ripening. Late-season infections are avoided by preventing early infections. Early disease lesions quickly add to the inoculum potential and hasten immense buildups of inoculum during the season. The importance of controlling disease during the early growing season cannot be overemphasized.

FUNGITOXICITY

Fungicides, although harmful to fungi, are safe to higher plants and animals. This specificity is based more or less on penetration to the site of action. Resistance to fungicides may be due to impermeability or detoxication. McCallan and Miller (1963) have emphasized the poor efficacy of fungitoxicants. The dose, 100 to 10,000 μg/g of fungal tissue, is far greater than that of antibiotics, insecticides, certain bactericides, and the newer herbi-

cides. However, the more recently introduced sterol inhibiting fungicides are potent at levels around 1 ppm or below. Previously, the high dosage has been ascribed to mechanisms of toxicity (Ferguson, 1939), but later work (Woodcock, 1964) suggested excessive detoxication by the cellular thiol pool, and in some cases, the cellular amino pool. Most metals and organic fungicides react with thiols. The potency of certain fungicides increases if the thiol pool within fungi is reduced first by pretreatment with sulfhydryl reagents (Lukens and Rich, 1959; Richmond and Somers, 1962b).

Except for antibiotics and newly discovered systemics, fungicides act as general metabolic inhibitors. They may affect many metabolic systems in fungal physiology, but only those systems essential for life are considered the ultimate sites of action. Locating these sites is analogous to finding a needle in a hay stack. Fungicides in common use or that have a unique application in crop production will now be discussed.

HEAVY METALS

Copper, first in Bordeaux mixture and later in "fixed coppers," is the most extensively used fungicide for control of foliar diseases. Large amounts of copper fungicides have been consumed to combat late blight disease of potato and tomato and Sigatoka disease of banana. Because copper often reduces crop yield, it was replaced by organic fungicides. However, the use of fixed copper is returning to replace those fungicides and bactericides that may be toxic to nontarget organisms or that show selected resistance with continued use. Organotin compounds have been used on edible crops in Europe and to a limited extent in the United States, but most uses have been discontinued because of possible toxicology.

Performance in the Field

It was fortunate for the early plant pathologist that the lime in Bordeaux mixture forms an insoluble copper complex with high tenacity. This residue weathers extremely well on most plant leaves. Appreciation of factors affecting performance of spray deposits was not needed until organic fungicides were developed. On smooth leaves, Bordeaux does not stick well unless the amount of lime in the mixture is reduced. In low-lime mixtures, a different type of crystal forms that contacts the leaf surface more intimately (Burchfield and Goenaga, 1957).

Copper is completely bound in aged deposits of Bordeaux mixtures. Germinating spores of copper-sensitive fungi excrete malic acid and amino acids (McCallan and Wilcoxon, 1936), which solubilize the metal (Goldsworthy and Green, 1936). Copper-resistant fungi fail to solubilize the metal from spray deposits.

Permeation

Heavy metals must permeate fungal cells in order to be toxic. Most metals are absorbed as cations, a few as anions through ion-exchange mechanisms. They may compete with magnesium, calcium, and potassium for receptor sites (Marsh, 1945). The amount of competition varies with fungal species (Miller and Russakow, 1964). Uptake of heavy metals by a physical mechanism may follow the Freundlich-Langmuir absorption isotherm (Parker-Rhodes, 1941). However, the work of Dassner and Esdorn (1923) with organomercurials, Horsfall et al. (1937) with copper ions, and Hartel (1958) with organotin compounds suggests that these fungitoxicants sometimes may permeate through lipophilic centers in the fungal membranes.

Metals can leak from spores when they are placed in water (Bodnar and Terenyl, 1932), dilute acid (Prevost, 1807), and solutions of chelating agents (Muller and Biederman, 1952).

Fungal spores can accumulate metals against a gradient. In an hour, spores of *Monilinia fructicola* accumulate mercuric ions at 7×10^6 times the rate of the ambient fluid (Owens, 1952). The extent of metal accumulation varies with fungal species (Miller et al., 1953b). Accumulation occurs within the fungal spore. This was first shown by Goldsworthy and Green (1936) for copper by using a copper dye, and later by Owens and Miller (1958) for silver and cesium radioisotopes and sonic disruption of spores.

The question of whether metals are adsorbed or absorbed becomes moot in light of invagination of the cell membrane within the protoplast (Miller, 1962). Fast uptake and release of metallic ions may occur via the interphases of these folding membranes, with storage of metals occurring in the overlapping lobes or free space within the protoplast (McCallan and Miller, 1963).

Chemical Mechanisms

Chemical bonding between metals and reactive groups is critical in the biologic activity of metals. Shaw (1954) drew attention to the metal-sulfur bond by showing that toxicity of heavy metals was related to the insolubility of metal sulfide. He suggested that metals act by taking up key functional thiol groups of enzymes.

Horsfall (1956) called attention to chelation as a toxic mechanism by relating the toxicity of metallic cations to the stability of their chelates. That amino acids are strong chelating agents would suggest proteins as principal targets of heavy metals.

The strength of covalent bonds of metals and organic residues that are operating in metal-sulfur and metal-chelate bonds is determined in part by the electronegativity of the metallic ion. For the fungi, Somers (1961) has verified Danielli and Davis's (1951) theory that toxicity of metals is correlated with their electronegativity.

Mode of Action of Metals

Fungitoxicity of heavy metals may occur through enzyme inhibition, altered cellular permeability, and nonspecific precipitation of proteins. Inhibition of enzymes by heavy metals is well known; metals may compete with metallic or organic cofactors for sites on an enzyme. Owens (1953) has discussed the specificity of several metals for certain enzyme systems that require iron, copper, amino, and thiol groups. Horsfall (1956) suggested that metals act by interfering with cell permeability. Such action may be of a physical nature, as suggested by Sommers (1961). Protein denaturation by metals is also a physical process. At high concentrations, metals affect proteins in enzymes and cellular membranes through this mechanism. Competitive enzyme inhibition may account for the static action of metals at low doses, but denaturation of protein results in permanent damage at lethal doses.

Detoxication of Metals

Numerous reports show that thiols can reverse the toxicity of metals (Yoder, 1951; Santelli and Katy, 1962; Fildes, 1940; Brewer, 1940). It is difficult to determine the exact nature of thiol reversal. Thiols could remove heavy metals from the sites of action or they could repair damaged thiols. They could also merely detoxify metals. Ashworth and Amin (1964) have shown that resistance to mercury of fungi lies in a large thiol pool. Resistance could be induced in sensitive fungi by growing them on a medium containing a reduced form of sulfur.

Organotin

Triphenyl tin compounds, having a broad spectrum of action, control diseases of many crops. The most commonly used forms are the acetate, chloride, hydroxide, and oxide salts. Slight phytotoxicity can occur, the extent of which varies with salt, crop, and weather. The acetate and chloride salts have been reported to act systemically in plants (Soilel, 1971; Mukhopadhyay and Thakur, 1972). Both triphenyl and trialkyl tin salts are fungitoxic, with maximum effectiveness of the latter occuring with the tributyl tin analog (Sisjpesteijn, 1959). However, the tributyl tin salts are too phytotoxic for use on crops. Little is known about the action of triphenyl tin on fungi. Apparently, there is more to its fungitoxic action than the inhibition of oxidative phosphorylation of the respirator inhibitor, thributyl tin sulfate (Aldridge and Cremer, 1955).

SULFUR-CONTAINING COMPOUNDS

Sulfur

Elemental sulfur has long been used for control of plant diseases. It remains important in the treatment of peaches for brown rot disease and is used against various powdery mildews. When mixed with lime, it forms an excellent spray residue with stability and tenacity that consists of calcium polysulfides. Elemental sulfur slowly arises from this complex mixture. Sulfur is formulated as a wettable colloid. Its activity on foliage is proportional to the number of particles rather than to its weight.

Sensitive fungi reduce sulfur to H_2S. In the process, extra oxygen is consumed and molar equivalents of CO_2 are given off (Miller et al., 1953a). The process may occur in the cytochrome system (Tweedy and Turner, 1966).

How sulfur kills fungi has been the subject of some

extensive debates. Horsfall (1956) describes the various theories of the fungitoxic action of the element. Fungitoxicity has been ascribed to hydrogen sulfide. Fungi resistant to sulfur succumb to H_2S. Their resistance to sulfur may lie in their inability to reduce the element. The H_2S theory was discarded by Miller et al. (1953a) because H_2S is about 1/50 as toxic as sulfur. They suggested that toxicity lay in proton-robbing of dehydrogenase-hydrogenase systems because the reduction process ($S > H_2S$) consumes protons. It is hard to accept the proton-robbing theory completely, because the reduction process is sensitive to sodium arsenite, whereas fungitoxicity is not (Miller et al., 1953a).

Tweedy and Turner (1966) have found that sulfur raises the respiratory quotient with subsequent curtailment of stored metabolites and cessation of energy-reacquiring syntheses. In cell-free systems, sulfur inhibits the reduction of cytochrome c and the oxidation of $NADH_2$. The apparent diversion of electrons between $NADH_2$ and cytochrome c by sulfur instead of oxygen may cause a loss in energy and depletion of high-energy phosphates.

Toxicity of sulfur has also been accredited to the formation of pantothenic acid (Young, 1922) and of free radicals (Owens, 1960). The former theory has been discounted by Wilcoxon and McCallan (1930), and the latter is yet to be demonstrated.

Dithiocarbamates

Dithiocarbamate fungicides are widely used in agriculture as soil and foliar protectants. Thiram (bis-dimethylthiocarbamyl disulfide) is used for seed treatment and control of diseases of turf and some fruit. Metal salts of dimethyldithiocarbamate and ethylene bisdithiocarbamates are fruit and vegetable fungicides. Zineb (zinc ethylenebisdithiocarbamate), maneb (manganese salt of the same), and a zinc complex of polyethylenethiuram disulfide have been extensively used to control late blight disease on potato, downy mildews on other crops, and several diseases of fruit. Vapam (sodium-N-methyldithiocarbamate) and Mylone (3,5-dimethyl-1,3,4,2-tetrahydrothiazine-2-thione) are used as soil fungicides before planting crops.

Fungi can distinguish the monoalkyl from the dialkyldithiocarbamates (Klopping, 1951). The monoalkyldithiocarbamates, having a mobile hydrogen atom attached to the nitrogen atom, can be converted to other toxic products, whereas the dialkyldithiocarbamates, lacking a mobile hydrogen atom, are stable in this respect. A detailed discussion on the fungitoxicity of both types of dithiocarbamates is given in several reviews (Ludwig and Thorn, 1960; Thorn and Ludwig, 1962; van der Kerk, 1959; Rich, 1960).

Thiram Group

Fungitoxicity of the dimethyldithiocarbamates (DDC) is characterized by the bimodal dosage-response (D-R) curve (Dimond et al., 1941). This type of response is also characteristic of other fungitoxic metal-binding agents such as oxine and pyridinethione (Sijpesteijn et al.,

1957). The deviation of the bimodal D-R curves of these fungitoxicants from those of other materials is due to differential effectiveness of divalent heavy metal DDC species. Copper and zinc appear to be the most critical metals involved (Sijpesteijn et al., 1957; Smale, 1957; Goksoyr, 1955). Materials, such as histidine, that can take metals from DDC destroy its fungitoxic action (van der Kerk, 1959).

Thiram

There is strong evidence that thiram is toxic via metal DDC, because it is reduced to the DDC anion by fungal constituents (Richardson and Thorn, 1961). Another interpretation of fungal reduction of thiram suggests that the DDC anion is a product of a toxic reaction of thiram, namely inhibition of thiols, e.g., coenzyme A (Owens and Rubinstein, 1964). That thiols can reverse inhibition of yeast fermentation by thiram (Sisler and Cox, 1955) supports the latter theory.

On the basis of the nature of metabolic inhibition induced in Neurospora conidia by fungitoxic doses, the DDC fungicides are separable into three groups: (1) those that prevent synthesis of citrate from acetate but have little effect on keto acid metabolism [thiram and ferbam Fe (DDC)$_3$], (2) those that cause citrate and keto acids to accumulate [ziram Zn (DDC)$_2$], and those that have no effect on synthesis or accumulation of citric acid (NaDDC) (Owens and Hayes, 1964). Apparently, these DDC fungicides differ in their mode of fungitoxic action. Because ferbam is bioconverted to thiram (Thorn and Richardson, 1964), the two fungicides can conceivably affect similar systems. Ferbam fails to affect keto acid metabolism because aconitase, which attacks citrate, is iron-dependent. Thiol reversal of activity could occur by removing metals as well as by reducing oxidized thiols.

Nabam Group

This group includes the ethylene bisdithiocarbamates, Vapam and Mylone. These fungitoxicants show a linear DR curve and display a spectrum of action toward fungal species different from that of DDC (Klopping, 1951). According to van der Kerk (1959), compounds of the nabam group give rise to isothiocyanates, which attack cellular thiols. The sequence postulated is nabam > ethylene thiuram monosulfide (ETM) > ethylene bisdiisothiocyanate (Ludwig et al., 1955). However, the effects of maneb on and within fungal cells differ from those of ETM (Moorehart and Crossan, 1962, 1964). Because manganese catalyzes the conversion of nabam to ETM, maneb would also be expected to give rise to ETM. Additional doubt of the isothiocyanate theory of toxicity was raised by Rich and Horsfall (1961), namely, a dithiocarbamate ester is the product of the reaction between isothiocyanate and cellular thiols, and the conversion of nabam to isothiocyanate has yet to be demonstrated under physiologic conditions. Nabam does produce toxic vapors (Rich and Horsfall, 1950), one of which is carbonyl sulfide (Moje et al., 1964).

Nabam

The formation of methyl isothiocyanate in soil treated with Vapan or Mylone is well established (Hughes, 1959; Turner and Corden, 1963; Torgeson et al., 1957). The toxic vapor probably is responsible for the fumigant action of these materials. However, its effects on fungal cells differ from those of Vapam. Vapam affects cell permeability, whereas methyl isothiocyanate fails to do so (Wedding and Kendrick, 1959).

By giving rise to fungitoxic vapors, compounds of the nabam type may have a toxic mechanism not found in dialkyldithiocarbamates. They could also possess mechanisms similar to that of the dialkyldithiocarbamates. Moorehart and Crossan (1964) found that spores of *Colletotrichum capsici* convert maneb to ethylene thiuram disulfide. The disulfide could act through a mechanism similar to that of thiram. Residues of the nabam type of fungicides give rise to trace amounts of ethylene thiourea, which readily permeates plant tissue (Vonk and Sijpesteijn, 1970). Ethylene thiourea persists for some time in plant material, with part of it being converted to 2-imidazoline (Vonk and Sijpesteijn, 1971).

QUINONES

Quinones are well known for their fungitoxic properties. Cloranil (tetrachloro-*p*-benzoquinone), introduced by Cunningham and Sarvelle (1940) for seed treatment, was the first nonmetallic organic fungicides since formaldehyde to be used for plant disease control. Dichlone (2,3-dichloro-1,4-naphthoquinone) is a successful foliar fungicide for fruit and tomato diseases. Both of these compounds may injure plant foliage at high temperature.

Their use as foliar sprays is limited also by sublimation (Rich, 1965). Chloranil, which sublimes at a low temperature (24°C), is effective only on cool-season crops such as crucifers. Dichlone, which sublimes at high summer temperatures (29 to 32°C), loses potency in the field as summer arrives. Formerly, loss of chloranil from foliage was attributed to destruction by photo-oxidation and hydrolysis. Though photoreactions and hydrolysis occur, sublimation of chloranil from residual surface films may be more important in the loss of fungicidal effectiveness.

Dichlone

Fungitoxicity of quinones has been reviewed by McNew and Burchfield (1951), Horsfall (1956), Woodcock (1959), Rich (1960, 1963, 1965) and Sisler (1963). Two mechanisms may account for biologic action of these materials, namely, alkylation and oxidation. Quinones, because they are alpha, beta-unsaturated ketones, alkalate thiols, and amino groups of enzyme systems, and because they are redox chemicals, rob protons from electron-transport systems. Because chlorination of alpha and beta carbons of quinones increase fungitoxicity (Byrde and Woodcock, 1953), alkylation may be important in fungitoxic reactions. Chlorination increases permeability of quinones to fungal cells and increases reactivity of alpha and beta carbons of the quinone ring.

At fungitoxic doses, dichlone affects metabolism of *Neurospora sitphila* at many sites (Owens and Novotny, 1958). It inhibits certain dehydrogenases and carboxylases. Coenzyme A may be the site of action for those enzymes requiring the coenzyme. Dichlone inhibits coenzyme A irreversibly, indicating that it does so by alkylation.

Dichlone inhibits phosphorylation in a manner similar to that of nitrophenol. Apparently, the quinone uncouples phosphorylation from oxidation systems by diverting electrons to an abnormal pathway. It may function in this way while bound to thiol or amino groups (Sisler, 1963).

HETEROCYCLIC NITROGEN FUNGICIDES

Many heterocyclic nitrogen compounds play important roles in the metabolism of microorganisms. Heterocyclic nitrogen compounds should also be potential metabolic inhibitors. Four heterocyclic fungicides containing nitrogen will be considered.

Glyodin

The fungitoxic properties of 2-heptadecyl-2-imidazoline acetate (glyodin) were discovered by Wellman and McCallan (1946). Glyodin is used primarily as a foliar fungicide against apple scab and cherry leaf spot diseases. It is an excellent protectant and has some eradicative action.

Maximum fungitoxicity of glyodin occurs with an alkyl chain of 17 carbons. Presumably, the carbon chain affects performance by influencing permeability (Rich and Horsfall, 1952). Uptake by sensitive fungi is rapid (Miller et al., 1953b). Other fungal spores hinder uptake, presumably by secretions (Miller et al., 1953b; Blumer and Kundert, 1960). Glyodin is concentrated in lipid fractions of fungal cells (Owens and Miller, 1958), and an ambient concentration is required for lethal activity.

Though glyodin destroys selective permeability of fungal membranes (Kottke and Sisler, 1962), other physiologic effects are considered more important in this fungitoxic activity. Glyodin prevents utilization of amino acid and prevents synthesis of tyrosine, gamma-aminobutyric acid, and cysteic acid (Siegal and Crossan, 1960). It inhibits nucleic acid and protein synthesis at fungitoxic levels (Kerridge, 1958). This inhibition can be reversed by guanine. Fungitoxicity can be reversed with xanthine in addition to guanine (West and Wolf, 1955). Apparently glyodin acts by inhibiting purine synthesis.

Glyodin

Dyrene

The *s*-triazines present an interesting group of agricultural pesticides. The anilino derivatives are highly fungitoxic and practically nonphytotoxic; aryloxy derivatives are weakly fungitoxic and highly phytotoxic. The 2,4-dichloro-6(*o*-chloranilino)*s*-triazine (Dyrene) has been developed for use as a fungicide (Schuldt and Wolf, 1956), and various alkylamino derivatives have been developed for use as weed killers (Gysin and Knusli, 1960). Dyrene shows promise as a wide-spectrum fungicide for vegetable crops and turf.

Dyrene

Apparently, Dyrene owes it biologic activity to its reactive chlorines. The compound enters nucleophilic substitution reactions with amino and thiol groups (Burchfield and Storrs, 1956). Although amino groups are preferably attacked, the reaction rates depend upon the dissociation of the biologic groups, as indicated by the effect of pH on the reactions. About 80% of a toxic dose is bound to cellular constituents (Burchfield and Storrs, 1957). The large quantity of Dyrene required for a toxic dose would suggest indiscriminate reaction with many cellular constituents.

At subtoxic concentrations, Dyrene alters permeability of fungal membranes, causing the fungicide and cellular constituents to leak out. At higher concentrations, it is toxic, but for completion of its toxic action, a high ambient concentration of the fungicide is required. Apparently, Dyrene attacks many sites and vital processes within fungi.

Captan

Captan (*N*-trichloromethylthio-4-cyclohexene-1,2-dicarboximide) ranks second to the dithiocarbamates in

importance as an organic fungicide in agriculture. It has a broad spectrum of action and is safe to spray on many crops. Its major use is against fruit diseases. The spectrum of folpet, the phthalimide analog of captan, extends to certain powdery mildews against which captan has little effect. Difolatan, an analog of captan in which the -SCCl₃ group is enlarged to a tetrachloroethylthio form, is more effective than captan against foliar diseases of tomato and potato.

Captan

Interest in the fungitoxicity of captan has approached that of the dithiocarbamates and oxine. Reviews have been frequent (Horsfall, 1956; Rich, 1960, 1963: Massing, 1955; Barbera, 1961; Lukens, 1969, 1971). Both fungitoxicity and detoxication of captan have centered on its reactions with thiols (Lukens and Sisler, 1958; Owens and Blaak, 1960a; Richmond and Somers, 1962a, b, 1963).

Captan and folpet are reduced by cellular thiols to the imides and trichlormethylmercaptan. In this reaction, the thiols are oxidized to disulfide. The trichloromethyl mercaptan can be transferred directly to thiol sites or it can decompose to thiophosgene. Thiophosgene reactions are of two types. It can hydrolyze rapidly to carbonyl sulfide, hydrochloric acid, and hydrogen sulfide, or it can combine with thiols and other functional groups of the cell to form addition products. With intact cells, the initial reaction must proceed on uptake because little free imide can be recovered from treated cells, whereas 11 to 35% of the sulfur of the mercaptan portion of the molecule accumulates in the cells (Siegel and Sisler, 1968).

Fungitoxic doses of captan strongly inhibit respiration of fungi (Hochstein and Cox, 1956; Owens and Novotny, 1959; Montie and Sisler, 1962), presumably by inhibiting certain respiratory enzymes. Inhibition of pyruvate decarboxylase by captan is competitive with cocarboxylase (Hochstein and Cox, 1956). Respiration of acetate to citrate inhibited by captan is due to inactivation of coenzyme A (Owens and Blaak, 1960a). Coenzyme A is reactivated by mild reducing agents.

Although captan causes these inhibitions in fungal cells and although these inhibitions may lead to death of the cells, other lethal actions must occur, too, because thiamine pyrophosphate and thiols fail to reverse fungitoxicity of captan (Hochstein and Cox, 1956; Lukens and Sisler, 1958). The sites of action of other R-SCCl₃ fungicides may be thiol-dependent systems because thiols can reverse fungitoxicity (Lukens et al., 1965).

Although folpet can react with protein thiols to cause inhibition of enzyme activity and resultant products of fungicide decomposition (Siegel, 1971a), low-molecular-weight thiols detoxify unreacted folpet and partially restore activity of inhibited enzymes. Reactions of fungicide with alpha-chymotrypsin, a nonthiol-containing protein, cause conformational changes and inhibition of enzyme activity (Siegel, 1971b). Histidyl groups at the catalytic center may be affected. The reversal of fungitoxicity of captan by histidine (Rich, 1959) and by enriched medium (Adams, 1960) both support the possibility of imide-SCCL$_3$ reacting with nonthiol groups.

Presumably, captan permeates fungal membranes by a lipoid route, because a threshold of lipid solubility is required by imide-SCCl$_3$ compounds for fungitoxicity (Richmond and Somers, 1963). The rate-determining factor for the net uptake of captan appears to be the reaction of captan with cellular thiols (Richmond and Somers, 1962b). Much of the captan removed from the ambient fluid by fungal cells is detoxified. By reducing the thiol content of fungal cells with low concentrations of thiol reactants, a reduction occurs in the amount of captan required for toxicity (Lukens and Rich, 1959; Richmond and Somers, 1962b).

SYSTEMIC FUNGICIDES

Fungicides that are taken up by plants and control disease at distant sites have become a reality with the introduction of ozathiins and benzimidazoles. Many newly discovered compounds show promise for successful application.

Oxathiins

Carboxin (2,3-dihydron-6-methyl-5-phenylcarbamoyl-1,4-oxathiin) is highly selective in the control of diseases that are caused by *Rhizoctonia solani*, smut fungi, and rusts (von Schmeling and Kulka, 1966). Oxycarboxin (in which the sulfenyl is oxidized to the sulfone) is more toxic than carboxin to the rusts. Any substitution or alteration of the phenyl ring, as well as partial oxidation of the sulfur atom, reduces toxicity. The actions of the oxathiins are highly limited to *Basidiomycetes*. With the exception of *Verticillium albo-atrum*, most *Deuteromycetes*, *Ascomycetes*, and *Phycomycetes* spp. are little affected (Edgington et al., 1966). The oxathiins have filled the void in many instances for seed treatment on the removal of mercurials from fungicidal use (Brooks, 1972).

Carboxin

The oxathiins are taken up by sensitive and insensitive fungi alike, with most of the fungicide accumulating in the ribosomal and soluble fractions of disrupted cells (Mathre, 1968). Although synthesis of protein and nucleic acids is strongly interrupted (Mathre, 1970; Rags-

dale and Sisler, 1970), the site of action is considered to be the inhibition of succinate dehydrogenase in the mitochondrial fraction (Mathre, 1971; Lyr et al, 1971; White, 1971). The action is noncompetitive and proceeds only when the enzyme is bound in the mitochondria. The hexose monophosphate shunt appears to be an important respiratory pathway in sensitive fungi (Lyr et al., 1971). Carboxin is highly fungistatic.

Benzimidazoles

Benomyl [1-(butylcarbamoyl)-2-(benzimidazole) carbamic acid, methyl ester] hydrolyzes in acidic solutions to methyl benzimidazolcarbamate (MBC). MBC has been shown to be the principal fungitoxicant of benomyl, which is systemic in plant tissue (Clemons and Sisler, 1969; Peterson and Edgington, 1970; Biehn and Dimond, 1969). Methyl thiophanate, another systemic fungicide, gives rise to MBC in basic solutions and in plant tissue (Vonk and Sijpesteijn, 1971). Thiabendazole [2-(4′-thiazolyl-benzimidazol)] is a fungicide systemic in plants, also. All three display similar fungitoxic action. They are highly effective against some basidiomycetes, ascomycetes, and imperfect fungi, especially those that cause powdery mildews, apple scab, and peach brown rot. Notable exceptions are phycomycete pathogens causing downy mildews and late blight of potato; *Helminthosporium* blights of turf grasses and grains; and tomato early blight caused by *Alternaria solani*.

MBC

The actions of benomyl and MBC are essentially the same in most fungi. Synthesis of DNA is severely inhibited before other systems are affected (Clemons and Sisler, 1971). However, in studies with synchronized cells, the inhibition of DNA synthesis occurs after a disruption in mitosis. Doublets formed contain only a single compact nucleus (Hammerschlag and Sisler, 1973). The compound inhibits the synthesis of tuberlin, an essential component of the tubercles involved in mytosis. Benomyl can affect primary metabolism, e.g., respiration and RNA and protein syntheses. These secondary actions can be attributed to butyl isocyanate, a coproduct with MBC on hydrolysis of benomyl.

Resistance to MBC Fungicides

Shortly after the introduction of benomyl, fungi tended to develop resistance where it was used exclusively throughout the disease period. Efforts to retard or delay the selection of resistance by combining benomyl with contact fungicides of dissimilar modes of action were met with little success. Where the use of the fungicide was restricted during the diseased period, resistance to the fungicide did not develop. Evidently, the selection for resistance to benomyl necessitates a constant exposure of the fungicide to a population of the pathogen within the crop. Contact fungicide with its sphere of action limited to the plant surface was insufficient in joint action with benomyl to retard the selection of resistance to benomyl (Szkolnik et al., 1978; McGee and Zuck, 1981).

Terrazole

Terrazole (5-ethoxy-3-trichloromethyl-1,2,4-thiadiazole) is highly toxic to the phycomycete fungi *Pythium* and *Phytophthora*, which cause rots and seedling and turf blights. The compound has some effect against *Rhizoctonia*, *Verticillium*, and *Fusarium* pathogens. Systemic action in plants has been reported (Al-Bleldawi and Sinclair, 1969). Little is known about the fungitoxic action. Fungitoxicity is retained if the 5-ethoxy group is replaced by chloro or amino groups, whereas members containing diethylamino, methoxy, or butoxy groups at the 5-position are herbicidal (Schroeder, 1966).

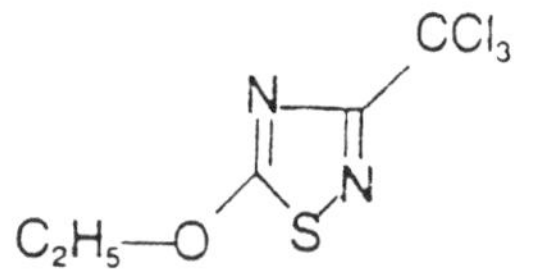

Terrazole

Chloroneb

This systemic fungicide (1,4-dichloro-2,5-dimethoxybenzene) is effective against root rots and seedling blights. Following application to soil, the fungicide accumulates in roots and lower stems (Fielding and Rhodes, 1967). Chloroneb acts synergistically with thiram to inhibit mycelial growth (Richardson, 1973). *Rhizoctonia solani*, a sensitive fungus, hydrolyzes chloroneb to its corresponding phenol (Hock and Sisler, 1969). Sensitivity to the fungicide is related neither to its uptake nor to conversion to other products (Tillman and Sisler, 1971). At growth-inhibiting concentrations, chloroneb inhibits the synthesis of DNA more than RNA or protein does. The action is directed against the polymerization of nucleotidase into DNA (Hock and Sisler, 1969).

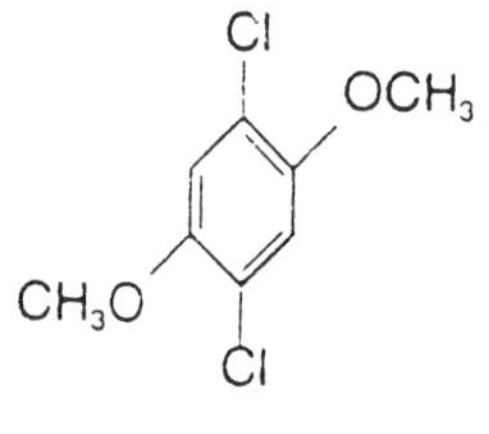

Chloroneb

Acetylanilines

Metalaxyl (*N*-(2,6-dimethyl)-*N*-(methoxyacetyl) alanine methyl ester) and Ofurace (2-chloro-*N*-(2,6-dimethyl phenyl-*N*-(2,6-dimethyl phenyl)-*N*-(tetrahydro-2-oxo-3-furanyl) acetamide) are curative systemic fungicides highly effective against phycomycete plant pathogens (Staug et al., 1978; Lukens et al., 1978). The fungicides tend to be 10 to 100 times more active on plants in controlling disease than they are on agar media in inhibiting fungal growth. Field resistance to these fungicides has occurred during exclusive use of metalaxyl, but not where either was used with other fungicides during the periods of active disease.

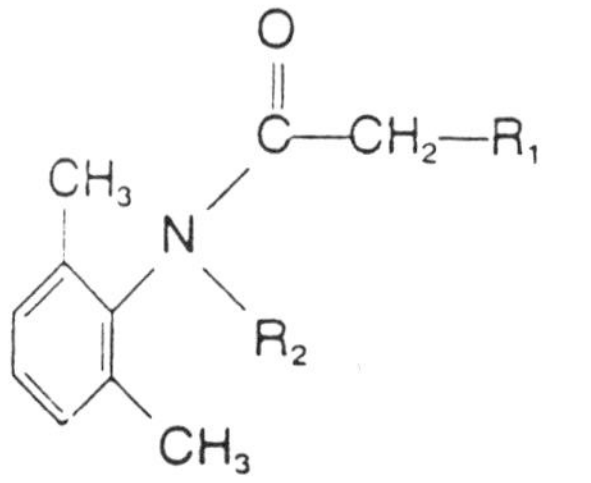

Metalaxyl: R₁ = methoxy, R₂ = methyl-2-propanate
Ofurace: R₁ = Cl, R₂ = *N*(tetrahydro-2-oxo-3-furanyl)

Structure-activity studies on disease control indicate a lock-and-key fit of the phenyl moiety with high efficacy restricted to 2,6-dimethyl or dichloro substituents in addition to a naphthylene structure as effective members. Some variation in R₂ is effective with active lactone or beta-alanine. Variation in the acetyl moiety is restricted to R₁ being (or giving rise to) a leaving group for Sn2 reactions (Lukens et al., 1978).

Little is known about the mode of action of the acetylanilines. Phytoalexins may play a role in the therapeutic action. Lukens (unpublished) found no indication of phaseolin in pinto beans following treatment with ofurace. However, metalaxyl has been reported to increase glyceollin synthesis in soybean once the phytoalexin has been elicited by an invading pathogen (Ward et al., 1980).

Fungitoxicity appears to involve the inhibition of RNA synthesis and, in turn, protein synthesis and reduction in mitosis with some effect on lipid synthesis (Fisher and Hayes, 1982).

Sterol Inhibitors

The new systemic fungicides, fenarimol (alpha-(4-chlorophenyl)-5-pyrimidinemethanol), triforine (*N*, *N'*-bis(1-formamido-2,2,2-trichloroethyl)piperdine), triadimefon (1-(4-chlorophenoxy) -3,3- dimethyl-1-(1-*H*-1,2,4-triazol-1-yl)-2-butanone), imazolil (1-2(2,4-dichlorophenyl)-2-(2-propenyloxy-ethyl))-1*H*-imidazole), and etaconazole (1 - (2 - (2,4 - dichlorophenyl) - 4 - ethyl - 1,3 - dioxolan - 2yl-methyl)-1*H*1,2,4-triazole), inhibit basidiomycete and ascomycete plant pathogens that require ergosterol for growth (Ragsdale, 1977; Siegel and Ragsdale, 1978; Buchenauer, 1977a, b; Henry and Sisler, 1981). Triadimefon is readily bioreduced to tridimenol, which also is a fungicide. In cells treated with fungicides, levels of C-4 desmethyl sterols decline with a concomitant increase in methyl and dimethyl sterols. The sites of inhibition appear to be the C-14 or C-4 demethylation. Other bioresponses to the fungicides have been noted, e.g., fungitoxicity reversed by sterols and fatty acids and differential sensitivities of mycelial growth and sporulation to individual fungicides. The basic site of fungitoxicity in growing cultures appears to be the inhibition of ergosterol synthesis.

P254 cytochrome system appears to be central to the bioactivity of these compounds. There is no chemical structure common to these fungicides that can be said to effect fungitoxicity. However, a carbonium ion appears to be a reactive intermediate common to all of these compounds.

The sterol-inhibiting fungicides are mobile within plants exerting curative action against disease, often at very low doses. However, these fungicides exhibit growth-regulating effects that may limit their usefulness on crops.

Among the newly introduced sterol-inhibiting type fungicides for the control of plant diseases are penconzole, diclobutrazole, diniconazle, triapenthenol, flusilazol, pyrifenox, and RH-7592 (2-cyno-2-phenyl-2-(beta-p-chlorophenethyl)-ethyl-1H-1,2,4-triazole).

MISCELLANEOUS FUNGICIDES

Dodine

Dodecylguanidine acetate (dodine), like glyodin, is a fungitoxic cationic surfactant. Its major use is on apple for controlling scab. Because of its eradicative properties and its control of powdery mildew, it has certain advantages over other scab fungicides.

$$C_{12}H_{25}-NHC-NH_3^{+-}O-C-CH_3$$
$$\overset{\|}{N}\,H$$

Dodine

Like glyodin, the alkyl carbon chain of dodine influences its toxic action. The 12-carbon homolog is the most effective (Brown and Sisler, 1960). Toxicity increases with rise in pH within the range of pH 5 to 8. Dodine is concentrated quickly within fungal cells, where it inhibits glucose oxidation. Although this inhibition may not be directly tied to toxicity, it illustrates the potential of dodine to inhibit enzymatic reactions. Dodine alters cell permeability to allow leakage of phosphorus and amino materials for poisoned cells. Toxicity is attributed to its surfactant activity at the cell membrane and inactivation of certain vital enzymes (Brown and Sisler, 1960; Forsyth, 1964). Affected vital enzymes have yet to be determined.

Chlorothalonil

Chlorothalonil (2,4,5,6-tetrachlorisophthalonitrile) is a broad-spectrum fungicide highly effective on a wide variety of crops (Turner et al., 1964; Didario et al., 1965). The compound is used as a fumigant (it sublimes when heated about 100°C) on greenhouse crops (Turner et al., 1965). Chlorothalonil reacts with thiols to form addition products. Such reactions involve detoxication of the compound as well as fungitoxicity. Addition products of chlorothalonil and glutathione are recovered from treated fungal cells. Thiols can reverse fungitoxicity. Chlorothalonil inhibits both oxidation of glucose at growth-inhibiting concentrations and activity of purified preparations of thio-dependent enzymes (Vincent and Sisler, 1968). Within a series of halogenated analogs of chlorothalonil, fungitoxicity was closely related to chemical reactions of the compound with thiols. Within the series examined, the hydrophobic bonding property of the compounds did not limit fungitoxicity (Turner and Battershall, 1970).

Chlorothalonil

Chlorinated Nitrobenzenes

Chlorinated nitrobenzenes are a unique group of fungicides that are toxic to a limited number of plant pathogens. Tetrachloronitrobenzene (TCNB) is a practical treatment on lettuce for *Botrytis*, on potato for *Fusarium*, and on cabbage for *Plasmodiophora* club root. When applied to soil, pentachloronitrobenzene (PCNB) combats damping-off diseases of seedlings caused by *Rhizoctonia solani* and *Sclerotinium rolfsii*.

Pentachloronitrobenzene

The uniqueness of the chlorinated nitrobenzenes extends to the types of resistance that fungi develop toward them. Here, resistance is clear-cut and is genetically controlled. Georgopoulos (1963b) has shown in *Hypomyces solani f. cucurbitae* that resistance to PCNB is found in three independent genes, one of which is linked with a locus for mating type. Apparently, it is linked with loci for pathogenicity, too, because fungal mutants resistant to PCNB have little pathogenicity (Georgopoulos, 1963a; Elsaid and Sinclair, 1964; Shalta and Sinclair, 1963). An exception is *Botrytis allii*, strains of which may be resistant to PCNB and still retain their pathogenicity to onions (Priest and Wood, 1961).

Fungal resistance to one chlorinated nitrobenzene fungicide extends to other chlorinated, brominated, and fluorinated nitrobenzenes as well as to 2,6-dichloro-4-nitroaniline, an effective material against *Botrytis* (Priest and Wood, 1961; Georgopoulos, 1963b). This may suggest a common mode of action for these materials.

Fungitoxicity increases with increase in chlorination of nitrobenzene with maximum effect in TCNB and PCNB (Eckert, 1962). Presumably, chlorination aids permeation by reducing water solubility of the compounds. With TCNB, the 2,3,5,6-tetrachloro isomer is far more effective than other isomers (Brooks, 1952). Because TCNB may act as a vapor, the difference in effect between isomers may be due to differences in modes of action or permeability rates. Phytotoxicity is minimal with PCNB. Because it persists in soil, PCNB is an excellent soil treatment for certain root pathogens. The material is only fungistatic. Eckert (1962) suggested that the chlorinated nitrobenzenes are nonspecific inhibitors. In view of the fungal resistance to these compounds, however, resistant fungi have a unique means for bypassing the inhibition, which could be an enzyme for detoxication. This is feasible in light of genetically controlled resistance to PCNB.

Fenaminosulf

Fenaminosulf is a common name for dimethylaminobenzenediazo sodium sulfonate, a fungicide with restricted action. It attacks the water mold pathogens, *Pythium*, *Phytophthora*, and *Aphanomyces*. Because fenaminosulf's potency is destroyed by light (Hills and Leach, 1962), its use is restricted to seed and soil treatments. Tolmsoff (1962) attributed the specificity of fenaminosulf to its attack on the pyridine nucleotide-cytochrome system, the major pathway for electron transport in *pythium*. This system is not present in *rhizoctonia*, a fungus resistant to fenaminosulf. However, because respiration of *pythium* is not affected by toxic doses of fenaminosulf (Torgeson, 1963), terminal oxidative systems may not be the primary site of toxic action.

Fenaminosulf

Dinitro Derivatives

Generally, dinitro derivatives are too phytotoxic for use on plants. Dinitro-*o*-cresol has been used as a ground spray to eradicate *Venturia inequalis* in litter beneath apple trees (Keitt et al., 1941), but the practice has since been discarded because it was not sufficiently effective.

Karathane (2-(1-methyl-*n*-heptyl)-4,4-dinitro phenyl crotonate), which is safe to plant foliage, is used to control powdery mildew diseases. It controls mites also. Its fungitoxicity was initially examined by Rich and Horsfall (1949). Though it was highly toxic to the pathogens tested, it lost its potency on drying. Fungitoxicity was ascribed to the crotonic acid moiety, because this was hydrolyzed in spray residues. However, toxicity has since been ascribed to the phenolic moiety because the free phenol is nearly as fungitoxic as Karathane (Kirby and Frick, 1958).

Karathane

SOIL DISINFECTANTS

Chloropicrin and several halogenated straight-chain hydrocarbons, together with Vapam and Mylone, are extensively employed to disinfect soil of plant pathogenic fungi and nematodes. These materials are phytotoxic and have to be applied to soil 1 to 3 months prior to planting crops. These materials are general toxicants and destroy plant pathogenic organisms as well as their competitors in soil. From lack of competition, plant pathogens could become severe if reinfestation occurs. The normal microcommunity may require up to 3 years for reestablishment when destroyed by soil treatments. Because intensive cultivation favors development of high amounts of plant pathogens in the soil, soil treatments are a necessity under continuous cultivation of a single crop.

Most soil disinfectants act through vapors. For a discussion of factors influencing fumigant action in soil, the reader is referred to Hemwell (1960). Moje (1959, 1960) related chemical structure of halogenated hydrocarbons to toxic reactions with nematodes. These compounds enter unimolecular and bimolecular nucleophilic displacement reactions. The type and rate of reaction that proceeds would depend upon hydrocarbon group, halogen, biologic reactive groups, and solvent conditions.

Formaldehyde has been used for many years as a sole disinfectant. Again, its toxicity is not limited to plant pathogens, and it is primarily a protein denaturant, possibly by combining with amino groups as it does in Sorenson formal titration of amino acids (Rich, 1960).

ANTIBIOTICS

The performance of antibiotics in plant disease control has not measured up to early expectations. Although antibiotics are our most potent toxicants, they have failed in practice because of phytotoxicity, instability, poor systemic activity, or cost. Streptomycin, griseofulvin, and cycloheximide have been used to a limited degree, the latter being the most widely used antifungal antibiotic.

Cycloheximide

The antifungal antibiotic cycloheximide (*beta*(2-(3,5-dimethyl-2-oxyxyxlohexyl)-2-hydroxyethyl)glutarimide) is another product of *Streptomyces griseus*, the streptomycin-producing actinomycete (Whiffen et al., 1946). The antibiotic attacks many plant pathogens, but is too phytotoxic for general use. For information about its use in agriculture, see Ford et al. (1958).

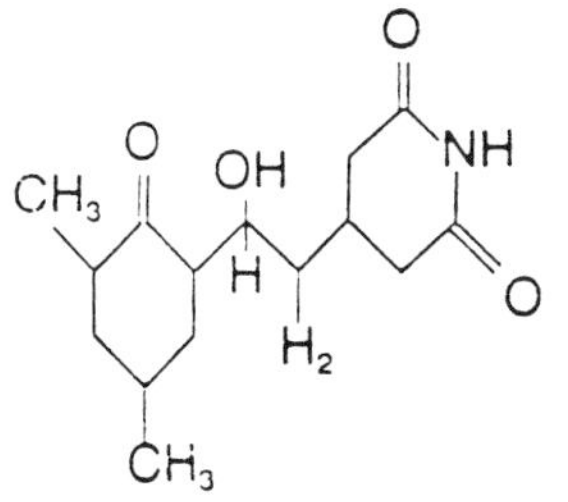

Cycloheximide

Cycloheximide is a highly specific inhibitor. Its effective innate toxicity is low (ED_{50} = 0.38 mg/kg fresh weight of *Saccharomyces pastorianus*) (Wescott and Sisler, 1964). The compound has little effect on energy-producing systems, but it inhibits synthesis of many diversified cellular constituents. See Sisler (1963), Sisler and Coursen (1960), and Coursen and Sisler (1960) for details. Cycloheximide inhibits protein synthesis at doses lower than those needed to inhibit DNA (Kerridge, 1958; Shepard, 1958; Siegel and Sisler, 1964a, b). In mammalian cells, it inhibits the transfer of amino acid from soluble RNA to polypeptide (Ennis and Lubin, 1964). In resistant organisms, *Escherichia coli* and *Streptococcus fragilis*, protein synthesis is not affected. The antibiotic permeates resistant yeast cells, but fails to accumulate as it does in susceptible yeast cells (Wescott and Sisler, 1964). Resistance can be attributed to the ribosome fraction of the resistant yeast. Protein-synthesizing systems from both resistant and susceptible yeast are not inhibited by cycloheximide when ribosomes for resistant yeast are present (Siegel and Sisler, 1964c).

Tetracycline

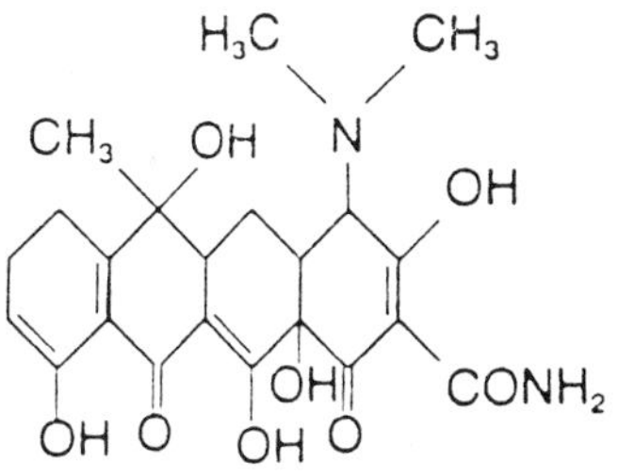

Tetracycline

This antibiotic is effective against plant disease caused by mycoplasma. Injection of tetracycline or oxytetracycline at concentrated solutions into tree trunks can inhibit symptoms of peach-X, pear decline, coconut palm yellows, and citrus greening (McCoy, 1972; Nyland and Moller, 1973; Capoor and Thirumalackar, 1973). However, problems of distribution in the tree limit the practical utility of the antibiotic against tree diseases. In sensitive bacteria, tetracycline inhibits protein synthesis by preventing the binding of AA*t*RNA to ribosome A-Site (Pestka, 1971). Other steps in protein synthesis may be affected at higher concentrations of the antibiotic.

NONFUNGITOXIC MATERIALS

Tricyclazole

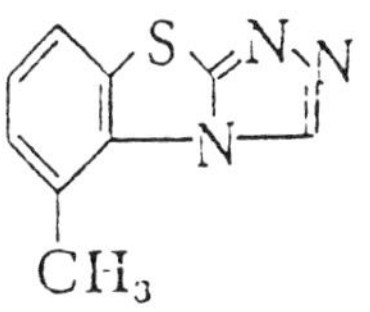

Tricyclazole

Tricyclazole was found to be highly effective in the control of rice blast disease. However, it is nontoxic to the pathogen *Piricularia oryzae*. On tricyclazole-amended media the fungus appears white, apparently lacking melanin pigmentation. Colorless mutants of the pathogen are commonly nonpathogenic. Biochemical studies, show that, indeed, tricyclazole inhibits the synthesis of melanin (Woloshuk, et al., 1981). The lack of pathogenicity of the pathogen when grown on tetrazole-amended media was shown to be ascribed to the lack of functioning of the appresoria (modified hyphal cells that are necessary for host penetration). Haline appresoria lack the rigidity required as back pressure to force the infection peg through the epidermis of the rice plant.

CONCLUSION

Though this discussion is by no means thorough, it gives a glimpse of the kinds of materials used, their role in disease control, and their biologic action. Although knowledge of the biologic action is far from complete, we have a workable understanding for wise use of the materials. The high capacity of protectant fungicides to enter chemical reactions provides an element of safety in their continued use, because it prevents development both of resistant fungi and of a high residual potency when that potency is no longer desired.

REFERENCES

Adams, A.M. 1960. Functional inhibition of Saccharomyces spp. by captan and phaltan. Rep. Hort. Exp. Sta. Prod. Lab., *15959–60*, 72–78.
Al-Beldawi, A.S., and Sinclair, J.B. 1969. Evidence for systemic activity of ter-

razole against *Rhizoctonia solani* in cotton seedlings. Phytopathology, 59, 68–70.

Aldridge, W.N., and Cremer, J.E. 1955. The chemistry of organo-tin compounds. Biochem. J., *61*, 406–418.

Ashworth, L.J., Jr., and Amin, J.V. 1964. A mechanism for mercury tolerance in fungi. Phytopathology, *54*, 1459–1463.

Barbera, C. 1961. Los fungicidas organicos. I. Trichlorometilsulfenil-derivados. Quim. Industr. Bibao, 7, 183–189.

Biehn, W.L., and Dimond, A.E. 1969. Reduction of tomato Fusarium wilt symptoms by 1-butylcarbamoyl-2-benzimidazole carbamic acid, methyl ester. Phytopathology, 59, 397.

Blumer, S., and Kundert, J. 1960. Uber den Einflub der Terperatur aud die Wirkung von Fungiziden. Landw. J.G. Schweig. N.F., *9*, 465–495.

Bodnar, J., and Terenyi, A. 1932. Biochemistry of the smut disease of cereals, Note 4. The mechanism of the action of mercury salts on the spores of wheat bunt (*Tilletra tritici*(bjeck)Winter). Hoppe-Seylers Z. Physiol. Chem., *207*, 78–92.

Brewer, J.H. 1940. Clear liquid medium for the "aerobic" cultivation of anaerobes. JAMA, *115*, 598–600.

Brook, M. 1952. Differences in the biological activity of 2,3,5.6-tetrachloronitrobenzene and its isomers. Nature, *170*, 1022.

Brooks, D.H. 1972. Results in practice. I. Cereals. In *Systemic Fungicides*. Edited by R.W. Marsh. London, Longman Group Ltd., pp. 186–205.

Brown, I.F., and Sisler, H.D. 1960. Mechanisms of fungitoxic action of n-dodecylguanidine acetate. Phytopathology, *50*, 830–839.

Buchenauer, H. 1977a. Mechanism of action of the fungicide imazilil in *Ustilago avenae*. Z. Pflanzenkeiten Pflanzenschutz, *84*, 440–450.

Buchenauer, H. 1977b. Mode of action of triadimefon in *Ustilago avenae*. Pestic. Biochem. Physiol., *7*, 309–320.

Burchfield, H.P., and Goenaga, A. 1957. Some factors governing the deposition and tenacity of copper fungicide sprays. Contrib. Boyce Thompson Inst., *19*, 141–156.

Burchfield, H.P., and Storrs, E. 1957. Effects of chlorine substitution and isomerism on the interactions of s-triazine derivatives with conidia of *Neurospora sitophila*. Contrib. Boyce Thompson Inst., *18*, 429–452.

Burchfield, H.P., Storrs, E. 1956. Chemical structures and dissociation constants of amino acids, peptides, and proteins in relation to their reaction rates with 2,4-dichloro-6-(*o*-chloroanilino)-*s*-triazine. Contrib. Boyce Thompson Inst., *18*, 395–418.

Byrde, R.J.W., and Woodcock, D. 1953. Fungicidal activity and chemical constitution. II. Compounds related to 2,3-dichloro-1,4-naphthaquinone. Ann. Appl. Biol., *40*, 675–687.

Capoor, S.P., and Thirumalackar, M.J. 1973. Cure of greening affected citrus plants by chemotherapeutic agents. Plant Dis. Reptr., *57*, 160–163.

Clemons, G.P., and Sisler, H.D. 1971. Localization of the site of action of a fungitoxic benomyl derivative. Pestic. Biochem. Biophys., *1*, 32–43.

Clemons, G.P., and Sisler, H.D. 1969. Formation of a fungitoxic derivative from benolate. Phytopathology, *59*, 705–706.

Coursen, B.W., and Sisler, H.D. 1960. Effect of the antibiotic, cycloheximide, on the metabolism and growth of *Saccharomyces pastorianus*. Am. J. Bot., *47*, 541–549.

Cunningham, H.S., and Sharvelle, E.G. 1940. Organic seed protectants for lime beans. Phytopathology, *30*, 4.

Daines, R.H., Lukens, R.J., Brennan, E., and Leone, L.A. 1957. Phytotoxicity of captan as influenced by formulation, environment, and plant factors. Phytopathology, *47*, 657–672.

Danielli, J.F., and Davis, J.T. 1951. Reactions at interfaces in relation to biological problems. Adv. Enzymol., *11*, 35.

DiDaria, A., Curry, T.L., Thayer, P., and Turner, N.J. 1965. The biological performance of tetrachloroisophthalonitrile as influenced by particle size and crystalline form. Phytopathology, *55*, 1055.

Dimond, A.E., Heuberger, J.W., and Stoddard, E.M. 1941. Role of the dosage-response curve in the evaluation of fungicides. Conn. Agric. Exp. Stat. Bull., *451*, 635–667.

Duyfjes, W. 1958. The formulation of pesticides. Philips Tech. Rev., *19*, 165–176.

Echert, J.W. 1962. Fungistatic and phytotoxic properties of some derivatives of nitrobenzene. Phytopathology, *52*, 642–649.

Edgington, L.V., Walton, G.S., and Miller, P.M. 1966. Fungicide selective for *Basidiomycetes*. Science, *153*, 307–308.

Elsaid, H.M., and Sinclair, J.B. 1964. Adapted tolerance to organic fungicides by isolates of *Rhizoctonia solani* from seedling cotton. Phytopathology, *45*, 518–522.

Ennis, H.L., and Lubin, M. 1964. Cyclohexidmide: Aspects of inhibition of protein synthesis in mammalian cells. Science, *146*, 1474–1476.

Ferguson, J. 1939. The use of chemical potentials as indices of toxicity. Proc. R. Soc., *127*, 387–404.

Fielding, M.J., and Rhodes, R.C. 1867. Studies with C14 labeled chloroneb fungicide in plants. Proc. Ann. Cotton Dis. Counc., *27*, 56–58.

Fildes, P. 1940. The mechanism of the antibacterial action of mercury. Br. J. Pathol., *21*, 67–73.

Fisher, D.J., and Hayes, A.L. 1982. Mode of action of the systemic fungicides furalaxyl, metaloxyl, and ofurace. Pestic. Sci., *13*, 330–339.

Ford, J.H., Klomparens, W., and Hammer, C.L. 1958. Cycloheximide (Actidion) and its agricultural uses. Plant Dis. Reptr., *42*, 680–695.

Forsyth, F.R. 1964. Surfactants as fungicides. Can. J. Bot., *42*, 1335–1347.

Fowler, D.L., and Mahan, J.N. 1973. *The Pesticide Review*. Washington, D.C., Agriculture Stabilization and Conservation Service, Washington.

Gassner, G., and Esdorn, I. 1923. Beitràge sur Frage der Chemotherapeutischen Bervertung gegen Weiznstreinbrand. Arb. Biol. Beichstanstalt. Land-u. Forstwirtsch Berlin-Dahlem, *11*, 373–385.

Georgopoulos, S.G. 1963a. Pathogenicity of chlorinated-nitrobenzene-tolerant strains of *Hypomyces solani* F. *cucurbitae* race 1. Phytopathology, *53*, 1081–1085.

Georgopoulos, S.G. 1963b. Tolerance to chlorinated nitrobenzene in *Hypomyces solani* F. *cucurbitae* and its mode of inheritance. Phytopathology, *53*, 1086–1093.

Goksyr, J. 1955. The effect of some dithiocarbamal compounds on the metabolism of fungi. Physiol. Plantar., *8*, 719–835.

Goldsworthy, M.C., and Green, E.L. 1936. Availability of the copper of Bordeaux mixture residues and its absorption by the conidia of *Sclerotinia fructicola*. J. Agric. Res., *52*, 517–533.

Gysin, H., and Knusli, E. 1960. Chemistry and herbicidal properties of triazine derivatives. In *Advances in Pest Control Research*. Edited by R.L. Metcalf. New York, Interscience Publishers, pp. 289–358.

Hammerschlag, R.S., and Sisler, H.D. 1973. Benomyl and methyl-2-benzimidazolecarbamate (MBC): Biochemical, cytological and chemical aspects of toxicity to *Ustilago maydis* and *Saccharomyces cerevisiae*. Pestic. Biochem. Physiol., *3*, 42–54.

Hartel, K. 1958. Organic tin compound as a crop fungicide. Q.J. Tin Res. Inst., *43*, 9–14.

Hemwall, J.B. 1960. Theoretical considerations of several factors influencing the effectivity of soil fumigants under field conditions. Soil Sci., *90*, 157–168.

Henry, M.J., and Sisler, H.D. 1981. Inhibition of ergosterol biosynthesis in *Ustilago maydis* by the fungicide 1-(2-(2,4-dichlorophenyl)-4-ethyl-1,3-dioxolan-2yl-methyl)-1*H*-1,2,4-triazole. Pestic. Sci., *12*, 98–102.

Hills, F.J., and Leach, L.D. 1962. Photochemical decomposition and biological activity of *p*-dimethylaminobenzenediazo sodium sulfonate (Dexon). Phytopathology, *52*, 51–56.

Hochstein, P.E., and Cox, C.E. 1956. Studies on the fungicidal action of N-(trichloromethylthio)-4-cyclohexene-1,2-dicarboximide (Captan). Am. J. Bot., *43*, 437–441.

Hock, W.K., and Sisler, H.D. 1969. Specificity and mechanism of antifungal action of chloroneb. Phytopathology, *59*, 627–632.

Horsfall, J.G. 1956. *Principles of Fungicidal Action*. Waltham, MA, Chronica Botanica, pp. 141–210.

Horsfall, J.G. 1945. *Fungicides and Their Action*. Waltham, MA, Chronica Botanica, pp. 42–96.

Horsfall, J.G., Marsh, R.W., and Martin, H. 1937. Studies upon the copper fungicides. IV. The fungicidal value of the copper oxides. Ann. Rev. Biol., *24*, 867–882.

Hughes, J.T. 1959. Preliminary observations on the conversion of sodium-N-methyldithiocarbamate (Metham-sodium) to methyl isothiocyanate in soil. Rept. Glassh. Crops Res. Inst., 108–111.

Keitt, G.W., Clayton, C.N., and Langford, M.H. 1941. Experiments with eradicant fungicides for combating apple scab. Phytopathology, *31*, 296–322.

Kerridge, D. 1958. The effect of Actidione and other antifungal agents on nucleic acid and protein synthesis in *Saccharomyces carlsbergensis*. J. Gen. Microbiol., *19*, 497–506.

Kirby, A.H.M., and Frich, E.L. 1958. Karathane: The relative importance of the phenolic and unsaturated acid components in toxicity towards certain plant pathogens. Nature, *182*, 1445–1446.

Klopping, H.L. 1951. *Chemical Constitution and Antifungal Action of Sulfur Compounds*. Utrecht, Schotamus and Jens, p. 142.

Kottke, M., and Sisler, H.D. 1962. Effect of fungicides on permeability of yeast cells to the pyruvate ion. Phytopathology, *52*, 959–961.

Ludwig, R.A., and Thorn, G.D. 1960. Chemistry and mode of action of dithiocarbamate fungicides. Adv. Pest Cont. Res., *3*, 219–252.

Ludwig, R.A., Thorn, G.D., and Unwin, C.H. 1955. Studies on the mechanism of fungicidal action of metallic ethylenebisdithiocarbamates. Can. J. Bot., *33*, 42–59.

Lukens, R.J. 1971. *Chemistry of Fungicides. Molecular Biochemistry and Biophysics*. Volume 10. New York-Heidelberg-Berlin, Springer-Verlag.

Lukens, R.J. 1969. Heterocyclic nitrogen compounds. In *Fungicides*. Volume II. Edited by D. Torgeson. New York, Academic Press, pp. 395–445.

Lukens, R.J., and Rich, S. 1959. Cobalt pretreatment of yeast cells increases toxicity of captan. Phytopathology, *49*, 228.

Lukens, R.J., and Sisler, H.D. 1958. Chemical reactions involved in the fungitoxicity of captan. Phytopathology, *48*, 235–244.

Lukens, R.J., Chan, D., and Etter, G. 1978. ORTHO 20615, a new systemic for the control of plant diseases caused by *oomycetes*. Phytopathol. News, *12*(9), 142.

Lukens, R.J., Rich, S., and Horsfall, J.G. 1965. Role of the R-group in the fungitoxicity of R-SCCl₃ compounds. Phytopathology, 55, 658–662.

Lyr, H., Luthardt, W., and Ritter, G. 1971. Wirkungsweise von Oxathiin-Derivaten auf die Physiologie sensitiver und insensitiver Hefearten. Z. Allg. Microbiol., 11, 373–385.

Lyr, H., Ritter, G., and Casperson, G. 1971. Wirkungsmechanisms des systemichen Fungicids Carboxin. Z. Allg. Microbiol., 12, 271–280.

Marsh, P.B. 1945. Salts as antidotes to copper in its toxicity to the conidia of Sclerotinia fructicola. Phytopathology, 35, 54–61.

Martin, H. 1964. The Scientific Principles of Crop Protection. 5th Edition. New York, St. Martin's Press, pp. 62–151.

Massing, W. 1955. Captan in Rehmen der anderen Fungizide. Möglichkeiten und Grenzen des Einstaze. Mitt. Biol. Bundesanstalt Land-u. Berlin-Dahlen, Forstwistach, 83, 59–68.

Mathre, D.E. 1971. Mode of action of oxathiin systemic fungicides. III. Effect of mitochondrial activities. Pestic. Biochem. Physiol., 1, 216.

Mathre, D.E. 1970. Mode of action of oxathiin systemic fungicides. I. Effect of carboxin and oxycarboxin on the general metabolism of several basidiomycetes. Phytopathology, 60, 671–676.

Mathre, D.E. 1968. Uptake and binding of oxathiin systemic fungicides by resistant and sensitive fungi. Phytopathology, 58, 1464–1469.

McCallan, S.E.A., and Miller, L.P. 1963. Uptake of fungitoxicants by spores. Conn. Agric. Exp. Stat. Bull., 663, 137–148.

McCallan, S.E.A., and Wilcoxon, F. 1936. The action of fungus spores on Bordeaux mixture. Contrib. Boyce Thompson Inst., 8, 151–165.

McCoy, R.E. 1972. Remission of lethal yellowing in coconut palm treated with tetracycline antibiotics. Plant Dis. Reptr., 56, 1019–1021.

McGee, D.C. and Zuck, M.G. 1981. Competition between benomyl-resistant and sensitive strains of Venturia inaequalis on apple seedlings. Phytopathology, 71, 529–532.

McNew, G.L., and Burchfield, H.P. 1951. Fungitoxicity and biological activity of quinones. Contrib. Boyce Thompson Inst., 16, 357–374.

Metcalf, R.L. 1971. Pesticides. J. Soil Water Conserv., 2, 57–60.

Miller, L.P. 1962. Natural membranes. In Diffusion and Membrane Technology. Edited by S.B. Turviner. New York, Reinhold, pp. 345–467.

Miller, L.P., and Russakow, N. 1964. Quantitative studies on possible competition of silver, cerium, and dodine for receptor sites in fungus spores. Phytopathology, 54, 900–901.

Miller, L.P., McCallan, S.E.A., and Weed, R.M. 1953a. Quantitative studies on the role of hydrogen sulfide formation in the toxic action of sulfur to fungus spores. Contrib. Boyce Thompson Inst., 17, 151–171.

Miller, L.P., McCallan, S.E.A., and Weed, R.M. 1953b. Rate of uptake and toxic dose on a spore weight basis of various fungicides. Contrib. Boyce Thompson Inst., 17, 173–195.

Moje, W. 1960. The chemistry and nematocidal activity of organic halides. In Advances in Pest Control Research. Volume 3. Edited by R.L. Metcalf. New York, Interscience Publishers, pp. 181–217.

Moje, W. 1959. Structure and nematocidal activity of allylic and acetylenic halids. J. Agric. Food Chem., 7, 702–707.

Moje, W., Munnecke, D.W., and Richardson, L.T. 1964. Carbonyl sulfide, a volatile fungitoxicant from nabam in soil. Nature, 202, 831–832.

Montie, T.C., and Sisler, H.D. Effects of captan on glucose metabolism and growth of Saccharomyces pastorianus. Phytopathology, 50, 94–102.

Moorehart, A.L., and Crossan, D.F. 1964. Isolation of ethylene bis(thiocarbamyl)disulfide from fungicide-exposed spores. Phytopathology, 54, 1278.

Moorehart, A.L., and Crossan, D.F. 1962. The effect of manganese ethylene bisdithiocarbamate (maneb) on some chemical constituents of Colletotrichum capsici. Toxicol. Appl. Pharmacol., 4, 720–729.

Mukhopadhyay, A.N., and Thakur, R.P. 1972. Systemic activity of triphenyltin chloride in sugar beet seedlings. Plant Dis. Reptr., 56, 776–778.

Muller, E., and Biedermann, W. 1952. Der Einfluss von Cu⁺⁺ Ionen auf den Keimungablouf von Alternaria tenuis. Phytopath. Z., 19, 343–350.

Nyland, G., and Miller, W.J. 1967. Control of pear decline with a tetracycline. Plant Dis. Reptr., 57, 634–637.

Ordish, G., and Mitchell, J.F. 1967. World fungicide usage. In Fungicides. Volume 1. Edited by D.C. Torgeson. New York, Academic Press, pp. 37–62.

Owens, R.G. 1960. Effects of elemental sulfur, dithiocarbamates, and related fungicides on organic acid metabolism of fungus spores. Dev. Ind. Microbiol., 1, 187–205.

Owens, R.G. 1953. Studies on the nature of fungicidal action. I. Inhibition of sulfhydryl, amino, iron, and copper-dependent enzymes in vitro by fungicides and related compounds. Contrib. Boyce Thompson Inst., 17, 221–242.

Owens, R.G. 1952. Spore uptake of fungitoxicants assayed by analyase inhibition. Phytopathology, 42, 471–472.

Owens, R.G., and Blaak, G. 1960a. Site of action of captan and dichlone in the pathway between acetate and citrate in fungus spores. Contrib. Boyce Thompson Inst., 20, 459–474.

Owens, R.G., and Blaak, G. 1960b. Chemistry of the reactions of dichlone and captan with thiols. Contrib. Boyce Thompson Inst., 20, 475–497.

Owens, R.G., and Hayes, A.D. 1964. Biochemical action of thiram and some dialkyldithiocarbamates. Contrib. Boyce Thompson Inst., 22, 227–240.

Owens, R.G., and Miller, L.P. 1958. Intracellular distribution of metal and organic fungicides in fungus spores. Contrib. Boyce Thompson Inst., 19, 117–188.

Owens, R.G., and Novotny, H.M. 1959. Mechanism of action of the fungicide captan (N-trichloromethylthio)-4-cyclohexene-1,2-dicarboximide). Contrib. Boyce Thompson Inst., 20, 171–190.

Owens, R.G., and Novotny, H.M. 1958. Mechanism of action of the fungicide dichlone (2,3-dichlorol,4-naphthoquinone). Contrib. Boyce Thompson Inst., 19, 463–482.

Owens, R.R., and Rubinstein, J.H. 1964. Chemistry of the fungicidal action of tetramethylthiuram disulfide (thiram) and ferbam. Contrib. Boyce Thompson Inst., 22, 241–257.

Parker-Rhodes, A.F. 1941. Studies on the mechanism of fungicidal action. I. Preliminary investigations of nickel, copper, zinc, silver, and mercury. Ann. Appl. Biol., 28, 389–405.

Pestka, S. 1971. Inhibitors of ribosome functions. Ann. Rev. Microbiol., 25, 487–550.

Peterson, C.A., and Edgington, L.V. 1970. Transport of the systemic fungicide, benomyl, in bean plants. Phytopathology, 60, 475–478.

Prevost, B. 1897. Memoire sur la cause immediate de la carie on charbon des bles et de plusiers autres maladies des plants, et sur le preservatifs de la carie. Phytopathology Classic, 6, 1-94 (translated by G.W. Keitt, 1939).

Priest, D., and Wood, R.K.S. 1961. Strains of Botrytis allii resistant to chlorinated nitrobenzene. Ann. Appl. Biol., 49, 445–460.

Ragsdale, N.N. 1977. Inhibitors of lipid synthesis. In Fungicides. Volume 2. Edited by M.C. Siegel and H.D. Sisler. New York, Dekker Press, pp. 333–363.

Ragsdale, N.N., and Sisler, H.D. 1970. Metabolic effects related to fungitoxicity of carboxin. Phytopathology, 60, 1422–1427.

Rich, S. 1965. Quinones. In Fungicides, An Advanced Treatise. Edited by D.C. Torgeson. New York, Academic Press, pp. 447–476.

Rich, S. 1963. Fungicides as metabolic inhibitors. In Metabolic Inhibitors. Edited by R.M. Hochester and J.H. Quastel. New York, Academic Press, pp. 263–284.

Rich, S. 1960. Fungicidal Chemistry. In Plant Pathology, an Advanced Treatise. Volume 2. Edited by J.G. Horsfall and A.E. Dimond. New York, Academic Press, pp. 553–602.

Rich, S. 1959. Reversal of captan fungitoxicity by l-histidine. Phytopathology, 49, 321.

Rich, S., and Horsfall, J.G. 1961. Fungitoxicity of carbamic and thiocarbamic acid esters. Conn. Agric. Exp. Stat. Bull., 639, 1–95.

Rich, S., and Horsfall, J.G. 1952. The relation between fungitoxicity, permeation, and lipid solubility. Phytopathology, 42, 457–460.

Rich, S., and Horsfall, J.G. 1950. Gaseous toxicants from organic sulfur compounds. Am. J. Bot., 37, 643–650.

Rich, S., and Horsfall, J.G. 1949. Fungicidal activity of dinitrocaprylphenylcrotonate. Phytopathology, 39, 19.

Richardson, L.T. 1963. Synergism between chloroneb and thiram applied to peas to control seed rot and damping-off by Pythium ultimum. Plant Dis. Rptr., 57, 3–6.

Richardson, L.T., and Thorn, G.D. 1961. The interaction of thiram and spores of Glomerella cingulata. Spald. and Schrenk. Can. J. Bot., 39, 531–540.

Richmond, D.V., and Somers, E. 1963. Studies of the fungitoxicity of captan. III. Relation between sulfhydryl content of fungal spores and their uptake of captan. Ann. Appl. Biol., 50, 33–43.

Richmond, D.V., and Somers, E. 1962a. Studies on the fungitoxicity of captan. I. The structure specificity of captan and six n-trichloromethylthio analogues. Ann. Appl. Biol., 50, 33–43.

Richmond, D.V., and Somers, E. 1962b. Studies on the fungitoxicity of captan. II. The uptake of captan by conidia of Neurospora crassa. Ann. Appl. Biol., 50, 45–56.

Santilli, V., and Katz, S. 1962. Inactivation of tobacco mosaic virus infectious ribonucleic acid by HgCl₂ and the reversal of this effect with cysteine. Phytopathology, 52, 750.

Schroeder, H. 1966. Thiadiazoles as fungicides, herbicides, and nematicides. U.S. Patent No. 3,260,588.

Schuldt, P.H., and Wolf, C.N. 1956. Fungitoxicity of substituted s-triazines. Contrib. Boyce Thompson Inst., 18, 377–393.

Shatta, M.N., and Sinclair, J.B. 1963. Tolerance to pentachloronitrobenzene among cotton isolates of Rhizoctonia solani. Phytopathology, 52, 1407–1411.

Shaw, W.H.R. 1954. Toxicity of cations toward living systems. Science, 120, 361–368.

Shepard, C.J. 1958. Inhibition of protein and nucleic acid synthesis in Aspergillus nidulans. J. Gen. Microbiol., 18, IV–V.

Siegel, M.R. 1970a. Reactions of the fungicide folpet (N-(trichloromethylthio)phthalimide) with a thiol protein. Pestic. Biochem. Physiol., 1, 225–233.

Siegel, M.R. 1970b. Reactions of the fungicide folpet (N-(trichloromethylthio)phthalimide) with a non-thiol protein. Pestic. Biochem. Physiol., *1*, 234–240.

Siegel, M.R., and Crosson, D.F. 1960. Effects of copper and glodin fungicides on amino acids, sugar content and oxygen use of *Colletotrichum capsici*. Phytopathology, *50*, 680–684.

Siegel, M.R., and Ragsdale, N.N. 1978. Antifungal mode of action of imazalil. Pestic. Biochem. Physiol., *9*, 48–56.

Siegel, M.R., and Sisler, H.D. 1968. Fate of the phthalimide and trichloromethylthio (SCCl₃) moieties of folpet in the toxic action of cells of *Saccharomyces pastorianus*. Phytopathology, *58*, 1123–1128.

Siegel, M.R., and Sisler, H.D. 1964a. Site of action of cycloheximide in cells of *Saccharomyces pastorianus*. I. Effect of the antibiotic on cellular metabolism. Biochim. Biophys. Acta, *87*, 70–82.

Siegel, M.R., and Sisler, H.D. 1964b. Site of action of cycloheximide in cells of *Saccharomyces pastorianus*. II. The nature of inhibition of protein synthesis in a cell free system. Biochim. Biophys. Acta, *87*, 83–89.

Siegel, M.R., and Sisler, H.D. 1964c. Basis of sensitivity and resistance to cycloheximide in two species of yeast. Phytopathology, *54*, 748.

Sijpesteijn, A.K. 1959. Organic tin compounds as potential agricultural fungicides. Medel. Landb. Hageschool Gent, *24*, 850–855.

Sijpesteijn, A.K., Janssen, M.J., and Dekhuyzen, H.M. 1957. Effect of copper and chelating agents on growth inhibition of *Aspergillus niger* by y 8-hydroxyquinoline and pyridine-*N*-oxide-2-thiol. Nature, *180*, 505–506.

Sisler, H.D. 1963. Fungitoxic mechanisms. Conn. Agric. Exp. Stat. Bull., *663*, 116–133.

Sisler, H.D., and Coursen, B.W. 1960. Effects of cycloheximide (Actidione) on metabolism and growth of fungi. Del. Ind. Microbiol., *1*, 181–186.

Sisler, H.D., and Cox, C.E. 1955. Effects of tetramethylthiuram disulfide on anaerobic breakdown of glucose by brewer's yeast. Am. J. Bot., *42*, 351–356.

Smale, B.C. 1957. Effects of certain trace metals on the fungitoxicity of sodium dimethyldithiocarbamate. Ph.D. thesis, University of Maryland.

Solel, Z. 1971. The systemic fungicidal activity of triphenyl tin acetate against *Cercospora beticola* on sugar beet. Phytopathology, *61*, 738–739.

Somers, E. 1961. The fungitoxicity of metal ions. Ann. Appl. Biol., *49*, 246–253.

Staub, T., Dahmen, H., and Schwrinn, F.J. 1978. Effect of ridomil on the development of target pathogens on their host plants. Abstracts of papers of the 3rd Int. Cong. Plant Pathol., Munchen, Germany, No. 336.

Szkolnik, M., et al. 1978. Impact of benomyl treatment on populations of benomyl-tolerant *Monilinia fructicola*. Phytopathology News, *12*(10), 239.

Thorn, G.D., and Ludwig, R.A. 1962. *The dithiocarbamates and related compounds*. New York, Elsevier, pp. 224–261.

Thorn, G.D., and Richardson, L.T. 1964. Decomposition of ferbam. Phytopathology, *61*, 914.

Tillman, R.W., and Sisler, H.D. 1971. A cloroneb-resistant mutant of *Ustilago maydis*. Phytopathology, *61*, 914.

Tolmsoff, W.F. 1962. Biochemical basis for biological specificity of Dexon (*p*-dimethylaminobenzenediaso sodium sulfonate) as a fungistat. Phytopathology, *52*, 775.

Torgeson, D.C. 1963. Effect of fungicides on the respiration of three species of soil fungi. Phytopathology, *53*, 891.

Torgeson, D.C., Yoder, D.M., and Johnson, J.B. 1957. Biological activity of Mylone breakdown products. Phytopathology, *57*, 536.

Turner, N.J. 1965. Fumigation with tetrachloroisophthalonitrile to control fungal diseases in greenhouse. Phytopathology, *55*, 1080.

Turner, N.J., and Battershell, R. 1970. The relationship between chemical reactivity, oil:water partitioning, and temperature on the rate of fungicidal action of tetrachloroisophthalonitrile and some of its analogues. Contrib. Boyce Thompson Inst., *24*, 203–212.

Turner, N.J., and Corden, M.E. 1963. Decomposition of sodium *N*-methyldithiocarbamate in soil. Phytopathology, *53*, 1388–1394.

Turner, N.J., et al. 1964. A new foliage protectant fungicide, tetrachloroisophthalonitrile. Contrib. Boyce Thompson Inst., *22*, 303–310.

Tweedy, B.G., and Turner, N. 1966. The mechanism of sulfur reduction by conidia of *Monilinia fructicola*. Contrib. Boyce Thompson Inst., *23*, 255–265.

Van der Kerk, G.J.M. 1959. Chemical structure and fungicidal activity of dithiocarbamates. In *Plant Pathology, Problems and Progress, 1908–1958*. Edited by C.S. Holten, et al. Madison, WI, University of Wisconsin Press, pp. 280–290.

Vincent, P.G., and Sisler, H.D. 1968. Mechanisms of antifungal action of 2,4,5,6-tetrachloroisophthalonitrile. Physiol. Plantar., *21*, 1249–1264.

Vonk, J.W., and Sijpesteijn, A.K. 1971. Tentative identification of 2-imidazoline as a transformation product of ethylenebisdithiocarbamate fungicides. Pestic. Biochem. Physiol., *1*, 163–165.

Vonk, J.W., and Sijpesteijn, A.K. 1970. Studies on the fate in plants of ethylenebisdithiocarbamate fungicide and their decomposition products. Ann. Appl. Biol., *65*, 489–496.

Von Schmeling, B., and Kulka, M. 1966. Systemic fungicidal activity of 1,4-oxathiin derivatives. Science, *152*, 659–660.

Ward, E.W., et al. 1980. Glyceolin production associated with control of *Phytophthora rot* of soybeans by the systemic fungicide metalaxyl. Phytopathology, *70*, 738–740.

Wedding, R.T., and Kendrick, J.B. 1959. Toxicity of *N*-methyl dithiocarbamates and methyl isothiocyanate to *Rhizoctonia solani*. Phytopathology, *49*, 557–561.

Wellman, R.H., and McCallan, S.E.A. 1946. Glyoxalidine derivatives as foliage fungicides. I. Laboratory studies. Contrib. Boyce Thompson Inst., *14*, 151–160.

Wescott, E.W., and Sisler, H.D. 1964. Uptake of cycloheximide by a sensitive and resistant yeast. Phytopathology, *54*, 1261–1264.

West, B., and Wolf, F.T. 1955. The mechanism of action of the fungicide, 2-heptadecyl-2-imidazoline. J. Gen. Microbiol., *12*, 396–401.

Whiffen, A.J., Bohonos, N., and Emerson, R.L. 1946. The products of an antifungal antibiotic by *Streptomyces griseus*. J. Bacteriol., *52*, 610–611.

White, G.A. 1961. A potent effect on 1,4 oxathiin systemic fungicides on succinate oxidation by a particulate preparation from *Ustilago maydis*. Biochem. Biophys. Res. Commun., *44*, 1212.

Wilcoxon, F., and McCallan, S.E.A. 1930. The fungicidal action of sulfur. I. The alleged role of pantothenic acid. Phytopathology, *20*, 391–417.

Woloshuk, C.P., Wolkow, P.M., and Sisler, H.D. 1981. The effect of three fungicides, specific for the control of rice blast disease, on the growth and melanin biosynthesis by *Pyricuaria oryzae*. Cav. Pestic. Sci., *12*, 86–90.

Woodcock, D. 1964. Microbial degradation of synthetic compounds. Ann. Rev. Phytopathol., *2*, 321–340.

Woodcock, D. 1959. The relation of chemical structures to fungicidal activity. In *Plant Pathology, Problems and Progress, 1908–1958*. Edited by C.S. Holten, et al. Madison, WI, University of Wisconsin Press, pp. 267–279.

Yoder, D.M. 1951. Reversibility of copper toxicity to conidia of *Sclerotinia fructicola*. Phytopathology, *41*, 39.

Young, H.C. 1922. The toxicity of sulfur. Ann. Mo. Bot. Gard., *95*, 403–435.

CHAPTER 45

FOOD- AND WATER-INFECTIVE MICROORGANISMS

John A. Lopes

Food- and water-borne infective microorganisms constitute a diverse group that includes viruses, bacteria, algae, protozoa, fungi, and helminths. These agents can cause acute, chronic, or latent infections with incubation periods of a few hours, days, or even weeks, the severity ranging from mild transient to fatal episodes. The illness may be manifested by preformed toxins or by the invading pathogens or both. The organism may be free-living and saprophytic in nature or fastidious, multiplying only in the host. The agent may show a single host specificity or may infect hosts of different species. The organism may be highly susceptible to physical-chemical agents or may form highly resistant spores. The pathogens may be highly aerobic or they may show extreme oxygen sensitivity and be anaerobic. Some of these agents may cause local intestinal infections, whereas others cause septicaemia. Some pathogens have a potential of causing explosive epidemics, others only localized outbreaks. However, all these pathogens use food and water as a common vehicle and the gastrointestinal tract as a common route of infection.

CHANGING PATTERN OF INFECTIONS

Food and water have been the most common sources of infectious diseases because the gastrointestinal tract offers pathogens direct access to the interior of the host. The pathogenic microorganisms often use food and water both as a vehicle and as a growth medium. Ingestion of contaminated food and water has been the cause of serious outbreaks, large epidemics, or waves of pandemics of diseases. One of the pathogens that has caused ravaging epidemics with high fatality rates is the etiologic agent of cholera, Vibrio cholerae. A brief historical perspective of this typical food- and water-infective pathogen is interesting. Cholera, as the term was used in Hippocratic writings 2400 years ago, represented sporadic gastrointestinal derangements of diverse origin (van

Heyningen and Seal, 1983). Since the late nineteenth century, however, cholera has designated the illness caused by V. cholerae. The illness represents most significantly an altered disease pattern resulting from industrialization without sanitation practices (Fenner, 1980). In seven pandemics, each starting from 1817, 1829, 1852, 1863, 1881, 1889, and 1961 respectively, it has claimed millions of lives in several countries. Transmission of cholera through water was discovered by Snow and York (1855) during the study known as "the cause of Broad Street Pump." The victims used well water contaminated by drainage. The epidemic was arrested by removal of the handle of the pump located on Broad Street! Sand filtration of water was found effective in containing the cholera epidemic in Altona, Germany, at the end of the nineteenth century. The original biotype of V. cholerae has been replaced by the El Tor strain in most parts of the world.

During the first half of the twentieth century, pathogens such as Salmonella typhi, Vibrio cholerae, Shigella species, Brucella species, Streptococcus pyogenes, Clostridium botulinum, Entamoeba histolytica, and polioviruses were known as primary food- and water-borne pathogens. These pathogens still cause widespread illnesses in the developing countries. Amebiasis claimed 40,000 to 110,000 lives around the world in 1984 (Walsh, 1988). Salmonella typhi was encountered in probably the largest recorded epidemic of typhoid fever, resulting from contaminated well water in Sangli, India, during 1975–1976 (Sathe et al., 1983). Incidence of typhoid and paratyphoid fever in Indonesia, the Philippines, Thailand, and Malaysia has been reported to be as high as 45, 89, 157, and 54, respectively, per 100,000 persons (Todd, 1987). Vibrio cholerae infections are still endemic in certain regions of the world. Shigella spp. was reported in large outbreaks of bacillary dysentery in Nigeria (Umoh et al., 1983) and in India (Kapadia et al., 1984). High incidence of brucellosis has been reported in Ar-

Table 45–1. *Food- and Water-Infective Bacteria*

Produce Toxins in Food
  Bacillus cereus
  Clostridium botulinum
  Staphylococcus aureus

Produce Infection
  Aeromonas hydrophila
  Brucella abortus, B. suis, B. melitensis
  Campylobacter jejuni, C. coli, C. fetus
  Clostridium botulinum
  Clostridium perfringens
  Escherichia coli (enteropathogenic strains)
  Klebsiella pneumoniae
  Legionella pneumophila
  Listeria monocytogenes
  Mycobacterium bovis
  Plesiomonas shigelloides
  Salmonella spp.
  Shigella sonnei, S. dysenteriae, S. flexneri
  Streptococcus pyogenes (Group A)
  Vibrio cholerae, V. mimicus, V. vulnificus, V. parahaemolyticus
  Yersinia enterocolitica, Y. pseudotuberculosis

Adapted from Madden, J.M., McCardell, B.A., and Archer, D.L. 1986. Virulence assessment of food borne microbes. In *Food Borne Microorganisms and Their Toxins: Developing Methodology.* Edited by M.D. Pierson and N.J. Stern. New York, Marcel Dekker, pp. 291–315.

gentina, Peru, Iran, Laos, Spain, Malta, and Italy (Thimm, 1981). With the implementation of control measures in developing countries, the above-mentioned pattern of infectious diseases will probably follow that observed in the developed countries. Tables 45–1, 45–2, and 45–3 present a list of food- and water-borne microorganisms pertaining to bacteria, viruses, and parasites, respectively. Each of these classes of microbes includes several genera and species of infective agents. A mention

Table 45–2. *Food- and Water-Infective Viruses*

Adenovirus
Astrovirus
Calicivirus
Coronavirus
Cytomegalovirus
Enteroviruses: Coxsackie, ECHO, Polio and Hepatitis A
Epidemic non-A, non-B hepatitis
Norwalk like viruses: Amulree, Hawaii, Montgomery County, Otofuke, Sapporo, Snow Mountain and Taunton
Papovavirus
Parvovirus
Pestivirus
Picobirnavirus
Rotavirus

Adapted from: Gerba, C.P. 1988. Viral disease transmission by seafoods. Food Technol., *42*, 99–103; Larkin, E.P. 1986. Detection, quantitation and public health significance of foodborne viruses. In *Food Borne Microorganisms and Their Toxins: Developing Methodology.* Edited by M.D. Pierson and N.J. Stern. New York, Marcel Dekker, pp. 439–451; Le Baron, C.W., et al. 1990. Viral agents of gastroenteritis. MMWR, *39*, 1–24.

should be made that there are over 45 types of parasites, and a number of toxin-producing fungi and algae, when considering food- and water-infective microorganisms. Parasitic infections are endemic and widespread in developing countries.

In developed countries a different pattern of food- and water-borne infections has been emerging because of previously little-noticed or newly discovered pathogens, often termed as "emerging" pathogens (Foster, 1988). The increasing incidence of emerging pathogens becomes more evident in developed countries against the background of declining incidence of previously recognized pathogens. Some of the emerging food- and water-borne pathogens are listed in Table 45–4. Some previously recognized pathogens such as *Staphylococcus aureus*, *Entamoeba histolytica*, and *Shigella* spp. are included with the emerging pathogens, because these pathogens either maintain a significant incidence or are sporadically encountered even in the developed countries. Therefore at the present time the term "emerging" should be assigned to the pathogens with significant incidence under apparently improved sanitary conditions.

RECOGNITION OF EMERGING PATHOGENS

A number of related or unrelated factors have been responsible for the recognition of emerging pathogens. Some of the pathogens, such as *Legionella pneumophila*, rotavirus, or the Norwalk agent have been relatively newly discovered, whereas others such as *Giardia lamblia* have been known for centuries. The incidence of psychrotrophic *Listeria monocytogenes* or *Yersinia enterocolitica* could be linked to certain practices in modern food industry such as longer storage of products at refrigeration temperature. Emergence of *Legionella pneumophila* and *Mycobacterium avium* complex bacteria has been associated with piped hot-water systems. Higher incidences of latent and otherwise uneventful infections with *Isospora belli*, *Cryptosporidium* spp., or *Sarcocystis* spp. have been associated with the increased population of immunocompromised individuals. Regardless of the factors associated with the recognition of the emerging pathogens, their emergence has been marked by a large outbreak that often has resulted in an "event" in the communications media.

Noteworthy Outbreaks and Events

Giardia lamblia is probably the earliest recognized pathogen, discovered or observed by Antony Van Leeuwenhoek in 1681 (Dobell, 1920). It was recognized as an important pathogen during the largest laboratory-confirmed outbreak in Rome, New York during 1974–1975 with an estimated 4000 to 5000 cases (Shaw et al., 1977). Giardiasis has accounted for the largest number of gastroenteritis cases due to protozoal infection in the United States (Craun, 1984). *Salmonella enteritidis* and *S. typhimurium* probably were the few earliest bacteria associated with food-borne infections (Gartner, 1888; de Nobele, 1898). The importance of these and other non-

Table 45–3. *Common Food- and Water-Infective Parasites*

Source	Agent	Comments
AMOEBA		
Fecal contamination of food and water	*Entamoeba histolytica*	Human pathogen. Incubation period is variable from a few days to several weeks. Invasion of colonic tissue results in acute diarrhea, abdominal pain, and bloody mucoid stools. Complication of lung, brain, or liver in severe cases.
Recreational water (swimming)	*Naegleria fowleri*	Free living. Found in soil, fresh water, sewage, and sludge. More common in lakes used for cooling water. Causes acute and fulminating primary amebic meningoencephalitis (PAM).
Recreational water (swimming)	*Acanthamoeba culbertsoni castellani polyphaga astronyxis*	Free living. Found in soil, fresh water, brackish water, and sea water. Causes chronic granulomatous amebic encephalitis that may be fatal. May cause eye infections. Immunocompromised individuals may get infection by inhalation of cysts from soil.
FLAGELLATES		
Community water and raw vegetables	*Giardia lamblia*	Both warm- and cold-blooded animals serve as carriers. Does not multiply outside the body. Causes diarrhea, flatulence, cramps, nausea, anorexia, and fatigue. Causes acute and chronic infection in the asymptomatic carriers. Multiplies in small intestine.
Oral fecal contamination of food and water	*Dientamoeba fragilis*	Flagellate without flagella and cyst form. Infection is associated with *Enterobiasis* (pin worm infection). Probably uses *Enterobius* eggs to bypass stomach acidity. Illness results in diarrhea, nausea, and vomiting.
CILIATES		
Food, water contaminated with pig feces	*Balantidium coli*	More common in tropics. Largest protozoan parasite. Both cyst and trophozoite found in the feces. Pig serves as a natural host. Inhabits colon. Symptoms include nausea, vomiting, and watery diarrhea. Both acute and chronic infections and colonic ulcers are observed.
COCCIDIA		
Fecal contamination of food and water by carnivorous host	*Isospora belli*	Inhabits mucosa of small intestine. Intracellular parasite. Can produce severe intestinal disease with diarrhea, nausea, and fever. Disease may persist for months or years. Fatal in immunocompromised individuals.
Fecal contamination of food and water	*Cryptosporidium* spp.	Infects brush border of intestinal epithelium. Infects other organs in immunocompromised individuals. Causes profuse and watery diarrhea, epigastric pain, and nausea that is prolonged in immunocompromised individuals.
Fecal contamination of cats and undercooked meat of intermediate hosts	*Toxoplasma gondii*	Causes acute and chronic infections. Disease may resemble mononucleosis. Congenital infection may involve CNS and ocular abnormalities, and may be fatal. Reactivated in immunocompromised individuals, resulting in encephalitis, pneumonitis, and myocarditis. Cats serve as primary host. Frequency of infection can be as high as 80% in regions of France to as low as 1% in the U.S.
HELMINTHS		
	Nematodes (tissue)	
Undercooked raw pork, bear meat	*Trichinella spiralis*	Develops in mucosa of small intestine. Nonspecific gastroenteritis, fever eosinophila, and myositis.
Ingestion of animal livers or food contaminated with eggs from soil	*Capillaria hepatica*	Develops in liver parenchyma.
Food contaminated with dog feces	*Toxocara canis*	Hyper-eosinophila, hepatomegaly, fever, and pneumonitis.
Consumption of raw fish dishes: sushi, sashimi, and ceviche	*Anisakiasis* *Anisakis* spp. *Phocanema* spp. *Terranova* spp.	Eosinophilic granuloma.

Table 45–3. *Common Food- and Water-Infective Parasites* Continued

Source	Agent	Comments
Raw or undercooked shrimp, crabs, large edible snails; improperly washed lettuce, fruits, and strawberries	*Angiostrongylus cantonensis*	Lungworms inhabiting pulmonary artery of rats and passed on to slugs and snails. Causes human eosinophilic meningitis or meningoencephalitis. Observed in Hawaii, Thailand, Indonesia, and other southeast Asian countries and Cuba. Worms migrate to brain, spinal cord, and eye, giving prolonged severe headache and other central nervous system complications.
	NEMATODES (intestinal)	
Fecal contamination of food and water	*Enterobius vermicularis*	Infections associated with gastrointestinal tract. Human pinworm. Primarily infects children. Eggs survive for prolonged periods in feces.
	Ascaris lumbricoides	Human large roundworm found in cecum.
	Trichuris trichuria	Human whipworm common in moist, warm regions.
Raw and poorly cooked fish	*Capillaria philippinensis*	Parasite of fish-eating birds and fish. Common in Philippines, Thailand, and areas around south China sea.
	CESTODES (tissue)	
Poorly cooked fish or the use of frog and snake poultices	*Spirometra mansoni*	Parasites of cats, dogs, wild canids, and wild felids common in China, Japan, Korea, and Vietnam.
	Spirometra mansonoides	Common in U.S.
Food contaminated by dog feces	*Teenia multiceps*	Parasite of dogs, cats, and fishes. Human infection through dog feces.
Consumption of undercooked meat	*Echinococcus granulosis*	Domestic and wild canids as primary host. Common in sheep and cattle raising areas. Forms hydatid cysts and CNS complications.
	Echinococcus multilocularis	Develops invasive cysts in liver. Common in Europe, Japan, North and South America, Australia, and New Zealand.
	Echinococcus vogeli	Primarily found in Latin America. Bush dogs and large rodents are primary hosts. Develops invasive cysts in liver.
	CESTODES (intestinal)	
Undercooked fish	*Diphyllobothrium latum*	Fish tapeworm found in cold, clear lakes of U.S., Canada, USSR, Japan, and Europe.
Beef	*Taenia saginata*	Cattle tapeworm.
Pork	*Taenia solium*	Pig tapeworm. Most prevalent in Latin America, India, China, Africa, and Europe. Can cause severe CNS and eye infections.
Grains and cereals	*Hymenolepsis nana*	Mice are primary host; grains and cereal infecting beetles are secondary host.
Food contaminated with dog and cat feces	*Dipylidium caninum*	Dogs and cats are primary hosts. Children are most susceptible.
	TREMATODES	
Consumption of undercooked water vegetables like water chestnut and water caltrop or watercress	*Fasciolopsis buski*	Largest and most pathogenic intestinal fluke. Common in China, India, Indonesia, Thailand, Taiwan, and Vietnam.
Water vegetables such as watercress	*Fasciola hepatica*	Worldwide in occurrence.
Undercooked and pickled fish	*Clonorchis sinensis*	Parasite found in bile duct of humans, cats, and dogs.
Poorly cooked crustaceans	*Paragonimus westermani*	Parasite of dogs, cats, and wild animals.

Adapted from: Healy, G.R., et al. 1984. Food borne parasites. In *Compendium of Methods for Microbiological Examination of Foods*. Edited by M.L. Speck. Washington, D.C., American Public Health Association, pp. 542–556; Korgstad, D.J., Visvesvara, G.S., Walls, K.W. and Smith, J.W. 1985. Blood and tissue protozoa. In *Manual of Clinical Microbiology*. 4th Edition. Edited by E.H. Lennette, A. Balows, W.J. Hausler and H. Jean Shadomy. Washington, D.C., American Society for Microbiology, pp. 612–630; Melvin, D.M., and Healy, G.R. 1985. Intestinal and urogenital protozoa. In *Manual of Clinical Microbiology*. 4th Edition. Edited by E. H. Lennette, A. Balows, W.J. Hausler and H. Jean Shadomy. Washington, D.C. American Society for Microbiology, pp. 631–650.

Table 45–4. *"Emerging" Pathogens*

Bacteria
    Aeromonas hydrophila
    Bacillus cereus
    Campylobacter jejuni
    Clostridium botulinum type E
    Clostridium perfringens
    Escherichia coli (enteropathogenic strains)
    Legionella pneumophila
    Listeria monocytogenes
    Mycobacterium avium complex
    Plesiomonas shigelloides
    Salmonella typhimurium (and other nontyphi spp.)
    Staphylococcus aureus
    Shigella spp.
    Vibrio parahaemolyticus
    Yersinia enterocolitica

Protozoa
    Cryptosporidium spp.
    Entamoeba histolytica
    Giardia lamblia
    Isospora belli
    Naegleria fowleri
    Sarcocystis spp.
    Toxoplasma gondii

Viruses
    Cytomegalovirus
    Hepatitis A
    Epidemic non-A, non-B hepatitis
    Norwalk-type viruses
    Rotavirus

typhoidal salmonellae was realized after the largest milk-borne outbreak due to *S. typhimurium* in Illinois in 1985 resulted in 16,000 cases (Ryan et al., 1987). Gastrointestinal infections due to *Campylobacter jejuni* outnumber those due to both *Salmonella* spp. and *Shigella* spp. However, the magnitude of these infections was only realized after improved isolation procedures during the early 1980s (Blaser, 1982). *Yersinia enterocolitica* was recognized as an emerging pathogen after an epidemic in New York State, which was marked by several unnecessary appendectomies (Black et al., 1978) and a multi-state outbreak in Arkansas, Tennessee, and Mississippi that involved several thousand cases (Lofgren et al., 1982). The pathogenic potential of *Listeria monocytogenes* was observed after the epidemics in Germany (Ortel, 1968), Canada (Schlech et al., 1983), and the U.S. (James et al., 1985). These epidemics involved several hundred cases and were marked by high mortality rates. The widespread nature of *Vibrio parahaemolyticus* infection became evident after its first isolation in Japan in 1950 (Fujino et al., 1950). The pathogen accounted for 40 to 50% of bacterial gastroenteritis cases in Japan (Sakazaki and Shimada, 1982). *Clostridium perfringens*, long known to be the causative agent of gas gangrene, was associated with food poisoning during the early 1960s (Hall et al., 1963). The ability of this bacterium to sporulate in the intestine results in poisoning from the spore-coat protein (Hobbs, 1979). *Clostridium botulinum*

(types A, B, and E) has been known as the classic toxin-producing bacterium in canned foods. During the 1960s the ability of *Cl. botulinum* types E, B, and F to grow and produce toxin under refrigeration conditions was recognized (Cann et al., 1965). The bacterium can also multiply in the gastrointestinal tract. Feeding of contaminated honey has resulted in development of botulism in infants (Midura and Arnon, 1976; Pickett et al., 1976). The pathogen has also been incriminated in botulism due to contaminated rain water in rural Australia (Sugiyama and Sofos, 1982). *Aeromonas hydrophila* was first described as an enteropathogen by Caselitz in 1955, and since then it has been associated with gastrointestinal infections (Atwegg and Geiss, 1989). Its ubiquitous nature and enhanced virulence for immunocompromised individuals makes it an important member of the emerging pathogens. *Plesiomonas shigelloides* has been associated with water-borne gastroenteritis in tropical countries in the past two decades (Bhat et al., 1974).

Escherichia coli has been known primarily as a nonpathogenic inhabitant of the intestine. However, pathogenic strains probably account for the largest number of diarrheal infections in developing countries (Kornacki and Marth, 1982). A particularly virulent strain, referred to as colihemorrhagic *E. coli* 0157:H7, has been isolated during rapidly spreading outbreaks of hemorrhagic colitis in Canada (Stewart et al., 1983) and in the U.S. (Taylor et al., 1982; Ryan et al., 1986). Unlike other strains of *E. coli*, colihemorrhagic *E. coli* failed to hydrolyze 4-methylumbelliferone glucuronide (MUG), commonly used for rapid detection of *E. coli* (Doyle and Schoeni, 1984). *E. coli* 0157:H7 is also unusual in its inability to ferment sorbitol, which is fermented by 93% of *E. coli* strains (Doyle, 1988). *Legionella pneumophila* is a fairly recent member of the emerging pathogens. Numerous outbreaks of infections due to *L. pneumophila* since 1977 give testimony to its virulence potential (Meyer, 1983). The discovery of *L. pneumophila* in an outbreak of respiratory illness associated with the American Legion convention in Philadelphia was unusual and widely publicized (McDade et al., 1977). The etiologic agent turned out to be a gram-negative bacterium and not a rickettsia-like agent as indicated by isolation procedures and the nature of illness. Since then *L. pneumophila* has been associated with past outbreaks of unknown cause in Washington, D.C. in 1965, in Pontiac, Michigan in 1968, in James River, Virginia in 1973, in Benidorm, Spain in 1973, and in Philadelphia in 1974. Interestingly, the last outbreak in Philadelphia was associated with the Odd Fellows convention in the same hotel as that of American Legion. Relatively less virulent *Mycobacterium avium* serovars have been found to cause enteritis and/or bacteremia or granulomata in liver and bone marrow in patients with acquired immunodeficiency syndrome (AIDS) (Young et al., 1986). A large percentage of the population (20 to 80%) has been found to be infected by *Toxoplasma gondii* through fecal contamination or by consumption of undercooked meat (Korgstad et al.,

1985). This uneventful infection is reactivated in AIDS or transplantation patients to give rise to encephalitis, pneumonitis, and myocarditis. Similarly, *Isospora belli*, *Sarcocystis* spp., and *Cryptosporidium* spp. cause severe and often fatal infections in immunocompromised individuals (Melvin and Healy, 1985). *Leptospira* spp. and *Coxiella burnetii* may emerge from time to time as food- and water-infective microorganisms. Several viral agents responsible for gastroenteritis have been discovered only recently (Blacklow and Cukor, 1985; Larkin, 1986). Rotavirus has now been recognized as a major cause of viral diarrhea in children. Small round viruses, such as the Norwalk agent, have been reported as causative agents for gastroenteritis from several countries.

Thus, a whole new spectrum of emerging pathogens ranging from viruses to protozoa has been observed during food- and water-borne outbreaks of infections. The emergence of new infectious diseases has been associated with changes taking place during human evolution (Mims, 1980). There have been multiple and sometimes similar factors responsible for these outbreaks.

Causative and Recognition Factors of Outbreaks Due to Emerging Pathogens

Inadequacy of Legislative Guidelines on Sanitation in the Food Industry

Automation of large-scale food processing facilities has resulted in elimination of contamination of food due to manual handling. The practices of pasteurization and refrigeration, and the use of sanitizers during processing, transportation, and storage, has increased shelf-life and improved organoleptic properties of food products. Early legislative guidelines on sanitation were directed toward control of infections caused by previously recognized pathogens. These measures also resulted indirectly in the production of desired organoleptic quality of food through the control of mesophilic spoilage microorganisms. Thus desired organoleptic properties and microbiologic safety became synonymous in the food industry; the microbiologic aspect apparently became secondary as long as the organoleptic quality of food product was maintained. The practice of using outdated but organoleptically acceptable pasteurized milk, "returned" from supermarket shelves, for the preparation of ice-cream and other frozen dairy products presented an underlying danger of contamination by psychrotrophic pathogens such as *Listeria monocytogenes*. Operation of the processing facilities for extended periods, poor sanitation of hard-to-reach dead spaces in the pipelines, and difficult-to-clean intricate mechanical parts (e.g., fillers) may result in an ill-defined loss in microbiologic quality. Mechanical parts also result in cross-contamination with pathogens. Defeathering rubber fingers were found to spread *Campylobacter jejuni* in poultry processing plants (Genigeorgis et al., 1986). Similarly, *Salmonella* spp. was spread by cross-contamination in a cattle slaughtering plant (Stolle, 1981).

Production of larger quantities of food requires pooling of small batches, i.e., comingling of milk. Thus a single contaminated source can spread pathogens to the bulk quantity. Legislative guidelines for monitoring pathogens in these situations were and probably are not adequate or are difficult to implement for the lack of time, techniques, economic resources, or some other factors (NRC, 1985b).

Storage, Packaging, and Distribution

Compromise, abuse, or ignorance of the temperature factor in food storage can lead to growth of pathogens in food. Storage temperature a few degrees above 4 to 5°C can permit the growth of pathogens such as *Clostridium botulinum* type E, salmonellae, *Staphylococcus aureus*, *Clostridium perfringens*, *Bacillus cereus*, and *Vibrio parahaemolyticus* (Corlett, 1989; Palumbo, 1986). Some pathogens can grow even at proper refrigeration temperatures. *Aeromonas hydrophila* was found to increase from 10^3 to 10^8 per milliliter in 14 days at 4°C (Palumbo et al., 1985). *Clostridium botulinum* type E was found to grow below 4°C (Schmidt et al., 1961). The generation time of *Listeria monocytogenes* in dairy food was reported to be 1.2 to 1.7 days at 4°C (Rosenow and Marth, 1986).

With better transportation facilities, food processed in a single plant has been distributed to larger sections of population over wide geographic areas. Large outbreaks of salmonellosis, listeriosis, and yersinosis have been traced to single dairy food processing facilities (Health Protection Bureau, 1985; CDC, 1985; James et al., 1985; Lofgren et al., 1982). Brie cheese produced in one factory in France caused outbreaks of *E. coli*-associated illness in Washington, D.C., Colorado, Georgia, Illinois, and Wisconsin in the U.S. (Bryan, 1988).

The center of hot food can remain at 50°F for 24 hrs even when stored in a refrigerator, thus resulting in optimal growth temperatures for pathogens in contaminated food (Smith et al., 1985). Pathogens have been found to survive on the surface of refrigerated packages (Stanfield et al., 1987). These contaminated surfaces can maintain their potential for transmission of pathogens. One of the largest epidemics of enteritis due to *Yersinia enterocolitica* resulted from contamination of the external surfaces of fresh milk cartons. The cartons in turn were contaminated by milk crates previously used to transfer outdated products to a pig farm. The crates were contaminated by runoff from the pig pens during heavy rains (Schiemann, 1987; Tacket et al., 1984).

Increasing Number of Immunocompromised Individuals

Immunosuppressive treatment has been used in modern medicine for cancer and transplantation patients. Such treatment often results in increasing the number of immunocompromised individuals in communities. These figures, when combined with ever-increasing number of patients with AIDS, present a section of population that is particularly vulnerable to infectious microorganisms. Less virulent and opportunistic microorganisms often produce severe illnesses in these individuals, whereas virulent pathogens may cause fatal infections (James et al., 1985; Johnson, 1987; Sperber and Schleupner, 1987).

Use of Antibiotics and Drugs

The use of antibiotics, either in animal feed or for therapy, can alter the pattern of food-borne infections. Antibiotics in animal feed have been associated with emergence of drug-resistant strains in food-borne salmonellosis (Holmberg et al., 1984). Therapeutic use of antibiotics appears to enhance the infectious process in individuals under treatment. Antibiotic-resistant *Salmonella newport* caused serious illness among persons taking antimicrobials. Intestinal flora may also initiate infection when shifted out of balance during therapy. *Clostridium difficile*, a normal intestinal inhabitant and a common soil and water bacterium, has been associated with diarrhea and pseudomembranous colitis (Bartlett, 1979). Gastric acidity is one of the natural defenses of the host against infection from food- and water-infective microorganisms. Hornick et al. (1971) reported that illness-inducing oral doses of *Vibrio cholerae* ranged from 10^3–10^4 to 10^8–10^{11} cells under buffered and unbuffered conditions, respectively. Ho et al. (1986) and Schlech et al. (1986) have reported protection against infections due to *Listeria monocytogenes* by gastric acidity. Antacid and cimetidine therapy, which reduced gastric acidity, was associated with listeria infections. Reduced gastric acidity also enhanced pathogenesis in salmonella infections (Gionella et al., 1971). These results indicate that altering gastric acidity by increasing use of antacids and other drugs may expose individuals to infections that otherwise could be naturally prevented. Thus the widespread use of antibiotics and drugs can alter the course of infection by food- and water-borne infective microorganisms.

Travel and Tourism

Movement of populations has been associated with the spread of infections since antiquity. Darius' campaigns against the Greeks (492 B.C.) and the British campaign in Gallipoli (1915) over the same ground suffered because of food- and water-infective microorganisms (Pearson and Hewlett, 1988). Modern transportation facilities have increased the exposure of susceptible populations to food- and water-borne infections many orders of magnitude. Tourism and increased traveling populations resulting from military movements, political refugees, pilgrimages, and international business expose individuals to food- and water-borne infective pathogens endemic in certain areas. It has been estimated that up to 50% of 500 million tourists traveling each year are likely to acquire traveler's diarrhea (WHO, 1984). Infections due to enteropathogenic *E. coli*, *Vibrio parahaemolyticus*, *Giardia lamblia*, and *Entamoeba histolytica* have been more commonly encountered by travelers.

Intercontinental travel or tourism often involves confinement in planes or cruise ships. Limitation of space, water, toilet facilities, mass catering, and improper stor-age temperatures can create hazardous conditions with respect to microbiologic safety. Food prepared in flight kitchens is often stored for prolonged periods at temperatures conducive for the growth of pathogens. *Staphylococcus aureus* and *Salmonella* spp. have been encountered in food-borne infection outbreaks on international flights (Jackson Tartakow and Vorperian, 1980; Todd, 1987). Food-borne outbreaks of gastroenteritis due to *Salmonella* spp., enteropathogenic *E. coli*, *Vibrio parahaemolyticus*, *Shigella* spp., *Trichinella spiralis*, and *Staphylococcus aureus* have been reported on cruise ships (Jackson Tartakow and Vorperian, 1980). Travelers may acquire local culinary habits and consume raw food dishes such as sushi and sashimi, which are more likely to be contaminated with pathogens than cooked dishes are.

Developments in Detection Methods

Newer and more sensitive detection methods have resulted in associating previously unknown or unsuspected pathogens with gastroenteritis outbreaks. The use of new isolation media has led to the realization of the widespread nature of *Campylobacter jejuni* infections (Dekeyser et al., 1972). The small round viruses such as the Norwalk agent were associated with gastroenteritis through the use of electron microscopy (Kapikian et al., 1972). Improvement in detection methods has reduced the time required for the isolation and identification of *Listeria monocytogenes* (Lovett, 1988; Datta et al., 1987). The application of fluorescent and immunofluorescent methods have expedited the identification of intestinal parasites (Gallard and Bueno, 1989). Improvements in isolation of sublethally injured bacteria in processed food have also resulted in increased frequency of isolating pathogens (Ray, 1986).

Role of Modern Communications Media

Instant communication through radio, television, and newspapers has often alarmed the general population about the outbreaks of illness due to food- and water-borne infectious agents. Thus modern communications media have played an important role in educating people about the emergence of new pathogens. Public interest about illness due to the emerging pathogens such as *Salmonella* spp., *Campylobacter* spp., and *Listeria* spp. could be compared to that of agents of cholera and typhoid early in this century (Prentice et al., 1989; Martelle and Tschirhart, 1988; Kendall, 1989).

FACTORS THAT INFLUENCE INFECTIONS THROUGH FOOD AND WATER

Survival and growth of pathogens in food and water primarily determine the course of the infectious process. Some of the factors that determine the survival and growth are pH, water activity, and resistance to radiation, temperature, osmotic pressure, and salt content, as well as the ability of the pathogens to form resistant cysts or spores. These factors have been individually

Table 45–5. *Number of Pathogens Required to Produce Illness*

Organism	Number
Bacillus cereus	$\geq 10^5$/g of food
Campylobacter jejuni	5×10^2 to 10^6
Clostridium perfringens	10^8 to 10^9 or $\geq 10^5$/g of food
Escherichia coli	10^6 to 10^{10}
Giardia lamblia	10^1 to 10^2
Hepatitis virus	10^3
Norwalk virus	10^1
Salmonella spp.	10^4 to 10^{10}
Shigella spp.	10^1 to 10^2
Staphylococcus aureus	$\geq 10^5$/g of food
Streptococcus faecalis	10^9 to 10^{10}
Vibrio cholerae	10^6 to 10^{11}
Vibrio parahaemolyticus	10^3 to 10^7 or $\geq 10^5$/g of food
Yersinia enterocolitica	10^9

Adapted from: Bryan, F.L. 1978. Factors that contribute to outbreaks of foodborne diseases. J. Food Protect., 41, 816–827; NRC. 1985a. Selection of pathogens as components of microbiological criteria. In *An Evaluation of the Role of Microbiological Criteria for Foods and Food Ingredients*. Washington, D.C., National Academy Press, pp. 72–103; Banwart, G.J. 1981. *Basic Food Microbiology*. New York, AVI; Rendtorff, R.C. 1954. The experimental transmission of human intestinal protozoa parasites II. *Giardia lamblia* cysts given in capsules. Am. J. Hyg., 59, 209–270.

discussed in great detail by Silliker et al. (1980) and Troller (1986). Some other parameters that determine the probability of infection are the nature and source of food and water; processing and handling; association of the pathogens with particulate matter, soil, or sediment; and environmental interaction with other microorganisms. The number of infecting organisms is also an important factor in determining the infectious process. Some virulent pathogens can initiate infections in lower numbers, whereas others require massive doses to cause illness (Table 45–5). However, host resistance should also be considered as an important aspect in determining the outcome of the infectious process.

Nature and Source of Food and Water

The sources of water, food, and food products are important factors in determining the type and number of infecting pathogens. Bryan (1977) reviewed worldwide medical and engineering literature and reported that typhoid fever, infectious hepatitis, fascioliasis, and cholera are the most frequently occurring food-borne diseases due to foods such as vegetables, fish, shrimp, and shellfish contaminated by sewage or irrigation water in agricultural or aquacultural practices. Todd (1987) reported in a review that infected food and farm animals were responsible for tuberculosis, brucellosis, salmonellosis, and parasitic infection in developing countries. Vasavada (1988) reviewed milk as a source of pathogens and reported occurrence of emerging pathogens such as *Listeria monocytogenes*, *Yersinia enterocolitica*, *Campylobacter jejuni*, enteropathogenic *E. coli*, and *Salmonella typhimurium* in milk and milk products in the U.S. Poultry, eggs, and beef have been common sources of *Cam-*

pylobacter and *Salmonella* infections (Genigeorgis, 1986; C.D.C., 1987). Droppings by nocturnal roosting gulls in winter on a water storage reservoir, supplying water to Glasgow, Scotland, resulted in deterioration of water quality (Benton et al., 1983). Contamination of water by bird feces corresponded with appearance of *E. coli* and salmonellae in untreated water and on three occasions in treated water samples. Thermal pollution of man-made lakes as well as that of rivers used for cooling electrical power plants has resulted in increased numbers of pathogenic *Naegleria fowleri* in water (Tyndall et al., 1989). Use of water from these sources either for recreational or drinking purposes presents a danger of infection by *N. fowleri*, which can cause fatal human primary amebic meningoencephalitis (PAM).

Processing and Handling

Food can become contaminated during processing and handling. The level of pathogens in contaminated food may increase depending on processing and handling practices. In decreasing order of frequency, the first ten most important factors found to result in food-borne infections were improper cooling (44%), delay of 12 or more hours between preparation and consumption of food (23%), food handlers as carriers of pathogens (18%), mixing of uncooked and cooked food or ingredients (16%), inadequate processing (16%), improper hot holding (14%), inadequate reheating (11%), unsafe sources (10%), cross-contamination (5%), and improper cleaning (5%) (Bryan, 1988).

Eight outbreaks of food-borne infections due to consumption of meat and meat products have been examined (Genigeorgis, 1986). Undercooking, improper cooling of cooked food, unsanitary handling practices, ingestion of raw products, delay of 24 hours or more between preparation and consumption, food handlers as carrier of pathogens, and improper thawing of raw food were important factors that contributed to 46, 34, 16, 15, 13, 12, and 10% of outbreaks, respectively. The restaurants, care institutions, and small food businesses were most often the suspected locations in which food became contaminated (Beckers, 1988).

Interaction of Pathogens with Other Environmental Microorganisms

The interaction between pathogens and nonpathogenic environmental microorganisms can determine the survival and virulence of pathogens in food and water. *Flavobacterium breve*, a common environmental water bacterium, probably supports the growth of *Listeria pneumophila* in sediments on taps, sinks, and other water distribution systems by providing L-cysteine to the fastidious pathogen (Wadowsky and Yee, 1983). Microorganisms interact more efficiently in sediments because of proximity to each other. Stewart and Koditscheck (1980) showed the transfer of antibiotic resistance between *E. coli* strains in marine sediments. Similar mechanisms were suspected in the appearance of multiple drug resistance in *E. coli* and *Staphylococcus aureus* present in marine and fresh recreational waters in the Northwestern U.S. (Vasconcelos and Anthony, 1985). Parasitic microorganisms present in the environment have been found to support the growth of pathogens. *Legionella pneumophila* was found to multiply intracellularly in an amoeba and two ciliates (Barbaree et al., 1986). On the other hand, a brachiopod was found to remove *E. coli* from a waste-water pond (Seaman, 1986).

Association of Pathogens with Sediment and Soil

Water-infective pathogens have been found concentrated on sediment particles, as compared to being found in the body of water. The concentration of *Vibrio parahaemolyticus* was found to be 436 per 100 g of sediment as compared to 36 per 100 ml of seawater near Alexandria, Egypt (El-Sahn et al., 1982). Similarly, the concentration of enteroviruses in sediment was found to be 10 times higher than that in water (Lewis et al., 1986). Compared to poliovirus I and ECHO virus 1, hepatitis A virus was found to be less readily adsorbed to soils (Sobsey et al., 1986). This could probably explain in part the cause of some outbreaks of hepatitis A infections due to drinking ground water (Bowen and McCarty, 1983). Enteroviruses have been found at 67 m and up to aquifer depth of 18 m from a subsurface leaching pool (Vaughn et al., 1980). Various factors such as type, pH, electrical charge, and moisture content of the soil can determine adsorption of pathogens on the sediments.

Increased concentration of pathogens in the sediment has accounted for increased risk of infection for young bathers in shallow waters of wading pools (Vasconcelos and Anthony, 1985).

Virulence Factors

Microbial toxins are important determinants of bacterial, fungal, and algal virulence. Some of the toxins produced by these organisms are presented in Tables 45–6, 45–7, and 45–8.

Besides toxin production, the ability of food- and water-infective microorganisms to cause illness depends on their survival under the hostile conditions present in the gastrointestinal tract. Gastric acidity, digestive enzymes, bile salts, peristalsis, osmolarity, and high temperatures may inhibit some pathogens. Successful pathogens not only survive but even use the unfavorable environment to their advantage. The enteroviruses, *Giardia* cysts, and *Dientameoba fragilis* all survive gastric acidity. *Giardia lamblia* probably uses gastric acidity for triggering excystment into the trophozoite form for growth in the small intestine (Bingham and Meyer, 1979). The trophozoite form of *Dientameoba fragilis* apparently escapes gastric acidity by hiding inside *Enterobius* eggs (Melvin and Healy, 1985). *Helicobacter* (previously *Campylobacter*) *pylori* has been associated with peptic ulcer (Goodwin et al., 1989). It probably resists gastric acidity by using urease to produce ammonium and bicarbonate, which raise the pH in the microenvironment around the ingested bacterium (Hornick, 1988).

To colonize, the pathogens must be able to attach to a suitable site in the intestinal tract. Therefore, the ability to attach is also a virulence-determining factor. The distribution of receptors to which pathogens attach on the host cells may influence tissue tropism and thus may determine the expression of certain virulence characteristics such as neurovirulence of poliovirus (Racaniello et al., 1990). Studies with Coxsackie viruses suggest that pathogens which exhibit wider host range may show specificity to more than one receptor (Hsu et al., 1990). Parasites use physical processes for attachment, e.g., ventral disc of *Giardia lamblia*. Bacterial and viral pathogens attach by means of chemical moieties and adhesins to the receptor sites on the host cells. In the case of pathogenic *Yersinia enterocolitica*, the adhesins are always expressed on the surface of the cells, whereas in *Salmonella typhimurium* and *S. choleraesius* the adhesins are induced by trypsin- and neuraminidase-sensitive structures on the epithelial cells (Finlay et al., 1989). In the case of *Vibrio* spp., the pilus needed for attachment is synthesized in response to environmental signals such as pH, temperature, and osmolarity (Miller et al., 1989).

Invasion of the host cells is an integral part of active pathogenesis. The pathogens are endocytosed and internalized by the epithelial cells in response to either constitutive or induced invasion factors present on the surface of the microorganisms (Finlay et al., 1989; Finlay and Falkow, 1989). Both *Shigella* spp. and *Listeria monocytogenes* respectively produce hemolysin and listeriolysin to lyse intracellular membrane-vacuole and enter the cell cytoplasm. *Salmonella* spp. use fused vacuoles to traverse the cell barrier (Fields et al., 1989). Both *Yersinia enterocolitica* and *Shigella* spp. use temperature-dependent (37°C) expression of the virulence factors (Portnoy et al., 1981; Maurelli et al., 1984). The expression of virulence factors to environmental signals is an important characteristic of some emerging pathogens.

Host range is also an important aspect of virulence. Wide host range is another feature of some emerging pathogens. Host-adapted pathogens such as *Salmonella typhi*, *Vibrio cholerae*, or polioviruses cannot maintain their infective cycle through animals used for food. Pathogens with wide host range, on the other hand, can maintain a continuous chain of growth from man to animals, and thus have greater infective potential. *Salmonella typhimurium*, *Listeria monocytogenes*, and *Campylobacter jejuni* can be transmitted from species to species with increasing numbers.

Intoxication of food by bacteria, fungi, and algae are also important virulence-determining factors of food- and water-borne pathogens. Accumulation of histamine-like metabolites during growth on scombroid fishes, such as tuna or mackerel, may be considered an aspect of pathogenicity of *Proteus morgani*, *Klebsiella pneumoniae*, and *Clostridium perfringens*.

CONTROL OF FOOD- AND WATER-INFECTIVE MICROORGANISMS

Control of food- and water-infective microorganisms has been a challenging problem for microbiologists as

Table 45–6. *Some Bacterial Pathogens and Their Toxins*

Organism	Location in G.I. Tract	Toxin/Virulence Determinant	Comment/Effect/Activity
Aeromonas hydrophila		Beta-hemolysin	Cytotoxic activity
		Cytotonic enterotoxin	Intestinal fluid secretion
		Cytotoxic enterotoxin	
		Invasive factors	
		Adhesins	
Bacillus cereus		Enterotoxin	Increased intestinal permeability, diarrhea, tissue necrosis
		Emetic toxin	Vomiting
		Edema factor	
		Lethal toxin	
		Hemolysin: heat-stable (HT) and heat-labile (LT)	
Campylobacter jejuni	Small intestine	Enterotoxin	Acts through cyclic AMP mediated adenylate cyclase
		Cytotoxin	Cell toxicity
		Motility due to spiral shape and flagellum	Facilitates movement through viscous mucin layer toward intestinal wall
		Chemotaxis	For mucin and L-fucose
		Adhesins: (outer membrane protein, lipopolysaccharide, and microcalyx material)	Attachment to cell receptors; specific for L-fucose, D-mannose, and D-fucose
Clostridium botulinum A, B, E, F	Colon	Neurotoxin	Respiratory paralysis, inhibits release of acetylcholine
Clostridium perfringens		Enterotoxin	Spore-coat protein alters transport of fluid and glucose; causes tissue damage and inhibits metabolic process
		Gamma and Eta toxin	Lethal activity
		Delta toxin (B and C strains)	Lethal activity, hemolysis
		Theta toxin	Lethal activity, hemolysis, and necrotizing activity
		Kappa toxin	Collagenase
		Lambda toxin (B, E, and D strains)	Protease
		Mu toxin	Hyaluronidase
		Nu toxin	Deoxyribonuclease
		Alpha toxin	Phospholipase C, lysis of cell membrane, intravascular hemolysis
		Beta and Iota toxins	Increased capillary permeability
		Epsilon toxin	Prototoxin converted by trypsin; increased vascular permeability leading to tissue necrosis
		Sialidase	
Escherichia coli	Small intestine	Heat-labile toxin (LT)	Cyclic AMP mediated fluid loss
		Heat-stable toxin (ST)	Cyclic GMP mediated fluid loss
		Cell-associated toxin	
		Cytotoxin	
		Colonization factors: CFA/I, CFA/II, CFA/III	Colonization in human intestine
		Pili adhesins type 1	Mannose-specific
		Pylonephritis-associated pili (PAP)	α Gal (1–4) β Gal-specific
		S pili	Sialic acid-specific
		Afimbrial adhesin	Specific for squamous and transitional epithelial cells

Table 45–6. *Some Bacterial Pathogens and Their Toxins* Continued

Organism	Location in G.I. Tract	Toxin/Virulence Determinant	Comment/Effect/Activity
Listeria monocytogenes		Listeriolysin	Facilitates entry of the pathogen into cytoplasm from endocytic vacuole
		Oxygen radicals	Survival in macrophages
Salmonella spp.	Terminal ileum: epithelium and Peyer's patches (M cells)	Enterotoxin (Cell associated) Delayed permeability factor	Probably fluid loss Cyclic AMP-mediated fluid loss
		Cytoxin	Inhibition of host protein synthesis
		Mannose-resistant hemagghtinin	
Shigella spp.	Colon: columnar mucosal epithelium	Exotoxin	Inhibition of hostprotein synthesis, cytotoxic and neurotoxic activity
		Hemolysin	Invasion of cytoplasm by lysis of endocytic vacuole
		Active metabolism Cell-associated invasive factors Aerobactin Lipopolysaccharide with O antigen	Required for invasion
Staphylococcus aureus		Enterotoxins (A,B,C,D,E,F)	Emetic
		Hemolysins (α, β, γ, δ)	Hemolytic
		Hemolysin α	Lethal and dermonecrotic
		Hemolysin δ	Enteric hemolytic
		Exfoliative toxin (AB)	Exfoliation
		Fibronectin binding protein	Attachment to epithelial cells
		Hyaluroniase	Invasive factor
		Coagulase	Plasma coagulation
		Staphylokinase	Fibrinolytic
		Leucocidin	Lethal to leucocytes
Vibrio cholerae		Cholera toxin	Cyclic AMP-mediated fluid loss
		A1	Acts on adenylate cyclase system
		A2 B (five subunits)	Facilitates entry of toxin into the cell Bind to cell receptors
		Invasive and adhesin factors	Pilus synthesized in response to pH, temperature, and osmolarity
		Flagellum	Facilitates colonization
Yersinia enterocolitica	Small intestine	Invasion factors	Ca^{++}-dependent and expressed at 37°C
	Peyer's patches	V (protein) W (lipoprotein) outer membrane protein Autoagglutination Heat-stable (ST) toxin	Mediates guanylate cyclase system
		Ail DNA (attachment invasion locus)	

Adapted from: Cato, E.P., Lance George, W., and Finegold, S.M. 1986. Genus clostridium. In *Bergey's Manual of Systematic Bacteriology.* Volume 2. Edited by P.H.A. Sneath, N.S. Mair, E.M. Charpe and J.G. Holt. Baltimore, Williams & Wilkins, pp. 1141–1200; Glatz, B.A. 1988. Genetic regulation of toxin production by foodborne microbes. In *Food Microbiology.* Volume 1. Concepts in physiology and metabolism. Edited by T.J. Montville. Boca Raton, FL, CRC press, pp. 103–130; Finlay, B.B. and Falkow, S. 1989. Common themes in microbial pathogenicity. Microbiol. Rev., 53, 210–230; Atwagg, M., and Geiss, H.K. 1989. *Aeromonas* as human pathogen. CRC Critical Rev. Microbiol. *16,* 253–286.

Table 45–7. *Food Poisoning by Algal Toxins*

Alga	Toxin	Comment
Gambierdiscus toxicus *Provocentrum concavum* *Provocentrum mexicana*	Ciguatoxin and maitotoxin	Ciguatera poisoning through reef- or bottom-feeding fishes: baracuda, grouper, red snapper, and sea bass
Gonyaulax catenella *Gonyaulax tamarensis*	Sagitoxins	Paralytic shellfish poisoning through clams, mussels, cockles, and scallops
Ptychodiscus brevis	Brevitoxins B and C	Neurotoxic shellfish poisoning associated with red tide
Dinophysis fortii *Dinophysis acuminata*	Okadaic acid, dinophysistoxins, and pectenotoxins	Diarrhetic shellfish poisoning

Adapted from Taylor, S.L. 1988. Marine toxins of microbial origin. Food Technol., *42*, 94–98.

Table 45–8. *Some Fungal Toxins Found in Food Products*

Organism	Toxin	Food Product
Aspergillus flavus *A. parasiticus*	Aflatoxins	Wheat, corn, soybean, flour, bread, barley, cornmeal, peanut, cheese, hops, moldy meats
Alternaria spp.	Alternariol Altenuisol Alternuene Tenuazonic acid	Processed tomato products, pecans
Penicillium citrinin *P. implicatum* *P. chrzaszczi* *P. citreo-sulfuratum* *P. lividum* *P. phaeo-janthinellum* *P. viridicatum* *Aspergillus terreus* *A. candidus* *A. niveus*	Citrinin	Cereal grains, barley, rice
Claviceps purpurea	Ergot alkaloids	Cereal grains, forage grasses
Aspergillus flavus *A. oryzae* *A. tamari* *A. glaucus*	Kojic acid	Foods stored in homes
Penicillium brevi-compactum *P. roquefortii* *P. viridicatum* *P. brunneum*	Mycophenolic acid	Cheese
Aspergillus nidulans	Nidulin	Corn
Aspergillus ochraceus *A. melleus* *A. sulphureus* *Penicillium viridicatum*	Ochratoxins	Corn, wheat, oats, barley, and green coffee
Aspergillus clavatus *A. giganteus* *A. terreus* *Penicillium patulum* *P. griseo-fulvum* *P. claviforme* *P. expansum, P. novae-zeelandiae* *P. melinii, P. leucopus* *P. equinum* *Gymnoascus* spp.	Patulin	Apple products

Table 45–8. *Some Fungal Toxins Found in Food Products* Continued

Organism	Toxin	Food Product
Penicillium viridicatum *Trichophyton megnini* *T. rubrum* *T. violaceum*	Xanthomegnin	Stored grains
Penicillium viridicatum *Aspergillus sulphureus* *A. melleus*	Viomellien	Stored grains
Penicillium puberculum *P. stoloniferum* *P. cyclopium* *P. martensii* *P. thomii* *P. suavolens* *P. palitans* *P. baarnense* *P. madriti* *Aspergillus ochraceus* *A. sulphureus* *A. guericinus* *A. melleus*	Penicillic acid	Corn-dried beans, moldy tobacco, cereal grains
Penicillium rubrum	Rubratoxins	Feedstuff
Aspergillus versicolor *A. flavus* *A. nidulans* *Penicillium luteum* *Bipolaris* spp.	Sterigmatocystins	Feed wheat, coffee, cheese
Fusarium spp. *Myrothecium* spp. *Trichothecium* spp.	Trichothecenes	Corn, wheat, mixed feeds
Gibberella zeae	Zearalenone	Corn, moldy hay, feed

Adapted from: Bullerman, L.B. 1986. Mycotoxins and food safety. Food Technol., *40*, 59–66; Stoloff, L. 1984. Toxigenic fungi. In *Compendium of Methods for the Microbiological Examination of Foods*. Edited by M. Speck. Washington, D.C. American Public Health Association, pp. 557–572.

well as for public-health scientists for over a century. New problems have come up after employing newer processing, storage, and transportation procedures in the food industry. Several measures are available to control food- and water-borne pathogens. Food- and water-borne infective agents can be controlled by prevention through the practice of cleaning, sanitation, and personal hygiene. The use of vaccines, antibiotics, and physical and chemical agents also can be used to control the pathogens. Prevention of intestinal colonization by pathogens through microbiologic, chemical, and genetic methods have potential to control these microorganisms.

An Integrated System

A preplanned integrated approach to control the pathogens in the food industry and related establishments was recommended by National Research Council (NRC, 1985a). This was termed as the Hazard Analysis and Critical Control Point (HACCP) system. The HACCP system is designed (1) to identify and to assess hazards associated with growing, harvesting, processing, marketing, preparation, and use of a given raw material or food product, (2) to determine specific measures (critical control points) to control an identifiable hazard, and (3) to establish systems to monitor critical control points. Microbiologic, chemical, and physical tests, as well as visual observations, are employed to monitor the critical control points.

Factors that are considered in hazard analysis include (1) epidemiologic evidence of food as a vehicle of disease, (2) the ability of pathogens to contaminate, survive, and grow in the food during manufacture, storage, distribution, preservice preparation, and serving, and (3) susceptibility of probable consumers to the infective agent or toxins.

Standards, guidelines, and specifications for both pathogens and indicator organisms are considered for evaluating microbiologic criteria during hazard analysis. Presence of pathogens relates directly to the risk, whereas presence of indicator organisms points to the probable presence of a pathogen or its toxins, improper practices adversely affecting safety or shelf-life, or unsuitability of food or an ingredient for its intended use.

When detection of pathogens is difficult or time-consuming, assessment of fecal contamination can be determined by the presence of indicator organisms such as

Table 45–9. *Preventive Practices for Food- and Water-Infective Microorganisms (Applicable for Poor Rural Areas of Developing Countries)*

Food preparation
Washing hands with soap and water before food handling
Avoidance of fecal contamination during food preparation
Safe preparation of dried or artificial milk
Short delay between preparation and consumption of food
Thorough cooking
Washing fruits and vegetables
Appropriate storage of left-over foods
Protection of food from insects and rodents

Feeding of children
Breast-feeding and delaying onset of weaning
Feeding safe supplements in clean bottles or by cups and spoons

Handling of water
Use of safe water supply
Treatment of unsafe water supply
Boiling water for drinking
Storage of drinking water in separate and clean containers

Toilet practices
Use of toilets and latrines
Washing hands with soap and water after toilet visits or after handling of human or animal feces

Adapted from WHO. 1984. The role of food safety in health and development. Report of a joint FAO/WHO expert committee on food safety. Geneva.

Table 45–10. *Risk of Development of Bacterial Resistance to Antibiotics*

Risk Rating*	Antibiotic(s)
1	Bacitracin, flavophospholipo, virginiamycin
2	Polymyxin, furans, lincomycin, tylosin, and related macrolides
3	Erythromycin, spiramycin, oleandomycin
4	Penicillins, tetracyclines
5	Ampicillin, cephalosporins
6	Sulphonamides, streptomycin, neomycin
7	Chloramphenicol

*Higher number indicates higher risk.
Adapted from Silliker, J.H., et al. 1980. *Microbial Ecology of Foods.* Volume 1. New York, Academic Press.

E. coli, Streptococcus faecalis or bacteriophages, commonly found in the intestine in large numbers. Sensitive and faster detection of indicator organisms can be used to implement sanitation procedures for the control of pathogens (Hartman et al., 1982). However, absence of indicator organisms does not always indicate absence of pathogens. Thus water that meets regulatory indicator standards may show presence of enteroviruses.

Some of the hazards or risk factors responsible for foodborne infections in industrialized countries have been mentioned previously in the section under processing and handling. Prevention or elimination of these hazards by appropriate measures can result in control of foodborne infections. Table 45–9 shows precautions and practices necessary for the control of food- and water-borne pathogens in poor rural areas of developing countries (WHO, 1984).

Physical and Chemical Agents

The application of heat and radiation, low-temperature storage, and desiccation are some of the physical methods used for control of pathogens in the food industry. Irradiation of food for the control of pathogens is likely to become one of the most versatile technologies in the near future (Urbain, 1989). Use of chemicals for preservation as well as for disinfection and sanitation can result in effective control of most of the water- and food-infective microorganisms. Commonly used food-plant sanitizers such as acid anionics, quaternary ammonium

compounds, iodophores, and organic and inorganic hypochlorites have been found effective against both grampositive and gram-negative bacteria (Lopes, 1986). Chlorine, ozone, and chlorine dioxide have broad disinfecting range against viruses, bacteria, and protozoa, and have been used in disinfection of drinking water (Logsdon and Hoff, 1986). Filtration of water prior to chemical treatment to remove particulate matter and many microorganisms by using sand and polymers effectively increases activity of disinfectants.

Role of Antibiotics

Antibiotics are the most effective class of agents used to control food- and water-infective microorganisms. However, widespread and indiscriminate use of antibiotics for therapy, prophylaxis, and growth enhancement in animal feeds has led to development of plasmid-mediated multiple-drug-resistant microorganisms (Levy et al., 1976). This raises both the possibility of transfer of drug resistance from nonpathogenic to pathogenic organisms and the fear of failure of antibiotic therapy (Swann Committee Report, 1969; FDA, 1972). Because man and animals live in a single ecologic system, the use of antibiotics in animal feed can result in the appearance of drug-resistant human pathogens (Holmberg et al., 1984). However, the use of antibiotics for therapy and in animal feeds has made possible successful modern farming with intense and crowded rearing conditions (Kiser et al., 1971).

The WHO working group (WHO, 1973) emphasizes that the benefit of feeding low levels of antibiotics far outweighs the hazards of their use in agriculture. This report classifies the antibiotics used for therapy, prophylaxis, and growth enhancement in order of increasing risk with respect to the development of bacterial resistance (Table 45–10). Regulated use of antibiotics is essential for the control of pathogens and for economic benefits. Because pathogens often cross national boundaries, a single unified global regulation is essential for the use of antibiotics.

Principle of Competitive Exclusion

The use of either microorganisms or chemicals for preventing attachment and subsequent colonization by pathogens in the intestine are comparatively new and upcoming concepts. This approach probably can be employed to protect the host from infection by some food- and water-infective pathogens. Stern and Meinersmann (1989) concluded that prevention of colonization of pathogens such as *Campylobacter jejuni* in poultry can be one of the most important approaches in the control of pathogens in food derived from animals. Use of genetics for breeding birds resistant to colonization by pathogens can also be considered one of the control measures.

"Nurmi" Concept

Commercial poultry flocks often become carriers of pathogenic microorganisms (Mead and Impey, 1987; Genigeorgis et al., 1986; Beery et al., 1988). Nonhost-specific salmonellae readily colonize the intestinal tracts of newly hatched chicks and turkey poults on commercial farms. Nurmi and Rantala (1973) showed that salmonellae colonization in chicks can be prevented by establishing mature intestinal microflora by feeding chicks with a suspension of gut contents of *Salmonella*-free adult birds. The "Nurmi" concept or the principle of competitive exclusion can be employed to prevent the carrier state of food-borne pathogens in birds. Birds receiving adult microflora become resistant to colonization by higher numbers of salmonellae. The treatment reduces the incidence of the carrier state and the number of salmonellae being shed. The birds also show increased resistance to colonization by other pathogens such as *Campylobacter jejuni*, *Clostridium botulinum* type C, *C. perfringens*, pathogenic *E. coli*, and *Yersinia enterocolitica* (Mead and Impey, 1987). The mechanism probably involves saturation of attachment sites by adult microflora on intestinal epithelium, resulting in exclusion and subsequent prevention of colonization of pathogens. Immunosuppressed chicks also exhibit colonization resistance when fed on gut flora, indicating direct saturation of epithelial attachment sites rather than activation of immune system.

Use of Chemical Moieties

Chemical moieties show potential for use in preventing the first major interaction and attachment of pathogens and the host. Small chemical molecules with high specificity can either bind to the adhesins of the pathogens or to the receptors on the host cells, thereby preventing attachment of pathogens or toxins to host cells (Paulson, 1985; Eidels et al., 1983; Finlay and Falkow, 1989). Of the numerous receptor sites present on the host cell, only a few serve as targets for the attachment of pathogens.

Many species of *Enterobacteriaceae* attach by means of adhesins that specifically bind to D-mannose residue on the host-cell receptors (Clegg and Gerlach, 1978; Eisenstein, 1988). Cholera toxin and heat-labile (LT) *E. coli* toxin bind to the same ganglioside receptors on mammalian cell surface (Eidels et al., 1983). *Staphylococcus aureus* and *Streptococcus pyogenes* (group A) use fibronectin, a glycoprotein molecule present on epithelial cell surface, as a receptor for attachment (Beachey and Courtney, 1987; Proctor, 1987). Lipoteichoic acid present on *S. pyogenes* (group A) cells acts as an adhesin to attach to fibronectin molecule (Courtney et al., 1988).

These specific binding characteristics can be useful in controlling infection processes. A mannose-containing glycoprotein (the Tam-Horsfall protein) produced in the kidney and present in urine, binds to type 1 pili of *Enterobacteriaceae*. It may protect the host from bacterial infection of the kidney (Finlay and Falkow, 1989). N-acetyl-D-galactosamine, L-fucose, D-galactose, L+ arabinose and D+ mannose were found to reduce attachment of *Salmonella typhimurium* to ceca of 1-week-old chicks (McHan et al., 1989). L-Fucose was found to inhibit adhesion of *Vibrio cholerae* to intestinal brush-borders of the adult rabbit in vitro (Jones et al., 1976; Jones and Freter, 1976). Fructose and tannin-like material from cranberry juice were reported to interfere in the attachment of *E. coli* cells to receptors through type 1 and P pili, respectively (Fox, 1979). P pili bind specifically to galactose disaccharide present on the host-cell receptors.

Economic Factors

Acceptance and implementation of measures at the national and community levels to control food- and water-infective microorganisms require cost-effectiveness and net benefit from these measures. The economic losses due to illness will vary with the infective agent and will differ from country to country. The annual cost of salmonellosis was reported to be 10.8 million deutsche marks, 4.5 million British pounds, 98 million Canadian dollars, and 1.9 to 2.3 billion U.S. dollars (WHO, 1986; Todd, 1989a, b). Maintenance of cleanliness, education of personnel associated with food processing and food service sectors, and use of chemical sanitizers were reported to be some of the least expensive control measures, whereas irradiation and competitive exclusion (Nurmi method) were found to be relatively more expensive control measures against human salmonellosis associated with poultry. On a large-scale and long-term basis, the last two measures would probably be more cost-effective. Implementation of more than one single control measure is necessary for success in preventing infections and illnesses due to food- and water-infective microorganisms.

ACKNOWLEDGMENT

The author thanks Dr. N.J. Stern, the U.S. Department of Agriculture, and Dr. M.V.N. Shirodkar, Indian Council of Medical Research, for reviewing the manuscript, and Dr. S.S. Block, University of Florida, for suggesting improvements.

REFERENCES

Ashenafi, M., and Busse, M. 1989. Inhibitory effect of *Lactobacillus palantarum* on *Salmonella infantis*, *Enterobacter aerogenes* and *Escherichia coli* during tempeh fermentation. J. Food Protect., 52, 169–172.

Atwegg, M., and Geiss, H.K. 1989. *Aeromonas* as human pathogen. CRC Crit. Rev. Microbiol., *16*, 253–286.

Banwart, G.J. (ed.) 1981. *Basic Food Microbiology.* New York, AVI.

Barbaree, J.M., et al. 1986. Isolation of protozoa from water associated with legionellosis outbreak and demonstration of intracellular multiplication of *Legionella pneumophila.* Appl. Environ. Microbiol., *51*, 422–424.

Bartlett, J.G. 1979. Antibiotic associated colitis. Clin. Gastroenterol., 8, 783–801.

Beachey, E.H., and Courtney, H.S. 1987. Bacterial adherence: the attachment of group A streptococci to mucosal surfaces. Rev. Infect. Dis., *9*(Suppl. 5), 475–481.

Beckers, H.J. 1988. Incidence of food borne diseases in the Netherlands: annual summary 1982 and an overview from 1979 to 1982. J. Food Protect., *51*, 327–354.

Beery, J.T., Hugdahl, M.B., and Doyle, M.P. 1988. Colonization of gastrointestinal tracts of chicks by *Campylobacter jejuni.* Appl. Environ. Microbiol., *54*, 2365–2370.

Benton, C., et al. 1983. The contamination of a major water supply by gulls (*Larus* spp.). Water Res., *17*, 789–798.

Bhat, P.B., Shanthakumari, S., and Rajan, D. 1974. The characterization and significance of *Pleisiomonas shigelloides* and *Aeromonas hydrophila* isolated from an epidemic of diarrhea. Indian J. Med. Res., *62*, 1051–1060.

Bingham, A.K., and Meyer, E.A. 1979. *Giardia* excystation can be induced in vitro in acidic solutions. Nature, *277*, 301–302.

Black, R.E., et al. 1978. Epidemic *Yersinia enterocolitica* infection due to contaminated chocolate milk. N. Engl. J. Med., *298*, 76–79.

Blacklow, N.R., and Cukor, G. 1985. Viral gastroenteritis agents. In *Manual of Clinical Microbiology.* 4th Edition. Edited by E.H. Lennette, A. Balows, W.J. Hausler, and H. Jean Shadomy. Washington, D.C., American Society for Microbiology, pp. 805–812.

Blaser, M.J. 1982. *Campylobacter jejuni* and food. Food Technol., *36*, 69–92.

Bowen, G.S., and McCarty, M.A. 1983. Hepatitis A associated with a hardware store water fountain and contaminated well in Lancaster County, Pennsylvania, 1980. Am. J. Epidemiol., *117*, 695–705.

Bryan, F.L. 1977. Diseases transmitted by foods contaminated by waste water. J. Food Protect., *40*, 45–56.

Bryan, F.L. 1978. Factors that contribute to outbreaks of foodborne diseases. J. Food Protect., *41*, 816–827.

Bryan, F.L. 1988. Risks of practices, procedures and processes that lead to outbreaks of foodborne diseases. J. Food Protect., *51*, 663–673.

Bullerman, L.B. 1986. Mycotoxins and food safety. Food Technol., *40*, 59–66.

Cann, D.C., et al. 1965. The incidence of *Clostridium botulinum* type E in fish and bottom deposits in the North Sea and off the coast of Scandinavia. J. Appl. Bacteriol., *28*, 426–430.

Caselitz, F.H. 1955. Ein neues Bacterium der Gattung: *Vibrio muller, Vibrio jamaicensis.* Z. Tropenmed. Parasitol., *6*, 52.

Cato, E.P., Lance George, W., and Finegold, S.M. 1986. Genus Clostridium. In *Bergey's Manual of Systematic Bacteriology.* Volume 2. Edited by P.H.A. Sneath, N.S. Mair, E.M. Charpe, and J.G. Holt. Baltimore, Williams & Wilkins, pp. 1141–1200.

CDC. 1985. Milk-borne salmonellosis—Illinois. Morbid. Mortal. Weekly Rep., *34*, 200.

CDC. 1987. Update: *Salmonella enteritidis* infections in the Northeastern United States. Morbid. Mortal. Weekly Rep., *36*, 204–205.

Clegg, S., and Gerlach, G.F. 1987. Enterobacterial fimbriae. J. Bacteriol., *169*, 934–938.

Coodwin, C.S., et al. 1989. Transfer of *Campylobacter pylori* and *Campylobacter mustelae* to *Helicobacter* gen. nov. as *Helicobacter pylori,* comb. nov. and *Helicobacter mustelae* comb. nov. respectively. Int. J. Syst. Bacteriol., *39*, 397–405.

Corlett, D.A. 1989. Refrigerated foods and use of hazard analysis and critical control point principles. Food Technol., *43*, 91–94.

Courtney, H.S., et al. 1988. Localization of a lipoteichoic acid binding site to a 24-kilodalton NH2-terminal fragment of fibronectin. Rev. Infect. Dis., *10*(Suppl. 2), 360–362.

Craun, G.F. 1984. Waterborne outbreaks of giardiasis, current status. In *Giardia and Giardiasis.* Edited by S.L. Erlandsen. New York, Plenum Press, pp. 243–261.

Datta, A.R., Wentz, B.A., and Hill, H.E. 1987. Detection of hemolytic *Listeria monocytogenes* by using DNA colony hybridization. Appl. Environ. Microbiol., *53*, 2256–2259.

Dekeyser, P., Gossuln-Detrain, M., Butzler, J.P., and Sternon, J. 1972. Acute enteritis due to related vibrio: first positive stool cultures. J. Infect. Dis., *125*, 390–392.

de Nobele, J. 1898. Du Séro-diagnostic dans les affections gastro-intestinales d'origine alimentaire. Ann. Soc. Med. Gand., *LXXVII*, 281–306.

Dobell, C. 1920. The discovery of intestinal protozoa of man. Proc. R. Soc. Med., *13*, 1–15.

Doyle, M.P. 1986. Detection and quantitation of food borne pathogens and their toxins: gram-negative bacterial pathogens. In *Food Borne Microorganisms and Their Toxins: Developing Methodology.* Edited by M.D. Pierson and N.J. Stern. IFT Basic Symposium Series, Marcel Dekker, New York, pp. 317–344.

Doyle, M.P., and Schoeni, J.L. 1984. Survival and growth characteristics of *Escherichia coli* associated with hemorrhagic colitis. Appl. Environ. Microbiol., *48*, 855–856.

Eidels, L., Proia, R.L., and Hart, D.A. 1983. Membrane receptors for bacterial toxins. Microbiol. Rev., *4*, 596–620.

Eisenstein, B.I. 1988. Type I fimbriae of *Escherichia coli*: genetic regulation, morphogenesis, and role in pathogenesis. Rev. Infect. Dis., *10*(Suppl. 2), 341–344.

El-Sahn, M.A., El-Banna, A.A., and El-Tabbey Shehata, A.M. 1982. Occurrence of *Vibrio parahaemolyticus* in selected marine invertebrates, sediment and seawater around Alexandria, Egypt. Can. J. Microbiol., *28*, 1261–1264.

Fields, P.L., Groisman, E.A., and Heffron, F. 1989. A *Salmonella* locus that controls resistance to microbial proteins from phagocytic cells. Science, *243*, 1059–1061.

Fenner, F. 1980. Sociocultural change and environmental diseases. In *Changing Disease Pattern and Human Behavior.* Edited by N.F. Stanley and R.A. Joske. New York, Academic Press, pp. 8–25.

Finlay, B.B., and Falkow, S. 1989. Common themes in microbial pathogenicity. Microbiol. Rev., *53*, 210–230.

Finlay, B.B., Heffron, F., and Falkow, S. 1989. Epithelial cell surfaces induce *Salmonella* proteins required for bacterial adherence and invasion. Science, *243*, 940–943.

Foster, E.M. 1988. A half century of food microbiology and a glimpse at the years ahead. Dairy Food Sanit., *8*, 586–592.

Fox, J.L. 1989. Bacterial lectins and the cranberry factor. ASM News, *55*, 657.

Fujino, T., et al. 1951. On bacteriological examination of shirasu food poisoning. J. Jap. Assoc. Infect. Dis., *25*, 11–12.

Gallard, L., and Bueno, H. 1989. Advances in laboratory diagnosis of intestinal parasites. Am. Clin. Lab., *8*, 18–19.

Gärtner. 1888. Ueber die Fleischvergiftung in Frankenhausen a. K. und dea Erreger derselben. Cor. Bl. d. allg. ärztl. Ver. v. Thüringen, Weimar. XVII, 573–600.

Genigeorgis, C., Hassuneh, M., and Collins, P. 1986. *Campylobacter jejuni* infection on poultry farms and its effect on poultry meat contamination during slaughter. J. Food Protect., *49*, 895–903.

Genigeorgis, C. 1986. Problems associated with perishable processed meats. Food Technol., *40*, 140–154.

Gerba, C.P. 1988. Viral disease transmission by seafoods. Food Technol., *42*, 99–103.

Gionella, R.A., Broitman, S.A., and Zamcheck, N. 1971. Salmonella enteritis: role of reduced gastric secretions in pathogenesis. Am. J. Dig. Dis., *16*, 1000–1013.

Glatz, B.A. 1988. Genetic regulation of toxin production by foodborne microbes. In *Food Microbiology.* Volume 1. Concepts in physiology and metabolism. Edited by T.J. Montville. Boca Raton, FL, CRC Press, pp. 103–130.

Grady, G.F., et al. 1987. Update: *Salmonella enteritidis* infections in the Northwestern United States. Mortal. Morbid. Weekly Rep., *36*, 204–205.

Hall, H.E., Angelotti, R., Lewis, K.H., and Foster, M.J. 1963. Characteristics of *Clostridium perfringens* strains associated with food and foodborne disease. J. Bacteriol., *85*, 1094–1103.

Hartman, P.A., Petzel, J.P., and Kaspar, C.W. 1982. New methods for indicator organisms. In *Foodborne Microorganisms and Their Toxins: Developing Methodology.* Edited by M.D. Pierson and N.J. Stern. New York, Marcel Dekker, pp. 175–217.

Healy, G.R., et al. 1984. Food borne parasites. In *Compendium of Methods for Microbiological Examination of Foods.* Edited by M.L. Speck. Washington, D.C., American Public Health Association, pp. 542–556.

Health Protection Bureau. 1985. Salmonellosis associated with cheese consumption—Canada. Morbid. Mortal. Weekly Rep., *33*, 387.

Ho, J.L., et al. 1986. An outbreak of type 4b *Listeria monocytogenes* infection involving patients from eight Boston hospitals. Arch. Intern. Med., *146*, 520–524.

Hobbs, B.C. 1979. *Clostridium perfringens* gastroenteritis. In *Food Borne Infections and Intoxications.* Edited by H. Riemann and F. Bryan. New York, Academic Press, pp. 131–171.

Holmberg, S.D., Osterholm, M.T., Senger, K.A., and Cohen, M.L. 1984. Drug resistant *Salmonella* from animals fed antimicrobials. N. Engl. J. Med., *311*, 617–622.

Hornick, R.B. 1988. *Campylobacter pylori*—a bacterial cause of peptic ulcer disease. Bull. N.Y. Acad. Med., *64*, 529–537.

Hornick, R.B., et al. 1971. The Broad Street pump revisited: response of volunteers to ingested cholera vibrios. Bull. N.Y. Acad. Med., *47*, 1181–1191.

Hsu, K.L., Paglini, S., Alstein, B., and Crowell, R.L. 1990. Identification of a second cellular receptor for a coxsackievirus B3 variant, CB3-RD. In *New Aspects of Positive-Strand RNA Viruses.* Edited by M.A. Brinton and F.X. Heinz. American Society for Microbiology, Washington, D.C., pp. 271–277.

James, S.M., et al. 1985. Listeriosis outbreak associated with Mexican-style cheese—California. Morbid. Mortal. Weekly Rep., *34*, 357–359.

Jackson Tartakow, L., and Vorperian, J.H. 1980. Gastrointestinal illness aboard cruise ships and aircraft. In *Food Borne and Water Borne Diseases.* Westpoint, CT, AIV Publishing, pp. 259–264.

Jones, G.W., Abrams, G.D., and Freter, R. 1976. Adhesive properties of *Vibrio cholerae*: adhesion to isolated rabbit brush-border membranes and haemagglutinating activity. Infect. Immun., *14*, 232–239.

Jones, G.W., and Freter, R. 1976. Adhesion properties of *Vibrio cholerae*: nature of the interaction with isolated brush-border membranes and human erythrocytes. Infect. Immun., *14*, 240–245.

Johnson, R.W. 1987. Microbial food safety. Dairy Food Sanit., *7*, 174–176.

Kapadia, C.R., Bhat, P., Baker, S.J., and Mathan, V.I. 1984. A common source epidemic of mixed bacterial diarrhea with secondary transmission. Am. J. Epidemiol., *120*, 743–749.

Kapikian, A.Z., et al. 1972. Visualization by immune electron microscopy of a 27 nm particle associated with acute infectious nonbacterial gastroenteritis. J. Virol., *10*, 1075–1088.

Kendall, D. 1989. One in three chickens contaminated, USDA Warns. *Detroit News*, July 1.

Kiser, J.S., Gale, G.O., and Kemp, G.A. 1971. Antibiotics as feedstuff additives: the risk-benefit equation for man. CRC Crit. Rev. Toxicol., *1*, 55–92.

Korgstad, D.J., Visvesvara, G.S., Walls, K.W., and Smith, J.W. 1985. Blood and tissue protozoa. In *Manual of Clinical Microbiology.* 4th Edition. Edited by E.H. Lennette, A. Balows, W.J. Hausler, and H. Jean Shadomy. Washington, D.C., American Society for Microbiology, pp. 612–630.

Kornacki, J., and Marth, E.H. 1982. Foodborne illness caused by *Escherichia coli*: A review. J. Food Protect., *45*, 1051–1067.

Larkin, E.P. 1986. Detection, quantitation and public health significance of foodborne viruses. In *Food Borne Microorganisms and Their Toxins: Developing Methodology.* Edited by M.D. Pierson and N.J. Stern. New York, Marcel Dekker, pp. 439–451.

LeBaron, C.W., et al. 1990. Viral agents of gastroenteritis. Morbid. Mortal. Weekly Rep., *39*, 1–24.

Levy, S.B., FitzGerald, G.B., and Macone, A.B. 1976. Spread of antibiotic-resistant plasmids to chicken and from chicken to man. Nature, *260*, 40–42.

Lewis, G.D., Austin, F.J., and Loutit, M.W. 1986. Enteroviruses of human origin and fecal coliforms in riverwater and sediments downstream from a sewage outfall in Taleri river, Otago. J. Mar. Freshwater Res., *20*, 101–105.

Lofgren, J.P., et al. 1982. Multistate outbreak of yersinosis. Morbid. Mortal. Weekly Rep., *31*, 505–506.

Logston, G.S., and Hoff, J.C. 1986. Barriers to the transmission of water borne disease. In *Water Borne Diseases in the United States.* Edited by G.F. Craun. New York, CRC Press, pp. 256–273.

Lopes, J.A. 1986. Evaluation of dairy and food plant sanitizers against *Salmonella typhimurium* and *Listeria monocytogenes*. J. Dairy Sci., *69*, 2791–2796.

Lovett, J. 1988. Isolation and enumeration of *Listeria monocytogenes*. Food Technol., *42*, 172–175.

Madden, J.M., McCardell, B.A., and Archer, D.L. 1986. Virulence assessment of food borne microbes. In *Food Borne Microorganisms and Their Toxins: Developing Methodology.* Edited by M.D. Pierson and N.J. Stern. New York, Marcel Dekker, pp. 291–315.

Martelle, S., and Tschirhart, D. 1988. Ailment is infectious, can be dangerous. *Detroit News*, October 15.

Maurelli, A.T., Blackmon, B., and Curtiss, R. 1984. Temperature-dependent expression of virulence genes in *Shigella* species. Infect. Immunol., *43*, 195–201.

McDade, J.E., et al. 1977. Legionnaire's disease: isolation of a bacterium and demonstration of its role in other respiratory disease. N. Engl. J. Med., *297*, 1197–1203.

McHan, F., Cox, N.A., Blankenship, L.C., and Bailey, J.S. 1989. In vitro attachment of *Salmonella typhimurium* to chick ceca exposed to selected carbohydrates. Avian Dis., *33*, 340–344.

Mead, G.C., and Impey, C.S. 1987. The present status of the Nurmi concept for reducing carriage of food-poisoning salmonellae and other pathogens in live poultry. In *Elimination of Pathogenic Organisms from Meat and Poultry.* Edited by F.J.M. Smulders. Amsterdam, Elsevier, pp. 57–77.

Melvin, D.M., and Healy, G.R. 1985. Intestinal and urogenital protozoa. In *Manual of Clinical Microbiology.* 4th Edition. Edited by E.H. Lennette, A. Balows, W.J. Hausler, and H. Jean Shadomy. Washington, D.C., American Society for Microbiology, pp. 631–650.

Meyer, R.D. 1983. *Legionella* infections: a review of five years of research. Rev. Infect. Dis., *5*, 258–278.

Midura, T.F., and Arnon, S.S. 1976. Identification of *Clostridium botulinum* and its toxins in faeces. Lancet, *2*, 934–935.

Miller, J.F., Mekalanos, J.J., and Falkow, S. 1989. Coordinate regulation and sensory transduction in the control of bacterial virulence. Science, *243*, 916–921.

Mims, C. 1980. The emergence of new infectious diseases. In *Changing Disease Pattern and Human Behavior.* Edited by N.F. Stanley and R.A. Joske. New York, Academic Press, pp. 231–250.

NRC. 1985a. Selection of pathogens as components of microbiological criteria.

In *An Evaluation of the Role of Microbiological Criteria for Foods and Food Ingredients.* Washington, D.C., National Academy Press, pp. 72–103.

NRC. 1985b. Current status of microbiological criteria and legislative bases. In *An Evaluation of the Role of Microbiological Criteria for Foods and Food Ingredients.* Edited by subcommittee on microbiological criteria for foods and food ingredients. Washington, D.C., National Academy Press, pp. 152–173.

Nurmi, E., and Rantala, M. 1973. New aspects of *Salmonella* infection in broiler production. Nature, *241*, 210–211.

Ortel, S. 1968. Bakteriologische serologische and epidemiologische untersuchungen warhend einer Listeriose-Epidemie. Dtsh. Gesundheitswes., *16*, 753–759.

Palumbo, S.A., Morgan, D.R., and Buchanan, R.L. 1985. The influence of temperature, NaCl and pH on the growth of *Aeromonas hydrophila*. J. Food Sci., *50*, 1417–1421.

Palumbo, S.A. 1986. Is refrigeration enough to restrain foodborne pathogens? J. Food Protect., *49*, 1003–1009.

Paulson, J.C. 1985. Interaction of animal viruses with cell surface receptors. In *The Receptors.* Volume II. Edited by P. Michael Conn. New York, Academic Press, pp. 131–219.

Pearson, R.D., and Hewlett, E.L. 1988. Amebiasis in travellers. In *Amebiasis.* Edited by J.I. Ravdin. New York, John Wiley & Sons, pp. 556–562.

Pickett, J., Berg, B., Chaplin, E., and Brunstetter-Shafer, M. 1976. Syndrome of botulism in infancy: clinical and electrophysiologic study. N. Engl. J. Med., *295*, 770–772.

Portnoy, D.A., Moseley, S.L., and Falkow, S. 1981. Characterization of plasmids and plasmid-associated determinants of *Yersinia enterocolitica* pathogenesis. Infect. Immunol., *31*, 775–782.

Prentice, T., Wood, N., and Ford, R. 1989. Health chief warns of new food danger. *London Times*, Feb. 11.

Proctor, R.A. 1987. The staphylococcal fibronectin receptor: evidence for its importance in invasive infection. Rev. Infect. Dis., *9*(Suppl. 4), 335–340.

Racaniello, V.R., et al. 1990. Molecular genetics of cellular receptors for poliovirus. In *New Aspects of Positive-Strand RNA Viruses.* Edited by M.A. Brinton and F.X. Heinz. American Society for Microbiology, Washington, D.C., pp. 278–294.

Ray, B. 1986. Impact of bacterial injury and repair in food microbiology: its past, present and future. J. Food Protect., *49*, 651–655.

Rendtorff, R.C. 1954. The experimental transmission of human intestinal protozoa parasites. II. *Giardia lamblia* cysts given in capsules. Am. J. Hyg., *59*, 209–270.

Rosenow, M., and Marth, E.H. 1987. Growth patterns of *Listeria monocytogenes* in skim, whole and chocolate milk and whipping cream at 4, 8, 13, 21, and 35°C. J. Food Protect., *50*, 452–459.

Ryan, C.A., et al. 1987. Massive outbreak of antimicrobial resistant salmonellosis traced to pasteurized milk. JAMA, *258*, 3269–3274.

Ryan, C.A., et al. 1986. *Escherichia coli* 0157:H7 diarrhea in a nursing home: clinical, epidemiological, and pathological findings. J. Infect. Dis., *154*, 526–529.

Sakazaki, R., and Shimada, T. 1982. *Vibrio* species as causative agents of foodborne infection. In *Development in Food Microbiology— 2.* Edited by R.K. Robinson. New York, Elsevier, pp. 123–151.

Sathe, P.V., et al. 1983. Investigation report of an epidemic of fever. Int. J. Epidemiol., *12*, 215–219.

Schiemann, D.A. 1987. *Yersinia enterocolitica* in milk and dairy products. J. Dairy Sci., *70*, 383–391.

Schlech, W.F., Chase, D.P., and Badley, A. 1986. A rat model of *L. monocytogenes* infection via the oral route. 1. Development and effect of gastric acidity on infective dose. Presented at 26th Interscience Congress on Antimicrobial Agents and Chemotherapy. New Orleans, LA, Sept. 29–Oct. 1.

Schlech, W.F., et al. 1983. Epidemic listeriosis: Evidence for transmission by food. N. Engl. J. Med., *308*, 203–206.

Schmidt, C.F., Lechowich, R.V., and Follinazzo, J.F. 1961. Growth and toxin production by type E *Clostridium botulinum* below 40°C. J. Food Sci., *26*, 626–630.

Seaman, M.T., Gophen, M., Cavari, B.Z., and Azoulay, B. 1986. *Brachionus calyciflorus* as an agent for removal of *E. coli* in sewage ponds. Hydrobiologia, *135*, 55–60.

Sharrar, R.G. 1985. Prior outbreaks of legionellosis. In *Legionellosis.* Volume 1. Edited by S.M. Katz. New York, CRC Press, pp. 12–18.

Shaw, P.K., et al. 1977. A community wide outbreak of giardiasis with evidence of transmission by a municipal water supply. Ann. Intern. Med., *87*, 426–432.

Silliker, J.H., et al. 1980. *Microbial Ecology of Foods.* Volume 1. New York, Academic Press.

Smith, M., et al. 1985. Turkey associated salmonellosis at an elementary school— Georgia. Morbid. Mortal. Weekly Rep., *34*, 707–708.

Snow, J., and York, J. 1855. Report on the cholera outbreak in the parish of James, Westminster, July, J. Churchill, London.

Sobsey, M.D., et al. 1986. Survival and transport of hepatitis virus in soils, ground water and wastewater. Water Sci. Technol., *18*, 97–106.

Sperber, S.J., and Schleupner, C.J. 1987. Salmonellosis during infection with human immunodeficiency virus. Rev. Infect. Dis., 9, 925–934.

Stanfield, J.T., Wilson, C.R., Andrews, W.H., and Jackson, G.J. 1987. Potential role of refrigerated milk packaging in the transmission of listeriosis and salmonellosis. J. Food Protect., 50, 730–732.

Stern, N.J., and Meinersmann, R.J. 1989. Potentials for colonization control of *Campylobacter jejuni* in the chickens. J. Food Protect., 52, 427–430.

Stewart, P.J., Desormeaux, W., and Chene, J. 1983. Hemorrhagic colitis in a home for the aged—Ontario. Can. Dis. Weekly Rep., 9, 29.

Stewart, K.R., and Kodistschek, L. 1980. Drug-resistance tranfer in *Escherichia coli* in New York Bight Sediment. Mar. Pollut. Bull., 11, 130–133.

Stolle, A. 1981. Spreading of salmonellas during cattle slaughtering. J. Appl. Bacteriol., 50, 239–245.

Stoloff, L. 1984. Toxigenic fungi. In *Compendium of Methods for the Microbiological Examination of Foods.* Edited by M. Speck. Washington, D.C., American Public Health Association, pp. 557–572.

Sugiyama, H., and Sofos, J.N. 1982. Botulism. In *Developments in Food Microbiology.* Edited by R.K. Robinson. New York, Elsevier, pp. 77–120.

Swann Committee Report. 1969. Report of joint committee on the use of antibiotics in animal husbandry and veterinary medicine. HM Stationery Off., London.

Tacket, C.O., et al. 1984. A multistate outbreak of infections caused by *Yersinia enterocolitica* transmitted by pasteurized milk. JAMA, 251, 483–486.

Taylor, S.L. 1988. Marine toxins of microbial origin. Food Technol., 42, 94–98.

Taylor, W.R., et al. 1982. A foodborne outbreak of enterotoxigenic *Escherichia coli* diarrhea. N. Engl. J. Med., 306, 1093–1095.

Thimm, B.M. 1982. Brucellosis—distribution in man, domestic and wild animals. New York, Springer-Verlag.

Todd, E.C.D. 1987. Impact of spoilage and foodborne diseases on national and international economies. Int. J. Food Microbiol., 4, 83–100.

Todd, E.C.D. 1989a. Preliminary estimates of costs of foodborne disease in Canada and costs to reduce salmonellosis. J. Food Protect., 52, 586–594.

Todd, E.C.D. 1989b. Preliminary estimates of costs of foodborne disease in the United States. J. Food Protect., 52, 595–601.

Troller, J.A. 1986. Water relations of foodborne bacterial pathogens—An updated review. J. Food Protect., 49, 656–670.

Tyndall, R.L., et al. 1989. Effect of thermal additions on the density distribution of thermophilic amoebae and pathogenic *Naegleria fowleri* in a newly created cooling lake. Appl. Environ. Microbiol., 55, 722–732.

Umoh, J.U. 1983. Epidemiological features of an outbreak of gastroenteritis/cholera in Kastina, Northern Nigeria. J. Hyg. (G.B.), 91, 101–111.

Urbain, W.M. 1989. Food irradiation: The past fifty years as prologue to tomorrow. Food Technol., 43, 76, 92.

US FDA. 1972. Report to the commissioner of the food and drug administration by the FDA task force on the use of antibiotics in animal feeds. FDA, Rockville, Maryland.

Van Heyningen, W.E., and Seal, J.R. 1983. *Cholera. The American Scientific Experience 1947–1980.* Boulder, CO, Westview Press.

Vasavada, P.C. 1988. Pathogenic bacteria in milk—a review. J. Dairy Sci., 71, 2809–2816.

Vasconcelos, G.J., and Anthony, N.C. 1985. Microbiological quality of recreational waters in the pacific northwest. J. WPCF, 57, 366–377.

Vaughn, J.M., Landry, E.F., and Thomas, M.Z. 1983. Entrainment of viruses from septic tank leach fields through a shallow, sandy, soil aquifer. Appl. Environ. Microbiol., 45, 1474–1480.

Wadowsky, R.M., and Yee, R.B. 1983. Satellite growth of *L. pneumophila* with an environmental isolate: *Flavobacterium breve.* Appl. Environ. Microbiol., 46, 1447–1449.

Walsh, J.A. 1988. Prevalence of *Entamoeba histolytica* infection. In *Amebiasis.* Edited by J.I. Ravdin. New York, John Wiley & Sons, pp. 93–105.

WHO. 1984. The role of food safety in health and development. Report of a joint FAO/WHO expert committee on food safety. WHO Technical Report Series 705, Geneva.

Young, L.S., Inderlied, B.C., George Berlin, O., and Gotlieb, M.S. 1986. Mycobacterial infections in AIDS patients, with an emphasis on *Mycobacterium avium* complex. Rev. Infect Dis., 8, 1024–1033.

CHAPTER 46

SANITATION IN FOOD MANUFACTURING OPERATIONS

H.W. Walker and W.S. LaGrange

The topic of sanitation in food manufacturing operations encompasses a wide array of subjects including food plant design and construction, process equipment, cleaning and sanitizing, hygienic practices of employees, control of pests including insects and rodents, packaging sanitation, sanitation of food storage facilities, food transport sanitation, water treatment, waste disposal, purity of air, and cleanliness of raw materials and other food ingredients. In past years, several books have been published that deal with the broad topic of sanitation in the food industry; among these are books by Parker and Litchfield (1962), Jowitt (1980), Katsuyama and Strachan (1980), and Troller (1983). In this chapter, only factors related to cleaning and sanitizing for reduction of microbial numbers in food processing operations will be emphasized.

LEGAL ASPECTS OF FOOD SANITATION

Keeping the work environment in a food processing plant clean and sanitary, and the maintenance and sanitization of equipment used for manufacturing and packaging of food, are important for several reasons. Probably the most compelling reasons for good food hygiene are that it is the *law* and it prevents or inhibits food poisoning and food spoilage. The Federal Food, Drug, and Cosmetic Act of 1938, with subsequent amendments, specifies that food manufacturing and packaging plants be maintained in a clean and sanitary condition. Following are some excerpts from the Federal Food, Drug, and Cosmetic Act that relate directly and indirectly with legal requirements of cleanliness and sanitation during the handling of food.

I. *Prohibited Acts*
   Sec. 301 (331) The following acts and the causing thereof are hereby prohibited:
   a. The introduction or delivery for introduction into in-
   terstate commerce of any food, drug device, or cosmetic that is adulterated or misbranded.
   b. The adulteration or misbranding of any food, drug device, or cosmetic in interstate commerce.
   c. The receipt in interstate commerce of any food, drug device or cosmetic that is adulterated or misbranded, and the delivery or proffered delivery thereof for pay or otherwise.
   d. The refusal to permit entry or inspection of a plant as authorized by section 704.

II. *Penalties*
   Sec. 303 (333)
   a. Any person who violates any of the provisions of section 301 shall be guilty of a misdemeanor and shall, on conviction thereof, be subject to imprisonment for not more than one year, or a fine of not more than $1,000, or both; but if the violation is committed after a conviction of such person under this section has become final, such person shall be subject to imprisonment for not more than three years, or a fine of not more than $10,000, or both.

III. *Seizure*
   Sec. 304 (334)
   a. Any article of food, drug device, or cosmetic that is adulterated or misbranded when introduced into or while in interstate commerce or while held for sale—after shipment in interstate commerce—shall be liable to be proceeded against while in interstate commerce, or at anytime thereafter.

IV. *Adulterated Food*
   Sec. 402 (342) A food shall be deemed to be adulterated:
   a. 1. If it bears or contains any poisonous or deleterious substance which may render it injurious to health;
      2. (a) If it bears or contains any added poisonous or added deleterious substance;
         (b) If it is a raw agricultural commodity and it bears or contains a pesticide chemical which is unsafe;
         (c) If it is, or it bears or contains, any food additive which is unsafe;
      3. If it consists in whole or in part of any filthy, putrid or decomposed substance, or if it is otherwise unfit for food;

4. If it has been prepared, packed or held under unsanitary conditions whereby it may have become contaminated with filth, or whereby it may have been rendered injurious to health;

5. If its container is composed, in whole or in part, of any poisonous or deleterious substance which may render the contents injurious to health;

b. 1. If any valuable constituent has been in whole or in part omitted or abstracted therefrom;

2. If any substance has been substituted wholly or in part;

3. If damage or inferiority has been concealed in any manner;

4. If any substance has been added thereto or mixed or packed therewith so as to increase bulk or weight or make it appear better or of greater value than it is.

V. *Factory Inspection*
Sec. 704 (374)

a. (FDA inspectors), upon presenting appropriate credentials and a written notice to the owner, operator or agent in charge, are authorized

1. To enter, at reasonable times, any factory, warehouse or establishment in which foods are manufactured, processed, packed or held for introduction into interstate commerce or after such introduction, or enter any vehicle and all pertinent equipment, finished and unfinished materials, containers and labeling therein.

b. Upon completion of any such inspection of a factory, warehouse or other establishment, and prior to leaving the premises, the officer making the inspection shall give to the owner, operator, or agent in charge a report in writing setting forth any conditions or practices observed by him which indicate that any food, drug, device or cosmetic in such establishment:

1. Consists in whole or in part of any filthy, putrid, or decomposed substance;

2. Has been prepared, packed, or held under unsanitary conditions whereby it may have been rendered injurious to health.

c. If the FDA inspector making any such inspection of a factory, warehouse, or other establishment has obtained any sample in the course of inspection, upon completion of the inspection and prior to leaving the premises he shall give to the owner, operator or agent in charge a receipt describing the samples obtained.

d. Whenever the FDA inspector obtains a sample of any such food, and an analysis is made of such sample for the purpose of ascertaining whether such food consists in whole or in part of any filthy, putrid, or decomposed substance, or is otherwise unfit for food, a copy of the results of such analysis shall be furnished promptly to the owner, operator, or agent in charge.

A listing of food regulatory agencies and their responsibilities is presented in Table 46–1.

ROLE OF SANITATION IN SAFETY AND SHELF-LIFE OF FOOD

Another reason, even more important than the legal ramifications, for stringent programs of cleanliness and sanitation is the protection of the pubic health—a major

Table 46–1. *Summary of Regulatory Agencies and Their Relationship to the Food Industry*

UNITED STATES DEPARTMENT OF AGRICULTURE
Inspection of meat, poultry, and egg processing plants
Nutritional research and educational programs
Grading of grain, fruits, vegetables, meat and poultry, and dairy foods

BUREAU OF ALCOHOL, TOBACCO, AND FIREARMS
(Department of Treasury)
Regulation of alcoholic beverages (< 7% alcohol)

CENTERS FOR DISEASE CONTROL
Investigation and reporting of food-borne illnesses and other health problems
Educational programs relating to food-borne illnesses

DEPARTMENT OF JUSTICE
Seizure of contaminated foods
Prosecution of food safety violators

ENVIRONMENTAL PROTECTION AGENCY
Regulation of pesticides—safety, setting of tolerance levels, and safety publications
Water quality

FEDERAL TRADE COMMISSION
Regulation of advertising of foods (Bureau of Consumer Protection)

FOOD & DRUG ADMINISTRATION
Administration of necessary programs and regulations for maintaining the safety and wholesomeness of all foods sold in interstate commerce, except meat, poultry, and eggs
Development of standards for composition, quality, nutrition, and safety of foods, food colors, and food additives
Collection of data on nutrition, food additives, and environmental factors that affect food
Establishment of some food standards
Enforcement of federal regulations on labeling, food and color additives, food sanitation, and food safety
Inspection of food plants involved in interstate commerce, imported foods, and animal feed plants
Monitoring food recalls

NATIONAL MARINE FISHERIES SERVICE
(Department of Commerce)
Voluntary inspection of fish products
Fisheries management and development

STATE AND LOCAL GOVERNMENT
Cooperation with federal government agencies on food safety and quality
Cooperation in standards and regulations with federal agencies
Inspection of restaurants, retail food stores, and food processing plants
Fish inspection taken within the state (28 states)
Adoption of FDA guidelines for dairy and restaurant requirements, and conduction of inspection

From Modeland, V. 1989. America's food safety team: a look at the lineup. Dairy Food Environ. Sanit., 9, 14–15.

consideration for all involved in food manufacturing and handling. The ultimate purpose of detergency and sanitation in the food industry is the reduction of numbers of potential food pathogens to a level that minimizes the risk of food-borne illness. In addition to the safety factor, the shelf-life of the food is extended by the reduction in total numbers of bacteria. These two factors, safety and extended shelf-life, result in quality foods that can be more readily marketed.

Other reasons for the need for a well supervised and executed sanitation program are that it provides a more pleasant work environment that encourages the employees to maintain high quality standards, discourages the presence of insects and rodents, and helps maintenance people do their job more efficiently in keeping equipment for manufacturing, packing, and storage of food in good condition.

The key to safe food manufacturing and marketing is the people directly involved. They are intimately involved with raw food and food ingredients, food processing equipment and environment, and the packaging, storage, delivery, and marketing of processed foods. People can be a major source of pathogenic microorganisms that contaminate food and cause food-borne illness among food consumers. People contribute to the occurrence of food-borne illness by not using good manufacturing practices throughout the manufacturing and marketing of safe and acceptable foods.

Recognizing that people are important in the manufacturing and marketing of safe food, the Federal Food, Drug, and Cosmetic Act As Amended includes regulations under the heading *Current Good Manufacturing Practice in Manufacturing, Processing, Packing, or Holding Human Food* that defines specifically personnel sanitation practices when involved in food processing. Commonly referred to as Umbrella GMPs, they have the force and effect of law. These regulations are detailed, specifying standards for all food manufacturing functions including processing, packaging, and storing (Troller, 1983).

The FDC Act relating to food appears in the United States Code of Federal Regulations, Code 21, published in the Federal Register. Part 110 of these regulations includes a section on personnel. The personnel section details the responsibility of the food plant manager to assure that the food plant personnel are not a source of disease; are clean and sanitary in appearance, work performance, and wear; receive education and training in safe food processing, packaging, storage; and are supervised by competent personnel.

SANITIZING AS IT PERTAINS TO THE FOOD INDUSTRY

Asbury (1983) has defined the term "sanitize" as the act of reducing the number of bacterial contaminants in the environment to a safe or relatively safe level as may be judged by public health requirements or at least to a significant degree where public health standards have not been established. Block (1983) qualifies the definition of a sanitizer in that such an agent is ordinarily used on an inanimate surface. These definitions emphasize the importance of the elimination of pathogenic or infectious agents to a safe level. Asbury, however, in his discussion includes the economic importance of food sanitation, noting that it controls organisms responsible for food spoil-

age and enhances the shelf-life of the food. In fact, the food industry, in most instances, stresses the reduction of noninfectious microorganisms that cause spoilage with the premise that infectious agents also will be controlled. Sanitization of a surface does not mean sterilization, because bacterial spores and some resistant vegetative bacterial cells may survive. Some of these survivors, particularly spores, can be of extreme importance to the food processor.

All authorities stress the importance of the thorough cleaning and rinsing for removal of loosened soil and cleaner residues on surfaces before sanitizing (Katsuyama and Strachan, 1980; Troller, 1983; Parker and Litchfield, 1962). These materials react with the sanitizers and reduce their effectiveness. Cleaning and rinsing also reduce microbial populations on equipment surfaces that, in turn, reduce the time required for exposure to the sanitizer. A number of factors, which are not always easily controlled, influence the efficiency of a sanitizer; a list would include concentration of sanitizer, time of exposure to the sanitizer, numbers of organisms present, pH, presence of organic matter, presence of minerals (water hardness), and temperature.

Katsuyama and Strachan (1980) have listed eleven characteristics of the ideal sanitizer: (1) rapid destruction of microorganisms, (2) safe and nonirritating to employees, (3) nontoxic for consumers and acceptable to regulatory agencies, (4) rinsable, (5) no adverse effects on the food being processed such as changes in odors, flavors, or appearance, (6) economical, (7) easily tested for concentration in use solutions, (8) stable when concentrated or in solution, (9) noncorrosive, (10) compatible with other chemicals, and (11) readily soluble in water. No single agent will possess these characteristics; the sanitarian, therefore, is responsible for selecting the sanitizer that is most effective for the specific operation.

CLEANING FOOD PROCESSING EQUIPMENT AND THE WORK ENVIRONMENT

Removing or cleaning soil from food processing and packaging equipment and the surrounding work areas is one of the more important and frequent activities associated with the food manufacturing industry. Food safety, regulatory standards, extended shelf-life, and minimal rework are among the key reasons for an effective cleaning and sanitizing program in food manufacturing.

Unclean processing and packaging equipment provides an excellent environment for metabolism and reproduction of microorganisms that can directly influence the safety and the expected shelf-life of the food being manufactured. In addition, unclean equipment may attract pests such as insects and rodents that can influence the safety, quality, and aesthetic aspects of the food. Equally important is that cleaned food processing and packaging equipment allows sanitizers to be more effective in reducing levels of microorganisms to an acceptable standard. Both food contact and noncontact surfaces of the equipment must be kept clean.

Unclean work environments also influence the safety and quality of food being processed and packaged. Dust, dirt, and aerosols from the processing and packaging environment can directly contaminate foods and ingredients. Pests are attracted to an unclean area. Personnel working in an unclean environment are influenced in job performance, including their sanitary habits and efficiency (Troller, 1983; Katsuyama and Strachan, 1980). Food industry managers must include cleanliness as a top priority in all areas of the food industry.

CLEANING FACTORS

Several factors must be considered by the managers of food manufacturing sanitation programs in order to make this important activity effective. The first factor is consideration of the type of soil to be removed from equipment and the work environment. Soil types are usually peculiar to both the type of food being manufactured and the manufacturing methods employed. In food manufacturing, soil is usually composed of some combination of sugar, fat, protein, and salts. Table 46–2 illustrates soil characteristics encountered in food manufacturing. This information has been published previously in Troller (1983), Guthrie (1988), and Cheow and Jackson (1982), among others.

The type of soil to be removed influences the composition of the cleaning compound, the concentration of the chemicals in the cleaning solution, the temperature of the cleaning solution, and the method of cleaning to be used to remove the soil.

WATER

Because water is the primary solvent for cleaning compounds, the hardness of the available water supply is an important influence on the ingredients included in the formulation of the cleaning compound. Water hardness caused by the salts of calcium and magnesium reduces the effectiveness of cleaners by binding with compounds in the cleaner. These salts also may be deposited on the equipment. Color deposits on equipment are frequently caused by soluble iron and magnesium salts in the water.

Incorporating a water softening treatment method within the food plant may be appropriate to facilitate an effective and efficient cleaning program. Water stone and other water mineral deposits must be avoided on food processing and packaging equipment. These types of deposits prevent visual evaluation of equipment cleanliness, protect microorganisms from cleaning and sanitizing agents, and may contribute to metal corrosion. The processing plant's water supply should be tested for hardness and, if necessary, include water-softening equipment or use specially formulated cleaners (Katsuyama and Strachan, 1980; Troller, 1983).

INGREDIENTS IN CLEANING COMPOUNDS

Water is essential to the cleaning process but, in most cases, is not a very efficient cleaning substance. Most cleaning compounds include several ingredients that help water become an efficient and effective cleaning agent. These various ingredients play their part in wetting and penetrating the soil to be removed from the equipment, dispersing the soil and keeping it in suspension until it can be flushed away, and preventing the precipitation of hard water minerals. Besides these duties, a cleaning compound should be noncorrosive to equipment, rinse freely, destroy microorganisms in the soil on equipment being cleaned, be economical, be biodegradable, have storage stability, and dissolve readily in water (Katsuyama and Strachan, 1980, Troller, 1983; Henderson, 1972). Some of the key basic types of ingredients included in most food equipment-cleaning compounds are presented in Table 46–3.

Two basic classes of cleaning compounds are used in the food industry. These include alkaline and acid cleaners. The alkaline cleaners, of which there are several formulations designed for specific cleaning jobs, make up the majority of the cleaners used in the food industry. The other major cleaner is the acid cleaner, used mostly to remove highly insoluble mineral salts in the soil on the equipment.

Alkaline Cleaners

Most alkaline cleaners consist of several chemical compounds. These may include basic alkalis, polyphosphates, chelating agents, wetting agents, and chlorine. Each compound is added for a specific purpose when a cleaner is formulated so it will have the cleaning capability needed for specific soil removal requirements. Usually alkaline salts plus one or more surfactants are blended together to make up a cleaner.

The *basic alkalis* form the bulk of many alkaline cleaners. Usually two or more are used in combination. The basic functions of the alkalis are peptization of proteins

Table 46–2. *Soil Characteristics*

Component on Surface	Solubility	Ease of Removal	Effect of Heating
Sugar	Water soluble	Easy	Carmelization, more difficult to clean
Fat	Water insoluble, alkali soluble	Difficult	Polymerization, more difficult to clean
Protein	Water insoluble, alkali soluble, sl. acid soluble	Very difficult	Denaturation, more difficult to clean
Salts			
Monovalent	Water soluble, acid soluble	Easy to difficult	Generally not significant
Polyvalent (i.e., CaPO₄)	Water insoluble, acid soluble	Easy to difficult	Interactions with other constituents

Table 46–3. *Classification and Function of Leading Compounds*

Class of Compound	Major Function
Basic alkalis	Soil displacement by emulsifying, saponifying, and peptizing
Complex phosphates	Soil displacement by emulsifying and peptizing; dispersion of soil; water softening, prevention of soil depositions
Surfactants	Wetting and penetrating soils; dispersion of soils and prevention of soil redepositions
Chelating compounds	Water softening; mineral deposit control; soil displacement by peptizing; prevention of redepositions
Acids	Mineral deposit control; water softening

From Guthrie, R. K. 1988. *Food Sanitation.* New York, Van Nostrand Reinhold.

and emulsification and saponification of fat. Following are alkaline cleaning chemicals often used in alkaline cleaners:

Sodium hydroxide (NaOH or lye or caustic soda)
Characteristics include saponification of fat and dissolving of protein. Provides inexpensive alkalinity. Used to clean heat exchange equipment, but is highly corrosive to metal and flesh. A 1% solution has a pH of 12.2.

Sodium carbonate (Na_2CO_3—soda ash)
Common alkali used in manual and automatic cleaners. Inexpensive, has air cleaning ability, provides some alkalinity, and serves as a buffering agent, but can precipitate out of solution as $CaCO_3$.

Sodium bicarbonate ($NaHCO_3$)
A weak cleaner.

Sodium metasilicate (Na_2SiO_3)
Provides high active alkalinity, is a good emulsifier, and helps suspend soil in solution. Relatively noncorrosive and protects metals against corrosion by other alkalis.

Trisodium phosphate (Na_3PO_4 or TSP)
Readily soluble in water, a good emulsifier, somewhat corrosive to metals unless metasilicate is included in the cleaner formulation, fairly expensive source of alkalinity, and a fair water softener by precipitating out the calcium.

Polyphosphates are added to alkaline cleaners to help soften the water used to make up the cleaning solution and to provide some cleaning force to the cleaner. The polyphosphates form complexes or sequester calcium and magnesium, so these cations do not interfere with cleaning and rinsing.

Water hardness is a critical consideration in formulating and selecting a cleaner. The water to be used for dissolving the cleaner should be tested for hardness. The softer the water to be used for cleaning, the smaller the amount of the chemicals in the cleaner that will be tied

up softening the water and that will not be available for cleaning. Efficiency and economics of cleaning may be bettered by softening the water. Calcium, magnesium, and iron are the cations of particular concern in water.

Examples of chemical water-softening polyphosphates that may be incorporated in cleaners for sequestering the hardness cations include sodium tetraphosphate, sodium hexametaphosphate, tetrasodium pyrophosphate, and sodium tripolyphosphate.

Chelating agents are organic sequestering agents. Like the polyphosphates, they combine with calcium and magnesium ions as well as other heavy metal ions to form molecules in which the ions are tightly held so they can no longer react. Some of the common chelating agents are ethylene diamine tetraacetate (EDTA), nitrilo triacetate (NTA), polyacylates, and citric acid.

Wetting agents or surface activating agents are widely used in cleaners to wet the soil to be removed and to form soil colloids so the soil can be rinsed away. Minimal concentrations of these compounds are used in a cleaner formulation because they cause foaming, a problem not needed in CIP (clean-in-place) systems. There are three general types of wetting agents. One is an anionic wetting agent with a negative charge, used in both acid and basic or alkaline formulations. Sulfated alcohols and alkyl arylsulfonates are examples of anionic wetting agents. Cationic and positively charged ions such as quaternary ammonium compounds work only fairly in cleaning compounds. They work best in detergent-sanitizers because they have good antimicrobial activity. Nonionic wetting agents are complex organic chemicals that do not ionize. These are used with most cleaning compounds and do not foam.

Chlorinated alkaline cleaners have become popular in CIP and spray ball cleaning systems. Chlorine is added to these cleaners, not as a sanitizer but to increase the peptizing efficiency of the alkaline compounds. Between 75 and 200 parts per million of chlorine are added to these cleaner compounds.

Acidic Cleaners

Certain types of soils, especially inorganic soils, are more easily removed with an acid cleaner. Acid cleaners frequently are used in heat exchange equipment cleaning and in hard water and high mineral deposit situations. Acid cleaners frequently are used in association with alkaline cleaners in heat exchange cleaning and periodically in many other cleaning jobs. Organic acids such as acetic, lactic, hydroxyacetic, citric, levulinic, and tartaric have been used in acid cleaner formulations. Phosphoric acid also is a popular and effective addition to a food plant acid cleaning compound.

GENERAL CLEANING SCHEDULE

Most food processing systems are sensitive to microbial growth and metabolic activity and must be wet cleaned and sanitized frequently. Other food systems such as milk powder manufacturing systems are basically dry processing systems. These systems are regularly dry cleaned to minimize microbial increases. Most any cleaning routine should usually start with dry cleaning whether or not the remaining routine will be dry or wet cleaning. By picking up, sweeping, or otherwise removing gross soil and contamination in the area or equipment to be cleaned, less water and cleaning solution will later be needed. In addition, macro-sized food particles will not enter the waste water system, thus easing the potential load on the waste treatment system.

Rinsing equipment and work areas soon after use will help prevent drying of soil and will make the cleaning easier. Rinsing of soiled equipment also will remove and flush away a fairly large portion of the microorganisms that may be present within the soil. Depending on soil type, lukewarm water (95 to 110°F) should be used to flush away most of the soil. If hot water is used as a rinse, soil protein may coagulate and make later soil removal difficult.

Wet cleaning methods used in sanitation programs include manual, soak, low- and high-pressure spray, foam-gel, and clean-in-place (CIP). These methods employ both physical and chemical factors. The proper selection of the method as well as the type of cleaner are important decisions in order to make cleaning efficient, thorough, and economical. Manual cleaning is a common task in all food processing plants. Because human skin usually comes in contact with the cleaning solution and the equipment to be cleaned, the temperature of the solution and chemical concentration must be moderate enough to prevent skin irritation. This means that the temperature of the cleaning solution should be maintained at 115 to 120°F and the alkalinity should be less than pH 10. Usually a pail of a mild alkaline cleaning solution and a brush are the tools required—aside from elbow grease of the person using the brush. Besides cleaning pieces of equipment, manual brush cleaning works well on cleaning work environment areas such as floors, walls, and drains.

Another important method of cleaning equipment that is employed in all food plants is the soak method. This procedure includes soaking equipment parts in a parts washer tank for 15 to 30 minutes at cleaning solution temperatures near 150°F. Usually a motor-drive pump circulates the cleaning solution and provides energy needed to help with soil removal.

Spray cleaning is a convenient method of cleaning hard-to-reach areas and equipment in food processing plants. These areas include the exterior of transportation trucks, conveyor belts, and walls of processing areas. Use of high-pressure spray cleaning must be restricted to areas in the food processing plant where aerosols created by the spraying are not a problem to later contamination of food ingredients and products.

Low-pressure foam and gel applications of cleaning compounds to the exterior of equipment and walls are gaining popularity. The foam and gel materials encapsulate the cleaning compound, holding it against the surface to be cleaned. A few minutes of contact time is one of the cleaning aids. After the cleaner has broken down the soil, the foam cleaner-soil mixture can be rinsed away with water. Do not, however, allow the foam cleaner to dry on surfaces.

Clean-in-place (CIP) is an effective and efficient method of cleaning food processing equipment. An important consideration in using this cleaning method is whether or not the equipment system has been engineered for CIP. Some older food processing systems were built at a time when CIP was not available. Trying to use CIP under these conditions may lead to false expectations. However, if the system is designed for CIP and the CIP system is monitored and managed properly, there is no more-efficient cleaning method available.

The success of a CIP system is keyed not only to proper engineering of all the component parts but to proper water velocity, solution temperature, and selection of the appropriate cleaning compound. When the interior of storage tanks and similar vessels are to be included in a CIP system, a properly designed spray ball or nozzle assembly with sufficient temperature, solution pressure, and concentration is an important consideration. The recirculating equipment is one of the primary elements to the CIP system and includes a cleaning solution tank, centrifugal pump, and automatic valves.

Although a fully automatic CIP system can fit the cleaning needs of a properly engineered food processing system and do a thorough cleaning job in a minimal amount of time, a fail-safe design must be included to prevent cleaning solutions from contaminating food in process or storage when adjoining equipment is being cleaned. Much of the previous information on the cleaning process can be found in Henderson (1971), Katsuyama and Strachan (1980), Troller (1983), Skaarup (1985), and Parker and Litchfield (1962).

CLEANING EVALUATION METHODS

Both cleaning and sanitizing results must be appraised daily. The company supplying the chemicals should not only service its account with each food processor on a frequent basis but instruct the appropriate plant personnel on the methods of using cleaning and sanitizing chemicals and systems properly. Testing solution strengths also must be part of the service.

Visual evaluation of cleaning is an excellent way to check on the results. There should be no obvious soil left on cleaned equipment surfaces under scrutiny of a good light. Cleaned surfaces should show no signs of excessive water beading when the surface is wet. Cleaned surfaces must not be rough or greasy. Also, cleaned equipment and environmental areas should have no objectionable smells. A person's eyes, hands, and nose are effective tools for evaluating cleaned surfaces and areas within food processing facilities.

Microbiologic methods also help in evaluation of cleaning results. Contact-plate methods reproduce the pattern of distribution of microorganisms present on the cleaned surface. The swab method can be used to estimate the number of microorganisms left on equipment surfaces after cleaning. Although no standards have been universally adopted by the food industry for these methods, low counts over a prescribed area do indicate satisfactory cleaning has taken place (Guthrie, 1988; Henderson, 1971; Skaarup, 1985).

SANITIZING AGENTS—PHYSICAL

The use of heat is a proven means of sanitizing and is used frequently in food processing. The heat transfer medium is generally air, water, or steam, but water or steam is normally used for food processing applications (Jennings, 1965). Jennings cites several advantages to the use of heat over the use of other means of sanitizing. Heat can effectively destroy microorganisms in small cracks and crevices into which chemical sanitizers may not penetrate. Heat is nonselective and effective against all microorganisms, depending on time and temperature of exposure. Also, heat leaves no residue that may be later classified as an unintentional food additive.

Katsuyama and Strachan (1980) point out that moist heat is much more efficient for killing microorganisms than dry heat. Nevertheless, the surface to be sanitized must reach the sanitizing temperature and remain there for an appropriate length of time. Generally, water temperatures of 75 to 95°C are used with exposure times of 2 to 20 minutes, depending on the type of equipment, the product, and the degree of microbial destruction needed (Jennings, 1965). Jennings also mentions that food residues may be baked or cooked onto surfaces by heat sanitization and become more difficult to remove. The residues can give thermal protection to microorganisms.

Steam is most useful for sanitizing in enclosed systems. The usefulness of steam when applied to exposed equipment or surfaces is limited. The Grade A Pasteurized Milk Ordinance, U.S. Public Health Service (1985 revision), states that when steam is used, each group of assembled piping must be treated separately, and after insertion of the steam hose into the inlet, steam flow should be continued for at least 5 minutes after the temperature of the drainage has reached 200°F (94°C). Hot water should be pumped through the system for at least 5 minutes after the temperature has reached 170°F (77°C).

SANITIZING AGENTS—CHEMICAL

Chlorine Compounds

The three most common classes of chemical sanitizers used in the food industry are chlorine, iodine, and quaternary ammonium compounds (QACs). Details of the chemistry and mode of action of these compounds are described in other chapters and will not be repeated here. Chlorine and its compounds are the most widely used sanitizers in the food industry. Mercer and Som-

mers (1957) reviewed the history of the use of chlorine and pointed out that Semmelweis in 1846 succeeded in controlling puerperal fever in his medical clinic by using hypochlorite. The dairy industry was probably the first among food processors to take advantage of the bactericidal and deodorant properties of chlorine; calcium hypochlorite was used as a sanitizer for milk bottles (Whittaker and Mohler, 1912). Chlorine was recommended in the U.S. Milk Ordinance and Code of 1939 for the sanitizing of dairy equipment between uses. Additional studies soon resulted in the addition of chlorine to water used for washing and rinsing equipment during routine cleaning and sanitizing. Scott (1937) reported that in 1931, the canning industry initiated the practice of adding chlorine to cooling water to control spoilage of canned foods due to leakage of small amounts of contaminated water through apparently normal seams. Vaughn and Stadtman (1946) demonstrated a reduction in bacterial counts in the finished food product after using chlorinated sprays at selected points during manufacturing operations. They also observed reduced build-up of bacterial slimes and reduced odors.

The addition of chlorine to the water used in the food processing plant causes a marked reduction in the number of microorganisms present in the water, on equipment surfaces, and in the final product (Mercer and Sommers, 1957). The practice of adding chlorine to the entire water supply of a plant is referred to as in-plant chlorination. Automatic injectors maintain an available chlorine level of approximately 5 to 7 ppm; during cleanup operations, however, the residuals may be increased to 15 to 20 ppm (Mercer and Sommers, 1959; Jennings, 1965; Malpas, 1971).

Chlorine compounds, when in solution, react in various ways to produce hypochlorous acid (HOCl), which is an extremely powerful oxidizing chemical and is the biocidal agent. Hypochlorite ion (OCl⁻) has little if any bactericidal activity (Gardner and Peel, 1986; Katsuyama and Strachan, 1980; Mercer and Sommers, 1957). Charlton and Levine (1937) and Rudolph and Levine (1941) used spores of *Bacillus metiens* to demonstrate that HOCl is the effective agent for biocidal activity and that pH of the solution was the paramount factor controlling the concentration of HOCl in solution. In solutions of pH 4.0 to 5.0, practically all the chlorine occurs in the form of HOCl; below pH 4.0, HOCl breaks down to release Cl_2. As the pH becomes more alkaline, increasing amounts of OCl⁻ occur. Dychdala (1983) has summarized the information establishing that the efficiency of hypochlorites decreases as the pH increases with the accumulation of a greater proportion of OCl⁻. At pH values of 5 or below, corrosion becomes a serious problem, and Katsuyama and Strachan (1980) recommend maintaining a pH range of 6.0 to 7.5 where corrosion and irritancy are minimal but the concentration of HOCl is sufficient for effective sanitizing.

The major sources of chlorine for use as sanitizers are sodium hypochlorite, granular calcium hypochlorite, granular chlorocyanurates, gaseous chlorine, chloramine T, and generation from sodium chloride. The last source is sometimes referred to as nascent chlorine and is produced on-site by electrolysis of 0.4% salt brine and addition of acid (Troller, 1983; Katsuyama and Strachan, 1980; Gardner and Peel, 1986).

Hypochlorites are available as powders or liquids (Gardner and Peel, 1986; Dychdala, 1983). Sodium hypochlorite is available as an aqueous solution usually containing 12 to 14% available chlorine. When preparing dilutions from this concentrated solution, allowance needs to be made for loss of available chlorine; a solution containing initially 14% available chlorine may contain 10% or less in about 4 weeks. Calcium hypochlorite dihydrate is available as a powder, granulated material, or tablet containing 65% available chlorine; these preparations have a strong chlorine odor. Lithium hypochlorite is a white, granulated material also having a strong chlorine odor and containing 35% available chlorine. The concentrated powders may be diluted with appropriate compounds to produce lower available chlorine compounds. These compounds may be combined with trisodium phosphate to produce chlorinated TSP containing about 3.25% available chlorine. These preparations in solution produce HOCl and also have the advantage of alkaline phosphate for detergency.

Probably the most frequently used concentration of available chlorine in the food industry is 200 ppm. However, concentrations ranging as low as 5 ppm to 5000 ppm are employed; the latter strength being used to control mold growth (Lesser, 1949; Gardner and Peel, 1986). In 1929, Prucha recommended solutions containing 50 to 100 ppm active chlorine for rinsing or pumping through large equipment, 70 to 100 ppm for dipping equipment, and 200 ppm for spraying. His recommendations were for cold or lukewarm water; effectiveness increases with temperature, but he did not advise using a temperature over 120°F. He stressed that hypochlorites were effective only on clean surfaces and that contact must be made with all surfaces for at least 10 seconds or long enough to produce an acceptable kill of microorganisms. Skaarup (1985) and Trueman (1971) also stressed the need for thorough cleaning of surfaces and recommended that 200 to 300 ppm of available chlorine be used for disinfecting surfaces in canneries. Other recommendations for use of hypochlorites are found in the Grade A Pasteurized Milk Ordinance (1985 revision); these guidelines of the U.S. Public Health Service recommend a solution of hypochlorite containing 50 ppm of available chlorine for sanitizing utensils and equipment with a minimal exposure of 1 minute at a minimal temperature of 75°F (24°C); for spraying, 100 ppm of available chlorine is recommended. Compounds other than hypochlorites may be used if they will produce biocidal activity commensurate with 50 ppm hypochlorite at a pH of 10 at 75°F (24°C) after an exposure of 1 minute.

Trueman (1971) has summarized some of the levels of hypochlorite recommended for use in various food processing operations. Some specific uses he mentioned were disinfecting knives in slaughter houses (20 ppm available chlorine) and general sanitation using in-plant chlorination (5 to 10 ppm), poultry processing (10 ppm for all process water), and chlorination of cooling water in canneries (2 to 5 ppm). Chlorine at these low levels (2 to 10 ppm) may be adequate to control microbial contamination in process water, but the chlorine can react rapidly with organic matter. Thus, levels of chlorine must be checked frequently.

Malpas (1971) emphasizes the need for treatment of water used in food processing. Even though the water may be treated to meet drinking water standards, it is possible that potable water may contain bacterial spores which, on gaining entry into a can, can grow and cause spoilage or food poisoning; for example, a botulism outbreak in canned tuna was attributed to entry of *Clostridium botulinum* spores into the cans during cooling (Eadie et al., 1964). Malpas also pointed out that the use of 10 to 20 ppm in the process water in poultry processing plants reduced the bacterial count and helped to control the presence of pathogenic organisms in the environment. High levels (200 ppm) of chlorine in the chill tanks for cooling the carcasses extended the shelf-life of the poultry meat and helped to control cross-contamination by destroying bacteria that were washed off the carcasses (Dixon and Pooley, 1961; Ranken et al., 1965; Patterson, 1968). Skaarup (1985) and Malpas (1971) recommend the use of hypochlorites and peracetic acid for most purposes in meat and fish processing for the same purposes as cited for poultry processing. Mrozek (1985) has presented data comparing halogens, QACs, and peracetic acid. He found peracetic acid to have the quickest and most complete inactivation against bacteriophages and also to be extremely effective against bacilli and clostridia. For yeasts and molds, it was more effective when in combination with a surface-active agent, preferably a QAC.

Other food products or processes for which chlorination of wash water has been advantageous are the prepackaging of vegetables, the sugar beet industry, dairy processing, and the soft drinks industry (Malpas, 1971). Others, however, have stated that treatment of beef, chicken, lamb, and Brussels sprouts with 200 ppm of chorine resulted in less than two orders of magnitude of reduction of microbial populations, and consider this treatment to be of limited value (Kelly et al., 1981; Marshall et al., 1977; Morrison and Fleet, 1985; Brackett, 1987).

The resistance of bacteria to chlorination is obviously an important factor. The usual chlorination procedures used in food plant operations are designed to destroy vegetative forms of bacteria (Mercer and Sommers, 1957). The concentration of chlorine in water for processing and sanitizing that would be required to kill bacterial spores within a reasonable time would not be practical. Both gram-positive and gram-negative organisms in the vegetative state are highly susceptible to chlorine.

Recently, considerable interest has been expressed concerning the effectiveness of chlorine for controlling *Listeria monocytogenes* because of its wide distribution and the seriousness of the food-borne disease it causes (Mustapha and Liewen, 1989; El-Kist and Marth, 1988). Brackett (1987) found that chlorine concentrations of less than about 50 ppm were not reliable for eliminating *L. monocytogenes* in vitro, but exposure to 50 ppm or above for less than 20 seconds was effective. El-Kist and Marth (1988) concluded that from a practical viewpoint *L. monocytogenes* is not particularly resistant to chlorine and that its control in the food industry through a good program of cleaning and sanitizing should be no more difficult to control than any other non-sporeforming bacteria. Mustapha and Liewen (1989) found sodium hypochlorite and quaternary ammonium compounds effective against this organism when used at levels recommended by the manufacturer. They observed that approximately 200 ppm of hypochlorite applied for 2 minutes was necessary for efficient destruction on smooth surfaces, and that approximately 400 ppm was needed for porous surfaces. With the use of quaternary ammonium compounds, 50 ppm applied for 1 minute was sufficient.

In addition to the hypochlorites, certain organic chlorine compounds have found use as sanitizers in the food industry. These include chloramine T, the chlorinated hydantoins, and the chlorinated isocyanurates. Chloramine T is available in a powdered form containing 25% available chlorine; dichlorocyanuric and trichlorocyanuric acids are also available in powdered form containing 70 to 90% available chlorine. These compounds, in general, have slower germicidal activity than hypochlorites, are affected by the same factors that influence the activity of hypochlorites, and are relatively nonirritating to the skin.

In the Grade A Pasteurized Milk Ordinance, U.S. Public Health Service, 1985 revision, it is stressed that pH has a profound effect on organic forms of chlorine. For example, for chloramine T solutions, a maximum pH of 7.2 is acceptable for suitable germicidal activity when 200 ppm of available chorine is present in solution. At 100 ppm, the maximum is pH 6.8, and at 50 ppm, the maximum is pH 6.4. Chloramine T is restricted to uses when long exposure times or low pHs are feasible. Chlorinated hydantoin formulations yield satisfactory results in solutions of pH 7.0 or below, and chlorinated isocyanuric acid solutions have suitable activity at pH values up to 9.5.

Iodophors

Iodine is an effective biocidal agent for a wide spectrum of microorganisms including enteric bacteria, enteric viruses, bacteriophages, protozoan cysts, and algae (Gottardi, 1983; Hoehn, 1976; Trueman, 1971). Aqueous and alcoholic preparations of iodine have characteristics that preclude their use in the food industry; namely, staining, toxicity, and corrosiveness. These disadvantages were overcome to a great extent when it was discovered that iodine could be complexed with surface active agents to form iodophors (Troller, 1983; Parker and Litchfield, 1962; Katsuyama and Strachan, 1980; Jennings, 1965). Advantages claimed for iodophors are that they have rapid germicidal activity in acid solutions of cold or hard waters; they are readily dissolved; they are nontoxic at concentrations recommended for sanitizing; they are nonirritating to skin and can be used as hand dips for food plant employees; they have detergent and surfactant properties in addition to germicidal activity; and they are tasteless and odorless in foods at recommended use levels (Parker and Litchfield, 1962; Katsuyama and Strachan, 1980). These compounds also aid in the removal or prevention of scale or films such as the formation of milkstone in the dairy industry (Troller, 1983; Gardner and Peel, 1986). Another advantage is that solutions of iodophors of 10 ppm or above have an amber color; when available iodine falls below this level, the solution becomes straw-colored or loses color, indicating the need for additional sanitizer (Katsuyama and Strachan, 1980).

Troller (1983) and Trueman (1971) have mentioned some disadvantages to the use of iodophors as disinfectants for food operations. Iodophors are more costly than chlorine compounds; they are corrosive to some metals such as galvanized iron, aluminum, and copper; they release free iodine at temperatures above 110°F (43.3°C); they form a purple complex with starches; and they stain some plastics.

Iodophors have been acknowledged in the food industry as general detergent-sanitizers (Trueman, 1971). When used as detergent-sanitizers, 25 ppm of iodine is recommended. These iodine complexes have been used for clean-in-place operations of food processing plants as well as for transportation equipment such as road and rail tankers. They are also useful for cleaning floors, work surfaces, and handling equipment in high-speed operations such as poultry processing. Other uses are as fogging agents in enclosed areas for control of airborne organisms, for treating surfaces of areas normally difficult to clean and sanitize, and for controlling yeast and mold growth in cold storage areas.

Molecular iodine (I_2) and hypoiodous acid (HOI) have biocidal activity, with I_2 being the most active in sanitizing solutions (Gottardi, 1983; Trueman, 1962; Katsuyama and Strachan, 1980). Iodophor preparations usually contain an acid (frequently phosphoric acid) to give a pH under 5.0 when diluted for sanitizing purposes. Iodophors are most active in an acid pH where I_2 predominates. Experimental results indicate that one part of available iodine is equivalent to 3 to 6 parts of available chorine (Trueman, 1972). The destructive capacity of 25 ppm iodine to vegetative bacterial cells at low pH is comparable to that of 200 ppm of chlorine at neutral pH (Jennings, 1965). The level of iodine in most commercial preparations of iodophors is from 0.5 to 1.75%; these preparations are diluted to obtain use dilutions of available iodine (Trueman, 1972).

Recommended use concentrations of iodophors usually are in the range of 12.5 to 25 ppm (Jennings, 1965). Hays et al. (1967), after a survey of germicidal activity at various concentrations, suggested that a concentration of 25 ppm might be more appropriate for iodophor solutions than 12.5 ppm. They found iodophors to be more effective against yeasts than hypochlorites, as did Mosley et al. (1976). Lopes (1986) reported that sanitizing solutions containing 12.5 and 25 ppm of titratable iodine had germicidal activity equivalent to 50 and 200 ppm of available chlorine, respectively, against *L. monocytogenes,* and 100 and 200 ppm of available chlorine, respectively, against *Salmonella typhimurium.* Dunsmore and Thomson (1981) used a cleaning simulator to determine changes in soil and bacterial numbers on stainless steel surfaces soiled with milk and found iodophors at 25 ppm to be most effective in reducing numbers of bacteria. Gardner and Peel (1986) stated that iodophors are suitable for disinfection of clean equipment and work surfaces, and that 50 to 100 ppm of available iodine is recommended.

Quaternary Ammonium Compounds

A third group of compounds that has found use as a sanitizer in the food industry is the quaternary ammonium compounds (QACs). These compounds have several advantages, as cited by Parker and Litchfield (1962) and Katsuyama and Strachan (1980). They are stable to heat over a long period; they leave a nonvolatile residue on surfaces rendering them bacteriostatic for some time after treatment; they are effective over a wide pH range but most effective at a slightly alkaline pH; they are noncorrosive and nonirritating to skin; they are less affected by organic matter than hypochlorites; and they are odorless and tasteless. They also have certain disadvantages, such as incompatibility with soaps, anionic detergents, pine oils, and inorganic polyphosphates such as sodium hexametaphosphate, sodium tetraphosphate, and sodium tripolyphosphate, but they are unaffected by trisodium phosphate, tetrasodium phosphate, and nonionic detergents. The QACs have been classified as Type A (alkyl dimethyl or dimethyl ethyl benzyl ammonium chloride) and Type B (diisobutyl phenoxy ethoxy ethyl dimethyl benzyl ammonium chloride or methyl dodecylbenzyl trimethyl ammonium chloride). Water hardness has no effect on Type A, but Type B needs a sequestrant in hard water (Katsuyama and Strachan, 1980). Earlier, Chambers et al. (1955) attributed variations in the bacterial effectiveness of QAC solutions to variations in the amount of calcium and magnesium bicarbonates, sulfates, and chlorides in the water. However, some QACs were effective in the presence of considerable water hardness, and others required a more alkaline pH or a sequestrant agent to have maximal activity. It is recommended that the limiting hardness be determined for each quaternary ammonium compound.

Another disadvantage for QACs is their selective ac-

tion for certain types of bacteria. They are effective against lactic organisms but not against bacteriophages or gram-negative organisms like *E. coli* or *Pseudomonas aeruginosa;* in fact, certain strains of *Ps. aeruginosa* are capable of growing in hand-dip solutions of QACs (Soprey and Maxcy, 1968; Adair et al., 1969). Elliker in 1958 reported that QACs are effective in destroying micrococci, including the thermoduric types of concern in the dairy industry, but are somewhat slow in the destruction of coliforms and gram-negative psychotrophic bacteria. He also reported them to be less effective for control of spores and bacteriophage than chlorine. In general, QACs are considered to be more efficient for destruction of gram-positive bacteria than for destruction of gram-negative bacteria.

Detergent-Sanitizers

Combinations of bactericidal agents and detergents are sometimes used for cleaning and sanitizing equipment in one step. This practice, however, has some limitations. The mixing of certain sanitizers and detergents can impair the effectiveness of either agent or both. Also, the activity of the detergent-sanitizer mixture tends to be reduced more rapidly in the presence of solids and organic matter than when the sanitizing step is a separate process after cleaning. Mrozek (1985) has stated that heavy fouling of pasteurizers and evaporators makes effective one-phase cleaners comparatively expensive. He is of the opinion that a good two-phase process with stored solutions may be cheaper.

CONCLUSIONS

Economics is a significant factor in food plant sanitation; modern cleaning and sanitizing aim for greatest effectiveness at the lowest cost (Mrozek, 1985). Important cost factors include the energy required to heat the solutions for circulation and for cleaning and sanitizing equipment; water used for prerinse, intermediate rinse, and preparation of cleaning and disinfection solutions; and labor costs. Labor costs have been reduced in some instances by converting to automation.

Mrozek (1985) also emphasizes that to obtain maximum benefits from a sanitation program, recontamination must be avoided. Some measures to accomplish this are disinfection procedures, which must include outer plant surfaces and surrounding areas; prevention of water-borne contamination of the processing lines; protection of outer surfaces of equipment by spraying with appropriate solutions; and supplying filtered sterile air to the work place. Mrozek summarizes strategies for cleaning and sanitizing for maintenance of a satisfactory hygienic environment as follows: for food contact areas, CIP-cleaning; for connected spaces, dismantling and treating; for outer surfaces, manual treatment; for workroom areas, automatic spray; for supplies, sterilization where feasible; and for germ carriers, exclusion.

The goals of an effective food sanitation program are designed to anticipate and eliminate potential hazards before they become serious problems. Several items common to successful sanitation programs are total management participation, a company sanitation manual, an effective training program, adherence to good manufacturing practices, good personal hygiene of employees, good communication and supervision, effective pest-control programs, self-inspection, and respect for the food being handled (Gravani, 1986; Bianco, 1987).

REFERENCES

Adair, T.W., Geftic, S.G., and Gelzer, J. 1969. Resistance of *Pseudomonas* to quaternary ammonium compounds. I. Growth in benzalkonium chloride solution. Appl. Microbiol., *18*, 299–309.

Asbury, E.D. 1983. Methods of testing sanitizers and bacteriostatic substances. In *Disinfection, Sterilization and Preservation*. Edited by S.S. Block. Philadelphia, Lea & Febiger, pp. 964–980.

Bianco, L.J. 1987. Good sanitation practices. Dairy Food Sanit., *7*, 566–568.

Block, S.S. 1983. Definition of terms. In *Disinfection, Sterilization and Preservation*. Edited by S.S. Block. Philadelphia, Lea & Febiger, pp. 877–881.

Brackett, R.E. 1987. Antimicrobial effect of chlorine on *Listeria monocytogenes*. J. Food Protect., *60*, 999–1003.

Chambers, C.W., et al. 1955. Bactericidal efficiency of Q.A.C. in different waters. Public Health Rpts., *70*, 545.

Charlton, D., and Levine, M. 1937. Germicidal properties of chlorine compounds. Iowa State College Eng. Expt. Sta. Bull., No. 132.

Cheow, C.S., and Jackson, A.T. 1982. Circulation of a plate heat exchanger fouled by tomato juice. I. Cleaning with water. J. Food Technol., *17*, 417–430.

Dixon, J.M.S., and Pooley, F.E. 1961. The effect of chlorination on chicken carcasses infected with salmonellae. J. Hygiene, *59*, 343.

Dunsmore, D.H., and Thomas, M.A. 1981. Bacteriological control of food equipment surfaces by cleaning systems. II. Sanitizer effects. J. Food Protect., *44*, 21–27.

Dychdala, G.R. 1983. Chlorine and chlorine compounds. In *Disinfection, Sterilization and Preservation*. Edited by S.S. Block. Philadelphia, Lea & Febiger, pp. 157–182.

Eadie, G.A., Molner, J.G., Solomon, R.J., and Aach, R.D. Type E botulism, report of an outbreak in Michigan. JAMA, *187*, 496–499.

El-Kest, S.E., and Marth, E.H. 1988. Inactivation of *Listeria monocytogenes* by chlorine. J. Food Protect., *55*, 520–524.

Elliker, P.R. 1958. Chemical sanitizers for the milk industry. Dairy Foods Rev., *62*, 14.

Gardner, J.F., and Peel, M.M. 1986. *Introduction To Sterilization and Disinfection*. Churchill Livingstone, Melborne.

Gottardi, W. 1983. Iodine and iodine compounds. In *Disinfection, Sterilization and Preservation*. Edited by S.S. Block. Philadelphia, Lea & Febiger, pp. 183–196.

Gravani, R.B. 1986. Sanitation in the food industry. Dairy Food Sanitat., *6*, 250–251.

Guthrie, R.K. 1988. *Food Sanitation*. New York, Van Nostrand Reinhold.

Hays, H., Elliker, P.R., and Sandine, W.E. 1967. Microbial destruction by low concentrations of hypochlorite and iodophor germicides in alkaline and acidified water. Appl. Microbiol., *15*, 575–581.

Henderson, J.L. 1971. *The Fluid-Milk Industry*. AVI Publishing, Westport, Connecticut.

Hoehn, R.C. 1976. Comparative disinfection methods. J. Am. Water Works Assoc., *68*, 302–308.

Jennings, W.G. 1965. Theory and practice of hard surface cleaning. Adv. Food Res., *14*, 325–458.

Jowitt, R. 1980. *Hygienic Design and Operation of Food Plant*. Chichester, Ellis Horwood.

Kaysuyama, A.M., and Strachan, J.P. 1980. *Principles of Food Processing Sanitation*. Washington, D.C., Food Processors Institute.

Kelly, C.A., Dempster, J.F., and McLaghlin, A.J. 1981. The effect of temperature, pressure and chlorine concentration of spray washing water on numbers of bacteria on lamb carcasses. J. Appl. Bacteriol., *51*, 415–424.

Lesser, M.A. 1949. Hypochlorites as sanitizers. Soap Sanit. Chem., *25*(8), 119–125, 139.

Lopes, J.A. 1986. Evaluation of dairy and food plant sanitizers against *Salmonella typhimurium* and *Listeria monocytogenes*. J. Dairy Sci., *69*, 2791–2796.

Malpas, J.F. 1971. The use of chlorine for water disinfection in industry. Chemistry Industry, *4*, 111–115.

Marshall, R.T., Anderson, M.E., Naumann, H.D., and Stringer, W.C. 1977. Experiments in sanitizing beef with sodium hypochlorite. J. Food Protect., *40*, 246–249.

Mercer, W., and Sommers, I.J. 1957. *Chlorine in Food Plant Sanitation*. New York, Academic Press.

Modeland, V. 1989. America's food safety team: a look at the lineup. Dairy Food Environ. Sanit., *9*, 14–15.

Morrison, G.J., and Fleet, G.H. 1985. Reduction of *Salmonella* on chicken carcasses by immersion treatments. J. Food Protect., *48*, 939–943.

Mosley, E.B., Elliker, P.R., and Hays, H. 1976. Destruction of food spoilage, indicator and pathogenic organisms by various germicides in solution and on a stainless steel surface. J. Milk Food Technol., *39*, 830–836.

Mrozek, H. 1985. Detergency and disinfection. J. Soc. Dairy Technol., *38*, 119–121.

Mustapha, A., and Liewen, M.B. 1989. Destruction of *Listeria monocytogenes* by sodium hypochlorite and quaternary ammonium sanitizers. J. Food Protect., *52*, 306–311.

Parker, M.E., and Litchfield, J.H. 1962. *Food Plant Sanitation*. New York, Reinhold.

Patterson, J.T. 1968. Bacterial flora on chicken carcasses treated with high concentrations of chlorine. J. Appl. Bacteriol., *31*, 544–550.

Prucha, M.J. 1929. Chemical sterilization of dairy utensils. Univ. Illinois Agric. Exp. Sta. Circular 332.

Ranken, M.D., Clemlow, G., Shrimpton, D.H., and Stevens, B.J.H. 1926. Chlorination in poultry processing. Bact. Poultry Sci., *6*, 331–337.

Rudolph, A.S., and Levine, M. 1941. Factors affecting germicidal efficiency of hypochlorite solutions. Iowa State Coll. Eng. Exp. Sta. Bull. No. 150.

Scott, G.C. 1937. Cooling tank contamination. Canning Age *18*(5), 190.

Skaarup, T. 1985. *Slaughter House Cleaning and Sanitation*. FAO Animal Production and Health Paper 53. Rome, Food and Agriculture Organization of the United Nations.

Soprey, P.R., and Maxcy, R.B. 1968. Tolerance of bacteria for quaternary ammonium compounds. J. Food Sci., *33*, 536–540.

Troller, J.A. 1983. *Sanitation in Food Processing*. New York, Academic Press.

Trueman, J.R. 1971. The halogens. In *Inhibition and Destruction of the Bacterial Cell*. Edited by W.B. Hugo. New York, Academic Press, pp. 137–183.

Vaughn, R.H., and Stadtman, T.C. 1946. Sanitation in the processing plant and its relation to the microbial quality of the finished product. Food Freezing, *7*, 334–336, 364.

Whittaker, H.A., and Mohler, B.M. 1912. The sterilization of milk bottles with calcium hypochlorite. Am. J. Public Health, *2*, 282.

CHAPTER 47

CHEMICAL FOOD PRESERVATIVES

P.M. Foegeding and F.F. Busta

FOOD SPOILAGE AND PRESERVATION

A food preservative is any agent that extends the storage life of food products by retarding or preventing deterioration of flavor, odor, color, texture, appearance, nutritive value, or safety. Deteriorative changes may result from microbial growth or from chemical or enzymatic reactions. This chapter is concerned only with control of microbial deterioration.

Some ancient methods of food processing and preservation include drying (dehydration), salting, smoking, and fermentation. Preserved foods could be used during periods when crop production and hunting were limited. As the human population increased, food preservation became more important, and added objectives were to diminish food waste and to maintain the wholesomeness and safety of food. Expansion of industrial production and distribution of foods, development of more perishable preserved food products, modifications in food processing and distribution approaches, centralization of food processing and distribution centers, greater acceptance of convenience foods, and reduction in numbers of people directly involved in food production, coupled with the increasing total world population, have resulted in greater potential for mishandling during various stages of food processing. Furthermore, the trend in food processing is toward production of high quality foods with long shelf-lives that resemble, to the greatest extent possible, fresh or freshly prepared foods. Production of this type of product demands knowledgeable, precise use of appropriate chemical and physical preservation treatments. Consequently, food preservation has recently attained greater significance.

Microbial proliferation and associated chemical and enzymatic activities in food may cause changes in the general appearance, color, flavor, texture, consistency, and nutritive value of the product or may affect the public health. Food that has supported undesirable microbial growth becomes unfit for consumption (contributing to our worldwide food shortage), creates health problems for the individuals consuming the food, and has adverse effects on private and national economies.

The main objectives of food preservation are to extend the shelf-life, retain nutritive value, and ensure safety by delaying or preventing microbial decomposition and by suppressing the growth of pathogenic microorganisms. Physical control processes such as dehydration, low-temperature storage, and heat processing constitute approved and widely used methods of food preservation. However, there are many foods for which such processes cannot be applied or have limited usefulness. In these instances, preservation by the application of chemical compounds becomes a possible alternative.

Chemical food preservation is defined as the inhibition or inactivation of undesirable microbial proliferation by chemical compounds in a food system. Chemical compounds may be used without concomitant physical treatment, although physical methods of food preservation often are used in combination with chemical compounds. Such combinations allow the processes or agents to be used at lower intensity or concentration while the food retains good keeping quality with only minor changes in product properties.

SELECTION OF FOOD PRESERVATIVES

Currently, no single food preservative is ideal for use in all food products and situations. The action of every food preservative is affected by a variety of factors (Ingram et al., 1964; Mossel, 1975; Jarvis and Burke, 1976; Branen and Davidson, 1983), which should be closely evaluated when a preservative is selected for a specific food. The antimicrobial activity of specific compounds varies and depends in part on the types of microorganisms and foods.

A broad antimicrobial spectrum frequently is desirable. Often, one group of microorganisms suppresses the growth of another. Inhibition of the first group may permit the second to predominate and cause spoilage or public health problems not previously encountered.

Therefore, the range of activity of the selected antimicrobial agent should include the full complement of unwanted microorganisms that may occur in the product. In certain instances, such as in useful lactic acid fermentations, it is necessary to choose a preservative that suppresses unwanted growth but does not interfere with desirable microbial growth.

Incorporation of a preservative in a food should guard against the development of resistant strains, especially in the species against which the preservative is intended to act. For example, some mold and yeast species have developed resistance to benzoate and sorbate (Marth et al., 1966). Concern over resistant strains has been one major hindrance to the direct addition of classic antibiotics as food preservatives.

Physical and chemical properties of the preservative and their relationship to the specific food product constitute a major factor in the compound efficacy. Properties such as solubility, pK_a (dissociation constant), toxic levels, and chemical reactivity are influential and should be examined carefully before a compound is considered for preservation of a specific product. Because the antimicrobial activity of weak acid preservatives is attributed mostly to their undissociated form, the pK_a or dissociation constant will predict the efficacy of such preservatives in a food system with a specified pH.

Different compounds of the same class may differ in antimicrobial activity as well as in physical and chemical properties. The most useful alternative should be chosen to suit the situation. Often, the salt forms of organic acids are more water soluble than is the acid itself. The salts are preferred if water solubility is important, such as in spray or brine applications. In applications made directly into the products, however, such as in emulsions, the acid form may be more useful. The antimicrobial activity of parabens increases with chain length, but water solubility decreases with increased chain length. In this case, a mixture of two or more compounds may improve effectiveness. Two or more compounds also can be used in cases in which activity over a wider pH range is required, or a broader spectrum of microorganisms must be controlled.

The aforementioned and other properties of a compound should be considered in relation to the general composition, physical and chemical processing, storage, and distribution of the food. In addition to pH, which has been identified as a major deterrent in selecting a preservative, other components of the system may be influential by exerting their own antimicrobial activity or by acting synergistically with the proposed preservative. Thermal processing or product dehydration to a lower water activity (A_w) may enhance the effect of preservatives and decrease the concentrations required for stability. Cured meat products are a dramatic example of complex interactions in food preservation (Ingram, 1974, 1976; Lechowich et al., 1978; Sofos et al., 1979c; Busta and Sofos, 1979). The microfloras of the products are also influential in selection of a food preservative.

The types of microorganisms present will determine which compound or compounds are most effective under the given conditions, and the extent of contamination will dictate what concentrations should be employed.

The requirements that a compound must meet for approval as a food preservative, as well as the complexity of foods and the variety of influential factors, demonstrate the difficulty in selecting an appropriate preservative for a product. Selecting a chemical preservative for a specific system is a long and tedious process, which is complicated by the fact that few compounds are currently in use as preservatives, the number of alternative preservatives has not increased recently, tighter restrictions are being imposed by regulatory authorities, all available food preservatives have certain disadvantages, and the demand for food preservation is greater today than at any time in the past.

APPLICATION OF CHEMICAL FOOD PRESERVATIVES

Chemical food preservatives are incorporated directly into food products or develop during processing (such as fermentation) of the food. Some chemical compounds have been used accidentally or intentionally in the preservation of foods for many centuries. These traditional preservatives include common salt, sugars, alcohols, acids, and components of smoke, which have been introduced through processes such as fermentation, salting, curing, and smoking. Meat and fish products were commonly preserved by such processes in ancient times.

Chemical food preservatives may be directly applied by dipping, spraying, gassing, or dusting onto the outside of the product. Preservatives may be included with other ingredients in the product formulation or in a brine that is applied to the food by soaking or injection. Some additives are incorporated in the packaging material rather than applied directly to the food itself.

REGULATORY ASPECTS OF CHEMICAL FOOD PRESERVATION

Use of chemical compounds in food is regulated by the appropriate authorities of each country, such as the Food and Drug Administration (FDA) of the Department of Health and Human Services in the United States. Internationally, the Food and Agriculture Organization (FAO) and the World Health Organization (WHO) are concerned with chemical food preservatives and recommend the acceptable daily intake of many preservatives. In the U.S., the Food Additives Amendment to the Food, Drug and Cosmetic Act specifies the conditions and the process under which any substance may be approved as a chemical additive. Assuming that the safety of the compound is established by the manufacturer, a regulation will be issued specifying applications, amounts used, and any other conditions necessary to protect the public well-being. The use of additives and preservatives in foods is controlled by legislation in all developed countries. Jarvis and Burke (1976) and Ahlborg et al. (1977) detail preservative legislation in several countries. For specific information about the legislation governing use of chemical food preservatives in a certain country, the appropriate domestic authorities and publications should be consulted. For example, in the U.S., for lists and conditions for use of substances generally recognized as safe (GRAS), the reader is referred to the Code of Federal Regulations, Title 21, part 182 (parts 180–189 and other parts are pertinent to use of chemical food preservatives).

Some chemical food preservatives (acetic acid, sorbic acid, sulfur dioxide) are GRAS in the U.S., hence, they are exempted from the food additive regulations. The intended use of a GRAS additive, however, must fall within the conditions for use and must be approved for the food product. The principles of good manufacturing practices must be followed when no limits on the use-concentration are set in the GRAS list. In the United States, every chemical food preservative used must be identified on the product label.

In the past, use of chemicals in food was often considered adulteration because they were used to increase the product volume or to conceal poor quality (Jarvis and Burke, 1976). Today, the major arguments against the use of chemicals for food preservation are that they may be harmful to the public, they may reduce nutritional quality of the food, they may make faulty food appear normal, and their use could be eliminated if good manufacturing procedures were followed. Regulatory authorities of each country are responsible for prevention of such abuses.

The use of chemicals or food preservatives is approved only when (1) there is need for preservation of the food concerned, (2) the chemical is proven capable of performing the described preservative action under the specific conditions of the described food product, (3) the compound is nontoxic and is proven safe and noncarcinogenic at concentrations above intended levels of use, (4) it does not damage the food identity by altering such qualities as flavor and appearance, (5) its food application is practical and its properties (e.g., solubility) do not interfere with application, (6) its cost is affordable, (7) it is adequately available, and (8) its total consumption (including that from existing uses) would not exceed specified safe levels.

These requirements have set strict controls on the approval of chemicals for use as food preservatives (Ingram et al., 1964). Few new preservatives have been approved recently because of these requirements. In some cases, it is even difficult to extend the application of commonly used preservatives to food products other than those currently approved. Thus, most of the initial preservatives, some of which were proven effective and safe by long accidental use, are still applied despite well known limitations.

PHYSICAL METHODS OF FOOD PRESERVATION

Food is commonly preserved by physical methods, including heat-processing (pasteurization and sterilization), low-temperature storage (refrigeration and freezing), and drying. Application of such processes is limited to certain types of food products, and the degree of application is limited in certain instances. Changes in product identity or function, energy requirements of the processes, available technology, and consumer acceptance are some major factors limiting use of these physical methods.

Irradiation, or radappertization, can be considered a physical control method in food preservation. Application is often restricted to the field of medicine, because in most countries irradiation is not approved as a method of food preservation, but only as a decontamination treatment for food constituents. Public concern about potential induction of mutagenic or carcinogenic compounds in the food through irradiation has restricted its food application, although no such alterations have been documented.

The mechanism, kinetics, applications, and usefulness of thermal processing and irradiation are discussed elsewhere in this volume. Direct removal of microorganisms by processes such as filtration is another physical method of preservation that may be applied to food products.

Dehydration and Reduced Water Activity

Dehydration is a process in which water activity (A_w) is lowered by removal of most of the water present in a product. Dehydration may be accomplished by vaporization or sublimation of the water in the product. The antimicrobial effect is based upon reduction of water activity to a level that prohibits microbial growth. Dehydration is a complex process; the reader is referred to Karel (1975a, b) for extensive discussions of dehydration. Dehydration is used to preserve sugar, starch, coffee, milk products, flour mixes, breakfast foods, snacks, pasta products, fruits, vegetables, and other foods.

Water activity may be depressed below the minimum for microbial activity by addition of a variety of chemical food preservatives that function as humectants. These include salt, sugar, and ethyl alcohol, which are discussed below, as well as other preservatives. Bacteria generally are more sensitive to reduced water activity than are yeasts or molds. The International Commission on Microbiological Specifications for Foods (1980) has provided an excellent introduction to the effect of water activity on microbial growth and food preservation.

Low-Temperature Storage

Refrigeration and freezing are used both in homes and commercially to preserve foods during transport and storage. Refrigeration, or chilling, is storage of foods below about 15°C and above freezing, whereas freezing is storage at temperatures below the freezing point. Low-temperature storage is used to reduce the rates of chemical reactions and of microbial metabolism. Generally, the lower the temperature, the slower the reaction rate. Low temperatures damage certain food tissues or systems, however, so the choice of storage temperature depends upon the particular food. Psychrotrophic or psychrophilic organisms may grow well at refrigerated temperatures; some of these organisms cause spoilage or public health problems in refrigerated foods.

Freezing also slows the rates of many chemical reactions because of the low temperature. Also, part of the antimicrobial mechanism of freezing is due to dehydration. Liquid water is removed from the system, and ice (crystallized water) is formed. Many textbooks and literature references deal extensively with preservation by refrigerated and frozen storage and the effects of low temperatures on microorganisms (Fennema, 1975a, b; Banwart, 1979).

Refrigeration is used to preserve many foods, including fresh meat, poultry, fish, eggs, dairy products, vegetables, fruits, and others. Freezing is used for preservation of meat, poultry, fish, meat products, ice cream, vegetables, fruits, and numerous other foods.

TRADITIONAL, NATURAL, OR FREQUENTLY USED PRESERVATIVES

Some food preservatives, such as common salt, have been added to foods for centuries, contributing considerably to safety and stability of the food. Often, application of such traditional food preservatives was accidental, and the initial purpose of addition was to improve flavor. Many food preservatives are naturally present and not added to certain foods, but may be added to other foods because of their antimicrobial properties. Some traditional, natural, and frequently used food preservatives are discussed below. Although many acids may be considered in these categories, they are discussed in a separate section.

Sugar

Sugars (glucose, fructose, sucrose, and syrups) are widely used in the food industry as sweeteners, flavorings, and fermentable materials. The sugars are highly water-soluble, usually sweet-tasting, white crystals. Sucrose, the most commonly used sugar, has the formula $C_{12}H_{22}O_{11}$ and a molecular weight of 342.30. Sugars are natural components of many foods and are used in the body as a carbohydrate for energy production. Their addition for preservation purposes is not subject to any food regulations.

The antimicrobial activity of sugars may be direct or indirect. The direct action is a result of lowering the water activity or increasing the osmotic pressure, because the moisture of the food is complexed by the sugar. Microorganisms are unable to grow and multiply in high osmotic pressures. High sugar levels are necessary for direct control of microorganisms. Typically, direct inhibition due to sugar concentration combined with other preservative factors such as heating, drying, or other added preservatives, is of practical importance more often than sugar alone is. In fermented foods, sugar provides the substrate for production of acid, alcohol, and other antimicrobial compounds resulting in indirect preservative action. Indeed, Smith and Palumbo (1981)

treated microorganisms as food additives in a review of fermentation preservation.

In small concentrations, sucrose is necessary for or promotes the growth of many spoilage organisms and pathogens (Hobbs, 1976). Because of osmotic effects, sucrose may increase the heat resistance of molds and other organisms (Doyle and Marth, 1975). Sugar-metal ion complexes, particularly of iron, also may influence bacterial growth and control (Charley et al., 1963; Sams and Carroll, 1966; Tompkin, 1978). Xylitol may have unique antimicrobial activity because it is not, or is only slowly, fermented by many food-borne microorganisms (Mäkinen and Söderling, 1981).

Bacteria are less tolerant of reduced water activity than are yeasts or molds; hence, bacteria are more susceptible to high sugar concentrations. Some yeasts and molds are especially osmotolerant. These include the yeasts *Saccharomyces rouxii* and *Torulopsis* species and the mold *Aspergillus glaucus*. *Zygosaccharomyces* species are saccharophilic. The direct antimicrobial activity of sugar is used in the preservation of several foods, including jams, jellies, candied fruits, candies, and sweetened condensed milk.

Salt

Salt, or sodium chloride (NaCl), is widely employed as a preservative and flavoring agent. Its use dates to ancient times (Jensen, 1954). Salt has retained its importance in food preservation, although it is used less today as a preservative alone than in combination with other preservation methods. It is the main ingredient of curing mixes or brines, and its use in meat preservation led to the initially accidental use of nitrate and nitrite in meat curing (Binkerd and Kolari, 1975). Sodium chloride has a molecular weight of 58.44 and is a highly water-soluble, white, cubic crystal. Salt is a vital dietary constituent that, when fed in excess, retarded growth and shortened the life span of laboratory animals (Meneely et al., 1953). Currently, the controversy concerning the health effects of dietary sodium continues. Thus, the trend is toward reduction of sodium (NaCl is only one source) in processed food. As a necessary dietary constituent and an ancient food additive, salt is subject to few legal restrictions. However, the controversy concerning health effects of dietary sodium has prompted a flurry of research to identify methods to reduce NaCl in food processing. For example, dry curing of meats traditionally has used high NaCl concentration as one component of the preservation process not only for protection against microbial problems but also for devitalization of the parasitic nematode, *Trichinella spiralis*. Recently, following of a study by Pinedo et al. (1987), the USDA (1989) has proposed partial replacement of NaCl by KCl in dry-cured meats as an alternative process.

The mode of bacterial inhibition by salt is complex. The antimicrobial effects of salt and applications in food preservation have been reviewed by Sofos (1983). Antimicrobial effects may include plasmolysis, dehydration, interference with enzymes, or cellular toxicity of high sodium or chloride ion concentrations. Sato et al. (1972) and Ito et al. (1977) reported evidence suggesting that the lethal effect of NaCl is related to loss of Mg^{++} from bacterial cells. Ten percent NaCl reduces the A_w of food systems to below 0.935, which is inhibitory to *Clostridium botulinum* and other microorganisms (Schmidt, 1964). Lower salt concentrations act synergistically with other preservatives and preservation methods (Rao et al., 1966; Deibel, 1979; Robach and Stateler, 1980; Robach, 1979b).

Tolerance of microorganisms to salt varies greatly. Generally, mesophilic gram-negative rods and psychrotrophic bacteria are the most salt-sensitive, tolerating no more than 4 to 10% salt. The lactic acid bacteria and spore-forming bacteria tolerate about 4 to 15% and 5 to 16%, respectively (Banwart, 1979). Halophiles (salt-loving organisms) need relatively high salt concentrations for growth and, if present, may spoil salted foods (Tanner, 1944; Walker, 1977). These include *Halobacterium* and *Halococcus* species. Yeasts and molds vary in their salt tolerance; some are extremely tolerant to salt.

Salt is used to preserve many foods either alone or in combination with other agents. Some foods in which it is a primary preservative include butter, margarine, cheese, dry salted meat and fish, sausage, ham, and brined vegetables.

Spices

Many spices, seasonings, and essential oils that are added to foods as flavoring ingredients have antimicrobial properties. Marth (1966) reviewed the antimicrobial activity of spices and their essential oils. Vaughn (1951), Johnson and Vaughn (1969), Al-Delaimy and Ali (1970), Bullerman (1974), Beuchat (1976), Bogen et al. (1979), Huhtanen (1980), Davidson et al. (1983), and Zaika (1988) have discussed the antimicrobial activity of spices and spice components. The amount of spices commonly added to foods is small, and the antimicrobial action of their components in preservation of the product may be synergistic.

Smoke

The use of smoke from an open fire is one of the oldest known methods of meat, fish, and poultry preservation. Knowledge of smoke constituents is not complete. Benzopyrene, a known carcinogen, is the main component of toxicologic relevance in smoke. It is possible to keep the concentration of benzopyrene low if smoking is carried out properly. In most countries, smoking is not governed by any food regulations.

Wood smoke contributes to flavor and has a preservative effect through heating, drying, and introduction of chemical components of smoke into the product. Phenolic compounds, formaldehyde, acetic acid, and creosote are components of smoke that have preservative action. Smoke from different wood sources differ in antimicrobial effectiveness (Boyle et al., 1988), apparently because of compositional differences. Components of smoke may lower the pH and have other antimicrobial

activity, such as prevention of spore formation and control of growth of certain organisms (Fiddler et al., 1966; Trujillo and Laible, 1970; Trujillo and David, 1972; Sink and Hsu, 1977). The antimicrobial action of smoke is relatively weak and mainly a surface phenomenon (Christiansen et al., 1968; Tatini et al., 1976). The antimicrobial activity of smoke is directed primarily against gram-negative bacteria. Spores of bacteria and molds are relatively resistant.

Lysozyme

Lysozyme is an enzyme that is naturally present in many biologic systems, including food. For example, lysozyme is present in milk and egg white. Egg white lysozyme has been suggested as a preservative for other foods and beverages. Lysozyme degrades the cell wall of bacteria and has maximum activity at pH 7.0. Hughey and Johnson (1987) recently evaluated the effectiveness of lysozyme for control of several pathogenic and spoilage bacteria associated with foods. Their data indicate a broad range of sensitivities to lysozyme. The relatively high cost of lysozyme currently limits its widespread use as a food preservative.

Lactoperoxidase

This enzyme is present in high concentrations in milk and other body fluids. In combination with thiocyanate (or halides) and hydrogen peroxide (each of which may be present in milk, the latter because of microbial activity), an effective antimicrobial system results. The system is not specifically used in the U.S. However, it has found application in developing countries to extend the shelf-life of milk. Its potential effectiveness for preservation of infant formulas has been demonstrated by Banks and Board (1985) and could find application for extending the shelf-life and safety of formula rehydrated with water of poor quality in developing countries, for example. However, the lactoperoxidase system is bacteriostatic but not cidal to *Listeria monocytogenes* (Earnshaw and Banks, 1989).

Other Natural Preservatives and Natural Preservative Systems

Many naturally occurring food components reportedly have some antimicrobial properties. Beuchat and Golden (1989) recently have reviewed antimicrobials occurring naturally in foods. Most of these are weak antimicrobial agents at the levels present in foods. These include hop resins, anthocyanins, flavenols, cocoa extracts, oleuropin or tyrosol of olives, polyamines of animal tissues, lactoferrin of milk, and conalbumin of egg. Banks and co-workers (1986) have suggested the interesting idea of further exploitation of natural antimicrobial systems for effective food preservation. The lactoperoxidase-thiocyanate-hydrogen peroxide system is one example. This system is used to preserve milk in developing countries where refrigeration is not available or reliable (Medina et al., 1989). Additionally, Banks et al. (1986) have reviewed other antimicrobial systems in animals, plants, and microorganisms that may find future application in food preservation.

ACIDS AND ACID DERIVATIVES

Several acids are added to foods or are formed in food through fermentation. In addition to their preservative function, these acids may also be flavoring agents, buffers, synergists to antioxidants, and curing adjuncts (Gardner, 1972). Many preservatives are more active at acidic pH levels; consequently, acidulants enhance the action of other preservatives.

Acidic pH values facilitate microbial destruction by heat, permitting shorter sterilization or pasteurization processing times and, therefore, minimizing heat damage of product quality. Low pH values prevent or delay spore germination and growth of spore-forming bacteria. To prevent growth and toxin production of *Clostridium botulinum*, a pH value of 4.6 or less is required. Thus, to avoid the requirement for extreme thermal processing and to enhance thermal inactivation, acidification is required in some countries for canning certain foods including figs, artichokes, and certain other vegetables and fruits.

Acids are effective preservatives for more reasons than just pH depression, however. Importantly, the active form of acids as preservatives is the undissociated acid. Thus to select an acid preservative it is useful to consider the pH of the food and the pK_a (pH at which 50% of the acid is dissociated) of the acid (Sauer, 1977). Ideally, the pH of the food should be less than the pK_a so that the majority of the acid is undissociated. In the undissociated form, the uncharged acid is free to diffuse through the membrane and into the cell cytoplasm. Microorganisms have mechanisms to maintain homeostasis so that the cytoplasmic pH generally is maintained near pH 7 and frequently is greater than the environmental pH. Thus, the acid will dissociate once it is inside the cell to reach an equilibrium of charged (dissociated) and uncharged (undissociated) acid. This equilibrium, and hence the degree of dissociation, is dictated by the pK_a of the acid and the pH of the environment, in this case the cytoplasm. Thus, acids that are uncharged in the food environment (pK_a is high, ideally greater than pH of the food environment) are able to penetrate the cell, where they are effective inhibitors by generally acidifying the cell as well as causing other specific inhibitory effects targeted at, for example, enzymatic reactions and transport systems. Microorganisms may expend a great deal of energy trying to maintain the intracellular pH and remove acid preservatives. The mode of action of organic acid preservatives has been reviewed by Doores (1983). Recently, Goodson and Rowbury (1989) suggested that prior exposure to acid may permit increased resistance to acid for *Escherichia coli*.

Organic acids are generally weak acids, as is reflected by their relatively high pK_a values, and tend to be excellent preservatives that find diverse application in foods. In addition to pK_a, efficacy and application are affected by carbon-chain length and degree of unsaturation. Antimicrobial activity of organic acids generally increases with chain length, but limited water solubility of long-chain acids restricts their use (Foster and Wynne, 1948; Roth and Halvorson, 1952; Nieman, 1954). The antimicrobial activity increases with the degree of unsaturation; *cis* isomers are more effective than are *trans* isomers (Kodicek, 1956). Some of the most common food preservatives are organic, lipophilic acids such as benzoic or sorbic acids. Many organic acids are natural components of foods and are considered GRAS in the U.S. They typically have low acute toxicity. Acute toxicity data and acceptable daily intake values have been tabulated by Doores (1983).

Acetic Acid

Acetic acid, CH_3COOH, is water soluble; it has a pK_a of 4.76, a molecular weight of 60.05, and low toxicity. It is inexpensive and is produced through oxidation of alcohol by bacteria of the genus *Acetobacter* (Derosier, 1970). Acetic acid, present at a concentration of 4% or greater in vinegar, is the principal organic component of vinegar. Vinegar is generally produced by the alcoholic fermentation (anaerobic step) of sugars, grapes, cider, wine, or malt, followed by oxidation (aerobic step) of the alcohol to acetic acid by *Acetobacter* (Derosier, 1970; Prescott and Dunn, 1959; Jacobs, 1958). Vinegar is one of the oldest preservatives and flavoring agents. Both vinegar and acetic acid are listed as GRAS in the U.S.

Acetic acid inhibits many species of bacteria, yeasts, and molds. Acetic acid is more effective against bacteria and yeasts than against molds (Chichester and Tanner, 1972). However, calcium acetate and calcium or sodium diacetate have been reported effective against molds in breads. An oxidized derivative of acetic acid, peracetic acid decomposes to acetic acid and oxygen in the presence of organic substrates. Peracetic acid has been suggested for disinfection of food contact surfaces.

The main application of acetic acids is in the form of vinegar. Vinegar or acetic acid is used in many foods, including catsup, prepared mustard, mayonnaise, salad dressings, pickles, and marinades. Other uses of acetic acid, such as spray sanitization with 4% acetic acid on beef surfaces, have been suggested. Bala et al. (1977) showed that this significantly reduced the microbial population without adversely affecting color or desirability of the beef. Similar treatment of poultry meat was undesirable because of the resultant pungent odor and tough meat surface (Mountney and O'Malley, 1965). Sodium diacetate does not introduce off-flavors in bread when used as a mold and ropiness inhibitor, and its action is not as pH-dependent as is the action of acetic acid.

Dehydroacetic Acid

Dehydroacetic acid, $C_8H_8O_4$, has a pK_a of 5.27. It inhibits bacteria, yeasts, and molds, but appears to be a better fungistatic than bacteriostatic agent. The toxicity data on this chemical tend to be contradictory (Spencer et al., 1950; Seevers et al., 1950). At 0.17%, dehydroacetic acid inhibits undesirable secondary fermentations in alcoholic beverages (Banwart, 1979). Dehydroacetic acid and its sodium salt are permitted in the U.S. for protecting cut or peeled squash from undesirable mold attack and for treatment of cheese wrappers.

Monohalogenacetic Acids

The antimicrobial action of monohalogenacetic acid has been known for a long time. Best known are monochloroacetic acid and monobromoacetic acid. Monobromoacetic acid and its ethyl ester have the most powerful antimicrobial effect. Their antimicrobial action is due to reaction with sulfhydryl-containing enzymes and interference with oxidation-reduction reactions in the cell. Yeasts are more susceptible than bacteria or molds. Monochloroacetic acid and monobromoacetic acid and its esters have been used to stabilize juices and wine. None of the monohalogenacetic acids are currently permitted in foods in any country (Lueck, 1980).

Propionic Acid

Propionic acid (CH_3CH_2COOH) is an aliphatic, monocarboxylic acid with a pK_a of 4.88 and a molecular weight of 74.08. Usually, the sodium or calcium salts are used in food because the acid itself is corrosive. These salts yield the free acid in the pH range of the foods in which they are used; optimum effectiveness is around pH 5.0 and below (Cruess and Irish, 1932). Both salts are white, free-flowing powders. The sodium salt is soluble at 150 g/100 ml water at 100°C, and the calcium salt is soluble at 55.8 g/100 ml water at 100°C. Propionic acid is produced by *Propionibacterium* during the manufacture of Swiss cheese, where its concentration may be as high as 1%. Propionic acid has a strong odor and flavor.

Propionic acid and its salts are readily absorbed by the digestive tract because of their high water solubility. There is no risk of accumulation in the body, because propionic acid is metabolized as a fatty acid. Propionic acid decomposition in mammals occurs by linkage with coenzyme A via methylmalonyl-CoA, succinyl-CoA, and succinate to yield CO_2 and H_2O. Propionic acid is normally formed by decomposition of several amino acids and by the oxidation of fatty acids containing odd numbers of carbon atoms. The FAO has not set a limit on the acceptable daily intake of propionic acid or its salts. Propionates are GRAS in foods in the U.S. They are permitted for food use in many countries, including Australia, Belgium, Brazil, Canada, Denmark, Finland, Germany, Italy, Japan, Soviet Union, Spain, Sweden, and the United Kingdom.

Several microorganisms, notably *Propionibacterium* spp., can produce propionic acid, whereas many others can metabolize it. Its antimicrobial action is partially due to nutrient transport inhibition (Eklund, 1980) and to the fact that it specifically inhibits metabolic enzymes. Propionic acid also inhibits microbial growth by competing with necessary growth substances such as alanine and other amino acids (Hesseltine, 1952). The action of propionates is directed primarily against molds (Hesseltine,

1952; Olson and Macy, 1945). Reportedly, calcium propionate is more effective against aflatoxin formation than against mold growth itself (Lueck, 1980). Propionates have essentially no activity against yeasts, and in fact, many yeasts metabolize propionic acid. Propionates are poorly active against bacteria, with the notable exception of their ability to inhibit *Bacillus mesentericus*, the organism that causes rope formation in bread.

The main application of the propionates is in the baking industry, where they are used to prevent rope formation and growth of mold in bread and cakes (O'Leary and Kralovec, 1941; Cathcart, 1951; Matz, 1972; Seiler, 1964). Propionates are also used to control mold on cheese, fruits, vegetables, tobacco, and malt extract (Olson and Macy, 1945; Jacobs, 1947; Ingram et al., 1956; Dunn, 1968; Chichester and Tanner, 1972; Gardner, 1972). Propionic acid was more effective than acetic acid for control of *A. parasiticus* aflatoxigenesis (Rusul et al., 1987). Propionate at pH 5 also is somewhat effective in controlling *Listeria monocytogenes* (El-Shenawy and Marth, 1989). The type and amount of propionate that may be employed depends upon the product and its acidity. Levels as high as about 0.38% may be added to food (Chichester and Tanner, 1972). Both calcium and sodium propionate mix well with emulsifying agents and dough ingredients. Calcium propionate is preferred in yeast-raised bread as a means of calcium enrichment. The sodium salt is preferred in cakes because calcium ions interfere with chemical leavening. Propionate may be added to wrappers and packages in addition to being added directly to the product as a mold inhibitor.

Lactic Acid

Lactic acid ($CH_3CHOHCOOH$) has a pK_a of 3.83 and is highly water-soluble. It may be manufactured through microbial fermentations and sold commercially. As a natural constituent of some foods, lactic acid is one of the oldest preservatives used. It is a GRAS substance of low toxicity and is nonmutagenic; indeed, as an end-product of anaerobic glycolysis, lactic acid is a normal body constituent. The FAO has set no limit for the acceptable daily intake of lactic acid and several of its salts.

The antimicrobial action of lactic acid is directed primarily against bacteria, including sporeformers such as putrefying anaerobes and butyric acid bacteria (Woolford, 1975). Lactate also inhibits *Bacillus cereus* spore germination (Wong and Chen, 1988). Many molds and yeasts are capable of growing at acidic pH values and can metabolize lactic acid. Consequently, lactic acid is frequently combined with an antimicrobial agent, such as benzoic or sorbic acid, aimed at inhibiting yeasts and molds (Melnick et al., 1954b; Costilow et al., 1957; Lueck, 1980). Both lactic and citric acids have been reported to specifically inhibit mycotoxin formation, including aflatoxin and sterigmatocystin (Reiss, 1976); however, El-Gazzar et al. (1987) reported that certain concentrations of lactic acid stimulated aflatoxin biosynthesis.

Lactic acid is produced by many bacterial species,

primarily of the genera *Lactococcus, Lactobacillus, Leuconostoc,* and *Pediococcus.* Other bacteria and some mold species also produce lactic acid. Lactic acid is the primary acid produced during microbial fermentation of sugar to produce cheeses, sauerkraut, pickles, sausage, and olives. The acid produced in such fermentations lowers the pH to levels unfavorable for the growth of spoilage organisms and inhibitory to *Clostridium botulinum* growth and toxin production. In the U.S., lactic acid production via fermentation of added sugar is allowed in bacon processing for faster nitrite depletion and botulinal protection due to lowered pH (USDA, 1979). Derivatives of lactic acid may be used as direct food acidulants. Glucono-delta-lactone, a permitted acidulant in certain meat products, hydrolyses to release lactic acid and functions identically to added lactic acid. Certain carbonated beverages are preserved by a combination of lactic acid and CO_2. Besides being an acidulant and exhibiting preservative action due to decreased pH, it may be used as a flavoring agent in frozen desserts (Gardner, 1972).

Benzoic Acid

Benzoic acid (benzenecarboxylic acid, phenylformic acid), C_6H_5COOH, is a granular or crystalline powder with a sweet or astringent taste. It is usually used in the form of sodium benzoate, because the sodium salt is considerably more water-soluble than the acid. Sodium benzoate, a white powder or flake, dissolves in water at a level of 50 g/100 ml at 25°C, in contrast to the acid form with water solubility of only 0.35 g/100 ml. Sodium benzoate is soluble in alcohol at a level of 1.3 g/100 ml. The pK_a of benzoic acid and its sodium salt is 4.2, and the molecular weights are 122.2 and 144.11, respectively. Sodium benzoate and benzoic acid are GRAS substances in the U.S. Sodium benzoate is inexpensive and one of the most extensively used food preservatives in the U.S. and other countries. Sodium benzoate is more toxic to rats than sodium sorbate is. Humans have high tolerance to sodium benzoate because of a detoxifying mechanism whereby benzoate and glycine or glycuronic acid are conjugated and excreted as hippuric acid or benzoyl glucuronide (Chichester and Tanner, 1972). An intermediate step in the detoxification is formation of benzoyl CoA at the expense of ATP. Benzoate is not mutagenic in *Drosophila* or *Salmonella* but reportedly interacts with nucleosides and DNA in vitro (Njagi and Gopalan, 1980).

Benzoate inhibits yeast more than it inhibits molds or bacteria. However, osmotolerant yeast resistant to benzoic acid often limit shelf-life of intermediate moisture foods preserved with this acid (Jermini and Schmidt-Lorenz, 1987). Food-poisoning and spore-forming bacteria are inhibited by undissociated benzoic acid concentrations of 0.01 to 0.02%, whereas many spoilage organisms show higher resistances. *Listeria monocytogenes* also is susceptible to the action of benzoic acid (El-Shenawy and Marth, 1988b). Rahn and Conn (1944) reported that benzoic, salicylic, and sulfurous acids were approximately 100 times more effective antimicrobial agents in acid than in neutral solution, that the antimi-

crobial activity was due to the undissociated acid, and that yeast multiplication was inhibited by 25 mg/ml undissociated benzoic acid. The undissociated, molecular form is able to pass through the cell membrane more readily than the charged form. Reviews by Bosund (1962) and Chipley (1983) present evidence showing that benzoic acid interferes with many enzymatic processes in microorganisms at concentrations that retard the growth rate. Altered membrane permeability may be another antimicrobial effect of benzoic acid. Eklund (1980), however, showed that inhibition of nutrient uptake could account for only part of the antimicrobial action of benzoate. *Zygosaccharomyces bailii* is resistant to benzoic and sorbic acids. Resistance of this yeast apparently is due to an inducible, energy-requiring system that transports preservative from the cell (Warth, 1977, 1988).

Benzoate is most effective from pH 2.5 to 4.0 (Cruess and Richert, 1929). At pH values above about 4.5, the antimicrobial activity of benzoate is low, and the addition of an acidulant or another preservative should be considered. Sodium benzoate, the form most widely used, is a common preservative for acid foods, including carbonated and still beverages, fruit juices and salads, syrups, icing, jams, jellies, preserves, margarine, mincemeat, pickles, relishes, pie fillings, and prepared salads. Sodium benzoate is used at concentrations of 0.03 to 0.10% in the U.S. Chipley (1983) tabulated benzoic acid concentrations permitted in foods produced in other countries. It is a natural component of many foods, including cranberries, prunes, plums, cinnamon, ripe cloves, and most berries. Because of the astringent flavor of benzoates, a lower level of benzoate, in combination with a second preservative such as sorbate or a paraben, may be desirable in some food products. Jermini and Schmidt-Lorenz (1987) have proposed concentrations of benzoate plus paraben to preserve intermediate moisture foods at pH values ranging from 3.0 to 4.8. Sulfurous acid may be used in combination with benzoate to avoid discoloration and oxidative changes due to benzoate. Benzoate may be added directly to foods by blending with the dry ingredients of the product, or applied by dipping foods or coating packaging films, especially for fish (Dunn, 1947).

Esters of Parahydroxybenzoic Acid

Alkyl (methyl, ethyl, propyl, butyl) esters of *p*-hydroxybenzoic acid (parabens, parasepts, or PHB esters) find use as food, cosmetic, and pharmaceutical preservatives. These esters have properties similar to benzoic acid, yet the modification enhances their utility. The methyl ester is the most water soluble: 0.25 g dissolves in 100 g of water at 25°C. Water solubility decreases as the number of carbon atoms increases, whereas the reverse is true for ethanol, propylene glycol, and oil solubility. Some salt forms are available for food use to provide higher water solubility. The parabens commonly used in food are white, free-flowing powders with a faint odor or no odor. The methyl and propyl parabens are GRAS in the U.S., with a total addition limit of 0.1%.

Other parabens are approved for use in other countries. Paraben toxicity is reportedly low, with an acute toxicity dose (LD_{50}) from 180 to over 8000 mg/kg of body weight, varying with the form of administration (Matthews et al., 1956; Chichester and Tanner, 1972). The acceptable average daily intake is 10 mg/kg of body weight.

The parabens are more active against molds and yeasts than against bacteria (Ingram et al., 1964; Davidson, 1983). Generally, gram-positive bacteria are more susceptible than gram-negative bacteria to parabens. Davidson (1983) has tabulated available literature information on the concentrations of the various parabens required to inhibit numerous genera of microorganisms. Parabens are used in food to prevent or inhibit the growth of all three microbial types. Robach and Pierson (1978) reported that 200 to 1200 µg/g methyl or propyl paraben will delay or inhibit *Clostridium botulinum* growth and toxin production in laboratory media. Deibel (1979), however, reported that methyl or propyl paraben was ineffective against *Clostridium botulinum* in a wiener system. Pierson et al. (1980) showed that 300 µg/g propylparaben slowed growth of *Salmonella typhimurium*, whereas 500 µg/g resulted in a gradual decline of viable cell numbers of *Staphylococcus aureus*. Antimicrobial activity has been reported against numerous species including *Escherichia coli, Staphylococcus aureus, Bacillus subtilis, Salmonella* species, *Saccharomyces cerevisiae, Rhizopus nigrificans, Aspergillus niger*, and *Aerobacter*.

Data reported by Eklund (1980) show a close parallel of growth inhibition and nutrient transport inhibition in *Escherichia coli, Pseudomonas aeruginosa*, and *Bacillus subtilis* in the presence of parabens. The data imply that transport inhibition is the primary mode of action of parabens. For benzoate, nutrient uptake inhibition appeared to be only part of the antimicrobial action. Inhibition of respiration (Shiralkar and Rege, 1978) and of DNA, RNA and protein synthesis (Nes and Eklund, 1983) may contribute to the mechanism of action of parabens. Parker (1969) indicated that germination of bacterial spores was inhibited by parabens.

An advantage of parabens over benzoate and other preservatives is their high pK_a (8.5). Because of this, the undissociated acid molecule can be retained over a wider pH range, extending the spectrum of activity of foods with pH values ranging from 3 to 8. The antimicrobial activity of branched chain esters is low, and activity increases with increasing chain length (Huppert, 1957; Dymicky and Huhtanen, 1979) indicating that the esterification has an effect other than just raising the pK_a. Solubility limits the use of esters larger than three or four carbons. Methyl and propyl benzoates are often combined to get good solubility and antimicrobial action.

Parabens may be used to preserve baked goods (non–yeast-leavened), soft drinks, fruit products, jams, jellies, pickles, olives, syrups, creams, pastas, and various intermediate moisture foods (Neidig and Burrell, 1944; von Schelhorn, 1951; Chichester and Tanner, 1972;

Jermini and Schmidt-Lorenz, 1987). The *n*-heptyl ester can be used to control secondary yeast fermentation in beer at a level of 12 µg/g (Banwart, 1979; Chichester and Tanner, 1972). They also may be used in fruit-based beverages and noncarbonated soft drinks at 20 µg/g. Parabens have been proposed as antibotulinal agents and suggested as an alternative to nitrite in a U.S. patent (Sweet, 1975). Parabens may be added to a food as part of the dry or liquid ingredients. By dipping the casing of dry sausage in a 3.5% solution, they may be used as mold inhibitors. Both methyl and propyl paraben are permitted as antimycotic agents in food-packaging materials. Experimental uses of *p*-hydroxybenzoic acid esters have been reported in margarine, butter, soy sauce, and syrup (Frank and Willits, 1961).

Ascorbic Acid and Isoascorbic Acid

Ascorbic acid (vitamin C), $C_6H_8O_6$, is present in many foods, notably citrus fruits, and has a molecular weight of 176.14. Its pK_a values are 4.17 and 11.57. It is highly soluble in water and less soluble in organic solvents. Ascorbic acid is safe to use as a food additive. Isoascorbic (erythrobic) acid is chemically related to ascorbic acid and has similar physical properties.

Ascorbates affect the anticlostridial action of nitrite in canned meats. They increase the antibotulinal activity when a proper ascorbate concentration is present (Schack and Taylor, 1963; Tompkin et al., 1978a, b, c; 1979b) or decrease the activity when the concentration is excessive because they may cause more rapid depletion of nitrite (Tompkin et al., 1979b). Their main purposes in cured meats are to serve as reducing and chelating agents. Ascorbates chelate iron, which is important in the antibotulinal activity of nitrite (Tompkin et al., 1978a, b; 1979a). Ascorbate alone does not appear to have any antibotulinal effect. Ascorbic acid reportedly inhibits pseudomonads in liquid substrate, but no measurable effect occurs when it is sprayed on meat surfaces (Banwart, 1979). Presumably, the meat buffers the pH or oxidizes the ascorbate so that the effectiveness is lost.

Citric Acid

Citric acid [$COOHCH_2C(OH)(COOH)CH_2COOH$], the main acid in citrus fruits, is an acidifying agent with unique flavor characteristics. It is highly water-soluble and has pK_a values of 3.1, 4.8, and 6.4. It is nontoxic. The acceptable daily intake suggested by the FAO is not limited.

Citric acid generally is a less effective antimicrobial agent than other acids partly because many organisms metabolize citrate and also because of the low pK_a that defined the equilibrium between the uncharged and monovalent anionic states. It has been reported that 0.3% citric acid lowered the level of salmonella on poultry carcasses (Thompson et al., 1967) and was effective in reducing the total microbial load of fish (Debevere and Voets, 1972). Citric acid is widely used in the production of carbonated beverages. It is a GRAS substance for miscellaneous and general-purpose use in the U.S.

Sorbic Acid

Sorbic acid $(CH_3-CH=CH-CH=CH-COOH)$, 2,4-hexadienoic acid, is a *trans-trans* unsaturated fatty acid with a molecular weight of 112.13. It was first manufactured by A.W. Hofmann in 1859 from rowan berry oil. The antimicrobial action of sorbic acid was discovered independently by E. Muller in 1939 and by C.M. Gooding in 1940 (Lueck, 1980).

Sorbic acid has a pK_a of 4.76. The maximum pH for antimicrobial activity of sorbate is about 6.0 to 6.5, whereas for propionate and benzoate, it is 5.0 and 4.5, respectively. Sorbic acid is a white crystalline powder which is only slightly soluble in water (0.16 g dissolves in 100 ml water at 20°C) with a distinctive odor and sour taste. The acid is more soluble in lipid materials than in water. The sodium, potassium, and calcium salts of sorbic acid are frequently used because of their high water solubilities. For example, potassium sorbate, the most frequently used salt form, is a white, fluffy powder that is soluble at a level of 139 g/100 ml water at 20°C. When added to acidic foods, the salts equilibrate to the acid form. The esters of sorbic acid with low-molecular-weight, aliphatic alcohols are of no importance in food processing owing to their strong odor.

Sorbic acid is considered nontoxic and is metabolized by beta- and omega-oxidation, as are long-chain fatty acids (Deuel et al., 1954a, b). Thus, feeding studies have reported minor weight gains in animals fed diets containing sorbic acid compared to controls. The LD_{50} for sorbic acid is in the range of 7 to 11 g/kg of body weight and about 6 to 7 g/kg of body weight for the sodium salt (Lueck, 1980). Sorbic acid irritates the mucous membranes in highly sensitive individuals. Potassium and calcium sorbates have no mutagenic action, nor is the potassium salt teratogenic. Sorbic acid and potassium sorbate administered in feed have no carcinogenic action. The FAO acceptable daily intake of sorbic acid and its salts is 25 mg/kg of body weight, which is the highest acceptable daily intake of the common food preservatives. In foods, sorbic acid and its salts are relatively tasteless and odorless, and they are inexpensive. They were first recommended as food preservatives in 1945 by Gooding and are permitted in nearly all countries of the world for preservation of a wide variety of foods. In the U.S., sorbic acid and sorbates are considered GRAS. The maximum permissible level of sorbic acid is usually between 0.1 to 0.2%.

Components of the antimicrobial action of sorbic acid appear to be due to inhibition of enzymes and nutrient transport. Eklund (1980) reported evidence that inhibition of nutrient transport was responsible for part, but not all, of the antibacterial action of sorbate. Many enzymes reportedly are strongly or weakly inhibited by sorbate. These include enolase (Azukas, 1962), lactate dehydrogenase, malate dehydrogenase, isocitrate dehydrogenase, alpha-ketoglutarate dehydrogenase (Lueck, 1980), fumarase, and aspartase (York and Vaughn, 1964). Additionally, sorbic acid bonds covalently with sulfhydryl groups, thereby inactivating sulfhydryl enzymes, and it may interact with catalase and peroxidase (Lueck, 1980; Martoadiprawito and Whitaker, 1963).

Sorbic acid and its salts inhibit yeasts, molds, and some bacteria, primarily catalase-positive bacteria. Certain molds are more resistant or can metabolize sorbic acid (Melnick et al., 1954a, b; Troller, 1965). Sorbic acid or the potassium salt has been found to be effective against *Staphylococcus aureus* in bacon, *Vibrio parahemolyticus* in fish, yeasts, and molds in ham, *Salmonella* species in poultry, *Listeria monocytogenes* in laboratory media, *Bacillus* species in rice pastry filling, *Moraxella* and *Arthrobacter* spp. from seafood, *Pseudomonas* species (although resistant species from seafood have been identified by Chung and Lee, 1982), yeast in Mexican hot sauce, *Aspergillus parasiticus* and *Penicillium commune* on laboratory media, and molds and coliform bacteria in butter (Kaul et al., 1979; Raevuori, 1976; Robach, 1978, 1979a; Robach and Hickey, 1978; Robach and Ivey, 1978; Bullerman, 1979; Kemp et al., 1979; Pierson et al., 1979a; Flores et al., 1988; El-Shenawy and Marth, 1988a). Additionally, sorbate is reported to extend the shelf life of poultry parts and fish sausage (Amano et al., 1968; Wada et al., 1975; Cunningham, 1979; Chung and Lee, 1982).

Early reports indicated that sorbic acid was ineffective against clostridia and could be used to select for such organisms (Emard and Vaughn, 1952; York and Vaughn, 1954, 1955; Hansen and Appleman, 1955). In 1974, Tompkin and coworkers published evidence that potassium sorbate delayed toxin production by *Clostridium botulinum* in an uncured sausage product. This report stimulated additional research on sorbate as an antibotulinal agent owing to concern over the carcinogenic properties of products generated by the heating of nitrite and related compounds and the resultant interest in reducing or eliminating nitrite in cured meat products. Several studies on sorbate as an antibotulinal agent in meat products, either alone or in combination with low levels of nitrite (40 to 80 µg/g), have demonstrated its effectiveness (Ivey and Robach, 1978; Ivey et al., 1978; Sofos et al., 1979a–d, 1980a, b; Pierson et al., 1979b, c; Price and Stevenson, 1979) and suggest inhibition of spore germination (Sofos et al., 1979; Sofos and Busta, 1980, 1981), perhaps due to a competitive mechanism (Smoot and Pierson, 1981). Sorbate dissipated the proton motive force of the membrane and inhibited phenylalanine uptake, decreased the rate of protein synthesis, and altered patterns of phosphorylated nucleotide accumulation, resulting in increased cellular concentrations of GTP and ppGpp in Putrefactive Anaerobe 3679 (Ronning and Frank, 1987). The phosphorylated nucleotide concentrations were partially reestablished in the presence of noninhibitory amounts of tetracycline. Thus, Ronning and Frank (1987) concluded that inhibition of PA 3679 by sorbate was due to a stringent-type response induced by the protonophoric activity of sorbate.

A review on botulinal control in cured meats by nitrite and sorbate has been published by Sofos et al. (1979c) and by Sofos and Busta (1983). Meat casings for dry sausages may be dipped in sorbate to prevent growth of molds. Some reports have shown synergistic effects of sorbate with salt and sugar (Kaul et al., 1979; Gooding et al., 1955; Robach, 1979a; Robach and Stateler, 1980). Response by Putrefactive Anaerobe 3679 to combination of sorbate and curing ingredients were used to express caution in modification of curing processes (Ronning and Frank, 1988). Antimicrobial effects of sorbate derivatives such as sorbohydroxamic acid, sorbic aldehyde, and others have been reported (Dudman, 1963; Troller and Olsen, 1967).

Sorbates are used to inhibit yeasts in applications such as cucumber fermentation, in which growth of the catalase-negative lactic acid bacteria is desirable (Phillips and Mundt, 1950; Jones and Harper, 1952; Costilow et al., 1956, 1957). Sorbates are used for mold and yeast inhibition and general shelf-life extension in cheese products, baked goods, fruits, vegetables, wines, soft drinks, fruit juices, pickles, jams, jellies, syrups, sauerkraut, salads, margarine, meat, and fish products. Reports dealing with such applications have been published by Jones and Harper (1952), Melnick and Luckmann (1954), Smith and Rollin (1954), Boyd and Tarr (1955), Salunkhe (1955), Bonner and Harmon (1957), Costilow et al. (1957), Ferguson and Powrie (1957), Weaver at al. (1957), Auerbach (1959), Geminder (1959), Nury et al. (1960), Perry and Lawrence (1960), Pederson et al. (1961), Kaloyereas et al. (1961), Seiler (1964), Perry et al. (1964), Harris and Rosenfield (1965), and numerous other investigators. Because sorbate inhibits yeasts, it is not used in yeast-raised bread. Sorbate may be applied by dipping, spraying, dusting, or impregnating wrappers and packaging materials, or it may be added directly to the food.

Formic Acid

Formic acid (HCOOH) has a molecular weight of 46.03 and a pK_a of 3.75. It is a colorless, transparent liquid with a pungent odor and is miscible with water. The LD_{50} of formic acid is 1 to 2 g/kg of body weight (Lueck, 1980). In high concentrations it may irritate the skin and mucous membranes. The sodium and potassium salts are less acutely toxic. The daily intake of formic acid in the usual applied concentrations reportedly causes no damage (von Oettingen, 1959). Neither formic acid nor formates are carcinogenic or teratogenic, but formic acid is mutagenic to Drosophila (Tracor-Jitco, Inc., 1974). Formic acid is readily absorbed by the gut or through skin or mucous membranes. It is a normal constituent of human tissue and blood and is metabolically important in transfer of one-carbon substances. The FAO-suggested acceptable daily intake of formic acid is 3 mg/kg of body weight. Formic acid is permitted for food preservation in some countries, but not in the U.S. or the United Kingdom.

Some of the antimicrobial action of formic acid is as an acidulant. Additionally, formic acid inhibits decarboxylases and heme enzymes, especially catalase (Lueck, 1980), even at pH values at which it is essentially totally dissociated. Formic acid is most effective at pH values below about 3.5. Formic acid is active primarily against yeasts and some bacteria. Lactic acid bacteria and molds are relatively resistant. Organisms that produce formic acid as a byproduct of carbohydrate metabolism through the mixed acid pathways are more resistant.

Where permitted, formic acid or its salts are used primarily in fish preserves, pickles, and fruit juices. Formates are frequently used in conjunction with a second preservative, such as benzoic or sorbic acids.

Phosphoric Acid and Hydrochloric Acid

Phosphoric acid (H_3PO_4) and hydrochloric acid (HCl) are strong acids that rely on low pH, and hence high external hydrogen ion concentration, for antimicrobial action. Phosphoric acid is the acidulant in carbonated beverages. The necessary low pH required for effective antimicrobial activity is usually undesirable in food. These are the only two inorganic acids that are GRAS for use as food acidulants.

Malic Acid

Malic acid ($COOHCH_2CHOHCOOH$), hydroxysuccinic acid, is a natural component of and the predominant acid in apples, cherries, apricots, grapes, peaches, oranges, bananas, broccoli, carrots, peas, potatoes, and rhubarb. It also occurs in citrus fruits, figs, tomatoes, and beans (Gardner, 1972). Its pK_a values are 3.4 and 5.1. It is GRAS in the U.S. and is primarily used as an acidifying ingredient and preservative in mayonnaise and other salad dressings, sherbets, fruit preserves, jams, jellies, and beverages. Malic acid is a microbiostatic agent against certain bacteria and yeasts (Banwart, 1979).

Tartaric Acid

Tartaric acid [$COOH(CHOH)_2COOH$] is one of the primary acids in grapes and is produced from the waste products of the wine industry. Monopotassium tartrate (cream of tartar) is commonly used in baking. Tartaric acid is GRAS in the U.S. It is used in fruits, jams, jellies, preserves, sherbets, and beverages.

Adipic Acid

Adipic acid [$COOH(CH_2)_4COOH$] is a poorly soluble, nonhygroscopic acid. This feature makes it advantageous for use as an acidulant in dry, powdered food products.

Succinic Acid

Succinic acid ($COOHCH_2CH_2COOH$) and its anhydride are used as acidulants primarily in bakery products. Its pK_a values are 4.2 and 5.6. Succinic acid effectively inhibited or reduced the microbial load on poultry carcasses (Mountney and O'Malley, 1965; Cox et al., 1974). It is GRAS in the U.S.

Caprylic Acid

Caprylic acid [$CH_3(CH_2)_6COOH$], octanoic acid, is an eight-carbon fatty acid with a pK_a of 4.9. It primarily is used as a mold inhibitor in cheese or on the wax coating or other cheese-packaging material.

Glutaric Acid

Glutaric acid [$COOH(CH_2)_3COOH$] is a five-carbon dicarboxylic acid that is a natural component of many foods. Its pK_a values are 4.3 and 5.2. It has been suggested for use as a food acidulant with preservative activities (Merten and Bachman, 1976). Bruce (1935) reported that it was effective over a wider pH range than other acidulants, and was effective for *Salmonella* control.

Salicylic Acid

Salicylic acid, *o*-hydroxybenzoic acid, has a molecular weight of 138.12 and is a white crystal that dissolves at a level of 0.2 g/100 g of water at room temperature. Because of its toxicologic properties, salicylic acid has been virtually abandoned as a food preservative. It is not permitted for this use in the U.S. The minimum lethal dose in dogs is approximately 0.5 g/kg of body weight (Spector, 1956), and organ damage may result from ingestion of lesser amounts.

Salicylic acid reacts with proteins, damaging the plasma of microbial cells and probably interfering with activities of a variety of enzymes (Lueck, 1980). Salicylic acid interferes with pantothenic acid formation, which is necessary for many microorganisms (Wyss, 1948). Salicylic acid was highly effective as a preservative only in acidic foods because of its dissociation behavior (pK_a of 2.97).

Salicylic acid has been used to preserve unsalted liquid egg yolk, fish marinades, anchovies, gherkins, pickled olives, fruit preserves, jellies, and jams. It is still used in a few countries at a concentration of about 0.04 to 0.06% to preserve pickled olives.

Boric Acid

Boric acid (H_3BO_3) and borax ($Na_2B_4O_7 \cdot 10H_2O$) have molecular weights of 61.8 and 381.4, respectively. They are white powders or crystals that will dissolve at a level of 5 g/100 ml of water at room temperature. The pK_a of boric acid is 9.14; thus, it is present in foods almost entirely in the undissociated state even at a neutral pH. Boric acid is acutely toxic, having an LD_{50} of 1 to 5 g/kg of body weight (Smyth et al., 1969). Both boric acid and borax are absorbed rapidly and completely and excreted slowly by the body; hence, accumulation of boric acid in the body is likely if quantities are ingested over a long period. High doses of boric acid reduce the utilization of food by the body (Lueck, 1980). Because of their toxicity, boric acid and borax are permitted for food use in few countries, and are not permitted in the U.S.

Boric acid reportedly blocks enzymes in the metabolism of phosphate (Lueck, 1980). Boric acid is more active against yeasts than against molds or bacteria.

In some countries, boric acid is permitted in caviar at concentrations of 0.3 to 0.5%. Boric acid and borax have been used as preservatives for butter, margarine, rennet, egg yolk, meat, fish, and citrus fruits.

Dicarbonic Acid Esters

Dicarbonic acid esters, or pyrocarbonic acid esters, have the formula $R_1O\text{-}CO\text{-}O\text{-}CO\text{-}OR_2$. The most common forms are the diethyl and dimethyl esters. Dicarbonic acid diethyl ester is also known as diethyl pyrocarbonate (DEPC), and the dimethyl ester is known as dimethyl dicarbonic acid (DMDC). DMDC has a molecular weight of 134.1, is miscible with ethanol, and dissolves in water at a level of 3.65%. DEPC has a molecular weight of 162.1, is miscible with ethanol, and will dissolve in water only up to 0.6%. Both are colorless, transparent liquids with fruity odors. In aqueous solutions, the esters hydrolyze to methanol and ethanol, respectively, and CO_2. The hydrolysis is governed by temperature and pH, proceeding more rapidly in acidic than in neutral solutions. The methyl ester hydrolyzes faster than the ethyl ester (Ough, 1983). Both DEPC and DMDC irritate the skin and mucous membranes, and eye contact with these compounds should be avoided. Because these compounds hydrolyze readily in solution, their toxicity may be less important than the toxicity of their reaction products. DMDC is not permitted for use in foods in the U.S. but is allowed for food use in several other countries. DEPC has not been permitted for food use in any country since about 1973 because of questions and controversy about the carcinogenicity of products produced in the presence of ammonia (Ough, 1983).

The antimicrobial action of dicarbonic acid esters is due to their interaction with nucleophilic groups of enzymes within the microbial cell (Genth, 1964). Because they kill microorganisms faster than conventional preservatives, dicarbonic acid esters may be considered to be disinfectants rather than preservatives and have been termed cold-sterilization agents, sterilization auxiliaries, or chemical sterilants. The effectiveness of dicarbonic acid esters against yeasts, molds, and bacteria has been summarized by Ough (1983). Yeasts generally are more sensitive than molds or bacteria. The effect on microorganisms depends on both concentration and microbial population, and may be inhibitory or lethal. The antimicrobial activity is best at pH values less than 4.0 (Chichester and Tanner, 1972) and is enhanced at elevated temperatures.

Diethyl pyrocarbonate was permitted in many countries, including the U.S., for use in wines, noncarbonated soft drinks, fruit juices, fermented malt beverages, and beer. In the Federal Republic of Germany, the dimethyl ester had been used in soft drinks. To be effective, the microorganisms present must be killed before hydrolysis occurs, and the product must be protected from recontamination. Use of a second preservative with a more lasting effect in conjunction with DMDC may be desirable.

Monolaurin

Monolaurin, or lauricidin, refers to the monoglycerides of lauric acid, the most effective of which appear to be the lower-weight monoglycerides. Monolaurin is reported to have some antimicrobial activity against psychrotrophic bacteria, *Clostridium sporogenes* PA3679, *Cl. perfringens, Cl. botulinum, Staphylococcus aureus, Aspergillus* spp., and osmophilic yeasts (Robach et al., 1981; Katz and Branen, 1981; Smith and Palumbo, 1980; Kato, 1981; Notermans and Dufrenne, 1981; Chipley et al., 1981; Kabara, 1984). Monolaurin will enhance the effectiveness of heat inactivation for control of *Bacillus subtilis* and *B. stearothermophilus* spores (Kimsey et al., 1981). Use of monolaurin in meat and other foods is attractive because it also has emulsifying properties. Kabara (1983) has reviewed applications of monolaurin and proposed inclusion of this antimicrobial as part of a three-component antimicrobial system for broad-spectrum, effective antimicrobial activity in foods (Kabara, 1981). Monolaurin is GRAS for use as an emulsifier in the U.S.

Fumaric Acid Esters and Maleic Acid Esters

Fumaric acid (*trans*-butenedioic acid) esters, primarily monomethylfumarate (methylfumarate) and dimethylfumarate, have some antifungal activity and antibotulinal activity in laboratory media and meat systems (Huhtanen et al., 1981). The *n*-mono-alkyl maleates and fumarates esterified with C_{13} to C_{18} alcohols have antibotulinal activity in laboratory media (Dymicky et al., 1987).

GASES

Several gases are used in food processing as antimicrobial agents or for other purposes. These gases may have direct or indirect antimicrobial effects.

Sulfur Dioxide and Sulfites

Sulfur dioxide is a colorless, nonflammable, pungent-smelling gas with a molecular weight of 64.06. In water, 80 L/L dissolves at 0°C and 40 L/L dissolves at 20°C. Sulfur dioxide is produced by heating sulfitic ores, by burning elemental sulfur or by other methods. Sulfur dioxide is employed as a liquid under pressure or in aqueous solution. Additionally, various sulfite salts containing 50 to 68% active SO_2 may be used in food processing and are easier to handle than the gas or liquid forms of SO_2. The sulfites include sodium sulfite (Na_2SO_3), sodium hydrogen sulfite ($NaHSO_3$), sodium metabisulfite ($Na_2S_2O_5$), potassium metabisulfite ($K_2S_2O_5$), and calcium sulfite [$Ca(SO_3)_2$]. The sulfites are produced by feeding sulfur dioxide into the appropriate alkaline solution. SO_2 and the sulfite salts dissolve in water at low pH to yield sulfurous acid, bisulfite, and sulfite ions.

Sulfur dioxide and sulfites in the body are oxidized to sulfate and rapidly excreted in the urine. Thus, there is no accumulation in the body. Feeding studies have in-

dicated that acute, subchronic, and chronic toxicities of sulfur dioxide and sulfites take the form of vomiting, vitamin B_1 deficiency, diarrhea, organ damage, and decreased use of dietary protein and fat (Hoppe and Goble, 1951; Bhagat and Lockett, 1964; Til et al., 1972; Shtenberg and Ignat'ev, 1970). In humans, fatal poisoning is not possible, because of vomiting (Lueck, 1980). Sulfite is not indicated to be carcinogenic (Lockett and Natoff, 1960; Shtenberg and Ignat'ev, 1970), but sulfur dioxide shows mutagenic effects in bacterial studies (Mukai et al., 1970; Hayatsu and Miura, 1970). Some reports suggest sulfites may trigger asthmatic episodes in susceptible individuals. This has led to concern over the common use of sulfites, especially in foods that do not typically carry ingredient labels (such as restaurant salads). Other acute responses in a small number of susceptible individuals have been reported. Walker (1985) has reviewed the current toxicologic status of sulfites and addressed risks and benefits of their use in foods.

Levels of application of sulfites are inherently restricted owing to flavor problems at concentrations above 500 μg/g (Chichester and Tanner, 1972). The FAO acceptable daily intake of sulfur dioxide and sulfites is 0.7 mg/kg of body weight per day, which is well below levels believed to cause mutagenic effects. Sulfur dioxide and the sulfites are not recommended or are not permitted for use in foods considered to be thiamine (vitamin B_1) sources, because they destroy this nutrient. In fact, many of the reported toxicity problems are symptoms of vitamin B_1 deficiency.

Because SO_2 is highly reactive, it may interact with many cell components; consequently, the precise cause of microbial inhibition or death may not always be known. Cell damage may result from interaction with thiol groups in structural proteins, enzymes, cofactors, vitamins, nucleotides and nucleic acids, and lipids (Clark and Takács, 1980). NAD-dependent enzyme reactions are sensitive. For example, blockage of the conversion of glyceraldehyde-3-phosphate to 1,3-diphosphoglycerate in yeasts and malate to oxaloacetate in *Escherichia coli* are the salient inhibitory features (Lueck, 1980).

Sulfur dioxide cleaves disulfide bonds in proteins, which may change the molecular conformation of enzymes, thus modifying the active site. The activity of thiamine is destroyed owing to cleavage; hence thiamine-dependent enzyme activity is lost. Lipid peroxidation due to SO_2 may interfere with membrane functioning, and evidence exists that the bisulfite ion may interact with pyrimidine bases. Furthermore, sulfur dioxide inhibits enzymes by binding enzyme intermediates or end-products, thus upsetting the reaction equilibrium. Microbial death or inhibition may be the result of a combination of these factors (Hammond and Carr, 1976).

The antimicrobial action of sulfite is pH-dependent. In water, SO_2 forms sulfurous acid (H_2SO_3), which has pK_a values of 1.8 and 7.2. The lower the pH, the higher the proportion of SO_2 or H_2SO_3. Molecular SO_2 or undissociated H_2SO_3 are more inhibitory than sulfite ions, so that the antimicrobial effect is greatest at pH values below 4 (Wyss, 1948). The undissociated acid (H_2SO_3) is approximately 100 times more effective than HSO_3^- or SO_3^{--} against mold (*Aspergillus niger*), 100 to 500 times more effective against yeast (*Saccharomyces cerevisiae*), and approximately 1000 times more effective against *Escherichia coli* (Cruess and Irish, 1932; Joslyn and Braverman, 1954; Ingram et al., 1956). Sulfur dioxide is active against only certain species of bacteria, yeasts, and molds. The sensitivity apparently depends primarily on the species and not the microbial type (Carr et al., 1976; Hammond and Carr, 1976; Clark and Takács, 1980). Duration of contact, pH, SO_2 concentration, and SO_2 binding influence the preservative action of SO_2.

Sulfur dioxide has been used for many centuries, especially as a wine preservative (Amerine and Joslyn, 1951; Joslyn and Braverman, 1954) where it is regulated by the Bureau of Alcohol, Tobacco, and Firearms of the Department of the Treasury in the U.S. It is added to the expressed juice (must) of grapes to control the natural but undesirable mold, bacteria, and yeast flora before the desirable fermentative yeast is added (Amerine and Joslyn, 1940, 1951; Joslyn and Braverman, 1954). In wine, sulfite is also important as an equipment sanitizer, a disinfectant for corks, barrels, and bottles, an antioxidant, and a clarifier, and is used to prevent undesirable changes and bacterial spoilage during storage. Currently, sulfur dioxide and the bisulfite salts are permitted in most countries for use in a wide variety of foods, except those that are major dietary sources of thiamine. These include fruit juices, soft fruits, dehydrated fruits and vegetables, acid pickles, syrups, and meat and fish products in some countries. Growth of *Botrytis, Cladosporium*, and other molds is controlled in soft fruits (cherries, gooseberries, grapes, raspberries, and strawberries), enabling production of jam over a longer period than would otherwise be possible (Roberts and McWeeny, 1972). For fruit juices and syrups, the compound is added to prevent fermentation during processing and storage. Sulfites are not permitted in fresh or processed meats in the U.S., because these foods are sources of thiamine, and sulfite may restore the color of old meat, which may mislead consumers. However, sulfites have been shown to delay outgrowth of *Clostridium botulinum* in meat (Tompkin et al., 1980). Sulfites have been used as sausage preservatives in the United Kingdom and as fish and shrimp preservatives in France. In sausage, sulfites delay growth of yeasts, molds, and gram-negative mesophilic bacteria. Sulfite favors the development of acid-producing bacteria, including *Lactobacillus* species and *Microbacterium thermosphactum*, especially during refrigerated storage (Dyett and Shelly, 1966). Proteolytic breakdown of meat may also be prevented by sulfites (Block and Bevis, 1963; Block and Taylor, 1964; Pearson, 1970). In addition to its antimicrobial effects, sulfur dioxide is added to foods to prevent enzymatic reactions, notably browning, to prevent nonenzymatic browning, and for its antioxidant and reducing properties. There is a trend toward decreased use of sulfur dioxide and sulfites in food, and increased labeling requirements, because of individual sensitivities and allergies to the compounds. The Institute of Food Technologists (1986) has prepared a concise summary of applications and regulations of sulfites in food as well as reported health problems from ingestion of sulfite.

Carbon Dioxide

Carbon dioxide (CO_2) has a molecular weight of 44.21. It is a noncombustible, colorless gas with an acidic odor and flavor. At room temperature, the water solubility of CO_2 is 1 L/L. CO_2 dissolved in water or the liquid phase of foods forms carbonic acid. CO_2 is generally used in the form of a liquefied gas. Solid CO_2 (dry ice) is used as a refrigerant. In the presence of 20% (by volume) O_2, 30 to 60% (by volume) CO_2 will rapidly produce death in animals (Lueck, 1980). Lesser concentrations inhaled over a long period may be dangerous. CO_2 is subject to almost no food law regulations.

The antimicrobial action of CO_2 is based on several factors. CO_2 displaces oxygen, a vital requirement for aerobic organisms. Thus, it intervenes in the respiratory metabolism of various microorganisms. If applied in high concentrations, CO_2 may lower the pH by forming carbonic acid (Koser and Skinner, 1922; Hays et al., 1959). CO_2 generally inhibits the growth of microorganisms rather than inactivating them. Its activity depends on concentration, the microorganisms under consideration and their stage of growth, the A_w of the system, and the storage temperature. Depending upon these factors, CO_2 may have a stimulative effect (Foegeding and Busta, 1983c), no effect, or an inhibitory effect, or it may inactivate the microorganisms (King and Nagel, 1967; Parekh and Solberg, 1970). The inhibitory effect of CO_2 is manifested by an increased lag phase and an increased generation time for both bacteria and fungi (Brown, 1922; Tomkins, 1932; Ogilvy and Ayres, 1951). The growth rate under CO_2 does not change with time, indicating that the metabolic systems of the organisms do not adapt during growth under CO_2, nor is there selection for more CO_2-resistant organisms (King and Nagel, 1967; Clark and Takács, 1980). The antimicrobial action of CO_2 in carbonated beverages increases with CO_2 pressure and decreases with sugar content (Insalata, 1952). Lowering the water activity increases the inhibitory effect of CO_2 (Scott, 1957).

Carbon dioxide acts mainly against obligate aerobic microorganisms, although some molds may be highly resistant (Tomkins, 1932). When the CO_2 content is 10 to 90% of the atmosphere, aflatoxin-forming molds produce less toxin with increasing CO_2 (Sanders et al., 1968; Shih and Marth, 1973). Yeasts are only slightly CO_2-sensitive. The antibacterial action of CO_2 is varied. *Pseudomonas*, "*Achromobacter*" (current taxonomic position is unknown according to *Bergy's Manual of Systematic Bacteriology*, Krieg and Holt, 1984), and *Escherichia coli* strains are particularly sensitive, whereas lactic acid bacteria and clostridia are fairly CO_2-resistant (King and

Nagel, 1975; Parekh and Solberg, 1970; Gill and Tan, 1979). Concentrations of 100% CO_2 are reported to have killed species of *Bacillus*, *Flavobacterium*, and *Micrococcus*, whereas species of *Proteus*, *Lactobacillus*, and *Clostridium perfringens* were only inhibited (Ogilvy and Ayres, 1951, 1953; Parekh and Solberg, 1970). CO_2 will enhance germination of *Clostridium botulium* spores (Foegeding and Busta, 1983c). Generally, CO_2 concentrations of 5 to 50% inhibit sensitive yeasts, molds, and bacteria (Hales, 1962; Smith, 1963).

Carbon dioxide is used to control psychrotrophic spoilage of meat and meat products, poultry, fish, eggs, fruits, and vegetables by addition of dry ice during storage and transportation of these products or by addition of CO_2 gas. The dry ice sublimes to form gaseous CO_2. Also, CO_2 gas is added directly to some beverages. Atmospheres high in CO_2 may be established passively by selection of oxygen-impermeable packages for use with fresh (respiring) fruits and vegetables. CO_2 is used in vacuum-packaged meats, in which it inhibits aerobic spoilage organisms while encouraging growth of lactobacilli. For vacuum-packaged meats, 10 to 20% CO_2 is common; higher concentrations may cause undesirable odors with only a slight increase in antimicrobial activity (Clark and Lentz, 1969; Silliker et al., 1977). In controlled-atmosphere storage of fruits and vegetables, respiration and ripening, as well as spoilage, are delayed if appropriate combinations of O_2 and CO_2 are used (von Schelhorn, 1951; Smith, 1963). CO_2 is used primarily in carbonated soft drinks, mineral waters, wines, beers, and ales, in which it functions as an antimicrobial and effervescing agent. Additionally, exclusion of oxygen prevents oxidative deterioration of beer and ale. CO_2 has been shown to increase the shelf-life of milk.

Nitrogen

Nitrogen (N_2) is a colorless and odorless gas with a molecular weight of 14.01. Nitrogen is practically insoluble in water. Because of its inert nature, nitrogen is not toxic, apart from the fact that it must not be inhaled in high concentrations, because it would displace oxygen. Nitrogen, the main component of air, is not subject to any food law regulations.

The antimicrobial action of nitrogen is based on its displacement of oxygen, which is essential to obligate aerobes. Liquid nitrogen indirectly inhibits or kills microorganisms by freezing or chilling the food. Nitrogen itself is reported to have no direct antimicrobial action (Huffman, 1974; Parekh and Solberg, 1970; Shih and Marth, 1973). Nitrogen is used as a protective gas in food packaging, and liquid nitrogen is used as a cryogenic agent.

Ozone

Ozone (O_3) is an unstable blue gas with a pleasant odor at concentrations below 2 ppm. Ozone is water-soluble and has a molecular weight of 48.00. Because of irritation to the mucous membranes, eyes, nose, and throat, a concentration of 0.1 μg/g is objectionable to all humans,

and 0.04 μg/g is the upper limit tolerable by humans. Ozone in solution will explode if warm. Ozone is produced by passing air between plate electrodes, causing an electric arc through air, and by UV light in wavelengths of 175 to 210 nm (Nagy, 1959). Because it decomposes rapidly in air and water to form O_2, it is usually generated at the point of use.

The antimicrobial action of ozone is due to its strong oxidizing effect. Because of its oxidizing ability, it is postulated that the main antimicrobial effect is due to oxidation of sulfhydryl groups in enzymes and oxidation of unsaturated cell-wall lipids, causing loss of enzyme activities and leakage of cellular components, respectively (Ingram and Haines, 1949; Scott and Lesher, 1963; Ingram and Barnes, 1954). Susceptibility to the antimicrobial activity of ozone is influenced by the stage of microbial growth, pH, temperature, relative humidity, and the amount of organic matter present. Resting cells are more sensitive than rapidly growing cells (Kefford, 1948; Ingram and Barnes, 1954). Acidity and decreased temperature appear to increase the biocidal effect. Increases in relative humidity from 45% to 60% or 80% increase the biocidal effect. The presence of organic matter decreases the biocidal effect (Clark and Takács, 1980).

Bacteria are more ozone-sensitive than are yeasts and molds, and bacterial spores are 10 to 15 times more resistant than vegetative bacterial cells (Ingram and Barnes, 1954; Broadwater et al., 1973; Foegeding, 1985). Gram-positive bacteria are more sensitive than gram-negative bacteria.

Ozone has been used mainly for water sterilization and to remove metals, off-odors, flavors, and colors from water in many countries. It is used as a maturing agent in ciders and wines and to sterilize beverage bottles (Torricelli, 1959). It can be used to preserve eggs, to retard the growth of spoilage organisms on surfaces of stored foods, and to detoxify mycotoxins. Because ozone is produced by UV treatment, it is considered to cause part of the germicidal effect of UV light.

Epoxides

Epoxides (ethylene oxide C_2H_4O, and propylene oxide C_3H_6O) are cyclic ethers. The molecular weights are 44.0 and 58.0 for ethylene oxide and propylene oxide, respectively. Both are highly reactive gases with slightly sweet odors. The condensed gases are highly miscible with water. Concentrations of ethylene oxide from 0.1 to 0.2 g per liter of air will be fatal to humans in a few seconds (Lueck, 1980). Concentrations above 100 μg/g cause lung and eye irritations and may result in nausea and mental disorientation. Propylene oxide is less biologically active than is ethylene oxide. Its toxicity was reported to be one-third that of ethylene oxide (Bruch, 1961).

The breakdown products of ethylene oxide include ethylene glycol and chlorohydrin (Bruch, 1972); propylene oxide yields propylene glycol on breakdown. Epoxides may be used to fumigate certain foods contained in closed chambers, and are removed from food by evacuation of the chamber accompanied by gentle heating. The remaining glycols are considered nontoxic, although chlorohydrin and the epoxides themselves are toxic. Low concentrations (3%) of ethylene oxide, and to a lesser extent, of propylene oxide, are explosive in air.

To facilitate handling, nonflammable mixtures of 10 to 20% ethylene oxide with 80 to 90% carbon dioxide, and similar mixtures of propylene oxide, are recommended for use. Also, mixtures of ethylene oxide and fluorinated hydrocarbons or methyl formate have found commercial application. Ethylene oxide does not lose its antimicrobial activity in such mixtures (Mayr and Suhr, 1972). Questions about the safety of ethylene chlorohydrin have limited the use of epoxides to spices in recent years. The U.S. has a gas residue regulatory limit in spices of 50 μg/g, and other countries have similar requirements. Besides potential toxicity, use of ethylene oxide in food is restricted because it affects adversely the stability of several vitamins and important amino acids (Windmueller et al., 1959). In many countries, propylene oxide is not permitted for use in foods, whereas in other countries, it often has replaced the more widely used and biologically active ethylene oxide.

Ethylene and propylene oxides have an alkylating effect on proteins, nucleic acids, and other organic compounds, which is believed to be related to the sterilizing effect (Winarno and Stumbo, 1971). Additionally, the epoxides are particularly reactive with sulfhydryl and other enzyme reactive groups (Phillips, 1952). The antimicrobial action is a function of time, concentration, temperature, relative humidity, and penetration of the gas through the treated material (Skinner and Hugo, 1976).

Microbial inactivation by epoxides follows first-order kinetics. Propylene oxide is less reactive and less penetrating than ethylene oxide. For similar sterilization effects, the required concentrations of propylene oxide (800 to 2000 mg/L) are two or more times the required concentrations of ethylene oxide (Bruch, 1961). The epoxides possess germicidal properties in both aqueous and gaseous phases (Marletta and Stumbo, 1970). Molds and yeasts are the least resistant to ethylene oxide, with nonspore-forming bacteria and vegetative cells approximately twice as resistant as yeasts and molds, and bacterial spores approximately 10 times as resistant as vegetative cells (Toth, 1959; Phillips and Kaye, 1949). Frequently, *Bacillus subtilis* var. *niger* is used to monitor the effectiveness of ethylene oxide sterilization.

Ethylene oxide gas has been used to decontaminate dried food products such as dried fruits, corn starch, potato and other flours, corn, wheat, barley, dried egg, gelatin, gums, and cereals (Whelton et al., 1946; Pappas and Hall, 1952; Bruch and Koesterer, 1961; Mayr and Kaemmerer, 1959). In this capacity, it reduces microbial contamination in addition to killing insects. Currently, in the U.S., use of ethylene oxide is permitted only for whole or ground spices, except in mixtures containing salt. The residue of the gas must not exceed 50 μg/g. In the U.S., propylene oxide may be used to control microorganisms and insects in dried products when these foods are to be processed further, such as cocoa, spices, starch, nuts, and gums. For this use, a residue of 300 μg/g has been set. Both epoxides have been used for equipment sterilization.

Chlorine

Chlorine has most commonly been used in the forms of Cl_2 (a green gas), sodium hypochlorite (NaOCl), calcium hypochlorite [$Ca(OCl)_2$], and chlorine dioxide gas (ClO_2), with molecular weights of 70.91, 74.44, 142.99, and 67.45, respectively. Elemental chlorine is highly corrosive. It causes a severe inflammatory reaction on the skin and mucous membranes. The inhalation of air containing 20 ppm chlorine for 15 minutes may be fatal (Lueck, 1980).

If present in adequate concentrations, chlorine rapidly inactivates microorganisms. The antimicrobial action is based on its strong oxidizing effect and involves penetration of the cell wall. There have been suggestions that the chlorine reacts with cellular protoplasm, enzyme systems, and cell membranes, causing oxidation or denaturation of proteins, inactivation of enzymes, inhibition of respiration, or altered membrane permeability. NaOCl may be capable of reacting with the DNA of cells, causing oxidation of purine and pyrimidine moieties (Rosenkranz, 1973; Wlodkowski and Rosenkranz, 1975). Wyatt and Waites (1975) and Foegeding and Busta (1983a, b) reported that chlorine disrupts the coat of *Bacillus* and *Clostridium* spores, resulting in damage to the germination mechanism, prevention of outgrowth of germinated spores, and leakage of spore contents. Spore heat resistance is reduced by chlorine treatment (Kulikovsky et al., 1975). Bacterial spore resistance to chlorine compounds has been reviewed by Foegeding (1983).

Chlorine is highly reactive; hence, the antimicrobial action of chlorine is severely reduced in the presence of organic matter. Chlorine acts best in the neutral to weakly acidic pH range, where the most biocidal (HOCl) form is present in the greatest amount. However, Foegeding et al. (1986) reported that pH had little effect on inactivation of *Bacillus* spores by ClO_2, whereas ClO_2 at pH 8.5 was more effective than at 4.5 or 6.5 for inactivation of *Clostridium perfringens* spores. Heat intensifies the antimicrobial action of chlorine. Chlorine is active against bacteria, including bacterial spores, yeast, molds, viruses, algae, and protozoa. Specific information on inactivation of *Listeria monocytogenes* by chlorine has been reported by El-Kest and Marth (1988a–c).

The most important use of chlorine is in the disinfection of drinking water, in which the concentration of active chlorine is usually not greater than 0.3 mg/L. Chlorine is also used to sanitize containers and equipment used in food processing. Typically, concentrations of 200 mg/L are used for this application.

NITRATE AND NITRITE

Nitrate (saltpeter, niter, nitre) and nitrite are typically used as the potassium or sodium salts and have the formulas NO_3^- and NO_2^-, respectively. Nitrate and nitrite are used either pure or in mixtures with common salt and other substances as a curing salt. Sodium nitrite has a formula weight of 69.00 and is a white to pale-yellow crystal that is readily soluble in water. Sodium nitrate has a formula weight of 84.99 and is also a white, highly water-soluble crystal. Both salts are produced by passing the nitrous gases from the combustion of ammonia through a caustic soda solution.

The lethal dose of nitrate for humans is 300 to 350 mg/kg of body weight. Smaller doses cause intestinal irritation and diarrhea. Nitrite, also, is highly toxic to humans; the lethal dose of nitrite for humans is approximately 300 mg/kg body weight. Long-term feeding studies with nitrite resulted in reduced hemoglobin and increased methemoglobin contents of the blood. Methemoglobinemia may result, leading to death due to oxygen shortage. Because of the nature of long-term feeding studies, nitrite had not been considered carcinogenic until the late 1970s. In 1979, Newberne presented evidence implicating nitrite as a carcinogen to laboratory animals, stimulating a flurry of research directed at identifying alternatives to nitrite for food preservation, particularly meat curing. Neither nitrate nor nitrite have teratogenic action. The FAO-acceptable daily intake is 0 to 5 mg/kg for nitrate and is temporarily 0 to 0.2 mg/kg for nitrite. Nitroso compounds (nitrosamines and nitrosamides), which may be formed in foods containing nitrite, are carcinogens.

The precise mechanism of antimicrobial action of nitrate and nitrite is not fully understood at this time. Nitrate does not appear to have a direct effect, but functions as a source of nitrite, and the action of nitrite is based mainly on the release of nitrous acid and oxides of nitrogen. An interesting chronological review of the research that has contributed to our understanding of the mechanism and antimicrobial activity of nitrate has been presented by Tompkin (1983).

Nitrite inhibited active transport of proline in *Escherichia coli*, aldolase from *E. coli* and *Streptococcus faecalis*, and active transport, oxidative phosphorylation, and oxygen uptake in *Pseudomonas aeruginosa* (Yarbrough et al., 1980). Nitrite may interfere with microbial metabolism by interaction with heme proteins such as cytochromes and sulfhydryl enzymes (Castellani and Niven, 1955). Spore outgrowth, but not germination, is inhibited by nitrite (Gould, 1964; Duncan and Foster, 1968; Pivnick et al., 1970). Germinated spores may grow or die slowly depending on the nitrite concentration (Christiansen et al., 1978; Tompkin et al., 1978c). Tompkin and coworkers (1978a, b; 1979a) propose that a reaction between nitric oxide formed from nitrite and an essential iron compound, for example the iron of a cidophore involved in electron transport in clostridia, may account for the anticlostridial action. They suggested the

nitric oxide-iron reaction product is reversible but stable as long as a reserve of nitrite is present. Kim et al. (1987) suggested that the reduction in botulinal inhibition when ionic iron was added to cured meat systems may be due to the formation of iron -NO- protein complexes, which deplete the amount of NO available to inhibit spore outgrowth. Inactivation is a function of nitrite concentration and pH, with pH levels of 4 to 5.5 being the most favorable (Tarr, 1942; Shank et al., 1962).

Perigo factor is a name given to antibacterial products putatively formed when nitrite is heated with laboratory media or meat systems (Pivnick and Chang, 1973; Lee et al., 1978). The Perigo factor in meat has only minor antibacterial activity, and its antimicrobial mechanism, as well as its actual existence, is not known and is difficult to study because of, among other reasons, its instability.

The action of nitrite is almost exclusively antibacterial. It is used in muscle foods primarily for its effect against *Clostridium botulinum*, which produces lethal neurotoxins. In general, concentrations of more than 100 μg/g in food are necessary for botulism control. The importance of nitrite to the botulinal safety of cured meat products has been reviewed by Busta and Sofos (1979), Sofos et al. (1979c), and Tompkin (1983). Presence of nitrite in a meat system does not inhibit *C. botulinum* outgrowth indefinitely. Protection against *C. botulinum* is the result of interactions of nitrite with salt, reduced A_w, sufficiently low pH, storage temperature, heating, and low microbial load of the food (Lee et al., 1978; Lechowich et al., 1978; Silliker, 1959; Roberts, 1975; Sofos et al., 1979c; Tompkin, 1983).

The antimicrobial effects of nitrite against several genera, including *Achromobacter*, *Aerobacter*, *Escherichia*, *Flavobacterium*, *Micrococcus*, and *Pseudomonas*, were observed early in its regular use (Tarr, 1941a, b, 1942). Nitrite does not have the same effect against all microorganisms. Some bacteria (bacilli, lactobacilli, salmonellae, *Clostridium perfringens*) are more resistant to nitrite than *C. botulinum* (Castellani and Niven, 1955; Grever, 1974). Slight inhibitory effects of high concentrations of nitrite have been demonstrated against *Staphylococcus aureus*, *Clostridium perfringens*, salmonellae, and total spoilage flora of meat products (Gough and Alford, 1965; Buchanan and Solberg, 1972; Bayne and Michener, 1975; Riha and Solberg, 1975a, b; Sauter et al., 1977). Nitrite effects are generally greater under vacuum packaging than under aerobic conditions (Barber and Deibel, 1972; Herring, 1973; Labots, 1977).

Sodium and potassium nitrate are permitted in many European countries, and in Canada and the U.S. as additives to certain meat, fish, and cheese products. In cheese, the objective is to prevent late blowing due to gas formation by *Clostridium butyricum* and *tyrobutyricum*. Sodium and sometimes potassium nitrite are permitted in nearly all countries as additives to fish and meat products. Because of nitrite's toxicity, some countries require use of a nitrite plus common salt mixture rather than nitrite alone, to prevent misuse.

Nitrite and nitrate salts have been used in meat processing for centuries as impurities of the salt were used to preserve meats during ancient times; their initial use was accidental (Binkerd and Kolari, 1975; Sofos et al., 1979c). The salts from desert and coastal areas contained saltpeter or nitre [$Ca(NO_3)_2$], a product of nitrifying bacteria. Observations that use of these salts resulted in a uniform, desirable, red meat color led to regular use of nitrate in cured meat. During the nineteenth century, nitrite, and not nitrate, was shown to be responsible for cured meat color formation through reaction with hemoglobin and myoglobin. In the beginning of the twentieth century, the use of nitrite in meat curing was officially permitted in the U.S. and other countries, and its functions were defined.

Nitrite added to meat results in both chemical and antimicrobial effects. It reacts with heme proteins to form the characteristic cured meat color, has a mild antioxidant effect that prevents rancidity and "warmed over" flavor in such products, and has an antimicrobial effect, especially against *Clostridium botulinum*. Experience and research have demonstrated these properties, and regulatory agencies have approved the use of nitrite and nitrate salts in meat-curing mixtures. During the twentieth century, nitrite and nitrate salts (primarily sodium and potassium) have been used regularly in many countries for meat processing. The good botulinal safety record of commercially processed, cured meat products is believed to be directly related to nitrite addition (Silliker et al., 1958; Ingram, 1974; Roberts, 1975; Busta and Sofos, 1979; Sofos et al., 1979c), although other processing and handling factors, including many of those mentioned previously, are important.

When nitrite is added to meat, it is involved in a variety of chemical reactions (Cassens et al., 1979), the rates of which are affected by product pH, temperature, composition, microbial contamination, and other factors. These reactions result in depletion of the added nitrite. As the pH declines, nitrite is depleted by increased formation of nitrous acid and nitric oxides, the reactive forms of nitrite. Because of this, addition of acidulants or inoculation with acid-forming bacteria will have a beneficial effect on the action of nitrite. For positive chemical effects (color, flavor), nitrite concentrations of 15 to 50 µg/g are needed, whereas antibotulinal activity requires concentrations of 100 µg/g or more. Research has indicated that lower nitrite concentrations (40 to 80 µg/g) in combination with sorbate may be sufficient for antimicrobial activity (Ivey and Robach, 1978; Ivey et al., 1978; Pierson et al., 1979b, c; Price and Stevenson, 1979; Sofos et al., 1979a–d, 1980a, b; Sofos and Busta, 1983). In the U.S. the content of sodium nitrite in cured meat products is limited to 200 µg/g, with the specific regulatory level varying with the particular product. In the United Kingdom, potassium and sodium nitrite are permitted in cured meat up to a maximum of 200 µg/g.

During the last decade, reports have demonstrated the occurrence of carcinogenic *N*-nitroso compounds (ni-

trosamines) in cured meat products (e.g., bacon) when cooked under certain conditions (e.g., temperatures over 171°C). A large number of nitrosamines (over 65) have been reported to be carcinogenic (Magee and Barnes, 1967). Reviews on nitrosamine formation and their importance and occurrence in meat products as well as in other foods are given by Sebranek and Cassens (1973), Crosby and Sawyer (1976), and Gray and Randall (1979). Nitrosamine incidence and level of occurrence in bacon products have decreased recently through research and product control. In the U.S., a maximum level of acceptance (16 µg/kg) has been set, monitored by strict regulations.

The effects on human health of amounts of nitrosamines that may occur in foods because of addition of nitrite, and their importance relative to higher concentrations of nitrate, nitrite, and nitrosamines from other food sources (e.g., vegetables), are unknown. The importance of nitrite in the control of botulism, as well as the extremely deleterious effects of botulinal toxins, have caused regulatory authorities to act cautiously on the subject. No major changes in nitrite regulations have been imposed. A compromise solution balancing botulism and nitrosamine risks and benefits has been sought. Such a compromise might be a reduction of ingoing nitrite levels coupled with simultaneous inclusion of other preservatives (e.g., sorbate), an increase in levels of existing product components (e.g., salt), addition of lactic-acid–producing bacteria, or irradiation. The Institute of Food Technologists (1987) has summarized the application and potential hazards and regulatory considerations of nitrate, nitrite, and nitroso compounds in foods.

ETHYL ALCOHOL

Ethyl alcohol, or ethanol (CH_3CH_2OH), is a colorless liquid with a molecular weight of 46.07. Ethyl alcohol used for food is obtained exclusively from the fermentation of sugar-containing liquids. It is highly miscible in water. The LD_{50} of ethanol after peroral administration is 5.5 to 13.7 g for the mouse, rat, rabbit, and dog (Spector, 1956). For humans, consumption of 200 to 400 ml of pure alcohol in a brief period is hazardous, whereas consumption of 40 to 80 g daily over the long term may be considered tolerable. Addition of alcohol to foods for the purpose of preservation is not subject to many food law controls because alcohol is an essential constituent of several foods. The exception to this is alcoholic drinks, which in many countries may not have the alcohol content increased by addition of extraneous alcohol.

The antimicrobial action of ethanol is due to nonspecific denaturation of the proteins of the protoplast. Ethanol concentrations of 60 to 80% are the most effective. Lower concentrations of ethanol (5 to 20%) have some preservative action due to lowered water activity of the food. In an intermediate moisture food system in which humectants were used to lower the water activity, 2 to 4% added ethanol had a preservative effect (Shapero et al., 1978). Because ethanol denatures proteins nonspecifically, alcohol is effective against all kinds of microorganisms, although bacterial spores are not affected or are affected much less than vegetative cells.

Alcohol is either added or naturally present in fruit products, alcoholic drinks such as liquors, wines, and beers, flavor extracts, and some intermediate-moisture foods.

HYDROGEN PEROXIDE

Hydrogen peroxide (H_2O_2) is a colorless, water-miscible liquid with a molecular weight of 34.01. It is obtained by the hydrolysis of other peroxides such as peroxidisulfuric acid. Hydrogen peroxide in concentrations of 30% and greater is caustic. Because it rapidly decomposes to oxygen and water in the presence of organic material and metal ions, it is not a toxicologic hazard. Hydrogen peroxide is approved for food use in many countries.

Hydrogen peroxide rapidly inactivates microorganisms, provided an adequate concentration is employed. The effectiveness is affected by concentration, bacterial population, temperature, pH, and time of contact (Smith and Brown, 1980). It does not have a long-lasting effect because it decomposes relatively rapidly. Hydrogen peroxide is a strong oxidizing agent, which accounts for its antimicrobial activity. Hydrogen peroxide is active against all types of microorganisms, but yeasts and molds are more resistant than bacteria. Aerobic spore-formers and gram-negative bacteria are more resistant than clostridia or *Staphylococcus aureus* (Toledo et al., 1973; Walker and Harmon, 1965).

Hydrogen peroxide has been approved for use in the U.S. as an antimicrobial agent in raw milk to be used to make certain types of cheese. This milk may be treated with no more than 0.05% H_2O_2. H_2O_2 may be added to liquid egg white as an aid in pasteurization. When treated with H_2O_2, milk and liquid egg can be pasteurized at a lower temperature than normally used. The excess H_2O_2 is destroyed by heat or by the addition of catalase, which enzymatically converts H_2O_2 to O_2 and H_2O. Addition of H_2O_2 to fish marinades suppresses bacterial spoilage. H_2O_2 may be used to treat packages used for aseptic processing of foods. Hydrogen peroxide treatment of food may result in undesirable, oxidized flavors, cause bleaching of color, or destroy nutrients such as vitamin C.

PHOSPHATES

Phosphates, such as sodium hexametaphosphate [$(NaPO_3)_6$], sodium tripolyphosphate ($Na_5P_3O_{10}$), and others are a group of closely related salts that are used in food processing for a number of reasons. The phosphates are highly soluble in water and relatively inexpensive. They have low toxicity or none at all, and most are GRAS in the U.S.

The antimicrobial action of phosphates has been known since 1864 (Morgan, 1864). The action is due to chelation of bivalent metal ions, particularly iron, calcium, and magnesium, which are essential to the microbial cell. This interferes with cell metabolism, and cell wall stability (Post et al., 1963). The antimicrobial effect is against bacteria, including *Staphylococcus aureus, Streptococcus faecalis, Bacillus subtilis,* and clostridia (Gould, 1964); yeasts and molds, including *Penicillium expansium, Rhizopus nigricans,* and *Botrytis* and *Saccharomyces* species; and viruses (Ellinger, 1972). The most effective phosphates have chain lengths ranging from 18 to 24 phosphate units (Ellinger, 1972).

The antimicrobial effect of phosphates is particularly important in the manufacture of processed cheese and meat products. The concentration of phosphate was more influential in prolonging shelf-life of a cooked meat system than was the type of phosphate (Marcy et al., 1988). Monobasic calcium phosphate [$CaH_4(PO_4)_2H_2O$] has been used as a rope inhibitor in bread.

ANTIBIOTICS

Antibiotics were widely tested and used for food preservation between 1945 and 1960, immediately after the discovery of penicillin and the successful use of antibiotics to treat bacterial disease. Application of classic antibiotics in food preservation has been either restricted or prohibited since their discovery. Only oxytetracycline and chlortetracycline were ever permitted for use in the U.S. In the U.S., on September 6, 1967 (Federal Register, Volume 32, p. 172), the FDA prohibited use of antibiotics and introduced specifications to eliminate antibiotic residues carried over from treated animals to food products. The major reason for restriction of the use of antibiotics for food preservation in the U.S. and other countries was the development and discovery of strains of microorganisms resistant to antibiotics. Microbial resistance to antibiotics may be the result of selection of existing resistant organisms or genetic mutation or modification. If antibiotic-resistant microorganisms colonize the host, the antibiotics used for medical purposes could become ineffective. Additionally, application of antibiotics in food preservation and development of resistant microorganisms could result in loss of their value as food preservatives.

Antibiotics have been used directly for the preservation of poultry, fish, meat, milk, milk products, fresh fruits and vegetables, and canned foods. The primary uses are as adjuncts to other preservation methods, such as to lengthen the shelf-life of refrigerated foods or to combine antibiotics with heat to reduce the thermal processing time of canned foods. Today, it is more likely that antibiotics would be present in foods as a result of their use in animal feeds. Thus, they may occur in milk or animal tissue. In the U.S., the presence of antibiotics due to direct addition or indirect addition from feed is not permitted, because such antibiotics are considered food additives. Marth (1966) gave an excellent review of antibiotics in foods. Other reviews of the use of antibiotics have been published by Anderson and Michener

(1950), Wrenshall (1959), Goldberg (1964), Fukusumi (1972), Katz (1983), and others.

Chlortetracycline and Oxytetracycline

Chlortetracycline (Aureomycin) and oxytetracycline (Terramycin) are two tetracyclines that had been used as food additives. The basic structure of all tetracyclines is a four-membered tetracycline ring with characteristically distributed polar side groups. Because the chemical structures of these two tetracyclines are similar, their physicochemical properties and modes of antimicrobial action are similar. Tetracyclines are weakly basic and poorly soluble in water (Kurytowicz, 1976). The tetracyclines are stable to heat. For example, chlortetracycline is only partially inactivated after brief boiling.

Tetracyclines are broad-spectrum antibacterial agents that are bacteriostatic or bactericidal at low or high concentrations, respectively. Tetracyclines inhibit binding of aminoacyl t-RNA to the acceptor site on the 30S ribosomal subunit. At high concentrations, the tetracyclines may exert their biocidal action by linkage with Mg^{++} in ribosomes. In effect, protein synthesis is inhibited along with interference with many enzyme reactions (Franklin and Snow, 1971; Fey and Kersten, 1972).

The tetracyclines had been used primarily to extend the storage stability of fresh meat, fish, and poultry (Goldberg, 1964). Many studies have reported that the shelf-life of fresh poultry or fish is extended by dipping the product in solutions of approximately 3 to 100 µg/g tetracycline for approximately 10 minutes to 2 hours, followed by holding at refrigerated temperatures, or by holding fish on ice containing 1 to 4 µg/g chlortetracycline (Kohler et al., 1954, 1955; Lennon, 1972; Lee et al., 1967; Boyd and Southcott, 1968; Tarr et al., 1954).

Tylosin

Tylosin is a macrolide (a class of antibiotics characterized by a large lactone ring in glycosidic linkage to rare sugars) produced by *Streptomyces fradiac*. Its water solubility is low. Tylosin is not used therapeutically and has slight acute toxicity. The LD_{50} is reported to be 12 g/kg of body weight (Shibasaki, 1970). Presently, residues of tylosin are not permitted in food in the U.S.

Tylosin has a broader spectrum than the bacteriocins, nisin, or subtilin. It is effective against gram-positive bacteria, including clostridia (Suzuki et al., 1970). Poole and Malin (1964) reported that the effectiveness of tylosin depended on the growth environment and on initial, postprocessing, and post-storage concentrations.

Because of its activity against spore-forming bacteria, especially clostridia, tylosin has been considered for use as a thermal processing adjuvant. It is more heat stable than nisin (Denny et al., 1961) and has been tested in many canned foods, including mushrooms, dog food, and various canned meats. Tylosin prevented botulinal toxin production in smoked fish when 100 µg/g was added to the brine (Segmiller et al., 1965).

Natamycin

Natamycin (WHO generic name), or pimaricin, is synthesized by *Streptomyces natalensis* (Clark et al., 1964). It is a macrolide, similar to tylosin, with the formula $C_{33}H_{47}NO_{13}$, and molecular weight 665.73. Natamycin appears as white crystalline needles, is soluble in water or alcohol at a level of only 0.005%, is highly soluble in propylene glycol, glycerol, and acetic acid, and is stable at pH 4 to 7 (Lueck, 1980). The LD_{50} of natamycin for the mouse, rat, and guinea pig is 1.5, 1.5 to 4.7, and 0.45 mg/kg of body weight, respectively (Struyk et al., 1957–1958; Levinskas et al., 1966). Subchronic toxicity tests conducted by Levinskas et al. (1966) showed no damage after 90 days with feedings of 45 mg/kg of body weight. Higher doses resulted in reduced weight gain due to vomiting and diarrhea.

Chronic toxicity studies by Levinskas and coworkers (1966) showed that rats fed 0.2% natamycin over a 2-year period had no appreciable damage compared to control animals but did have a smaller weight gain. Natamycin is permitted in some western European countries for surface preservation of cheese and as an additive to cheese coating. The FAO acceptable daily intake of natamycin is 0.3 mg/kg of body weight. It is not permitted in the U.S., United Kingdom, or the Federal Republic of Germany. It is used medically to treat fungi that grow on skin.

Natamycin is an antifungal antibiotic, effective against yeast and mycotoxin-producing fungi. Its antimicrobial action is ineffective against bacteria, viruses, or actinomycetes. Some molds, including *Aspergillus flavus*, produce enzymes that inactivate natamycin, resulting in loss of its effectiveness if applied after growth has developed. At some concentrations, *A. parasiticus* was inhibited yet was able to grow and produce aflatoxin (Rusul and Marth, 1988). The mode of antimicrobial action of natamycin on *Candida* species is similar to that of surface-active substances, indicating interaction with the cell membrane (Lueck, 1980). Microbial cells treated with natamycin lose cellular components such as amino acids and nucleic acids, preventing reproduction. The effective pH range is 3.0 to 9.0.

Because of its action against molds, aqueous suspensions of natamycin are used for the surface treatment of cheese and have been proposed for use on sausage, with the primary purpose of restricting the growth of mycotoxin-producing molds (Bullerman, 1977; Holley, 1981). During ripening and storage of the cheese, natamycin may be decomposed. Natamycin has been used to retard yeast and mold spoilage of fruit, fruit juices and drinks, cottage cheese, poultry, and sausage. The antibiotic may be applied by mixing with the food, dipping, spraying, dusting, or by treating the packaging material.

Bacteriocins

Bacteriocins are proteins or protein complexes with bactericidal activity. The antimicrobial activities of lactic acid bacteria have long been known, although only recently have the bacteriocins produced by the lactic acid bacteria been identified and characterized. These bacteriocins, which are used as direct or indirect (produced during fermentation of food) food preservatives, have been reviewed recently by Klaenhammer (1988). Daeschel (1989) also has surveyed antimicrobial substances including bacteriocins from lactic acid bacteria for use as food preservatives. Nisin, a bacteriocin produced by *Lactococcus lactis* (formerly *Streptococcus lactis*), is the only bacteriocin that has realized commercial application as a directly added food preservative. Bacteriocins may be present in food because of production during fermentation processes or growth of spoilage organisms. Bacteriocins are produced by numerous gram-positive and gram-negative bacteria. Owing to their proteinaceous nature, their toxicity is likely to be low in all cases because they would be susceptible to digestive enzymes.

Nisin

Nisin is a family of polypeptide antibiotics produced by *Lactococcus lactis*. It contains a high concentration of sulfur-containing amino acids and contains the unique amino acids lanthionine, dehydroalanine, and beta-methyl lanthienine (Kurytowicz, 1976; Hurst, 1981). Nisin exists as a stable dimer or tetramer of the 3500-dalton protein. Nisin is stable at 100°C for 10 minutes under acid conditions; at higher pH values, the stability decreases. Nisin is sensitive to alpha-chymotrypsin, but is resistant to pronase and trypsin.

The toxicity of nisin is low (Frazer et al., 1962; Shtenberg and Ignat'ev, 1970; FDA, 1988). In the U.S., the FDA recently affirmed that nisin is GRAS for use in pasteurized cheese spreads. Nisin is permitted in many countries, including the United States, United Kingdom, Belgium, Finland, France, Israel, Italy, India, and Portugal, chiefly for the preservation of processed cheeses or other dairy products. In countries where its use in food is permitted, there is often no limit on the amount used, or there is a limit of about 100 to 500 μg/g. Nisin is not employed in human or animal medicine.

The antimicrobial action of nisin is directed against the cytoplasmic membrane. The action of nisin against spores is greater than that against vegetative cells (Gould, 1964), and it appears that nisin inhibits spore germination (Gupta et al., 1972). The action of nisin occurs after the heating process (Tramer, 1964), at which point it enhances the heat sensitivity of bacterial spores. Nisin is effective against *Bacillus* and *Clostridium* spores. In meat slurries, nisin (75 μg/g) was superior to nitrite (150 μg/g) in inhibiting *Clostridium sporogenes* PA3679 outgrowth (Rayman et al., 1981). In a laboratory medium, 2000 IU nisin/ml prevented outgrowth of *C. botulinum* to an extent similar to that shown by 120 μg/g nitrite (Scott and Taylor, 1981a). Nisin was more effective against *C. botulinum* spore outgrowth at pH 6 than at pH 7 or 8 (Scott and Taylor, 1981b), and its optimal activity is reportedly at pH 6.5 to 6.8 (Lueck, 1980). Nisin-producing *Lactococcus lactis* will inhibit *Listeria monocytogenes* (Harris et al., 1989). Nisin acts exclu-

sively against gram-positive bacteria. Yeasts and molds are not inhibited by nisin; in fact, many yeasts and molds decompose nisin. The preservative effect of nisin has been reviewed by Hurst (1978, 1981).

Nisin is used in dairy products, primarily in processed cheese, in which its action is directed against spore-forming bacteria, particularly butyric acid bacteria and clostridia. The antibotulinal effectiveness of nisin in pasteurized process cheese spreads was reported by Somers and Taylor (1987). Because it appears to increase the heat sensitivity of many bacterial spores, nisin may be used in canned products as a sterilizing auxiliary. It is permitted in canned foods in Italy, Singapore, Malta, the United Kingdom, and the USSR. The primary purpose for use is its action against *C. botulinum* and other *Clostridium* spores.

Subtilin

Subtilin is a polypeptide produced by *B. subtilis*. It is poorly water-soluble. Subtilin is not presently permitted in foods in the U.S. It is not used for medical purposes.

Subtilin is effective against gram-positive bacteria, including spores, thermophiles, and clostridia, and against some gram-negative bacteria (Banwart, 1979). It may be bacteriostatic or bactericidal, depending on the concentration.

Because it is stable to heat and active against clostridial spores, subtilin has been suggested to reduce the intensity of sterilization conditions for canned foods. Inoculated pack studies conducted by the National Canners Association indicated that it was not effective in this role (Chichester and Tanner, 1972).

Other Bacteriocins Produced by Lactic Acid Bacteria

Other bacteriocins are produced by many species and strains of lactic acid bacteria, including lactocin and helviticin J of *Lactobacillus helviticus*, lactacin B and F of *L. acidophilus*, plantaricin A of *Lactobacillus plantarum*, Las 5 and diplococcin of *Lactococcus cremoris*, formerly *Streptococcus cremoris*, and pediocin A of *Pediococcus pentosaceus*. For a review of the biochemical and genetic aspects of these bacteriocins, which may be present in a wide variety of fermented foods, the reader is referred to Klaenhammer (1988).

OTHER ANTIMICROBIALS

Some of the other antimicrobial agents that are currently used, have been used, or have been proposed for use in various countries and foods are described in the following.

Butylated Hydroxyanisole

Butylated hydroxyanisole (BHA; $C_{11}H_{16}O_2$) is added to foods as an antioxidant. It also has antimicrobial properties that have been reviewed by Branen et al. (1980), Davidson (1983), and Raccach (1984). Chang and Branen (1975) reported that 0.1% BHA prevented growth and aflatoxin production by *Aspergillus parasiticus* spores. Rusul and Marth (1988) reviewed these and other food additives for control of aflatoxingenic aspergilli. BHA also has been reported to inhibit growth of *Clostridium perfringens* vegetative cells, *Staphylococcus aureus*, *E. coli*, *Salmonella typhimurium* and *Vibrio parahaemolyticus* (Chang and Branen, 1975; Pierson et al., 1980; Ayaz et al., 1980; Robach et al., 1977; Klindworth et al., 1979), as well as *Saccharomyces cerevisiae* growth, sporulation, and pseudomycelium production (Eubanks and Beuchat, 1982). Dawson and coworkers (1975) found, however, that ground turkey containing BHA had increased microbial counts.

Butylated Hydroxytoluene

Butylated hydroxytoluene (BHT; $C_{15}H_{24}O$) has been used in foods as an antioxidant. Some reports indicate that BHT has antimicrobial properties (Ward and Ward, 1967; Branen et al., 1980; Ayaz et al., 1980).

Tertiary Butylhydroquinone

Tertiary butylhydroquinone (TBHQ) is commonly used as an antioxidant in foods. It is reported to have some antimicrobial effect against *Salmonella typhimurium*, *Staphylococcus aureus*, *Pediococcus pentosaceus*, and *Saccharomyces cerevisiae* (Robach and Stateler, 1980; Branen et al., 1980; Eubanks and Beuchat, 1982; Davidson et al., 1981; Raccach and Henningsen, 1982).

Ethylenediaminetetraacetic Acid

Ethylenediaminetetraacetic acid (EDTA, versene) is a chelating agent with the chemical formula $(HOOCCH_2)_2$-NCH_2CH_2N-$(CH_2COOH)_2$. Along with its sodium and calcium salts, EDTA is used as a synergist for antioxidants in foods. EDTA and its salts are tasteless, odorless, and colorless. There are conflicting reports on the toxicity of EDTA (Krum and Fellers, 1952; Anonymous, 1972). Considering that EDTA can form complexes with vital metal cations, making them unavailable to the body, excessive ingestion of EDTA should be avoided. EDTA and its sodium and calcium salts are approved as food additives in many countries, including the U.S.

By chelating trace metals that are necessary to microorganisms, EDTA has some antimicrobial activity. Metals may be necessary for activities of certain metal-containing enzymes or for germination and outgrowth of spores. Germination, outgrowth, and toxin production of *Clostridium botulinum* type A in fish homogenate was inhibited by 5mM EDTA (Winarno et al., 1971). The inhibitory action increased as pH increased and was eliminated by the addition of $CaCl_2$ and $MgCl_2$. Kuusi and Löytömaki (1972) reported that the total bacterial count of fresh fish was only slightly increased by EDTA, but that the shelf-life was lengthened. The formation of trimethylamine and hypoxanthine is suppressed in fresh fish by dipping in EDTA or its salts (Levin, 1967; Kuusi and Löytömaki, 1972). EDTA reportedly has antiviral activity (Ward and Ashley, 1980).

In the U.S., EDTA and its salts are approved for use in several foods. In some countries, EDTA dips are used to preserve fish and shrimp.

Bromates

By increasing the oxidation-reduction potential, potassium bromate ($KBrO_3$) has some antibacterial action. It has been used in processed cheeses at concentrations of 0.04% and below to prevent spoilage by anaerobic butyric acid bacteria (Lueck, 1980). It is not used currently because it imparts an off-flavor to and lowers the quality of the cheese.

Fluorides

Sodium and potassium fluorides (NaF, KF) inhibit bacteria, yeasts, and molds, probably by inhibiting various enzyme systems. They have been used to preserve milk, butter, margarine, egg, meat, beer, and wine. Fluorides are toxic in the concentrations used for food preservation.

Thiourea

Thiourea (H_2NCSNH_2) had been used in a 2 to 10% aqueous solution or a 4 to 6% wax emulsion to preserve citrus fruits. It is effective primarily against molds. Because of its toxicity, thiourea is no longer used.

Allyl Isothiocyanate

Allyl isothiocyanate ($CH_2=CHCH_2NCS$), or volatile oil of mustard, is poorly soluble in water and has an undesirable odor. In Italy, it has been used to stabilize large containers of wine.

8-Oxyquinoline

8-Oxyquinoline (C_9H_7NO), 8-hydroxyquinoline, or hydroxybenzopyridine has been used to preserve primarily tobacco and some foods. For tobacco preservation, it was used in the form 8-oxyquinoline sodium hydrogen sulfate at concentrations of 0.03 to 0.05% (Lueck, 1980).

Nitrofurans

Two common nitrofuran derivatives are furyl furamide ($C_{11}H_8O_5N_2$; AF-2) and nitrofuryl acrylamide (nitrofuran Z). Like many nitrofurans, these have been found to be mutagenic and carcinogenic (Tazima et al., 1975; Takayama and Kuwabara, 1977; Sugiyama et al., 1975). Nitrofuran derivatives inhibit electron transfer. Furyl furamide has more antimicrobial activity than nitrofuryl acrylamide. Nitrofurans are not affected significantly by the pH value of food, and their antimicrobial effect is directed primarily against bacteria, especially aerobic bacteria. The effective concentration is between 5 and 50 µg/g (Matsuda, 1966). Use of furyl furamide was permitted for a limited time in certain foods in eastern Asia, including Japan. The maximum allowable concentration was 20 mg/kg of food. It has never been permitted in the U.S. or Western Europe. It was used to preserve tofu, bean paste, and meat.

Glycols

Low-molecular-weight glycols, notably propylene glycol ($CH_3CHOHCH_2OH$) and butylene glycol

(CH$_3$CHOHCHOHCH$_3$), are humectants that have some antimicrobial action. The glycols that are permitted in foods have low LD$_{50}$ values and are not carcinogenic. As a humectant, the antimicrobial activity is based on reduction in the water activity. Consequently, the concentration of glycol must be high, usually greater than 1%. A major application is in intermediate-moisture foods. In laboratory medium, *Staphylococcus aureus* grew more slowly and reached a tenfold-lower maximum population in the presence of propylene or butylene glycol at concentrations permitted in foods. Cells grown in the presence of these preservatives showed reduced enterotoxin synthesis, with higher levels of intracellular enterotoxin accumulated than in controls (McIver et al., 1978).

Thiabendazole

Thiabendazole, C$_{10}$H$_7$N$_3$S, is a white crystalline powder with a molecular weight of 201.25. It is poorly water-soluble, its maximum water solubility being 3.84% at pH 2.2. The LD$_{50}$ of thiabendazole is 3.1 to 3.8 g/kg of body weight for mice, rats, and rabbits. Dosages of 200 mg daily for 180 days do not affect the growth of rats; twice this quantity retards their growth only slightly (Robinson et al., 1965). In light of the small quantities ingested, thiabendazole is considered a safe food preservative. Use of thiabendazole is permitted in several countries for the preservation of citrus fruits and bananas.

Thiabendazole has primarily fungistatic action. It is especially effective against *Penicillium italicum*, *P. digitatum*, and *Gloeosporium* species (Robinson et al., 1964). The mechanism of antimicrobial action is not known. Thiabendazole is used in food processing to prevent mold growth on citrus fruits and bananas. It is added to wax emulsions used to treat the fruit concentrations of 0.1 to 0.45% (Rizk and Isshak, 1974; Isshak et al., 1974). Apple growers use thiabendazole to reduce fruit rot by *Gloeosporium* species (Edney, 1973).

Silver

Silver (Ag) has a molecular weight of 107.87. Silver treatment involves the use of colloidal silver or silver adsorbed to colloidal carriers. No thorough, systematic investigations on the toxicology of colloidal silver are available. Silver treatment is permitted for drinking water and other drinks in some countries.

The mode of action of silver is speculated to be due to adsorption of silver onto the negatively charged bacterial cell surface or interaction of silver with microbial enzymes. Suspended matter, proteins, chlorides, and calcium ions reduce the effectiveness of silver (Lueck, 1980). Silver is most active against bacteria; yeasts and molds are inactivated to a lesser extent.

Silver is primarily used to disinfect drinking water and has also been used for vinegar, fruit juices, effervescent drinks, and wine. Silver concentrations of 0.025 to 10 mg/L have been used.

Hexamethylenetetramine

Hexamethylenetetramine (HMTA), C$_6$H$_{12}$N$_4$, has a molecular weight of 140.19 and is a white crystalline powder with a sweet flavor and bitter aftertaste. It is highly water-soluble and more soluble in cold than in hot water. It is produced by reacting ammonia and formaldehyde in aqueous solution, and is nontoxic in small doses. HMTA is not considered teratogenic, but is mutagenic to *Drosophila* larvae and bacteria (Hurni and Ohder, 1973; Englesberg, 1952; Natvig et al., 1971). HMTA was employed in several countries, especially in northern and central Europe, but its use has been largely discontinued because of its toxicity. It is not permitted in the U.S.

The antimicrobial action of HMTA is based on release of formaldehyde in acidic medium. Formaldehyde reacts with and denatures proteins in the microbial cell (Linko and Kikkilä, 1959). The proteins and amino acids of foods react with HMTA; hence, larger concentrations of HMTA are needed to inactivate microorganisms in food systems than in a nutrient laboratory medium. Because the action with proteins is nonspecific, all types of microorganisms are inhibited by HMTA.

HMTA has been used to preserve caviar, provolone cheese, and fish products, including fish marinades, shrimp, and mussel. Excess quantities of HMTA may cause hardening of the fish flesh due to denaturation of the fish proteins by formaldehyde. Typically, 0.01 to 0.1% HMTA has been used to preserve food, often in conjunction with benzoic or sorbic acid to increase the antifungal activity.

o-Phenylphenol

o-Phenylphenol (o-hydroxybiphenyl, orthoxenol, Dowicide 1, SOPP, 2-phenylphenol) has a molecular weight of 170.21 and molecular formula of C$_6$H$_5$C$_6$H$_4$OH. o-Phenylphenol is poorly soluble in water, whereas the sodium salt dissolves readily. It is sold under the trade names Dowicide A and Preventol ON Extra. There have been no serious acute, subchronic, or chronic toxicities detected by animal feeding studies. The LD$_{50}$ of o-phenylphenol is 0.5 and 3 g/kg of body weight for the cat and rat, respectively (Macintosh, 1945; Hodge et al., 1952). o-Phenylphenol is permitted in foods in many countries.

o-Phenylphenol nonspecifically denatures microbial cell wall components and inhibits various enzyme systems, including NADH-oxidase (Lueck, 1980). Because the dissociated compound is a more powerful antimicrobial agent than the undissociated compound, the antimicrobial action of o-phenylphenol increases as the pH increases. The antimicrobial action of o-phenylphenol, like that of most phenol derivatives, has a broad spectrum. As a food preservative, however, its fungistatic action is more important than its bacteriostatic action. Molds are inhibited by 10 to 50 µg/g, whereas bacterial inhibition requires higher concentrations (Lueck, 1980). o-Phenylphenol is used for preservation of citrus fruit, which is immersed in 0.5 to 2% aqueous solutions for 0.5 to 1 minute.

Esters of Phenylalanine

Some aliphatic esters of phenylalanine may inhibit bacteria and molds in foods and beverages.

Diphenyl

Diphenyl, biphenyl, or phenylbenzene, $C_6H_5C_6H_5$, has a molecular weight of 154.21, is colorless with a pleasant odor, and is poorly soluble in water. The LD_{50} is 2.4 to 5 g/kg of body weight for rats, rabbits, and cats (Lueck, 1980). Chronic and subchronic toxicity studies in animals indicate that kidney and liver damage may result upon prolonged feeding. Fertility and litter size may also be reduced (Macintosh, 1945; Ambrose et al., 1960). Rats, rabbits, and dogs convert diphenyl to substances that are excreted in the urine (West, 1940). Diphenyl is permitted in many countries, including the United Kingdom.

Diphenyl inhibits a large number of microorganisms. Most important is its action against molds, including *Penicillium italicum* and *P. digitatum* (Lueck, 1980).

Diphenyl is used to preserve citrus fruits by application to the material used to wrap the fruits during storage and transportation (Hopkins and Loucks, 1947). Usually the applied concentration is 1 to 5 g/m^2 of the wrapping material. Diphenyl may migrate into the peel, but little is found in the citrus juice.

Captan

Captan ($C_9H_8Cl_3NO_2S$), or *N*-trichloromethyl mercapto-4-cyclohexene-1,2-dicarboximide, is used on raisins as a fungicide.

Cinnamylphenol and Cinnamic Aldehyde

Both cinnamylphenol and cinnamic aldehyde are components of cinnamon that have antimicrobial properties. Cinnamylphenol may be used to preserve fruit juices.

Hinokitiol

Hinokitiol (*m*-isopropyltropolon, 2-hydroxy-4-isopropylol, or 2,4,6- cycloheptatriene) may enhance the keeping quality of fish. The preservative action may be due to protease inhibition.

Glutaraldehyde

Glutaraldehyde [$OHC(CH_2)_3CHO$] may be used to inactivate viruses and other microorganisms (Saitanu and Lund, 1975). It is a natural component of many foods.

Glycine

Glycine (NH_2CH_2COOH) is an amino acid that is a natural component of many plant and animal systems. It has been shown to have antibacterial action against several bacteria (Hammes et al., 1973).

COMBINATIONS

The preceding discussion details the actions and uses of many food preservatives. It is not uncommon to have more than one preservative incorporated into a food product. As indicated by Wagner and Moberg (1989), the approach of combining food preservatives and preservation systems undoubtedly will continue and likely will grow. This chapter is concerned for the most part with the use, effectiveness, and mode of action of individual food preservatives used singly for preservation. Combinations of preservatives, frequently called hurdles or barriers, may be effective in food products to produce the desired preservative effect. Roberts (1989) has reviewed models for predicting the responses of microorganisms to various combinations of antimicrobials and processing methods. Such combinations are desirable because they frequently result in synergistic or additive effects, although they may cause antagonistic actions. Combinations of preservative systems provide unlimited preservation alternatives that are especially useful in meeting consumer demands for new products.

REFERENCES

Ahlborg, U.G., Dich, J., and Ericksson, H.-B. 1977. Data on food preservatives. Var Foda, 29(2), 41–96.

Al-Delaimy, K.S., and Ali, S.H. 1970. Antibacterial action of vegetable extracts on the growth of pathogenic bacteria. J. Sci. Food Agric., 21, 110–112.

Amano, K., Shibasaki, I., Yokoseki, M., and Kawabata, T. 1968. Preservation of fish sausage with tylosin, furylfuramide, and sorbic acid. Food Technol., 22, 881–885.

Ambrose, A.M., Booth, A.N., DeEds, F., and Cox, A.J. 1960. Toxicological study of biphenyl, a citrus fungistat. Food Res., 25, 328–336.

Amerine, M.A., and Joslyn, M.A. 1951. *Table Wines: The Technology of Their Production.* Berkeley, University of California Press.

Amerine, M.A., and Joslyn, M.A. 1940. Commercial production of table wines. Calif. Agric. Exp. Stat. Bull. No. 639.

Anderson, A.A., and Michner, H.D. 1950. Preservation of foods with antibiotics. I. The complementary action of subtilin and mild heat. Food Technol., 4, 188–189.

Anonymous, 1972. The complexities of EDTA. Food Cosmet. Toxicol., 10, 697–700.

Auerbach, R.C. 1959. Sorbic acid as a preservative agent in wine. Wines and Vines, 40 (August), 26–28.

Ayaz, M., Luedecke, L.O., and Branen, A.L. 1980. Antimicrobial effect of butylated hydroxyanisole and butylated hydroxytoluene on *Staphylococcus aureus*. J. Food Protect., 43, 4–6, 18.

Azukas, J.J. 1962. Sorbic acid inhibition of enolase from yeast and lactic acid bacteria. Ph.D. Thesis, Michigan State University.

Bala, K., Stringer, W.C., and Naumann, H.D. 1977. Effect of spray sanitization treatment and gaseous atmospheres on the stability of prepackaged fresh beef. J. Food Sci., 42, 743–746.

Banks, J.G., Board, R.G., and Sparks, N.H.C. 1986. Natural antimicrobial systems and their potential in food preservation of the future. Biotech. Appl. Biochem., 8, 103–147.

Banks, J.G., and Board, R.G. 1985. Preservation by the lactoperoxidase system (LP-S) of a contaminated infant formula. Lett. Appl. Microbiol., 1, 81–85.

Banwart, G. 1979. *Basic Food Microbiology.* Westport, AVI Publishing.

Barber, L.E., and Deibel, R.H. 1972. Effect of pH and oxygen tension on staphylococcal growth and enterotoxin formation in fermented sausage. Appl. Microbiol., 24, 891–898.

Bayne, H.G., and Michener, H.D. 1975. Growth of *Staphylococcus* and *Salmonella* on frankfurters with and without sodium nitrite. Appl. Microbiol., 30, 844–849.

Beuchat, L.R. 1976. Sensitivity of *Vibrio parahaemolyticus* to spices and organic acids. J. Food Sci., 41, 899–902.

Beuchat, L.R., and Golden, D.A. 1989. Antimicrobials occurring naturally in foods. Food Technol., 43(1), 134–142.

Bhagat, B., and Lockett, M.F. 1964. The effect of sulphite in solid diets on the growth of rats. Food Cosmet. Toxicol., 2, 1–13.

Binkerd, E.F., and Kolari, O.E. 1975. The history and use of nitrate and nitrite in the curing of meat. Food Cosmet. Toxicol., 13, 655–661.

Block, S.S., and Bevis, J. 1963. Investigation of chemical agents for the canning preservation of meat. Dev. Ind. Microbiol., 4, 201–212.

Block, S.S., and Taylor, J., Jr. 1964. Storage tests of bisulfite-preserved canned beef. Dev. Ind. Microbiol., 6, 277–283.

Bogen, D.W., Naglik, O.A., and Shelef, L.A. 1979. Sensitivity of some common food-borne bacteria to spices sage, rosemary, and allspice. Presented at the Institute of Food Technologists Annual Meeting. St. Louis, Missouri, June, 1979.

Bonner, M.D., and Harmon, L.G. 1957. Characteristics of organisms contributing to spoilage of cottage cheese. J. Dairy Sci., 40, 1599–1611.

Bosund, I. 1962. The action of benzoic and salicylic acids on the metabolism of microorganisms. Adv. Food Res., 11, 331–353.

Boyd, J.W., and Southcott, B.A. 1968. Comparative effectiveness of ethylene-diaminetetraacetic acid and chlortetracycline for fish preservation. J. Fish Res. Board, Canada, 25, 1753.

Boyd, J.W., and Tarr, H.L.A. 1955. Inhibition of mold and yeast development in fish products. Food Technol., 9, 411–412.

Boyle, D.L., Sofos, J.N., and Maga, J.A. 1988. Inhibition of spoilage and pathogenic microorganisms by liquid smoke from various woods. Lebensmittel-Wissenschaft Technol., 21, 54–58.

Branen, A.L., and Davidson, P.M. (eds.). 1983. *Antimicrobials in Foods.* New York, Marcel Dekker.

Branen, A.L., Davidson, P.M., and Katz, B. 1980. Antimicrobial properties of phenolic antioxidants and lipids. Food Technol., 34(5), 42–53, 63.

Broadwater, W.T., Hoehn, R.C., and King, P.H. 1973. Sensitivity of three selected bacterial species to ozone. Appl. Microbiol., 26, 391–393.

Brown, W. 1922. On the germination and growth of fungi at various temperatures and in various concentrations of oxygen and carbon dioxide. Ann. Bot., 36, 257–283.

Bruce, W.F. 1935. Some relationships between molecular structure, pH, and the ability of bacteria to grow in solutions of salts of organic acids. J. Am. Chem. Soc., 57, 1495–1503.

Bruch, C.W. 1972. Sterilization of plastics: Toxicity of ethylene oxide residues. In Industrial Sterilization. Edited by G.B. Phillips and W.S. Miller. Durham, Duke University Press, pp. 49–77.

Bruch, C.W. 1961. Gaseous sterilization. Annu. Rev. Microbiol., 15, 245–262.

Bruch, C.W., and Koesterer, M.G. 1961. The microbicidal activity of gaseous propylene oxide and its application to powdered or flaked foods. J. Food Sci., 26, 428–435.

Buchanan, R.L., and Solberg, M. 1972. Interaction of sodium nitrite, oxygen, and pH on growth of *Staphylococcus aureus.* J. Food Sci., 37, 81–85.

Bullerman, L.B. 1979. Effects of potassium sorbate on mycotoxin production and growth of *Aspergillus parasiticus, Penicillium commune* and *Penicillium patulum* in broth substrates. Presented at the Institute of Food Technologists Annual Meeting. St. Louis, Missouri, June, 1979.

Bullerman, L.B. 1977. Incidence and control of mycotoxin producing molds in domestic and imported cheeses. Ann. Nutr. Aliment., 31, 435–446.

Bullerman, L.B. 1974. Inhibition of aflatoxin production by cinnamon. J. Food Sci., 39, 1163–1165.

Busta, F.F., and Sofos, J.N. 1979. Alternatives to the use of nitrite as an antibotulinal agent. Presented at the Institute of Food Technologists Annual Meeting. St. Louis, Missouri, June, 1979.

Carr, J.G., Davies, P.A., and Sparks, A.H. 1976. The toxicity of sulphur dioxide towards certain lactic acid bacteria from fermented apple juice. J. Appl. Bacteriol., 40, 201–212.

Cassens, R.G., Greaser, M.L., Ito, T., and Lee, M. 1979. Reactions of nitrite in meat. Food Technol., 33(7), 48–57.

Castellani, A.G., and Niven, C.F., Jr. 1955. Factors affecting the bacteriostatic action of sodium nitrite. Appl. Microbiol., 3, 154–159.

Cathcart, W.H. 1951. Baking and bakery products. In The Chemistry and Technology of Food and Food Products. Volume II. 2nd Edition. Edited by M.B. Jacobs. New York, Interscience Publications, pp. 1195–1203.

Chang, H.C., and Branen, A.L. 1975. Antimicrobial effects of butylated hydroxyanisole (BHA). J. Food Sci., 40, 349–351.

Charley, P.J., Sarkar, B., Stitt, C.F., and Saltman, P. 1963. Chelation of iron by sugars. Biochim. Biophys. Acta, 69, 313–321.

Chichester, D.F., and Tanner, F.W., Jr. 1972. Antimicrobial food additives. In Handbook of Food Additives. 2nd Edition. Edited by T.E. Furia. Cleveland, The Chemical Rubber Co., pp. 137–208.

Chipley, J.R. 1983. Sodium benzoate and benzoic acid. In Antimicrobials in Foods. Edited by A.L. Branen and P.M. Davidson. New York, Marcel Dekker, pp. 11–35.

Chipley, J.R., Story, L.D., Todd, P.T., and Kabara, J.J. 1981. Inhibition of Aspergillus growth and extracellular aflatoxin accumulation by sorbic acid and derivatives of fatty acids. J. Food Safety, 3, 109–119.

Christiansen, L.N., Deffner, J., Foster, E.M., and Sugiyama, H. 1968. Survival and outgrowth of *Clostridium botulinum* type E spores in smoked fish. Appl. Microbiol., 16, 133–137.

Christiansen, L.N., Tompkin, R.B., and Shapiris, A.B. 1978. Fate of *Clostridium botulinum* in perishable canned cured meat at abuse temperatures. J. Food Protect., 41, 354–355.

Chung, Y.-M., and Lee, J.S. 1982. Potassium sorbate inhibition of microorganisms isolated from seafood. J. Food Protect., 45, 1310–1313.

Clark, D.S., and Lentz, C.P. 1969. Microbiological studies in poultry processing plants in Canada. Can. Inst. Food Sci. Technol. J., 2, 33–36.

Clark, D.S., and Takács, J. 1980. Gases as preservative. In *Microbial Ecology of Foods.* Volume I. *Factors Affecting Life and Death of Microorganisms.* International Commission on Microbiological Specifications of Foods. New York, Academic Press, pp. 170–192.

Clark, W.L., Shirk, R.J., and Kline, E.F. 1964. Pimaricin, a new food fungistat. In Microbial Inhibitors in Food. Edited by N. Molin. Stockholm, Almqvist and Wiksell, pp. 167–184.

Code of Federal Regulations. 1990. Title 21, Part 182—Substances generally recognized as safe. Office of Federal Register, National Archives and Records Administration. Washington, D.C., U.S. Government Printing Office.

Costilow, R.N., Coughlin, F.M., Robach, D.L., and Raghed, H.S. 1956. A study of the acid-forming bacteria from cucumber fermentations in Michigan. Food Res., 21, 27–33.

Costilow, R.N., Coughlin, F.M., Robbins, E.K., and Hsu, W.-T. 1957. Sorbic acid as a selective agent in cucumber fermentations. II. Effect of sorbic acid on the yeast and lactic acid fermentation in brined cucumbers. Appl. Microbiol., 5, 373–379.

Cox, N.A., et al. 1974. Evaluation of succinic acid and heat to improve the microbiological quality of poultry meat. J. Food Sci., 39, 985–987.

Crosby, N.T., and Sawyer, R. 1976. N-nitrosamines: A review of chemical and biological properties and their estimation in foodstuffs. Adv. Food Res., 22, 1–71.

Cruess, W.V., and Irish, J.H. 1932. Further observations on the relation of pH value to toxicity of preservatives to microorganisms. J. Bacteriol., 23, 163–166.

Cruess, W.V., and Richert, P.H. 1929. Effects of hydrogen ion concentration on the toxicity of sodium benzoate to microorganisms. J. Bacteriol., 17, 363–371.

Cunningham, F.E. 1979. Shelf-life and quality characteristics of poultry parts dipped in potassium sorbate. J. Food Sci., 44, 863–864.

Daeschel, M.A. 1989. Antimicrobial substance from lactic acid bacteria for use as food preservatives. Food Technol., 43(1), 164–166.

Davidson, P.M. 1983. Phenolic compounds. In Antimicrobials in Foods. Edited by A.L. Branen and P.M. Davidson. New York, Marcel Dekker, pp. 37–74.

Davidson, P.M., Brekke, C.J., and Branen, A.L. 1981. Antimicrobial activity of butylated hydroxyanisole, tertiary butylhydroquinone and potassium sorbate used in combination. J. Food Sci., 46, 314–316.

Davidson, P.M., Post, L.S., Branen, A.L., and McCurdy, A.R. 1983. Naturally occurring and miscellaneous food antimicrobials. In Antimicrobials in Foods. Edited by A.L. Branen and P.M. Davidson. New York, Marcel Dekker, pp. 371–419.

Dawson, L.E., Stevenson, K.E., and Gertonson, E. 1975. Flavor, bacterial and TBA changes in ground turkey patties treated with antioxidants. Poultry Sci., 54, 1134–1139.

Debevere, J.M., and Voets, J.P. 1972. Influence of some preservatives on the quality of prepackaged cod fillets in relation to the oxygen permeability of the film. J. Appl. Bacteriol., 35, 351–356.

Deibel, R.H. 1979. Parabens. Presented at the Meat Industry Research Conference, March, 1979. American Meat Institute Foundation, Washington, D.C.

Denny, C.B., Sharpe, L.E., and Bohrer, C.W. 1961. Effects of tylosin and nisin on canned food spoilage bacteria. Appl. Microbiol., 9, 108–110.

Derosier, N.W. 1970. The Technology of Food Preservation. Westport, AVI Publishing.

Deuel, H.J., Jr., Alfin-Slater, R., Weil, C.S., and Smyth, H.F., Jr. 1954a. Sorbic acid as a fungistatic agent for foods. I. Harmlessness of sorbic acid as a dietary component. Food Res., 19, 1–12.

Deuel, H.J., Jr., et al. 1954b. Sorbic acid as a fungistatic agent for foods. II. Metabolism of β-unsaturated fatty acids with emphasis on sorbic acid. Food Res., 19, 13–19.

Doores, S. 1983. Organic acids. In Antimicrobials in Foods. Edited by A.L. Branen and P.M. Davidson. New York, Marcel Dekker, pp. 75–108.

Doyle, M.P., and Marth, E.H. 1975. Thermal inactivation of conidia from Aspergillus flavus and Aspergillus parasiticus. II. Effects of pH and buffers, glucose, sucrose and sodium chloride. J. Milk Food Technol., 38, 750–758.

Dudman, W.F. 1963. Sorbic hydroxamic acid, an antifungal agent effective over a wide pH range. Appl. Microbiol., 11, 362–367.

Duncan, C.L., and Foster, E.M. 1968. Effect of sodium nitrite, sodium chloride and sodium nitrate on germination and outgrowth of anaerobic spores. Appl. Microbiol., 16, 406–411.

Dunn, C.G. 1968. Food preservatives. In Disinfection, Sterilization, and Preservation. 1st Edition. Edited by C.A. Lawrence and S.S. Block. Philadelphia, Lea & Febiger, pp. 632–651.

Dunn, C.G. 1947. Chemical agents give quality improvements in fisheries. Food Technol., 1, 371–384.

Dyett, E.J., and Shelly, D. 1966. The effects of sulphite preservative in British fresh sausage. J. Appl. Bacteriol., 29, 439–446.

Dymicky, M., Bencivengo, M., Buchanen, R.L., and Smith, J.L. 1987. Inhibition of *Clostridium botulinum* 62A by fumarates and maleates and relationship of activity to some physicochemical constants. Appl. Environ. Microbiol., 53, 110–113.

Dymicky, M., and Huhtanen, C.N. 1979. Inhibition of *Clostridium botulinum* by *p*-hydroxybenzoic acid *n*-alkyl esters. Antimicrob. Agents Chemother., *15*, 798–801.

Earnshaw, R.G., and Banks, J.G. 1989. A note on the inhibition of *Listeria monocytogenes* NCTC 11994 in milk by an activated lactoperoxidase system. Lett. Appl. Microbiol., *8*, 203–205.

Edney, K.L. 1973. Post harvest deterioration of fruit. Chem. Ind., *1973*, 1054–1056.

Eklund, T. 1980. Inhibition of growth and uptake processes in bacteria by some chemical food preservatives. J. Appl. Bacteriol., *48*, 423–432.

El-Gazzer, F.E., Rusul, G., and Marth, E.H. 1987. Growth and aflatoxin production by *Aspergillus parasiticus* NRRL 2999 in the presence of lactic acid and at different initial pH values. J. Food Protect., *50*, 940–944.

El-Kest, S.E., and Marth, E.H. 1988a. Inactivation of *Listeria monocytogenes* by chlorine. J. Food Protect., *51*, 520–524.

El-Kest, S.E., and Marth, E.H. 1988b. *Listeria monocytogenes* and its inactivation by chlorine: a review. Lebersm. -Wiss. u.-Technol., *21*, 346–351.

El-Kest, S.E., and Marth, E.H. 1988c. Temperature, pH, and strain of pathogen as factors affecting inactivation of *Listeria monocytotgenes* by chlorine. J. Food Protect., *51*, 622–625.

Ellinger, R.H. 1972. Phosphates in food processing. In *Handbook of Food Additives*. 2nd Edition. Edited by T.E. Furia. Cleveland, The Chemical Rubber Co.

Elliot, J.M., Hogue, D.E., Myers, G.S., and Loosli, J.K. 1965. Effect of acetate and propionate on the utilization of energy by growing-fattening lambs. J. Nutr., *87*, 233–238.

El-Shenawy, M.A., and Marth, E.A. 1989. Behavior of *Listeria monocytogenes* in the presence of sodium propionate. Int. J. Food Microbiol., *8*, 85–94.

El-Shenawy, M.A., and Marth, E.H. 1988a. Inhibition and inactivation of *Listeria monocytogenes* by sorbic acid. J. Food Protect., *51*, 842–847.

El-Shenawy, M.A., and Marth, E.H. 1988b. Sodium benzoate inhibits growth of or inactivates *Listeria monocytogenes*. J. Food Protect., *51*, 525–530.

Emard, L.O., and Vaughn, R.H. 1952. Selectivity of sorbic acid media for the catalase-negative lactic acid bacteria and clostridia. J. Bacteriol., *63*, 487–494.

Englesberg, E. 1952. The mutagenic action of formaldehyde on bacteria. J. Bacteriol., *63*, 1–11.

Eubanks, V.L., and Beuchat, L.R. 1982. Effects of antioxidants on growth, sporulation and pseudomycelium production by *Saccharomyces cerevisiae*. J. Food Sci., *47*, 1717–1722, 1733.

Fennema, O.R. 1975a. Preservation of food by storage at chilling temperatures. In *Principles of Food Science*. Part II. *Physical Principles of Food Preservation*. Edited by O.R. Fennema. New York, Marcel Dekker, pp. 133–171.

Fennema, O.R. 1975b. Freezing preservation. In *Principles of Food Science*. Part II. *Physical Principles of Food Preservation*. Edited by O.R. Fennema. New York, Marcel Dekker, pp. 173–215.

Ferguson, W.E., and Powrie, W.D. 1957. Studies on the preservation of fresh apple juice with sorbic acid. Appl. Microbiol., *5*, 41–43.

Fey, G., and Kersten, H. 1972. Fluorescence analysis of tetracycline binding to ribosomes. Adv. Antimicrob. Antineoplast. Chemother., *1*(2), 827.

Fiddler, W., Doerr, R.C., Wasserman, A.E., and Salay, J.M. 1966. Composition of hickory sawdust smoke. Furans and phenols. J. Agric. Food Chem., *14*, 659–662.

Flores, L.M., Palomar, L.S., Roh, P.A., and Bullerman, L.B. 1988. Effect of potassium sorbate and other treatments on the microbial content and keeping quality of a restaurant-type Mexican hot sauce. J. Food Protect., *51*, 4–7.

Foegeding, P.M. 1985. Ozone inactivation of *Bacillus* and *Clostridium* spore populations and the importance of spore coat to resistance. Food Microbiol., *2*, 123–134.

Foegeding, P.M. 1983. Bacterial spore resistance to chlorine compounds. Food Technol., *37*(11), 100–104, 110.

Foegeding, P.M., and Busta, F.F. 1983a. Hypochlorite injury of *Clostridium botulinum* spores alters germination responses. Appl. Environ. Microbiol., *45*, 1360–1368.

Foegeding, P.M., and Busta, F.F. 1983b. Proposed mechanism for sensitization by hypochlorite treatment of *Clostridium botulinum* spores. Appl. Environ. Microbiol., *45*, 1374–1379.

Foegeding, P.M., and Busta, F.F. 1983c. Effort of carbon dioxide, nitrogen and hydrogen gases on germination of *Clostridium botulinum* spores. J. Food Protect., *46*, 987–989.

Foegeding, P.M., Hemstapat, V., and Giesbrecht, F.G. 1986. Chlorine dioxide inactivation of *Bacillus* and *Clostridium* spores. J. Food Sci., *51*, 197–201.

Food and Drug Administration. 1988. Nisin preparation; affirmation of GRAS status as a direct human food ingredient. Fed. Reg., *53*, 11247–11250.

Foster, J.W., and Wynne, E.S. 1948. Physiological studies on spore germination with special reference to *Clostridium botulinum*. J. Bacteriol., *55*, 495–501.

Frank, H.A., and Willits, C.O. 1961. Prevention of mold and yeast growth in maple syrup by chemical inhibitors. Food Technol., *15*, 1–3.

Franklin, T.J., and Snow, G.A. 1971. *Biochemistry of Antimicrobial Action*. London, Chapman and Hall.

Frazer, A.C., Sharratt, M., and Hickman, J.R. 1962. The biological effects of food additives. I. Nisin. J. Sci. Food Agric., *13*, 32–42.

Fukusumi, E. 1972. Preservatives in the future. Properties and uses. Shokuhin Kogyo, *15*, 40–45.

Gardner, W.H. 1972. Acidulants in food processing. In *Handbook of Food Additives*. 2nd Edition. Edited by T.E. Furia. Cleveland, CRC Press, pp. 225–270.

Geminder, J.J. 1959. Use of potassium and sodium sorbate in extending shelf-life of smoked fish. Food Technol., *13*, 459–461.

Genth, H. 1964. On the action of diethylpyrocarbonate on microorganisms. Proc. 4th Int. Symp. Food Microbiol., Göteborg, Sweden, pp. 77–84.

Gill, C.O., and Tan, K.H. 1979. Effect of carbon dioxide on growth of *Pseudomonas fluorencens*. Appl. Environ. Microbiol., *38*, 237–240.

Goldberg, H.S. 1964. Non-medical use of antibiotics. Adv. Appl. Microbiol., *6*, 91–117.

Gooding, C.M. 1945. Process of inhibiting growth of molds. U.S. Patent No. 2,379,294.

Gooding, C.M., Melnick, D., Lawrence, R.L., and Luckmann, E.H. 1955. Sorbic acid as a fungistatic agent for foods. IX. Physicochemical considerations in using sorbic acid to protect foods. Food. Res., *20*, 639–648.

Goodson, M., and Rowbury, R.J. 1989. Resistance of acid-habituated *Escherichia coli* to organic acids and its medical and applied significance. Lett. Appl. Microbiol., *8*, 211–214.

Gough, B.J., and Alford, J.A. 1965. Effect of curing agents on the growth and survival of food-poisoning strains of *Clostridium perfringens* J. Food Sci., *30*, 1025–1028.

Gould, G.W. 1964. Effect of food preservatives on the growth of bacteria from spores. In *Microbial Inhibitors in Food*. Edited by N. Molin. Stockholm, Almqvist and Wiksell, pp. 17–24.

Gray, J.I., and Randall, C.J. 1979. The nitrite/N-nitrosamine problem in meats: An update. J. Food Protect., *42*, 168–179.

Grever, A.B.G. 1974. Minimum nitrite concentrations for inhibitions of clostridia in cooked meat products. In *Proceedings of the International Symposium on Nitrite in Meat Products*. Edited by B. Krol and B.J. Tinbergen. Wageningen, Netherlands, Pudoc.

Gupta, K.G., Sidhu, R., and Yadav, N.K. 1972. Effect of various sugars and their derivatives upon the germination of *Bacillus* spores in the presence of nisin. J. Food Sci., *37*, 971–972.

Hales, K.C. 1962. Refrigerated transport on shipboard. Adv. Food Res., *12*, 147–152.

Hammes, W., Schleifer, K.H., and Kandler, O. 1973. Mode of action of glycine on the biosynthesis of peptidoglycan. J. Bacteriol., *116*, 1029–1053.

Hammond, S.M., and Carr, J.G. 1976. The antimicrobial activity of SO_2^- with particular reference to fermented and non-fermented fruit juices. In *Inhibition and Inactivation of Vegetative Microbes*. Edited by F.A. Skinner and W.B. Hugo. Society of Applied Bacteriology Symposia Series, No. 5. New York, Academic Press, pp. 89–110.

Hansen, J.D., and Appleman, M.D. 1955. The effect of sorbic, propionic, and caproic acids on the growth of certain clostridia. Food Res., *20*, 92–96.

Harris, L.J., Daeschel, M.A., Stiles, M.E., and Klaenhammer, T.R. 1989. Antimicrobial activity of lactic acid bacteria against *Listeria monocytogenes*. J. Food Protect., *52*, 384–387.

Harris, N.E., and Rosenfield, D. 1965. Protection of cheese with calcium sorbate treated wrappers. Food Technol., *19*, 656–658.

Hayatsu, H., and Miura, A. 1970. The mutagenic action of sodium bisulfite. Biochem. Biophys. Res. Comm., *39*, 983–988.

Hays, G.L., Burroughs, J.D., and Warner, R.C. 1959. Microbiological aspects of pressure packaged foods. II. The effect of various gases. Food Technol., *13*, 567–570.

Herring, H.K. 1973. Effect of nitrite and other factors on the physicochemical characteristics and nitrosamine formation in bacon. In *Proceedings of the Meat Industry Research Conference*. American Meat Institute Foundation, Washington, D.C., pp. 47–60.

Hesseltine, W.W. 1952. Sodium propionate and its derivatives as bacteriostatics and fungistatics. J. Pharm. Pharmacol., *4*, 577–581.

Hobbs, G. 1976. *Clostridium botulinum* and its importance in fishery products. Adv. Food Res., *22*, 135–185.

Hodge, H.D., Maynard, E.A., Blanchet, H.J., and Rowe, V.K. 1952. Toxicological studies of orthophenyphenol (Dowicide 1). J. Pharmacol. Exp. Ther., *104*, 202–210.

Holley, R.A. 1981. Prevention of surface mold growth on Italian dry sausage by natamycin and potassium sorbate. Appl. Environ. Microbiol., *41*, 422–429.

Hopkins, E.F., and Loucks, K.W. 1947. The use of diphenyl in the control of stem-end rot and mold in citrus fruits. Citrus Ind., *28*, 5–11.

Hoppe, J.O., and Goble, F.C. 1951. The intravenous toxicity of sodium bisulfite. J. Pharmacol. Exp. Ther., *101*, 101–106.

Huffman, D.L. 1974. Effect of gas atmosphere on microbial quality of pork. J. Food Sci., *39*, 723–724.

Hughey, V.L., and Johnson, E.A. 1987. Antimicrobial activity of lysozyme against bacteria involved in food spoilage and food-borne disease. Appl. Environ. Microbiol., *53*, 2165–2170.

Huhtanen, C.N. 1980. Inhibition of *Clostridium botulinum* by spice extracts and aliphatic alcohols. J. Food Protect., 43, 195–196.

Huhtanen, C.N., Dymicky, M., and Trenchard, H. 1981. Methyl and ethyl esters of fumaric acids as substitutes for nitrite for inhibiting *Clostridium botulinum* spore outgrowth in bacon. Presented at the Institute of Food Technologists Annual Meeting. Atlanta, Georgia, June, 1981.

Huppert, M. 1957. The antifungal activity of homologous series of parabens. Antibiot. Chemother., 7, 29–36.

Hurni, H., and Ohder, H. 1973. Reproduction study with formaldehyde and hexamethylenetetramine in beagle dogs. Food Cosmet. Toxicol., 11, 459–462.

Hurst, A. 1978. Nisin: Its preservative effect and function in the growth cycle of the producer organism. In *Streptococci*. Edited by F.A. Skinner and L.B. Quesnel. The Society for Applied Bacteriology Symposium Series No. 7. New York, Academic Press, pp. 297–314.

Hurst, A. 1981. Nisin. In *Advances in Applied Microbiology*. Volume 27. Edited by D. Perlman and A.I. Laskin. New York, Academic Press, pp. 85–123.

Ingram, M. 1976. The microbial role of nitrite in meat products. In *Microbiology in Agriculture, Fisheries, and Food*. Edited by F.A. Skinner and J.G. Carr. London, Academic Press, pp. 1–18.

Ingram, M. 1974. The microbiological effects of nitrite. In *Proceedings of the International Symposium on Nitrite in Meat Products*. Edited by B. Krol and B.J. Tinbergen. Wageningen, Netherlands, Pudoc.

Ingram, M., and Barnes, E.M. 1954. Sterilization by means of ozone. J. Appl. Bacteriol., 17, 246–271.

Ingram, M., Buttiaux, R., and Mossell, D.A.A. 1964. General microbiological considerations in the choice of antimicrobial food preservatives. In *Microbial Inhibitors in Food*. Edited by N. Molin. Stockholm, Almqvist and Wiksell, pp. 381–392.

Ingram, M., and Haines, R.B. 1949. Inhibition of bacterial growth by pure ozone in the presence of nutrients. J. Hyg., 47, 146–158.

Ingram, M., Ottoway, F.J.H., and Coppock, J.B.M. 1956. The preservative action of acid substances in food. Chem. Ind., 42, 1154–1163.

Insalata, N.F. 1952. CO$_2$ versus beverage bacteria. Food Eng., 24(7), 84–85, 190.

Institute of Food Technologists. 1987. Nitrate, nitrite, and nitroso compounds in foods. Food Technol., 41(4), 127–134, 136.

Institute of Food Technologists. 1986. Sulfites as food ingredients. Food Technol., 40(6), 47–52.

International Commission on Microbiological Specifications for Foods. 1980. Reduced water activity. In *Microbial Ecology of Foods*. Volume 1. New York, Academic Press.

Isshak, Y.M., Rizk, S.S., Khalil, R.I., and Fahmi, B.A. 1974. Long term storage of Valencia orange treated by thiabendazole. Agric. Res. Rev., 52, 85–98.

Ito, K., Nakamura, K., Izaki, R., and Takahashi, H. 1977. Degradation of RNA in *Escherichia coli* induced by sodium chloride. Agric. Biol. Chem., 41, 257–263.

Ivey, F.J., and Robach, M.C. 1978. Effect of potassium sorbate and sodium nitrite on *Clostridium botulinum* growth and toxin production in canned comminuted pork. J. Food Sci., 43, 1782–1785.

Ivey, F.J., Shaver, K.J., Christiansen, L.N., and Tompkin, R.B. 1978. Effect of potassium sorbate on toxinogenesis of *Clostridium botulinum* in bacon. J. Food Protect., 41, 621–625.

Jacobs, M.B. 1958. Vinegar. In *The Chemical Analysis of Foods and Food Products*. 3rd Edition. Princeton, D. Van Nostrand.

Jacobs, M.B. 1947. *Synthetic Food Adjuncts*. New York, D. Van Nostrand.

Jarvis, B., and Burke, C.S. 1976. Practical and legislative aspects of the chemical preservatives in food. In *Inhibition and Inactivation of Vegetative Microbes*. Edited by F.A. Skinner and W.B. Hugo. London, Academic Press, pp. 345–367.

Jensen, L.B. 1954. *Microbiology of Meats*. Champaign, IL, Garrard Press.

Jermini, M.F.G., and Schmidt-Lorenz, W. 1987. Activity of Na-benzoate and ethyl-paraben against osmotolerant yeasts at different water activity values. J. Food Protect., 50, 920–927.

Johnson, M.G., and Vaughn, R.H. 1969. Death of *Salmonella typhimurium* and *Escherichia coli* in the presence of freshly reconstituted dehydrated garlic and onions. Appl. Microbiol., 17, 903–905.

Jones, A.H., and Harper, G.S. 1952. A preliminary study of factors affecting the quality of pickles on the Canadian market. Food Technol., 5, 304–308.

Joslyn, M.A., and Braverman, J.B.S. 1954. The chemistry and technology of the pretreatment and preservation of fruit and vegetable products with sulfur dioxide and sulfites. Adv. Food Res., 5, 97–160.

Kabara, J.J. 1984. Inhibition of *Staphylococcus aureus* in a model agar-meat system by monolaurin: a research note. J. Food Safety, 6, 197–201.

Kabara, J.J. 1983. Medium-chain fatty acids and esters. In *Antimicrobials in Foods*. Edited by A.L. Branen and P.M. Davidson. New York, Marcel Dekker, pp. 109–140.

Kabara, J. 1981. Food-grade chemicals for use in designing food preservative systems. J. Food Protect., 44, 633–647.

Kaloyereas, S., Crown, R.M., and McCleskey, C.S. 1961. Experiments on pres-ervation with a new ice containing glycol diformate and sorbic acid. Food Technol., 15, 361–364.

Karel, M. 1975a. Dehydration of foods. In *Principles of Food Science*. Part II. *Physical Principles of Food Preservation*. Edited by O.R. Fennema. New York, Marcel Dekker, pp. 309–357.

Karel, M. 1975b. Freeze dehydration of foods. In *Principles of Food Science*. Part II. *Physical Principles of Food Preservation*. Edited by O.R. Fennema. New York, Marcel Dekker, pp. 359–395.

Kato, N. 1981. Antimicrobial activity of fatty acids and their esters against a film-forming yeast in soy sauce. J. Food Safety, 3, 121–126.

Katz, S.E. 1983. Antibiotic residues and their significance. In *Antimicrobials in Foods*. Edited by A.L. Branen and P.M. Davidson. New York, Marcel Dekker, pp. 353–370.

Katz, B., and Branen, A.L. 1981. Inhibition of *Clostridium perfringens* by 1-monolaurin. Presented at the Institute of Food Technologists Annual Meeting. Atlanta, Georgia, June, 1981.

Kaul, A., Singh, J., and Kuila, R.K. 1979. Effect of potassium sorbate on the microbiological quality of butter. J. Food. Protect., 42, 656–657.

Kefford, J. 1948. Effect of ozone on microbial growth on beef muscle, and on the flavor of beef fat. J. Counc. Sci. Ind. Res., 21, 116–121.

Kemp, J.D., Langlois, B.E., Solomon, M.B., and Fox, J.D. 1979. Quality of boneless dry-cured ham produced with or without nitrite, netting or potassium sorbate. J. Food Sci., 44, 914–915.

Kim, C., Carpenter, C.E., Cornforth, D.P., Mettanant, O., and Mahoney, A.W. 1987. Effect of iron form, temperature, and inoculation with *Clostridium botulinum* spores on residual nitrite in meat and model systems. J. Food Sci., 52, 1464–1470.

Kimsey, H.R., Adams, D.M., and Kabara, J.J. 1981. Increased inactivation of bacterial spores at high temperatures in the presence of monoglycerides. J. Food Safety, 3, 69–82.

King, A.D., and Nagel, C.W. 1975. Influence of carbon dioxide upon the metabolism of *Pseudomonas aeruginosa*. J. Food Sci., 40, 362–366.

King, A.D., and Nagel, C.W. 1967. Growth inhibition of *Pseudomonas* by carbon dioxide. J. Food Sci., 32, 575–579.

Klaenhammer, T.R. 1988. Bacteriocins of lactic acid bacteria. Biochimie, 70, 337–349.

Klindworth, K.J., Davidson, P.M., Brekke, C.J., and Branen, A.L. 1979. Inhibition of *Clostridium perfringens* by butylated hydroxyanisole. J. Food Sci., 44, 564–567.

Kodicek, E. 1956. The effect of unsaturated fatty acids, of vitamin D and other sterols on gram-positive bacteria. In *Biochemical Problems of Lipids*. Edited by G. Popjak and E. LeBreton. London, Butterworths, pp. 401–406.

Kohler, A.R., Broquist, H.P., and Miller, W.H. 1954. Chlortetracycline and the control of poultry spoilage. Food Technol., 8, 19.

Kohler, A.R., Miller, W.H., and Broquist, H.P. 1955. Aureomycin chlortetracycline and the control of poultry spoilage. Food Technol., 9, 151–154.

Koser, S.A., and Skinner, W.W. 1922. Viability of the colon-typhoid group in carbonated water and carbonated beverages. J. Bacteriol., 7, 111–121.

Krieg, N.R., and Holt, J.G. 1984. *Bergy's Manual of Systematic Bacteriology*. Baltimore, Williams & Wilkins.

Krum, J.K., and Fellers, C.R. 1952. Clarification of wine by a sequestering agent. Food Technol., 6, 103–106.

Kulikovsky, A., Pankratz, H.S., and Sadoff, H.L. 1975. Ultrastructural and chemical changes in spores of *Bacillus cereus* after action of disinfectants. J. Appl. Bacteriol., 38, 39–46.

Kurytowicz, W.A. (ed.). 1976. *Antibiotics: A Critical Review*. Warsaw, Polish Medical Publishers.

Kuusi, T., and Löytömaki, M. 1972. On the effectiveness of EDTA in prolonging the shelf-life of fresh fish. Z. Lebensmittel-Untersuch Forsch., 149, 196–204.

Labots, H. 1977. Effect of nitrite on development of *Staphylococcus aureus* in fermented sausage. In *Proceedings of the Second International Symposium on Nitrite in Meat Products*. Edited by B.J. Tinbergen and B. Krol. Wageningen, Netherlands, Pudoc.

Lechowich, R.V., Brown, W.L., Deibel, R.H., and Somers, I.I. II. 1978. The role of nitrite in the production of canned cured meat products. Food Technol., 32, 45–58.

Lee, S.H., Cassens, R.G., and Sugiyama, H. 1978. Factors affecting inhibition of *Clostridium botulinum* in cured meats. J. Food Sci., 43, 1371–1374.

Lee, J.S., Willett, C.L., Robinson, S.M., and Sinnhuber, R.D. 1967. Comparative effects of chlortetracycline, freezing and γ-radiation on microbial populations of ocean perch. Appl. Microbiol., 15, 368–372.

Lennon, R.E. 1972. Chemicals in fish farming, what's cleared, what isn't. Fish Farming Ind., 3, 15.

Levin, R.E. 1967. The effectiveness of EDTA as a fish preservative. J. Milk Food Technol., 30, 277–283.

Levinskas, G.J., Ribelin, W.E., and Shaffer, C.B. 1966. Acute and chronic toxicity of pimaricin. Toxicol. Appl. Pharmacol., 8, 97–109.

Linko, R.R., and Kikkilä, O.E. 1959. Chemical preservatives in foodstuffs. III. Hexamethylenetetramine as mold inhibitor and the antagonistic action of amino acids. Maataloustieteellinen Aikakauskirja, 31, 162–173.

Lockett, M.F., and Natoff, I.L. 1960. A study of the toxicity of sulphite. I. J. Pharm. Pharmacol., 12, 488–496.

Lueck, E. 1980. *Antimicrobial Food Additives*. Berlin, Springer-Verlag.

Macintosh, F.C. 1945. The toxicity of diphenyl and o-phenyl-phenol. Analyst, 70, 334–335.

Magee, P.N., and Barnes, J.M. 1967. Carcinogenic nitrosocompounds. Adv. Cancer Res., 10, 163–246.

Mäkinen, K.K., and Söderling, E. 1981. Effect of xylitol on some food-spoilage microorganisms. J. Food Sci., 46, 950–951.

Marcy, J.A., et al. 1988. Effects of selected commercial phosphate products on the natural bacterial flora of a cooked meat system. J. Food Sci., 53, 391–393, 577.

Marletta, J., and Stumbo, C.R. 1970. Some effects of ethylene oxide on *Bacillus subtilis*. J. Food Sci., 35, 627–631.

Marth, E.H. 1966. Antibiotics in foods—naturally occurring, developed and added. Residue Rev., 12, 65–161.

Marth, E.H., et al. 1966. Degradation of potassium sorbate by *Penicillium* species. J. Dairy Sci., 49, 1197–1205.

Martoadiprawito, W., and Whitaker, J.R. 1963. Potassium sorbate inhibition of yeast alcohol dehydrogenase. Biochim. Biophys. Acta, 77, 536–544.

Matsuda, T. 1966. Review on recent nitrofuran derivatives used as food preservatives. J. Ferment. Technol., 44, 495–508.

Matthews, C., et al. 1956. *p*-Hydroxybenzoic acid esters as preservatives. II. Acute and chronic toxicity in dogs, rats, and mice. J. Am. Pharmaceut. Assoc. Sci. Ed., 45, 260–267.

Matz, S.A. 1972. Minor ingredients. In *Bakery Technology and Engineering*. 2nd Edition. Westport, AVI Publishing, pp. 149–164.

Mayr, G., and Kaemmerer, H. 1959. Fumigation with ethylene oxide. Food Manufact., 34, 169–170.

Mayr, G.E., and Suhr, H. 1972. Preservation and sterilization of pure and mixed spices. *Proceedings of the Conference on Spices*. London, Tropical Products Institute, pp. 201–207.

McIver, R., Noren, P., and Tatini, S.R. 1978. Influence of certain food preservatives on growth and production of enterotoxins by *Staphylococcus aureus*. Abst. Annu. Meet. Am. Soc. Microbiol., 1978, 187.

Medina, M., Gaya, P., and Nuñez, M. 1989. The lactoperoxidase system in ewe's milk: levels of lactoperoxidase and thiocyanate. Lett. Appl. Microbiol., 8, 147–149.

Melnick, D., and Luckmann, F.H. 1954. Sorbic acid as a fungistatic agent for foods. IV. Migration of sorbic acid from wrapper into cheese. Food Res., 19, 28–32.

Melnick, D., Luckmann, F.H., and Gooding, G.M. 1954a. Sorbic acid as a fungistatic agent for foods. V. Resistance of sorbic acid in cheese to oxidative deterioration. Food Res., 19, 33–43.

Melnick, D., Luckmann, F.H., and Gooding, G.M. 1954b. Sorbic acid as a fungistatic agent for foods. VI. Metabolic degradation of sorbic acid in cheese by molds and the mechanism of mold inhibition. Food Res., 19, 44–58.

Meneely, G.R., Tucker, R.G., Darby, W.J., and Auerbach, S.H. 1953. Chronic sodium chloride toxicity: Hypertension, renal and vascular lesions. Ann. Int. Med., 39, 991–998.

Merten, H.L., and Bachman, G.L. 1976. Glutaric acid: a potential food acidulant. J. Food Sci., 41, 463–464.

Morgan, J. 1864. On a new process of preserving meat. J. Soc. Arts, 12, 347–363.

Mossel, D.A.A. 1975. *Microbiology of Foods and Dairy Products*. Utrecht, Netherlands. The University of Utrecht, Faculty of Veterinary Medicine.

Mountney, G.J., and O'Malley, J. 1965. Acids as poultry meat preservatives. Poultry Sci., 44, 582–586.

Mukai, F., Hawryluck, I., and Shapiro, R. 1970. The mutagenic specificity of sodium bisulfite. Biochem. Biophys. Res. Comm., 39(5), 983–988.

Nagy, R. 1959. Application of ozone from sterilamp in control of mold, bacteria and odors. In *Ozone Chemistry and Technology*. Edited by H.A. Leedy. Adv. Chem. Ser., No. 21. American Chemical Society, Washington, D.C.

Natvig, H., Andersen, J., and Rasmussen, E.W. 1971. A contribution to the toxicological evaluation of hexamethylenetetramine. Food Cosmet. Toxicol., 9, 491–500.

Neidig, C.P., and Burrell, H. 1944. The esters of parahydroxybenzoic acid as preservatives. Drug. Cosmet. Ind., 54, 408–415.

Nes, I.F., and Eklund, T. 1983. The effect of parabens on DNA, RNA and protein synthesis in *Escherichia coli* and *Bacillus subtilis*. J. Appl. Bacteriol., 54, 237–242.

Newberne, P.M. 1979. Nitrite promotes lymphoma incidence in rats. Science, 204, 1079–1081.

Nieman, C. 1954. Influence of trace amounts of fatty acids on the growth of microorganisms. Bacteriol. Rev., 18, 147–163.

Njagi, G.D.E., and Gopalan, H.N.B. 1980. DNA and its precursors might interact with the food preservatives, sodium sulphite and sodium benzoate. Experientia, 36, 413–414.

Notermans, S., and Dufrenne, J. 1981. Effect of glycerol monolaurate on toxin production by *Clostridium botulinum* in meat slurry. J. Food Safety, 3, 83–88.

Nury, F.S., Miller, M.W., and Brekke, J.E. 1960. Preservative effect of some antimicrobial agents on high-moisture dried fruits. Food Technol., 14, 113–115.

Ogilvy, W.S., and Ayres, J.C. 1953. Post-mortem changes in stored meats. V. Effects of carbon dioxide on microbial growth on stored frankfurters and characteristics of some microorganisms isolated from them. Food. Res., 18, 121–130.

Ogilvy, W.S., and Ayres, J.C. 1951. Post-mortem changes in stored meats. II. The effect of atmosphere containing carbon dioxide in prolonging the storage life of cut-up chicken. Food Technol., 5, 97–102.

O'Leary, D.K., and Kralovec, R.D. 1941. Development of *B. mesentericus* in bread and control with calcium acid phosphate and calcium propionate. Cereal Chem., 18, 730–741.

Olson, J.C., Jr., and Macy, H. 1945. Observations on the use of propionate-treated parchment in inhibiting mold growth on the surface of butter. Science, 28, 701–710.

Ough, C.S. 1983. Dimethyl dicarbonate and diethyl dicarbonate. In *Antimicrobial in Foods*. Edited by A.L. Branen and P.M. Davidson. New York, Marcel Dekker, pp. 299–325.

Pappas, H.J., and Hall, L.A. 1952. Control of thermophilic bacteria. Food Technol., 6, 456–458.

Parekh, K.G., and Solberg, M. 1970. Comparative growth of *Clostridium perfringens* in carbon dioxide and nitrogen atmospheres. J. Food Sci., 35, 156–159.

Parker, M.S. 1969. Some effects of preservatives on the development of bacterial spores. J. Appl. Bacteriol., 32, 322–328.

Pearson, D. 1970. Effect on various spoilage values of the addition of sulphite and chlortetracycline to beef stored at 5°C. J. Food Technol., 5, 141–147.

Pederson, C.S., Albany, M.N., and Christensen, M.D. 1961. The growth of yeasts in grape juice stored at low temperature. IV. Fungistatic effects of organic acids. Appl. Microbiol., 9, 162–167.

Perry, G.A., and Lawrence, R.L. 1960. Preservative effect of sorbic acid on creamed cottage cheese. J. Agric. Food Chem., 8, 374–376.

Perry, G.A., Lawrence, R.L., and Melnick, D. 1964. Extension of poultry shelf-life by processing with sorbic acid. Food Technol., 18, 891–897.

Phillips, C.R. 1952. Relative resistance of bacterial spores and vegetative bacteria to disinfectants. Bacteriol. Rev., 16, 135–143.

Phillips, C.R., and Kaye, S. 1949. The sterilizing action of gaseous ethylene oxide. Am. J. Hyg., 50, 270–279.

Phillips, G.F., and Mundt, J.O. 1950. Sorbic acid as inhibitor of scum yeast in cucumber fermentations. Food Technol., 4, 291–293.

Pierson, M.D., Ivey, F.J., Smoot, L.A., and van Tassel, K.R. 1979a. Potassium sorbate inhibition of *Clostridium botulinum* in bacon. Abstr. Annu. Meet. Am. Soc. Microbiol., 1979, 214.

Pierson, M.D., Robach, M.C., van Tassel, K.R., and Smoot, L.A. 1979b. Sodium nitrite and potassium sorbate inhibition of *Clostridium botulinum* as influenced by storage temperature variation. Presented at the Institute of Food Technologists Annual Meeting. St. Louis, Missouri, June, 1979.

Pierson, M.D., Smoot, L.A., and Stern, N.J. 1979c. Effect of potassium sorbate on growth of *Staphylococcus aureus* in bacon. J. Food Protect., 42, 302–304.

Pierson, M.D., Smoot, L.A., and van Tassel, K.R. 1980. Inhibition of *Salmonella typhimurium* and *Staphylococcus aureus* by butylated hydroxyanisole and the propyl ester of p-hydroxybenzoic acid. J. Food Protect., 43, 191–194.

Pinedo, R., Pilkington, D., and Foegeding, P. 1987. KCl in dry cured hams: effect on trichinae devitilization and chemical and physical properties. J. Food Sci., 52, 554–557, 563.

Pivnick, H., and Chang, P.C. 1973. Perigo effect in pork. In *Proceedings of the International Symposium on Nitrite in Meat Products*. Edited by B. Krol and B.J. Tinbergen. Wageningen, Netherlands, Pudoc.

Pivnick, H., Johnston, M.A., Thacker, C., and Loynes, R. 1970. Effect of nitrite on destruction and germination of *Clostridium botulinum* and putrefactive anaerobes PA 3679 and 3679h in meat and in butter. Can. Inst. Food Technol. J., 3, 103–109.

Poole, G., and Malin, B. 1964. Some aspects of the action of tylosin on *Clostridium* species PA 3679. J. Food Sci., 29, 475.

Post, F.J., Krishanmurty, G.B., and Flanagan, M.D. 1963. Influence of sodium hexametaphosphate on selected bacteria. Appl. Microbiol., 11, 430–435.

Prescott, S.C., and Dunn, C.G. 1959. *Industrial microbiology*. 3rd Edition. New York, McGraw-Hill.

Price, J.F., and Stevenson, K.E. 1979. Effects of sorbate and nitrite in bacon on color, flavor, and *Clostridium botulinum* toxigenesis. Presented at the Institute of Food Technologists Annual Meeting. St. Louis, Missouri, June 1979.

Raccach, M. 1984. The antimicrobial activity of phenolic antioxidants in foods: a review. J. Food Safety, 6, 141–170.

Raccach, M., and Henningsen, E.C. 1982. Antibacterial effect of tertiary butylhydroquinone against two genera of gram-positive cocci. J. Food Sci., 47, 106–109.

Raevuori, M. 1976. Effect of sorbic acid and potassium sorbate on growth of *Bacillus cereus* and *Bacillus subtilis* in rice filling of Karelian pastry. Eur. J. Appl. Microbiol., 2, 205–213.

Rahn, O., and Conn, J.E. 1944. Effect of increase in acidity on antiseptic efficiency. Ind. Eng. Chem., 36, 185–187.

Rao, G.K., Malathi, M.A., and Vijayaghavan, P.K. 1966. Preservation and packaging in Indian foods. II. Storage studies on preserved chapaties. Food Technol., 20, 1070–1073.

Rayman, M.K., Aris, B., and Hurst, A. 1981. Nisin: a possible alternative or adjunct to nitrite in the preservation of meats. Appl. Environ. Microbiol., 41, 375–380.

Reiss, J. 1976. Prevention of the formation of mycotoxins in whole wheat bread by citric acid and lactic acid (mycotoxins in foodstuffs, IX). Experientia, 32, 168–169.

Riha, W.E., Jr., and Solberg, M. 1975a. Clostridium perfringens inhibition by sodium nitrite as a function of pH, inoculum size and heat. J. Food Sci., 40, 439–442.

Riha, W.E., Jr., and Solberg, M. 1975b. Clostridium perfringens growth in a nitrite-containing defined medium sterilized by heat of filtration. J. Food Sci., 40, 443–445.

Rizk, S.S., and Isshak, Y.M. 1974. Thiabendazole as a post harvest disinfectant for citrus fruits. Agric. Res. Rev., 52, 39–46.

Robach, M.C. 1979a. Influence of potassium sorbate on growth of Pseudomonas putrefaciens. J. Food Protect., 42, 312–313.

Robach, M.C. 1979b. Interaction of salt, potassium sorbate and temperature on the outgrowth of Clostridium sporogenes (PA 3679) spores in a pre-reduced medium. Presented at the Institute of Food Technologists Annual Meeting. St. Louis, Missouri, June, 1979.

Robach, M.C. 1978. Effect of potassium sorbate on the growth of Pseudomonas fluorescens. J. Food Sci., 43, 1886–1887.

Robach, M.C., and Hickey, C.S. 1978. Inhibition of Vibrio parahaemolyticus by sorbic acid in crab meat and flounder homogenates. J. Food Protect., 41, 699–702.

Robach, M.C., Hickey, C.S., and To, E.C. 1981. Antimicrobial effects of monolaurin and sorbic acid. Presented at the Institute of Food Technologists Annual Meeting. Atlanta, Georgia, June, 1981.

Robach, M.C., and Ivey, F.J. 1978. Antimicrobial efficacy of potassium sorbate dip on freshly processed poultry. J. Food Protect., 41, 284–288.

Robach, M.C., and Pierson, M.D. 1978. Influence of para-hydroxybenzoic acid esters on the growth and toxin production of Clostridium botulinum 10755A. J. Food Sci., 43, 787–789, 792.

Robach, M.C., Smoot, L.A., and Pierson, M.D. 1977. Inhibition of Vibrio parahaemolyticus 04:K11 by butylated hydroxyanisole. J. Food Protect., 40, 549–551.

Robach, M.C., and Stateler, C.L. 1980. Inhibition of Staphylococcus aureus by potassium sorbate in combination with sodium chloride, tertiary butylhydroquinone, butylated hydroxyanisole or ethylenediamine tetraacetic acid. J. Food Protect., 43, 208–211.

Roberts, T.A. 1989. Combinations of antimicrobials and processing methods. Food Technol., 43(1), 156–163.

Roberts, T.A. 1975. The microbial role of nitrite and nitrate. J. Sci. Food Agric., 26, 1755–1760.

Roberts, A.C., and McWeeny, D.J. 1972. The uses of sulfur dioxide in the food industry. A review. J. Food Technol., 7, 221–238.

Robinson, H.J., Phares, H.F., and Graessle, O.E. 1964. Antimycotic properties of thiabendazole. J. Invest. Dermatol., 42, 479–482.

Robinson, H.J., Stoerk, H.C., and Graessle, O.E. 1965. Studies on the toxicologic and pharmacologic properties of thiabendazole. Toxicol. Appl. Pharmacol., 7, 53–63.

Ronning, I.E., and Frank, H.A. 1988. Growth response of Putrefactive Anaerobe 3679 to combinations of potassium sorbate and some common curing ingredients (sucros, salt, and nitrite), and to non-inhibiting levels of sorbic acid. J. Food Protect., 51, 651–654.

Ronning, I.E., and Frank, H.A. 1987. Growth inhibition of Putrefactive Anaerobe 3679 caused by stringent-type response induced by protonophoric activity of sorbic acid. Appl. Environ. Microbiol., 53, 1020–1027.

Rosenkranz, H.S. 1973. Sodium hypochlorite and sodium perborate; preferential inhibitors of DNA polymerase-deficient bacteria. Mutat. Res., 21, 171–174.

Roth, N.G., and Halvorson, H.O. 1952. The effect of oxidative rancidity in unsaturated fatty acids on the germination of bacterial spores. J. Bacteriol., 63, 429–435.

Rusul, G., and Marth, E.H. 1988a. Food additives and plant components control growth and aflatoxin production by toxigenic aspergilli: a review. Mycopathologia, 101, 13–23.

Rusul, G., and Marth, E.H. 1988b. Growth and aflatoxin production by Aspergillus parasiticus in a medium at different pH values and with or without pimaricin. Z. Lebensm. Unters Forsch., 187, 436–439.

Rusul, G., El-Gazzar, F.E., and Marth, E.H. 1987. Growth and aflatoxin production by Aspergillus parasiticus NRRL 2999 in the presence of acetic or propionic acid and at different pH values. J. Food Protect., 50, 909–914.

Saitanu, K., and Lund, E. 1975. Inactivation of enterovirus by glutaraldehyde. Appl. Microbiol., 29, 571–574.

Salunkhe, D.K. 1955. Sorbic acid as a preservative for apple juice. Food Technol., 9, 590.

Sams, W.M., Jr., and Carroll, N.V. 1966. Prediction and demonstration of iron chelating ability of sugars. Nature, 212, 404–405.

Sanders, T.H., Davis, N.D., and Diener, U.L. 1968. Effect of carbon dioxide, temperature and relative humidity on production of aflatoxin in peanuts. J. Am. Oil. Chem. Soc., 45, 683–685.

Sato, T., Izaki, K., and Takahashi, H. 1972. Recovery of cells of Escherichia coli from injury induced by sodium chloride. J. Gen. Appl. Microbiol., 18, 307–317.

Sauer, F. 1977. Control of yeasts and molds with preservatives. Food Technol., 31(2), 62–65.

Sauter, E.A., Kemp, J.D., and Langlois, B.E. 1977. Effect of nitrite and erythorbate on recovery of Clostridium perfringens spores in cured pork. J. Food Sci., 42, 1678–1679.

Schack, W.R., and Taylor, R.E. 1963. Extending shelf life of cured meats. Canadian Patent No. 674,171.

Schmidt, C.F. 1964. Spores of Clostridium botulinum: formation, resistance, germination. In Botulism, Proceedings of a Symposium. Edited by K.H. Lewis and K. Cassel. U.S. Department of Health, Education, and Welfare, Public Health Service, No. 999-FP-1. Washington, D.C., p. 69.

Scott, D.B.M., and Lesher, E.C. 1963. Effect of ozone on survival and permeability of Escherichia coli. J. Bacteriol., 85, 567–576.

Scott, V.N., and Taylor, S.L. 1981a. Effect of nisin on the outgrowth of Clostridium botulinum spores. J. Food Sci., 46, 117–120, 126.

Scott, V.N., and Taylor, S.L. 1981b. Temperature, pH and spore load effects on the ability of nisin to prevent the outgrowth of Clostridium botulinum spores. J. Food Sci., 46, 121–126.

Scott, W.J. 1957. Water relations of food spoilage microorganisms. Adv. Food Res., 7, 83–127.

Sebranek, J.G., and Cassens, R.G. 1973. Nitrosamines: a review. J. Milk Food Technol., 36, 76–91.

Seevers, M.H., et al. 1950. Dehydroacetic acid (DHA). II. General pharmacology and mechanism of action. J. Pharmacol. Exp. Ther., 99, 69–83.

Segmiller, J.L., Xezones, H., and Hutchings, I.J. 1965. The efficacy of nisin and tylosin lactate in selected heat-sterilized food products. J. Food Sci., 30, 166–171.

Seiler, D.A.L. 1964. Factors affecting the use of mould inhibitors in bread and cake. In Microbial Inhibitors in Food. Edited by N. Molin. Stockholm, Almqvist and Wiksell, pp. 211–220.

Shank, J.L., Silliker, J.H., and Harper, R.H. 1962. The effect of nitric oxide on bacteria. Appl. Microbiol., 10, 185–189.

Shapero, M., Nelson, D.A., and Labuza, T.P. 1978. Ethanol inhibition of Staphylococcus aureus at limited water activity. J. Food Sci., 43, 1467–1469.

Shibasaki, I. 1970. Antibacterial activity of tylosin on Hiochi-bacteria. J. Ferment. Technol., 48, 110–115.

Shih, C.N., and Marth, E.H. 1973. Aflatoxin produced by Aspergillus parasiticus when incubated in the presence of different gasses. J. Milk Food Technol., 36, 421–425.

Shiralkar, N.D., and Rege, D.V. 1978. Mechanism of action of p-hydroxybenzoates. Indian Food Packer, 32, 34–41.

Shtenberg, A.J., and Ignat'ev, A.D. 1970. Toxicological evaluation of some combinations of food preservatives. Food Cosmet. Toxicol., 8, 369–380.

Silliker, J.H. 1959.. The effect of curing salts on bacterial spores. In Proceedings of the Meat Industry Research Conference. American Meat Institute Foundation, Washington, D.C., pp. 51–60.

Silliker, J.H., et al. 1977. Preservation of refrigerated meats with controlled atmospheres: treatment and post-treatment effects of carbon dioxide on pork and beef. Meat Sci., 1, 195–204.

Silliker, J.H., Greenberg, R.A., and Schack, W.R. 1958. Effect of individual curing ingredients on the shelf stability of canned comminuted meats. Food Technol., 12, 551–554.

Sink, J.D., and Hsu, L.A. 1977. Chemical effects of smoke processing on frankfurter manufacture and storage characteristics. J. Food Sci., 42, 1489–1491.

Skinner, F.A., and Hugo, W.B. (eds.). 1976. Inhibition and Inactivation of Vegetative Microbes. London, Academic Press.

Smith, D.P., and Rollin, N. 1954. Sorbic acid as a fungistatic agent for foods. VII. Effectiveness of sorbic acid in protecting cheese. Food Res., 19, 59–65.

Smith, J.L., and Palumbo, S.A. 1981. Microorganisms as food additives. J. Food Protect., 44, 936–955.

Smith, J.L., and Palumbo, S.A. 1980. Inhibition of aerobic and anaerobic growth of Staphylococcus aureus in a model sausage system. J. Food Safety, 2, 221–233.

Smith, Q.J., and Brown, K.L. 1980. The resistance of dry spores of Bacillus subtilis var. globigii (NCIB 8058) to solutions of hydrogen peroxide in relation to aseptic packaging. J. Food Technol., 15, 169–179.

Smith, W.H. 1963. The use of carbon dioxide in the transport and storage of fruits and vegetables. Adv. Food Res., 12, 96–118.

Smoot, L.A., and Pierson, M.D. 1981. Mechanisms of sorbate inhibition of Bacillus cereus and Clostridium botulinum 62A spore germination. Appl. Environ. Microbiol., 42, 477–483.

Smyth, H.F., et al. 1969. Range-finding toxicity data: List VII. Am. Ind. Hyg. Assoc. J., 30, 470–476.

Sofos, J.N. 1983. Antimicrobial effects of sodium and other ions in foods: a review. J. Food Safety, 6, 45–78.

Sofos, J.N., and Busta, F.F. 1983. Sorbates. In *Antimicrobials in Foods*. Edited by A.L. Branen and P.M. Davidson. New York, Marcel Dekker, pp. 141–175.

Sofos, J.N., and Busta, F.F. 1981. Antimicrobial activity of sorbate. J. Food Protect., 44, 614–622.

Sofos, J.N., and Busta, F.F. 1980. Alternatives to the use of nitrite as an antibotulinal agent. Food Technol., 34(5), 244–251.

Sofos, J.N., Busta, F.F., and Allen, C.E. 1980a. Influence of pH on *Clostridium botulinum* control by sodium nitrite and sorbic acid in chicken emulsions. J. Food. Sci., 45, 7–12.

Sofos, J.N., et al. 1980b. Effects of various concentrations of sodium nitrite and potassium sorbate on *Clostridium botulinum* toxin production in commercially prepared bacon. J. Food. Sci., 45, 1245–1292.

Sofos, J.N., Busta, F.F., and Allen, C.E. 1979a. Sodium nitrite and sorbic acid effects on *Clostridium botulinum* spore germination and total microbial growth in chicken frankfurter emulsions during temperature abuse. Appl. Environ. Microbiol., 37, 1103–1109.

Sofos, J.N., Busta, F.F., and Allen, C.E. 1979b. Botulism control by nitrite and sorbate in cured meats: A review. J. Food Protect., 42, 739–770.

Sofos, J.N., Busta, F.F., and Allen C.E. 1979c. *Clostridium botulinum* control by sodium nitrite and sorbic acid in various meat and soy protein formulations. J. Food Sci., 44, 1662–1667, 1671.

Sofos, J.N., Busta, F.F., Bhothipaksa, K., and Allen, C.E. 1979d. Sodium nitrite and sorbic acid effects on *Clostridium botulinum* toxin formation in chicken frankfurter-type emulsions. J. Food Sci., 44, 668–675.

Somers, E.B., and Taylor, S.L. 1987. Antibotulinal effectiveness of nisin in pasteurized process cheese spreads. J. Food Protect., 50, 842–848. (Also see J. Food Protect., 52, 525.)

Spector, W.S. 1956. *Handbook of Toxicology*. Volume 1. Philadelphia, W.B. Saunders, pp. 262–263.

Spencer, H.C., Rowe, V.K., and McCollister, D.D. 1950. Dehydroacetic acid (DHA). I. Acute and chronic toxicity. J. Pharmacol. Exp. Ther., 99, 57–68.

Struyk, A.P., et al. 1957–1958. Pimaricin, a new antifungal antibiotic. Antibiot. Annu., 1957–1958, 878–885.

Sugiyama, T., Goto, K., and Uenaka, H. 1975. Acute cytogenetic effect of 2-(2-furyl)-3-(5-nitro-2-furyl)-acrylamide (AF-2, a food preservative) on rat bone marrow cells *in vivo*. Mutat. Res., 31, 241–246.

Suzuki, M., Okazaki, M., and Shibasaki, I. 1970. Mode of action of tylosin. J. Ferment. Technol., 48, 525–532.

Sweet, C.W. 1975. Additive composition for reduced particle size meats in the curing thereof. U.S. Patent No. 3,899,600.

Takayama, S., and Kuwabara, N. 1977. The production of skeletal muscle atrophy and mammary tumors in rats by feeding 2-(2-furyl)-3-(5-nitro-2 furyl) acrylamide. Toxicol. Lett., 1, 11–16.

Tanner, F.W. 1944. *The Microbiology of Foods*. 2nd Edition. Champaign, IL, Garrard Press.

Tarr, H.L.A. 1942. The action of nitrites on bacteria. Further experiments. J. Fish Res. Board, Canada, 6, 74–89.

Tarr, H.L.A. 1941a. The action of nitrites on bacteria. J. Fish. Res. Board, Canada, 5, 265–275.

Tarr, H.L.A. 1941b. Bacteriostatic action of nitrites. Nature, 147, 417–418.

Tarr, H.L.A., Boyd, J.W., and Bissett, H.M. 1954. Experimental preservation of fish and beef with antibiotics. J. Agric. Food Chem., 2, 372–375.

Tatini, S.R., Lee, R.Y., McCall, W.A., and Hill, W.M. 1976. Growth of *Staphylococcus aureus* and production of enterotoxins in pepperoni. J. Food Sci., 41, 223–225.

Tazima, Y., Kada, T., and Murakami, A. 1975. Mutagenicity of nitrofuran derivatives, including furylfuramide, a food preservative. Mutat. Res., 32, 55–80.

Thompson, J.E., Banwart, G.J., Sanders, D.H., and Murcuri, A.J. 1967. Effect of chlorine, antibiotics, propiolactone, acids and washing on *Salmonella typhimurium* on eviscerated fryer chickens. Poultry Sci., 46, 146–151.

Til, H.P., Feron, V.J., and deGroot, A.P. 1972. The toxicity of sulphite. II. Short- and long-term feeding studies in pigs. Food Cosmet. Toxicol., 10, 463–473.

Toledo, R.T., Escher, F.E., and Ayres, J.C. 1973. Sporicidal properties of hydrogen peroxide against food spoilage organisms. Appl. Microbiol., 26, 592–597.

Tomkins, R.G. 1932. The inhibition of the growth of meat-attacking fungi by carbon dioxide. J. Soc. Chem. Ind., 51, 261T–264T.

Tompkin, R.B. 1983. Nitrite. In *Antimicrobials in Foods*. Edited by A.L. Branen and P.M. Davidson. New York, Marcel Dekker, pp. 205–256.

Tompkin, R.B. 1978. The role and mechanism of the inhibition of *C. botulinum* by nitrite—is a replacement available? In *Proceedings of the 31st Annual Reciprocal Meat Conference*, June 18–22. National Livestock and Meat Board, Chicago, pp. 135–147.

Tompkin, R.B., Christiansen, L.N., and Shaparis, A.B. 1980. Antibotulinal efficacy of sulfur dioxide in meat. Appl. Environ. Microbiol., 39, 1096–1099.

Tompkin, R.B., Christiansen, L.N., and Shaparis, A.B. 1979a. Iron and the antibotulinal efficacy of nitrite. Appl. Environ. Microbiol., 37, 351–353.

Tompkin, R.B., Christiansen, L.N., and Shaparis, A.B. 1979b. Isoascorbate levels and botulinal inhibition in perishable canned cured meat. J. Food Sci., 44, 1147–1149.

Tompkin, R.B., Christiansen, L.N., and Shaparis, A.B. 1978a. Antibotulinal role of isoascorbate in cured meat. J. Food Sci., 43, 1368–1370.

Tompkin, R.B., Christiansen, L.N., and Shaparis, A.B. 1978b. The effect of iron on botulinal inhibition in perishable canned cured meat. J. Food Technol., 13, 521–527.

Tompkin, R.B., Christiansen, L.N., and Shaparis, A.B. 1978c. Enhancing nitrite inhibition of *Clostridium botulinum* with isoascorbate in perishable canned cured meat. Appl. Environ. Microbiol., 35, 59–61.

Tompkin, R.B., Christiansen, L.N., Shaparis, A.B., and Bolin, H. 1974. Effects of potassium sorbate on salmonellas, *Staphylococcus aureus*, *Clostridium perfringens*, and *Clostridium botulinum* in cooked, uncured sausage. Appl. Microbiol., 28, 262–264.

Tompkins, R.G. 1932. The inhibition of the growth of meat-attacking fungi by carbon dioxide. J. Soc. Chem. Ind., 51., 261T–264T.

Torricelli, A. 1959. Sterilization of empty containers for food industry. In *Ozone Chemistry and Technology*. Edited by H.A. Leedy. Adv. Chem. Ser. No. 21. Washington, D.C., American Chemical Society.

Toth, L.Z.J. 1959. The sterilization effect of ethylene oxide vapor on different microorganisms. Arch Mikrobiol., 32, 409–410.

Tracor-Jitco, Inc. 1974. Scientific literature reviews on generally recognized as safe (GRAS) food ingredients—formic acid and derivatives. PB-228 558. National Technical Information Service, U.S. Dept. of Commerce, Springfield, MA.

Tramer, J. 1964. The inhibitory action of nisin on *Bacillus stearothermophilus*. Proc. 4th Int. Symp. Food Microbiol. Göteborg, Sweden, pp. 25–33.

Troller, J.A. 1965. Catalase inhibition as a possible mechanism of the fungistatic action of sorbic acid. Can. J. Microbiol., 11, 611–617.

Troller, J.A., and Olsen, R.A. 1967. Derivatives of sorbic acid as food preservatives. J. Food Sci., 32, 228–231.

Trujillo, R., and David, T.J. 1972. Sporostatic and sporocidal properties of aqueous formaldehyde. Appl. Microbiol., 26, 618–622.

Trujillo, R., and Laible, N. 1970. Reversible inhibition of spore germination by alcohols. Appl. Microbiol., 20, 620–623.

United States Department of Agriculture. 1989. Additional methods for destroying trichinae. Fed. Reg., 54, 15946–15951.

United States Department of Agriculture. 1979. Acid producing microorganisms in meat products for nitrite dissipation. Fed. Reg., 44, 9372–9373.

Vaughn, R.H. 1951. The microbiology of dehydrated vegetables. Food Res., 16, 429–438.

Von Oettingen, W.F. 1959. The aliphatic acids and their esters—toxicity and potential dangers. The saturated monobasic aliphatic acids and their esters. Formic acid and esters. Am. Med. Assoc. Arch. Ind. Health, 20, 517–531.

Von Schelhorn, M. 1951. Control of microorganisms causing spoilage in fruit and vegetable products. Adv. Food Res., 3, 429–482.

Wada, S., et al. 1975. The preservative effects of sorbic acid for fish sausage. J. Food Hyg. Soc. Jap., 17, 95–100.

Wagner, M.K., and Moberg, L.G. 1989. Present and future use of traditional antimicrobials. Food Technol., 43(1), 143–147, 155.

Walker, R. 1985. Sulphiting agents in foods: some risk/benefit considerations. Food Addit. Contam., 2, 5–24.

Walker, H.W. 1977. Spoilage of food by yeast. Food Technol., 31(2), 57–61, 65.

Walker, G.C., and Harmon, L.G. 1965. Hydrogen peroxide as a bactericide for *Staphylococcus* in cheese milk. J. Milk Food Technol., 28, 36–40.

Ward, M.S., and Ward, B.Q. 1967. Initial evaluation of the effect of butylated hydroxytoluene upon *Salmonella seftenberg*. Poultry Sci., 46, 1601–1603.

Ward, R.L., and Ashley, C.S. 1980. Comparative study on the mechanisms of rotavirus inactivation by sodium dodecyl sulfate and ethylenediaminetetraacetic acid. Appl. Microbiol., 39, 1148–1153.

Warth, A.D. 1988. Effect of benzoic acid on growth yield of yeasts differing in their resistance to preservatives. Appl. Environ. Microbiol., 54, 2091–2095.

Warth, A.D. 1977. Mechanism of resistance of *Saccharomyces bailii* to benzoic, sorbic and other weak acids used as food preservatives. J. Appl. Bacteriol., 43, 215–230.

Weaver, E.A., Robinson, J.F., and Hills, C.H. 1957. Preservation of apple cider with sodium sorbate. Food Technol., 11, 667–669.

West, H.D. 1940. Evidence for the detoxification of diphenyl through a sulfur mechanism. Proc. Soc. Exp. Biol. Med., 43, 373–375.

Whelton, R., Phaff, H.J., Mark, E.M., and Fisher, C.D. 1946. Control of microbiological food spoilage by fumigation with epoxides. Food Ind., 18, 23–25, 174–176, 318–319.

Winarno, F.G., and Stumbo, C.R. 1971. Mode of action of ethylene oxide on spores of *Clostridium botulinum* 62A. J. Food Sci., 36, 892–895.

Winarno, F.G., Stumbo, C.R., and Hayes, K.M. 1971. Effect of EDTA on the germination and outgrowth from spores of *Clostridium botulinum* 62A. J. Food Sci., 36, 781–785.

Windmueller, H.G., Ackerman, C.J., Bakerman, H., and Mickelson, O. 1959.

Reaction of ethylene oxide with nicotinamide and nicotinic acid. J. Biol. Chem., *234*, 889–894.

Wlodkowski, T.J., and Rosenkranz, H.S. 1975. Mutagenicity of sodium hypochlorite for *Salmonella typhimurium*. Mutat. Res., *31*, 39–42.

Woolford, M.K. 1975. Microbiological screening of food preservatives, cold sterilants, and specific antimicrobial agents as potential silage additives. J. Sci. Food Agric., *26*, 229–237.

Wong, H-C., and Chen, Y-L. 1988. Effects of lactic acid bacteria and organic acids on growth and germination of *Bacillus cereus*. Appl. Environ. Microbiol., *54*, 2179–2184.

Wrenshall, C.L. 1959. Antibiotics in food preservation. In *Antibiotics. Their Chemistry and Non-Medical Uses.* Edited by H.S. Goldberg. Princeton, D. Van Nostrand, pp. 449–527.

Wyatt, L.R., and Waites, W.M. 1975. The effect of chlorine on spores of *Clostridium bifermentans, Bacillus subtilis* and *Bacillus cereus*. J. Gen. Microbiol., *89*, 337–344.

Wyss, D. 1948. Microbial inhibition by food preservatives. Adv. Food Res., *1*, 373–393.

Yarbrough, J.M., Rake, J.B., and Eagon, R.G. 1980. Bacterial inhibition of nitrite: inhibition of active transport, but not of group translocation, and of intracellular enzymes. Appl. Environ. Microbiol., *39*, 831–834.

York, G.K., and Vaughn, R.H. 1964. Mechanisms in the inhibition of microorganisms by sorbic acid. J. Bacteriol., *88*, 411–417.

York, G.K., and Vaughn, R.H. 1955. Resistance of *Clostridium parabotulinum* to sorbic acid. Food Res., *20*, 60–65.

York, G.K., and Vaughn, R.H. 1954. Use of sorbic acid enrichment media for species of *Clostridium*. J. Bacteriol., *68*, 739–744.

Zaika, L.L. 1988. Spices and herbs: their antimicrobial activity and its determination. J. Food Safety, *9*, 97–118.

CHAPTER 48

ASEPTIC PACKAGING

B. von Bockelmann

The goal of aseptic packaging is to maintain the high microbiologic quality of a commercially sterile product. Consequently, prior to the aseptic packaging operation, the food product needs to be sterilized, i.e., subjected to a suitable in-flow sterilization process: a UHT (ultra high temperature) treatment. Furthermore, the product rendered commercially sterile in the product sterilizer must be transferred to an aseptic filler without any re-infection, i.e., under aseptic conditions.

The actual aseptic filling operation has been defined as sterilization of the packaging material or container food contact surface, filling of a commercially sterile product in a sterile environment, and production of containers that are tight enough to prevent reinfection, i.e., that are hermetically sealed (Hallström, 1979; B. von Bockelmann and I. von Bockelmann, 1986; Food and Drug Administration, 1980) (Fig. 48–1).

The term "aseptic" implies the absence or exclusion of any unwanted organisms from the product, package, or other specific areas (Carlson, 1980); the term "hermetic" is used to indicate suitable mechanical properties to exclude the entrance of bacteria (microorganisms) into a package or more stringently to prevent the passage of microorganisms and gas or water vapor into or from the package (Food and Drug Administration, 1980).

UHT-treated and aseptically packaged products are commercially sterile and intended for longer periods (months) of unrefrigerated storage. Consequently, the packaging operation as such must be aseptic and the packaging material must maintain the following aspects of the packaged product throughout its intended shelf life:

Microbiologic integrity
Nutritional value
Flavor

To this end, protection against light, oxygen penetration, or both must be provided for.

The microbiologic performance level (unsterility rate) of a plant producing long-life products is controversial

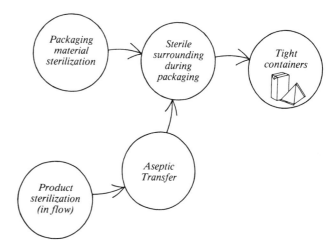

Fig. 48–1. Principle of UHT-processing—aseptic packaging.

(von Bockelmann, B., 1985; von Bockelmann and von Bockelmann, 1986). As stated above, aseptic packaging procedures should maintain the high level of microbiologic quality of the sterilized product, i.e., the state of commercial sterility. It needs to be stressed that unsterile packages in an aseptic operation (product sterilization, aseptic transfer, aseptic packaging) originate not only from the packaging operation but also from the product sterilization process as well as from any reinfection of the properly sterilized product on its way from sterilizer to packaging machine (von Bockelmann, I., 1985). The performance level of an aseptic plant must be looked on as a performance level of the entire process rather than that of a single component of the production line (Cerf and Brissende, 1981). This opinion is questioned (Burton, 1988): "It can be generally assumed that the spoilage rate of a combined UHT-aseptic filling system is determined by the performance of the aseptic filler." Even though the aseptic filling operation is usually technically more complicated and complex than the actual process of product sterilization and the aseptic transfer system, the ac-

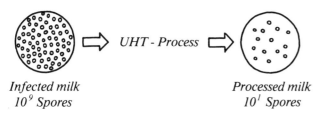

Infected milk
10^9 *Spores*

Processed milk
10^1 *Spores*

Fig. 48–2. Principle of sterilizing effect.

tual defective rate of a long-life product production line is determined by (1) the sterilization efficiency of the product sterilizer, (2) the microbial load of the product fed into the sterilizer, (3) cleaning and plant sterilization procedures applied, (4) efficiency of the packaging material sterilization process, (5) microbial load on the packaging material food contact surface, (6) cleaning and filler-sterilization procedures, (7) service and maintenance of the plant, and (8) operational care (von Bockelmann, I., 1985).

Two more points should be added to the list of factors contributing to the defective rate in a long-life product production line: (9) complexity of the total installation, and (10) the physical arrangement and connection of the different parts in the installation (e.g., piping and valves).

The resulting picture is complex, and the situation will be different from production plant to production plant. During the planning stage of a long-life product production line, careful attention should be paid to the above points in order to create the best precondition possible. Often unnecessary defective rates are already designed into such production lines.

The state of commercial sterility has been defined as "the absence of microorganisms capable of reproducing in the food under normal nonrefrigerated conditions of storage and distribution" (Food and Drug Administration, 1980). This definition implies the *total* absence of possible spoilage microorganisms and thus becomes absolute. However, the absolute absence of all microorganisms cannot be achieved (Heim and Jud, 1973). Statements like "the destruction of all microorganisms" should be avoided (Cerf and Brissende, 1981). The logarithmic order of death makes it impossible to destroy all microorganisms (Cerny, 1978; Kelsey, 1974a).

Sterilization processes should not be looked at in absolute terms but should rather be regarded as procedures achieving a certain process-specific *reduction* in the number of possible product spoilage organisms. This is accounted for by introducing the term "sterilizing effect" as a means to describe a sterilization process. The "sterilizing effect" has been defined as the log proportion of surviving microorganisms (Fig. 48–2).

Consequently, "maximal acceptable defective rates" have been discussed for this technology. A maximal acceptable defective rate of 1:1000 (0.1%) has been suggested (Cerf and Brissende, 1981; Dtsch. Molk.-Ztg., 1982; Rippen, 1970; Samuelsson and Kristiansen, 1970; Swartling and Lindgren, 1962). An overall spoilage level of 1:5000 (0.02%) should be attainable in commercial

practice (Hermsom, 1985). The general rejection rate of aseptically packaged products was estimated to be 1:10,000 (0.01%) (Lembke, 1972). Even a "sterile guarantee" of 1:10,000 (0.01%) has been offered for one aseptic packaging system (Lütkemeyer, 1983). As indicated above, the actual defective rate achieved depends on a large number of factors. As far as maximal acceptable defective rates are concerned, the following more general classification can be made (von Bockelmann, B., 1987):

1:	100:	too high: unacceptable
1:	1000:	for some products realistic
1:	10,000:	ambitious
1:	100,000:	difficult to achieve
1:	1,000,000:	impossible, theoretical limit has been passed

Maximal acceptable defective rates cannot be stated generally. What is acceptable depends on a number of factors, such as (1) legislation, (2) kind of product in question, (3) consumer group, (4) quality policy of the commercial processor, (5) competitive situation. Consequently, such maximum acceptable defective rates have to be decided on from case to case.

It should be underlined that the above stated defective rates relate to the result achieved by a *total* production line and not by single components. Especially when low defective rates are being discussed, i.e., anything at about 1:1000 or lower, it becomes impossible to determine the contribution of individual components. Furthermore, from a practical point of view, the overall performance of a line is of interest.

MICROBIOLOGIC ASPECTS OF ASEPTIC PACKAGING

With regard to the sterilization of the container food-contact surface, the following equation has been developed to calculate the risk of defectives originating from this source (Cerf and Brissende, 1981):

$$R = C_0 S \times 10^{-\frac{t}{D}}$$

where R = risk, C_0 = number of the most resistant organisms per cm^2, S = 2 cm of the food-contact area, t = time of the sterilization process, and D = decimal reduction time of the most resistant organisms. A somewhat different equation permits the calculation of the defective rate resulting from the sterilization of the packaging material food contact surface (Reuter, 1987):

$$F_s = \frac{N}{R} \times A$$

where F_s = unsterility rate, R = decimal reduction rate of the sterilization process, N = number of microorganisms per area unit (m^2), and A = the area of the food contact surface in square meters.

The risk or unsterility rate resulting from the packaging material food-contact surface sterilization process becomes strictly proportional to the initial contamination level, and the area of the unit container and depends on the efficiency of the lethal treatment.

Prior to the start of an aseptic packaging operation, the filler must be sterilized. Sterilization of the packaging equipment involves surface sterilization procedures applying heat, chemicals, or both. Time might be necessary to reach temperature equilibrium, but once such an equilibrium is reached, the sterilization process can be described by the following formula (Toledo, 1978):

$$\log\left(\frac{N_0}{N}\right) = \frac{\text{contact time with sterilant}}{D}$$

where N_0 = initial number of viable organisms, N = viable count after a given time of contact with the sterilant, and D = decimal reduction time of the organisms.

In aseptic packaging machines, valves, pipes, and like materials are usually sterilized by live steam at temperatures of 120 to 140°C (248 to 284°F) (Buchner, 1980; Dtsch. Milchwirtsch., 1973; Linke, 1971; Voss, 1974; Zimmermann, 1974). Chambers, tunnels, cabinets, and such materials are often sterilized by a spray of a suitable disinfectant, usually hydrogen peroxide, and subsequently dried with hot sterile air (Buchner, 1980; Dtsch. Milchwirtsch., 1974; Kelsey, 1974b; Toledo and Chapman, 1973; Voss, 1974).

In the production of shelf-stable, aseptically packaged food products, usually four separate processes of sterilization are involved: (1) sterilization of the process equipment, (2) sterilization of the food product, (3) sterilization of the filler, and (4) sterilization of the packaging material (food-contact surface). In addition, sterile air often is required in the aseptic filling operation necessitating (5) an air-sterilization procedure.

Depending on the installation, i.e., whether or not a sterile tank is included in the process line, two further sterilization procedures might be needed: (6) sterilization of the sterile tank (and pipeline), and (7) sterilization of air to maintain overpressure in the sterile tank.

Thus, operation of an aseptic process line can incorporate up to seven different sterilization procedures. In this connection, attention will mainly be paid to the sterilization of the packaging material (food-contact surface).

Sterilization Processes Involved in the Production of Long-Life Products

1. Sterilization of the process equipment
2. Sterilization of the food product
3. Sterilization of the filler
4. Sterilization of the packaging material
5. Sterilization of air
6. Sterilization of a sterile tank
7. Sterilization of air (sterile tank)

Procedures that can be used for the sterilization of packaging material (food-contact surfaces) depend, of course, to a large extent on the type of material in question. Rigid containers such as metal cans or glass bottles can be sterilized by heat alone. This also includes some

plastic materials, such as polystyrene. Polystyrene cups have been successfully sterilized by using saturated steam under high pressure (Cerny, 1982a, 1983). In this connection, the heat of extrusion as applied in the manufacture of some plastic bottles should also be mentioned: depending on the type of plastic material used, the heat of extrusion often ranges from 230 to 240°C (446 to 464°F), which is considered sufficient for sterilization (Ashton, 1972; Ed., Dairy Ind., 1972; Mann, 1975b; Zimmermann, 1975). For most flexible or semirigid packaging materials, the suitability of sterilization by heat alone has been questioned (Kelsey, 1974a; Voss, 1974), and other means of sterilization should be looked for, such as irradiation or chemical sterilization. In general, the following characteristics must be fulfilled by such sterilization procedures (Toledo, 1975): (1) sporicidal activity, (2) applicability in aseptic packaging systems, (3) compatibility with packaging material, (4) ease of removal from treated food contact surface, and (5) tolerance for residues (lack of toxicity).

A perfect sterilant should be easy to use, be part of an in-line operation, and be residue-free after application. It must have a sufficient kill rate in the shortest possible time; it should be inexpensive; and it should not be toxic to the user or damage the equipment (Farahnik, 1982).

In microbiologic terms, the result obtained from any sterilization process is a function of two parameters: (1) the effectiveness (i.e., sterilizing effect) of the process, and (2) the microbiologic load (often spore count) of the object (e.g., food product, packaging material food contact surface) to be sterilized.

In a heat sterilization process, the sterilizing effect is determined by the time-temperature treatment applied. An increase in temperature as well as longer exposure times result in an increase in the sterilizing efficiency of the process. On the other hand, a larger load of temperature will damage the object: chemical changes in the product (flavor, vitamin content, deposit formation) or the packaging material (food-contact surface, sealability, migration, flavor). Thus limits exist: a suitable compromise has to be established between the desired increase in sterilizing effect—more-severe heat treatment—and changes in the object to be sterilized—less-severe heat treatment.

In the same way, chemical sterilization procedures used must be regarded as a compromise. Increased concentration, higher temperatures, and prolonged time of exposure to the sterilizing agent will usually increase the sterilizing effect of the treatment. However, interaction of the process with the packaging material limits its severeness. A sterilizing effect is *not* a means in itself but rather a means to an end: it relates to the result that is achieved by a certain specified process. This result can be defined by maximal acceptable defective rates but must take into account possible and realistic microbial loads of or on the object to be sterilized.

The aspect of the impossibility to achieve sterility in

its absolute sense has been recognized and used to define the term "commercial sterility." Commercial sterility implies that the defective rate due to the procedures applied is low enough to permit marketing of the product in question.

The efficiency of a sterilization process can be expressed by the number of decimal reductions in spore counts achieved. If highest acceptable failure rates are decided on, minimal decimal reduction rates can be calculated. The failure rate of a sterilization process is mainly determined by the number of the most resistant microorganisms present—i.e., bacterial spores—and not by the total count. Little is known about spore counts on packaging material food-contact surfaces. Consequently, calculations of minimum sterilization effects (decimal reductions) necessary are often based on the assumption that all microorganisms on food contact surfaces are bacterial spores, and furthermore, that infection levels at the site of operation are not accounted for. Sterilization of such surfaces has been defined as a reduction of the microbial load from 10^4 to 10^0, i.e., four-decimal reduction cycles. For aseptic packaging of milk and milk products in plastic containers, procedures should be chosen that reduce the number of possible spoilage organisms by four to six decimals (Gruber and Ziemba, 1970; Hahn, 1981). Four- to five-decimal reductions are regarded as necessary to obtain a maximal spoilage rate of 5 in 10,000 (Heim and Jud, 1973). Four-decimal reductions (as tested with spores of a strain of *Bacillus subtilis*) are stated to be a minimum requirement of the U.S. FDA for the chemical sterilization of food-contact surfaces (Lütkemeyer, 1983). This opinion is shared by others (Cerny, 1985; Swartling and Lindgren, 1962). To meet the requirements of aseptic filling of low-acid food products, five- to six-decimal reductions are considered necessary (Cerny, 1983).

A clear distinction needs to be made between a sterilization process as such and the result obtained by such a process. The process in question can be described by certain parameters, such as (1) concentration of a chemical applied, (2) time of exposure, and (3) temperature of the solution. These critical parameters depend on the process in question and will, of course, vary from aseptic packaging system to aseptic packaging system. If these critical points are controlled and recorded, a controlled, scheduled process is in operation: a requirement raised by the FDA (CFR 21, §113) for filing of a process intended for the production of shelf-stable (nonrefrigerated) handling of low-acid food products. However, the result of a process depends actually on two factors: (1) the application of the actual process *and* (2) the microbial load fed into the process.

In this connection it appears therefore appropriate to discuss the microbial load on food-contact surfaces. The actual subject of interest is, of course, the number of bacterial spores fed into the process of packaging material food-contact surface sterilization. This count is determined by two factors: (1) the spore load on the surface due to the manufacturing process *and* (2) the infection of this surface at the site of operation.

Data available in the literature refer to microbial counts on food-contact surfaces as determined after the process of manufacturing. Strictly speaking, they do not represent a clear picture of what is being fed into the sterilization process. Average microbial counts on plastic food-contact surfaces range from 0 to 10 microorganisms per 100 cm² (Brody, 1971; Buchner, 1978a; Cerny, 1982a; Heim and Jud, 1973; Lisiecke, 1971; Swartling and Lindgren, 1962; von Bockelmann, B., 1971, 1978, 1980; Woss, 1974) (Fig. 48–3).

Though the total microbial load on food-contact surfaces to be sterilized is of some interest, the kind of microorganisms and their counts are even more so. Very few data are available, and all originate from the same source (von Bockelmann, B., 1970, 1978, 1980). The following microflora was found on polyethylene food-contact surfaces of paperboard-based laminates: Average total count: 0 to 5 organisms/100 cm², 10.6% yeast, 20.6% molds, 68.8% bacteria.

The bacterial flora was further differentiated as follows (based on the total microbial count): 44.4% *Micrococci*, 3.1% *Bacillus* spores, 3.7% *Streptococci*, 1.2% *Pseudomonas*, 6.9% gram-positive rods, and 9,4% gram-negative rods.

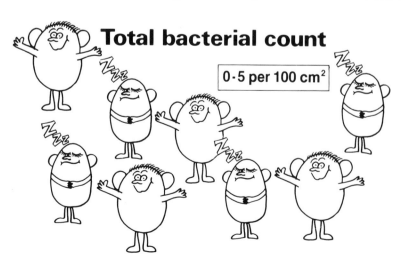

Total bacterial count

0·5 per 100 cm²

Fig. 48–3. Load of microorganisms after converting of packaging material.

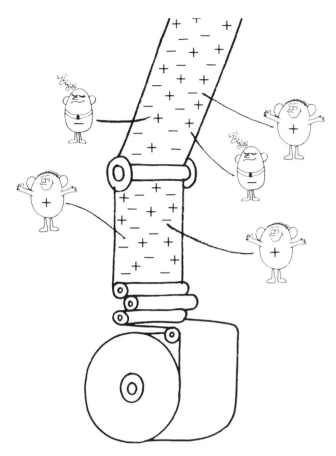

Fig. 48–4. Additional load of microorganisms prior to sterilization.

. All the above counts were obtained immediately after producing the packaging material, not accounting for further infection of the food-contact surface at the site of the commercial processor where the filling equipment is operated. The microbial data on food-contact surfaces clearly indicate an airborne infection. Nothing is published on changes in number and composition of this flora during storage of the packaging material. It seems unlikely that gram-negative rods (*Pseudomonas*) and yeasts will survive longer periods. Considering the goal of aseptic packaging, the bacterial spore count appears to be of predominant interest because these are the microorganisms most difficult to eliminate (Toledo, 1973).

To minimize, reduce, or limit infection of the packaging material food-contact surface at the site of production, suitable measures should be taken (Fig. 48–4).

In a number of countries guidelines for the construction of food plants in general and of those intended for the production of shelf-stable low-acid food specifically are given in "Good Manufacturing Practices" (GMPs) regulations or guidelines. It should be borne in mind that although "the application of these hygienic design principles can be relatively easy during the project stage of a new processing area or factory, it is more complicated when the concepts have to be applied to an existing working environment" (Duke, 1988). Careful attention should be paid right from the beginning of a project.

Such installations should be kept as straightforward as possible. Unnecessary complications must be avoided. As far as the aseptic packaging operation is concerned, the following should be observed: (1) aerosols, (2) outer wrapping equipment, (3) personal hygiene, (4) traffic in the filling area, (5) cleanabilityof walls and floors, (6) ventilation, and others.

As a general rule, the filling area should be physically separated from other areas. To reduce the chances of cross contamination, the postprocess area and its personnel should be segregated from other sections, particularly from the preparation area of the plant (Food and Drink Manufacture—Good Manufacturing Practice: A Guide to Its Responsible Management, The Institute of Food Science & Technology, UK, 20 Queensberry Place, London SW7 2DR).

Aerosols are an effective means of concentrating microorganisms. As a consequence, they can contribute heavily to the level of infection on packaging material food-contact surface. Aerosols originate from many different sources, such as (1) splashing when removing product residues from the floor, (2) the use of air guns for removal of water from different objects, (3) drains in the sewage system, particularly when hot liquids are discharged—such drains should preferably be placed outside the filling area—and (4) any unnecessary discharge of water in general.

Outer wrapping equipment in which cardboard is handled can create larger amounts of dust originating both from the cardboard itself and from dust collected during storage. Environmental regulations have limited the use of biocides in paper mills. Restrictions are being placed on the cleanliness of water discharged from such mills. To an increasing extent, recycled paper is being used in the manufacture of cardboard. All these measures, as understandable as they may be from an environmental point of view, result in an increased microbiologic load on the cardboard. Particularly, the count of bacterial spores increases. For this very reason, it is recommendable to separate outer wrapping equipment handling cardboard from the filling area by a partition wall.

Personal hygiene relates to activities in which operating staff handles packaging material. Infection can be passed from the machine operators to the food-contact surfaces in packaging material splicing operations and so on. A training program should be implemented to increase the awareness of the operators. Suitable instructions should be given to minimize this type of infection.

Traffic in the filling area should be kept to a minimum. Only authorized staff should be permitted in the filling area. The introduction of a special color on working clothes to identify operating staff for such an area might be considered. Particularly, passage of vehicles should be banned, such as forklifts. Wooden pallets are usually heavily infected with molds. Often they are dirty from soil and other sources. Usually, soil has a high content of bacterial spores (mainly *Bacillus*) and can thus significantly contribute to the spore count in the air where pallets are handled.

Cleanability of walls and floors is essential. "Floors in manufacturing areas should be made of impervious materials, laid to an even surface and free from cracks and open joints. They should be of adequate construction and material for the wear and tear and conditions of manufacture encountered. Walls should be sound and finished with a smooth, impervious and easily cleaned surface. Ceilings should be so constructed and finished that they can be maintained in a clean condition. The coving of junctions between walls, floors and ceilings in critical areas is recommended" (Food and Drink Manufacture—Good Manufacturing Practice: A Guide to its Responsible Management, the Institute of Food Science & Technology (UK), 20 Queensberry Place, London SW7 2DR). Aside from the direct microbiologic impact of an unclean area, the effect on the working force should not be underestimated: a "clean" performance will only result in clean surroundings.

Ventilation and—depending on climatic conditions— air conditioning should be planned carefully. Filter systems should be used in the air supply. An overpressure should be maintained in the filling room, sealing this area from the surrounding area by an airflow from the filling room into the surrounding area.

STERILIZATION OF THE PACKAGING MATERIAL FOOD-CONTACT SURFACE

Different procedures are being used today for the sterilization of the packaging material food-contact surface in aseptic packaging machines. The choice of suitable methods depends to a large extent on characteristics of the packaging material in question.

Heat has been used for the sterilization of cans. Superheated steam has been applied to sterilize metal containers (Ito, 1984). The temperatures applied range from about 274 to 300°C (525 to 575°F) (Brody, 1971). Glass bottles have been sterilized using heat. Applying flame sterilization, temperatures of 200 to 400°C (392 to 752°F) could be reached at different parts of the bottle (Fink and Cerny, 1988; Gössel, 1986, 1988). Using polystyrene cups, saturated steam under high pressure has been applied. Bacterial spore counts were reduced by 5.5 to almost 7 logarithmic cycles when exposed for 4 to 6 seconds to saturated steam at a temperature of 147°C (297°F) and 3.5 bar overpressure. As mentioned above, the temperature of extrusion as applied in the manufacture of some bottles is considered sufficient.

Irradiation has been advocated as a suitable sterilant for packaging material food-contact surfaces. Brown Boveri has developed high-intensity ultraviolet (UV) irradiation equipment (Mayer, 1975). Statements on the efficiency of the sterilization of food-contact surfaces vary. Good killing efficiencies are reported by some researchers. A dose of 30 mW/cm² is stated to result in four-decimal reductions in the count of *Bacillus subtilis* spores after 0.3 seconds of exposure, whereas fungal spores re-

quired 1 second of exposure time to achieve the same killing effect. A few seconds of exposure were needed to accomplish four- to six-decimal reductions in microbial counts on flat surfaces when using a dose of 250 mW/cm² (Verpack.-Rundsch., 1981). For sterilization of preformed cups, about 5 times this dose was required. UV-C irradiation is regarded to be sufficient for use in aseptic filling systems provided that the irradiated materials are smooth, UV-resistant, and rather free from dust particles (Cerny, 1977). Dust as well as "shadows" interfere with UV sterilization procedures (Cerny, 1978; Verpack.-Rundsch., 1981).

The following lethal irradiation values are given (Reuter, 1987): vegetative bacteria: 2 to 6 mW/cm², grampositive bacteria requiring about twice as much as gram-negative bacteria. Spores of *Bacillus* tolerate about 5 to 10 times that dose, whereas spores of molds—particularly colored species such as *Aspergillus*—can survive 20 to 100 times of that dose. Generally, colored microorganisms such as yellow or red *Micrococci* are more resistant against the action of UV irradiation. Maximal killing action is achieved at a wavelength of 253.7 nm. The killing efficiency of UV irradiation is influenced by a number of factors, such as dust particles, agglomerates of microorganisms, shape of the container, and humidity. Thus, only 90 to 99% reduction of the microbial load on plastic cups is reported after UV irradiation with up to 1500 mW/cm²; the limited sterilizing effect is explained by dust particles and microbial cell aggregation (Gasti Informiert, 1980). With *Aspergillus niger* as the test organism, only two-decimal reductions resulted after UV-C irradiation (Dtsch. Molk.-Ztg., 1982). This limited killing efficiency is regarded as insufficient for aseptic packaging operations (Reuter, 1987).

Though UV irradiation alone hardly provides the safety of operation needed when sterilizing food-contact surfaces for aseptic packaging of low-acid foods, a combination of relatively low concentrations of hydrogen peroxide and UV irradiation very well might. UV irradiation of *Bacillus subtilis* spores in the presence of hydrogen peroxide produced a rapid kill that was up to 2000 times faster than the one produced by irradiation alone (Bayliss and Waites, 1979a, 1979b). More-resistant strains of *Bacillus* and *Clostridium* required a mild heating—60 seconds at 80°C (176°F)—to achieve a minimum of four-decimal reductions in spore counts after UV irradiation in a 2.5% solution of hydrogen peroxide (Bayliss and Waites, 1979a, 1979b). UV irradiation and hydrogen peroxide act synergistically when used together but not when applied separately. Irradiation of spores in the presence of higher concentrations of hydrogen peroxide reduced the kill, which is explained by absorption of the UV light. The lethal effects of UV irradiation alone or in combination with hydrogen peroxide against spores of *Bacillus subtilis* on paper-based packaging material laminates with no aluminium foil was greater than on boards with aluminium in the laminate (Stannard, 1985). The sporicidal action of hydrogen peroxide is seen in the formation of hydroxyl radicals, which are produced when hydrogen peroxide is irradiated with light of wavelengths below 400 nm (Bayliss and Waites, 1979a). Under practical conditions of use, the combined application of hydrogen peroxide and UV irradiation was found to be less effective than expected. As compared to UV irradiation alone, only a five-fold increase in sterilization efficiency was observed when sterilizing erected carton blanks having a polyethylene coating. This effect is explained by the hydrophobic characteristics of the polyethylene resulting in only 35 to 40% coverage of the food contact surface after application of hydrogen peroxide by spraying (Cerny, 1985).

Particle irradiation techniques using cobalt-60 and the like are regarded as too expensive (Kelsey, 1974a, 1974b). A sterilizing procedure using high-energy electron irradiation has been described (Mod. Packag., 1972). The advantages of low-energy (100 keW), large-area electron beams for the surface sterilization of packaging/container materials have been pointed out (Nablos and Hippel, 1972). However, such particle irradiation procedures often affect plastic coatings resulting in loss of sealability as well as in migration products, which can give rise to off-flavors in the packaged product.

Chemical sterilization of food contact surfaces is the most frequently applied procedure in aseptic packaging. Toledo's review (1974) covers gaseous as well as liquid sterilants. The action of gases (ethylene oxide, propylene oxide, β-propiolactone, formaldehyde, methyl bromide) is too slow to be used in filling machines. Such gases can, however, be useful in presterilization of the packaging material. Halogen solutions, hydrogen peroxide, peracids, and aldehyde solutions can be used in liquid form. Hypochlorite at a concentration of 4000 ppm has been tested (Swartling and Lindgren, 1962). Though good sterilizing effects are reported, corrosion problems prevented practical application. Peracetic acid as well as aldehyde solutions have been shown to have sporicidal properties; however, pungent and irritating odor or vapors, off-flavor problems resulting from residuals, and relatively long exposure times required rendered these compounds less suitable (Toledo, 1974).

Ethyl alcohol was used in some early aseptic filling systems for the treatment of plastic films. At 80% concentration, ethyl alcohol is an effective sterilant against vegetative organisms. However, it is ineffective against bacterial spores and is no longer used (Burton, 1988).

Hydrogen peroxide appears to be the most promising sterilant. At ambient temperatures hydrogen peroxide possesses very slow sporicidal activity. However, at elevated temperatures the D values decrease rapidly in a logarithmic order (Toledo, 1974). Chemical sterilization of food-contact surfaces requires fast microbiocidal action (even against bacterial spores), no negative effects on the packaging material, good possibilities for elimination, no corrosive action of the filling equipment, and no danger in handling; these demands are met by hydrogen peroxide (Heim and Jud, 1973).

Today, most aseptic packaging systems are using hydrogen peroxide as a sterilant of the food-contact surface. Literature reviews have been published on the microbiocidal action of hydrogen peroxide (Stevenson and Schafer, 1983) covering the effect of concentration, exposure times, temperature of exposure, and pH. The resistance of bacterial spores to hydrogen peroxide solutions bears no relation to their thermal resistance (Toledo, 1973). In practice, the sterilizing effectiveness of hydrogen peroxide in relation to aseptic filling is usually assessed against spores of either *Bacillus subtilis* or *Bacillus subtilis* var. *globigii* because of their relatively high resistance (Burton, 1988). However, the killing efficiency of hydrogen peroxide as used under practical conditions in aseptic filling systems is difficult to predict because the mode of use usually is rather complex; heating results in increased concentration and temperature as well as the development of hydrogen peroxide gas. As a consequence, the effectiveness of such systems is usually tested empirically.

Hydrogen peroxide is regarded as a suitable sterilizing agent for treatment of food-contact surfaces in aseptic packaging of low-acid foods, provided it is heated to a temperature of at least 85 to 90°C (185 to 194°F) and the time of exposure is at least 3 to 4 seconds (Ed., Gasti Informiert, 1980). A 15 to 20% solution of hydrogen peroxide was found to meet the theoretical and practical requirements if followed by a heating to 125°C (257°F) (Swartling and Lindgren, 1962); the killing effect was explained by a combined action of liquid and gaseous (vapor) hydrogen peroxide. Others (Gruber and Ziemba, 1970; Hahn, 1981) claim that a safe killing rate (at least four-decimal reductions) of bacterial spores can be achieved in seconds only if the concentration of the hydrogen peroxide used is at least 30% and the temperature on the food-contact surface reaches at least 80 to 90°C (176 to 194°F). Organic material—provided it is free from catalase—has little effect on the sporicidal action of hydrogen peroxide (Ito, 1973).

After inactivating *Bacillus subtilis* spores with hydrogen peroxide, reactivation could be observed by heating the treated spores (30% hydrogen peroxide, 5 minutes, 24°C [75°F]) to 50 to 80°C (122 to 176°F). Above and below this temperature range, no reactivation was observed.

Surfaces of packaging material have been treated within an ultrasonic bath or blown with sterile air under high pressure. Such precleaning procedures in aseptic filling machines prior to sterilization should lead to a considerable increase in efficiency of the sterilization process (Cerny, 1985).

ASEPTIC PACKAGING SYSTEMS

A large number of different aseptic filling systems are being offered today. Various types of materials and packages are being produced: (1) cans, (2) glass bottles, (3) plastic bottles, (4) plastic pouches, (5) plastic cups, and (6) paper based laminates. A detailed description of all the different systems on the market would be very lengthy. In the following, a short presentation is given of the principles involved in aseptic packaging.

Metal *cans* have been used for aseptic packaging of presterilized liquid (pumpable) food products for a long time. A more detailed description of such filling systems can be found in the literature (Brody, 1971, 1973; Burton, 1988; Lange, 1987).

In the aseptic Dole canning system, the filler, the can, and the lids are sterilized by superheated steam permitting operation at normal atmospheric pressure. With gas burners, saturated steam at a temperature of 110 to 120°C (230 to 248°F) is rapidly superheated to 316°C (601°F). When reaching the cans, the temperature of the superheated steam has dropped to about 220 to 226°C (428 to 439°F). At this temperature, an exposure time of 40 seconds is sufficient for sterilization of the cans. The lids are sterilized in a similar manner.

Sterility of the equipment is maintained by a slight overpressure obtained by the superheated steam in the can sterilization tunnel, the lid sterilization cabinet, and the filling station. Prior to filling, the cans having a temperature of about 225°C (401°F) are cooled down either by sterile condensate, water, or air. Product is continuously admitted through a slit-type filler or a sterile rotary piston filler into cans passing below the filling head. About 1% of product losses are encountered when using the slit-type filling principle.

A more recent development of the Dole filling system operates with hot air sterilization. The cans are heated to 143°C (289°F) and sterilized at this temperature for 4 minutes.

A further use of aseptic filling is in aerosol cans. Whipping cream is filled in such containers using nitrous oxide (N$_2$O) as expelling gas. Sterilization of the cans is done by superheated steam (45 seconds at 225°C [401°F], Dole) or by hot air (20 minutes at 230°C [446°F], Coster), or by hydrogen peroxide (Serac) (Burton, 1988).

Aseptic filling in *glass bottles* has been tried for a long time. However, none of the prototype aseptic fillers for glass bottles reached commercial operation. Recently there has been a revival of interest, and several new systems have been developed (Buchner, 1988; Dtsch. Milchwirtsch., 1986; Dtsch. Molk.-Ztg., 1986; Gössel, 1988; Grundy, 1974; Schreyer, 1985).

Aseptic processing of glass bottles poses a complex problem because of thermal shock characteristics. Some years ago, Dole applied its superheated steam sterilization concept (metal cans) to glass aseptic packaging. Containers were introduced into a nonpressurized superheated steam chamber and the entire mass of glass was brought to a sterilizing temperature of about 216°C (421°F). Because of thermal shock characteristics it was necessary to remove heat energy to reduce temperature to about 33°C (60°F) differential between temperature at point of fill and cold sterile product. The result was successful but cumbersome and slow, and not acceptable for commercial use.

Pressurized steam and hydrogen peroxide have been shown to be more successful sterilants. Glass containers entering the sterilization section in a rotating pressurized chamber are subjected to pressurized steam at approximately 4.0 atmospheres at a temperature of 135°C (275°F). It has been proven empirically that with wet steam at 135°C (275°F) sterilization is effected by exposure for 1.5 to 2.0 seconds.

Using hydrogen peroxide as a sterilant, the glass bottles are wetted with a 30% solution at 50 to 60°C (122 to 140°F) and subsequently dried with hot air (130°C, 266°F) in a tunnel drier. A killing effect of 5.2-decimal reductions was determined using spores of *Bacillus subtilis*. Plastic–aluminium-foil laminates served as closures. These lids are sterilized in wet steam at 5 bar for 5 seconds. The drying tunnel and filling station are presterilized by hydrogen peroxide and steam while the filling device is steam-sterilized.

One aseptic filling system for glass bottles applies hot air as a means of sterilization. The bottles pass a heating tunnel where air at a temperature of 270°C (518°F) is circulated. Heat transfer is by convection and is determined by air temperature, air speed, mass of the container, surface of the container, and heat-transfer value.

Aseptic filling systems using blow-molded *plastic bottles* are of three different types: (1) a standard, nonsterile bottle is sterilized and then filled and sealed aseptically, (2) a bottle is first blown in such a way that it is sterile, and then filled and sealed aseptically, and (3) a bottle is blown aseptically, filled, and sealed consecutively at the same station so that sterility is maintained (Burton, 1988).

Plastic bottles are produced from granulate, usually low- or high-density polyethylene or polypropylene. The transperity and oxygen permeability of these materials can cause oxidation problems in the filled products intended for a long storage life. Developments in blowmolding techniques and materials have now made it possible to mold bottles from multilayered material (Ed., Verpack.-Rundsch., 1985) that has satisfactory light and oxygen barrier properties, though the costs are somewhat higher. It is assumed that the pressure (ca. 400 atmospheres) and the temperature of extrusion (ca. 230 to 240°C, 446 to 464°F) are sufficient to sterilize the material (Ashton, 1972; Ed., Dairy Ind., 1972; Mann, 1975; Zimmermann, 1975a).

If plastic bottles are produced under standard, nonaseptic conditions, the blow-molded bottles are usually sterilized by hydrogen peroxide in combination with heat. The heat treatment serves to increase the killing effect and, at the same time, to remove the hydrogen peroxide. A rinse with sterile water can also be included. After being sterilized, the bottles are fed to an aseptic filling unit and finally closed with separately sterilized caps. Prior to operation, the unit is sterilized by hydrogen peroxide spraying and drying with hot air. Sterility is maintained during production by an overpressure of sterile air, usually obtained by filtration.

Production of plastic bottles and aseptic filling in one

operation is a technically complex operation. In this form-fill-seal operation only the filling device needs to be sterilized prior to start of the aseptic filling process because the sterile surrounding is obtained and maintained by the extruded plastic tube itself. Sterilization of the parts of the filling pipe coming into contact with the product is done by wet steam at a temperature of about 140°C (284°F) (Zimmermann, 1974). Using sterile air, the bottles are blow-molded in the conventional way. The product filling pipe is concentric with the air-blowing tube, product being admitted by a piston filler. When filling is completed, the blowing and filling nozzles retract, and jaws in the mold head close to seal the bottle.

Separating blow-molding and filling of plastic bottles is thought to simplify the operation from a technical point of view and makes it easier to adapt the two processes to each other (Dtsch. Milchwirtsch., 1982). Such a procedure, however, requires a separate aseptic filling unit.

Plastic bottles are blow-molded using sterile air. The temperature of extrusion is sufficient to sterilize the inner surfaces of the bottle, which leaves the extruder hermetically sealed. The bottles are then either stored or directly transported to a separate aseptic filling station. This fill-seal unit is sterilized by a suitable disinfectant, usually hydrogen peroxide. Valves and pipes coming into contact with the sterile filling product are sterilized by wet steam. Sterility in the unit is maintained by an overpressure of a laminar sterile air flow.

Entering the filling station, the outside of the plastic bottles is sterilized by either passing through a hydrogen peroxide bath or by a hydrogen peroxide spray. The closure is cut-off and the bottle is filled and reclosed by a suitable laminate usually containing aluminium foil. Sterilization of the closure foil is done either by passage through a bath containing hydrogen peroxide and subsequent heating or by UV irradiation.

Aseptic *plastic pouches* are a simple, cheap form of container for liquids. The plastic material used may either be simple polyethylene or coextruded material containing polyvinylidene chloride (PVDC) or ethylene vinyl alcohol (EVOH) to improve barrier characteristics. Pigments can be included in the laminate serving as a light barrier.

Two different procedures are being used for the sterilization of the plastic food-contact surface: chemical sterilization executed in the filling equipment and the heat of extrusion of a tubular material outside the filler.

Prior to production, the filler cabinet is sterilized by spraying hydrogen peroxide alone or with other suitable disinfectants such as formaldehyde (Mann, 1977, 1978), or by the use of a germicidal soap (Kelsey, 1974a) with subsequent drying by hot sterile air. The sterility of the system thus achieved is maintained by an overpressure of filtered sterile air fed into the enclosed superstructure of the filler (Ed., Dairy Ind., 1967; Dtsch. Milchwirtsch., 1974; Uteschill, 1971). Piping and valves of the filling device are usually sterilized by saturated, live steam.

The packaging material is supplied in one (Ed., Dairy Ind., 1972; Kelsey, 1974a) or two webs (Ashton, 1972; Mann, 1977, 1978). Sterilization of the packaging material is accomplished by passage through a hydrogen peroxide bath followed by UV irradiation or by "active agents on alcohol bases," such as ethyl alcohol at 95°C (203°F), followed by high-intensity UV irradiation. The liquid used for sterilization is subsequently dried off by hot, sterile air. However, application of ethyl alcohol as a sterilant must be regarded as an unsuitable film sterilizing system; its practical application has resulted in some problems.

Using a tubular extrusion process, the heat applied (over 200°C, 392°F) is sufficient for sterilization of the intended food-contact surface, i.e., the inner side of the plastic tube. The extruded plastic layer is thick enough to prevent penetration of any potential spoilage organisms from the outside. In the aseptic filling operation, only the infected outside of the material tube needs to be sterilized to maintain sterility in the filling equipment. Before entering the sterile chamber of the filler, the flat web of tubular packaging material passes through a bath of hydrogen peroxide followed by UV irradiation.

A relatively large number of aseptic fillers using *plastic cups* are on the market. Some of these are intended for high-acid (pH < 4.6) food products, often only applying simplified sterilization systems that must be regarded as insufficient for low-acid foods. Normally polystyrene or polypropylene serve as packaging material but more-sophisticated co-extruded materials with better barrier characteristics can also be used. Two different types of aseptic cup filling machines can be distinguished: those using prefabricated cups and those working from a roll stock.

All aseptic cup fillers operate with a sterile chamber or tunnel. Prior to the actual filling operation, these chambers are sterilized, usually by a hydrogen peroxide spray and subsequent drying by hot sterile air. During production, sterility in this area is maintained by an overpressure of sterile air. Sterile air is produced in the equipment by filtration, incineration, or both. Usually piston fillers dose the product into the cup. Sterilization of these devices is done by wet live steam.

In fillers using prefabricated cups, sterilization of the cups is achieved either by steam, hydrogen peroxide and heat, or UV irradiation.

Sterilization by heat (Amman, 1987; Burton, 1988; Cerny, 1983; Dtsch. Milchwirtsch., 1985) is done by steam in a pressurized chamber. Eighteen to 20 inverted polypropylene cups are fed into a vertical, cylindrical sterilizing chamber. A vacuum is applied to remove air that would interfere with heat transfer. Saturated steam at 3 to 3.5 bar, corresponding to 140 to 147°C (284 to 297°F) or a steam air mixture heated to about 200°C (392°F) is admitted. These sterilization conditions are maintained for 1.2 seconds, whereafter the pressure is released. Lids are sterilized in the same manner. Applying 3 bar, 5.5-decimal reductions were obtained using spores of *Bacillus subtilis*. This killing effect increased to 7-decimal reductions when the pressure was raised to 3.5 bar. The total time for the sterilization cycle—evacuation, pressurizing, and depressurizing—amounts to about 6 seconds.

Hydrogen peroxide is the sterilant most frequently used in aseptic filling machines for cups. A 30 to 35% solution is applied either by spraying, condensation of hydrogen peroxide gas, or by passage through a hydrogen peroxide bath (Burton, 1988; Dtsch. Milchwirtsch., 1974; Dtsch. Molk.-Ztg., 1988; Mann, 1975a; Neue Verpackg., 1987; Tolasch, 1987; Turtschan, 1987).

Spraying the inside of the cup with hydrogen peroxide solution with subsequent removal by hot sterile air is considered the conventional method. The inside of the cup covered with hydrogen peroxide needs to reach a temperature of at least 70°C (158°F) in order to accomplish satisfactory sterilization. The sterilization performance is stated to be a minimum of 3 decimal reductions as tested with spores of *Bacillus globigii*. Some systems claim a killing rate of 5 decimal reductions and more. To a certain extent, the killing efficiencies of such systems depend on coverage of the inner surface of the hydrophobic plastic cup with hydrogen peroxide. It has been shown that this coverage very much depends on the size of droplets. Conventional spraying devices produce droplets of about 30 to 80 μm in diameter. With such a procedure, only 30 to 40% of the surface area is covered with the hydrogen peroxide solution. An ultrasonic system can be used by which the diameter of the droplets is reduced to about 3 μm and an average surface coverage of about 60% is achieved.

Evaporation of hydrogen peroxide and recondensation on plastic food-contact surfaces also results in a droplet size of 3 to 4 μm in diameter and, consequently, good coverage of the surfaces. A disadvantage of this procedure is that comparatively large amounts of hydrogen peroxide are being used up because only part of the vapor condenses. Furthermore, because of the heat applied in the process of evaporation, some of the hydrogen peroxide decomposes, resulting in a drop in concentration.

In one aseptic filling system, the cups are put on a conveyor belt and passed through a bath containing a 35% solution of hydrogen peroxide heated to 85 to 90°C (185 to 194°F). Exposure time is adjusted to about 2 seconds. The hydrogen peroxide is removed from the cups by heating, by passage through a bath containing sterile water, and finally by drying with hot, sterile air.

Other aseptic cup filling systems work from roll stock. In these form-fill-seal machines hydrogen peroxide is usually used as a sterilant (Burton, 1988; Dtsch. Milchwirtsch., 1973; Dtsch. Molk.-Ztg., 1987; Lütkemeyer, 1987; Verpack., Rundsch., 1983). The flat packaging material web passes through a bath containing a 30 to 35% solution of hydrogen peroxide often at a temperature of 60 to 80°C (140 to 176°F). Passage time through the bath is about 15 seconds. Under these conditions a sterilizing effect of more than 4-decimal reductions of *Bacillus* spores is achieved. In some systems, high-velocity ("jet-

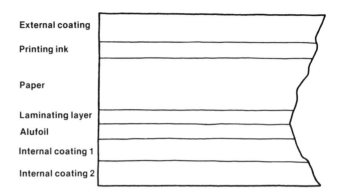

Fig. 48–5. Structure of packaging material.

stream") washing of both the body and lid foil is applied by rapid circulation of the hydrogen peroxide solution. By such a procedure air bubbles are removed from the surface and the microbial load is reduced by a "wash-off" effect. Removal of the hydrogen peroxide from the food-contact surface is done by heat applied in the thermoform station as well as by a flow of hot sterile air. The temperature reached in the process contributes to the sterilization efficiency of the hydrogen peroxide treatment.

In one system polystyrene cups are produced from roll stock and subsequently sterilized by saturated steam under a pressure of 3 to 6 bar corresponding to a temperature of 153 to 165° (275 to 329°F). An exposure time of 1.5 seconds results in a sterilizing effect of 5- to 6-decimal reductions of *Bacillus* spores. The lid foil is sterilized in the same manner.

An alternative version avoids the need of packaging material sterilization. Co-extruded multilayer films are used in which one outer layer can be peeled away, leaving a surface that has been sterilized in the process of extrusion.

Two different principles can be distinguished with regard to aseptic packaging systems using *paper-based laminates*: machines using prefabricated blanks and fillers operating from roll stock. Hydrogen peroxide is the predominant sterilant in both systems.

The packaging material consists of multilayered laminate usually having the following layers, from the outside: (1) polyethylene, (2) base paper, (3) polyethylene (4) aluminium foil, (5) polyethylene, (6) polyethylene (Fig. 48–5).

The grammages and to a certain extent the exact composition are determined by the size (volume) of the package and by the kind of product packaged.

In aseptic filling systems operating from prefabricated blanks, the longitudinal or side seams are completed and the creases are applied by the manufacturer of the packaging material. The blanks are fed into the filling machine in lay-flat form, erected, and bottom sealed. Such filling machines are usually adjustable within a certain range of filling volume (Dtsch. Milchwirtsch., 1983). For certain aseptic operations, the boxed blanks are presterilized with gas, i.e., ethylene oxide (Burton, 1988).

Filling machines of this kind have a sterile chamber in which the cartons are sterilized, filled, and sealed. Prior to the start-up of the actual filling operation, this chamber is sterilized using hydrogen peroxide or a combination of hydrogen peroxide and peracetic acid (Oxonia active), which is stated to be more efficient (Stephenson, 1986). The solution is usually sprayed into the chamber and dried by hot sterile air. During production, sterility is maintained by an overpressure obtained by a laminar flow of sterile air. Air sterilization is usually done by filtration, incineration, or both.

The erected, bottom-sealed cartons enter the chamber and are sprayed with a 30 to 35% solution of hydrogen peroxide. The amount needed depends on the size of the container, 0.1 to 0.2 ml being used per 1-liter carton. Total coverage of the food-contact surface is desirable. Depending on the size of droplets in the hydrogen peroxide mist, this coverage will be more or less complete. Special "nebulizers" have been developed to improve coverage of the food-contact surface (Food Eng., 1981; Farahnik, 1982). Checking coverage of the inner carton surface, only 30 to 60% of the surface was found to be covered by hydrogen peroxide. In spite of this observation, good killing efficiency is reported on the entire surface due to the action of hydrogen peroxide in the gas phase created during evaporation (Ashton, 1972; Cerny, 1978). In this process, only the inside (food-contact) surface is sterilized. Microorganisms on the outside of the container can enter the sterile zone, and careful adjustment of the sterile air flow is necessary to prevent such microorganisms from entering the product in the filling operation. Application of the hydrogen peroxide solution takes 2 to 4 seconds, and its removal by hot sterile air 4 to 8 seconds. The temperature of the air used to complete sterilization and to remove the hydrogen peroxide falls in the range of 170 to 200°C (338 to 392°F). In this process, an inside surface temperature of about 85°C (185°F) is reached (Cerny, 1978).

The sterilized cartons are moved to the filling station where product is dosed into the containers, usually by specially devised piston pumps that have been sterilized by live, wet steam prior to the filling operation. Foam resulting from filling is removed by a defoaming device using suction procedures (Doublas, 1981).

Finally, the top seam is effectuated either by sealing with sterile hot air (Verpack.-Rundsch., 1982) or by ultrasonic welding (Dtsch. Milchwirtsch., 1975, 1983). The sealed cartons leave the sterilized chamber, and the process of aseptic packaging is terminated.

Aseptic packaging systems using paperboard-based laminates from roll stock are form-fill-seal machines using hydrogen peroxide as a sterilizing agent. Heat is applied to increase the sterilizing efficiency of the hydrogen peroxide as well as to eliminate the agent from the food-contact surface. If necessary, a stainless steel superstructure protects the sterilized packaging material from

reinfection. Prior to production, this housing is sterilized, usually using a spray of hydrogen peroxide that is subsequently dried by hot sterile air. During production, sterility is maintained by an overpressure of sterile air.

To sterilize the packaging material food-contact surface, two different procedures of hydrogen peroxide application are being used: application onto the food-contact surface only, or passage of the material through a dip-in bath in which both the food-contact surface and the outside of the packaging material are treated with hydrogen peroxide.

When applying hydrogen peroxide onto the food-contact surface only, concentration of the sterilant ranges from 15 to 35%. A wetting agent is needed to achieve total coverage of the hydrophobic (polyethylene) food-contact surface with a thin film of hydrogen peroxide. Depending on food legislation, different wetting agents can be used such as polyoxyethylene-sorbitane-mono-laurate (PSM, Tween 20) and sugar esters. The sterilizing solution (hydrogen peroxide containing about 0.2 to 0.3% wetting agent) is applied onto the food-contact surface by a system of transfer rollers.

By pressure rollers excessive hydrogen peroxide is removed, leaving a very thin layer on the food-contact surface, its thickness being on the order of magnitude of micrometers. By subsequent heating, the sterilizing efficiency of the hydrogen peroxide is increased, and simultaneously evaporated. To achieve this effect a temperature of about 105 to 110°C (221 to 230°F) is necessary. This heating can be accomplished by passing the material over a surface of a heated drum (Mann, 1977, 1978; Packag. Technol., 1983), by radiation heating (Buchner, 1978a; von Bockelmann, B., 1978), by air (Cerny, 1978; Kelsey, 1974a), or by hot air (Brody, 1971; Dtsch. Milchwirtsch., 1975; Dtsch. Molk.-Ztg., 1975; Hansen, 1975; Mann, 1975a; Schulte, 1987). Often, combinations of above procedures are applied. Sterile air is usually produced by incineration to temperatures of 360 to 380°C (662 to 716°F).

To sterilize the packaging material food-contact surface by liquid hydrogen peroxide in a bath, elevated temperatures are needed. In such systems, the hydrogen peroxide solution is usually heated to 60 to 80°C (140 to 176°F) with exposure times of 6 to 8 seconds (Ashton, 1972; Brody, 1971; Buchner, 1978a, 1978b; Dtsch. Milchwirtsch., 1975; Dtsch. Molk.-Ztg., 1975; Hansen, 1975; Mann, 1978; Samuelsson, 1970; Schulte, 1987). Excessive hydrogen peroxide is usually removed by pressure rollers in combination with air knives fed with hot sterile air or by hot sterile air alone.

REFERENCES

Anonymous. 1967. Aseptic filling of plastics sachets. Dairy Ind., 32, 739.
Anonymous. 1972. DLG International Dairy Equipment Exhibition, part 2. Dairy Ind., 32, 608.
Anonymous. 1973. Reinfektionsfreies formen, füllen und verschliessen. Dtsch. Milchwirtsch., 24, 1559.
Anonymous. 1974. Aseptische becherfüllung auf benhil-formseal-maschinen. Dtsch. Milchwirtsch., 25, 822.

Anonymous. 1975. Zwei neue verpackungssysteme für H-milch. Dtsch. Milchwirtsch., *26*, 563.

Anonymous. 1982. H-Produkte in kunststoff-flaschen. Dtsch. Milchwirtsch., *33*, 1197.

Anonymous. 1983. Das PKL combibloc-System mit Ultraschallverschluss mit Kopfstegnaht. Dtsch. Milchwirtsch., *34*, 609.

Anonymous. 1985. Keimarme abfüllmaschine mit dem Heissluft/ Heissdampf-Sterilisationsverfahren von Ampack-Ammann in Königsbrunn. Dtsch. Milchwirtsch., *36*, 1640.

Anonymous. 1986. H-Milch im glas? Dtsch. Milchwirtsch., *37*, 501.

Anonymous. 1975. Zwei neue Aseptik-Verpackungssysteme für H-Milch. Dtsch. Molk.-Ztg., *94*, 552.

Anonymous. 1982. Abhängigkeit der Anzahl unsteriler Packungen von der Ausgangskeimzahl des Packmittels und dem keimabtötungseffekt des Packmittels-Sterilisationsverfahren. Dtsch. Molk.-Ztg., *103*, 1216.

Anonymous. 1986. Glasaseptik—Symposium der Firmen Bosch und Oberland Glas. Dtsch. Molk.-Ztg., *107*, 556.

Anonymous. 1987. UHT-Kaffeesahne, aseptisch verpackt. Dtsch. Molk.-Ztg., *108*, 177

Anonymous. 1988. Aseptische Verpackung mit hoher Ausbringung. Dtsch. Molk.-Ztg., *109*, 1201

Anonymous. 1980. Food and Drug Administration, CRF 21, §113.

Anonymous. 1981. System controls sterilant application in aseptic packaging process. Food Eng., *53*, 63.

Anonymous. 1980. Stand der Packmittelsterilisation mittels UV-C-Strahlen und mittels H_2O_2. Gasti Informiert, 3.

Anonymous. 1972. Container sterilization by radiation for aseptic food packaging. Mod. Packag., 62

Anonymous. 1987. Packmittelentkeimung und aseptische Abfüllung. Neue Verpackg., *40*, 58.

Anonymous. 1983. International Paper Company's extended shelf-life packaging. Packag. Technol., March/April.

Anonymous. 1981. Aseptisches Verpacken von Lebensmitteln (I). Verpack.-Rundsch., *32*, 1368.

Anonymous. 1982. Flüssigkeitsverpackungen auf dem neuesten Stand der Technik—das Combibloc-System. Verpack.-Rundsch., *33*, 500.

Anonymous. 1983. Neue Technologien bestimmen den Markt von morgen. Verpack.-Rundsch., *34*, 1212.

Anonymous. 1985. Aseptik und Coextrusion verbessern die Lagerfähigkeit. Verpack.-Rundsch., *36*, 966.

Ammann, S. 1987. Aseptisches Verpacker im Bechern aus Polypropylen und deren Sterilisation mit einem Heissluft Heissdampf-Gemisch. In *Aseptisches Verpacken von Lebensmitteln*, Hamburg, Behr's Verlag, p. 207.

Ashton, T.R. 1972. IDF Monogr. UHT Milk, 100.

Bayliss, C.E., and Waites, W.M. 1979a. The combined effect of hydrogen peroxide and ultraviolet irradiation on bacterial spores. J. Appl. Bacteriol., *47*, 263.

Bayliss, C.E., and Waites, W.M. 1979b. The synergistic killing of spores of *Bacillus subtilis* by hydrogen peroxide and ultra-violet irradiation. PEMS Microbiol. Lett., *5*, 331.

Brody, A.L. 1971. Food canning in rigid and flexible packages. CRC Crit. Rev. Food Technol., July, 187.

Brody, A.L. 1973. Current issues in aseptic packaging. Techhnical/Engineering, Dec., 47.

Buchner, N. 1978a. Die aseptische Verpackung von Lebensmitteln—Entwicklungsstand und Entwicklungsaussichten (I). Verpack.-Rundsch., *24*, 36.

Buchner, N. 1978b. Die aseptische Verpackung von Lebensmitteln—Entwicklungsstand und Entwicklungsaussichten (II). Verpack.-Rundsch., *24*, 788.

Buchner, N. 1980. Aseptische abgefüllte Kaffee-Sahne in tiefgezogenen Einzelpackungen. Neue Verpack., *33*, 588.

Buchner, N. 1988. Anlagen zur aseptischen Befüllung von Flaschen aus Glas und Kunststoff. Dtsch. Molk.-Ztg., *109*, 1522.

Burton, H. 1988. Ultra High Temperature Processing of Milk and Milk Products. London, Elsevier Applied Science Publishers Ltd.

Carlson, R. 1980. Aseptic packaging. Am. Dairy Rev., April, 38.

Cerf, O., and Brissende, C.H. 1981. IDF Monogr. UHT Milk, *133*, 93.

Cerny, G. 1977. Entkeimen von Packstoffen beim aseptischen Abpacken. Verpack.-Rundsch., *28*, 77.

Cerny, G. 1978. Microbiologische Aspekte der Lebensmitteltechnologie und verpackung. Verpack.-Rundsch., *29*, 49.

Cerny G. 1983. Entkeimen von Packstoffen beim aseptischen Abpacken. Verpack.-Rundsch., *34*, 55.

Cerny, G. 1985. Entkeimen von Packstoffen beim aseptischen Abpacken. Verpack.-Rundsch., *36*, 49.

Doublas, J. 1981. Proceedings, Seminar on UHT Processing, Australian Society of Dairy Technology, Melbourne, Technical Publication, No. 26, p. 11.

Duke, M. 1988. Good manufacturing practices an essential ingredient of quality and safety. Bulletin of the IDF 229, 27.

Farahnik, S. 1982. A new method of hydrogen peroxide application "Nebulization". Dairy Food Sanitation, *2*, 136.

Fink, A., and Cerny, G. 1988. Entkeimen von Packstoffen beim aseptischen Abpacken. Verpack.-Rundsch., *39*, 63.

Gössel, K. 1988. Glasaseptik in Allugäu. Dtsch. Milchwirtsch., *39*, 1639.

Gruber, E.J., and Ziemba, J.V. 1970. Packs aseptically in milk-style cartons. Food Eng., *42*, 72.

Grundy, C. 1974. Aseptic filling of liquids into glass containers under strictly commercial conditions. Pira Sem., March.

Hahn, G. 1981. Reinfektionsfreies Abfüllen von Milchprodukten in Bechern mit H_2O_2. Dtsch. Molk.-Ztg., *102*, 518.

Hallström, B. 1979. Proceedings: International Conference on UHT Processing and Aseptic Packaging of Milk and Milk Products, Department of Food Science, North Carolina State University, Raleigh, NC, p. 133.

Hansen, R. 1975. Compak aseptik. Nordeuropeisk Mejeri-tidsskrift, *41*, 435.

Heim, W., and Jud, W. 1973. Möglichkeiten zum Herstellen aseptischer Packungen. Verpack.-Rundsch., *24*, 1104.

Hermsom, A.C. 1985a. Plenary lecture: Technical and scientific arguments. Proceedings, Symposium on Aseptic Processing and Packaging of Foods. IUFoST, Tylösand, Sweden, p. 9.

Ito, K. et al. 1973. Resistance of bacterial spores to hydrogen peroxide. Food Technol., *27*, 58.

Ito, K. et al. 1984. Sterilization of packaging materials using aseptic systems. Food Technol., *38*, 60.

Kelsey, R.J. 1974a. Aseptic-packaging-machine design. Mod. Packag., *2*, 37.

Kelsey, R.J. 1974b. Methods of sterilization. Mod. Packag., *8*, 39.

Lange, H.J. 1987. Aseptisches Prozessieren und Packen (APP) von Lebensmitteln in Dosen. In *Aseptisches Verpacken von Lebensmitteln*, Behr's Verlag, Hamburg, p. 227.

Lembke, A. 1972. IDF Monogr. UHT Milk.

Linke, A. 1972. Das aseptische Abfüllen von Molkereiprodukten in tiefgezogene Kunststoffpackungen. Dtsch. Milchwissensch., *26*, 543.

Lisiecki, R.E. 1971. Aseptic carton system. Mod. Packag., 77.

Lütkemeyer, B. 1983. Marktbedeutung der aseptisch arbeitenden Thermoform-, Füll- und Verschliessmaschinen Servac 78 sowie TFA 241 AS der Robert Bosch GmbH. Dtsch. Molk.-Ztg., *104*, 1263.

Lütkemeyer, B. 1987. Aseptisches Verpacken in Kunststoffbechern, die von der Rolle gefertigt werden. In *Aseptisches Verpacken von Lebensmitteln*, Hamburg, Behr's Verlag, p. 163.

Mann, E.J. 1975a. Aseptic packaging of milk and milk products, part 1. Dairy Ind., *40*, 94.

Mann, E.J. 1975b. Aseptic packaging of milk and milk products, part 2. Dairy Ind., *40*, 134.

Mann, E.J. 1977. Aseptic packaging, part 1. Dairy Ind., *42*, 46.

Mann, E.J. 1978. Aseptic packaging, part 2. Dairy Ind., *43*, 19.

Mayer, P. 1975. UV-C-Strahler, ein neuer Hochleistungs-Quecksilberdampf Niederdruckstrahler. BBC-Nachr., *57*, 11.

Nablo, V., and Hippel, J.E. 1972. Low energy electron beams for surface sterilization and aseptic practice. Proceedings, 30th Annual Technical Conference Society of Plastics Engineers, Chicago, May.

Reuter, H. 1987. Kriterien zur Beurteilung von aseptischen Abfüll- und Verpackungssystemen. In *Aseptisches Verpacken von Lebensmitteln*, Hamburg, Behr's Verlag, p. 121.

Rippen, A.J. 1970. Aseptic packaging of Grade A dairy products. Dairy Sci., *53*, 111.

Samuelsson, E.G., and Kristiansen, N. 1970. Aseptisk emballering af konsummaelk. N. Maelkeritidende, *83*, 319.

Schreyer, G. 1985. Die umweltfreundliche Alternative: H-Milch in der Glasflasche. Dtsch. Molk.-Ztg., *106*, 482.

Schulte, G. 1987. Aseptisches Verpacken in Kartonverpackungen von der Rolle. In *Aseptisches Verpacken von Lebensmitteln*, Hamburg, Behr's Verlag, p. 137.

Stannard, C.J. et al. 1985. Efficiency of treatments involving ultraviolet irradiation for decontaminating packaging board of different surface compositions. J. Food Prot., *48*, 786.

Stephenson, K. 1986. The aseptic equation. Packaging Today, Sept., 71.

Stevenson, K.E., and Shafer B.D. 1983. Bacterial spore resistance to hydrogen peroxide. Food Technol., *37*, 111.

Swartling, P., and Lindgren, L.N. 1962. Aseptic filling in Tetra Pak sterilization of the paper. Milk Dairy Res. Rep., Report No., 66.

Tolasch, G. 1987. Hochwirksames Peroxid-Aerosol-Abscheidings verfahren zum Sterilisieren von Kunststoffbecherpackungen. In *Aseptisches Verpacken von Lebensmitteln*, Hamburg, Behr's Verlag, p. 195.

Toledo, R.T. 1978. Proceedings, Conference on Aseptic Processing and Bulk Distribution of Food. Indianapolis, Purdue University, p. 16.

Toledo, R.T., and Chapman, J.R. 1973. Aseptic packaging in rigid plastic containers. Food Technol., *27*, 68.

Toledo, R.T. et al. 1973. Sporicidal properties of hydrogen peroxide against food spoilage organisms. J. Appl. Microbiol., *26*, 592.

Toledo, R.T. 1974. Trends in Packaging. Proceedings of Ninth Annual Symposium, New York State Agriculture Experiment Station, p. 6.

Toledo, R.T. 1975. Chemical sterilants for aseptic packaging. Food Technol., *29*, 103.

Turtschan, A. 1987. Aseptisches Verpacken in vorgefertigten Kunststoffbechern—Vergleich verschiedener Sterilisationsverfahren und der dabei entstehenden Kosten. In *Aseptisches Verpacken von Lebensmitteln*, Hamburg, Behr's Verlag, p. 175.

Uteschill, H. 1971. Use of the "Bertopack" system for packaging milk of long keeping quality. Dairy Sci. Abstr., *33*, 4468.

von Bockelmann, B. 1971. Aseptische Verpackungen für Milch und Milchprodukten. Dtsch. Milchwirtsch., *22*, 136.

von Bockelmann, B. 1978. Proceedings, Conference on Aseptic Processing and Bulk Storage and Distribution of Food, Indianapolis, Purdue University, p. 66.

von Bockelmann, B. 1980. Aseptic packaging of liquid food in Tetra Pak systems: microbiological aspects. S. Afr. Food Rev., Feb/March, 36.

von Bockelmann, B. 1985. Quality control of aseptically packaged food products. Proceedings, Symposium on Aseptic Processing and Packaging of Foods, IUFoST, Tylösand, Sweden, p. 150.

von Bockelmann, B. 1987. Qualitätskontrolle aseptisch verpackter Lebensmittel. In *Aseptisches Verpacken von Lebensmitteln*, Hamburg, Behr's Verlag, p. 277.

von Bockelmann, B. and von Bockelmann, I. 1986. Aseptic Packaging of Liquid Food Products: A literature review. J. Agri. Food Chem., *34*, 384.

von Bockelmann, I. 1985. Aseptic in-plant transportation. Proceedings, Symposium on Aseptic Processing and Packaging of Foods, IUFoST, Tylösand, Sweden, p. 134.

von Bockelmann, I. and von Bockelmann, B. 1972. The sporicidal action of hydrogen peroxide—a literature review. LWT-Ed., *5*, 221.

Voss, E. 1974. Fortschritte in der aseptischen Abfüllung von Lebensmitteln. Zbl. Bakt. Hyg., I Abt. Orig. B, *159*, 335.

Zimmermann, L. 1974. Das Abpacken von verderblichen und haltbaren Milcherzeugnissen in Kunststoff-Flaschen. Dtsch. Molk-Ztg., *95*, 274.

Zimmermann, L. 1975. Verfahren zur aseptischen Verpackung von stillen Fruchtsaft-getränken in umweltfreundliche Kunststoff-Flaschen. Dtsch. Lebensmitteltechnol., *26*, 195.

CHAPTER 49

DISINFECTION AND DISEASE PREVENTION IN VETERINARY MEDICINE

P.J. Quinn

The frequency and severity of infectious diseases in food-producing animals are major obstacles to increased production, especially in intensively reared animals. Estimates of the losses attributable to infectious diseases through mortality, subclinical disease or lost productivity vary from 15 to 20%. Once it gains entry into a group of susceptible animals, an infectious agent can spread and multiply leading to clinical or subclinical disease. The outcome of such a series of events will be determined by the susceptibility of the animals, the virulence of the infectious agent and the influence of management, nutrition, and chemotherapy on the course of the disease. The development of intensive livestock production, the increased value of individual animals and the emergence of new or recently recognized diseases have created many challenges for the veterinary profession, especially in the area of disease control.

Vaccination, when successful, is one of the preferred methods for preventing infectious diseases. However, there are still many major diseases of animals which cannot be controlled by this means. Consequently, vaccination is the answer to a limited number of diseases caused by specific agents. Increasingly, "complex" diseases often of uncertain etiology, are being recognized in intensively reared animals. The measures appropriate for controlling endemic infectious diseases, therefore, range from vaccination and disinfection to effective management and chemoprophylaxis, while exotic diseases are controlled by test and slaughter policies followed by thorough disinfection.

TRANSMISSION OF INFECTIOUS AGENTS

Infected animals shed pathogenic organisms, often in large numbers, and environmental contamination frequently follows. Contaminated biological materials, such as feces, urine, and exudates, and contaminated transport vehicles or buildings may harbour infectious agents for long periods and perpetuate infections in groups of animals unless the cycle of infection is interrupted by effective control measures. Figure 49–1 illustrates the various ways in which infectious agents may become disseminated in the environment and the control measures which apply. Survival of pathogenic organisms in the environment is determined, in part, by the number shed and their ability to withstand adverse environmental conditions. Pathogenic mycobacteria, a number of animal viruses, bacterial spores, coccidial oocysts, and parasitic ova are capable of prolonged survival in animal products, in feces, soil, water, animal dwellings, and on pasture. Strategies for preventing or controlling infectious diseases of animals are illustrated in Figure 49–2. These include measures appropriate for exotic diseases and endemic diseases. Disinfection plays an important role in the implementation of test and slaughter policies and in the destruction of infectious agents in contaminated biological products, buildings, transport vehicles, equipment, footwear, and clothing of personnel working with contaminated material. Many diseases of animals are transmissible to man (zoonoses) and disinfection is used to limit the spread of zoonotic agents during the production phase of food-producing animals and subsequently in meat plants and dairies.

SURVIVAL OF INFECTIOUS AGENTS IN THE ENVIRONMENT

Many infectious agents of animals, some of zoonotic importance, are capable of surviving for long periods in soil, feces, water, animal products, hay, straw, grain, and fomites. Spores of *Bacillus anthracis* can survive for decades in soil unless appropriate measures are taken to destroy them when burying carcasses of animals which have died from anthrax. Flood waters, earthworms, scavenging animals, subsidence, or erosion may allow spores

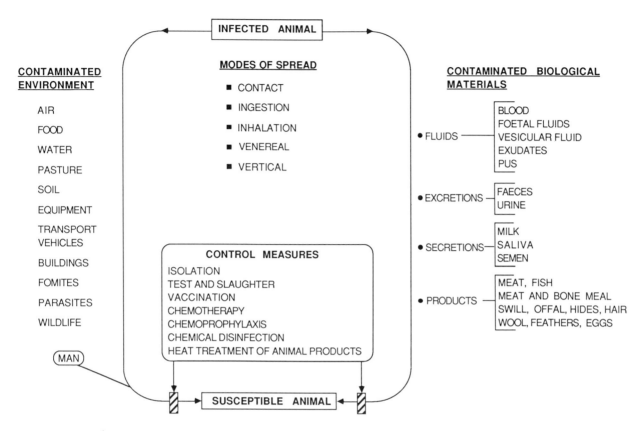

Fig. 49–1. Modes of transmission of infectious agents from infected to susceptible animals via contact, fluids, excretions, secretions, meat, and other products. Infection may be spread by environmental contamination by farm workers, or others visiting farms or production units. Control measures are aimed at breaking the cycle of infection either by preventing contact between host and agent, treating infected or in-contact animals, through raising the host's immune status by vaccination, or by appropriate disinfection procedures.

to reach the surface and subsequently infect susceptible animals.

Wastes from dairies, dairy factories, and from meat plants are being increasingly disposed of on agricultural land. Cattle and pig slurry is usually spread on arable land or pasture. Many pathogenic organisms are excreted in feces and urine, and others shed in the immediate vicinity of animals may contaminate slurry. Although slurry is usually stored for at least one month prior to spreading, this may be an insufficient interval to ensure loss of infectivity. In cattle slurry, salmonella organisms may survive up to 286 days and in soil up to 140 days (Jones, 1980). Their survival time on pasture is not well documented.

Experiments with *Brucella abortus* shed into liquid manure following abortions, show that high numbers of organisms can survive in slurry for at least 8 months (Verger, 1982). *Mycobacterium bovis* is capable of surviving for up to 300 days when mixed with blood, urine, and feces and shielded from direct sunlight, and for up to 2 years in soil (Wray, 1975). The pattern of survival of *M. bovis* is influenced by sunlight, dehydration, and temperature. Although there are differences in the data available, it is clear that pathogenic mycobacteria may

survive for months in slurry and for many weeks on shaded pasture (Wray, 1975; Jones, 1980).

Table 49–1 lists factors that influence the survival of infectious agents in the environment. Coccidial oocysts, parasitic ova, bacterial spores, and mycobacteria are among the infectious agents most resistant to desiccation, pH changes, extremes of temperature, and other environmental factors.

PRINCIPLES OF DISEASE CONTROL

Maintaining animals free from infectious diseases relies on well established procedures which may be employed nationally, locally or by individual animal owners. These procedures vary with the status of the disease in the country, its public health significance and its importance internationally. Diseases which are endemic in a country may be dealt with in different ways depending on their impact on the animal industry or on human health.

Prevention and control of infectious diseases of animals generally rely on four distinct approaches:
1. Control of animal movement
2. Testing suspect groups of animals, slaughtering

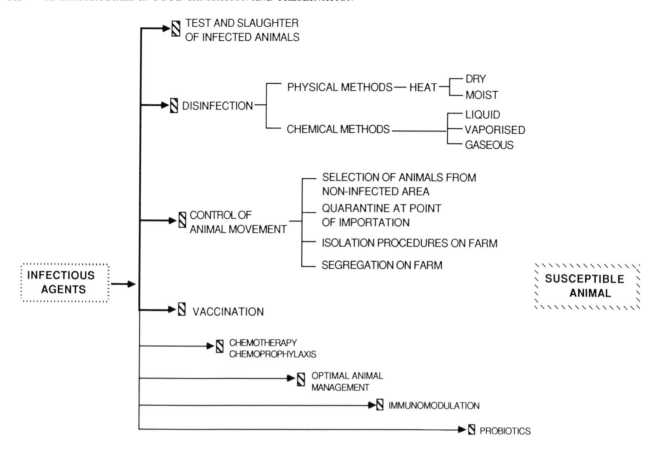

Fig. 49–2. Measures used for the prevention and control of infectious disease in domestic animals. The relevance and efficiency of individual measures vary with the nature of the infectious agent, its mode of transmission and, the suitability of the measure being employed. The ▨ symbol denotes methods of preventing transmission of infection or limiting its impact.

Table 49–1. *Factors Influencing the Survival of Infectious Agents in the Environment*

1. Method of shedding into the environment
2. Duration of shedding, number of infectious particles shed and their infectivity
3. Stability of the infectious agent to:
   Dehydration
   Ultraviolet light
   Temperature changes
   pH changes
   Disinfection procedures
4. Survival pattern of the infectious agent in:
   Faeces
   Slurry
   Urine
   Aerosols
   Water
   Pasture
   Soil
   Feed
   Fomites
   Transport vehicles
   Buildings
5. Route of infection for susceptible animals and the number of infectious particles required to produce disease

those infected, and disposing of the carcasses by burial or burning
3. Disinfection of premises, transport vehicles, or other contaminated sources of infection
4. Vaccination of susceptible animals

Additional measures may involve chemotherapy, chemoprophylaxis, or improving management systems. The measures appropriate for dealing with an outbreak of an infectious disease depend on whether it is exotic or endemic; whether it is being eradicated from an entire country or part of a country, its significance in international trading, and the nature and lability of the causative agent. Figure 49–2 illustrates measures appropriate for the prevention and control of infectious diseases in general. Long incubation periods, the development of a carrier state or sub-clinical disease with the likelihood of intermittent shedding, together with the possibility of insect vectors render effective control of many animal diseases somewhat uncertain. Land frontiers and wildlife reservoirs of infection further diminish the chances of success for some diseases such as rabies.

Inactivation of Infectious Agents

Infectious agents vary widely in their susceptibility to physical and chemical disinfection procedures. Ranked

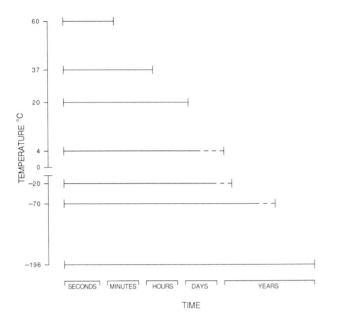

Fig. 49–3. The influence of temperature on the survival pattern of animal viruses. Some viruses, such as parvoviruses, are relatively heat-resistant and may survive temperatures in the region of 80°C for several minutes. Pasteurization, therefore, cannot always be relied on as an effective method for inactivating all animal viruses. The heat resistance of infectious agents associated with transmissible encephalopathies such as scrapie and bovine spongiform encephalopathy (BSE) is remarkable.

according to their susceptibility to chemical disinfectants, mycoplasmas, gram-positive bacteria, and gram-negative bacteria are usually highly susceptible; rickettsiae, enveloped viruses, chlamydiae, and fungal spores show a greater degree of resistance, while nonenveloped viruses, such as parvoviruses and bacterial spores, exhibit considerable resistance not only to chemical disinfectants but also to heat. The effect of temperature on the survival of viruses in general is shown in Figure 49–3. While many viruses are labile at temperatures in excess of 60°C, parvoviruses may survive temperatures in excess of 80°C for 30 min. They are, however, inactivated within one min at 100°C (Saknimit, et al., 1988). Foot-and-mouth disease virus can survive pasteurization at 72°C for 15 sec in milk and 93°C for 15 sec in cream (Blackwell and Hyde, 1976). The virus can be reliably inactivated at 148°C for 3 sec (Cunliffe, et al., 1979; Walker, et al., 1984).

Another group of infectious agents, sometimes referred to as unconventional etiological agents (prions), associated with encephalopathies in sheep, cattle, goats, and other species, are extremely resistant to standard decontamination procedures. Strain variation is noted, with some strains retaining infectivity after exposure to dry heat at 160°C for 24 hrs (Taylor, 1989). Resistance of these agents to chemical disinfectants is as remarkable as their resistance to physical decontamination procedures. Sodium hypochlorite, giving 2% available chlorine, has been recommended for disinfecting the environment after an outbreak of bovine spongiform

encephalopathy, but experimental evidence is required to support the efficacy of this procedure.

The mode of action of chemical disinfectants varies with their composition, concentration, and the nature and state of the infectious agent present. Table 49–2 indicates the probable sites of action of chemical disinfectants under optimal conditions. Irrespective of the method of inactivation used, when infectious agents are exposed to a lethal procedure such as disinfection, the kinetics of cell (or particle) death are usually exponential. Because of this inactivation pattern, the larger the initial number of infectious agents present, the more intense or prolonged the treatment required to ensure their destruction.

THE ROLE OF DISINFECTION IN DISEASE PREVENTION

Increased reliance on disinfection procedures for the control of infectious diseases in animals derives in part from the trend towards intensive rearing of livestock with the consequent build-up of infectious agents in units. The emergence of "complex" diseases and the necessity to have expensive buildings restocked soon after completion of a production cycle, highlight the necessity for efficient disinfection programs to deal with the residual infectious agents. These considerations apply particularly to the pig and poultry industries. The losses incurred by producers through clinical and subclinical disease combined with the cost of chemotherapy and chemoprophylaxis, and the limited effect of these measures on viral diseases encourage producers to implement thorough cleaning and disinfection programs for their buildings and to use animal isolation, transport vehicle disinfection, and footbaths at the entrance to their premises to prevent disease transmission. In the dairy industry, teat dipping has become an established method for reducing the incidence of bovine mastitis. The emergence of strains of mastitis-producing bacteria resistant to antimicrobial chemotherapy has refocused attention on the central role of teat dipping and disinfection of milking machine clusters for preventing or reducing new infections.

Despite sustained progress in vaccine production techniques, especially with subunit vaccines, many economically important diseases still cannot be controlled through immunization. Equine infectious anemia, a viral disease of horses in which biting flies act as mechanical vectors, and African swine fever, a viral disease of pigs with soft ticks acting as biological vectors, are examples of major viral diseases for which vaccines are not yet available. Control of animal movement, serological testing and slaughter of positive animals, boiling of swill in the case of African swine fever, control of vectors, and efficient disinfection are the principal control methods employed for these two diseases.

Disinfection also plays a role in eradication programs for diseases such as foot-and-mouth disease, brucellosis in ruminants and pigs, and transmissible gastroenteritis

Table 49–2. *Sites of Action of Chemical Agents with Antimicrobial Activity*

	Sites of Action					
Agent	Cell Wall	Cell Membrane	Proteins	Nucleic Acids	Enzymes with -SH Groups	Amino Acids
Acid (Mineral)		+	+		+	
Alcohols		+	+		+	
Alkalis		+	+		+	
Alkylating agents		+		+	+	+
Biguanides		+				
Dyes, e.g., acridine dyes				+		
Halogens		+			+	+
Heavy metals			+		+	
Phenolic compounds	+	+	+			
Quaternary ammonium compounds		+	+			

Adapted from Hugo, W.B. 1982. Disinfection mechanisms. In *Principles and Practice of Disinfection, Preservation and Sterilization.* Edited by A.D. Russell, W.B. Hugo and G.A.J. Ayliffe. Oxford, Blackwell Scientific Publications, pp. 158–185; van Oss, C.J. 1982. Action of physical and chemical agents on microorganisms. In *Medical Microbiology.* Edited by F. Milgrom and T.D. Flannagan. New York, Churchill Livingstone, pp. 69–79; Willett, H.P. 1984. Sterilization and disinfection. In *Zinsser Microbiology,* 18th Edition. Edited by W.K. Joklik, H.P. Willett and D.B. Amos. Norwalk, Appleton-Century-Crofts, pp. 233–249; Gardner, J.F., and Peel, M.M. 1986. Principles of chemical disinfection. In *Introduction to Sterilization and Disinfection.* Edited by J.F. Gardner and M.M. Peel. Melbourne, Churchill Livingstone, pp. 150–168; and Pelczar, M.J., Chan, E.C.S., and Krieg, N.R. 1986. Control by chemical agents. In *Microbiology,* 5th Edition. New York, McGraw-Hill, pp. 488–509.

of pigs. The availability of disinfectants of known potency has improved consumer confidence and allowed the selection of compounds effective against specific infectious agents not only for routine use on the farm but also for strategic use in the event of an epizootic of an exotic disease. Some problems have emerged in recent years with the recognition of new and potentially serious diseases of animals. One of these, bovine spongiform encephalopathy, a slowly progressive neurological disorder of adult cattle, has many features in common with a group of transmissible spongiform encephalopathies affecting animals and man caused by unconventional etiological agents. These agents, apparently, do not stimulate a specific immune response and have incubation periods measured in years. Confirmation of these diseases relies initially on their clinical recognition and subsequent histopathological examination of brain tissue post mortem. The unusual resistance of these unconventional etiological agents to heat and chemical disinfectants warrants further investigation so that effective disinfection procedures can be instituted to ensure their destruction.

Selection and Use of Disinfectants

There are diverse applications for chemical disinfectants in limiting the spread of infectious agents: on farms, in intensive production units, in dairies, meat plants, and food processing units. Table 49–3 lists the potential applications of disinfectants in disease prevention. The selection and use of a disinfectant for a particular application in veterinary medicine requires consideration of the range of infectious agents likely to be present or the actual infectious agents involved in a disease outbreak. If uncertainty exists about the infectious agents present, disinfectants with a wide spectrum of activity should be

selected. Surfaces should be thoroughly cleaned before the application of disinfectants. This process alone removes the majority of infectious agents if carried out in a competent manner. Personnel responsible for cleaning and disinfecting buildings should be properly trained to understand the specific needs of the entire procedure. When dealing with major zoonoses such as anthrax, workers should wear protective clothing, rubber gloves, waterproof footwear and masks; immediate disinfection without precleaning should be carried out.

Table 49–3. *Disinfection in the Control of Infectious Diseases: Potential Role*

1. To prevent transmission of disease by:
   lateral spread
   animals to man
   man to animals
2. As a routine measure to eliminate build-up of infectious agents in farm buildings
3. To maintain farms or animal production units free from disease with footbaths and wheel baths
4. To prevent the spread of mastitis-producing organisms by the application of teat dips
5. To decontaminate water systems
6. To render transport vehicles free from infectious agents
7. To prevent a build-up of infectious agents in lairages
8. To maintain boarding kennels and laboratory animal units free of infectious agents
9. To ensure that zoological parks and wildlife reserves do not transmit infectious diseases to native animal populations and to safeguard the health of exotic species from endemic diseases
10. To strengthen the role of quarantine stations by decontaminating effluent and all equipment and vehicles used for imported animals

Cleaning Prior to Disinfection

To avoid the generation of dust which may harbour infectious agents, it is advisable to spray the premises with water, preferably containing detergent. This also facilitates removal of dried feces, urine, milk or other adherent biological material. Initially, all portable equipment should be removed and, where appropriate, soaked in detergent solution and cleaned separately.

All organic matter—manure, bedding, litter, feed—should be removed and disposed of in an appropriate manner. Small amounts of bedding and litter may be burned, or if damp, composted. Gross dirt should be removed either manually, or, if the building is suitably designed, by mechanical methods. It is usual to wet all surfaces first with water containing either a nonfoaming detergent or 4% sodium carbonate (washing soda). A pressure hose, preferably a high pressure, low volume system, should then be employed to clean all surfaces capable of withstanding the pressure used. Steam cleaners are particularly effective for cleaning greasy areas, but rapid cooling on surfaces limits their antimicrobial effectiveness.

Cleaning should commence at the highest parts of the building—ceilings, then walls and finally floors, starting at the points furthest from the drain. In a large building with separate divisions, it is important to ensure that newly cleaned areas are not recontaminated as cleaning proceeds.

Movable items should be hand-cleaned by brushing or hosing before disinfection. Particular attention should be given to feeding equipment and drinkers. Tanks supplying the drinking water should be emptied and cleaned prior to disinfection of the entire water system with sodium hypochlorite.

Disinfection

The selection and use of chemical disinfectants for individual situations should be related to the practical conditions in which they are being used and the infectious agents present. Because it is difficult to clean all parts of an animal house equally well, it is generally advisable to select disinfectants that remain active in the presence of considerable amounts of organic matter. Halogen disinfectants, particularly sodium hypochlorite, are readily inactivated by organic matter, whereas phenolic disinfectants retain much of their activity in similar circumstances. Disinfectants suitable for building disinfection are listed in Table 49–4. Surfaces of a building may be treated with a disinfectant solution by brushing or by spraying under low or high pressure. Portable items should be soaked in a tank of disinfectant. For a disinfection program to succeed, the correct dilution of a disinfectant should be allowed sufficient time to act at the appropriate temperature. Traces of inhibitory substances such as soaps and detergents may interfere with the bactericidal or virucidal activity of quaternary ammonium compounds or biguanides. Environmental factors which may interfere with the activity of disinfectants in field applications are listed in Table 49–5. When buildings are of a suitable design, fumigation may be used as a final step in the procedure.

In a routine disinfection program, failure to inactivate the infectious agents may relate to the selection and use of the disinfectant or to environmental factors. Table 49–6 lists the spectrum of antimicrobial activity of some commonly used disinfectants. Apparent failure may result from the re-introduction of infection via carrier animals or from other sources. Table 49–7 lists the factors contributing to the failure of a disinfection program.

Table 49–4. *Disinfectants Suitable for Use in Farm Buildings after Routine Cleaning**

Part of Building	Phenols	Coal Tar Derivatives	Halogens Cl₂	Halogens I₂	Aldehydes	Quaternary Ammonium Compounds	Comments
Floor: Concrete	+ [a]	+	+	+	+	−	Disinfection of
Wood	+	+	±	±	±	−	infectious agents in
Earth	±	±	−	−	±	−	soil is unreliable
Walls and Roof	+	+	+	+	+	±	QACs and iodophors
Water supply	−	−	+	±	−	−	are expensive
Fittings: Wood	+	+	±	+	−	−	
Metal	+	±	±	±	−	±	
Plastic	+	±	+	+	−	±	
Air space [c]	± [b]	−	−	−	+	−	Fumigation possible only if building design suitable
Footbaths	+	+	−	±	± [d]	−	

[a] +, suitable; ±, of limited suitability; −, unsuitable

[b] Some aerosolized phenols suitable

[c] Application of an aerosolized acaracide and chemoattractant may be necessary for poultry houses with mite infestations.

[d] also suitable for use in footbaths for animals.

*An outbreak of a known infectious disease in a group of housed animals may further limit the choice of disinfectant suitable for a building (see Table 49–6).

Table 49–5. *Environmental Factors Which May Interfere with the Activity of Disinfectants in Field Applications*

Disinfectant	Organic Matter	pH	Relative Humidity	Soaps and Detergents	Water Hardeners
Acids	+	+	−	−	±
Alcohols	+	−	−	−	−
Alkalis	+	+	−	−	±
Alkylating Agents:					
Formaldehyde ╱ Gas dissolved in water (Formalin)	±	−	±	−	−
Formaldehyde ╲ Gas	+	−	+	−	−
Glutaraldehyde	±	+	−	−	±
Ethylene oxide	+	−	±	−	−
Biguanides	±	+	−	+	±
Halogens	+	+	−	−	±
Oxidizing agents	+	−	−	−	−
Phenolic compounds	±	+	−	−	±
Quaternary ammonium compounds	±	+	−	+	±

+, activity adversely affected; −, activity unaffected; ±, activity partially affected

Building design features may militate against the implementation of effective disinfection. Uneven, cracked, or pitted surfaces are difficult to disinfect, as are old wooden fittings. The drainage and ventilation systems may also present special difficulties in a disinfection program. The factors influencing the activity of chemical disinfectants in practical situations include the composition of the disinfectant, the temperature at which it is being used, and the type of infectious agents present (Table 49–8).

Safety Aspects of Disinfection

Some chemicals used in disinfection procedures are corrosive, toxic, irritant, or potentially carcinogenic. All disinfectants should be handled with care; manufacturers' instructions should be followed, and trained personnel should supervise the dilution of disinfectant prior to use. Acid and alkaline solutions should not be mixed; rubber gloves and a face shield should be worn while working with strong acids or alkalis. Both formaldehyde and methyl bromide are highly toxic for man and animals, so fumigation with these compounds should only be carried out by experienced personnel.

Electrical appliances used for disinfection should be well maintained and plugs should be fitted with a fuse of the correct rating. The electricity supply should be disconnected in buildings prior to power hosing and an alternative supply from an adjacent building should be used with a cable fitted with a circuit breaker.

Footbaths

Footbaths are likely to be effective only if all staff wear waterproof footwear and immerse clean footwear for at least one minute in disinfectant. Absorbent material, such as sponge soaked in disinfectant, is an unreliable substitute for a footbath. Waterproof protective clothing, that can be easily hosed down, should also be worn when dealing with exotic or highly infectious diseases.

Table 49–6. *The Antimicrobial Spectrum of Disinfectants, Classified According to Their Chemical Composition[a]*

Microorganisms Listed in Order of Increasing Resistance to Disinfectants	Acids (Mineral)	Alcohols	Aldehydes	Alkalis	Biguanides	Halogens Cl₂	Halogens I₂	Oxidising Agents	Phenolic Compounds	QACs
Mycoplasmas	+ +	+ +	+ +	+ +	+ +	+ +	+ +	+ +	+ +	+ +
Gram-positive bacteria	+ +	+ +	+ +	+	+ +	+ +	+ +	+ +	+ +	+ +
Gram-negative bacteria	+ +	+ +	+ +	+	+	+ +	+	+	+ +	+
Rickettsiae	+	+	+	+	±	+	+	+	+	±
Enveloped viruses	+	+	+ +	+	±	+ +	+	+	±[b]	±
Chlamydiae	±	±	+	+	±	+	+	+	±	−
Fungal spores	±	±	+	+	±	+	+	±	±	±
Nonenveloped viruses	±	−	+	±	−	+	±	±	−	−
Acid-fast bacteria	−	+	+	±	−	+	+	±	±	−
Bacterial spores	±	−	+	±	−	+	+	+[c]	−	−
Coccidial oocysts	−	−	−	±[d]	−	−	±[e]	−	±[f]	−

+ +, highly effective; +, effective; ±, limited activity; −, no activity; a, individual members may vary from the activity listed for that category; b, varies with the composition of disinfectant; c, peracetic acid, a strong oxidising agent is sporicidal; d, ammonium hydroxide is coccidiocidal; e, methyl bromide is coccidiocidal; f, some have activity against coccidia.

Table 49–7. *Factors Contributing to the Failure of a Disinfection Program*

Failure Relating to the Selection and Use of the Disinfectant	Failure Relating to Environmental and Other Factors	Apparent Failure
Selection of a disinfectant lacking activity against the infectious agent(s).	Presence of organic matter due to inadequate cleaning prior to disinfection.	Reintroduction of infectious agents to the disinfected area via carrier animal
Application of a suitable disinfectant at the incorrect dilution.	Synthetic materials such as plastics reduce the activity of QACs and biguanides. Lack of penetration of some materials, such as blankets, by gaseous disinfectants.	drinking water airborne infection personnel fomites food
Insufficient time allowed for the disinfectant to inactivate the infectious agent(s).	Inactivation of QACs and biguanides by soaps and detergents; partial inactivation of some compounds by the pH, or other characteristics of the material being treated.	transport vehicles insects rodents wildlife other sources
Temperature too low for optimal activity of disinfectant.	Incorrect application. Inadequate treatment of the water supply.	
Relative humidity too low for gaseous disinfectants.	Disinfection of slurry tanks containing large volumes of contaminated fluid is a difficult and often an uncertain measure, especially where resistant infectious agents are present.	

Suitable disinfectants for footbath use include phenols, cresols, and iodophors. If a specific infectious agent is identified in a disease outbreak, a disinfectant with known activity against that agent should be used at the appropriate concentration. The disinfectant in footbaths should be changed frequently. On large units, the disinfectant solution should be replaced daily or more frequently if there is evidence of gross contamination with organic matter. On smaller units with fewer staff, replacement of the disinfectant solution at three day intervals may suffice.

In circumstances where gross soiling of footwear is unavoidable, a second footbath containing dilute detergent for preliminary washing should be located alongside the footbath with disinfectant. This avoids rapid depletion of the disinfectant solution by organic matter.

Contaminated footwear and clothing may transfer infectious agents from one area to another, especially

Table 49–8. *Factors Influencing the Activity of Disinfectants in Practical Situations*

Factors Relating to the Disinfectant	Environmental Factors	Factors Relating to the Microorganisms Present
Chemical composition and stability of formulation	Temperature Relative humidity pH	*Type* Number, strain, and state (if spore-bearing); stability in adverse environmental conditions
Spectrum of activity	Presence of organic matter or other interfering substances such as water hardeners, soaps or detergents.	*Location:* On surfaces Floors, walls, ceilings, ventilators,
Mode of action	Nature and state of surfaces being disinfected:	permanent fittings, water tanks
Concentration employed	stone, concrete, tile, synthetic material, metal, wood, earth, or fabric	*In fluids* Such as slurry, water, blood, milk, saliva, amniotic and allantoic fluid, semen, urine, exudates, pus, vesicular fluid
Ability to penetrate		*On inanimate objects* On soil, bedding, transport vehicles, feed or fomites *Airborne* Either as an aerosol, or in association with dust or debris *Accessibility* of microorganisms to the disinfectant applied

agents shed in feces or urine such as salmonellae, coccidial oocysts, transmissible gastroenteritis virus, and leptospires. Footbaths serve to alert personnel to the risks of transferring infectious agents on footwear, but if they are to be effective their purpose and method of use should be made clear.

In view of the time taken to inactivate infectious agents by disinfectants, brief immersion of footwear in a footbath cannot be regarded as an adequate approach for limiting the spread of infectious agents. Immersion of clean footwear to a depth of 15 cm for at least one minute should ordinarily suffice. Footwear design, especially corrugations on the soles and heels which form angles, may retain organic matter even after routine washing. Parallel corrugations on the soles and heels are more easily cleaned than complex patterns.

The importance of other methods of transferring infection, such as clothing, wheels of transport vehicles, and the vehicles themselves, varies with the nature, number and virulence of the infectious agents and the susceptibility of exposed animals.

Footbaths should be located at suitable entry points to the unit or farm and be protected from flooding by surface water or heavy rainfall. Suggested dimensions for a footbath are shown in Figure 49–4. In frosty weather, antifreeze compatible with the disinfectant should be added at an appropriate concentration.

To ensure strict adherence to disinfection concentrations, it may be necessary for farm managers or supervisors to prepare appropriate dilutions of disinfectants not only for footbaths but also for general disinfection programs. Employees should also be instructed to dispose of used disinfectant solutions in a manner that minimizes the risk of environmental pollution.

Wheel Baths

Infection may be introduced into a farm or production unit by transport vehicles either on the body of the vehicle or on its wheels. Drivers and their vehicles visiting successive farms may inadvertently transfer infection on wheels or footwear.

To be effective, the design, construction, and use of wheel baths should ensure adequate contact with disinfectant for sufficient time to destroy the infectious agents on the surface of the wheels. Construction should be to strict specifications and conform to local planning and pollution control regulations. They should be sited in a location that will minimize the risk of flooding, contamination by surface water or subsidence. Design features should ensure the accommodation of the largest vehicles entering the farm. The dimensions of a wheel bath should be such that they allow for thorough immersion of one complete revolution of the largest circumference wheel passing through it. Since tractor wheels may have a circumference of approximately 6 m, it is essential that bath dimensions allow for this variation in wheel size. Baths should be waterproof, free of structural defects such as cracks and have no openings or valves which might allow accidental pollution of water courses. Capacity should allow for heavy rainfall without the risk of disinfectant overflow. A plan and elevation for a wheel bath with suggested dimensions is shown in Figure 49–5.

Wheel baths should only be installed if their use is justified and all other systems of disease control are func-

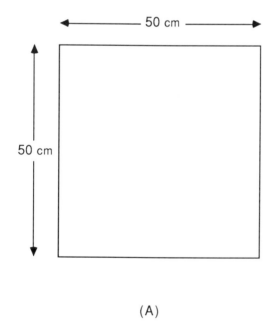

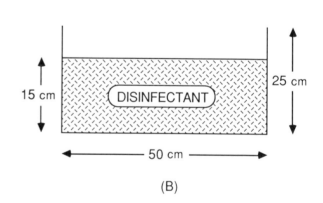

(A)   (B)

Fig. 49–4. Plan (A) and elevation (B) for a footbath for personnel. If gross soiling of footwear is unavoidable, a second footbath with diluted detergent and washing system should be placed alongside for the removal of organic matter prior to immersion of footwear in the disinfectant solution.

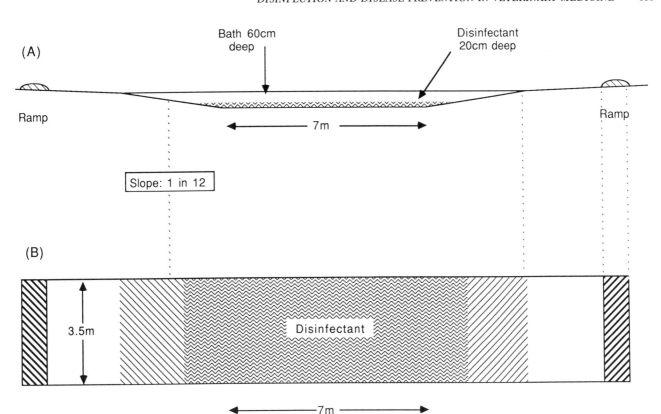

Fig. 49–5. Elevation (A) and plan (B) for a wheel bath, with suggested dimensions. The bath should be constructed to the highest specifications to ensure that no leaks of disinfectant occur. The dimensions may be modified in accordance with the type of vehicles for which it is intended. The disinfectant should be environmentally safe.

tioning optimally. The large volume of diluted disinfectant required (approximately 5000 l for the dimensions shown in Figure 49–5) and the cost of maintaining the disinfectant in an active state are serious limitations on their routine use for disease prevention. In addition, it is imperative that a vacuum tanker (slurry tanker) be available for routine filling and emptying and that the used disinfectant can be discarded in an environmentally acceptable manner. Disposal of used disinfectant into a large slurry tank, followed by agitation of slurry, is one possible on-farm method. If necessary a sump, or gradual slope on the floor of the bath towards one corner could be incorporated in the design to allow for complete emptying using a wide diameter hose fitted to a vacuum tanker. Concentration and type of disinfectant used in the wheel bath are important; although phenolic-based disinfectants are comparatively cheap and are active against many of the infectious agents likely to be transferred on wheels, disposal of a large volume could be difficult. Iodophor disinfectants are more environmentally safe, more readily neutralized than phenolic disinfectants and are more stable than hypochlorite-based disinfectants. Used at a concentration of 0.5%, changed at frequent intervals (at least when visibly contaminated by organic matter), and replenished if diluted by heavy rain, iodine-based disinfectants have a wide spectrum of activity and are usually nontoxic to man, domestic animals, and wildlife.

The siting of a wheel bath requires careful planning so that it cannot be bypassed by vehicles entering the farm. It should not, however, interfere with free movement of animals, pedestrians or cyclists. For the safety of drivers, a luminous warning sign should be displayed on either side of the bath, at a distance of approximately 20 m.

The success or failure of wheel baths is difficult to assess in practical farming circumstances. Their use and application should be considered as part of an overall disinfection program when all other aspects of the program are in place.

Design of Disinfection Programs

Intensive animal production systems frequently result in high numbers of animals occupying the same air space with attendant problems of occasional overcrowding and competition for floor or trough space. Frequently the environment is dusty with airborne microorganisms and gaseous contaminants challenging the optimal functioning of immune and physiological mechanisms of the upper and lower respiratory tract. In such circumstances it is unrealistic to expect a disinfection program to compensate for inefficient management, unsuitable building design, inadequate ventilation and low standards of hygiene, all of which may contribute to disease outbreaks. Disinfection is but one method of preventing transmission of infectious agents (Fig. 49–2) and its role is to complement optimal animal management and other control measures appropriate for the species, age and purpose for which the animals are being produced. The objectives of a disinfection program should be to provide an environment in which the animals' health can be maintained and their productivity sustained with minimal inconvenience to staff and at reasonable cost to management. The design and implementation of an efficient disinfection program requires an evaluation of the disease status of the farm, an accurate record of disease problems, including laboratory reports if available, details of animal purchases, review of isolation facilities for replacement animals, the type of vaccination program in operation, and the type of building and its suitability for a particular disinfection routine. Consideration should also be given to the water supply and periodic disinfection of the water system, the use of foot baths and wheel baths, the cleaning equipment available on the farm, and the suitability of the disinfectants to be used for the infectious agents identified on the farm. The management policy regarding disinfection procedures and the personnel implementing the cleaning and disinfection of the premises should also be examined.

Factors Which Limit the Impact of a Disinfection Regime

Structural features and other characteristics of buildings may render them difficult to clean and disinfect. Houses with slatted floors, buildings with open ridge ventilation, ill-fitting doors and windows, and damaged roofs make fumigation inefficient. Calf pens with pallets used as slats, buildings with extensive old timber fittings, with cobblestone, cracked or earth floors, or with unplastered walls are difficult to clean and disinfect. In addition, the absence of electricity, a power hose, and a mains water supply on remote farms or "out-farms," may make efficient cleaning impossible.

Certain management systems make no provision for appropriate action in sudden, explosive outbreaks of disease in large groups of animals. In such systems, isolation of suspect cases and proper disinfection are often difficult to implement. Problems of this nature may be encountered in farrowing units in which a sudden outbreak of Aujeszky's disease may result in multiple abortions. When an outbreak of acute infectious disease resulting in abortion occurs in cows, such as at a self-feed silage face, the accumulation of slurry hampers implementation of a proper cleaning regime. If no alternative feeding location is available, the time during which such animals can be removed from their only food source is limited. Removal of slurry from yards also requires considerable manpower, together with appropriate agricultural equipment, such as tractors fitted with scrapers.

Slurry Disposal

A serious difficulty arising from infectious diseases in groups of intensively reared animals on slatted floors, particularly in winter, is the utilization or dispersal of slurry known to contain pathogenic organisms. Some pathogenic bacteria such as *Brucella abortus* and *My-*

cobacterium bovis can survive many months in slurry tanks (Verger, 1982; Wray, 1975; Jones, 1980).

A number of viruses, such as those causing swine vesicular disease, foot-and-mouth disease, and Aujeszky's disease, may also be capable of surviving for extended periods in slurry. The continued survival of helminth ova and coccidial oocysts in fecal matter is well established. Storage with a view to natural loss of infectivity, therefore, is an uncertain measure to adopt for many animal pathogens. Chemical disinfection of slurry has received limited attention, but should be considered where exotic infectious agents are present or where the disease agent is the subject of an eradication program. Application of slurry to arable land or to land unsuitable for grazing can be considered for agents of endemic infectious diseases. The possibility of wildlife such as deer or badgers acquiring infection from such sources should also be borne in mind.

THE ACTIVITY OF DISINFECTANTS AGAINST SPECIFIC PATHOGENS OF VETERINARY IMPORTANCE

There are still many important infectious diseases of animals, some of considerable economic significance, that cannot be controlled by vaccination. Examples of these are mastitis in dairy cattle, African swine fever in pigs, equine infectious anemia of horses, and feline infectious peritonitis of cats. Infectious agents also vary widely in their susceptibility to physical and chemical methods of disinfection, and although some structural and biochemical features of pathogens correlate with their resistance to disinfection, well defined experimental procedures, incorporating appropriate controls, are required to determine the efficacy of particular disinfectants against particular infectious agents.

VIRUSES

Virucidal tests present several difficulties not encountered with bactericidal tests. Demonstration of virus survival requires either tissue culture, chick embryo, or animal inoculation. Different numbers of virus particles, depending on their virulence, may be required to produce disease in susceptible animals or induce cytopathic effects in tissue culture. Accordingly, complete inactivation of a virus suspension cannot normally be determined, since the destruction of the last infectious virus particle cannot be readily detected. The toxicity of disinfectants for tissue cultures is an additional difficulty in testing virucides. Methods of overcoming the cytotoxic effects induced by disinfectants have been reviewed (Quinn, 1987).

Foot-And-Mouth Disease Virus (FMDV)

This virus was rapidly inactivated in the presence of acids and alkalis, and provided the pH value was sufficiently acid or alkaline, a 5 log reduction in virus titer was found in 15 sec (Sellers, 1968). Virus inactivation in the presence of phenolic disinfectants was slow. FMDV was rapidly inactivated by sodium hypochlorite, but the addition of organic matter reduced the activity of this disinfectant and allowed virus survival.

Pasteurization cannot be relied on for the destruction of FMDV as virus was recovered from whole milk of infected cows following heating at 72°C for 5 minutes (Blackwell and Hyde, 1976). FMDV also survived in the cream component following heating at 93°C for 15 sec. Heating at 148°C for 3 sec inactivated the virus (Cunliffe et al., 1979; Walker et al., 1984).

African Swine Fever Virus

Ten commercially available disinfectants, representative of the common classes of disinfectants and detergents, were tested at a high pH in 2% sodium hydroxide and at a low pH in 2% acetic acid, for their ability to inactivate the virus of African swine fever (Stone and Hess, 1973). All were evaluated by their ability, at a 1% concentration, to inactivate the virus of African swine fever in a protein-rich medium. Although a number of the compounds used had marked virucidal activity in laboratory-based tests, a phenolic compound containing *o*-phenylphenol was the only disinfectant with virucidal activity when virus-disinfectant mixtures were tested in pigs. The inactivation by *o*-phenylphenol was attributed to solubilization of the lipid segment of the virus envelope.

Swine Vesicular Disease Virus

Acids, alkalis, oxidizing agents, detergents, and a range of other chemicals were tested for their activity against swine vesicular disease virus (Herniman, et al., 1973). Organic matter interfered with many of the disinfectants except formalin, acetic acid, and ethyl alcohol. Sodium hydroxide was more effective than acids and raising the temperature increased the rate of inactivation.

Of 13 compounds tested against swine vesicular disease virus at 25°C for 30 minutes, only 5 completely inactivated the virus (Blackwell, et al., 1975). Only sodium hydroxide, sodium hypochlorite, and formaldehyde inactivated the virus in less than 2 min under test conditions. The activity of sodium hypochlorite was markedly decreased in the presence of high concentrations of organic material.

Porcine Parvovirus, Pseudorabies Virus, and Transmissible Gastroenteritis Virus

Fourteen disinfectants were evaluated for their virucidal activity against porcine parvovirus, transmissible gastroenteritis (a coronavirus), and pseudorabies (a herpesvirus) by Brown (1981). The disinfectants used included ethyl alcohol, iodophors, aldehydes, quaternary ammonium compounds, phenolic compounds, sodium hydroxide and sodium hypochlorite. Only sodium hypochlorite and sodium hydroxide inactivated porcine parvovirus after 5 min incubation, while pseudorabies and transmissible gastroenteritis viruses were inactivated by all of the disinfectants tested in the same time interval.

When the incubation time was increased to 20 min, both 2% glutaraldehyde and 8% formaldehyde inactivated porcine parvovirus.

Talfan Virus and Porcine Adenovirus Type 2

Ten disinfectants were tested for their activity against Talfan virus (a porcine enterovirus) and a strain of porcine adenovirus type 2 by Derbyshire and Arkell (1971). Cetrimide and a phenolic disinfectant were active against the adenovirus, but not against the Talfan virus. Chlorhexidine and an ampholytic surface active agent had little activity against either virus. Inactivation of the viruses by formaldehyde was slow, while an iodophor preparation had some virucidal activity. Sodium hypochlorite and ethyl alcohol were the most efficient disinfectants under the conditions of the test.

Equine Infectious Anemia

A study on the efficiency of inactivation of equine infectious anemia virus by 12 disinfectants was reported by Shen et al. (1977). All the compounds inactivated 4 $\log_{10}$ of virus within 5 min at 23°C in the presence of 10% bovine serum. Sodium hydroxide, formalin and glutaraldehyde took longer to inactivate the virus than substituted phenolic disinfectants, halogen derivatives, chlorhexidine and 70% ethyl alcohol. The authors concluded that the susceptibility of the equine infectious anemia virus to chemical disinfectants was similar to that of other enveloped viruses.

Feline Viruses

Thirty-five commonly used commercial disinfectants were evaluated for their virucidal activity against feline viral rhinotracheitis (a herpesvirus), feline calicivirus, and feline panleukopenia (a parvovirus) (Scott, 1980). Of 22 tested against feline viral rhinotracheitis, all were virucidal; 11 of 35 were virucidal for feline calicivirus, but only 3 of 27 were effective against feline panleukopenia. Sodium hypochlorite at a 0.175% concentration was the most effective and practical virucidal product used.

Newcastle Disease Virus

Five phenolic-based commercial disinfectants were tested for their virucidal activity at concentrations ranging from 0.39% to 1.56% (Wright, 1974). All were effective virucides at the manufacturers' recommended concentrations.

Aleutian Disease Virus of Mink

The virucidal activity of 9 disinfectants against Aleutian disease virus of mink was investigated by Shen, Leendertsen and Gorham (1981). Sodium hypochlorite, an iodophor, glutaraldehyde and a commercial (phenol-based) disinfectant inactivated 4 $\log_{10}$ of virus within 10 min at 23°C. Formalin took 30 min to inactivate the virus.

Eight Virus Groups Affecting Different Species

The efficacy of 9 compounds, representing the major classes of disinfectants, against 8 virus groups was assessed by a comparison of titers of the viruses before and after exposure to each disinfectant (Evans, Stuart, and Roberts, 1977). The viruses used were, an enterovirus, coronavirus, reovirus, myxovirus, adenovirus, herpesvirus, togavirus, and poxvirus. Formalin, glutaraldehyde, hypochlorite and peracetic acid were effective against all the viruses.

Coronaviruses and Parvoviruses of Laboratory Animals

The virucidal efficacy of chemical disinfectants, heating and ultraviolet irradiation against mouse hepatitis virus, canine coronavirus, Kilham rat virus and canine parvovirus was evaluated by Saknimit et al. (1988). Coronaviruses were inactivated by ethanol, isopropanol, benzalkonium chloride, iodophor, sodium hypochlorite, cresol soap, and formaldehyde. The authors reported that the parvoviruses appeared to be inactivated by formaldehyde, iodophor, and sodium hypochlorite. Coronaviruses were destroyed by heating at 60°C for 15 min, whereas parvoviruses were stable up to 80°C for 30 min. When heated to 100°C, parvoviruses were inactivated within 1 min. Ultraviolet irradiation inactivated all viruses within 15 min.

San Miguel Sea Lion Virus and Vesicular Exanthema of Swine Virus

A total of 12 test compounds were used against these 2 viruses (Blackwell, 1978). The 2 caliciviruses were inactivated rapidly by a number of chemical formulations including sodium hypochlorite, sodium carbonate, sodium hydroxide, citric acid, and acetic acid. Resistance to an iodophor, formaldehyde and a substituted phenol was greater with vesicular exanthema of swine virus than San Miguel virus.

Pseudocowpox

The effect of 3 commercial teat dips, chlorhexidine, an iodophor, and linear dodecyl benzene sulphonic acid on pseudocowpox was investigated by Puddle, Pulford and Ralston (1986). In a series of teat-dipping experiments, the iodophor was the only sanitizer which significantly decreased the incidence of pseudocowpox lesions, compared to controls. The authors concluded that teat dipping with an iodophor would be a practical method of limiting the spread of pseudocowpox in a dairy herd, but once virus lesions appeared on the teats, teat dipping was unlikely to enhance remission of lesions.

SUSCEPTIBILITY OF PATHOGENIC FISH VIRUSES TO VARIOUS DISINFECTION PROCEDURES

The virucidal properties of iodophor, sodium hypochlorite, formalin, thiomersal (an organic mercurial), malachite green, and acriflavine were tested on infectious pancreatic necrosis virus (IPNV), isolated from rainbow trout (Elliot and Amend, 1978). Iodine and chlorine compounds showed good activity, but efficacy depended on the concentration of virus, the presence of organic matter, and water pH. The virus was not inactivated by exposure to 0.2% formalin for 60 min or by thiomersal or malachite green. Acriflavine in cell culture media prevented the development of cytopathology caused by the virus.

The effect of ultraviolet irradiation on selected pathogenic fish viruses including infectious haematopoietic necrosis virus (IHNV), was evaluated by Yoshimizu, Takizawa and Kimura (1986). IHNV was sensitive to ultraviolet irradiation, but other viruses varied in their susceptibility to this disinfection procedure.

The disinfectant effect of an ultraviolet-ozone water sterilizer on viruses and bacteria in water was examined by Sako and Sorimachi (1985). IPNV was resistant to the treatment, whereas IHNV was inactivated. Three species of pathogenic bacteria were also inactivated by this method.

BACTERIA

Mycobacteria

Mycobacteria are considered separately from other vegetative bacteria for several reasons: most pathogenic mycobacteria grow slowly, are more resistant to desiccation and chemical disinfection than other vegetative bacteria, and their survival time outside the body is relatively long. They possess an unusually high content of cell wall lipid, including waxes, which impede penetration of aqueous solutions and the resultant hydrophobic nature of the envelope may be partly responsible for their high resistance to chemical disinfection.

Mycobacterium bovis, the cause of tuberculosis in cattle and other species, is still of considerable importance in many countries, not only because of its pathogenicity for animals but also for its public health significance. Generally, the most effective method of inactivating mycobacteria is by heat.

Treatment of *M. bovis* in meat products for one hr with 0.3% benzalkonium chloride did not reduce the number of organisms present (Merkal and Whipple, 1980). Treatment with a phenolic disinfectant, followed by formaldehyde vapor, was effective in disinfecting equipment contaminated with meat emulsion containing *M. bovis*.

The tuberculocidal activity of phenol and a phenolic compound containing o(2)-phenylphenol against *M. bovis* in milk was investigated using five strains of the organism (Richards and Thoen, 1979). The phenolic disinfectant diluted ⅛ and phenol diluted ¹⁄₃₂, killed each of 5 strains of *M. bovis* suspended in untreated milk during a 6 hour exposure at 23°C.

Chlorhexidine gluconate inhibited the growth of saprophytic mycobacteria such as *Mycobacterium phlei*, *Mycobacterium smegmatis* and *Mycobacterium marinum*, but did not affect *Mycobacterium avium*, *Mycobacterium kansasii* and *Mycobacterium scorfulaceum* (Fodor and Szabó, 1980).

The antitubercular action of 10 commercially available disinfectants was determined using *Mycobacterium tuberculosis* derived from active cases of tuberculosis as test organism (Bergan and Lystad, 1971). Neither quaternary ammonium compounds nor 2% glutaraldehyde proved effective. Phenolic disinfectants were more tuberculocidal than most of the others tested.

Brucella abortus

Brucellae are unique among nonspore-forming bacteria in their resistance to different environmental conditions. In liquid manure, they can survive for at least 8 months without much loss of viability (Verger, 1982). These organisms are primarily found in fetal membranes, the aborted fetus, uterine secretions, raw milk, and milk products. Hall (1979) reported that chlorhexidine gluconate gave a 5 log reduction in *B. abortus* after 60 sec exposure. No organic matter was added to the test system and the initial concentration of organisms was not specified.

Gayot and Ursache (1976) tested the bacterial activity of sodium hypochlorite, formol, phenol, and sodium hydroxide on *B. abortus* for 10 min at room temperature and concluded that sodium hypochlorite was the most active disinfectant. The effects of various phenol concentrations, incubation temperature and time on the viability of *B. abortus* was investigated by Scanlan, Hannon and Matthews (1982). They concluded that a reference strain at a concentration of 1×10^{11}/ml in broth, with 5% serum, survived in 1.0, 2.0, 5 and 10% phenolized saline for 24 hrs.

The activity of 7 disinfectants, which included phenolic, halogen, quaternary ammonium, and aldehyde groups of disinfectants, were evaluated against *B. abortus* in vitro (Quinn, 1984). These disinfectants performed well against high concentrations of the organisms at 0.5% and 1% concentrations in the absence of organic matter. The addition of serum had a marked inhibitory effect on their bactericidal activity, apart from 1% formalin which proved consistently reliable even in the presence of serum.

Bacterial Spores

Bacterial spores are recognized as one of the more resistant forms of microbial life. They are much more resistant to adverse environmental conditions, heat and chemical disinfectants than their corresponding vegetative cells. Many antimicrobial compounds have limited activity against spores and the ability of certain bacteria to form spores, gives them a separate status in relation to other microorganisms. Temperatures exceeding 100°C are usually required to kill bacterial spores but the level of heat resistance varies widely according to the species. Disinfectants such as alcohol, biguanides, phenols, and quaternary ammonium compounds may be sporostatic but not sporicidal.

In veterinary medicine, diseases caused by spore-forming bacteria are of considerable significance. *Bacillus anthracis* is one example of an organism which produces spores of high resistance, and environmental pollution by these resistant microbial structures presents special difficulties in relation to disinfection procedures. Clostridia, a group of anaerobic spore-forming bacteria whose habitat is soil, are associated with many diseases of animals but their impact is lessened through vaccination rather than disinfection.

The sporicidal activity of a wide range of hospital disinfectants was investigated using *Bacillus subtilis* as test organism (Kelsey, Mackinnon and Maurer, 1974). Alcoholic hypochlorite and glutaraldehyde had some sporicidal activity, while iodophors, formalin and phenolic disinfectants were less effective. Chlorhexidine showed no sporicidal activity.

When buffered hypochlorite and buffered alcohol-hypochlorite mixtures were tested against *B. subtilis* spores, high sporicidal activity was achieved with low concentrations of alcohol and hypochlorite by buffering in the pH range 7.6 to 8.1 (Death and Coates, 1979).

The bactericidal, fungicidal, and sporicidal properties of hydrogen peroxide and peracetic acid were compared by Baldry (1983). Peracetic acid was rapidly sporicidal for spores of *B. subtilis* especially under acidic conditions; hydrogen peroxide was more effective as a sporicide than as a bactericide.

The sporicidal effect of peracetic acid on spores of *Bacillus anthracis* has been investigated by Hussaini and Ruby (1976). A complete sporicidal effect was observed on spores in soil, treated with 3% peracetic acid for 10 min at 4°C.

Lensing and Oei (1984) studied the efficacy of a chlorine-containing compound, peracetic acid, formaldehyde, glutaraldehyde, and other veterinary disinfectants against spores of *B. anthracis*. After 30 min at 20°C, the chlorine-containing compound (2400 ppm active chlorine) and 0.25% peracetic acid had significant sporicidal effect in the presence of 4% horse serum. Under the same test conditions, 4% formaldehyde and 2% glutaraldehyde were sporicidal after two hrs exposure.

Fungal Agents

Peracetic acid exhibited rapid fungicidal activity against the yeast *Saccharomyces cerevisiae*, especially under acidic conditions (Baldry, 1983). The antifungal properties of glutaraldehyde have been investigated using *Aspergillus niger, Rhizopus stolonifer, Penicillium chrysogenum, Mucor hiemalis, Saccharomyces cerevisiae* and *Trichophyton mentagrophytes* (Gorman and Scott, 1977). Alkaline glutaraldehyde in concentrations greater than 0.1% prevented growth of all the species examined, while 0.5% acid glutaraldehyde was necessary to achieve this effect. After 90 min contact with 0.5% alkaline glutaraldehyde, a 99.99% reduction in viable counts was achieved. A considerable drop in spore production was also observed after treatment with alkaline glutaraldehyde.

DISINFECTION AND DISEASE PREVENTION IN POULTRY

The poultry industry, since it moved from extensive small units to the intensive industry that operates in many countries today, has employed disinfection to great advantage for controlling infectious diseases. Disease control programs for poultry usually employ (1) vaccination, (2) hygiene and disinfection, (3) chemoprophylaxis, (4) optimal nutrition, and (5) efficient management. All of these approaches are needed to ensure good feed conversion rates and profitability. Vaccination for specific infectious disease such as Marek's disease and infectious bronchitis are routine and effective procedures, while chemoprophylaxis for coccidiosis is standard practice in most poultry units. However, vaccination and medication are only effective for a limited number of infectious diseases. Intelligent use of disinfectants can limit the impact of poultry pathogens at every phase of production, from the hatchery stage to laying units.

A disinfection program, like a vaccination program, should be designed to suit the needs of a particular unit. Points to be considered include the known disease risks, the management system, the production cycle, the structure of the buildings and equipment and any other relevant data available from flock records. The program should contain advice to personnel on good hygiene practices, movement of equipment, the use of footbaths, and the selection and use of detergents and disinfectants for the terminal cleaning and disinfection of poultry units after depopulation.

Hatcheries

Even assuming proper construction to facilitate routine cleaning and disinfection, the opportunity for disease transmission through the hatchery must be regarded as a serious potential risk for the poultry industry because of the many sources of eggs and the wide distribution of chicks to poultry farms. There are numerous ways whereby infection may be introduced onto the premises. These include the surface of eggs, egg boxes, transport vehicles, rodents, flies and other insects, footwear, clothing and hands of hatchery staff, customers or other visitors to the hatchery. Return of sick birds for consultation or diagnosis should not be permitted.

Boxes used for chick transportation should be nonreturnable. If chick boxes are designed for re-use, they should be thoroughly cleaned and disinfected after each shipment. Transport vehicles belonging to the hatchery should be hosed down and washed with disinfectant on completion of deliveries each day. Visitors to the hatchery should, ideally, be provided with clean outer clothing such as boiler suits at point of arrival, wear waterproof footwear, and use a footbath for at least one minute before entering active sections of the hatchery. Workers in the hatchery should be advised to avoid contact with poultry farms and should be provided with clean outer clothing on a regular basis. Maintaining the premises free of rodents should be a priority. Flies, cockroaches,

and wild birds, especially starlings and other potential vectors of disease, should be kept under effective control. Unless there is a concerted effort made to maintain the premises free of infection by education of staff, suppliers, customers, and visitors, with the full cooperation of all personnel involved, a hatchery disinfection program, however thorough, may not achieve its objective.

Incubator Hygiene

Incubator trays and removable fittings should be cleaned, washed, and disinfected each time they are used. All other equipment coming in contact with eggs should be cleaned and disinfected at regular intervals. These include trolleys and containers used for transport or storage of eggs. To minimize the dispersal of dust and its associated pathogens, vacuum cleaning should be employed where possible. Alternatively, dust and debris particularly on metal surfaces, should be sprayed with an iodine-based disinfectant prior to cleaning. Chlorine-based disinfectants may also be used, but they are rapidly inactivated by organic matter and may corrode metal surfaces.

Formaldehyde Fumigation of Incubators. Under carefully controlled conditions, fumigation with formaldehyde gas is an effective method of disinfecting the shells of hatching eggs at the flock farm and at the hatchery. Purpose-built fumigation cabinets are used on some farms to disinfect the shell surface as soon as eggs are collected and before bacteria have had time to penetrate into the egg through the shell and shell membranes. Eggs are also fumigated routinely in purpose-built units on arrival at the hatchery.

Methods commonly used for generating formaldehyde gas are (1) the potassium permanganate method, (2) the paraformaldehyde method, and (3) evaporation of formalin solution. When potassium permanganate crystals are added to 40% formalin solution, there is a rapid and violent reaction with the release of formaldehyde gas. The reaction generates a substantial amount of heat; metal containers should be used for this procedure. The addition of 35 ml of 40% formalin to 10 g potassium permanganate crystals per meter cubed (m^3) generates a satisfactory concentration of formaldehyde gas. For safety reasons, this method of fumigation is discouraged on farms.

Using paraformaldehyde powder or pellets (prills), formaldehyde gas can be generated in sufficient concentration by heating 10 g of powder per m^3 in an electric pan with a thermal cut-out switch. It is advisable to raise the relative humidity above 70% by adding some water to the prills before heating.

Evaporation of 40% formalin at a rate of 60 ml per m^3 of hatchery space is another procedure sometimes used to control microbial contamination of eggs.

It is important that eggs are not fumigated between the twelfth and ninety-sixth hour after setting as the embryo is sensitive to formaldehyde at this stage. Some workers question the safety of fumigation of eggs at any time after incubation begins (Harry and Binstead, 1961).

Special precautions apply to formaldehyde fumigation since the gas is toxic for man and animals. Doors should be locked and notices posted when fumigation is in progress. A respirator should be available for use by staff in the event of an emergency and formaldehyde gas should *not* be used along with chlorine-containing compounds because a potent carcinogen may be formed if the two chemicals interact.

Poultry Houses: Cleaning and Disinfection Procedure

Some variation in procedures will apply depending on design features and the purpose for which the building is being used. The general approach to such an operation has common features. Following depopulation, feed bags and other refuse should be removed and if dead birds are discovered, they should be incinerated. All movable equipment, such as feeders and drinkers, should be removed and soaked in a tank of detergent. If the building design allows for it, a tractor can be used to remove most of the bedding and the remainder can be removed manually by brushing and scraping. If the building is dry and dusty, it should be sprayed with water, preferably containing nonfoaming detergent, to control dust during cleaning and to soften adherent organic matter on surfaces. The building should be isolated from the electricity supply before spraying commences.

Acaricide Application

If *Dermanyssus gallinae* has been detected in the house, immediately after the litter has been removed and before the house has cooled, the interior of the house should be sprayed with a chemoattractant, followed by an acaricide such as pyrethrum or dichlorvos. The use of a chemoattractant is necessary as the mites are found in cracks or crevices in timber fittings where they may be inaccessible to acaricides. The same treatment should be applied one week later as the life cycle from egg to adult takes seven days and the second application of acaricide is required to ensure destruction of nymphal or adult stages that emerge after the first application.

Washing Procedure

Starting at the ceiling and walls, the surfaces should be washed, preferably with a power hose, paying particular attention to all areas where dust accumulates, such as ledges and ventilator shafts. It is important to ensure that all organic matter in the vicinity of the building outside is also removed.

When visibly clean, a disinfectant active in the presence of organic matter should be applied to all surfaces and allowed to act for several hours before being washed off. Portable fittings should be hand-washed and disinfected separately. The water system should then be disinfected.

Disinfection of the Water System

The water supply should be turned off and the system drained. The header tank should be cleaned, drained, and filled with sodium hypochlorite at a concentration of 500 ppm. All drinking lines should be flushed through and the disinfectant left to act in the entire system for 12 hrs. The disinfectant solution should be drained, each line flushed through with clean water and the header tank refilled with mains water.

Formaldehyde Fumigation

The house, with bedding and fittings in place, can be fumigated using either formaldehyde or methyl bromide. Both chemicals are potentially dangerous and require experienced staff to ensure safety and success. For successful fumigation, the building should be capable of being sealed against the escape of gas, the temperature should be close to 20°C and the relative humidity should be above 70%, without pools of water on the floor or in drains. Fumigation can be carried out by heating paraformaldehyde, a safe method if heated pans are available, by adding formalin to potassium permanganate, or with a formalin aerosol using aerosol generators. The latter is probably the least satisfactory of the three methods.

Paraformaldehyde Method. The air space of the building should be calculated and the amount of paraformaldehyde distributed at a maximum rate of 500 g per pan. These specially designed electrically heated pans should reach a temperature of 200°C and they should be placed not more than 30 m (approximately 100 feet) apart. All ventilators, windows, drains, and spaces along pipes should be securely sealed. Plastic sheets or clean strong plastic bags can be fitted over ventilators and taped in position. This method can also be used to seal spaces in ill-fitting windows or doors. All doors, except the exit door for the operators, should be closed, locked, and sealed with tape.

Power switching should be from outside the building once the exit door is locked. A notice indicating that fumigation is in progress should be displayed on all doors. The building should remain closed for at least 24 hrs before being ventilated.

Formalin-Potassium Permanganate Method. This method requires close supervision and experienced personnel. It is potentially dangerous, especially if operators slip on wet floors as formaldehyde gas is being released. Deep metal containers should be used for the reacting chemicals. As the reaction between these two compounds is rapid and violent, not more than 500 g of potassium permanganate and one liter of formalin should be added to each container. Considerable heat is generated by these reacting chemicals and containers should be placed at least 2 m (6 feet) away from combustible material. Containers with the weighed quantities of potassium permanganate required should be distributed evenly along the length of the building at intervals of 30 m. The exit door of the building should be securely fixed in an open position, whereas all other doors should be sealed, locked, and warning notices posted on them. The operator, wearing a respirator, should pour the formalin over the potassium permanganate crystals from a wide-mouthed container, starting at the end of the building furthest from the open door. A second person, also wearing a respirator, should supervise the procedure in case of mishap. The addition of formalin to the crystals should take place quickly but smoothly. When the operation is complete, the exit door should be closed, locked, and sealed. The building should be left sealed for 24 hrs before being thoroughly ventilated. A respirator must be worn if the building has to be entered to open windows and switch on fans.

Aerosol Fumigation. Aerosol generators are sometimes used for fumigation at a rate of 100 ml of formalin per 10 m³. In large buildings a number of generators are required as the droplets produced have directional effects. Trials with aerosol generators indicate that this method may give variable results.

Drinking bowls and food containers should be rinsed with water before poultry are moved in after fumigation. Footbaths should be placed in position at major access points for use by all staff visiting the building.

Formaldehyde gas is pungent, and irritating to mucous membranes even at low concentrations; personnel should not be exposed to concentrations above 2 ppm. At higher concentrations, it is rapidly toxic and the long-term effects of constant exposure, even to low doses, may present some health risks.

Evaluation of Formaldehyde Fumigation

The efficacy of formaldehyde fumigation of calf houses, using different methods of gas generation under standard farming conditions, was investigated by Scarlett and Mathewson (1977). By sampling one square foot of various surfaces before and after fumigation, it was concluded that if the house could be effectively sealed, releasing the gas by heating paraformaldehyde, mixing formalin with potassium permanganate, or by boiling formalin gave a significant reduction in bacterial numbers. Aerosol generation yielded unsatisfactory results. Efficient precleaning and sealing were deemed to be of much greater importance than relative humidity and temperature. The formalin-potassium permanganate method gave satisfactory results at a rate of 500 ml of formalin and 250 g potassium permanganate per 10 m³.

The infectivity of suspensions of avian viruses, including reovirus, adenovirus, infectious bronchitis, Newcastle disease, poxvirus, avian encephalomyelitis, and infectious laryngotracheitis virus, was reduced by over 99% by one fumigation cycle of formalin using a commercial insecticide fogger at a flow rate of 40 ml per min and a volume of 36 ml per m³ (Ide, 1979). A second fumigation cycle was necessary to ensure loss of infectivity of Newcastle disease virus and reoviruses. The effect of formaldehyde fumigation on dried virus preparations in dust or on surfaces, as occurs under natural conditions, was not determined.

Fumigation with Methyl Bromide

Methyl bromide has greater penetrating power than formaldehyde and will kill a wide range of infectious agents including bacteria, viruses, and coccidia. It is, however, extremely toxic and fumigation should be undertaken only by trained and fully equipped personnel familiar with the hazards and the precautions to be taken. Attention has been directed towards the effectiveness and practicability of the use of methyl bromide fumigation for the disinfection of litter in situ, so that it can be re-used (Harry and Brown, 1974). It has been shown to be a more effective fumigant than formaldehyde when subsurface layers of porous material, such as litter, are being disinfected. Although extremely toxic, it can be readily dispelled from a building by ventilating for a few hours. This facilitates rapid re-use of disinfected premises and no adverse effects have been detected in trials of commercial poultry houses where two successive batches of broilers were reared on litter which had been fumigated on two occasions (Harry and Brown, 1974). Methyl bromide has also been used for fumigation of poultry food but residues of inorganic bromide in the tissues and eggs of poultry fed fumigated food, raise questions about safety aspects for consumers.

CLEANING AND DISINFECTION OF CALF HOUSES

When calf houses are used continuously, there is a high probability that infectious agents will accumulate, leading to an increased prevalence of enteric and respiratory disease. The pathogenic agents likely to be present include bacteria, viruses, mycoplasmas, fungi, and coccidia. Two approaches may be used to prevent a build-up of disease-producing agents: (1) leaving the houses vacant after calves are moved out, or (2) cleaning and disinfecting between each batch of calves. Leaving expensive housing vacant after cleaning is not usually a realistic way of dealing with a disease problem, neither can it be relied on to ensure natural loss of infectivity by the pathogenic agents distributed throughout the building.

Cleaning Procedure

Work should commence immediately after the calves have been moved out. All movable equipment should be dismantled, removed from the house and soaked in a tank of detergent for subsequent cleaning and disinfection. All gross organic matter—bedding, manure, hay, feed, or litter—should be removed. Small amounts of bedding and litter may be burned; larger amounts should be stacked for composting and disposed of at a later stage on arable land. Electricity should be disconnected before washing commences. All surfaces should be cleaned by scraping or brushing, or with a steam cleaner or power hose. A nonfoaming detergent or a 4% solution of sodium carbonate, preferably as a hot solution, facilitates cleaning greasy surfaces. If the building is dry and dusty, all surfaces should be sprayed with water before cleaning commences. Particular attention should be given to ceilings, ventilators and food troughs if respiratory and enteric diseases were recorded in previous occupants of the building.

Tanks supplying drinking water should be drained,

cleaned, and disinfected with 500 ppm sodium hypochlorite.

If automatic feeding equipment has been used, it should be dismantled, soaked in a dairy detergent, brushed, and rinsed clean with water. When assembled it should be flushed with a dilute solution of hypochlorite (approximately 0.05%). Manufacturer's instructions should be followed regarding the type and concentration of disinfectants suitable for use in the equipment.

When the building is visibly clean, it can be disinfected. The type of disinfectant selected depends on the infectious agents being eliminated, the method of application available, the building design, and the cost of the disinfection procedure. Other factors to be considered include the safety of the procedure and the experience of staff carrying out the disinfection program. The building can be disinfected by spraying with phenolic disinfectants, iodophors, or sodium hypochlorite if surfaces are entirely free from organic matter, or it can be fumigated with formaldehyde. The latter option applies only if the building can be sealed securely. Fumigation is labor saving, and, in many instances, more effective than the application of chemical solutions by spraying. (Details of the procedure have been presented in the section on poultry house disinfection.)

If the calf house is old with timber fittings, decontamination for spores of *Trichophyton verrucosum*, the common cause of ringworm in cattle, may not be achieved by fumigation. These spores are resistant to many of the commonly used disinfectants and because of their location may be inaccessible to disinfectants. Creosote has been found to be effective when painted on contaminated surfaces but toxicity for animals limits its usefulness. Thorough scrubbing of infected timber with hot detergent followed by rinsing and the liberal application of 2% iodine-based disinfectants on two occasions may inactivate these fungal spores. On completion of a disinfection program, the building should be well ventilated before animals are moved in.

Disinfection of calf houses is just one method which may be used to reduce the risk of infectious diseases in calves. Although the building should be free of infectious agents immediately after it is disinfected, additional precautions should be taken to ensure that infection is not introduced by using footbaths at all access points, and the general standard of management and hygiene should ensure that the next batch of healthy calves are reared in a clean, well-ventilated environment.

TEAT DIPS AND MASTITIS PREVENTION

Infection of the bovine udder is usually the result of microorganisms gaining entry through the teat duct. Transfer of pathogens occurs primarily during milking. The most important sources of infection are the milking cluster, udder cloths, and the milker's hand. Important aspects of mastitis prevention are the reduction of transfer of pathogens between cows, between teats, and their removal from the regions surrounding the teat orifice.

Decreasing the microbial population on teat skin, therefore, decreases the probability that the udder will become infected with a mastitis pathogen.

The organisms commonly transmitted through contact with milking machines or during the milking procedure are *Staphylococcus aureus, Streptococcus agalactiae* and *Streptococcus dysgalactiae.* Transmission of these organisms outside the milking parlor is less frequent and usually of little consequence. Some other bacteria may contaminate the teats between milkings because they are more widespread in the environment. Prominent among these are *Escherichia coli, Streptococcus uberis* and pseudomonads. These bacteria may be isolated from feces, bedding, sawdust used as bedding, water, and from sites on the body of the cow. Good milking hygiene techniques including post-milking teat disinfection, combined with antibiotic therapy at drying-off, culling of cows with recurring clinical mastitis, and regular tests on milking machines with correction of faults, form the basis of mastitis control programs in most countries.

Properties and Activity of Teat Dips

For a teat dip to be of benefit to the dairy farmer and acceptable to the consumer, certain criteria need to be met. The preparation should have demonstrable persistent antimicrobial activity on the teat skin after milking. It should be non-irritant, non-toxic and promote healing of lesions on the teats. It should act in the presence of organic matter such as milk, and be cost effective. It should not be absorbed into the tissues or leave undesirable residues in milk. Few of the many commercially available teat dips satisfy all of these requirements.

The majority of teat dips are based on a limited range of chemical disinfectants: sodium hypochlorite, iodophors, and chlorhexidine gluconate, often with emollients added to reduce the incidence of skin lesions. In recent years, preparations containing natural germicides have been developed in an attempt to overcome residues and avoid teat irritation.

Evaluation of Teat Dips

Since their promotion by scientists at the turn of the century for the prevention of mastitis, teat dips have become an established part of good milking hygiene. The ultimate test of these preparations, however, is their ability to prevent new intramammary infections under natural conditions.

A comparison of the effectiveness of iodophor and hypochlorite disinfectant teat dips in reducing new intramammary infection in dairy cows was made by O'Shea, Meaney, Langley and Palmer (1975). They conducted in vitro tests, simulated in vivo tests on teat skin, and in vivo tests measuring new infections in lactating cows. In vitro tests showed that a hypochlorite dip containing 1% available chlorine was more effective as a bactericidal agent than an iodophor containing 0.6% available iodine. In simulated in vivo tests, 1% chlorine was as effective as 0.6% available iodine. Neither 1% nor 1.2% chlorine was effective in reducing new infections in vivo, but a

50% reduction in new infections was achieved with either 4% chlorine or 0.6% iodine. Teat dips containing chlorhexidine, ethanol, and iodophor were evaluated for their persistence against *Streptococcus uberis* and *Escherichia coli* in lactating cows at 15 min and 15 hrs after application (Godinho and Bramley, 1980a). All three dips showed marked bactericidal activity 15 min after application, but only chlorhexidine retained this activity after 15 hrs. When the same three preparations were tested for their ability to prevent infection in the early dry period using the same challenge organisms, 15 hrs after teat dips were applied, chlorhexidine-dipped quarters again had the lowest infection rate. The authors suggested that teat dips with increased persistence on teat skin might improve the control of environmental mastitis in lactating cows.

A teat dip containing chlorhexidine and cetrimide was compared with two iodophor solutions, one containing the recommended concentration of 0.5% iodine and the other diluted ten fold (King, Morant, and Bramley, 1977). The test organisms were *S. aureus* and *E. coli*. The 0.5% iodophor was significantly more bactericidal than either the diluted iodophor or the combined chlorhexidine/cetrimide teat dip. A quaternary ammonium teat dip used at 0.5% concentration under natural conditions was judged to be 77% effective against *S. aureus* and 18% effective against *Streptococcus* species of environmental origin (Stewart and Philpot, 1982).

Nine post-milking teat dips containing sodium hypochlorite, sodium dichloro-s-triazene-trione, chlorhexidine gluconate, and povidine iodine were evaluated by an experimental challenge model against *S. aureus*, *Streptococcus agalactiae*, or both (Pankey, Philpot, Boddie, and Watts, 1983). The chlorhexidine and povidine iodine products reduced *S. agalactiae* infections by approximately 70%. Sodium dichloro-s-triazene-trione, chlorhexidine gluconate and povidine iodine reduced *S. aureus* infections by 76%, 92%, and 78% respectively, while the other teat dips gave less favorable results.

The addition of glycerol to iodophor teat dips as an emollient, has been shown to be both effective in healing and preventing teat lesions. The addition of 10 to 33% glycerol to an iodophor solution did not reduce titratable iodine present and did not reduce its bactericidal activity (Godinho and Bramley, 1980b).

An iodophor teat dip, containing 5000 mg available iodine/l, when used in a lactating herd reduced the number of new outbreaks of *S. aureus* significantly (Sheldrake and Hoare, 1980). When diluted to 1000 mg available iodine/l, no significant reduction was observed.

An increase in the iodine content of milk resulting from the use of iodophors in teat dips has caused consumer concern in many countries. Some systemic transfer of iodine from the teat skin to milk has been observed but the greater amount of iodine residue in milk seems to be of direct teat skin origin (Sheldrake, Hoare, Chen, and McPhillips, 1980). Drying teats with a paper towel for at least 10 seconds after dipping with a 1% iodophor

disinfectant reduced iodine residues in milk (Galton, et al., 1983). Reducing the iodophor concentration in teat dips from 1% to 0.5% also reduced iodine residues in milk.

The efficacy of a postmilking teat germicide containing fatty acids and lactic acid was evaluated at two concentrations against new udder infections caused by *S. aureus* and *S. agalactiae* (Boddie and Nickerson, 1988). At the higher concentration, it was 68% effective against *S. aureus* and 77% effective against *S. agalactiae*.

Teat dipping has been recognized as one of the most important procedures in dealing with residual contamination and colonization of teat ducts and lesions. Its applications, however, are of limited value in controlling contamination and infections with pathogens that are prevalent in the environment of the cow rather than confined to the infected udder. If teat dips with greater persistence of bactericidal activity were available, control of mastitis resulting from environmental pathogens such as *S. uberis* and *E. coli* might be possible. Whether this can be achieved without increasing disinfectant residues in milk remains to be determined.

DISINFECTION PROCEDURES FOR FOOT-AND-MOUTH DISEASE

Although the precise regulations that apply may vary from country to country in accordance with their animal health status and the resources available for controlling infectious diseases, some general guidelines can be considered. These may be modified to take into account local farming, social conditions, climatic and environmental factors, and the impact of the disease on international trade. Control measures rely on rapid and reliable laboratory diagnosis, slaughter of infected and in-contact animals, disposal of carcasses by burial or burning, and a thorough disinfection regime. In countries where the disease is endemic, a stamping out policy is not realistic and the prevalence of disease is reduced by national vaccination programs.

Foot-and-mouth disease virus (FMDV) infects a wide variety of cloven-hoofed domestic and wild animal species. An outbreak of disease on a farm usually involves all susceptible species. The incubation period is short. The disease is highly contagious, and the main route of infection in ruminants is by inhalation, but ingestion of infected food and contact with infected material can readily produce disease. Milk secreted during the prodromal stage of the disease contains large amounts of virus (Blackwell and Hyde, 1976).

When informed of a suspicious case, the veterinarian should proceed promptly to the premises suitably equipped with waterproof protective clothing, rubber boots, containers suitable for use as footbaths, disinfectant active against the virus, a stirrup pump, and the necessary veterinary diagnostic supplies. The transport vehicle used should not enter the property.

If suspicious of the case, the veterinarian should inform the police and request immediate surveillance of the premises. Footbaths should be positioned at all exit points and a detailed history of relevant facts should be recorded. Movement of people in or out of the premises should be prohibited or restricted, the central veterinary authority should be informed, and the regional veterinary office should be alerted. Appropriate samples should be collected in duplicate for transmission to a diagnostic laboratory. Meanwhile the necessary legal steps to prevent movement of animals, usually within a 16 km (10 mile) radius of the outbreak, are implemented.

If foot-and-mouth disease is confirmed, the national government usually implements a well-defined plan. This forbids movement of people and animals into the infected place, authorizes slaughter of infected and in-contact animals, and describes in detail procedures to be followed. Apart from footbaths at all exit points, a bed of straw 20 cm deep, 7 m long and 2 m wide soaked in a prescribed disinfectant should be placed at all gateways to ensure that all vehicles leaving disinfect their wheels. In stormy weather, fine sand can be used around the edges and interspersed with the straw to hold it in place.

Slaughter of infected and in-contact animals is followed by deep burial, or if for geographic or climatic reasons that is not possible, by burning. Disinfection begins with the removal of material of little value such as wooden fittings, for burning. All drains should be blocked to prevent dispersal of infected material and the building disconnected from the electricity supply. The entire building and its contents should be soaked in a prescribed disinfectant. After the disinfectant has been allowed sufficient time to act, the drains are opened and cleaning proceeds. The FMDV is highly susceptible to pH changes; acids and alkalis rapidly inactivate it. Alternative disinfectants include formaldehyde and glutaraldehyde.

Manure, bedding, hay, silage concentrates, and all other organic matter should be removed for deep burial if present in small quantities, or for composting if present in larger amounts. Material for composting should be collected into heaps, sprayed with disinfectant, fenced off and left to compost for some weeks before dispersal on land used for tillage. Hay, straw, or silage faces should be cut back 15 cm (6 inches) and removed for burning or burial. The fresh surface should then be sprayed to a height of 200 cm with 4% sodium carbonate. Implements used for cleaning and vehicles used for moving infected material also require thorough disinfection.

The building should be sprayed with a hot solution of 4% sodium carbonate and thoroughly cleaned with a power hose or by brushing and scraping. Movable objects should be soaked in a tank of 4% sodium carbonate for handwashing and disinfection. The water supply should be disinfected by turning off the supply, cleaning the header tank, and draining the entire system. The tank should be refilled with sodium hypochlorite at a concentration of 10,000 ppm; all outlets should be opened and the disinfectant allowed to flow from each line until all air locks are removed. Each line is then closed off

and the disinfectant is left to act for 12 hrs in the tank and lines before being drained from the system. Finally, the tank should be refilled with clean water and the entire system flushed through with mains water. Surfaces should be sprayed with a prescribed disinfectant, but not sodium hypochlorite if formaldehyde fumigation is to be used later. If the building is capable of being sealed against the escape of gas it should then be fumigated by heating paraformaldehyde at a rate of 40 g per 10 m³ (approximately 4 oz per 100 cubic feet) with heating pans not more than 30 m apart, or by adding formalin to potassium permanganate at a rate of 500 ml formalin and 250 g potassium permanganate per 10 m³. The building should be kept sealed for 24 hrs. Footwear, clothing, gloves, and all implements used for cleaning should be thoroughly disinfected before removal from the premises. Clothing not suitable for chemical disinfection should be boiled.

The building and farm should be left unstocked for six months. Sentinel animals may be used to monitor the reliability of disinfection. It is essential that animals selected for this purpose are immunologically naive.

DISINFECTION PROCEDURES FOR ANTHRAX

In veterinary medicine, diseases caused by spore-forming bacteria are of considerable significance. *Bacillus anthracis* is one example of an organism that produces spores of high resistance. Outbreaks of disease, originating from soil-borne infection, tend to occur after a major change of climate and usually in warm weather when the temperature is over 15°C. The disease is typically peracute and is characterized by septicemia and sudden death with exudation of tarry blood from body orifices. If vegetative *B. anthracis* is exposed to oxygen, spore formation may follow with environmental contamination the likely outcome. For this reason, postmortem examinations should *not* be carried out on suspect carcasses. These spores are resistant to most external influences, including dehydration, sunlight, and standard disinfectants. They can survive for many years in soil, particularly in alkaline soil. The organism may be ingested, inhaled, or may enter the body through the skin. Because of the high resistance of anthrax spores, disinfection is difficult and the normal contact time for all disinfectants should therefore be increased.

Animals infected with *B. anthracis* are likely to die suddenly. The absence of rigor mortis and the presence of tarry exudate should alert the veterinarian to the possibility of anthrax. If the animal is found dead in a building, other animals close by should be moved and kept in isolation for observation until cases cease. If found dead at pasture, the area surrounding the dead animal should be immediately fenced off and a designated person appointed to ensure that no scavenger animals approach the area.

The procedure followed in the event of an anthrax outbreak varies according to the status of the disease in that country. When the disease is normally absent from a country, the attending veterinarian should inform the police of the suspected case and also inform the central veterinary authority and the regional veterinary office. All personnel dealing with the suspect case should wear waterproof clothing, rubber boots, and, if necessary, face masks, as anthrax is a zoonotic disease. A footbath containing 5% formalin or another sporicide should be placed in position at access points and used by all staff leaving the infected building. The necessary legal steps relating to control of animal movement, sale of animal produce from the infected farm and other measures aimed at preventing the spread of the disease should be implemented without delay.

Diagnosis of the disease should be confirmed by smears of peripheral blood collected with a syringe and needle from the unopened carcass. Blood or edema fluid should be collected in a similar manner for guinea pig or mouse inoculation and for blood culture. A postmortem examination, carried out inadvertently, showing failure of the blood to clot, the presence of ecchymotic hemorrhages throughout the body tissues, and tarry exudates at all natural orifices is strongly suggestive of anthrax.

Disinfection Procedures

If anthrax is confirmed on the farm, the carcass should be removed for burning or deep burial together with bedding, feed, or soil contaminated with discharges. Burial should be at least two meters deep with copious amounts of quicklime added.

The infected building should be disinfected initially with all fittings in place and all drains blocked. A 5% solution of formalin or a hot 10% solution of sodium hydroxide should be sprayed over all surfaces and left to act for at least 3 hrs before cleaning commences and drains are opened. Movable items should be soaked in detergent for cleaning and subsequent disinfection in formaldehyde, glutaraldehyde, peracetic acid, or halogen disinfectants. A steam cleaner or a power hose should be used to clean all surfaces. All solid debris should be buried and the entire building sprayed twice with a sporicidal disinfectant at a rate of 1 liter per m³ with an interval of 2 hrs between each application. As an alternative to spraying, the building if suitably constructed, should be sealed and fumigated either by heating paraformaldehyde at a rate of 40 g per 10 m³, or by adding formalin to potassium permanganate at a rate of 250 g potassium permanganate and 500 ml of formalin per 10 m³.

All items moved from the infected building and all equipment used for cleaning should be disinfected in a sporicidal solution for at least 4 hrs. Transport vehicles, excavating vehicles, and other items, such as ropes or chains, should likewise be thoroughly disinfected before being removed from the infected farm. As yet there are few if any satisfactory methods for decontaminating soil polluted with anthrax spores. A flame gun applied to the area of ground where blood or exudates from an anthrax carcass have been spilled should clear the area of the infective agent. In the absence of a flame gun, the top 20 cm of soil should be removed, mixed with combustible material such as sawdust or peat moss and burned. Hussaini and Ruby (1976) suggested that 7.85 l (1.7 gallons) of a 3% aqueous solution of peracetic acid would effectively sterilize one square meter area of pasture soil. If liquid manure in a slurry tank requires decontamination it should be treated with undiluted formalin (40% W/V formaldehyde in water) at a rate of 40 l of formalin per m³ of slurry for at least 6 hrs. This procedure is usually only realistic for small quantities of slurry because of the cost involved.

Any material of animal origin likely to be contaminated, such as wool, hair, or hides should be either decontaminated or incinerated. Formaldehyde vapor can be used for wool, 2.5% hydrochloric acid can be used for hides, and autoclaving at 121°C for 20 minutes is suitable for hair.

EVALUATION OF DISINFECTION PROGRAMS

Evaluation of a disinfection program under field conditions requires a simple and reliable sampling procedure for surfaces, equipment, and air space to determine if infectious agents have survived. When dealing with animal pathogens, sentinel animals susceptible to the infectious agents may be used to determine if there is residual infectivity.

Marker Organisms

The use of marker organisms is a useful method of validating results, especially when dealing with resistant infectious agents. It is essential that the marker organisms selected be as closely matched as possible to the infectious agent in terms of resistance to disinfectants and numbers present.

Sentinel Animals

Sentinel animals may be used to monitor the reliability of disinfection programs following an outbreak of an exotic disease. Animals selected for this purpose should (1) be susceptible to the infectious agent being eradicated; (2) be immunologically naive; (3) be in the appropriate age category to show clinical signs or other effects on performance. Under practical conditions, local conventional animals are often selected for this purpose. If the disease has been present in the surrounding district for some time, however, the immune status of local animals may render them unsuitable. Animals selected from the local population may have recovered from disease induced by the infectious agent or from a subclinical form of the disease. Passive immunity transmitted via colostrum in calves, lambs, foals, piglets, puppies, or kittens, or via the yolk sac in birds, may protect against challenge, thereby leading to erroneous conclusions. The presence of an active immune response, either humoral or cell-mediated, may also mask the true situation. Some infectious diseases have age-related characteristics. To ensure that surviving infectious agents are being detected, it may be necessary to select animals of suitable ages to demonstrate the presence of such pathogenic agents.

The presence of infectious agents following disinfection does not necessarily result in susceptible animals becoming clinically affected. The number of surviving organisms, the route of infection and the possibility of latent or chronic infection should also be considered when interpreting results of such trials. If sentinel animals fail to show clinical signs of disease shortly after occupying a suspect building, their health status should be monitored for some months in a location free of the infectious agent to exclude a latent infection or a slowly progressing disease. A particular difficulty arises with those infectious agents associated with the spongiform encephalopathies of cattle, sheep and goats which have incubation periods measured in years.

Specific pathogen-free animals offer many advantages over conventional farm animals, but their cost and availability limit their usefulness. When investigating diseases of poultry, such as Newcastle disease, the use of specific pathogen-free birds adds to the reliability of the test procedure.

In-Use Tests

These tests are performed to assess the efficiency of disinfection under actual conditions of use. The quality of surfaces following a disinfection program is assessed using contact plates, sterile adhesive tapes, or by swabbing surfaces with sterile cloths or sponges. The site of sampling in a building and the surface area swabbed should be based on statistically valid sampling procedures. The area of surface sampled should bear a realistic relationship to the total surface area of the building.

Equipment, such as that used in food processing, may be sampled by swabbing and rinsing. To get a reliable picture of the true number of organisms present, it may be necessary to resort to spray-rinse techniques, or to operating the equipment to circulate sampling fluid, thus simulating actual conditions of use.

CONCLUSION

If carried out in an efficient manner, a disinfection program when combined with appropriate test-and-slaughter policies can control and ultimately eradicate many infectious diseases from animal populations and thereby have a direct impact on their health status and performance. The strategic application of a thorough cleaning and disinfection program at an appropriate point in the production cycle can shorten the time between depopulation and repopulation to a matter of days. When combined with control of animal movement, including quarantine of imported animals, disinfection can play a major role in limiting the spread of disease between farms and between countries.

Applications for chemical disinfectants are diverse. They are used in every phase of animal production, surgical procedures, mastitis control programs, in meat plants, and in dairies. The ready availability of these compounds, however, does not necessarily ensure their proper use in the control of pathogenic microorganisms. Many decisions relating to the selection and use of disinfectants require professional advice, particularly when dealing with resistant infectious agents such as mycobacteria, non-enveloped viruses, and spore-forming bacteria. Success in a disinfection program calls for strict adherence to basic guidelines that ensure safety for those implementing the program, profit for the producer through improved feed conversion or performance, and improved quality of animal produce for the consumer. The environment, too, must not be neglected when considering the selection, use, and disposal of disinfectants. Education of the public, especially the farming community, on the careful selection, proper use, and safe disposal of disinfectants is a role which the veterinary profession should be competent to fill.

ACKNOWLEDGMENTS

I wish to thank my colleagues for constructive criticism, Mrs. D. Maguire for preparing the illustrations, Mrs. L. Doggett for typing the manuscript, and the Library staff for assistance with data base searches.

REFERENCES

Baldry, M.G.C. 1983. The bactericidal, fungicidal and sporicidal properties of hydrogen peroxide and peracetic acid. J. Appl. Bacteriol., 54, 417–423.

Bergan, T., and Lystad, A. 1971. Antitubercular action of disinfectants. J. Appl. Bacteriol., 34, 751–756.

Blackwell, J.H. 1978. Comparative resistance of San Miguel sea lion virus and vesicular exanthema of swine virus to chemical disinfectants. Res. Vet. Sci., 25, 25–28.

Blackwell, J.H., Graves, J.H., and McKercher, P.D. 1975. Chemical inactivation of swine vesicular disease virus. Br. Vet. J., 131, 317–322.

Blackwell, J.H., and Hyde, J.L. 1976. Effect of heat on foot-and-mouth disease virus (FMDV) in the components of milk from FMDV-infected cows. J. Hyg. Camb., 77, 77–83.

Boddie, R.L., and Nickerson, S.C. 1988. Efficacy of a fatty acid-lactic acid post-milking teat germicide in reducing incidence of bovine mastitis. J. Food. Prot., 51, 799–801.

Brown, T.T. 1981. Laboratory evaluation of selected disinfectants as virucidal agents against porcine parvovirus, pseudorabies virus, and transmissible gastroenteritis virus. Am. J. Vet. Res., 42, 1033–1036.

Cunliffe, H.R., Blackwell, J.H., Dors, R., and Walker, J.S. 1979. Inactivation of milkborne foot-and-mouth disease virus at ultra-high temperatures. J. Food. Prot., 42, 135–137.

Death, J.E., and Coates, D. 1979. Effect of pH on sporicidal and microbiocidal activity of buffered mixtures of alcohol and sodium hypochlorite. J. Clin. Pathol., 32, 148–153.

Derbyshire, J.B., and Arkell, S. 1971. The activity of some chemical disinfectants against Talfan virus and porcine adenovirus type 2. Br. Vet. J., 127, 137–142.

Elliot, D.G., and Amend, D.F. 1978. Efficacy of certain disinfectants against infectious pancreatic necrosis virus. J. Fish Biol. 12, 277–286.

Evans, D.H., Stuart, P., and Roberts, D.H. 1977. Disinfection of animal viruses. Br. Vet. J., 133, 356–359.

Fodor, T., and Szabó, I. 1980. Effect of chlorhexidine gluconate on the survival of acid fast bacteria. Acta Microbiol. Hung., 27, 343–344.

Galton, D.M., et al. 1983. Effects of premilking udder preparation on bacterial population, sediment, and iodine residue in milk. J. Dairy Sci., 67, 2580–2589.

Gardner, J.F., and Peel, M.M. 1986. Principles of chemical disinfection. In Introduction to Sterilization and Disinfection. Edited by J.F. Gardner and M.M. Peel. Melbourne, Churchill Livingstone, pp. 150–168.

Gayot, G., and Ursache, R. 1976. Étude du pouvoir bactéricide de quelques désinfectants usuels. Rec. Med. Vét., 152, 299–304.

Godinho, K.S., and Bramley, A.J. 1980a. The efficacy of teat dips of differing persistence on teat skin in preventing intramammary infection by Streptococcus uberis and Escherichia coli in dry cows. Br. Vet. J., 136, 574–579.

Godinho, K.S., and Bramley, A.J. 1980b. The interaction of glycerol and an iodophor teat dip. J. Appl. Bacteriol., *48*, 449–453.

Gorman, S.P., and Scott, E.M. 1977. A quantitative evaluation of the antifungal properties of glutaraldehyde. J. Appl. Bacteriol., *43*, 83–89.

Hall, R. 1979. The activity of chlorhexidine gluconate against *Brucella abortus*. Vet. Rec., *105*, 305–306.

Harry, E.G., and Binstead, J.A. 1961. Studies on the disinfection of eggs and incubators. V. The toxicity of formaldehyde to the developing embryo. Br. Vet. J., *117*, 532–539.

Harry, E.G., and Brown, W.B. 1974. Fumigation with methyl bromide–applications in the poultry industry—a review. World's Poultry Sc. J., *30*, 193–216.

Herniman, K.A.J., Medhurst, P.M., Wilson, J.N., and Sellers, R.F. 1973. The action of heat, chemicals and disinfectants on swine vesicular disease virus. Vet. Rec., *93*, 620–624.

Hugo, W.B. 1982. Disinfection mechanisms. In *Principles and Practice of Disinfection, Preservation and Sterilization*. Edited by A.D. Russell, W.B. Hugo and G.A.J. Ayliffe. Oxford, Blackwell Scientific Publications, pp. 158–185.

Hussaini, S.N., and Ruby, K.R. 1976. Sporicidal activity of peracetic acid against *B. anthracis* spores. Vet. Rec., *98*, 257–259.

Ide, P.R. 1979. The sensitivity of some avian viruses to formaldehyde fumigation. Can. J. Comp. Med., *43*, 211–216.

Jones, P.W. 1980. Health hazards associated with the handling of animal wastes. Vet. Rec., *106*, 4–7.

Kelsey, J.C., Mackinnon, I.H., and Maurer, I.M. 1974. Sporicidal activity of hospital disinfectants. J. Clin. Pathol., *27*, 632–638.

King, J.S., Morant, S.V., and Bramley, A.J. 1977. The bactericidal activity of a teat dip containing chlorhexidine and cetrimide. Vet. Rec., *101*, 421–423.

Lensing, H.H., and Oei, H.L. 1984. A study on the efficiency of disinfectants against anthrax spores. Tijdschr. Diergeneeskd., *109*, 557–563.

Merkal, R.S., and Whipple, D.L. 1980. Inactivation of *Mycobacterium bovis* in meat products. Appl. Environ. Microbiol., *40*, 282–284.

O'Shea, J., Meaney, W.J., Langley, O.H., and Palmer, J. 1975. Comparison of the effectiveness of iodophor and hypochlorite disinfectant teat dips in reducing new intramammary infection in dairy cows. Ir. J. Agric. Res., *14*, 99–105.

Pankey, J.W., Philpot, W.N., Boddie, R.L., and Watts, J.L. 1983. Evaluation of nine teat dip formulations under experimental challenge to *Staphylococcus aureus* and *Streptococcus agalactiae*. J. Dairy Sci., *66*, 161–167.

Pelczar, M.J., Chan, E.C.S., and Krieg, N.R. 1986. Control by chemical agents. In *Microbiology*, 5th Edition. New York, McGraw-Hill, pp. 488–509.

Puddle, B.M., Pulford, H.D., and Ralston, M.J. 1986. Efficacy of different teat sanitizers for control of pseudocowpox. N.Z. Vet. J., *34*, 16–18.

Quinn, P.J. 1984. An investigation of the activity of selected disinfectants against *Brucella abortus*. Ir. Vet. J., *38*, 86–94.

Quinn, P.J. 1987. Evaluation of veterinary disinfectants and disinfection processes. In *Disinfection in Veterinary and Farm Animal Practice*. Edited by A.H. Linton, W.B. Hugo, and A.D. Russell. Oxford, Blackwell Scientific Publications, pp. 66–116.

Richards, W.D., and Thoen, C.O. 1979. Chemical destruction of *Mycobacterium bovis* in milk. J. Food Prot., *42*, 55–57.

Saknimit, M., Inatsuki, I., Sugiyama, Y., Yagami, K. 1988. Virucidal efficacy of physico-chemical treatments against coronaviruses and parvoviruses of laboratory animals. Exp. Anim., *37*, 341–345.

Sako, H., and Sorimachi, M. 1985. Susceptibility of fish pathogenic viruses, bacteria and fungus to ultraviolet irradiation and the disinfectant effect of u.v.-ozone water sterilizer on the pathogens in water. Bull. Natl. Res. Inst. Aquaculture, *8*, 51–58.

Scanlan, C.M., Hannon, S.S., and Matthews, M.R. 1982. Effects of phenol concentration, incubation temperature and time on cell viability of *Brucella abortus* in phenolized saline. *Proceedings of the Twenty-Fifth Annual Meeting of the American Association of Veterinary Laboratory Diagnosticians*. pp. 197–202.

Scarlett, C.M., and Mathewson, G.K. 1977. Terminal disinfection of calf houses by formaldehyde fumigation. Vet. Rec., *101*, 7–10.

Scott, F.W. 1980. Virucidal disinfectants and feline viruses. Am. J. Vet. Res., *41*, 410–414.

Sellers, R.F. 1968. The inactivation of foot-and-mouth disease virus by chemicals and disinfectants. Vet. Rec., *83*, 504–506.

Sheldrake, R.F., and Hoare, R.J.T. 1980. Post-milking iodine teat skin disinfectants. 2. New intramammary infection rates. J. Dairy Res., *47*, 27–31.

Sheldrake, R.F., Hoare, R.J.T., Chen, S.C., and McPhillips, J. 1980. Post-milking iodine teat skin disinfectants. 3. Residues. J. Dairy Res., *47*, 33–38.

Shen, D.T., Crawford, T.B., Gorham, J.R., and McGuire, T.C. 1977. Inactivation of equine infectious anaemia virus by chemical disinfectants. Am. J. Vet. Res., *38*, 1217–1219.

Shen, D.T., Leendertsen, L.W., and Gorham, J.R. 1981. Evaluation of chemical disinfectants for Aleutian disease virus of mink. Am. J. Vet. Res., *42*, 838–840.

Stewart, G.A., and Philpot, W.N. 1982. Efficacy of quaternary ammonium teat dip for preventing intramammary infections. J. Dairy Sci., *65*, 878–880.

Stone, S.S., and Hess, W.R. 1973. Effects of some disinfectants on African swine fever virus. Appl. Microbiol., *25*, 115–122.

Taylor, D.M. 1989. Scrapie agents decontamination: implications for bovine spongiform encephalopathy. Vet. Rec., *24*, 291–292.

van Oss, C.J. 1982. Action of physical and chemical agents on microorganisms. In *Medical Microbiology*. Edited by F. Milgrom and T.D. Flannagan. New York, Churchill Livingstone, pp. 69–79.

Verger, J.M. 1982. Prevalence and survival of *Brucella* species in manures. In *Communicable Diseases Resulting from Storage, Handling, Transport and Landspreading of Manures*. Edited by J.R. Walton and E.G. White. EUR 7627. Luxembourg, Commission of the European Communities. pp. 157–160.

Walker, J.S., de Leeuw, P.W., Callis, J.J., and van Bekkum, J.G. 1984. The thermal death time curve for foot-and-mouth disease virus contained in primarily infected milk. J. Biol. Stand., *12*, 185–189.

Willett, H.P. 1984. Sterilization and Disinfection. In *Zinsser Microbiology*, 18th Edition. Edited by W.K. Joklik, H.P. Willett, and D.B. Amos. Norwalk, Appleton-Century-Crofts, pp. 233–249.

Wray, C. 1975. Survival and spread of pathogenic bacteria of veterinary importance within the environment. Vet. Bull., *45*, 543–550.

Wright, H.S. 1974. Virucidal activity of commercial disinfectants against velogenic viscerotropic Newcastle disease virus. Avian Dis., *18*, 526–530.

Yoshimizu, M., Takizawa, H., and Kimura, T. 1986. U.V. susceptibility of some fish pathogenic viruses. Fish Path., *21*, 47–52.

PART VII

Antimicrobial Preservatives and Protectants

CHAPTER 50

PRESERVATION OF MEDICINES AGAINST MICROBIAL CONTAMINATION

Reza A. Fassihi

Most drug delivery systems are associated with undesirable side effects. These are largely inherent in the active component of the formulation and thus difficult to avoid. However, side effects such as infection and pyrexia caused by microbiologically contaminated dosage forms are easily avoided. In recent years reports of clinical complications arising from microbial contamination of oral and topical products in several European countries and the United States has resulted in product recalls. Tightened regulatory and compendia limits have reemphasized the need for the drug formulator to carefully and thoroughly consider all aspects of formulation design.

The formulation of an elegant, efficacious medicine that is both stable and acceptable may necessitate the use of a wide variety of ingredients in a complex physical state. This could create conditions conducive to the survival, and even extensive replication, of contaminant microorganisms that might enter the product either during its manufacture or with use by the patient or medical staff.

Microbial contamination of pharmaceuticals has been studied extensively and various methods have been discussed whereby the microbial content of dosage forms may be limited, and their susceptibility to microbial spoilage reduced (Ringertz and Ringertz, 1982; Spooner, 1985). In addition Good Manufacturing Codes of Practice (GMPs) have been widely adopted. Many drug preparations for parenteral administration, and preparations likely to contact broken skin or internal organs must be sterile in order to avoid the possibility of infection arising from their use. Injections, ophthalmic preparations, irrigation fluids, dialysis solutions, sutures, implants, surgical dressings, and instruments necessary for their administration are presented in a sterile condition and should remain sterile throughout the period of use.

The quality of non-sterile pharmaceuticals has so improved, that today the majority contain only minimal microbial populations. In spite of this, the incidence of product contamination with unacceptable levels and types of contaminant has accumulated over the past 25 years (Crompton, 1973; Kuehne and Ahearn, 1971; Noble and Savin, 1966; Beveridge, 1975; Kallings et al., 1966; Pederson and Ulrich, 1968).

Many of the ingredients used in drug formulations become suitable substrates for microorganisms when conditions of water availability, pH, and temperature are favorable for growth. Pharmaceutical preparations may be contaminated by molds, yeasts, or bacteria, with the latter generally favoring a slightly alkaline medium and the others an acid medium. Although few microorganisms can grow outside the pH range 4 to 9, most pharmaceutical preparations are within the vulnerable pH range and must be protected against microbial growth.

Several studies have illustrated the wide range of raw materials (colors, dyes, pigments, talcs, starches, clays, fillers, natural gums, and thickening agents) and finished products that may contain viable microorganisms. Although the United States Pharmacopeia (USP) XXI has procedures for determining the microbial content of raw materials and finished products, limits on the number and types of microorganisms have not been officially specified. However, all materials must be free of the "harmful microorganisms" listed in the USP XX. Most of the manufacturers have set up their own microbiologic specifications suitable to their raw materials and finished products. In addition to the use of contaminated raw materials, contamination may occur during manufacture (contaminated equipment, water, operators, air, and packaging materials) and, after manufacture, by the user (Baird, 1987; Denyer, 1987; Fassihi and Parker, 1987; Parker and Fassihi, 1988). Living organisms, by virtue of their growth potential, metabolic versatility, and ability to act in concert, propagate at the expense of their environment, leading to product spoilage and subsequent loss of drug efficacy. If this is uninhibited by any restraining influence, it often causes rapid and profound changes in the chemical environment. In the synthesis of new protoplasm, many complex chemical reactions are accomplished within a remarkably short period.

Substances added to medicines to prevent microbial spoilage, retard deterioration, and restrain organismic growth to low levels are known as preservatives. Governmental regulatory agencies require the use of a preservative whenever a formulation will be used more than once from the same container. They must be nontoxic because they are included in oral, topical, and some parenteral injections. They are used primarily in multiple-dose containers to inhibit the growth of microorganisms that may be introduced during or subsequent to the manufacturing process. Antimicrobial agents should not be used solely to reduce the viable microbial count as a substitute for GMPs. All useful preservative agents are toxic. For maximum protection of the consumer, the concentration of the preservative shown to be effective in the final packaged product should be considerably below the toxic level for humans. It should also be recognized that the presence of living microorganisms or fragments of dead microorganisms may produce pyrogenic reactions or may cause adverse reactions in sensitized persons.

It has been known for many years that microbial contaminants may effect the spoilage of pharmaceutical products through chemical, physical, or aesthetic changes, thereby rendering them unfit for use. Active drug constituents may be metabolized to less-potent or chemically inactive forms. Therapeutic agents as diverse as morphine, barbiturates, aspirin, paracetamol, thalidomide, atropine, steroids, and mandelic acid, and pharmaceutical ingredients such as surfactants, polymers, fats, oils, sweetening agents, flavoring agents, and coloring agents can be metabolized by microorganisms and serve as substrates for microbial growth (Marshall and Wiley, 1982; Grant et al., 1970; Grant, 1971; Bucherer, 1965; Brookes et al., 1981). Physical changes commonly seen are due to breakdown of emulsions, visible surface growth on solids, or the formation of slimes, pellicles, or sediments in liquids. These changes are sometimes accompanied by the production of such things as gas, odors, or unwanted flavors. Chemical reactions are catalyzed by a wide variety of enzymes produced by microorganisms, and include hydrolysis, dehydration, oxidation, reduction, decarboxylation, deamination, phosphorylation, and dephosphorylation (Wedderburn, 1964). The metabolic pathways employed by bacteria differ between different genera and species and depend on the environmental conditions. For example, *Aerobacter aerogenes* will attack pyruvic acid at pH 8 to give acetic and formic acids.

$$CH_3COCOOH + H_2O \rightleftharpoons CH_3COOH + HCOOH$$

At pH 6 the same organism will decarboxylate pyruvic acid.

$$2CH_3COCOOH \rightleftharpoons CH_3COCHOH + 2CO_2$$

By decomposing constituents of the environment many of these metabolic processes yield end-products that have a growth-limiting effect on the organisms (Wedderburn, 1964). A further consequence of the establishment of primary invaders in a pharmaceutical preparation is a reduction in the efficiency of the preservative system. A variety of genera can cause breakdown of preservatives (Beveridge and Hugo, 1964; Hugo and Foster, 1964; Dagley, 1971; Beveridge, 1975). The growth of microorganisms in a product may produce obvious spoilage and may influence the stability and even the release patterns of the pharmaceutical preparations. More important from the clinical point of view is that microbial growth may be associated with the production of toxins, resulting in food poisoning from an orally administered preparation. The microorganisms capable of producing toxins, including certain strains of *Bacillus cereus* and *Staphylococcus aureus* and mycotoxin-producing fungi, constitute a potential hazard.

FORMULATION DESIGN AND PRESERVATION

Pharmaceutical preparations are manufactured in a clean environment by following the GMP recommendations. Most ophthalmic and injectable preparations are sterilized by physical methods during their manufacture. To enable multidose drug preparations to cope adequately with contaminants gaining access during repeated withdrawal of doses, presence of a potent antimicrobial preservative is essential. It must be noted that only the undissociated fraction or molecular form of a preservative is active, because the ionized portion is incapable of penetrating the microorganism. Thus the preservative selected must be largely undissociated at the pH of the formulation. Consequently, the preservation of medicines involves formulation (including preservative agents), quality control of ingredients and packaging, good manufacturing practice, and storage under appropriate conditions.

Many compatible combinations of preservative agents and other formulation components have been reported in recent years. Conversely, incompatibilities that result in preservative inactivation involve macromolecules such as various cellulose derivatives, polyvinylpyrrolidone, polyethylene glycols, Tween 80, Myrj 52, and sucrose mono-oleate (Kazmi and Mitchell, 1976; Parker and Barnes, 1967). Product storage temperature, as well as interaction with surfactants or other active substances, may change the concentration of unbound preservative in the aqueous phase.

Plastic containers, metal ointment tubes, rubber or plastic caps, or liners may absorb the preservative, thereby decreasing the quantity available for antimicrobial activity.

In almost every drug formulation there are factors predisposing it to or inhibiting microbial growth—e.g., pH, osmotic effects, and the presence of toxic molecules. The balance among these factors, including the presence of a preservative, will determine the microbial growth or bactericidal rate. As noted, the efficiency of the preservative is itself subject to favorable and unfavorable influences of the formulation components.

Appreciable chemical or physicochemical spoilage probably requires significant growth of microbial contaminants within the formulations. Early indicative signs will often be organoleptic, with the release of unpleasant tasting or smelling metabolites such as "sour" fatty acids, ketones, "fishy" amines, "rotten eggs" (H_2S), ammonia, and bitter, sickly, or alcoholic tastes and smells. Products frequently develop unappealing discoloration because of various microbial pigments, and even polythene may exhibit a pink discoloration when colonized by fungi (Beveridge, 1987). Depolymerization of thickening agents or polymerization of sugar or surfactant molecules will result in a rapid loss of stabilizing efficacy; the accumulation of acidic or basic metabolites can produce marked shifts in product pH.

An effectively designed preservative system must retain its antimicrobial activity for the shelf-life of the product (Sykes, 1971). To ensure compliance with this requirement, the preservative characteristics of the product in its final form must be studied as a function of time.

Most aqueous preparations, especially emulsions, suspensions, and some creams, are excellent media for microbes. Syrups containing approximately 85% sugar resist bacterial growth by virtue of their exosmotic effect on microorganisms. Syrups containing less than 85% sucrose, but sufficient polyol (e.g., sorbitol, glycerin, propylene glycol) to be hypertonic similarly resist bacterial growth. Hydroalcoholic and alcoholic preparations containing more than 15% alcohol may not require the addition of a chemical preservative; hence, elixirs, spirits, and tinctures are self-sterilizing.

MICROBIAL ORGANISMS ASSOCIATED WITH PHARMACEUTICAL PRODUCTS

To determine whether a specific organism is hazardous in given circumstances, one must consider the nature of the product, its dose, the probable state of health of the user, and clinical reports on the frequency and severity of infections caused by the microorganism in question. The FDA recognizes the categories "harmful," "objectionable," and "opportunistic" in respect of microorganisms. "Harmful" refers to those microbial organisms or their toxins responsible for human disease or infection. Examples of organisms that must not be present in a product are given, e.g., *Salmonella* species, *Escherichia coli*, certain species of *Pseudomonas*, including *P. aeruginosa*, *Staphylococcus aureus*, *Candida albicans*, and *Aspergillus niger*. An "objectionable" organism can cause disease, inactivate the drug, or lead to the deterioration of the product. The following are objectionable organisms and should not be present in a pharmaceutical or cosmetic product: *Pseudomonas putida*, *P. multivorans*, *P. maltophilia*, *Proteus mirabilis*, *Serratia marcescens*, *Klebsiella spp.*, *Acinetobacter anitratus*, and *Candida*

spp. (Bruch, 1972). Organisms are defined as "opportunistic" if they produce disease in immunocompromised patients, such as the newborn, patients with AIDS, and patients undergoing immunosuppressive therapy.

A medicine may be considered microbiologically spoiled if low levels of acutely pathogenic microorganisms or higher levels of opportunist pathogens are present, or if toxic microbial metabolites persist even after death of the original contaminants, or if microbial growth has initiated significant physical or chemical deterioration of the product. Such spoilage may well have serious financial consequences for the manufacturer, either in the immediate loss of product or in the increasingly expensive process of litigation should the spoilage cause harm to the user.

Contaminants isolated from products range from true pathogens, such as *Clostridium tetani*, to opportunistic pathogens, such as *Pseudomonas aeruginosa* and many other free-living organisms. Some of the microorganisms more frequently isolated from medicinal products are shown in Table 50–1.

The main problem with these organisms is that their simple nutritional requirements enable them to survive in a wide range of pharmaceuticals. They tend to be present in high numbers, sometimes in excess of 10^6 cfu g^{-1} or ml^{-1}. In spite of this the product may itself show no visible sign of contamination.

CONTAMINATED MEDICINES AND CLINICAL IMPLICATIONS

Although isolated outbreaks of drug-related infections have been reported for many decades, it is only in the past 20 years that the significance of these infections has been properly understood. The infection dose of microorganisms is not only largely unknown but variable; furthermore, it varies not only between and within species but also between individual patients. The symptoms and outcome of a medicament-borne infection may be diverse. Clinical reactions may range from local infections of wounds or broken skin following contact with a contaminated cream, to serious systemic infections such as bacteriemia or septicaemia from contaminated parenteral products. Gastrointestinal infections can follow the ingestion of contaminated oral products. The most serious outbreaks of infection have been seen in the past where contaminated products have been injected into the bloodstream of patients whose immunity is already compromised by their underlying disease or therapy.

During the 1970s there were reports of septicaemia following infusion of contaminated solutions (Phillips et al., 1972; Felts et al., 1972; Meers et al., 1973). The contaminating microorganisms were mainly of gram-negative bacilli that grow readily in water, such as *Pseudomonas* and *Enterobacter spp.*, as well as fungi (Robertson, 1970; Goldmann and Maki, 1973). Various antimicrobial agents, usually quaternary ammonium compounds, contaminated with *Pseudomonas*, have repeatedly caused septicaemia when used as skin cleanser

Table 50–1. *Examples of the Organismic Contaminants Isolated from Pharmaceutical and Cosmetic Products**

Bacteria	Molds	Yeasts
Clostridium tetani	Absidia	Candida spp.
Achromobacter spp.	Aspergillus spp.	Torulopsis
Aerobacter spp.	Cladosporium spp.	Zygosaccharomyces
Klebsiella pneumoniae	Dematium	
Pseudomonas aeruginosa	Fusarium	
Pseudomonas cepacia	Geotrichum	
Pseudomonas stutzeri	Helminthosporium	
Staphylococcus aureus	Hormodendrum	
Streptococcus spp.	Mucor	
Micrococcus spp.	Paecilomyces	
Salmonella muenchen	Penicillium spp.	
Salmonella agona	Rhizopus	
Salmonella cubana	Stemphylium	
Serratia marcescens	Thamnidium	
Enterobacter spp.	Trichothecium	
	Verticillium	

*Some of the various genera are reported by Manowitz (1961), Kallings et al. (1966), and Baird (1985).

prior to parenteral therapy. Although this mechanism has been known for decades (Plotkin and Austrian, 1958), new outbreaks still occur (Frank and Schaffner, 1976). The clinical outcome varies considerably and depends on the type of organism involved and the patients receiving the infusion. If the degree of contamination is high there is usually an immediate reaction of endotoxic shock, which may be fatal. If the patient survives, the reaction is usually followed by pyrexia and signs of bacteraemia.

Injectable and ophthalmic solutions are often simple preparations and provide gram-negative opportunist pathogens with sufficient nutrients to multiply during storage. If such preparations are contaminated, numbers in excess of 10^6 cfu/ml and endotoxins should be expected. Crompton (1973) reported that 33% of eye ointments tested in Australia were contaminated. Later the dangers of using contaminated creams in British hospitals were highlighted by Noble and Savin (1966) and Savin (1967).

P. aeruginosa, the notorious contaminant of eyedrops, has caused serious ophthalmic infections, including loss of sight in some cases (Bruch 1972; Wilson and Ahearn, 1977). The problem is compounded when the eye is damaged following trauma or ophthalmic surgery.

In Sweden the gravity of the problem was demonstrated in an outbreak where a hydrocortisone eye ointment caused eight cases of *P. aeruginosa* infection, resulting in impaired vision in five of the patients and necessitating enucleation of the eye in one. In this outbreak the ointment contained from 20 to more than 2000 microorganisms g^{-1} (Ringertz and Ernerfeldt, 1965). Eye cosmetics have also been found to be contaminated with various yeasts and moulds, such as *Candida albicans, C. parapsilosis, Fusarium* spp., *Penicillium* spp., and others (Kuehne and Ahearn, 1971; Wilson et al., 1975; Ahearn and Wilson, 1976).

Investigations carried out by the Swedish National Board of Health in 1965 produced some startling findings on overall microbiologic quality immediately after manufacture of nonsterile products made in Sweden. A wide range of products was routinely found to be contaminated with *Bacillus subtilis, Staphylococcus epidermidis* (formerly *S. albus*), yeasts, and molds; also, large numbers of coliforms were found in a variety of tablets. An outbreak of salmonellosis (Kallings et al., 1966) was related to thyroid tablets containing millions of bacteria per gram (200 cases of infection with *Salmonella muenchen, Staphylococcus bareilly,* or both were reported). Of 150 other tablet types examined, 20 had counts in the range of 10^4 to 10^6 per tablet. Those batches of thyroid tablets subsequently examined contained as many as 10^5 microorganisms per tablet.

Topical preparations are often used on damaged skin. For most such preparations the presence of a small number of microorganisms (less than 100 g^{-1}) is probably harmless as long as potential pathogens are absent (Ringertz and Ringertz, 1982). Bruch (1972) categorized the following microorganisms as objectionable in this type of product: *Pseudomonas aeruginosa, Pseudomonas cepacia, Pseudomonas putida, Serratia marcescens, Klebsiella* spp., *Staphylococcus aureus, Clostridium perfringens, Clostridium tetani,* and *Clostridium novyi. Aspergillus* spp. and *Candida albicans* might be added to this list. If a topical preparation contains a corticosteroid it may considerably increase the patient's susceptibility to infection. Such preparations should therefore be sterile.

Accumulated evidence has provided a better understanding of why and how contamination occurs, the extent and frequency of contamination, the factors determining the outcome for the patient, and finally what preventive measures may be taken to control the problems.

PRESERVATIVE REQUIREMENTS

Pharmaceutical formulations often contain a number of ingredients, such as carbohydrates, proteins, phosphatides, emulsifiers, thickeners, solubilizers, opacifiers, suspending agents, and "active ingredients," that readily support the growth of a variety of microorganisms. Inclusion of a preservative is thus a necessary part of the formulation process. It is essential for the formulation pharmacist to examine all formulative ingredients to ensure that each agent is free to serve its intended purpose. The early selection of the preservative in the development of new formulations should be considered as an integral part of it, rather than an ad hoc addition.

The formulator must be aware of potential detrimental interaction between ingredients. Many of the recognized incompatible combinations that result in preservative inactivation involve macromolecules such as cellulose derivatives, polyethylene glycols, and natural gums. These attract and hold preservative agents, such as the parabens and phenolic compounds, rendering them inactive. An example of such interaction is the complexation of nonionic surfactants, such as polysorbate 80, with parabens.

An ideal preservative can be qualitatively defined as one meeting the following criteria (Gershenfeld and Perlstein, 1939; Gladhart et al., 1955; Gottfried, 1962):

The preservative should

1. Be free of toxic or irritant effect at the concentrations used on the skin, mucous membranes, and gastrointestinal tract, depending on the administration route
2. Be effective in preventing the growth of microorganisms most likely to contaminate the preparation
3. Be sufficiently soluble in water to achieve adequate concentrations in the aqueous phase of a system of two or more phases
4. Have adequate stability to heat and prolonged storage, with no chemical decomposition or volatilization during the desired shelf-life
5. Be chemically compatible with all other formulation components and retain the undissociated form at the pH of the preparation
6. Not adversely affect the preparations container or its closure.
7. Have an acceptable odor and color and a reasonable cost

At present no single antimicrobial agent has emerged as a universally acceptable preservative for pharmaceutical preparations. A study of the principles involved in preventing growth in these systems indicates that no such preservative is likely to be found.

The more important groups of preservatives, and some popular examples used in pharmaceuticals, are shown in Table 50–2. The activities of the antimicrobial agents listed in the table vary widely and depend on the microorganisms involved. Reviews deserving the reader's attention include those by Russell et al. (1967), Jaconia (1972), and Happel (1983).

MECHANISM OF ACTION OF PRESERVATIVES

Different substances have different specific effects, depending on the molecular structure or the chemical nature of the attack. Preservatives may act at various sites and inhibit different biochemical pathways within the microorganisms. Amongst the factors influenced by chemical substances are modification of membrane permeability or electrical potential; enzymes and other proteins; oxidation or reduction of cellular constituents (or both); hydrolysis; and other interference with essential metabolites. The possible modes of action of preservatives are listed in Table 50–3.

FACTORS MODIFYING THE EFFICIENCY OF PRESERVATIVES IN PHARMACEUTICAL FORMULATIONS

pH

The activity of ionizable preservatives is usually influenced markedly by the pH of the formulation, because activity resides in the neutral or undissociated molecules of preservatives. The weakly acidic preservatives such as benzoic acid ($pK_a = 4.2$) and sorbic acid ($pK_a = 4.75$) are effective only at low pH, where neutral molecules will predominate. These weak acids will therefore dissociate incompletely to give the three entities HA, H^+, and A^- in solution. Because the undissociated form, HA, is the active agent, the ionization constant, K_a, is important, and the pK_a of the acid must be considered in a particular formulation.

Conversely, the p-hydroxybenzoate esters with their nonionizable, esterified carboxyl group and poorly ionized hydroxyl group ($pK_a = 8.5$) are active at neutral pH. The quaternary ammonium preservatives (chlorhexidine) are ionized under all pH conditions, and activity probably resides mainly with their cations.

If the ionization of a weak acid is represented as

$$HA \rightleftharpoons H^+ + A^-$$ (1)

we may express the equilibrium constant as

$$K_a = \frac{(H^+)(A^-)}{(HA)}$$ (2)

K_a is variously referred to as the ionization, dissociation, or acidity constant for the weak acid. The negative logarithm of K_a is referred to as pK_a. Thus,

$$pK_a = -\log K_a$$ (3)

Taking logarithms of the expression for the dissociation constant of a weak acid (equation 2),

$$-\log K_a = -\log(H^+) - \log \frac{(A^-)}{(HA)}$$ (4)

Therefore

$$pH = pK_a + \log \frac{(A^-)}{(HA)}$$ (5)

Table 50–2. *Some Pharmaceutically Useful Preservatives*

Class	Usual Concentration (%)	Antimicrobial Spectrum
Acidics and Phenolics		
Benzoic acid and salts	0.05 – 0.1	Antifungal agent
Sorbic acid and salts	0.05 – 0.2	
Propionic acid and salts	*	
Boric acid and salts	0.5 – 1.0	
Dehydroacetic acid	*	
Sulphurous and vanillic acids	*	
Phenol	0.2 – 0.5	Broad spectrum
Cresol	0.1 – 0.5	
Chlorocresol	0.05 – 0.1	
O-phenylphenol	0.005 – 0.01	
Chlorothymol	*	
Parabens		Broad spectrum and synergist
Alkyl esters of parahydroxybenzoic acid	0.001 – 0.2	
Methyl, ethyl, propyl, benzyl, and butyl-p-hydroxybenzoates		
Mercurials		
Thiomersal	0.001 – 0.1	Broad spectrum
Phenylmercuric acetate and nitrate	0.002 – 0.005	
Nitromersol	0.001 – 0.1	
Sodium ethylmercurithiosalicylate	*	
Quaternary Ammonium Compounds		
Benzalkonium chloride	0.004 – 0.02	Broad spectrum
Cetylpyridinium chloride	0.01 – 0.02	
Benzethonium chloride	*	
Cetyltrimethyl ammonium bromide	0.01	
Miscellaneous		
Alcohols	15.0 –20.0	Broad-spectrum eye preparations Parenterals
Chlorobutanol	0.5	
Phenoxy-2-ethanol	*	
Benzyl alcohol	0.5 – 5.0	
β-phenylethyl alcohol	0.2 – 1.0	
Chlorhexidine	0.0025– 0.01	
Chloroform	*	
6-Acetoxy-2,4-dimethyl-m-dioxane 2,4,4′ Trichloro-2′-hydroxy-diphenylether	*	Active against gram-positive bacteria
Imidizolidinyl urea compound	0.1 – 0.5	Broad spectrum
Bromo-2-nitropropanediol-1,3	*	
5-Bromo-5-nitrol-1,3 dioxane		
2-methyl-4-isothiazolin-3-one and 5 chloro derivative		
1-(3-chloroallyl)-3,5,7-triazo 1-azoniaadamantane chloride (Dowicil 200)ᴿ	0.02 – 0.3	

Use of some of these antimicrobial agents is prohibited in some countries, and formulators must consult the relevant regulations.
*Effective concentration in each case should be determined for a particular drug preparation.

This of course is the familiar Henderson Hasselbalch equation.

Equation 5 may be rearranged to facilitate the direct determination of the molar percentage ionization as follows:

$$(HA) = (A^-) \text{ antilog } (pK_a - pH) \quad (6)$$

Thus, percentage ionization equals

$$\frac{(A^-)}{(HA) + (A^-)} \times 100 = \frac{100}{1 + \text{antilog } (pK_a - pH)} \quad (7)$$

The influence of pH of the formulation on the percentage ionization may be determined for preservatives of known pK_a. For example, the proportions of dissociated sorbic acid at various pH levels are given in Table 50–4. Thus at pH 7 approximately 64 times as much sorbic acid is required then at pH 3.

Bell et al. (1959), studying the effect of sorbic acids on the growth of various species of bacteria yeasts and molds, found that sorbic acid was most effective at the highest concentration of undissociated acid. On the other

Table 50–3. *Possible Modes of Action of Some Preservatives*

Alcohols and 2-phenoxyethanol	Inhibit active transport by uncoupling oxidation from phosphorylation, and protein coagulation
Mercurials and bronopol	Inhibit enzymes in the membrane and cytoplasm and have toxic effect on cell thiol groups
Cetrimide, phenol, and hexylresorcinol	Lyses cytoplasmic membrane, resulting in leakage of amino acids, purines, pyrimidines, potassium ions, and pentoses
Acridine dyes	React specifically with nucleic acid, interfering with its function
Sulphur dioxide	React with amino groups essential for metabolic activity
QACs and chlorhexidine	General coagulation and disruption of the permeability barrier of the cell
Benzoic acid and esters of *p*-hydroxybenzoic acid	Membrane action and competition with coenzymes, inhibit folic acid synthesis
Boric acid	Inhibit phosphate enzymes
Sorbic acid	Suppression of fumarate oxidation in catalase-positive organisms

Much more detailed treatment of the subject is given by Hugo (1967, 1971, and 1982)

Table 50–4. *Proportion of Dissociated Sorbic Acid* at Various pH Levels*

pH	Ionized Sorbic Acid (%)
2	0.16
3	1.56
4	13.68
5	61.31
6	94.06
7	99.37

*pK_a of sorbic acid = 4.8.

hand Wolf and Westveer (1950) found that dehydroacetic acid enolizes to give a weak acid. They tested dehydroacetic acid at pH 5, 7, and 9 against *Micrococcus pyogenes* var. *aureus* and *Salmonella typhosa* and found no change in the minimum bactericidal concentration at the three pH levels. It was concluded that the anion must be as active as the undissociated acid. This is in contrast to the true organic acids, which are more active in the acid pH range. Other reports indicate that 100 times as much dehydroacetic acid is required to inhibit *Aspergillus niger* at pH 7 as is required at pH 3.5 (Von Schelhorn, 1953). Bandelin (1958) has reported that the antimicrobial activity of esters of *p*-hydroxybenzoic acid and vanillin were only slightly influenced by pH. Many cases are known in which ionization is essential for initiation of antibacterial activity. Albert (1945) found that the most important factor in the action of the acridines at any pH is the amount of the cationic moiety. This relationship between cationic concentration and antibacterial activity holds not only for the acridine series, but also for the three series of benzacridines, the three series of benzquinolines, and the phenanthridines.

Distribution of Preservative in Multiphase Drug Formulation

In complex formulations such as an o/w pharmaceutical emulsion, cream, or other semisolid preparation, dissolved preservative molecules distribute themselves between all phases. This distribution may take a consid-

erable time to reach equilibrium. Conversely, agents that reduce preservative efficiency by various bonding attractions, surfactant micelles by solubilization, polymeric suspending agents by competitive displacement of water of solvation, or solid particles by adsorption, or the presence of microorganisms, will influence the preservative's thermodynamic activity even though its original concentration remains constant. The selection of a preservative with suitable physicochemical characteristics and estimation of the overall concentration necessary to give adequate levels of active preservative in drug formulation present considerable problems.

Certain preservatives are more soluble in oil than in water, and when these are used, additional preservative must be added to maintain the required concentration in the aqueous phase. Bean et al. (1969) derived an equation for determining the amount of preservative (C_w) that remains (active) in the aqueous phase. The equation relates this value to the total amount (C) of preservative with partition coefficient P, added to an emulsion with an oil/water phase ratio of ϕ:

$$C_w = \frac{C\,(\phi + 1)}{R\,(P\phi + 1)} \quad (8)$$

where R is the preservative/emulsifier ratio or interaction ratio. If the volume of oil is V_o and the total volume of the emulsion is V_t, then the volume of the aqueous phase is $V_t - V_o$, and therefore

$$\phi = \frac{V_o}{V_t - V_o} \quad (9)$$

and

$$V_o = \frac{\phi V_t}{(1 + \phi)} \quad (10)$$

Because V_o or ϕ is known from the composition of the emulsion, only P and R need be determined experimentally. The presence of surfactant micelles alters the native partition coefficient of the preservative molecules. Partition then occurs between the oil globule and the aqueous micellar phases. Distribution of phenol in o/w dispersion has been determined. In liquid paraffin-water dispersion P < 1; thus a fixed overall concentration of phenol is partitioned so that as the ratio of oil to water is increased, the concentration in both phases increases. In the case of arachis oil-water systems with P > 1, increase in the oil/water ratio leads to a reduction of preservative concentration in the aqueous phase. This is the case with phenol and chlorocresol in arachis oil emulsions (data for which are presented by Konning, 1974) containing 60% arachis oil (ϕ = 1.5) and 1% polysorbate 80 as stabilizer. Phenol and chlorocresol are present in 2.5% concentration. Nearly 9.6% of the phenol resides in the free water phase, but only 0.3% of the more lipophilic chlorocresol is free in the water phase. As much as 93% of the phenol and 99.9% of chlorocresol are trapped in the oily phase. The use of equation 8 has, however, been criticized because of the manner in which R has been measured and defined. For further discussion of complex emulsified systems see Mitchell and Kazmi (1975).

One method for determining available preservative is to determine the proportion of preservative that is readily dialyzable from the complex formulation through a cellophane membrane into water (Kazmi and Mitchell, 1978). It is, however, essential to evaluate the formulation against a direct microbial challenge.

Preservative Concentration

To be effective a sufficient concentration of preservative must be available in the aqueous phase. Effectiveness depends mainly on the types and numbers of microorganisms likely to contaminate the product, and the rate at which it is necessary to kill them. In the case of multidose parenteral, ophthalmic, and nasal preparations, sterility is essential and hence the rate of kill must be high. In emulsions and other preparations used externally, however, a low rate is acceptable. The rate of kill is a kinetic process and usually depends on the "availability and efficacy" of the antimicrobial preservatives. There is generally an exponential relationship between microbicidal activity and preservative concentration. Thus, if the log of a death time (that is, the time to kill a standard inoculum) is plotted against log concentration, a straight line is usually obtained, the slope of which is the concentration exponent (η) and expressed as an equation:

$$\eta = \frac{\text{(log death time at concentration } C_2)}{\log C_1 - \log C_2}$$

Thus, η may be obtained by substitution in the above equation. Some numerical values of η are given in Table 50–5.

The practical meaning of the concentration exponent is demonstrated by the following: Parabens have a concentration exponent of 2.5; therefore, threefold dilution will result in a decrease in activity of $3^{2.5}$, or 15.6, times.

Temperature Effect

Temperature increase almost always increases antimicrobial activity. This may be expressed quantitatively

Table 50–5. *Concentration Exponents (η) for Some Preservatives*

Preservative	η
Mercurials	0.03–3.0
Quaternary ammonium compounds	0.8 –2.5
Acridines	0.7 –1.9
Parabens	2.5
Sorbic acid	2.6 –3.2
Bronopol	0.7
Chlorhexidine	2.0

by means of a temperature coefficient: either the temperature coefficient per degree rise in temperature, denoted by θ, or the temperature coefficient per 10° rise, the Q_{10} (rate of change of activity per 10°). θ may be calculated from the equation

$$\theta^{(T_2 - T_1)} = \frac{t_1}{t_2}$$

where t_1 is the extinction time at T_1°C, and t_2 the extinction time at T_2°C (i.e., T_1 + 1°C). Values may be easily calculated by determining the extinction time at two temperatures differing by 10°C.

$$Q_{10} = \frac{\text{Time to kill at } T°}{\text{Time to kill at } (T + 10)°}$$

The value of the temperature coefficient (Q_{10}) may vary with preservative, type of organism, and temperature range (Hugo and Russell, 1987).

Thus, if the value of θ for an antimicrobial agent is 3, the increase in activity for a 3°C rise in temperature is 3^3 or 27-fold. On the other hand, if the value of Q_{10} for phenol is 5, a drop in temperature from 30 to 20°C can result in a fivefold reduction in the killing rate of the antimicrobial agent. The temperature effect is highly important when evaluating preservative action in challenge-testing procedures.

Surfactant Effect

Susceptibility of organisms to preservatives varies with the nature of ingredients and the possibility of interactions between them. Even though a normally active concentration of preservative may be present, it may not be fully effective because the microorganisms are protected from its action.

In most instances, before an antibacterial agent can act on a cell, it must combine with it. This process often follows the pattern of an adsorption isotherm. Factors that affect the state of the cell surface must affect, to some extent, the adsorption process. The addition of low concentrations of cationic detergents has been shown to potentiate the biologic effect of antibacterial agents such as phenols. However, nonionic surfactant can inhibit the interaction between preservative and cell membrane.

Judis (1962) studied the mechanism of action of phenolic disinfectants by measuring the release of radioactivity from cells of *E. coli* labeled with C^{14}. Tween 80 was found to protect *E. coli* from the lethal effects of O-chloro-m-xylenol and prevent in part the leakage of the cell contents, as indicated by release of radioactivity. Beckett and Robinson (1958) found that the addition of extremely low concentrations of polyethylene glycol 1000 monocetylether (cetomacrogol) reduces the amount of hexylresorcinol taken up by *E. coli* at several different concentrations. The amount of cetomacrogol present was too small to have interfered with the availability of hexylresorcinol to the bacteria, and it was concluded that the nonionic surfactant interfered with the interaction of the drug at the cytoplasmic membrane of the organism. Similar findings have shown that Tween 80 and polyethylene glycol 400 laurate protect the cells of *E. coli, Pseudomonas fluorescens,* and *Streptococcus bovis* from the inhibitory effects of the preservative.

Degree of Binding of Preservatives

Preservatives are also removed from solution and used up during their inactivation of microorganisms. Nonspecific interactions of preservative with the general organic component of drug preparations usually reduces preservative capacity more significantly than interaction with the microbial component does because of the relatively larger mass of the former (Beveridge, 1987). Volatile preservatives, such as chloroform, are readily lost by the routine opening and closing of bulk containers, and phenolic preservatives can easily permeate rubber closures with consequent marked decline in preservative concentrations of the preparations. The United States Pharmacopeia (1985) directs that the container must not interact physically or chemically with the article placed in it so as to alter the strength, quality, or purity of the article beyond the official specification. Appreciable interactions have been observed between certain plastics and preservatives by surface adsorption; adsorption onto glass surfaces has significant effect in removing quaternary ammonium preservatives and sorbic acid (McCarthy, 1971). McCarthy examined the behavior of a wide range of preservative solutions during storage in brown glass, polyvinyl chloride, polyethylene, and polypropylene containers at ambient temperatures during periods of up to 12 weeks. In general, polyethylene was the least suitable material, allowing substantial loss of phenolics and dehydroacetic acid. Loss of the widely used *p*-hydroxybenzoate was shown to be negligible. The other plastics presented fewer problems, although sorbic acid and dichlorophenol were rapidly lost from polypropylene. The multiplicity of factors that influence preservative-plastic interaction make it difficult to assess information published by individual laboratories (Parker, 1982). Dean (1978) has emphasized that differences between grades of plastic surfaces, thickness, and degree of crystallinity, and the presence of fillers, accelerators, vulcanizing agents, pigments, and plasticizers all have their effects.

The degree of binding of various preservatives by macromolecules has been investigated by several workers (Blaug and Ahsan, 1961; Deluca and Kostenbauder, 1960; Kostenbauder, 1962). There is overwhelming evidence that for a given preservative the thermodynamic activity is equivalent to the preservative activity. When binding between a preservative and a macromolecule occurs, an equilibrium is set up so that when some of the preservative is adsorbed or otherwise removed by its action on microorganisms, there will be a shift in equilibrium, making more preservative available (Allawaha and Riegelman, 1954). Thus a system in which the reservoir of preservative exists (bound preservative) could be more efficient than a simple aqueous solution of similar thermodynamic activity. The preservative molecules must not, however, be "irreversibly bound" to other components of the formulation that will render the preservatives inactive. Only the concentration of free, or unbound, preservative is effective. The efficacy of a particular preservative is also influenced by formulation type, nutritive value of the product, and manufacturing operations. These factors are discussed by Wedderburn (1964).

The influence of the manufacturing procedure in the preservation of tablets against microbial spoilage has been examined by Fassihi et al. (1978). They present interesting methods of incorporating preservative into tablet formulation for maximum protection against microbial growth. In direct compression tableting fine particles of preservative may be added to the dry powders, which are then mixed and immediately compressed. When wet granulation is required the preservative should be dissolved in the granulation liquid. Alternatively, final granules may be sprayed with preservative while rotating in either a coating pan or a fluidized bed unit. The dry-mix technique and wet granulation procedures yield the highest levels of preservative (parabens) in the finished tablets. The lowest levels were found in tablets produced from sprayed granules. The tablets produced from granules sprayed with preservative solution were the most resistant to microbial challenge. It is likely that in the dry-mix and wet granulation situations there is no loss of preservative or interaction between preservative and tablet ingredients, so that final measured levels of preservative are high. In the spray technique losses of preservative can occur during the spraying procedure, as can surface interaction in the wet state. These losses are, however, compensated for by the greater surface availability and preservative activity. Microbial spoilage of tablets is usually due to surface growth; preservative coated externally onto the granules migrates more readily to the surface than preservative incorporated into the core does.

Several workers have reported that macromolecules without surface active properties reduce the efficacy of certain preservatives, and because many hydrophilic polymers are used in pharmaceuticals, their effects must be considered. Miyawaki et al. (1959) studied the effect of polyethylene glycol 4000 on methyl and propyl parabens using both solubility and equilibrium dialysis methods. Their results showed that in a solution of 5% polyethylene glycol 4000, approximately 1.6 times as much of the methyl ester would be required to effect adequate preservation as would be needed in the absence of the macromolecule, and that the propyl ester was bound to a greater extent than the methyl was. Eisman et al. (1957) examined the effectiveness of chlorbutanol, phenylmercuric acetate, merthiolate, a mixture of methyl and propyl parabens, benzalkonium chloride, and phenol in 3% gum tragacanth jellies. By contaminating the variously preserved jellies with a standard inoculum of *Staphylococcus aureus* organisms and determining survival rates, they found the activity of all the above components reduced in comparison with their activity in water. A neutralizing effect by gum tragacanth, probably as the result of physical adsorption, was suggested by the authors. Polyvinylpyrrolidone contains an amido group; Kostenbauder and Higuchi (1956) demonstrated that compounds such as phenols, which are capable of acting as proton donors, tend to form complexes with amides. These degrees of binding might, under some conditions, necessitate the action of a supplementary amount of preservative.

Combinations of Preservatives

A combination of two preservatives may be synergistic. Synergy is measured against a single microorganism and may be evaluated by preparing mixtures of the two compounds and determining their growth inhibitory power in terms of minimum inhibitory concentration (MIC). The results may be plotted in the form of an isobologram (Hugo and Russell, 1987). Combinations may extend the spectrum of a preservative system. The preservative Germall II (an imidazolidine urea compound) has an essentially antibacterial activity but no antifungal action. If combined with parabens, which possesses antifungal activity, a broader-spectrum preservative system with antibacterial/antifungal properties is obtained.

Combinations of hexachlorophane and esters of *p*-hydroxybenzoic acid together provide a widening of the antimicrobial spectrum and allow the hexachlorophane to be used in low concentrations to minimize toxicity. The justifications for using combinations of preservatives have been summarized as follows (Garrett, 1966):

1. The spectrum of antimicrobial activity is increased and the resistance of an organism to one preservative may be prevented
2. The toxic effects of the greater concentration of one preservative may be averted if a synergistic effect is achieved
3. Formulation problems such as solubility may be prevented

An alternative to the use of preservative combinations is the use of potentiating agents, which are not usually used as antimicrobial agents per se, but which enhance antimicrobial efficacy (Parker, 1982). These agents act in a variety of ways. For example, propylene glycol increases the aqueous solubility of lipophilic preservatives (Prickett et al., 1961; Woodford and Adams, 1972); the

disodium salt of ethylenediamine-tetraacetic acid (EDTA) utilizes hydrophilic groups to chelate metal ions, yielding water-soluble complexes, and so augmenting bactericidal effects (Brown and Richards, 1965; Sheikh and Parker, 1972); phenylethyl alcohol, phenoxyethanol, and surfactants potentiate antimicrobial activity by interfering with membrane permeability (Clausen and Raugsted, 1965; Richards and McBride, 1971a).

Type of Compound

Benzoic Acid and Salts

The organic acid, C_6H_5COOH, is either included alone as the sodium salt, or in combination with other preservatives, in many oral pharmaceutical preparations. The nonionized acid is the active substance; thus a limitation in its use is imposed by the pH of the final product as the pK_a of benzoic acid is 4.2. It is advisable to limit use of the acid to the preservation of pharmaceuticals having a final pH of less than 4.0. The other disadvantage of these compounds is that some organisms develop resistance to them.

Sorbic Acid and Salts

This compound is a widely used preservative, both in the food industry and in pharmaceutical products such as gels, mucilages, and syrups. Both the acid and its potassium salts are useful as mold and yeast inhibitors. The pK_a is 4.8 and, as with benzoic acid, activity decreases with increasing pH. The compound is one of the least toxic preservative agents.

Dehydroacetic Acid

This compound, although included in USP XX, Second Supplement, is only occasionally used as a preservative, primarily in oral preparations. It is much more active at acidic pH range and is inactive at available concentrations in neutral or alkaline preparations (Wickliffe and Entrekin, 1964).

Sulphur Dioxide, Sodium Sulphite, Sodium Metabisulphite

Sulphur dioxide is extensively used as a preservative in the food and beverage industries. In a pharmaceutical context sodium sulphite and metabisulphite have a dual role acting as preservatives and antioxidants.

Phenols

Phenols are widely used as disinfectants and preservatives. A 0.5% aqueous phenol solution will rapidly kill most vegetative bacteria. The activity of phenols is markedly diminished by dilution and by organic matter. The use of phenols has decreased because of their odor, volatility, toxicity, and numerous incompatibilities (Elowe, 1955).

Cresol

Cresol is a mixture of *o*-, *m*-, and *p*-methylphenol. Because of its poor solubility, it is solubilized with a soap prepared from linseed oil and potassium hydroxide. It forms a clear solution on dilution, and is used in concentrations of 0.3 to 0.5%. Spectrum of activity is similar to that of phenol but is less caustic and less poisonous. Cresol has found some use in immunologic products, because its activity is not reduced in the presence of organic matter (Russell et al., 1967).

Chlorocresol

Chlorocresol, which is approximately ten times more active than phenol, is used as a preservative for pharmaceutical preparations. It is recommended for use by the British Pharmacopoeia (BP) at a concentration of 0.1% w/v for preservation of injections, and of 0.2% w/v when included as a part of the sterilization procedure by heating with a bactericide. It has the same limitations as phenol. It is highly soluble in rubber with a distribution ratio between rubber and water of 85 to 15 (Royce and Sykes, 1957). Other phenolic compounds such as xylenols, ethylphenol, chloroxylenol, bisphenols, and phenylphenol have not gained wide acceptance.

Esters of p-Hydroxybenzoic Acid (Parabens)

The methyl, ethyl, propyl, and butyl esters of p-hydroxybenzoic acid are used in combination with one another because of their synergistic action as preservatives of emulsions, creams, and lotions. Parabens are less readily ionized than the parent acid. They have pK_a values in the range of 8 to 8.5, and exhibit good preservative activity even at pH levels of 7 to 8. Optimum activity is displayed in acidic solutions. They are generally employed at concentration levels approaching saturation in water. Combinations of esters are most successful in products in which two phases exist. The more water-soluble methyl ester protects the aqueous phase, whereas the propyl or butyl esters usually dissolve and protect the oil phase. The parabens are popular preservatives. They are odorless, do not discolor, are nonirritating and are of low toxicity. The major disadvantages of parabens are their low water solubility and tendency to hydrolyze and vaporize upon heating. They are less effective against gram-negative bacteria than against molds and yeast. Preservation has traditionally been effectively accomplished by use of the p-hydroxybenzoate esters, although failures have been known to occur. These may have been due to a variety of causes, such as loss of the preservative from the aqueous to the oil phase because of unstable solubility characteristics, the use of insufficient concentrations relative to optimal dissociation, or physical incompatibility between the preservative and other formulation components.

Although it has been reported that the surface-active sorbitan esters and polyoxyethylene sorbitan esters reduced the effect of methyl-p-hydroxybenzoate, the addition of propylene glycol to simple pharmaceutical syrups potentiates the effect of methyl and propyl esters of p-hydroxybenzoate. This enables their effective concentration to be reduced. In order to establish the effects of propylene glycol and glycerol on the partition coeffi-

cient of methyl p-hydroxybenzoate, Hibboth and Monks (1961) used a mixture of water, oleyl alcohol, and preservative with increasing amounts of either propylene glycol or glycerol. Their results indicate that the presence of more than 5% propylene glycol in the aqueous phase changes the solubility of the preservative, making it more available. Phenolic preservatives are, however, especially susceptible to interaction with compounds containing polyoxyethylene groups. Practically all nonionic surfactants based on ethylene and propylene oxide condensed with each other or with fatty esters, alcohols, or acids, and inactivate nearly all the preservatives currently considered suitable for pharmaceuticals. The extent of the adverse effect has been related to the hydrophile-lipophile balance of the surfactant and the chemical structure of the preservative (Wedderburn, 1958).

The interaction of parabens with several nonionic macromolecules has been reported (Blaug and Ahsan, 1961). In determining the binding tendencies of the esters with Tween 80 (polyoxyethylene sorbitan mono-oleate), Myrj 52 (polyoxyethylene monostearate), polyethylene glycol 4000 and 6000, and Pluronic F-68 (polyethylene propylene glycol), the authors confirmed that the greater lipophilic tendencies reduced the effectiveness of esters more than the more hydrophilic macromolecules. Combining the parabens with phenoxyethanol (Boehm and Maddox, 1970) or with imidazolidinyl urea (Germall II) has been shown to improve their activity against bacteria, yeast, and molds (Berke and Rosen, 1980).

Another preservative that may be combined with parabens is 1-(3 chloroallyl)-3,5,7-triazo-1-azoniaadamantane chloride (Dowicil 200). This combination is effective against bacteria, yeast, and molds and is not inactivated by nonionic, anionic, or cationic formulation ingredients. It is extremely water-soluble but is virtually insoluble in oils and organic solvents and should not be heated above 50°C. It is stable in the pH range 4 to 10.

In the series of parabens, water solubility decreases in the following order: methyl, ethyl, propyl, and butyl esters. By combining these products it is possible to protect both aqueous and oil phases of the formulation.

Mercurials

The industrial and agricultural applications of mercurials have greatly declined, because of their potential environmental pollution hazard. Plasmid-mediated resistance has also resulted in many pathogenic microorganisms becoming insensitive to the antimicrobial effects of mercurials (Scott and Gorman, 1987). The phenylmercuric salts (0.002%) are recommended for preservation of eyedrops and injections as well as for sterilization by heating with a bactericide. The cation of the phenylmercuric salts is the active portion, whereas the anion, usually nitrate or acetate, provides the desired water solubility. Thiomersal, in a concentration range of 0.001 to 0.004%, is employed as a preservative for contact lens solutions, either alone or in combination with potentiating agents such as EDTA. Although mercurials are powerful biostatic compounds, they are relatively slow-acting bactericides (Lawrence, 1955; Eriksen, 1970). Their use in ophthalmic preparations when rapid bactericidal effects are required has been questioned (Riegelman et al., 1955; Kohn et al., 1963). Mercurials are absorbed from solution to a significant extent on exposure to rubber closures, polyethylene, and plastic containers (Jaconia, 1972; Lachman, 1968). Thiomersal is often considered the preservative of choice for biological products, vaccines, antitoxins, and immune serum in which inactivation of the active principle must be avoided (Jaconia, 1972). Because the compound is a basic salt of a weak organic acid, its use is limited to alkaline and neutral solutions (Eriksen, 1970). These solutions are, however, subject to a variety of incompatibilities, with mercurials being readily reduced to free mercury and the quaternary compounds being inactivated by a variety of anionic substances (Lachman, 1968).

Quaternary Ammonium Compounds (QACs)

The QACs are water-soluble cationic surface-active agents that are nontoxic, are well tolerated, and inhibit microorganisms in low concentrations. These are organically substituted ammonium compounds, as shown, where the R substituents are alkyl or heterocyclic radicals to give compounds such as cetyltrimethylammonium bromide (cetrimide), cetylpyridinium chloride, and benzalkonium chloride. Inspection of the structures of these compounds indicates that for good antimicrobial activity it is important to have a chain length in the range C_8 to C_{18} in at least one of the R substituents (Merck Index, 1983).

$$\text{General structure of QACs} \quad \left[\begin{array}{c} R_1 \\ | \\ R_4{-}N{-}R_2 \\ | \\ R_3 \end{array} \right]^+ X^-$$

The QACs are most effective against microorganisms at neutral or slightly alkaline pH and become virtually inactive below pH 3.5. They are incompatible with anionic detergents such as soap, and demonstrate a high degree of binding with nonionic surfactants. This is possibly due to the formation of micelles (Deluca and Kostenbauder, 1960). The presence of significant amounts of organic matter such as serum, feces, milk, and certain salts such as nitrates will also adversely affect their activity. QACs exhibit activity against gram-positive bacteria at concentrations as low as 1:200,000. Gram-negative bacteria are more resistant, requiring a level of 1:20,000 or higher still if Pseudomonas aeruginosa is present (1:5000). The QACs have not been shown to possess any useful antiviral, sporicidal, or fungicidal activity. This rather narrow spectrum of activity limits the usefulness of the compounds. Benzalkonium chloride and cetrimide are employed extensively in surgery, urology, and gynecology as aqueous and alcoholic solutions, as creams, and sometimes in conjunction with biguanide disinfectants such as chlorhexidine.

The QACs are frequently used in ophthalmic solutions; several authors have reported benzalkonium chloride as the agent of choice for such preparations (Lawrence, 1955; Kohn et al., 1963; Brown et al., 1964). Ethylenediaminetetraacetate (EDTA) has been demonstrated to increase the activity of benzalkonium chloride against gram-negative organisms, especially P. aeruginosa (MacGregor and Elliker, 1958). A similar effect has been confirmed by Brown and Richards (1965) with chlorhexidine and polymyxin. It appears that EDTA is synergistic with these compounds. Jaconia (1972) reported that the addition of EDTA would prevent the growth of P. aeruginosa resistant to benzalkonium chloride.

Chlorhexidine

Chlorhexidine containing the biguanide structure could be expected to have a good antibacterial effect, as has been described by Davies (1954). Chlorhexidine base is not readily soluble in water and so the freely soluble salts, acetate, gluconate, and hydrochloride are used in pharmaceuticals. Chlorhexidine is effective at ambient temperatures. It exhibits the greatest antibacterial activity at pH 7 to 8 where it exists exclusively as a dication. Organic matter and anionic compounds, including soaps and anions, will reduce chlorhexidine's activity because of the formation of insoluble salts. It is particularly active against gram-positive bacteria, whereas gram-negatives are somewhat less sensitive to it. A concentration of 1:2,000,000 prevents growth of Staphylococcus aureus, whereas a 1:50,000 dilution prevents growth of Pseudomonas aeruginosa (Scott and Gorman, 1987). Anderson et al. (1964) stated that the compound in concentrations of 0.005 to 0.01% most closely approximates the ideal bacteriostatic agent for ophthalmic preparations. Pseudomonad contamination of aqueous chlorhexidine solutions has prompted the inclusion of small amounts of ethanol or isopropanol. In general chlorhexidine is well tolerated and nontoxic when applied to skin or mucous membranes. A limited antifungal activity has been demonstrated, which restricts its use as a general preservative.

Alcohols

Ethanol and isopropanol, which are used for disinfection, are bactericidal against vegetative forms, including Mycobacterium species, but are not sporicidal. Ethanol is widely used as a solvent and is a highly effective preservative. It is useful only in oral preparations, where it is limited by taste, cost, volatility, and lack of consumer acceptance. Gabel (1921) recommended 15% ethanol in acid solutions and 17.5% in neutral or mildly alkaline preparations for preservation purposes. It has bactericidal action at concentrations between 60 and 95%, but is usually employed as a 70% solution for the disinfection and cleansing action of skin prior to injection or surgical procedures.

Isopropanol (isopropyl alcohol) has slightly greater bactericidal activity, but is approximately twice as toxic. It is used at concentrations of 70% and above in preoperative skin treatment and as a preservative for cosmetics.

Propylene glycol has preservative activity at concentrations of 10% in syrups and 20% in gelatin preparations. When used in combination, 2 to 5% propylene glycol has enhanced the bactericidal activity of the parabens (Prickett et al., 1961).

Benzyl alcohol has antibacterial and weak local anesthetic properties. A 1% concentration is used and recommended by the BP in preparations intended for injections, in which benzyl alcohol's anesthetic properties are useful (Nogneira, 1962). Benzyl alcohol is neutral in reaction, has a pleasant odor, is stable to heat, is active over a broad pH range, and is soluble in water up to 4% (Elowe, 1955), but is volatile and may penetrate closures (Russell et al., 1967).

Chlorobutanol has been used as a preservative in injections and eyedrops. It is normally used at 0.5%, which is near to saturation limits; problems can arise because of crystallization at low temperatures. Unfortunately, the compound is not stable except under acid conditions, which has curtailed its use. Chlorobutanol is volatile and may be absorbed by rubber stoppers or lost through plastic containers during storage (Nair and Lach, 1959; Lachman, 1962).

Phenylethanol is reported to have greater activity against gram-negative than against gram-positive organisms and is primarily bacteriostatic in action (Berrah and Konetzka, 1962). It is used as a preservative, usually in conjunction with benzalkonium chloride, phenylmercuric nitrate, or chlorhexidine (Richards and McBride, 1971b).

Phenoxymethanol is more active against *P. aeruginosa* than against other bacteria. It is employed as a preservative at a concentration of 1%, which is nontoxic, usually in combination with ether preservatives to broaden the spectrum of antimicrobial activity (Scott and Gorman, 1987).

Bronopol (2-bromo-2-nitropropan-1,3-diol) has a broad spectrum of antibacterial activity. It has been widely used as a preservative in pharmaceutical and cosmetic preparations at concentrations of 0.01 to 0.02%. It possesses high aqueous solubility and is effective over a wide pH range in the presence of surfactants. It decomposes at an alkaline pH, particularly with an increase in temperature.

Chloroform

Chloroform ($CHCl_3$) has a narrow spectrum of activity. It has been extensively used since the last century as a preservative of pharmaceuticals. Recently limitations have been placed on its use (Scott and Gorman, 1987). It is highly volatile, which can lead to reductions in concentration, resulting in possible microbial growth.

Dowicil

Dowicil 200 is extremely water-soluble and has a broad-spectrum antimicrobial effect at concentrations of 0.02 to 0.3%. It is not inactivated by nonionic, anionic,

Table 50–6. *USP XX Procedure for Determination of Preservative Efficacy*

Organisms Used
Candida albicans, Aspergillus niger, Escherichia coli, Staphylococcus aureus, Pseudomonas aeruginosa

Inoculum
0.1 ml/20 ml; 100,000 to 1,000,000 cfu/ml

Medium
TAT broth consisting of tryptone (2%), azolectin (0.5%), and polysorbate 20 (4%) has been found suitable

Sampling
At 7, 14, 21, and 28 days after inoculation

Determination of Effectiveness
The preservative system is deemed effective if the number of viable organisms is reduced to not more than 0.1% of the initial inoculum, the viable count of yeast and molds remains unchanged or falls during the first 14 days, and the concentration of each test organism remains at or below these levels after 28 days.

or cationic formulation ingredients. It should not be heated above 50°C and is unstable below pH 4 and above pH 10. Discoloring may occur, but can be prevented by the addition of sodium sulfite.

Determination of Preservative Efficacy in Preserved Pharmaceuticals

An essential part of the quality control procedure is to determine the efficacy of preservatives in a final product. According to the British Pharmacopoeia (1980) recommendation this is done by inoculating the product with four stock cultures of bacteria, yeast, and a mold, and then assessing its ability to withstand microbial contamination. A colony count of the initial inoculum is determined and expressed as colony-forming units (cfu) per milliliter. A multiple-challenge test may be used if considered necessary. The inclusion of known spoilage organisms (e.g., osmotolerant yeasts) is recommended where this is thought to be a possible in-use problem.

The BP (1980), in its 1986 Addendum, Appendix XVI, contains a test for efficacy of preservatives. The product is challenged separately by the fungi *Aspergillus niger* and *Candida albicans* and the bacteria *Pseudomonas aeruginosa* and *Staphylococcus aureus* with details provided of type, maintenance, and subculturing of organisms. Different performance criteria are laid down for multidose injectable, ophthalmic, otic, nasal, topical, and oral liquid preparations. Variation in the end-point required is allowed according to the product tested. Multidose injections and ophthalmic preparations have to reduce the bacterial challenge (number of challenging organisms, 10^6 ml^{-1} or g^{-1}) by a factor of not less than 10^3 within 6 hours, whereas topical and oral liquid forms are allowed 48 hours to achieve a similar reduction. The BP Appendix should be consulted for full details of the experimental procedures to be used. Table 50–6 gives the USP XX procedure for topicals, including the organisms

Table 50–7. *Neutralizing Agents for Some Preservatives**

Preservative	Neutralizing Agent
Benzoic acid and esters of p-hydroxybenzoic acid	Tween 80, polysorbate 20, or dilution
Mercurials	Thioglycollic acid
QACs and chlorhexidine	Tween 80 and lecithin or Azolectin
Phenolic disinfectants	Tween 80 or dilution
Alcohols	Dilution
Bronopol	Cysteine hydrochloride
Hexachlorophane	Tween 80

*By performing viable counts at selected time intervals, care must be taken to ensure that at the moment of sampling, the antibacterial action is immediately arrested by the use of above specific inactivators, which are nontoxic to microorganisms.

used, inoculum size, sampling periods, and measure of effectiveness. When performing viable counts care must be taken to ensure that, at the moment of sampling, the preservative is inactivated by dilution or the use of a suitable neutralizer (Table 50–7). The United States Pharmacopeia (1985, 21st Edition) also gives procedures for evaluating the efficacy of antimicrobial preservatives in other types of pharmaceutical preparations and should be consulted for experimental procedures.

An alternative method for rapid determination of preservative efficacy utilizes the so-called D-value, or decimal reduction time, which is calculated from a plot of the log number of surviving organisms per gram or milliliter against time following inoculation of the product with specific organisms. The D-value can be used to compare the rate of inactivation of different organisms in one or more products and permits the calculation of the time required for the complete destruction of any population size of organisms (Idson and Lazarus, 1986). For example: if the mean D-value for *S. aureus* in a pharmaceutical product is 3.0 hours, the time for 10^6 *S. aureus* per milliliter to be totally inactivated is given by the product of the log number of the organisms per milliliter multiplied by the D-value, or 6×3.0 hours = 18 hours.

There has been extensive debate on challenge testing (Cowen and Steiger, 1967; Moore, 1978). The criticisms of these challenge tests are many and center upon the choice of challenge organisms, number of challenges, microbial load in challenge, preparation of microorganisms, ambient temperature of test, end-point stipulated, and sampling and recovery techniques. Answers to some of these questions are offered in the Third Joint Report (Laboratory and Drug Control Services and FIP, 1984).

CONCLUSIONS

Pharmaceuticals may be contaminated during manufacture mainly through contaminated raw materials or improper handling, during dispensing in the pharmacy, or during use. If the product allows microbial multipli-

cation following any of these modes of contamination, it may result in high bacterial counts at the time of use. This may cause deterioration of the product, loss of potency, pyrogen reactions, infection or colonization of the patient with risk of secondary spread, loss of patient compliance, inadequate drug delivery, and transformation of therapeutic agents, which may alter pharmacologic activity.

The quality of pharmaceutical products must be maintained throughout their storage and use. They should therefore be presented in a form that as far as possible excludes contamination during use. The increasing emphasis on the microbiologic attributes of nonsterile products has generated additional responsibility in the quality control of raw materials, especially those derived from animal or botanical origin. In recognition of this, USP XXI has included microbiologic quality control test procedures to monitor nonsterile preparations for possible contamination with *E. coli*, *S. aureus*, and certain species of *Pseudomonas* and *Salmonella*. The absence of pathogens is important, and the total count gives a measure of microbiologic normality. Nonsterile pharmaceuticals susceptible to microbial attacks should have antimicrobial properties (e.g., they could contain preservative).

In the case of multidose containers such as injectables, eye drops, and otic and nasal preparations, it is desirable that the product be so effectively preserved that any microbial contamination likely to be introduced into the preparation during use is eliminated before the next dose is taken out. Many pharmaceutical preparations are strongly antimicrobial in themselves and do not need the addition of a preservative. Bacteraemia associated with intravenous therapy is rarely caused by contaminated infusion solutions; more frequently it is due to intravenous infusion catheters being left in the blood vessel too long. This practice is known to involve a high risk of thrombophlebitis and septicaemia, usually caused by coagulase-negative *Staphylococci* (Fisher, 1988). However, *S. aureus*, *Corynebacterium*, *Bacillus* species, gram-negative bacteria, and fungi have all been implicated in catheter-associated infections. As a result of the increasingly stringent regulations worldwide with greater emphasis placed on formulation of products and standards of manufacture, the quality of pharmaceutical preparations has improved considerably during the last decade.

REFERENCES

Ahearn, D.G., and Wilson, L.A. 1976. In *Developments in Industrial Microbiology*. Edited by L.A. Underkofler. Vol. 17, 23–28.

Albert, A. 1945. Influence of chemical constitution on antibacterial activity; general survey of acridine series. Br. J. Exp. Pathol., *26*, 60.

Allawala, N.A., and Riegelman, S. 1954. Phenol coefficients and the Ferguson principle. J. Am. Pharm. Ass., Sci. ed. 43, 93.

Anderson, K., Lillie, S., and Crompton, D. 1964. Efficacy of bacteriostats in ophthalmic solutions. Pharm. J., *192*, 593–594.

Baird, R.M. 1985. Microbial contamination of pharmaceutical products made in a hospital pharmacy. Pharm. J., *234*, 54–55.

Baird, R.M. 1987. Contamination of non-sterile pharmaceuticals in hospital and community environments. In *Pharmaceutical Microbiology*. 4th Edition. Edited by W.B. Hugo and A.D. Russell. Oxford, Blackwell Scientific, p. 381.

Bandelin, F.J. 1958. The effect of pH on the efficiency of various mould inhibiting compounds. J. Am. Pharm. Assoc., 47, 691.

Bean, H.S., Konning, G.K., and Malcolm, S.M. 1969. A model of the influence of emulsion formulation on the activity of phenolic preservatives. J. Pharm. Pharmacol., 21, 173.

Beckett, A.H., and Robinson, A.E. 1958. The inactivation of preservatives by non-ionic surface active agents. Soap Perfum. Cosm., 31, 454–459.

Bell, T.A., Etchells, J.L., and Borg, A.F. 1959. Influence of sorbic acid on the growth of certain species of bacteria, yeasts, and filamentous fungi. J. Bacteriol., 77, 573.

Berke, P.A., and Rosen, W.E. 1980. Are cosmetic emulsions adequately preserved against Pseudomonas? J. Soc. Cosm. Chem., 31, 37–40.

Berrah, G., and Konetzka, W.A. 1962. Selective and reversible inhibition of the synthesis of bacterial deoxyribonucleic acid by phenethyl alcohol. J. Bacteriol., 83, 738–744.

Beveridge, E.G. 1975. The microbial spoilage of pharmaceutical products. In Microbial Aspects of the Deterioration of Materials. Edited by R.J. Gilbert and D.W. Lovelock. London, Academic Press, pp. 213–235.

Beveridge, E.G. 1987. Microbial spoilage and preservation of pharmaceutical products. In Pharmaceutical Microbiology. 4th Edition. Edited by W.B. Hugo and A.D. Russell. Oxford, Blackwell Scientific, pp. 360–380.

Beveridge, E.G., and Hugo, W.B. 1964. The resistance of gallic acid and its alkyl esters to attack by bacteria able to degrade aromatic ring structures. J. Appl. Bacteriol., 27, 304–311.

Blaug, S.M., and Ahsan, S.S. 1961. Interaction of sorbic acid with nonionic macromolecules. J. Pharm. Sci., 50, 138.

Boehm, E.E., and Maddox, D.N. 1970. Preservative failures in cosmetics with special reference to combating contamination by Pseudomonas using binary and tertiary systems. Am. Perf. Cosm., 85, 31–34.

British Pharmacopoeia. 1980. Addendum 1986. London, Pharmaceutical Press.

Brookes, F.L., Grant, D.J.W., Hugo, W.B., and Denyer, S.P. 1981. Degradation of Hydrocortisone by Pseudomonas Testosteroni. J. Pharm. Pharmacol., 33, 74P.

Brown, M.R.W., Foster, J.H.S., Norton, D.A., and Richards, R.M.E. 1964. Preservation of ophthalmic solutions. Pharm. J., 192, 8.

Brown, M.R.W., and Richards, R.M.E. 1965. Effects of ethylenediamine tetraacetate on the resistance of Ps. aeruginosa to antibacterial agents. Nature, 207, 1391–1393.

Bruch, C. 1972. Objectionable microorganisms in nonsterile drugs and cosmetics. Drug. Cosmet. Ind., 111(4), 51–54, 150–156.

Bucherer, H. 1965. Uber den mikrobiellen Abbau von Giftshoffen, 4, Uber den mikrobiellen Abbau von Phenylacetat, Strychnin, Brucin, Vomicin und Tubocurarin. Zbl Bakt [Naturwiss] 119, 232–238.

Clausen, O., and Raustad, K. 1965. The bactericidal combination effect of propylene glycolβ-phenylether plus aminacrine hydrochloride. Norges Apotek Tidskrift, 73, 16, 365–370.

Cowen, R.A., and Steiger, B. 1976. Antimicrobial activity—a critical review of test methods of preservative efficiency. J. Soc. Cosm. Chem., 27, 467–481.

Crompton, D.O. 1973. Sterility of eye medicaments. Lancet, ii, 150.

Dagley, S. 1971. Catabolism of aromatic compounds by microorganisms. In Advances in Microbial Physiology. Volume 6. Edited by A.H. Rose and J.F. Wilkinson. London, Academic Press, pp. 1–46.

Davies, G.E. 1954. 1:6-Di-4'-chlorophenyldiguanidohexane (Hibitane). Br. J. Pharmacol., 9, 192–196.

Dean, D.A. 1978. Some recent advances in the packaging of pharmaceuticals. Drug Dev. Ind. Pharm., 4, v–vi.

Deluca, P.P., and Kostenbauder, H.B. 1960. Interaction of preservatives with macromolecules. IV. Binding of quaternary ammonium compounds by nonionic agents. J. Am. Pharm. Assoc., 46, 144.

Denyer, S.P. 1987. Factory and hospital hygiene and good manufacturing practice. In Pharmaceutical Microbiology. 4th Edition. Edited by W.B. Hugo and A.D. Russell. Oxford, Blackwell Scientific, p. 433.

Eisman, P.C., Cooper, J., and Jaconia, D. 1957. Influence of gum tragacanth on the bactericidal activity of preservatives. J. Am. Pharm. Assoc., 46, 144.

Elowe, L.N. 1955. Preservation of pharmaceuticals. Part II. Preservatives used in pharmacy. Ontario Coll. Pharm. Bull., 4, 45–47.

Eriksen, S.P. 1970. Preservation of ophthalmic, nasal and otic products. Drug Cosmet. Ind., 107, 36–40.

Fassihi, A.R., Parker, M.S., and Dingwall, D. 1978. The preservation of tablets against microbial spoilage. Drug Dev. Ind. Pharm., 4, 217–221.

Fassihi, A.R., and Parker, M.S. 1987. Inimical effects of compaction speed on microorganisms in powder systems with dissimilar compaction mechanisms. Pharm. Sci., 76, 6, 466–470.

Felts, S.K., Schaffner, W., Melley, M.A., and Koenig, M.G. 1972. Sepsis caused by contaminated intravenous fluids. Epidemiologic, clinical, and laboratory investigation of an outbreak in one hospital. Ann. Intern. Med., 77, 881–890.

Fisher, G.B. 1988. In Hospital-Acquired Infection in the Pediatric Patient. Edited by L.G. Donowitz. Baltimore, Williams & Wilkins, p. 99.

Frank, M.J., and Schaffner, W. 1976. Contaminated aqueous benzalkonium chloride: an unnecessary hospital hazard. JAMA, 236, 2418–2419.

Gabel, L.F. 1921. The relative action of preservatives in pharmaceutical preparations. J. Am. Pharm. Assoc., 10, 767–768.

Garrett, E.R. 1966. A basic model for the evaluation and prediction of preservative action. J. Pharm. Pharmacol., 18, 589–601.

Gershenfeld, L., and Perlstein, D. 1939. Preservatives for preparations containing gelatin. Am. J. Pharm., 111, 277–287.

Gladhart, W.R., Jr., Wood, R.M., and Purdum, W.A. 1955. An evaluation of certain bacteriostatic agents used in multiple dose vials sterilized by autoclaving. Bull. Am. Soc. Hosp. Pharm., 12, 534–539.

Goldman, D.A., and Maki, D.C. 1973. Infection control in total parenteral nutrition. JAMA, 223, 1360–1364.

Gottfried, N.S. 1962. Alkyl p-hydroxybenzoate esters as pharmaceutical preservatives. A review of the parabens. Am. J. Hosp. Pharm., 19, 310–314.

Grant, D.J.W. 1971. Degradation of acetylsalicylic acid by a strain of Acinetobacter lwoffii. J. Appl. Bacteriol., 34, 689–698.

Grant, D.J.W., De Szoes, J., and Wilson, J.V. 1970. Utilization of acetylsalicylic acid as sole carbon source and the induction of its enzymatic hydrolysis by an isolated strain of Acinetobacter lwoffii. J. Pharm. Pharmacol., 22, 461–464.

Happel, J.A. 1983. Antimicrobial preservatives in pharmaceuticals. In Disinfection, Sterilization and Preservation. 3rd Edition. Edited by S.S. Block. Philadelphia, Lea & Febiger, pp. 579–588.

Hibbot, H.W., and Monks, J. 1961. Preservation of emulsion p-hydrobenzoic ester partition coefficient. J. Soc. Cosmet. Chem., 12(2), 1–10.

Hugo, W.B., and Foster, J.H.S. 1964. Growth of Pseudomonas aeruginosa in solutions of esters of p-hydroxybenzoic acid. J. Pharm. Pharmacol., 16, 209.

Hugo, W.B. 1967. The mode of action of antiseptic. J. Appl. Bacteriol., 30, 17–50.

Hugo, W.B. (ed). 1971. The Inhibition and Destruction of the Microbial Cell. London, Academic Press.

Hugo, W.B. 1982. Disinfection mechanisms. In Principle and Practice of Disinfection, Preservation and Sterilisation. Edited by A.D. Russell, W.B. Hugo, and G.A.J. Ayliffe. Oxford, Blackwell Scientific, pp. 158–185.

Hugo, W.B., and Russell, A.D. 1987. Evaluation of non-antibiotic antimicrobial agents. In Pharmaceutical Microbiology. Edited by W.B. Hugo and A.D. Russell. London, Blackwell Scientific, p. 279.

Idson, B., and Lazarus, J. 1986. Semisolids. In The Theory and Practice of Industrial Pharmacy. 3rd Edition. Edited by L. Lachman, H.A. Liberman, and J.L. Kanig. Philadelphia, Lea & Febiger, pp. 553–554.

Jaconia, D. 1972. Preservatives in pharmaceutical products. In Quality Control in the Pharmaceutical Industry. Volume 1. New York, Academic Press.

Judis, J. 1962. Studies on the mechanism of action of phenolic disinfectants. I. Release of radioactivity from carbon-14-labelled Escherichia coli. J. Pharm. Sci., 51, 261.

Kallings, L.O., Ringertz, O., Silverstone, L., and Ernerfeldt, F. 1966. Microbial contamination of medical preparations. Acta Pharmaca Suecica, 3, 219–228.

Kazmi, S.J.A., and Mitchell, A.G. 1976. The interaction of preservative and nonionic surfactant mixtures. Can. J. Pharm. Sci., 11, 10–17.

Kazmi, S.J.A., and Mitchell, A.G. 1978. Preservation of solubilised and emulsified systems. Int. J. Pharm. Sci., 67, 1260–1265.

Kohn, S.R., Gershenfeld, L., and Barr, M. 1963. Effectiveness of antibacterial agents presently employed in ophthalmic preparations as preservatives against Pseudomonas aeruginosa. J. Pharm. Sci., 52, 967–974.

Konning, G.K. 1974. Stability of medicaments in shea butter ointments and creams. Can. J. Pharm. Sci., 9, 103.

Kostenbauder, H.B. 1962. Developments in Industrial Microbiology. Volume 3. New York, Plenum Press, p. 286.

Kostenbauder, H.B., and Higuchi, T. 1956. Formation of molecular complexes by some water-soluble amides, I: interaction of several amides with p-hydroxybenzoic acid, salicylic acid, chloramphenicol and phenol. J. Am. Pharm. Assoc. 45, 518–522.

Kuehne, J.W., and Ahearn, D.G. 1971. Incidence and characterization of fungi in eye cosmetics. Dev. Indust. Microbiol., 12, 173–177.

Lachman, L. 1962. Stability of antibacterial preservatives in parenteral solutions. I. Factors influencing the loss of antimicrobial agents from solutions in rubber stoppered containers. J. Pharm. Sci., 51, 224–232.

Lachman, L. 1968. The instability of antimicrobial preservatives. Bull. Parent. Drug Assoc., 22, 127–144.

Lawrence, C.A. 1955. An evaluation of chemical preservatives for ophthalmic solutions. J. Am. Pharm. Assoc., 44, 457–464.

Manowitz, M. 1961. Developments in Industrial Microbiology. Volume 2. New York, Plenum Press, p. 65.

MacGregor, D.R., and Elliker, P.R. 1958. A comparison of some properties of strains of Pseudomonas aeruginosa sensitive and resistant to quaternary ammonium compounds. Can. J. Microbiol., 4, 499–503.

Marshall, V.P., and Wiley, P.F. 1982. In Microbial Transformation of Bioactive Compounds. Volume 1. Edited by J.P. Rosazza. Boca Raton, FL, CRC Press, pp. 45–80.

McCarthy, T.J. 1971. Aspects of preservative in aqueous systems. S. Afr. Pharm. J., 219, 507–510.

Meers, P.D., Calder, M.W., Mazhar, M.M. and Lawrie, G.M. 1973. Intravenous infusion of contaminated dextrose solution. Lancet, *ii*, 1189–1192.

Merck Index. 1983. 10th Edition. Rahway, N.J., Merck & Co., pp. 281–282.

Mitchell, A., and Kazmi, S.J.A. 1975. Preservative availability in emulsified systems. Can. J. Pharm. Sci., *10*, 67–68.

Miyawaki, G.M., Patel, N.K., and Kostenbauder, H.B. 1959. Interaction of preservatives with macromolecules III. Parahydroxy-benzoic acid esters in the presence of some hydro-philic polymers. J. Am. Pharm. Assoc., *48*, 315.

Moore, K.E. 1978. Evaluating preservative efficacy by challenge testing during the development stage of pharmaceutical products. J. Appl. Bacteriol., *44*(3), Sxliii-Slv, June, 1978.

Nair, A.D., and Lach, J.L. 1959. The kinetics of degradation of chlorobutanol. J. Am. Pharm. Assoc., *48*, 390–395.

Noble, W.C., and Savin, J.A. 1966. Steroid cream contaminated with *Pseudomonas aeruginosa*. Lancet, *i*, 347–349.

Nogueira, A.L. 1962. Os conservantes em farmacia. Rev. Part. Farm., *12*, 168–190.

Parker, M.S., and Fassihi, A.R. 1988. First Anglo-Egyptian Conference of Pharmaceutical Sciences, Nov. 15, p. 70.

Parker, M.S., and Barnes, M. 1967. The interaction of non-ionic surfactants with preservatives. Soap. Perfum. Cosm., *40*, 163–170.

Parker, M.S. 1982. The preservation of pharmaceuticals and cosmetic products. In *Principle and Practice of Disinfection, Preservation and Sterilisation*. Edited by A.D. Russell, W.B. Hugo, and G.A.J. Ayliffe. Oxford, Blackwell Scientific, pp. 287–305.

Pederson, E.A., and Ulrich, K. 1968. Microbial content in nonsterile pharmaceuticals. Dansk Tidsskrift Farmaci, *42*, 71–83.

Phillips, I., Eyken, S., and Laker, M. 1972. Outbreak of hospital infection caused by contaminated autoclaved fluids. Lancet, *i*, 1258–1260.

Plotkin, S.A., and Austrian, R. 1958. Bacteremia caused by *Pseudomonas* Sp. following the use of materials stored in solutions of a cationic surface-active agent. Am. J. Med. Sci., *235*, 621–627.

Prickett, P.S., Murray, H.L., and Mercer, N.H. 1961. Potentiation of preservatives (parabens) in pharmaceutical formulations by low concentrations of propylene glycol. J. Pharm. Sci., *50*, 316–320.

Richards, R.M.E., and McBride, R.T. 1971a. Phenylethanol enhancement of preservatives used in ophthalmic preparations. J. Pharm. Pharmacol., *23*(Suppl.), 141S–146S.

Richards, R.M.E., and McBride, R.J. 1971b. The preservation of ophthalmic solutions with antibacterial combinations. J. Pharm. Pharmacol., *23*(Suppl.), 234S–235S.

Riegelman, S., Vaughan, D.G., Jr., and Okumoto, M. 1955. Rate of sterilization as a factor in the selection of ophthalmic solutions. Arch. Ophthalmol., *54*, 725–732.

Ringertz, O., and Ernerfeldt, F. 1965. Report to the Royal Medical Board, Stockholm: "Microbiological Contamination of Medical Products."

Ringertz, O., and Ringertz, S.H. 1982. The clinical significance of microbial contamination in pharmaceutical products. In *Advances in Pharmaceutical Sciences*. Volume 5. Edited by H.S. Bean, A.H. Beckett, and J.E. Carless. London, Academic Press, pp. 202–226.

Robertson, M.H. 1970. Fungi in fluids—a hazard of intravenous therapy. J. Med. Microbiol., *3*, 99.

Royce, O., and Sykes, G. 1957. Losses of bacteriostats from injections in rubber-closed containers. J. Pharm. Pharmacol., *9*, 814–822.

Russell, A.D., Jenkins, J., and Harrison, I.H. 1967. The inclusion of antimicrobial agents in pharmaceutical products. Adv. Appl. Microbiol., *9*, 1–38.

Savin, J.A. 1967. The microbiology of topical preparations in pharmaceutical practice. 1. Clinical aspects. Pharm. J., *199*, 285–288.

Scott, E.M., and Gorman, S.P. 1987. Chemical disinfectants, antiseptics and preservatives. In *Pharmaceutical Microbiology*. Edited by W.B. Hugo and A.D. Russell. London, Blackwell Scientific, p. 226.

Sheikh, M.A., and Parker, M.S. 1972. The influence of ethylenediamine tetra-acetate and phenylethanol upon the fungistatic action of aminacrine hydrochloride. J. Pharm. Pharmacol., *24*(Suppl.), 158S.

Spooner, D.F. 1985. Microbiologic criteria for non-sterile pharmaceuticals. Manuf. Chemist, *56*, 42–45, 71–75.

Sykes, G. 1971. Microbial contamination in pharmaceuticals for oral and topical use: Society's working party report. Pharm. J., *207*, 400–402.

1984. Third joint report, Laboratory and Drug Control Services and FIP. In *Cosmetics and Drug Preservation*. Edited by J.J. Kabara. New York, Marcel Dekker, p. 423.

United States Pharmacopeia. 1985. 21st Edition. Easton, PA, Mack Publishing.

Wedderburn, D.L. 1964. Preservation of emulsions against microbial attack. Adv. Pharm. Sci., *1*, 195–268.

Wedderburn, D.L. 1958. Preservation of toilet preparations containing nonionics. J. Soc. Cosmet. Chem., *9*, 210–228.

Wickliffe, B., and Entrekin, P.N. 1964. Relation of pH to preservative effectiveness. II. Neutral and basic media. J. Pharm. Sci., *53*, 769–773.

Wilson, L.A., and Ahearn, D.G. 1977. *Pseudomonas*-induced corneal ulcers associated with contaminated eye mascaras. Am. J. Ophthalmol., *84*, 113–119.

Wilson, L.A., Julian, A.J., and Ahearn, D.G. 1975. The survival and growth of microorganisms in mascara during use. Am. J. Ophthalmol., *79*, 596–601.

Wolf, P.A., and Westveer, W.M. 1950. The antimicrobial activity of several substituted pyrones. Arch. Biochem., *28*, 201–206.

Woodford, R., and Adams, E. 1972. Effects of ethanol and propylene glycol, and a mixture of potassium sorbate with either, on *Pseudomonas aeruginosa* contamination of an oil-in-water cream. Am. Perfum. Cosmet., *87*, 53–56.

CHAPTER 51

PRESERVATION OF COSMETICS

F. Sharpell and M. Manowitz

Traditionally, cosmetics have been defined as that huge category of products that are applied to the human body for the purpose of beautifying or altering appearance. Although the definition still holds, the functions, ingredients, and claims of the products have become significantly more aggressive in the past decade and frequently have placed the industry in conflict with the FDA. The composition of these formulations can vary from a few simple ingredients to a long list of components selected from a continually expanding variety of synthetic and natural products. Cosmetics are prepared in a large assortment of physical forms from solids to low-viscosity liquids as essentially anhydrous products or products containing greater than 90% water, using packaging and delivery systems that range from the very simple to the highly sophisticated. Thus, cosmetics are a highly diversified group of products that require protection against microbial attack during manufacture and use by the consumer.

The sparsity of published literature on cosmetic preservation prior to 1968 was followed by a period of more extensive study of this subject and the emergence of new antimicrobials and methods of preventing microbiologic infestation. It was during this period that the FDA intensified the pressure on the industry to preserve the microbial integrity of their products not only at the time of manufacture but during use and abuse by the public. A major additional problem of increasing intensity has been introduced in recent years: the question of the toxicologic safety of some of the more effective preservatives. Organic mercurials are restricted in their use, formaldehyde and formaldehyde donors are under continuous attack, bromonitro preservatives are of concern because of their involvement in nitrosamine formation, and the highly active isothiozolidinone compounds are the subject of an increasing number of published reports on their sensitization potential. It would appear that the expanding demands for preservative protection of cosmetic products from cradle through final use are on a collision course with the limitations on the number and uses of effective preservatives that are available. A partial solution to this dilemma might be found in designing packaging that limits consumer access to no more than a single application of the cosmetic at one time. This would protect the bulk of the product from contamination by the user, a major source of contamination.

MICROBIAL CONTAMINATION OF COSMETICS

Microbial spoilage of cosmetic preparations was the major concern of manufacturers in former years (Manowitz, 1961). Spoilage in this context is defined as microbial growth that results in various deleterious effects such as noxious odors and gases; changes in pH, viscosity, and color; and the destruction of emulsions. The presence of a visible mass of fungal growth or bacterial slime on the surface of a product obviously renders it unsuitable for marketing. Smart and Spooner (1972) critically re-examined this subject and graded the various types of cosmetics on their relative susceptibility to microbial deterioration. Liquids, including aqueous solutions and suspensions, syrups, emulsions, and creams were in the high risk category.

The organisms that have been identified in cosmetic compositions by various investigators through the years make a rather formidable list. Among those reported were species of the following (deNavarre, 1962): *Absidia, Alternaria, Aspergillus, Citromyces, Cladosporium, Dematium, Fusarium, Helminthosporium, Hormodendrum, Mucor, Geotrichum, Paecilomyces, Penicillium, Phoma, Aureobasidium, Rhizopus, Thamnidium, Trichothecium, Verticillium, Archomobacter, Aerobacter, Bacillus, Enterococcus, Escherichia, Micrococcus, Proteus, Pseudomonas, Sarcina, Serratia, Staphylococcus, Streptococcus, Candida, Saccharomyces, Torula, Zygosaccharomyces*. Without doubt, the organisms most frequently identified and the most difficult to control are the ubiquitous pseudomonads. Bruch (1971) described various members of the genus *Pseudomonas* whose presence in topical products should be considered objectionable. The many problems encountered in controlling *Pseudomonas* is cosmetics were reviewed by Tenenbaum (1967). These organisms alone, especially *Ps. aeruginosa*, are probably responsible for a major portion of the microbiologic problems in cosmetics as well as for those in topical and ocular drugs. Detailed procedures for enumerating, isolating, and identifying pseudomonads and other microorganisms in cosmetics have been presented in the literature (Woodward and McNamara, 1971; Evans et al., 1972; Tenenbaum, 1972; Scott, 1973). The FDA, in its Bacteriological Analytical Manual (1984), devotes a chapter (25) to the isolation and identification of cosmetic contaminants. This is probably the most comprehensive discussion of the topic.

Sources of Contamination

Microorganisms can be introduced into cosmetic products from a variety of sources: raw materials, water, air, processing equipment, packaging materials, and operating personnel. Raw materials of animal or vegetable origin normally have far greater possibilities of being contaminated than the highly refined or synthetic compounds (Lennington, 1969). Goldman (1969) showed that egg-white powder used in formulating a new product was the greatest source of its microbial contamination. The combination of certified specifications by the raw ingredient supplier and retesting of these components by the manufacturer should control most of the raw material problems. Kano et al. (1976) discuss a quality control program used for the entire manufacturing procedure with emphasis on raw materials and equipment. Water supplies are probably the major source of contamination during the manufacture of cosmetics. Demineralized water is contaminated more often than not, and the resin beds of ion exchangers are usually responsible (Wedderburn, 1965; Cruickshank and Braithwaite, 1949; Eisman et al., 1949). The importance of this problem prompted The Cosmetic Toiletry and Fragrance Association to develop a set of guidelines to control the microbial quality of water used in the manufacture of cosmetics (CTFA Quality Assurance Microbiology Subcommittee, 1972). The use of ultraviolet radiation, chemical disinfection, heat, and membrane filtration to control microbial growth in water systems has been comprehensively discussed (Olson, 1967; Woodward, 1971; Dawson, 1973; Schenk, 1979).

Various sterilization procedures, including the use of gamma irradiation and ethylene oxide treatment (Prince and Welt, 1971; Lazier and Galand, 1975; Gilmour, 1978; Alguire and Yeung, 1979), have been used or proposed for contaminated raw materials. The importance of plant and personnel hygiene, the design and sanitizing of manufacturing equipment, and the various other factors fundamental to the production of uncontaminated cosmetics have been described in several publications (Wedderburn, 1965; Van Abbe et al., 1970; Most and Katz, 1970; Davis, 1972; Yablonski, 1978).

Incidence and Hazards of Contaminated Cosmetics

The incidence of contaminated cosmetics has been the subject of several investigations. Wolven and Levenstein (1969) performed bacterial counts on a total of 250 cosmetic products purchased on the open market and found that 61 were contaminated. Eyeliners, cake eye shadow, and hand and body lotions were most frequently contaminated, and *Pseudomonas* was the predominant organism found. A similar study conducted 3 years later showed that only 8 of 223 products sampled contained bacteria (Wolven and Levenstein, 1972). Pseudomonads again proved to be the major problem. Contamination of various samples of shampoos was demonstrated by Baker (1959), who found *Pseudomonas, Aerobacter,* and molds among the invading microorganisms. Wilson et al. (1971) examined 233 samples of new and used eyeliner, eye shadow, and mascara for the presence of bacteria and fungi. The incidence of fungal and bacterial contamination among the used materials was 12 and 43% respectively, whereas the new cosmetic samples were essentially free of microorganisms. Anderson and Ayers (1972) demonstrated the proliferation of microorganisms in unpreserved cosmetic products attributable to contamination by the consumer. Their investigations indicated that anhydrous stick makeups and dry applied pressed products did not require a preservative. A bacteriologic survey of a large number of new and used cosmetic products also was conducted by Myers and Pasutto (1973). Twenty of 165 new products showed the presence of bacteria, whereas 110 of 222 used samples were contaminated. The CTFA (1977) surveyed almost 4000 cosmetics over a 3-year period and found no eye or baby products to be outside the CTFA guidelines of less than 500 microorganisms, and only 0.5% to be outside the guidelines of less than 1000 microorganisms per gram for other products.

Although the incidence of contamination of cosmetic formulations has been demonstrated, the public health hazards that such products present have not been well documented. Answers to questions posed by these relationships are elusive and are complicated by the millions of bacteria normally present on the skin and the constant exposure of the human integument to contaminating organisms in the environment. Eye cosmetics are a category of serious concern because of reported past experiences with ophthalmic solutions. (Theodore and Feinstein, 1952; Ayliffe et al., 1966). Wilson and Ahearn (1977) documented seven cases of *Pseudomonas* infection resulting from contaminated mascaras. Parker (1972) suggested that application of cosmetics to the intact skin of healthy subjects should not cause disease from the microorganisms commonly found in these products. Certain hand and body creams and lotions, however, are generally used in hospitals, and their microbial integrity then becomes a matter of great concern. Reports on the contamination of such products from hospitals in the United States and abroad reveal a potential hazard to individual patients and possibly to the entire hospital environment

(Ayliffe et al., 1969; Kallings et al., 1966; Knights and Harvey, 1964). Morse and coworkers (1967) described an outbreak of septicemia due to *Klebsiella pneumoniae* that was traced to a heavily contaminated hand cream dispenser. In further studies, Morse and Schonbeck (1968) found that 4 of 26 brands of hand lotion had significant populations of identifiable gram-negative bacteria present, including *Pseudomonas aeruginosa*, *Klebsiella pneumoniae*, and *Serratia marcescens*. They recommended that all hospitals be alerted to the potential hazard of the use of contaminated hand lotions.

The FDA's position concerning the legal basis for classifying contaminated cosmetics as adulterated under Section 601 of the Food, Drug and Cosmetic Act was described by Olson (1970). The presence of specific infectious bacteria such as *Pseudomonas aeruginosa* or of an excessive, nondescript microbiologic population would be considered adulteration. On this basis, there were 25 recalls of cosmetic products from 1966 to 1968 (Dunnigan, 1968). Sixteen of the recalls were lotions, and 14 of these contained *Ps. aeruginosa*. As yet, there are no official standards concerning permissible numbers of microorganisms in cosmetics, and each case is judged individually on the basis of many factors. It has been suggested that any preparation placed directly on the skin should contain less than 100 microorganisms per gram with no tolerance for pathogens (Dunnigan, 1968). Leyden et al. (1980) evaluated *Ps. cepacia* and *Ps. aeruginosa* on human skin. They concluded that *Pseudomonas* contamination does not pose a serious problem on intact skin, because concentrations of 10,000 pseudomonads per gram had no effect on scarified skin. The potential for cosmetic products to produce skin infections is still a matter of controversy, however. No product should have a microbial content recognized as harmful to the user (Tenenbaum, 1972).

PRESERVATIVES

Although numerous preservatives are available for use in cosmetics, the market continues to be dominated by only a few. Recent introductions have made only a minor contribution to the overall frequency of preservative use. For comprehensive lists of preservatives, see Wallhäusser (1984) and Anonymous (1985).

Esters of *p*-Hydroxybenzoic Acid—Parabens

$$R = CH_3, C_2H_5, \text{etc.}$$

Introduced into Europe over 50 years ago (Sabalitschka, 1924), the parabens remain by far the most pop-ular preservatives. In a listing of antimicrobial ingredients in order of frequency of use in cosmetic formulations, the parabens, particularly methyl and propyl, occupy the top 10% of all products used (Decker and Wenninger, 1987).

The physical and chemical properties of the parabens were described by Aalto et al. (1953), who also tested their antibacterial and antifungal properties. With 22 different microorganisms, it was shown that the parabens were more effective against fungi and gram-positive bacteria than against gram-negative bacteria. In general, the activity of the parabens increased with increasing chain length. The methyl and ethyl esters, however, were more effective against *Ps. aeruginosa* and *Ps. flourescens* than the propyl and butyl esters. Although higher esters are even more active than the butyl, decreasing solubility in aqueous solutions diminishes their usefulness.

The parabens most widely used are the methyl, propyl, and butyl esters, primarily in combination with each other. Concentrations up to 0.4% are considered acceptable for the single esters, whereas a concentration of 0.8% is acceptable for the combined esters.

The parabens are effective over a pH range of 4 to 8 (Aalto et al., 1953). As the pH rises above 8, the parabens become less effective because of ionization of the molecule (Gucklhorn, 1969a). At a pH of 8.5, 50% of the compound is ionized and considerable loss of activity occurs. Parrott (1968) calculated the theoretical rate constant at 25°C for the hydrolysis of methyl paraben to the inactive *p*-hydroxybenzoic acid. He predicted that hydrolysis occurs slowly at pH 6.0 but is accelerated at a pH of 8.0.

In many ways, the parabens are ideal cosmetic preservatives. They are essentially colorless, odorless, stable, effective over a wide pH range, and relatively active against a full spectrum of microorganisms. Their cost is low in relation to the use-concentration, and they are readily available. Numerous studies have indicated that the parabens have a low order of acute and chronic toxicity (Sokol, 1952; Jones et al., 1956), although some cases of contact dermatitis were reported (Rudner, 1966). Various other investigators have described and commented upon the adverse reactions associated with parabens (Wuepper, 1967; Schamberg, 1967; Schorr, 1968; Epstein, 1968; Fisher, 1975, 1980). Nevertheless, considering the widespread use of the parabens and the low incidence of adverse reactions, the parabens obviously are among the safest of all preservatives. The antimicrobial activity of the parabens is reduced by the incorporation of nonionic surfactants into cosmetic formulations (deNavarre and Bailey, 1956; Patel and Kostenbauder, 1958). Various other agents are also capable of inactivating the parabens (Guttman and Higuchi, 1956; Miyawaki et al., 1959; Tillman and Kuramoto, 1957; Bryce and Smart, 1965). Despite these difficulties, the parabens are still the preservatives of choice in many cosmetic formulations.

Imidazolidinyl Urea (Germall 115)

Germall 115 is an odorless, tasteless, water-soluble white powder that is stable and effective over a wide pH range (Berke and Rosen, 1970). It has the particular advantage of being compatible with almost all cosmetic ingredients.

Germall 115 appears to be equally effective against gram-negative and gram-positive bacteria (Berke and Rosen, 1970). Of note is its activity against *Pseudomonas*. Germall 115 is good against some fungi and yeast and poor against others (Rosen and Berke, 1973). These inconsistencies are overcome by using Germall 115 in combination with the parabens (Jacobs et al., 1975). Synergetic effects have also been noted with sorbic acid, dehydroacetic acid, quaternaries, and Triclosan (Wallhäusser, 1985). In most cases, a concentration of 0.3% is adequate to protect most cosmetic products (Berke and Rosen, 1978).

In-depth toxicity testing of Germall 115 indicates that this preservative is safe when incorporated in cosmetic products in amounts similar to those currently marketed (Elder, 1980).

Diazolidinyl Urea (Germall II)

In the mid-1980s Germall II was introduced as a cosmetic preservative, and has since gained increasing acceptance. Like Germall 115, Germall II is a fine, white, free-flowing powder with a characteristically mild odor. Its antibacterial spectrum is superior to that of Germall 115 (Wallhäusser, 1981), buts its antifungal activity is only marginally better. Concentrations of 0.1 to 0.3% are recommended. Germall II is compatible with other cosmetic ingredients and is not affected by nonionic surfactants, ethoxylated compounds, or proteins (Sutton Laboratories, Inc., undated Technical Bulletin). The safety

of Germall II has been established by extensive safety and toxicity testing. The incorporation of the parabens with Germall II in formulations provides additional antimicrobial protection.

2-Bromo-2-Nitropropane-1,3-Diol (Bronopol)

Although the synthesis of Bronopol was first reported in 1897 by Henry, its potential as an antimicrobial agent was not recognized until the 1960s. Bronopol is available in three grades—Bronopol-Boots (BNPD), Myacide BT, and Myacide AS—differing only in purity (The Boots Company PLC Technical Bulletin, 1986). Bronopol-Boots is a cosmetic-grade product, whereas Myacide BT is used for wash-off toiletries and Myacide AS for industrial applications. Laboratory testing of Bronopol showed that bacteria were inhibited by concentrations of 12.5 to 50 ppm and that yeast and fungi were inhibited by 50 to 400 ppm (Croshaw et al., 1964). Of particular interest is its activity against the gram-negative *Pseudomonads*, showing inhibition at 50 ppm. It is recommended that Bronopol be used at a concentration range of 0.01 to 0.1% in liquid and cream cosmetics.

Bronopol is effective at acid pH levels at which optimum chemical stability occurs. Although Bronopol is chemically less stable in alkaline systems (Bronopol-Boots, 1986), its antimicrobial activity appears to be equal if not better than at acid pH. Bronopol is unaffected by most nonionic, cationic, and anionic surfactants. Sulphydryl compounds, however, cause significant reduction in activity, as do reducing agents such as sodium thiosulphate.

Dimethylol Dimethylhydantoin-1,3-bis (hydroxymethyl)-5,5-dimethyl-2,4-imidazolidine-dione (Glydant)

Glydant, a 55% solution of dimethylol dimethylhydantoin (DMDMH), is another preservative whose use has dramatically increased—approximately 20-fold between 1977 and 1987. Glydant demonstrates broad-spectrum antimicrobial activity, but is less effective against fungi and yeast than against bacteria. In some applications, antifungal activity must be fortified by using other antimicrobial agents such as the parabens. The recommended range of use is between 0.15 and 0.4%.

Glydant is in many ways the perfect shampoo preservative (Rosen, 1985). It is stable over a wide pH range and at a temperature of 80°C. The inhibitory level of DMDMH was found to be 0.1% in acidic and alkaline anionic lotions and in an alkaline nonionic lotion. Its MIC was greater than 0.1% in an acidic nonionic lotion. Although compatible with almost all cosmetic ingredients, Glydant belongs to that group of compounds known as formaldehyde donors, which may restrict its use in many products.

Phenoxyethanol

Phenoxyethanol is an oily liquid with a faint aromatic odor. It is not as effective as many of the antimicrobials previously discussed, but its stability and wide pH range may make it suitable for some applications. The recommended use concentration is 0.5 to 2.0%. Although compatible with anionics and cationics, it may lose activity with nonionics. The use of the parabens to supplement the overall activity is recommended.

Dowicil 200 (Quaternium 15) 7-(cis-3-Chloro-2-propenyl)-1,3,5-triaza-7-azoniatricyclo[3.3.1.1]decane

Dowicil 200 is a highly active broad-spectrum antimicrobial designed specifically for the preservation of cosmetics. Its major features have been summarized by Marouchoc (1984). Dowicil 200 is effective against bacteria, yeast, and molds at concentrations normally between 0.02 and 0.3%. It is particularly effective against *Pseudomonas*. Dowicil 200 is not inactivated by nonionic, anionic, or cationic formulation ingredients, nor by proteins. It is highly soluble in water but virtually insoluble in oils and organic solvents. Dowicil 200 is active over a wide pH range. Extensive studies have demonstrated that Dowicil 200 has favorable toxicologic properties for cosmetic use and should present no hazards during manufacturing operations.

Another advantage of Dowicil 200 is its compatibility with other biocides, producing an additive effect. In some acidic formulations, Dowicil 200 produces a yellow discoloration. Small quantities (0.05 to 0.1%) of sodium borate or sodium sulfite may be effective in preventing discoloration.

Kathon CG (5-chloro-2-methyl-3(2H)isothiazolone and 2-methyl-3-(2H)-isothiazolone

First introduced in 1975, Kathon CG is gaining increasing acceptance as a cosmetic preservative. Formulated at a 1.5% concentration in water with magnesium salts, Kathon CG is one of the few antimicrobials sold as a liquid. It is readily miscible in water, lower alcohols, glycols, and other hydrophilic organic solvents (Law et al., 1984). Kathon CG possesses a broad antimicrobial spectrum, being equally effective against gram-positive and gram-negative bacteria and against fungi and yeasts. Recommended use levels are 0.02 to 0.1% (3 to 15 ppm active ingredients). Kathon CG is compatible with proteins, emulsifiers, and cationic, anionic, and nonionic surfactants. Kathon has a wide pH range and imparts neither color nor odor to most finished formulations.

In depth toxicological testing showed that Kathon CG is safe at use concentrations in cosmetic formulations.

Formaldehyde

Formaldehyde is another prominent and potent antimicrobial agent that has been used in cosmetics. Toxicologic concerns, however, have substantially reduced its use as a cosmetic preservative. Other applications include the disinfection of ion-exchange columns for the preparation of deionized water and the sterilization of cosmetic manufacturing equipment (Wallhäusser, 1974). In high concentrations, formaldehyde is sporicidal and bactericidal; at low concentrations, it is bacteriostatic. *Escherichia coli* and *Staphylococcus aureus* can be inhibited by as little as 20 μg/ml of formaldehyde (Hamilton, 1971), whereas a 3 to 8% solution of formaldehyde is actively sporicidal even in the presence of organic matter (McCulloch, 1945).

Formaldehyde is used as a preservative in shampoos and other products that are applied to the skin for brief periods. Formalin, an aqueous solution of 37% formaldehyde, can easily be incorporated into cosmetic products. Although economically the most attractive of all the preservatives, formaldehyde is pungent, volatile, and incompatible with a number of materials, such as coloring matter and proteins. The original concentration of formaldehyde is rapidly lost once the container is opened. Although a concentration of 0.05% formaldehyde is toxicologically acceptable (Eurotox Report, 1962), concentrated solutions can be irritating to the manufacturing personnel who prepare the formulations (Henley and Sonntag, 1970).

Essential Oil, Natural Products, and Perfume Compounds

The antimicrobial properties of essential oils and their constituents have been the subject of many investigations during the past 70 years. Their activity is attributable to their high content of phenolics, such as thymol and eugenol.

Kellner and Kober (1955) examined the antibacterial action of 175 ethereal oils against 9 organisms and classified 21 of the most active oils according to chemical composition. The following constituents were reported to have strong antibacterial properties: p-cymene, linalool, geraniol, nerol, thymol, carvacrol, eugenol, safrole, benzaldehyde, cumic aldehyde, cinnamic aldehyde, salicylaldehyde, pulegone, thujone, ascaridole, and cineol.

Maruzzella and coworkers (1956, 1958, 1960, 1961, 1962, 1963) conducted extensive investigations of the antibacterial and antifungal properties of essential oils, perfume oils, and aromatic chemicals. They reported a high incidence of activity among these materials both as contact and vapor-phase antimicrobial agents.

Munzing and Schels (1972) examined a number of essential oils for antimicrobial activity and suggested that mixtures of essential oils might replace conventional preservatives in certain preparations.

Nadal and associates (1973) investigated the antimicrobial activity of bay and other phenolic essential oils. Both the essential oils and their phenolic constituents were effective against gram-positive and gram-negative bacteria, acid-fast bacteria, and fungi.

Dabbah et al. (1970) investigated the antimicrobial activity of citrus fruit oils using four species of bacteria including *Pseudomonas aeruginosa*. Terpineol was the most active ingredient of the oils evaluated. Morris et al. (1979) summarized the antimicrobial activity of 212 common soap fragrance raw materials and concluded that a practical antimicrobial soap fragrance does not appear to be possible. Isacoff (1981) reviewed aromatics as bactericides and provided a comprehensive list of references and a bibliography.

Blakeway (1986) studied the antimicrobial properties of essential oils using agar diffusion tests. He concluded that essential oils have generally little activity against gram-negative bacteria, although white and red thyme oils have strong selective activity, probably because of phenolic components. With the exception of tree-trunk oils or plant-root oils, practically all oils tested had activity against *Bacillus subtilis*, a known spore former. There was wide effectiveness against yeast and molds. Several oils had activity against *Staphylococcus aureus* and *Escherichia coli*.

The antibacterial activity of essential oils from Turkish spices and citrus were evaluated by Kivouc and Akgül (1986). Results varied, but *Pseudomonas aeruginosa* was the most resistant and *Staphylococcus aureus* and *Proteus vulgaris* the most sensitive. Zemak et al. (1987) evaluated antimicrobial properties of aromatic chemicals

of plant origin. Eugenol was found to be the most effective inhibitor against bacteria and yeast-like organisms.

It is obvious from these studies that a relatively large number of fragrance materials possess at least a mild degree of antimicrobial activity. Because almost all cosmetics contain significant quantities of perfume ingredients, it might be assumed that the perfumes would protect these products. Experience has shown, however, that this is not so, and the addition of synthetic preservatives is required. At present, the use of perfume materials as cosmetic preservatives is mainly of academic interest, but their activity in combination with other antimicrobials might be a fruitful field for investigation.

Alcohols

Methyl, ethyl, n-propyl, isopropyl, n-butyl, and higher alcohols all possess antimicrobial activity, but only ethyl and isopropyl alcohol are widely used as preservatives in cosmetic products. The optimum bactericidal activity of ethyl alcohol diluted with water is 50 to 90% (Lockemann et al., 1941; Price, 1950). A 15 to 18% ethyl alcohol content, depending on the pH of the substrate, has generally been considered acceptable for preservation.

Isopropyl alcohol, although similar in antimicrobial activity to ethyl alcohol, has several advantages. It kills many types of bacteria more rapidly, has a lower surface tension, and is a better fat solvent (von Fenyes, 1970). The optimum bactericidal activity of isopropyl alcohol is 30 to 80% (Lockemann et al., 1941).

Benzyl alcohol has occasionally been employed as a cosmetic preservative. Its antimicrobial activity against gram-negative and gram-positive bacteria and fungi is in the range of 0.3 to 0.5%. Phenylethyl alcohol, a perfume material with a rose-like character, has similar antimicrobial activity (Carter et al., 1958), and its use in cosmetics may contribute to the overall preservative effect.

Glycols are frequently incorporated as humectants into hand and body lotions and other cosmetics. Osipow et al. (1968) compared the antimicrobial activity of 1,3-butylene glycol and propylene glycol in a cosmetic lotion. Microbial growth was significantly retarded by 5% concentrations of both glycols.

The use of the lower aliphatic alcohols and benzyl and phenylethyl alcohol as preservatives in cosmetics has been reviewed by Bandelin (1977). Despite their effectiveness, however, the alcohols are generally used for special purposes or as solubilizing agents.

Dehydroacetic acid—DHA

Dehydroacetic acid (3-acetyl-6-methyl-2H-pyran-2,4(3H)-dione) and its sodium salt have been used as preservatives in various cosmetic formulations. The chemical, physical, and antimicrobial properties of this compound were described by Wolf (1950). The activity of DHA is reduced with increasing pH, but it is more effective than benzoic or sorbic acid at higher pH levels (Bandelin, 1958). Antimicrobial activity is also negated by the presence of nonionic surfactants in the media (Wedderburn, 1958). DHA discolors in the presence of iron (Henry and Jacobs, 1981). DHA is often used in combination with other antimicrobial agents as a cosmetic preservative (Winkler, 1955).

Other Cosmetic Preservatives

Numerous other chemicals have been used throughout the years as cosmetic preservatives. Some (benzoic acid, sorbic acid) are best known as food preservatives. Others are used in specialized applications. Comprehensive lists and descriptions have been compiled by Wallhäusser (1984) and by the trade magazine *Cosmetics and Toiletries* (Anonymous, 1985).

COMBINATIONS AND SYNERGISTS

Deficiencies in the spectrum of one preservative frequently may be overcome by combining it with another. Mixtures of parabens are commonly used and are commercially available. One of these, Liquipar, is an emulsified blend of paraben esters for which are claimed formulation advantages (Mallinkrodt Technical Bulletin, 1981). Numerous papers have described the antimicrobial properties of these combinations (Boehm, 1960; Littlejohn and Husa, 1955; Schimmel and Husa, 1956). Combinations of the parabens were generally found to be more effective against gram-positive and gram-negative bacteria, molds, and yeast than the single esters were. Particularly noteworthy was the effectiveness of paraben mixtures against pseudomonads. These mixtures take advantage of the fact that each ester is independently soluble. As a result, a higher combined concentration can effectively be introduced into a formulation. The claims for paraben mixtures have varied from simple additive effects to potentiation. There is also evidence that the mechanism of the antimicrobial action of each paraben may be different (Gerrard et al., 1962).

Mixtures of the parabens with other preservatives have also been described. A commercial product, Phenonip, is a liquid preservative consisting of a mixture of parabens and phenoxyethanol (Parker, 1972b). Its broad-spectrum activity was demonstrated by Parker et al. (1968). In addition to discussing the properties of Phenonip, Boehm and Maddox (1971) used capacity tests in various cosmetics to determine the potential of this product. They also combined Phenonip with cetylpyridinium chloride and thiomersal and claimed synergism against *Pseudomonas aeruginosa*. The synergistic effect of imidazolidinyl urea (Germall 115) and the parabens has been amply demonstrated (Jacobs et al, 1975; Rosen et al., 1977; Rosen and Berke, 1978, 1980). This combination is widely used throughout industry. A basic preservative

system consists of 0.3% Germall 115, 0.2% methyl paraben, and 0.15% propyl paraben. The proportion of each can be varied, depending upon the specific cosmetic formulation involved. Mixtures of the parabens with dehydroacetic acid and sorbic acid are the subject of a patent by Winkler (1955). Various agents have been reported to potentiate the parabens—e.g., phenylethanol (Richards and McBride, 1971) and propylene glycol (Prichett et al., 1961). Poprzan and deNavarre (1959) also claimed that the inactivation of the parabens by nonionics can be prevented by the addition of 10% or less of ethanol or various glycols. Other combinations and synergistic systems include the following:

1. Dehydroacetic acid and sorbic acid esters (Wells and Lubowe, 1964)
2. Benzalkonium chloride, chlorbutol, chlohexidine, and chlorocresol with phenylethanol (Richards and McBride, 1971)
3. Fentichlor (2,2'-thiobis (4-chlorophenol) and phenylethanol (Richards and Hardie, 1972)
4. Benzalkonium chloride and ethylenediaminetetraacetate (Brown and Richards, 1965)

With the increasing complexity of cosmetics, mixtures no doubt will play a more important part in the preservation of formulations.

FACTORS INFLUENCING ACTIVITY

An imposing number of antimicrobial agents have been recommended as cosmetic preservatives, but most of these compounds have proved inadequate. Some are effective in one or a few formulations but fail miserably in others. This lack of activity on the part of so many potent compounds can be caused by the influence of various physical and chemical elements present in the cosmetic potpourri. The more notable factors that can significantly influence activity are pH, oil-to-water ratio, type and concentration of surfactant, and the presence of certain macromolecules or other potential binding solids (Wedderburn, 1970). A thorough summary of methods used to study antimicrobial interactions in cosmetics has been published (Coates and Woodford, 1973).

Ionization and pH

The role of ionization and the effect of pH on the activity of certain antimicrobial compounds are well known phenomena (Albert, 1951). Rahn and Conn (1944) demonstrated that only the undissociated molecules of benzoic and salicylic acids were toxic to microorganisms and that the concentration of nonionized molecules depend on the pH of the medium. Bandelin (1958) determined the antifungal activity of various preservatives at several pH levels and found that the organic acids such as benzoic, salicylic, propionic, and sorbic acids all lost activity with increasing pH. The concentration of undissociated molecules of acid preservatives present at various levels is readily calculated from their dissociation constants. Thus, the percentage of un-ionized material existing at two pH levels is shown below:

	% Undissociated	
	pH 4.0	pH 6.5
Salicylic acid	9	0.03
Benzoic acid	61	0.5
Sorbic acid	86	2.0

It is obvious, then, that the use of these preservatives in formulations with a pH of 6.5 or higher would result in unsatisfactory protection unless massive quantities were used.

The pH effect is also related to other factors such as oil-water partition coefficients. Garrett and Woods (1953) studied the distribution of benzoic acid in a peanut oil-water system as a function of pH. They found greater quantities of benzoic acid present in the aqueous phase as the pH was increased. The pH factor also effects solubility, and the solubility of antimicrobial agents can be reduced below effective levels at certain pH values (Manowitz, 1964).

Partition Coefficients

Partition coefficients are a significant factor in determining the activity of antimicrobial agents in oil-in-water systems. Protection of these emulsions requires that lethal levels of the preservative contact the microorganisms in the aqueous phase. Preservatives with high oil-water partition coefficients concentrate in the oil and are made unavailable to the organisms. Partitioning properties often explain the inability of inherently potent compounds to preserve various oil-in-water emulsions. This is particularly true in the various creams and lotions that contain significant quantities of emulsified oils. Atkins (1950) measured the solubility of the methyl and propyl esters of p-hydroxybenzoate in the oil phase and in the aqueous phase of a cosmetic cream. He found that the methyl ester was twice as soluble in the aqueous phase as in the oil phase, whereas the propyl ester was nine times more soluble in the oil phase than in the water phase. Tests on the finished creams containing these esters demonstrated that the methyl ester was more effective than the propyl ester as a preservative in this product. Hibbot and Monks (1961) determined the oil-water partition coefficient of methyl p-hydroxybenzoate in a number of oils and waxes. Then they tested the activity of this preservative in a series of creams prepared from the oils covering a range of calculated partition coefficients, indicating that this property can be used to estimate a preservative's performance in an emulsion. The investigations of Bean and Heman-Ackah (1964) demonstrated that the activity of bactericides in oil-water dispersion depend on their concentration in the aqueous phase and at the oil-water interface, both of which are controlled by the oil-water ratio. Activity was also governed by the oil-water partition coefficient, which was influenced by temperature. Bean et al. (1970) determined the partition coefficients of methyl paraben in aqueous mixtures and emulsions of mineral oil, safflower oil, isopropyl palmitate, and lanolin. The oil-water coefficient for the preservative in mineral oil was 0.11, because of its limited solubility in this vehicle. The partition coefficients in the other oils were about 100 to 150 times greater than in mineral oil.

Surfactants

The introduction and subsequent widespread use of nonionic surfactants in cosmetics enhanced the problems of cosmetic preservation. Bolle and Mirimanoff (1950) demonstrated that these surfactants decrease the fungistatic action of some antiseptics and predicted that this would lead to problems in the cosmetic field. Extensive investigations by deNavarre with large numbers of nonionics and preservatives led to the conclusion that any soluble ethoxylated nonionic surfactant would inactivate the commonly used preservatives at use concentrations in agar media (deNavarre and Bailey, 1956; deNavarre, 1957b). Results of studies by Wedderburn (1958) with 26 different preservatives and many nonionic surfactants showed that the nonionics reduced the efficiency of all preservatives when the ratio of surfactant to preservation exceeded a critical value. The critical ratio was different for each combination of nonionic and preservative and varied with the test organisms. Numerous additional studies and reviews in the literature have confirmed the ability of nonionic surfactants to reduce preservative activity (Beckett and Robinson, 1958; deNavarre, 1960; Nowak, 1963; Marx et al., 1968; Schmolka, 1973).

The mechanism of nonionic inactivation of preservatives has also received considerable study. Higuchi and coworkers demonstrated the complexing of phenolic preservatives with polyethylene glycols, which are attributed to the association of acidic hydrogen groups of the phenol with electrophilic oxygen in the glycols (Higuchi and Lach, 1954; Guttman and Higuchi, 1956). Rieger (1981) assumed, however, that the presence of polyethylene glycol macromolecules does not affect the preservative activity of the parabens, because the low-energy hydrogen bonding may be readily broken. Dyer (1958) attributed inactivation to a partitioning of the preservative between the micelles of the nonionic surfactant and the aqueous phase. Compounds with high micellar solubility would be present in insufficient quantities in the aqueous phase to inhibit microbial growth. Evans (1964) also explained inactivation on the basis of solubilization of the preservative in the nonionic micelles and suggested that complex formation played an unimportant role in this phenomenon. Kostenbauder (1960) stated that it was unnecessary to distinguish between the two mechanisms, because micellar solubilization would fall within the broad scope of complex formation.

The quantitative aspects of inactivation were investigated by Patel and Kostenbauder (1958), who measured the amount of p-hydroxybenzoate bound by nonionics using a dialysis method. Pisano and Kostenbauder (1959) presented evidence that the activity of p-hydroxybenzoate esters in the presence of nonionics was a function of the unbound preservative. They suggested that the total concentration of preservative required to protect a nonionic formulation could be estimated from predetermined binding data. Models and methods of determining or predicting the quantity of free preservatives available in cosmetic systems have been described in the literature (Parker and Barnes, 1967a; Bean et al., 1969; McCarthy, 1973). Although most nonionic inactivation studies were conducted in relatively simple aqueous systems, Charles and Carter (1959) determined the activity of *p*-hydroxybenzoates and sorbic acid in 18 typical nonionic cosmetic emulsions. They found the preservatives more effective in these products than would be anticipated from results obtained with simpler systems. Their results again indicate the need for testing the final finished product with all components present.

Schuster and Modde (1969, 1971) reported on the inactivating effect of anionic surfactants on preservatives with low water solubility. Inactivation occurred only after a certain ratio of surfactant to preservative, which varied with the nature of both the preservative and the surfactant, was reached. A review of the interaction of anionic, cationic, and nonionic surfactants with preservatives was presented by Coates (1973).

Other Inactivating Agents

In addition to the influence of pH, partitioning, and nonionics, specific components of cosmetic formulations have been cited for their effect on preservatives (Eisman et al., 1957; Tillman and Kuramoto, 1957). Horn et al. (1971) studied the effect of suspended solids often present in formulations on preservative activity. Results of their tests with 15 powders and 9 different preservatives demonstrated the importance of examining these interactions. McCarthy (1970a and b) investigated the stability of preservatives stored as aqueous solutions in polyethylene polyvinyl chloride, and glass containers. Polyethylene proved unsuitable for substituted phenols, phenylmercuric nitrate, and benzoic acid. Studies also have indicated that rubber closures can effect activity by absorbing significant quantities of the preservative from solution (Lachman et al., 1963).

Obviously, many factors in cosmetic formulations can reduce the activity of preservatives. The presence of these factors and the degree to which they exert their influence vary with the composition of the formulation and the nature of the preservative. Their magnitude often can be estimated on the basis of data obtained in simple systems and overcome by the addition of greater quantities of preservative. Final judgment of preservative performance, however, remains with tests on the finished cosmetic product.

EVALUATION OF PRESERVATIVES

Stringent controls and good manufacturing procedures have significantly reduced but not eliminated the incidence of microbial contamination of susceptible cosmetic products. The addition of an effective antimicrobial agent is a necessary adjunct to sound manufacturing operations. The presence of an effective preservative prevents the growth of any undetected organisms remaining after manufacture and provides protection against the gross contamination introduced by the consumer during use.

Selection of an effective preservative for use in cosmetic products depends on many factors in addition to antimicrobial activity (Gershenfeld, 1963). The compound must be relatively nontoxic, nonirritating, and nonsensitizing. In addition, the preservative should be stable, compatible with all ingredients in the formulation, and have no effect on color and odor. The cost of the compound and its ease of incorporation also are considerations.

The method selected for preservative efficacy testing is determined by a number of factors, including the following (Orth, 1989):

Time available for testing
Reliability of the method
Ability to maintain control of the method
   by use of statistical treatment of the data
"Need" for rechallenge testing
Type of product to be examined
Test organisms used
Acceptance criteria

The CTFA (1973) and USP (1985) procedures have generally been accepted as standards in industry. The American Society for Testing and Materials (1978) has published similar testing procedures. Recently, rapid screening tests have been proposed to obviate the lengthy time required for the completion of the CTFA, USP, and ASTM procedures. Mulberry et al. (1987) discussed three procedures designed to shorten the time to determine the adequacy of preservation of cosmetics. These are the Linear Regression Method of Orth (1979), the Accelerated Preservation Test of O'Neill (1981), and the Presumptive Challenge Test and Rapid Kill Curve Test of Chan and Prince (1981). Orth, in a series of publications, elaborated on a linear regression method for the rapid determination of cosmetic preservative efficacy.

This test uses decimal-reduction time (D-values) to determine the preservative efficacy of a cosmetic product. The D-value is the time required to inactivate 90% of the microorganisms exposed to a biocide and is calculated from the logarithmic death rate of an inoculated culture. D-values allow preservative efficacy to be determined in 2 days for bacteria and 7 days for fungi. The total time required for destruction of any size of microbial population may be estimated.

The Presumptive Challenge Test and Rapid Kill Curve Test are in reality two tests. The first involves serially diluting a test product in an inoculum, incubating for 24 hours, and then streaking a transfer onto neutralizing agar and incubating. The number of colonies recovered indicates the activity of the product for each dilution. The second test uses frequent sampling over 24 hours of an inoculated test product to determine the time required for a l-log kill. Efficacy can be determined in 48 hours.

The Accelerated Preservation Test uses "in-house" and *Pseudomonas* organisms as well as fungi to challenge a "nutrified" product. Microbiologic assays are performed at 2 days and 7 days for bacteria, and at 2, 7, and 12 days for fungi. A 2- to 3-log reduction by day two and no recoveries at day 7 are the passing criteria for bacteria. Fungal acceptance requires significant die-off of the population.

Mulberry et al. (1987) concluded that rapid screening tests are a useful time-saving tool for screening product formulations but cautions that rapid methods should not be used in place of standard (CTFA, USP) methods without validation. Orth (1985) recommends the linear regression method as the method of choice over the CTFA and USP procedures because it requires less time, provides quantitative data on death rates, and has been shown to be reliable. Although rapid tests are undoubtedly a useful tool for screening preservatives and evaluating products, microbiologists are reluctant to leave their traditional evaluation procedures. The reams of data accumulated over the years have provided confidence in the standard test procedures. It may take many years and much validation before rapid testing becomes generally acceptable.

MICROORGANISMS AND PRESERVATIVES

Testing the activity of a preservative in a cosmetic formulation entails inoculation with microorganisms and incubating the finished product containing the compound. Periodic reinoculation of the samples during incubation is helpful in revealing unstable compounds or those with borderline activity. The microorganisms used as inocula have varied with the investigators conducting the tests (Olson, 1967; Parker and Barnes, 1967b; Butler, 1968; Barnes and Denton, 1969; Anderson and McConville, 1973). Specific organisms have been suggested by the CTFA (1973) and the USP (1985). Often the organisms isolated from a spoiled product are used for testing the activity of a preservative in the same or related formulations. It is advantageous to test against as large a spectrum of microorganisms as possible to ensure a wide range of protection. The inclusion of *Aspergillus niger* and *Pseudomonas aeruginosa* in the inocula is recommended because these ubiquitous organisms grow in a large variety of formulations and are relatively resistant to antimicrobial agents.

It is also advisable to challenge a product after long-term storage to determine if interactions between the container, the cosmetic, and the preservative may have deactivated the preservative system. Elevated temperatures may help to accelerate stability studies.

Recently, increasing interest has developed in the adaption and resistance of microorganisms to preservatives. Orth and Lutes (1985) evaluated the ability of laboratory cultures of *Ps. aeruginosa*, *Staphylococcus aureus*, and *Escherichia coli* to adapt to a series of preservatives in culture media. Tested products included methyl paraben, Germall 115, Dowicil 200, Kathon CG, phenoxyethanol, DMDH hydantoin, Germaben, and Phenonip. It was found that the cultures were able to adapt in various degrees to all preservatives tested except phenoxyethanol, although it was stressed that many factors may effect adaption. As a result of their testing, the authors recommended that a combined preservative system be used.

Fauet et al. (1987) used procedures similar to those of Orth and Lutes to determine if *E. coli*, *S. aureus*, and *Ps. aeruginosa*, as well as *Micrococcus luteus*, *Bacillus subtilis*, *Clostridium sporogenes*, *Candida albicans*, *Penicillium notatum*, and *Aspergillus niger* could be adapted to Kathon CG and Germall II alone and in combination. Adapted gram-negative bacteria can survive in the presence of low levels of preservatives, but the adaptions are unstable. The danger of using low levels of preservatives also exists with *S. aureus*. It was concluded, however, that despite the survival of bacteria in low concentrations of these preservatives, adaption does not play an important role when using normal concentrations.

The perseverance of preservatives in microbially contaminated products has not been studied by analytical methods. Recently, using methyl and propyl paraben, Scott and Jungermann (1987) compared a laboratory *Pseudomonas aeruginosa* with a "wild" strain. The "wild" *Ps. aeruginosa* was able to grow rapidly, reducing the paraben concentration by approximately 30% over 28 days. The ATCC organisms neither grew nor affected the paraben level. It was postulated that the "wild" organisms may have been able to acetylate or conjugate the *p*-hydroxy group of the parabens, thereby deactivating them.

The survival strategies used by bacteria under adverse conditions have been discussed by Levy (1987). The ability of *Pseudomonas* to adapt to different conditions is well known. Biochemically, *Pseudomonas* microorganisms are the most diverse encountered in the cosmetic industry. Discrepancies may exist between results obtained using standard microbiologic tests and actual in-use observations. This is, in part, due to differences between laboratory and wild microorganisms. Furthermore, laboratory and in-use conditions can differ substantially. Levy states that the acquisition or reshuffling of genetic elements can enable bacteria to successfully overcome inhibitor conditions in a preserved product. This period of adaption, in which resistant cells appear, may last longer than the testing period. As a result, quick test methods based on short-term death rates may not give an accurate picture of these problems.

TOXICOLOGIC ASPECTS—CIR PROGRAM

The Cosmetic Ingredient Review (CIR) program was established in 1976 by the Cosmetic, Toiletry and Fragrance Association (CTFA) to have the safety of ingredients used in cosmetics evaluated in an unbiased, expert manner (Elder, 1980). An Expert Panel of scientists review and assess the available published and unpublished data for ingredients to arrive at conclusions and recommendations relevant to the safety of the use of these ingredients in cosmetics. The Panel's reports are generally recognized as authoritative, scientific documents concerning the safety of individual ingredients. To date, most of the more widely used cosmetic preservatives have been evaluated and reported on by this program.

Parabens

The esters of *p*-hydroxybenzoic acid probably have the longest history of safe use among the cosmetic preservatives. After reviewing the expansive literature covering the toxicologic and experiential data with these materials, the CIR concluded that they were safe as cosmetic ingredients in the present practices of use, up to 1.0% (CIR, 1983).

The benzyl ester was also reviewed by the CIR panel of experts. They reported, in 1986, that the available data was *insufficient* to support the safe use of Benzyl-paraben in cosmetics (CIR, 1986).

Imidazolidinyl Urea

This preservative has been widely used through the years in combination with other preservatives such as the parabens. The published review on the safety of this material in 1980 indicated that the product was safe to use at concentrations up to 5.0% (CIR, 1980). It was also suggested at that time that additional toxicologic studies be conducted on this preservative.

Diazolidinyl Urea

This is one of the formaldehyde releasing agents, structurally related to imidazolidinyl urea, that is widely used in cosmetics alone or in combination with other preservatives. The major consideration concerning safety is its sensitization potential on formaldehyde allergic subjects. The recommendation of the CIR expert panel is that it can be used safely at a concentration not to exceed 0.5% (CIR, 1989).

2-Bromo-2-nitropropane-1,3-diol (Bronopol)

Bronopol, one of the more effective gram-negative and gram-positive preservatives, was originally approved safe for use up to a level of 0.1% by the Panel in 1980 (CIR, 1980). However, because of the nitrosating properties of Bronopol, the Panel cautioned against its use in formulations in which its action could lead to the formation of nitrosamines. A subsequent review by the CIR group in 1984 concurred with its original conclusion of safe use up to 0.1% and mentioned possible sensitization to subjects with sensitive or damaged skin (CIR, 1984).

DMDM Hydantoin

This is another formaldehyde donor in the hydroxymethyl imidazolidenedione series of preservatives that is used in cosmetics. Concerns of its safe use are again related to its release of formaldehyde. The CIR panel, after reviewing the extensive toxicologic data for DMDM hydantoin, concluded that it was safe as a cosmetic ingredient at its present levels of use, up to 1.0% (CIR, 1988).

Phenoxyethanol

Phenoxyethanol has been used in cosmetics, alone or in combination with other preservatives, for many years. The Expert Panel's safety assessment in 1989 concluded that phenoxyethanol was safe to use in cosmetics at presently used concentrations, 0.1 to 1.0% (CIR, 1989).

Quaternium-15

Quaternium-15 is an antibacterial agent that has been extensively used as a preservative in food packaging and industrial products as well as in cosmetics. It is considered a potential skin sensitizer especially for formaldehyde-sensitized subjects. The CIR Panel concluded that it was safe as a cosmetic ingredient at currently used concentrations, less than 0.1% to 1.0% (CIR, 1986).

Methylisothiazolinone and Methylchloroisothiazolinone (Kathon)

This antimicrobial agent is supplied to cosmetic manufacturers as an aqueous solution containing 1.5% of a mixture of the two isothiazolinones. It is by far the most potent new preservative to be used in cosmetics during the last decade. A major concern with its use, however, is its strong potential for skin sensitization. Because of this adverse effect, the Expert Panel concluded that Kathon was safe to use *only* at a maximum level of 15 ppm (active) and only in rinse-off products (CIR, 1988). The risk of sensitization to Kathon is a controversial problem that continues to receive prominent attention in the literature (CIR, 1988). This publicity alone and not the scientific data could lead ultimately to the decreased use of this preservative in cosmetic products.

Formaldehyde

Formaldehyde, usually in the form of an aqueous solution (formalin), was widely used as an effective cosmetic preservative, especially in wash-off products such as hair shampoos, until the early 1980s. Safety concerns about this preservative at that time were mainly directed to its sensitization potential for a certain segment of the population (Jordan et al., 1979). During the early 1980s reports and warnings of the potential carcinogenic properties of formaldehyde vapors for the nasal mucosa (NIOSH, 1981) have reduced the cosmetic use of this antibacterial agent. The CIR Expert Panel concluded that formaldehyde was safe for use in cosmetics for the great majority of the public. Because of the skin sensitivity of some consumers to this compound, the panel recommended that the level used should not exceed 0.2% as free formaldehyde (CIR, 1984).

5-Bromo-5-Nitro-1,3-Dioxane

This is a preservative closely related to Bronopol in structure and in activity that has been used to a lesser extent than Bronopol in cosmetics. As with Bronopol, there is major concern relevant to nitrosamine formation. The panel concluded that this preservative is safe for use in cosmetics up to a level of 0.1%, with a caveat concerning formulations in which nitrosamines might form (CIR, 1989).

Chloroacetamide

This preservative was widely used in the past in European cosmetics but was only one of the minor antibacterials in the U.S. The EEC Cosmetic Directive in 1986 limited its use to a maximum of 0.3% with a warning label on the product. The Expert Panel concluded that chloroacetamide was unsafe for use as a cosmetic product (CIR, 1988).

REFERENCES

Aalto, T.R., Firman, M.C., and Rigler, N.E. 1953. p-Hydroxybenzoic acid esters as preservatives. I. J. Am. Pharm. Assoc., Sci. Ed., 42, 449–457.

Albert, A. 1951. *Selective Toxicity.* New York, John Wiley & Sons.

Alguire, D.E., and Yeung, A.C. 1979. Making cosmetics microbiologically safe. Cosmet. Toil., 94, 77–80.

Anderson, D.W., Jr., and Ayers, M. 1972. Microbiological profile of selected cosmetic products with and without preservatives after use. J. Soc. Cosmet. Chem., 23, 863–873.

Anderson, D.W., Jr., and McConville, J.F. 1973. Microbiological profile of used eye cosmetics by examination of product only. Cosmet. Perf., 88(8), 25–27.

Anonymous. 1985. Cosmetic preservatives encyclopedia. Cosmet. Toil., 100, 85–88, 90–92, 94, 97–101.

ASTM. 1978. Standard test method for preservatives in water-containing cosmetics. ANSI/ASTM E640–78.

Atkins, F. 1950. Some aspects of creams in cosmetics. Mfg. Chem., 21, 51–54.

Ayliffe, G.A. Barrowcliff, D.F., and Lowbury, E.J. 1969. Contamination of disinfectants. Br. Med. J., 1, 505.

Ayliffe, G.A., et al. 1966. Postoperative infection with *Pseudomonas aeruginosa* in an eye hospital. Lancet, 1, 1113.

Baker, J.H. 1959. The unwanted cosmetic ingredient—bacteria. J. Soc. Cosmet. Chem., 10, 133–143.

Bandelin, F.J. 1977. Antibacterial and preservative properties of alcohols. Cosmet. Toil., 92, 59–70.

Bandelin, F.J. 1958. The effect of pH on the efficiency of various mold-inhibiting compounds. J. Am. Pharm. Assoc., Sci. Ed., 46, 691–694.

Barnes, M., and Denton, G.W. 1969. Capacity tests for the evaluation of preservatives in formulations. Soap Perf. Cosmet., 42, 729–733.

Bean, H.S., and Heman-Ackah, S.M. 1964. Influence of oil:water ratio on the activity of some bactericides against *Escherichia coli* in liquid parrafin and water dispersions. J. Pharm. Pharmacol., 16(Suppl.), 58T–67T.

Bean, H.S., Konning, G.H., and Malcom, S.A. 1969. A model for the influence of emulsion formulations on the activity of phenolic preservatives. J. Pharm. Pharmacol., 21(Suppl.), 173S–181S.

Bean, H.S., Konning, G.H., and Thomas, J. 1970. Significance of the partition coefficient of a preservative in cosmetic emulsions. Am. Perf. Cosmet., 85, 61–65.

Beckett, A.H., and Robinson, A.E. 1958. The inactivation of preservatives by nonionic surface active agents. Soap. Perf. Cosmet., 31, 454–459.

Berke, P.A., and Rosen, W.E. 1978. Imidazolidinyl urea activity against *Pseudomonas*. J. Soc. Cosmet. Chem., 29, 757–766.

Berke, P.A., and Rosen, W.E. 1970. Germall, a new family of antimicrobial preservatives for cosmetics. Am. Perf. Cosmet., 85, 55–59.

Blakeway, J. 1986. The anti-microbial properties of essential oils. Soap Perfum. Cosmet., 59, 201, 203, 207.

Blaug, S.M., and Ahsan, S.S. 1961. Interaction of sorbic acid with nonionic macromolecules. J. Pharm. Sci., 50, 38–141.

Boehm, E. 1960. Combination of the esters of parahydroxybenzoic acid. Am. Perf. Aromat., 1st Doc. Ed., 104–105.

Boehm, E., and Jones, E. 1957. Nipa-ester combinations as preservatives and disinfectants. J. Soc. Cosmet. Chem., 8, 30–40.

Boehm, E., and Maddox, D. 1971. Problems of cosmetic preservation. Mfg. Chem. Aerosol News, 42, 41–43.

Bolle, A., and Mirimanoff, A. 1950. Antagonism between nonionic detergents and antiseptics. J. Pharm. Pharmacol., 2, 685–691.

Bronopol-Boots (BNPD) and Myacide BT. 1986. Technical Bulletin 5, The Boots Company PLC, Nottingham, England.

Brown, M.R.W., and Richards, E.M.E. 1965. Effect of polysorbate Tween 80 on the resistance of *Pseudomonas aeruginosa* to chemical inactivation. Nature, 207, 1391.

Bruch, C.W. 1971. Microbiological products of topical quality-types vs. numbers of microorganisms. Drug Cosmet. Ind., 109, 26–29, 105.

Bryce, D.M., and Smart, R. 1965. The preservation of shampoos. J. Soc. Cosmet. Chem., 16, 187–201.

Butler, N.J. 1968. The microbiological deterioration of cosmetics and pharmaceutical products. In *Biodeterioration of Materials.* Edited by A.W. Walters and J.S. Elphick. New York, Elsevier, pp. 269–280.

Carter, P.V., et al. 1958. Preparation and the antibacterial and antifungal properties of substituted benzyl alcohols. J. Pharm. Pharmacol., 10, 149T–159T.

Chan, M., and Price, H.N. 1981. A rapid screening test for ranking preservative efficacy. Drug Cosmet. Ind., 129, 34–37, 80, 81.

Charles, R.D., and Carter, P.J. 1959. The effect of sorbic acid and other preservatives on organism growth in typical nonionic emulsified commercial cosmetics. J. Soc. Cosmet. Chem., 10, 383–394.

Coates, D. 1973. Interaction between preservatives and surfactants. Mfg. Chem. Aerosol News, 44, 41–42.

Coates, D., and Woodford, R. 1973. Methods available for studying antimicrobial interaction in cosmetics. Cosmet. Perfum., 88, 43–48.

Cosmetic Ingredient Review 1980. Final report of the safety assessment for the imidazolidinyl urea. J. Environ. Pathol. Toxicol., 4, 133–146.

Cosmetic Ingredient Review 1980. Final report on the safety assessment for 2-bromo-2-nitropropane-1,3-diol. J. Environ. Pathol. Toxicol., 45, 48–64.

Cosmetic Ingredient Review 1984. Addendum to the final report on the safety assessment of 2-bromo-2-nitro-propane-1,3-diol. J. Am. Coll. Toxicol., 3, 139–155.

Cosmetic Ingredient Review 1984. Final report on the safety assessment of formaldehyde. J. Am. Coll. Toxicol., 3, 157–184.

Cosmetic Ingredient Review 1986. Final report on the safety assessment of quaternium-15. J. Am. Coll. Toxicol., 5, 61–101.

Cosmetic Ingredient Review 1988. Tentative report on methylisothiazolinone and methylchloroisothazolinone (April 15, 1988). Prepared by the Expert Panel of the CIR. Unpublished.

Cosmetic Ingredient Review 1988. Tentative final report on chloroacetamide (August 31, 1988). Prepared by the Expert Panel of the CIR. Unpublished.

Cosmetic Ingredient Review 1988. Final report on the safety assessment of DMDM hydantoin. J. Am. Coll. Toxicol., 7, 245–277.

Cosmetic Ingredient Review 1989. Tentative final report on Phenoxyethanol (February 3, 1989). Prepared by the Expert Panel of the Cosmetic Ingredient Review. Unpublished.

Cosmetic Ingredient Review 1989. Final report on 5-bromo-5-nitro-1,3-dioxane (February 17, 1989). Prepared by the Expert Panel of the CIR. Unpublished.

Cosmetic Ingredient Review 1989. Final report on Diazolidinyl urea (March 30, 1989). Prepared by the Expert Panel of the CIR. Cosmetic, Toiletries and Fragrance Association, Inc. Washington, D.C.

Croshaw, B., Grove, M.J., and Lessel, B. 1964. Some properties of Bronopol, a new antimicrobial agent active against *Pseudomonas aeruginosa*. J. Pharm. Pharmacol., 16, 127T–130T.

Cruickshank, G.A., and Braithwaite, D.G. 1949. Sterilization of cation exchange resins. Ind. Eng. Chem., 41, 472–473.

CTFA Preservation Subcommittee of the CTFA Microbiological Committee. 1973a. A guideline for the determination of adequacy of preservation of cosmetics and toiletry formulations. Cosmetics, Toiletries and Frangrance Association, Inc., Washington, D.C.

CTFA 1973b. Microbiology preservative bibliography. CTFA Cosmetic J., 5, 13–15.

CTFA Microbial Content Subcommittee. 1977. The CTFA national microbiological survey of cosmetics and toiletries 1972–75. CTFA Cosmetic J., 9(3), 24–31.

CTFA Preservation Subcommittee. 1973. Evaluation of methods for determining preservative efficacy. CTFA Cosmetic J., 5, 2–7.

CTFA Quality Assurance Microbiology Subcommittee. 1972. Microbiological quality assurance guidelines for the manufacture of cosmetics. CTFA Cosmetic J., 4, 20–23.

Dabbah, R., Edwards, V.M., and Moates, W.A. 1970. Antimicrobial action of some citrus fruit oils on selected food-borne bacteria. Appl. Microbiol., 19, 27–31.

Davis, J.G. 1972. Fundamentals of microbiology in relation to cleansing in the cosmetic industry. J. Soc. Cosmet. Chem., 23, 45–71.

Dawson, F.W. 1973. Some techniques for microbial controls in manufacturing plants. J. Soc. Cosmet. Chem., 24, 655–662.

Decker, R.L., Jr., and Wenninger, J.A. 1987. Frequency of preservative use in cosmetic formulas as disclosed to the FDA—1987. Cosmet. Toil., 102, 21–24.

DeNavarre, M.G. 1962. *The Chemistry and Manufacture of Cosmetics.* Volume I. New York, D. Van Nostrand.

DeNavarre, M.G. 1960. The interferences of nonionic emulsifiers with preservatives. Am. Perf. Aromat., 1st Doc. Ed., 99–100.

DeNavarre, M.G. 1957. The interferences of nonionic emulsifiers with preservatives with special reference to cosmetics. J. Soc. Cosmet. Chem., 8, 371–380.

DeNavarre, M.G., and Bailey, H.E. 1956. The interferences of nonionic emulsifiers with preservatives. II. J. Soc. Cosmet. Chem., 7, 427–433.

Dow Chemical Company. 1970. Dowicil 200 Technical Bulletin.

Dunnigan, A.P. 1968. Microbiological control of cosmetics. Drug Cosmet. Ind., 102, 43–45, 152–158.

Dyer, D.L. 1958. A review of detergent-germicide interactions. Soap Chem. Spec., 34, 53–55, 139–141.

Eisman, P.C., Cooper, J., and Jaconia, D. 1957. Influence of gum tragacanth on the bactericidal activity of preservatives. J. Am. Pharm. Assoc., Sci. Ed., 46, 144–147.

Eisman, P.C., Kull, F.C., and Mayer, R.L. 1949. The bacteriological aspects of deionized water. J. Am. Pharm. Assoc., Sci. Ed., 48, 88–91.

Elder, R.L. 1980. Cosmetic ingredients and their safety assessment. J. Environ. Pathol. Toxicol., 4, 2–3, 147–170.

Elder, R.L. (ed.). 1980. Final report on the safety assessment for imidazolidinyl urea. J. Environ. Pathol. Toxicol., 4(4), 133–146.

Entrekin, D.N. 1961. Relation of pH to preservative effectiveness. I. J. Pharm. Sci., 50, 743–746.

Epstein, S. 1968. Paraben sensitivity: subtle trouble. Ann. Allergy, 26, 185–189.

Eurotox Report. 1962. The prevention of hazards from chronic toxicity of cosmetics and toilet preparations. J. Soc. Cosmet. Chem., 13, 322–331.

Evans, J.R., Gilden, M.M., and Bruch, C.W. 1972. Methods for isolating and identifying objectionable gram-negative bacteria and endotoxins from topical products. J. Soc. Cosmet., 23, 549–564.

Evans, W.P. 1964. The solubilization and inactivation of preservatives by nonionic detergents. J. Pharm. Pharmacol., 16, 323–331.

Fisher, A.A. 1975. Allergic paraben and benzyl alcohol hypersensitivity relationship of the "delayed" and "intermediate" varieties. Contact Dermatitis, 1, 281–284.

Fisher, A.A. 1980. Cosmetic dermatitis. Part II. Reaction to some commonly used preservatives. Cutis, 26, 136, 141–142, 147–148.

Fuet, J., et al. 1987. Adaption of Escherichia coli, Pseudomonas aeruginosa and Staphylococcus aureus to Kathon CG and Germall II in an o/w cream. 1987. Cosmet. Toil., 102, 75–76, 78–80, 82–85.

Garrett, E.R., and Woods, O.R. 1953. The optimum use of acid preservatives in oil-water systems: benzoic acid in peanut oil-water. J. Am. Pharm. Assoc., Sci. Ed., 42, 736–739.

Gerrard, H.N., Parker, M.S., and Bullock, K. 1962. Fungistatic activity of methyl and propyl p-hydroxybenzoates and a mixture of these against Penicillium spinulosum. J. Pharm. Pharmacol., 14, 103.

Gershenfeld, L. 1963. Antimicrobial agents in cosmetic preparations. Am. Perf. Cosmet., 78, 55–67.

Gilmour, R.H. 1978. Ethylene oxide treatment of cosmetics. Soap Perfum. Cosmet., 51, 498–499.

Goldman, C.L. 1969. A microbiological case history of a cosmetic product. TGA Cosmet. J., 1, 42–43.

Gucklhorn, I.R. 1969. Antimicrobials in cosmetics, Part 3. Mfg. Chem. Aerosol News, 40, 71–75.

Guttman, D., and Higuchi, T. 1956. Possible complex formation between macromolecules and certain pharmaceuticals. X. J. Am. Pharm. Assoc., Sci. Ed., 45, 659–664.

Hamilton, W.A. 1971. Membrane active antibacterial compounds. In Inhibition and Destruction of the Bacterial Cell. Edited by W.B. Hugo. New York, Academic Press, p. 78.

Henley, W.O., and Sonntag, N.O.V. 1970. Formaldehyde and its donors as preservatives in cosmetic formulations. Am. Perf. Cosmet., 85, 95.

Henry, L. (1897). Zur Kenntnis der Nitritten Alkohole. Gesellschaft, 30, 2206.

Henry, S.M., and Jacobs, G. 1981. Cosmetic preservatives—1981. Cosmetic. Toil., 96, 29–37.

Hibbot, H.W., and Monks, J. 1961. Preservation of emulsions—p-hydroxybenzoic ester partition coefficient. J. Soc. Cosmet. Chem., 12, 2–8.

Higuchi, T., and Lach, J.L. 1954. Study of the possible complex formation between macromolecules and certain pharmaceuticals. J. Am. Pharm. Assoc., Sci. Ed., 44, 465–470.

Horn, N.R., McCarthy, T.J., and Price, C.H. 1971. Interaction between preservatives and suspension systems. Am. Perf. Cosmet., 86, 37–40.

Isacoff, H. 1981. Aromatics as bactericides. Cosmet. Toil., 96, 69–76.

Jacobs, G., Henry, S.M., and Cotty, V.R. 1975. The influence of pH, emulsifier, and accelerated aging upon preservative requirements of O/W emulsions. J. Soc. Cosmet. Chem., 26, 105–117.

Jones, P.S., Thigpen, D., Morrison, J.L., and Richardson, A.P. 1956. o-Hydroxybenzoic acid esters as preservatives. III. J. Am. Pharm. Assoc., Sci. Ed., 45, 268.

Jordan, W.P., Sherman, W.T., and King, S.E. 1979. Theshold response in formaldehyde-sensitive subjects. J. Am. Acad. Dermatol., 1, 44–8.

Kallings, L.O., Ringertz, O., Silverstolpe, L., and Enerfeldt, F. 1966. Microbiological contaminations of medical preparations. Acta Pharm. Suec., 3, 219–228.

Kano, C., Nakata, O., Kurosaki, S., and Yanagi, M. 1976. Microbial quality

control for the manufacture of cosmetic emulsions. J. Soc. Cosmet. Chem., 27, 73–86.

Kellner, W., and Kober, W. 1955. Possibilities of the use of ethereal oils for room disinfection. II. Arzneim. Forsch., 5, 224–229.

Kivanc, M., and Akgul, A. 1986. Antibacterial Activities of Essential Oils from Turkish spices and citrus. Flav. Frag. J., 1, 175–179.

Klauder, J.V. 1960. The closed, open, prophetic and repeated insult patch tests in study of cutaneous reaction. J. Soc. Cosmet. Chem., 11, 249–262.

Knights, H.T., and Harvey, J. 1964. Hand creams containing hexachlorophene and cross infection with gram-negative bacteria. N. Z. Med. J., 63, 653.

Kostenbauder, H.B. 1960. Some physico-chemical aspects of phenolic preservatives in the presence of macromolecules. Am. Perf. Aromat., 75, 28–29, 32–33.

Lachman, L., Urbanyl, T., and Weinstein, S. 1963. Stability of antibacterial preservatives in parenteral solutions. IV. Contribution of rubber closure composition on preservative loss. J. Pharm. Sci., 52, 244–249.

Law, A.B., Moss, J.N., and Lashen, E.S. 1984. In Cosmetic and Drug Preservation. Edited by J.J. Kabara. New York, Marcel Dekker, pp. 129–141.

Lazier, J., and Galand, G. 1975. La décontamination microbiologique des cosmétiques et produits de beauté par irradiation. Parfums, Cosmetiques, Aromes, 3, 133–120.

Lennington, K.R. 1969. The FDA's viewpoint. Drug Cosmet. Ind., 104, 44–47, 163–165.

Letters to the Editor 1989. Risk of sensitization to Kathon CG. Contact Dermatitis, 20, 76–79.

Levy, E. 1987. Insights into microbial adaption to cosmetic and pharmaceutical products. Cosmet. Toil., 102, 69–74.

Leyden, J.J., Stewart, R., and Kligman, A.M. 1980. Experimental inoculation of Pseudomonas aeruginosa and Pseudomonas cepaciae on human skin. J. Soc. Cosmet. Chem., 31, 19–28.

Littlejohn, O.M., and Husa, W.K. 1955. The potentizing effect of anti-molding agents in syrups. J. Am. Pharm. Assoc., Sci. Ed., 44, 305–308.

Lockemann, G., et al. 1941. Ueber die keimtotende Wirkung von Alkoholen. (The sterilization effects of alcohols.) Zentrabl. Bakteriol., 147, 1–15.

Mallinkrodt Technical Bulletin, 1981. Mallinkrodt Inc., St. Louis, Mo.

Manowitz, M. 1964. The antifungal properties of G-11. Sindar Reporter, 2.

Manowitz, M. 1961. Preservation of cosmetic emulsions. In Developments in Industrial Microbiology. 2. New York, Plenum Press, pp. 65–71.

Marouchoc, S.R. 1984. Dowicil 200 preservative. In Cosmetic and Drug Preservation. Edited by J.J. Kabara. New York, Marcel Dekker, pp. 143–164.

Maruzella, J.C. 1963. Antifungal properties of perfume oils. J. Pharm. Sci., 52, 601–602.

Maruzella, J.C. 1962. The germicidal properties of perfume oils and perfumery chemicals. Am. Perf., 77, 67–70.

Maruzella, J.C., and Henry, P.A. 1958. The antimicrobial activity of perfume oils. J. Am. Pharm. Assoc., Sci. Ed., 47, 471–476.

Maruzella, J.C., and Lichtenstein, M.B. 1956. The in vitro antibacterial activity of oils. J. Am. Pharm. Assoc., Sci. Ed., 45, 378–381.

Maruzella, J.C., and Sicurella, N.A. 1960. Antibacterial activity of essential oil vapors. J. Am. Pharm. Assoc., Sci. Ed., 49, 692–694.

Maruzella, J.C., Chiaramonte, J.S., and Garofalo, M.M. 1961. Effects of vapors of aromatic chemicals on fungi. J. Am. Pharm. Assoc., Sci. Ed., 50, 665–668.

Marx, H., Sabalitschka, T., and Boehm, E.E. 1968. Behavior of antimicrobial materials in nonionic systems. Am. Perf. Cosmet., 83, 39–42, 44, 47.

McCarthy, T.J. 1970a. Interaction between aqueous preservative solutions and their plastic containers. I. Pharm. Weekbl., 105, 557–563.

McCarthy, T.J. 1970b. Interaction between aqueous preservative solutions and their plastic containers II. Pharm. Weekbl., 105, 1139–1146.

McCarthy, T.J. 1973. Preservatives released from creams and emulsions—a dissolution method. Cosmet. Perf., 88, 61–63.

McCulloch, E.C. 1945. Disinfection and Sterilization. Philadelphia, Lea & Febiger.

Miyawaki, G.M., Patel, N.K., and Kostenbauder, H.B. 1959. Interaction of preservatives with macromolecules. III. Parahydroxybenzoic acid esters in the presence of hydrophilic polymers. J. Am. Pharm. Assoc., Sci. Ed., 48, 315.

Morris, J.A., Khettry, A., and Seitz, E.W. 1979. Antimicrobial activity of aroma chemicals and essentials oils. J. Am. Oil Chem. Soc., 56, 595–603.

Morse, L.J., and Schonbeck, L.E. 1968. Hand lotions—a potential nosocomial hazard. N. Engl. J. Med., 278, 376–378.

Morse, L.J., et al. 1967. Septicemia due to Klebsiella pneumoniae originating from hand-cream dispenser. N. Engl. J. Med., 277, 472.

Most, S., and Katz, S. 1970. Cosmetic manufacturing sanitation. Am. Perf. Cosmet., 85, 67–71.

Mulberry, G.K., Entryup, M.R., and Agin, U.R. 1987. Rapid screening methods for preservative efficacy evaluations. Cosmet. Toil., 103(12), pp. 47–53.

Munzing, H.P., and Schels, H. 1972. Uber die Moglichkeiten die ersatzes von Konservierungs-mitteln in kosmetischen Praparaten durch atherische Ole. J. Soc. Cosmet. Chem., 23, 841–852.

Myers, G.E., and Pasutto, F.M. 1973. Microbial contamination of cosmetics and toiletries. Can. J. Pharm. Sci., 8, 19–22.

Nadal, N.G.M., Montalvo, A.E., and Seda, M. 1973. Antimicrobial properties of bay and other phenolic essential oils. Cosmet. Perf., *88*, 37–38.

NIOSH. 1981. Department of Health and Human Services. Formaldehyde: Evidence of Carcinogenicity. Current Intelligence Bulletin 34. Washington, D.C., U.S. Government Printing Office.

Nowak, G.A. 1963. The preservation of nonionic emulsions. Soap Perf. Cosmet., *36*, 914–924.

Olson, J.C., Jr. 1970. Some considerations relative to microbial contamination of cosmetics. Am. Perf. Cosmet., *85*, 43–46.

Olson, S.W. 1967. The application of microbiology to cosmetic testing. J. Soc. Cosmet. Chem., *18*, 191–198.

O'Neill, J., Mead, C.A., and Scibienski, E.J. 1981. A presentation at the Society of Chemists annual meeting, Dec. 1981.

Orth, D.S. 1989. Microbiological considerations in cosmetic formula development and evaluation. 1. Microbiological quality of a product. Cosmet. Toil., *104*, 49–64.

Orth, D.S. 1979. Linear regression method for rapid determination of cosmetic preservative efficacy. J. Soc. Cosmet. Chem., *30*, 321–332.

Orth, D.S., and Lutes, C.M. 1985. Adaption of bacteria to cosmetic preservatives. Cosmet. Toil., *100*, 57–59, 63–64.

Osipow, L.I., Morra, D., and Resmansky, N. 1963. 1,3-Butylene glycol in cosmetics. Drug Cosmet. Ind., *103*, 54.

Parker, M.S. 1972. A new generation of preservatives. Soap Perf. Cosmet., *45*, 621–624.

Parker, M.S., and Barnes, M. 1967a. The interaction of nonionic surfactants with preservatives. Soap Perf. Cosmet., *40*, 163–170.

Parker, M.S., and Barnes, M. 1967b. Microbiological quality control of cosmetics and pharmaceutical preparations. Soap Perf. Cosmet., *40*, 875–878.

Parker, M.S., McCafferty, M., and MacBride, S. 1968. Phenonip: a broad spectrum preservative. Soap Perf. Cosmet., *41*, 647–649.

Parker, M.T. 1972. The clinical significance of the presence of microorganisms in pharmaceutical and cosmetic preparations. J. Soc. Cosmet. Chem., *23*, 415–426.

Parrott, E.L. 1968. Stability of methyl paraben. Am. Perf. Cosmet., *83*, 27.

Patel, N.K., and Kostenbauder, H.B. 1958. Interaction of preservatives with macromolecules. I. J. Am. Pharm. Assoc., Sci. Ed., *47*, 289–293.

Pisano, F.D., and Kostenbauder, H.B. 1959. Interaction of preservatives with macromolecules. II. J. Am. Pharm. Assoc., Sci. Ed., *48*, 310–314.

Poprzan, J., and DeNavrre, M.G. 1959. The interference of nonionic emulsifiers with preservatives. VIII. J. Soc. Cosmet. Chem., *10*, 81–87.

Price, P.B. 1950. Re-evaluation of ethyl alcohol as a germicide. Arch. Surg., *60*, 492–502.

Prichett, P.S., Murray, H.L., and Mercer, N.H. 1961. Potentiation of preservatives (parabens) in pharmaceutical formulations by low concentrations of propylene glycol. J. Pharm. Sci., *50*, 316–320.

Prince, H.N., and Welt, M.A. 1971. Microbiological studies on pressed powders and the sterilizing effect of gamma irradiation. Am. Perf. Cosmet., *86*, 49–52, 54.

Rahn, O., and Conn, J.E. 1944. Effect of increase in acidity on antiseptic efficiency. Ind. Eng. Chem., *36*, 185–187.

Richards, R.M.E., and Hardie, M.P. 1972. Effect of polysorbate 80 and phenylethanol on the antibacterial activity of Fentichlor. J. Pharm. Pharmacol., *24*, 90P–93P.

Richards, R.M.E., and McBride, R.J. 1971. Phenylethanol enhancement of preservatives used in ophthalmic preparations. J. Pharm. Pharmacol., *23*, 141S–146S.

Rieger, M.M. 1981. The inactivation of phenolic preservatives in emulsions. Cosmet. Toil., *96*, 39–43.

Rosen, M. 1985. Glydant and MDMH as cosmetic preservatives. In *Cosmetic and Drug Preservation*. Edited by J.J. Kabara. New York, Marcel Dekker, pp. 165–190.

Rosen, W.E., and Berke, P.A. 1980. Are cosmetic emulsions adequately preserved against Pseudomonas? J. Soc. Cosmet. Chem., *31*, 37–40.

Rosen, W.E., and Berke, P.A. 1973. Modern concepts of cosmetic preservation. J. Soc. Cosmet. Chem., *24*, 663–675.

Rosen, W.E., Berke, P.A., Matzin, T., and Peterson, A.F. 1977. Preservation of cosmetic lotions with imidazolidinyl urea plus parabens. J. Soc. Cosmet. Chem., *28*, 83–87.

Rudner, E.J. 1966. Contact sensitivity to para-hydroxybenzoate esters. Dermatol. Dig., *5*, 51–54.

Sabalitschka, T. 1924. Chemische Konstitution und Consiervierungsvermogen. Chem. Ztg., *48*, 703.

Schamberg, I.L. 1967. Allergic contact dermatitis to methyl and propyl paraben. Arch. Dermatol., *95*, 626.

Schenck, G.O. 1979. Moglichkeiten des einsatzes der Ultra-violett-Bestrahlung zur Entkeimung von Brauchwasser. Parfumerie Kosmetik, *60*, 397–406.

Schimmel, J., and Husa, W.J. 1956. The effect of various preservatives on microorganisms isolated from deteriorated syrups. J. Am. Pharm. Assoc., Sci. Ed., *45*, 204–208.

Schmolka, I.R. 1973. Synergistic effects of nonionic surfactants upon cationic germicidal agents. J. Soc. Cosmet. Chem., *24*, 577–592.

Schorr, W.F. 1968. Paraben allergy. JAMA, *204*, 859.

Schorr, W.F., Keran, E., and Plotka, E. 1974. Formaldehyde allergy. Arch. Dermatol., *110*, 73–76.

Schuster, G., and Modde, H.K. 1971. Examination of the efficacy of preservatives in anion-active surfactants. Part II. Am. Perf. Cosmet., *86*, 37–41.

Schuster, G., and Modde, H.K. 1969. Examination of the efficacy of preservatives in anion-active emulsifiers. Am. Perf. Cosmet., *84*, 37–46.

Scott, H.M.G. 1973. Methods for counting and testing for microorganisms in raw materials, topical and oral products. J. Soc. Cosmet. Chem., *24*, 65–78.

Scott, R.A., and Jungermann, E. 1985. The fate of parabens in a contaminated surfactant product. Soap Cosmet. Chem. Spec., Jan., pp. 24–26, 87.

Smart, R., and Spooner, D.F. 1972. Microbiological spoilage in pharmaceuticals and cosmetics. J. Soc. Cosmet. Chem., *23*, 721–737.

Sokol, H. 1952. Preservation of pharmaceuticals. Drug Stand., *20*, 89.

Sutton Laboratories, Inc. Undated. Germall II and Germaben II Sales Bulletin.

Tenenbaum, S. 1972. Microbiological limit guidelines for cosmetics and toiletries. CTFA Cosmet. J., *4*, 25–31.

Tenenbaum, S. 1967. Pseudomonas in cosmetics. J. Soc. Cosmet. Chem., *18*, 797–807.

Theodore, F.H., and Feinstein, R.R. 1952. Practical suggestions for the preparation and maintenance of sterile ophthalmic solutions. Am. J. Ophthalmol., *35*, 656.

Tillman, W.J., and Kuramoto, R. 1957. A study of the interaction between methylcellulose and preservatives. J. Am. Pharm. Assoc., *46*, 211–214.

U.S. Government Code of Federal Regulations, 1987. Title 21, Parts S 184.1490 and S 184.1670.

USP. 1985. Microbiological tests, antimicrobial preservatives—effectiveness. United States Pharmacopeia XXI. Easton, PA, Mack Publishing.

Van Abbe, N.J., Dixon, H., Hughes, O., and Woodroffe, R.C.S. 1970. The hygienic manufacture and preservation of toiletries and cosmetics. J. Soc. Cosmet. Chem., *21*, 719–800.

van Fenyes, C.K. 1970. Alcohols as preservatives and germicides. Am. Perf. Cosmet., *85*, 91–93.

Wallhäusser, K.H. 1984. Appendix B. In *Cosmetic and Drug Preservation*. Edited by J.J. Kabara. New York, Marcel Dekker, pp. 605–745.

Wallhäusser, K.H. 1981. Einwandfreie Kosmetika aus mikrobiologischer Sicht. Parfümerie Kosmetik, *62*, 379–387.

Wallhäusser, K.H. 1974. Die Konservung von Kosmetika. Seifen-Öle-Fette-Wachse, *100*, 11–16.

Wedderburn, D.L. 1970. Interactions in cosmetic preservation. Am. Perf. Cosmet., *85*, 49–53.

Wedderburn, D.L. 1965. Hygiene in manufacturing plant and its effect on the preservation of emulsions. J. Soc. Cosmet. Chem., *9*, 210–222.

Wells, F.V., and Lubowe, I.I. 1964. *Cosmetics and the Skin*. New York, Reinhold, pp. 586–598.

Wilson, L.A., and Ahearn, D.G. 1977. *Pseudomonas*-induced corneal ulcers associated with contaminated eye mascaras. Am. J. Ophthalmol., *84*, 112–118.

Wilson, L.A., Kuehne, J.W., Hall, S.W., and Ahearn, D.G. 1971. Microbial contamination in ocular cosmetics. Am. J. Ophthalmol., *71*, 1298–1302.

Winkler, J. 1955. Dehydroacetic acid and its salts for inhibition of the growth of microorganisms. U.S. Patent No. 2,722,483.

Wolf, P.A. 1950. Dehydroacetic acid, a new microbiological inhibitor. Food Technol., *4*, 294–297.

Wolven, A., and Levenstein, I. 1972. Microbiological examination of cosmetics. Am. Cosmet. Perf., *87*, 63–65.

Wolven, A., and Levenstein, I. 1969. Cosmetics—contaminated or not. CTFA Cosmet. J., *1*, 34–37.

Woodward, C.R., Jr. 1971. Some microbiological aspects of cosmetic manufacturing. Am. Perf. Cosmet., *86*, 45–48.

Woodward, C.R., and McNamara, T.F. 1971. A practical method for the microbiological examination of cosmetics. Am. Perf. Cosmet., *86*, 29–32.

Yablonski, J. 1978. Microbiological aspects of sanitary cosmetic manufacturing. Cosmet. Toil., *93*, 37–40, 43–46, 48, 50.

Zemek, J., et al. 1987. Antimicrobial properties of aromatic compounds of plant origin. Folia Microbiol. (Praha), *32*, 421–425.

CHAPTER 52

PRESERVATIVES FOR INDUSTRIAL AND MISCELLANEOUS PRODUCTS

Seymour S. Block

Microorganisms, as well as chemical and physical agents, cause degradation and deterioration of materials. In this respect microorganisms are a formidable enemy. They are ubiquitous, being found everywhere on the earth, in the water, and in the air. They are found in dust, in the clouds, in hot springs with nearly boiling water, and in the Dead Sea with a salt concentration of 30%. They live and propagate in air or without air, in light or darkness, and with small or large amounts of moisture, and a wide range of nutrients. This is because there are so many different kinds of bacteria, fungi, algae, and protozoa, and because of their ability to adjust to a wide range of different conditions. In this chapter we are interested in the saprophytes, those that grow on non-living matter. They are useful when they destroy unwanted materials but deleterious when they attack products we want to preserve. In some cases they degrade materials by decomposing them and in other cases by merely producing an unsightly appearance or offensive odor.

The art of preservation goes back thousands of years, as demonstrated by the expert mummification of human bodies by the Egyptians in the time of the pharaohs, 5000 years ago.

The use of preservatives for industrial products was practiced on a small scale all through history, cedar oil having been used by the ancients and mentioned in the Apocrypha, by Horace, Ovid, and Pliny the Elder, but it was not until recent times—the period of World War II—that their use was begun on a massive scale.

Because of the shortages of almost all types of goods, substitutes had to be made to fill requirements for which they were never intended, and ordinary products and materials had to be treated to make them outlast their normal service lives. In addition, replacement of articles that deteriorated when in military use was often difficult and sometimes impossible. But the most serious loss of all was in the lives lost in combat because of rotted tow

ropes, fungus-etched telescopes, and faulty radio insulation. The armed services set up specifications that demanded *tropicalization* of electronic equipment, mildew-proofing of binocular cases, and rot-proofing of rifle covers, camouflage nets, life preservers, barrage balloons, and numerous other items. The war in Viet Nam also created a demand for preservative treatment. Having witnessed the benefits derived from preservative treatment, manufacturers have continued to incorporate these procedures as part of their regular industrial practice.

The economic savings thus obtained are greater than generally appreciated. Hueck-van-der-Plas (1965) estimated economic losses due to microbial activities to be 2% of the value of all technical materials. The cost of replacement of the damaged material, however, may greatly exceed the cost of the material. Wessel and Bejuki (1959) collected figures on the damage to materials caused by microorganisms and the savings brought about by preservative treatments. In New Guinea, for the first 2 years of the Allied South Pacific campaign, the Australian Army reported a loss of $5 to $10 million from tropical effects. Microbiologic damage to the tents of the United States Army during World War II amounted to $4 million per month. (In considering these dollar amounts and those to follow in this chapter one must translate them into today's values taking into account the inflation factor and the increased production of preservative-treated products.) In the Korean War, the service life of shoes subject to microbiologic deterioration was reduced to about 10 days, and nearly 0.5 million pairs of shoes shipped to Korea were used up in a 2-month period. In normal times, approximately a million dollars are spent annually for leather finish preservatives. It has been estimated that at least 1 billion dollars worth of damage is done by fungi to wood products in the United States each year (Levi, 1977), and this does not include damage to standing trees. Loss from cotton and textile

Table 52–1. *U.S. Consumption of Specialty Biocides by End Use 1989 (Manufacturers' Dollars)*

End Use	$ Million	% Of Total
Wood preservation	$150	18%
Swimming pools and spas	150	18
Food and feed preservatives	115	14
Paint	60	7
Disinfectants and sanitizers	60	7
Cosmetics and toiletries	60	7
Plastics	35	4
Paper	35	4
Hospital and medical antiseptic	35	4
Cooling water	30	4
Metalworking fluids	20	2
Petroleum production	20	2
Other*	80	9
Total	$850	100%

*Includes latex, adhesives, slurries, pharmaceuticals, and leather.

decay is approximated at $100 million annually. Decay organisms take a toll of $18.5 million annually from fishing nets and fishing equipment. According to a survey by Charles H. Kline and Co., Farfield, NJ. (Marisca, 1991), the estimated sales of biocides in the United States for consumer and industrial products in 1989 was $850 million (Table 52–1), compared to $380 million in 1977 and $159 million in 1973 (see Chapter 56 for more economics and business information).

In 1962, the Committee for Scientific Research of the Organization for Economic Cooperation and Development calculated that materials subject to biodeterioration amounted to $50 billion per year's production and they estimated an annual loss from this type of deterioration of $1 billion annually. They noted that this figure may be low since it uses values for raw products rather than finished materials and, further, that no figure is included for indirect losses as in the deterioration of joints in pipelines, the occurrence of microbial slime in paper mills, etc. (Anon., 1965).

Sharpell (1980) divides industrial preservatives into two categories. One includes biocides that are put into a manufactured product to prevent its deterioration. This category includes wood, wood veneers, textiles, waxes, leather, hides, linseed oil-based paints, water-based paints, paper, paperboard, plastics, optical equipment, hoses, cords, rubber, hydrocarbon fuels, cement, inks, glues, adhesives, and liquid polishes. The other category is made up of biocides used in an industrial process to ensure the proper operation of that process. Products or processes in this category are metalworking fluids, latexes, resins, polymer emulsions, pigment slurries, lignosulfonates, textile lubricants, spin finishes, antistatics, cooling tower waters, pulp and paper waters and suspensions, secondary and tertiary petroleum oil recovery systems, casein solutions, gum solutions, silicone emulsions, and printing solutions. Some of the industrial biocides currently offered in the trade are given in Table

52–2, and some of the compounds mentioned in this chapter are shown in Figure 52–1.

WOOD PRESERVATION

Wood utilizes a greater quantity of chemical preservatives than all other industrial preservatives together.

According to statistics (Micklewright, 1989), in 1987 576 million cubic feet of wood were treated with chemicals to prevent damage by decay, insects, marine worms, and fire. Assuming a rate of treatment of 5 lbs of preservative per cubic foot of wood, an estimated 2.9 billion lbs of chemicals were used for this purpose. Specific figures give a total consisting of 97.8 million cubic feet of creosote solution, 48.6 million cubic feet of pentachlorophenol, 419 million cubic feet of waterborne preservatives, and 10.6 million cubic feet of fire retardant chemicals. Compounds of copper, zinc, boron, chromium, fluorine, arsenic, and phenols were used. Treated with these chemicals were 372.8 million cubic feet (6412.8 million board feet) of lumber and timbers, 96% treated with water-borne preservatives; 68.9 million cubic feet of crossties, practically all treated with creosote solutions; and 75.3 million cubic feet of poles, 57.7% treated with pentachlorophenol, 21.7% treated with creosote solutions, and 20.6% treated with water-borne preservatives. The balance was used to treat fence posts, plywood, and miscellaneous products. About 587 plants for treating wood with preservatives are presently operating in the United States. The wood preservation industry began in earnest about 100 years ago, although mercuric chloride was reported to protect wood from decay as early as 1705.

Wood has the capacity for great durability (Borgin, 1971). There are wooden churches in Norway that are still in use after 900 years, and a Viking ship was found almost intact after having been buried for almost 1100 years. Figure 52–2 shows one of the oldest frame houses in the United States, built in 1683 and still standing. The design, which did not allow water to collect, has protected the wood for three centuries. Wood withstands most chemical and physical forces well, but is quite vulnerable to biologic attack. Being composed of lignin, cellulose, hemicellulose, pentosans, and many other organic products, wood provides a source of nutrients to certain fungi, insects, and sea worms.

Bacteria also play a role in the deterioration of wood, which has only recently been appreciated (Greaves, 1971). They generally have an auxiliary rather than a primary effect in fiber breakdown, however, as is the case with certain fungi and insects. Different species of woods may be more or less vulnerable to attack (Southwell et al., 1962) owing to their content of extractives, which are toxic to attacking organisms (Rudman, 1963). In olden times, only the more resistant heartwood of trees was used in construction, while the more susceptible sapwood was discarded, but today we employ the whole tree, and most wood products must rely upon added preservatives to extend their normal serviceabil-

Table 52–2. *Industrial Biocides*

Composition	Trade names	Applications
Alkyl benzyldimethyl ammonium bromides	Onyxide (Onyx)	Textiles
2-[(Hydroxymethyl)amino]-2-methylpropanol	Troysan 192 (Troy)	Latex paints, resin emulsions
β-Bromo-β-nitrostyrene (9.2%) and methylene bisthiocyanate (4.9%)	Slime-Trol, RX 41 (Betz)	Pulp and paper mills
3,5-Dimethyl-tetrahydro-1,3,5-2H-thiadiazine-2-thione (Mylone)	Various	Leather, paint, glue, casein, starch, paper mill
Hexahydro-1,3,5-tris(2-hydroxyethyl)-5-triazine (78%)	Grotan (Lehn & Fink) Onyxide 200 (Onyx)	Cutting oils and diluted coolants
2-n-Octyl-4-isothiazolin-3-one (45%)	Skane M-8 (Rohm & Haas) Micro-chek (Ferro)	Latex and oil-based in-can paint preservative
2-n-Octyl-4-isothiazolin-3-one (5%)	Kathon LM (Rohm & Haas)	Fabrics
2-n-Octyl-4-isothiazolin-3-one (8.1%)	Kathon LP (Rohm & Haas)	Wet processing of hides
5-Chloro-2-methyl-4-isothiazolin-3-one (10.1%) and 2-methyl-4-isothiazoline-3-one (13.9%)	Kathon 886 MW (Rohm & Haas)	Wood veneer, cutting fluids and coolants, paste, slimes, cooling towers, paper and paperboard
Methylene bisthiocyanate	Metasol T-10 (Merck) Biosperse 284 (Drew) MBT (Various)	Paper slimes, recirculating cooling water systems, latexes, emulsions
2-[(Hydroxymethyl)-amino]ethanol	Troysan 174 (Troy) Cosan 91 (Cosan)	Paints, resin emulsions
Hexachloro dimethyl sulfone	Stauffer N-1386 (Stauffer)	Industrial emulsions
Diiodomethyl-p-tolyl sulfone	Amical 48 (Abbott) (Angus)	Paint
p-Chlorophenyl diiodomethyl sulfone	Amical 77 (Abbott) (Angus)	Paint
2,4,5,6-Tetrachloroisophthalonitrile	Nopcocide N-96 (Diamond Shamrock)	Latex paints
Poly[oxyethylene(dimethyliminio)ethylene-(dimethyliminio)ethylene dichloride] (60%)	Busan 77 (Buckman)	Cooling water systems, cutting fluids
3-Iodo-2-propynyl butyl carbamate (40%)	Troysan Polyphase Anti-mildew (Troy)	Interior and exterior coatings
p-Chloro-m-cresol	PCMC (Cosan)	Various emulsions
4,4-Dimethyloxazolidine and 3,4,4-trimethyloxazolidine	Bioban CS-1135 (Angus) Cosan 101 (Cosan)	Emulsions
1,1′-(2-Butenylene)bis(3,5,7-triaza-1-azoniaadamantane chloride)	Cosan 265 (Cosan)	Latex paints, resin emulsions, adhesives, dispersed colors
10,10′-Oxybisphenoxarsine 5% in a polymeric resin carrier	Vinyzene SB-1 (Ventron)	PVC, polyurethane and other polymeric compositions
10,10′-Oxybisphenoxarsine in various non-volatile plasticizer carriers	Vinyzene BP series (Ventron)	Film and sheeting, extruded plastics, plastisols, molded goods, organosols, fabric coatings, etc.
Copper oleate	Various	Wood, cordage, textiles
Copper naphthenate	Uversol (Harshaw) Nuodex Copper 6%, 8% (Nuodex)	Wood, cordage, textiles
Solubilized copper 8-quinolinolate	Culinate series (Ventron) Quinosol (Napp-Lemke) Quindex (Nuodex)	Wood and wood products, glues and adhesives, paper products
Rosin amine D-pentachlorophenate	Cumimene series (Ventron)	Paper, textiles, rope, emulsion systems
2,2′-Methylenebis (4-chlorophenol)	Cuniphen series (Ventron) Preventol GDC (GAF) Nuophene (Nuodex)	Textiles, rubber products, hoses
6-Acetoxy-2,4-dimethyl-m-dioxane	Giv-Gard DXN (Brand of Dimethoxane) (Givaudan) Socci 7350 (Ventron)	Textile lubricants, polymer emulsions, other aqueous emulsions
o-Phenylphenol	Dowicide I (Dow)	Protein-based paints, metalworking fluids, polishes, adhesives, gums, latexes, textiles
o-Phenylphenate (sodium-o-phenylphenate tetrahydrate)	Dowicide A (Dow)	Protein-based paints, metalworking fluids, polishes, adhesives, gums, latexes, textiles
Pentachlorophenol (88%) and 2,3,4,6-tetrachlorophenol (12%)	Dowicide EC-7 (Dow)	Wood preservation
2,4,5-Trichlorophenol	Dowicide 2 (Dow)	Paper mills, paint, wood, adhesives, textiles
Sodium pentachlorophenate	Dowicide G-ST (Dow)	Paper making, pulp, paper and paper products, leather, hides, drilling muds

Table 52–2. *Industrial Biocides* (continued)

Composition	Trade names	Applications
1-(3-Chloroallyl)-3,5,7-triaza-1-azoniaadamantane chloride plus sodium bicarbonate	Dowicil 75 (Dow)	Adhesives, metalworking fluids, latex paints, textile emulsions, water-based coating formulations
2,2-Dibromo-3-nitrilopropionamide (DBNPA) (20%, 10% or 5%) in polyethylene glycol	Dow Antimicrobials 7287, 8536 and XD-8259 (Dow) Biosperse 240, 244 (Drew)	Water cooling towers, pulp and paper mills, metalworking fluids, oil recovery
Pentachlorophenol	Penta (Reichold)	Wood, leather, latex
1,2-Dibromo-2,4-dicyanobutane	Tektamer 38 (Merck)	Aqueous paints, latex emulsions, joint cements, adhesives
2-(4-Thiazolyl)-benzimidazole	Metasol TK 100, TK-50 50% (Merck)	Paint
1,2-Benzisothiazolin-3-one (30%)	Proxel CRL (ICI)	Adhesives, latex, paper coatings, aqueous emulsions
4-(2-Nitrobutyl) morpholine (70%) and 4,4'-(2-ethyl-nitrotrimethylene) dimorpholine (20%)	Bioban P-1487 (Angus)	Metalworking fluids, pulp and paper industry, petroleum production, jet fuels
Tris(hydroxymethyl)nitromethane	Tris Nitro (Angus)	Oil in water emulsions, pulp and paper industry, water treatment
2-Mercaptobenzothiazole	Thiotax (Monsanto) M-B-T (Uniroyal) Captax (Vanderbilt) (Buckman)	Aqueous systems, textiles, leathers
Sodium dimethyldithiocarbamate (27.6%) and sodium 2-mercaptobenzothiazole (2.4%)	Vancide 51 (Vanderbilt)	Paper mills, cooling towers, paper and paperboard, cotton fabrics, paste, wood, veneer, cutting oils
Zinc dimethyldithiocarbamate (87.0%) and zinc 2-mercaptobenzothiazole (7.5%)	Vancide 51Z (Vanderbilt)	Adhesives, cooling water, paper mills, paper and paperboard, textiles
trans-1,2-bis(n-propyl sulfonyl) ethene	Vancide PA (Vanderbilt)	Paints, textiles
N-trichloromethylthio-4-cyclohexene-1,2-dicarboximide (Captan)	Vancide 89 (Vanderbilt)	Paint, plasticizers, lacquer
Zinc naphthenate	Various	Wood, textiles
N-(trichloromethylthio) phthalimide (Folpet)	Various	Nonaqueous paints and caulking compounds
Tributyl tin oxide	TBTO (Carlisle) (M&T) Keycide X-10 (Witco)	Paint, plastic
Organotin, quaternaries and amines	Biosperse 201 (Drew)	Cooling water systems
Polychlorophenates, organosulfurs	Biocide 207 (Drew)	Cooling towers
Polychlorophenates, alcohol and amines	Biosperse 209 (Drew)	Cooling towers and evaporative condensers
Dioctyl dimethyl ammonium chloride and ethanol	Biosperse 216 (Drew)	Cooling water systems
Organic chlorine releasing compound	Biosperse 230 (Drew)	Industrial recirculating water
Organosulfur compound blend	Biosperse 280 (Drew)	Cooling towers, air washer systems
Methylene bisthiocyanate, polychlorophenol	Biocide 285 (Drew)	Water cooling tower systems
Barium metaborate	Busan 11-M-1 (Buckman)	Paints
2-(Thiocyanomethylthio)benzothiazole (30%)	Busan 30 (Buckman)	Wood
Potassium N,N-dimethyl dithiocarbamate	Busan 1009 (Buckman)	Latex paint
Potassium N-hydroxymethyl-N-methyl-dithiocarbamate (32%) and sodium 2-mercaptobenzothiazole (8%)	Busan 52 (Buckman)	Water-thinned colloids, emulsion resins, emulsion paints, waxes, cutting oils, adhesives
2-(Thiocyanomethylthio)benzothiazole (32%) and 2-hydroxypropyl methanethiosulfonate (28%)	Busan 74 (Buckman)	Paint films
2-Bromo-4'-hydroxyacetophenone	Busan 90 (Buckman)	Pulp and paper mills, paper-making chemicals, felt
Poly[hydroxyethylene(dimethyliminio)-ethylene(dimethyliminio)]methylene dichloride (60%)	Busan 79 (Buckman)	Industrial water systems
Hexahydro-1,3,5-triethyl-s-triazine	Vancide TH (Vanderbilt)	Cutting oils, synthetic rubber latexes, adhesives, latex emulsions
Benzyl bromoacetate	Merbac-35 (Merck)	Paint raw materials (cellulose, casein)
5-Hydroxymethoxymethyl-1-aza-3,7-dioxabicyclo(3.3.0)octane (24.5%), 5-hydroxymethyl-1-aza-3,7-dioxabicyclo(3.3.0)octane (17.7%) and 5-hydroxypoly [methyleneoxy(74% C_2, 21% C_3, 4% C_4, 1% C_5)]methyl-1-aza-3,7-dioxabicyclo(3.3.0)octane (7.8%)	Nuosept 95 (Nuodex)	Latex paints

Table 52–2. *Industrial Biocides* (continued)

Composition	Trade names	Applications
Di(phenylmercuric)dodecenyl succinate	Super Ad-It (Nuodex)	Latex paint
Organic mercurials	Various	Paints
Ethyl p-hydroxybenzoate	Ethyl Parasept (Tenneco and others)	Adhesives, starch and gum solutions, inks, polishes, latexes, other emulsions
Methyl p-hydroxybenzoate	Methyl Parasept (do.)	
Propyl p-hydroxybenzoate	Propyl Parasept (do.)	
Butyl p-hydroxybenzoate	Butyl Parsept (do.)	
Sodium salt of 2-mercaptobenzothiazole	Nuodex 84 (Nuodex)	Adhesives, textiles, paper rug backings, waxes
β-Bromo-β-nitrostyrene (25%)	Giv-Gard BNS (Givaudan)	Water systems, lignosulfonates
Chloroxylenol	Ottasept (Ferro)	Vinyl emulsions
Chlorethylene bisthiocyanate 10%	Cytox 3810 (American Cyanamid)	Water systems, emulsions
Zinc 2-pyridinethiol-N-oxide 20%), 5,4'-dibromosalicylanilide (36%), 3,5,6-tribromosalicylanilide (36%) and other brominated salicylanilides (7%)	Omadine 645 (Olin)	Water-based latex, acrylic and PVA paints, joint cement, PCV plastic, adhesives
Zinc 2-pyridinethiol-1-oxide powder (95%), aqueous dispersion (48%)	Zinc Omadine (Olin)	Metalworking fluids, PCV plastic
Sodium 2-pyridinethiol-1-oxide powder (90%), aqueous solution (40%)	Sodium Omadine, Triadine 10 (Olin)	Metalworking fluids, vinyl and latex emulsions
2-2'-Oxybis-(4,4,6-trimethyl-1,3,2-dioxaborinane)-2,2'-(1-methyltrimethylenedioxy)-bis-(4-methyl-1,3,2-dioxaborinane) (95%)	Biobor JF (U.S. Borax)	Hydrocarbon fuels, ship fuels and marine storage, home heating fuels

From Sharpell, F. 1988. Biocides in specialty products. Chemspec USA '88 Symposium, pp. 79–82.

ity. Service records of good crossties of 20 different kinds of woods showed untreated ties to have an average life of 5.5 years. Those treated with zinc chloride at the rate of 0.5 lb/ft³ lasted 15 years, whereas those receiving 10 to 12 lb/ft³ of coal-tar creosote lasted about 30 years (Burton, 1944). In Great Britain, 8000 creosote-treated telegraph poles were still in service 70 years after their installation (Bennett and Bins, 1951).

Wood is invaded by a number of insects including powder-post beetles, carpenter ants, and the better-known dry wood and subterranean termites. In water environments, marine borers, which are worm-like animals related to shellfish, may destroy untreated wood pilings in less than a year. The fungi that produce rot and decay of wood are mainly related to the mushrooms and belong to the higher fungi, mainly to the class known as *Basidiomycetes*. Spore-forming bodies bearing toadstools or brackets appear on the side of rotting trees or stumps, while the mycelium inside the wood attacks and rots the wood fibers.

The decay fungi are of three main groups: the white rots, the brown rots, and the soft rots. The white rots attack mainly the lignin of the wood, leaving cellulose in pockets or streaks separated by areas of firm wood. The brown rots favor the cellulose and leave a brownish residue that can be readily crumbled into powder. Brown rots often cause decay in building timbers. The so-called dry rot is a brown rot. Dry rot is a misnomer since wood does not rot unless it has at least 30% moisture. Soft rots, which are made up of *Ascomycetes* and members of the *Fungi Imperfecti,* take their toll of cut timber in cooling water towers, house siding, and boats. Lower fungi may grow superficially on fresh lumber and pro-

duce colored sap stain, which is an important economic liability where appearance is a factor in the marketability of the lumber. It has been estimated that there is a loss of $5 to $25 per thousand board feet in upper grades of pine because of staining (Krause, 1950).

Types of Treatment

Wood preservatives are applied by impregnation methods, or by surface treatments such as dipping or brushing. The former are preferable, since the latter are suitable only for a short duration of service or less strenuous conditions. Windowsills and floorboards of a house may receive brush or spray treatments, but fence posts, telephone poles, and crossties are usually treated by pressure impregnation. Dipping is the most effective of the surface treatments since the preservative has an opportunity to reach the whole surface and penetrate into the wood to a small extent. Cracks and checks are penetrated, and the preservative helps to protect the interior of the wood, which otherwise would be vulnerable to penetration by fungi and termites. Millwork is often dipped for a few minutes with a clean, paintable preservative such as pentachlorophenol in a volatile oil. Green lumber may be steeped for days in a bath of a water-soluble preservative such as 5% zinc chloride. Another procedure for treating green lumber utilizes the diffusion process, whereby water-soluble salts such as chromates and fluorides are applied to the surface of the wood in the form of paste or cream and held in place by waterproof paper, permitting the salts to diffuse into the sap of the wood.

Better than surface application, but not as effective as pressure impregnation, is the hot and cold bath treatment. It requires little more than a soaking tank and

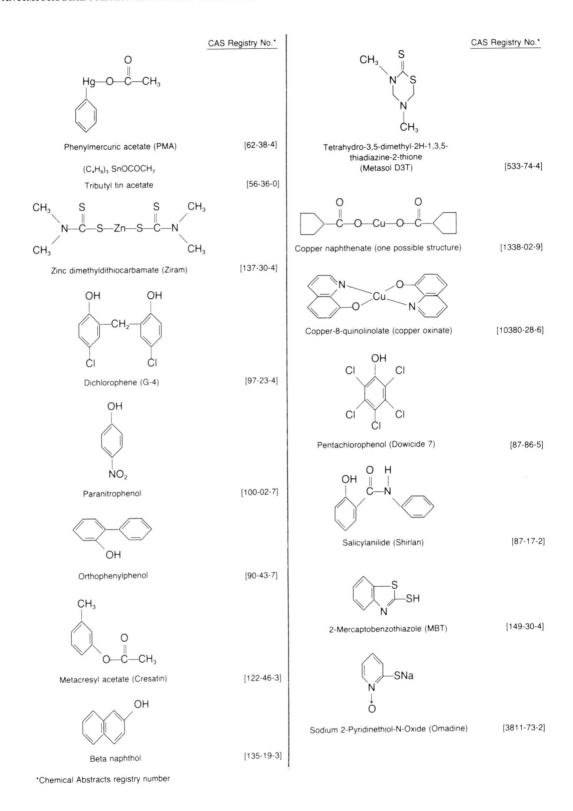

Fig. 52–1. Some organic compounds that serve as industrial biocides.

CAS Registry No.*

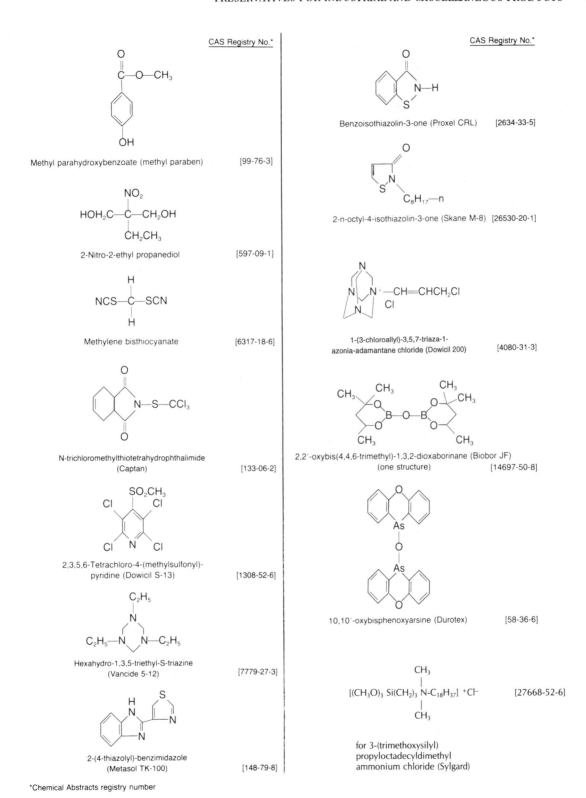

Methyl parahydroxybenzoate (methyl paraben)   [99-76-3]

2-Nitro-2-ethyl propanediol   [597-09-1]

Methylene bisthiocyanate   [6317-18-6]

N-trichloromethylthiotetrahydrophthalimide
(Captan)   [133-06-2]

2,3,5,6-Tetrachloro-4-(methylsulfonyl)-
pyridine (Dowicil S-13)   [1308-52-6]

Hexahydro-1,3,5-triethyl-S-triazine
(Vancide 5-12)   [7779-27-3]

2-(4-thiazolyl)-benzimidazole
(Metasol TK-100)   [148-79-8]

CAS Registry No.*

Benzoisothiazolin-3-one (Proxel CRL)   [2634-33-5]

2-n-octyl-4-isothiazolin-3-one (Skane M-8)   [26530-20-1]

1-(3-chloroallyl)-3,5,7-triaza-1-
azonia-adamantane chloride (Dowicil 200)   [4080-31-3]

2,2'-oxybis(4,4,6-trimethyl)-1,3,2-dioxaborinane (Biobor JF)
(one structure)   [14697-50-8]

10,10'-oxybisphenoxyarsine (Durotex)   [58-36-6]

$[(CH_3O)_3 Si(CH_2)_3 N-C_{18}H_{37}]^+Cl^-$ [27668-52-6]

for 3-(trimethoxysilyl)
propyloctadecyldimethyl
ammonium chloride (Sylgard)

*Chemical Abstracts registry number

Fig. 52-1 *continued.*

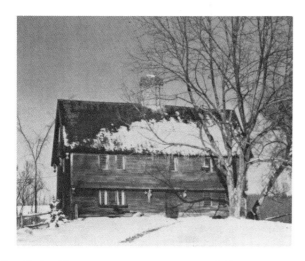

Fig. 52–2. The Parson Capen House in Topsfield, Massachusetts, built in 1683 and still standing, shows the potential durability of wood.

brings about appreciable penetration of the preservatives into the wood. Either oils or water-soluble preservatives may be employed. The lumber or poles are submerged in the liquid that is heated to about 100°C to expand the air in the cells of the wood. After several hours, the heating is discontinued and as the wood cools, the preservative is pulled into the wood to replace the air that was displaced during heating.

Pressure treatment requires more elaborate equipment, such as a pressure cylinder and pump, but it makes possible controlled penetration deep into the wood so as to afford maximum protection (Figs. 52–3, 52–4). Seasoned or green timber may be employed in the full-cell or empty-cell processes. In the full-cell process, a vacuum is first applied, then the hot preservative solution is released into the cylinder and is driven into the cells of the wood with pressure. This fills the wood with preservative.

In the empty-cell process, the cells in the wood, in effect, are just painted with preservative. This is accomplished by forcing the preservative solution into the wood against the pressure of the air in the cells (Lowry process) or by forcing more air into the wood prior to adding the preservative solution (Rueping process), and then withdrawing the excess preservative by the expansion of the entrapped air as the external pressure is removed. In all processes, a final vacuum treatment helps to remove excess liquid preservative from the surface of the lumber.

Another method of treatment of recent development might be called volatile solvent impregnation. In this method, a solution of the preservative in a volatile organic solvent is forced deeply into the wood fibers using a pressure-treating cycle. Upon release of the pressure and use of a vacuum, the solvent rapidly evaporates, leaving the nonvolatile preservative impregnated in the wood. The solvent is recovered by distillation for reuse. This treatment does not interfere with the dimensional stability of the wood or its ability to be painted or glued. One such process based upon this development employs

pentachlorophenol dissolved in butane, which is a liquid when under pressure (American Wood Preservers Association, 1963). Another process employs pentachlorophenol in methylene chloride. The solvent, which boils at 104°F, is removed from the wood with water vapor and recovered for reuse (Marouchoc, 1972).

Many different chemicals have been employed as wood preservatives. A chemical so used should have certain characteristics: It should be toxic to fungi, termites, marine borers, and other destructive organisms, but relatively safe to humans in normal handling and use. It should be liquid or capable of solution in common, cheap solvents. It should be stable, nonvolatile, and resistant to leaching. Of course it must not deteriorate the wood and should not corrode nails and metals used in the wood. It must be cheap at its effective concentration. Other characteristics that are desirable but not essential are that the preservative at its use-concentration provides no odor or color and no interference with the physical structure of the wood or its paintability. Creosote, for example, which is the preservative used in greatest volume, meets the former but not the latter criteria. One method of classifying wood preservatives is to divide them into three groups: (1) preservative oils, (2) water-soluble compounds, and (3) organic solvent-soluble compounds.

Preservative Oils

The preservative oils include coal tar creosote, petroleum oils, wood tar creosote, and water-gas tar creosote. Of these oils, coal tar creosote is the most important. It has been the No. 1 wood preservative of commerce for many years. Coal tar creosote is "a distillate of coal tar produced by high temperature carbonization of bituminous coal, consisting principally of liquid and solid aromatic hydrocarbons and contains appreciable quantities of tar acids and tar bases. It has a continuous boiling range of at least 125°C, beginning at about 200°C." The tar acids are phenolics—naphthols, cresols and xylenols; the bases include pyridines, quinolines, and acridines; and the hydrocarbons are made up of benzene, toluene, naphthalene, anthracene, and many other higher and lower ring structures (Roche, 1952). Creosote has the toxicity, longevity, resistance to leaching, and other desirable properties of a wood preservative, except for the aesthetic features. It is sometimes diluted with petroleum oil and sometimes fortified with pentachlorophenol, but usually is employed without admixture at retentions of 6 to 20 lb/ft³. Coal tar contains carcinogens and should be used with proper caution.

Water-Soluble Preservatives

Preservatives that are soluble in water have no fire or explosion hazard and as solids may be transported cheaply to the treatment plant. On the other hand, the treated wood has to be dried after treatment. Further, the wood swells in the presence of the water and shrinks and cracks as the water evaporates. Some water-borne treatments are easily leached out and may be employed

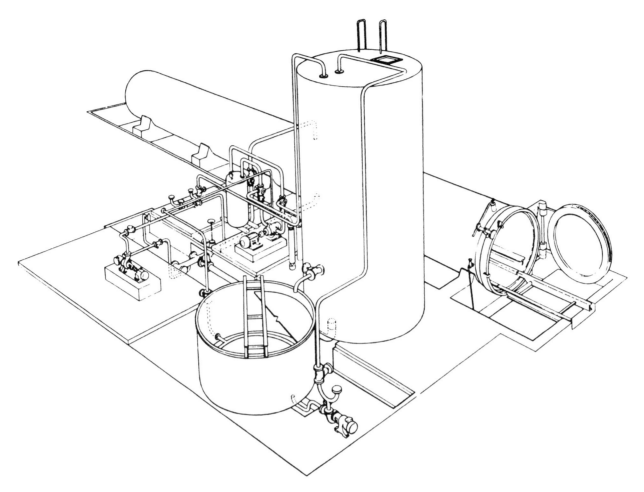

Fig. 52–3. Layout of a conventional pressure impregnation plant showing the cylinder fitted with quick-locking doors and rails for the feed bogies, the storage tank, the salt mixing tank, and the pipework. Courtesy of Hickson's Timber Products Ltd. From Richardson, B.A. 1978. *Wood Preservation*. Lancaster, England, The Construction Press.

where weathering is not a problem, as for example inside buildings. Some treatments become insoluble with evaporation of the water and give weather resistance. This may be accomplished by using complexes of salts with ammonia or acetic acid, as in the case of copper chromate, where the ammonia or volatile acid evaporates during drying, thus destroying the complex and precipitating the insoluble salt. Chromium salts, as in the case of chromated zinc chloride and chromated copper arsenate, are said to improve resistance to leaching over compounds without the chromium. Chromates are also toxic to fungi and help to prevent corrosion. Among the more commonly used water-soluble compounds are zinc chloride, copper sulfate, borax, copper chromate, sodium fluosilicate, sodium arsenate, sodium fluoride, sodium dinitrophenate, and sodium pentachlorophenate. These materials are often found in combination in trade name products such as Wolman salts, Tanalith, Boliden, Celcure, and Greensalts, to name a few. Very popular is CCA, chromated copper arsenate. Another formulation known as Chemonite, which is ammoniacal copper ar-

senate (ACA), has shown excellent service in use (Table 52–3) as reported by Morgan (1989). Boron compounds are favored in certain applications because they donate some resistance to fire in addition to decay and insect resistance. Further, they are less toxic than arsenic compounds for which they have been substituted. In fact, Curtis and Williams (1990) state that there is a current revolution toward the use of borates. In addition to providing rot and insect preservation, borates are promising in sap stain control in combination with other fungicides such as quaternary ammonium compounds. They have the disadvantage, however, of being more readily leached by water than other water-soluble treatments that become chemically fixed to the wood.

Solvent-Soluble Preservatives

The major preservatives applied in organic solvents other than creosote are pentachlorophenol and copper naphthenate. Pentachlorophenol is a powerful fungicide and deterrent to insects and has been a popular preservative for both surface applications and pressure impregnation. It gives a clean, colorless, and paintable finish.

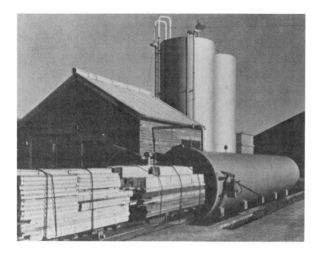

Fig. 52–4. Typical pressure impregnation plant with bogies for the charge, quick-locking doors, pump house, and storage tanks for two different preservatives. Courtesy of Hickson's Timber Products Ltd. From Richardson, B.A. 1978. *Wood Preservation*. Lancaster, England, The Construction Press.

Its volatility and solubility in water are both low. It is irritating on contact with the skin, but with normal precautions it is regularly handled without difficulty. In applications undergoing heavy weathering, pentachlorophenol may be dissolved in a heavy oil or in creosote, whereas in wood to be painted, it is dissolved in light petroleum solvents such as Stoddard solvent. A 5% solution is generally used to give 0.4 to 0.6 lb/ft³ of wood.

Like pentachlorophenol, copper naphthenate provides excellent protection against fungi and insects but ordinarily does not give a paintable surface. It has a blue-green color and a petroleum-like odor. For pressure impregnation, it is dissolved in a petroleum oil to give a 5% solution, but for surface treatment, four or five times this concentration is required. Copper naphthenate has been used a great deal for wood used in boats. Another copper wood preservative applied in volatile solvents is copper-8-quinolinolate (in solubilized form) which, although expensive compared to other preservatives used for wood, has the advantage of low mammalian toxicity and may be used to treat wood in contact with food, such as in fruit crates and in railroad cars.

A solvent-soluble material finding use as a wood preservative is tributyltin oxide. It is expensive but highly

Table 52–3. *Wood Preservation Tests of Ammoniacal Copper Arsenate (ACA). Forest Products Laboratory Stake Tests in Mississippi on 2.4 Inch Southern Yellow Pine, 39-Year Service*

Retention (lb/cu. ft)	% Destroyed	% Servicable*	% Good
0.24	50	50	0
0.51	10	70	20
0.97	0	0	100

*Shows some decay, termite attack, or both.

Morgan, J. III. 1989. The evaluation and commercialization of a new wood preservative. Am. Wood Preserv. Assoc. Proc., 85, 16–26.

active, so that it can be used in low concentration (0.06 lb/ft³). In contact with soil, it fails, but is useful in above-ground application. It is colorless and does not influence paint properties (Evans, 1973).

Among new biocides for wood preservation are alkylammonium compounds (AAC) (Barnes, 1985). Didecyldimethylammonium chloride was shown to be particularly effective. Other compounds showing promise include 3-iodo-2-propynl butyl carbonate, isothiazolinones, benzothiazoles, salicyanilide derivatives, sulfonamides, ammoniacal copper-fatty acids, and tetrachloroisophthalonitrile (Nicholas, 1983).

As in all cases where toxic agents are used, the government has imposed regulations. The EPA has classified creosote, pentachlorophenol, and inorganic arsenicals for "restricted use." This means that these products may no longer be sold to the general public, but are limited to certified applicators or persons under their direct supervision. An applicator certification program has been set up under the Federal Insecticide, Fungicide, and Rodenticide Act.

Other Methods

Gaseous fumigants have shown possibilities for protective treatment of wood. Hand et al. (1970) reported successful control of decay fungi and insects with Vapam (sodium-*N*-methyldithiocarbamate) poured into holes drilled in poles above the ground level. Vorlex (methylisothiocyanate) and chloropicrin (trichloronitromethane) also demonstrated effectiveness in stopping decay (Graham, 1973).

Fungal deterioration of wood may be prevented without fungicides by merely eliminating moisture or oxygen. In practice, the former is accomplished by drying the timber in kilns and storage above ground in covered shelters. The latter is practiced by storing fresh timber submerged under water (ponding) or in a container in which air is displaced by an inert gas such as carbon dioxide.

An interesting development is the resistance to fungi, termites, and marine borers of wood from pine trees treated with the herbicide paraquat (1,1'-dimethyl-4,4'-bipyridinium dichloride). When injured mechanically or by insects or disease, pine trees tend to seal off the damaged area by producing oleoresin and turpentine. It was discovered that paraquat treatment greatly increased the amount and speed of resin formation by the tree (Roberts, 1973) over that caused by injury. Trees treated with paraquat were cut 18 months later and field-tested for 2 years in soil and marine exposures. The untreated controls were destroyed completely in the terrestrial experiments, whereas only about 12% of the treated stakes were appreciably damaged by fungi or insects. Similar resistance to marine borers was demonstrated in marine exposure (Beal et al., 1979).

Particle board, made from wood and resins, is susceptible to biodeterioration, although less so than is solid wood (Toole and Barnes, 1974). Sodium pentachlorophenate was demonstrated to be protective when added to the resin on the basis of 0.3 to 0.65% of the dry weight of wood.

Tests of Effectiveness

Field service tests provide the only sure way to determine the effectiveness of a wood preservative, but proving a new material by this method may take a lifetime. For this reason, accelerated test methods are employed. Treatment and exposure of small stakes will often give satisfactory indication of the activity of a preservative in 1 to 5 years. The laboratory soil block method, using pure cultures of fungi (Smith and Gjovik, 1972) reduces the time to 3 months. The blocks are weighed before and after exposure to determine the amount consumed. An automatic respiratory analysis procedure claims to give results like the soil method in only 1 month (Smith, 1975). A strength test of wooden strips in a similar laboratory test is said to indicate decay in as little as 2 weeks (Connolly, 1961).

COTTON PRESERVATION

During World War II mile upon mile of cotton tent cloth was treated to prevent rotting. Tarpaulins, awnings, and tobacco shade cloth are a few of the hundreds of cotton items that receive preservative treatment. In addition jute, hemp, and flax, like cotton, are cellulosic fibers susceptible to rotting. Sandbags, ropes, and nets are among other fabrics that are treated to extend their useful life.

The cost of deterioration of cellulosic textiles was estimated to be as high as $100 million per year in 1924, and in World War II spoilage of tentage was claimed to be $48 million per year. Material losses due to spoilage in Viet Nam were estimated at $240 million per year (David and Barr, 1972). Being cellulosic in composition, cotton can be readily deteriorated by cellulose-decomposing fungi and bacteria. Although there is evidence that bacteria may play an important role in the biologic deterioration of cotton (Reuszer, 1945) in above-ground applications it is generally agreed that the fungi are the most active agents of decomposition. Fungi such as the rapid cellulose fermenter *Chaetomium globosum* (Thom et al., 1934) and the slow-growing angiocarpous fungi (Zuck and Diehl, 1946) have definitely been shown to be associated with the rotting of cotton fabrics in field exposure, and there are many other cellulose-decomposing fungi on the fabric that undoubtedly contribute to the deterioration. Untreated 10-ounce cotton duck lost 67% of its tensile strength in 1 year and 93% in 2 years in shade tests in Florida (Block, 1949). Similar results were obtained in tests in New Orleans (Dean and Worner, 1947) and in the Canal Zone (Barghoorn, 1945).

Types of Treatment

The Coppers

The most effective single group of compounds in protecting cotton and other cellulosic textile fibers such as jute, sisal, and hemp from microbiologic breakdown are the copper fungicides, and the most prominent copper fungicide is copper naphthenate. This bluish-green, waxy solid is one of the cheapest yet most effective preservatives for cellulosic fibers. It is more widely used than any other textile preservative. It has a low order of toxicity to humans and does not cause dermatitis. Derived from naphthenic acids of petroleum, copper naphthenate is not a pure compound, but a mixture of salts of related acids. It has the advantage of being soluble in many common organic solvents.

There is considerable evidence of the effectiveness of copper naphthenate. In service tests of copper-treated sandbags, Dean et al. (1946) rated different copper treatments and found copper naphthenate most effective on a basis of 1% copper metal. In Florida, copper naphthenate-treated cotton duck with 0.1%, 0.2%, and 0.5% of copper lost only 39%, 24%, and 13%, respectively, of its original strength after 2 years' outdoor exposure (Block, 1949). Most preservatives are much more effective when the material is in above-ground service than when it is in contact with or buried in the soil. The copper compounds, and copper naphthenate in particular, maintain their superiority in soil contact and soil burial. There are many reports in the literature attesting to the efficacy of copper naphthenate on soil-buried cotton (Siu, 1951). Marsh et al. (1944) showed that copper naphthenate prevents rotting of cotton fabric in soil at lower concentrations on the fabric than does copper oleate, copper "tallate," or copper hydrogenated resinate. The high preservative capacity of copper naphthenate was related to the fact that naphthenic acid is itself a fungicide. Copper-resistant fungi, such as *Aspergillus niger*, were shown to solubilize and permit leaching of copper from fabric treated with copper oleate and copper "tallate." The fungitoxicity of the naphthenic acid inhibited *Aspergillus* and *Penicillium* organisms and prevented this loss of copper through solubilization.

A combination of preservatives giving excellent results in service tests of rot-proofed sandbags was copper naphthenate plus creosote (Dean et al., 1946). Based on the rating of copper naphthenate alone as 100, copper naphthenate plus creosote rated 176, while the untreated control rated 9. Creosote, no doubt, functioned both as a fungicide and as a water repellent.

In practice, an amount of copper naphthenate equivalent to 0.6 to 0.8% copper is generally applied to fabric by a bath containing a volatile solvent such as mineral spirits. In military service, fabric may require treatment to render it rot proof, water repellent, and fire retardant. An example of such a fabric treatment, the Jeffersonville Quartermaster Depot #242 finish, was used by Barghoorn (1945) in rotting tests in the Canal Zone (Table 52-4).

There is some question as to whether copper naphthenate accelerates the oxidation of cellulose in the presence of sunlight. It is known that sunlight alone will deteriorate cotton fabric, and by measurement of cuprammonium fluidity, it is possible to distinguish be-

Table 52–4. *A Rot-Proof, Water-Repellent, and Fire-Retardant Finish Formula for Cotton Fabrics*

	%
42% chlorinated paraffin	26
70% chlorinated paraffin	13
Amberol M-88 (phenolic resin)	6.66
Rubbery pitch (asphalt)	3.7
Antimony oxide	20
Calcium carbonate	12
Copper naphthenate (as copper metal)	0.35
Hydrocarbon solvent	As needed

tween degradation resulting from biologic attack and that resulting from photochemical effects. In the case of biologic attack, the fluidity is lower than in the latter case (Dean and Worner, 1947). Copper sulfate appears to accelerate breakdown (Barlett and Goll, 1945), but there is considerable conflicting literature on copper naphthenate (Weatherburn, 1947). The conclusion expressed by Shanor et al. (1945) is that, even though a slight loss in the tensile strength of treated cloth might be experienced as a result of copper-accelerated oxidation, the great value of copper naphthenate in preventing degradation by microorganisms overbalances the other drawback. Screening pigments such as those used in the formulation in Table 52–4 function to prevent actinic degradation, as shown by Barghoorn (1945). On this subject, Bayley et al. (1965), who have studied the effect of pigments on actinic degradation, showed that, whereas the chromates of lead and zinc protect cellulose over a range of treatment concentrations, the chromates of copper and barium enhanced actinic degradation when used in low concentrations. Thus copper may be suspected as being a catalyst for this type of breakdown of cellulose textiles. A significant exception is the case of copper-8-quinolinolate.

Copper-8-quinolinolate is unique as an industrial preservative. Although it is many times more costly than copper naphthenate and other common preservatives, its high toxicity to microorganisms and other desirable properties have brought it into prominence. On laboratory media, "copper-8" in concentrations of fractions of a part per million will completely prevent the growth of many fungi. It is low in toxicity to humans, does not irritate the skin, and does not stiffen fabric. Its solubility in pure water is 0.8 ppm (Benignus, 1948). It has no odor, but has a characteristic yellow-green fluorescent color. It does not tender fabrics when exposed to actinic radiation. In fact, a study of photodegradation of cotton tentage treated with flame-, water-, weather-, and mildew-resistant finish (Reagan, 1975) showed that copper-8-quinolinolate was actually protective against photodegradation in addition to donating water repellancy and flame retardation to fabric exposed to extensive arc-light illumination. Despite its low solubility in water, it requires formulation with a repellent for best performance. "Copper-8" is not soluble in cheap solvents, and fabric treatment with it has been accomplished by dispersion

of the chemical in water or organic solvents, or by the two-bath process. In the two-bath process, the compound is formed in situ on the fabric by first dipping the cloth into a solution of 8-quinolinol (8-hydroxyquinoline) and then into a bath of copper acetate. Fortunately, a process was developed (Kalberg, 1951a and b) for solubilizing "copper-8" for use in common organic solvents. With solubilized "copper-8," better penetration of the preservative is obtained. Despite its relatively high cost, "copper-8" is required in many government specifications. It is used as 0.5 to 1.0% (0.1 to 0.2% copper) on the cloth.

Other copper preservatives for textiles are the copper soaps of fatty or oleoresinous acids, copper oleate, copper stearate, copper resinate, and copper tallate. They have many of the same characteristics of copper naphthenate, but in tests of treated sandbags, they were found to be inferior (Dean et al., 1946).

The copper ammonium complexes, cuprammonium hydroxide, cuprammonium carbonate, and cuprammonium fluoride, can be used where application with an inflammable solvent is undesirable. The basic copper compounds and salts dissolve in aqueous ammonia to give complexes stable in alkaline solution. The fabric is treated by the one-bath process, and ammonia is driven off by heating the cloth to approximately 80°C, thus rendering the treatment resistant to leaching. When proofing with cuprammonium compounds, a range of 1 to 1.5% copper is desirable, which is approximately twice that necessary with copper naphthenate.

Still other copper preservatives for cotton textiles include copper formate, copper phenyl salicylate, copper pentachlorophenate, copper chromate, and copper cupferron. The latter is a chelate and has shown many of the properties of copper-8-quinolinolate (Klens and Stewart, 1957). Copper borate has been incorporated in a zirconium complex, whereby it may be applied in water solution. Such a treatment containing 1% of copper and 2.4% of zirconyl acetate protected cotton cloth in outdoor weathering in New Orleans for 14 months with only 28% loss of tensile strength and no mildew stains (Conner et al., 1964). Another evaluation of the copper borate-zirconium treatment showed it to provide good microbial protection relative to copper-8-quinolinolate (Greenberger and Kaplan, 1977). For further information on copper and zinc preservatives see Chapter 21.

Other Metals

Preservatives with metals other than copper have a limited use, in applications in which copper may be undesirable. For example, zinc naphthenate is colorless and may be employed where the blue-green color of copper naphthenate is objectionable. Zinc naphthenate is only about half as effective as copper naphthenate (Cavill et al., 1949); therefore it must used in higher concentration to afford the same protection. Copper compounds catalyze the oxidation of rubber and cannot be used in any products containing rubber. Zinc dimethyldithiocarbamate, a vulcanization catalyst, is used in such applications.

A number of organic mercury salts have been tested as preservatives for cotton. They have strong fungicidal action but tend to break down in weathering. An organic lead compound, N-(tributylplumbyl)imidazole, was shown to be an effective preservative for cotton fabric in soil burial tests. The treated fabrics were colorless and odorless and had a good hand (Donaldson et al., 1970), but the possibility of toxicity due to the lead would seem to be a deterrent to acceptance. Tributylin oxide at 0.1% was shown to be as effective in exposure tests as 2.0% pentachlorophenol laurate (Miller, 1972), but this treatment suffers from deterioration by ultraviolet radiation and loss of activity in soil contact.

Cadmium selenide is an interesting protectant for cotton fabric. After 2 years of outdoor weathering, fabric containing only 0.13% of selenium as cadmium selenide, plus sun-screening pigments, retained 60% of its initial strength (Brysson et al., 1963). The selenide, which is inactive against fungi, is apparently converted by sunlight to the active selenite. The sun-screening pigments control the rate of this reaction.

Organic Preservatives

Nonmetallic, organic preservatives for cotton include the phenolics, the amine salts, and the sulfur compounds. Of these, the phenolics have received greatest attention.

Dichlorophene, chemically 2,2'-methylene-bis (4-chlorophenol), is one of the fungicides that appeared and gained popularity during World War II. A relative of hexachlorophene, dichlorophene showed its excellent protective properties in tests on cotton fabric.

Marsh and Butler (1946) tested a large number of other bisphenols as cotton fabric preservatives, but none was superior to dichlorophene. In the Canal Zone (Barghoorn, 1945) cotton duck treated with 2% dichlorophene and water repellent showed no loss in strength after ground contact for 7 weeks and after soil burial for 4 weeks. There was 59% loss after 13 weeks in the soil. Dichlorophene is insoluble in water but may be applied to cloth by first dissolving it in an alcohol and diluting this solution with a petroleum solvent. As with other similar preservatives, a water repellent is desirable to help prevent leaching. The compound is colorless and nonirritating to the skin, has low toxicity, and is active against both mildew and rot fungi.

Salicylanilide, or "Shirlan," has given satisfactory service in textiles for many years. Selected from many compounds, salicylanilide was found to have the best combination of desirable properties (Fargher et al., 1930). It is effective against both rotters and mildews, has practically no odor, does not color fabrics, and is not hazardous to use. Like other phenolic compounds, it is susceptible to leaching in outdoor weathering and should be used with a water repellent.

Esters of pentachlorophenol, particularly pentachlorophenyl laurate, have had considerable use for rot-proofing cotton textiles, applied as 2% on the cloth. They are quite resistant to leaching but sensitive to photochemical breakdown (Hueck et al., 1968). Dichlorophen oxychlorophenol at 1% concentration in laboratory tests against cellulolytic fungi was shown to be more inhibitory than 1% dichlorophene or 1% ziram. The protection was improved when the fungicide was used with melamine formaldehyde copolymer (Szostak-Kotowa et al., 1979).

Mercaptobenzothiazole is an effective organic sulfur fungicide, toxic to superficial molds and cellulose-decomposing fungi. Application may be made from alcohol or by preparing a concentrate in Cellosolve, which may be diluted with volatile petroleum solvents. This compound has been used in combination with zinc dimethyldithiocarbamate (Somerville, 1957).

An area of interest for potential protectants are organic compounds that break down slowly to release formaldehyde. Tests with several such compounds (Amin et al., 1975) demonstrated that cotton fabrics subject to soil burial had rot resistance in relation to the amount of formaldehyde released.

A fundamentally different approach for textile preservation does not use antiseptic chemicals, but chemically modifies the cellulose so that it cannot be digested by microorganisms. Such processes include acetylation, cyanoethylation, and methylol-melamine resin treatment. These treatments have their advantages and disadvantages. Among the latter is that although they impart rot resistance, they do not prevent the growth of molds and algae that grow on the surface of fabric and stain it. Evidence indicates that reaction of the resin polymer with the cellulose is preferable but not essential for protection (Kaplan et al., 1972).

Northrop and Rowe (1987) are interested in the deterioration of textile fibers from a different angle, namely the use of these fibers as trace evidence in criminal investigations. They buried textiles composed of man-made fibers, acrylic, polyester, polyamide, and cellulose acetate in soil. The cellulose acetate fibers were completely degraded in 4 to 9 months, whereas the others showed no alteration in 12 months. Singer and Rowe (1989), following this forensic work, showed that rayon fibers decomposed even more rapidly than cellulose acetate and triacetate; microscopic examination then could not be used for their identification.

WOOL PRESERVATION

Wool is a protein fiber and is much more resistant to attack by fungi than is cotton. It can be deteriorated by the "athlete's foot" fungus, *Trichophyton interdigitale*, as Rogers et al. have shown (1940), but deterioration, when it does occur, is generally brought about by proteolytic bacteria such as *Bacillus mesentericus*, *B. subtilis*, and *B. fusiformis* (Burgess, 1924; Shaposhnikov et al., 1964). Because bacteria require much higher quantities of moisture than fungi, there is little deterioration of wool unless it is wet. Soil-buried wool is quickly decomposed, as is soil-buried cotton. From a microbiologic standpoint, however, the important economic problem in wool preservation is the prevention of the growth of surface molds that do not decompose the wool but that spot and stain it and frequently make it unmarketable.

Mildew or bacterial infection may also result in uneven dyeing of the wool. Pure scrubbed wool is practically nonsusceptible to mildew, but there is usually sufficient organic matter in the wool in the form of oils, soaps, conditioning agents, and dust to support mold growth (Burgess, 1929). Wool is more hygroscopic than cotton and will mildew in an atmosphere of lower relative humidity, for, as has been shown (Block, 1953a), the higher the equilibrium moisture content of a material, the lower is the relative humidity at which it will mildew, other things being equal. Chemical degradation of wool and increased water solubility caused by ultraviolet radiation increase the susceptibility to mildew (Burgess, 1934).

Burgess (1924, 1928, 1930, 1931, 1934) made a thorough study of the problems associated with the growth of microorganisms in wool. He tested 150 preservatives and found only sodium fluoride, sodium fluosilicate, and salicylanilide to be satisfactory. Sodium fluosilicate was not as effective against molds as was salicylanilide, but it was more active as a bactericide. In addition, it imparted some moth-repelling properties to the wool.

Chromium in a concentration of 1% prevents mildew. Bayley and Weatherburn (1945) recommended the use of 1% of potassium dichromate on the goods as a preservative for woolen blankets, sleeping bags, and socks for use in the jungle. As used in the dyeing of wool, chromium gives resistance to mildew, but it apparently acts by removing the degradation products that support mold growth and not as an antiseptic, for the concentration of potassium dichromate is insufficient to stop mildew. Nitschke (1961) reported that, although chromium compounds gave inferior antibacterial and antifungal resistance than does fluorodinitrobenzene or bis (chloromethyl) dimethylbenzene, the application is simpler and more economical.

Woolen felts used in the papermaking process are continually wet and subject to microbial plugging and deterioration caused by bacterial and fungal growth. *Sphaerotilus natans* and other filamentous bacteria were found to accumulate a deposit of ferric hydroxide around them, which agglomerates with the clay and fiber in the circulating paper mill water to destroy the filtering properties (Drescher, 1957). Treatment with any of the better cotton biocides is effective. In some mills woolen felts have been replaced with synthetics made of polyester or polypropylene to alleviate this problem.

Deterioration of wool by microorganisms is serious in storage and shipment and in the processing mills. For the first problem, Burgess (1931) recommended ventilation of the storage containers and the holds of the ships, in addition to a preservative treatment with salicylanilide. In the mill, fungus is more difficult to control than bacterial growth, for the latter is no problem if the water is kept slightly acid. Preservatives may be added at several stages of the processing of wool in the plant (Burgess, 1931). In the winding process, 2% of salicylanilide may be applied with the water for conditioning the cloth. In mill runs, 0.6% of salicylanilide and 0.67% of sodium o-phenylphenate were satisfactory. During the oiling process, 0.2% of salicylanilide on the wool, applied in the olive oil-water mixture, gave protection for over 22 days. Undyed wool was kept free of mildew and in good condition at 100% humidity for 2 years in a closed container with p-dichlorobenzene crystals (Block, 1951).

ANTIBACTERIAL TEXTILE FINISHES

Aside from use in the prevention of deterioration, antimicrobial agents have been used on textiles to reduce odors from bacterial decomposition and to reduce the risk of infection resulting from fabrics that are contaminated with pathogenic microorganisms. Materials that have been treated or are proposed for treatment include personal items such as undergarments, bedding, shoe liners, towels, sanitary napkins, bandages, handkerchiefs, diapers, and nonpersonal materials such as upholstery, rugs, and draperies. Turner (1967) states that in 1959 more than 1 billion dollars worth of fabrics with bacteriostatic finishes were sold in the United States.

Hurst et al. (1958) demonstrated that air in hospital laundry chutes contained pathogenic bacteria presumably coming from the contaminated laundry. Stuart (1957) cited the treatment of surgical drapes with a residual bacteriostat prior to heat sterilization as having been shown to keep down the bacterial count during long operations. He also noted that treatment of diapers and bed pads with antibacterial agents has been demonstrated to be of practical value in preventing the formation of ammonia from urea by bacteria in the urine of infants and incontinent patients. Textile finishes on the market go under such names as antibacterial finishes, biostatic fabrics, sanitizing finishes, odor preventers, and fabric fresheners.

Gagliardi (1962) grouped antibacterial finishes into nondurable and durable finishes. The nondurable finishes were produced by treating the fabric with antibacterial chemicals. Some of the chemicals that have been used or recommended are bithionol, trichlorocarbanilide, neomycin, silver thiocyanate, rosin amine pentachlorophenate, phenylmercuric acetate, tributyltin oxide, hexachlorophene, pentachlorophenol, lauryl pyridinium chloride, and t-octylphenoxyethoxy-ethyldiethylbenzylammonium chloride.

The durable finishes were listed as five general types: (1) fiber reaction and metastable bond, (2) thermosetting antibacterial agents, (3) coordination compounds, (4) ionic bonding, and (5) regenerative principle. These methods include various ways to bind a toxic agent to the fabric through the use of resins, complexing reactions, etc. For example, Hg, Ag, R_3Sn, or PhHg as 3% of the cation salts of bis(methoxymethyl) carboxymethylamino-methyl triazine that was heat-cured on cotton resisted ten standard alkaline washes. Two percent of the silver derivative of a nitrogen heterocyclic compound, as levulinic acid hydantoin, which was reacted with the fibers and a thermosetting resin (urea-formaldehyde) resisted 25 washes. A bactericidal finish for cotton and cotton-polyester textiles employing zinc acetate and hydrogen peroxide that claims to retain activity through 50 launderings was developed by the USDA (Dana et al., 1979). With 4.2% on the fabric, the analysis shows 2.7% zinc and 0.74% H_2O_2. After 20 launderings, the zinc was reduced to 0.6% and the peroxide to 0.23%.

For bacteria to be killed on a fabric, even in the presence of antibacterial agents, some moisture must be present. Otherwise, the bacteria or spores are not killed by the chemical agent. Thus, the environmental conditions play a large part in determining effectiveness of antibacterial fabric treatments. These factors must be taken into account in testing procedures, as considered by Hoffman et al. (1955) for so-called self-sterilizing and self-disinfecting surfaces. More methods are considered by Lashen (1971).

Treated stockings and shoe linings are claimed to have cured athlete's foot and reduced foot odor according to a patent (Yamanchi, 1980). The items to be protected were treated with binder (100 parts) containing 60 parts of polyvinyl acetate emulsion, foaming agents (30 parts), ethylene glycol (5 parts), antifoam agent (0.1 part), 50-μm size copper powder (25 parts), copper-silver alloy (1 part), and enough water to give a viscosity of 8000 centipoises. This was then screen-printed on the soles of cotton-nylon socks and heated for 1 minute at 120°C.

In hospitals the spread of *Staphylococcus aureus* infections has been a problem. It has been shown that this organism is able to survive laundering and can be transferred to different items in the laundry. The impregnation of woolen blankets with 0.5% cetyltrimethylammonium bromide to give 0.125% on the weight of the blanket was recommended to render the blanket sterile and self-disinfecting (Barnard, 1952). Goldsmith et al. (1956) reported that cotton was rendered bacteriostatic more readily than wool or nylon.

A major development in the market came with the fixing of the quaternary to the fabric, or other surface, with an organic silicon compound. This treatment, developed by Dow Corning Corporation under the name Sylgard or antimicrobial agent 5700, is chemically 3-trimethoxysilypropyloctaecyldimethylammonium chloride. According to Gettings and Triplett (1978), this treatment imparts a durable antimicrobial finish to textiles that is active against bacteria, fungi, yeasts, and algae. Treated with this finish are odor-resistant socks, under the Bioguard trademark of Burlington Industries. Other textile items treated by Sylgard to combat the deleterious effects of microorganisms, foul odor, mildew, and rot, were cotton and polyester sheeting, carpets, underwear, outerwear, nylon hosiery, mattress ticking, filter fabrics, and nonwoven fabrics.

For odor abatement, Bioguard-treated orlon/nylon socks were tested against bacteria isolated from used,

Table 52–5. *Surface Test of Antibacterial-Treated Nonwoven Surgical Drape Cloth*

| Sample | % Reduction in Bacterial Count[1] in Minutes | | | | |
	3	5	30	60	120
A[2]	0	0	0	0	0
B[3]	2	5	0	0	0
C[4]	0	0	0	0	0
D[5]	3	17	59	62	72

[1]Inoculum: 90% defibrinated sheep blood contaminated with *Klebsiella pneumoniae* ATCC 4352
[2]Green surgical linen
[3]Nonwoven table cover from J&J Laparotomy Pack
[4]HiLoft-untreated control
[5]HiLoft with Dow Corning 5700 antibacterial agent (Sylgard)-ISO-BAC fabric

White, W.C. and Olderman, J.M. 1983. Antimicrobial techniques for medical nonwovens. Dow Corning Corp. and American Converters.

untreated socks. Above 90% reduction in bacterial numbers was obtained with *Micrococcus* spp., *Staphylococcus epidermidis*, *Acintobacter calcoaceticus*, and *Staphylococcus aureus*. *Enterobacter aglomerans* was reduced 69%. After 40 wash cycles Bioguard-treated socks were reduced 98.1% over the count on untreated socks. This was true whether water alone or a number of commercial detergents were used in the washing (Gettings and Triplett, 1978).

Aseptic surgery followed some years after Lister's introduction of antiseptic surgery, and surgeons have been using surgical gowns and drapes since before the turn of this century. The purpose, of course, is to prevent infective microorganisms from entering the field of surgery. A major advance was made when Beck (1952) showed that bacteria pass through layers of absorbent linen with "instantaneous rapidity," but that a nonwoven fabric treated with a water-repellent finish resisted bacterial transmission and appeared to be "ideal as a bacterial barrier." A series of research papers, reviewed by White and Olderman (1983), confirm Beck's finding in tests of woven and nonwoven fabric for surgical drapes and gowns. With the use of Sylgard, Dow Corning and American Converters have taken the nonwoven fabric one step further by treating it with a durable antimicrobial finish, as shown in Table 52–5 (White and Olderman, 1983; Hayes and White, 1984). In addition to surgical drapes, this material (ISO-BAC) is recommended for treated bandages, sponges, surgical masks, baby diapers, and adult incontinent pads. The Sylgard treatment was approved by the EPA and the FDA.

LEATHER PRESERVATION

Leather, like wool, is a proteinaceous material. Its susceptibility to attack by microorganisms in some ways resembles that of wool and in some ways differs. The differences result in part from the unique processing that leather undergoes. This includes salting, pickling, bating, tanning, and finishing. Before they are tanned, skins to be used for leather are susceptible to rotting by bacteria, but the finished leather is not rotted even in soil burial (Kanagy et al., 1946). When army shoes fell apart in the New Guinea campaign (Anon., 1942) the difficulty was traced to deterioration of the cotton stitching rather than to damage to the leather itself (Abrams, 1948).

The same superficial mold flora that contaminates wool grows on leather. Most common are the penicillia and aspergilli.

While mildew does not cause any appreciable deterioration of the hide substance in leather, there may be an increase in stiffness and loss in tensile strength. The grain also is weakened and tends to crack, according to tests made at the Bureau of Standards (Kanagy et al., 1946). It has been demonstrated that, in addition to the water-soluble constituents, the fatty oils and particularly the stuffing grease make finished leather susceptible to mildew (Abrams, 1948). The deleterious changes in the physical properties of leather after mold growth have been attributed, at least in part, to the removal of the grease.

Much work has been done on preservatives for leather. For the finished leather, the organic mercurials successfully control mildew when employed in low concentration. Concentrations of 0.05 to 0.1% of phenylmercuric stearate, phenylmercuric oleate, or phenylmercuric 2-ethyl hexoate prevented mold growth on leather at 100% relative humidity, whereas 0.5% of the best nonmercury fungicide, pentachlorophenol, was required under the same conditions (Block, 1953b). Cordon et al. (1949) found 0.03% of phenylmercuric acetate or phenylmercuric lactate complex to be effective, as were also 0.2% of a phenylmercuric octadecanoic complex and 3% of pentachlorophenol.

The mercurials have not been used extensively because they may cause dermatitis on prolonged skin contact, as shown by Lollar (1944) for leather bearing 0.75% of three mercurials.

Paranitrophenol is the compound workers have found most suitable as a leather antiseptic, and consequently it has been employed more extensively than any other material for this purpose. Jordan (1934) reported p-nitrophenol more effective than beta-naphthol in preventing mildew. For chrome-tanned leather, which is more resistant to fungi than vegetable-tanned leathers, 0.1% p-nitrophenol or a similar concentration of chlorophenol salts was satisfactory (Richardson, 1940). In tests of ten fungicides on two kinds of leather by the agar plate, soil burial, and tropical chamber methods, the highest activity was shown by p-nitrophenol in all cases (Hollingsworth, 1976). Based on tests of 40 selected fungicides, Lollar (1944) recommended 0.5% p-nitrophenol or p-chloro-m-xylenol in commercial leathers where maximum resistance to molds is desired. In patch tests for dermatitis, he found no irritation with 0.75% p-nitrophenol in 48 hours. Reporting on tests of fungicide-treated leather conducted cooperatively at four different

laboratories, Kanagy et al. (1948) concluded that p-nitrophenol and pentachlorophenol were most effective. No mercurials were included in these tests. Pentachlorophenol was even more fungitoxic than p-nitrophenol (0.25% compared to 0.35% for protection) but was not favored because of its tendency to cause skin irritation. With a combination of p-nitrophenol and pentachlorophenol, however, the quantity of pentachlorophenol and p-nitrophenol may be cut to 0.1% each, and the leather dressing will control the growth of Aspergillus niger (Abrams, 1948). At this concentration of 0.2% total fungicides, the leather may be used on articles that come in contact with the body. This fungicidal composition, developed at the National Bureau of Standards, was the basis for a mixture for use on leathers supplied to soldiers in the tropical regions during the latter part of World War II. Except in the case of white leathers, where other compounds must be substituted, the yellow color of p-nitrophenol is no drawback because it is masked by the natural color of the leather. Although p-nitrophenol is fairly soluble in water, it has been shown to be effective even after vigorous washing of the treated leather in distilled water.

Second to p-nitrophenol in order of preference, the British Leather Manufacturers Research Association (1945) named beta-naphthol. It is an old-line antiseptic and fungicide that has been recommended for leather by many workers. Orthman and Higby (1929) found beta-naphthol to be both economical and effective in keeping molds from growing on hides during tanning and dyeing. Abrams (1948) found that, after leaching, it took 0.82% beta-naphthol to eliminate Aspergillus niger, compared to 0.65% for p-nitrophenol. Other compounds that have been recommended include p-chloro-m-xylenol and salicylanilide (Lollar, 1944), tetrachlorophenol (Greene and Lollar, 1944), 2-methyl-1,4-naphthoquinone (Cordon et al., 1949), and cresylic acid (British Leather Manufacturers Association, 1945).

Dahl and Kaplan (1957, 1958, 1960, 1961) made an extensive examination of chemicals that might serve as preservatives for leather. They found chloro-p-nitrophenol to be less water soluble and more fungicidal than p-nitrophenol. Almost as active against fungi but less irritating to the skin, colorless, and insoluble in water was tetrachlorohydroquinone. Esters of p-nitrophenol such as bis(p-nitrophenol) carbonate and bis(o-chloro-p-nitrophenol) carbonate were found to demonstrate about the same activity of the free phenols but were colorless and insoluble in water. An effective nonphenolic fungicide for leather, 5,6-dichloro-2-benzoxazolinone, was found to have the desirable physical properties and to protect vegetable-tanned sole leather at 0.4% and chrome-tanned leather at lower concentrations. In the preservation of military leather, Prentiss and Sigafoos (1979) reported the fungicide Kathon LP (n-octyl-4-isothiazol-3-one) provided good protection to wet blue leather.

Work has also proceeded toward treatments to render leather antibacterial. Leather used in fabricating pros-

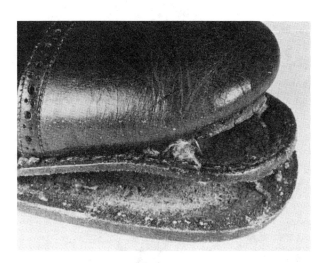

Fig. 52–5. Leather-soled shoe showing separation of the sole due to biodeterioration of the welt thread. From Pettit, D., and Abbott, S.G. 1975. Biodeterioration of footwear. In *Microbial Aspects of the Deterioration of Materials.* Edited by R.J.G. Gilbert and D.W. Lovelock. London, Academic Press, pp. 237–253.

theses for amputees is subject to attack by skin bacteria and by chemicals in the sweat. The leather retains odors, undergoes cracking and degradation, and stains clothing. Chrome-tanned horsehide harnesses used in prostheses have been shown to have a useful life as short as 1 month. Leonard and DeFries (1955) found that a coating of alcohol-soluble nylon prevented deterioration of the leather for periods of over 1 year of use. Treatment of the coating with 2,2′-methylenebis(3,4,6-trichlorophenol), i.e., hexachlorophene, or 2,2′-thiobis(4,6-dichlorophenol), i.e., actamer, produced bacteriostatic properties. In a review of bacteriostatic and fungistatic finishes, the types of compounds needed to achieve a permanent bactericidal effect were discussed (Centres de Recherches, 1965).

Although leather is resistant to microbiologic deterioration, other components of footwear such as the linen welt threads (Fig. 52–5), cotton vamp linings, and bonded cellulose insole boards undergo degradation caused by microorganisms. Figure 52–6 shows linings from a pair of shoes worn in a 6-month trial. The lining on the left was badly rotted, whereas that on the right, treated with a fungicide, showed only a few small holes due to abrasion (Pettit and Abbott, 1975).

Preservatives not only are important for the finished leather but are employed in many stages of leather processing, where skins, hides, and some tanning materials may be damaged by microorganisms. Mold may grow on dried hides and skins, and fungicides have been incorporated in salt used in curing (Stuart and Frey, 1934). During the soaking process, bacteria and molds damage skins and hides, causing offensive odor, excessive hair slippage, and some destruction of the collagen fibers (Buckman Laboratories, 1949).

Cordon and co-workers (1961) showed that in the unhairing process both the enzyme employed and the leather itself could be attacked and degraded if the bacterial population in the bath exceeded 10^8 per ml. Phenol-type bactericides and organic mercurials in less than 0.1% effectively suppressed bacterial growth, whereas without these agents the bacteria exceeded 3×10^8 per ml in 1 day.

Although pickling is designed to preserve skins, in this process mold and yeasts may stain and damage skins. If pickling is effected at a sufficiently high acidity, pH 2.4, with the proper quantity of sodium chloride, and preferably with acetic acid, mold growth is prevented (Pleass, 1935). Acetic acid was found better for this purpose than formic, salicylic, or benzoic acids. Vegetable tanning liquors are subject to attack by bacteria, yeasts, and molds. Of these, the molds are the most important, for certain molds, as *Aspergillus niger* and certain of the penicillia, produce an enzyme, tannase, which destroys tannin and causes the tanner to suffer economic loss (Richardson, 1941). A selective disinfectant is desirable to prevent mold and yeast growth but to permit the lactic acid bacteria to continue their desired fermentative activities. The British Leather Manufacturers Association (1945) has recommended treatments for use at different stages of leather processing and has given specific directions.

Woods et al. (1973) have found that the great losses from decay of leather result from bacterial action on the raw hide prior to penetration by the salt curing. Money (1974) describes a treatment that is said to give short-term preservation eliminating salt curing, at considerably less cost, allowing time for transport or for hide packs to be built up before processing. The fresh hides are treated with a dilute solution of sodium chlorite, calcium hypochlorite, or zinc chloride plus sodium pentachlorophenate or phenol and can then be held for several days without damage. Zinc chloride was safest and cheapest. Busan 72, 2-(thiocyano-methylthio)benzothiazole, at less than 0.025%, prevented fungal growth on wet blue hides for over 90 days, while methylene bisthiocyanate and beta-naphthol gave the same protection at 0.1% (Galloway and Cooper, 1974).

For sterilization, cleaning, and reconditioning of used army shoes, Greene (1945) recommended treatment with aqueous formaldehyde, followed by a wash with soap and a treatment with an oil containing pentachlorophenol.

There is a potential health hazard in working with hides and skins in tanneries, especially those that are imported. In such cases, it is essential that the materials be sterilized, for which a solution of sodium fluoride or sodium silicofluoride is recommended. This helps to prevent the spread of anthrax and foot-and-mouth disease (O'Flaherty and Doherty, 1939).

Greene and Lollar (1944) developed a formula for an army dubbing containing for its preservative 0.8% each of *p*-nitrophenol, *p*-chloro-*m*-xylenol, and tetrachlorophenol. Kanagy et al. (1948) give a formula for a fungicidal leather dressing employing *p*-nitrophenol, which was adopted by the Office of the Quartermaster General.

Since most leather fungicides are fat soluble and are

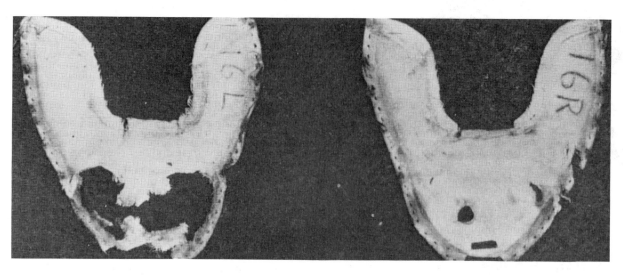

Fig. 52–6. Linings from a pair of shoes worn in a 6-month trial. The untreated lining from the left shoe is badly rotted; the other lining, treated with a fungicide, shows only two small holes, which are due to abrasion. From Pettit, D., and Abbott, S.G. 1975. Biodeterioration of footwear. In *Microbial Aspects of the Deterioration of Materials.* Edited by R.J.G. Gilbert and D.W. Lovelock. London, Academic Press, pp. 237–253.

lost when the grease migrates to the surface, work was performed to bind the agent to the collagen, releasing the fungicide only under warm, moist conditions favoring mold growth (Bowes et al., 1970).

PAINT PRESERVATION

In water-emulsion paints, preservatives are required to prevent decomposition of certain ingredients by bacteria, with resulting gas formation that may cause the can to swell or blow up. The paint film, after it has been applied, may be susceptible to mildew attack and should be preserved. Antifouling paints for ship bottoms must discourage the growth of the many types of micro- and macrobiologic plant and animal forms in order to keep the hulls as free as possible from fouling organisms. For breweries, packing houses, and hospitals, antiseptic paints are desirable. Lacquers and other coatings for electronic equipment should be inhibitory or inert to fungi that, in growth, produce moisture that causes electrical leakage and faulty operation of the equipment.

Mildew of painted surfaces has received considerable attention. The reason is self-evident. A house painted white may be gray and dingy in appearance in 6 months to 1 year under conditions favorable to mildew, and the cost of repainting is many times greater than the cost of the paint itself. The composition of the paint to a great extent determines its susceptibility to mildew. Natural oils, plasticizers, emulsifying agents, thickening agents, etc., serve as sources of carbon for fungi. Impurities and some organic constituents supply nitrogen and other essential nutrients. Substitution of inert resins increases resistance to mildew. In general, it can be said that a quick-drying, hard film will be more resistant to mildew than a tacky, soft film. The hard film not only catches less dirt and fewer mold spores, but also has a lower moisture content under equal conditions of humidity

(Harnden, 1945). In exposure tests in New Guinea, chlorinated rubber was the best vehicle for mildew resistance, alkyds and polyvinyl alcohol were intermediate, and linseed oil was by far the worst (Rischbieth et al., 1974).

In outdoor exposure of paint films, the most common fungus is *Aureobasidium (Pullularia) pullulans.* This ubiquitous scavenger has the ability to adhere tenaciously to the surface, to withstand extremes of temperature, and to resist desiccation. Furthermore, due to melanin production, which gives it a black color resembling dirt, the fungus is also resistant to ultraviolet radiation. Other black-colored fungi that do not produce melanin are not able to withstand the ultraviolet rays of sunlight. Thus, *Aureobasidium pullulans* competes successfully with other fungi such as *Aspergillus, Cladosporium, Alternaria,* and *Mucor* that colonize the film. Zabel and Terracina (1980) showed that this organism does not feed upon or break down the paint film, but disfigures it by using it as an inert sponge to derive moisture and obtains its carbon from detritus that deposits on the paint. Although it resists desiccation, it would not grow at 100% relative humidity, but required liquid water. Certain algae have been shown to grow on painted surfaces and resist desiccation. They are light green when moist and actively growing but dark green, almost black, when old and dry (Block, 1982). Paint films that are water resistant, such as chlorinated rubber, mentioned previously, are more resistant to fungi. Zinc oxide in paint serves to harden the paint and make it water resistant.

Data show that bacteria multiply at the interface between a wooden surface and the paint. The presence of large numbers of bacteria at this interface of weathered paint that failed by peeling implicates the microorganisms in the deterioration of the coating (Ross, 1964).

Zinc Oxide

Perhaps the chemical most widely used as a mold inhibitor for paint has been zinc oxide (Gardner et al., 1934; Vannoy, 1948). This compound is not specifically a preservative but is a normal component of the pigment formulation of paint. Gardner et al. (1934) reported that white lead paint formulations containing zinc oxide always showed inhibition of mildew, while those without zinc oxide did not. The quantity of zinc oxide is important since, in tests extending over 5 years, Vannoy (1948) showed that paint with only 30% of the pigment as zinc oxide become badly mildewed, whereas paint with 50% zinc oxide had no mildew. Harnden (1945) stated that zinc pigments are poor mildewcides but that zinc oxide is effective because of its property of hardening the paint film. Salvin (1944), on the other hand, demonstrated that zinc oxide inhibits respiration of fungus spores and prevents mycelial growth, although it does not kill the fungus.

In tropical Africa, mildew tests demonstrated not only the superiority of zinc oxide, but also that it promoted chalking, checking, and loss of gloss (Whitely, 1965). For reducing checking, chalking, and flaking with zinc oxide, Vannoy (1956) recommended leaded zinc oxide or zinc oxide with larger-size pigment particles. In exposure tests in New Guinea, 15% zinc oxide improved paints, but the chalking product did better than the chalk-resistant (Rischbieth et al., 1974). In varnish-based paints in which 45% of the pigment was chalk-resistant ZnO, the mildew was not less than on the controls with no ZnO.

It is reported that zinc oxide is incompatible with many binders (Pauli, 1972) and that it may increase viscosity, causing brushing problems and possible embrittlement of the dry film (Coleman and Hall, 1972). On the plus side, its opacity makes it possible to reduce the titanium dioxide content (Werthan, 1968), and its antifungal activity permits a reduction of many fungicides to one-half (Hart, 1971; Lederer, 1971; Keith, 1971; Scott and Dickert, 1972; Hoffman, 1972).

Barium Metaborate

Ross (1964) presented evidence that barium metaborate used in paint in high quantities provided mildew protection without chalking. Under conditions that initiated chalking, zinc oxide was found superior to barium metaborate in keeping the paint surface free of fungal growth, but in places where the paint was protected and did not chalk, barium metaborate was reported to be a better mildew inhibitor. Unfortunately, barium metaborate does not have the hiding power required of a paint pigment. A modified barium metaborate (Ross, 1971) is presented as a broad-spectrum bactericide-fungicide for both preservation of water-thinned emulsion paints and fungus resistance in oil paint films. Recommended at 5 to 20% of the weight of the dry solids, it keeps an alkaline environment in the film, discouraging growth and corrosion. It cannot be used in high-gloss paints.

Mercurials

Mercurials have been popular paint preservatives for they retard mildew in paints when used in low concentration. After years of testing preservatives for paint, Gardner and coworkers (1933, 1934 1938, 1939) concluded that the mercurials were the best preservatives for outside paint. Although mercurials are effective as mildew inhibitors in paints, reports (Ross, 1964; Whitely, 1965; Taylor and Hunter, 1972) indicate that their effectiveness is limited to less than 2 years in outdoor exposure. Nevertheless, hundreds of millions of gallons of paint have employed phenylmercuric compounds as a bactericide for in-can preservation of water-thinned paints and fungicide for applied paint films. Their activity at low concentration, lack of color and odor, and relatively low cost at the rate employed made them the major paint biocides for many years. In 1969 and 1970, about 700,000 pounds of mercury per year were used in this way (Goll, 1970) at a cost of $10 million. The safety of mercurials has been at issue in recent years (Goll, 1970; Mann, 1971) and the threat of the Environmental Protection Agency canceling registration for mercury pesticides (Scott and Dickert, 1972) directed attention toward other materials (see Mann, 1971, for list). At present, mercurials are restricted by the EPA to in-can preservation of water-based paints and to their outdoor application (Environmental Protection Agency, 1976), although they might be entirely eliminated (Chapter 19).

Phenols

In large-scale tests under practical use conditions in the Canal Zone, Shapiro (1958) found tetrachlorophenol effective when employed as 4% of the dry weight of the paint. Pentachlorophenol is employed as an in-can preservative for protein paints at 0.6%. In stains and penetrating wood treatments, it is employed for mold control at a level of 5%. Phenol preservatives discolor in ultraviolet light (Keith, 1971) and in the presence of iron, which limits their use.

Copper-8-Quinolinolate

The only treatment found equivalent to 4% tetrachlorophenol in the Canal Zone tests (Shapiro, 1958) was 0.5% copper-8-quinolinolate. In outdoor exposure tests, Vannoy (1956) found "copper-8" still effective against mold when phenylmercurials had failed. This chemical has a strong greenish-brown color that restricts its use where color is important, but its low toxicity and high activity in paints have won it a place for paints in meat packing houses, food freezer rooms, dairies, and breweries (Richardson and Del Guidice, 1952; Herman and Reed, 1952; O'Connor, 1969; Hoffman, 1972).

Nitrogen-Sulfur Compounds

A fungicide widely used in agriculture, N-(trichloromethylthio)phthalimide (Phaltan), has been shown to be a good mildew preventative in interior and exterior solvent-based paints when used at 3% (Hoffman, 1971). In latex paints, it undergoes slow hydrolysis (Pauli, 1972). Other chemically related compounds, N-(fluorodichloromethylthio)phthalimide and N-dimethyl-N-phenyl-N-(fluorodichloromethyl thiosulfamide) have similar application but need only to be used at 1.5 to 2.0%. The latter compound was said to have kept paints free from mold at humid sites for 4 years (Pauli, 1972).

A highly active fungicide, 2-(4-thiazolyl) benzimidazole (Metasol TK-100), is said to be cost-equivalent to the phenylmercurials (Snyder, 1972). It is said to have been incorporated in millions of gallons of paint without deleterious action to the paint. Stable to acid and alkali, it does not discolor with sulfide fumes. It is recommended for exterior use at 1.0% and less for interior coatings. It is not a bactericide and cannot be used as an in-can preservative for water-thinned paints (Lederer, 1971).

A mold inhibitor used for latex paints is a mixture of the zinc salts of dimethyldithiocarbamate and 2-mercaptobenzothiazole. Two percent is suggested for outdoor use (Hart, 1971). This compound combination has low mammalian toxicity and does not cause discoloration in sulfide atmospheres. It cannot be used for oil and alkyd paints, as it interferes with drying.

Arsenical

An organic arsenic compound, 10,10′-oxybisphenoxarsine, was shown to be about as active antimicrobially as phenylmercurials in outdoor weathering tests of latex coatings, but was more persistent than the mercurials and tetrachlorophenol (Wolf and Riley, 1965). With 3% oxybisphenoxarsine, no mildew appeared after 20 months' exposure in Texas. With 1%, it held up for 12 to 18 months. The mercurials at 2% gave 6 to 7 months of mildew-free service and 3% tetrachlorophenol only 4 to 6 months. The arsenical was also shown to be superior in asphalt coatings. It has been used extensively as a mildew preventative in vinyl plastics. Although it is potentially toxic owing to the arsenic atom, no toxicologic hazards have been demonstrated for the uses approved by the regulatory agencies, which include preservation of adhesives, ink bases, latex, tapes, wallpaper, pipe wrapping fabrics, and emulsions. It is marketed as a 2% concentrate under the name Durotex.

Newer Compounds

Three new compounds serve as preservatives for latex and other water-emulsion paints rather than as mildewcides. One claiming 6 years of service is 1-(3-chloroallyl)-3,5,7-triaza-1-azonia-adamantane (Dowicil 100) (Keith, 1971). It is employed at 0.05 to 0.2% in latex paints, in which it acts by gradually releasing formalin into the aqueous solution. Another is 1,2-benzisothiazolin-3-one (Proxel CRL), which has been used in Europe and England (Carter and Huddart, 1974). It has a mammalian toxicity of 1250 mg/kg and is used in average concentrations of 0.05% in polyvinylacetate and polyacrylic emulsions. It is supplied as a brown liquid and may cause discoloration if concentrations far above those recom-

mended are employed. Another can preservative offered for latex paints is hexahydro-1,3,5-triethyl-s-triazine (Vanicide 512) (Hart, 1971). It is water soluble and stable at pH 6.5 or higher. Suggested concentration for use is 0.02 to 0.05%.

A fungicide for oils and alkyd paints that has been applied to several hundred thousand houses is trans-1,2,-bis(n-propylsulfonyl) ethene (Hart, 1971). It is a white insoluble powder, low in toxicity, stable in solvents but not stable above pH 7, as exists in some water-thinned paints. It is recommended for use at 0.5 to 1.0%.

A new wide-spectrum biocide for paint use as an in-can preservative and mildew inhibitor in the film is 2-n-octyl-4-isothiazolin-3-one (Skane M–8) (Scott and Dickert, 1972). It has an LD_{50} of 1470 mg/kg as compared to 90 for phenylmercurials. Stable over a wide pH range, it undergoes slow decomposition in the presence of high concentration of ammonia or amines. Protection against such decomposition is said to be afforded by the use of zinc oxide. In 2 years of tests, it was found to be more effective than phenylmercurials when it was used at a level of 0.4%. With 5% zinc oxide, only 0.1 to 0.2% was necessary. The product was labeled with ^{14}C, and traces were found to be biodegradable in nature.

Another promising new paint antimicrobial agent, 2,3,5,6-tetrachloro-4-(methyl sulfonyl)-pyridine (Dowicil S-13) is primarily a fungicide but at 0.5% will serve also as a bactericide for can storage protection. It is recommended at 0.5 to 1.0% in oil-based and latex paints. In a latex paint, the pH must be stabilized at neutrality or slight alkalinity. A higher pH will result in hydrolysis to a product with lower fungicidal activity (Keith, 1971).

Grant et al. (1986) tested fungicidal paints employing a number of commercial fungicides in a white gloss emulsion paint. They also tested a number of commercially produced fungicidal emulsion paints. Each was tested and compared employing laboratory tests, site trials, and a high-humidity test chamber. The fungicides used were diiodomethyl p-tolyl sulphone (Amical 50), dithio-2,2′ bis benzmethylamide (Densil P), 2,4,5,6-tetrachloroisophthalonitrile (Nopcocide N96), 2-n-octyl-4-isothiazolin-3-one (Skane M–8), tributyl tin compound (Stannicide M), 3-iodo-2-propynlbutyl carbamate (Troysan Polyphase Antimildew), heterocyclic compounds (Algon 100), tetramethyl thiuramdisulphide (TMTD) (Robac TMT), and N-dimethyl-N′-phenyl-(N-fluorodichloromethylthio) sulphamide (Preventol A4). Their tests showed that paints containing TMTD and a commercial paint believed to contain barium metaborate performed "extremely well," superior to the others.

Chemically Anchored Fungicides

An attempt to obtain permanent mildew resistance in paints has recently been reported (Pittman et al., 1978). It was claimed that vinyl acetate and ethyl acrylate polymers containing 0 to 5 mol percent of fungicidal groups gave coatings that resist fungi. These coatings were prepared by copolymerizing vinyl acetate or ethyl acrylate with 2-(4-thiazolyl)-1-benzimidazolyl acrylate, pentachlorophenyl acrylate, 8-quinolinolyl acrylate, or 2-(phenylaminocarbonyl) phenylacrylate, using 5-butyl peroxide as catalyst.

In-Can Preservatives

With the advent of water-based latex emulsion paints came the problem of spoilage of the paint in the can. The main spoilage problem, due to growth of bacteria (principally of the genus *Pseudomonas*), is the enzymatic hydrolysis by cellulases of the cellulose ethers used as thickeners to cause a loss of viscosity (Carman and Goll, 1970). Cellosize (hydroxyethyl cellulose) is an example of such a thickening agent that is adversely affected. Other problems are gas production in the can and bad odor due to bacterial activity.

Machemer (1979) tested a number of mercurial and nonmercury in-can preservatives with various water-based decorative paints. These were challenged with *Pseudomonas aeruginosa, Escherichia coli, Bacillus subtilus,* and *Enterobacter aerogenes.* The best of five mercury compositions was chloromethoxypropyl mercury acetate, which gave sterility at 0.005% Hg, compared to 0.01 to 0.02% for the others. In comparison, a nonmercurial 1-(3-chlorallyl)-3,5,7-triaza-1-azonia adamantane chloride required 0.15 to 0.2%. On a cost basis, the mercurials were superior and faster in sterilizing the contents of the can. Those nonmercurials that gave protection were the adamantane chloride just cited, K *N*-hydroxymethyl-*N*-methyldithiocarbamate, Na 2-mercaptobenzothiazole, hexahydro-1,3,5-triethyl-S-triazine, and 2-[(hydroxymethyl)amino] ethanol. The nonmercurials were considered suitable candidates, should mercurials be completely banned.

Antifouling Paints

Antifouling paints employ considerable quantities of biocides to discourage the growth of microbial and higher forms of plant and animal life such as barnacles, hydroids, sea-squirts, tube-worms, and mussels on the bottoms of ships below the water line. The sinking of the German warship *Graf Spee* in World War II has been ascribed to a reduction in its speed due to fouling. Increased drag produced by fouling for 6 months necessitates the use of 40% more fuel to maintain the same speed. Other costs are for cleaning and painting and time out of service. Antifouling paints traditionally have employed copper, principally cupric oxide. Copper acetoarsenite (Paris green) has the combined toxicity of copper and arsenic. Mercury compounds add to the toxicity when mixed with copper. Tributyltin oxide has been the subject of much recent interest for this application. It is used as 10% of the film and has given promising results against plant and animal fouling (Evans, 1970). In sea water, organotin compounds are leached out of the paint as the organotin chloride or hydroxide (Monaghan et al., 1980). Among the organic biocides used in antifouling paints, which include herbicides, algicides, and molluscicides, are chlorophenyl ureas, polychlorinated hydrocarbons, thia-

diazoles, nitrothiazoles, chloronaphthoquinones, and dithiocarbamates (de la Court, 1977).

Lacquers and Varnishes

For fungus-proofing lacquers and varnishes for electrical circuitry, the mercurials were the most effective (Leonard and Pitman, 1951). However, they found salicylanilide also to be effective when used as 10 to 15% of the film, and it was designated in specifications for antimildew lacquers for electrical equipment (Ezekiel, 1950).

Antiseptic and Germicidal Paints

Antiseptic and germicidal paints have been a goal of researchers for many years, but the fruits of their labors have been minimal. In general, the germicidal properties brought about by active antimicrobial compounds are short lived. The nature of the surface is important. Bacteria are more easily killed, for example, on coated glass than on coated wood. The humidity is also a significant factor: Bacteria are much harder to kill at relative humidity levels below 50% than those above. In many cases, the active agent is trapped in the film and cannot exert its antimicrobial activity. A notable exception is the case of volatile agents such as formaldehyde, which produce "self-sterilizing" coatings. But being volatile, the potency dissipates quickly. For a longer discussion of this subject and references, refer to pages 807 to 808 in the second edition of this book (Block, 1977).

PAPER PRESERVATION

Slimicides

Preservatives are required in many stages of the process for manufacturing paper. Bacteria, molds, and yeasts may grow in the pulp to sour and stain it and to reduce the quality of the paper. In the processing equipment, a complex microbiologic slime clogs pipes, screens, and filters, causes spots in the sheet, sometimes a break in the roll of paper, and an appreciable loss of production time. The different microorganisms contributing to the formation of slime are fully discussed by Appling (1955). Oppermann and Wolfson (1961) describe how the slime grows and attaches to wooden and metal components used in the aqueous system employed in paper making.

Buckman Laboratories (1982) estimate that the economic loss caused by slime in a paper mill may be up to $5 per ton of pulp processed. It is further estimated that a mill may pay $0.10–2.50 per ton for chemical control of slime. Sanborn (1944, 1951) studied the slime problem and stressed the importance of cleanliness and found (as did Appling et al., 1951) that the large masses of slime must be removed before chemical agents are effective. This is done manually, after which a hot solution of an alkaline slime remover is circulated. Technologists refer to slime control as being 60% housekeeping in the mill, 15% plant design, and 25% choice of an effective biocide.

There have been many changes in slime control in the

past 50 years. Chlorine was first depended upon and used at a level of 1 to 2 ppm of free, residual chlorine. Sometimes 1 to 2 ppm of copper sulfate was also used to control the fungi not checked by the chlorine. Where there was considerable organic matter, the free chlorine was ineffective, and chloramines were employed for a time. A chloramine residual of 0.2 to 0.3 ppm was used for acid systems, and twice as much for alkaline systems. Excellent control was given at 1 to 2 cents per ton of paper produced (Schirtzinger, 1963). Hypochlorites were also used in wash-ups, but after a time, more resistant bacteria and fungi became prevalent in the slime (Sanborn, 1965).

By this time, organic mercurials had been introduced and were found to give economic slime control. But these slimicides also had problems. The results with them were often spotty and local to the area of introduction. Halliday (1950) demonstrated that phenylmercuric ions are adsorbed by cellulose fibers and may not be distributed evenly throughout the processing system. Despite the high biostatic activity of these mercurials, new government restrictions on paper products used for food and new regulations concerning pollution have militated against their continued use.

The sodium salts of trichlorophenol and pentachlorophenol are broad-spectrum antimicrobials that have been used in paper mills for many years. Their low cost-effectiveness, activity in the presence of organic matter, and persistence in the mill system have earned them popularity. Environmental and possible health problems, however, led to the introduction of new agents. Introduced in 1963, methylenebis-thiocyanate has been making its way into the field. It has powerful action against slime-forming bacteria and is active against spore-formers and fungi; however, yeasts are better controlled with the chlorinated phenols (Starnes, 1969). Other organic sulfur slimicides include chloromethyl- and methylenebis-butanethiolsulfonate, and disodium cyanodithioimidocarbonate with potassium n-methyldithiocarbonate and ethylenediamine. Bromohydroxyacetophenones are another broad-spectrum antimicrobial group being used in paper plants. Chlorine dioxide, in a stabilized form of 4 to 5% ClO_2, has been made available to the paper industry for use as a slime control agent. It is an effective bactericide that is not absorbed by the fibers and removed from the water system. β-Bromo-β-nitrostyrene is one of the newer chemicals finding use as a slime-control agent (Sharpell, 1988) (see Table 52–2).

Many of the slimicides are most effective when different chemicals are used alternately, giving the microorganisms a one-two punch. Rather than using a level concentration that, for economic reasons is necessarily dilute, best results are produced by slugging the system intermittently with large doses, which penetrate the slime and kill the organisms rather than just inhibiting them.

Wood Pulp and Chips

Wood pulp that is stored in a wet condition for future use in making paper, paperboard, and boxes is attacked by fungi, which stain and rot the pulp. A combination of fungicides is preferred, since one fungus, *Penicillium roqueforti* Thom, is resistant to mercury and produces a violet stain in groundwood treated with phenylmercuric acetate (Appling et al., 1950). This is often followed by "red rot," which causes decay as well as staining, which has been shown to result from inactivation of the mercurial, making it inactive against mercury-sensitive rot fungi (Russel, 1961). Phenylmercuric acetate in combination with 8-quinolinol and sodium pentachlorophenate found use in pulp preservation. A combination of sodium pentachlorophenate and sodium trichlorophenate was found to give complete protection to groundwood at 0.1% of the dry weight of the fibers and was not detrimental to the strength of the fibers (Osanov et al., 1964). Because these chemicals are being phased out, other agents currently employed include dithiocarbamates, benzothiazole, benzisothiazolone, dichlorophen, and sodium metaborate.

Another problem is the deterioration of wood chips, used in making paper pulp, that are stored outdoors. The chips sustain considerable damage through enzymatic, chemical, and microbiologic action, in which they heat up to 70° to 80°C (Chalk, 1968). The financial loss is estimated at $4 a ton. Among the chemicals that have been tested to prevent damage by the thermophilic bacteria and fungi are chlorinated phenols, organic mercurials, paper-mill black liquor, borax, and nickel sulfate. It is claimed that the latter selectively prohibits wood-rotting fungi but permits the growth of molds that are antagonistic to the wood rotters (Anon., 1969). Other chemicals that have been the subject of laboratory tests are sulfur dioxide (King et al., 1971), propionic acid (Eslyn, 1973), and sodium n-methyl dithiocarbamate with dinitrophenol (Springer et al., 1973). The cost of chemical treatment at 25 cents per ton of dry wood would be $5 million a year just for the Canadian markets alone. This market for biocides, however, may not develop, for Eslyn and Laundrie (1973) report that chips stored anaerobically under water or in an atmosphere of 95% nitrogen and 5% carbon dioxide remained in good condition for up to 26 months.

Treated Paper

Finished paper with antibacterial and antifungal treatments has stimulated considerable interest and investigation. Preservative-treated paper to prevent food spoilage has filled important needs. Citrus fruit wrappers treated with biphenyl are used commercially for controlling stem end rot and *Penicillium* mold in the shipment of the fruit (Fletcher, 1954). Propionates (Macy and Olsen, 1939) and sorbic acid (Smith and Rollin, 1954) have been employed successfully in paper wrappers for dairy products such as butter and cheese. Tests have also shown the effectiveness of dimethyl dichlorosuccinate in an antimycotic cheese wrapper (Mottern, 1954). An interesting development was the food wrapper containing a silver coating (Goetz, 1944) that was found to protect fruit pastes and dried fruits from spoilage under tropical storage conditions. Mold-resistant paperboard egg crate fillers and flats containing sodium pentachlorophenate keep eggs free of mold during cold storage, according to Mallmann and Michael (1940).

Soap wrappers, gummed tape, and insulation board have been protected from fungus attack with sodium o-phenylphenate and sodium pentachlorophenate (Ballman and Smith, 1943). Crandall (1955) indicated the need for preservative-treated paper in fertilizer packaging, paper sandbags, and wrapping for electrical cable.

In military shipment, it is essential that materials be packaged to withstand outdoor weathering. Waterproof barrier materials are used as baling, case liners, wrappers, and temporary tarpaulins during transit or storage. They consist of paper or cotton scrim as the supporting material, and wax, polyethylene, asphalt, or metal foil for the waterproof coating. After exposure to fungi, paper-asphalt barriers were severely degraded, with a complete loss of water resistance and a great loss in breaking strength. Polyethylene or aluminum foil laminated materials retained their water resistance but decreased considerably in breaking strength. Copper pentachlorophenate, at a concentration of 0.3% copper on paper that was coated with polyethylene, gave a fungus-resistant barrier showing little loss in breaking strength (Ross et al., 1956).

Based upon fungus-resistance tests using six commercial fungicides for treating the kraft paper portion of the barrier material, three of the fungicides appear to be suitable (Ross and Teitell, 1966; Teitell and Ross, 1966). They are copper-8-quinolinolate, copper pentachlorophenate, and sodium pentachlorophenate. They must be used at concentrations of 4% or greater to be expected to give permanent protection under severe exposure conditions. Sodium pentachlorophenate must be restricted to uses where rain will not fall on the paper portion of the barrier. In a screening of 15 selected fungicides, the compounds were applied to filter paper in concentrations of 0.25 to 4.0% and subjected to soil burial and agar plate tests. Those compounds showing greatest strength retention were 2,2'-dithiopyridine-1,1'-dioxide and 1-fluoro-2,4-dinitrobenzene.

The literature indicates other interest in paper with antimicrobial properties. Meat packaged in paper with 5 to 25 mg of chlortetracycline per square meter was reported to have an extended shelf life (Hartshorne, 1962). Propylene oxide, not to exceed 700 ppm, was approved for use as a package fumigant with dried prunes and glacé fruit (Anon., 1961a). Volatile corrosion inhibitors, cyclohexylamine carbonate and dicyclohexylamine nitrite, have been shown to have antifungal properties and can prevent early degradation of paper, cardboard, and packaging materials that are used in conjunction with metals (Evans and Levisohn, 1964). Crepe-paper tow-

eling with 0.5% alkylaryl polyether benzyl ammonium chloride (Hyamine 1622) is claimed to be resistant to *Staphylococcus aureus* (Pattilloch, 1962). Paper for food wrapping impregnated with sodium benzoate plus p-hydroxybenzoic acid and its methyl ester was more effective against selected bacteria, yeast, and fungi than sodium pentachlorophenate or sorbic acid, according to tests by Bomar (1961). The literature mentions other chemicals such as orthophenyl phenol, acetaldehyde, and dehydroacetic acid for paper wraps to inhibit fungus growth. For protecting individual fruits in storage and shipping, wraps treated with biphenyl and with iodine have been used.

ELECTRONICS AND MISSILES

In the South Pacific area in World War II, General Douglas McArthur said: "Tropicalization prevents mold and fungus, brings inaccurate equipment up to specifications, and puts back in operation equipment thought to be useless." Communication equipment used in jungles, swamps, and foxholes was rarely dry and soon became infested with fungi and inoperative. Field reports stated that these organisms in some cases caused equipment to break down in as little as 6 hours, and as much as 50% of some types of ground signal mechanisms failed within 30 days (Benignus and Rogers, 1945). Moreover, fungus growth on electrical equipment was restricted not only to jungles: the United States Ordnance Department discovered that the electrical portions of the power drive for 90-mm antiaircraft guns stored in this country were found sometimes so profusely overgrown with fungi as to make them unfit for combat operation. Many such instances of fungus growth on electrical equipment stored in this country were found. Something had to be done about it.

The immediate answer was "tropicalization." The Signal Corps required equipment manufacturers to treat with fungicides, or fungicide-containing waxes, lacquers and varnishes, assemblies that contained organic substances that served as fungus nutrients. In 1945, Leutritz of Bell Telephone Company noted: "The overall spraying of apparatus with fungicidal varnishes has helped as an emergency measure to keep much military equipment in operative condition in the field. It will soon be restricted, however, to critical parts of circuits because equipment will be engineered to avoid the injurious effects of moisture and fungus growth." Twenty-one years and two wars later, research reports entitled "Microbial Deterioration of Electronic Components" (Gauger et al., 1966), showed that the problems had not been engineered away.

Equipment failed to function and, on examination, fungus growth was much in evidence, but was the fungus just an indicator of the real cause of the trouble, i.e., moisture, or did the fungus itself contribute to the electrical leakage, breakdown, and corrosion of metal parts? The significance of the fungus to the operation of the equipment became a matter of some controversy, which is mentioned by Teitell et al. (1955). Their work and other investigations preceding it show convincingly that fungi serve as conducting bridges causing electrical leakage and cessation of performance. Electrical insulating tapes inoculated with fungus spores and exposed to 100% relative humidity became covered with fungus mycelium, producing an increase of direct current surface conductance from less than 1 to as high as 10^4 to 10^5 microhos. When the conditions were the same except that the spores had been killed with ethylene oxide, the surface conductance did not increase. The electrical properties of hookup wire deteriorated long before there was visible mold growth (Luce and Mathes, 1951); did this mean that fungi were not involved? No, microscopic examination showed fungus hyphae making interlacing pathways all over the equipment long before they were visible to the naked eye.

Of the materials supporting fungus growth, braid-covered hookup wire is one of the worst offenders. Fungal filaments growing vigorously on the cotton braid spread rapidly to other elements. In recent studies of susceptible materials (Gauger et al., 1966) polyvinyl chloride clear or black insulation, Tygon (polyvinyl acetate chloride) insulation, a phenolic terminal connector board, a phenolic printed circuit board, and polyvinyl hookup wire insulation supported growth of fungal cultures in laboratory culture media. Under high-humidity storage conditions, evidence was obtained of deterioration of epoxy boards. Military and space missiles contain many electrical and electronic components that have been found to be infected with fungus (Lee, 1961). While the growth in many cases was light, the presence of fungi was considered a source of potential difficulty in the tactical operation of missiles. Whole missiles such as the Honest John rocket were placed in high-humidity chambers to ascertain their susceptibility to fungus attack.

To prevent fungus growth, with its concomitant problems, four methods are possible: (1) to sterilize and hermetically seal the unit, (2) to encase the component in plastic or "pot" it, (3) to employ nonsusceptible or "funginert" materials, and (4) to use fungistatic chemicals, either alone or in organic coatings. Numerous technical considerations as well as cost influence the selection of the method. The first two methods are excellent when they can be used. The simplest method is substituting a nonsusceptible material for a susceptible one. For example, cotton braid-covered wire was replaced by wire with a polyvinyl-chloride primary insulation and a thin nylon extruded jacket over it. Nylon being funginert and resistant to moisture showed resistance of over 1000 megohms as compared to 2 megohms for cotton braid wire after 1 year's exposure at Key West on gun directors (Ezekiel, 1950).

Unfortunately, the problem is not always one of easy substitution. Some components are fabricated of a number of different materials, one or more of which may be susceptible. Further, dust, oil, or fingerprints may provide, on the surface of an inert material, sufficient nutrient to permit fungus growth, provided growth conditions are ideal. While working at the Frankford Arsenal in Philadelphia, I saw missile components containing a funginert material, silicone rubber, that supported luxuriant mold growth when they were exposed in a tropical chamber. The Office of Scientific Research and Development prepared a summary report of the wartime studies on the problem of fungus growth on synthetic resins, plastics, and plasticizers, which are the fabricating materials for much of the electrical and electronic equipment (Brown, 1945). Although this report is too detailed to review here, it may be noted that, whereas most synthetic resins and plastics, excepting those based upon cellulose, were resistant to fungi, the composition materials containing plastics were much more susceptible. To a great extent, this can be attributed to the plasticizer—the better plasticizers generally being the more susceptible ones.

Fungistatic coatings of wax, varnishes, and lacquers used with funginert materials appear to provide the greatest insurance against trouble. Interestingly enough, many of the excellent antifungal compounds do not perform well when incorporated in plastic compositions, even when in high concentrations. For example, Leonard and Bultman (1955) reported the indifferent merits of copper-8-quinolinolate in a phenolic resin and tung oil varnish. Some materials are deleterious to the components, as illustrated by the injurious effect of organic mercurials on selenium rectifiers. The use of pentachlorophenol likewise was discontinued because it tended to cause corrosion.

In general, thermoplastic materials have been made more resistant to fungi by incorporating antifungal chemicals in the plastics. With phenolic materials, however, the incorporation of fungus inhibitors has generally not met with success, probably due to the reactivity of formaldehyde with the added chemicals at the high thermosetting temperatures. In exposure tests in a mangrove swamp in Florida, plastic samples coated with treated varnish or lacquer showed best results with a combination of salicylanilide and an organic mercurial, phenylmercuric-o-benzoic sulfimide, which evidenced only light fungus growth. Salicylanilide was just as good alone in the varnish but showed slightly more growth than the combination in the lacquer. The mercurial alone was inferior to salicylanilide but better than the coating without any fungistat or the uncoated plastic, which had profuse growth (Ezekiel, 1950).

In their tests of cotton braid wire coated with a treated varnish, Leonard and Bultman (1955) used six different fungistats singly and in binary mixtures and exposed the samples in a closed hut in a Panama jungle for 33 months. The compounds tested included pentachlorophenol, salicylanilide, phenylmercuric phthalate, uranyl nitrate, copper-8-quinolinolate, and p-toluene sulfonamide, which were tested as 2%, 4%, and 8% of the dry weight of the varnish. The p-toluene sulfonamide was much superior to the other compounds, giving complete protection for 33 months at even the 2% concentration. This is the more surprising when it is considered that this compound shows no antifungal activity in the ordinary laboratory tests.

A patent of a microbicidal film for electronic printed circuits (Inoue and Morita, 1977) says it protects the circuits from the effects of bacteria and fungi. It employs Dowicil S-13 and *N*-dimethyl-*N'*-phenyl (fluorodichloromethylthio)sulfonamide, and is dispersed in a 0.05-mm-thick polyethylene film. The film is placed over the printed circuit, the dispersed side inward, and the circuit is tightly sealed by the film.

PETROLEUM

Engine Fuels

It has long been known that certain microorganisms can attack petroleum and utilize its hydrocarbons as a source of energy and nutrition. This property is currently employed in refining petroleum and in producing microorganisms for cattle feed. When petroleum products are stored in large tanks, there is usually some water in the bottom of the tank, and microbial growth occurs at this interface. This has long been known, and antimicrobial agents such as sodium borate have been used in the water layer to discourage the microbial growth.

In 1956, however, the problems attached to microbial growth on petroleum products suddenly received major scrutiny when the Air Force first became aware that malfunction of refueling equipment in a jet tanker aircraft was due to sludge formation of microbial origin in JP-4 jet fuel. Work by the Air Force, Navy, Army, and aircraft companies demonstrated that microorganisms in turbine fuels have been implicated in filter and fuel line blockage, malfunction of fuel probes, degradation of fuel tank coatings, and corrosion of wing tanks and bulk storage tanks. Hydrocarbons of the fuel are metabolized by the organisms and altered in the process. Growth of the microorganisms is associated with the presence of sludge, slimes, and soaps, which act to plug filters and other equipment. Whereas fuels containing aromatic hydrocarbons are resistant to microorganisms, the turbine fuels contain mainly paraffinic hydrocarbons and are susceptible. Growth of microorganisms does not occur in the absence of water but, while the fuel may dissolve only 0.01 to 9.02% of water at 34°C (Kereluk and Baxter, 1963), this is ample, particularly when it is condensed out into a separate phase as the aircraft gains altitude and the temperature decreases.

Leathen and Kinsel (1963) made 184 isolates of microorganisms from jet-fuel storage tanks at 9 Air Force bases. They took their samples from the water bottoms of these tanks. Both bacteria and fungi were represented, and 61% of the isolates survived and grew abundantly at the water-oil interface in substrates containing jet fuel as the only source of carbon. The predominant bacteria were *Pseudomonas*, and the most prevalent fungi belonged to the *Hormodendrum*. Other bacteria were

members of the genera *Aerobacter* and *Bacillus*. Later work suggested *Cladosporium resinae* to be the most important fungus encountered in wing tanks and was considered responsible for filter blockage and metal corrosion (Berner and Ahearn, 1977). According to Hill (1976) this is only in subsonic aircraft. In supersonic aircraft, a higher temperature prevails and the predominant flora found are *Aspergillus fumigatus*, gram-negative bacteria, yeasts, and other fungi.

The most obvious method for preventing problems arising from microbial growth in fuel would be to remove the water from the fuel, but unfortunately this is impractical. Filtration of the fuel to remove fine particles is practiced in refueling, and this is helpful, as indicated by London et al. (1964). Chemical preservatives have been generally suspect, not from the standpoint of antimicrobial effectiveness, but in regard to lack of knowledge of their effect on the combustion of the fuel and the possibility of their causing damage to the engine. Churchill and Leathen (1961) tested 178 water-soluble chemicals in a fuel-water system for their effect on microbial growth. Those that prevented growth included bromoacetic acid at 1000 ppm, an alkyl quaternary ammonium acetate at 5000 ppm, a mixture of sodium ethyl mercuric thiosalicylate and sodium orthophenylphenate at 5000 ppm, and an *n*-alkyl (C_{12} to C_{18}) dimethyl benzyl ammonium chloride at 500 ppm. Of the boron compounds tested, diethylamine borane and tri-*n*-butyl borate were found effective in laboratory tests, but sodium tetraborate was not. DeGray and Fitzgibbons (1965) found that organoborates kill hydrocarbon-ingesting microorganisms at lower dosages of boron in the aqueous phase of a fuel-water system than does boric acid. The rate of kill of the organoborates increases with the lyophilicity of the compound.

Biobor J.F., a mixture of 2,2'-(1-methyltrimethylenedioxy)bis(4-methyl-1,3,2-dioxaborinane) and 2,2'-oxybis(4,4,6-trimethyl)-1,3,2-dioxaborinane at 135 to 270 ppm has been demonstrated to be an excellent biocide for jet fuel. It is highly effective in controlling organisms associated with sludge build-up and is useful not only for jet fuel but for all hydrocarbon fuels in storage, such as diesel and kerosene (but not gasoline and aromatics), and has been successful in preventing filter plugging, producing cleaner injector nozzles, and reducing fuel tank corrosion (Stormont, 1962). It is suggested that it be used during engine maintenance and then drained or burned off so as not to damage the jet engine (Elphick, 1970). A new boron preservative shown to have higher fungicidal activity was 4-hydroxymethyl-2-phenyl-2-bora-1,3-dioxacyclopentane (Singer, 1976).

Organic boron compounds are of interest because they were already used as gasoline additives; therefore, they are thought not to be deleterious to the engine and its performance. Fortuitously, an anti-icing additive of aircraft fuel was found to possess biocidal properties. This fuel additive, referred to as PFA 55 MB, is a two-component blend of ethylene glycol monomethyl ether (methyl Cellosolve) and glycerol in a mixture of 99.6 to

0.4%. This additive in the fuel at 0.15 to 2% has been used in military service since 1962 and is approved for use in commercial aircraft.

Hitzman (1964) has conducted tests on this additive and reports that the ethylene glycol monomethyl ether is the dominant biocidal component, and organisms isolated from various sources have been found to be susceptible to its biocidal action. With a low concentration of this additive in a large volume of the fuel in contact with a small volume of the water, the additive partitions predominantly into the water phase to give equilibrium concentrations in the water of 200 to 800 times the amount in the fuel phase. This high concentration results in the biocidal activity of this compound, which is not normally considered a biocide, since it is not antimicrobially active in the low concentrations of common biocides. A report by London of the Air Force and his co-workers (1964) states that the efficacy of ethylene glycol monomethyl ether as a microbial inhibitor has been well documented in practice. Based on a number of field surveys at Air Force bases, they note that although a low level of viable microorganisms continues to be observed in Air Force fuel systems, the application of good "housekeeping" and the effect of this additive appear to have controlled their activity. Continuous use of this agent might be feared lest adaptive microbial forms become resistant to it, but experimental work (Hitzman, 1964) showed no adaptation in his tests.

Hill conducted experiments on fuel biocides with ethylene glycol monomethyl ether (EGME), an organoborate, and mixtures of EGME with various parahydroxybenzoates (1970). The mixtures produced sterility in the fuel in a few hours, whereas with EGME alone, sterility took several days to achieve. To "debug" fuel systems and rid them of the dead organisms, a quaternary ammonium salt at 0.15% both cleaned and sterilized surfaces in 2 hours. Agitation and a trace of water accelerated the action.

One of the more serious problem areas of microbial growth in aircraft fuel is the corrosion of the wing tanks of jet aircraft. Subsequent to the contamination and corrosion problems in commercial wet wing aircraft, the Air Force in 1960 became cognizant of similar conditions in tanker and bomber aircraft. Inspection of the integral wing tanks of these aircraft in bases in Florida and Puerto Rico revealed significant corrosion of aluminum members and the presence of large quantities of ill-defined debris. The sealant and top coating materials also showed degradation (London et al., 1964). When further investigations emphasized that the problem was more general than had been realized, numerous studies were authorized.

A study by Crum et al. (1966) explored the effect of surfactants in the fuel on the microbiologic deterioration of aluminum fuel tank systems. Surfactants find their way into fuels from various sources. They are present in crude petroleum and fuel additives and may be picked up from pipelines through which the fuel is transported. By lowering the interfacial tension between the fuel and water, surfactants interfere with the functioning of filter separators, thus permitting fine particles of solid contamination and dispersed droplets of water to enter the fuel. This mixture and the surfactant itself may be utilized as food by the bacteria and fungi present. Reports have indicated that when the surfactant-induced water problem was corrected growth of microorganisms ceased. In laboratory tests, Crum et al. (1966) found some correlation between the presence of the surfactant and anti-icing additive, the growth of microorganisms, and the extent of corrosion. The degree of corrosion and microbial growth was greatest when Tween 20 surfactant was employed in the system, less with Triton X-100 surfactant, and least with the ethylene glycol monomethyl ether. Thus the type of surfactant, as relating to its effect on microbial growth, appears to be a contributing factor to the corrosion.

Blanchard and Goucher (1965), investigating the corrosion of aluminum, reported that a pseudomonad isolated from an aircraft wing tank derived all its essential nutrients from a mineral growth medium, a source of nitrogen, and JP-4 jet fuel. It produced a water-soluble yellow pigment that was found to corrode aluminum alloys. The fuel tank coatings are penetrated by the microorganisms, and corrosion is found underneath. This is noted especially in the case of Buna-N coating, which provides nitrogen for the growth of the organisms (Kereluk and Baxter, 1963; Reynolds et al., 1966). Smith (1966) reported that a polyurethane-based tank lining was essentially non-nutritional for microorganisms, and, although they could penetrate it, it was far superior to Buna-N as a coating for the fuel tanks. Further, the addition of an antimicrobial agent to the urethane would prevent penetration by microorganisms. To prevent adaptation of the organism to the antimicrobial agent and increased tolerance to it, Smith showed that the addition of 10^{-8} moles per liter of a mutagenic agent, 8-azaguanine, prevented the development of a resistant population. Hedrick et al. (1966) found, in laboratory corrosion tests, that two alloys lost 73 and 57% more aluminum by corrosion when the system was inoculated with microorganisms. In tests of several different alloys, it was found that those that corroded the most were those with the greatest percentage of magnesium. The researchers concluded that the microorganisms that contaminate fuels utilize metals in the aluminum alloys, particularly magnesium, and that other types of alloys might be more resistant to such corrosion. Other methods for control include (1) removing water by draining, (2) heating the fuel and centrifuging the entrained water, and (3) heating the fuel to 160 to 180° C to distill the water and kill any organisms in the system (Hill, 1982, 1987).

A number of biocides for the control of microorganisms in various petroleum fuels have been proposed by different workers in the past decade. These include 8-hydroxyquinoline, sodium pentachlorophenate, dimethylethylalkylbenzyl ammonium chloride, alkylammonium salts of 2-pyridinethiol-1-oxide, 1,3,5-triethylhexahydro-1,3,5-triazine, and strontium chromate.

Microbial problems with aircraft occur mainly during storage, because the low temperatures encountered in upper atmospheres during flight are not conducive to microbial proliferation. With ships, however, the problems are worse because the temperature is often high and the fuel is usually in contact with water.

Secondary Oil Recovery

Petroleum crude oil is obtained from wells that tap pools of oil deep in the ground. When these wells are pumped dry, it is still possible to obtain considerably more oil from isolated pockets by a process known as secondary recovery or water-flooding. Fresh or salt water is pumped into the well to displace the oil that is trapped in the interstices of the formation. Bacteria that are introduced with water may proliferate and interfere with this process by clogging the porous sands through which the water must pass. There is another problem—that of microbially induced corrosion of the pipes and equipment used in the flooding process.

While many types of microorganisms play a role in this unhappy drama, the generally recognized villain is the sulfate-reducing bacterium, *Desulfovibrio desulfuricans*. This organism is an anaerobic autotroph found in lakes, marshes, and rivers. It obtains energy for survival by reducing the inorganic sulfate present in water to hydrogen sulfide, which reacts with iron to produce black iron sulfide and the pitting type of corrosion in iron pipes.

Corrosion may be produced in several ways. Hydrogen sulfide itself is corrosive, especially in the presence of oxygen. More important is the electrochemical corrosion brought about by the bacteria. Iron and steel pipe in water develops anodic and cathodic areas but an equilibrium is reached when no further corrosion occurs. Under the anaerobic conditions in which the sulfate reducer grows, the organisms utilize the hydrogen in their metabolism, thereby acting as cathodic depolarizers and thus accelerating the electrochemical degradation. Iron sulfide that is produced is cathodic to metallic iron, and this further aids in the corrosion (Wolfson, 1960). This corrosive damage is by no means limited to oil wells, but is found in all types of wells and underground pipes and tanks exposed to water. The sulfate-reducing bacteria do not restrict their activities to iron but attack underground cables and concrete pipe and tanks. See Chapter 53 for further information on microbial corrosion.

Other types of bacteria are also involved in corrosion. The sulfur-oxidizing bacterium *Thiobacillus suboxydans* oxidizes sulfur to produce sulfuric acid, the concentration of which has been known to reach 10%. Iron bacteria, which are found in water systems, remove iron from the water and deposit a sheath of iron hydroxide around themselves. They may clog filters, screens, and sand beds, and they may provide anaerobic conditions that permit the growth of the corrosion-causing bacteria. Where the water used in flooding is stored in open tanks and ponds, algae are almost sure to grow and, while they will cause plugging and fouling in themselves, they can also serve as a source of nutrient for nonautotrophic bacteria.

Biocidal chemicals have two primary requirements; they must be effective in great dilution and they must be cheap, for a great quantity of water is employed. Most of the chemicals that have been considered as slimicides in paper mills have received consideration in floodwater operations. Halogenated phenols, for example, have found use in this application. In a study of 63 phenolic compounds for their inhibition of *Desulfovibrio desulfuricans*, 3 compounds at 25 ppm completely inhibited hydrogen sulfide production for 28 days. These were 2-bromo-4-phenylphenol, 4-chloro-2-cyclo-hexylphenol, and 2-chloro-4-nitrophenol (Bennett et al., 1958). A number of germicidal quaternary ammonium salts and fatty primary amine salts have been effective in low concentration (Lagarde, 1961). Lagarde also found formaldehyde to be active at 10 ppm. Tris(hydroxymethyl) nitromethane slowly releases formaldehyde and is marketed for oil-well flooding systems (Commercial Solvents Corp., 1958). Sulfur bacteria were found to be more sensitive to substituted nitroparaffins than to mercurials or phenols. Of 200 tested, the following 7 compounds completely inhibited *Desulfovibrio* for 28 days: 3-chloro-3-nitro-2-butanol, 2-chloro-2-nitro-1-butanol stearate, 2-chloro-2-nitrobutyl acetate, 4-chloro-4-nitro-3-hexanol, 1-chloro-1-nitro-1-propanol, and 2-chloro-2-nitro-1-propanol (Bennett et al., 1960). Glutaraldehyde has been found to be effective in field and laboratory tests in concentrations as low as 3 to 5 ppm (Union Carbide Chemicals Co., 1958). It is economical and completely water miscible. Triethyltin chloride, 1 to 10 ppm, is claimed for the protection of ferrous oil-well casings in oil-well brine from corrosion due to *Desulfovibrio* (Thompson, 1963).

For controlling sulfate reducers and other bacteria, Woods (1973) discussed the use of various chemical agents such as acrolein and hexachlorodimethylsulfone. The importance of using germicides in well-drilling fluid is stressed by Smith and Ritter (1968). They say a reservoir can be contaminated soon after a well is fractured or flooded with water containing sulfate-reducing bacteria. The bacteria utilize the hydrocarbon source for energy and multiply, producing hydrogen sulfide corrosion. However, 0.1% bactericide in the drilling mud is said to control the bacteria during drilling.

Brunt (1987) reported that the following biocides were used in the oil-producing industry at these concentrations: glutaraldehyde, 5 to 80 ppm; arolein, <1 ppm; 1,2-benzoisothiazolin-3-one, 1 to 10 ppm; 5-chloro-2-methyl-4-isothiazolin-3-one plus 2-methyl-4-isothiazolin-3-one, 1 ppm; oxazolidines, 5 to 50 ppm; biguanidines, 500 to 2000 ppm; 2-nitropropane-1,3-diol, 1 to 50 ppm; 2-hydroxyethyl-2,3-dibromopropionate, 8 to 30 ppm. Other biocides included dichlorophen, 2,2-dibromo-3-nitrilopropionamide and 2-hydroxyethoxylmethane. Maxwell et al. (1987) noted that in waterflood system one of the most common treatments is a weekly dose for 6 hours of 50 ppm of glutaraldehyde. This works fine for the planktonic bacteria but in recent years it has been found that the sessile bacteria require slug treatments of higher concentrations. To remain cost-effective, the duration was reduced. These workers experimented with 150 ppm for 2 hours, up to 600 ppm for 1 hour. These treatments appeared to control the general aerobic bacteria as well as the sulfate reducers. The importance of prior chlorination with 0.5 to 0.8 ppm chlorine was stressed.

A novel method for protecting pipelines, posts, and tanks buried or partially buried in the ground from bacterial corrosion involves the use of (1) a protective coating such as polyvinyl chloride or bitumen-impregnated wrapping containing a suitable germicide, and (2) the treatment of a 1- to 6-inch contiguous layer of fill with a different germicide. A double defense is thereby provided against the organisms, by preventing acquired resistance to the germicide. Arsenicals, chlorophenols, and cresols are mentioned as germicides (Hitzman and Schneider, 1961).

Lubricating Oils

Cutting oils are used for lubricating and cooling the cutting and grinding surfaces of metals in metal-working machines. They are supplied to the machines from tanks holding about 50 gallons or dispensed centrally in large shops from tanks holding as much as 100,000 gallons. There are over a million machinists in the United States using a total of about 100 million gallons of cutting oils per year at an estimated cost of 50 million dollars. Straight oils are mainly mineral oil and are used in low-speed work principally for lubrication. The synthetic types are water solutions or dispersions and are used mainly for cooling with high-speed work where great heats are generated. The soluble oils are principally mineral oil (up to about 15%) with emulsifying agents that produce an emulsion on dilution with 20 to 40 parts of water. This type gives both lubrication and cooling and is also more susceptible to microbial spoilage. Spoilage is not the only microbially induced problem with cutting oils, however. These fluids come in contact with workers' hands and are reported to account for 25% of all cases of industrial dermatitis (Braun and Sitgreaves, 1958). Some investigators have attributed this condition to bacteria in the oils, but others see the oil as clogging the ducts in the hair follicles, resulting in irritation (Lee and Chandler, 1941).

Many different pathogens have been isolated from emulsion oils in commercial use. These are mostly gram-negative bacteria, suggesting a potential health hazard (Tant and Bennett, 1956). Whether or not the fluid itself is spoiled (from the standpoint of operation) the metabolism of bacteria in numbers of 15 to 50 million per ml (Lee and Chandler, 1941) may produce products that will stain or corrode the metal or, as commonly occurs, the oil becomes so foul smelling that it must be discarded (Flemming and Baker, 1960). At a dilution of the soluble oil with water of 40 to 1, there could be, in the United States, a total of 1 to 2 billion gallons of bacterially contaminated water containing 2 to 5 million pounds of antimicrobial chemicals to be disposed of annually. This could be a serious problem for those concerned with pollution prevention.

While a variety of different microorganisms have been found in cutting oil emulsions, the principal types are aerobic gram-negative bacteria, coliform bacteria, pseudomonads, and anaerobic sulfate reducers. Rossmoore (1962) found that the coliform bacteria were not correlated with spoilage of the oil, but that deterioration was always accompanied by large numbers of the sulfate reducers. Isenberg and Bennett (1959) suggested that spoilage of the oil as indicated by a blue to black color (FeS), odor of H_2S, and breaking of the emulsion is the result of a commensal relationship between aerobic heterotrophic bacteria belonging to the *Pseudomonas* and the anaerobic sulfate-reducing bacteria such as *Desulfovibrio desulfuricans*. The aerobic bacteria are thought to oxidize components of the emulsion that are toxic to the sulfate-reducing bacteria and to lower the oxidation-reducing potential to favor growth of the latter.

To control spoilage, which they attribute to the sulfate-reducing bacteria obtaining energy through electrochemical action involving iron, Flemming and Baker (1960) recommended the following procedures: (1) good housekeeping and plant sanitation, (2) use of a bactericide, (3) keeping the emulsion about pH 9.0 to 9.5, (4) avoiding anaerobic conditions, (5) prompt removal of metal cuttings, (6) periodic aeration, (7) use of soft water for the emulsion, (8) periodic pasteurization, (9) refrigeration of coolant to 18°C, and (10) use of low sulfur content metals and minimum use of sulfurized oils. On the subject of bactericides, they commented that no bactericide was found that would give protection without periodic additions. They suggested periodic change in the type of bactericide, and multiple bactericides rather than single ones.

In practice, the use of antibacterial agents is relied upon almost exclusively over other methods. The chemical must be compatible with oil and water in the emulsion system, and it must not be harmful to the worker or the work. Bennett (1956) gave a compilation of data on inhibitors for aerobic bacteria in emulsion oils. In tests of several commercial cutting oil inhibitors, none successfully controlled bacterial growth (Wheeler and Bennett, 1956). They tested 51 inhibitors in both open and closed systems, and only 5 gave complete inhibition for 60 days at 1000 ppm. These were 2,4,5-trichlorophenol; 2,4,6-trichlorophenol; 2,2'-thiobis(3,4,6-trichlorophenol); 1,3-dichloro-5,5-dimethylhydantoin; and tris(hydroxymethyl) nitromethane.

The nitroparaffins have proved to be highly effective in cutting fluids as well as low in cost and toxicity. Those found to be protective for 50 to 100 days with only 50 ppm were 2-nitro-2-ethyl-1,3-propanediol dipropionate; 2-nitro-2-ethyl-1,3-propanediol, and 2-nitro-2-methyl-

1,3-propanediol (Carlson and Bennett, 1960). Sodium ethyl mercuric thiosalicylate was the most effective inhibitor in these tests, but because of possible toxicity, the use of mercurials has been prohibited.

A patented cutting fluid of the synthetic type said to be resistant to bacterial decomposition (Davis and Laug, 1963) has the following composition: alkanolamine organic acid reaction product, 1.5 to 3.0%; castor oil fatty acids, 2.5 to 7.5%; KOH, 0.23 to 0.7%; triethanolamine, 8.5 to 11.5%; 85% H_3PO_4, 1.69 to 2.25%; $NaNO_2$, 0.3 to 1.0%; phenol, 0.1 to 1.0%; methyl p-hydroxybenzoate, 1.5 to 2.0%; and o-phenylphenol, 0.5% to 1.0% (and the rest water). The two last-mentioned chemicals are the principal microbial inhibitors.

Watson and Sowden (1972) give a favorable report on hexahydro-1,3,5-tris(2-hydroxyethyl)-s-triazine with consideration of its activity, cost economy, and toxicity to fish on disposal in bodies of water. This chemical was able to control growth of *Fusarium* at 0.05% when added immediately after inoculation, but 0.2% did not control previously established populations (Rossmoore and Holtzman, 1974).

Grier and co-workers (1980) found an even better triazine in 1,3,5-tris(tetrahydro-2-furanyl)-methyl)-hexahydro-s-triazine. Over a 9-week period, 0.05 to 0.1% of this compound in a cutting oil emulsion, as a single initial dosing, produced sterility after 48 hours upon weekly challenges with pure cultures of organisms and with spoiled emulsions. The tris(2-hydroxyethyl) analog failed under these conditions. The superiority of the furanyl analog was thought to stem from its fivefold-greater lipophilicity, although both compounds were hydrophilic.

An increase in the activity of the 2-hydroxyethyl-s-triazine and seven other cutting oil preservatives was found when EDTA or its sodium salts were added. With the EDTA, the inhibition of growth was more or less uniform with all of the compounds. The EDTA alone showed practically no activity (Izzat and Bennett, 1979). Hill (1982) gave examples of preservatives in use for cutting oil emulsions. These include 2-phenylphenol, 2-benzyl-4-chlorophenol, 2,4,6-trichlorophenol, dichlorophane, 2,2'-thiobis (3,4,6-trichlorophenol), 6-acetoxy-2,4-dimethyl-1,3-dioxane (Dioxin), 1,3-di(hydroxymethyl)-5,5-dimethyl-2,4-dioxoimidazole (Dantoin, DMDMH-55), N,N-methylenebis-5'-(1-hydroxymethyl)-2,5-dioxo-4-imidazolidinyl urea (Germall 115), 5-chloro-2-methyl-4-isothiazolin-3-one plus 3-methyl-4-isothiazolin-3-one (Kathone 886MW), cis-1-(3 chloroally 1-3,5,7-triaza-1-azonia) adamantine chloride (Dowicil 200), hexahydro-1,3,5-triethyl-s-triazine, and 1,3-dichloro-5-dimethyldioxomimidazole (Halane). Hill notes that when bacteria are killed by germicides that do not control fungi or yeast, which is often, these organisms proliferate. In this case, he suggests that the latter organisms be countered by a mixture of agents such as a formaldehyde releaser and a phenolic preservative. Other methods of control, such as filtration and use of gamma radiation, have been investigated, but these measures have not proved to be practical.

In addition to the cutting oils, ordinary petroleum oil lubricants may be subject to deterioration in the presence of small amounts of moisture. For example, lubricant greases, oil for optical instruments, and engine oils have received attention in recent years from the standpoint of microbial spoilage, and preservatives similar to those in cutting oils were recommended. Hill (1976) comments on the hazard of the degradation of engine oils. Where their protective function is lost, the viscosity is affected, the acidity increases, and water becomes permanently entrained in the oil, leading to corrosion, especially in the presence of microbial products such as acids, sulfide, and ammonia. The source of water and infections is the water-cooled pistons. An oil-soluble quaternary ammonium disinfectant was shown to be effective in controlling this problem.

WATER-COOLING TOWERS

Industries that use large quantities of water for cooling purposes often conserve the water by cooling it in large evaporative cooling towers and recycling it. The water and the system will become contaminated with microorganisms unless a biocide is employed (Fig. 52–7). The biocide must be effective at great dilution, inexpensive, nonvolatile, and noncorrosive, and it must have a broad spectrum of activity. Biocides that have been employed include quaternary ammonium compounds, chlorinated phenols, organic tin compounds, dithiocarbamates, and other sulfur species. A more recent constraint is environmental, namely, the toxicity of the cooling-tower effluent. Friend and Whitekettle (1980) studied three biocides currently in use that act quickly to kill microorganisms, then hydrolyze at neutral pH to give products that are much less toxic to aquatic animals. These compounds are methylene bisthiocyanate (MBT), 2,2-dibromo-3-nitrilopropionamide (DBNPA), and β-bromo-β-nitrostyrene (BNS). According to their data, MBT was active against a spectrum of bacteria, yeasts, molds, and algae at roughly 1 to 3 ppm, DBNPA at 5 to 100 ppm, and BNS at 0.5 to 5 ppm. As the pH of the water was increased from 7 to 9 the half-lives of these compounds ranged from 19 hours to 1 hour or less.

Cooling tower sanitation has always been considered an economic necessity, but a possible health aspect may be involved in the newly-revealed Legionnaires' disease. The organism associated with this fatal illness, *Legionella pneumophila*, has been isolated from aquatic habitats including air-conditioning water-cooling towers and evaporative condensers. In outbreaks of the disease, aerosols from these sources have been strongly implicated as the source of infection (see Chapter 45 and Chapter 65). While there are still many unknown factors on the relationship of this organism to the onset of the disease, the fact that air-conditioning water-cooling towers are widely used by hotels, hospitals, office buildings, and industries makes their sanitation of much greater im-

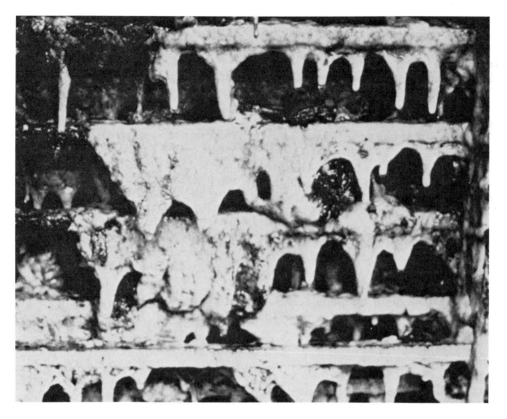

Fig. 52–7. Microbial slime on water-cooling tower slats from a citrus processing plant in Florida.

portance than if economic criteria were the only consideration. Wang et al. (1979) tested the organism in laboratory culture against a number of common disinfectants. With a concentration of 10^4 organisms per ml and an exposure of 1 minute, the following disinfectants were inhibitory: phenolic (Amphyl) at 0.05%, iodophor (Betadine) at 10 ppm, quaternary ammonium salt (Zephiran) at 1:8000, glutaraldehyde (Cidex) at 0.031%, hypochlorite (Chlorox) at 5.0 ppm, formalin at 2.0%, ethanol at 70% (lower concentrations not tested), and hydrochloric acid at pH 1.7. Greater dilutions of the disinfectants were not inhibitory under these conditions.

Miller et al. (1981) tested two biocides commonly used to prevent slime formation in cooling water systems against the Legionnaires' disease bacterium. These were Bio-Guard DCM which contained the quaternary ammonium compound, alkyl dimethyldichlorobenzylammonium chloride, and Bio-Guard CWT-100, a mixture of alkyldimethylammonium chlorides, alkyldimethylethylammonium bromide, and tributyltin neodecanoate. These chemicals were bacteriostatic at less than 1 ppm of active ingredients with 3.6×10^9 bacteria per ml. Bactericidal activity was shown for both products at 62 ppm in the presence of 750 ppm calcium hardness and 1% horse serum after 120 minutes of exposure.

PLASTICS

Most plastics contain synthetic polymers, which are mostly resistant to microbial degradation (Heap and Mor-

rell, 1968). There are exceptions in the case of low-molecular-weight polyethylenes, some polyesters, and some polyester polyurethanes. Plastics may also contain plasticizers, fillers, pigments, stabilizers, and lubricants that may serve as nutrients for bacteria and fungi. Even though the plastic itself does not degrade, it may fail in its function—as in the case of electrical insulation supporting fungus growth. Luce and Mathes (1948) showed that fungi provided a moisture bridge, lowering the resistivity of the plastic.

Of the additives to the polymer the plasticizer, which may make up to 50% by weight of the plastic, is the ingredient most susceptible to bacteria and fungi. Plasticizers vary in susceptibility, and it is desirable to obtain one that is as bioinert as possible while still possessing other desirable properties. For example, to obtain flexibility, polyvinyl films employ vegetable oils and esters of fatty acids as plasticizers, which are readily attacked by fungi. Fungi grow in the plastic and on its surface and disfigure it. Bacterial growth may cause plastic films to become brittle and crack. It may also produce foul odors. Algae grow on the surface of moist plastic in outdoor exposure and make it unsightly.

The two types of plastic that have suffered the most from microorganisms are the vinyls and the polyurethanes. Vinyl plastics have been used widely for many products such as raincoats, tents, shower curtains, hospital sheets, and inflatable boats. They use large quantities of plasticizer to obtain the necessary flexibility. Previously they were preserved with phenylmercurials and copper-8-quinolinolate at 1% concentrations. The latter was undesirable for its color and the former for its toxicity. The compound, 10,10'-oxybisphenoxyarsine, however, has found favor in vinyl formulations. It gives spectacular zones of inhibition against most organisms and is employed with a heat stabilizer and ultraviolet screening agent (Yeager, 1977). Other biocides for plastics include diphenylantimony ethylhexoate, zinc dimethyldithiocarbamate, tetramethylthiuram disulfide, dithiopyridine dioxide, dodecyldimethylbenzylammonium naphthenate, and dibromosalicylanilide (Klausmeier and Andrews, 1981). Hopfenberg and Tulis (1970) investigated antibacterial plastics for hospital supplies such as draw sheets, pillow covers, mattress covers, toilet seats, etc. They demonstrated that a low-density polyethylene film containing 0.25% hexachlorophene exhibited antibacterial activity for a year without lessening. It was proposed that a reservoir of antibacterial chemical will ensure that the antibacterial properties of the polymer will exceed the life of the finished product. It was discovered that the zone of inhibition of the treated polyethylene was larger than that of the pure hexachlorophene. This was explained by the small particle size of the crystals emerging from the plastic. A toilet seat made of high-impact polystyrene incorporating 3% hexachlorophene was shown to be relatively sterile, whereas without the hexachlorophene, the bacterial count was in the thousands. In a nursery for the newborn, reduction in infection rate was attributed primarily to the use of antibacterial bassinet covers used over a 3-year period.

Work to develop antimicrobial polymers for self-sanitizing medical articles such as catheters, sutures, and drainage bags has been performed by binding the antimicrobial agent to the copolymer backbone, rather than by simply mixing in the chemical, as is usually done. This way it was hoped that the plastic would serve as a reservoir of the germicide for extended lengths of time. Employing carboxyl-containing ethylene copolymers such as poly(ethylene-co-acrylic acid), the salts were made with basic nitrogen-containing antimicrobial agents. Of a number tested, the two most successful were benzalkonium chloride and 8-hydroxyquinoline. The polymers prevented bacterial growth but were not bactericidal (Ackart et al., 1975).

The introduction of plastic contact lenses for eye glasses in recent years has introduced microbiologic problems as well. Being in direct contact with the eyeball, the lenses accumulate protein from the eye fluid, which is susceptible to microbial growth unless carefully removed by cleansing. Failure to do so may produce irritation and infection of the eyes and also microbial attack of the plastic lenses, especially the hydrophilic, soft contact lenses. Kimmerer and Szabocsik (1978) found that daily cleaning and disinfection of hydroxyethyl methacrylate lenses as prescribed by the manufacturer was effective in preventing fungal growth. Where this is not done, fungi grew and the lenses were etched. Treatment of the lenses has included cleaning, disinfection with heat, treatment with chemicals including thimerosal, quaternary ammonium compounds, iodine, and hydrogen peroxide. According to Bruch (1976), only disinfection with near-boiling water received FDA approval. For lenses of materials that cannot be disinfected with heat, Levine et al. (1981) suggest that 6% hydrogen peroxide is suitable. Whereas 3% H_2O_2 has been marketed in Canada and Great Britain, the U.S. FDA has not approved it. Six-percent H_2O_2, according to the investigators, is at least twice as effective as the 3% solution in reducing the bioburden.

RUBBER

Natural rubber was the first elastomer and plastic. The latex is readily attacked by microorganisms, but vulcanized rubber is much more resistant, although it can be partially degraded by actinomycetes (Cundell and Mulcock, 1975). As in other plastic materials, the chemical additives for increasing plasticity and mold release increase the susceptibility to microorganisms. Rubber accelerators used in the processing of rubber, such as mercaptobenzothiazole and tetramethylthiuram disulfide, have seen double duty as antimicrobial agents for rubber.

Phaltan and sodium pentachlorophenate have served as rubber antimicrobials. Yeager (1977) states that dehydroabietylamine (rosin amine) pentachlorophenate is the most widely used microbicide in rubber manufacturing. It is combined with the mineral oil plasticizer and provides the protection of pentachlorophenol without its fugitive characteristics. Dayal et al. (1965) reported that rubber condoms packaged in airtight aluminum foil in the tropical climate of India were found to have supported growth of *Aspergillus niger*. Talcum powder containing 1.75% boric acid applied to the sheaths or 2% boric acid added to the lubricant controlled the problem. Cundell and Mulcock (1973), seeking a solution to the microbial deterioration of vulcanized natural rubber pipe joints in underground pipelines conveying sewage and stormwater, studied the protection afforded by four microbicides as 2% of the rubber. They did not suppress microbial activity. It was suppressed, however, by surface chlorination of the rubber, which the authors felt would prevent deterioration. Zyska (1981), in a thorough review of the microbiology of rubber, listed many biocides that have been tested as rubber preservatives. He observed that as rubber requires vulcanization at 135 to 175° C only a small group of microbiocides can be considered, and an ideal preservative that can act as a bactericide and fungicide has not yet been found. Among those giving good results were cresylic acids at 2%. Williams (1986) conducted soil burial experiments on rubber. He found that soil microorganisms preferentially attack the stearic acid component of vulcanized rubber. Levels of 2 to 4% of sulfur accelerators protected the rubber. These included tetramethylthiuram disulfide, mercaptobenzothiasole, mercaptobenzothiazole sulfonamide, and cyclohexylbenzo-thiazole. High levels of carbon black (70%) made it protective, whereas paraffin wax (0.4 to 3%) made it more susceptible.

Hofmann (1969) discusses another problem with rubber goods, e.g., rubber boots, gloves, and mats in bathrooms, that is, the carrying and nurturing of pathogenic microorganisms such as the athlete's foot fungus. He cited statistics showing that as high as 75% of miners suffered from this ailment caused by moist feet from rubber footwear. The solution he proposed was to make the rubber antimicrobial with antiseptic chemicals. He showed that tetramethylthiuram disulfide, ortho- and parabenzyl phenol and salicylanilide in 0.5 to 2.0% concentrations had activity in this direction. He performed experiments with a commercial product containing a mixture (said to be of the ingredients just mentioned, according to Cundell and Mulcock, 1973) called Antimy-kotikum A, for which he claimed antimicrobial properties of rubber. Hofmann found that the treated rubber was not only inhibitory, but actually killed bacteria and fungi rapidly. Some antimycotic action was reported in a treated rubber bath mat after several years of use. He recommended this treatment for tennis shoes, rubber sponge insoles, rubber bed sheeting, and various hospital items made of rubber.

OPTICAL EQUIPMENT

Damage to lenses and optical equipment caused by the growth of fungi in tropical climates has long been a problem (Fig. 52–8). Cameras and microscopes require expensive cleaning to remove the fungus mycelium. The problem was especially serious in World War II in the South Pacific area for binoculars and gun sights, where inspection indicated that half of the instruments were overgrown with fungi, interfering with vision to a greater or lesser extent. Mold obtains no nourishment from the glass itself but from the organic dust and grease and the leather case. The best solution to the problem is storage of the equipment in dehumidified containers, but where this has not been feasible, chemical methods have been

employed. Best control was given with metacresyl acetate (Cresatin). This is a volatile fungicide employed by mixing with an equal quantity of ethyl cellulose resin and enclosing the resultant taffy-like product in an aluminum capsule which is placed in the instrument case. One-half million of these capsules were procured by Frankford Arsenal and distributed throughout the Pacific area for application to instruments during servicing and repair (N.D.R.C., 1946). In Panama Canal zone exposure tests, the m-cresyl acetate capsules were the only means found to be completely effective in controlling fungus inside binocular cases (Teitell and Berk, 1952).

In Australian investigations (N.D.R.C., 1945), the recommended use of sodium ethylmercuric thiosalicylate is referred to. This compound was incorporated to the extent of 0.2% in lacquer used to paint interior surfaces of instruments and was mixed with the cement and luting compounds. It has been noted to cause some deterioration of plastics and rubber (Baker, 1967). In Canal Zone tests, however, Teitell and Berk (1952) found that sodium ethylmercuric thiosalicylate-treated binoculars became moldy in large numbers. Vicklund (1946) reported on an interesting method for prevention of the fungus fouling of optical instruments. Metal foil treated with 15 µg per square inch of radium sulfate and used to surround the lenses prevented fungus growth as a result of the alpha radiation. Teitell and Berk confirmed the protective properties of the radioactive foil but indicated a possible health hazard in the storage of foil-treated instruments. Use of a quaternary ammonium salt in an antifogging compound applied to the lens surfaces kept the lenses mold-free for over a year in Panama (N.D.R.C., 1946). Inner lens surfaces should be protected by hermetically sealing the lenses so that moisture or dust cannot penetrate.

Adams (1969) reports that glasses that contained trace amounts of heavy metals were less severely affected by fungi. Saxena et al. (1963) found that satisfactory protection could be afforded by incorporating fungicides such as m-cresyl acetate (Cresatin), thimerosal (Merthiolate), copper naphthenate, and pentachlorophenol in lacquers, waxes, lutings, greases, and paints applied to

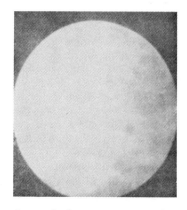
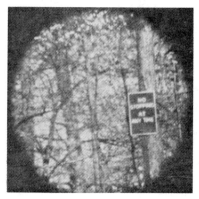

Fig. 52–8. The effect of alpha radiation of radium in preventing fungus fouling of optical instruments. *Left,* View through an untreated telescope after 2 months in a tropical testing chamber. *Right,* View through a telescope protected with radium foil.

various components of the instruments. A controlled-release volatile fungicide preparation was developed and tested by Upsher (1985) for protection of optical equipment and electronic circuitry. He employed 2.5% each of tributyltin acetate and tributyltin chloride in 400-mg disks of polyurethane foam. These were placed in closed 50-L vessels at 95% R.H. and room temperature with eight species of fungi applied to nutrient-treated paper. The vapor concentration was 200 μg/L for each chemical. The vapors suppressed growth of all the fungi for 6 months and for four species for 12 months.

Russian workers have shown interest in the prevention of mold growing on glass and optical materials for use in the tropics. Baigozhin (1980) reported on chemisorbed fungicidal siloxane coatings on optical glasses. With other coworkers (1981), he reported on the fungicidal treatment of mirrors. Aluminized mirrors were coated with $(EtO)_4Ti$ and $Et_3[2-CH_3-(1-oxo-2-propenyl)oxy)]$ stannate, which increased the reflection 2 to 4%.

CONCRETE AND STONE

Concrete, like stone and glass, is inorganic and generally thought to be impervious to attack by microorganisms. This is not true, for concrete floors in dairies and breweries and concrete pipes and ducts carrying sewage are attacked and degraded by the action of microorganisms. Concrete is composed of hydrated portland cement with an inert aggregate of sand or crushed stone. The calcium silicates and aluminates making up the cement may be dissolved by the organic and inorganic acids produced by microorganisms, thus "corroding" the concrete. This condition occurs in food plants where the floors and walls are contaminated with organic matter and continually wet. The bacteria and fungi grow on the food in the crevices of the concrete where acids and metal complexing agents are produced and dissolve the cement surrounding the pieces of aggregate, causing the floor surface first to roughen and then to crumble away.

Sewage, particularly that with large quantities of undigested organic matter, such as industrial wastes and garbage from home disposal units, supports the growth of sulfur bacteria, which produce sulfides under anaerobic conditions. While it is doubtful whether H_2S and the sulfides have any direct damaging effect on concrete, they are converted under aerobic conditions to sulfuric acid, which dissolves the calcium salts in the cement, and the pipes are badly damaged.

In food plants, an antibacterial cement that is troweled onto the floor surface in a half inch coating has been shown to have given protection in a number of trials (Levowitz, 1952). Concrete floors said to have required replacement every 3 to 4 months in a brewery and sugar refinery held up for 13 and 9 months, respectively, with the antibacterial product.

A magnesium oxychloride cement containing 10% fine copper powder is said to produce copper oxychloride, which has been shown to be antibacterial and antifungal.

It produced a reduction in number of bacteria in a 15-minute interval, and the growth of mold cultures was completely inhibited in this period. Covering the cement with dirt or washing with water for 6 hours did not reduce the antiseptic properties, and similar results were demonstrated under actual service conditions during a 6-months test (Farrell and Wolff, 1941). Mallman (1941) demonstrated that fragments of this cement in broth or water suspensions of bacteria, yeasts, and molds had lethal effects. *Epidermophyton interdigitale* was isolated from ordinary concrete floors in a locker room but not from the copper oxychloride-covered floor, and Mallman considered this cement to be an aid in the control of floor-borne infections of the feet.

In the corrosion of concrete sewer and water pipes, the use of protective coatings and linings is recommended (Munger, 1960). A heavy toweled vinyl polymer in several coats totaling one-eighth inch gave protection for 15 years where brick and tile had failed. High-polymer vinyl chloride linings are said to be most effective.

There is considerable interest in the decay of stone statuary and monuments and the part that may be played by microorganisms. Fusey and Hyvert (1966) studied the deterioration of monuments in Cambodia. They discounted the effect of sulfur-oxidizing bacteria and nitrifying bacteria but blamed a complex cycle of physical, chemical, and biologic agents, with actinomycetes, algae, and fungi involved in the process. They suggest architectural modifications to divert rain and note that organometallic salts have given good results. Studying the deterioration of masonry art works in Venice, Paleni and Curri (1972) implicate microorganisms and play down the effect of sulfur dioxide from industrial pollution. They believe that carbon dioxide and water vapor have an important part in the dissolution of limestones.

A related problem is the staining of pebble-encrusted roof shingles, which has been demonstrated to result primarily from algal growth. Insoluble zinc and copper compounds coated on the pebbles have shown inhibitory effects (Block, 1982) and shingles utilizing a band of zinc metal have been in commercial use for several years. Work by Amburgey (1974) indicates that the deterioration of the shingles may in part by caused by fungal breakdown of the wood fibers in the asphalt.

An asbestos-cement building board treated to give antifungal properties claimed no black mold after 7 years of outdoor exposure (Kubota Ltd., 1980). The board was coated with cement, Fe_2O_3, 0.2% copper powder, then spray-coated with colored sand containing 0.2% copper powder, and coated with an acrylic resin emulsion containing 100 ppm copper powder.

To protect concrete against biologically active agents in sea water, a German patent (Moraru, 1980) prescribes a three-layered protective coating consisting of a 3.5% aqueous solution of fluosilic acid or the sodium or zinc salt, a 40 to 50% solution of water-insoluble biocidal agents in an organic solvent containing a quantity of polyester or epoxy resin, followed by a 5 to 10% solution of the resin. The biocides recommended were copper naphthenate, pentachlorophenol, and tributyltin oxide, individually or as a mixture.

ADHESIVES

In 1961, almost half of the 0.5 billion pounds of adhesives produced contained some preservative, which in an average amount of 0.25% by weight amounted to an estimated 625,000 pounds of preservatives (Yeager, 1962). These included pentachlorophenol, formaldehyde, sodium pentachlorophenate, phenol, sodium o-phenylphenate, methyl p-hydroxybenzoate, propyl p-hydroxybenzoate, copper-8-quinolinolate, 2,2'-methylenebis (4-chlorophenol), and sodium and potassium propionates.

Adhesives require preservation of the aqueous solution prior to application and for the dried film after use. In solution, adhesives are attacked mostly by bacteria and yeasts, whereas the dried product is attacked by fungi. Whereas synthetic polymers, some of which are bioinert, are making inroads in the adhesives business, costs and tradition prevail in utilizing mainly natural products like gums, starch, and protein. For preservatives, traditional additives such as formalin, phenol, and sodium benzoate continue to be used (Yeager, 1977). Among the more active biocides employed are sodium pentachlorophenate, and sodium-o-phenylphenate. For preservation of the liquid product, protein, starch, or dextrin, 0.1 to 0.2% will usually suppress growth of the microorganisms, but under severe conditions of some products as much as 2 to 3% has been found necessary. For the dried film 2% p-nitrophenol was found to give the best protection of many fungicides tested, with 3,5-dinitro-o-cresol a close second (Berk, 1948). For food packaging, those most commonly used (Yeager, 1977) are 2,2-methylenebis(4-chlorophenol) and copper-8-quinolinolate, the latter being particularly effective in protein glues. Also effective for protein-based glues (Hovey, 1959) is 1000 ppm pyridinethione stabilized with 1000 to 2500 ppm borax. Thermosetting glues for plywood containing alkaline-condensed phenolic resins can be rendered fungistatic by the inclusion of 2 to 10% isosafrole(1,2-methylenedioxy-4-propenylbenzene), according to Brown (1960). A Czech patent (Rabas et al., 1980) describes preserved solutions of water-soluble adhesives such as carboxymethyl cellulose, polyvinyl alcohol, and soybean flour. A typical formula contains 500 parts of carboxymethyl cellulose, 490 parts dextrin, 10 parts 8-hydroxyquinoline, and 1 part each of zinc salts of trichloroisocyanurates and perfume.

A Japanese patent (Nichiden Kaguku Co., 1980) describes the use of a hydroxyethyl acrylate-starch copolymer as an adhesive. When 100 g of the polymer was heated with 300 g of water and 20 g KOH was added to give 42% saponification, and this neutralized with 17 g benzoic acid, an adhesive product resulted that remained free of mold during 4 weeks of storage in a tropical chamber.

BUILDING MATERIALS

The deterioration of building materials is touched on in many sections of this chapter. The rotting of wood, microbial attack of paints, plastics, adhesives, rubber, cement, and stone have already been discussed. The effect of microorganisms, like algae and lichens on buildings and monuments, will be mentioned under the discussion of art objects. Bravery (1982) presents an excellent review on preservation in the construction industry in which he tabulates different chemicals employed, their trade names and producers, and literature references mentioning them. This information has been reproduced here in Tables 52–6 and 52–7.

BEDDING

Foter (1960) surveyed the work on disinfectants for bedding. Data on disinfection of mattresses and pillows showed that dry heat alone at 110° C for 2 hours or a combination of dry heat and formalin (1 quart per 1000 cubic feet) in commercial chambers did not accomplish sterilization. Gibbons et al. (1945), however, found that formalin vapors at 80 pounds per 1000 cubic feet gave excellent results in 6 hours. With reduced pressure, penetration was much more rapid, so that using the same dosage and 10 inches of vacuum, the bacteria inoculated into the mattress were killed in 3 hours. With 20 inches of vacuum, it took a little more than an hour for sterilization. Using moist heat alone at 135° C, 24 to 30 hours were required for sterilization. Foter (1960) notes that ethylene oxide and beta-propiolactone have been found to be effective sterilants for bedding materials and clothing.

Commercial laundering followed by ironing of bedding and clothing was effective in lowering numbers of microorganisms. Germicidal rinses are recommended to greatly reduce counts and prevent recontamination. Germicides studied include o-phenylphenol, p-tertiary amylphenol, and potassium ricinoleate (Ravenholt et al., 1958), chlorine, and quaternary ammonium compounds (Goldsmith et al., 1954). Other products used include chlorophenols, hydrogen peroxide, perborates, and hypochlorites. Home automatic washers with water at 63°C and a 10- to 20-minute wash cycle, with a germicide in the rinse cycle, effected a 99% reduction of bacteria in bedding linen and clothes (Procter and Gamble Co., through Foter, 1960). Foter (1960) gives instructions on the use of germicidal rinses of different compositions.

BOOKS

Bookbinding fabrics, sizings, and leather, as well as the bookbinding adhesives and the paper itself, are all susceptible to attack by fungi under certain conditions,

Table 52–6. *Inorganic Chemicals for Controlling Growths on Masonry**

Active Chemical	Application rate/ Concentration (%)	Product	Application*	Reference
Alkali fluorides			I	Nicot, 1951
Ammonium fluoride			I	Roizin, 1951
Barium metaborate			P	Drisko, 1973
Chromium trioxide			C	Forrester, 1959
Copper (metallic)			C	Forrester, 1959
Copper (II) aceto-arsenite (plus many other Cu compounds including oxychloride)	10		C	Robinson & Austin, 1951
Copper (II) carbonate			C	Gilchrist, 1953
Copper (II) carbonate in dilute ammonia	0.2 5		I	Rechenberg, 1972 BRE, 1972 Genin, 1973
Copper (II) cyanide or arsenate + copper (II) oxide			IE	Norddeutsche Affinerie, 1953
Copper (II) naphthenate			E	Stinson, 1956
Copper (II) 8-quinolinolate				Richardson & Ogilvy, 1955
Copper (II) oxide	0.2 (by wt in cement)		EC	Rechenberg, 1972 Lurie & Brookfield, 1948
Copper (II) sulphate	(2 in limewash) 0.1 (by wt in cement)		CE P	Aslam & Singh, 1971 Rechenberg, 1972 Kauffmann, 1960
Disodium octaborate tetrahydrate†	5 4–10	Polybor		Genin, 1973 Anon., 1972 Richardson, 1973
Iron fluoride			I	Roizin, 1951
Mercuric chloride (mercury (II) chloride)			E	Sadurska & Kowalik, 1966
Magnesium fluorosilicate‡	4–10	Lithurin	IE	Genin, 1973 Keen, 1976 Anon., 1972
Potassium permanganate				Rechenberg, 1972
Selenium metal			C	Gilchrist, 1953
Silver nitrate				Sadurska & Kowalik, 1966
Sodium fluoride				Roizin, 1951
Sodium hypochlorite	5	Bleach	CI	Rechenberg, 1972 Keen, 1976 Anon., 1972
Sodium salicylate	2		I	Rechenberg, 1972
Sodium silicofluoride			IC	Roizin, 1951 Gilchrist, 1953
Zinc fluorosilicate‡	4	Lithurin	IE	Genin, 1973 Keen, 1976 Anon., 1972
Zinc naphthenate			E	Stinson & Keyes, 1953
Zinc oxychloride			I	Anon., 1977 Savory, 1980

*I, toxic wash (interior use); C, cement additive; E, toxic ash (exterior use); P, plastics product.

†Supplied by Borax Consolidated Ltd., Borax House, Carlisle Place, London SW1.

‡Supplied by Laporte Industries Ltd., General Chemicals Division, Moorfields Road, Widnes WA8 0HE, England and Chemical Buildings Products Ltd., Cleveland Road, Hemel Hempstead, Herts. HP2 7PH, England.

Bravery, A.F. 1982. Preservation in the Construction Industry. In *Disinfection, Preservation, and Sterilization*. Edited by A.D. Russell, W.B. Hugo, G.A.J. Ayliffe. Oxford, Blackwell Scientific, p. 385.

Table 52–7. *Organic Chemicals Used to Control Growths in the Construction Industry*

Key to coding

A = adhesives	F = fillers, stoppers, groutings	O = wet state protection concrete additives
B = bitumen products	I = toxic wash (interior use)	P = plastic products
C = cement additive	J = jointing compounds, sealants, putty	R = rubbers (synthetic and natural)
E = toxic wash (exterior use)		

Active Chemical	Application Rate/ Concentration (%)	Product	Source of Supply	Application	Reference(s)
Aqueous cresol (cresylic acid)		Lysol		I	Rechenberg, 1972 Keen, 1976
Alkoxysilane: 3(trimethoxy-silyl)-propyldimethyl-octadecyl ammonium chloride	0.1	Si-QAC	Dow Corning Corp.	E	Isquith et al., 1972
Benzimidazole derivative + chloracetamide	0.5–2	Mergal 592	Hoechst UK Ltd	PF	
1,2-Benzisothiazolin-3-one	0.01–0.1	Proxel AB, CRL, HL	ICI Organics	AO	
Benzyl-hemiformals mixture		Preventol D2	Bayer UK	A (liquids)	
Bis(trichloromethyl sulphone)		Chlorosulphone	Tenneco Organics Ltd	AO	
Chloracetamide + polyglycols + heterocyclic compounds	2–5 0.1–0.3	Mergal K6	Hoechst UK Ltd	EI A	
Chloracetamine + quaternary ammonium compound + fluorides	0.1–0	Mergal AF	Hoeschst UK Ltd	A	
Cresylic acids	2			R	Pitis, 1972
Copper 8 hydroxy-quinolinolate				P	Kaplan et al., 1970
Dichlorophen [2,2′-methylene-bis(4-chlorophenol)]	1 free phenol in isopropanol	Panacide	BDH	EC	Rechenberg, 1972 Keen, 1976
2,3-Dichloro 1.4 naphthoquinone				I	Morgan, 1959
Diisocyanate				I	Sponsel, 1956
Dimethylbenzylammonium chloride		Hyamine 3500	Rohm & Haas (UK) Ltd	IE	
Dimethyl aminomethyl phenol				R	Anon., 1974
3,5-Dimethyl-tetra-hydro 1,3,5-2H-thiadiazine-2-thione			Tenneco Organics Ltd	AP	
Diquat 1-1 ethylene-2.2 dipyridiylium				ME	Rechenberg, 1972
Dithio 2,2-bis benzmethylamide	0.2–2	Densil P	ICI Organics	A	
Dithiocarbamates + benzimidazole derivatives	0.05–0.6	Mergal AT30	Hoechst UK Ltd	AFJ	
Dodecylamine salicylate	2–5	Nuodex 87	Durham Chemicals	EI	
Fluorinated sulphonamide	0.2	Acticide APA	Thor Chemicals Ltd	F	
Formaldehyde	5 2			IE	Rechenberg, 1972 Keen, 1976
Halogenated acid amide derivatives	0.1–0.3	Parmetol A23	Sterling Industrial	AO	
Halogenated acid amide derivatives + aldehyde + Heterocyclic compounds	0.05–0.3	Parmetol K50	Sterling Industrial	O	
Halogenised acid amide derivatives + heterocyclic compounds	1.0–3.0	Parmetol DF12	Sterling Industrial	I	
Hexaminium salt	0.1–0.3	Preventol DI	Bayer UK	A	
2-Hydroxybiphenyl potassium salt	3–20	Acticide 50	Thor Chemicals Ltd	E	
2-Hydroxydiphenyl sodium salt		Preventol ON	Bayer UK	A	
5-Hydroxymethoxmethyl 1-aza-3,7-dioxabicyclo (3,3,0) octane + other substituted oxazolidines		Nuosept 95	Durham Chemicals Tenneco Organics Ltd	AFO	
Lead phenolate and other lead salts of synthetic fatty acids				P	Wexler et al., 1971
3-Methyl-4-chlorophenol		Preventol CMK	Bayer UK	A (powder) F	

Table 52–7. *Organic Chemicals Used to Control Growths in the Construction Industry* (continued)

Key to coding

A = adhesives	F = fillers, stoppers, groutings	O = wet state protection concrete additives
B = bitumen products	I = toxic wash (interior use)	P = plastic products
C = cement additive	J = jointing compounds, sealants, putty	R = rubbers (synthetic and natural)
E = toxic wash (exterior use)		

Active Chemical	Application Rate/ Concentration (%)	Product	Source of Supply	Application	Reference(s)
Methylene-bisthiocyanate			Tenneco Organics Ltd	APFO	
2-Mercaptobenzothiazole	0.1–1	Mystox MB	Catomance Ltd	AO	
2-Mercaptobenzothiazole sodium salt	0.1–0.5	Nuodex 84	Nuodex UK Ltd; Tenneco Organics Ltd	A	
N-dimethyl-N′-phenyl-(N′-fluorodichloromethylthio) sulphamide	1.5–2	Preventol A4	Bayer UK Ltd	EIJ	
N(fluorodichloromethylthio) phthalimide	1–2	Preventol A3	Bayer UK Ldt	EIPJ	
N(trichloromethylthio)phthalmide		Folpet	Murphy Chemical Ltd (UK)	PEI	Kaplan et al., 1970 Rechenberg, 1972
N(Trichloromethylthio)-4-cyclohexene 1,2-dicarboximide	0.5–2.5	Captan	Murphy Chemical Ltd (UK)	P	Kaplan et al., 1970
2,n-Octyl-4-isothiazolon-3-one		Kathan 893	Rohm & Haas UK Ltd	EI	
Organic acid amine	1–5	Nuodex 87	Nuodex Ltd UK	EI	
Organic-ethoxy compound	0.1–0.5 0.3–0.8	Acticide BG THP	Thor Chemicals	AFO AO	
Organo-mercury				I R	Nicot, 1951 Zyska et al., 1972
Organo-tin	0.2–0.5	Acticide FPF	Thor Chemicals	AF	
Ortho-phenyl phenol				E	
10,10′-Oxybisphenoxarsine				P	Darby & Kaplan, 1968 Cadmus, 1976
Oxyquinoline					Nicot, 1951
Oxyquinoline sulphate					Nicot, 1951
Paraquat		Gramoxone		E	Powell, 1975
Pentachlorophenol	2 0.1–0.3	Mystox G	Catomance Ltd	ECR A (starch pastes)	Kaplan et al., 1970 Rechenberg, 1972 Gilchrist, 1953 Purkiss, 1972 Zyska et al., 1972
Pentachlorophenyl laurate	1–3.5	Mystox LPL LSL	Catomance Ltd	APOR	Zyska et al., 1972
Phenoxy fatty acid polyester	0.4–1.5	Preventol B2	Bayer (UK) Ltd	JB	
Phenyl mercury acetate			Tenneco Organics Ltd	A	
Phenyl mercury nonane	0.05–0.3	Acticide MPM	Thor Chemicals	AO	
Phenyl mercury oleate					Drisko, 1973
Quaternary ammonium compounds	1	Gloquat C	ABM Chemicals; Glover (Chemicals) Ltd	E I	Keen, 1976 Genin, 1973 Anon., 1972 Richardson, 1973 Nicot, 1951
	0.3–0.2	Preventol R Vantoc HL, CL, IB	Bayer UK Ltd ICI Organics		
Quaternary ammonium salt: di-isobutyl cresoxyethoxyethyl dimethyl benzyl ammonium chloride monohydrate		Hyamine 10x	Rohm & Haas	IE	Paleni & Curri, 1973
Quaternary ammonium salt: di-isobutyl phenoxyethoxyethyl dimethylbenzyl ammonium chloride monohydrate	0.5	Hyamine 1622	Rohm and Haas	IE	Paleni & Curri, 1973

Table 52–7. *Organic Chemicals Used to Control Growths in the Construction Industry* (continued)

Key to coding

A = adhesives	F = fillers, stoppers, groutings	O = wet state protection concrete additives
B = bitumen products	I = toxic wash (interior use)	P = plastic products
C = cement additive	J = jointing compounds, sealants, putty	R = rubbers (synthetic and natural)
E = toxic wash (exterior use)		

Active Chemical	Application Rate/ Concentration (%)	Product	Source of Supply	Application	Reference(s)
Quaternary ammonium compound + lauryl pentachlorphenate		Mystox QL	Catomance Ltd	E	Barr, 1977
Quaternary ammonium salt with tri-*n*-butyl tin oxide		Thaltox O Stannicide AQ	Wykamol Limited; Thomas Swan & Co Ltd	E	Genin, 1973 Keen, 1976 Richardson, 1973
Salicylamide	5–8		Bayer UK Ltd	JP (cable insolation)	Cadmus, 1976
Sodium *o*-phenyl phenate	2 2.5	Brunsol con	Stanhope Chemical Products Ltd	E	Genin, 1973 Rechenberg, 1972 Keen, 1976
	5	Mystox WFA	Catomance Ltd	EI	
Sodium pentachlorophenate	2 0.2 on wt on cement	Santobrite	Monsanto Ltd	EI C	Genin, 1973 Rechenberg, 1972 Keen, 1976 Sponsel, 1956
		Preventol PN	Bayer UK Ltd	AFJ	
	2	Brunobrite	Stanhope Chemical Products Ltd	E	Anon., 1972
Sodium salicylanilide	1–5 0.5–1.5	Shirlan NA	ICI Ltd	I A	Keen, 1976
2,4,5,6-Tetrachloro-isophthalonitrile	0.5–1.5	Nopcocide N96	Diamond Shamrock UK	APJ	
2,4,5-Tetrachloro-isophthalonitrile (aq.)	0.3–1.8	Nopcocide N54D	Diamond Shamrock UK	AP	
3,3,4,4-Tetrachloro-tetrahydrothiophene 1,1-dioxide		Nopcocide 170	Diamond Shamrock UK	EI	
Thiadiazine	0.1–1.0	Thion 66	Thor Chemicals	A	
Thinned tar oil					Rechenberg, 1972 Keen, 1976
Tri-*n*-butyl-tin acetate	0.005–1			C P	Bartl and Valecky, 1971 Cadmus, 1976
Tri-*n*-butyl tin oxide	1	Stannicide M Stannicide A	Thomas Swan & Co. Ltd	IEO	Drisko, 1973 Richardson, 1973 Sadurska & Kowalik, 1966
Tri-*n*-butyl tin oxide + non-ionic emulsifier		Stannicide O	Thomas Swan & Co. Ltd		
Trifluoromethyl-thiophthalmide					Rechenberg, 1972
α,α-Trithiobis (*N,N*-dimethylthio formalite)				I	Morgan, 1959
Zinc dithiocarbamate + benzimidazole derivatives	0.5–1.0	Mergal S88	Hoechst UK Ltd	AFJ	
Zinc-8-hydroxyquinolinolate			Ward Blenkinsop	A	

From Bravery, A.F. 1982. Preservation in the construction industry. In *Disinfection, Preservation and Sterilization*. Edited by A.D. Russell, W.B. Hugo, and G.A.J. Ayliffe. Oxford, Blackwell Scientific, pp. 386–390.

with the resultant degradation of the materials and impairment of the appearance of the books. Air conditioning, dehumidification, and use of synthetic resin coatings and adhesives represent solutions to the problem when they are employed, but antifungal treatments are valuable when susceptible materials are employed and the environment cannot be controlled.

Evans (1966) reported tests of bookbinding materials in the tropics. After 2 years on bookshelves in an office, all books were in good condition except for slight mold growth on the spines. When the books were left in crates in an open shelter, however, none of the treatments, including 1% phenylmercuric acetate and 5% pentachlorophenate, afforded adequate protection. In prolonged storage tests in a tropical room, glue with 2% o-phenylphenol and 2% pentachlorophenol failed in 2 months but with 2% dichlorophene was effective for 1 year. Paperbacks with this glue and o-phenylphenol and pentachlorophenol that were shipped to the tropics were returned with *Aspergillus glaucus* on their spines after 6 months in storage. Records kept in the House of Lords in London are reported to be preserved by wrapping and interleaving them with a tissue impregnated with sodium pentachlorophenate; sheets of this paper are put into deed boxes to protect documents stored for long periods against fungal attack (Anonymous, 1960).

Thymol, tetramethylthiuram disulfide, dinitrothiocyanobenzene, and formalin were effective at 0.005 to 0.05% in book paste used for manuscript restoration (Aleksi-Meskhishvili, 1978). Manuscripts and archival material are treated with fumigants such as methyl bromide, ethylene oxide, formaldehyde, and p-dichlorobenzene. Gamma radiation also has been shown to kill microorganisms and insects that attack books.

ART OBJECTS

Paintings, watercolors, sculpture, and murals are subject to microbial damage. They contain organic nutrients for microorganisms such as starch, gums, sucrose, glucose, glycerine, egg, and oils, which are used as paints, pastes, glues, binders, plasticizers, and sizings. Attention was more recently directed to the conservation and restoration of works of art as a result of the flood in Florence, Italy in 1966. In the years following that episode fungal damage to art masterpieces was reported (Gargani, 1968). Many frescoes were seriously damaged where fungi were found around the pigment grains in the paint film, which became detached from the wall. The subject of art conservation and restoration has been reviewed by Strzelczyk (1981). Damage can be attributed to physical and chemical agents and insects as well, but microbiologic agents play a major part when moisture is a factor in the deterioration.

The Metropolitan Museum of Art in New York recommends keeping the humidity at 45 to 55% for storing organic materials, noting that relative humidity above 65% may permit mold growth and relative humidity below 45% leads to embrittlement (Shelley, 1987). Figure

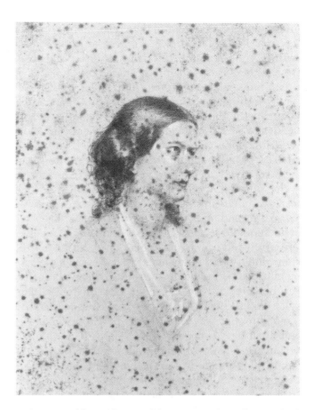

Fig. 52–9. Mold growth caused by excessive humidity resulted in the foxing on this chalk drawing. Drawing is by George Fuller (1882–1884), *Portrait of a Lady.* M. and M. Karolik Collection. From F.W. Dolloff and R.L. Perkinson. 1985. *How to Care for Works of Art.* 4th Ed. Boston, Museum of Fine Arts.

52–9 shows a drawing attacked by mold. Illustrations of miniature Indian paintings damaged by fungi in locations where the humidity reached 78% are given by Dhawan and Agrawal (1986). Temperature is less important than humidity. A temperature of 68 to 72° F (20 to 22° C) is recommended, with the note of caution that extremes of temperature result in extremely damp or extremely dry conditions (Shelley, 1987). Because bacteria generally require liquid moisture for growth, the damage done to stored art usually results from molds.

For objects that have been attacked by microorganisms Strzelczyk (1981) recommends that they be disinfected by either fumigation or treatment with fungicide solutions by spraying, brushing, or injecting. The chemicals used must be carefully selected so that they will not damage the object. For instance, pentachlorophenol, which is a powerful fungicide, is said to hydrolyze and damage canvas. For other reasons, sodium fluoride is not approved for preservation of paintings. Plenderleith and Werner (1973) recommended 0.5% o-phenylphenol for textiles and leather. For fumigation they prefer the use of thymol, which they say may be safe for pastels, prints, drawings, books, parchment, and vellum. However, they warn that thymol softens oil paints and varnishes. Other workers question the effectiveness of thymol and prefer ethylene oxide. For spraying or brushing, Strzelczyk (1981) recommends p-chloro-m-cresol with phenylmercuric acetate, using 0.3 g of the cresol and 0.01 g of the mercurial in a solution of 33 ml acetone and 67 ml turpentine. He has found this solution to be effective for disinfection of canvas paintings, paintings on wood, mural paintings, and sculptures. Jeffries (1986) disinfected mural paintings in Canterbury Cathedral that had been infected with the fungus, *Beauvaria alba*, which produced powdering and flaking of the paint surface. He used three spray applications of 0.3% p-chloro-m-cresol and 0.1% of phenylmercuric acetate in absolute ethanol, which removed the fungus and had no adverse effects on the mural. Strzelczyk (1981) stated that he tested these two fungicides for their effect on paper on 56 water color paints and on 96 crayons from different firms without unfavorable results. He stated also that the art objects were protected against microbial attack for a long time. Where fungi were determined to be damaging frescoes in a church, six fungicides were tested and three, Florasan, Benlate, and Bavistin, controlled the fungi (Bianchi et al., 1980). Fungal damage to art masterpieces in Florentine churches was observed in 1961 to 1965 and particularly after the flood of 1966 (Gargani, 1968). Many frescoes were seriously damaged, and fungi were found around the pigment grains in the paint film, which became detached from the wall. Spraying the water-soluble antibiotic nystatin on the painted wall was effective in stopping the damage. At a concentration of 10 to 100 μg/ml, however, its activity was reduced to half after 1 day.

With murals, sculptures, and monuments that are outdoors and exposed to the weather, algae and lichens can be serious agents of deterioration. Algae can be harmful in several ways. Being photosynthetic they grow without organic matter and attach themselves firmly to exposed surfaces, defacing them. In their metabolism they produce organic acids that may react with the surface, or when they die they provide organic nutrition, enabling bacteria and fungi to grow. An example of the latter case was reported by Bassi et al. (1986) in which marble carvings that decorate the facade of the Certosa of Pavia, a fifteen to sixteenth century monument in North Italy (Fig. 52–10), were covered with orange-red stains. These stains were determined to be produced by two bacteria that live in the stone on a substrate of green unicellular algae. These bacteria, *Micrococcus* spp. and *Flavobacterium* spp., produced this red pigment, which was diffused by water over the stone. Biocidal experiments with the bacteria showed that Bradophen (Ciba Geigy), a 90% solution of dodecyl-(oxyethyl)-benzylammonium chloride, at 0.005% stopped their growth. The authors recommended treating the contaminated surfaces with 0.1 to 0.2% Bradophen.

One further way that algae can be harmful is when they are hooked up in symbiotic relationship with a fungus in a union we call a lichen. Lichens grow on stone surfaces and produce oxalic and chelating organic acids that react with the minerals in the stone, leading to granular disintegration of the statuary or carving. The mechanical motion generated by the alternate wetting

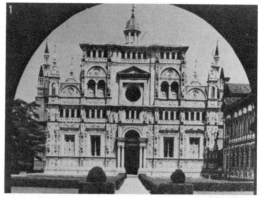

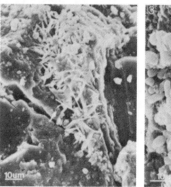

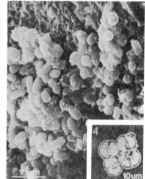

Fig. 52–10. *1*, Microorganisms staining a building, the Certosa of Pavia in northern Italy. From M. Bassi, A. Ferrari, and C. Sorlini. 1986. Red stains on the Certosa of Pavia. A case of biodeterioration. Int. Biodeter., *23*, 201–205. *2*, Surface of stained Carrara marble. A few cells are visible (SEM–scanning electron microscope). *3*, Inner surface of the marble shown in *2*, showing the presence of many cells (SEM). *3*, *Chlorella*, a green alga found in a powdered piece of stained Carrara marble.

and drying of the lichen may cause the detachment of the loosened mineral fragments, exposing new surfaces to attack by the acids (Jones and Wilson, 1985). The sculptured walls of Barabadur, a world-famous Buddhist monument in central Java, and the sculptured surfaces of the Mayan ruins in Mexico are examples of priceless monuments that are disintegrating because of the penetration of the tough lichen rhizoids, which attach tightly to stone surfaces and crevices. How to prevent this damage is a difficult problem that has yet to be solved. Polymer coatings have been attempted without success. Strzelczyk (1981) reports the best results were obtained with algicides by spraying or brushing stone surfaces with a 3% ethanol solution of either Lastanox TA (Lachema, Brno, Czechoslovakia), Alalon 50 (Farbwerke Hoest AG, Germany), a urea derivative, or Atrazin 50 (Fixn. Pest Control Ltd., U.K.), a derivative of atrazin.

MISCELLANEOUS PRODUCTS

Photographic film was protected from mold by treatment with 1% alcoholic solutions of dinitrochlorobenzene, dinitrothiocyanobenzene, and tetramethylthiuram disulfide, and a 1% aqueous solution of sodium phenolate. The fungicides had no effect on the silver image of black and white film but caused some distortion of the color image of multilayered photocopies (Yeremenko and Shapiyevskaya, 1958). Jump and Hutchinson (1945) tested a number of fungicidal baths for dipping processed film. An alkyldimethylbenzylammonium chloride (Roccal) gave the most satisfactory results in dilutions of 0.1 to 1.0% for preserving negatives. The mold-free storage life of inoculated Ektachrome X film was increased to 127 days in a humid chamber with treatment of an aqueous solution of 0.01% chloramphenicol and 0.05% dodecyldimethylbenzylammonium chloride compared to 27 to 36 days with either of the ingredients alone (Saito, 1973). The authors thought that this material used in conjunction with a waterproofing lacquer might prevent tackiness of the film as well. Shirk (1954) gives instructions on cleaning up fungus-fouled negatives where the gelatin has not been destroyed. Photographic paper is packaged in moisture-proof packages to prevent fungus damage when stored in tropical regions.

In the printing industry, fountain etch fluids are used to flood the plates to permit the selective adherence of inks. The fluids are made up of inorganic salts and organic dispersing agents. They are recirculated over and over and become contaminated with microorganisms that build up on the screens, causing blockage and expensive shutdown. A preservative must be water-soluble, active with nonionic surfactants, and nondiscoloring. According to Yeager (1977), a uniquely suitable compound for this purpose, low in toxicity, and chemically degradable for disposability, is 2,6-dimethyl-m-dioxan-4-ol-acetate.

Flowers and ornamental plants delivered to hospitals were found to be reservoirs of bacteria causing nosocomial infections (McLary and Layne, 1977). These include *Pseudomonas aeruginosa, Escherichia coli, Serratia marcescens,* and *Enterobacter cloacae.* They may be found on the foliage, in the vase water, and in the soil of potted plants. *Pseudomonas aeruginosa* was most commonly isolated and found to be the same strain isolated from clinical specimens. Disinfection with benzalkonium chloride (1.5 ml Roccal per gallon or 30 ml Zephiran per gallon) prevented bacterial growth for 72 hours. In different studies, commercial solutions that are used in vase water to prolong the life of cut flowers contain sugar and organic nutrients and require preservation. Various preservatives were useful, but 8-hydroxyquinoline was preferred.

In the art of embalming, formaldehyde has been the principal preservative employed. Certain dialdehydes have been claimed to have certain advantages over formaldehyde. Dialdehydes react with proteins to make them more resistant to decomposition and there is less dehydration than with formaldehyde. The embalmed tissues are said to be firm yet pliable (Anon., 1962). These dialdehydes include glyoxal, glutaraldehyde, 2-hydroxydipaldehyde, and pyruvic aldehyde. The antibacterial activity of glutaraldehyde is also useful in preventing the foul odors from decomposing fish waste, etc., in the bilge water of ships (Anon., 1961b).

REFERENCES

Abrams, E. 1948. Microbiological deterioration of organic materials. National Bureau of Standards Miscellaneous Publication 188.

Ackart, W.B., Camp, R.L., Wheelwright, W.L., and Byck, J.S. 1975. Antimicrobial polymers. J. Biomed. Mater. Res., 9, 55–68.

Adams, P.B. 1969. The biology of glass. New Scientist, 41, 25–27.

Aleksi-Meskhishvili, L.G. 1978. Testing of fungicides in paste used in manuscript restoration. Soobshch Akad. Nauk Gruz SSR, 91, 717–719.

Amburgey, T.L. 1974. Organisms causing discoloration and deterioration of asphalt roofing shingles. Forest Prod. J., 24 (6), 52–54.

American Wood Preservers Association, 1980. Statistics. Proceedings, 76, 330.

American Wood Preservers Association, 1966. Laboratory soil block method for testing wood preservatives. Am. Wood Pres. Assoc., Washington.

American Wood Preservers Association, 1963. Appendix A. Pentachlorophenol-liquefied petroleum gas wood preservative solution. Am. Wood Pres. Assoc. Proc., 59, 49–52.

Amin, S.A., Kharadly, E.A., and Kamel, M. 1975. Rot-proofing properties of chemically-modified cotton fabrics. Am. Dyestuff Rep., 64, 21–22.

Anonymous, 1978. Unsettled market for biocides in U.S. says Kline. Soap Cosmet. Chem. Spec., 54, June 74B.

Anonymous, 1977. Decay in buildings: recognition, prevention and cure. Building Research Establishment, Princes Risborough Laboratory. Technical Note No. 44.

Anonymous, 1974. Latex preservation. Dimethylaminomethyl phenol. Annual Report of the Rubber Research Institute of Malaya 1972, pp. 128–129.

Anonymous, 1972. Antimicrobial paint proves effective against broad range of bacteria and fungi. Paint Varnish Prod., 62, 67–69.

Anonymous, 1972. Control of lichens, moulds and similar growths. Building Research Establishment, Digest No. 139. London: HMSO.

Anonymous, 1969. The growing market for chemicals in chip treatment. Pulp Paper Mag. Can., 70, 45–49.

Anonymous, 1968a. Search for an ideal slimicide. Can. Pulp Paper Ind., 21, 45–46.

Anonymous, 1968b. Antifouling agents. Cont. Paint Resin News, 6, 7–9.

Anonymous, 1965. A cooperative approach. Int. Biodeter. Bull., 1, 2–4.

Anonymous, 1962. Dialdehyde based fluids improve embalming procedures. Chemical Progress (Union Carbide Chemicals Co.), February.

Anonymous, 1961a. Food additives. Propylene oxide. Federal Register, 26, 11799–117800.

Anonymous, 1961b. Odor corrector. Chemical Progress (Union Carbide Chemicals Co.), March.

Anonymous, 1960. Chem. Trade J. Chem. Eng., 146, 910.

Anonymous, 1957. Cutting fluids poise for new sales splash. Chem. Week, 81, 91, 92, 94–95.

Anonymous, 1942. Claims shoes defective in New Guinea campaign. Hide Leath. Shoes, 104, 9.

Appling, J.W. 1955. *Microbiology of Pulp and Paper.* Technical Association, Pulp and Paper Industry, New York, 282 pp.

Appling, J.W., Buckman, S.J., and Cash, C.D. 1950. Some further observations on *Penicillium roqueforti* Thom. Tappi, 33, 346–349.

Appling, J.W., Ridenour, N.J., and Buckman, S.J. 1951. Pink slime in paper mills. Tappi, 34, 347–352.

Army-Navy-National Defense Research Committee. 1944. Preservation of leather for use in the armed services. Army-Navy-National Defense Research Committee Tropical Deterioration Report No. 2.

Aslam, M., and Singh, S.M. 1971. Copper sulphate as an algicide in limewash. Paintindia, 21, 21–22.

Baigozhin, A. 1980. Grafting of biologically active compounds to the surface of optical materials. Usp. Khim, 1980, 49(11), 2241–2254.

Baigozhin, A., et al. 1981. Fungicidal compounds and coatings developed from them for aluminized mirrors. Opt.-Melkh Promst., 1981, 28–30.

Baker, P.W. 1967. An evaluation of some fungicides for optical instruments. Int. Biodeter. Bull., 3, 59–64.

Ballman, D.K., and Smith, F.B. 1943. Fungicides and germicides in the pulp and paper industry. Paper Ind. Paper World, 25, 143–148.

Barghoorn, E.S. 1945. Deterioration of textiles under tropical conditions in the Canal Zone. Office of Scientific Research and Development Report No. 4807.

Barnard, H.F. 1952. The sterilization of woolen fabrics. Br. Med. J., 1, 21–24.

Barnes, H.M. 1985. Trends in the wood-treating industry: State of the art report. Forest Prods. J., 35, 13–22.

Bartlett, A.E., and Goll, M. 1945. Does copper naphthenate oxidize cellulose? Am. Dyestuff Rep., 34, 225–227.

Barr, A.R.M. 1977. Comparative studies on the inhibition of lichen and algal growth on asbestos paving slabs. International Biodegradation Research Group, Constructional Materials Working Group. April 1977.

Bartl, M., and Velecky, R. 1971. The fungicidal effect of organic tin in cements, limes and plasters. Cement Technology, 51, 54–57.

Bassi, M., Ferrari, A., Realini, M., and Sorlini, C. 1986. Red stains on the Certosa of Pavia. A case of biodeterioration. Int. Biodeter., 23, 201–205.

Bayley, C.H., and Weatherburn, M.W. 1945. The effect of accelerated weathering on cotton thread proofed by the cutch-copper-ammonia process and the chrome process. Report to National Research Council of Canada Coordinating Committee on Protective Equipment (Research), March 24.

Bayley, C.H., Rose, G.R.F., Clifford, J.B., and Cooney, J.D. 1965. The effect of noncellulosic material on the actinic degradation of cotton fabric. Part III: Some inorganic chromate pigments. Text. Res. J., 35, 180–184.

Beal, R.H., Amburgey, T.L., Bultman, J.D., and Roberts, D.R. 1979. Resistance of wood from paraquat-treated southern pines to subterranean termites, decay fungi, and marine borers. Forest Prod. J., 29, 35–38.

Beck, W.C., and Collette, T.S. False faith in the surgeon's gown and surgical drape. Am. J. Surgery, 83, 125–126.

Belyakova, L.A., and Kozulina, O.V. 1961. Book preservation in USSR libraries. Unesco Bull. Libr., 15, 198–202.

Benignus, P.G. 1948. Copper-8-quinolinate industrial preservative. Ind. Eng. Chem., 40, 1426–1429.

Benignus, P.G., and Rogers, D.F. 1945. Foxholes and fungicides. Monsanto Mag., 24, 22–23.

Bennett, E.O. 1956. Bacterial spoilage of emulsion oils. Soap Chem. Spec., 32, 47–49, 46–48, 155.

Bennett, E.O., Guynes, G.J., and Isenberg, D.L. 1960. The sensitivity of sulfate-reducing bacteria to antibacterial agents-III. The nitro-paraffin derivatives. Prod. Mthly., 24, 26–27.

Bennett, E.O., Guynes, G.J., and Isenberg, D.L. 1958. The sensitivity of sulfate-reducing bacteria to antibacterial agents (phenolic compounds). Prod. Mthly., 23, 18–19.

Bennett, R.G., and Binns, E.J. 1951. The preservation of wooden transmission poles. Record of British Wood Preserving Association, 1st Annual Convention, 37–40.

Berk, S. 1948. Fungicides for fungus-proofing glue-glycerol-bonded cork gaskets. Ind. Eng. Chem., 40, 262–267.

Berner, N.H., and Ahearn, D.C. 1977. Observations on the growth and survival of Cladosporium resinae in jet fuel. Dev. Ind. Microbiol., 18, 705–710.

Bertolet, R. 1943. The finishing of army ducks with special reference to mildewproofing. Am. Dyestuff Rep., 32, 214–219.

Bianchi, A., Favali, M.A., Barbieri, N., and Bassi, M. 1980. The use of fungicides on mold covered frescoes. Int. Det. Bull., 16, 45–51.

Blanchard, G.C., and Goucher, C.R. 1965. Metabolic products formed by hydrocarbon oxidizing microorganisms. Dev. Ind. Microbiol., 7, 343–353.

Block, S.S., 1982. Unpublished data.

Block, S.S. 1977. Preservatives for industrial products. In Disinfection, Sterilization, and Preservation. 2nd edition. Philadelphia, Lea & Febiger.

Block, S.S. 1953a. Humidity requirements for mold growth. Appl. Microbiol., 1, 287–294.

Block, S.S. 1953b. Unpublished work.

Block, S.S. 1951. Experiments in mildew prevention. Mod. Sanit., 3(12), 61–67.

Block, S.S. 1949. Fungicide-treated cotton fabric outdoor exposure and laboratory tests. Ind. Eng. Chem., 41, 1783–1789.

Bomar, M. 1961. Viability of microorganisms on microbiocidal wrapping paper. Prumysl Potravin, 12, 564–568.

Borgin, K. 1971. Why wood is durable. New Scientist and Sci. J., 50, 200–203.

Bowes, J.H., Carter, C.W., and Taylor, J.E. 1970. Substantive fungicides. J. Am. Leath. Chem. Assoc., 65, 85–96.

Braun, D.C., and Sitgreaves, R. 1958. Dermatitis in industry. Arch. Ind. Health, 17, 259–271.

Bravery, A.F. 1982. Preservation in the construction industry. In Disinfection, Preservation, and Sterilization. Edited by A.D. Russell, W.B. Hugo, and G.A.J. Ayliffe. Oxford, Blackwell Scientific Publications, pp. 385–390.

British Leather Manufacturer's Research Association, 1945. Mold-resistant leathers for use in tropical conditions. Mthly. Dig., February.

Brown, A.E. 1945. The problem of fungal growth on synthetic resins, plastics, and plasticizers. U.S. Office of Scientific Research and Development Report No. 6067.

Brown, J.P. 1960. Fungistatic plywood glues. British Patent Spec. 854, 156.

Bruch, M.K. 1976. The regulation of hydrophilic contact lenses by the Food and Drug Administration. Dev. Ind. Microbiol., 17, 29–47.

Brunt, K.D. 1987. Biocides for the oil industry. In Microbial Problems in the Offshore Oil Industry. I. Edited by E.C. Hill, J.L. Shennan, and R.J. Watkinson. London, Wiley, pp. 201–207.

Brysson, R.J., Reeves, W.A., and Piccolo, B. 1963. The cadmium selenides. New outdoor fabric fungicides. Am. Dyestuff Rep., 52, 642–646, 652.

Buckman Laboratories, Inc., 1982. Personal communication, Mr. Ray Thornton.

Buckman Laboratories, Inc., 1949. Microorganism control in leather manufacture. Bulletin 3L.

Buckman, S.J. 1949. Microorganism control in mechanical pulp and its relation to paper manufacture. Tappi, 32, 129–144.

Burgess, R. 1934. Causes and prevention of mildew on wool. J. Soc. Dyers Colour., 50, 138–142.

Burgess, R. 1931. Development of mildew on wool. J. Soc. Dyers Colour., 47, 96–99.

Burgess, R. 1930. Liability of dyed wool to mildew with special reference to the resistance resulting from chroming. J. Text. Inst., 21, T441–452.

Burgess, R. 1929. Microbiology of wool: The enhancement of mildew in soaps and vegetable oils. J. Text. Inst., 20, T333–372.

Burgess, R. 1928. Microbiology of wool. J. Text. Inst., 19, T315–322.

Burgess, R. 1924. Bacteriology and mycology of wool. J. Text. Inst., 15, T573–583.

Burton, W.J. 1944. Tie service record. Report of committee 7–1. Proc. Am. Wood Pres. Assoc., 36, 170.

Carlson, V., and Bennett, E.D. 1960. The relationship between the oil-water ratio and the effectiveness of inhibitors in oil-soluble emulsions. Lubric. Eng., 16, 572–574.

Cadmus, E.L. 1976. Biodeterioration in the United States: A review. Proceedings of the 3rd International Biodegradation Symposium. Edited by J.M. Sharpley and A.M. Kaplan. London: Applied Science Publishers, pp. 343–346.

Carman, J.R., and Goll, M. 1970. The role of industrial hygiene in the manufacture of latex paint. Dev. Ind. Microbiol., 11, 327–329.

Carter, G., and Huddart, G. 1974. Preservation of water-thinned paints in metallic containers. Double Liason-Chim. Peint. 21(225), 219–226.

Cavill, G.W.K., Phillips, J.N., and Vincent, J.M. 1949. Relation between fungistatic activity and structure in a series of simple aromatic compounds. J. Soc. Chem. Ind., 68, 12–16.

Centre de Recherches et de Controles Techniques, 1965. Teint. Appret., 89, 111–123.

Chalk, R. 1968. Wood deterioration during outside chip storage. Pulp Paper Mag. Can., 69, 75–85.

Chemical Warfare Service Development Laboratory, Massachusetts Institute of Technology. 1945. Comparative evaluation of commercial fungicides. Miscellaneous 12, Tropical Deterioration Information Center.

Churchill, A.V., and Leathen, W.W. 1961. Development of microbiological sludge inhibitors. ASD Technical Report 61–193. Aeronautical Systems Division, Wright-Patterson Air Force Base.

Coleman, L.J., and Hall, J.F. 1972. Some side effects of fungicides in paints. In Biodeterioration of Materials. Volume 2. Edited by A.H. Walters and E.H. Hueck-Van Der Plas. London, Applied Science Publishers, pp. 360–369.

Commercial Solvents Corp. 1948. Bacteria and fungi can't pass this protector. Chem. Week, 85, 84.

Conner, J.C., Cooper, A.S., Jr., Reeves, W.A., and Trask, B.A. 1964. Some microbial-resistant compounds of zirconium and their effect on cotton. Text. Res. J., 34, 347–357.

Connolly, R.A. 1961. Measurements of strength reduction reveal wood decay. Bell Labs. Rec., 39, 317–320.

Cordon, T.C., Everett, A.L., and Windus, W. 1961. The influence of bacteria on depilation of hides by enzymes. J. Am. Leath. Chem. Assoc., 56, 164–173.

Cordon, T.C., Rogers, J.S., Mann, C.W., and Teitell, L. 1949. Protection of army ordnance leather equipment from molds. J. Am. Leath. Chem. Assoc., 44, 472–503.

de la Court, F.H. 1977. Fouling resistant coatings: Their functioning and future developments. Proc. 3rd Int. Conf. on Organic Coatings, pp. 97–137.

Crandall, H.C. 1955. Fungus proofing of paper and paperboard. Appl. Microbiol., 3, 89–94.

Crum, M.G., Reynolds, R.J., and Hedrick, H.G. 1966. Effect of surfactants and additives on the progress of microbiological corrosion of aluminum alloys. Dev. Ind. Microbiol., 8, 253–259.

Cundell, A.M., and Mulcock, A.P. 1975. The biodegradation of vulcanized rubber. Dev. Ind. Microbiol., 16, 88–96.

Cundell, A.M., and Mulcock, A.P. 1973. Effects of microbiocides on the microbial deterioration of vulcanized natural rubber. Dev. Ind. Microbiol., 14, 253–257.

Curtis, A.B. Jr., and Williams, L.H. 1990. Borates offer effective protection with less hazard to the environment. Forest Service, USDA, Utilization Rept. R8–UR6.

Dahl, S., and Kaplan, A.M. 1961. 5,6-Dichloro-2-benzoxazolinone as a leather fungicide. J. Am. Leath. Chem. Assoc., 56, 686–698.

Dahl, S., and Kaplan, A.M. 1960. 4-Nitrophenyl esters, including mixed carbonates and bis carbonates, as leather fungicides. J. Am. Leath. Chem. Assoc., 55, 480–500.

Dahl, S., and Kaplan, A.M. 1958. Studies of leather fungicides. J. Am. Leath. Chem. Assoc., 53, 103–120.

Dahl, S., and Kaplan, A.M. 1957. Fungicidal effectiveness of compounds applied to leather. J. Am. Leath. Chem. Assoc., 52, 536–549.

Dana, C.F., Vigo, T., and Welch, C.M. 1979. Antibacterial textile finishes utilizing zinc acetate and hydrogen peroxide. U.S. Patent Application 974,171, August 31. 33 pp.

Daoust, D.B., Meloro, F.A., and Boor, L. 1951. Studies on degradation of plastic films by fungi and bacteria II. Res. Serv. Test Rept. C&P-259-F. U.S. Quartermaster Depot, Philadelphia.

Darby, R.T., and Kaplan, A.M. 1968. Fungal susceptibility of polyurethanes. Applied Microbiol., 16, 900–905.

David, J., and Barr, A.R.M. 1972. Textiles and microorganisms. Text. Inst. Ind., 10, 173–176.

Davis, R.H., and Laug, E. 1963. Cutting fluid. U.S. Patent 3,017,545.

Dayal, H.M., Nigam, S.S., and Agarwal, P.N. 1965. Prevention of mould growth on sheaths protective rubber (condoms). Res. Ind., 10, 1–3.

Dean, J.D., and Worner, R.K. 1947. The degradation of untreated cotton fabrics exposed to weather in a subtropical climate. Am. Dyestuff Rep., 36, 405–410, 423–424.

Dean, J.D., Strickland, W.B., and Berard, W.N. 1946. Service test of copper-treated cotton sandbags. Am. Dyestuff Rep., 35, 346–348.

DeGray, R.J., and Fitzgibbons, W.O. 1965. Mechanisms of microbiocidal action of organoborates in fuel-water systems. Dev. Ind. Microbiol., 7, 384–391.

Dhawan, S., and Agrawal, O.P. 1986. Fungal flora of miniature paper paintings and lithographs. Int. Biodeter., 22, 95–99.

Dolloff, F.W., and Perkinson, R.L. 1985. How to Care for Works of Art. 4th Ed. Boston, Museum of Fine Arts.

Donaldson, D.J., Guice, W.A., and Drake, G.L., Jr. 1970. Fungicidal agent for cotton. Text. Ind., 134, 171, 173, 180, 185.

Drisko, R.W. 1973. Control of algal growths on paints at tropical locations. US Dept. Commerce, National Technical Information Service. Naval Civil Engineering Laboratory, California, December 1973.

Eisenschiml, O., and Kalberg, V. 1948. Fungicides in protective coatings. Paint Oil Chem. Rev., 111, 17–19, 29–30.

Elphick, J.J. 1970. Microbial corrosion in aircraft fuel systems. In Microbial Aspects of Metallurgy. Edited by J.D.A. Miller. New York, Elsevier, pp. 157–172.

Environmental Protection Agency, 1976. Federal Register, 41, 27953–28253.

Epstein, S.S. 1937a. Mind your paint. Food Ind., 9, 386–387, 419–420.

Epstein, S.S. 1937b. Tests in breweries show germicidal paints retain protective powers. Food Ind., 9, 513, 541–543.

Epstein, S.S. 1937c. Paint and brewery operation. Am. Brewer, 70, 41–46.

Epstein, S.S., and Snell, F.D. 1941. Antiseptic and germicidal paints. Ind. Eng. Chem., 33, 398–401.

Eslyn, W.E. 1973. Propionic acid—A potential control for deterioration of wood chips stored in outside piles. Tappi, 56, 152–153.

Eslyn, W.E., and Laundrie, J.F. 1973. How anaerobic storage affects quality of Douglas fir pulpwood chips. Tappi, 56, 129–131.

Evans, C.J. 1973. Tin chemicals in the roof. Tin and its Uses, 97, 7–9.

Evans, C.J. 1970. The development of organotin-based anti-fouling paints. Tin and its Uses, 85, 3–7.

Evans, D.M. 1966. The deterioration of book-binding materials. Microbiology in the tropics. Science Monograph No. 23. Society Chemical Industry, London, pp. 179–184.

Evans, D.M., and Levisohn, I. 1964. Fungitoxic properties of volatile corrosion inhibitors. Chem. Ind., 1964, 1386–1387.

Ezekiel, W.N. 1950. Problems in fungus and moisture deterioration. Elec. Mfg., 45, 78–85, 178–190.

Fargher, R.G., Galloway, L.D., and Probert, M.E. 1930. Inhibitory action of certain substances on the growth of mould fungi. J. Text. Inst., 21, T245–260.

Farrell, M.A., and Wolff, R.T. 1941. The effect of cupric oxychloride cement on microorganisms. Ind. Eng. Chem., 33, 1185–1188.

Flemming, C.D., and Baker, R.J. 1960. Controlling spoilage of water-soluble cutting fluids. Lubric. Eng., 16, 414–419.

Fletcher, W.A. 1954. Use of diphenyl wraps against decay in New Zealand lemons. N.Z. J. Agric., 88, 115–117, 119–120.

Flieder, F. 1959. Fungicidal and insecticidal adhesive. French Patent 1,189,189.

Forrester, J.A. 1959. Destruction of concrete caused by sulphur bacteria in a purification plant. Surveyor, 118, 881–884.

Foter, M.J. 1960. Disinfectants for bedding I, II. Soap Chem. Spec., 36, 73–76, 103, 127–133, 141.

Friend, P.L., and Whitekettle, W.K. 1980. Biocides and cooling towers. Dev. Ind. Microbiol., 21, 123–132.

Fusey, P., and Hyvert, G. 1966. Biological deterioration of stone monuments in Cambodia. Microbial deterioration in the tropics. Science Monograph No. 23. Society of Chemical Industry, London, pp. 125–129.

Gagliardi, D.D. 1962. Antibacterial finishes. Am. Dyestuff Rep., 51, 49–58.

Gagliardi, D.D., Shippee, F.B., and Jutras, W.J., Jr. 1963. Silver containing reaction products, methods for their production and use in forming permanent materials. U.S. Patent 3,085,909.

Galloway, A.C., and Cooper, D.R. 1974. Fungicides for treating wet blue hides. J. Soc. Leath. Technol. Chem., 58, 67–71.

Gardner, H.A., and Hart, L.P. 1939. Mildew prevention. Natl. Paint Varnish Lacquer Assoc., Sci. Sect. Circ., 579, 52–55.

Gardner, H.A., Hart, L.P., and Sward, G.G. 1938. Further study on mildew prevention. Natl. Paint Varnish Lacquer Assoc., Sci. Sect. Circ., 558, 112–132.

Gardner, H.A., Hart, L.P., and Sward, G.G. 1934. Mildew prevention on painted surfaces. Second report. Natl. Paint Varnish Lacquer Assoc., Sci. Sect. Circ., 448, 11–32.

Gardner, H.A., Hart, L.P., and Sward, G.G. 1933. Mildew prevention on painted surfaces. Natl. Paint Varnish Lacquer Assoc., Sci. Sect. Circ., 442, 242–265.

Gardner, H.A., Sward, G.G., and Hart, L.P. 1937. Mildew tests at Panama Canal Zone. Natl. Paint Varnish Lacquer Assoc., Sci. Sect. Circ., 536, 194–199.

Gargani, G. 1968. Fungus contamination of Florence art masterpieces before and after the 1966 disaster. In Biodeterioration of Materials. Volume 1. Edited by A.H. Walters and J.S. Elphic. New York, Elsevier, pp. 252–257.

Gauger, G.W., et al. 1966. Microbial deterioration of electronic components: I. Selected components and materials of construction. II. Printed circuit boards and polyurethane wrapped capacitors. Dev. Ind. Microbiol., 8, 372–416.

Genin, G. 1973. Control of lichens, fungi and other organisms. Paint Pigments Vernis, 49, 3–6.

Gettings, R.L., and Triplett, B.L. 1978. A new durable antimicrobial finish for textiles. 1978 Book of Papers, Am. Assoc. Text. Chemists Colorists Natl. Tech. Conf., pp. 259–261.

Gibbons, E.H., Harris, W.D., and Zeller, P.J.A. 1945. Disinfection of mattresses. Agric. Mech. Coll. Tex. Bull., 87, 1–26.

Gilchrist, F.M.C. 1953. Microbiological studies of the corrosion of concrete sewers by sulphuric acid-producing bacteria. South African Industrial Chemist, 7, 214–215.

Goetz, A. 1944. S-coating . . . a self-sterilizing surface for packing materials. Mod. Packag., 18, 113–115.

Goetz, A., Tracy, R., and Goetz, S. 1942. Self-sterilizing surfaces. Science, 95, 537–538.

Goldsmith, M.T., Latlief, M.A., Friedl, J.L., and Stuart, L.S. 1956. The effect of quaternary treatment under varied ratios of weight-volume-concentration on the bacteriostatic property of fabrics. Appl. Microbiol., 4, 91–94.

Goldsmith, M.T., Latlief, M.A., Friedl, J.L., and Stuart, L.S. 1954. Adsorption of available chlorine and quaternary by cotton and wool fabrics from disinfecting solutions. Appl. Microbiol., 2, 360–364.

Goll, M. 1970. Current status of mercury biocide usage by the paint industry. Am. Paint. J., 55, 14, 16, 18.

Graham, R.D. 1973. Fumigants can stop internal decay of wood products. Forest Prod. J., 23, 35–38.

Grant, R.D., Bravery, A.F., Springle, W.R., and Worley, W. 1986. Evaluation of fungicidal paints. Int. Biodeter., 22, 179–194.

Greaves, H. 1971. The bacterial factor in wood decay. Wood Sci. Technol., 5, 6–16.

Greenberger, M., and Kaplan, A.M. 1977. An evaluation of some zirconium-containing finishes as fungicides for the preservation of cotton fabric. U.S. NTIS Report AD—AO43074.

Greene, H.S. 1945. Report on the microbiological flora and sterilization of used shoes. J. Am. Leath. Chem. Assoc., 40, 96–110.

Greene, H.S., and Lollar, R.M. 1944. Report on preservatives in army dubbings. J. Am. Leath. Chem. Assoc., 39, 209–218.

Grier, N., Witzel, J.A., Jakubowski, A., and Dulaney, E.L. 1980. A broad spectrum hexahydro-s-triazine inhibitor of microbial deterioration in cutting fluids. Dev. Ind. Microbiol., 21, 411–418.

Halliday, W.J. 1950. Control of slime in paper mills. Aust. Pulp Paper Ind. Tech. Assoc. Proc., 242–249. (Through Chemical Abstracts, 45, 4925i.)

Hand, O.F., Lindgren, P.A., and Wetsch, A.F. 1970. The control of fungal decay in transmission poles by gas phase treatment. Branch of laboratories, Bonneville Power Administration, Vancouver, Washington, 28 pp.

Harnden, R.C. 1945. Mildew control in the paint industry. Paint Oil Chem. Rev., 108, 32–34.

Hart, L.P., and Gardner, H.A. 1940. Mildewproofing of red and other dark colors. Natl. Paint Varnish Lacquer Assoc., Sci. Sect. Circ., 589, 1–6.

Hart, S. 1971. Non-mercurial microbiocides for coating. Am. Paint J. (Mar. 1), 55, 21–22.

Hartshorne, E. 1962. Meat wrapper containing antibiotic. U.S. Patent 3,041,184.

Hayes, S.F., and White, W.C. 1984. How antimicrobial treatment can improve nonwovens. Am. Dyestuff Rep., 73, 35–40, 44–45.

Heap, W.M., and Morrell, S.H. 1968. Microbiological deterioration of rubbers and plastics. J. Appl. Chem., 18, 189–194.

Hedrick, H.G., Reynolds, R.J., and Crum, M.G. 1966. Factors influencing the mechanism of corrosion of aluminum by aerobic bacteria. Dev. Ind. Microbiol., 8, 267–274.

Herman, L.G., and Reed, C.L. 1952. New coating agent promises mold-free surfaces. Food Eng., 24, 71–72, 201, 202, 203.

Hill, E.C. 1982. Biocides for cutting oil emulsions. In Principles and Practice *of Disinfection, Preservation and Sterilization.* Edited by A.D. Russell, W.B. Hugo, and G.A.J. Ayliffe. Oxford, Blackwell Scientific, pp. 343–351.

Hill, E.C. 1982. Fuels and lubricants. In *Principles and Practice of Disinfection, Preservation and Sterilization.* Edited by A.D. Russell, W.B. Hugo, and G.A.J. Ayliffe. Oxford, Blackwell Scientific, pp. 352–357.

Hill, E.C. 1987. Fuels. In *Microbial Problems in the Offshore Oil Industry.* I. Edited by E.C. Hill, J.L. Shennan, and R.L. Watkinson. London, Wiley, pp. 219–229.

Hill, E.C. 1976. Evaluation of biocides for use with petroleum products. Process Biochem., *11*, 36–38, 48.

Hill, E.C. 1970. The control of microorganisms in aircraft fuel systems. J. Inst. Petrol., *56*, 138–146.

Hitzman, D.O. 1964. The control of bacterial and fungal growth in jet fuels. Dev. Ind. Microbiol., *6*, 105–116.

Hitzman, D.O., and Schneider, R.P. 1961. Microbiological corrosion protection by germicidal zone and protective coating. U.S. Patent 2,979,377 (to Phillips Petroleum Co.).

Hoffman, E. 1972. The development of fungus-resistant paints. In *Biodeterioration of Materials.* Volume 2. Edited by A.H. Walters and E.H. Hueck-Van Der Plas. London, Applied Science Publishers, pp. 370–375.

Hoffman, E. 1971. Inhibition of mold growth by fungus resistant coatings under different conditions. J. Paint Technol., *43*, 54–59.

Hoffman, R.K., Kaye, S., and Feazel, C.E. 1959. Sporicidal surface coatings. Fed. Paint Varnish Prod. Clubs, Off. Dig., *31*, 1095–1106.

Hoffman, R.K., Yeager, S.B., and Kaye, S. 1955. A method of testing self-disinfecting surfaces. Soap Chem. Spec., *31*, 135–138, 163, 165.

Hofmann, W. 1969. Rubber articles with antimicrobial treatment. Indian Rubber Bull., *246*, 13–19.

Hollingsworth, B.S. 1976. Some methods for the evaluation of fungicides, particularly for the leather industry. Rev. Tech. Ind. Cuir, *68*, 310–317.

Hopfenberg, H.B., and Tulis, J.J. 1970. Advances in antibacterial plastics. Mod. Plast., *47*, 110–111, 113, 116.

Hovey, A.G. 1959. Preservative composition comprising pyridine-thione and a soluble borate. U.S. Patent 2,909,459.

Hueck, H.J., LaBrijn, J., Copper, J.A., and Van Ham, J. 1968. Investigations on the biological activity of pentachlorophenyl esters. In *Biodeterioration of Materials.* Volume 1. Edited by A.H. Walters and J.J. Elphick. New York, Elsevier, pp. 539–545.

Hueck-van-der-Plas, E. 1965. Cooperative research in biodeterioration. Int. Biodeter. Bull., *1*, 1.

Hurst, V., Grossman, M., Ingram, F., and Lowe, A. 1958. Hospital laundry and refuse chutes as a source of cross infection. JAMA, *167*, 1223–1229.

Inoue, M., and Morita, M. 1977. Microbiocides for industrial products. Japanese Patent Kokai 77 07, 435. Jan 20, 1977.

Isenberg, D.L., and Bennett, E.O. 1959. Bacterial deterioration of emulsion oils. II. Nature of the relationship between aerobes and sulfate-reducing bacteria. Appl. Microbiol., *7*, 121–125.

Isquith, A.J., Abbot, E.A., and Walters, P.A. 1972. Surface-bonded antimicrobial activity of an organo–silicon quaternary ammonium chloride. Applied Microbiol., *24*, 859–863.

Izzat, I.N., and Bennett, E.O. 1979. The potentiating effects of different sodium salts of EDTA upon cutting fluid preservatives. Dev. Ind. Microbiol., *20*, 683–686.

Jeffries, P. 1986. Growth of *Beauvaria alba* on mural paintings in Canterbury Cathedral. Int. Biodeter., *22*, 11–13.

Jones, D., and Wilson, M.J. 1985. Chemical activity of lichens on mineral surfaces—A review. Int. Biodeter., *21*, 99–104.

Jordan, L.D. 1934. Troubles in leather manufacture caused by molds. Leath. Trades Rev., *67*, 197–198.

Jump, J.A., and Hutchinson, W.G. 1945. The fungus fouling of photographic film. U.S. OSRD Report No. 5685.

Kalberg, V.N. 1951a. Aluminum carboxylic acid soap-heavy metal salt of hydroxyquinoline fungicidal composition and preparation thereof. U.S. Patent 2,561,379 (assigned to Scientific Oil Compounding Co., Inc.).

Kalberg, V.N. 1951b. Water insoluble carboxylic acid soap-heavy metal salt of hydroxyl quinoline fungicidal composition and preparation thereof. U.S. Patent 2,561,380 (assigned to Scientific Oil Compounding Co., Inc.).

Kanagy, J.R., Charles, A.M., and Abrams, E. 1948. Development of a fungicidal dressing for leather. J. Am. Leath. Chem. Assoc., *43*, 14–31.

Kanagy, J.R., Charles, A.M., Abrams, E., and Tener, R.F. 1946. Effects of mildew on vegetable tanned strap leather. J. Am. Leath. Chem. Assoc., *41*, 198–213.

Kaplan, A.M., Mandels, M., and Greenberger, M. 1972. Mode of action of resins in preventing microbial degradation of cellulosic textiles. In *Biodeterioration of Materials.* Volume 2. Edited by A.H. Walters and E.H. Hueck-Van Der Plas. London, Applied Science Publishers, pp. 268–278.

Kaplan, A.M., Greenberger, M., and Wendt, T.M. 1970. Evaluation of biocides for treatment of polyvinyl chloride film. Polymer Engineering Science, *10*, 241–246.

Kauffmann, J. 1960. Corrosion et protection des pierres calcaires des monuments. Corrosion et Anticorrosion, *8*, 87–95.

Kaye, S. 1971. Evaluating algistatic activity of films. Mod. Plast. *48*, 78, 81.

Keen, R. 1976. Controlling algae and other growths on concrete. Advisory Note 45–020. London: Cement and Concrete Association.

Keith, J.R. 1971. Non-mercurial antimicrobial agents for the paint industry. Am. Paint J. (Mar. 1)., *55*, 28–30.

Kereluk, K., and Baxter, R.M. 1963. Microbial activity in integral fuel tanks. II. The effects of Buna-N on the growth of *Pseudomonas aeruginosa* and *Hormodendron.* Dev. Ind. Microbiol., *4*, 235–244.

Kimmerer, R.W., and Szabocsik, J.M. 1978. Consideration of fungal deterioration of hydrophilic contact lenses. Dev. Ind. Microbiol., *19*, 237–244.

King, A.D., Jr., Stanley, W.L., Jurd, L., and Boyle, F.P. 1971. Wood chip microbiological control with sulfur dioxide. Tappi, *54*, 262.

Klausmeier, R.E., and Andrews, C.C. 1981. Plastics. In *Microbial Biodeterioration.* Edited by A.H. Rose. London, Academic Press, pp. 431–472.

Klens, P.F., and Koda, C.F. 1958. Self sanitizing paint surfaces. Fed. Paint Varnish Prod. Clubs, Off. Dig., *30*, 408–413.

Klens, P.F., and Stewart, W.J. 1957. New developments in textile preservation. Am. Dyestuff Rep., *46*, 346–350.

Krause, R.L. 1950. Reducing blue stain losses in lumber. South. Lumberm., *181*, 45–46, 48–51, 53–54.

Kubota, Ltd. 1980. Building materials with improved black mold resistance. Japan Tokkyo Koho 80, 85, 756. June 28, 1980.

Lagarde, E. 1961. Studies on the bacteriostatic and bactericidal activities of certain compounds against a pure strain of *Desulfovibrio desulfuricans.* Ann. Inst. Pasteur, *100*, 368–376.

Lashen, E.S. 1971. New method for evaluating antibacterial activity directly on fabric. Appl. Microbiol., *21*, 771–773.

Leathen, W.W., and Kinsel, N.A. 1963. The identification of microorganisms that utilize jet fuel. Dev. Ind. Microbiol., *4*, 9–16.

Lederer, S.J. 1971. A new nonmetallic fungicide for all coatings systems. Am. Paint J., *55*, 31–33.

Lee, C.B. 1961. The role of fungi in the deterioration of missiles and missile components. Dev. Ind. Microbiol., *2*, 55–64.

Lee, M., and Chandler, A.C. 1941. A study of the nature, growth, and control of bacteria in cutting compounds. J. Bacteriol., *41*, 373–386.

Leonard, F., and DeFries, M.G. 1955. Nylon-coated leather. Industrial Microbiological Proceedings, Society for Industrial Microbiology, p. 27.

Leonard, J.M., and Bultman, J.D. 1955. Tropical performances of fungicidal coatings. Part II. Naval Research Laboratory. NRL Report 4563, 1–8.

Leonard, J.M., and Pitman, A.L. 1951. Tropical performance of fungicidal coatings: a statistical analysis. Ind. Eng. Chem., *43*, 2338–2341.

Leutritz, J., Jr. 1945. Protecting communications equipment for the tropics. Bell Labs. Rec., *23*, 105–107.

Levi, M.P. 1977. Fungicides in wood preservation. In *Antifungal Compounds.* Volume 1. Edited by M.R. Siegel and H.D. Sisler. New York, Marcel Dekker.

Levine, S.L., Litsky, W., and Lamm, R.A. 1981. Disinfection of hydrophilic contact lenses with commercial preparations of 3 percent and 6 percent hydrogen peroxide. Dev. Ind. Microbiol., *22*, 813–819.

Levowitz, D. 1952. Antibacterial cement gives longer lasting floors. Food Eng., *24*, 57–60, 134, 135.

Lochhead, A.G., and Farrell, M.A. 1930. The effect of preservatives on fermentation by sugar-tolerant yeasts from honey. Can. J. Res., *3*, 95–103.

Lollar, R.M. 1944. Mold resistant treatment for leather. J. Am. Leath. Chem. Assoc., *39*, 12–24.

London, S.A., Finefrock, V.H., and Killian, L.N. 1964. Microbial activity in Air Force jet fuel systems. Dev. Ind. Microbiol., *6*, 61–79.

Luce, R.H., and Mathes, K.N. 1951. The effect of moisture and mold on the electrical properties of electronics hook up wire insulations. Annual Report, 1950 Conference on Electrical Insulation, National Research Council, pp. 27–29.

Luce, R.H., and Mathes, K.N. 1948. Studies in the deterioration of electrical insulation; the effect of moisture and mold on the d.c. resistance characteristics of low voltage hookup wires. Final Report, Rensselaer Polytechnic Institute Contr. W28–099-ac69.

Lurie, H.I., and Brookfield, E. 1948. Copper impregnated concrete floors. South Africa Medical Journal, *22*, 487–489.

Machemer, W.E. 1979. Use of mercury in protective coatings. Dev. Ind. Microbiol., *20*, 25–39.

Macy, H., and Olson, J.C. 1939. Preliminary observations on the treatment of parchment paper with sodium or calcium propionate. J. Dairy Sci., *22*, 527–534.

Mallmann, W.L. 1941. A bacteriologic study of a sanigenic flooring. JAMA, *117*, 844–847.

Mallmann, W.L., and Michael, C.E. 1940. The development of mold on cold storage eggs and methods of control. Mich. State Coll. and Agric. Stat. Tech. Bull., *174*, 1–34.

Mann, A. 1971. Mercurial biocides: paint's problem material. Paint Varnish Prod., *61*, 26–37.

Manowitz, M., and Gump, W.S. 1962. Antibacterial textile fabrics. U.S Patent 3,061,469.

Marouchoc, S.R. 1972. A new process for the clean treatment of wood. Am. Wood Pres. Assoc., 68, 148–153.

Marsh, P.B., and Butler, M.L. 1946. Fungicidal activity of bisphenols as mildew preventives on cotton fabric. Ind. Eng. Chem., 38, 701–705.

Marsh, P.B., Greathouse, G.A., Bollenbacher, K., and Butler, M.L. 1944. Copper soaps as rotproofing agents on fabrics. Ind. Eng. Chem., 36, 176–181.

Maxwell, S., McLean, K.M., and Kearns, J. 1987. Biocide application and monitoring in a waterflood system. In Microbial Problems in the Offshore Oil Industry. I. Edited by E.C. Hill, J.L. Shennan, and R.J. Watkinson. London, Wiley, pp. 209–218.

McLary, C.L., and Layne, J.S. 1977. Flower vase water and ornamental potted plants as reservoirs for gram-negative pathogenic bacteria. Dev. Ind. Microbiol., 18, 731–739.

Merrick, G.D. 1964. Wood preservation statistics. Proc. Am. Wood Pres. Assoc., 60, 201–218.

Miller, G. 1972. Tributyltin oxide: Some factors influencing its development and application as a preservative. In Biodeterioration of Materials. Volume 2. Edited by A.H. Walters and E. H. Hueck-Van Der Plas. London, Applied Science Publishers, pp. 279–285.

Miller, J.J., Brown, W.E., and Krieger, V.J. 1981. Laboratory methods for testing bacteriostatic and bactericidal effects of water-treatment biocides on Legionella pneumophila (Legionnaires' disease bacterium). Dev. Ind. Microbiol., 22, 763–770.

Minich, A., and Goll, M. 1946. Mildew-proofing protective coatings. Paint Oil Chem. Rev., 109, 6–7, 36–37.

Monaghan, C.P., O'Brien, E.J., Jr., Reust, H., and Good, M.L. 1980. Current status of the chemical speciation of organotin toxicants in antifoulants. Dev. Ind. Microbiol., 21, 211–215.

Money, C.A. 1974. Short term preservation of hides. II. Use of zinc chloride or calcium hypochlorite as alternatives to sodium chlorite. J. Am. Leather Chem. Assoc., 69, 112–30.

Money, C.A. 1970. Short term preservation of hides. J. Am. Leath. Chem. Assoc., 65, 64–77.

Moraru, D.S. 1980. Protecting concrete against the action of seawater and other biologically active waters. German Offen. 2,904,932. August 14, 1980.

Morgan, J. III. 1989. The evaluation and commercialization of new wood preservative. Am. Wood Preserv. Assoc. Proc., 85, 16–26.

Morgan, O.D. 1959. Chemical control of algae and other nuisance growths on greenhouse benches, pots and potting soil. Plant Disease Reporter, 43, 660–663.

Mottern, H.H. 1954. Cheese keeps longer in antimycotic wrapper. Food Eng., 26, 93–94.

Munger, C.G. 1960. Sewer corrosion and protective coatings. Civil Eng., 30, 57–59.

National Defense Research Committee. 1945. Prevention of deterioration of optical instruments in the tropics. Office of Scientific Research and Development Report No. 6055.

National Defense Research Committee. 1946. Tropical deterioration of equipment and materials. Dept. Commerce Office of Technical Services P.B.-L-81801.

Nette, I.T., Pomortseva, N.V., and Kozlova, E.I. 1959. Destruction of rubber by microorganisms. Mikrobiologiia, 28, 821–827.

Nichiden Kaguku Co., Ltd. 1980. Modified starch adhesives. Japan Kokai Tokkyo Koho 80 112,203. August 29, 1980.

Nicholas, D.D. 1983. Trends in the use of chemicals for preservative treatment of wood. Advances in the production of forest products. AIChE Symp. Series, 79, 75–78.

Nicot, J. 1951. Degradation des mur de plâtre par les moissisures. Revue Mycologique, 16, 168–172.

Nitschke, G. 1961. Investigations on the use of chrome salts to improve the resistance of wool to moisture and microbiological attack. Melliand Textilber., 42, 818–821, 941–943.

Nordeutsche Affinerie. 1953. Preventing the development of animal and plant life on water-soaked surfaces. German patent 870 340. Chemical Abstracts, 52(1958), 20775f.

Northrop, D.M., and Rowe, W.F. 1987. Effect of the soil environment on the biodeterioration of man-made textiles. Biodeterioration Research 1. Edited by G.C. Llewellyn and C.E. O'Rear. New York, Plenum Press, pp. 7–17.

O'Connor, J.C. 1969. Surface mold growth. Food Eng., 41, (9), 92–93.

O'Flaherty, F., and Doherty, E.E. 1939. Foot and mouth disease. I. A problem of international concern. II. A method for sterilizing skin and hides against the virus of foot-and-mouth disease. J. Am. Leath. Chem. Assoc., 34, 325–336.

Oppermann, R.A., and Wolfson, L.L. 1961. Mechanisms of slime formation. Fimbriae. Tappi, 44, 905–909.

Orthman, A.C., and Higby, W.M. 1929. Mold growth on leather and its prevention. J. Am. Leath. Chem. Assoc., 24, 657–663.

Osanov, B.P., Zubkovskii, E.P., Oshchepkova, E.P., and Domozhirova, V.P. 1964. Preservation of market groundwood. Bumazhn Prom., 1964, 11–13.

Paleni, A., and Curri, S. 1973. The attack of algae and lichens on stone and means of their control. Proceedings of the 1st International Symposium on the Deterioration of Building Stones, pp. 157–166. La Rochelle: Centre de Rechercher et d'Études Oceanographiques.

Paleni, A., and Curri, S. 1972. Biological aggression of works of art in Venice. In Biodeterioration of Materials. Volume 2. Edited by A.H. Walters and E.H. Hueck-Van Der Plas. London, Applied Science Publishers, pp. 392–400.

Pattilloch, D.K. 1962. Germicidal paper. U.S. Patent 3,060,079.

Pauli, O. 1972. Paint fungicides—a review. In Biodeterioration of Materials. Volume 2. Edited by A. H. Walters and E.H. Hueck-Van Der Plas. London, Applied Science Publishers, pp. 355–359.

Pettit, D., and Abbott, S.G. 1975. Biodeterioration of footwear. In Microbial Aspects of the Deterioration of Materials. Edited by R.J.G. Gilbert and D.W. Lovelock. London, Academic Press, pp. 237–253.

Phillip, A.T. 1972. Underwater marine coatings. I. Modern trends in marine antifouling paint research. Rep. Def. Stand. Labs. Aust., No. 526, 44 pp.

Pickelesimer, L.G. 1959. Investigation of a fungicidal tannage. U.S. Wright Air Development Center. Technical report 59–250. (Through Wessel, C.J., and Lee, R.W.H. 1964. Microbiological aspects of leather and fabrics. Dev. Ind. Microbiol., 5, 36–49.)

Pitis, I. 1972. Mycological protection of rubber for industrial products. Proceedings of the 2nd International Biodeterioration Symposium, pp. 294–300. London: Applied Science Publishers.

Pittman, C.U., Stahl, G.A., and Winters, H. 1978. Synthesis and mildew resistance of vinyl acetate and ethyl acrylate films containing chemically anchored fungicides. J. Coat. Technol., 50, (636) 49–56.

Pleass, W.B. 1935. The pickling of sheep skins. II. Pickling in the presence of certain organic acids. J. Int. Soc. Leath. Trades Chem., 19, 4–13.

Plenderleith, H.J., and Werner, A.E.A. 1974. The Conservation of Antiquities and Works of Art. London, Oxford University Press.

Prentiss, W.C., and Sigafoos, C.R. 1979. Isothiazolones for leather preservation. II. Military leather. J. Am. Leath. Assoc., 74, 322–328.

Powell, J.M. 1975. Use of gramoxone to control mosses and liverworts in greenhouse pots. Bi-monthly Research Note, Vol. 31, No. 5. Sept.–Oct. Department of the Environment of Canada.

Procter and Gamble Co., through Foter 1960. Unpublished data. Cincinnati. (See Foter, M.J.)

Purkiss, B.E. 1972. Biodeterioration of multiple phase systems. Proceedings of the 2nd International Biodeterioration Symposium, pp. 99–102. London: Applied Science Publishers.

Rabas, V., et al. 1980. Adhesives for paper, textiles, and leather. Czech Patent 181,377.15 Jan., 1980.

Ravenholt, O.H., Baker, E.F., Wrysham, D.N., and Geidt, W.R. 1958. Disinfection of blankets with a synthetic phenolic compound. U. Minn. Med. Bull., 29, 421.

Reagan, B.M. 1975. An evaluation of the photodegradation of cotton tentage fabrics finished with selected combinations of flame, water, weather, and mildew resistant finishes. Ph.D. Dissertation, Department of Home Economics, Purdue University.

Rechenberg, W. 1972. The avoidance and control of algae and other growths on concrete. Betontechnische Berichte, 22, 249–251.

Reynolds, R.J., Crum, M.G., and Hedrick, H.G. 1966. Studies on the microbiological degradation of aircraft fuel tank coatings. Dev. Ind. Microbiol., 8, 260–266.

Reuszer, H.W. 1945. The role of bacteria in the deterioration of cotton duck under tropical conditions. Office of Scientific Research and Development Report No. 4806.

Richardson, B.A. 1973. Control of biological growths. Stone Industries, 8, 2–6.

Richardson, J.H., and Ogilvy, W.S. 1955. Antimicrobial penetrant sealers. Applied Microbiol., 3, 277–288.

Richardson, J.F. 1941. Chlorophenols as antiseptics in vegetable tanning liquors. Shoe Leath. Rep., 221, 17–21.

Richardson, J.F. 1940. The disinfectant properties of phenol derivatives. Hide Leath., 99, 28, 38.

Richardson, J.H., and Del Giudice, J.V. 1952. The testing and use of fungicidal paints in food processing plants. Modern Sanit., 4, (3) 32–37; (4), 32–35.

Rischbieth, J.R., Freeman, L.O., Bussel, K.R., and Hill, M. 1974. Practical evaluation of antifungal paints in the tropics. J. Oil Col. Chem. Assoc., 57, 228–40.

Roberts, D.R. 1973. Inducing lightwood in pine trees by paraquat treatment. U.S. Dept. Agric. Forest Serv. Res. Note SE—191, SE Forest Exp. Stat., Asheville, NC.

Robinson, R.F., and Austin, C.R. 1951. Effect of copper-bearing concrete on moulds. Industrial and Engineering Chemistry, 43, 2077–2082.

Roche, J.N. 1952. Coal tar creosote—its composition and how it functions as a wood preservative. J. Forest Prod. Res. Soc., 2, 75–79.

Rogers, R.E., Hirschmann, D.J., and Humfeld, H. 1940. Comparison of growth of Trichophyton interdigitale on wool fabric with and without additional nutritive media. Proc. Soc. Exp. Biol. Med., 45, 729–733.

Roizin, M.B. 1951. A whitewash that prevents moulding in storage houses for fruit, vegetables and potatoes. Doklady Vshesoyuznoy Akademii Nauk imeni V.I. Lenina, 16, 39–41. In Chemical Abstracts, 1952. 46, 224.

Romanelli, F.H. 1972. An in-can preservative with a 6-year history. Am. Paint J. (May 1), 56, 56–57.

Ross, R.T. 1971. Modified barium metaborate. Am. Paint. J., 55, 23–37.

Ross, R.T. 1964. Microbial deterioration of paint films. Dev. Ind. Microbiol., 6, 149–163.

Ross, S.H., and Teitell, L. 1966. Factors in the development of fungus-proof barrier materials. I. Treatments for kraft paper. Dev. Ind. Microbiol., 7, 179–191.

Ross, S.H., Rosenwasser, E.S., and Teitell, L. 1956. Effects of fungi on barriers. Mod. Packag., 29, 180–184, 237–241.

Rossmoore, H.W. 1962. Correlation of coliform activity and anaerobic sulfate reduction with deterioration of cutting fluids. Lubric. Eng., 18, 226–229.

Rossmoore, H.W., and Brazin, J.G. 1968. Control of cutting oil deterioration with gamma radiation. In Deterioration of Materials. Volume 1. Edited by A.H. Walters and J.J. Elphick. New York, Elsevier, pp. 386–401.

Rossmoore, H.W., and Holtzman, G.H. 1974. Growth of fungi in cutting fluids. Dev. Ind. Microbiol., 15, 273–280.

Roth, P.B., and Hallows, L.B. 1963. Durable antibacterial textile finish for cellulosic fibers. U.S. Patent 3,072,534.

Rubbo, S.D., Albert, A., and Gibson, M.I. 1950. The influence of chemical constitution on antibacterial activity. Part V: The antibacterial action of 8-hydroxyquinoline (oxine). Br. J. Exp. Pathol., 31, 425–441.

Rudman, P. 1963. The causes of natural durability in timber. Part XI. Some tests on the fungi toxicity of wood extractives and related compounds. Holzforschung, 17, 54–57.

Russell, P. 1961. Microbiological studies in relation to moist groundwood pulp. Chem. Ind., No. 20, 642–649.

Sadurska, I., and Kawalik, R. 1966. Experiments on control of sulphur bacteria active in biological corrosion of stone. Acta Microbiologica Polonica, 15, 199–202.

Saito, K. 1973. Photographic film antimold agent. Japanese Patent Kokai 73, 83,820. November 8, 1973.

Salvin, S.B. 1944. Influence of zinc oxide on paint molds. Ind. Eng. Chem., 36, 336–340.

Sanborn, J.R. 1965. Selection of slimicides. Nature of problems dictates control agent. Paper Trade J., 149, 59–62.

Sanborn, J.R. 1951. Relation of red slimes to general paper mill slime control. Tappi, 34, 490–493.

Sanborn, J.R. 1944. Progress in methods of slime control. Paper Trade J., 119, 37–42.

Savory, J.G. 1980. Treatment of outbreaks of dry rot Serpula lacrymans. Newsletter, British Wood Preservation Association, News sheet No. 160, May 1980.

Saxena, B.B.L., Nigam, S.S., and Sengupta, S.R. 1963. Fungal attack of optical instruments and its protection. Indian J. Technol., 1, 283–286.

Schirtzinger, M. M. 1963. Chlorine compounds for microbiological control. Paper Mill News, 86, 18, 22–25.

Schroder, H. 1958. Objects made from glass. German Patent 1,032,899.

Scott, J.D., and Dickert, A.D. 1972. A non-metallic paint mildewcide and can preservative for the seventies. Am. Paint J. (May 22), 56, 66, 68–74.

Shanor, L., and The Sub-Committee on Textile and Cordage, National Defense Research Committee, 1945. Fungus-proofing of textiles and cordage for use in tropical service. Office of Scientific Research and Development Report No. 4513.

Shapiro, S. 1958. The evaluation of fungicides for use in paints. Fed. Paint Varnish Prod. Clubs, Off. Dig., 30, 414–430.

Shaposhnikov, V.N., Kozlova, E.I., and Azova, L.G. 1964. Destruction of wool by microorganisms. Vestn. Moskov Univ. Ser. VI Biol. Pochv., 19, 58–63.

Sharpell, F. 1988. Biocides in specialty products. Chemspec USA '88 Symposium, pp. 77–82.

Shelley, M. 1987. The Care and Handling of Art Objects. New York, The Metropolitan Museum of Art.

Shirk, H.G. 1954. Optical instruments and photographic equipment. In Deterioration of Materials. Edited by G.A. Greathouse, and C. J. Wessel, New York, Reinhold Publishing Co., pp. 702–715.

Singer, M. 1976. Laboratory procedures for assessing the potential of antimicrobial agents as industrial biocides. Process Biochem., 11, 30–35.

Singer, S.M., and Rowe, W.F. 1989. Biodeterioration of man-made textiles in various soil environments. Biodeterioration Research 2. Edited by C.E. O'Rear and G.C. Llewellyn. New York, Plenum Press, pp. 81–91.

Siu, R.G.H. 1951. Microbial Decomposition of Cellulose. New York, Reinhold Publishing Co.

Smith, C.L., and Ritter, J.E. 1968. Engineered formation cleaning. Prod. Mthly., 32, 14–18.

Smith, D.P., and Rollin, N.J. 1954. Sorbic acid as a fungistatic agent for foods. VII. Effectiveness of sorbic acid in protecting cheese. Food Res., 19, 59–65.

Smith, R.L. 1966. The control of microbial damage to fuel tank linings with 8-azaguanine. Dev. Ind. Microbiol., 8, 360–366.

Smith, R.S. 1975. Automatic respiration analysis of the fungitoxic potential of wood preservatives, including an Oxathiin. Forest Prod. J., 25, (1), 48–53.

Smith, R.S., and Gjovik, L.R. 1972. Interlaboratory testing of wood preservatives using ASTM D1413–61. Wood and Fiber, 4, 170–178.

Smith, T.H.F. 1969. Toxicological and microbiological aspects of cutting fluid preservatives. Lubric. Eng., 8, 313–320.

Snyder, H.D. 1972. Fungicides without mercury. Chem. Technol., 2, 609–613.

Somerville, A.A. 1957. Synergistic fungicides. U.S. Patent 2,776,731.

Southwell, C.R., et al. 1962. Natural resistance of woods to biological deterioration in tropical environments. Part I. Screening tests of a large number of wood species. Naval Research Laboratory, NRL Report 5673.

Springer, E.L., Feist, W.C., Zoch, L.L., Jr., and Hajny, G.J. 1973. New and effective chemical treatment to preserve stored wood chips. Tappi, 56, 157.

Sponsel, K. 1956. Vermeidung von Pilz-und Schimmelbildung in Textilbetrieben. Zeitschrift für die gesamte Textil-Industrie, 58, 596–597.

Starnes, W.D. 1969. What are the latest developments in paper mill slime control? Paper Trade J., 153, 37–38.

Stinson, R.F. 1956. Algal growth and the performance of flowering plants in clay pots treated with copper naphthenate. Proceedings of the American Society of Horticultural Science, 68, 564–568.

Stinson, R.F., and Keyes, G.G. 1953. Preliminary report on copper and zinc naphthenate treatments to control algae on clay flower pots. Proceedings of the American Society of Horticultural Science, 61, 569–572.

Stormont, D.H. 1962. Boron additive helps NYC combat bacterial fouling of diesel fuel. Oil Gas J., 60, 133–134.

Strzelczyk, A.B. 1981. Painting and sculptures. In Microbiological Deterioration. Edited by A.H. Rose. London, Academic Press, pp. 203–233.

Stuart, L.S. 1957. Antimicrobial additives. Soap Chem. Spec., 33, 95, 97, 99, 101, 233.

Stuart, L.S., and Frey, R.W. 1934. Molding of pickled sheepskins. J. Am. Leath. Chem. Assoc., 29, 113–118.

Sweitser, D. 1968. The protection of plasticized PVC against microbial attack. Rubber Plast. Age, 49, 426–430.

Szostak-Kotowa, J. et al., 1979. Evaluation of biocides used to protect cotton fabrics. II. Resistance of impregnated fabric to the effects of pure strains of cellulytic fungi. Przegl. Wlok., 33, 634–6.

Tant, C.O., and Bennett, E.O. 1956. The isolation of pathogenic bacteria from used emulsion oils. Appl. Microbiol., 4, 332–338.

Taylor, C.G., and Hunter, G.H. 1972. Radiometric studies of mercury loss from fungicidal paints. J. Appl. Chem. Biotechnol., 22, 711–718.

Teitell, L., and Berk, S. 1952. Prevention of mold growth in optical instruments. Ind. Eng. Chem., 44, 1088–1095.

Teitell, L., Berk, S., and Kravitz, A. 1955. The effects of fungi on the direct current surface conductance of electrical insulating materials. Appl. Microbiol., 3, 75–81.

Teitell, L., and Ross, S.H. 1966. Factors in the development of fungus-proof barrier materials. II. Plastics and asphalt laminates. Dev. Ind. Microbiol., 7, 192–200.

Thom, C., Humfeld, H., and Holman, H.P. 1934. Laboratory tests for mildew resistance of outdoor cotton fabrics. Am. Dyestuff Rep. 23, 581–586.

Thompson, R.N. 1963. Inhibiting bacterial growth. U.S. Patent 3,089,847 (to Hagan Chemicals & Controls, Inc.)

Toole, E.R., and Barnes, H.M. 1974. Biodeterioration of particle board. Forest Prod. J., 24, 55–57.

Tsunoda, J., and Nishimoto, K. 1986. Evaluation of wood preservatives for surface treatment. Int. Biodeter., 22, 27–30.

Turner, J.N. 1967. The Microbiology of Fabricated Materials. Boston, Little Brown, p. 154.

Union Carbide Chemicals Co. 1958. Glutaraldehyde. Technical Information F-40005B.

Upsher, F.J. 1985. Development of a controlled release volatile fungicide preparation. Int. Biodeter., 21, 211–214.

Valentine, E. 1936. Bactericidal power of dried painted surfaces. I. Proc. Soc. Exp. Biol. Med., 34, 166–170.

Vallée, M.J. 1934. Concerning bactericidal paints and a new means of preparation of these paints. Chim. Ind., 31 (Special No.), 962–968.

Vannoy, W.G. 1956. Development in exterior house paints–oil types. Am. Paint J., 40, (30), 80–93, (26), 16–30, (27), 76–88.

Vannoy, W.G. 1948. Mildew inhibitors for house paints. Fed. Paint Varnish Prod. Clubs, Off. Dig., 277, 163–175.

Vicklund, R.E. 1946. Preventing the fungus fouling of optical instruments. Ind. Eng. Chem., 38, 774–779.

Vicklund, R.E., and Manowitz, M. 1950. Mechanism of action of copper 8-quinolinate. CADO, Tech. Data Dig., 15, 18–21.

Waksman, S.A., et al. 1944. Fungi and Tropical Deterioration. 3rd Edition. Office of Scientific Research and Development Report No. 4101.

Walchli, O. 1962. Paper-damaging pests in libraries and archives. Textil-Rundschau, 17, 63–76.

Wang, L.W., Blaser, M.J., Cravens, J., and Johnson, M.A. 1979. Growth, survival and resistance of Legionnaires' disease bacterium. Ann. Intern. Med., 90, 614–18.

Watson, E.T., and Sowden, R.H. 1972. The way Gray products meets customer requirements in the field of industrial biocides. J. Inst. Petrol., 58, 263–267.

Weatherburn, M.W. 1947. The rotproofing of textiles and related materials—a survey of literature. Natl. Res. Coun. Can., NRC No. 1601.

Werthan, S. 1968. Zinc oxide and modern exterior latex paint. Am. Paint. J., *53*, 88, 90.

Wessel, C.J., and Bejuki, W.M. 1959. Industrial fungicides. Ind. Eng. Chem., *51*, 52A–63A.

Wexler, T., Ortenberg, E., and Pitis, I. 1971. New fungistatic agents and their activity in mixtures PVC. Chim. Ind.-Genie Chim., *104*, 201–206.

Wheeler, H.O., and Bennett, E.D. 1956. Bacterial inhibitors for cutting oil. Appl. Microbiol., *4*, 122–126.

White, W.C., and Olderman, J.M. 1983. Antimicrobial techniques for medical nonwovens. Dow Corning Corp. and American Converters.

Whitely, P. 1965. Mold resistant decorative paint in the tropics. J. Oil Colour Chem. Assoc., *48*, 172–204.

Williams, G.R. 1986. The biodeterioration of vulcanized rubbers. Int. Biodeter., *22*, 307–311.

Wolf, P.A. and Riley, W.H. 1965. Fungistatic performance of 10,10′-bis-phenoxarsine in exterior latex and asphalt coatings. Appl. Microbiol., *13*(1), 28–33.

Wolfson, L.L. 1960. Microbiology in secondary recovery systems. Corrosion, *16*, 298–300t.

Woods, D.R., Rawlings, D.E., Cooper, D.R., and Galloway, A.C. 1973. Collagenolytic activity of hide bacteria and leather decay. J. Appl. Bacteriol., *36*, 64–77.

Woods, G.A. 1973. Bacteria: friends or foes? Chem. Eng., *80*, 81–84.

Yamanchi, A. 1980. Sanitary footwear articles. British Patent 1,581,586. December 17, 1980.

Yeager, C.C. 1977. Fungicides in industry. In *Antifungal Compounds*. Edited by M.R. Siegel and H.D. Sisler. New York, Marcel Dekker, pp. 381–387.

Yeager, C.C. 1962. Pink staining in polyvinyl chloride; nature, cause, and how to deal with it. Plastics World, *20*, (Dec.) 14–15.

Yeremenko, K.F., and Shapiyevskaya, V.P. 1958. Fungicidal treatment of films attached by mold. Trudy Vses N.-1. Kinfoto In-ta, *3*, (26), 27–36.

Zuck, R.K., and Diehl, W.W. 1946. On fungal damage to sun exposed cotton duck. Am. J. Botany, *33*, 374–382.

Zyska, B.J. 1981. Rubber. In *Microbial Deterioration*. Edited by A.H. Rose. London, Academic Press, pp. 323–379.

Zyska, B.J., Rytych, B.J., Zankowicz, L.P., and Fudalej, D.S. 1972. Microbiological deterioration of rubber cables in deep mines and the evaluation of some fungicides in rubber. Proceedings of the 2nd International Biodeterioration Symposium. London: Applied Science Publishers, pp. 256–267.

CHAPTER 53

PRESERVATION OF METALS
FROM MICROBIAL CORROSION

Jose Rafael Sifontes and Seymour S. Block

Microbial corrosion (MC), as part of the general corrosion problem, is a widely recognized phenomenon in most industrial processes worldwide. The objectives of this chapter are to present the state of the art information on the understanding of the mechanisms of the corrosion process caused or influenced by these prolific microorganisms, and how to prevent this pervasive problem.

Although the actual cost of corrosion is difficult to ascertain, some recent estimates have been made. Poff (1985) indicated that metallic corrosion represents, in the United States alone, an approximately $140 billion per year problem. Based on a National Bureau of Standards Study (1978), the national cost of metal corrosion in the United States was estimated to be in the range of $170 billion for the year 1985. As for microbial corrosion, a study performed in England by the National Corrosion Service (Wakerly, 1979) estimated that about 10% of metallic corrosion is caused by microbial intervention. However, several authors have reported MC costs to be on the order of 50 to 77% of the total corrosion problem, in a wide range of industrial applications. For instance Booth (1964) estimated it to be the cause of at least 50% of all pipeline failures in the United Kingdom. Butlin et al. (1952) associated MC with 70% of all corrosion of water mains in the United Kingdom. Allred et al. (1959) reported MC to be the cause of 77% of the corrosion in a group of producing wells, and Paternaude (1985) reported that 50% of the steel culvert pipe corrosion in Wisconsin was due to the sulfate-reducing bacteria (SRB). Assuming the level of 10% of corrosion caused specifically by microbial action, this would represent $14 to $17 billion per year in the United States. These costs include replacement, prevention, and maintenance; but they do not include losses of time, money, natural resources, human suffering, and death due to equipment failure such as occurs in gas pipeline ruptures.

Metallic corrosion is a natural process in which metals return to their natural, oxidized states. During the man-ufacturing process of extracting metals from their ores, much energy is put into the process, which makes it thermodynamically unstable. Most corrosion processes are essentially surface electrochemical mechanisms, common to all metals in aqueous or at least humid environments. This conclusion was first reached by Whitney (1903). *Microbial* corrosion (MC) is the deterioration of a material by corrosion processes that occur directly or indirectly as a result of the activity of microorganisms. MC is a diverse, complex problem, and the literature associated with it tends to be just as diverse and complex. It requires the understanding of several scientific disciplines (in particular microbiology, thermodynamics, metallurgy, chemistry, chemical engineering, and physics) in order to gain an optimal insight into its study. Only in the last decade was it well recognized and established that MC is a serious problem. Corrosion-influencing microorganisms generally do not lead to a new form of corrosion, but to a stimulation of the classic electrochemical corrosion process. Metal dissolution takes place at anodic sites, with the electrons being accepted in cathodic reactions at separate sites (Table 53–1).

EXTENT OF DAMAGE

All engineering materials in general use, with few exceptions, are susceptible to some forms of MC, which usually arises from the activity of a wide range of microorganisms and their metabolic products. MC has been identified in many areas and industries around the world such as wastewater facilities, nuclear power plants, water flood systems, oil production equipment, cooling water systems, underground structures and pipelines, aircraft fuel tanks, ships and marine structures, chemical process industries, power generation industries, and paper mills. Among the metals and alloys reported as being susceptible to MC are iron and its alloys, copper and its alloys, aluminum and its alloys, nickel and its alloys, cobalt-based alloys, and titanium alloys (Zamandeh et al., 1989;

Table 53–1. *The Cathodic Depolarization Theory*

Component	Reaction	
(1) Metal dissolution	$4Fe = 4Fe^{++} + 8e$	Anode
(2) Hydrogen reduction	$8H^+ + 8e = 8H$	Cathode
(3) Water dissociation	$8H_2O = 8H^+ + 8 OH^-$	
(4) Microbial activity	$SO_4^= + 8H = S^- + 4H_2O$	
(5) Corrosion product	$Fe^{++} + S^= = FeS$	
(6) Corrosion product	$3Fe^{++} + 6 OH^- = 3Fe(OH)_2$	
(7) Total reaction	$4FE + SO_4^= + 4H_2O = 3Fe(OH)_2 + FeS + 2OH^-$	

Griffin et al., 1989; Gabrielli, 1988; von Wolzogen Kuhr, 1934).

It is indicated that the forms of corrosion that are stimulated by the interaction of microorganisms with metals are numerous. They range from general pitting corrosion, crevice corrosion, and stress corrosion cracking, to enhancement of corrosion fatigue, intergranular stress cracking (of sensitized austenitic stainless steel), and hydrogen embrittlement with cracking.

BIOFILM DEVELOPMENT

Most cells will stick to most surfaces, whether the surfaces are those of other cells or merely inert material such as metals. In nutrient-poor environments (e.g., water transmission pipelines) most bacteria grow attached to surfaces mainly because of hydrophobicity. Initially, sessile bacteria adhere randomly to metal surfaces by means of their production of extracellular polysaccharides. The continued production of the polysaccharide and the reproduction of the bacteria leads to the development of biofilms in which a consortium of cells interact in a hydrated matrix of anionic polysaccharide polymers that provide protection from natural or synthetically produced antimicrobial agents (Costerton and Geesey, 1985). Within biofilms, as a bacterium begins to proliferate, its metabolic products stimulate the growth of other organisms. As the different microorganisms develop, molecular or proton exchanges occur; consortia such as this have been detected in association with microbial corrosion. The corrosion process can be initiated by the formation of either differential concentration cells or by local electrochemical corrosion cells within the biofilm in which the concentration of protons and other cations is formed.

METALLIC SURFACES AND CORROSION

In many neutral solutions the corrosion of the common structural metals appears to be associated with the flow of electric currents between various parts of the metal surface at finite distances from one another. This statement is supported by much qualitative evidence in the case of steels, where the quantities of current flowing during corrosion account for the amount of corrosion that occurs. In other words, the corrosion of metals and their alloys in neutral solutions appears to be electrochemical in nature (Mears and Brown, 1941). When the corrosion current is controlled, the corrosion process is governed. This control is satisfied when any one of four elements

of electrochemical corrosion is regulated: (1) electrodes, (2) electrolyte, (3) potential difference, and (4) electrical continuity.

Localized attack of metals is often the result of MC. However, in general, corrosion engineers and scientists have associated corrosion with any of the following non-biologic factors: (1) impurities in the corroding metal, (2) grain boundaries, (3) orientation of grains, (4) differential grain size, (5) differential thermal treatment, (6) surface roughness, (7) local scratches and abrasions, (8) differences in shape, (9) differential strain, (10) differential pre-exposure to air or oxygen, (11) differential concentration or composition of the corroding solution, (12) differential aeration, (13) differential heating, (14) differential illumination, (15) differential agitation, (16) contact with dissimilar metals, (17) externally applied potential, and (18) complex cells.

The eight known forms of corrosion are uniform, galvanic, crevice, pitting, intergranular, dealloying, erosion, and stress.

HISTORICAL REVIEW

To provide a historical perspective for the development of an understanding of biocorrosion, emphasis will be placed on the anaerobic microbial corrosion by sulfate reducing bacteria (SRB). It was accepted, as early as the late nineteenth century, that microorganisms play a role in the corrosion of metals and alloys buried in the ground or immersed in water. Probably the first reported suggestion that microbes might be involved in the corrosion of metals was made by Garret (1891). He attributed the corrosion of the lead-sheathed cable to the action of bacterial metabolites (ammonia, nitrates, and nitrites). In the early twentieth century, Gaines (1910) produced evidence that iron and sulfur bacteria were involved in the corrosion of the interior and exterior of water pipes by demonstrating the presence of abnormally large quantities of sulfur. He suggested that *Gallionella* and *Sphaerotilus* and SRB were responsible for the corrosion of ferrous alloys buried in soil. *Caulobacter* and *Gallionella* (iron-depositing bacteria) were later reported to be associated with deposits in pipes (Ellis, 1919; Harder, 1919). During 1924, Bengough and May reported on the effect of ammonia produced by bacteria on the corrosion of copper alloys. Later in 1934, von Wolzogen Kuhr and van der Vlugt proposed for the first time a mechanism for MC, which initiated systematic studies on MC, and differentiated the different components of the microbial corrosion process (namely metal, liquid, and microorganisms). They proposed that the SRB accelerated the corrosion of ferrous metals by cathodic depolarization, that is, by removing adsorbed hydrogen from the cathodic surfaces of the metal. The theory appeared to be relatively simple to confirm by conventional electrochemical techniques. However, confirmation has been obtained only for specific combinations of SRB species and experimental conditions. Evidence for bacterially associated corrosion continued to accumulate from around the world and was reviewed by Starkey and Wright (1945).

One of the first studies that demonstrated cathodic depolarization with SRB was conducted by Booth and Tiller (1960). They indicated that depolarization occurred with a hydrogenase-positive strain of *Desulfovibrio vulgaris,* and did not occur with a pure strain of hydrogenase-negative *Desulfotomaculum orientis.* Furthermore, they made additional observations that complicated matters: (1) Depolarization was observed only when the culture was in active growth. (2) The stimulation of corrosion was approximately similar for both microbes. (3) The FeS film formed on the iron samples had an apparent inhibitory effect on corrosion rates. (4) The corrosion rates reported were much lower than reported rates for similar alloys in a natural anaerobic environment in the presence of SRB. A possible explanation for the low rates was the low biologic activity in the bath culture they used with low concentration of nutrients. This hypothesis was later tested by Booth et al. (1967a) who reported corrosion rates in the order of 40 mils per year (mpy) and an absence of the protective FeS film. They noted the growth of a bulky black envelope of corrosion products around the metal specimens. The results were confusing because there was no correlation between corrosion rates and hydrogenase activity. Booth et al. (1967b) demonstrated that cathodic depolarization was also affected by precipitated FeS. Once formed, depolarizing activity continued even in the absence of bacteria. Booth and Tiller (1962) had previously indicated experimental evidence that the structure of the FeS film played a part in the corrosion process. In the presence of *Desulfovibrio salexigens,* they observed cathodic depolarization, and there was little reduction in the rate of anodic reaction accompanying formation of the FeS film. Although the anodic activity remained high, they could not detect a chemical difference between that film and a normally protective FeS film, so they attributed the difference to the film structure.

More recent research on the MC of ferrous metal by SRB is cited by Miller (1981). The results reported by Mara and Williams (1972), King et al. (1973), Smith and Miller (1975), and King et al. (1976) suggest the following: precipitated FeS might initially form a protective film on a ferrous metal surface in the presence of SRB. As the MC process continues, the film thickens and changes stoichiometrically, and as the ratio of Fe to S in the film changes from a sulfur-deficient to a sulfur-rich structure, the film becomes less protective and eventually spalls. Once spalled, the film does not reform, and vigorous anodic activity proceeds at the exposed metal surfaces. According to Smith and Miller (1975), the FeS film, re-

gardless of structure, is cathodic to iron, and the corrosion process continues galvanically. Smith (1980) indicated that the FeS film would not remain permanently cathodic in the absence of bacteria. The role of the SRB, he suggests, could be either to depolarize the FeS, enabling it to remain cathodic, or to produce more FeS by their metabolism. Iverson (1981) discounts the FeS argument in his paper. He reported corrosion rates above 210 mpy for mild steel specimens exposed to filtered media from actively growing cultures of *Desulfovibrio* (API strain). He also filtered media of growing cultures after 9 days to remove bacteria, then precipitated all free sulfide by treating with excess ferrous ion. Thus, only soluble products in the filtrate were present from the original media. Iverson reports that the SRB produce a highly corrosive compound (phosphine) in addition to hydrogen sulfide. The process appears to depend on whether FeS forms a protective film before the highly corrosive product contacts the metal surface. Thus, it is apparent that a number of factors from the metal and the solution are involved in the process of MC by SRB. As a result, measurement and control of the process variables will significantly affect the outcome of experimental results from one experiment, and one laboratory, to another. Postgate (1979) rather concisely accounted for the variety of factors involved in MC: (1) nature of metal surface, (2) dissolved ions, organic matter, or both, (3) biofilm formation, (4) FeS precipitate forms, and (5) other ions (sodium, chloride) present.

A large amount of literature up to the last decade has been influenced by the theory of cathodic depolarization and has referred to it, either to prove it or to criticize it. The use of electrochemical techniques allowed Horvath and Solti (1959) to discover an anodic effect in addition to the cathodic effect of the theory. They studied this effect as a function of pH, environmental regulatory conditions, and the concentration of FeS present. According to those results, the SRB have an indirect role in MC, which would be the stabilization of the sulfide compounds over the metal surface by modification of the redox potential. One of the most conclusive findings was reported by Costello (1974). He indicated a cathodic effect due to the hydrogen sulfide produced by the SRB. Thus, the hydrogen utilization by the SRB becomes secondary, and so does the participation of these bacteria in the corrosion process.

The role of microorganisms in aerobic corrosion was postulated by Olsen and Saybalski (1949) to be due in part to the formation of tubercles in conjunction with microbial growth, which initiates oxygen concentration cells. This mechanism, along with others, was proposed as the cause of the worldwide problem of microbiologically associated aluminum wing tank corrosion, which surfaced in the late 1950s and early 1960s. Both commercial and military aircraft were affected. Many microorganisms were reported to be present in significant numbers in the fuel tank sludge (Churchill, 1963). The same year Leathen and Kinsel made 184 isolates of microorganisms from jet fuel storage tanks at nine Air Force bases. Results indicated the presence of bacteria and fungi. The predominant bacteria were *Pseudomonas,* and the most abundant fungi were of the genus *Hormodendrum*. This case showed the presence of a variety of species of fungi, bacteria, and yeast that participated in the process of microbial corrosion. Furthermore the medium was complex because of the presence of the two liquid phases in contact, water and fuel. Later work suggested that *Cladosporium resinae* was the most important fungus encountered in wing tanks; this organism was considered responsible for filter blockage and metal corrosion (Berner and Ahearn, 1977). In 1976, Hill indicated that *C. resinae* is only found in subsonic aircraft. In supersonic aircraft, a higher temperature prevails, and the predominant flora found were *Aspergillus fumigatus*, gram-negative bacteria, yeast, and other fungi. Recent evidence appears to indicate that organic acids, produced by fungi, were primarily involved in this corrosion (Miller, 1981).

During the 1980s, a number of corrosion-induced equipment failures in the chemical process industries occurred. For example, serious problems caused by the activities of SRB have arisen in offshore oil operations (Hamilton and Sanders, 1986). Two other problems have arisen in the legs and storage cells of offshore structures; these are the production of hydrogen sulfide, which is a serious personnel safety hazard, and the production of bacterial metabolites that give rise to accelerated concrete deterioration (Wilkinson, 1983). MC (internal and external) of long, large-capacity subsea pipelines, which transmit oil and gas to shore from offshore production fields, also appears to be a major problem (King et al., 1986). In the last decade substantial advances have been made in microbiology, including the understanding of the SRB (Postgate, 1982) and the biochemistry of dissimilatory sulfate reduction in *Desulfovibrio*. This has revealed enzymes and electron carriers of special character and structure whose functions and intracellular distribution are beginning to be revealed, throwing light on the curious features of energy generation in these bacteria (Peck and LeGall, 1982). Corrosion science has also contributed to this advancement. Electrochemical investigations have given us a positive understanding of the corrosive activity of the biotic and inorganic sulfide ions and their derivatives (Shoesmith et al., 1978; Salvarezza et al., 1983). Their action in the disruption of the passivity of iron and steels by pitting have been investigated (Salvarezza and Videla, 1980, 1982, 1984; Videla, 1985). For these studies, FeS was defined as the metal passive film: the sulfite activity was different if the passive film was iron hydroxide (easier to break than FeS) or iron oxide. In the case of iron oxide, the passive film broke at passive film discontinuities or inclusion zones, because of the difficulty of transport of the aggressive species through the passive film. These workers reported also the synergistic effect of chloride ion with the sulfide ion in the corrosion of steels. Other sulfur species have been studied to complement the forementioned sulfide ion effect (Vasquez et al., 1984). Different sulfur species are produced at different concentrations during the dissimilatory sulfate reduction by SRB (Cragnolino and Tuovinen, 1984). In addition, volatile metabolites have been reported to be responsible for MC of steels in en-

vironments free of sulfate and sulfide (Iverson, 1985). Iron phosphide was detected among the corrosion products found. It seems that the chemical reaction is the result of the competition between the sulfide that would passivate the metal and the volatile phosphorous (phosphine) that would replace the sulfide. Finally, there is no experimental evidence on the chemical nature of the corrosion product. Iverson (1985) and Costello (1974) considered the activity of volatile compounds in the corrosion of the metal excluding the direct contact between the bacteria and the metal.

CASE HISTORIES

Case histories of microbial corrosion are presented in Table 53–2.

MICROORGANISMS INVOLVED IN MICROBIAL CORROSION

The microorganisms that have been associated with microbial corrosion involve many genera and species. Microorganisms are anatomically simple yet biochemically complex. They may be divided into three groups: (1) protists (e.g., algae, fungi), (2) protozoa, and (3) monera (e.g., bacteria). Many of these organisms have been firmly established as having roles in the corrosion process as a result of laboratory and field studies, whereas others have merely been isolated from suspected corrosion sites.

Some characteristics of many of the microorganisms involved in corrosion are as follows: (1) they are generally very small, starting from less than 0.2 μm, which allows them to penetrate crevices down to several hundred micrometers in length very easily; (2) they are motile, which aids them in migrating to more favorable environments; (3) they have the ability to establish themselves in sites that offer distinct advantages to their growth. For instance, microbes colonize metal surfaces where, in the case of cooling water systems, higher concentrations of substrates accumulate because of their hydrophobic properties. (4) They can withstand a wide range of environmental conditions: pH values from 0 to 11, temperatures from 30 to 180° F, and oxygen concentrations from 0 to 100%. (5) They can adhere to a surface and form colonies of different species. This consortium once formed can sustain survival of at least some members under adverse conditions. (6) They can reproduce themselves to a great number in a short time. This fact allows them to bloom and take over an environment quickly. (7) They are easily dispersed in air, water, animals, etc. and adapt to other environments that might be easier for them to grow in. (8) They can adapt to a wide variety of substrates. Some species of *Pseudomonas*, for example, can use well over 100 compounds as sole carbon and energy sources. (9) They can produce extracellular polysaccharides or slime layers where a consortia of bacteria can develop and consequently influence corrosion. These layers attract food and other microorganisms and cause several other well known problems in the process industry, such as filter plugging and poor heat transfer.

Table 53–2. *Case Histories of Microbial Corrosion*

Metals Attacked	Industry Affected	Microorganisms and Problems	Preservation and Control (See Refs)	References
Copper: Nickel alloy 90:10 (CDA706) 70:30 (CDA710)	Sea water piping system	SRB. MC at crevices, occlusions, and surface irregularities of bolt and socket welds	$FeSO_4$ and Na_2SO_3 evaluated as inhibitors. 50 ppm $FeSO_4$ did not alter attack of sulfide on the heat affected zones. 10 ppm Na_2SO_3 lessens sulfide attack	Little et al., 1988
Aluminum AA7075 AA2024 pure Al	Aircraft wing tanks, fuel storage and distribution systems	*Cladosporium resinae, Serratia marscescens.* Biologic sludge at tank bottoms and sides. Pitting corrosion. Plugging of fuel pump, filter, and coalescer	Eliminate ammonium and nitrate ions from aqueous phase, then control with chlorine	Ayllon and Rosales, 1988; Videla et al., 1988
Stainless steel 904L. (UNS N08904) Austenitic SS	Sulfuric acid heat exchanger system	SRB. Corrosion pitting at crevices and welds in the water box	Chlorine control and good management. Upgrade material with higher Mo austenitic stainless steel with higher critical crevice temperature	Scott and Davies, 1989
Stainless steel AISI 304	Metal coupons in sea water	*Vibrio natriegens.* Biofilm increased corrosion rate >10 fold	Biofilm removed by sonication and washing	Nivens et al., 1986
Stainless steel AISI 316L AISI 304L	Metal coupons in rich nutrient bacterial culture	SRB. Corrosion pitting and intergranular attack	Biofilm removal by HCl pickling	Ringas and Robinson, 1988
Galvanized steel	Air conditioning cooling tower basin	*Thiobacillus* and *Desulfovibrio.* Discrete deposits and pitting corrosion	Use no Zn-containing inhibitor. Use organic phosphonated triazolemolybdate or brominated biocide. Epoxy coating best solution	Tatnall et al., 1981
Steel pipe Carbon steel 300 series SS and Cu alloys	Waterflood pipeline	SRB, corrosion	Use glutaraldehyde 50–100 ppm for 2 hrs, 3 times per week	Eagar et al., 1988
Stainless steel AISI 409 Cast iron aluminum	Wastewater treatment plant system: impeller, doors, windows, bolts, nuts, etc.	SRB. Corrosion failures above and below the water surface. Severe pitting at weld metal	Use superior material against MC, i.e., use nickel alloy impellers instead of ductile-cast iron	Licina, 1989
Stainless steel 300 series	Water and steam pipes in power generating plants	*Gallionella.* Pitting corrosion at or near welds	Avoid sensitization of stainless steel, change to a low carbon grade steel	Borenstein, 1988
Stainless steel AISI 304	Utility condenser	SRB. Massive failure due to pitting corrosion on tubes	Use epoxy coating for 12-month periods	Puckorius, 1983
Stainless AISI 304	Portable water piping system	*Gallionella.* Pitting corrosion after hydrostatic test	Not given	Tatnall, 1981
Monel metal	Heat exchanger tubes in cooling water system	SRB and *Pseudomonas.* Ni leaching and intergranular corrosion	Not given	Stoecker, 1984, 1985
Nickel 201	Tubing joints, hot water system	Filamentous thermophilic bacterium. Breaking up of metal passivation	Not given	Little, 1986

Table 53–2. *Case Histories of Microbial Corrosion* (continued)

Metals Attacked	Industry Affected	Microorganisms and Problems	Preservation and Control (See Refs)	References
Stainless steel AISI 304 Carbon steel	Closed cooling water system in paper mill	*Pseudomonas, Aerobacter,* SRB, *Clostridium,* and *Flavobacter*	Select better materials and better housekeeping. Thiocyanate biocide reduces odors but does not control MC	Tatnall, 1981
Stainless steel	Waste treatment tank	SRB and iron bacteria. Mound-like deposits along bottom half with deep pitting on most pipes, anchor bolts consumed by corrosion	Use AISI 304 anchor instead of AISI 303. Coat with epoxy resin after sandblasting. Cathodically protect equipment	Tatnall 1981
Carbon steel	Bloomcaster closed loop cooling water system in a continuous casting	SRB, SOB, and iron bacteria. Tubercules, nodules, and stalks	Eliminate the use of reclaimed wastewater. Use phosphonate/poly-acrylate dispersant. Use dimethylamide of fatty acid as penetrant/biodispersant. Use organo sulfur microbiocide such as Na-2-mercaptobenzothiazole	Honneysett et al., 1985

(10) They produce spores that resist severe environmental conditions, and are capable of surviving dormant for long periods. They can quickly colonize surfaces when the environment changes. (11) They can resist antimicrobial agents by virtue of their ability to degrade them or by being impermeable to them. Such resistance might be acquired by genetic mutation or acquisition of a plasmid. (12) They produce a variety of organic acids that promote corrosion of alloys even at low concentration. (13) They produce mineral acids that are extremely corrosive (e.g., *Thiobacillus thiooxidans* produces sulfuric acid). (14) They metabolize nitrite, sometimes used as corrosion inhibitor (e.g., *Pseudomonas* spp. reduces nitrate and nitrite to nitrogen gas). Other organsms convert nitrate to nitrite, ammonia to nitrite (e.g., *Nitrosomonas*) and still others nitrite to nitrate (e.g., *Nitrobacter*). (15) They form ammonia from the metabolism of amino acids. This forms ammonium ions, which might play a role in the corrosion of copper alloys. (16) They produce enzymes, which are excreted outside the cell, and which can act on substances outside the cell. Hydrogenase, for example, has been reported as responsible for depolarizing cathodic sites during the microbial corrosion of iron and steel. (17) They produce carbon dioxide and hydrogen as a result of their fermentative metabolism. Carbon dioxide in acidic solutions becomes carbonic acid, which is corrosive. Hydrogen can depolarize surfaces of stainless steel and cause hydrogen embrittlement. (18) Although they use organic compounds as carbon and energy sources, some can use hydrogen as their energy source and carbon dioxide as their carbon source, living chemoautotrophically. This can cause depolarization of cathodic sites on steel and promote corrosion (e.g., methanogens). (19) They can oxidize or reduce metals or metallic ions directly. For example, the iron-oxidizing bacteria (*Gallionella, Spherotillus*) oxidize ferrous ion to ferric ion. The ferric compounds precipitate in a sheath around the cells and form tubercules in pipes and cause plugging. Concentration cells are easily formed under those deposits. On the other hand, ferric ion can be reduced to ferrous ion by *Pseudomonas* spp. from oil wells and marine sediments. It has been suggested that the ferric film, which normally stabilizes the surfaces of mild steel toward corrosion, is destroyed, leaving the surface susceptible to corrosion attack. Other bacteria can oxidize or reduce other metals such as manganese. (20) They can form synergistic communities (e.g., algae and bacteria). These consortia can accomplish things that individually would be difficult if not impossible. Another example is the case of fungi and *Desulfovibrio* spp.; fungi break down wood to organic acids and consume oxygen, which provides the nutrients and anaerobic conditions for *Desulfovibrio*.

Microorganisms are sustained by chemical reactions. Organisms ingest a reactant and eliminate waste products. These processes can influence corrosion in the following ways: (1) directly influencing anodic and cathodic reactions, (2) influencing protective surface films, (3) producing deposits, (4) producing corrosive metabolites, and (5) destroying corrosion inhibitors.

Bacteria

The most important bacteria that play a role in the corrosion process are those involved in the sulfur cycle (Pfennig and Widdel, 1982; Williams, 1985). These include those involved in the oxidation as well as the reduction of sulfur compounds (Jorgensen, 1982; Trudinger, 1982; Bos and Kuenen, 1983). Of those two groups, the SRB are the most significant bacteria in the corrosion process (Iverson, 1987).

Sulfate-Reducing Bacteria (SRB)

The SRB are a group of strict anaerobes that are taxonomically diverse but physiologically and ecologically similar. Although they are anaerobes, they can survive for long periods in the presence of oxygen. They are distinguished by their ability to conduct dissimilatory sulfate reduction, using sulfate as the terminal electron acceptor and reducing it to sulfide (Peck and LeGall, 1982; Thauer, 1982). A few recently discovered species, such as *Desulfomonas acetooxidans*, use sulfur instead of sulfate as the electron acceptor (Widdel and Pfennig, 1977). The biochemical physiology of SRB has been reviewed by Postgate (1984). Organisms in the genus *Desulfovibrio*, which contains seven species, are non–spore-forming bacteria that are spirals or curved rods (Bergey's Manual, 1984). They have been associated with anaerobic corrosion in laboratory and field isolation studies, probably more than any other genus of SRB. Until recently, this genus and the spore-forming genus *Desulfotomaculum*, with five species, were considered to be the only two genera of SRB. Because of the work of Widdel and Pfennig (Bergey's Manual), seven additional genera of SRB have now been recognized. These are *Desulfuromonas, Desulfomonas, Desulfobacter, Desulfobulbus, Desulfoccoccus, Desulfosarsina,* and *Desulfonema*. The most unusual feature of these new bacteria, aside from their morphologic differences, is the wide range of carbon sources they can use. Usable carbon sources for *Desulfovibrio* and *Desulfotomaculum* are primarily restricted to lactate, pyruvate, and malate, whereas with the new genera, carbon dioxide and fatty acids, from acetate to stearate, can be used.

Sulfur-Oxidizing Bacteria (SOB)

In stressing the importance of anaerobic corrosion by SRB, corrosive effects of acids produced by other microorganisms should not be overlooked. The most important active acids are those produced by SOB. Primarily these acid-producing bacteria are acidophilic, aerobic chemolithotrophs in the genus *Thiobacillus*. The mechanisms by which these motile, gram-negative organisms produce sulfuric acid from inorganic sulfur has been reviewed by Purkiss (1971), Kelly (1982), and Kuenen and Bendeker (1982). *Thiobacillus thiooxidans* and a variant, *T. concretivorous*, are the most common organisms associated with corrosion. *T. ferrooxidans*, in addition to oxidizing sulfur, also oxidizes ferrous to ferric ions. This is of economic value in biohydrometallurgy, because of the property of *T. ferrooxidans* to leach metal sulfide ores and, in the case of pyrite, to oxidize both the sulfur and ferrous moiety. Bos and Kuenen (1983) recently reviewed the SOB and their relationship to corrosion and leaching.

Iron Bacteria

A third group of bacteria, the aerobic iron bacteria, has also been associated with microbial corrosion. Two types are included: (1) the stalked bacteria in the genus *Gallionella*, and (2) the filamentous bacteria in the genera *Sphaerotilus, Crenothrix, Leptothrix, Clonotrix,* and *Lieskeela* (Ehrlich, 1981). Both types contain chemolithotropic autotrophs, obtaining energy from the oxidation of ferrous to ferric ions, which results in deposition of ferric hydroxide. They have been associated with the formation of tubercules, hard deposits of iron oxides in water pipes. Filamentous iron bacteria have been associated with hollow, hemispheric tubercles in stainless steel equipment (Tatnall, 1981). *Gallionella* has also been reported to be associated with the corrosion of stainless steel, particularly at or near weld seams, where bacterial deposits are rich in both iron and manganese (Tatnall, 1981).

Miscellaneous Bacteria

In addition to the already mentioned bacteria, there have been reports of other bacteria related to microbial corrosion of metals and alloys. Bacteria in the genus *Pseudomonas* and *Pseudomonas*-like organisms have been reported in connection with cases of corrosion. A strain of *Pseudomonas*, isolated from pipe systems carrying crude oil, was found to reduce ferric ion to soluble ferrous ion, thus continually exposing a fresh surface to a corrosive environment (Obuekwe et al., 1981). *Pseudomonas* species are most prevalent in industrial water environments alone and with other slime-forming bacteria, where their primary role appears to be colonizing metal surfaces, thereby creating oxygen-free environments that harbor SRB. Any microorganism with this capacity can be considered potentially corrosive. A variety of hydrogenase-positive, photosynthetic, and non-photosynthetic bacteria have been tested in the laboratory for their corrosive effects by cathodic depolarization (Mara and Williams, 1971, 1972) and by measurement of ion loss (Umbreit, 1976) following formation of rust. Only small effects were noted. In laboratory studies, however, several heterotrophic bacteria that form hydrogen, carbon dioxide, and acids (Frenzel, 1965) have been reported to play an important role during the corrosion of iron. Moreau and Brison (1972) classified heterotrophic aerobic and facultative bacteria into four groups, based on their proteolytic, nitrate-reducing, and carbohydrate-breakdown properties, with respect to the corrosion of copper and nickel. Some groups inhibited corrosion and others caused limited or extensive corrosion. Recently, a new group of bacteria has been included in the corrosion-causing microorganisms, namely, the methanogens (Daniels et al., 1987). These authors suggested that methanogens can be significant contributors to the corrosion of iron-containing materials in anaerobic environments. Furthermore, they indicated that methanogens, which normally use molecular hydrogen and carbon dioxide to produce methane and are the major inhabitants of most anaerobic ecosystems, use either pure elemental iron or iron in mild steels as a source of electrons in the reduction of carbon dioxide to methane. They also suggested that this mechanism of iron oxidation is cathodic depolarization. Belay and Daniels (1990) reported that besides iron, there are other metals (aluminum, zinc, nickel, arsenic) that methanogens use as electron sources for biologic methane formation, which results in their corrosion.

Fungi

Fungi can be divided into two major types, the molds and the yeasts. The molds, which can be filamentous or colonial, are nonphotosynthetic and require oxygen and organic compounds for growth. The pH range for growth is from 2 to 8; temperature ranges for growth are from 32 to 140° F. They can reproduce by cellular division, fragmentation, and asexual spore formation, and many by sexual means. The yeasts, also nonphotosynthetic, are unicellular, generally reproducing by budding, and are relatively large. The yeasts (along with the protozoans) appear to be of minimal importance in the context of MC of metals, because they are rarely found involved in corrosive systems (Sequeira et al., 1988).

One of the most significant fungi in MC is *Cladosporium resinae*, which is involved in the corrosion of aluminum fuel tanks of subsonic aircraft, leading to wing perforation and loss of fuel. This organism grows at the water/fuel interface at the bottom of fuel tanks and uses components of the fuel (C3 to C16 alkanes) and inorganic constituents dissolved in the water for nutrients (Miller, 1981; Tiller, 1982). It is now believed that the aluminum corrosion is caused by carboxylic acid production by *C. resinae* (Miller, 1981). In supersonic aircraft fuel tanks, an albino mutant strain of *Aspergillus fumigatus* has been shown to be the primary corrosive agent because of its ability to grow at higher temperatures in the tanks (Hill and Thomas, 1975). In an earlier report, a *Cerestomella* organism was reported to have caused the corrosion of steel- and aluminum-clad aircraft parts that were still inside the original wooden cases (Copenhagen, 1950). Later, Al'bitskaya and Shaposhnikova (1960) demonstrated the corrosion of copper, aluminum, and steel using five acid-producing species of fungi: *Aspergillus niger*, *A. amstelodami*, *Penicillium brevicompactum*, *Penicillium cyclopium*, and *Paecilomyces varioti*. A recent report describes the corrosion of a ship's hold by fungi (Stranger-Johannesen, 1986).

Algae

Algae are eucaryotic, photosynthetic organisms that are relatively large, sometimes motile, and usually colored. They can tolerate conditions of high to very low light intensity, and are even able to grow in the dark with organic nutrients. They can grow over a pH range of 5.5 to 9.0, although rare strains tolerate a wider range. The temperature range for survival is from much less than 30° F to well over 100° F. The algae, along with the cyanobacteria, are widely recognized as agents that can cause severe fouling problems that in turn cause such problems as reduction in heat transfer rate and plugging of tubes. These fouling problems can also be the source of many problems related to MC. Algae, along with the higher plants, are primary producers of the food necessary to support the growth of bacteria and fungi in the biosphere (Sequeira et al., 1988).

There are relatively few reports of direct corrosion by algae, although they would appear to have the potential for inducing corrosion by virtue of their production of oxygen, corrosive organic acids (Prescott, 1968), and nutrients for corrosion-inducing microorganisms, as well as their role in slime formation (concentration cells). Das and Mishra (1986) have reported on the corrosion of various types of welded mild steel and 304 stainless steel by a species of red algae (*Graciollasia* spp.) and two

species of *Cyanobacteria* (*Nostoc parameloides* and *Anabaena sphaerica*) from the Bay of Bengal. Cathodic polarization studies of these three strains of hydrogenase-positive Chlorophyta indicated that the organisms were able to utilize cathodic hydrogen (Mara and Williams, 1972). It has been found, however, that under healthy microalgal mats composed of *Oscillatoria* spp., colonial diatoms, and *Enteromorpha* spp., the pH was raised to high values, which tends to reduce the corrosion rate (Edyvean and Terry, 1983). In areas where there was a decay of the mat the pH was lowered, probably because of the production of corrosive organic acids, causing differential pH corrosion cells as well. Conditions were also found to be rendered favorable to the growth of SRB.

Other Organisms

The study of MC has tended to consider processes in isolation rather than actual cases of MC. For instance, many studies deal with the effect of a single species of microorganism on metal corrosion. Although such investigations are valuable in elucidating mechanisms, they give little insight into the wider biologic, metal-fluid interaction. Although recent reappraisal for the role of bacterial consortia, together with studies of the effect of such consortia, have improved our knowledge of the MC process, few studies of MC look beyond bacterial consortia and surface corrosion effects to wider biologic, metal-fluid interactions. Edyvean (1988) in his recent work discusses the interaction of both bacteria and macro and micro algae in the fouling community on steel substrata in sea water. Of particular importance is the enhancement of corrosion fatigue crack growth rates, where the larger, frondose algae increase hydrodynamic loading, and algal bacterial interactions at the metal surface can increase hydrogen embrittlement.

Furthermore, any living or even a dead organism that becomes associated with a metal surface immersed in an electrolyte has the potential ability to influence the corrosion of that metal. Marine barnacles are another example of organisms that are well known for the differential aeration cells they produce. A wide range of differential concentration cells can be originated by organisms such as seaweeds that can produce, in addition, potentially corrosive metabolites, including H_2SO_4. Of the hydrogenase enzyme found in algae, there are little data on its effect in anaerobic corrosion. Considerable physical disruption can be caused by larger organisms. The roots and holdfasts of plants and marine algae and the burrowing of some mollusks and sea urchins are known to damage both coatings of metals and the metal itself. The very strong attachment developed by some of these organisms will often resist mechanical cleaning, even on bright metal surfaces.

MECHANISMS OF MICROBIAL CORROSION

For the proper selection of methods to prevent or control MC, it is necessary to know the mechanisms by which microbial activity affects the deterioration of metals. The mechanisms of MC in some cases are well defined, but where environments encourage the activity of

SRB, the corrosion processes are more complex and still not fully understood. The mechanisms of MC can be subdivided into direct and indirect mechanisms. If a microbe interlinks an electrode process with its own metabolism or presence, it is a direct effect; otherwise it is an indirect effect.

Even though the mechanisms of MC are not well understood, microbes that cause or influence corrosion have been classified into the following groups (Kobrin, 1976):

Acid Producers. Some microbes can oxidize sulfur compounds to sulfuric acid. Very low pH has been reported in places where SOB are active. Many species produce a wide variety of organic acids (e.g., acetic, butyric, succinic, formic), which might promote corrosion of many metals and their alloys.

Protective Coating Destroyers. Protective coatings ranging from polymeric materials to passive films can be broken by the activity of microorganisms, after which corrosion of bare metal starts rapidly.

Producers of Corrosion Cells. Differential aeration and ion concentration cells are notable examples. These are due to the growth of biofilms on the metal surface.

Sulfur Reducers (SRB) and Oxidizers (SOB). SRB are the most publicized class of corrosive microbes. They reduce sulfates to sulfides and can depolarize cathodic sites by consuming hydrogen. Most SOB fall into the category of acid producers.

Concentrators of Anions, Cations, or Both. Iron and manganese bacteria are examples of this category. They generally form thick, bulky deposits that create concentration cells or harbor other corrosive microbes. This group is also known as metal ion oxidizers or reducers.

Hydrocarbon Feeders. Certain microorganisms have been observed that destroy organic coatings or linings in the presence of hydrocarbon fuels. Some others destroy metals such as aluminum and feed on hydrocarbon fuels.

Slime Formers. Certain algae, yeast, bacteria, and fungi form deposits that foul heat-transfer equipment and produce concentration cells on metal surfaces.

Combination of Mechanisms. Under natural conditions, the MC phenomena include several of the above mechanisms. Figure 53–1 represents an example in which at least five MC mechanisms in anaerobic environment are involved: difference concentration cells, sulfur reduction, slime formers, producers of corrosion cells, and acid producers.

These categories can be grouped into three general modes of microbial attack based on their metabolism: corroded material that serves as substrate for microbial growth, microbes that colonize the material surface but feed on something else, and microbes that produce metabolites that corrode material. Figure 53–2 depicts some of the MC environments as well as some of the mechanisms enumerated above.

CATHODIC DEPOLARIZATION

Cathodic depolarization has been the source of considerable controversy since it was postulated in 1934 by von Wolzogen Kuhr and van der Vlugt. The systematic study of MC began after the publication of the cathodic depolarization theory. The idea of the authors resulted from their interpretation of the electrochemical theory of the anaerobic corrosion of cast iron pipe in wet soils near Amsterdam. Because the soil was clay with a near-neutral pH, they could not explain the phenomenon of the severely corroded pipe. The alternative cathodic reactions for the reduction of hydrogen or oxygen were not feasible under those conditions.

This famous theory separates for the first time the three components of the MC system: microorganisms, metal, and fluid. It is presented in Table 53–1.

Figure 53–3 illustrates the mechanism for cathodic depolarization of iron by sulfate-reducing bacteria.

Research shows that the mechanism is not entirely correct. Equation (4) (Table 53–1) is the controversial one in the theory. Some of the problems with the theory are:

1. The stoichiometry of the overall reaction (7) (Table 53–1) indicates that 4 moles of Fe are oxidized to produce 3 moles of $Fe(OH)_2$ and 1 mole of FeS. This relationship has not been demonstrated. Furthermore, the values reported so far range from 1 to 20 times as many moles of $Fe(OH)_2$ as FeS (Hamilton, 1985).
2. The ability of bacteria to assimilate hydrogen directly from the reaction site and produce a cathodic depolarization effect has not been proven (Booth, 1971).
3. The role of FeS in the corrosion reaction at different concentrations and its cathodic effect has not been considered (King and Wakerly, 1973).
4. The role of the bacterial consortia through the formation of tubercules or associations within biofilms has not been taken into account (Costerton, 1984).
5. The direct effect of the SRB metabolites in the breaking of the passivity of carbon steel in natural habitats as has been indicated recently by Salvarezza and Videla (1980) was not considered.
6. The importance of the ionic composition of the environment during the breakdown of the biogenic sulfides' passivity was not taken into account (Salvarezza and Videla, 1984).
7. Other alternative metabolic pathways, other than by SRB, that might affect the corrosion of steel were not mentioned (Cragnolino and Touvinen, 1984).
8. The roles of the biofilm or inorganic films on the passivity of the metal and its breakdown were not clarified (Videla, 1985).
9. The effect of the hydrogen produced on the steel itself was not discussed (Walch and Mitchell, 1985).
10. The effect of elemental sulfur on the corrosion of the metal was not considered (Schaschl, 1980).

According to the literature, five other theories exist to explain the involvement of SRB in the corrosion process. These include (1) the cathodic depolarization theory, (2) the theory of corrosion by sulfide ion, (3) the theory of galvanic corrosion through FeS film formation, (4) the theory of corrosion through formation of elemental sul-

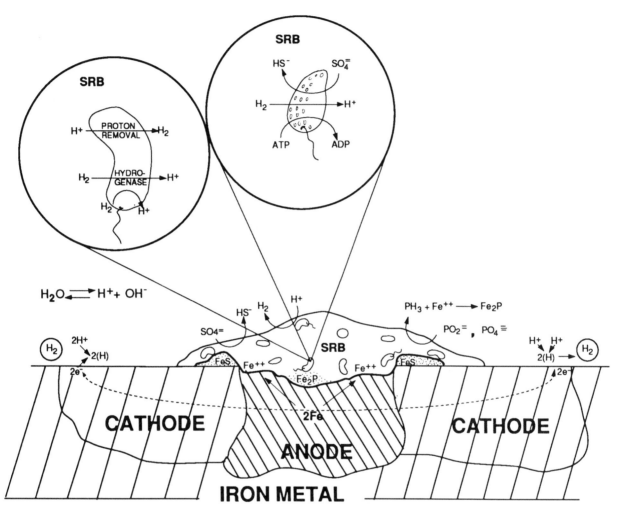

Fig. 53–1. Corrosion mechanisms by sulfate-reducing bacteria (SRB) in anaerobic environments.

fur, and (5) the theory of corrosion through the production of a corrosive volatile phosphorous compound.

DETECTION

An effective treatment to prevent MC requires the assurance that microorganisms are a factor in corrosion. The diagnosis of MC must begin with the capability of determining the cause and the mechanisms associated with the corrosion problem, which includes the proper detection and identification of microorganisms.

The detection process is not simple and requires some judgment to determine the appropriate method and the relevance of the data obtained. Detection may include electrochemical means, complemented by microbiologic methods, physical and metallurgic methods, in-system monitoring techniques, and other useful techniques.

Electrochemical Techniques

All electrochemical techniques are indirect methods based on Faraday's law. The electrochemical methods are marked by the extremely high accuracy for measuring

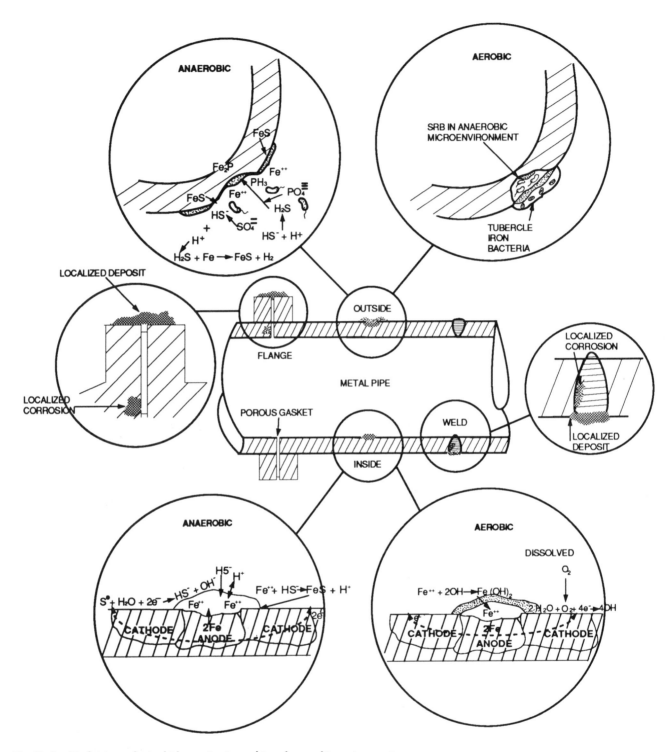

Fig. 53–2. Mechanisms of microbial corrosion in aerobic and anaerobic environments.

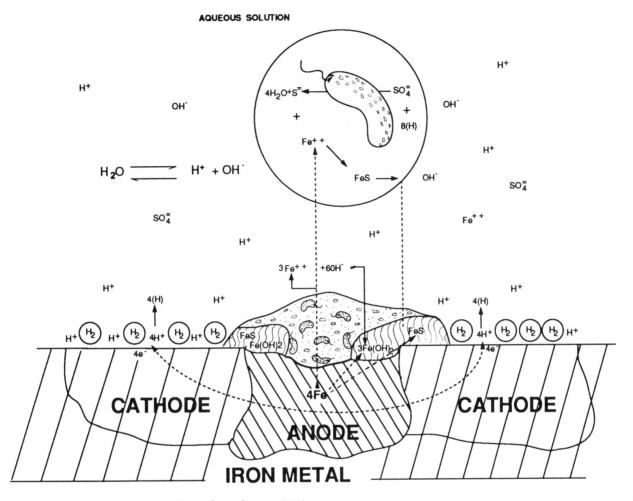

Fig. 53–3. Cathodic depolarization by sulfate-reducing bacteria (SRB).

the electrical potential and the current density. This technique can be useful in identifying the onset of corrosion. If simultaneous measurements of corrosion rate and pitting index are obtained, MC can be associated from their divergence. Basic electrochemical procedures can be found in any standard textbook on electrochemistry.

Microbiologic Methods

The emergency of some cases of MC requires the implementation of rapid techniques to identify the microorganisms involved in the MC process. Basic methods for the identification and enumeration of microorganisms can be found in the literature. Within the last few years

increasing interest has been shown in developing rapid techniques (Gaylarde, 1990) such as the following:

Dip Slides (Bailey and May, 1979). These medium-coated slides allow the enumeration of microorganisms without the necessity for making dilutions of the sample. The slide is dipped briefly into the test fluid, or placed firmly on the surface to be sampled, before replacing it in its sterile container for incubation. Often a fungal growth medium is placed side-by-side with a bacterial growth medium. This way, bacteria and fungi can be enumerated simultaneously. The incorporation of indicators, such as tetrazolium salts, in the media enhances the visibility of colonies produced on the agar, and allows

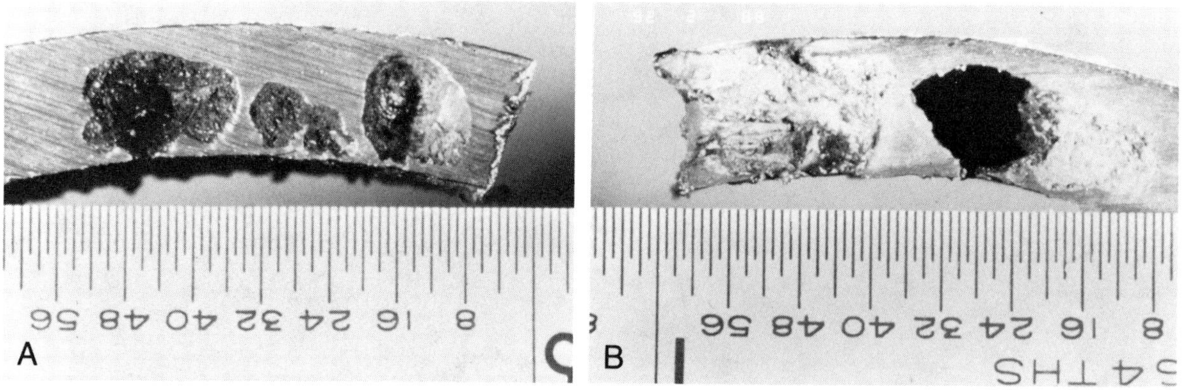

Fig. 53–4. Pitting biocorrosion of steel pipe in gas transmission pipeline by sulfate reducing bacteria (SRB). A, Intermediate stages. B, Final stage showing hole in pipe.

results to be obtained earlier than would otherwise be the case. The limitation of this method is determined by the media; only microbes capable of living on the media will be detected. This method is ideal for field use to obtain rough measurements of microorganisms present.

Epifluorescence (Hoff, 1988). The use of fluorescent stains facilitates the identification of microorganisms by direct microscopic examination. Cells have to be stained, using acridine orange or diamidinophenylindole, after having been filtered in an appropriate membrane filter in order to be detected. A fluorescence microscope is used for this simple and quick method. Most cells can be detected unless biofilms or other deposits are present. In addition, if fluorescent specific antibodies are used, particular species within the consortia of microbes can be identified and enumerated.

Adenosine Triphosphate (ATP) (Stanley, 1988). All living organisms have ATP. This substance can be extracted by several methods and can be analyzed using high-performance liquid chromatography or by the luciferin luciferase reaction. The test itself takes about 5 minutes, but the amount of ATP does not specify the microbe or the number of cells present. This technique is used for the detection of the presence of microorganisms.

Respiratory Activity (Staley and Konopka, 1985). Several tests such as the methylene blue and resazurine dye tests, based on the respiratory activity of microbes reducing the colored dye to a colorless form, have been in use for a long time. However, this technique lacks sensitivity and can be unreliable. Recent methods use radiolabeled products (radiorespirometry) to determine the activity of microorganisms by measuring the reacted product in scintillation counters. This method is sensitive and accurate, but expensive and possibly hazardous.

Nonrespiratory Activity (Chrzanowski et al., 1984). This technique is used especially to determine enzymatic activity of microorganisms. It employs fluorescein diacetate, which microbes can metabolize, and acetate and fluorescein (yellow fluorescent material) are released. This is a cheap and semiquantitative method. A fluorom-

eter is used and the sample may be assayed with or without prior solvent extraction.

Modified General Methods. Some of the above general methods can be made selective by simple changes to the medium. Dip slide is made selective by using specific media such as MacConkey agar for enterobacteria. Enzyme assays are selective if the enzyme detected is found in a certain group of organisms. The radiorespirometry can be made selective if a specific radiolabeled product is used (e.g., $^{35}SO_4^=$ to measure SRB activity).

Immunoassay (Gaylarde and Cook, 1987). The most selective methods known are those involving specific antibodies for the organisms of interest. SRB can be detected within hours by various modifications of the enzyme-linked immunosorbent assay (ELISA) technique. *Thiobacillus thiooxidans* can be detected within minutes by the fluorescent antibody staining technique. These techniques are best used for detection but not for enumeration.

Other Selective Methods. Oxygen-specific electrodes can be used to determine general aerobic activity by direct measurement of oxygen utilization. Micrometer-sized probes offer great potential for making measurements within biofilms (Revsbech, 1988). Biomass sensors are recent developments that use potentiostatic electrochemical techniques to measure the electron transport activity of microorganisms (Turner et al., 1989). These systems still lack sensitivity. Gas liquid chromatography has been used to identify specific fatty acids of SRB in sediments and biofilms (White et al., 1986). This method is costly and requires experience for the interpretation of results. Gene probes are powerful tools for the detection of microbes. They are produced by isolating and cloning a segment of DNA, which is labeled either radioactively or with an enzymatically detectable molecule. Microbes are detected after blotting or transfer by other means onto a solid support such as a nylon filter where DNA is released after cell lysis (Festl et al., 1986).

Physical and Metallurgic Methods

These methods involve the identification of the type of corrosion occurring (e.g., pitting, crevice, hydrogen

Table 53–3. *Microorganisms Identified during Microbial Corrosion*

Bacteria

Achromobacter spp.	*Micrococcus* spp.
Aerobacter spp.	*Microspira* spp.
A. aerogenes	*Nocardia* spp.
Alcaligenes spp.	*Paracolobacterium* spp.
Bacillus spp.	*Proteus* spp.
B. cereus	*P. morganis*
B. subtilis	*P. vulgaris*
Beggiatoa spp.	*Pseudomonas* spp.
Chromobacterium spp.	*P. aeruginosa*
Clostridium spp.	*P. oleovorans*
Crenothrix spp.	*Salmonella* spp.
Desulfotomaculum spp.	*Sarcina* spp.
D. nigrificans	*Shigella* spp.
D. orientis	*Sphaerotilus* spp.
Desulfovibrio spp.	*Spirillum* spp.
D. africannus	*Sporovibrio* spp.
D. desulfuricans	*Staphylococcus* spp.
D. salexigens	*S. albus*
D. vulgaris	*S. aureus*
Diplococcus spp.	*S. citreus*
D. pneumoniae	*Streptococcus* spp.
Escherichia spp.	*Thiobacillus* spp.
E. coli	*T. concretivorous*
E. freundii	*T. thiooxidans*
Ferrobacillus ferrooxidans	*T. thioparus*
Flavobacterium spp.	*Thiothrix* spp.
F. hydrophilium	*Vibrio* spp.
Gallionella ferruginea	*Desulfomonas* spp.
Klebsiella spp.	*D. acetooxidans*
K. pneumoniae	*Clonothrix* spp.
Lactobacillus spp.	*Lieskeella* spp.
Leptothrix spp.	*Clostridium* spp.
Nitrosomonas spp.	*C. acetobutilicum*
Nitrobacter spp.	Methanogens
Caulobacter spp.	

Fungi

Cladosporium resinae	*Aspergillus fumigatus*
Cerostomella spp.	*Aspergillus niger*
Penicillium buricompactum	*Aspergillus amstelodami*
Penicillium cyclopium	*Paecilomyces varioti*
Yeast	

Algae

Nostoc parameloides	*Anabaena sphaerica*
Graciollasia spp.	*Oscillatoria* spp.
Diatoms	*Enteromorpha* spp.
Chlorophyta	Cyanophyta

embrittlement), employing metallography, macroanalysis, and microanalysis. In macroanalysis, the techniques include the use of special devices such as atmosphere-controlled autoclaves and special sensors capable of monitoring the environmental pressure, temperature, shear stress, pressure and temperature gradients, and cycles. In microanalysis the methods include the use of scanning electron microscopy (SEM), transmission electron microscopy (TEM), scanning transmission analytical electron microscopy (STAEM), quantitative radiographic microanalysis using energy dispersive spectrometry (EDS), and electron probe microanalysis (EPMA) using wavelength dispersive spectrometry (WDS) techniques, with x-ray mapping. For more information on those techniques see Marquis (1988) or the appropriate metals handbook.

In-System Monitoring Techniques

There are no established methods to detect or monitor MC in an operating system. However, techniques have been developed for the study of actual cases of MC. Such techniques must be located in the system at strategic places in order not to cause interruptions of the process being performed. Two examples follow: (1) *Isolated metal coupons and pipe segments*. These devices should be placed at locations where MC is suspected to occur, at sites that have previously experienced MC. The design should enable the coupon or pipe segment to be removed for periodic inspection and analysis. *(2) Side stream monitors*. This technique can involve several types of equipment and devices such as heat exchangers and pilot scale components that can be used to study corrosion and functional performance of the component. Side stream monitors are sometimes designed to hold racks of coupons that may be removed or inserted periodically in water-treatment programs for the prevention of MC.

Other Useful Techniques

Fourier transformed infrared spectroscopy has the potential for identifying "fingerprints" for certain bacteria on a surface. Unfortunately, this technique has most of the disadvantages of the fatty acid analysis technique, such as the need for expensive equipment and trained personnel. There is also the difficulty with preparation of field samples without disrupting the samples.

Other techniques, such as gas chromatography, ion chromatography, high-performance liquid chromatography, nuclear magnetic resonance, and electron spin resonance, can also be used to analyze corrosion and metabolic products.

PREVENTION

There is no universal approach to the prevention of MC, and the problem is usually tackled more from the corrosion standpoint than from the microbiologic point of view. The solution is generally difficult, time-consuming, and expensive. One should be content if MC can be controlled to an acceptable degree. If possible, MC should be prevented rather than cured, and prevention should be a matter of top priority in the process industry. The proper control technology depends basically on the materials of construction, the water quality requirements, and the environmental conditions of the process.

The methods available include chemical treatment, physical and chemical cleaning, and materials selection.

For an effective chemical treatment the system needs to be cleaned and free from corrosion products, biofilms, and debris that can prevent biocides from doing their job. Typical chemicals used are corrosion inhibitors, biocides, surfactants, defloculants, chelating agents, and dispersants. Chemical treatment refers also to the control and prevention of scales and deposits. Physical cleaning methods include the use of high-pressure jetting, pigging, brushing, jet mole, sand blasting, and other such devices. These methods will remove scale, deposits, and biofilms. It is important during the cleaning operation that most if not all foreign material be removed to avoid the continuation of corrosion. These methods are used in conjunction with the chemical treatment programs to minimize the input and activity of organisms in the system and effectively control MC.

Chemical cleaning includes chemical filling, cascading, emulsion cleaning, foaming, and other related methods. These methods are usually more effective than mechanical cleaning methods; however, more caution is required during their application because the equipment can be damaged if the proper chemicals are not selected. These methods are used like the mechanical ones in conjunction with chemical treatment.

The system should provide control of flow velocity to a range that will be a limiting factor in the growth of sessile microorganisms. Continuous flow is preferred to intermittent flow conditions. Dead legs and bypass circuits should be avoided to allow for drainage. Provisions should be included for drains, traps, recycle circuits, monitoring equipment, and the capability for allowing periodic draining and cleaning. Provision should be made for circulating water periodically in those components that typically remain stagnant for long periods (e.g., fire safety water systems). For additional details consult Uhlig and Revie (1985) and Fontana and Greene (1987).

Long ago the selection of materials of construction was done without consideration for preventing MC because other criteria, such as cost, were given higher priority. Nowadays, this is the most common method used to prevent corrosion, in which the proper metal or alloy is selected for a particular environment.

In many instances, better or more economic materials are available. For many years tantalum was favored when minimal corrosion was required, such as for implants in the human body. For reducing environments and aqueous solutions, nickel, copper, and their alloys are used. For extremely powerful oxidizing conditions, titanium and its alloys have shown superior corrosion resistance. The corrosion resistance of a pure metal is usually better than that of one containing impurities or small amounts of other elements. However, pure metals are usually expensive and are relatively soft and weak.

Nonmetallic materials, particularly composite fiber reinforced resin systems, are now gaining ground in substituting for metals. The seven general classes of nonmetallics are

Rubbers
Concrete
Plastics
Carbon and graphite
Ceramics
Wood
Composites

In general, rubbers and plastics, as compared with metals and alloys, are much weaker, softer, and more resistant to chloride ions and hydrochloric acid, but less resistant to strong sulfuric acid and oxidizing acids such as nitric. They are less resistant to solvents, and have relatively low temperature limitations. Small-diameter polymeric pipes are now frequently used for water distribution systems. Ceramics possess excellent corrosion and temperature resistance. Their main disadvantages are that they are brittle and have low tensile strength. Carbon shows good corrosion resistance as well as electric and heat conductivity, but it is fragile. Wood is attacked by a host of organisms including fungi, bacteria, insects, and marine organisms; the most common attackers are termites and fungi. Nowadays many of the problems associated with strength and durability of these products appear to have been overcome by the composite fiber reinforced resin systems. These composite materials are available for use in a wide spectrum of environments.

Cement products are widely used, including spur concrete and other reinforced or prestressed concrete. Systems are also available in which fine concrete is sprayed onto both internal and external surfaces of a thin tubular iron pipe. Pipes of very large diameter can be fabricated by this technique, which has had some success in aggressive soils. Large-diameter cement and asbestos-cement pipes are satisfactory for use in unpressurized systems provided there is no possibility for SOB, which attack concrete, transforming it into a soft chalky material through the production of sulfuric acid.

The problem of MC could be avoided altogether if chemically inert materials of adequate strength were available at a cost competitive with that of mild steel. Nonmetallic materials, such as polyvinyl chloride (PVC), fiberglass-reinforced PVC, concrete, and various coatings and linings, have been used to provide some degree of prevention of MC-related failures. Each of these materials has limitations as a substitute for metallic materials (Uhlig and Revie, 1985; Fontana and Greene, 1987).

The environment in which metals are to be used should be assessed for corrosivity. Selection of a less corrosive environment would thereby alleviate corrosion and the need for corrosion control. For example, soil corrosivity can be assessed, resistivity being the most favored single test used.

Electrochemical Applications

The application of electrical current to metals counteracts the natural corrosion process. Two well-known techniques accomplish this—cathodic and anodic protection.

Cathodic Protection

Cathodic protection theoretically is the most important of all approaches to corrosion control by itself. By means of an externally applied electric current, corrosion is reduced virtually to zero, and the metal surface can be maintained in a corrosive environment without deterioration for an indefinite time. The principle of cathodic protection is to make the metal environment potential so negative that cations cannot escape into solution from the metal. The mechanism of protection depends on external current polarizing cathodic elements of local action cells to open circuit potential of the anodes. The surface becomes equipotential and corrosion currents no longer flow. Cathodic protection can be accomplished in two ways: one way is by the use of metal sacrificial anodes such as aluminum, magnesium, or zinc, that corrode and thereby supply the electrons to the protected metal. The other way is by the use of an inert anode with the electrons supplied from the rectifier.

Anodic Protection

In contrast to cathodic protection, anodic protection is a relatively new technique. It was developed using electrode kinetic principles and requires advanced concepts of electrochemistry theory in order to be described properly. Simply, it is based on the formation of a protective film on metals by externally applied anodic currents. In general, the application of anodic currents to a structure should tend to increase the dissolution rate of a metal and decrease the rate of hydrogen evolution in aqueous systems. However, this usually does not occur in metals with active passive transitions such as nickel, chromium, iron, titanium, and their alloys. If carefully controlled anodic currents are applied to these materials, they are passivated and the rate of metal dissolution is decreased. A potentiostat (electronic device that maintains constant potential of a metal with respect to a reference electrode) is required to supply anodic currents. It is typical of anodic protection that corrosion rates, although small, are not reduced to zero, as opposed to cathodic protection. Anodic protection can reduce corrosion 100,000 fold in corrosive attack in some systems. The primary advantages of anodic protection are its applicability to extremely corrosive environments and its low current requirements.

See Uhlig and Revie (1985) and Fontana and Greene (1987) for further information.

Corrosion Inhibitors

A corrosion inhibitor (CI) is a chemical substance that effectively decreases the corrosion rate when added in a small concentration to an environment. A CI may be introduced via liquid or vapor phase or both. CIs must affect the metal side of the metal-fluid interface and, to function effectively, they must be transported to the interface.

There are two classes of CIs: passivators and organic inhibitors. Passivators are usually inorganic, oxidizing substances (e.g., chromates, nitrites, molybdates) that passivate the metal surface and shift the corrosion potential several tenths of a volt in the noble direction. In general they reduce corrosion rates to low values; consequently they are considered the best inhibitors for selected metal-environment combinations. The organic inhibitors have only a small effect on the corrosion potential in either direction, noble or active. Such an effect is on the order of a few millivolts.

Corrosion inhibitors can also be classified according to the corrosion process they control. If they impede the cathodic reaction as in the case of oxygen reduction, they are called cathodic inhibitors and are represented by the organic class mentioned above. If they affect the anodic reaction they are called anodic inhibitors. In this case they reduce the rate at which metal ions are dissolved in the solution, and are represented by the passivators. When a mixed mode of inhibition of the cathodic and anodic reaction is in effect, they are called mixed inhibitors.

Protective Coatings

The use of protective coatings to provide a barrier between the metal and its corrosive environment is an old but effective measure of protection. Materials that have been employed include metallic coatings, inorganic coatings, and organic coatings. In many cases, the failures reported for coated metals are due to poor application or to mechanical damage from handling and backfilling. The application of electrical current to metals counteracts the natural corrosion processes in those cases. Two well-known techniques accomplish this—namely cathodic and anodic protection. For further information on these techniques refer to Uhlig and Revie (1985) and Fontana and Greene (1987).

The desirable qualities of a protective coating are coherence, adherence, nonporosity, mechanical resistance, and chemical resistance. An ideal coating does not exist. However, the most effective corrosion protection system, particularly for large-diameter pipelines, uses coatings that ensure protection as well as impressed current cathodic protection where breaks occur in the coating.

Metallic Coatings

Relatively thin coatings of metallic materials provide a satisfactory barrier between the metal and its environment. Metal coatings are applied by electrodeposition, electroless deposition, flame spraying, cladding, hot dipping, or vapor deposition.

Inorganic Coatings

Vitreous enamels, glass lining, or porcelain enamels are all essentially glass coatings of suitable coefficient of thermal expansion fused on metals. Glass in powdered forms is applied to a pickled or otherwise prepared surface, then heated in a furnace at a temperature that allows the glass to soften and bond to the metal surface. Several coats may be applied. These coatings are used mostly on steels, but are also possible on copper, brass, and aluminum. In addition to the decorative utility, vitreous enamels protect base metals against corrosion. Pores in the coating are acceptable when cathodic protection supplements the glass coating. For other applications the coating must be perfect without a single defect.

Some other types of inorganic coatings are portland cement coatings with steel reinforcement and chemical conversion coatings such as anodized aluminum.

Organic Coatings

These types of coating provide a relatively thin barrier between the substrate material and its environment. Paints, varnishes, lacquers, and similar coatings doubtless protect more metal against corrosion attack than any other material. Exterior coated surfaces are more familiar, but inner coatings or linings are also widely used.

Biologic Control

Simple, routine microbiologic, chemical, and corrosion monitoring programs can be combined with detailed surveys to minimize microbiologic problems in industrial systems. This approach is of great value in identifying trends in both microbiologic contamination and MC. Such an approach, backed up by laboratory simulations, also allows the selection of appropriate, effective, remedial measurements such as an effective treatment program using antimicrobial agents.

Most microbiologic problems associated with the process industry are caused by a mixed population of microorganisms. As indicated earlier the microorganisms involved in the problems are algae, bacteria, and fungi. Typically, the problems are the result of interactions between groups of microorganisms. The most common microbiologic problems in the process industry are related to the following, each leading to the next: (1) biologic slime, (2) plugging and fouling, and (3) microbial corrosion.

The first fundamental to recognize in this section is that the application of prevention and control techniques to a microbial problem is cheaper than trying to repair it. Second, the use of antimicrobial agents is still the most popular method for the prevention and control of microbiologic problems.

Biocide Treatment

Routine chemical preventative treatment is generally ineffective for the control of MC. Some inhibitors such as chromates, hydrazine, and benzothiazoles have a degree of biocidal activity, but at the dosages used for corrosion inhibition do not provide the proper control of microorganisms. In addition, some corrosion inhibitors are susceptible to degradation by microbial growth (e.g., nitrite- and phosphate-based inhibitors).

As indicated earlier a necessary condition for a good biocide treatment is that the system be cleaned from scale, debris, and biofilms. Initial biocide treatment is effective in preventing the establishment of microorganisms in such areas as cooling water systems, circulating water systems, and fire protection systems. Once a bacterial colony has been established, a biofilm or nodule can be formed, and the biocide has difficulty in penetrating it. Stainless steel equipment is compatible with most biocides. The chemical corrosion from the biocide is minimal in comparison to the pitting corrosion induced or caused by microorganisms. Stainless steel is susceptible to corrosion attack by chlorine.

Typical water systems that require the use of demineralized water are made of stainless steel and are susceptible to MC. Demineralized water is relatively pure but not sterile. The use of most biocides for these systems is undesirable because of the changes in the water quality that can result. A satisfactory solution for these systems is treatment with hydrogen peroxide, at doses as high as 100 ppm for 24 hours, or with ozone or ultraviolet light. None of these treatments affects water quality to any significant extent.

For systems of carbon steel that operate at stagnant conditions, a nonoxidizing biocide with pH adjusted to 10.5 can be effective in controlling bacteria. Nonoxidizing biocides have longer periods of decomposition than oxidizing biocides, and the high pH also helps to inhibit the growth of the microbes. These biocides also produce lower rates of corrosion in carbon steel than the oxidizing biocides. This approach can also be applied to closed loop systems. Additionally, for best results, pH, residual biocide, and biofilm development should be monitored.

In all events, the selection of biocides should be performed, taking into consideration the compatibility with the materials of construction, so that biocides will not increase the corrosion. With some materials the dosage of an oxidizing biocide to achieve a desired level of disinfection can produce an increased rate of corrosion. In testing the system for MC, stagnant, low-flow, and full-flow environments should be evaluated, and the materials employed should be typical of those used in the actual system.

Environmental System Considerations

The use of wide-spectrum microbiocides is necessary to control microbiologic problems over a wide range of conditions. A thorough understanding of the dynamics of the microbial population and the conditions that control the population growth is also important. In a dynamic environment many of the growth-controlling conditions constantly change, and the microflora respond to such changes.

Antimicrobial Agents

The use of antimicrobial agents in process industries for various operational activities such as preoperational cleaning, hydrostatic testing, operation turnarounds, and routine operations is of great importance in providing protection to the system against MC.

Most antimicrobial agents are susceptible to environmental conditions such as pH. Practical experience indicates that a chlorine treatment of pH less than 7.8 is effective in the water. At pH greater than 7.8 bromine compounds and chlorine dioxide are more effective than chlorine. Above pH 8.5 most oxidant materials are not sufficiently effective in providing control of microbial growth (Lamot, 1988; Sequeira et al., 1988; The Nalco Water Handbook, 1979).

Recently the use of surfactants (penetrants/biodispersants) has been shown to improve the effectiveness of antimicrobial agents (Tiller, 1988; Costerton and Lashen, 1983; Honneysett et al., 1985). Chemically, these substances are composed of nontoxic organic compounds with penetrating and dispersing properties. The biodispersants allow the sessile colonies to be penetrated by the antimicrobial agents; thus the latter may be used at lower dosages with improved effectiveness. The dispersants prevent the biomass from becoming so massive that antimicrobial agents cannot penetrate the consortia of microbes. Some penetrants are hydrophobic, causing a film to form on the metal surfaces, which permits less deposition of sessile microbial colonies and less MC. Successful corrosion control in a cooling water system

Table 53–4. *Chemicals that Affect Microorganisms*

Chemical Name	Trade Name	Manufacturer	Reference
Antibiotics			
Albomycin			Pomortseva, 1963
Chloramphenicol		Parke, Davis & Company	Report 1952; Report 1959
Chlortetracycline		Lederle Laboratories	Report 1952; Report 1959; Pomortseva, 1963
Citrinin			Report 1950
Colimycin			Pomortseva, 1963
Dihydrostreptomycin			Pomortseva, 1963
Erythromycin		Abbot Laboratories	Pomortseva, 1963
Mycerin			Pomortseva, 1963
Neomycin		Armour & Company	Report 1952; Pomortseva, 1963
Nystatin		Lederle Laboratories	Report 1952; Pomortseva, 1963
Oxytetracycline		Pfizer Laboratories	Anderson et al., 1958; Pomortseva, 1963
Penicillin		Wyeth Laboratories	Starka, 1951
Phenoxymethyl penicillin		Bristol Laboratories	Pomortseva, 1963
Phytobacteriomycinhydrochloride			Pomortseva, 1963
Phytobacteriomycin sulphate			Pomortseva, 1963
Polymycin		Burroughs Wellcome Co.	Pomortseva, 1963
Polymyxin B		Burroughs Wellcome Co.	Saleh, 1964
Polymyxin E		Burroughs Wellcome Co.	Report 1951
Streptomycin			Report 1948
Streptomycin sulphate			Saleh, 1964
Tetracycline		Lederle Laboratories	Pomortseva 1963
Dyes			
	Acridinium 914		Barton-Wright, 1945; Postgate, 1952; Rogers, 1940, 1945
	Aeriflavine		Rogers, 1940
	Proflavine		Rogers, 1940; Report 1959
	Benzyl viologen		Saleh, 1964
	Brillian green		Davis, 1962
	Crystal violet		Davis, 1962
	Gentian violet		Rogers, 1940
	Methylene blue		Saleh, 1964
	Nile blue		Rogers, 1940
Diamines			
Formic acid salt of coco-diamine	Chemicide 2-C	Chemical Additives	Farquhar, 1969
Glycollic acid salt of coco-diamine	Magna 434	Magna Corporation	Farquhar, 1969
Salicylic acid salt of coco-diamine	CM-47	Betz Laboratories	Farquhar, 1969
	CM-48	Betz Laboratories	Farquhar, 1969
	Magna 4066-2	Magna Corporation	Farquhar, 1969
Adipic acid salt of coco-diamine	Magna 404	Magna Corporation	Farquhar, 1969
	Aquanul 808	Milchem	Farquhar, 1969
	Aquanul 819	Milchem	Farquhar, 1969
Coco-diamine derivative	Corexit 7674	Enjay Chemical Co.	Farquhar, 1969
	Visco 1150	Nalco Chemical Co.	Farquhar, 1969
	Aquanul 801	Milchem	Farquhar, 1969
	Aquanul 810	Milchem	Farquhar, 1969
Coco-diamine monotartrate	4155-B	Armour & Company	Farquhar, 1969
Active coco-diamine	Coco-diamine	Petrolite Corp.	Farquhar, 1969
Benzoic acid salt of coco-diamine	Aquanul 809	Milchem	Farquhar, 1969
	PD 3238	Armour & Company	Farquhar, 1969
	Magna 4066-3	Magna Corporation	Farquhar, 1969
Glycollic acid salt of coco-diamine	Magna 4066-4	Magna Corporation	Farquhar, 1969
Acetic acid salt of coco-diamine	Magna 424	Magna Corporation	Farquhar, 1969
Adipic acid salt of coco-diamine	Magna 4066-1	Magna Corporation	Farquhar, 1969
Stearic acid salt of coco-diamine	Duomeen CS	Armour & Company	Farquhar, 1969
Diacetate salt of coco-diamine	Visco 1151	Nalco Chemical Co.	Farquhar, 1969
Coco-diamine mono benzoate	Corexit 7675	Enjay Chemical Co.	Farquhar, 1969
	Corexit 7673	Enjay Chemical Co.	Farquhar, 1969

Table 53–4. *Chemicals that Affect Microorganisms* (continued)

Chemical Name	Trade Name	Manufacturer	Reference
Coco-diamine diacetate	Corexit 7672	Enjay Chemical Co.	Farquhar, 1969
Diamine with ether linkage	EP 8960-1-1	Archer-Midland-Daniels	Farquhar, 1969
	EP 8960-1-3	Archer-Midland-Daniels	Farquhar, 1969
Tallow diamine	Xcide XJ-8107	Petrolite Corp.	Farquhar, 1969
Octa decyl diamine mono-gluconate	Demcide 705	W.R. Grace & Co.	Farquhar, 1969
Quaternary ammonium compounds			Farquhar, 1969
	Arquad	Armour & Co.	Saleh, 1964; Report 1959
Cetylpyridinium bromide			(Unpublished) Nat. Chem.
			Lab., Teddinton
Cetyltrimethylammonium bromide			Report 1959
Dimethyl-benzyl-lauryl-ammonium chloride			Lagarde, 1961
Dimethyl-dilaurylammonium chloride			Lagarde, 1951
	RBS 25	Shandon	Saleh, 1964
Stearyl-dipolyglycol benzyl-ammonium chloride			Lagarde, 1951
Tetradecylpyridinium bromide			Report 1948
Methyl dodecyl benzyl trimethyl ammonium chloride	Hyamine 2389	Rohm-Haas	Farquhar, 1969
Di-isobutyl ethoxy ethyldimethyl benzyl ammonium chloride	Hyamine 1622	Rohm-Haas	Farquhar, 1969
Alkyl dimethyl benzyl ammonium chloride	Dichem 112-6	Diversified Chemicals Corp.	Farquhar, 1969
	Hyamine 3500	Rohm-Haas	Farquhar, 1969
Quaternary ammonium chloride	Visco 1149	Nalco Chemical Co.	Farquhar, 1969
	B-24	Petronics	Farquhar, 1969
	P-5	Petronics	Farquhar, 1969
	AT	Petronics	Farquhar, 1969
Cis-1-(3-chlorallyl-3,5,7-triaza-1-azonia)	Dowicil 200	Dow Chemical Company	Farquhar, 1969
1-(3-chloroallyl)-3,5,7-triaza-1-azonia adamantane chloride	Dowicil 100	Dow Chemical Company	Farquhar, 1969
Tallow, trimethyl ammonium chloride	Aquanul 811	Milchem	Farquhar, 1969
Coco, trimethyl ammonium chloride	Aquanul 812	Milchem	Farquhar, 1969
Soya trimethyl ammonium chloride	Aquanul 813	Milchem	Farquhar, 1969
Alkyl dimethyl benzyl ammonium chloride	Aquanul 802	Milchem	Farquhar, 1969
Dicoco dimethyl ammonium chloride	Aquanul 805	Milchem	Farquhar, 1969
	Magna 500	Magna Corporation	
	Dearcide	W.R. Grace & Co.	Farquhar, 1969
N-alkyl methyl iso-quinolinium chloride			
Diquaternary ammonium chloride	Xcide XC-370	Petrolite Corp.	Farquhar, 1969
Mixture of soya, trimethyl ammonium chloride and ethoxylated soya amine	482-B	Armour & Company	Farquhar, 1969
Mixture of Xcide XC-370 and butylene oxide	Xcide XP-8152	Petrolite Corp.	Farquhar, 1969
Mixture of coco-diamine monoadipate and soya trimethyl ammonium chloride	481-B	Armour & Company	Farquhar, 1969
Mixture of diquaternary ammonium chloride and tallow diamine	Xcide XJ-1130	Petrolite Corp.	Farquhar, 1969
Mixture of diamine salts, quaternary ammonium chloride, and ethoxylated amine	Jetcore 60-A	Jetco Chemicals, Inc.	Farquhar, 1969
Mixture of Xcide XC-370, wetting agent and corrosion inhibitor	Xcide XJ-6710	Petrolite Corp.	Farquhar, 1969
Mixture of alkyl diamine and n-alkyl dimethyl benzyl ammonium chloride	Dearcide 706	W.R. Grace & Co.	Farquhar, 1969
Mixture of dicoco dimethyl ammonium chloride and coco-diamine mono adipate	Aquanul 816	Milchem	Farquhar, 1969
Mixture of soya trimethyl ammonium chloride and tartaric acid	4124-B	Armour & Company	Farquhar, 1969
Soya trimethyl ammonium chloride ethoxylated primary soya amine	Aquanul 818	Milchem	Farquhar, 1969
Mixture of glycollic acid salt of coco-diamine and dicoco, dimethyl ammonium chloride	Magna 405	Milchem	Farquhar, 1969

Table 53–4. *Chemicals that Affect Microorganisms* (continued)

Chemical Name	Trade Name	Manufacturer	Reference
Mixture of dicoco dimethyl ammonium chloride and coco-diamine mono adipate	Aquanul 817	Milchem	Farquhar, 1969
Mixture of quaternary ammonium chloride and reducing agent	Jetcide 9023B	Jetco Chemicals, Inc.	Farquhar, 1969
Mixture of soya trimethyl ammonium chloride and coco diamine mono adipate	483-B	Armour & Company	Farquhar, 1969
Phenols			
Chlorinated phenols	Surflo B-33	National Lead Co.	Farquhar, 1969
	1-DS-174	Betz Laboratories	Farquhar, 1969
Mixture of Na salts of chlorinated phenols	B-20	Calgon Corporation	Farquhar, 1969
Chlorinated bis phenol	Cronox 45	Aquaness Chemical Corp.	Farquhar, 1969
	Aquanul 803	Milchem	Farquhar, 1969
Isomers of para-chloro-meta cresol	Octafect 7L	Ottawa Chemical Co.	Farquhar, 1969
Mixture of chlorinated phenates	Biomaster 132	Betz Laboratories	Farquhar, 1969
Mixture of chlorinated phenols, dispersants, and wetting agents	Nalco 201	Nalco Chemical Co.	Farquhar, 1969
Mixture of phenols and wetting agent	Magna 440	Magna Corporation	Farquhar, 1969
Mixture of glycollic acid salt of coco-diamine and chlorinated phenols	Magna 414	Magna Corporation	Farquhar, 1969
Mixture of coco diamine mono acetate and 2,4,5 trichlorophenol	Nalco 322	Nalco Chemicals, Inc.	Farquhar, 1969
Mixture of chlorinated phenols and coco diamine	ADS-173	Betz Laboratires	Farquhar, 1969
Mixture of coco diamine salt, quaternary ammonium chloride, and chlorinated phenol	Magna X326-48-6	Magna Croporation	Farquhar, 1969
Mixture of chlorinated phenols, primary and secondary amines	Dichem 625	Diversified Chemicals Corp.	Farquhar, 1969
Mixture of chlorinated phenols and diadipate of coco diamine	Jetcide 5200	Jetco Chemicals, Inc.	Farquhar, 1969
Chlorinated phenol			Starka, 1951
6-chlorothymol			Saleh, 1964
m-cresol			Report 1949
Dinitro-o-cresol			Report 1948
8-hydroxyquinoline			Bufton, 1964, Saleh, 1964
β-naphthol			Bufton, 1964, Saleh, 1964
Octyl cresol			Report 1949
N-acetyl-p-amino-phenol			Bennett et al., 1958
4-allyl-2,6-dimethyl-phenol			Bennett et al., 1958
o-amino-phenol			Bennett et al., 1958
m-amino-phenol			Bennett et al., 1958
p-amino-phenol			Bennett et al., 1958
2-amino-4-chloro-phenol			Bennett et al., 1958
2-amino-4-nitro-phenol			Bennett et al., 1958
p-anilino-phenol			Bennett et al., 1958
o-benzyl-p-chloro-phenol			Bennett et al., 1958
p-bromo-phenol			Bennett et al., 1958
2-bromo-4-phenyl-phenol			Bennett et al., 1958
o-chloro-phenol			Starka, 1951
m-chloro-phenol			Starka, 1951
p-chloro-phenol			Starka, 1951
4-chloro-2-cyclohexyl-phenol			Bennett et al., 1958
4-chloro-3-methyl-phenol			Bennett et al., 1958
2-chloro-4-nitro-phenol			Bennett et al., 1958
4-chloro-2-nitro-phenol			Bennett and Bauerle, 1960
2-chloro-4-phenyl-phenol			Bennett et al., 1958
p-chloro-thio-phenol			Bennett et al., 1958
o-cyclohexyl-phenol			Bennett et al., 1958
p-cyclohexyl-phenol			Bennett et al., 1958

Table 53–4. *Chemicals that Affect Microorganisms* (continued)

Chemical Name	Trade Name	Manufacturer	Reference
2,4-dichloro-phenol			Bennett et al., 1958
2-4-dichloro-phenol			Starka, 1951
N,N-diethyl-m-amino-phenol			Bennett et al., 1958
2-6-dimethoxy-4-propenyl-phenol			Bennett et al., 1958
Dimethylaminomethyl-phenol			Bennett et al., 1958
2-4-dinitro-phenol			Bennett and Bauerle, 1960
Dinonyl-phenol			Bennett and Bauerle, 1960
Di-sec-amyl-phenol			Bennett and Bauerle, 1960
2,4-di-sec-butyl-phenol			Bennett and Bauerle, 1960
2,4-di-tert-amyl-phenol			Bennett and Bauerle, 1960
2,4-di-tert-butyl-phenol			Bennett and Bauerle, 1960
p-(3-methyl-2-butenyl)-phenol			Bennett and Bauerle, 1960
2,2'-methylenebis-(6-bromo-4-chloro)-phenol			Bennett and Bauerle, 1960
2,2'-methylenebis-(6-bromo-4-methyl)-phenol			Bennett and Bauerle, 1960
2,2'-methylenebis-(4,6-dibromo)-phenol			Bennett and Bauerle, 1960
2,2'-methylenebis-(4-chloro)-phenol			Bennett and Bauerle, 1960
2,2'-methylenebis-(4-chloro-6-methyl)-phenol			Bennett and Bauerle, 1960
2,2'-methylenebis-(4,6-dichloro)-phenol			Bennett and Bauerle, 1960
2,2'-methylenebis-(3,4,6-trichloro)-phenol			Bennett and Bauerle, 1960
o-nitro-phenol			Bennett and Bauerle, 1960
p-nitro-phenol			Bennett and Bauerle, 1960
p-nitroso-phenol (Na salt)			Bennett et al., 1958
Nonyl-phenol			Bennett et al., 1958
Octyl-phenol			Bennett et al., 1958
Pentachloro-phenol (Na salt)			Bennett et al., 1958
Pentachloro-phenol			Report 1959
o-phenyl-phenol			Williams, 1958
o-sec-amyl-phenol			Williams, 1958
o-sec-butyl-phenol			Williams, 1958
p-sec-butyl-phenol			Williams, 1958
4-tert-butyl-2-chloro-phenol			Williams, 1958
4-tert-butyl-2-phenyl-phenol			Williams, 1958
2,3,4,6-tetrachloro-phenol			Williams, 1958
2,2'-thiobis-(4-bromo)-phenol			Bennett et al., 1958
2,2'-thiobis-(4-chloro)-phenol			Bennett et al., 1958
2,2'-thiobis-(4,6-dichloro)-phenol			Bennett et al., 1958
2,2'-thiobis-(3,4,6-trichloro)-phenol			Bennett et al., 1958
			Bennett et al., 1958
2,4,6-tribromo-phenol			Bennett et al., 1958
2,4,5-trichloro-phenol			Williams, 1958
2,4,6-trichloro-phenol			Bennett and Bauerle, 1960
2,2'-(2,2,2-trichloroethylidene)bis-(4-chloro)-phenol			Bennett et al., 1958
			Bennett et al., 1958
			Bennett et al., 1958
2,4,6-tri(dimethyl-aminomethyl)-phenol			Bennett et al., 1958
			Bennett et al., 1958
Tannins			Booth, 1960
2-phenyl phenol			Hill, 1982
2-benzyl-4-chlorophenol			Hill, 1982
2,4,6-trichlorophenol			Hill, 1982
2,2'-thiobis(3,4,6-trichloro-phenol)			Hill, 1982

Formaldehyde and Aldehyde Mixtures

Chemical Name	Trade Name	Manufacturer	Reference
Soya trimethyl ammonium chloride and formaldehyde	Jetcide 9022B	Jetco Chemicals, Inc.	Farquhar, 1969
	Jetcide 9202		Farquhar, 1969
	Jetcide 9200	Jetco Chemicals, Inc.	Farquhar, 1969
Formaldehyde	Formalin 40% NF	W.H. Curtin & Co.	Farquhar, 1969
Chlorinated phenols and aldehyde	1-DS-175	Betz Laboratories	Farquhar, 1969
Complex amine compound and aldehyde	Surflo B-19	National Lead Co.	Farquhar, 1969

Table 53–4. *Chemicals that Affect Microorganisms* (continued)

Chemical Name	Trade Name	Manufacturer	Reference
Heavy Metals and Mixtures			
Tributyl tin linoleate	Carsan T-18	Carlyle Chemical Works	Farquhar, 1969
Tributyl tin acetate	Carsan T-2	Carlyle Chemical Works	Farquhar, 1969
Bis (tributyl tin) oxide	Carsan T-0	Carlyle Chemical Works	Farquhar, 1969
Tributyl tin neo decanoate	Carsan T-10	Carlyle Chemical Works	Farquhar, 1969
Organo tin and quaternary ammonium	Magna X-326-47-5	Magna Corporation	Farquhar, 1969
chloride	Magna X-326-47-5	Magna Corporation	Farquhar, 1969
	Aquanul 804	Milchem	Farquhar, 1969
Organo-tin, quaternary ammonium chloride and complex amine	Biocide 201	Drew Chemical Company	Farquhar, 1969
N-alkyl, dimethyl benzyl ammonium chloride and complex amine	Dearcide 717	W.R. Grace & Co.	Farquhar, 1969
Organo-tin, organo-mercurial, and	Magna X-326-47-4	Magna Corporation	Farquhar, 1969
quaternary ammonium chloride	Magna X-326-47-3	Magna Corporation	
Na-tri and penta chlorophenates, n-alkyl dimethyl benzyl ammonium chloride, and tributyl tin chloride	Dearcide 704	W.R. Grace & Co.	Farquhar, 1969
o-chloromercuriphenol			Guynes et al., 1958
			Bennett and Bauerle, 1960
p-chloromercuritoluene			Guynes et al., 1958
Dibromoxymercurifluorescein (Na salt)			Guynes et al., 1958
Ethylmercuric acetate			Guynes et al., 1958
Ethylmercuric phosphate			Guynes et al., 1958
Ethylmercurithiosalicylate			Bennett and Bauerle, 1960
Mercuric chloride			Anderson and Liegey, 1956
Mercury naphthenate			Guynes et al., 1958
Mercury oleate			Guynes et al., 1958
Methaphen (4-nitro-5-hydroxy-mercuri-o-cresol anhydride)			Guynes et al., 1958
Methyoxyethylmercuric acetate			Guynes et al., 1958
Methylethylmercuric acetate			Guynes et al., 1958
Methylmercuric acetate			Guynes et al., 1958
Phenylmercuric acetate			Bennett and Bauerle, 1960
Phenylmercuric borate			Guynes et al., 1958
Phenylmercuric bromide			Guynes et al., 1958
Phenylmercuric chloride			Guynes et al., 1958
Phenylmercuric lactate			Bennett and Bauerle, 1960
Phenylmercuric linoleate			Guynes et al., 1958
Phenylmercuric monoethyl-ammonium acetate			Guynes et al., 1958
Phenylmercuric naphthenate			Bennett and Bauerle, 1960
Phenylmercuric octoate			Guynes et al., 1958
Phenylmercuric oleate			Guynes et al., 1958
Phenylmercuric salicylate			Guynes et al., 1958
Phenylmercuric stearate			Guynes et al., 1958
A-phenylmercuriethylenediamine			Guynes et al., 1958
Phenylmercuri-2-ethyl hexoate			Guynes et al., 1958
Phenylmercuri-8-hydroxyquinolinolate			Bennett and Bauerle, 1960
Phenylmercuri-monoethanol-ammonium acetate			Guynes et al., 1958
Phenylmercuri-triethanol-ammonium lactate			Guynes et al., 1958
Primary fatty amines			
Primary coco-amine acetate	Aquanul 815	Milchem	Farquhar, 1969
Primary coco-amine	1-DS-186	Betz Laboratories	Farquhar, 1969
	1-DS-187		
Fatty amine compound	Nalco 321	Nalco Chemical Co.	Manufacturer Catalog
Na-salt of 1-hydroxypyridine 2-thione	Sodium Omadine	Olin Matheson Chemical Corp.	Manufacturer Catalog

Table 53–4. *Chemicals that Affect Microorganisms* (continued)

Chemical Name	Trade Name	Manufacturer	Reference
Organic sulfur, bis-chlorophenol and complex amine	Biocide 270 Biocide 270-B	Drew Chemical Company	Manufacturer Catalog
Thimersal and o-phenylphenate in aqueous solution	Elcide 75	Elanco	Manufacturer Catalog
Nitro compounds			
2-bromo-2-nitropropyl acetate			Bennett and Bauerle, 1960
m-dinitrobenzene			Allen, 1949
Nitrobenzene			Allen, 1949
2-nitro-1-butanol			Bennett and Bauerle, 1960
2-nitro-2-ethyl-1,3-propanediol			Bennett and Bauerle, 1960
2-nitro-2-ethyl-1,3-propanediol dipropionate			Bennett and Bauerle, 1960
5-nitro-2-furaldehyde semicarbazone	Furacin		Report 1959
2-nitro-2-methyl-propanol			Bennett and Bauerle, 1960
Picric acid			Allen, 1949
Trinitrotoluene			Allen, 1949
Miscellaneous			
Carbolic acid	Phenol	Mallinkrodt Chem. Works	Manufacturer Catalog
Triazo dye	Jetcide 9026B	Jetco Chemicals, Inc.	Manufacturer Catalog
Cationic amine	Surflo B-11	National Lead Co.	Manufacturer Catalog
Ethylene imine	Jetcide 9020B	Jetco Chemicals, Inc.	Manufacturer Catalog
	Aquanul 814	Milchem	Manufacturer Catalog
	O.D. Bactericide	Robbint Chemical Co.	Manufacturer Catalog
	B-12	Calgon Corporation	Manufacturer Catalog
	B-3	Calgon Corporation	Manufacturer Catalog
	Biomaster 133	Betz Laboratories	Manufacturer Catalog
	Surflo B-1400	National Lead Co.	Manufacturer Catalog
Na-pyridinethione	Sodium omadine	Olin Matheson Chemical Corp.	Manufacturer Catalog
Inorganic compounds			
Chlorine dioxide			NACE 1972
Chlorine gas			NACE 1972
Sodium hypochlorite			NACE 1972
Calcium hypochlorite			NACE 1972
Hydrogen peroxide			NACE 1972
Copper sulfate			NACE 1972, Booth, 1963
Copper carbonate			NACE 1972, Miller, 1950b
Zinc sulfate			NACE 1972
Sodium selenate			NACE 1972
Potassium tellurate			NACE 1972
Potassium chromate			NACE 1972
Chromate ion			NACE 1972
Ammonium nitrate			Vamos, 1958
Potassium nitrate			Vamos, 1958
Potassium cyanide			Sorokin, 1954
Sulfide ion			Miller, 1950a
Other organic compounds			
Arsenic-organic salts			NACE 1972
Chlorinated isocyanurates			NACE 1972
Chlorhexidine			Marrie, 1981
Silver-organo complex			NACE 1972
Copper acetate salts			NACE 1972
Copper-8-quinolinolate			NACE 1972
Laurylaminoacetate, copper complex			NACE 1972
Organo-tin oxides			NACE 1972
Butylene tin oxides			NACE 1972
Trichloroacetic acid			NACE 1972
Acrolein			NACE 1972

Table 53–4. *Chemicals that Affect Microorganisms* (continued)

Chemical Name	Trade Name	Manufacturer	Reference
Glutaraldehyde		Union Carbide	NACE 1972
Acetylenic derivatives			NACE 1972
Phenol			NACE 1972
Pentachlorophenol			NACE 1972
Sodium phenates			NACE 1972
Chlorophenols			NACE 1972
Hexachlorophene			NACE 1972
Dichlorophene			Hill, 1982
Quaternary ammonium chlorides			NACE 1972
Benzyl quaternary ammonium compounds			Drummond, 1955
Cetyl pyridinium chlorides			Drummond, 1955
Diisobutylphenoxy ethoxyethyl dimethyl benzyl			Report 1952, 1959
Ammonium chloride			Drummond, 1955
Ammonium monofluro-phosphate			Postgate, 1952
Ethylene oxide			NACE 1972
Ethylene amine			NACE 1972
Na-benzene sulphonate			Report 1948
Na-α-naphthalene sulphonate			Report 1948
Naphenide			Saleh, 1962
Sulphanilamide			Report 1949
Sulphathiazole			(Unpublished) Nat. Chem. La. Teddington 1962
Methyl bromide			NACE 1972
Diamines			NACE 1972
Tertiary butylamine pyridinethione			Andrykovitch and Neihof, 1989
Acetate, propionate, adipate salts of various alkyl diamines			NACE 1972
Acetate salts of various polyamines			NACE 1972
Dioxaborinones			Andrykovitch and Neihof, 1989
Imidazoline acetates			NACE 1972
Imidazoline quats			NACE 1972
Isothiazolones			Andrykovitch and Neihof, 1989
Methylene bis-thiocyanate			NACE 1972
Hexachlorodimethylsulfone			NACE 1972
Sulfamide derivatives			NACE 1972
Alkyl dithiocarbamates			NACE 1972
Alkylene bisthiocarbamates			NACE 1972
2-nitro-2-ethyl-1,3-dimorpholino propane			NACE 1972
N-(2-nitroluithyl)morpholine			NACE 1972
Hydantoin dichloride			NACE 1972
3,5-dimethyltetrahydro-1,3,5-2H-thiadiazine-2-thione			NACE 1972
Dimethyl amide of fatty acid and Na-2-mercaptobenzothiazole			Honneysett et al., 1985
Na-dimethyldithiocarbamate			Honneysett et al., 1985
Methylene-bis(thiocyanate)			Honneysett et al., 1985
2(thiocyanmethylthio)benzothiazole			Honneysett et al., 1985
6-acetoxy-2,4-dimethyl-1,3-dioxane	Dioxin		Hill, 1982
1,3-di(hydroxymethyl)-5,5-dimethyl-2,4-dioximidazole	Dantoin DMDMH-55		Hill, 1982
N,N-methylenebis-5'-(1-hydroxy-methyl)-2,5-dioxo-4-imidazolidinyl urea	Germall 115		Hill, 1982
5-chloro-2-methyl-4-isothiazolin-3-one	Kathone 886 MW		Hill, 1982
2-methyl-4-isothiazolin-3-one	Kathone 886 MW		Hill, 1982
2-methyl-4-isothiazolin-3-one	Kathone 886 MW		Hill, 1982
Hexahydro-1,3,5-triethyl-5-triazine			Hill, 1982
1,3-dichloro-5-dimethyldioxoimidazole	Halane		Hill, 1982

was obtained by employing an organic corrosion inhibitor, a polyacrylate/phosphonate dispersant, and a combination of two microbiocides used simultaneously (Honneysett et al., 1985).

An important consideration during the application of antimicrobial agents is the persistence of the compound in the system. This refers to the duration of the chemical activity of the antimicrobial agent and the mode of system operation. If the system is operating normally, the application of the chemical can be made on a routine basis as determined by the treatment schedule. However, if the system is to be shut down (e.g., for periodic maintenance), alternative procedures must be used to prevent MC. A large dose of a persistent antimicrobial agent prior to shutdown may be used in order to adequately distribute the chemical in the system.

Other Considerations

A large number of chemicals are available to inhibit or kill planktonic microorganisms, but few, if any, are able to penetrate sessile colonies. If they do, they require much higher concentrations than are required to control planktonic microrganisms (Sanders, 1988). For laboratory studies, see Costerton and Lashen (1983); for field tests see Lunden and Stastny (1985). The use of surfactants to disperse biofilms and improve the penetration of antimicrobial agents is now an accepted practice. Presently, a number of antimicrobial agents are in use in industrial processes. These include oxidizing agents, phenolics, aldehydes, metal organic compounds, heavy metal salts, and quaternary ammonium compounds. Table 53–4 lists a number of chemicals that inhibit microorganisms. They represent more than 23 different manufacturers.

In 1964, Saleh et al. published a list of some 200 antimicrobial agents for the control of SRB activity. Later in 1972, the National Association of Corrosion Engineers (NACE) listed a group of antimicrobial agents that could be used to control and prevent MC in oil field equipment. In 1974, McCoy published a review of commercial antimicrobial agents for use in water systems that are subject to MC. Some antimicrobial agents effective in preventing fungal corrosion of aircraft fuel tanks were reported by Miller in 1981. Further, in 1983, Bessems gave an assessment of some antimicrobial agents for use in oil recovery systems. Hill (1984) published a review of antimicrobial agents for use in cutting oil and other types of oils.

REFERENCES

Al'bitskaya, O.N., and Shaposhnikova, N.A. 1960. Mikrobiol. USSR, 29, 725–730.

Allen, L.A. 1949. The effect of nitro-compounds and some other substances on production of hydrogen sulfide by sulphate-reducing bacteria in sewage. Proc. Soc. Appl. Bact., 12, 26.

Anderson, K.E., et al. 1958. The development of new bactericides and flood water treatment based upon the physiology of the sulfate reducing bacteria. Prod. Mon., 22, 20.

Anderson, K.E., and Liegey, F. 1956. Bactericidal screening using the strict anaerobe Desulfovibrio desulfuricans. Prod. Mon., 20, 36.

Andrykovitch, G., and Neikof, R.A. 1989. Control of sulfate-reducing bacteria in hydrocarbon fuel tanks. In Biodeterioration Research 2. Edited by C.E. O'Rear and G.C. Llewellyn. New York, Plenum Press, pp. 61–66.

Ayllon, E.S., and Rosales, B.M. 1988. Corrosion of AA 7075 aluminum alloy in media contaminated with Cladosporium resinae. Corrosion Sci., 44, 638–643.

Allred, R.C., Sudbury, J.D., and Olsen, D.C. 1959. Corrosion is controlled by bactericide treatment. World Oil, 149, 111.

Bailey, C.A., and May, M.E. 1979. Evaluation of microbiological test kits for hydrocarbon fuel systems. Appl. Environ. Microbiol., 37, 871–877.

Barton-Wright, E.C. 1945. Treatment of sulphate-reducing bacteria in a flour mill. J. Soc. Chem. Ind., 64, 295.

Belay, N., and Daniels, L. 1990. Elemental metals as electron sources for biological methane formation from CO_2. Antonie van Leeuwenhoek, 57, 1–7.

Bennett, E.O., and Bauerle, R.H. 1960. The sensitivities of mixed populations of bacteria to inhibitors. Aust. J. Biol. Sci., 13, 142.

Bennett, E.O., Guynes, G.J., and Isenberg, D.L. 1958. The sensitivity of sulfate-reducing bacteria to antibacterial agents (phenolic compounds). Prod. Mon., 23, 18.

Bengough, G.D., and May, R. 1924. Seventh Report to the Corrosion Research Committee of the Institute of Metals. J. Inst. Met., 32, 81–269.

Bergey's Manual of Systematic Bacteriology. 1984. VI. Baltimore, Williams & Wilkins.

Berner, N.H., and Ahearn, D.C. 1977. Observations on the growth and survival of Cladosporium resinae in jet fuel. Dev. Ind. Microbiol., 4, 9–16.

Bessems, E. 1983. Biological aspects of the assessment of biocides. In Microbial Corrosion. London, Metals Society, pp. 84–89.

Bos, P., and Kuenen, J.G. 1983. Microbiology of sulfur oxidizing bacteria. In Microbial Corrosion. London, Metals Society, pp. 8–27.

Booth, G.H. 1971. Microbiological Corrosion, M&B Monographs. London, CE/1 Mills and Boon Ltd.

Booth, G.H. 1964. Sulphur bacteria in relation to corrosion. J. Appl Bacteriol., 27, 174–181.

Booth, G.H. 1960. A study of the effect of tannins on the growth of sulphate-reducing bacteria. J. Appl. Bacteriol., 23, 125.

Booth, G.H., Cooper, A.W., and Cooper, P.M. 1967a. Rates of microbial corrosion in continuous culture. Chem. Ind., 86, 2084–2085.

Booth, G.H., Robb, J.A., and Wakerly, D.S. 1967b. The influence of ferrous ions on the anaerobic corrosion of mild steel by actively growing cultures of sulfate-reducing bacteria. Proc. Int. Conf. Met. Corrosion, 3rd 2, 542–554.

Booth, G.H., and Mercer, S.J. 1963. Resistance to copper of some oxidizing and reducing bacteria. Nature, 199, 622.

Booth, G.H., and Tiller, A.K. 1962. Polarization studies of mild steel in cultures of sulfate reducing bacteria. Part 3: Halophilic organisms. Trans. Faraday Soc., 58, 2510–2516.

Booth, G.H., and Tiller, A.K. 1960. Polarization studies of mild steel in cultures of sulfate reducing bacteria. Trans. Faraday Soc., 56, 1689–1696.

Borenstein, S.W. 1988. Microbiologically influenced corrosion failures of austenitic stainless steel welds. Mtls. Perform., 8, 62–66.

Butlin, K.R., Vernon, W.H.J., and Whiskin, L.C. 1952. Investigation on underground corrosion. Water & Water Eng., 56, 15–18.

Chrzanowski, T.A., Crotty, R.D., Hubbard, J.G., and Welch, R.P. 1984. Applicability of the fluorescein diacetate method of detecting active bacteria in fresh water. Microb. Ecol., 10, 179–185.

Churchill, A.V. 1963. Microbial fuel tank corrosion-mechanisms and contributory factors. Mater. Prot. Perform., 2, 18–20, 22, 23.

Copenhagen, W.J. 1950. Pathology of metals—corrosion of steel and alclad parts by fungus. Metal Ind., 77, 137.

Costello, J.A. 1974. Cathode depolarization by sulphate reducing bacteria. S. Afr. J. Sci., 70, 202.

Costerton, J.W. 1984. Influence of biofilm on efficacy of biocides on corrosion-causing bacteria. Materials Performance, 23, 13–17.

Costerton, J.W., and Geesey, G.G. 1985. The microbial ecology of surface colonization and of consequent corrosion. Proc. of the International Conference on Biology. Gaithersburg, MD, 1985, 223–232.

Costerton, J.W., and Lashen, E.S. 1983. The incident biocide resistance of corrosion-causing biofilm bacteria. Corrosion 83. Paper No 246. Anaheim.

Cragnolino, G., and Touvinen, O. 1984. The role of sulphate-reducing and sulphur-oxidizing bacteria in the localized corrosion of iron-base alloys. A review. Int. Biodeter., 20, 9.

Daniels, L., Belay, N., Rajagopal, B.S., and Weimer, P.J. 1987. Bacterial methanogenesis and growth from carbon dioxide with elemental iron as a sole source of electrons. Science, 237, 509–511.

Das, C.R., and Mishra, K.G. 1986. Biological corrosion of welded steel due to marine algae. Int. Conf. Biol. Induced Corrosion, pp. 114–117.

Davis, N.S. 1962. Isolation and growth studies of sulfate reducing bacteria. Ph.D. Thesis, University of Texas, Austin.

Drummond, J.P., and Postgate, J.R. 1955. A note on the enumeration of sulphate-reducing bacteria in polluted water and on their inhibition by chromate. J. Appl. Bacteriol., 18, 307.

Eagar, R.G., Leder, J., Stanley, J.P., and Theis, A.B. 1988. The use of glutaraldehyde for microbiological control in waterflood systems. Mater. Perf., 8, 40–45.

Edyvean, R.G.J. 1988. Algal-bacterial interactions and their effects on corrosion and corrosion fatigue. In *Microbial Corrosion 1*. Edited by C.A.C. Sequeira and A.K. Tiller. London, Elsevier.

Edvvean, R.G.J. and Terry, L.A. 1983. The influence of micro-algae on corrosion of structured steel used in the North Sea. In *Biodeterioration 5*. Edited by T.A. Oxley and S. Barry. New York, pp. 336–347.

Ehrlich, H.L. 1981. *Iron Bacteria*. London, Methuen.

Eliassen, R., Heller, A.N., and Kish, G. 1949. The effect of chlorinated hydrocarbons on hydrogen sulfide production. Sewage Wks. J., *21*, 457.

Ellis, D. 1919. *Iron Bacteria*. London, Methuen.

Farquhar, G.B. 1969. A manual for field engineers. The sulface reducing bacteria. Superior Oil Co., Drilling and Production Dept., Engineering section, Houston, TX.

Festl, H., Ludwig, W., and Schleifer, K.H. 1986. DNA hybridization probe for the pseudomonas fluorescens group. Appl. Environ. Microbiol., *52*, 1190–1194.

Fontana, M.G., and Greene, N.D. 1987. *Corrosion Engineering*. 3rd. Ed. New York, McGraw-Hill.

Frenzel, von, H.J. 1965. Investigation of the corrosion of iron by bacteria. Mater. Org., *1*, 75–80.

Gabrielli, F. 1988. An overview of water-related tube failures in industrial boilers. Mater. Perf., *6*, 53–56.

Gaines, R.H. 1910. Bacterial corrosion as a corrosion influence in the soil. J. Eng. Ind. Chemistry, *2*, 128–130.

Garret, J.H. 1891. *The Action of Water on Lead*. London, Lewis.

Gaylarde, C.C. 1990. Advances in detection of microbiologically induced corrosion. Int. Biodeter., *26*, 11–22.

Gaylarde, C.C., and Cook, P.E. 1987. ELISA techniques for the detection of sulphate-reducing bacteria. In *Immunoassay Techniques for the Detection of Bacteria*. Edited by J.M. Grange, A. Fox, and N.L. Morgan. Society for Applied Bacteriology Technical Series No 24. Oxford, Blackwell Scientific, pp. 231–244.

Griffin, R.B., Cornwell, L.R., Seitz, W., and Estes, E. 1989. Localized corrosion under biofouling. Mater. Perf., *3*, 71–74.

Guynes, G.J., and Bennett, E.O. 1958. The sensitivity of sulfate-reducing bacteria to antibacterial agents (the mercurials). Prod. Mon., *23*, 15.

Hamilton, W.A. 1985. Sulphate-reducing bacteria and anaerobic corrosion. Ann. Rev. Microb., *39*, 195–217.

Hamilton, W.A., and Sanders, P.F. 1986. In *Biodeterioration 6*. Edited by S. Barry and D.R. Houghton. Slough, England, C.A.B. International Mycological Institute, pp. 202–206.

Harder, E.C. 1919. Iron depositing bacteria and their geologic relations. Washington, D.C., U.S. Government Printing Office.

Hill, E.C. 1984. Biodegrading of petroleum products. In *Petroleum Microbiology*. Edited by R.M. Atlas. New York, Macmillan, pp. 579–617.

Hill, E.C. 1982. Cutting oil emulsions. In *Disinfection, Preservation and Sterilization*. Edited by A.D. Russel, W.B. Hugo, and B.A. Ayliffe. Oxford, Blackwell Scientific Publications, p. 349.

Hill, E.C. 1976. Evaluation of biocides for use with petroleum products. Process Biochem., *11*, 36–38, 48.

Hill, E.C., and Thomas, A.R. 1975. Proc. Int. Biodegrad. Symp. 3rd. London, Applied Science Publ., pp. 151–174.

Hoff, K.A. 1988. Rapid and simple method for double-staining of bacteria with 4',6-diamidino-2-phenylindole and fluorescein isothiocyanate-labelled antibodies. Appl. Environ. Microbiol., *54*, 2949–2952.

Honneysett, D.G., van der Berg, W.D., and O'Brien, P.F. 1985. Microbial corrosion control in a cooling water system. Mtls. Perf., *24*, 34–39.

Horvath, J., and Solti, M. 1959. Mechanism of anaerobic microbiological corrosion of metals in soils. Werkst. Korros., *10*, 624.

Iverson, W.P. 1987. Microbiol corrosion of metals. In *Advances in Applied Microbiology*. Volume 32. Edited by A.I. Laskin. New York, Academic Press.

Iverson, W.P. 1985. Anaerobic corrosion mechanisms. In Anales de la Reunion Argentino-Estadounidense sobre Biodeterioro de Materiales (CONICET-NSF), La Plata, Argentina.

Iverson, W.P. 1981. An overview of the anaerobic corrosion of underground metallic structures, evidence for a new mechanism. ASTM Special Technical Publication 741, pp. 33–52.

Jorgensen, B.B. 1982. Ecology of the bacteria of the sulphur cycle with special reference to anoxic-oxic interface environments. Phil. Soc. Roy. London, *B294*, 543–561.

Kelly, D.P. 1982. Biochemistry of the chemolithotrophic oxidation of inorganic sulfur. Phil. Trans. R. Soc. London, *B298*, 499–528.

Kemmer, F.N., ed. 1979. *Nalco Water Handbook*. New York, McGraw-Hill.

King, R.A., and Wakerly, D.S. 1973. Corrosion of mild steel by ferrous sulphide. Br. Corros. J., *8*, 41.

King, R.A., Miller, J.D.A., and Stott, J.F.D. 1986. Subsea pipelines: Internal and external biological corrosion. Proc. Int. Conf. Biol. Induced Corrosion, *6*, 268–274.

King, R.A., Dittmer, C.K., and Miller, J.D.A. 1976. Br. Corros. J., *11*, 105.

King, R.A., Miller, J.D.A., and Smith, J.S. 1973. Br. Corros. J., *8*, 137.

Kobrin, G. 1976. Corrosion by microbiological organisms in natural waters. Mater. Perf., *15*, 38–43.

Kuenen, J.G., and Bendeker, R.F. 1982. Microbiology of Thiobacilli and other sulphur-oxidizing autothrophs, mixotrophs, and heterotrophs. Phil. Trans. R. Soc. London, *B298*, 473–496.

Lagerde, E. 1961. Etude du pouvoir bacteriostatique et bactericide de quelques composses vis-a-vis d'une souche pure de bacteries sulfato-reductrices. Ann. Inst. Pasteur, *100*, 368.

Lamot, J.E. 1988. Role of biocides controlling microbial corrosion. In *Microbial Corrosion 1*. Edited by C.A.C. Sequeira and A.K. Tiller. London, Elsevier.

Leaden, W.W., and Kinsel, N.A. 1963. The identification of microorganisms that utilize jet fuel. Dev. Ind. Microbiol., *4*, 4–16.

Licina, G.J. 1989. An overview of microbiologically influenced corrosion in nuclear power plant systems. Mater. Perf., *10*, 55–60.

Little, B., Wagner, P., and Jacobus, J. 1988. The impact of sulfate-reducing bacteria on welded copper-nickel seawater piping systems. Mater. Perf., *8*, 57–61.

Little, B., et al. 1986. The involvement of thermophilic bacterium in corrosion process. Corrosion, *42*, 533–536.

Lunden, K.C., and Stanstny, T.M. 1985. NACE Corrosion 85, Paper No. 296.

Mara, D.D., and Williams, D.J.A. 1972. Polarization studies of pure Fe in the presence of hydrogenase positive microbes—II. Photosynthetic bacteria and microalgae. Corros. Sci., *12*, 29–34.

Mara, D.D., and Williams, D.J.A. 1971. Polarization studies of pure Fe in the presence of hydrogenase-positive microbes—I. Non-photosynthetic bacteria. Corros. Sci., *11*, 895–900.

Marquis, F.D.S. 1988. Strategy for macro and microanalysis in microbial corrosion. In *Microbial Corrosion 1*. Edited by C.A.C. Sequeira and A.K. Tiller. London, Elsevier, pp. 125–151.

Marrie, T.J., and Costerton, J.W. 1981. Prolonged survival of Serratia marcescens in chlorhexidine. Appl. Environ. Microbiol., *42*, 1043.

McCoy, J.W. 1974. *The Chemical Treatment of Cooling Water*. New York, Chem. Publ. Co.

Mears, R., and Brown, R.H. 1941. Causes of corrosion currents. Ind. Eng. Chem., *33*, 1001–1010.

Miller, J.D.A. 1981. Microbial biodeterioration. In *Economic Microbiology*. Volume 6. Edited by A.H. Rose. London, Academic Press, pp. 149–202.

Miller, L.P. 1950. Tolerance of sulfate-reducing bacteria to hydrogen sulfide. Contr. Boyce Thomson Inst., *16*, 73.

Miller, L.P. 1950. Formation of metal sulfides through the activities of sulfate-reducing bacteria. Contr. Boyce Thomson Inst., *16*, 85.

Moreau, R., and Brison, J. 1972. Quelques aspects de la corrosion des métaux par les bactéria. Applications aux aciers. Mem. Sci. Rev. Metallu., *69*, 829.

National Association of Corrosion Engineers (NACE). 1972. The role of bacteria in the corrosion of oil field equipment. TPC Publication No. 3. Houston, NACE.

National Bureau of Standards. 1978. Economic effects on metallic corrosion in the United States. NBS Special Pub. 511–1. Washington, D.C., National Bureau of Standards.

Nievens, D.E., et al. 1986. Reversible acceleration of the corrosion of AISI 304 stainless steel exposed to seawater induced by growth and secretion of the marine bacterium *Vibrio natriegens*. Corrosion, *42*, 204–210.

Obuekwe, C.O., Westlake, D.W.S., Cook, F.D., and Plambeck, J.A. 1981. Surface changes in mild steel coupons from the action of corrosion causing bacteria. Appl. Environ. Microbiol., *41*, 766–774.

Olsen, E., and Szybalski, W. 1949. Acta Chem. Scand., *3*, 1094–1105.

Paternaude, R. 1985. Microbial corrosion of culvert pipe in Wisconsin. Int. Conf. Biol. Induced Corrosion, June 10–12. Gaithersburg, Maryland, pp. 92–95.

Peck, J.R., and LeGall, J. 1982. Biochemistry of dissimilatory sulphate reduction. Phil. Trans. R. Soc. London, *B298*, 433–466.

Pfennig, N., and Widdel, F. 1982. The bacteria of the sulfur cycle. Phil. Trans. R. Soc. London, *B298*, 433–441.

Poff, W. 1985. A new era of corrosion awareness and education. Mater. Perf., *3*, 56.

Pomortseva, N.V., and Senyukov, V.M. 1963. The effect of antibiotics on desulphating bacteria. Mikrobiologiia, *32*, 131.

Postgate, J.R. 1984. *The Sulphate Reducing Bacteria*. 2nd Ed. London, Cambridge University Press.

Postgate, J.R. 1982. Sulphur bacteria. Phil. Trans. R. Soc. Lond., *B298*, 583–600.

Postgate, J.R. 1979. *The Sulfate Reducing Bacteria*. London, Cambridge University Press.

Postgate, J.R. 1952. Competitive and non-competitive inhibitors of bacterial sulphate reduction. J. Gen. Microbiol., *6*, 128.

Prescott, G.W. 1968. *The Algae: A Review*. Boston, Houghton Mifflin.

Prince, H.N. 1960. Specific inhibition of obligate anaerobes. Nature, *186*, 816.

Puckorius, P. 1983. Massive utility condenser failure caused by sulfide producing bacteria. Matls. Perform., *22*, 12, 19.

Purkiss, B.E. 1971. Corrosion in industrial situations by mixed microbial flora. In *Microbial Aspects of Metallurgy*. Edited by J.P.A. Miller. New York, Elsevier, pp. 107–128.

Report (1948). Chemistry Research 1947. London: HMSO.

Report (1949). Chemistry Research 1948. London: HMSO.

Report (1950). Chemistry Research 1949. London: HMSO.

Report (1951). Chemistry Research 1950. London: HMSO.

Report (1952). Chemistry Research 1951. London: HMSO.

Report (1957). Chemistry Research 1956. London: HMSO.

Report 1959 to the National Chemical Laboratory, 1958. London: HMSO.

Revsbech, N.P. 1988. Microsensors: Spatial gradients in biofilms. Proceedings of the Dahlem Workshop on Structure and Function of Biofilms, Berlin.

Ringas, C., and Robinson, F.P. 1988. Corrosion of stainless steel by sulfate-reducing bacteria—total immersion test results. Corros. Eng., *44*, 671–678.

Rogers, T.H. 1945. The inhibition of sulphate-reducing bacteria by dyestuffs. Part II. Practical applications in cable storage tanks and gas holders. J. Soc. Chem. Ind., *64*, 292.

Rogers, T.H. 1940. The inhibition of of sulphate-reducing bacteria by dyestuffs. J. Soc. Chem. Ind., *59*, 34.

Saleh, A.M., Macpherson, R., and Miller, J.D.A. 1964. The effect of inhibitors on sulphate reducing bacteria: A compilation. J. Appl. Bacteriol., *27*, 281–293.

Salvarezza, R.C., and Videla, H.A. 1984. Corrosion of carbon steel induced by sulphate reducing bacteria. Effect of chloride and sulfide ions. Marine Biol., Proc. VI Int. Cong. on Marine Corrosion and Fouling. Atens, 429.

Salvarezza, R.C., and Videla, H.A. 1980. Passivity breakdown of steel induced by sulphate reducing bacteria. Corrosion, *36*, 550.

Salvarezza, R.C., Videla, H.A., and Arvia, A.J. 1983. The electrochemical behavior of mild steel in phosphate-borate-sulphide solutions. Corros. Sci., *23*, 717.

Salvarezza, R.C., Videla, H.A., and Gariboglio, M.A. 1982. Importancia de los sulfuros en la iniciacion de la corrosion microbiologica del acero. Corrosion Proteccion, *13*, 5–6, 21.

Sanders, P.F. 1988. Monitoring and control of sessile microbes: Cost effective ways to reduce microbial corrosion. In *Microbial Corrosion 1*. Edited by C.A.C. Sequeira and A.K. Tiller. London, Elsevier.

Scheschl, E. 1980. Elemental sulfur as a corrodent in degenerated, neutral, aqueous solutions. Materials Performance, *19*, F:9.

Scott, P.J., and Davies, M. 1989. Microbiologically influenced corrosion of alloy 904L. Matls. Perform., *5*, 57–60.

Sequeira, C.A.C., Carrasquinho, P.M.N.A., and Cebola, C.M. 1988. Control of microbial corrosion in cooling water systems by the use of biocides. In *Microbial Corrosion 1*. Edited by C.A.C. Sequeira and A.K. Tiller. London, Elsevier, pp. 240–255.

Shoesmith, D.W., Bailey, M.G., and Ikeda, B. 1978. Electrochemical formation of mackinawite in alkaline sulphide solutions. Electrochem. Acta, *23*, 1329.

Smith, J.S. 1980. Corrosion of mild steel by mineral sulphides. Ph.D. Thesis. University of Manchester, England.

Smith, J.S., and Miller, J.D.A. 1975. Nature of sulphides and their corrosive effect on ferrous metals: A review. Br. Corros. J., *10*, 136.

Sorokin, Yu. I. 1954. Concerning the role of phosphate in chemosynthesis by sulphate-reducing bacteria. C. R. Acad. Sci. URSS, *95*, 661.

Staley, J.T., and Konopka, A.E. 1985. Measurements of insitu activities of non-photosynthetic microorganisms in aqueous and terrestrial habitats. Ann. Rev. Microbiol., *43*, 1256–1261.

Stanley, P.E. 1988. Rapid microbiology: The use of luminescence and ATP for enumerating microbes and checking effectiveness of biocides: Present status and future prospects. In *Biodeterioration 7*. Edited by D.R. Houghton, R.N. Smith, and H.O.W. Eggins. Barking, U.K., Elsevier, pp. 664–668.

Starka, J. 1951. Nove poznatky o mikrobialni reducki sulfatu pri vzniku leciveho bahna. Cas. Lek. Ces. Suppl. (Biol. Listy), *32*, 108.

Starkey, R.L., and Wright, K.M. 1945. Anaerobic corrosion of iron in soil. New York, Am. Gas Assoc.

Stoecker, J.G. 1985. Overview of industrial biological corrosion: Past, present, and future. In Proceedings of the International Conference on Biologically Induced Corrosion. Edited by S.C. Dexter. Houston.

Stoecker, J.G. 1984. Waterside corrosion of monel heat exchanger tubes. Matls. Perform., *23*, 48.

Stranger-Johannessen, M. 1986. In *Biodeterioration 6*. Edited by S. Barry and A.R. Houghton. Slough, England. C.A.B. International Mycological Institute, pp. 218–223.

Tatnall, R.E. 1981. Fundamentals of bacteria induced corrosion. Mater. Perf., *9*, 32–35.

Tatnall, R.E. et al. 1981. Pitting of galvanized steel in a cooling tower basin. Matls. Perform., *19*, 41.

Tatnall, R.E., Stanton, K.M., and Ebersole, R.C. 1988. Testing for the presence of sulfate-reducing bacteria. Mater. Perf., *8*, 71–80.

Thauer, R.K. 1982. Dissimilatory sulphate reduction with acetate as electron donor. Phil. Trans. R. Soc. London, *B298*, 467–471.

Tiller, A.K. 1988. The impact of microbially induced corrosion on engineering alloys. In *Microbial Corrosion 1*. Edited by C.A.C. Sequeira and A.K. Tiller. London, Elsevier, pp. 3–9.

Tiller, A.K. 1982. Aspects of microbial corrosion. In *Corrosion Processes*. Edited by R.N. Parkins. London, Applied Science Publ., pp. 115–159.

Trudinger, P.A. 1982. Geological significance of sulphur oxidoreduction by bacteria. Phil. Trans. R. Soc. London, *B298*, 563–582.

Turner, A.P.F., et al. 1989. An inexpensive method for ultra-rapid detection of microbial contamination in industrial fluids. Int. Biodeter., *25*, 137–146.

Uhlig, H.H., and Revie, R.W. 1985. *Corrosion and Corrosion Control: An Introduction to Corrosion Science and Engineering*. 3rd Ed. New York, John Wiley.

Umbreit, W. 1976. The oxidation of metallic iron by *Escherichia coli* and other common heterotrophs. Dev. Ind. Microbiol., *17*, 265–268.

Vamos, R. 1958. Inhibition of sulphate reduction in paddy soils. Nature, *182*, 1688.

Vasquez Moll, D.V., Salvarezza, R.C., Videla, H.A., and Arvia, A.J. 1984. A comparative pitting corrosion study of mild steel in different alkaline solutions containing salts with sulfur-containing anions. Corros. Sci., *24*, 751.

Videla, H.A. 1985. Corrosion of mild steel by sulphate reducing bacteria. A study of passivity breakdown by biogenic sulphides. In Proceedings of the International Conference on Biologically Induced Corrosion, NACE, Gaithersburg, Maryland.

Videla, H.A., Guiamet, P.S., DoValle, S., and Reinoso, E.H. 1988. Effects of fungal and bacterial contaminants of kerosene fuels on the corrosion of storage and distribution systems. Corrosion 88, Paper 91. St. Louis, NACE.

von Wolzegen Khur, C.A.H. 1961. Unity of anaerobic and aerobic iron corrosion process in the soil. Corrosion, *17*, 293t–299t.

von Wolzegen Khur, C.A.H., and van der Vlugt, L.S. 1934. Graphitization of cast iron as an electro-biochemical process in anaerobic soils. Water, The Hague, *48*, 147.

Wakerly, D.S. 1979. Microbial corrosion in the UK industries: A preliminary survey of the problem. Chem. Ind., *19*, 657–659.

Walch, M., and Mitchell, R. 1985. Microbial influence on hydrogen uptake by metals. In Proceedings of the International Conference on Biological Induced Corrosion, NACE, Gaithersburg, Maryland.

White, D.C., et al. 1986. Role of aerobic bacteria and their extracellular polymers in the facilitation of corrosion: Use of Fourier transforming infrared spectroscopy and "signature" phospholipid fatty acid analysis. In *Biologically Induced Corrosion*. Houston, NACE-8, pp. 233–243.

Whitney, W.R. 1903. The corrosion of iron. J. Am. Chem. Soc., *22*, 394–406.

Widdel, F., and Pfennig, N. 1977. A new anaerobic, sporing, acetate-oxidizing, sulfate-reducing bacterium. Desulfotomaculum (emend.) acetoxidous. Arch. Microbiol., *112*, 119–122.

Wilkinson, T.G. 1983. Offshore Monitoring. In *Microbial Corrosion*, London, Metal Society, pp. 117–123.

Williams, O.B. 1958. A comparison of the susceptibility of various strains of sulfate reducing bacteria to the action of bactericides. Prod. Mon., *22*, 12.

Williams, R.E. 1985. Sulfate simulated increases in hydrogenase production by sulfate-reducing bacteria. Consequences in corrosion. In Proceedings of the International Conference on Biologically Induced Corrosion. Gaithersburg, Maryland, pp. 184–192.

Zamanzadeh, M., O'Connor, K., and Bavarian, B. 1989. Case histories of corrosion problems in waste-water facilities. Mater. Perf., *9*, 43–46.

PART VIII

Miscellaneous Topics

CHAPTER 54

FEDERAL REGULATION OF ANTIMICROBIAL PESTICIDES IN THE UNITED STATES

Arturo E. Castillo

In the United States, certain antimicrobial agents are regarded as pesticides because of their intended uses. As such, they fall under the regulatory authority of the Federal Insecticide, Fungicide, and Rodenticide Act (FIFRA), and must be registered with the U.S. Environmental Protection Agency (EPA) before they can be legally marketed in the United States or in any of its territorial jurisdictions. In the rest of this chapter the term *antimicrobial agent* will be used synonymously with the term *disinfectant*.*

The purpose of this chapter is to identify those antimicrobial agents or disinfectants that are considered pesticides and to familiarize the reader with the requirements for registering them with the EPA.

Before proceeding with this task, it seems appropriate to briefly trace the history of pesticide legislation up to the current law, and the regulations by which the EPA registers pesticides—in particular, certain antimicrobial agents.

Federal regulation of pesticides began as the Insecticide Act of 1910, which prohibited the interstate sale of any pesticide or fungicide that was adulterated or misbranded. The Act was concerned with the effectiveness of products and deceptive labeling. The Federal Insecticide, Fungicide, and Rodenticide Act of 1947 mandated that pesticides be registered before being marketed, but did not provide authority to deny registration until 1964. Like the 1910 Act, the 1947 FIFRA was also primarily concerned with protection of consumers from ineffective products.

The Federal Environmental Pesticide Control Act of 1972, Public Law 92-516, enacted October 21, 1972, drastically transformed the FIFRA from a labeling law into a comprehensive regulatory statute with many new provisions and requirements aimed at controlling the manufacture, distribution, and uses of pesticides. This law was later amended by Public Law 94-140 on November 28, 1975, again by Public Law 95-396 on September 30, 1978, and most recently by Public Law 100-460, -464, -526, and -532, enacted on October 25, 1988. Throughout the rest of this chapter these important amendments will be referred to as the 1972, 1975, 1978, and 1988 FIFRA amendments. Their substance and far-reaching impact will become clear as we discuss the regulations resulting from these laws.

One of the mandates of the 1972 FIFRA was that regulations be issued by the EPA for implementing its provisions, as well as guidelines specifying the types of data necessary for the registration of pesticides, and the protocols for producing such data. For the first time in the regulatory history of pesticides, the Administrator of the EPA issued regulations for the registration, re-registration, and classification of pesticides. These were originally published in the Federal Register, Volume 40, No. 129, July 3, 1975, and were later codified in Title 40 of the Code of Federal Regulations (40 CFR), Pesticide Programs, Part 162, Regulations for the Enforcement of the Federal Insecticide, Fungicide, and Rodenticide Act, Subpart A, Registration, Re-registration, and Classification Procedures.

Data Requirements for the Registration of Pesticides were published in the Federal Register Volume 49, No. 207, October 24, 1984. They have since been codified in the Code of Federal Regulations for Pesticides at 40 CFR Part 158. It lists the data required for the registration of any pesticide based on the uses proposed by the applicant for the pesticide.

After undergoing several revisions the guidelines for data requirements and the protocols for conducting the

---

*The term disinfectant is used broadly here in a catch-all way to include various types of antimicrobial agents such as sanitizers, fungicides, preservatives, and slimicides, as well as for disinfectants as strictly defined in Chapter 2. Not included as disinfectants are antiseptics, preservatives for cosmetics, drugs, and other items used on or in the human body, or preparations used to combat diseases of man and animals. These are regulated by the Food and Drug Administration under the Bureaus of Medicine and Veterinary Medicine.

tests to generate the data required to register a pesticide have been published as advisory documents. They are available in microfiche form or as hard copies from the National Technical Information Service, 5285 Port Royal Road, Springfield, VA, 22161, Telephone Number 703-487-4650. The reader is referred to Part 158 of 40 CFR for a clearer understanding of the relationship of the guidelines to the data requirements, and for an itemized list of the various guidelines available.

The 1978 amendment to the FIFRA gave rise to the regulations for conditional registration of pesticides that are identical or substantially similar to previously registered products, the so-called "me-too" pesticides. Regulations for registering pesticides can be found at 40 CFR Part 162. The 1978 FIFRA amendments did not change the basic mandate of the 1972 FIFRA, which requires that before a pesticide is registered, neither the product nor any of its uses will cause any unreasonable risk to human health or the environment. However, the 1978 law established a different timetable for carrying out that mandate. The substance of the 1978 FIFRA and the ensuing regulations for conditional registration of pesticides are summarized below.

A registrant who wishes to register a product that is identical or substantially similar to one that is already registered can obtain a conditional registration by satisfying only minimal data requirements, such as product chemistry, acute toxicity data, and microbiologic efficacy data for the product proposed for registration. This is the so-called "me-too" product registration. Additional data such as teratogenicity data, mutagenicity data, and chronic effect studies are deferred, until such time as all products containing a particular active ingredient are called in for re-registration. At that time, the financial burden of providing all items of data necessary for complete evaluation of health and environmental effects of the active ingredient and all its uses would have to be shared by the registrants of all products containing that active chemical ingredient (see 40 CFR Part 162).

An application for registering a new use of a previously registered chemical active ingredient must undergo a five-step procedure for assessing the incremental risk posed by the new use prior to making a risk-benefit decision. If the benefits of the new use exceed the additional risks posed by the new use, the product is registered conditionally for the new use. Only data necessary for assessing the incremental risk are required from the registrant (40 CFR Section 158.30).

An application for registration of a new chemical active ingredient that has never been registered previously for any pesticidal use must undergo a complete evaluation against the no-unreasonable-adverse-effects provision of section 3(c)(5) of the FIFRA. This means that the applicant must provide all of the necessary items of data specified at Part 158 of 40 CFR for the uses proposed for the product.

A plan for re-evaluating pesticides and their uses prior to their re-registration by groups according to the pes-

ticide chemical contained in each group was published as the Registration Standard System in the Federal Register Volume 44, No. 248, December 26, 1979. Consistent with that plan a system for grouping some 600 or more pesticidally active ingredients found in 38,000 or more registered pesticides into 48 clusters was published in the Federal Register, Volume 45, No. 222, November 14, 1980. The EPA estimated that it would take 10 to 15 years to issue the registration standards for all generic chemical active ingredients. That meant that those clusters with the highest exposure to humans and the environment and the highest volume of production would be re-evaluated ahead of the lower-ranked clusters. Since the publication cited above the total number of pesticides currently registered has increased considerably.

As of this date, all of the pesticide regulations previously published in the Federal Register have been codified in Title 40 of the Code of Federal Regulations, except for the very recent regulations resulting from the 1988 amendments to the FIFRA. Those regulations were published as final rules in the Federal Register, Volume 53, No. 86, May 4, 1988, under the title Pesticide Registration Procedures and Pesticide Data Requirements, 40 CFR Parts 152, 153, 156, 158, 162, and 163. The reader should realize that those regulations do not replace previously issued regulations; they simply clarify or modify certain sections of the regulations, and in some instances provide additional regulatory authority for the EPA to deal with new concerns or issues that have arisen since the previous amendments to the FIFRA.

The 1988 amendments strengthen the EPA's authority in several major areas. Among other things, the amendments require the EPA to speed up the re-registration of pesticides, and authorize the collection of fees to support re-registration activities. It also changes the EPA's responsibilities and funding requirements for the storage and disposal of suspended and canceled pesticides, and changes the indemnification of holders of remaining stocks of canceled pesticides. Currently, a registrant must pay a yearly maintenance fee for each registered product to maintain its registration.

Of particular interest to persons applying for registration of a pesticide is the new provision of the law that requires the EPA to expedite consideration of an application for the registration of a pesticide that is identical or substantially similar to one that is already registered (me-too product registration). Under the expedited review provision, an applicant will be notified, within 45 days after the EPA receives an application, whether the application is complete. Within 90 days after the EPA has received a complete application, the registrant must be notified in writing whether the request is granted or denied. If it is denied the specific reasons for denial must be stated. See PR Notice 89-2, June 6, 1989, for more details for submitting an application under the expedited review procedures.

ORGANIZATIONAL STRUCTURE OF THE REGISTRATION DIVISION

The Registration Division of the Office of Pesticide Programs is composed of three branches: the Insecticide-

Rodenticide Branch, the Herbicide-Fungicide Branch, and the branch responsible for the registration of antimicrobial agents. For many years that branch was known as the Disinfectants Branch, but recently it has been renamed the Antimicrobial Program Branch. Each branch is composed of a Technical Support Section and a Product Management Section. In the Antimicrobial Program Branch the Technical Support Section includes several microbiologists and an acute toxicity data and precautionary labeling reviewer, supervised by the Section Head. Until recently that unit also included a chemist. As a result of a reorganization all chemists have been placed in a special section called the front-end review section. As part of the expedited review the chemists do a front-end review of the Confidential Statement of Formula and chemistry data before an application is forwarded to the product manager for a complete review of the label, precautionary statements, use recommendations, and any microbiologic efficacy data submitted.

The Product Management Section consists of two or more teams, each under a Supervisory Product Manager. Each Product Manager is in charge of a segment of registered products based on the pesticidally active ingredient contained in those products.

The Supervisory Product Manager is responsible for processing an application from the time it is received in the branch until the application for registration is denied or issued. The Technical Support Section provides guidance on data requirements for the various disciplines, reviews data submitted by applicants in support of registrations, and makes scientific recommendations. Such recommendations almost always result in prescribed revisions to the label proposed by the applicant.

The product manager is responsible for making sure that a prospective registrant satisfies all of the regulatory and scientific requirements before registering a pesticide. Upon request the reader can obtain a registration package from the EPA. Among other things, such as pertinent regulations, Pesticide Registration Notices, and application forms, the package includes a list of the senior staff members of the Registration Division, including the names of the Product Managers, their telephone numbers, and a broad indication of the types of products under each product manager's charge.

ANTIMICROBIAL AGENTS (DISINFECTANTS) CONSIDERED PESTICIDES

For a comprehensive discussion of the types of products that are considered pesticides, the reader should refer to the regulations at 40 CFR Part 162, and to the recent amendments to the regulations published as final rules in the Federal Register, Vol. 53, No. 86, May 4, 1988. For this chapter, those antimicrobial agents recommended or sold to kill microorganisms or to inhibit their growth on inanimate objects, surfaces, or other media are considered pesticides. The EPA considers such products pesticides whether the recommendations are made by means of a label, collateral literature, or advertising material, and whether they are written, implied, or made by word of mouth. Even if no representations are made for a product, if its major or only use is as a pesticide, and it is sold to someone who uses it as a pesticide, the EPA can cite the seller or user for a violation of the FIFRA.

Antimicrobial agents used on or in the living body of man or animals are not considered pesticides. Those products fall under the purview of the Food and Drug Administration (FDA), Bureaus of Medicine or Veterinary Medicine. Products represented to the consumer under a label or claims that fall under the authority of both agencies are regulated in accordance with a memorandum of understanding between the FDA and the EPA, published in the Federal Register, Volume 38, No. 172, September 6, 1973.

The following are some examples of disinfectants that are pesticides under the FIFRA that are intended to provide public health benefits, thus requiring efficacy data to support their registrations:

Household products represented as sanitizers, disinfectants, etc.

Products recommended to kill or control bacteria or algae in swimming pools, hot tubs, or spas

Aerosol products represented as air sanitizers or spray disinfectants

Products recommended for use in municipal or private water supplies for treating water to make it safe to drink

Sanitizers recommended for use in public food-handling establishments as final sanitizing rinses for articles, equipment, and surfaces that will come in contact with food or beverages after treatment

The following are examples of products that require registration under the FIFRA but are not intended to provide public health benefits. Therefore, the label recommendations do not have to be supported by microbiologic efficacy data:

Slimicides recommended to control slime-producing microorganisms in recirculating cooling-water systems, such as cooling-water towers, cooling water in brewery pasteurizers, and canning operations

Miscellaneous specialty products, such as preservatives for paints, adhesives, cutting oils, and products intended to be incorporated into fabrics, textiles, and other such materials to prevent growth of microorganisms that may cause spoilage of the materials

Certain household products recommended strictly to inhibit the growth of odor-causing bacteria such as in bathrooms and garbage cans

One of the main concerns of a prospective registrant of a disinfectant is determining what needs to be done to get a label for a product accepted and to obtain a registration notice, which is the license issued by the EPA to market a product legally within the United States and its territorial jurisdictions under the approved label.

From procedural considerations an applicant for a registration of a pesticide must submit a complete application for each product proposed for registration. The application must include all of the required forms properly completed, the proposed label with the use directions and recommendations for the product, and the supporting data for the registration. Assuming that the applicant qualifies for the formulator's exemption (see Section 152.85 of 40 CFR), and that the product is identical or substantially similar to one that has been previously registered by the EPA (a me-too product), the supporting information will most probably be Product Chemistry (40 CFR Section 158.120), Acute Toxicity Data (40 CFR Section 158.135, Guideline Series 81), and Product Performance Data (40 CFR Section 158.160). For antimicrobial pesticides, product performance data means microbiologic efficacy data developed with the specific product proposed for registration to support all claims or recommendations for the product intended to provide health benefits from its use. The data must be conducted at the dilutions and under the conditions recommended for the product in the proposed label. For more details on data requirements to support registration of pesticides the reader should consult the EPA guidelines previously described. Also, the efficacy data requirements for antimicrobial products are available from the Antimicrobial Program Branch of the EPA in the form of DIS/TSS Enclosures. Throughout the rest of this chapter they will be referred simply as "DIS/TSS No. 1" and so on. A complete list of those advisory documents appears in the bibliography of this chapter.

From the foregoing considerations the prospective registrant should note the importance of submitting a carefully prepared typewritten label with complete use directions and dosage recommendations for all the uses proposed for the product. The various levels of activity recommended for a disinfectant dictate the amount and types of product performance data required to support the registration of the product.

EXAMPLES OF DISINFECTANTS WITH DIFFERENT LEVELS OF ACTIVITY

Bacteriostat or Deodorizing Agent

The DIS/TSS No. 16 explains the difference between health-related and non–health-related claims. Certain products lend themselves to a consumer market in which the product is sold strictly for economic or aesthetic benefits and is not intended to provide health benefits. For such products the EPA only allows bacteriostatic claims and does not require microbiologic efficacy data to register them. Typical examples of such products are those recommended to inhibit the growth of slime-producing bacteria in cooling water in air conditioning systems, and those recommended to inhibit the growth of odor-causing bacteria in garbage cans or rest rooms.

Limited Level of Effectiveness

A typical and common example of this type of product is one containing pine oil, soap, and alcohol. The label recommends the product as a disinfectant for hard, non-porous surfaces such as floors, walls, and ceilings in rest rooms and such areas. It must be diluted with water and applied with a rag or mop. The label also recommends the product as a one-step cleanser disinfectant, meaning that the surfaces do not need a precleaning step to remove gross filth before treatment.

Experience with this type of product shows that it can be recommended only as a limited disinfectant because it can be expected to be effective only against gram-negative microorganisms (such as *Escherichia coli*, a typical intestinal tract microorganism) at the use dilutions generally recommended on labels for such products. Therefore, the EPA requires that the limited activity of such a product be qualified with label language such as "to inhibit the growth of odor-causing germs" or similar language that meets with the EPA's approval. Currently there is an EPA Label Improvement Program Notice for pine oil products that addresses these requirements. It is available from the Antimicrobial Program Branch.

General Level of Effectiveness

A typical example of this type of product is one containing as active ingredients, pine oil, a quaternary ammonium compound, soap, and alcohol. The "quat" is added to the product to fortify it, thus making it effective against gram-positive, as well as gram-negative, bacteria. Such a product can be recommended as a general broad-spectrum disinfectant that will provide health benefits from its use. The product must be supported by acceptable data against *Salmonella choleraesuis* and *Staphylococcus aureus* as specified in DIS/TSS No. 1.

In some cases the label for such a product may have additional claims such as "rapid acting," "cleans and disinfects in one application," and "treated articles or surfaces can be wiped dry immediately after treatment." These are examples of the subtleties that can exist in the language registrants propose on labels for their products. Such a product must be supported by microbiologic efficacy data for broad-spectrum activity (DIS/TSS No. 1). But because of the additional claims, the tests conducted with the product must be modified as prescribed by DIS/TSS No. 2 to include both a soil-load handicap and exposure periods shorter than those recommended in the standard tests to support the claim of rapid action. The data must be reported in accordance with DIS/TSS No. 3.

Hospital Disinfectants

This type of product is usually recommended for use in hospitals and other health care facilities. Such a product is usually represented on the label by language such as "hospital disinfectant," "extra-strength disinfectant," or "health care disinfectant." The registrant of this type of product must provide a label with use directions adequately prepared to comply with the recommendations of DIS/TSS No. 15. The label claims must be supported by microbiologic efficacy data against three microorganisms—*Salmonella choleraesuis*, *Staphylococcus aureus*, and *Pseudomonas aeruginosa*, as specified in the DIS/TSS No. 1 for this higher level of activity. The data must be developed according to the requirements of DIS/TSS No. 2, and carefully reported to comply with DIS/TSS No. 3.

Sanitizers for Food Handling Equipment and Utensils

A typical product in this category is a multiple-active-ingredient product such as one containing an iodine complex (iodofor), an organic acid, and a surfactant. The label usually recommends the product for use in public food-handling establishments, such as in restaurants and fast-food outlets, as a final sanitizing rinse for eating utensils, dishes, food-handling equipment, and surfaces that will come in contact with food or beverages after the treatment. The label may bear additional recommendations for the product such as for use in dairies to sanitize milking machines, tubulatures, and other equipment used in the dairy industry, and to treat equipment used in food processing plants and breweries.

Such a product must comply with the requirements of two agencies, the FDA and the EPA. The applicant must register the product with the EPA under a label with adequate use directions as specified in DIS/TSS No. 17. The directions for treating utensils and dishes in public eating establishments must include several important sequential steps: precleaning to remove gross soil or food particles by flushing with water, scraping, or if necessary presoaking; thorough washing with a good detergent or compatible cleanser; rinsing with potable water to wash away the detergent; and finally treating the articles with a freshly prepared solution of the sanitizer as a terminal sanitizing rinse for at least 1 minute and allowing the articles to drip dry or to dry in hot air before reusing them.

The label directions for the treatment of articles and equipment in other food or beverage preparation establishments mentioned on the label, such as breweries or dairies, must appear as separate directions for each establishment. The label must specifically identify the articles and equipment to be sanitized, and provide appropriate and adequate use directions for their treatment. In some states, all of those establishments are subject to local public health ordinances, as well as to the FDA's laws. It is not unusual, therefore, for a registrant to submit to the EPA a label for such a product that includes the recommendations of those agencies.

It is important to note that the only claim that the EPA will approve for such a product is as a sanitizer, not a disinfectant, and more specifically as a final sanitizing rinse for food contact articles or surfaces. As such only 99.999%, equivalent to a 3-log reduction, of all microorganisms present can be expected to be killed. The reason for this is that in public eating establishments, eating utensils and dishes cannot be allowed to remain in contact with the sanitizing rinse for an unreasonable long period. The washing operations must be rapid because the dishes and utensils are in constant demand. Another factor is that the concentration of the sanitizer in the final rinse is limited, owing to the residue consideration, to a low concentration that cannot be expected to disinfect the articles, i.e., to achieve a 100% kill of all microorganisms present.

The use of this type of product in treating articles, equipment, and machinery in other establishments engaged in the preparation of food or beverages for public consumption, such as dairies, breweries, food-canning plants, and meat-processing plants, is similarly limited to a sanitizing level of performance owing to the limitation in the concentration of the product used in the final sanitizing rinse. The underlying considerations in those situations are residues from the sanitizing solution remaining on the treated surfaces and the fact that such items as equipment, machinery, and piping cannot be disinfected, only sanitized, no matter how long the surfaces stay in contact with the sanitizing solution, because of the size and complexity of the external and internal surfaces that come in contact with the prepared food or beverage. For example, milking machines, ice cream vending machines, soft drink machines, milk tanks, and piping systems cannot be effectively disinfected, only sanitized, unless they are completely disassembled, and the internal surfaces throughly scrubbed clean of adhering soil or food deposits before they are treated with the solution.

Assuming then that a prospective registrant of such a product has prepared a draft label consistent with the foregoing considerations, the registrant must support the uses of the product in those establishments with efficacy data as specified in DIS/TSS No. 4. For a product containing an iodine complex, as described above, or a hypochlorite, a bromine derivative, or a chlorinated derivative of cyanuric acid, the supporting data must be developed against *Salmonella typhi*. For a sanitizer containing any other active ingredient, the data must be developed against *Escherichia coli* and *Staphylococcus aureus*.

Besides complying with the foregoing requirements, an applicant must obtain a provisional approval for those uses from the FDA, Division of Food and Color Additives (DFCA), because public eating establishments, food-processing plants, dairies, breweries, and similar establishments that process food or beverages for public consumption must comply with the laws of that agency relating to their sanitary operation for the protection of the public health. Thus, the registrant must provide the FDA with some kind of toxicologic data or other information to satisfy the FDA's concern that humans can safely ingest any residue from the product used in the final sanitizing rinse that the food or beverage might pick up from the treated articles or surfaces.

Assuming then that the registrant provides the FDA with the necessary information to obtain a provisional approval for a final sanitizing rinse and also satisfies the EPA's requirements, the product manager would register the product and request that the FDA amend its regulations for sanitizing solutions under Section 178.1010 of Title 21 of the Code of Federal Regulations to include a special entry authorizing the product for the sanitizing uses proposed on the label. It should be evident that this type of product must be individually cleared by the FDA for each proposed use with respect to both the active ingredients as declared on the label, and the inert ingredients contained in the product that are not disclosed on the label, at the dosages recommended in the final rinse solutions. The exception to this preclearance requirement is a product that is identical in every detail to one that has been previously approved: the same active ingredients, the same undeclared inert ingredients and the same amounts of the components of the product in the final sanitizing rinse for the same uses.

In past years registrants proposed labels for sanitizers of food contact surfaces with directions to rinse off the treated surfaces or articles with potable water prior to their use, thus avoiding the residue concerns of the FDA. Many products were registered by the EPA with such label recommendations. Currently, the EPA has gone on record that such sanitizers are in violation of the FDA's regulations. Therefore, registrants of sanitizers with such uses must comply with both agencies' requirements or delete those uses from the EPA-approved label that fall under the FDA's requirements. The rationale for this is that if a product is used as a sanitizer of food contact surfaces in public eating establishments and subsequently rinsed, the surfaces are recontaminated by the water rinse because the water contains bacteria. This procedure defeats the purpose of the final sanitizing rinse. There would be no need for the final sanitizing rinse if rinsing the utensils with potable water as the last step in the dishwashing operation would be enough to protect the public health.

Sterilizers

A sterilizer is a product that when used according to the label recommendations will kill all forms of microorganisms present on the treated articles or surfaces, including spores present from spore-forming bacteria. Such products by their very nature are generally recommended to treat contaminated articles in hospitals or other similar medical environments. The registrant of such a product usually proposes it as one that is unique or innovative in either design, uses, or mode of action, particularly if it requires specially designed equipment for its use. Sometimes even the preparation of the use solution, if there is one, is proposed as unique. Usually the prospective registrant has conducted some type of performance test at every stage in the development of the product, which may, at best, be presumptive evidence of the product's potential as a sterilizing agent. The registrant nevertheless assumes that those tests will be adequate to support the registration of the product.

Experience has shown that the registrant of a steri-

lizing agent can prevent unnecessary delays, difficulties, and misunderstandings in getting the product registered by acknowledging that this type of product may require more time to register than any of those described in the previous examples because of the complex demands of the data requirements, and the difficulties that can be encountered in developing the supporting data. Therefore, the prospective registrant of a sterilizer should consider several suggestions:

Be reasonably certain of the final formulation that will be proposed for registration. All operating parameters should have been finalized. A product still in its developmental stages should not be proposed for registration.

The sterilizing claims for the product should be such that they can be substantiated and duplicated in a medical environment. Articles and equipment that by their physical or structural nature are impossible to sterilize, should be excluded from the claims for the product.

Finally, the registrant of a sterilizer should not be surprised if informed that any tests that may have been conducted during the development of the product must be repeated according to criteria and guidelines prescribed by the Antimicrobial Program Branch of the Registration Division of the EPA.

With those considerations in mind, the registrant of a sterilizer should request a preregistration conference with the microbiologists of the Antimicrobial Program Branch to establish the criteria for developing the supporting data. The registrant should be prepared to present as much detailed information as is required about the product and any specialized equipment or apparatus associated with its use at this early stage of the proposed registration. The next step should be to submit a written testing procedure (protocol) for review and concurrence by the EPA microbiologists before proceeding with the development of the supporting data.

Assuming then that the registrant has heeded those suggestions, the proposed product is one recommended by its label as a sterilizing agent for surgical or dental instruments, articles, and hard, nonporous surfaces in critical medical or dental areas such as hospitals, operating rooms, dental offices, clinics, contagious disease wards, and similar critical health-related areas. Such a product must be able to deliver an absolute level of performance by killing all forms of microorganisms, spores as well as vegetative cells, that may be present on the treated article and that can present a serious health hazard by cross-contamination from those inanimate surfaces. The claims and use directions for such a product must be worded carefully to comply with the requirements of DIS/TSS No. 15. The label recommendations must be supported by efficacy data against *Bacillus subtilis* and *Clostridium sporogenes* as specified in DIS/TSS No. 9. In developing the data for a sterilizer, it is most important that the requirements of DIS/TSS No. 2 be taken into account wherever they are pertinent, and that the supporting data be reported in strict adherence to the criteria and requirements of DIS/TSS No. 3.

In past years, after the supporting data for a sterilizer have been reviewed by the EPA and determined to be scientifically valid, the agency required that a representative sample of the product from a pilot production batch be tested at the EPA's microbiology laboratory as a confirmatory step before registering the product. Currently, because of budgetary considerations, this practice has been discontinued as a routine procedure. The EPA reserves the option of requiring confirmatory testing by an independent laboratory on a case-by-case basis. Any questions about this matter should be directed to the product manager in charge of the proposed product, well in advance of the final plans to market a sterilizer.

Before leaving this area of microbiologic efficacy data, I will mention two other important points. DIS/TSS No. 6 specifies the microbiologic efficacy data requirements for claims against *Mycobacterium tuberculosis*, and for phenol coefficient claims. Any of those claims appearing on the label for a product must be supported by the appropriate data as specified in that enclosure. DIS/TSS No. 7 specifies the requirements for supporting label claims of effectiveness against specific viruses. Registrants wishing to make virucidal claims for a product should be aware that unqualified virucidal label claims are not acceptable to the EPA. Such a label claim must specify the virus or viruses for which the product has been tested and found effective, and must support the specific virucidal claims by data developed with the product against each virus specified on the label in accord with EPA guidelines.

DATA COMPENSATION PROVISIONS OF THE FIFRA

Given the enormous task of having to re-evaluate all chemical active ingredients and to re-register all pesticides, the EPA, early on, established a policy whereby it will register a me-too product based on the now famous Cite-All Method of Support, coupled with the Formulator's Exemption. In considering a me-too product for registration the EPA will use any data or information previously submitted by other registrants, with or without permission of the data submitters, as long as the registrant of the me-too product signs a statement and submits it with the application whereby the registrant acknowledges reliance on such data, and is prepared to offer compensation for their use to the original data submitters, to the extent that the owners are entitled to compensation under the law. Although the data compensation provisions of the FIFRA apply to all kinds of data, they impact mostly on toxicologic data required to assess potential adverse effects of pesticides.

About the time the data compensation provisions were first implemented by the EPA, some firms sued the EPA, challenging the agency's right to use data belonging to one firm in support of the registration of another firm's product without permission of the owner of the data. This prompted the EPA to put into effect elaborate and complicated procedures that allowed the agency to continue the policy of using previously submitted data with or without the original submitter's permission, and at the same time preserving the owners' right to compensation, until the courts settled the suit.

Shortly thereafter, the United States courts ruled in favor of the EPA, upholding the data compensation provisions of the FIFRA. Currently, the regulations for data compensation and protection of data submitters' rights have been codified in Part 152 of 40 CFR, Subpart E.

The impact of the data compensation provisions of the regulations to an applicant for registration of a pesticide can be summarized as follows. If a registrant purchases a registered source of an active ingredient from a supplier that is not affiliated with the registrant or with the firm of the registrant, and uses that purchased registered product to blend it with other ingredients or to repackage it as a pesticide, the registrant qualifies for the formulator's exemption as defined at 40 CFR Section 152.85. This means that the EPA will defer leveling any data requirements against the purchased registered technical grade of the active ingredient, even if there are data gaps for the active ingredient in the product, until such time that those requirements are imposed across the board for all pesticides containing that active ingredient. The registrant of the formulated or repackaged me-too product would only be responsible for satisfying the particular data requirements necessary to register the me-too product for the uses proposed for registration by the applicant. If an applicant does not qualify for the formulator's exemption, the applicant is responsible for two sets of data requirements—those data necessary to register the technical grade of the active ingredient, and those necessary to register the formulated product.

Assuming then that an applicant of a me-too product qualifies for the formulator's exemption, the applicant can obtain a registration with minimal data by using the now-famous Cite-All Method of Support (40 CFR Section 152.86). Under this method of support the applicant, in effect, requests the EPA to use any data within the agency in support of the application with the understanding that the applicant is prepared to compensate the owners of any data used by the EPA in support of the registration, to the extent that the owners are entitled to compensation under the law.

The other option is to use the Selective Method of Support (40 CFR Section 152.90). Under this method the applicant restricts the amount of data to be used in support of the application, and in so doing the potential compensation, by submitting or specifically citing those items of data that are to be used by the EPA in support of the registration. The data must be specifically identified, and if the data do not belong to the applicant, he must have written permission from the owners of the cited data for their use, or be liable for compensation for their use.

Regardless of the method of support used by an applicant, certain requirements and conditions must be satisfied, and certain forms dealing with this aspect of the registration process must be properly completed and submitted with each application. For more details on the data compensation procedures and the different obligations of registrants under the two methods of support for registration of pesticides the reader should refer to Pesticide Registration Notice (PRN) 85-3 of May 14, 1985, and 40 CFR Part 152: Section 152.85, Formulator's Exemption; Section 152.86, Cite-All Method of Support; and Section 152.90, Selective Method of Support. PR Notice 85-3 contains complete instructions and the forms necessary to satisfy the data compensation requirements.

TOXICOLOGIC DATA REQUIREMENTS

The toxicologic data requirements for the registration of a new chemical active ingredient can include acute toxicity data, mutagenicity data, teratogenicity data, and chronic effect studies as indicated in Part 158 of 40 CFR. The reader should note that unlike acute toxicity data, which are product-specific, and therefore are routinely required to support the registration of every pesticide product proposed for registration, the other items of toxicologic data mentioned here are generally required to be conducted with the purest grade of an active ingredient or with the technical grade of an active ingredient that is proposed for reformulating use. Thus, for a me-too type of product the minimal requirements are a battery of acute toxicity data as specified in Section 158.135 of 40 CFR: Guideline Series 81-1, Acute Oral Toxicity (rat); 81-2, acute dermal toxicity (rabbit); 81-3, Acute Inhalation Toxicity; 81-4, Primary Eye Irritation (rabbit); 81-5, primary dermal irritation; and 81-6, Dermal Sensitization. The reader should refer to the footnotes of 40 CFR Section 158.135 for more details as to when some of these requirements do not apply to a particular product.

The basic reason for requiring acute toxicity data for a pesticide is to establish its toxicity categories according to data developed with the product, as formulated and proposed for registration, through the various routes of exposure. The data determine the appropriate signal word and associated precautionary statements that will be required on the label for the product, consistent with the regulations for labeling requirements at Section 156.10 of 40 CFR. The data also determine whether the product must be marketed in child-resistant packaging.

Whether a prospective registrant needs to submit toxicologic data in support of an antimicrobial pesticide depends on several factors. From foregoing discussions in this chapter, the reader should be aware that, without any exception, an applicant for a pesticide registration must submit product chemistry as prescribed in Part 158 of 40 CFR, which includes complete disclosure of all the ingredients in the product. This is a prerequisite to a determination as to whether the product in question is indeed identical or substantially similar to one that has been registered by the EPA. Assuming then, that the proposed product is a bona fide me-too product, and that the applicant qualifies for the formulator's exemption as specified in 40 CFR Section 152.85, the applicant can use the Cite-All Method of Support (40 CFR Section 152.86), and thus avoid having to submit acute toxicity data developed with the proposed product. If all other requirements are satisfied the EPA will prescribe precautionary labeling for the product based on the results of data previously submitted by other registrants for products substantially similar to the proposed product, and register the product. Acceptance of a registration on that basis is an acknowledgment on the part of the registrant that he is liable for compensation to the data submitters for the use of the data, in accordance with the data compensation provisions of Part 152 of 40 CFR.

Registrants are reluctant to sign the Cite-All Method of Support Form and the Certification Statement with Respect to Citation of Data prescribed by PR Notice 85-3 because they believe that in so doing they are committing themselves to pay for unspecified sums of money for unidentified data. There are several ways by which an applicant can reduce or eliminate this uncertainty: examine the agency's data catalogs to identify the data for a particular chemical active ingredient and the submitter of the data; make arrangements for compensation before the registration is issued; appeal all claims of compensation for arbitration as to their validity and worth under the arbitration provisions of Section 3(c)(1)(D)(ii) of the FIFRA. Rules for arbitration of claims for data compensation of pesticide data were published in the Federal Register, Volume 44, No. 143, July 24, 1979. If a registrant receives a claim for compensation for the use of data to obtain his registration, and the claim is determined to be a valid claim, and if the claim is arbitrated and a fee for compensation is established that the registrant believes to be excessive, the registrant has the alternative option described below. The reader should take some comfort in the fact that the compensation provisions of the FIFRA are not intended to inflate the cost of data.

Alternatively, the prospective registrant may submit acute toxicity data developed with the product, or cite a specific set of acute toxicity studies under the Selective Method of Support as specified in Section 152.90 of 40 CFR with the owner's permission.

Regardless of the Method of Support that a prospective registrant selects in submitting an application for registration, the applicant must observe the procedures, and submit the necessary forms, for complying with the data compensation provisions of the EPA as specified in Pesticide Registration Notice 85-3 (May 14, 1989).

There are some situations in which an applicant for a registration must use a combination of the two methods of support. The reason for this is that the product may contain one or more chemical active ingredients, as declared on the proposed label, for which the applicant does not qualify for the formulator's exemption (Section

152.85 of 40 CFR). An example of this is the registration of a toilet bowel disinfectant containing hydrochloric acid, a chemical active ingredient that is not registered as a pesticide in its technical concentrated form, and a quaternary ammonium compound, which is registered as a pesticide for manufacturing and reformulating of end-use antimicrobials. Each of these chemicals contributes appreciably to the performance of the product as a toilet bowel disinfectant, and therefore both must be declared on the product's label as active ingredients. The manufacturer of the quaternary ammonium compound has registered it, in concentrated form, as the technical grade of the active ingredient. Because of the popularity of that two-ingredient consumer product, the manufacturer of the quat has developed a so-called "prototype" product according to a prescribed recipe, and developed the necessary product chemistry, acute toxicity data, and microbiologic efficacy data for the prototype. His clients in turn may cite the data under the Selective Method of Support to register their products. The only obligation of the registrant of the prototype formulation is to submit confirmatory microbiologic efficacy data for his particular product in accordance with DIS/TSS No. 5. This amount of data is considerably smaller than would be required for a product that is not a replica of the registered prototype. In some instances, the manufacturer of the prototype will perform the confirmatory testing as a customer service at no expense.

However, because hydrochloric acid is an unregistered technical pesticide, the clients do not qualify for the formulator's exemption for that particular active ingredient. Therefore, they must use the Cite-All Method of Support for that unregistered active ingredient. In this particular example hydrochloric acid is a chemical with old established multiple uses. Therefore, there is considerable literature in the public domain to satisfy the EPA's concerns for use of the product in toilet bowls. Consequently, a registrant can obtain a registration for this type of product using the Cite-All Method of Support for that active ingredient and not have to submit data on hydrochloric acid. This would not be true for other unregistered technical pesticides. In that case the applicant would have to address the data requirements for the unregistered active ingredient. Here again PR Notice 85-3 gives instructions on how to fill out the necessary forms in dealing with that situation.

LABELING REQUIREMENTS (SECTION 156.10 OF 40 CFR)

As mentioned earlier, each application for registration of a pesticide must be accompanied by several copies of the typewritten or otherwise-prepared draft label proposed for the product. Formerly the EPA had codified certain essential elements that must appear on a pesticide label at Section 162.10 of 40 CFR. In the 1988 amendment to the regulations those labeling requirements were redesignated as Section 156.10 of 40 CFR. An applicant should make sure that the product's label complies with the general requirements prescribed therein as thoroughly as possible. Among other things the label must bear the brand name that will be used in marketing the product, an ingredient statement, an appropriate signal word and associated precautionary statements consistent with the product's toxicity categories based on acute toxicity data, and storage and disposal statements. Another important labeling element is a complete set of adequate use directions. For antimicrobial pesticides the prospective registrant should consult DIS/TSS No. 15. Use directions that do not comply with those requirements will be found deficient by the EPA.

In this context, experience has demonstrated that the EPA will almost always prescribe changes to the label before issuing a registration. If nothing else the EPA will assign a registration number, which must appear on the finished printed label that will accompany the product in channels of trade.

Until a few years ago the registration of a pesticide involved at least two complete cycles of review. In some instances, depending on the complexity of the product, or whether the EPA review results in extensive revisions to the label or data deficiencies, the registration may take several more cycles of submissions and review. As the final step of the registration process, the registrant was formerly required to submit five copies of the finished printed label incorporating any revisions prescribed by the agency prior to the issuance of the registration. The registration notice was then issued together with a copy of the finished printed label bearing the EPA's acceptance stamp and date of acceptance. Until the registrant received those two documents he could not legally market the product.

Several years ago, as one of the EPA's regulatory relief initiatives, the agency announced a change in procedures in PR Notice 82-2, June 18, 1982, whereby it would no longer routinely require submission of finished printed labels as a prerequisite to the issuance of the registration notice (see also 40 CFR Section 162.6). Instead, the EPA now issues registration notices for me-too products on the basis of draft labels, which may be typewritten or mock-up labels. Any revisions prescribed by the EPA are itemized in the registration notice as part of the conditions for issuing the registration notice, with the understanding that the registrant will make the revisions when the label is printed and before the product is released for shipment or placed in channels of trade. A copy of the draft label before revisions is returned to the registrant bearing the agency's stamp "accepted with comments." As the final step of the registration the registrant is required to submit five copies of the revised finished printed labels for placement in the registration records for the product. PR Notice 85-2 states that the EPA will not review the printed label, nor will the agency return a copy with another stamp of acceptance to the registrant. The EPA will simply place the labels in the registration records for the product for future reference as needed. If at some later date it is established that the registrant did not show good faith by making the prescribed changes on the finished printed labels, or that the registrant failed to submit the revised finished printed labels, the registration will be subject to regulatory action by the agency.

This chapter has provided a broad summary of the regulatory and scientific requirements for registering disinfectants. This information is not intended to preempt the original sources from which most of the information presented in this chapter was obtained. For this reason, frequent and appropriate references to the original sources have been provided, so that the reader can readily refer to them for more information. The prospective registrant with questions about a particular product should consult the appropriate product manager. The product manager is the official representative for the EPA in registration matters.

BIBLIOGRAPHY

Federal Pesticide Control Act of 1972. Amendments to the Federal Insecticide, Fungicide, and Rodenticide Act, (USC 135 et seq.), (86 Stat. 973-999). Public Law 92-516, 92nd Congress, H.R. 10729, October 21, 1972.

The 1975 Amendment to the Federal Insecticide, Fungicide, and Rodenticide Act, (7 USC 136 et seq.), (86 Stat. 973-999). Public Law 94-140, 94th Congress, H.R. 8841, November 28, 1975.

The 1978 Amendment to the Federal Insecticide, Fungicide, and Rodenticide Act, (7USC 163 et seq.), (86 Stat. 973-999). Public Law 95-396, 95th Congress, S. 1678, September 30, 1978.

Regulations for Child Resistant Packaging of Pesticides, Federal Register, Volume 44, No. 48, p. 27932-27954, May 11, 1979.

Federal Mediation and Conciliation Service (29 CFR 1440). Proposed Rules for Mediation and Conciliation of Claims for Compensation of Pesticides Data by Arbitrators as provided by Public Law 95-396, September 30, 1978, FIFRA, Sections 3(c)(1)(D)(ii) and 3(c)(2)(B)(iii). Federal Register, Volume 44, No. 143, pp. 43292-43297, July 24, 1975.

Registration Standards for the Registration of Pesticides. The Registration Standard System for Registering Pesticides. Federal Register, Volume 44, No. 248, pp. 76312-76322, December 26, 1979.

Pesticide Chemical Active Ingredients; Proposed Registration Standards Ranking Scheme by Chemical Active Ingredient Clusters. Federal Register, Volume 45, No. 222, pp. 75488-75497, November 14, 1980.

Pesticide Assessment Guidelines. The guidelines contain the standards for conducting acceptable tests, guidance on the formulation of a pesticide that must be used to do each test, and guidance on evaluation and reporting of data, definition of terms, further guidance on when data are required, and examples of protocols. Various subdivisions according to disciplines are listed at 40 CFR Section 158.115. Many more are currently available from the National Technical Information Service, 5285 Port Royal Road, Springfield, Virginia, 22161. The telephone number is 703-487-4650.

CODE OF FEDERAL REGULATIONS—DESCRIPTIONS OF PERTINENT PARTS

Title 21 of the Code of Federal Regulations, Section 178.1010. Sanitizing solutions used as terminal rinses in food handling establishments.

Title 40 of the Code of Federal Regulations (July 1, 1987). Chapter I—Protection of the Environment (parts pertinent to registration of antimicrobial pesticides):

Part 152 Pesticide Registration and Classification Procedures
Part 153 Statements of Policies and Interpretations
Part 154 Special Review Procedures
Part 155 Registration Standards
Part 156 Labeling Requirements for Pesticides and Devices
Part 157 Special Packaging Requirements for Pesticides and Devices
Part 158 Data Requirements for Registration of Pesticides
Part 160 Good Laboratory Practice
Part 162 Regulations for the Enforcement of the Federal Insecticide, Fungicide, and Rodenticide Act
Part 165 Regulations for the acceptance of certain pesticides and recommended procedures for the disposal and storage of pesticides and pesticide containers

Pesticide Registration Procedures and Pesticide Data Requirements; Final Rule; 40 CFR Parts 152, 153, 156, 158, and 162. Amendments to the regulations resulting from the 1988 FIFRA Amendments. Federal Register, Volume 53, No. 86, May 4, 1988, pp. 15952-15999.

DISINFECTANTS (ANTIMICROBIAL PROGRAM) BRANCH/TECHNICAL SUPPORT SECTION ENCLOSURES: MICROBIOLOGIC EFFICACY DATA REQUIREMENTS

DIS/TSS Enclosure No. 1 (July 10, 1979). Specific data requirements for limited disinfectants, general or broad-spectrum disinfectants, and hospital disinfectants.

DIS/TSS Enclosure No. 2 (January 25, 1979). Supplemental requirements: specifies necessary modification of the standard tests to support claims of effectiveness for short exposure periods, effectiveness on porous surfaces, in hard water, and on soiled surfaces, without a precleaning step, etc.

DIS/TSS Enclosure No. 3 (January 30, 1979). Criteria and requirements for reporting microbiologic efficacy data.

DIS/TSS Enclosure No. 4 (January 30, 1979). Data requirements for final sanitizing rinses of food contact surfaces. See also Title 21 of the Code of Federal Regulations, Section 178.1010: Sanitizing solutions used as terminal rinses in food handling establishments.

DIS/TSS Enclosure No. 5 (August 18, 1980). Confirmatory data requirements for a duplicate of a registered prototype disinfectant and for minor formulation changes for limited disinfectants, broad-spectrum disinfectants, hospital disinfectants, and sanitizers for food contact surfaces.

DIS/TSS Enclosure No. 6 (February 1, 1979). Data requirements to support claims of effectiveness against pathogenic fungi and against *Mycobacterium tuberculosis*, and to support phenol coefficient claims.

DIS/TSS Enclosure No. 7 (February 6, 1979). Data requirements to support claims of effectiveness against viruses.

DIS/TSS Enclosure No. 8 (February 6, 1979). Recommendations for developing a protocol to test effectiveness of carpet sanitizers.

DIS/TSS Enclosure No. 9 (April 15, 1981). Data requirements for sterilizers.

DIS/TSS Enclosure No. 10 (February 6, 1979). Data requirements to support sanitizers on non–food-contact surfaces.

DIS/TSS Enclosure No. 11 (September 3, 1980). Air sanitizers: requirements for products with label claims for the treatment of air to reduce the number of airborne microorganisms.

DIS/TSS Enclosure No. 12 (April 23, 1979). Efficacy data requirements for swimming pool water disinfectants.

DIS/TSS Enclosure No. 13 (April 4, 1980). Efficacy data requirements for laundry additives; disinfection and sanitization; labeling requirements.

DIS/TSS Enclosure No. 14 (May 7, 1979). Laundry additives; residual self-sanitization and bacteriostasis.

DIS/TSS Enclosure No. 15 (March 24, 1981). Label requirements for antimicrobials used on hard surfaces.

DIS/TSS Enclosure No. 16 (June 26, 1979). Criteria for determining health-related uses and non–health-related uses.

DIS/TSS Enclosure No. 17 (December 2, 1979). Label requirements for use directions of pesticides recommended as final sanitizing rinses on food contact surfaces.

DIS/TSS Enclosure No. 18 (January 17, 1980). Label requirements for use directions of disinfectants recommended for use on farm premises.

DIS/TSS Enclosure No. 19 (January 17, 1980). Label requirements for use directions of disinfectants recommended for use in poultry houses.

PESTICIDE REGISTRATION NOTICES

PRN 82-2 (June 18, 1982). Change in procedures for approval of applications with regards to submission of finished printed labels.

PRN 83-3 (March 29, 1983). Label Improvement Program; Storage and Disposal Label Statements.

CHAPTER 55

FACILITIES FOR CONTROL OF MICROBIAL AGENTS

G. Briggs Phillips and Robert F. Morrissey

The design features of a facility have an important relation to the validity of the operations being carried out. Good design and equipment are valuable in containing or eliminating microbial agents. Indifferent or inconsistent arrangements complicate or limit efforts to control microorganisms and their environments. Facility design for microbial control includes any building feature or equipment, or a combination of these, that contains, confines, or destroys microorganisms. Although the possible features are numerous, their proper selection is all-important in achieving a facility that will provide adequate and efficient control at the lowest cost while maintaining an adequate degree of flexibility for future operational changes.

CONTAMINATION CONTROL SCHEME

It is useful to view the design of a facility for contamination control in the context of a general scheme to achieve that control (Phillips and Brewer, 1968). This scheme is shown in Figure 55–1.

The plan starts with an identification of the problem and the establishment of criteria, followed by activities, including facility design, that are designed to meet the criteria. It puts the features of the facility in proper perspective in relation to equipment, techniques, and other control measures. The following presents, as an example, a greatly simplified outline for a sterility testing laboratory.

Problem—Organize a laboratory for efficient sterility testing of sterile products.

Control Criteria—Sterility testing to be carried out at the rate of 100 tests per day and with a negligible incidence of false-positive results.

Control Methods
1. Facility Design
   Provide positive air pressure in sterility test laboratory, with a ventilation rate of 6 changes of air per hour and HEPA filtration of air entering room. All surfaces, including ceiling, must be impervious and capable of being washed with disinfectant solution.
   Provide suitable air locks and equipment pass locks to allow the donning of sterile outer garments and to pass in materials and supplies with a minimum ingress of contamination.
   Provide ceiling germicidal ultraviolet lamps to use during periods of nonoccupancy.
   Provide viewing windows, speaking diaphragms, and intercommunication system to reduce traffic into laboratory.
2. Containment Equipment
   Provide horizontal laminar airflow benches for sterility testing procedures. Placement of the benches should not disrupt airflow patterns.
3. Operational Technique
   Persons entering the sterility test room will don sterile lint-free gowns, head covers, and shoe covers.
   Sterile surgical gloves will be worn while working at the laminar airflow bench.
   The placement of the sterile devices in the culture media will be done only in the laminar airflow bench by a two-person team.
   The placement of materials in the bench should be controlled to minimize disruption of airflow patterns. Following each series of tests, all surfaces will be washed with a disinfectant.
   Once each week the entire room will be decontaminated.

Evaluate Results—Tests were conducted that showed that all HEPA filters were operating correctly and that the UV lamps met specification. Air-sampling studies never revealed organisms in the laminar benches, and the air-borne count in the room air never exceeded five microorganisms per liter. Surface sampling showed most surfaces to be sterile with only an occasional sample showing one to five colonies.

Under these conditions, a sterility testing evaluation was performed that did not reveal any false-positive results.

Certify and Standardize—Arrangements are made to pe-

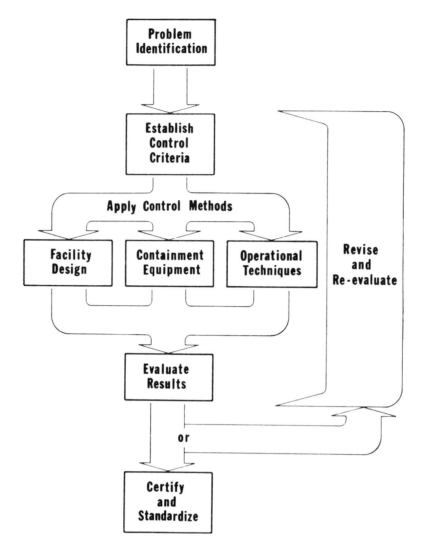

Fig. 55–1. General scheme for contamination control.

riodically retest or replace all HEPA filters and UV lamps. A program of periodic testing of air and surfaces is established and the results are reviewed to ensure that standard conditions are being met.

The foregoing is obviously a fictitious example, but it illustrates the extent to which the control facilities provided in such a situation relate to and depend on other control measures.

In general, whenever possible, it is desirable to establish specific standards prescribing the level of control needed. The degree of microbial control, for example,

needed to fill empty sterile vials with sterile solutions is obviously of a different order of magnitude than that needed to prevent excessive contamination of food products with specific pathogens during processing. It is useful to establish specific microbial standards that the facility design should help to achieve. This can be expressed in terms such as number of microorganisms allowed in an environment and types of organisms allowed or not allowed. Such criteria could also specify the methods for locating or detecting microbial contamination.

PLANNING CONSIDERATIONS

When a new facility or a major renovation of an existing facility is being considered, it is recommended that thought be given to the establishment of a planning team and the development of a formal program of requirements document. The detailed procedures related to such planning have been discussed in detail by Runkle and Phillips (1969). Planning and design features of laboratories using infectious disease agents are a part of a comprehensive book called *Laboratory-Acquired Infections* by Collins (1988).

A properly selected planning team should first provide a description of all activities that are to take place in the facility and those contemplated in the future. From this description it should be possible to identify numbers of personnel, major equipment requirements, space allocations, and other information needed in initial design activities. It should also be possible to establish the general environmental control criteria needed for the functions to take place in the facility. The planning team can use these functional descriptions to establish basic policy decisions concerning the facility control features, techniques, methods, and procedures. The policy decisions will often deal with tradeoffs between inflexible and costly building features and means of achieving microbial control more cheaply by alternate methods that rely more on equipment and techniques. Some typical policy questions are:

1. Is the facility for a single specific project? If so, is it suitable for the probable next use, or will remodeling be necessary?

2. How will predictable future changes in governmental regulations affect the adequacy of the facility? Will more stringent environmental controls be required?

3. How much flexibility in design is needed? Should the facility be designed for easy expansion, easy conversion to alternate use, or both?

4. Will pathogenic microorganisms be used now or later that will require special facility features for personnel protection?

5. Are quarantine areas needed for the isolation of incoming or outgoing goods while validating their biologic content?

6. If animals are used, will requirements for the number and types of animals change or will there be changes in the ways that the animals are used?

7. Will work be done now or later that will require the treatment of air or liquid effluents discharged from the facility?

The preceding information forms the basis of a program of requirements for a facility. A program of requirements includes an analysis of all current and projected needs of the facility. We will not deal here with the normal architectural/engineering requirements such as site location, soil conditions, seismic state, reliability of water and electrical sources, and effects on the ecology of the community. Rather, special considerations will be mentioned relative to contamination control requirement.

It is recommended that the planning team, which reports to the program director, function not only in preparing the program requirements, but also in reviewing the final facility design plans and in following construction through all stages, including facility checkout and acceptance. It is advantageous to have one member of the team handle all relations and communications with the architectural/engineering firm.

DESIGN CONCEPTS FOR MICROBIAL CONTROL

A major design concept to be considered early in the planning is whether or not there should be functional zones within the facility that will have a higher degree of environmental control than other zones. These may be thought of in terms of protected versus nonprotected areas. From a cost point of view, it is better to limit contamination control features to those zones or areas where they are needed. Space used for administrative functions, storage, and facility support equipment usually needs no special treatment with regard to ventilation, air filtration, water supply, and discharge of effluents. Areas requiring higher degrees of environmental control have more costly engineering and design requirements. The concept recommended in dealing with the zoning of a facility is discussed in the following and illustrated in Figure 55–2.

Identify those areas that do not require any unusual facility arrangement nor any type of protected internal environment. These generally include the entrance areas to the building, offices, libraries, cafeterias, shipping and receiving areas, storage rooms, and areas for mechanical equipment.

Identify those areas that are to be protected and that require some degree of environmental control. These include product areas, laboratory areas, hospital operating rooms, central sterile supply areas, packaging rooms, and sterility testing rooms.

Identify the necessary transitional areas. Transitional areas are those in which people or materials pass back and forth between protected and nonprotected areas. They are needed to ensure a minimum transfer of contamination between the two types of areas. Transitional spaces may include change rooms containing showers, toilets, and storage space for clothing; walk-through air locks with germicidal ultraviolet, double-access sterilization chambers installed in walls between protected and nonprotected areas; and UV pass boxes or liquid dunk baths for the transfer of materials. The need for transitional rooms can often be minimized by installing view panels and speaking diaphragms in doors and walls between zones and by providing communication systems.

Once the areas that need special environmental control are identified, the next considerations are the specific design features that should be included to achieve the required level of microbial contamination control. In ap-

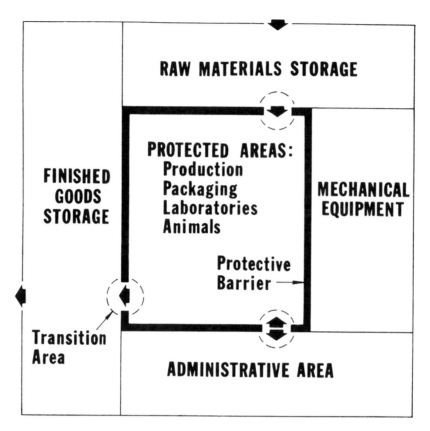

Fig. 55–2. Typical protected and unprotected areas of a facility.

proaching these decisions, the concept of primary and secondary barriers should be considered (Fig. 55–3). Enclosures, barriers, or other containment devices that provide microbial control immediately around the procedure or operation are considered primary barriers. The extent of their use is related to the extent of the control devices that are a part of the building. These are designated as secondary barriers. In general, efficient use of primary barriers is less expensive and provides greater flexibility than dependence on secondary barriers. There are obvious trade-offs between the use of primary and secondary barriers in any particular design situation. Examples of primary barriers are the use of ventilated negative-pressure cabinets for work with infectious microorganisms and the use of laminar airflow cabinets to provide a protected environment during sterility testing or sterile assembly operations.

Secondary barriers are those features of the protected zones that ensure the adequate separation of zones and a separation from the outside community. Such features include the floors, walls, and ceilings, control of air pressures and air movements between zones, filtration of supply air, exhaust air or both, provisions for water supplies, provisions for the treatment of liquid effluents, and the use of germicidal ultraviolet.

Primary Barriers

The more effective the primary barrier, the less elaborate will be the required secondary barrier systems. Primary barriers are designed to *contain* or *exclude* microbial contaminants. Containment systems often aim at protecting humans or animals in situations in which infectious microorganisms are used. These are operated at a negative air pressure. Systems to exclude contamination are used to provide product protection and are operated at a positive air pressure. In some situations, a barrier system is needed that provides both product and personnel protection.

Because biologic safety cabinets are the most frequently used and best standardized primary barriers, three classes are described in the following. More complete discussions have been presented by Barkley (1981) and Collins (1988).

A *Class I* biologic safety cabinet (Fig. 55–4) is an open-

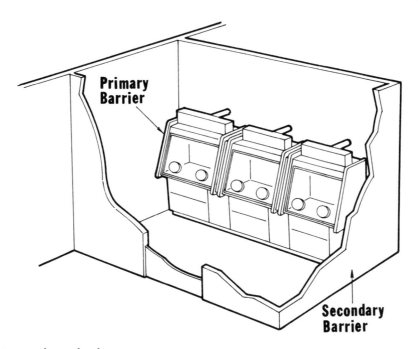

Fig. 55–3. Concept of primary and secondary barriers.

fronted, negative-pressure, ventilated cabinet with a minimum inward airflow velocity at the work opening of at least 75 feet per minute. Exhaust air from the cabinet is filtered by a high-efficiency particulate air (HEPA) filter. A Class I cabinet may be used in three modes: with an open front, with a front closure panel not equipped with gloves, and with the panel but equipped with arm-length rubber gloves.

The *Class II* biologic cabinet (Fig. 55–5) utilizes vertical laminar airflow and has an open front with an average inward face velocity at the work opening of at least 75 feet per minute. This cabinet provides HEPA-filtered, recirculated, laminar airflow within the work space. Exhaust air from the cabinet is also HEPA filtered. Design, construction, and standards of performance for Class II cabinets have been developed by the National Sanitation Foundation, Ann Arbor, Michigan (1976).

The *Class III* cabinet (Fig. 55–6) is a totally enclosed, ventilated cabinet of gas-tight construction. Operations are conducted through attached rubber gloves. In use, the Class III cabinet is maintained under negative air pressure of at least 0.5 inches of water. Supply air is admitted to the cabinet through HEPA filters. Exhaust air is treated by two HEPA filters installed in series. The exhaust fan for the Class III cabinet is generally separate from the exhaust fans of the ventilation system of the building.

Personnel protection provided by Class I and Class II cabinets depends on the inward airflow. Because the face velocities are similar, they generally provide an equivalent level of personnel protection. The use of these cabinets alone, however, is not appropriate for containment of highest-risk infectious agents because aerosols may escape accidentally through the open front during operations such as centrifuging.

The Class II cabinet offers the additional capability and advantage of protecting materials contained within the cabinet from extraneous air-borne contaminants. This protection is provided by the filtered, recirculated mass airflow within the work space.

The Class III cabinet gives the highest level of personnel and product protection. This protection is provided by the physical isolation of the space in which the laboratory work is done. When these cabinets are required, all procedures involving dangerous agents are contained within them. Several Class III cabinets therefore are typically set up as an interconnected system. All equipment required by the laboratory activity, such as incubators, refrigerators, and centrifuges, should be an integral part of the cabinet system. Double-door autoclaves and chemical dunk tanks are also attached to the cabinet system to allow introduction and removal of supplies and equipment.

In addition to the three classes of biologic safety cabinets, the use of laminar airflow provides an excellent tool for protective environments where personnel safety is not a consideration (Phillips and Runkle, 1973). Figure 55–7 shows the basic design of a horizontal laminar air-

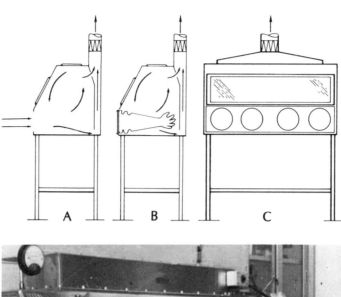

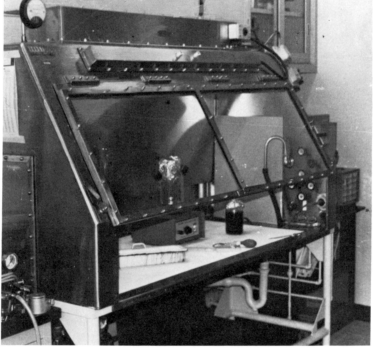

Fig. 55–4. Class I cabinet. A, Cutaway view showing airflow at work opening. B, Cutaway view showing closure panel and attached gloves. C, Front closure panel with access ports.

flow work bench often used in product protection situations such as sterility testing or sterile filling and assembly.

Secondary Barriers

Detailed descriptions of all facility design considerations for the control of microbial agents are beyond the scope of this chapter. However, it is useful to discuss some elements of design and of facility systems that should be considered.

Floors, Walls, and Ceilings

The design criteria will depend upon the procedures to be carried out. If a washdown of the walls and ceiling

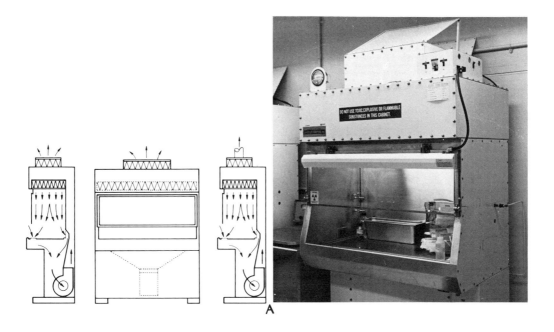

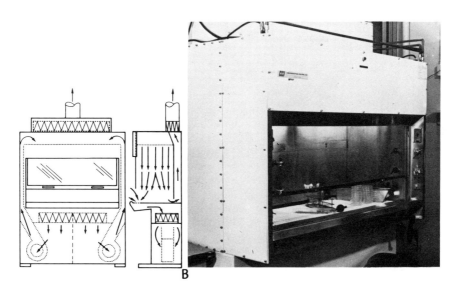

Fig. 55–5. A and B, Class II cabinets.

at intervals is needed, waterproof construction is necessary, with finishes resistant to the germicides to be used. Floors in protected areas should always be continuous and waterproof. To prevent the seepage of water under walls, it is recommended that concrete wall curbs, approximately 4 inches high, be poured integral with the floor. The face of the curb should be flush with the face of the wall above. Coved corners are recommended for easy cleaning. Expansion joints in concrete floors should

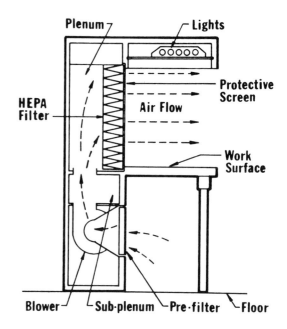

Fig. 55–7. Horizontal laminar airflow bench.

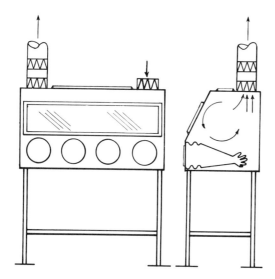

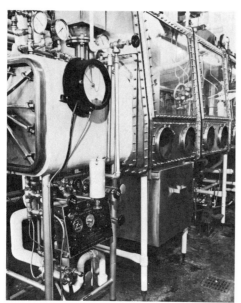

Fig. 55–6. Class III cabinets.

be provided with a continuous water stop and should be filled to a depth of ½ inch with a two-component polysulfide sealant or a one-part silicone sealant. A watertight seal should be provided at each floor level around all pipes, conduits, instrument tubing, and ducts whenever they pass through floors, walls, or ceilings.

Various floor finishes are available; their utility and unit cost vary over a wide range. Tile and sheet linoleum should be avoided for rooms that are to be washed frequently with disinfectants and water. A satisfactory floor finish for many purposes can be obtained by using a nonslip metallic aggregate top layer for concrete that is steel-troweled to a glass finish. In this process, it is necessary to treat the uncured surface with a concrete hardener, seal it, and finish it with a nonskid wax. Such a floor will withstand almost any use or abuse, from flooding with disinfectants to the heavy traffic of carts and hand trucks. Another satisfactory finish can be obtained by applying an epoxy-aggregate floor topping (approximately ⅛ inch thick) to the finished concrete.

Obviously, walls and ceilings in protected areas should be as smooth and free of cracks and crevices as possible. If waterproof ceilings are required, waterproof light fixtures must also be provided. Modern epoxy paints provide a finish with good resistance to most disinfectants.

Floor Drains

Floor drains present several problems. Unless liquid disinfectants are used, the traps become breeding places for microorganisms and insects. If the traps dry out, sewer gas may create contamination or an explosive hazard. In areas under substantial negative air pressure, the liquid may be pulled from the traps of the drains. Because of these considerations, it is recommended that floor drains be installed only where needed. Drains from protected and nonprotected areas should not be interconnected or have common vents. When floor drains are installed, it is recommended that they have extra-deep traps and be provided with a piped priming water supply to each trap and screw-type plugs for use when a drain is not used for long periods.

Windows

Outside windows that open are not desirable in biologically protected areas. Even nonopening windows create problems because of heat or cooling loss unless double-pane insulating units are used. Any type of window detracts from the available wall area in any work situation. If outside windows must be used for protected areas, they should be nonopening and properly insulated.

Sealing

An important aspect of facility design is the sealing of pipes, ducts, etc., that penetrate walls, floors, and ceilings. For control of the movement of contaminants, for easy cleaning and decontamination, and for related reasons, seals must be air- and liquid-tight and resistant to environmental agents. Some typical methods of sealing are shown in Figure 55–8. These provide tight seals for wall or floor penetrations separating protected and nonprotected areas.

Services

Compressed Air. Although there is little danger of reverse flow or cross-contamination in these systems, there is often a need to filter the air to avoid contamination of items or areas. Compressors used should be of the oil-free type.

Vacuum. A vacuum system for protected areas should not be common with one for nonprotected areas unless the two legs of the system are separated with HEPA filters. Vacuum systems accumulate liquids in the vacuum receiving tank, and these can be a source of contamination. Where pathogenic organisms are in use, arrangements should be made to sterilize or decontaminate liquids collecting in the vacuum system.

Gas. A common system for the delivery of propane or natural gas to protected and nonprotected areas of a facility poses no problems.

Electricity. Conduits providing electric service to protected areas should be internally sealed at each entrance to a room to avoid the possibility of transfer of contamination from air moving through the conduit.

Venting. Careful design of vent lines from sinks, toilets, etc., is necessary to avoid cross-contamination. In areas where pathogens are to be handled, all vent lines should have welded joints. Common vents or cross-venting between protected and nonprotected areas should not be allowed. In critical instances, to avoid the escape

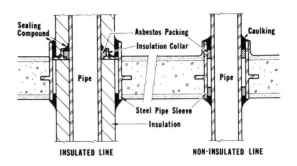

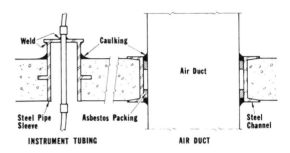

Fig. 55–8. Typical methods of sealing penetrations through floors, walls, and ceilings to separate protected and nonprotected areas.

of contamination, it is possible to place biologic filters on vent lines.

Water Service

If a sufficient level of hazard exists that undesirable microbiologic agents used in a facility will contaminate the central water supply system, the need for preventive measures should be considered. A break tank is the most reliable method, although certain types of backflow preventors may be used if properly tested and serviced. According to the type of work being carried out, it may be desirable to have a separation of water services according to function. In some instances, for example, the water used for laboratory, plant, or animal room cleaning and processing may be a separate system from the water used for drinking, showers, or for deionizers or stills. One arrangement is to have the water for drinking or personal use come directly from the water main, with all other water going through a break tank or backflow preventor.

When systems to make and deliver deionized or distilled water are used, the need to control microbiologic contamination should be considered. One way is to minimize the amount of delivery piping involved. UV is often useful in limiting the growth of microorganisms in water storage tanks. It is recommended that a deionized or distilled water system be designed for easy cleaning and decontamination at appropriate intervals. Improperly

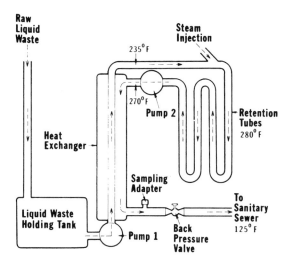

Fig. 55–9. Constant flow heat exchanger liquid waste sterilization system.

maintained deionizing columns are potent sources of microbiologic contamination.

Liquid Wastes

There can be three categories of liquid wastes from a biologic facility. Storm sewage consists of normal runoff water from rain and ordinarily poses no problems in the control of microbial agents. Sanitary sewage is the liquid waste from nonprotected areas that is usually disposed of in a conventional sewage treatment plant (e.g., municipal water treatment system). Contaminated sewage is that liquid from the protected areas of a facility if it contains infectious microorganisms, radioactive materials, or toxic substances. This sewage may require sterilization or decontamination before discharge into conventional sanitary sewage lines.

Two methods for sterilizing sewage have been found most acceptable. A continuous-flow system utilizing heat exchangers is shown in Figure 55–9. Another method is that of batch sterilization of the liquids collected in a pressure vessel by the injection of steam. Both methods are relatively expensive, and their use is justified only when no other method can adequately avoid the discharge of sewage containing undesirable contaminants.

Although heat is the most desirable method of treating contaminated sewage, other methods such as chemical treatment or treatment with ozone are feasible.

Air-Handling Systems

This system is important because air is the most common ingredient for spreading contamination. Although air systems have other functions, we will cover here only considerations related to ventilation rates and methods of delivery, recirculated versus nonrecirculated air, and treatment of supply and exhaust air.

Ventilation rates and the method of delivering air to occupied areas provide opportunities for controlling contamination. While recommended ventilation rates vary according to the demands for control of temperature and relative humidity, it is obvious that higher rates will remove air-borne contamination faster. However, the placement of air supply and exhaust ducts is also important. Improperly placed supply and exhaust grills often result in a shortcutting of the air and incomplete mixing. Properly located grills can do much to affect the efficiency of contamination control, no matter what the ventilation rate. In animal rooms or in areas where dust is produced, it is often better to introduce air at the ceiling and to remove it at the floor level. Animal rooms generally require about 20 changes of air per hour as compared to 6 changes per hour for ordinary occupied spaces.

The most complex and expensive method of room ventilation is the laminar airflow method. Ventilation rates may approach 600 to 700 changes per hour, and one third of the floor-ceiling-wall area is given over to exhaust and supply grills.

Many occupied areas requiring biologic contamination control use only outside supply air with no recirculation. The primary justification for 100% outside supply air is that it allows the maximum isolation of a room or area with minimum chance of cross-contamination via the air. Although 100% outside air systems are expensive, they are sometimes recommended for rooms or areas that require periodic decontamination. With a single-pass air system, vapor decontamination can be accomplished without interrupting activities in surrounding areas. Except for the reason just given, the availability of reliable HEPA filters provides a good method of preventing air cross-contamination without resorting to 100% outside air. Wherever possible, HEPA filtration of recirculated air should be considered an alternate to 100% outside supply air. According to the microbial control requirements, supply air, exhaust air, or both can be subjected to microbial filtration. Other methods of air treatment, such as incineration or electrostatic precipitation, are not recommended.

Transition Methods

These minimize the transfer of contamination due to the movement of people or materials back and forth from protected to nonprotected areas.

Change Rooms. As a maximum these provide for a complete change of clothing and shoes when entering a protected area. Showers can be required for persons entering or leaving. Very often, however, change rooms are designed for the donning of overgarments, shoes, and hair covers.

Air Locks. Air locks are frequently used for the passage of personnel in and out of protected areas. They are generally not ventilated, and UV lamps are often placed on the ceiling. To be effective, only one door of the air lock should be opened at a time; this is sometimes accomplished by use of electric interlocks. A typical air lock is shown in Figure 55–10. (Wedum et al., 1956).

Shoe Treatment Devices. Such devices can play an important role in reducing the amount of contamination tracked into protected spaces on the shoes of personnel. They are particularly needed in clean rooms and related areas where change-room procedures are not used and when shoe covers are not worn over street shoes. A variety of devices have been used. For rubber shoes or boots, as often worn in animal rooms, a shallow foot bath with a liquid disinfectant can be used. In other instances, a sponge mat outside of the entrance to an area can be kept moistened with a disinfectant. Tacky mats and air showers have also been used to remove gross contamination from shoes.

Communication Through Barriers. Communication between areas with different levels of contamination serves to reduce traffic and reduce chances of contamination breaching the barrier. The easiest and most inexpensive method uses clear plastic (Saran or Mylar) speaking diaphragms and glass viewing panels. Effective speaking diaphragms are available commercially. Figure 55–11 shows a speaking diaphragm in a wall to a sterility testing room.

In some instances, telephone communication may be desirable to reduce traffic in and out of an area. Another concept is the use of television cameras for monitoring containment areas where there is a danger of accidents, or for monitoring control panels from a remote location. These devices are also employed for monitoring patients under strict isolation.

It is often advisable to have arrangements for transition

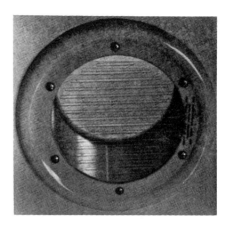

Fig. 55–11. Speaking diaphragm.

of materials and supplies between protected and non-protected areas. Through-the-wall autoclaves, ethylene oxide gas chambers, and pass boxes utilizing UV have been used in such situations. UV pass boxes are also frequently used for passing materials in and out of cabinet systems.

FACILITY DESIGN GUIDELINES AND REGULATIONS

Guidelines and regulations relating to facility design have become increasingly important in recent years. Agencies such as the Food and Drug Administration, the Occupational Safety and Health Administration (OSHA), and the Environmental Protection Agency have finalized regulations that affect facility design requirements. Others, such as the Centers for Disease Control and the National Cancer Institute, have promulgated guidelines with important recommendations for facility design criteria.

Facilities in which ethylene oxide gas sterilization chambers are to be used present a special situation because of worker safety and environmental considerations. To use this effective gas to control microbial agents and sterilize products, certain design standards are needed. OSHA (1984) has established limits for worker safety at 1 ppm based on an 8-hour time-weighted average and has specified required engineering controls. The Environmental Protection Agency is currently addressing emissions regulations that will require attention to facility attributes. Other sterilization agents to be used in a facility may require certain engineering features for containment.

Those concerned with laboratory and animal testing of new drugs, devices, or diagnostic products will find that "good-laboratory-practice" type regulations (21 CFR) contain requirements for practices of microbial isolation and control that relate in a real sense to the attributes of the facility. Firms in the health care field

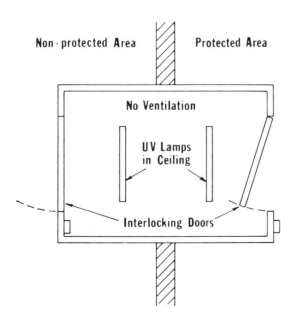

Non-protected Area   **Protected Area**

No Ventilation

UV Lamps in Ceiling

Interlocking Doors

Fig. 55–10. Typical air lock for personnel passage.

Table 55–1. *Proposed Containment Equipment and Facilities for Four Levels of Biosafety*

Biosafety Level	Containment Equipment	Facilities
Level 1— Basic Facility	Not required	Sink, easily cleaned benches and furniture, screens on open windows. Autoclave in same building.
Level 2— Containment Facility	Class I, II, or III biologic safety cabinets, special containment for centrifugation and aerosol-producing operations	Same as Level 1
Level 3— High Containment Facility	Same as Level 2, with some additions	Same as Level 1 plus limited access to laboratory through change room or air lock. Design to prevent entrance of arthropods. Special handwashing sinks. Closed and sealed windows. Self-locking, self-closing access doors. Autoclave. Specific HVAC requirements for ventilation, filtration, and air-pressure balance.
Level 4— Maximum Containment Facility	Class III cabinets or Class I or II cabinets plus one-piece, positive-pressure ventilated suits.	Same as Level 3, but should be a separate building, isolated and marked. Inner and outer change/showing rooms, air locks, sealed floors, walls and ceilings resistant to liquids and chemicals. Double-door autoclaves. Provision for filter isolation of sewer and ventilation lines. Minimize dust-collecting flat surfaces. Foot- or elbow-operated handwashing sink. Isolation of central vacuum and other services. Special arrangements for water, including backflow prevention. Treatment of liquid effluents, special air systems with alarms, and microbial filtration.

whose products come under FDA regulation will find that regulations on good manufacturing practices, product sterilization, and sterility testing in many ways will dictate required design features of the research and manufacturing facility.

Also, guidelines for biosafety in microbiologic and biomedical laboratories handling infectious organisms and safety during genetic manipulations exist.

Although these guidelines originally were developed by different committees, they have been combined to define 4 biosafety and containment levels (USPHS, 1984). The approach is to equate facility design and equipment for containment to varying levels of risk created by laboratory operations.

Table 55–1 defines the levels of containment and indicates the recommended types of equipment and facilities.

CONCLUSIONS

The physical facility in which sterilization, disinfection, or preservation activities are being carried out is important to the success of these operations. Environmental control to eliminate or reduce the ingress or egress of microbial contamination is best arrived at by a combination of primary and secondary barriers, where the primary barrier is the enclosure most immediately around the procedure and the secondary barrier is the control added by the features of the building.

This chapter contains a number of suggestions related to planning such a facility and the identification and selection of primary and secondary barriers. Two additional areas that are needed in a well founded facility with microbial contamination control objectives were not covered. There must be valid methods of monitoring the physical and biologic aspects of the environment, and there must be a training and management program to control and standardize the specific techniques and procedures carried out by the human occupants of the facility.

REFERENCES

Barkley, W.E. 1981. Containment and Disinfection. In *Manual of Methods for General Bacteriology*. Am. Soc. Microbiol., pp. 487–503.

Collins, C.H. 1988. *Laboratory Acquired Infections*. 2nd Edition. London, Butterworth & Co.

Guidelines for Research Involving Recombinant DNA Molecules. National Institutes of Health, November, 1980.

National Sanitation Foundation Standard 49, 1976. Class II (Laminar Flow) Biohazard Cabinetry. Ann Arbor, Michigan.

OSHA, 1984. Occupational Exposure to Ethylene Oxide. Final Standard, CFR 29, 1910.19. Washington, D.C., Government Printing Office.

Phillips, G.B., and Brewer, J.H. 1968. Recent advances in microbiological environmental control. Dev. Ind. Microbiol., 9, 105–121.

Phillips, G.B., and Runkle, R.S. 1973. *Biomedical Applications of Laminar Airflow*. Cleveland, CRC Press.

Proposed Biosafety Guidelines for Microbiological and Biomedical Laboratories. Center for Disease Control, Atlanta, Georgia.

Runkle, R.S., and Phillips, G.B. 1969. *Microbial Contamination Control Facilities*. New York, Reinhold Book Corporation.

21 Code of Federal Regulations, Parts 210, 211, and 820.

USPHS, 1984. CDC/NIH. Biosafety in Microbiological and Biomedical Laboratories. Washington, D.C., Government Printing Office.

Wedum, A.G., Hanel, E., Jr., and Phillips, G.B. 1956. Ultraviolet sterilization in microbiological laboratories. Public Health Rep., 71, 331–336.

CHAPTER 56

MARKETING OVERVIEW OF SPECIALTY BIOCIDES

Anthony J. Marisca

The terms performance chemicals and specialty chemicals often have been used interchangeably by the chemical industry. Simply defined, performance chemicals are differentiated products sold to performance specifications for what they will do rather than to composition specifications for what they contain. In this regard, antimicrobial and specialty biocide products would fall into the area of performance chemicals.

Two categories of chemical products are classified as performance chemicals: pseudocommodities and specialty chemicals. Both are differentiated end products. Differentiated products cannot be characterized by chemical formulas or statement of chemical content alone, but are either produced with real differences between products of different suppliers or are marketed with imputed differences.

Pseudocommodities can be characterized as follows:

1. Synthesized (or, more rarely, formulated), in large volume, often from captive sources of raw material
2. Produced to generally accepted specifications of performance in several related end uses
3. Widely used but often sold chiefly to a relatively few large volume buyers

Examples of biocide pseudocommodities would be chlorine, sodium hypochlorite, ethylene oxide, formaldehyde, creosote and acid anionics.

Specialty chemicals are differentiated end products that are formulated or synthesized in low volume, generally from purchased raw materials, designed to solve specific customer problems, and often distributed to a relatively large number of small-volume buyers. Specialty chemicals are classified into three major groups: functional chemical products, multipurpose additives, and end-use additives. Biocides fall into the category of multipurpose additives because they perform a particular function, i.e., microbial control, in a variety of end-use industries ranging from leather tanning to plastics. Market estimates presented here involve only specialty bio-

cides and do not include commodity and pseudocommodity items.

PRODUCT CATEGORIES AND END-USES

Kline and Company, an international business consulting firm headquartered in Fairfield, NJ, has tracked and analyzed the specialty biocides business for nearly 20 years and has completed numerous proprietary and syndicated studies addressing various aspects of the biocides industry and its ultimate end uses. Market figures reported here have been developed for Kline's latest biocides annual service entitled *Specialty Biocides USA*.

There are over 130 different chemical compounds used as biocides with the greatest variety of materials classified as quaternary compounds. The other six major classifications are halogens, inorganics, nitrogen compounds, organometallics, organosulfurs, and phenolics. Each of these major types can be further subdivided, and the most significant products in each classification are shown in Figure 56–1.

In 1989, U.S. consumption of specialty biocides was estimated at $850 million at the manufacturers' level, equivalent to approximately 60% of the worldwide total of $1.5 billion. Much as with other specialty chemicals, biocides are sold on the basis of their performance in specific applications. Other similarities with the basic profile of specialty chemicals include high degree of technical service and marketing intensiveness, relatively low price competition, high profitability, and use by comparatively few customers in many different applications. In many applications biocides are essential for adequate performance of finished products, even though the consumer is unaware of their presence. In other applications, the biocide provides the primary function of the finished product (Messinger and Wittig, 1983).

In terms of sales volume, halogens are the largest group of biocides, primarily because of chloroisocyanurates, a group of products used as swimming pool sanitizers and industrial and institutional (I&I) cleaning com-

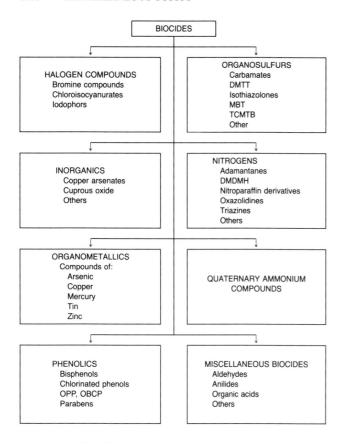

Fig. 56–1. Classification of specialty biocides by chemical group. Courtesy of Kline and Company, Fairfield, NJ.

pounds. Other products making up the halogen category include iodophors and bromine compounds. Sales of halogenated biocides were estimated at $210 million in 1989, with chloroisocyanurates accounting for nearly three-quarters of the total. Chloroisocyanurates are supplied by Monsanto and Olin domestically and are also available from a host of foreign suppliers, including Nissan, Shikoku, Sigma (Italy), and Delsa (Spain). The increased cost of chloroisocyanurates over inexpensive hypochlorites is offset by significant advantages in storage and formulation stability, ease of handling and dispensing, and improved solubility (Burakevich, 1979).

Halogenated hydantoin compounds produced domestically by Great Lakes Chemical and Lonza are crystalline compounds that hydrolyze in water to release halogens for biocidal activity. Hydantoins are one of the fastest growing segments of halogen biocides, offering improved performance and advantages in solubility and handling.

Organosulfur compounds range from such established generic items as methylene bisthiocyanate (MBT), thiocarbamates, and 3,5 dimethyl-tetrahydro-1,3,5-2H-thiadiazine-2-thione (DMTT or Thione) to proprietary compounds based on isothiazolones (Kathon, Proxel), pyrithiones (Omadine) and 2-(thiocyano-methylthio) benzothiazole (TCMTB). The superior performance of the newer proprietary products enabled this product group to achieve double-digit growth in the 1980s. In

1989, organosulfur compounds sales were estimated at $130 million, with isothiazolones and thiocyanates accounting for more than half the total.

The principal inorganic compounds used to control microorganism growth are the copper arsenates, used extensively in wood preservation. These high-volume products account for approximately 90% of the inorganic biocide market, estimated at roughly $100 million. Other inorganic products include cuprous oxide and barium metaborate, which are used primarily in paint applications.

Historically, chlorinated phenolics have been the most cost-effective biocides, but environmental concerns have dramatically reduced the consumption of these products. Chlorinated phenolics were used extensively in cooling water, paper, leather tanning, and metalworking fluids, but stringent government regulations have virtually eliminated their use in these industries. Wood preservation remains as the major application of pentachlorophenol. Other less toxic phenolic compounds include orthophenyl phenol (OPP) and orthobenzylchlorophenol (OBCP), used primarily as disinfectants, and hydroxybenzoic acid esters or parabens. Relative safety and ease of handling make parabens leading preservatives for cosmetic, pharmaceutical, food, and adhesive products. In 1989, the phenolic market was estimated at $75 million. Because of large volumes consumed for wood preservation, pentachlorophenol is the leading product, accounting for approximately half of the total.

Quaternary ammonium compounds (quats) became commercially significant as concerns regarding phenolics forced consumers to seek alternate products. The major application for quats is in formulated disinfectant cleaners. Other important uses include cooling water, swimming pools, and petroleum production. EPA reports that 211 registered technical-grade active-ingredient products contain varying concentrations of quats, each coded separately on the basis of alkyl chain length and percentage carbon distribution within the chain (EPA, 1988). Alkyl dimethyl benzyl ammonium chloride (AD-BAC) is the most widely used type of quat for various applications. Other popular quats include dialkyl dimethyl ammonium ("Dialkyls") and alkyl dimethyl/ethyl benzyl ammonium chlorides ("Duals"). Polymeric quaternary compounds are gaining favor for their low-foaming characteristics. In 1989, the quat market was estimated to be $70 million.

Similar to organosulfurs, nitrogen-based biocides consist of a wide variety of generic and proprietary chemistries. Most nitrogen compounds in this category can be described as formaldehyde condensate products (Rossmoore and Sondossi, 1988). Chemistries range from such cyclic compounds as triazines, oxazolidines, and azoniaadamantanes to such N-methylol derivatives as 1,3-dimethylol-5,5-dimethyl-hydantoin (DMDMH). Other nitrogen compounds include imadazolidinyl ureas and nitroparaffin derivatives. The wide selection of ni-

Table 56–1. *Estimated U.S. Consumption of Specialty Biocides by Chemical Class in 1989 (Manufacturer's Dollars)*

Class	$ Million	% of Total
Halogens	210	25
Organosulfurs	130	15
Inorganics	100	12
Nitrogen	70	9
Phenolics	75	9
Quaternaries	70	8
Organometallics	50	6
Miscellaneous	145	16
Totals	850	100

Courtesy of Kline and Company, Fairfield, NJ.

Table 56–2. *U.S. Consumption of Specialty Biocides by End Use in 1989 (Manufacturer's Dollars)*

End Use	$ Million	% of Total
Wood preservation	150	18
Swimming pools and spas	150	18
Food and feed preservatives	115	14
Paint	60	7
Disinfectants and sanitizers	60	7
Cosmetics and toiletries	60	7
Plastics	35	4
Paper	35	4
Hospital and medical antiseptics	35	4
Cooling water	30	4
Metalworking fluids	20	2
Petroleum production	20	2
Other*	80	9
Totals	850	100

*Includes latex, adhesives, slurries, pharmaceuticals, and leather.
Courtesy of Kline and Company, Fairfield, NJ

trogen-based biocides is used in many end-use applications, including paints and coatings, metalworking fluids, wood preservation, latexes, oil production, and cosmetics. In 1989, the nitrogen biocides market was estimated at $70 million.

Organic compounds of mercury, arsenic, tin, zinc, and copper are a small and generally specialized group of biocides. U.S. consumption of organometallic biocides was approximately $50 million in 1989. Over 60% of the market is attributed to 10,10′ oxybisphenoxarsine (OBPA), an arsenic compound used extensively in the plastic industry. Mercury and tin compounds including phenyl mercuric acetate (PMA) and tributyltin oxide (TBTO) continue to decline as a result of regulatory pressure. Copper compounds are used primarily in mildew-proofing of textile products. The only organozinc compound of importance is zinc undecylenate, used in such pharmaceutical applications as athlete's foot remedies.

The principal miscellaneous biocides are organic acids and their salts, anilides, and aldehydes. Organic salts include sorbates, benzoates, and propionates, which are used extensively for food preservation. Glutaraldehyde is used in various industrial applications including medical instrument sterilization, secondary oil recovery, cooling waters, and metalworking fluids.

U.S. consumption of specialty biocides by major chemical category is shown in Table 56–1.

APPLICATIONS

Of the total U.S. consumption of biocides, three applications account for 50% of the dollar value as well as a major portion of the physical volume. Wood preservation and swimming pool sanitizers are the largest end uses for specialty biocides, both estimated at $150 million. Food and feed preservation is the third largest application, accounting for $115 million or 14% of the total. These three end uses dominate the industry with large volumes of commodity-like chemicals. A summary of major biocide markets is shown in Table 56–2.

Biocides are most widely used in industrial applications to preserve the integrity of such finished products as paints, adhesives, latexes, and pigment slurries. Biocides used for preserving industrial products accounted

for an estimated $415 million in 1989, or 49% of the total. Industrial processes that require large volumes of water and organic matter are susceptible to microbial attack and employ biocides to increase process efficiency, protect equipment or structure, and even protect workers from pathogenic organisms. Such dynamic aqueous systems as cooling water towers, metalworking fluid sumps, papermaking machines, and secondary oil recovery processes are subject to continuous exposure to microorganisms and provide essential nutrients for their survival. Considerable amounts of biocides are used in these industries to enhance productivity. Overall, processing applications of specialty biocides accounted for $105 million in 1989, or 12% of the total. A third industrial application is direct disinfection and sanitization. Biocides are formulated into industrial and institutional disinfectants and sanitizers for use in general janitorial applications as well as the more demanding areas of food processing sanitization and health-care disinfection.

Such consumer products as cosmetics, food, and swimming pool chemicals account for 28% of all biocides sales as shown in Table 56–3.

SUPPLIERS

The U.S. market for biocides is diffuse and extremely fragmented with many suppliers. Large multinational

Table 56–3. *Applications of Specialty Biocides*

Application	$ Million	% of Total
Industrial		
Preservatives	415	49
Processing	105	12
Disinfection	95	11
Subtotals	615	72
Consumer	235	28
Totals	850	100

Courtesy of Kline and Company, Fairfield, NJ.

firms involved in diverse areas of the chemical industry are some of the major biocide suppliers. Generally, biocides constitute a relatively small but important business unit or product line for such multibillion-dollar giants as Monsanto, Dow Chemical, ICI, Bayer, Rohm and Haas, and Merck. Most companies supply one or two product groups based on a chemistry where they have an expertise in either agricultural or pharmaceutical chemistry. These companies have the resources, time, and expertise necessary to develop new antimicrobial products. Many suppliers of biocides do not produce these allied products but are producers of other chemicals. Included in this group are Lonza, Olin, Morton International, Huls, and Union Carbide. A third group consists of smaller companies, often privately held, which are successfully involved in biocides including Buckman Laboratories, Troy Chemical, and Stepan Company, among others.

Formulators play an important part in the distribution of biocides into such diffuse and fragmented industries as cooling water, paper, metalworking fluids, and I&I cleaners, which are populated by a large number of small-volume users. Selling direct to these customers would require a large sales force and often local or regional warehouses, which would be impractical for most biocide products. There are approximately 350 companies formulating biocides for the cooling water industry in the United States. These water service companies generally purchase biocides from a variety of suppliers and either blend, formulate, react, or otherwise modify them for specific needs of their customers. Smaller water management companies simply repackage the ready-to-use formulated products for resale. Major water treatment companies distributing biocides include Betz, Nalco, Calgon, Dearborn, and Mogul. Similarly, such metalworking fluid formulators as Quaker Chemical, Castrol, Cinncinati Milicron, and E.F. Houghten buy biocides directly from suppliers. These products are then blended into formulated cutting oils as well as supplied to end users for tankside addition. Phenolics, quats, iodophors, and chloroisocyanurates are formulated into disinfectants and sanitizers by such I&I cleaning products companies as EcoLab, Chemed, and Calgon-Vestal. Paper, petroleum, and swimming pools are other applications for which biocides are supplied to the end-use markets by formulators and distributors. Formulated biocides are usually part of a complete line of products offered by service companies to meet the requirements of their customers.

Biocide producers sell directly to industries where the biocide is used to preserve the integrity of a manufactured product. Such applications as paints and coatings, cosmetics, latex emulsions, and adhesives are serviced directly by biocide manufacturers who provide necessary technical service to support their products. In these industries, there are generally a few large consumers who purchase a major portion of the products plus many other smaller purchasers. To these customers, biocides are key raw materials, and technical service requirements are

very high. Technical skills required by biocide suppliers include in-depth knowledge of the customer's technology and processing, formulating know-how, and the microbiology affecting the finished product.

GOVERNMENT REGULATIONS

The sale of biocides in the United States is subject to a number of federal, state, and local regulations. In general, these regulations are intended to protect the consumer against exposure to potentially hazardous materials and to prevent damage to the environment and to wildlife.

The Federal Insecticide, Fungicide, and Rodenticide Act (FIFRA), originally passed in 1947, regulates the marketing of economic poisons, which are defined as any substance intended to control or destroy pests, including bacteria, fungi, and other microorganisms. Under the original law, federal control of pesticides focused primarily on the licensing of pesticide products intended for interstate shipments, adequate labeling directions for use, and warnings adequate for safe use. EPA enforces these codes by requiring product registration, efficacy testing, toxicity testing, and various other data. FIFRA has evolved substantially from the 1947 statute, with major amendments in 1972, 1975, 1978, 1980, and most recently in 1988. Other important legislation related to biocides include the Federal Water Pollution Control Act; the Food, Drug, and Cosmetic Act; the Federal Hazardous Substances Labeling Act; the Williams-Steiger Occupational Safety and Health Act; and various state and local regulations including California's Proposition 65 (Messinger and Wittig, 1983).

The bulk of the regulatory burden in the biocides industry is the responsibility of the suppliers of active material. Costs associated with regulatory compliance are a large barrier to entry for new biocide products. Unlike agricultural pesticides, which have greater market potential, biocide products generate relatively low revenues, and regulatory costs are not recouped quickly.

In 1987, EPA issued a Data Call-In Notice (DCI) for chronic and subchronic toxicologic data for antimicrobial pesticide active ingredients. Before this time, EPA required only acute toxicologic studies for biocide products, assuming exposure to antimicrobial products involved short-term exposure of low concentrations of active ingredients (EPA, 1987). EPA evaluations of potential hazards posed by biocides are now treated in the same manner as pesticides other than antimicrobials. The Antimicrobial Data Call-In of 1987 is basically unaffected by the FIFRA Amendments of 1988. The mammalian toxicology data developed for this Data Call-In will be used to support the re-registration of antimicrobials as outlined by the new amendment.

The focal point of the 1988 FIFRA Amendment is the acceleration of re-registration. Re-registration is the process of re-examining previously registered pesticides to ensure that they are supported by a complete database and that their use will not cause unreasonable adverse effects on man or the environment. Under the old FIFRA laws, it was estimated that EPA would not have completed the re-registration process until early in the next century. The amended bill outlines a plan that estimates completion in approximately 9 years.

The FIFRA Amendments of 1988 have placed greater burdens on registrants to maintain pesticide registrations. The additional costs involved in providing the details required are substantial, and it can be expected that these costs will be passed through the manufacturing and distribution chain, ultimately affecting prices at the end-users level. Biocide manufacturers are faced with significant costs to maintain registrations of products that do not generate the volume and revenue that agricultural pesticides earn. As a result, it is expected that many marginal biocide products will be abandoned, thinning out the number of actives and formulations on the market.

Historically, environmental factors have had tremendous effects on the nature of the biocides industry. The concern of the hazards associated with phenolics and mercurials has reshaped the markets in wood preservatives, paints, disinfectants and sanitizers, and paper-making, to name a few. Traditional products have been replaced by newer chemistries, which have taken advantage of EPA mandates.

Today, there is rising concern of levels of formaldehyde in the workplace, jeopardizing the position of certain chemicals known as "formaldehyde-releasers."

Formaldehyde-releasers get their name from the proposed mechanism that in active material breaks down to liberate formaldehyde, which is biocidal to most microorganisms. The actual levels of formaldehyde that are released are small and still subject to debate. These products are used in various end-uses, including metalworking fluids, paints, pigments, and latexes. The controversy surrounding these chemicals has allowed other suppliers of "non-formaldehyde release" products to penetrate the marketplace. Such products as Rohm & Haas' Kathon, ICI's Proxel, Troy's Polyphase, and Angus' Bioban line have capitalized on their unique chemistries and have begun to replace the formaldehyde releasers as the biocides of choice in certain industries.

Recently, EPA has issued regulations restricting the continued use of tributyltin (TBT) compounds, which are used primarily as marine antifoulants. Antifouling agents inhibit growth of organisms on ship bottoms and other surfaces that are partially or totally submerged for extended periods. A wide variety of biocides have been tried as antifoulants, but the market is dominated by cuprous oxide and TBT compounds. Cuprous oxide is more widely used because it is relatively economical and efficient, but TBT provides better protection and is more easily formulated with colors. The EPA has determined that TBT is extremely toxic and is potentially fatal to aquatic organisms at parts-per-trillion concentrations. The restrictions imposed by the new regulations will primarily affect the use of paints for recreational boats, which account for a minor part of the antifoulant market.

In 1990, a reported case of mercury poisoning of a four-year-old child in Michigan prompted EPA to re-examine the use of mercury compounds in paints. As a result of this study, EPA and the registrants of mercury paint preservatives have agreed to eliminate the use of mercury in interior paints. Additionally, exterior paints formulated with mercury biocides are required to include a warning label stating the presence of mercury.

R&D AND PRODUCT DEVELOPMENT

Research and development of industrial biocides can be better described as development and research. The exorbitant costs involved in discovering novel biocides prohibits manufacturers from devoting dollars to pure research. Basic "molecule bending" is left to the pharmaceutical and agricultural industries, where revenues can provide funds necessary for basic research. In the biocides industry, development is key. Laboratories focus on improving existing products and formulations and emphasizing technical service to customers. It is estimated that R&D expenditures account for 4.5 to 5% of sales. Expenditures are increasing because of the toxicology studies required by the EPA's Data Call-In.

Another means of product development is through screening of chemicals purchased from pharmaceutical and agricultural laboratories. These compounds are tested for antimicrobial efficacy, and promising candidates are further developed. This is an economical alternative for biocides manufacturers to explore new active ingredients.

OPPORTUNITIES

In 1990, the specialty biocides industry began to exhibit changes that typify the competitive environment of a mature business. Limited growth increases competition for market share, and experienced end users enjoy a stronger buying position. As a result, firms will seek differentiation through technical service. Industry growth stage is marked by rapid introduction of new products and applications. In the late 1970s and early 1980s, such new biocide products as Kathon (Rohm and Haas), DBNPA (Dow Chemical), Polyphase (Troy), and glutaraldehyde (Union Carbide) experienced healthy growth at the expense of phenolics, mercurials, and less effective chemistries. As the industry matures, established technologies reduce the likelihood of new products entering the market. Regulatory constraints are much more stringent in today's business environment, adding to the barriers to entry and further reducing growth potential.

Opportunities to enter or expand operations in the biocides market have resulted from a variety of factors, including the need for more effective biocides in applications in which currently available products need improvements in efficacy or cost effectiveness. Industries in which human exposure to biocides is high seek less-toxic biocides where efficacy can be sacrificed for safety, or where legislation may restrict the more-toxic products. Conversely, certain markets will welcome improved performance in applications in which biocide costs account for a small portion of a product's manufacturing expenditures or a particular biocide is a critical component of the final product.

The diversification of product lines will be a key factor to future success in a mature market. With the constraints involved in research and development, companies will tend toward acquisitions as a means to expansion. Several important acquisitions were completed in the 1980s that helped to concentrate the industry. In many cases, the acquiring firm was able to build on an established technology base, using an acquired product line to expand market strengths.

Lonza Inc., the leading supplier of germicidal quaternary compounds, headquartered in Fairlawn, NJ, fortified its leading position in the specialty chemicals area with acquisitions of Bio-Lab in 1979, Rohm and Haas' Hyamine line of quaternary compounds in 1984, and Glyco Inc. in 1985. These acquisitions enabled Lonza to become a dominant supplier of specialty biocides for Industrial and Institutional, personal care, and swimming pool chemicals. In 1988, Angus Chemical Company of Northbrook, IL, the primary producer of nitroparaffins and their derivatives, acquired Abbott Laboratories' industrial biocide business, including its flagship product line, Amical. This purchase allows Angus greater penetration into the coatings and adhesives businesses with a non-nitroparaffin product. Stepan Company, located in Northfield, IL, became a supplier of biocide products with the 1986 acquisition of Onyx Chemical of Millmaster Onyx, a major supplier of quaternary ammonium compounds. The addition of Onyx's line of cationic surfactants complemented Stepan's position as a leading producer of surfactants and specialty chemicals. Other important acquisitions occurring in the biocide industry in the 1980s include GAF's purchase of Sutton Laboratories (1989), Olin's acquisition of FMC's chloroisocyanurate business (1985), and Cambrex's buyout of Cosan Chemical (1985).

Another means for better strategic position is through corporate reorganizations. Morton International restructured its Ventron Division, combining two business units, Ventron, the leading supplier of biocides for synthetic polymers, and Carstab, manufacturer of specialty chemicals for the plastics industry. As a result of this merger, Ventron is now a full-service plastics additive supplier, much like its competitors, Akzo and Ferro.

When Ventron's patent on formulated liquid OBPA expired in 1984, its position as the leading plastics biocide supplier was threatened. To counter the presence of new sources of OBPA, Ventron continues to develop and patent new formulations of the arsenic-based active material. By examining different plastic materials and testing their susceptibility to microbial attack, Ventron has developed new products that are compatible with various plastic formulations, protecting its position in the market place.

FOREIGN COMPETITION

In Western Europe, the large multinationals control approximately 80% of the biocides business. These firms also are involved in basic pharmaceutical and agricultural research, which may provide serendipitous discovery of new biocidal actives. The remaining 20% of the business is highly fragmented, consisting of a large number of formulators of either biocides or products for specific end-use applications.

The largest entry barrier facing foreign firms is EPA compliance. Like U.S. firms, internationals attempting entry into the U.S. market are frustrated by the extensive requirements needed for EPA registration. In the past, foreign manufacturers attempted to introduce new biocides in the United States, but decided to abandon efforts as a result of EPA requirements.

International companies have successfully used acquisitions to enter the valuable U.S. market. Huls AG, Akzo Chemicals, and LaPorte Industries became significant competitors in the biocide industry by acquiring established U.S. concerns. In 1985, Huls AG acquired Nuodex, Inc., a supplier of coatings and vinyl additives including an extensive biocide product line, giving the German specialty chemicals manufacturer a base for expanding its U.S. businesses. The 1987 acquisition of Stauffer's specialty chemicals business expanded Akzo's biocide product line to include such technical grade organosulfurs as MBT, DMTT, sulfones, and folpet. In 1987, LaPorte Industries purchased Vinings Chemical of Atlanta, GA, a basic producer of organosulfur compounds used for paper and water treatment.

FUTURE OUTLOOK

Overall growth in biocide consumption depends principally on (1) growth of the end-use industries, (2) government regulations, (3) consumer preference, and (4) development of new technology. It is expected that in the 1990s biocides will grow at an overall rate equal to GNP growth. Wood preservation will be an interesting segment, as new products enter the industry in response to government restrictions on creosote and pentachlorophenols. As more and more paper mills convert to alkaline processing, increased demand for more tolerant biocides will spur above-average growth in this booming end-use market. New areas of antimicrobial applications include hydrocarbon fuels and household cleaning products. Industries that are labeled as low-growth areas for specialty biocides include disinfectants and sanitizers and leather biocides.

The development of many new active biocide ingredients is unlikely because of the rising costs of research and regulatory compliance. Therefore, suppliers will continue to develop new formulations and applications of existing products. Technical service will be key, because formulators and end-users will rely on basic producers for input and assistance concerning formulations, microbiology, and registration compliance with a high degree of expertise and confidentiality.

To assure continued success in the specialty biocide market, industry competitors, including basic suppliers and formulators, should emphasize enhancing their ability to help customers reduce costs, improve quality, and respond to market challenges. Improving these areas will require a greater interaction between the research and development, technical service, and marketing groups of an organization. Lastly, access to timely and objective information on target market dynamics, customer needs and perceptions, and company image will help shape a successful strategic marketing plan.

ACKNOWLEDGMENTS

Appreciation is expressed to acknowledge the contributions of the following people: Joseph V. Tarantola, Vice President, Kline & Company, Inc., and Sandra L. Pisek, Administrative Assistant, Kline & Company, Inc.

BIBLIOGRAPHY

Burakevich, J. 1979. Cyanuric and isocyanuric acids. In *Kirk-Othmer Encyclopedia of Chemical Technology.* 3rd Edition. New York, Wiley Interscience. 397–409.

Ebner, L., et al. 1987. *Pesticide Regulation Handbook.* Revised Edition. Washington, D.C., Executive Enterprise Publications.

EPA. 1988. Pesticide Registration Notice 88–2. Washington, D.C., Environmental Protection Agency.

Greene, J.L. 1989. Regulation Pesticides: FIFRA Amendments of 1988. Washington, D.C., Bureau of National Affairs.

Messinger, A.R., and Wittig, W.F. 1983. Specialty Biocides: A Profile of High Performance Chemicals. Chemical Purchasing, Denver, Cahners Publishing, p. 29.

Rossmoore, H.W., and Sondossi, M. 1988. Applications and mode of action of condensate biocides. Adv. Appl. Microbiol., 33, 233.

Specialty Biocides. 1979. Kline and Company, Fairfield, NJ.

Specialty Biocides. 1984. Kline and Company, Fairfield, NJ.

Specialty Biocides USA Annual Service. 1988 and 1989. Kline and Company, Fairfield, NJ.

PART IX

Methods of Testing

CHAPTER 57

METHODS OF TESTING DISINFECTANTS

A. Cremieux and J. Fleurette

When developing a method of disinfectant testing, the scientist is faced with contradictory criteria. The technique selected must be precise, reproducible, and standardized; microbial strains, inoculum, and culture conditions must be clearly defined; and materials must be described with precision. For interpretation of results, data (active concentration, period of activity, sensitive microbial strains) must be directly reproducible or at least must give sufficiently precise information.

The scientific and technical criteria just described must fit in with other elements. The method selected must be easy to reproduce routinely and to apply under various conditions. For instance, in industry it will be used to monitor the manufacturing and verification of a product; for the official testing laboratory it serves for complex formulation disinfectants; for the consumer it checks whether the product will be adequate for specific requirements. Any method that includes all these criteria must be inexpensive. Obviously, no method that takes into account such conflicting criteria exists at present. This is because of the variety of active compounds and formulations used, of organisms tested, and especially of application conditions of the disinfectants.

A rapid lethal antimicrobial effect is expected of disinfectants, because they are for practical use. Evaluation of inhibitory effect (e.g., bacteriostasis, fungistasis) can be useful in preliminary testing for active substances and mixtures. The bacteriostatic techniques are adequately standardized, and one can refer to those applied for antibiotics. This has led us to consider here only methods with lethal effects.

In spite of the numerous studies carried out in the virology laboratories, to our knowledge, no generally accepted methods of testing disinfectants on viruses have been established as yet. This is most unfortunate, considering the role of these infectious agents in human and animal pathology. However, recent technical improvements have been described and experimental standards have been proposed.

Bacterial spores are a special case. Because of their strong resistance to chemicals, physical procedures (heat, gamma rays) are required for their destruction. It must be mentioned, however, that standardized methods to determine the action of a preparation on bacterial spores do exist (Van Klingeren et al., 1977; AOAC, 1980; AFNOR 1981, NF T 72-230 and 72-231).

Because disinfectants are widely used in public health, veterinary medicine, the food industry, and many categories of commercial and industrial activities, the procedures for in-situ use are varied and specific. A number of regulations exist in certain fields of activity. This chapter describes solely the general laboratory methods of in-vitro testing of disinfectants and those that simulate certain conditions of use in situ.

HISTORY

Since the beginning of the twentieth century, a large number of scientific publications have been devoted to methods of testing disinfectants; however, most of them have done a critical evaluation and have proposed improvements on two techniques, one by Koch (1881) and the other by Rideal and Walker (1903). This is due in part to the evolution of communicable diseases. Before the antibiotic era, disinfectants and antiseptics played an important role in the prevention and treatment of infections. The role of phenol, introduced in therapeutics by Lister, was essential, and the new (and rare) disinfectant molecules had to prove their value through comparison with phenol, which was considered the reference standard.

The introduction of antibiotics in therapy raised hopes that were amply justified, and relegated disinfectants to the background in the fight against disease. With the partial failure of antibiotics, revealed by the selection of resistant strains and the onset of new disease provoked by opportunistic microorganisms, antisepsis and disinfection made a comeback. Moreover, the steady rise in hygiene standards in, for instance, the food industry, catering, swimming pools, and conference halls led the official agencies to require reliable methods for testing disinfectants. Because of this, the methods of testing are currently updated in parallel with the appearance of numerous new products.

Since the times of Pasteur, the methods of testing disinfectants have evolved along two parallel and complementary lines: development of in-vitro tests (specific activity of the product) and development of methods that simulate, in the laboratory, the conditions of practical use. The Rideal-Walker test (1903) determines the highest dilution of disinfectant required to kill an organism within specified time intervals and under rigorous conditions. The particularity of this broth dilution technique is that it uses phenol (5% concentration) as the reference disinfectant.

The efficiency of the disinfectant is not evaluated per se, but in relation to that of phenol, and thus the phenol coefficient of the tested product is determined. In spite of undeniable advantages (in particular, a relative standardization), the serious disadvantages of the Rideal-Walker method have rendered it unacceptable. The test organism used, *Salmonella typhi*, is no longer relevant and can contaminate the laboratory technicians. Certain conditions, such as organic matter and hard water, were not considered, and these can reduce disinfectant activity. During assessment of survivors, the disinfectant is diluted, but the residual bacteriostatic activity is not neutralized. Also, it is difficult to extrapolate from the results to the choice of useful or practical concentrations with a sufficient safety margin.

The major drawback, however, is the fact that phenol is compared with disinfectants whose active molecule, and hence mode of action, can differ widely. The role played by the concentration exponent is completely left out, and erroneous results may be obtained with products that have a high residual bacteriostatic action after dilution.

In consequence, some authors have proposed modifications to the phenol coefficient procedure. Chick and Martin (1908) and the original authors (Rideal and Walker, 1921) introduced organic matter (yeast extract). A new species, *Staphylococcus aureus*, was added to the test because of its role in hospital infections (British Standard 2462 1961—AOAC Phenol Coefficient Test). The Association of Agricultural Chemists (AOAC) test also introduced *Pseudomonas aeruginosa*. Since quaternary ammonium compounds could not be evaluated by the phenol coefficient because of their high-dilution bacteriostatic effect, a quantitative suspension test was developed that could be used later for any disinfectant; this test was reported in 1960 (British Standard 32 86).

Three bacterial species were tested (*Staphylococcus aureus, Escherichia coli,* and *Pseudomonas aeruginosa*) in the presence of organic matter (whole milk), at varying temperatures and at contact times of up to 30 minutes. A neutralizing agent was added to the subculture medium. However, evaluation of bactericidal effectiveness was not stipulated. Sykes (1962) and Kelsey and Sykes (1969) developed an adequate quantitative suspension

test that is applicable in hospitals and can be used for most products, although its reproducibility is limited.

Drawing from these tests, the Deutsche Gesellschaft für Hygiene und Mikrobiologie (DGHM) in 1972 described a so-called quantitative suspension test, and in 1974 the Dutch Committee on Phytopharmacy devised a quantitative suspension test. That same year, the Association Française de Normalisation (AFNOR) published the first French Standard for the determination of bactericidal activity using a dilution-neutralization method.

Robert Koch (1881) introduced the first method of testing disinfectants that simulates practical conditions. He impregnated silk threads with the spores of *Bacillus anthracis* and soaked them in disinfectant solution for varying periods; the threads were washed, then used for inoculating nutrient. Two deficiencies were observed: the spores were protected against the action of the disinfectant by the dried proteins derived from the medium, and a certain quantity of disinfectant remained on the threads even after washing, resulting in a residual bacteriostatic effect during subculture.

Following Koch, a number of studies were developed, all tending to establish methods that could corroborate the results obtained by the phenol coefficient method and determine the lowest concentration of product required to provide adequate disinfection in actual use. Several so-called "carrier" methods were published successively. One is the AOAC Use-Dilution method, with its successive amendments (Stuart et al., 1953), in which the carriers are metal rings, and the three following test strains are used: *Salmonella choleraesuis, Staphylococcus aureus,* and *Pseudomonas aeruginosa*. After incubation with the disinfectant, the carrier is transferred into a neutralizing medium, and the results obtained are of the pass-fail type. Large-scale testing of the same product provides a result within 95% confidence limits.

Other carrier methods have been described in Germany and France; the German method was modified by Reybrouck (1974). As increasing numbers of bactericidal sprays are being used for surface disinfection, experimental test methods have been established (AOAC Method of Testing Germicidal Spray Products, AFNOR method). A novel method was developed in 1965 by Kelsey et al., the capacity-use-dilution test, the aim of which was to estimate the disinfection capacity of a product by adding repeated increments of cultures. This experimental protocol was intended to simulate certain practical applications. Following numerous criticisms (Croshaw, 1981) the method was improved and a standard was published recently (British Standards, 1987).

Recently, after numerous preliminary studies, Reybrouck in Belgium and workers in Germany developed a new test, the in-vitro test, which is a quantitative, standardized, and reproducible suspension test (Reybrouck, 1975; Reybrouck et al., 1979). Independently, in 1974 a group of French microbiologists proposed standardized tests for disinfectants and antiseptics, published in 1981 in one volume. The revision of the AFNOR methods undertaken in 1987 led to the publication of new standards in 1987, 1988, and 1989.

Under the supervision of the Council of Europe, a number of laboratories in eight European countries published the results of a collaborative study on a quantitative suspension test for the evaluation of the antimicrobial activity of disinfectants in food hygiene. The recommended method is currently being tested by other laboratories for further evaluation.

PRINCIPLES OF PRESENT METHODS

The methods available at present were designed to meet three main objectives: (1) to allow evaluation of the effectiveness of water-miscible disinfectants (no standardized widely used method exists at present to test nonwater-miscible emulsions that have antimicrobial activity; these are used mainly in antisepsis), (2) to be available for testing of solutions of simple, elementary, or molecular substances or of complex formulations whose active product or products are associated with others that play a precise role in the activity of the end product (the evaluation of the specific role played by each of the constituents in the stability of the product is essential), and (3) to eliminate all residual bacteriostatic action during counting of surviving microorganisms. This essential technical step is in fact delicate, because it is often difficult to find adequate inactivating agents.

Analysis of Technical Factors

With a view to precision, exactitude, repeatability, and reproducibility, all the test conditions must be defined. They must take into account not only the two main elements, the microorganism and the disinfectant, but also the physicochemical factors that may interfere, such as transport conditions of product to site of action (Dony and Millet, 1973; Fleurette, 1988).

Microbial Strains

The number and type of representative strains of microbial species depend on the type of evaluation of the product, because for practical and financial reasons, it is not possible to test large numbers of strains. An overall test includes strains from the main bacterial groups, bacilli and cocci, gram-positive and gram-negative, and mycobacteria in certain standards. Yeast and fungi can also be used. It is sometimes useful to include microorganisms of different species involved in specific applications.

Strain Selection. Strains are selected from international collections; their genetic stability is checked regularly. The media for preservation procedures must be described with precision. In the case of large-scale use of disinfectants (e.g., in hospitals), it may be necessary to evaluate the sensitivity of bacterial species causing nosocomial infections. These species are often different from the proposed reference species: *Serratia spp.*, *Klebsiella spp.*, *Enterobacter spp.* For example, certain *Proteus* and *Providencia* species are intrinsically resistant to

chlorhexidine. For the mycobacteria, several species have been proposed: *Mycobacterium bovis*, *M. smegmatis*, and *M. tuberculosis*; a recent study proposed *M. terrae* (Van Klingeren, 1987).

Preparation of Inoculum. Culture medium (broth or agar) contains all the elements required for abundant growth of strains. In the absence of an adequate chemically defined medium, an empirically selected medium will be used; its components will be detailed, especially the source of peptones. The medium recommended for survivor assessment is often rich: 18- to 24-hour cultures have been found to be the most suitable. In some cases it is advisable to test the disinfectant on cultures at an exponential phase of growth. Certain methods recommend two or three subcultures in the same medium before the final test. Size of inoculum is an essential element of the technique. Reybrouck (1975) has shown that size varied greatly in each of the four methods he studied. In terms of number of bacteria per milliliter, inocula range from 3.16×10^5 to 5.02×10^7 for *Staphylococcus aureus* and from 6.3×10^5 to 7.94×10^7 for *Pseudomonas aeruginosa*. French Standards require 10^7 cells/ml for all strains.

The size of the inoculum must allow an assessment of survivors of significant statistical value. It is therefore important to specify beforehand the bactericidal (or fungicidal) level required for a disinfectant. In most methods, it corresponds to a minimum decrease of 10^5 in the initial inoculum.

Contact Conditions. Conditions of contact between microorganisms and disinfectant differ in the carrier and in the suspension methods. In the first case, controlled inoculum is added to the carrier and dried briefly. The disinfectant is then dropped on the carrier. Similarly prepared controls establish the spontaneous mortality of bacteria, especially gram-negative bacteria, under the influence of desiccation. In the suspension method, the liquid phase is used for contact; the disinfectant is diluted in distilled water. Bacterial suspension is done under conditions that are a compromise between conflicting requirements: because the distilled water and 8.5% saline solution are sometimes bactericidal, the suspension is prepared in peptonic water, in broth, or buffer. However, the presence of organic matter may interfere with the activity of the disinfectant. The other physicochemical factors must also be defined with precision.

Volume of Microbial Inoculum and Disinfectant. The influence of the volume ratio has not been studied and varies considerably from one technique to another. In general, inoculum volume is much smaller than that of disinfectant, except in carrier methods. It is essential that these volumes be measured precisely.

Influence of Temperature

The higher the activity of a disinfectant, the greater its sensitivity to changes in temperature; this is measured by temperature coefficient θ:

$$\theta (T_2 - T_1) = \frac{t_1}{t_2}$$

where t_1 and t_2 are duration of killing action at temperatures T_1 and T_2. Generally, coefficient θ_{10}, which corresponds to change in activity for a temperature variation of 10°C, is measured; however, the changes observed are valid for certain concentration and temperature margins only. The reaction temperature usually selected is +20°C.

Disinfectant Concentration and Contact Period

The activity of a disinfectant is proportional to its concentration and action time, according to a law established by Watson (1908):

$$C^n \times t = k$$

where C is the disinfectant concentration, t is the time required for lethal action, n is the concentration exponent, and k is a constant.

Although the concentration exponent is difficult to determine in practice, the principle of the relation is interesting: disinfectants with elevated concentration exponents have a poor safety margin. When diluted, their action time must be increased to retain the same activity. In practice, the latter criterion is important; certain disinfections must be carried out rapidly, and the product is therefore expected to have a rapid lethal action. That is why most of the in-vitro (suspension) methods have a 5- to 10-minute contact time. The carrier method contact times range from 5 to 360 minutes.

Interfering Substances

Electrolytes. For many weak acids, antimicrobial activity is linked to the undissociated molecule: hypochlorous acid is weakly dissociated at pH 5 (0.30%) and strongly dissociated at pH 9 (91%). Some industrial applications of disinfectants require the verification of efficiency at determined pH. The salts found in hard water have an effect on many disinfectants, especially those that form chelates with metallic ions. In other cases, the electrolytes, together with the disinfectant, form insoluble salts or an inactive complex. Consequently, with hard water, the use-concentration of those disinfectants ought to be increased, especially with the gram-negative bacteria (Crémieux, 1986).

Organic Matter. The reduction in disinfectant activity in the presence of organic matter is linked to complex physicochemical phenomena in which molecule reactivity (oxidants, reductants) and adsorption mechanisms are involved. These substances differ widely, but because they are often proteins, a number of tests employ yeast extract, or animal and human serum. The reproducibility of these tests is improved by using standardized products such as bovine albumin.

In industry, disinfectants are required for a variety of specific uses, and it is advisable to carry out the tests in the presence of existing interfering substances, even if their standardization is not possible at the time (Gelinas et al., 1983).

Other Interfering Substances. Besides the incompatibilities due to their specific components, disinfectants may be inactivated by macromolecules such as polyvinylpyrrolidone or other polymers and by surfactants. One must not forget the role played by detergents used for cleaning, the residues of which may modify considerably the activity of the surface disinfectants.

Elimination of Inhibitory Residual Disinfecting Activity

This fundamental step in the evaluation of the test method is usually difficult. Technically, three procedures are possible: dilution, neutralization, and washing.

Dilution alone is normally not sufficient to suppress the antimicrobial residual activity: quaternary ammonium compounds and heavy metallic salts may have a bacteriostatic activity against certain species, even when highly diluted.

Neutralization probably corresponds to a complex phenomenon. Sometimes it is a purely chemical neutralization (e.g., for thiosulfate and iodic compounds, thiol radicals, and mercurials) and sometimes the chemical reactivity of the molecules is not involved. The inactivating agents generally mentioned contain phospholipids, such as lecithin, or nonionic surfactants such as polysorbates and polyoxyethylene fatty alcohols (Bergan and Lystad, 1972; Crémieux et al., 1981; Reybrouck, 1979). Nonpolar groups on these molecules probably lead to uptake of antiseptics and disinfectants, which often possess lipophilic structures. It is advisable that the inactivating agent have no antimicrobial activity, although this is not systematically verified (Reybrouck, 1978).

Washing procedures imply mechanical separation of microbial cells and of disinfectant-containing suspension liquid; this can be done by centrifugation or by membrane filtration. Centrifugation must not alter cell viability, even of those cells that have become fragile following disinfectant action. It is generally easier to use membrane filtration. It is essential to check that there is no disinfectant uptake on the membrane that will later be transferred to culture medium and on which an inhibitory effect might persist.

Two or three of the procedures can be used in conjunction. In numerous methods, the disinfectant-microorganism mixture is diluted in a neutralizing agent. Membrane filtration normally requires several washings. Its efficacy in removing the disinfectant can be improved by adding inactivating compounds in washing fluid, but such an addition in the culture medium is not suitable because, in these conditions, the contact time is not exactly limited.

For testing virucidal activity, the same principles must be applied and complemented by a preliminary check of the aptitude of the host cells to multiply the viruses in presence of the residual concentration of the disinfectant.

Interassociation of Antimicrobials and Association with Other Types of Molecules (Detergents)

Most present-day disinfectants are complex formulations that associate several antimicrobial substances. This is done to result in a synergy or an addition of antimicrobial properties or to limit the toxicity or corrosion of materials.

Surface-active agents are commonly added to facilitate the solubilization of non-water-soluble substances and to provide stable emulsions. Moreover, simultaneous disinfection and cleaning are often required; a number of disinfectants have detergent properties that are due to surfactants. In numerous instances antimicrobial activity is highly modified. Sometimes bactericidal efficacy is improved, but more frequently there is a significant decrease in the activity, especially with nonionic and amphoteric surface-active agents (Gershenfeld and Stedman, 1949; Crémieux et al., 1983). This phenomenon has received more attention for antiseptic formulations in which the role of thickening compounds was pointed out (Crémieux, 1985). It involves numerous antimicrobials and all classes of surfactants. In such associations varying effects (inhibition or potentiation) may be observed, depending on the microbial species (Crémieux et al., 1983). It is likely that it occurs above a certain critical micellar phase, which reduces the con-

Table 57–1. *Principal Official Methods of Disinfectant Testing*

Country	Published by	Principal Methods and Types of Disinfectants
U.S.A.	AOAC 14th Edition 1984	Phenol-coefficient methods Use-dilution methods Chlorine (available) in disinfectants Fungicidal activity of disinfectants Germicidal and detergent sanitizing action of disinfectants Germicidal spray products as disinfectants Sporicidal activity of disinfectants Tuberculocidal activity of disinfectants Bacteriostatic activity of laundry-additive disinfectants Disinfectants (water) for swimming pools
France	AFNOR 1986	Methods of airborne disinfection of surfaces (NF T 72–281)
	1987	Bactericidal activity (NF T 72–150, NF T 72–151)
	1987	Fungicidal activity (NF T 72–200, NF T 72–201)
	1988	Sporicidal activity (NF T 72–230, NF T 72–231)
	1988	Bactericidal activity in the presence of specific interfering substances (NF T 72–170, NF T 72–171)
	1988	Germ-carrier method (NF T 72–190)
	1989	Suspension test (NF T 72–300, NF T 72–301)
	1989	Virucidal activity (viruses of vertebrates) (NF T 72–180)
	1989	Virucidal activity (bacteriophages) (NF T 72–181)
Germany	DGHM 1981	Bacteriostatic and fungistatic activities Bactericidal and fungicidal activities Influence of proteins and detergents Carrier method (bacteria, tuberculous bacilli, fungi) Control of disinfection of hands, clothes, surfaces Control of disinfection of tuberculous sputum, feces, instruments
U.K.	British Standards Institution 1960	Disinfectant activity of quaternary ammonium compounds (B.S. 3286)
	1984	Antimicrobial value of QAC disinfectant formulations (B.S. 6471)
	1985	Rideal-Walker coefficient (B.S. 541)
	1986	Modified Chick Martin Test (B.S. 808)
	1986	Antimicrobial efficacy of disinfectants for veterinary and agricultural use (B.S. 6734)
	1987	Modified Kelsey-Sykes Test (disinfectants used in dirty conditions in hospitals—B.S. 6905)
Netherlands	Dutch Committee of Phytopharmacy	5-5-5 Suspension Test Method (bactericidal, fungicidal, sporicidal activity)
European Countries	Council of Europe 1987	Test methods for the antimicrobial activity of disinfectants in food hygiene

Table 57–2.

Method and Reference		Phenol Coefficient Methods AOAC 1984 Suspension Test	Use-Dilution Method AOAC 1984 Germ-Carrier Test
Objective		Bactericidal activity compared to phenol	Maximum dilutions effective for practical disinfection—to confirm phenol coefficient results
Preliminary Conditions		Disinfectant miscible with water The bacteriostatic effects can be neutralized by the subculture medium or overcome by suitable sub-transfer procedures	Disinfectant miscible with water
Strains		*Salmonella typhi* ATCC 6539 *Staphylococcus aureus* ATCC 6538 *Pseudomonas aeruginosa* ATCC 15442 (Preliminary check of resistance to phenol)	*Salmonella choleraesuis* ATCC 10708 ⎫ Final action *Staphylococcus aureus* ATCC 6538 ⎭ *Pseudomonas aeruginosa* ATCC 15442—First action
Inoculum		Broth culture obtained under specific conditions	The carriers are immersed in broth culture obtained under specified conditions.
Experimental Test Conditions	Contact Time and Temperature	5, 10, and 15 minutes 20°C	5, 10, 15 minutes 20°C
	Interfering Substances	Organic matter from broth	Organic matter from broth
	Germ Carriers		Stainless steel cylinders
Elimination of Disinfectant		None or possibility of neutralizing medium —fluid thioglycollate medium —letheen broth	None or possibility of neutralizing media —fluid thioglycollate medium —letheen broth
Subculture		Transfer with a calibrated loop into the medium and incubation 48 hours at 37°C—macroscopic and occasionally microscopic examination of growth.	Transfer of the carrier into medication tube with medium (48 hours of 37°C) If a bacteriostatic effect is suspected, transfer the carrier into a new tube of sterile medium 30 minutes after initial transfer, and incubate the two subcultures.
Interpretation		Phenol-coefficient number: ratio of (greatest dilution killing test organisms in 10 minutes but not in 5) to (greatest dilution of phenol giving the same results)	Safe use-dilution: maximum dilution that kills test organism on ten carriers in 10-minute intervals

Table 57–3.

Method and Reference		Chlorine (available) in disinfectants AOAC 1984 Capacity Test
Objective		Bactericidal activity of available chlorine of the disinfectant compared to a standard solution of hypochlorite
Strains		*Salmonella typhi* ATCC 6539 *Staphylococcus aureus* ATCC 6538 (Preliminary check of resistance to phenol and simultaneous check of resistance to NaOCl)
Inoculum		Broth culture obtained under specified conditions
Experimental Test Conditions	Contact Time	The capacity test requires ten additions of inoculum at 1.5 minute intervals and a subculture 1 minute after each addition (ten subcultures)
	Interfering Substance	Organic matter from broth
Elimination of Disinfectant		None or possibility of neutralizing media —fluid thioglycollate medium —letheen broth
Subculture		Transfer with a standard loop into the medium Incubation 48 hours at 37°C
Interpretation		Compare the activity of the disinfectant to disinfecting activity of 200, 100, and 50 ppm available chlorine. Determine germicidal equivalent concentration.

Table 57–4.

Method and Reference		Fungicidal Activity AOAC 1984 Suspension Test
Objective		Fungicidal activity
Strains		*Trichophyton mentagrophytes* isolated from dermatophytosis ATCC 9533 (with simultaneous control of resistance to phenol)
Inoculum		Conidial suspension from agar plate culture prepared under specified conditions and stored at 2° to 10°C. (5×10^5 conidia/ml in the assay)
Experimental Test Conditions	Contact Time and Temperature	5, 10, and 15 minutes 20°C
Elimination of Disinfectant		None or neutralizing medium
Subculture		Transfer with a calibrated loop into the medium. Subtransfer into a new tube of medium if fungistatic activity is suspected. Incubation 10 days at 25° to 30°C.
Interpretation		The highest dilution that kills spores within 10 minutes is considered effective for disinfection of inanimate surfaces

Table 57–5.

Method and Reference			Germicidal and Detergent Sanitizing Action of Disinfectants AOAC 1984 Suspension Test
Objective			Bactericidal activity of the disinfectant diluted in hard water. The hard-water tolerance is checked with reference quaternary compounds.
Strains			*Escherichia coli* ATCC 11229 *Staphylococcus aureus* ATCC 6538 (Preliminary check of resistance to phenol)
Inoculum			Spectrophotometer-adjusted suspension of agar culture giving 10×10^9 organisms/ml
Experimental Test Conditions	Contact Time and Temperature		30 and 60 seconds 25°C
	Interfering Substances		Synthetic hard water prepared and checked for hardness
Elimination of Disinfectant			Transfer into a neutralizer (Azolectin-Polysorbate) and subculture in a neutralizing agar medium.
Subculture			Inclusion in agar medium, including or not the neutralizer. Incubation 48 hours at 35°C. Confirm that surviving organisms are *E. coli* and *S. aureus*
Interpretation			The concentration giving 99.999% reduction in organism count in 30 seconds is considered effective.

Table 57–6.

Method and Reference		Germicidal Spray Products AOAC 1984 Carrier Test
Objective		Antibacterial and antifungal activity of sprays
Strains		*Trichophyton mentagrophytes* ATCC 9533 *Salmonella choleraesuis* ATCC 10708 *Staphylococcus aureus* ATCC 6538 *Pseudomonas aeruginosa* ATCC 15442 (Preliminary check of resistance to phenol)
Inoculum		0.01 ml of conidial suspensions of *T. mentagrophytes* or broth cultures of bacteria spread on slides and dried 30 to 40 minutes at 37°C
Experimental Test Conditions	Contact Time and Temperature	10 minutes Room temperature
	Interfering Substances	Organic matter from inoculum
	Germ Carriers	Microscopic slides (distances and time of spraying specified)
Elimination of Disinfectant		None
Subculture		Transfer of the slide into broth. Possible subculture in fresh tube if cloudy. Incubation of all cultures 48 hours at 37°C. If a bacteriostatic or fungistatic effect is suspected, check the fertility of the tube by inoculation of respective test culture and reincubate.
Interpretation		Killing of test organism in ten out of ten trials is presumptive evidence of disinfecting action.

Table 57–7.

Method and Reference		Sporicidal Activity AOAC 1984 Carrier Test
Objective		Sporicidal activity and potential efficacy as sterilizing agent
Preliminary Conditions		Applicable to liquids and gases
Strains		*Bacillus subtilis* ATCC 19659 *Clostridium sporogenes* ATCC 3584 Various spore-forming species: *B. anthracis, C. tetanis,* others
Inoculum		Spore suspension obtained under specified conditions and filtered. Carriers are immersed in the suspension, then dried. The resistance of dried spore to 2.5N HCl is determined.
Experimental Test Conditions	Contact Time and Temperature	Liquids: Immersion of the carriers at 20°C for the time specified Gases: Exposure of the carriers with rehydrated spores to gas for the time specified
	Interfering Substance	Organic matter from broth
	Germ Carriers	—Suture loop (size 3 surgical silk) —Penicylinders (porcelain)
Elimination of Disinfectant		Select medium containing the most suitable neutralizer and subtransfer into fresh fluid thioglycollate medium.
Subculture		Incubation of the subculture 21 days at 37°C. If no growth, heat the tubes 20 minutes at 80°C and reincubate 72 hours at 37°C.
Interpretation		According to the number of carriers and strains, and results: (1) sporicidal efficacy against one spore, (2) unqualified sporicidal efficacy, and (3) sterilizing efficacy, can be demonstrated.

Table 57–8.

Method and Reference		Tuberculocidal Activity AOAC 1984 Carrier Test	
Objective		I—Presumptive test for tuberculocidal activity	II—Confirmative test for determining tuberculocidal activity
Strains		*Mycobacterium smegmatis* PRD 1	*Mycobacterium bovis* BCG (Preliminary check of resistance to phenol)
Inoculum		Spectrophotometer-adjusted suspension from broth cultures obtained under specified conditions. Immersion of the carriers 15 minutes; drying under specified conditions.	
Experimental Test Conditions	Contact Time and Temperature	10 minutes 20°C	
	Interfering Substance	Gelatin from inoculum	Organic matter from inoculum
	Germ Carriers	Penicylinders (porcelain)	
Elimination of Disinfectant		None or by use of a neutralizer in the subculture medium	Transfer of the carrier into horse serum or into a suitable neutralizer
Subculture		Transfer of the carrier into broth tubes. Incubation 12 days at 37°C	Transfer of carrier into broth tubes. Subculture in broth, of portions horse serum or neutralizers. Incubation 60 days at 37°C. If no growth, incubate 30 days more before final reading.
Interpretation		Calculate for the three dilutions of disinfectant the percentage of carriers (30) on which organism is killed. Using log % probit paper, draw a line through the three points and extend to 99% kill line. The corresponding dilution is the presumed 95% confidence end point.	The maximal dilution killing the test organism on ten carriers represents the safe use-dilution for practical tuberculocidal disinfection.

Table 57–9.

Method and Reference		Disinfectants (water) for Swimming Pools AOAC 1984 Suspension Test
Objective		Bactericidal activity compared to hypochlorite
Strains		*Escherichia coli* ATCC 11229 *Streptococcus faecalis* PRD
Inoculum		Spectrophotometer-adjusted suspension from agar cultures obtained under specified conditions (10^6 cells/ml in presence of disinfectant)
Experimental Test Conditions	Contact Time and Temperature	0.5, 1, 2, 3, 4, 5, and 10 minutes 20° or 25°C
	Interfering Substance	None
Elimination of Disinfectant		Transfer into suitable neutralizer (thiosulfate, azolectine, other)
Subculture		Subculture into agar medium and broth. Incubation 48 hours at 37°C
Interpretation		The lowest concentration of disinfectant providing results equivalent to those of NaOCl solution (containing ≥ 0.58 but ≤ 0.62 ppm available chlorine at zero time and < 0.4 ppm after 10 minutes) is considered effective.

Table 57–10. *AFNOR Methods for Testing Antiseptics and Disinfectants (applies to Tables 57–11 through 57–18)*

1. Basic tests to qualify the antiseptic or the disinfectant
   as bactericidal—(NF T 72-150 and 72-151)
   as fungicidal—(NF T 72-200 and 72-201)
   as sporicidal—(NF T 72-230 and 72-231)
   as virucidal—(NF T 72-180 and 72-181)
   At the present state, these virucidal test methods allow the determination of the use-concentration of antiseptics and disinfectants.
2. Basic tests for bactericidal activity in presence of interfering substance and determination of use-concentration for common use (NF T 72-170 and 72-171).
3. Tests aimed at determining the use-concentrations and required time of application (for bacteria, yeasts and molds, and bacterial spores)
   germ carrier-test—NF T 72-190
   germ carrier-test—NF T 72-281
   suspension tests—NF T 72-300 and 72-301

centration available for fixation on microorganisms (Russel, 1981).

Determining Virucidal Activity

Determination of virucidal activity consists of measuring the loss of infective titer of a viral suspension under the effect of a disinfectant at a given concentration and temperature during a given time (AFNOR, 1985, 1986; Bundesgesundheitsamtes and Deutschen Vereinigung zur Bekämpfung der Viruskrankheiten, 1982). The viral infective potency is determined by the cytopathic effect observed on eukaryotic cells in culture or by the lytic effect of bacteriophages on host bacteria.

Most (if not all) of the disinfectants are more or less toxic for living cells. Even at infracytotoxic concentration, they can modify the structure of the cell membrane and therefore alter viral penetration in the cell.

The most difficult steps in the method are to neutralize the effect of the disinfectant after its contact with the viral suspension and to ensure that there is no virucidal residual activity as well as no infracytopathic effect. Various methods are proposed to reach this objective (Garrigue et al., 1984; Quéro et al., 1984; Damery et al., 1986). The choice of viral species is debatable. Animal viruses are the most representative for the purpose of hospital disinfection but they are sometimes difficult to produce in large amounts; certain bacteriophages are easier to produce and more stable. In addition they can be used in screening tests and in industrial applications.

Another approach has been proposed and consists of testing disinfectant activity on viral structural components such as hepatitis B Virus HBS antigen or enzymatic activities such as those of DNA polymerase or reverse transcriptase.

TYPES OF METHODS

Taking into account the restrictions mentioned in the introductory paragraph, one may classify the methods of testing disinfectants into two main categories.

Table 57–11.

Method and Reference	Dilution-Neutralization AFNOR NF T 72-150 (1987) Suspension Test	Membrane Filtration AFNOR NF T 72-151 (1987) Suspension Test
Objective	Classification as bactericidal	
Strains	*Pseudomonas aeruginosa* CIP A 22 *Escherichia coli* (ATCC 10536) *Staphylococcus aureus* ATCC 9144 *Enterococcus faecium* ATCC 10541 } Spectrum 4 *Mycobacterium smegmatis* CIP 7326	} Spectrum 5
Inoculum	Spectrophotometer-adjusted suspension of agar culture obtained under specified conditions. Number of viable cells in presence of antiseptic or disinfectant: 1–3 × 10^7/ml	0.5–1.5 × 10^7/ml
Contact Time and Temperature	5 minutes 20°C	
Elimination of Antiseptic or Disinfectant	Transfer of microorganism-disinfectant mixture into suitable neutralizer determined by preliminary test	Transfer of microorganism-disinfectant mixture into filtration apparatus. Wash under conditions defined by preliminary test with possible use of neutralizer
Count of Survivors	Survivor count in the neutralized mixture by inclusion in agar medium Incubation at 37°C for 48 hours (7 days for *M. smegmatis*)	Membrane placed on agar medium Incubation at 37°C for 48 hours (7 days for *M. smegmatis*)
Interpretation	Determine if the antiseptic or disinfectant is able to reduce by at least 10^5, in 5 minutes, at 20°C, the number of cells of each of the four or five strains. According to the results, the disinfectant is classified as bactericidal Spectrum 4 or bactericidal Spectrum 5.	

Table 57–12.

Method and Reference	Dilution-Neutralization AFNOR NF T 72-200 (1987) Suspension Test	Membrane Filtration AFNOR NF T 72-201 (1987) Suspension Test
Objective	Classification as fungicidal	
Strains	*Absidia corymbifera* CIP 1129-75 *Cladosporium cladosporioides* CIF 1232-80 *Penicillium verrucosum* var. *cyclopium* CIP 1231-80 *Candida albicans* ATCC 2091	
Inoculum	Suspensions adjusted by microscopic count, obtained from agar cultures according to strains and under specified conditions. Number of viable micromycetes cells in presence of disinfectant or antiseptic: 1–3×10^6/ml	0.5–1.5×10^6/ml
Contact Time and Temperature	15 minutes at 20°C	
Elimination of Antiseptic or Disinfectant	Transfer of microorganism-disinfectant mixture into suitable neutralizer determined by preliminary test	Transfer of microorganism-disinfectant mixture into filtration apparatus. Washing under conditions defined by preliminary test with possible use of neutralizer.
Count of Survivors	Inclusion in agar medium	Membrane placed on agar medium
	4-day incubation at 24°C (72 hours at 30°C for *C. albicans*, 40 to 70 hours at 30°C for *A. corymbifera*	
Interpretation	Determine if the disinfectant is able to reduce by at least 10^4 in 15 minutes at 20°C the number of fungi spores or yeast cells of each of the four strains. According to the results, the disinfectant is classified as fungicidal.	

Table 57–13.

Method and Reference	Dilution-Neutralization AFNOR NF T 72-230 (1988) Suspension Test	Membrane Filtration AFNOR NF T 72-231 (1988) Suspension Test
Objective	Classification as sporicidal	
Strains	*Bacillus cereus* CIP 7803 *Bacillus subtilis* var. *niger* ATCC 9372 *Clostridium sporogenes* 51 CIP 7939	
Inoculum	Titrated suspensions of spores obtained from cultures prepared under specified conditions. Number of viable spores in presence of disinfectant: 1–3×10^7/ml	
Contact Time and Temperature	1 hour at 20°C or 5 minutes at 75°C	
Elimination of Disinfectant	Transfer of microorganism-disinfectant mixture into suitable neutralizer as determined by preliminary test	Transfer of microorganism-disinfectant mixture into filtration apparatus. Washing under conditions defined by preliminary tests with possible use of neutralizer.
Subculture	Inclusion in agar medium	Membrane placed on agar medium
	72 hours incubation at 30°C (in anaerobiosis and at 37°C for *C. sporogenes*)	
Interpretation	Determine if the disinfectant is able to reduce by at least 10^5, in 1 hour at 20°C or 5 minutes at 75°C, the number of bacterial spores of the three strains. According to the results, the disinfectant is classified as sporicidal.	

Table 57-14.

Method and Reference		AFNOR NF T 72-180 (1989)	AFNOR NF T 72-181 (1989)
Objective		Virucidal Activity (Animal Viruses) Classification as virucidal and determination of the use-concentration	Virucidal Activity Toward Bacteriophages Classification as virucidal toward phages and determination of the use-concentration
Strains		Enterovirus Polio I (Sabin strain) and VERO cells Human Adenovirus, type 5, and KB cells Vaccinia virus and VERO cells	Phage T_2 and *Escherichia coli* B Phage MS_2 and *Escherichia coli* Hfrh Phage X 174 and *Escherichia coli* ATCC 13706 Phage n° 66 and Streptococcus lactis diacetylactis 1.l.56
Inoculum		Unpurified and titrated stock suspensions stored at $-80°C$. Titers required are 10^6 to 10^9 I.U./ml, and protein content is determined (Lowry method). Viral titer determined by cell suspension technique	Unpurified and titrated stock suspensions stored at $-18°C$ (at 4°C for a week) and diluted in broth to 10^9 PFU/ml for use
Experimental Test Conditions	Contact Time and Temperature	15, 30, 60 minutes at 20°C (32°C for antiseptics)	15 minutes at 20°C (disinfectants only).
	Interfering Substances	Organic matter from inoculum	Organic matter from inoculum
Elimination of Disinfectant or Antiseptic		Dilution or Gel-filtration methods are chosen in function of results of preliminary tests: —Subcytotoxic concentration of the disinfectant: maximal concentration allowing the cells to remain intact —Stop dilution: at the stop dilution, the disinfectant is ineffective on viruses —Efficacy of gel-filtration: in the filtrate, the disinfectant is ineffective on viruses	Dilution or neutralization plus dilution determined by preliminary test
Count of Survivors		—Count of surviving viruses by the technique used for inoculum titration (Preliminary check of aptitude of cells treated by the disinfectant in the experimental conditions of the method to multiply the virus)	—Plating of the treated phages-bacteria mixture on an agar medium and incubation at 37°C for 18 to 24 hours (Preliminary check of aptitude of bacterial cells treated by the disinfectant to multiply the phage)
Interpretation		Determine the lowest concentration required for the disinfectant to reduce by at least 10^4 in 15, 30 and 60 minutes at 20°C the viral count of each of the three viral strains. Retain as virucidal the highest of the three concentrations determined in this manner.	Determine the lowest concentration required for the disinfectant to reduce by at least 10^4 in 5 minutes at 20°C the PFU number of each of the four phages. Retain as virucidal toward bacteriophages the highest of the four concentrations determined in this manner.

Methods that Evaluate the Specific Activity of the Product

These techniques estimate the in-vitro bactericidal activity of the disinfectant under precise experimental conditions that take into account the parameters described in the preceding section. They are considered to be the primary methods and are generally suspension tests. A fixed volume of disinfectant solution is mixed with the bacterial suspension. After a defined contact time, the microbicidal capacity is evaluated using one of two possibilities: all or a sample of the mixture is subcultured in nutrient broth (the qualitative test), or survivors are counted in a sample of the mixture (the quantitative test). The latter test is now generally used, because it gives valuable information on the disinfectant and its killing rate. But the test implies that no residual bacteriostatic capacity remain when counting survivors. To attain this objective, two procedures are suggested: (1) dilution of disinfectant, combined with neutralization by one or by several given chemicals (neutralizers); the inactivation effect must be checked; and (2) membrane filtration of disinfectant-microorganism mixture, followed by washing in a fluid that does not attack the microorganisms and that may contain a neutralizer. The efficacy of the procedure must be checked.

In-Vitro Methods that Attempt to Simulate Conditions of Practical Applications of Disinfectants

The Kelsey-Sykes-Maurer capacity test is designed to estimate the ability of the disinfectant to destroy growing numbers of microorganisms in the presence or absence of organic matter. The most recent revised form of the capacity test is given in Table 57-22.

The carrier techniques attempt to reproduce surface disinfection conditions. Several conditions are reproduced, including direct application of liquid disinfectant

Table 57–15.

Method and Reference	Dilution-Neutralization AFNOR NF T 72-170 (1988) Suspension Test	Membrane Filtration AFNOR NF T 72-171 (1988) Suspension Test
Objective	Bactericidal activity in the presence of interfering substances. Determination of use-concentration for common use.	
Preliminary Conditions	The antiseptic or disinfectant must conform to test standards 72-150 or 72-151	
Strains	*Pseudomonas aeruginosa* CIP A 22 *Escherichia coli* ATCC 10536 *Staphylococcus aureus* Oxford ATCC 9144 } Spectrum 4 *Enterococcus faecium* ATCC 10541 *Mycobacterium smegmatis* CIP 7326 } Spectrum 5	
Inoculum	Spectrophotometer-adjusted suspension of solid medium culture obtained under specified conditions. Number of viable cells in presence of antiseptic or disinfectant: $1–3 \times 10^7$/ml	$0.5–1.5 \times 10^7$/ml
Experimental Test Conditions — Contact Time and Temperature	5 minutes 20°C	
Experimental Test Conditions — Interfering Substances	Albumin-yeast extract Hard water Buffer solution pH 5 Buffer solution pH 9 Any other possibly interfering substances	
Elimination of Antiseptic or Disinfectant	Transfer into suitable neutralizer determined during preliminary test	Transfer into filtration apparatus. Washing under conditions defined by preliminary test with possible use of neutralizer
Count of Survivors	Inclusion in agar medium	Membrane placed on agar medium
	Incubation at 37°C for 48 hours (7 days for *M. smegmatis*)	
Interpretation	Determine the lowest concentration required for antiseptic or disinfectant to reduce by at least 10^5, in 5 minutes, at 20°C, in the presence of interfering substances, the number of cells of each of the four or five strains. Retain as bactericidal concentration in the presence of the interfering substance (use-concentration for common uses) the highest of four of five concentrations determined in this manner.	

Table 57–16.

Method and Reference	Germ Carrier Test AFNOR NF T 72-190 (1988)
Objective	Bactericidal, fungicidal, and sporicidal activity for surface disinfection
Preliminary Conditions	The disinfectant must conform to test standards 72-150 or 72-230 or 72-151 (bactericidal); 72-200 or 72-201 (fungicidal); 72-231 (sporicidal)
Strains	4 or 5 bacteria strains as in 72-150 or 72-151 4 fungi strains as in 72-200 or 72-201 3 spore-forming strains as in 72-230 or 72-231
Inoculum	Adjusted suspension of solid medium culture obtained under specified conditions, or titrated spore suspension, diluted in skimmed milk Place on germ carrier—Dry at 37°C Number of viable cells on germ carrier $\geq 10^6$ (checked on control carriers kept at room temperature during testing)
Experimental Test Conditions — Contact Time and Temperature	15 minutes at room temperature Other times or temperatures to be precised
Experimental Test Conditions — Carriers	Watch glasses Steel disks Plastic carriers Any other
Experimental Test Conditions — Interfering Substances	Hard water and milk from inoculum
Elimination of Disinfectant	Dilution and membrane filtration under conditions defined by a preliminary test
Count of Survivors	Transfer of membrane and inclusion of germ carrier in agar Incubation at 37°C, as specified for each strain in standards mentioned above
Interpretation	Determine the lowest concentrations required for disinfectant to reduce by at least 10^5, 10^4, and 10^3, respectively, the number of bacteria, yeast and fungal spores, or bacterial spores of each of the tested strains. Retain as bactericidal, fungicidal, or sporicidal concentration for surface disinfection the highest of the various concentrations determined in this manner for each kind of microorganism.

Table 57–17.

Method and Reference	Germ Carriers Exposed to Vapor or Sprays AFNOR NF T 72-281 (1986)
Objective	Bactericidal, fungicidal, and sporicidal activity for airborne disinfection of surfaces
Preliminary Conditions	The method is applicable to both a disinfectant and an apparatus, and results concern the whole system
Strains	*Pseudomonas aeruginosa* CIP A 22 *Staphylococcus aureus* Oxford ATCC 9144 *E. faecium* ATCC 10541 *Bacillus subtilis* (spores) ATCC 6633 *Candida albicans* CIP 1180-79 *Penicillium verrucosum* var. *cyclopium* CIP 1186-79
Inoculum	Adjusted bacteria or yeast suspension, or titrated spore suspension from solid culture medium obtained under specified conditions, diluted in skimmed milk Place on germ-carrier, dry at 37°C Number of bacterial cells or spores on germ carrier: $\geqslant 10^6$ (checked on control carriers kept at room temperature during testing)

Experimental Test Conditions	Contact Time and Temperature	At the start: room at 21°C, relative humidity: 60% (other possible conditions to be precised) Contact time: Less than 12 hours
	Carriers	Watch glasses Any other support (avoid porous carriers)
	Interfering Substances	None, apart from milk in inoculum

Elimination of Disinfectant	Dilution and membrane filtration under conditions defined by a preliminary test
Subculture	Transfer of membrane and inclusion of germ carrier in agar. Incubation for 3 days at 37°C for bacteria and 30°C for yeast; 7 days at 24°C for mold
Interpretation	Determine contact time required to reduce, under test conditions, by at least 10^5, 10^4, and 10^3, respectively, the number of bacteria, yeast and fungal spores or bacterial spores of each of the tested strains. Retain as effective application time for bactericidal, fungicidal, and sporicidal effect the longest of times determined for each type of microorganism.

Table 57–18.

Method and Reference	Dilution-Neutralization AFNOR NF T 72-300 (1989) Suspension Test	Membrane Filtration AFNOR NF T 72-301 (1989) Suspension Test
Objective	Bactericidal, Fungicidal, and Sporicidal Activity with or without Interfering Substances. Determination of the use-concentration in specified conditions	
Preliminary Conditions	The disinfectant must conform to test standards —72-150 or 72-151 (bactericidal) —72-200 or 72-201 (fungicidal) —72-230 or 72-231 (sporicidal)	
Strains	Any strain or strains belonging to the panel of strains retained by the standards mentioned above	
Inoculum	Adjusted or titrated suspension obtained under specified conditions Number of viable cells in presence of disinfectant: $2 \pm 1 \times 10^7$/ml ($2 \pm 1 \times 10^6$ for fungi: $2 \pm 1 \times 10^5$ for bacterial spores)	$1 \pm 0.5 \times 10^7$/ml ($1 \pm 0.5 \times 10^6$ for fungi: $1 \pm 0.5 \times 10^5$ for bacterial spores)

Experimental Test Conditions	Contact Time and Temperature	Conditions set in function of the use foreseen	
	Interfering Substances	Added or not and chosen in function of the foreseen use. Proposed: —Specific interfering substances (NF T 72-170 or 72-171) —"Clean" and dirty" conditions (European Suspension Test)	

Elimination of Disinfectant	Transfer into suitable neutralizer determined during preliminary test	Transfer into filtration apparatus. Washing under conditions defined by preliminary test with possible use of neutralizer
Count of Survivors	Inclusion in agar medium	Membrane placed on agar medium
	Incubation in conditions suitable for the test strain	
Interpretation	Determine the lowest concentration required for disinfectant to reduce by at least 10^5, 10^4, or 10^3, respectively, the number of bacteria, yeast, and fungal spores or bacterial spores of each of the tested strains. Retain as use-concentration for the use corresponding to the experimental conditions the highest of the concentrations determined in this manner.	

Table 57–19.

Method and Reference		Suspension Test Method DGHM 1981 Qualitative Test	Suspension Test Method DGHM 1981 Quantitative Test
Objective		Bactericidal, tuberculocidal, and fungicidal activities (After test on bacteriostatic, tuberculostatic, and fungistatic efficiency)	Bactericidal and fungicidal activities
Strains		*Staphylococcus aureus* ATCC 6538 *Escherichia coli* ATCC 11229 *Proteus mirabilis* ATCC 14153 *Pseudomonas aeruginosa* ATCC 15442 *Mycobacterium tuberculosis* ATCC 25618 *Candida albicans* ATCC 10231 (Preliminary check of resistance to phenol)	*Staphylococcus aureus* ATCC 6538 The most resistant strain of gram-negative bacteria in the qualitative test *Candida albicans* ATCC 10231
Inoculum		Bacteria: broth culture (10^8–10^9 cells/ml) *Mycobacterium tuberculosis*: Loewenstein-Jensen culture, harvested homogenized, in broth 1 mg/ml (wet weight) Fungi: agar culture, harvested, diluted in broth (10^7–10^8 cells/ml) (0.1 ml in 10 ml of disinfectant dilution in hard water 300 ppm)	Broth culture ($\geq 10^9$ cells/ml) (0.1 ml in 10 ml of disinfectant dilution in hard water 300 ppm)
Experimental Test Conditions	Contact Time and Temperature	5, 15, and 30 minutes 20° ± 2°C	5, 30, 60 minutes at room temperature for disinfectant; 0.5, 1, 5 minutes for hand antiseptics
	Interfering Substances	Organic matter from broth Hard water from disinfectant dilution	Organic matter from broth. Test performed both with and without albumin (0.2%). Hard water from disinfectant dilution.
Elimination of Disinfectant		Possible inclusion of neutralizers in medium	Transfer (1/10) into a suitable neutralizer and dilution in distilled water
Subculture		Transfer of microorganism-disinfectant mixture into broth with or without neutralizer (Loewenstein-Jensen for mycobacteria)	Subculture (0.1 ml) of the neutralizer and of two dilutions on agar medium 48 hours at 37°C (72 hours for *Candida*)
Interpretation		Determination of concentrations required for "pass" or "fail" results Check of subculture medium fertility in test tubes with no growth	Determination of the microbicidal effect (ME) for each contact time ME = long Nc − log Nd Nc = number of viable cells in the inoculum in presence of hard water Nd = number of viable cells in the inoculum after contact with the disinfectant

and indirect spray application (see Tables 57–1 through 57–18).

MAIN OFFICIAL METHODS OF ANALYSIS— EVOLUTION

Some of the Official Methods previously reviewed have been revised, and two experimental standards for testing virucidal efficacy have been published in France. In Europe, a first step toward an international standard was published in 1987 by the Council of Europe. The most commonly used of these methods are listed and analyzed in the accompanying tables.

During the last few years, numerous methods presented as "modified methods" or "improved tests" have been reported (Ascenzi et al., 1987; Terlekys et al., 1987). They are characterized by a precise description of all technical factors that are known to be important

for reproducibility of results and consequently for the results' value. These studies concerned suspension-tests (including capacity-tests) as well as carrier-tests.

Suspension-tests are proposed for determining bactericidal, sporicidal, fungicidal, and virucidal activities. Most of them are quantitative tests requiring a 10^{-5} or 10^{-4} killing of the initial suspension of microorganisms or viruses. To determine the effective use-concentrations, capacity-tests and carrier-test are commonly applied, but their accuracy is debated. A collaborative study performed under the supervision of the AOAC pointed out the problems linked to the standardization of bacterial numbers on germ carriers (Cole et al., 1987).

A recent study (Robinson, 1988) showed that a quantitative suspension test may give an acceptable evaluation of disinfectant efficacy, as compared with the AOAC use-dilution method. This agrees with the observations of the French Standard Organization (AFNOR), which de-

Table 57–20.

Method and Reference		Germ Carrier Test DGHM 1981		
Objective		Bactericidal, tuberculocidal, and fungicidal activities		
Strains		*Staphylococcus aureus* ATCC 6538 *Escherichia coli* ATCC 11229 *Pseudomonas aeruginosa* ATCC 15442 *Proteus mirabilis* ATCC 14153	*Mycobacterium tuberculosis* ATCC 25618 (Preliminary check of resistance to phenol)	*Candida albicans* ATCC 10231
Inoculum		Agar culture harvested (cell density measured). The carriers are immersed in suspension (15 minutes)		
		10^9 cells/ml bacteria	1 mg/ml mycobacteria	10^7–10^8 cells/ml yeast
Experimental Test Conditions	Contact Time and Temperature	5, 15, 30, 60, 90, and 120 minutes Room temperature		
	Interfering Substances	Organic matter from nutrient broth for bacteria test. None for *M. tuberculosis* and fungi. Hard water from disinfectant dilution.		
	Germ Carriers	Linen squares (1 cm × 1 cm), washed, dried, ironed, immersed in 10 ml disinfectant dilution in hard water		
Elimination of Disinfectant		Washing (in duplicate) in broth or Middlebrook medium, with or without neutralizer		
Subculture		Immersion in liquid medium with or without neutralizer (78 hours at 37°C).	Place and rub on surface of egg medium (6 weeks at 37°C). Place and rub on surface of medium (in duplicate) (7 days at 37°C).	
Subculture		Immersion in liquid medium with or without neutralizer (78 hours at 37° C).	Place and rub on surface of egg medium (6 weeks at 37° C).	Place and rub on surface of medium (in duplicate) (7 days at 37° C).
Interpretation		Microscopic examination Check of subculture medium fertility	0 = growth neither on carriers nor on medium + = isolated colonies + + = > 10 colonies	

Table 57–21.

Method and Reference		Determination of the Rideal-Walker Coefficient of Disinfectants BS 541 (1985) Phenol coefficient method	Assessing the efficacy of disinfectants by the modified Chick-Martin Test BS 808 (1986) Phenol coefficient method	Suspension Test for Evaluation of Quaternary Ammonium Compounds (BS 3286)
Objective		Bactericidal activity compared to phenol of coaltar derivatives and/or substituted phenols	Bactericidal activity in the presence of yeast extract compared to phenol	Bactericidal activity
Strains		*Salmonella typhi* NCTC 786	*Salmonella typhi* NCTC 786	*Escherichia coli* *Pseudomonas aeruginosa* *Staphylococcus aureus* Plus yeast and fungi if required
Inoculum		24-hour broth culture (at least three successive daily subculturings—0.2 ml in 5 ml of disinfectant)	24-hour broth culture diluted 1/25 in 5% yeast suspension (2.5 ml of mixture added to 2.5 ml of disinfectant)	24-hour agar or broth culture
Experimental Test Conditions	Contact Time and Temperature	2.5, 5, 7.5, and 10 minutes 17°–18°C	30 minutes 20° ± 0.5°C	30 seconds or between 2 and 30 minutes 22°, 37°, or 44° ± 0.5°C
	Interfering Substances	None	Fresh yeast suspension (5% m/m dry mass) prepared in specified conditions	Organic matter
Elimination of Disinfectant		None	None	Dilution (at least 1/10 up to 1/100) in a neutralizer (as indicated)
Subculture		Loop transfer of disinfectant microorganism mixture into nutrient broth. Incubation for 48 to 72 hours at 37° ± 1°C	Loop transfer as in Rideal-Walker Test (in duplicate) into nutrient broth. Incubation for 48 hours at 37° ± 1°C	Inclusion in agar medium
Interpretation		Determine the disinfectant and phenol concentrations that give survivors in 2.5 and 5 minutes and no survivors after 7.5 and 10 minutes. Divide the phenol concentration by the disinfectant concentration to obtain the Rideal-Walker coefficient.	Divide the mean of the highest concentration of phenol permitting growth and the lowest concentration of phenol showing absence of growth by the corresponding mean concentration of the disinfectant to calculate phenol coefficient.	Results are expressed in terms of percentage survival or of numbers of survivors per million cells inoculated in relation to time of disinfection and concentration of disinfectant.

Table 57–22.

Method and Reference		Antimicrobial Efficacy of Disinfectants for Veterinary and Agricultural Use B.S. 6734 (1986) Suspension Test	Antimicrobial Value of QAC Disinfectant Formulations B.S. 6471 (1984)	Modified Kelsey-Sykes Test B.S. 6905 (1987)
Objective		Efficacy of general-purpose disinfectants and disinfectants intended for use against tuberculosis	Evaluation of quaternary ammonium compounds and disinfectant formulations containing QAC	Determination of use-dilution of disinfectant for hospitals in dirty conditions
Strains		*Salmonella choleraesuis* NCTC 10653 or *Mycobacterium fortuitum* NCTC 8573	*Escherichia coli* ATCC 11229 NCIB 9517	The most resistant (in a growth inhibition test) of the following strains: *Escherichia coli* NCTC 8196 *Pseudomonas aeruginosa* NCTC 6749 *Proteus vulgaris* NCTC 4635 *Staphylococcus aureus* NCTC 4163
Inoculum		Broth culture obtained under specified conditions (more than 10^8 CFU/ml) diluted 1/25 in 5% yeast suspension (2.5 ml of the mixture added to 2.5 ml of disinfectant dilution)	Broth culture obtained under specified conditions (2 parts by volume) diluted with 5 parts of horse serum and 3 parts of hard water (from 5.10^7 to 5.10^8 CFU/ml) (1 ml of the mixture is added to 9 ml of disinfectant dilution)	Broth culture (6 ml) obtained under specified conditions and mixed to yeast suspension (4 ml). Viable count: more than 10^8 and less than 10^{10} per/ml) (1 ml of the mixture added to 3 ml of disinfectant dilution)
Experimental Test Conditions	Contact Time and Temperature	30 minutes at $4 \pm 0.5°C$ (*S. choleraesuis*) 60 minutes at $4 \pm 0.5°C$ (*M. fortuitum*)	600 ± 5 seconds at $22 \pm 0.5°C$	The capacity test requires three additions of inoculum at 10-minute intervals and a subculture 8 minutes after each addition. 20 to 22°C
	Interfering Substances	Yeast suspension Hard water (342 mg/Kg) for dilutions of the disinfectant	Horse serum Hard water (200 ± 10 mg/Kg)	Organic matter from yeast and hard water (342 mg/Kg)
Elimination of Disinfectant		Horse serum in broth (1/20)	Soya lecithin (2% m/V) Tween 80 (3% m/V)	Tween 80 (3%) in subculture broth
Subculture		Transfer in the neutralizer (0.1/10) and then in broth (1/10–5 replicates) Incubation for 48 hours at 37°C	Transfer in the neutralizer (1/10) Inclusion of serial dilutions into agar medium	Transfer 20 μl in 10 ml broth (5 replicates) Incubation for 48 hours at 37°C
Interpretation		Record the antibacterial efficacy in terms of the greatest dilution of the product that produces absence of growth in two or more of the five subcultures. (99.99% reduction in the initial count)	Record the antimicrobial value as the greatest dilution of the product that gives a colony count not greater than 0.01% of the control colony count.	Record the initial concentration of disinfectant showing no growth in at least two out of the five subcultures after contact times of 8 and 18 minutes. Repeat the test on two subsequent days or until three similar growth patterns are obtained.

cided to retain suspension tests for the classification of disinfectants as bactericidal, fungicidal, or sporicidal, and to retain both suspension and germ-carrier tests for the determination of effective use-concentration in 1987 (Tables).

Two main questions must be raised when suspension tests are used to determine effective use-concentrations for practical disinfection:

1. Are the interfering substances included in the test suitable? For example, are they representative of the environment of bacteria targeted by the disinfection?

2. Are the criteria retained to define the disinfectant effect judicious? For example, are the differences in the nature and the physiologic state of the cells being taken into account? Is the log reduction required for the experimental population of microorganisms representative of the log reduction expected for the natural population of microorganisms?

An additional point concerns the choice of the test strains that ought to be representative of the resistance of the whole class to which they belong. The selection of strains retained for their high resistance to disinfect-

Table 57–23.

Method and Reference		5-5-5 Suspension Test Method Dutch Committee on Phytopharmacy		
Objective		Bactericidal, fungicidal, and sporicidal activities		
Strains		Food industry	Veterinary	Hospitals
		Pseudomonas aeruginosa *Salmonella typhimurium* *Staphylococcus aureus* *Saccharomyces cerevisiae* *Bacillus cereus*	*Pseudomonas aeruginosa* *Salmonella typhimurium* *Staphylococcus aureus* *Streptococcus faecalis* *Asperillus fumigatus* *Candida albicans* *Bacillus cereus*	*Pseudomonas aeruginosa* *Proteus mirabilis* *Salmonella typhimurium* *Staphylococcus aureus* *Candida albicans* *Bacillus cereus*
Inoculum		Bacteria and yeast: broth culture medium, centrifuged, washed, suspension adjusted: 10^8 cells/ml in test Bacterial spores: agar culture, spores harvested, centrifuged, washed, heated to 80°C, suspension adjusted: 10^5 cells/ml in test		
Experimental Test Conditions	Contact Time and Temperature	5 minutes 20° ± 1°C	5 minutes 20° ± 1°C	5 minutes 20° ± 1°C
	Interfering Substances	Bovine albumin	Horse serum	Bovine albumin
Elimination of Antiseptic or Disinfectant		Dilution and neutralization: preliminary test with:		
		Pseudomonas aeruginosa *Staphylococcus aureus*	*Salmonella typhimurium* *Staphylococcus aureus*	*Salmonella typhimurium* *Streptococcus aureus*
Subculture		Inclusion in agar medium		
Interpretation		Determine the lowest concentration required for disinfectant to reduce by 5 logs (bacteria and yeasts) and 1 log (spores) the number of microorganisms.		

Table 57–24.

Method and Reference		Test Method for the Antimicrobial Activity of Disinfectants in Food Hygiene Council of Europe—Strasbourg (1987) Suspension test
Objective		Bactericidal and Fungicidal Efficacy Determination of the potential efficacy of the disinfectant
Strains		*Staphylococcus aureus* ATCC 6538 *Streptococcus faecium* DVG 8582 *Pseudomonas aeruginosa* ATCC 15442 *Proteus mirabilis* ATCC 14153 *Saccharomyces cerevisiae* ATCC 9763
Inoculum		Spectrophotometer-adjusted suspension of solid medium culture obtained under specified conditions Bacteria: 10^7 cells/ml in test Yeast: 10^6 cells/ml in test
Experimental Test Conditions	Contact Time and Temperature	5 minutes at 20 ± 1°C
	Interfering Substances	Standard hard water ("clean" conditions) Standard hard water + albumin ("dirty" conditions)
Elimination of Disinfectant		Transfer of microorganism-disinfectant mixture into suitable neutralizer determined by preliminary test
Count of Survivors		Inclusion into agar medium
Interpretation		Calculate the microbiocidal effect: Me = Log Nc − Log No (Nc = control count; No = test count). The use-dilution recommended by the manufacturer must show by Me>5 for each of the 5 test-strains.

ants has been proposed and is justified in some special cases. For general purposes, however, the choice of the most resistant strains would lead to an increase in the use-concentration and consequently to higher costs and toxic risks.

BIBLIOGRAPHY

American Public Health Association. 1918. Report of committee on standard methods of examining disinfectants. Ann. J. Public Health, 8, 506–521.

Ascenzi, J.M., Ezzell, R.J., and Wendt, T.M. 1987. A more accurate method for measurement of tuberculocidal activity of disinfectants. Appl. Environ. Microbiol., 53, 2189–2192.

Association Française de Normalisation (AFNOR). 1981. Recueil de normes françaises des antiseptiques et désinfectants. Edition bi-lingue. Antiseptics and Disinfectants. 1st Edition. Paris, AFNOR.

Association Française de Normalisation—Official French Standards (NF). T 72–150 (1987); T 72–151 (1987); T 72–170 (1988); T 72–171 (1988); T 72–180 (1985); T 72–181 (1986); T 72–190 (1988); T 72–200 (1987); T 72–201 (1987); T 72–230 (1988); T 72–231 (1988); T 72–281 (1986); T 72–300 (1989); T 72–301 (1989). AFNOR Ed., 92080 Paris la Défense.

Association of Official Agricultural Chemists (AOAC). 1984. Disinfectants. Official Methods of Analysis of the Association of Agricultural Chemists. 14th Edition. Arlington, VA, AOAC, pp. 65–77.

Bergan, T., and Lystad, A. 1972. Evaluation of disinfectant inactivators. Acta Pathol. Microbiol. Scand., B 80, 507–510.

Bundesgesundheitsamtes und Deutschen Vereinigung zur Bekämpfung der Viruskrankheiten. 1982. Richtlinie zur prüfung von chemischen desinfektionmitteln auf wirksamkeit gegen viren. Bundesgesundhbl., 25(12), 397–398.

British Standard (BS 541). 1985. Determination of the Rideal-Walker coefficient of disinfectants. London, British Standard Institution.

British Standard (BS 808). 1986. Assessing the efficacy of disinfectants by the modified Chick-Martin test. London, British Standard Institution.

British Standard (BS 3286). 1960. Method for laboratory evaluation of disinfectant activity of quaternary ammonium compounds by suspension test procedure. London, British Standard Institution.

British Standard (BS 6471). 1984. Determination of the antimicrobial value of QAC disinfectant formulation. London, British Standard Institution.

British Standard (BS 6905). 1987. Estimation of concentration of disinfectants used in "dirty" conditions in hospitals by the modified Kelsey-Sykes test.

Chick, H. and Martin, C.J. 1908. The principles involved in the standardization of disinfectants and the influence of organic matter upon germicidal value. J. Hyg. (Cambridge), 8, 654–697.

Cole, E.C., Rutala, W.A., and Samsa, G.P. 1987. Standardization of bacterial numbers on penicylinders used in disinfectant testing: Interlaboratory study. J. Assoc. Off. Anal. Chem., 70, 635–637.

Commissie voor Fytofarmacie. 1974. Waardebepaling van desinfectie—middelen voor materiaal—ontsmetting in ziekenhmizen. cf. Von Klingeren, B. and Mossel D.A.A. 1978 Zentralbl. Bakteriol. Mikriobiol Hyg. Orig. B., 166, 540–541.

Cremieux, A. 1985. Unpublished results.

Cremieux, A. 1986. Factors affecting the bactericidal action of disinfectants. Implications for selection of resistant strains. Drugs Exp. Clin. Res., 12(11), 899–903.

Cremieux, A., Guiraud-Dauriac, H., and Dumenil, G. 1981. Neutralisation des antiseptiques et désinfectants. J. Pharm. Belg., 36, 223–226.

Cremieux, A., Guiraud-Dauriac, H., and Bendjelloul, D. 1983a. Influence des tensio-actifs non ioniques et ampholytes sur l'activité bactéricide de l'hexachlorophène, du glutaraldéhyde et de la chlorhexidine. J. Pharm. Belg., 38, 22–36.

Cremieux, A., Guiraud-Dauriac, H., and Bendjelloul D. 1983b. Interférence de deux surfactants anioniques sur l'activité bactéricide de quelques antiseptiques. J. Pharm. Belg., 38, 101–104.

Croshaw, B. 1981. Disinfectant testing, with particular reference to the Rideal-Walker and Kelsey-Sykes Tests. In Disinfectants. Their Use and Evaluation of Effectiveness. Edited by C.H. Collins, M.C. Allwood, S.F. Bloomfield, and A. Fox. London, Academic Press, pp. 1–15.

Damery, B., and Cremieux, A. 1986. Etude de l'activité virucide in vitro du dichloroisocyanurate de sodium. Ann. Inst. Pasteur/Virol., 137 E, 327–331.

Deutsche Gesellschaft für Hygiene und Mikrobiologie (DGHM). 1972. Richtlinien für die prüfung chemischer desinfektons-mittel. 2. Autl. Stuttgart, G. Fisher Verlag.

Deutsche Gesellschaft für Hygiene und Mikrobiologie (DGHM). 1981. Richtlinien für die prüfung und bewertung chemischer desinfectionverfarhen. Stuttgart, New York, G. Fisher Verlag.

Dony, J., and Millet, M. 1973. Réflexions sur la mesure de l'action germicide des substances antiseptiques ou désinfectantes. J. Pharm. Belg., 28, 721–734.

Fleurette, J., et Groupe de Travail "Antiseptiques" de la Société Française de Microbiologie. 1978. In Antiseptiques. Rev. Inst. Pasteur Lyon, 11, 3.

Fleurette, J. 1988. Les antiseptiques. In Pharmacologie Clinique: Bases de la Thérapeutique. Edited by J.P. Giroud, G. Mathé, and G. Meyniel. Paris, Expansion Scientifique Française, pp. 1584–1603.

Garrigue, G., et al. 1984. Activité virucide des antiseptiques et désinfectants. III. Technique par dilution-ultrafiltration-reconcentration. Pathol. Biol., 32 (5 bis), 647–650.

Gelinas, P., and Goulet, J. 1983. Neutralization of the activity of eight disinfectants by organic matter. J. Appl. Bacteriol., 54, 243–247.

Gershenfeld, L., and Stedman, R.L. 1949. The potentiating effects of various compounds on the antibacterial activities of surface active agents. Ann. J. Pharm., 121, 249–266.

Kelsey, J.C., Beeby, M.M., and Whitehouse, C.W. 1965. A capacity use-dilution test for disinfectants. Mth. Bull. Minist. Hlth., 24, 152–160.

Kelsey, J.C., and Sykes, G. 1969. A new test for the assessment of disinfectants with particular reference to their use in hospitals. Pharm. J., 202, 607–609.

Kelsey, J.C., and Maurer, I. 1974. An improved (1974) Kelsey-Sykes test for disinfectants. Pharm. J., 213, 528–530.

Koch, R. 1981. Uber Disinfektion. Mittheilungen aus dem kaiserlichen gesundheitsamte, 1, 234–282.

Myers, T. 1988. Failing the test: germicides or use-dilution methodology? A.S.M. News, 54, 19–21.

Quero, A.M., et al. 1984. Détermination de l'activité virucide des antiseptiques par une méthode de filtration sur gel. Pathol. Biol., 32 (5 bis), 636–639.

Reybrouck, G. 1974. Uber die standardisierung der wettbestimmung von Flächen desinfectionmitteln. Zentralbl. Bakteriol Mikrobiol. Hyg. [B], 158, 465–478.

Reybrouck, G. 1975. A theoretical approach of disinfectant testing. Zentralbl. Bakteriol. Mikrobiol. Hyg. [B], 160, 342–367.

Reybrouck, G. 1978. Bactericidal activity of 40 potential disinfectant inactivators. Zentralbl. Bakteriol. Mikrobiol. Hyg. [B], 167, 528–534.

Reybrouck, G. 1979. Efficacy of inactivators against 14 disinfectant substances. Zentralbl. Bakteriol. Mikrobiol. Hyg. [B], 168, 480–492.

Reybrouck, G., Borneff, J., Van de Woorde, H., and Werner, H.P. 1979. A collaborative study on a new quantitative suspension test, the in vitro bactericidal activity of chemical disinfectants. Zentralbl. Bakteriol. Mikrobiol. Hyg. [B], 168, 463–479.

Reybrouck, G. 1980. A comparison of the quantitative suspension tests for the assessment of disinfectants. Zentralbl. Bakteriol. Mikrobiol. Hyg. [B], 170, 449–456.

Reybouck, G. 1986. Uniformierung der prüfung von desinfektionsmitteln in Europa. Zentralbl. Bakteriol. Mikrobiol. Hyg. [B], 182, 485–498.

Rideal, S., and Walker, J.T.A. 1903. The standardization of disinfectants. J. R. Sanit. Inst., 24, 424–441.

Rideal, S., and Walker, J.T.A. 1921. An approved technique of the Rideal-Walker test. London, H.K. Lewis and Co.

Robinson, R.A., Bodily, H.L., Robinson, D.F., and Christensen, R.P. 1988. A suspension method to determine reuse life of chemical disinfectants during clinical use. Appl. Environ. Microbiol., 54, 158–164.

Russel, A.D. 1981. Neutralization procedures in the evaluation of bactericidal activity. In Disinfectants, Their Use and Evaluation of Effectiveness. C.H. Collins, M.C. Allwood, S.F. Bloomfield, and A. Fox. London, Academic Press.

Stuart, L.S., Ortenzio, L.F., and Friedl, J.L. 1953. Use dilution confirmation tests for results secured by phenol coefficient methods. J. Assoc. Off. Agr. Chem., 36, 466–480.

Sykes, G. 1962. The philosophy of the evaluation of disinfectants and antiseptics. J. Appl. Bacteriol., 25, 1–11.

Terlecky, S.B., and Axler, D.A. 1987. Quantitative neutralization assay of fungicidal activity of disinfectants. Antimicrob. Agents Chemother., 31, 794–798.

Van Klingeren, B., Leussink, A.B., and Van Wijngaarden, L.J. 1977. A collaborative study on the repeatability and the reproducibility of the Dutch Standard. Suspension-test for the evaluation of disinfectants. Zentralbl. Bakteriol. Mikrobiol. Hyg. [B], 164, 521–548.

Van Klingeren, B., and Pullen, W. 1987. Comparative testing of disinfectants against Mycobacterium tuberculosis and Mycobacterium terrae in a quantitative suspension-test. J. Hosp. Infect., 10, 292–298.

CHAPTER 58

METHODS OF TESTING ANTISEPTICS: ANTIMICROBIALS USED TOPICALLY IN HUMANS AND PROCEDURES FOR HAND SCRUBS

M.K. Bruch

The term antiseptic for both professionals and lay people has become a substitute word for antimicrobial. Every kind of product, from tincture of iodine to sunburn remedies and impregnated toilet seats, is called an antiseptic. As emphasis on handwashing and disinfection has intensified in the hospital environment, largely encouraged by the AIDS epidemic, there has been more concern about effectiveness; universal use of the term antiseptic, however—regardless of the degree of activity or intended use—still impedes acceptance of degrees of or differences in effectiveness. The FDA OTC Antimicrobial Panel moved strongly to limit the definition, but the term's present unrestrained use testifies to their failure.

The origin of the term antiseptic (see Chapter 1) predates the work of Semmelweis and Lister in references to elimination of purulent infection.

Recent attempts have limited the official use of the term antiseptic to products used on living tissue, usually topically applied (Bruch and Bruch, 1971; Sykes, 1965; Hugo, 1971; Code of Federal Regulations, 1981). An even more rigorous definition by the FDA OTC panel not only limits use to the skin but requires clinical verification of prevention of infection (Food and Drug Administration, 1974).

When a manufacturer chooses identification of a product as an antiseptic, it presumably identifies it as a drug, most especially with agents applied to living tissue.

Section 201 (0) of the Federal Food, Drug and Cosmetic Act states, "For the purpose of this Act—The representation of a drug in its labeling as an antiseptic should be considered to be a representation that it is a germicide, a bacteriostatic antiseptic drug requiring prolonged contact such as surgical dressing."

This chapter is directed to the testing of antimicrobial products applied on or in the living body of man or other animals. These drug products are regulated under the Food, Drug and Cosmetic Act, whereas disinfectant products for use on inanimate surfaces are regulated by the Environmental Protection Agency under the Federal Environmental Protection Act, which incorporates the earlier Federal Insecticide, Fungicide and Rodenticide Act.

Participants in the Second International Colloquium concerning the Evaluation of Disinfectants in Europe (Knorr, 1973) reasonably attempted to incorporate antisepsis as a gradation of disinfection into their stricter and more comprehensive definition of disinfection. Their discussions viewed disinfection as a substitute procedure for sterilization. Historical definitions of disinfectants limited the desired activity to pathogenic microorganisms, but with the ever-increasing difficulty in strictly defining a potential pathogen, this qualification loses its meaning.

The Colloquium defined disinfection as "the selective elimination of certain undesirable microorganisms in order to prevent their transmission"; this elimination is "achieved by action on their structure or metabolism, irrespective of their functional state," whereas they defined antisepsis as "destruction of vegetative forms of microorganisms but not their permanent forms." The generic term "Entkeimung" (elimination of germs) was introduced by this group and actually comes closer in meaning and perception to antimicrobial, but perhaps connotes a higher level of activity in elimination rather than "anti" activity. The derivation and analysis of definitions and testing procedures warrants further expansion, attention, and thought.

The distinction between disinfection and antisepsis can still be made in the United States because legal definitions are made by the Food and Drug Administration and by the Environmental Protection Agency and reg-

1028

ulation is administered by two different agencies. The European community has promoted the use of skin disinfection for antiseptics aimed at skin microflora. Skin degerming is also popular. Skin disinfection is more descriptive of actual use.

Obviously, the ideas from all of these sources are grounded in the same principles, that is, to kill or reduce microorganisms on the skin or other body surfaces. Such a reduction has long been regarded as desirable and prudent. Significant data from controlled studies relating reduction in microbial count to reduction in the incidence of infection or in transmission of infection are not conclusive. Although no one seriously considers abandoning the use of hand degerming procedures or preoperative preparation, it is time to seriously consider the goal for which the product is to be used and the concomitant activity required to achieve this goal. Surely we all recognize that there is probably not a single product that will do everything. Certain chemicals have properties such as substantivity, whereas others may have rapid activity; users must begin to make the correlation between activity and use.

Some justification exists for disparity between the common usage and usage that is appropriate for regulatory distinctions. The regulatory distinctions may be strained and become confusing because of various requirements of the Food, Drug and Cosmetic Act and the Federal Environmental Protection Act.

The most recent attempt to define and separate categories of usage of antimicrobials for topical use has·been made by the FDA Over-The-Counter (OTC) Drug Review (Food and Drug Administration, 1974).

The FDA OTC Antimicrobial Panel, in their review of the safety and effectiveness of antimicrobial products for repeated use on the skin, defined usage categories for a variety of product types that otherwise would all be called antiseptics. Their breakdown of terms associated with specific uses and specific levels of activity was as follows. The Panel distinguished between effectiveness in preventing or combating clinical infection (sepsis) and the reduction of resident or transient microorganisms on the skin. In so doing, it became obvious that the requirements for effectiveness would not, and should not, be the same.

The definitions proposed by the Antimicrobial I Panel report to the FDA as published in the Federal Register of September 13, 1974 (Food and Drug Administration) are presented below. There may eventually be changes in the final definitions. No Tentative Final Monograph has been published yet. One change may be in the Panel's stringent definition of antiseptic requiring proof of prophylaxis, or possibly the contradictions that exist in the Panel's definition of a skin wound cleanser. Furthermore, there seems to be a need for added definition in at least two areas of use that were neglected by the OTC Panel. These areas include a food-handlers' handwashing product, a germicidal hand rinse or rub, and a site-preparation product for invasive therapeutic and diagnostic procedures.

DEFINITIONS

Skin Antiseptic: A safe, nonirritating, antimicrobial-containing preparation that prevents overt skin infection. Claims stating or implying an effect against microorganisms must be supported by controlled human studies that demonstrate prevention of infection.

Patient Preoperative Skin Preparation: A safe, fast-acting, broad-spectrum, antimicrobial-containing preparation that significantly reduces the number of microorganisms on intact skin.

Surgical Hand Scrub: A safe, nonirritating, antimicrobial-containing preparation that significantly reduces the number of microorganisms on the intact skin. A surgical hand scrub should be broad-spectrum, fast acting, and persistent.

Health-Care Personnel Handwash: A safe, nonirritating preparation designed for frequent use that reduces the number of transient microorganisms on intact skin to an initial baseline level after adequate washing, rinsing, and drying. If the preparation contains an antimicrobial agent, it should be broad-spectrum, fast acting and, if possible, persistent.

Skin Wound Cleanser: A safe, nonirritating, liquid preparation (or product to be used with water) that assists in the removal of foreign material from small superficial wounds and does not delay wound healing.

Skin Wound Protectant: A safe, nonirritating preparation applied to small cleansed wounds that provides a protective barrier (physical, chemical, or both) and neither delays healing nor favors the growth of microorganisms.

Antimicrobial Soap: A soap containing an active ingredient with in-vitro and in-vivo activity against skin microorganisms. *Note:* Soaps without antimicrobial ingredients (as defined in 21 CFR 3.652) are exempt from regulation under the Federal Food, Drug and Cosmetic Act (Food and Drug Administration, Code of Federal Regulations, 1981).

ORAL ANTISEPTICS

The use of oral antimicrobial agents must be regarded in a different light from those used on the skin. Mucosal surfaces and the microorganisms that inhabit them form an ecosystem different from that of the bacteria/skin combination. The persistent use of antimicrobial chemicals to reduce oral bacteria continues to be a controversial subject, as does the ultimate question of what the effect of their use is on infection or oral disease processes. Chemicals such as phenol and quaternary ammonium compounds seem to show greater effectiveness when given orally than when used on the skin. For more details of testing procedures for oral antimicrobial products and information on the chemicals used, the reader is referred to the Federal Register report of the FDA OTC Oral Cavity Panel (Food and Drug Administration, 1979).

TEST PROCEDURES

Basic information about the antimicrobial activity of a given chemical is essential. At the same time there is every chance that this same chemical, although giving positive results in vitro, may not show significant activity when formulated and used topically. Release of the active ingredient from the formulation and the interaction, partition, and solubility of the ingredient when in contact with skin can influence activity significantly. Particularly with reference to topical antimicrobials, in vitro testing has been relied on heavily in the past, although even now, its exclusive use receives undue emphasis. Correlation of the in vitro tests that are done with actual use conditions or recognition of the specific areas of the body where products will be used is now regarded as essential. Current thinking is more and more in the direction that basic in vitro data are required to show that the ingredient and/or product is truly antimicrobial and the probable range of activity. Subsequently, in vivo tests must establish effectiveness for a given indication.

A step between a strictly in vitro and a frank in vivo clinical test is discussed in the OTC Panel report and can be useful in formulation testing and in screening for active chemicals or as a prelude to full-blown clinical testing. These procedures are based on several publications by Kligman and coworkers at the Department of Dermatology at the University of Pennsylvania (Singh et al., 1971; Marples and Kligman, 1972, 1974; Leyden et al., 1979). Several methods of producing a small controlled wound (by tape-stripping or the production of ammonium hydroxide blisters) that can be inoculated with known levels of selected bacteria have been reported. The normal skin flora (usually of the arm) can be manipulated by wrapping the site with saran wrap, thereby producing, in the originator's terms, flora expanded in both numbers and types. These two variable factors can be orchestrated so that a variety of testing conditions can be designed. The future undoubtedly will produce further refinements that ultimately may permit this type of skin model to be used in place of naturally occurring skin infections. A clinical study of superficial wound infections is becoming increasingly difficult to execute and frequently must now be done overseas because of the low wound infection rate in this country. Cost is high and monitoring difficult under these circumstances.

Recommendations for In Vitro Testing

The FDA OTC Panel outlined a basic set of tests that would provide information necessary to proceed to in vivo tests and would form technical support data.

An outline was published to be used as a basic guide when characterizing in vitro the activity of an antimicrobial agent. It was not meant to be exhaustive or final but simply to provide a guide that was appropriate at the time. The minimal inhibitory concentration (MIC) should be determined under standard conditions and against standard organisms that have known phenol coefficients and susceptibilities to other antimicrobials.

A series of mesophilic strains that have been recently isolated, including cutaneous pathogens and normal flora (100 isolates), were suggested for in vitro tests. The following groups should be represented (special environmental conditions and/or media may be required for some of the groups selected):

1. Staphylococci—5 groups
2. Micrococci
3. Pyogenic streptococci (Groups A, C, and D should be included)
4. Diphtheroids-lipophilic, nonlipophilic, and anaerobic (*Propionibacterium*)
5. Gram-negative enteric bacilli: *Escherichia, Enterobacter, Klebsiella, Proteus,* and *Serratia* should be included
6. *Neisseria* species
7. Aerobic spore formers
8. Atypical mycobacteria—fast-growing strains
9. Fungi—yeast-like species, *Pityrosporum ovale, Pityrosporum orbiculare, Candida albicans, Candida parapsilosis,* and *Torulopsis glabrata*
10. Selected filamentous dermatophytic species
11. Viruses—hydrophilic, lipophilic

The determination of development of resistance to the chemical being tested was suggested. One mechanism mentioned was the selection of sublethal levels of the active ingredient(s) incorporated into the culture medium for an extended series of exposures. Standard methods to determine the emergence of resistance were encouraged.

Phenol Coefficient

In an attempt to characterize the antimicrobial chemical, the routine determination of the phenol coefficient was included. A standard procedure with and without a specific neutralizer was recommended. If no neutralizer is known or available, 10% serum was to be used. Secondary subcultures, to determine the viability of the strain, were also encouraged.

Other tests were suggested for antimicrobial effectiveness based on the phenol coefficient test, providing data to substantiate antimicrobial activity with tests such as the Kelsey-Sykes procedure (Kelsey and Sykes, 1969) or others. The inclusion in the in vitro tests of a chemical or chemicals with recognized antimicrobial activity for comparative purposes was also recommended.

Although phenol coefficient testing is recommended as a basic test by the Panel, and it has a long and honorable history, it has little relevance for topically used antimicrobials. Many antimicrobials have substantive activity, that is, some amount of the applied chemical remains in the stratum corneum and continues to exert an antimicrobial effect. Furthermore, the majority of the newer chemicals are inhibitory to bacteria and may not be rapidly bactericidal at use concentrations. The reader is referred to numerous other descriptions of the phenol coefficient test, particularly those in previous editions of this book (Block, 1977; Lawrence and Block, 1968). Its use without interpretation may give possibly misleading information.

The use of a specific neutralizer for the antimicrobial chemical being tested is mentioned in the outline for in vitro testing (Food and Drug Administration, 1974), but the importance of stopping or otherwise counteracting the activity of the antimicrobial cannot be overestimated.

In Vivo Animal and Human Testing

Specific tests for the defined product categories were recommended in the OTC Panel's guidelines (Food and Drug Administration, 1974). Experts agree with the Panel's conclusion that a human in vivo test is to be preferred over animal in vivo data or in vitro data. The Panel's comments were particularly directed toward the use of a clinical trial as support for an antiseptic claim.

Recommendation for the specific in vivo testing procedures outlined in the OTC Antimicrobial I report are discussed for the claim to which they apply (Food and Drug Administration, 1974). A description of these tests follows, and now includes experiences with these tests and critiques of them.

Skin Antiseptic

A human clinical trial in skin infection demonstrating prevention of infection is required, although this type of study probably cannot be executed in the United States because of unusually low infection rates. Such a study has already been designed and executed in Central America (Taplin, 1981). Critical attention must be given to the design and statistical interpretation of results.

The continued misuse of the term antiseptic continues unrestricted in the void created by lack of finalization of the OTC Monographs.

Patient Preoperative Preparation

Few testing procedures for a preoperative preparation are published. Although clinical trials demonstrating a reduction in postoperative infection are probably impossible, prudence dictates as low a microbial count as can be achieved for a patient skin site marked for surgical procedure.

A variety of skin sampling procedures are described in the literature, from fingerprint cultures, tape contact, and velvet imprinting to glove fluid sampling. In general, fingerprint or contact plate or fabric culturing samples mostly superficial skin flora. A procedure utilizing a skin scrubbing procedure with a surfactant solution has been shown to give the highest counts and reproducible results (Williamson, 1965; Williamson and Kligman, 1965; Selwyn, 1972; Updegraff, 1964). One criterion of effectiveness is the $\log_{10}$ reduction from an established baseline microbial count. Part of the criteria of effectiveness should be evaluation of persistence or substantivity of a preparatory product. Microbial sampling of wounds

helps determine the source and number of potentially pathogenic bacteria.

In their report, the OTC Panel made specific recommendations concerning in vivo testing, in general, and a preoperative product in particular. Bilateral paired comparison, that is, the use of a variety of skin sites on half of the body with control sites on the matching side, was suggested as reasonable. A maximum of 30 minutes should be used as the time for testing activity, because the definition states that rapid activity is required.

The baseline count at the control site matching the test area should be established using the cup-scrubbing or possibly other appropriate sampling techniques. It is important that the same procedure be employed for other skin test areas. The Panel emphasized selection of a skin area where an adequate population exists, and sampling skin areas on various parts of the body, including the genital areas.

The Panel stressed the requirement for rapid and complete neutralization of the chemicals in the sample from the skin to inactivate active chemical carried over from the skin. The neutralizer selected should also be tested for neutralizing effectiveness and toxicity for cells. Both the culture conditions and the volume of the sample must be adequate to determine the range of organisms that might be isolated from the skin. (See published guidelines for suggested media.) Establishing efficacy for a product labeled as a preoperative skin preparation requires at least a 3-log reduction.

Artificial contamination of the skin with cultured organisms for testing of preoperative skin preparations has been attempted, but the results hardly seem applicable.

Sampling of the operative wound has been improved using some of the contact methods with agar plates or velvet blocks. Geelhoed (1983a,b) and Rhodeheaver (1988) have published studies and recommend that the correct sampling procedure for a preoperative preparation is a contact plate impression of the skin area. They reasoned that the microbial flora of concern is that which can move across the skin when it is wet under the drapes or dressings to the wound boundaries. This procedure is significantly different from the standardized cup-scrub recommended by the OTC Panel.

When the skin is sampled using a contact method, the transient and superficial organisms are dispersed in a layer of microcolonies. In contrast, the scrubbing sampling techniques disperse microcolonies, disturb layers of stratum corneum, and increase the count compared to assessment with the surface contact culture.

Surgical Hand Scrub

Historically, the results of standard handwashing trials such as those of Price (1938), Cade (1951), and Quinn et al. (1954) have been extrapolated to estimate the activity of surgical scrub procedures. The inadequacy of these routine handwashing tests in relation to actual use was recognized. Some investigators suggested that the count of organisms on the hand after the surgical gloves were donned was an important factor, rather than just the number of bacteria removed after scrubbing (Walter, 1965; Michaud et al., 1972; Walter, 1971).

The change from using an open basin sampling technique as Price popularized for handwashing effectiveness to a glove washing or sampling procedure has several almost simultaneous origins.

Acting on suggestions by others, including Reid et al. (1950) and Walter and Kundsin (1969), Michaud et al. (1972) reported a glove washing technique that was integrated into a formalized technique. They published this procedure just as the OTC Panel was convening. Michaud and a coauthor, Goss, in a far-sighted and predictive summary, cited as an asset of the test the ability to accumulate data on substantivity with this protocol, and commented that no real difference existed between using a brush and just sponging and washing the hands.

Bruch, the OTC Antimicrobial Panel I, and several consultants designed a testing procedure to examine the initial reduction of count from an estimated baseline when the hands are initially scrubbed and then subsequently over a 6-hour period after the surgical gloves are donned. The full test is repeated three times over 5 days. Initial reduction is a critical element and may differ among different types of products. A normal baseline count is established with three determinations prior to the test. Evidence of substantivity of the antimicrobial chemical can be drawn from observation of the initial count reduction over the 5-day period. It is expected that the count on the hands will rise during the wearing of the gloves. This rise can be precipitous, slow, and gradual, or the count level can remain constant during the 6-hour period. Comparative studies (Rosenberg et al., 1976; Peterson et al., 1978) can and do show differences in the various aspects of the test—that is, the initial reduction, the re-establishment of the count in the glove over 6 hours, and the presence of substantive activity.

The long-term effect on the microbial flora is important in a surgical hand scrub product; it is even more important today for a Health Care Personnel Handwash (HCPH) product because of the increased imposition of Universal Precautions, which involve the wearing of gloves for many tasks previously executed without gloves. The persistent effect of an antimicrobial is exhibited in a lowering of the level of the flora over days of use while at the same time exerting a suppression of the regrowth of the deep flora to re-establish the initial count.

The current testing guidelines do not address the practical and important effect of repeated and consistent use over an extended period (weeks), but really reflect an artificially constructed situation to provide a test acceptable to regulatory agencies.

The emphasis on certain results for acceptability of the test has led to considerable manipulation and free-wheeling alterations in protocol to achieve desired results. There is always this danger with a set protocol; vigilance is required to provide adequate controls.

Clearly, the testing of surgical scrubs must involve testing of the initial reduction and the subsequent re-establishment of the skin's microbial flora on the hands.

Both aspects of scrubbing are important, but the ultimate purpose of the scrub is to reduce the level of organisms in the glove in the event that the glove is either cut or torn.

Standardization of skin testing will be hard to achieve because investigators relish adding their own innovations to the test procedure. When the impact of these changes is added to the difficulty of a highly variable population among the subjects selected, and when it is recognized that the final test measurement is a small fraction of the population removed or released from the skin, it is not surprising that results are confusing. There is a wide variation in test results between investigators using the same formulation (Rotter, 1981; Peterson, Rosenberg and Alatary, 1978; Soulsby, Barnett and Maddox, 1986; and Bartzokas et al., 1983). The cited investigators have found a difference of as much as $3 \log(s)_{10}$ in initial reduction and in subsequent estimates of the persistent effect using the same formulations. These discrepancies can be attributed to variations in methods and neutralization, but it is clear that this test is open to manipulation of results, if the investigator chooses that course.

Because the microbial population varies so often in subjects, the three-time estimation of baseline prior to the actual study must be questioned. The pre-test baseline estimate in the current test is used for all pre- and post-scrub estimations, so that on the second and fifth days the baseline count is in reality much lower than the pre-test baseline estimate. Comparisons of the counts or reduction factors are unnecessarily exaggerated. The test must be refined by making the baseline estimate on one hand and the test procedure on the opposite hand because there is no significant variation in the microbial level between hands.

At least two alternative protocols have been proposed for our own and other regulatory purposes, ASTM procedure and in France (Cremieux et al., 1988).

1. The American Society of Testing Materials Committee (ASTM) has published a revised Glove Juice Test with several alterations in the original protocol. This procedure is a recommendation for changes, but the FDA has not made any official comments on it. The major elements of the protocol are appended with the Federal Register Glove Juice Test.

2. Dr. Cremieux of France also presented a testing procedure at the 1988 ICAAC Meeting in Los Angeles (Cremieux, 1988). This procedure is similar to the Glove Juice Test. Dr. Cremieux, recognizing the variation in repeated tests, reported an in vivo test in which subjects scrubbed three times per day for 5 days. No prewash is used, and as suggested elsewhere, the left hand is the control hand, and the right, the test hand. She recognizes the difficulty and variation in the recovery of the microbial flora for assessment. 400 ml of neutralizer

fluid was used in a plastic bag providing dilution and neutralization. She recommended at least 50 ml of solution with neutralizer in it.

The French effort has also recognized the variation in test results, and attributed it to the specific handwashing procedure and the mode of recovery. An evaluation is made each day for immediate recovery, cumulative effect, and remnant effect.

The test as described in the third edition of this book has been executed in numerous trials. Conflicting data have been collected by different investigators, especially when the results of this testing are compared with handwashing tests with the same compound (chlorhexidine) but with a different protocol for testing (Rotter, 1981). A truly excellent protocol should be reproducible in the hands of different investigators. Elements of a protocol that can be manipulated to reach predetermined values must be replaced. Any procedure must have the assurance that the active ingredient is neutralized or quenched.

Many studies listed by Rotter (1981) recorded an initial scrub reduction of 1 to 2 logs, whereas many studies performed in the United States have reported initial 2-plus reductions followed by exaggerated values reaching a 4 to 5-log reduction after donning gloves. Rotter attributes the difference to the use of neutralizers in the stripping solution used to sample the gloves.

No other element is as uncertain in obtaining consistent results as the selection of an effective neutralizing agent (a chemical or a combination of chemicals that will stop or quench the antimicrobial action of the test product). The neutralizer must be effective without killing the bacterial cells of the skin flora.

This selection is especially critical when the activity of the chemical is inhibitory at very low concentrations, as occurs with chlorhexidine, so that cells are inhibited by carry-over of the antimicrobial and do not grow to form colonies when recovery techniques are used. These effects are seen in the extremely varied and numerous formulas for neutralizing chlorhexidine—eight different formulas in ten studies, including the statement that chlorhexidine cannot be neutralized. At present, there is no standard for neutralizer testing. High dilution coupled with neutralization may be required to solve the problem with chlorhexidine.

The work with chlorhexidine is particularly perplexing because of the range of different neutralizers and reports of complete failure (Brandberg and Andersson, 1981). The commonly used Tween or polysorbate 80 was used in concentrations from 1 to 15%. These formulas cannot all be equally effective. Some reports claim that chlorhexidine cannot be neutralized (Rahaave, 1975).

This difficulty with chlorhexidine is complicated by the fact that chlorhexidine is bacteriostatic at concentrations of 1 to 10 ppm, making the likelihood of carry-over higher.

An effective protocol for testing neutralizers is needed. Routine high dilution combined with the presence of a neutralizer for the test sample may be necessary. Filtration of the sample probably would be required.

Some recent publications have contributed information from tests that relate to surgical scrub testing or provide a means to do preliminary or intermediate testing in vivo prior to a full-blown Glove Juice Test.

A recent study by Leyden and McGinley (1989) emphasized the importance and contribution of the microbial contamination under the fingernails. In the test, a significant reduction in count was observed when the nail area and nailbed were occluded with polymethylmethacrylate. Sampling was done using a glove wash procedure with agitation with a brush added. This procedure seems highly effective and reproducible in the assessment of under-nail accumulation.

Because this hidden flora can be highly variable, recognition of this source of variation may ultimately be used to normalize the baseline or pre-test counts.

Health-Care Personnel Handwash

Testing for health-care personnel handwash and a germicidal hand rinse or rub (if this category is defined) are similar, but testing both is quite different from a surgical hand scrub.

These products are probably the most important ones used in the hospital and other health-care facilities. The Second International Conference on Nosocomial Infections (1981) reinforced the central importance of personnel and their hands as the primary means of transferring infection. The quintessential characteristics are acceptance and the implementation of a repeated-use regimen. A product that meets the definition and that is acceptable in use must have rapid action in reduction or removal of transient flora acquired as part of patient care. Physical removal plays a part in the action of this type of product. Therefore, the vehicle for such a product is as important as the antimicrobial. This washing product differs from a product such as an alcohol-based hand rinse in that the detergent/surfactant constituents contribute to physical removal, whereas with the hand-rinse or hand-rub type of product, the volatile alcohol or other vehicle dries on the hands.

The testing guidelines suggested by the Panel have developed into specific testing procedures that now incorporate the following concepts (Food and Drug Administration, 1974):

1. Only the formulated product was initially required, but there is now general agreement that the vehicle alone must be tested.
2. The form of the test is to apply to the hands several types of bacterial contamination at a high level and test the removal with repeated washings.
3. Marker strains with easily identifiable cultural characteristics, such as color, are used for contaminating the hands.

When a health-care personnel handwash is tested, the major concern is the transient skin flora. The accepted procedure has been to artificially apply a "contamination" of transient bacteria. Because only one type of bacteria is applied in these procedures, this testing is only a simulation at best.

The original testing recommendations for an HCPH did not contain a control for the effect of the soap vehicle without the antimicrobial. This serious deficiency needs to be remedied in any future protocol. Friction and the detergency of the vehicle are both effective in removing the artificially applied organisms. The control is needed to recognize the contribution of the vehicle.

The method of applying organisms needs to be assessed and the most efficient one finally chosen. Rotter (1984) has used a method of rotating the hands while drying after dipping in a large volume of liquid culture. Lowbury (1975) has suggested applying the culture with rubber gloves with thorough rubbing-in of the culture. Either of these systems probably would give more-consistent contamination than applying a small high-count volume of culture into the palm of the hand, as is now recommended.

Antimicrobial Soaps

The effectiveness and testing of these products is actually not applicable to the present subject but traditionally has been included with this group of products. Antimicrobial soaps are of significant interest to the consumer because of widespread use, and to the microbiologist because of a suspected influence of repeatedly using antimicrobial chemicals with action against only gram-positive skin flora. Fears have been expressed that a potentially pathogenic gram-negative flora could form a replacement population for the normal gram-positive skin flora (Food and Drug Administration, 1974; Marples, 1969; Leyden et al., 1979). Testing should correlate the deodorant effect (using sniff tests) and the degree of microbial reduction where this is the basic claim. Some data showing this correlation have been accumulated. It is safe to say that the generally accepted reduction in flora achieved from using antimicrobial soaps is approximately 1 log. This is the figure quoted by the OTC Panel and is substantiated by data in FDA files.

First Aid Products

The definition and testing of these products is difficult and enters into the realm of psychologic well-being. Products of this type (which include skin wound cleansers and protectants) actually are used prophylactically. The flora against which activity is required, however, is always variable and unknown. Effectiveness such as that required for a skin antiseptic is not necessary, yet activity against pathogenic bacteria on the skin must be shown. This is best and most easily demonstrated using the human skin models described by Kligman and coworkers (Marples and Kligman, 1972, 1974; Leyden et al., 1979). The use of inoculated, small, artificially made wounds is most desirable. These products are often used only once or twice and should have some degree of lasting activity.

Summary

Mary Marples, in her 1965 book *The Ecology of the Human Skin* and in a later article (1969) prophetically urged the study of the normal human flora of the skin. She presented what is probably still the best picture of the balance of this particular ecosystem, stating in 1969 that

> Only recently have studies been undertaken of the natural cutaneous organisms, microbes that live in large numbers on the skin of most human beings. Some of these organisms are potential pathogens; although they are harmless on the skin surface, they may cause disease if they penetrate the deep cutaneous layers. The study of skin ecology is thus essential to the control of skin and wound infections, and it may also help to elucidate problems that classical ecology has failed to solve.

Although interest in the normal balance of the microbial flora of the skin has been stimulated, the work is tedious, time-consuming, and expensive. Yet the products and testing procedures described here all interrupt the normal balance, and it is essential to stop and consider the use, goals, and effects of antimicrobial products on the skin. Emphasis must be placed on killing and reduction in count, but the effect on the skin environment and the flora of the repeated users may well hold the key to effective control of infection in the closed environmental conditions in which antimicrobials are most often used.

In summary, antiseptic is a term everyone believes they can easily define. It has become so general, popularized, and overused that it seems uncertain whether strict definition will decrease its almost slang, generic use in favor of "antibacterial" or some more specific term. Certainly, restriction to products for use on human tissue should be made. It seems rational to restrict the term to products designed to prevent infection in the prophylactic sense. I certainly believe that it should not be used for inanimate objects that have been disinfected and that are intended for use in contact with body surfaces or tissue.

The testing procedures discussed depend on reliable skin sampling procedures. New and improved techniques have been and are consistently being developed and used, but other methods, particularly to sample difficult skin sites or topical sites, are needed. The multi-layered nature, varied environment, and seemingly clinging attachment of the flora to the skin layers is disturbed when sampling procedures intrude. We need methods that will give the truest reflection of the existing microenvironment.

TESTING PROTOCOLS AND DESIGNS

It must be emphasized that the following tests are the state of the art at the time of this writing. Certain nuances, details, and improvements in technique can be added at the time of use. Perhaps some of the adaptations that have been suggested by the American Society of Testing Materials (ASTM) Committee will be implemented. This protocol is also included, but it has not been made official. It seems that because there has been such a long period since introduction, there will certainly be changes when the OTC Antimicrobial Tentative Final Monograph is published by FDA.

It is always prudent to check the latest versions of testing procedures, protocols, and requirements, particularly if they are the basis of regulatory submission.

Minimal Inhibitory Concentration

This procedure is required to supply basic antimicrobial data before further specific testing is undertaken. When MIC determination was adapted to test antibiotic activity, zone of inhibition testing flowed from the need to rapidly determine the suspectibility of clinical isolates for a series of antibiotics. Whether tests are performed in a liquid or solid medium, results determining the bactericidal concentration are more pertinent for antimicrobials.

There are numerous descriptions and refinements of test procedures for MIC determinations, but the basic information here is taken from Youmans et al. (1975). The concentration of antimicrobial ingredient required to inhibit or kill a range of bacteria is considered against the amount that should be applied or levels that are achievable topically or systemically. The always uncertain element is the multiple of the MIC that should be used in formulation for assurance of effectiveness.

The determination is usually made by incorporating antimicrobial agents in a culture medium and then determining if the microorganism is inhibited from growing or is killed at different concentrations of the test agent. Most susceptibility testing is carried out by either of the two dilution methods or by measuring a zone of growth inhibition of the test microorganism surrounding a paper disk containing the antimicrobial agent. Youmans et al. (1975) list the advantages and disadvantages associated with the different techniques (Table 58–1).

Quantitative susceptibility testing by broth or agar dilution is performed by making twofold dilutions of the test antimicrobial agent in a culture medium by inoculating a standard number of microorganisms and incubating for 18 hours. The amount of the test agent that will inhibit visible growth of the test organism is termed the minimal inhibitory concentration (MIC). If the culture medium is broth, subcultures from tubes showing inhibition of growth after 18 hours are made to a medium free of antimicrobial agents and reincubated for an additional 18 hours to determine the minimal lethal concentration when the antimicrobial chemical is removed. The minimum lethal concentration is defined as the smallest concentration of antimicrobial agent that, on subculture, either fails to show growth or results in a 99.9% decrease in the initial inoculum—this is also known as minimal bactericidal concentration (MBC). Broth dilution studies traditionally have been carried out by the serial twofold dilutions of a single antimicrobial agent to produce eight to ten separate concentrations. Mechanized and automated procedures have been de-

Table 58–1. *Characteristics of Different Types of Susceptibility Test Procedures*

| | Type of Susceptibility Test | | |
| | Dilution | | Agar Disk |
Characteristic	Broth	Agar	Diffusion
Provides minimal inhibitory concentration	+	+	−
Can provide determination of lethal action	+	−	−
Accurate to within ± 1 dilution	+	+	−
Requires little effort (cost)	−	−	+
Information on large number of organisms easy to obtain	−	+	+
Contamination easily recognized	−	+	+

From Youmans, G.P., Paterson, P.Y., and Sommers, H.M. 1975. Drug susceptibility testing in vitro: monitoring of antimicrobial therapy. In *Biologic and Clinical Basis of Infectious Diseases.* Philadelphia, W.B. Saunders, p. 750.

veloped and continue to be improved for rapid determinations, especially for multiple clinical specimens. These can be valuable tools, but their limitations should be considered.

Agar dilution susceptibility testing is easily adapted to multiple bacterial or fungal isolates by using a replicator device, the "Steers replicator," which will inoculate 32 to 36 test drugs on a single plate. Serial twofold dilutions of the test chemical can be made, and it is possible to select concentrations of drug that are of interest but are outside of the twofold regimen.

The information derived from this type of test is basic and is useful in planning and designing future tests. The range of organisms to be tested is suggested elsewhere in this chapter. The characteristics of a particular antimicrobial may dictate the type of MIC determination, and its antimicrobial spectrum may focus on particular groups of test organisms a reasoned selection of organisms for type and use of the product is urged. Solubility of an ingredient may determine the type of test. Much MIC determination has become highly automated and mechanized in hospital use.

Kelsey-Sykes Procedure

The Kelsey-Sykes procedure is included in place of the more familiar, standardized phenol coefficient determination, which can be found in detail in previous editions of this book (Block, 1977; Lawrence and Block, 1968). Some chemical antimicrobials are not tested appropriately by methods utilizing a comparison to the action of phenol. Where this method is used, however, this test, using an organic load as part of the challenge, is more appropriate. Most topical antimicrobial product uses involve the presence of organic material or skin debris, simulating an inactivation influence that may occur in use.

In their description of the test, Kelsey and Sykes (1969)

state that numerous attempts have been made during the past 20 years to overcome the now universally recognized deficiencies in the Rideal-Walker, Chick-Martin, and similar phenol coefficient tests for determining the value of disinfectants. The major points of criticism are the absence of realism in the test conditions and the low level of reproducibility of the tests.

Absence of realism arises mainly from the choice of organisms used in the tests and the linking of the performance of the disinfectant with that of phenol. This results in the need for a fairly large correction factor to derive what is considered to be a satisfactory use-dilution. Frequently, no attempt is made to confirm the value derived by comparison with phenol.

The following test described by Kelsey and Sykes (1969) is taken from their original publication.

Materials

Standard hard water. Standard water of 300 ppm hardness, made by adding 17.5 ml of a 10% (w/v) solution of $CaCl_2·6H_2O$ and 5 ml of a 10% (w/v) solution of $MgSO_4·7H_2O$ to 3300 ml of distilled water and sterilizing in the autoclave in suitable small volumes.

Media. A good nutrient broth or agar (such as Oxoid CM 67 or CM 3) should be used. When necessary, an appropriate inactivator should be added and its efficacy checked as in British Standard 3286: 1960.

Yeast suspension. This is prepared as a 5% (dry weight) suspension of bakers' yeast in water as in the British Standard for determining the Chick-Martin coefficient of disinfectants (British Standard 808: 1938). For use in the test, 2 ml of this suspension are added to each 3 ml of distilled water to give a working concentration of 2%.

Horse serum. Inactivated horse serum (Burroughs Wellcome No. 2) at an initial concentration of 20% is the recommended culture suspension. Four organisms may be used: *Staphylococcus aureus* NCTC 4163, *Escherichia coli* NCTC 8196, *Pseudomonas aeruginosa* NCTC 6749, and *Proteus vulgaris* NCTC 4635. Other strains can be added as the occasion requires. These organisms should be maintained in the freeze-dried state and used throughout, preferably from normal 24-hour broth cultures, although cultures on slopes may also be used. Incubation is at 30 to 32°C. The current cultures should be renewed frequently at, say, monthly intervals from the freeze-dried stocks to avoid undue changes in resistance and other characteristics.

The viable counts from these cultures are normally in the range of 10^8 to 10^9/ml, and they should not be used if the count is less than 10^8/ml. If agar slope cultures are used, the 24-hour growth should be washed from the surface with a small amount of broth, yeast suspension, or horse serum, as appropriate, and diluted in the same liquid to give a concentration of about 10^9 organisms/ml. All cultures should be shaken with Ballotini beads immediately before counting to remove clumps. For tests simulating clean conditions, the organisms are suspended in broth; for those simulating dirty conditions, the organisms are suspended in yeast or horse serum.

Dilutions of the Disinfectant

Any number of a range of dilutions of the disinfectant may be tested, but probably the most suitable number is three: (1) the concentration recommended by the manufacturer, (2) a concentration 25% weaker than this, (3) a concentration that is an equal amount stronger than this. Such a choice gives some measure of the margin of safety when the disinfectant is used at the concentration recommended. The choice of concentrations differing from the recommended one by ±25% is arbitrary and can be varied according to requirements. All dilutions should be made in the standard hard water, and they should be freshly prepared.

Test Procedure

To 3 ml of each disinfectant dilution add 1 ml of the bacterial suspension prepared in broth, yeast, or serum, as required, and shake gently. After 8 minutes, remove a sample of the mixture with a "50 dropper" pipette and transfer one drop to each of five tubes of the liquid recovery medium. Alternatively, five drops may be placed separately on a nutrient agar plate. Two minutes later, i.e., 10 minutes after the first inoculation, reinoculate the disinfectant mixture with a further 1 ml of the bacterial suspension, and 8 minutes later subculture as before. A further 2 minutes later, i.e., 20 minutes after the first inoculation, repeat the process again. The initial test is carried out at 20 to 22°C, and all subcultures are incubated at about 32°C for 48 hours. Record the number of tubes showing growth in the liquid medium or the numbers of colonies growing on the surface plate cultures.

Interpretation of Results

No growth of the test organisms in two or more of the five subculture tubes after the second incremental addition signifies that the disinfectant is satisfactory for use at the initial concentration used in the test. It must not be assumed, however, that a reliable result can be obtained from a single test. The test should be repeated several times on different occasions and the mean response calculated for each disinfectant dilution employed. A satisfactory concentration is that in which there is no growth in 40% or more of the total number of tubes after the second increment. In terms of the surface-plate recovery technique, the satisfactory dilution is that which gives not more than five colonies from the five drops subcultured or in a series of tests, that dilution which gives a mean of not more than one colony from each drop cultured after the second incremental addition.

It can be readily seen that alterations in the specific details of this test may be necessary. For instance, disinfectant-resistant cultures available in the United States (ATCC-American Type Culture Collection) probably will need to be substituted. Consideration must be given to the chemical being tested, its recognized antimicrobial spectrum to determine which organisms may be resistant, and the specific conditions of use for the product being tested.

The same concepts expressed in this test have been incorporated into a preservative test described in a series of testing guidelines for contact lenses and solutions (Bruch, 1975). Often, antimicrobial products to be used on the human body do not require that an additional preservative be added to a formulation. Because of the limited antimicrobial spectrum of some topically applied antimicrobials, however, a preservative is often required. If testing of the preservative effectiveness of such a formulation is required, a preservative test such as the one I have described previously (Bruch, 1975) is recommended. This included the addition of organic load and a rechallenge with microorganisms during the time of the test, making it more appropriate for multiple-use commercial products than the conventional USP test. The additions in this preservative testing procedure flow directly from the Kelsey-Sykes procedure by considering the actual conditions of use.

Human Skin Model Studies

The tests described here derive from two basic procedures, that is, the discovery that wrapping the skin tightly with saran wrap (occlusive dressing) greatly expands the number of microorganisms per square centimeter and that relatively uniform small wounds can be produced by blistering the skin of volunteers with ammonium hydroxide. These tests have been developed by Leyden et al. (1979) at the University of Pennsylvania School of Medicine, Department of Dermatology, in an attempt to both quantify and simplify antimicrobial testing on the skin. Although there is potential for clinical evaluation in these tests, they are currently regarded as intermediate between strict in vitro testing and a full-blown clinical trial.

These tests can be used to evaluate antibacterial claims for first aid products, skin wound cleansers or protectants, and topical antibiotic products. Some precise time period for sampling and microbiologic evaluation should be established so that whatever time period is required for demonstration of duration of activity is bracketed.

Occlusion Test

The occlusion test measures the ability of an agent to prevent expansion of the resident microflora that occurs when an impermeable dressing is applied to the skin (usually the forearm, though not always). The expanded flora test measures the ability of an agent to suppress a dense population of microorganisms produced by expansion of the resident flora of the forearm by prior application of an impermeable occlusive dressing. The persistence test measures the ability of an agent to establish a reservoir in the skin and exert an antimicrobial effect up to 3 days after the last application of the test material. The ecologic shift test determines any major alteration in cutaneous microbial ecology following several applications of the material under occlusive dressings. The serum inactivation test determines whether the presence of serum proteins interferes with antimicrobial activity.

The 1979 publication by Leyden et al. summarizes the use of these various model tests. This updated summary relies on a number of earlier publications describing the use of skin models. References are made to the human model for inducing localized controlled infections with *Staphylococcus aureus* (Marples and Kligman, 1972) and a description of the cup-scrubbing technique developed by Williamson (1965).

Microbiologic Methods

Cup-Scrubbing Procedure. This method is integral in the testing outlines that follow and is also suggested as a sampling method for other tests described here. It is fairly simple and relatively reproducible; results are reported in organisms per square centimeter, and can be used on irregular skin surfaces. The Cup-Scrub has evolved for quantitative investigation of the skin flora. An area of skin (3.8 cm²) is delineated by a glass cup. One milliliter of wash solution (0.1% Triton X-100 in 0.075M phosphate buffer, pH 7.9) is pipetted in, and the area is scrubbed with moderate pressure for 1 minute. The fluid is replaced with a fresh 1 ml and the scrub repeated. An aliquot of the pooled sample is then diluted in tenfold steps using as diluent 0.05% Triton in 0.037M phosphate buffer to prevent any reaggregation of organisms and the appropriate dilutions plated in trypticase soy agar. After 48 hours of aerobic incubation at 37°C, colonies are counted and the number of viable cells in the original sample calculated by standard methods. I suggest the addition of specific neutralizer to the diluent where known and recommend incubation of the cultures at 32 to 35°C instead of 37°C, reflecting the lower temperature of the skin surface. The inclusion of an added specific neutralizer for the test agent in the stripping or releasing solution is recommended. Triton X-100 is nonionic, but may itself react with some antimicrobials but not with others. (Bergen and Lystad, 1972) is also widely used as a stripping or, better, a releasing agent in the United Kingdom and Europe.

Sampling for the various skin model studies is performed by the detergent scrub method in which the surface within a glass cup 3.8 cm² in area is scrubbed with a Teflon policeman using 0.1% Triton X-100 (a nonionic fluid detergent) as the wash fluid. After serial dilutions in half-strength buffered Triton X-100, single drops (0.025 ml) are allowed to fall on plates of trypticase soy agar (BBL) with and without lecithin and polysorbate 80 (Tween 80) as detoxicants. MacConkey's Agar Medium (BBL) is used for gram-negative organisms and Sabouraud's medium for fungi. Bacterial plates are incubated aerobically at 35°C for 2 days; plates for yeast and fungi are incubated at room temperature.

A potential source of error is the transfer of the antimicrobial substances from the skin to the culture system. This is monitored by assaying for residual antimicrobial activity in the sampling fluid. One drop (0.025 ml) of the original scrub sample is placed on a lawn plate inoculated with a susceptible strain of *Staphylococcus epidermidis*. Inhibition of bacterial growth at the drop sites indicates "carry-over." To evaluate the extent to which this invalidates the results, the survival of a sensitive strain of *S. epidermidis* in the undiluted scrub sample is determined as follows: 0.9 ml of the undiluted culture fluid and 0.1 ml of fresh saline suspension of *S. epidermidis* are mixed and allowed to stand for 4 hours. Quantitative subcultures are made from a mixture of 0.1 ml of inoculum of the *S. epidermidis* suspension in 0.9 ml of Triton X-100. If the counts decline in relation to the control, the test is invalidated. To test which agents carry over, either a neutralizer must be found or sampling must be done at a time when the residue of antimicrobial agent on the skin is insignificant.

When an antibiotic is tested, one must also take into account the possibility of false-negative results through the selection and overgrowth of organisms that are resistant to the test agent. This can be assessed by simultaneously culturing samples on media containing appropriate concentrations of the test antibiotic. Growth of organisms on plates containing the antibiotic demonstrates the presence of resistant strains.

Test Procedures

Occlusion Test. The principle of this test is that the microflora of the forearm skin is sparse (10^1 to 10^3 organisms per cm^2). An impermeable dressing will increase surface moisture by preventing diffusional water loss and thus enhance bacterial growth. The density of resident organisms increases significantly, with counts frequently reaching millions per cm^2 in 48 hours. The organisms involved in the expansion are primarily gram-positive cocci and diphtheroids. In earlier studies, Marples and Kligman (1974) compared antimicrobial agents for 48-hour time periods. This measures not only antibacterial activity but persistence and stability as well. An unstable or rapidly cleared substance would be judged falsely as ineffective. Hence, sampling is now done at 24 and 48 hours.

The procedure is as follows: On each arm, 0.1 ml of the test material is delivered to each of two 5-cm squares (25 cm^2) by a plastic tuberculin syringe (0.1 ml). Each site is covered immediately with a 5-cm square of impermeable plastic film (saran wrap). The site is sealed occlusively by encircling the limb with plastic tape (Dermiclear). A strip of white-backed adhesive tape ½ inch wide (Zonas, Johnson & Johnson) is placed between each test site to prevent the possibility of translocation of test agents and organisms from one site to another. A third site on each arm is treated with 0.1 ml of the vehicle. The control site is always prepared first to prevent its potential contamination by the test substances. After 24 hours of occlusion, the three sites on one arm are sampled quantitatively. The opposite arm is sampled after 48 hours.

Expanded Flora Test. This test measures the ability of an agent to suppress a dense and flourishing population of organisms. The forearm is wrapped with several layers of impermeable plastic film and then sealed at the wrist and below the elbow for 24 hours to expand the resident aerobic flora. After expansion of the resident flora, the procedures are identical to those described in the occlusion test. Two 25-cm^2 sites on each arm are treated with 0.1 ml of the test agent, while a third is treated with a vehicle control. Sites are cultured at 6, 24, and 48 hours, depending on the stability of the test agent. For agents designed to produce immediate bactericidal action, e.g., preoperative preparation (my term), cultures are performed 10 minutes after application. In such cases, care must be taken to rule out carry-over of the test material into the culture fluid as mentioned previously.

Persistence Test. The property evaluated in this procedure is the ability of the agent to establish a reservoir in the horny layer (stratum corneum). Substantive agents that diffuse into the horny layer or bind chemically to it will not be readily removed either by loss from the surface or by absorption, although both factors occur and should be considered.

The test agent (0.5 ml) is applied with a pipette twice daily for 4 days to one entire volar forearm. Twenty-four hours after the last application, occlusive dressings (as before) are applied to three sites on the chemically treated arm as well as to the other arm treated only with the vehicle. If an antimicrobial effect is demonstrable, the test is repeated, and the post-treatment interval is extended to 72 hours.

Ecologic Shift Test. Many agents, particularly antibiotics, have restricted in vitro antibacterial spectra. In vivo, this may bring about replacement of the resident microflora by potential pathogens (such as gram-negative organisms and yeasts) that normally do not inhabit the site except in low numbers. Ecologic displacements of this kind can be assessed as follows: three 5-cm squares are marked on each forearm, one site serving as a control. The other two sites are treated every 48 hours with the test agent for a total of three applications (1 week of continuous occlusion). The dressings are replaced after each application. Quantitative cultures are obtained after the third 48-hour period of occlusion.

Serum Inactivation Test. Certain antimicrobial agents may be inactivated if their use involves application to exudative lesions or to superficial injuries that produce serum on the surface. The effect of serum on antimicrobial activity is assessed as follows: volunteers who have given informed consent have 50% ammonium hydroxide applied to their forearms within a glass cylinder 1 cm in diameter according to the method of Frosch and Kligman (1977a). Within 15 minutes, intraepidermal blisters are produced: they are immediately unroofed with sterile scissors, producing an injury that mimics an abrasion. The blister is then inoculated with a marker strain of *Staphylococcus epidermidis*, a nonpathogenic resident coccus that grows readily and can be recognized by its red pigment. This ensures that the microbial population will be roughly the same at each site and also counteracts invasion of virulent organisms such as *Staphylococcus aureus*. The wounds are covered for 6 hours with impermeable plastic film to encourage growth of the implanted coccus. The test material (0.02 ml) is applied occlusively for 24 hours.

These same investigators have also employed the ammonium hydroxide wound and a scarification procedure described by Frosch and Kligman (1977b) to simulate clinical infections of minor wounds. They have used selected, antibiotic-susceptible strains of *Staphylococcus aureus* and *Streptococcus pyogenes* to inoculate the specially prepared types of artificially produced, superficial wounds. These procedures offer a convenient and inexpensive preliminary to performance of a clinical trial.

Comparative studies must be done to determine whether the adaptations required to perform the test alter the comparison of an actual wound with this artificially produced and inoculated one. Volunteers have been used in the studies executed to date, and great care must be taken that serious infection does not occur.

Testing Guidelines for a Health-Care Personnel Handwash

Testing of products for repeated application to remove or reduce transient flora have often been assessed by standard handwashing procedures, but these procedures often lack connection to the real conditions of use of the products.

Simulation of contamination of the hands that normally occurs during work in patient care or in other work situations has usually involved using artificially grown culture applied to the hands. No point-by-point protocol has been adopted for this testing. However, the factors required in this test can be enumerated.

Culture

Marker cultures that can be easily identified by color, morphology, or metabolic reaction with dye in the culture medium need to be used. *Bacillus subtilis* var. *niger* (*globigii*), *Serratia marcescens* (red pigmented strain), a pigmented strain of *Micrococcus*, and *Escherichia coli* have been used. Quantitative assessment of the number of organisms applied must be known, but the number removed by repeated washings also must be estimated. In some situations the number of the marker strain organisms remaining after the test regimen is applied has also been used to determine effectiveness.

Application

High counts per milliliter (10^8 to 10^{10}) have been used so that a small volume of culture may be spread evenly over the hands. Dipping of the hands into a volume of the culture has also been used as a means of contaminating the hands. Uniformity in application of high numbers of organisms is most important. Rotter's (1984) technique of dipping the entire hand into liquid culture with air drying is effective, but a better drying system could be used. Application by rubbing into the skin with a gloved finger tip has been cited (Lowbury, 1975).

Sampling

The glove juice procedure using a surfactant stripping solution in the glove (see later section on Glove Juice Test) has been used to sample hands after washing to determine removal of transients. Standard washing in a bowl after use of the test regimen, such as that employed in the Price handwashing procedure (Price, 1938), can be used. Selwyn (1972, 1985), in a comparison of sampling procedures, showed that all sampling methods tested recovered less than 20% of the total skin flora, and that the cup-scrub was the most efficient. Only full-thickness biopsy could recover the entire count. Ayliffe et al. (1978) utilizes a bowl with stripping solution (neu-

tralizer) and glass beads to effectively remove the fraction of the microbial count remaining. Casewell (1988) has adopted this technique to sampling inoculated fingers in a medicine vial with fluid and glass beads to assay the counts on individual fingers.

Controls

It is critically important that a control group utilizing the product (vehicle) without the active ingredient be tested. Some testing has been conducted without this control in the past and does show significant reduction after repeated contamination and washing of the hands. It must be remembered, however, that mechanical washing removes significant amounts of contamination acquired in the work process.

Subjects and Number of Applications

The testing performed to date has employed 25 to 30 subjects per group using 25 applications of the test regimen spaced at uniform intervals.

A substantive antimicrobial may show a decrease in the number of organisms remaining on the skin as time increases. The important criteria are rapid activity and removal of organisms, suggesting that surfactant activity and antimicrobial activity may be equally important.

Casewell et al. (1988) described a model for testing antimicrobials for hygienic hand disinfection. Hygienic hand disinfection is a term described by Rotter for testing our type of HCPH product. It is based on artificial contamination of the hands and is recognized as an official way of testing products in Germany, Austria and other European countries. Casewell reports that he does not believe it reflects the actual contamination/disinfection dynamic as it occurs in the hospital ward setting. Casewell replaces the much criticized test organism (*Escherichia coli*) with *Klebsiella aerogenes* (K21) which he recognizes as more clinically relevant.

The inoculum procedure was designed to be more clinically relevant. The most distal phalanges of the palmer surface of one hand are inoculated with culture from a Pasteur pipette. The fingertips are opposed and the inoculum evenly distributed. Each finger can then be sampled in a timed sequence (a valuable asset to eliminate variation).

To sample, the finger is washed and rotated for 30 seconds in a sterile galley pot containing 30 ml of sterile glass beads and 20 ml of 0.1% tryptane in phosphate buffer at pH 7.0 or neutralizer broth. An uninoculated finger is counted as a control. Finger tests for carry-over of the test product into the sampling fluid are tested. Samples are taken at 0, 1, 3, 10, and 30 minutes after inoculation. The target inoculum level for study is 10^3. The authors believe that fingertips become contaminated and are the means of transmission, and have tested them accordingly. Residual activity was demonstrated after several variations in scrubbing regimen.

**Testing Guideline for a Patient
Preoperative Preparation**

Specific protocols have not been formalized, but certain requirements for testing have emerged:

1. A variety of body sites must be tested, including the groin area.
2. A cup-scrubbing procedure (Williamson, 1965) for skin sampling is most efficient in quantitative recovery and can be used on some irregular areas of skin.
3. Alternate sides of the selected body area can be used for the control (baseline determination).
4. A criterion of a 3-$\log_{10}$ reduction from the pretreatment baseline count has been established for the definition of a preoperative preparation. A statistical test based on a hypothesis test confirming a 3-$\log_{10}$ reduction in microbial count comparing test site to control site should be made.
5. Often, a preoperative preparation is used after initial washing of the skin with an antimicrobial soap or a surgical scrub product. The testing procedures should be executed with the test preparation alone, because pretreatment of the skin area would reduce the count to an initial level that would prohibit showing a 3-$\log_{10}$ reduction. The goal of a preoperative preparation is removal or killing of as much of the skin microflora as possible prior to a surgical procedure. The addition of precleansing of the skin site simply adds to the effectiveness of the preoperative preparation.

**Effectiveness Test for a Surgical Hand Scrub:
Glove Juice Test**

The FDA OTC Antimicrobial I Panel members, working with Food and Drug Administration personnel and other microbiologists, recommended the following test, which is required by the Food and Drug Administration and which must be performed to support the efficacy of a product labeled as a surgical hand scrub.

The determination of the microbial counts found in the accumulated fluid in the surgeon's gloves has been suggested in the literature as a method for the determination of the efficacy of surgical scrub products. The characteristics of routine handwashing procedures derive from the Price test described in 1938 (more recently, the Cade and Quinn tests) and have their place, but the results of these tests are easily manipulated by changes in the routine, timing, and recovery procedures. The development of improved sampling (sampling solution) procedures and recovery techniques has greatly improved the reliability of skin sampling data. An effectiveness test that more closely simulates the actual procedures carried out by the surgeon is desirable and necessary.

This protocol is meant to be a guideline for performing tests to support claims of effectiveness as a surgical hand scrub. Undoubtedly it will be modified with experience.

Criteria for Subject Selection

(1) Mixed male and female. Race should be recorded. (2) Adults. (3) Subjects will vary greatly in the number of microorganisms carried on the skin. Subjects with a high hand count as measured by sampling with the glove juice procedure should be used for the test. Counts should be in the range from 1.5×10^6 to 4×10^6 per hand. (4) Medication: Subjects receiving antibiotics or taking oral contraceptives should be excluded from the test. (5) Thirty subjects per test.

Pretest Period

The subjects for this test should not use any products containing antimicrobials for at least 2 weeks prior to the test. This restriction includes antimicrobial antiperspirants and deodorants, shampoos, creams, lotions, soaps, or powders. Subjects receiving antibiotic therapy or taking oral contraceptives should be disqualified.

Subjects should be issued rubber gloves to be worn during their daily routine when they come in contact with detergents, acids, bases, or solvents.

Gloves for Test

Gloves should be washed with sterile distilled water before use and applied wet. Gloves that are prepowdered should be carefully washed free of powder, since many of these powders contain antimicrobials.

Baseline Period and Sampling

The baseline period should be 1 week following the 2 weeks of the pretest period. The baseline counts should begin on Day 1 of the baseline period. This initial count is a screen to determine eligibility.

The Day 1 count is also one count to be included for the mean baseline count. The counting procedure should be performed on Day 7 and also on either Day 3 or Day 5, for a total of three estimations of the baseline count.

The baseline counts should be performed using exactly the same sampling and recovery techniques used for the test products under the testing procedure. This information will also be used to provide evidence to assess the assumption that the right and left hand gave comparable results.

Both hands should be sampled for the baseline count. Subjects should not wash prior to the counting procedure on the day of the test.

The baseline procedure is as follows: Hands, including two-thirds of the forearm, are washed for 30 seconds with Camay soap and sterile distilled water at 35 to 40°C. The excess water is shaken from the hands and the gloves are donned with the hands wet. Sampling solution (see *Appendix* to this chapter) is added to the gloves (the volume of sampling solution should remain constant for all tests). The subject holds the glove closed at the wrist while the attendant massages the hand for 1 minute. A measured volume is withdrawn for the count.

Testing Procedure

Scrubbing Procedure. The scrubbing procedure should be exactly as directed on the label of the product being tested, including the use of a nail cleaner and/or a brush if indicated. The hand and two-thirds of the forearm should be scrubbed.

Sampling Technique and Times. After the scrub is performed, loose-fitting surgeon's or examining gloves are donned. Leave the hands wet by shaking off excess water when the gloves are put on. Immediately, the designated control hand is sampled for the 1-minute count as follows: Sampling solution containing buffer and surfactant is added to the glove, the hand massaged for 1 minute, and a measured sample removed for plating. The volume of the sampling solution added to the glove should be kept constant for all tests. The fluid should be shaken vigorously prior to dilution or culturing. If diluent is used, neutralizer should be added to dilution blanks.

The glove is to remain on the other hand for the duration of the time of the test. It is suggested that tests be done at least 1, 2, 3, 4, 5, and 6 hours after the scrub.

The times for which a glove remains on one of the hands after the scrub should be allocated by random selection among the subjects in groups of five. This procedure is performed on Day 1 and Day 2 of the test period. The procedure should be repeated on Day 5 after scrubbing with the product according to directions two additional times on Day 2 and three times per day on Days 3 and 4 at 1-hour intervals. One scrub should be performed on Day 5 and the gloves allowed to remain on the left hand for 1, 2, 3, 4, 5, and 6 hours.

The number of subjects used for the test should be 30, with randomization into 6 groups (n = 5 per group) corresponding to 1, 2, 3, 4, 5, and 6 hours. The allocation of subjects to groups remains constant after initial randomization.

Recovery Media. A medium containing a neutralizer specific for the antimicrobial being tested must be used. Media that have been used in the past include Letheen medium and trypticase soy agar with Tween 80 and serum added.

The neutralizing system used for antimicrobial agents must be tested and the data from the tests submitted. The neutralizer should not be toxic to cells and must be effective in neutralizing the specific chemical. These data must be submitted.

The cultures should be incubated at $30 \pm 2°C$ for 48 to 72 hours. If culturing is undertaken for specific organisms such as fungi or anaerobes, appropriate culturing procedures should be instituted.

Duplicate plates have been used routinely for plating in the past. Because of the inherent variability in counts and the presence of clumps of cells from skin sampling, it is suggested that a minimum of triplicate plating be used. A larger number may be required, depending on the variability. The counts should be reported as count per hand.

Variations of this procedure are in use. For instance, instead of sampling directly from the glove, the glove is removed and turned inside out into stripping fluid, and the hand is rinsed with sampling solution as well. If variations of this test are to be used, and if there is to be regulatory use of data, the protocol should be checked with Food and Drug Administration personnel first.

Data Handling: Design and Statistical Aspects

It is assumed that there are no differences in microbial count between the right and left hand. It is known that microbial handedness (a difference in count between hands) exists; however, this apparently has no relationship with whether the subject is left- or right-handed. The possible difference in count should be compensated for with the initial random allocation of subjects.

This will be tested using the baseline count to validate assumptions about the influence of handedness. It is necessary, therefore, to keep data for the left and right hand distinct. The assignment of hands is as follows:

Test the right hand at 1 minute as observation of reduction from baseline (right hand baseline) on all (30) subjects.

The objective of the design will be to test as follows:

1. Test the log_{10} reduction from baseline 1 minute after scrubbing with fast-acting, broad-spectrum antimicrobials.
2. Test the initial log_{10} reduction from baseline 1 minute after scrubbing with a substantive antimicrobial.
3. Test the log_{10} reduction from baseline 1 minute after scrubbing following 3 days with three consecutive scrubs per day performed at 1-hour intervals.

A Test of the Assumption. A test of the assumption that the agent produces a given log_{10} reduction, such as 1-, 2-, or 3-log_{10} reduction, should be made using the data from the 1-minute result from the right hand compared to the average baseline (right-hand baseline). A method like a paired t-test could be used.

Left-Hand Comparison. The left hand, at a time designated by random assignment to one of six time periods (five subjects in each of six groups), should be compared to the left-hand baseline.

The objective here is to characterize the trend (in microbial growth) with time up to 6 hours. It is desirable that the count not exceed the baseline over the 6 hours with fast-acting, broad-spectrum antimicrobials. It is expected that the count will not exceed the baseline in 6 hours in the testing of substantive antimicrobials.

The analyses should be performed first on each replication. There is replication of the entire test on Day 2 and on Day 5 after three consecutive washes at hourly intervals on Days 3, 4, and 5. Use the original group assignments of subjects observed for the same time periods as determined by random allocation.

Tests of trends may be done using either an orthogonal procedure or some suitable regression method. A combined analysis using the results of the three replications is possible using an appropriate analysis of variance technique, for example, an analysis of variance on the total set of experimental results using the model described by Winer (1961), where hours correspond to factor A and replications correspond to factor B. The baseline could be introduced as a covariant. Tests of trends using the orthogonal procedures should be employed.

Comments on the use of multiple plates in the culturing procedures and on the evaluation of specific neutralizers for use in the testing of antimicrobial agents apply to all in vivo testing.

Analyses of tests that have been performed have pointed to a needed addition in the analysis to compare the baseline/1-minute count reduction on Days 1, 2, and 5 in order to show substantive activity on the skin and effect on the resident microflora of the hands as the product is used over the 5-day test period.

The results from this testing procedure have shown it to be a good discriminating test for various aspects of the surgical scrubbing procedure, including the time the gloves are worn.

APPENDIX

1. Sampling solution (Williamson, 1965). Triton X-100: 0.1% in 0.075M phosphate buffer, pH 7.9.
2. Sampling fluid (Petersen, 1971, 1978). Potassium phosphate (monobasic)-0.4 g
   Sodium phosphate (dibasic)-10.1 g
   Triton X-100-1.8 g
   Distilled water-1 L
   Final pH: 7.8

Example of Glove Juice Test Data Demonstrating Artifact Problem

LOG_{10} REDUCTION IN COUNT*

	2% chlorhexidine product	4% chlorhexidine product	Hibiclens product
Immediate Reductions			
Day 1	1.7963	2.5371	1.5031
2	1.9459	2.7833	2.0726
5	4.1381	2.8057	2.9480
3 Hours After Scrub			
Day 1	1.1369	1.6547	0.9313
2	2.2000	2.2784	2.3111
5	2.6009	3.2950	4.0467
6 Hours After Scrub			
Day 1	1.4883	0.8324	0.7081
2	2.2632	1.4423	1.4931
5	4.3728	2.2619	2.1451

*Baseline determined −3 value estimate 1 week before the trial.
Baseline counts were 10^6 to 10^7 (log_{10} ranged from 6.1073 to 7.2279).

In reality, the initial reduction does not change over time as the test (Days 1 to 5) is now performed, the baseline is estimated the week before the test. On the first test day, the initial reduction (baseline minus time count) averages a 1 + log_{10}, but in these results presented above, it appears that the initial reduction increases over the test days. However, this is an artifact. When the antimicrobial is substantive or persistent, and to some extent even when it is not, the baseline count (count prior to exposure to antimicrobial) itself is reduced, but that initial reduction most likely does not change significantly—it only appears that the reduction increases.

Consequently, we believe when looking at data that the reduction increases when, in fact, the initial reduction stays the same; the real level of the count is reduced on Days 2 and 5 (we do not know to what degree). The reduction achieved may be maintained over the 6-hour period or may be gradually lowered with increasing count. We do not know these as facts, but test results mitigate to a change in the test to a one-hand baseline estimation at the time of the test.

Antimicrobial Soaps

These products are involved only peripherally in the subject of this chapter. These products are used widely for their deodorant effect. Entire-body exposure occurs in use; however, testing has been done almost exclusively with handwashing tests. Where deodorancy is the goal, correlation with deodorancy testing is important. Handwashing tests are still used, but modifications should be incorporated into the Cade handwashing test if it is to be used in the future.

The following comments from the OTC Antimicrobial Panel I report (Food and Drug Administration, 1978) are applicable.

Modified Cade Procedure

The Cade handwashing test was developed to standardize exposure to a given test product, usually an antimicrobial soap. The washing period was standardized in Cade's original publication (1951). The techniques for sampling and recovery of microbial flora have been refined over the years since the original publication. Some of these refinements are incorporated into the following discussion of the Cade test.

The data that can be derived from a Cade handwashing test are greatly expanded if a baseline level is established prior to the controlled washing with the test antimicrobial product. Thus, the analyses can be expanded to give reduction from a baseline with samples from the first basin, with subsequent basins or combinations from subsequent basins.

Some adaptations of the test employ a technique for this study that involves utilizing the numbers of microorganisms determined in the first basin used for washing as a representation of the level of the transient flora. They also use the fourth and fifth basins to average what is considered to be the reduction of the resident flora achieved by the repeated handwashings. Any protocol with significantly altered procedures should be checked with FDA personnel. A proposed statistical analysis and interpretation of the data should be planned as part of the protocol. Particular care should be taken that both the soap and the antimicrobial are adequately neutralized in the test procedures. Adequate selective media should be utilized to enumerate both gram-positive and gram-negative organisms.

The following outline contains only those modifications deemed necessary to approximate the Cade handwashing procedure (Cade, 1951):

(a) Baseline: A baseline should be established prior to test with at least three determinations with either the Cade procedures or the Glove Juice procedures for quantitative recovery.
(b) Standardized handwashing:
   1. Exposure to bar handling (at least 30 seconds).
   2. Work lather on hands (at least 60 seconds).
   3. Rinse, using a standardized treatment (at least 30 seconds).
(c) Microbial enumeration:
   1. Trypticase soy agar.
   2. Adequate neutralization in either broth or solid medium.
   3. At least triplicate samples.
   4. Millipore filter sampling of fluid as an alternative to plating.
   5. 3-day minimum incubation at 32 to 35°C.
   6. 1- to 2-L basin sterile water without added chlorine.
(d) Washing of hands plus two-thirds of forearm.
(e) Analysis of either:
   1. First basin or
   2. First and/or fourth and/or fifth basin;
   3. Reduction from baseline to first basin;
   4. Reduction from baseline to fourth and/or fifth basin.
(f) Duration of test: At least 10 consecutive days, optimally 14 days.
(g) Frequency of exposure: Three times daily. Washout period before subjects are used in another test should be established so that no substantial residual action remains. Periods from 2 weeks to 2 months have been proposed, but actual time should be established.
(h) At least 35 subjects in test with a selected high-count subject population. If groups are split, the analysis should specify this prior to the test and should be statistically acceptable.
(i) Correlation of microbial reduction on the hands is an indication of microbial population reduction. Actual claims of deodorancy should correlate such a microbial reduction to an adequately designed and executed deodorancy test, such as a controlled sniff test.

Data Analysis. Much of the data derived from this study have been analyzed with analysis of variance or other procedures to determine if a significant reduction has occurred after known exposure to the test soap. A more desirable procedure for analysis is to set a null hypothesis that a given reduction, i.e., a 1- or 2-$\log_{10}$ reduction, has taken place and then to test that hypothesis. Determination of a statistically significant reduction alone when dealing with microbial count is a naive approach, since a significant reduction can be achieved with a small reduction. Therefore, the approach just described should be used.

This model has potential for use in studying products for HCPH, and especially for analysis of substantivity or persistent action.

Summary of ASTM Method for Evaluation of Surgical Hand Scrub Formulations

This test method is conducted on panels of selected volunteers who have not used any antimicrobials for at least 2 weeks prior to the test. Twelve panelists are selected on the basis of high initial bacteria count, that is, $\geq 1 \times 10^5$ per hand determined by baseline measurements of bacteria on their hands.

The panelists perform a simulated surgical scrub under supervision. One hand, either right or left, of each of the panelists is sampled for microorganisms immediately after the scrub (within 5 minutes). The other hand of each of the panelists is sampled either 3 or 6 hours after scrubbing. Six panelists are sampled at each time interval.

Ten additional scrubs are performed with test formulation over the 5-day test period following the initial scrub. The hands are sampled two additional times, once after the second scheduled use of the product, and again after the last scheduled scrub.

This procedure should be used to evaluate the ability of a test formulation to reduce the bacterial population immediately after a single or multiple use and to determine the trend in growth over a 6-hour period whether a single or multiple use is tested.

Apparatus Appropriate

Colony Counter—Any of several types may be used.
Incubator—Any incubator capable of maintaining a temperature of $30 \pm 2°C$ may be used.
Sterilizer—Any suitable steam sterilizer capable of producing the conditions of sterility is acceptable.
Time (stop-clock)—One that can be read for minutes and seconds.
Hand Washing Sink—A sink of sufficient size to permit panelists to wash without touching hands to sink surface or other panelists.
Water Faucet(s)—Faucets should be located above the sink at a height that permits the hands to be held higher than the elbows during the washing procedure. [It is desirable for the height of the faucet(s) to be adjustable.]
Tap Water Temperature Regulator and Temperature Monitor—To monitor and regulate water temperature to $40 \pm 2°C$.

Materials and Reagents

Petri Dishes—100 mm by 15 mm. Required for performing standard plate count.
Bacteriologic Pipets—10.0 and 2.2 or 1.1 ml capacity.
Water-Dilution Bottles—Any sterilizable glass con-

tainer with a 150 to 200 ml capacity and tight closures may be used.

Baseline Control Soap—A liquid castile soap or other liquid soap containing no antimicrobial.

Gloves—Sterile loose-fitting gloves of latex, unlined, possessing no antimicrobial properties.

Test Formulation—Directions for use of test formulation should be included if available. If none are available, use directions provided in this test method.

Sampling Solution—Dissolved 0.4 g KH_2PO_4, 10.1 g Na_2HPO_4, and 1.0 g isooctylphenoxypolyethoxyethanol[10] in 1 L distilled water. Adjust to pH 7.8. Dispense in 75-ml volumes into water dilution bottles, or other suitable containers, and sterilize for 20 minutes at 121°C. Include an antimicrobial inactivator specific for the test formulation being evaluated in the sampling solution used to collect the bacterial samples from the hand following the final wash with the test formulation.

Important—A definitive recommendation regarding the inclusion of an inactivator in sampling solution used for bacterial collections prior to the final wash cannot be made. (*Author's note*—standardization is served as is consistency. If the concern is inactivation on the skin and spacing subsequent sampling, the difficulties could be rectified.) The following two questions should be considered in making a decision: (1) If an inactivator is included in the sampling solution used prior to the final wash, will residual inactivator on the skin reduce the efficacy of the test formulation in subsequent washes and result in higher-than-expected bacterial counts? (2) Can samples collected without an inactivator be processed quickly enough to avoid decreased bacterial count due to continued action of the test formulation? Whatever the decision, to facilitate the comparison of results across studies, the investigator should indicate whether or not an inactivator has been included.

Dilution Fluid—Butterfield's phosphate buffered water adjusted to pH 7.2 and containing an antimicrobial inactivator specific for the test formulation.

Soybeam-Casein Digest Agar—The agar with supplemental polysorbate 80 (0.5 to 10 g/L) to stimulate growth of lipophilic organisms is used.

Fingernail Cleaning Pics or Sticks—These should be used only if directions for use include.

Sterile Hand Scrub Brushes (required if specified for use with test formulation).

Test Panelists

Panelists should be healthy adult volunteers with no clinical evidence of dermatosis, who have not received antibiotics or taken oral contraceptives 2 weeks prior to the test, and who agree to abstain from these materials until the conclusion of the test.

Preparation of Volunteers

At least 2 weeks prior to start of the test, select approximately 20 volunteers as potential test subjects.

Instruct the volunteers to avoid contact with antimicrobials for the duration of the test. This restriction includes antimicrobial-containing antiperspirants, deodorants, shampoos, lotions, soaps, and materials such as acids, bases, and solvents. Bathing in chlorinated pools and hot tubs is to be avoided. Volunteers are to be provided with a kit of nonantimicrobial personal care products for exclusive use during the test and rubber gloves to be worn when contact with antimicrobials cannot be avoided.

Test Procedure

After panelists have refrained from using antimicrobials for at least 2 weeks, perform wash with baseline control soap. Volunteers are not to have washed their hands on this day 2 hours prior to baseline determination. After washing, determine first estimate of baseline bacterial population by sampling hands and enumerating the bacteria in the sampling solution. This is Day 1 of the Baseline Period. Repeat this baseline determination procedure on Days 3 and 7, Days 3 and 5, or Days 5 and 7 of Baseline Period to obtain three estimates of baseline population. After obtaining the first and second estimates of the baseline populations, select panelists who exhibited at each sampling interval counts $\geq 1 \times 10^5$. The three estimates of the baseline population, obtained for each of the 12 selected subjects, are averaged to obtain the mean baseline counts.

Divide the selected panelists into two groups of equal size. One group will represent a 6-hour post-scrub quantitative sample, the other group a 3-hour post-scrub quantitative microbiologic sample.

Between 12 hours and 4 days after completion of the baseline determination, panelists perform the initial scrub with the test formulation. Determine bacterial population on one hand of all panelists immediately after scrub (within 5 minutes) with test formulation. Determine the bacterial population of the other hand of one-half of the panelists 3 hours after scrub and that of the remaining panelists 6 hours after scrub. Determine bacterial population by sampling hands and enumerating the bacteria in the sampling solution as specified.

Repeat this scrubbing and sampling procedure the next day (Day 2). On Day 5, repeat the sampling procedure after scrubbing with the test material two additional times on Day 2 and three times per day on Day 3 and Day 4 with at least a 1-hour interval between scrubs. Perform one scrub on Day 5 prior to sampling. In summary, the panelists scrub a total of 11 times with the test formulation. Collect bacterial samples following 3 of the 11 scrubs. Collect the samples following the single scrubs on Days 1 and 5 and following the first scrub on Day 2.

Washing Technique for Baseline Determinations

Volunteers clean under fingernails with nail stick and clip fingernails to ≤ 2 mm of free edge. Remove all jewelry from hands and arms.

Rinse hands including two-thirds of forearm under running tap water at 38 to 42°C for 30 seconds.

Maintain hands higher than elbows during this procedure and other steps outlined.

Wash hands and forearms with baseline control soap for 30 seconds under tap water.

Don rubber gloves used for sampling the hands and secure gloves at wrist.

Surgical Scrub Technique

Repeat washing procedure above.

Perform surgical scrub with test formulation in accordance with directions furnished with the formulation.

Note: If no instructions are provided with the test formulation, use the 10-minute scrub procedure described herein.

Ten-Minute Scrub Procedures. Dispense formulation into hands.

Set and start timer for 5 minutes (time required for the steps).

With hands, distribute formulation over hands and lower two-thirds of forearms.

If scrub brush is to be used, pick up with fingertips and pass under tap to wet without rinsing formulation from hands.

Alternatively scrub right hand and lower two-thirds of the forearm and left hand and lower-two thirds of forearm.

Rinse both hands, the lower two-thirds of forearms, and the brush for 30 seconds.

Place brush in sterile dish within easy reach.

Repeat the scrub so that each hand and forearm is washed twice. The second wash and rinse should be limited to the lower one third of the forearms and the hands.

Perform final rinse. Rinse each hand and forearm separately for 1 minute per hand.

Don rubber gloves used in sampling hands and secure at wrist.

Surgical Scrub Technique When Bacterial Samples Are Not Included

Perform technique as described. Panelists dry hands with a clean paper towel after final rinse of hands.

Sampling Techniques

At specified sampling times, aseptically add 75 ml of sampling solution to the glove and hand to be sampled and occlude glove above wrist.

After adding sampling solution, uniformly massage all surfaces of the hand for 1 minute.

After massaging, aseptically sample the fluid of the glove.

Enumeration of Bacteria in Sampling Solution

Enumerate the bacteria in the sampling solution by a standard plate count procedure such as that described in Standard Methods for the Evaluation of Dairy Products but using soybean-casein digest agar and a suitable inactivator for the antimicrobial. Prepare sample solutions in dilution fluid. Plate in duplicate. Incubate plated sample at $30 \pm 2°C$ for 48 hours before reading.

Determination of Reduction Obtained

Determine changes from baseline counts obtained with test material at each sampling interval.

For a more realistic appraisal of the activity of products, all raw data should be converted to common (base 10) logarithms. Reductions should be calculated from the average of the logarithms. This will also facilitate statistical analysis of data.

Comparison of Test Materials with a Control Material

It may be desirable to compare the test material with a control material. If this is the case, an equivalent number of panelists should be assigned to the control product on a random basis. All test parameters will be equivalent for both products, although the scrub procedure for an established product may be different. Both products should be run concurrently. The identity of products used by panelists should be blinded from those counting plates and analyzing data. A suggested positive control is a surgical scrub formulation approved by the U.S. Food and Drug Administration.

Compare, at each sampling interval, changes from baseline counts obtained with test material to changes obtained with control material.

The reader is referred to the complete protocol published by ASTM (First edition, 1987) for Surgical Hand Scrub, HCPH, and Preoperative Skin Preparation.

REFERENCES

Ayliffe, G.A.J., Babb, J.R., and Quoraishi, A.H. 1978. A test for "hygienic" hand disinfection. J. Clin. Pathol., *31*, 923–928.

Bartzokas, C.A., Gibson, M.F., Graham, R., and Pinder, D.C. 1983. A comparison of triclosan and chlorhexidine preparations with 60 percent isopropyl alcohol for hygienic hand disinfection. J. Hosp. Infect., *4*, 245–255.

Bergen, T., and Lystad, A. 1972. Evaluation of disinfectant inactivators. Acta Pathol. Microbiol. Scand., *B80*, 507–510.

Block, S.S. 1977. *Disinfection, Sterilization, and Preservation.* 2nd Edition. Philadelphia, Lea & Febiger.

Brandberg, A., and Andersson, I. 1981. Preoperative whole body disinfection by shower bath with chlorhexidine soap: Effect on transmission of bacteria from skin flora. In *Skin Microbiology: Relevance to Clinical Infection.* New York, Springer-Verlag.

Bruch, M.K. 1975. The regulation of hydrophilic contact lenses by the Food and Drug Administration. In *Developments in Industrial Microbiology.* Volume 17. Monticello, NY, Lubrecht & Cramer, pp. 29–47.

Bruch, C.W., and Bruch, M.K. 1971. Sterilization. In *Husa's Pharmaceutical Dispensing.* Edited by E.W. Martin. Easton, PA, Mack Publishing, pp. 592–623.

Cade, A.R. 1951. A method for testing the degerming efficiency of hexachlorophene soaps. J. Soc. Cosmet. Chem., *2*, 281–290.

Casewell, M.W., Law, M.M., and Desai, N. 1988. A laboratory model for testing agents for hygienic hand disinfection: handwashing and chlorhexidine for removal of klebsiella. J. Hosp. Infect., *12*, 163–175.

Centers for Disease Control. 1981. Proceedings of the International Conference on Nosocomial Infections. Aug. 1981.

Code of Federal Regulations (21 CFR) Title I. 1981. Food and Drugs. Washington, D.C., Government Printing Office, pp. 130–end.

Cremieux, A., et al. 1988. A standardized method for the evaluation of hand disinfection. Presented at the Interscience Conference on Antimicrobial Agents and Chemotherapy. Los Angeles, CA, October 24–27.

Dixon, R.E. (ed.) 1981. *Nosocomial Infections.* New York, Yorke Medical.

Food and Drug Administration. 1979. OTC Oral Cavity Panel Report. Oral Health Care Drug Products for Over-the-Counter Human Use. Federal Register, Jan. 27, 1988. 53(17):2436–2461.

Food and Drug Administration. 1978. OTC Topical Antimicrobial Products. Tentative Final Monograph (21 CFR Part 33), 43, (4). Federal Register, Jan. 6, pp. 1210–1249.

Food and Drug Administration. 1974. OTC Topical Antimicrobial Products and Drug and Cosmetic Products. Federal Register, Sept. 13. 39(179). Part II. 33102–33141.

Frosch, P.J., and Kligman, A.M. 1977a. Rapid blister formation in human skin. Br. J. Dermatol., 96, 461–473.

Frosch, P.J., and Kligman, A. 1977b. The Chambers scarification test for assessing irritancy of topically applied substances. In *Cutaneous Toxicity— Proceedings of the Third Conference on Cutaneous Toxicity.* Washington, D.C., May 16–18, 1976. Edited by V.A. Drill and P. Lazar. New York, Academic Press, pp. 127–154.

Geelhoed, G.W., Sharpe, K. 1983. The rationale and ritual of preoperative skin preparation. Contemp. Surg., 23, 31–36.

Geelhoed, G.W., Sharpe, K., Simon, G.L. 1983. A comparative study of surgical skin preparation. Surg. Gynecol. Obstet., 157, 265–268.

Gove, P.B. 1963. *Webster's Third New International Dictionary.* Springfield, MA, G & C Merriam, p. 96.

Hugo, W.B. 1971. *Inhibition and Destruction of the Microbial Cell.* New York, Academic Press.

Kelsey, J.C., and Sykes, G. 1969. A new test for the assessment of disinfectants with particular reference to their use in hospitals. Pharm. J., 202, 607–609.

Knorr, M. (ed.) 1973. The 2nd International Colloquium about the Evaluation of Disinfectants in Europe. Translated from the German by D. Groschel. Zentralbl. Bakteriol. Mikrobiol. Hyg. [B], 157(5–6), 411–551.

Lawrence, C.A., and Block, S.S. 1968. *Disinfection, Sterilization, and Preservation.* 1st Edition. Philadelphia, Lea & Febiger.

Leyden, J.J., Stewart, R., and Kligman, A.M. 1979. Updated in vivo methods for evaluating topical antimicrobial agents on human skin. J. Invest. Dermatol., 72, 165–170.

Leyden, J.J., and McGinley, K. 1989. Regional variations in the cutaneous bacterial flora of the hand. Methodologies for evaluating antimicrobial agents. Presentation at the ICAAC, Houston, Texas. Sep., 1989.

Lowbury, E.J.L., and Lilly, H. 1975. A gloved hand as applicator of antiseptic to operation site. Lancet ii, 153–156.

Marples, M.J. 1969. Life on the human skin. Sci. Am., 220(1), 108–115.

Marples, M.J. 1965. *The Ecology of the Human Skin.* Springfield, IL, Charles C Thomas.

Marples, R.R., and Kligman, A.M. 1974. Methods for evaluating topical antibacterial agents on human skin. Antimicrob. Agents Chemother., 5, 323–329.

Marples, R.R., and Kligman, A.M. 1972. Bacterial infection of superficial wounds: a human model for *Staphylococcus aureus.* In *Epidermal Wound Healing.* Edited by H. Maibach and D. Rovee. Chicago, Yearbook.

Meleney, F.L., and Lopez-Mayor, J. 1964. A comparison of the antiseptic value of certain surgical scrub-up preparations. Am. Surg., 30, 77–82.

Michaud, R.N., McGrath, M.B., and Goss, W.A. 1972. Improved experimental model for measuring skin degerming activity on the human hand. Antimicrob. Agents Chemother., 2(1), 8–15.

Peterson, A. 1971. Personal communication.

Peterson, A., Rosenberg, A., and Alatary, S. 1978. Comparative evaluation of surgical scrub preparations. Surg. Gynecol. Obstet., 146, 63–65.

Price, P.B. 1938. The bacteriology of normal skin: a new quantitative test applied to a study of the bacterial flora and the disinfectant action of mechanical cleansing. J. Infect. Dis., 63, 301–318.

Quinn, H., Voss, J.G., and Whitehouse, H.S. 1954. A method for the in vivo evaluation of skin sanitizing soaps. Appl. Microbiol., 2, 202–204.

Reid, D.E., Walter, C.W., and Buch, A.S. 1950. Surgical scrubbing with pHisoderm G-11 as applied to a maternity hospital. Surg. Gynecol. Obstet., 91, 537–544.

Rhodeheaver, G. 1988. Personal communication.

Rosenberg, A. Alatary, S., and Peterson, A. 1976. Safety and efficacy of the antiseptic chlorhexidine gluconate. Surg. Gynecol. Obstet., 143, 789–792.

Rotter, M.L. Mittermayer, H., and Kundi, M. 1974. Studies on the model of the artificially contaminated hand. Proposal for a test method. Zbl. Bakt. Hyg. Orig B, 1959, 560.

Rotter, M. 1981. Povidone-iodine and chlorhexidine gluconate containing detergents for disinfection of hands. J. Hosp. Infect. 2:273–276.

Rotter, M.L. 1984. Hygienic hand disinfection. Infect. Control, 5(1), 18–22.

Rotter, M.L., et al. 1986. Evaluation of procedures for hygienic hand-disinfection: controlled parallel experiments on the Vienna Test Model. J. Hygiene, 96, 27–37.

Selwyn, S. 1972. Skin bacteria and skin disinfection reconsidered. Br. Med. J., 1, 136–140.

Selwyn, S. 1985. Evaluating skin disinfectants *in vivo* by excision biopsy and other methods. J. Hosp. Infec. 6(Suppl.):37–43.

Singh, G., Marples, R.R., and Kligman, A.M. 1971. Experimental *Staphylococcus aureus* infections in humans. J. Invest. Dermatol., 57, 194–162.

Soulsby, M.E., Barnett, J.B., and Maddox, S. 1986. Brief report: The antiseptic efficacy of chloroxylenol-containing vs. chlorhexidine gluconate-containing surgical scrub preparations. Infect. Control, 7(4), 223–226.

Stutard, I.W. 1961. Release of bacteria from surgeon's hands. Br. Med. J., 1, 591.

Sykes, G. 1965. *Disinfection and Sterilization.* 2nd Edition. Philadelphia, J.B. Lippincott.

Taplin, D. 1981. Antibacterial soaps: chlorhexidine and skin infections. Chap. 15. In: *Skin Microbiology: Relevance to Infection.* New York, Springer Verlag.

Updegraff, D.M. 1964. A cultural method of quantitatively studying the microorganisms on the skin. J. Invest. Dermatol., 43, 129–137.

Walter, C.W. 1965. Disinfection of hands [Editorial]. Am. J. Surg., 109, 691–693.

Walter, C.W., and Kundsin, R. 1969. The bacteriologic study of surgical gloves from 250 operations. Surg. Gynecol. Obstet., 129, 949–952.

Walter, G. 1971. Personal communication.

Williamson, P. 1965. Quantitative estimation of cutaneous bacteria. In *Skin Bacteria and Their Role in Infection.* Edited by H.I. Maibach, and G. Hildick-Smith. New York, McGraw-Hill.

Williamson, P., and Kligman, A.M. 1965. A new method for the quantitative investigation of cutaneous bacteria. J. Invest. Dermatol., 45, 498–503.

Winer, B.J. 1961. *Statistical Principles in Experimental Design.* New York, McGraw-Hill, p. 519.

Youmans, G.P., Paterson, P.Y., and Sommers, H.M. 1975. Drug susceptibility testing in vitro: Monitoring of antimicrobial therapy. In *Biologic and Clinical Basis of Infectious Diseases.* Philadelphia, W.B. Saunders, p. 750.

CHAPTER 59

STERILITY TESTING—VALIDATION OF STERILIZATION PROCESSES, AND SPORICIDE TESTING

Gordon S. Oxborrow and Robert Berube

Sterilization processes have been discussed in previous chapters. However, at the risk of repeating others, a brief discourse on the term "sterile" must be given as an introduction to this chapter.

The classic definition of "sterile," according to Webster's *Seventh New Collegiate Dictionary,* is "free from living organisms and esp. microorganisms." We have no argument concerning the literal state of sterility, but having said something is sterile does not prove it to be so. The process of sterilization is designed to render a product sterile. However, the effectiveness of any sterilization process depends upon several factors, any of which may render some or all of the product units nonsterile. An ethylene oxide sterilization process, for example, may fail because of inadequate humidification of some units within a load of product.

If it is not known that a sterilization process has been effective, then how can the state of sterility be measured? This chapter provides basic information on the requirements for performing a valid sterility test and the validation of a sterilization process. The use and testing of biologic indicators and the use of chemical indicators are discussed. An introduction to sporicidal testing of sterilants is also included.

The classic approach has been to test a product for sterility by exposing it to microbial growth media and observing the media for microbial growth; this method has limitations that will be discussed later. The dependency on sterility testing to determine if a sterilization process has been efficacious is gradually changing as the process of sterilization moves away from a "classic art" and becomes a "science." This change has been made possible by the technologic improvements in process control and monitoring equipment. The concept of what "sterile" means has now become a matter of degree, i.e., there is a certain probability of sterility for each unit of product being sterilized. This probability is commonly referred to as the sterility assurance level (SAL) of the product, and is defined as the $\log_{10}$ number of the probability of a survivor on a single unit; e.g., if the probability of a survivor is one in one million, the SAL would be 6.

To determine the SAL, it is necessary to obtain more information about the microbial load on the product (bioburden) and the physical parameters of the sterilization process than is normally known when releasing a product based on sterility testing. The development, accumulation, and documentation of these data is called "sterilization validation." When sterilization validation is done, the degree of sterility assurance can be determined. This concept requires the manufacturer to build sterility into a product as opposed to building a product and testing it for sterility.

Although it is desirable to build sterility into a product, it may not always be possible or practical. A product that is manufactured infrequently and in small lot sizes may not be amenable to sterilization validation because of inconsistencies in manufacturing. Where products are manufactured for in-house use, such as in hospitals or other health-care facilities, sterility testing together with sterilization load monitoring using biologic and chemical indicators may better serve to demonstrate an acceptable process. In some instances where single units are sterilized, sterility testing can't be done, and process indicators (physical, chemical, and biologic) must be relied upon to assure the effectiveness of the sterilization process for that product.

Four commonly used methods of sterilization have been thoroughly addressed in other chapters of this book, i.e., dry heat, steam, ethylene oxide, and ionizing radiation.

Other less commonly used methods of sterilization

have been developed. Among these are liquid sporicides, gaseous sterilants such as ozone, chlorine dioxide, low-temperature steam formaldehyde, vapor phase hydrogen peroxide, and formaldehyde-induced-plasma processes. These methods have a narrow range of application (Porner and Hoffman, 1968; Hennebert et al., 1986). Liquid sporicides are considered sterilants because they are capable of destroying spores of bacteria and fungi and vegetative cells of yeasts, molds, bacteria, and viruses. These liquid sporicides are routinely used to sterilize single-use medical devices such as hollow fiber dialyzer cartridges for blood purification that are to be reused in a clinical setting. Because there is no known nondestructive test for sterility, previous knowledge concerning the effectiveness of the process must be accumulated prior to assuming that the units can be sterilized with a sporicide. New sterilization processes, as well as the ones mentioned previously, may become applicable to unique product niches in the health-care industry. It is not likely, however, that these methods will become sterilants for a wide variety of products or that they will replace any of the four commonly used methods of sterilization.

STERILITY TESTING

Sterility testing of medical products, as described in the U.S. Pharmacopeia (USP), is the legal referee for determining if a product is sterile or not (USP-NF, 1985). The test protocols described are used by both the manufacturers and the regulatory agency—the U.S. Food and Drug Administration (FDA)—to determine the microbiologic safety of medical products and their components. These protocols are not mandatory, but they are reference tests, and when there is a difference of opinion between the manufacturer and the FDA, the USP tests become the legal basis for comparison, and other tests must be shown to be as good or better if the manufacturer is to avoid litigation (Guilfoyle and Yager, 1984). All of the sterility test protocols outlined in the USP are of two basic types; "direct inoculation" or "membrane filtration." Direct inoculation tests are simply the placement of a product, a portion of a product, or a rinse from a product directly into microbial growth media. All or part of the product may be used, depending on the consistency, the size, or the shape. Membrane filtration is the flushing of a product, a component of a product, or a wash from a product through a membrane filter where any microorganisms are collected. The membrane is then placed in growth media.

These methods sound simplistic, and in design they are. The performance of the test, however, is quite different. Five important factors affect the reliability of a sterility test. The first of these are (1) the sample itself and (2) the portion of each unit tested. The last three are testing factors: (3) the environment, (4) the equipment, and (5) the technique of the personnel doing the test. Each of the five points is now discussed.

Sample

Obtaining a sample that is representative of the sterilization lot with the number of units that is statistically valid for the degree of sterility assurance required, is frequently overlooked or ignored in product sterility testing. It is impossible to test enough units to assure a 100% probability of sterility; that would require a test of all of the product produced. Therefore, a sampling plan must be developed that will provide an acceptable probability of not finding a contaminated unit if one is present. The risks associated with sampling have been well understood for many years. The tables published by Brewer (1957) provide a characterization of these risks. Table 59–1 describes the probability of finding a number of positive units out of 10 test units when the true level of contamination is known. For example, if the true percentage of contamination of a product lot was 1%, then the probability of finding all test units negative for growth would be 90%; one positive unit would be found 1% of the time and two positive units would be found 0.4% of the time. It is obvious from this table that testing 10 units does not give great assurance of sterility unless there is gross failure of the sterilization process and most of the units are contaminated. Table 59–2 shows the relationship of the probability of accepting lots of varying assumed degrees of contamination for various sample sizes.

If the sample size commonly specified by the USP (20 units) is used, it can be seen that the probability of accepting a lot as sterile that has a contamination rate of 1% would be 82 out of every 100 lots tested. When contamination rates are low (1 per 1000), the probability

Table 59–1. *Probability of Designated Positives Out of Ten Samples Tested*

"True" % Contamination	0	1	2	3	4	5	6	7	8	9	10
0.1	.990	(Total = .010)									
0.5	.960	(Total = .040)									
1.0	.904	.091	.004	.000	.000						
2.0	.817	.167	.015	.001	.000						
5.0	.599	.315	.075	.010	.001						
10.0	.349	.387	.194	.057	.011	.001					
20.0	.107	.268	.302	.201	.088	.026	.005	.001			
30.0	.028	.121	.233	.267	.200	.103	.037	.009	.001		
40.0	.006	.040	.121	.215	.251	.201	.111	.042	.011	.001	
50.0	.001	.010	.044	.117	.205	.246	.205	.117	.044	.010	.001

Table 59–2. *Methods of Testing for Stability: Relationship of Probabilities of Acceptance of Lots of Varying Assumed Degrees of Contamination to Sample Size*

N*	% Contaminated													
	0.1	0.3	0.5	1	2	3	4	5	10	15	20	30	40
10	.99	.98	.96	.91	.82	.74	.67	.60	.34	.19	.10	.02	.006
20	.98	.94	.90	.82	.67	.54	.44	.35	.11	.04	.01	.001	
50	.95	.86	.78	.61	.36	.22	.13	.08	.005				
100	.91	.74	.61	.37	.13	.05	.02	.01	.00				
200	.82	.55	.36	.13	.05	.02	.002						
300	.74	.41	.22	.05	.002								
400	.67	.30	.13	.02	.000								
500	.61	.22	.08	.01									

*N = Number of samples tested

of accepting a contaminated lot is still greater than 60% of a 500-unit sample. Table 59–2 also shows that the probability of accepting a contaminated lot does not decrease significantly for a lot with a low level of contamination when the sample size increases from 20 units to 100 units.

Sampled Item Portion (SIP)

When the entire contents of a viral or a complete medical device can be placed into a growth media, the SIP is said to be 1.0. When half of a unit is tested, the SIP is 0.5, etc. This concept is important when sterility testing is used to release a product. If the level of contamination on a product is low, and only a portion of the unit is tested, the reliability of the test is decreased by the same ratio as the SIP; e.g., when testing a large surgical drape for sterility, it is common practice to remove two to four 2-in.² sections taken from various areas throughout the drape. These sections may represent only 8 in.² of a drape. Assuming that four sections were taken from a drape that is 1600 in.² the ratio would be 1:200. The reliability of the sterility test is significantly reduced, particularly when the contamination level is low and random.

Environment

A sterility test must be conducted in a controlled environment. A controlled environment is one that limits access to those persons doing the analysis. It is usually designed as a class 100 clean room to meet Fed. Std. 209-D specifications for particulate control and air flow characteristics. Some clean rooms have conventional (turbulent) air flow systems, whereas others have vertical or horizontal laminar air flow patterns.

High Efficiency Particulate Air (HEPA) filters are generally used regardless of the air flow patterns. HEPA filters are designed to remove particles 0.3 μm or larger from the duct air with a 99.999% efficiency. Because microorganisms are generally larger than 0.3 μm, the air supplied to the room is considered sterile and particle-free. When packages or containers are opened in a clean room, the risk of contaminating the product to be tested is less than if it was opened in a room with a conventional

filtration system. Properly designed clean rooms are easy to clean and maintain (Fed. Std. 209-D), but cleaning and maintenance procedures and schedules must be established and followed. Rooms may be designed to be disinfected with ultraviolet light or disinfecting aerosols. When ultraviolet is used, there must be a positive alarm to warn when ultraviolet is on. Sterility tests can not be conducted under ultraviolet light or in the presence of disinfecting aerosols.

Soft walled clean room modules are used in many instances to provide complete environmental control. These modules are similar to gnotobiotics modules in that all equipment and supplies are passed through a double-door sterilizer attached to the module. The person or persons who perform the sterility test do so through glove ports from the outside. These modules are especially effective for testing sterile-fill pharmaceuticals.

Equipment

Equipment, supplies, materials, and test media that are to come in contact with the product being tested or the environment must be sterile prior to initiating a sterility test. Instruments must be wrapped in a way that allows them to be removed from the package without contaminating them. It is usually desirable to wrap each unit individually, because it is difficult to remove a single instrument from a bulk pack without touching others in the pack. When membrane filtration is being used, great care must be taken to assure sterility of all of the components, including the membranes. A new disposable device for membrane filtration ("Steritest" by Millipore) has proven to be an effective device for reducing inadvertent contamination when sterility-testing filterable liquid products (Gee et al., 1985). It is provided in a sterile condition with filters in place, and is disposable after the test.

It is frequently desirable to conduct sterility tests in a laminar flow hood, even if they are being conducted in a clean room. These hoods are equipped with HEPA filters and provide a controlled area within the clean room environment (Fed. Std. 209-D, 1988). Selection of either a vertical or horizontal flow hood for a specific application can enhance the reliability of the test.

Attached gowning areas, as well as toilet and wash facilities, are necessary components of a sterility test suite. Transporting equipment or samples within the clean room must be done by dedicated carts that are not removed from the room. Equipment that is moved into or out of the room must be transferred to a cart outside the room. Carts must be easily cleaned and noncorrosive.

Personnel

The sterility test analyst is the single most important factor affecting the success or failure of a sterility test. Most false-positive sterility tests can be attributed to the analyst. The false-positive rate for sterility tests in conventional sterility test suites is considered acceptable when one positive is found for each 1000 units tested. The contamination rate is lower, however, in soft walled sterility test modules. The frequency of false-positives in conventional test rooms varies a great deal and depends on the complexity of the test, the technique of the analyst, the type of gowning used, and the amount of microbial shedding from the analyst. Some people shed greater numbers of microorganisms than others. This should be taken into consideration when assigning an analyst to do sterility testing. Anyone with open sores, colds, or other health problems that may contribute to microbial shedding or discharge should not be allowed to do sterility testing. Cosmetics and jewelry worn by the sterility test analyst may also contribute to product contamination, particularly rings with sharp projections that may puncture holes in gloves; these should be minimized. Adherence to good personal hygiene habits is an essential part of contamination control in a sterility test suite. Gowning procedures should be established and carefully adhered to by everyone entering the sterility test suite.

United States Pharmacopeia Sterility Tests

The USP is the standard by which industrial sterilization is legally judged. Although the tests were originally developed to control the quality of and provide test procedures for drugs, they are being applied more actively in the control and testing of medical devices. The USP Convention, Inc. recognizes that the tests described in this section may not be the only procedures that adequately test the sterility of a medical product when they state, "Alternative procedures may be employed to demonstrate that an article is sterile; provided the results obtained are at least of equivalent reliability."

Two basic media are described in the USP for recovery of microorganisms from inadequately sterilized products. They are Fluid Thioglycolate Medium (FTM) and Soy Bean Casein Digest Medium (SCD). A third medium, Alternative FTM, is also identified. Alternative FTM is the same as FTM without the agar and the resazurin sodium solution, and is used for products with lumens that must be flushed. The media used in the USP for sterility testing is adequate to detect most mesophilic, aerobic microorganisms. It can also support the growth of some mesophilic, anaerobic microorganisms. We have found that some thermally stressed or chemically stressed microorganisms may not grow in the media spec-

Table 59–3. *Microorganisms Used for Growth Promotion Testing*

Medium	Microorganism	ATCC No.	Temperature (°C)
FTM	*Bacillus subtilis*	6633	30–35
	Candida albicans	10231	30–35
	Bacteroides vulgatus	8482	30–35
Alt. FTM	*Bacteroides vulgatus*	8482	30–35
SCD	*Bacillus subtilis*	6633	20–25
	Candida albicans	10231	20–25

ified, and that other media formulations may be better for recovery. SCD that has been diluted to 50% of the recommended strength has been used for this application. Many of the fungi will not grow because of the pH, which is close to 7 for both media. Also, any psychrophilic or thermophilic microorganisms will not grow at the specified incubation temperatures of 20 to 25°C for SCD or 30 to 35°C for FTM. When the presence of these microorganisms is suspected in the production environment, other media and or incubation conditions should be used in conjunction with the required USP tests.

Growth promotion testing of the media is required by the USP and provides the user with the assurance that the media will support growth of most unstressed organisms and most contaminants that may get into the product or media. Table 59–3 provides a list of the microorganisms used for growth promotion testing.

For specific applications, *Micrococcus luteus* (ATCC No. 9341) and *Clostridium sporogenes* (ATCC No. 11437) may be used in place of or in conjunction with *Bacillus subtilis* and *B. vulgatus*, respectively.

Bacteriostasis and Fungistasis

Many drug products contain microbial inhibitors, and some drugs and medical devices are inhibitory because of their inherent chemistry. To properly sterility-test a product it is necessary to first determine if the product inhibits microbial growth.

The product to be tested is placed into the growth media in the appropriate quantities and inoculated with the organisms described in Table 59–2 using not more than 100 viable microorganisms. If growth occurs in 7 days, the product is not considered bacteriostatic or fungistatic. If growth does not occur in 7 days, the culture may be reinoculated with a comparable number of microorganisms, and observed for growth at the end of the next 7 days. If growth still does not occur, then the culture must be made noninhibitory. This may be done in some cases simply through the use of additional media to dilute the inhibitory component to a concentration at which it is not inhibitory, or by reducing the amount of the product to reduce the inhibitory substance. Sometimes, however, the inhibitory substance in the product may have to be neutralized, or testing of the product may require membrane filtration followed by a neutralizing rinse. Sterility testing of antibiotic solutions is a good example of a product requiring membrane filtration, followed by a neutralizing rinse. Although specific quantities of product to be tested are specified in the USP, the effect of inhibition on the outgrowth of the test microorganisms must be taken into consideration, and the amount of the product to be tested must be adjusted to assure a valid test.

Preparation for Sterility Testing

Prior to initiating a sterility test, it is necessary to prepare the environment, the analyst, the sample, and the equipment to be used for the test.

Environmental Controls

Cleaning procedures for the environment should be carried out well in advance of any sterility test, and records should be maintained for reference at the time of the test. The work surfaces should be checked for microbiologic cleanliness on a routine basis and the results maintained for reference by the analyst at the time of the test. A record of the maintenance schedule and the acceptability of the air handling equipment such as filter changes, particulate challenge tests, and air velocity checks should be available. Air sampling for viable and nonviable particles should be done on a routine basis, and the results should be received by the analyst. This information helps the analyst determine the validity of any positive results, should they occur.

The Analyst

Handling of samples for identification and preparation for placing them in the sterility test suite should be done using sterile gloves. Care should be taken to keep samples from coming in contact with other body parts or dirty work surfaces. Prior to entering the sterility test site the analyst must be appropriately gowned. Before initiating the actual test, the analyst should change to fresh sterile gloves. The analyst must display good personal hygiene habits and be able to conduct the test using good aseptic technique.

The Sample

Samples should be collected with a minimum of handling to avoid any additional microbial contamination on the packaging. Any secondary packaging should be removed just prior to placing the units into the sterility suite. Decontamination procedures should be accomplished prior to placing the sample into the sterility test field. This may include disinfectant wipes, submersion into disinfectants, or merely air washes, depending on the packaging and the need for cleaning. It is important to note that fumes from some disinfectants such as paracetic acid may enter porous packages and affect any viable organisms that may be there, thus invalidating the test. Ultraviolet light may also pass through some packaging materials, potentially killing any viable microorganisms. Care should be taken not to saturate porous packages with liquid disinfectants.

Equipment

Any equipment entering the sterility test field should be sterilized. It is often sterilized in double packaging. The outer package is removed as it enters the test suite, and the inner wrap is removed as it enters the sterility test field. Care must be taken to maintain the equipment in a clean, operational condition in order to assure smooth operation during the test. Equipment that must be sterilized is easier to sterilize if kept clean and relatively free from microbial contamination.

Sterility Test

The USP describes tests for specific product types using the two primary methods of sterility testing: direct inoculation and membrane filtration. The tests described are general enough for a wide range of products. The analyst, however, must select tests that are most appropriate for the specific product. Prefilled syringes, for instance, are included in the section on direct inoculation, but testing their contents with membrane filtration techniques may be more appropriate, especially if the contents are bacteriostatic or fungistatic. The analyst must also select the most appropriate portions of a drug or medical device to test, even though the USP specifies the portions in its tests. The portions specified may be impractical or toxic to microbial growth, and smaller portions or a greater dilution may be more appropriate.

Interpretation of Results

The USP allows two stages of testing using the procedures outlined above.

First Stage

If all sample units remain negative for growth throughout the incubation period, the sample meets the requirements of the sterility test. When positives occur and it can be demonstrated that the growth may have been due to the environment or faulty test procedures, the test can be repeated. If growth occurs and it cannot be attributed to a cause, then stage two can be initiated.

Second Stage

Testing of the product sample at the second stage requires double the number of units to be tested using the same procedures used in the first stage. If no positive tests are observed, the sample meets the requirements of the test. If positive units occur and it can be shown that the positives were due to the environment or to a faulty test procedure, the test can be repeated. If positives occur that cannot be attributed to an outside cause, the test fails to meet the requirements of the test and the product is considered contaminated. The interpretation of this test allows a great deal of latitude to the manufacturer, especially when the probability of accepting a nonsterile lot with a low level of contamination is considered. The manufacturer must carefully balance the probability of rejecting a lot that is truly sterile.

Other sterility tests for specific products are included

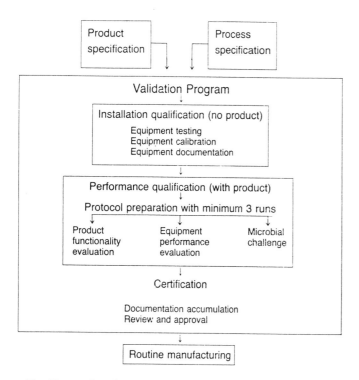

Fig. 59–1. Flow diagram of sterilization process validation. From AAMI. 1988. Guideline for Industrial Ethylene Oxide Sterilization of Medical Devices. Arlington, VA, AAMI.

in the Code of Federal Regulations. Tests for antibiotics and biologics are included in CFR 21, chapters 436.20 and 610.12, respectively (1980). Although these tests require some specific steps, the general procedures are comparable to those identified in the USP.

Product sterility testing is essential to assure that a product has been through a sterilization process, even though the probability of a nonsterile product can't be determined. It is also used during sterilization process validation to determine if the parameters of a process will reduce the microbial population to a nondetectable level.

STERILIZATION PROCESS VALIDATION

Validation is defined in the AAMI "Guideline for Industrial Ethylene Oxide Sterilization of Medical Devices" (1988) as "Establishing documented evidence that provides a high degree of assurance that a specific process will consistently produce a product meeting its predetermined specification and quality characteristics." This is a procedure that requires detailed knowledge of the equipment and its ability to perform in a consistent way, the sterilant/product interaction, and the documentation necessary to show that the process was repetitive and effective. A flow diagram extracted from the AAMI document cited above is presented in Figure 59–1.

There are three basic validation methods:
1. Overkill cycles, in which the process is challenged with Biologic Indicators (BIs) at sterilization times

that are equal to or less than one-half of the full cycle. This procedure is used when little is known about the microbial resistance or numbers of microorganisms on the product. The full cycle is usually considered acceptable when the BIs are killed and the product tested is found to be negative for growth at the half-cycle. Because the BIs have 10^6 spores per unit, and the resistance is considered to be greater than the microorganisms on the product (bioburden), the probability of nonsterility of the product is considered to be less than 1 in 1,000,000 following a 12-log reduction of the BI.
2. Combined biologic indicator–bioburden validation is used when the resistance and population of the bioburden on a product is known and the relationship between the total resistance of the bioburden and the BI is established. When these values are known, the probability of a nonsterile unit can be established. This type of process requires more knowledge of the bioburden than the overkill method does. The advantage of this cycle is that it allows the manufacturer to shorten the cycle time or design a cycle to minimize product exposure to the sterilant.
3. Pure bioburden validation is used only when BIs are not appropriate and the sterilization process must be kept to a minimum. To use pure bioburden validation, the microbial load and resistance of the bioburden to the sterilization process must be determined. This may be used, for example, on a product that is to be steam sterilized, but may become deformed when temperatures are maintained for extended times and where the bioburden level is less than one per unit with relatively low resistance (D-values less than 0.5 min). This requires extensive testing and control of the bioburden in order to establish and maintain an acceptable probability of a nonsterile unit.

The References section of this chapter supplies listings of AAMI documents that describe in detail the necessary steps to validate products using the Overkill method and the Combined Biologic Indicator/Bioburden method and the proper use of the BI.

Biologic Indicators

Biologic Indicators are defined in the AAMI standard for BIER/EO Gas Vessels as "A calibration of microorganisms (of high resistance to the mode of sterilization being monitored) in or on a carrier, put up in a package that maintains the integrity of the inoculated carrier and is of convenience to the ultimate user, which serves to demonstrate that sterilization conditions were met." Several standards developed by the AAMI Sterilization Standards Committee provide guidance for the testing and the use of BI for steam and ethylene oxide sterilization (AAMI, 1982, 1986, 1989). The USP XXI also provides monographs for testing Paper Strip BIs for dry heat, steam, and ethylene oxide. There are four basic commercial types of BIs: paper carrier packaged in glassine envelopes, self contained units, sealed ampules, and spore suspensions. Not all types of BIs are appropriate for a specific application; e.g., a BI made up of spores inside a hermetically sealed ampule should not be used to evaluate the sterilization of dry goods, because the liquid in the hermetically sealed container produces its own steam and does not indicate whether the product has had sufficient exposure to steam to allow sterilization to take place. Each type of BI is designed for use in specific applications. The AAMI "Guideline for the Use of Industrial Ethylene Oxide and Steam Biological Indicators" describes the proper use of BIs.

The AAMI Standards for BIER vessel design and operation are the foundation documents that allow calibration of the BI for the AAMI Standards, USP Monographs, and evaluation of inoculated medical products. The BIER vessel standards provide the tolerances and operating parameters that allow comparative resistance values to be obtained. The USP XXI monographs allow a 20% variability in the D-value from the initial test time through the expiration date. Oxborrow et al. found, however, that when 17 BIER vessels that met the AAMI BIER vessel standards were used, there was considerable variation between the determined D-values (Oxborrow et al., 1983). The variation in D-values was found to be 18% for ethylene oxide BIs when tested with one medium. When steam BIs were tested using three different media, the variation was found to be 20, 31, and 38%, respectively, indicating that the specifications in the USP are unrealistic. The variation due to the three different media lots was much greater than the variation due to the test vessel. The calibration of BIs should refer to a specific process using a specified medium if the BIs are to be used for product release or validation (Boris and Graham, 1985).

Other things can cause variation in the resistance of BI. The way the spores are produced including the sporulation media, the incubation temperature, the suspending solution, and the cleanliness of the spore suspension, can influence the D-value. Other factors such as the carrier material, the packaging, and the storage conditions can also affect the D-value. Several studies have been performed comparing one type of BI to another; not surprisingly, significant differences were found.

The species of spore-forming microorganisms most commonly used are *Bacillus subtilis* sub species *niger* for dry heat and ethylene oxide processes; *B. sterothermophilis* for steam; and *B. pumilus* for radiation. Although these are the most commonly used microorganisms, others may be used, provided their resistance characteristics are determined for the intended sterilization process.

When BIs are used to evaluate a sterilization process, there is always a problem of interpretation of the results. This is particularly important when validating a sterilization process. Two methods of evaluating a sterilization process can be used. One is to expose the BI to a partial cycle that would allow spores to survive, and then recover the surviving spores (survivor curve). The rate of kill can then be determined by counting the survivors for each exposure time and comparing the count to the initial population. A cycle time can then be established by extrapolating the kill rate (D-value) to the desired SAL. The second method is to expose BIs to a process that would reduce the population to a point at which only some units were positive (fraction negative). A most probable number of survivors can be determined using methods described in the AAMI standards or the USP Monographs. The D-value can be determined and the cycle time established. When BIs are used in overkill processes or for monitoring, the results are usually a negative response from the BIs, assuming the sterilization process was adequate. A negative biologic indicator tells the operator two things: (1) the process was adequate to kill the BI and (2) a product in the location within the load where the BI was placed should also be sterilized. *Note:* The BI must be placed in one or more of the most difficult places in the load to sterilize. It cannot be expected that because the BIs are negative that the entire load is sterile unless preliminary studies have shown the BI positions to be the most difficult to sterilize, and the relative resistance of the bioburden to the BI is known, or assumed to be greater.

Positive BIs, on the other hand, indicate a failed process, and the product is probably not sterile. False-positive BIs are rare, and any positive should be considered a process failure.

The USP XXI, Supplement Five, included three monographs for testing and evaluation of BIs: BIs for dry heat sterilization on paper strips, BIs for ethylene oxide sterilization on paper strips, and BIs for steam sterilization on paper strips (USP-NF, 1987). The monographs on steam and ethylene oxide BI are comparable to the AAMI Standards for health-care BIs but do not specify the strain of *Bacillus stearothermophilis* or *B. subtilis* to use. Also, the strain of *B. subtilis* is not specified for BIs that are to be used for the dry heat sterilization process. This is appropriate because any strain that has the necessary resistance will provide an equivalent challenge to the sterilization process.

To meet requirements of the USP BI Monographs, it is necessary to label the BIs according to the Monograph. Among the requirements of the labeling are the resistance values. The D-value and the exposure times to the sterilant required to obtain all survivors and the time to achieve complete kill are required along with the procedure used to determine the resistance—i.e., spore count or fraction negative. The USP also requires the labeling to state that ". . . the stated D-value is reproducible only under the exact conditions under which it was determined. . ." This serves as a warning to the users that the BIs may not be suitable for applications in which sterilization processes with other physical parameters are used.

Specific test parameters and test protocols for determining resistance are defined in the Monographs, along with a specific cultivation technique. The medium and incubation conditions for the BI species appropriate for each Monograph are specified. Although the USP Monographs describe the calculations for determining the BI D-value, the calculations are described much more clearly in the AAMI "Guideline for the Use of Industrial Ethylene Oxide and Steam Biological Indicators." Methods for determining the total spore count are also included in both documents. The USP requires the BI to meet the requirements for survival and kill based on the following calculations: "Survival time (in minutes) = not less than (labeled D-value) $\times$ ($\log_{10}$ labeled spore count per carrier $-$ 2); and Kill time (in minutes) = not more than (labeled D-value) $\times$ ($\log_{10}$) labeled spore count per carrier $+$ 4)."

Requirements for stability, purity, and disposal are also included in the Monographs.

Chemical Indicators

Chemical Indicators (CIs) are another way to monitor sterilization processes (AAMI, 1982). CIs are used in all types of sterilization and are specific to the mode of sterilization being monitored. Ionizing radiation uses dosimeters of various types and is specific to the dose range being monitored and the sensitivity required. Dry heat uses chemical indicators that indicate that the strip and the product it is attached to have reached the desired sterilization temperature. It does not indicate that the elapsed time or temperature of exposure was sufficient to sterilize. This type of indicator is called a "through-put" indicator. Through-put indicators are available for all types of sterilization processes and may indicate that some specific process parameter has been met. A common type of chemical indicator is one that changes color when the pH of the environment changes. These indicators will change when they contact steam or ethylene oxide and are used as through-put indicators.

"Temperature-specific" indicators are specific to steam sterilization processes and are frequently used as through-put indicators. These indicators have the ability to indicate when there is a cold spot in a steam sterilizer that may be due to entrapped air. They are not capable of integrating all of the parameters of the process, however. "Bowie-Dick" Indicators are a special CI designed to be used to detect entrapped air or air leaks in pre-vacuum steam sterilizers. These indicators are made up of inks that readily change color in the presence of steam and are usually contained in packs of towels or other test materials that challenge the penetration of steam. When air is present, the steam does not penetrate readily, and the color change is incomplete.

"Multi-parameter" indicators are designed to indicate some or all of the parameters of a sterilization process. There are numerous claims from various manufacturers as to what their product will do (Lee et al., 1979). Some multi-parameter indicators provide the user with additional assurance that the process was adequate and that

the product exposed at that position was exposed to sterilizing conditions. Some of these CIs are similar to BIs in their response to the sterilization process—i.e., the color change responds to a change in temperature simular to a "Z" value for BIs. The Z values may not be the same, however (Bunn and Sykes, 1980; Danielson, 1982; Hirsch and Manne, 1984; Hoborn, 1975).

CIs should be used as BIs are used—i.e., they should be placed in the most difficult to sterilize positions in the sterilizer load. They may also be used on each package to indicate exposure of the product to the sterilization process. Interpretation of the result may not be as specific as that of BIs because there is usually some incomplete response near the end-point of the CI, and the end-point is not easy to detect.

CIs are similar to BIs in their ability to indicate the state of sterility of a processed product. They only indicate that the sterilization parameters were achieved, not that the entire load is sterile. As discussed with BIs, CIs are only one part of the data package that supports the adequacy of a sterilization process. The entire package includes the physical, chemical, and biologic data, and these data must be considered in order to determine the probability of a nonsterile product.

Physical Indicators

Physical indications of an adequate sterilization process must include the temperature, pressure, gas concentration, steam purity, relative humidity, or delivered dose, whichever is appropriate, and the time of exposure to the specific set of conditions or the integrated time of exposure. These parameters may be accumulated by automated systems, electromechanical devices, or manual observation. However the data are accumulated, the instrumentation must be calibrated to national or international standards. Physical data are usually the first indicator of the adequacy of a sterilization process. Any deviation from the expected normal readings should alert the operator to potential problems.

When a well documented process has sufficient controls and read-out redundancy, the process does not need to be monitored with BIs or CIs and may be released based on the data from the physical parameters alone. This is called "process release" or "parametric release." There are few processes that meet the criteria for release in this way, and consideration of governmental regulatory concerns must be addressed before beginning a parametric release program.

EFFICACY TESTS FOR STERILIZING AND SPORICIDAL AGENTS

These tests have been specified by the Association of Official Analytical Chemists procedures for many years (AOAC, 1980). There has been a great deal of criticism concerning the adequacy of the test, much of which is founded. This test, however, is considered the reference test by which all new sporicides or sterilization processes are challenged and evaluated. One of the greatest concerns related to this test is the variability and inconsistency of the results. Several obvious reasons for the inconsistencies exist. The test is run using penicylinders of porcelain, stainless steel, or glass as carriers for the spores (Asconzi et al., 1985; Cole et al., 1987). Suture loops are also used. It has been found that the different materials retained the various test organisms at different levels, and consequently the sterilizing effect for a specific disinfectant was different. Although this study was done on disinfectants, the same problems can be expected for sporicidal tests.

Loading of spores on a carrier by submerging the carrier into a broth culture provides a major opportunity for variation among carriers of the same material, and particularly from test to test. The growth media, the amount of sporulation, and the extent to which the spores are coated by the dried media can significantly affect the kill response. Danielson et al. found significant differences between survival curve D-values when clean spore suspensions of *B. subtilis* with different ATCC numbers were prepared from different growth media (Danielson and Oxborrow, 1989). Both suspensions met the HCl resistance criteria specified in the method, but presented different challenges to the sporicide being tested. Another factor that affects the variability of the sporicidal test results is the degree to which the spore suspension is desiccated following inoculation. Generally, the more an inoculated carrier is desiccated, the greater the resistance to the sporicide.

MAINTAINING STERILITY (PACKAGING)

Regardless of the SAL at the conclusion of the sterilization process, the sterilized products may become contaminated if the packaging is insufficient or faulty. Placencia and Oxborrow (1984, 1986) have developed tests to evaluate the biobarrier integrity of medical packaging to assure that the materials used will maintain the sterility of the product. Most manufacturers state that the product will remain sterile as long as the package integrity is maintained. It is necessary, therefore, to assure that the materials are adequate for their application (Stellon, 1986).

CONCLUSIONS

Sterilization processes are getting more sophisticated as knowledge is accumulated on the control and monitoring of sterilization processes. The present standards of process control using physical, chemical, and biologic systems provides the SAL we expect for sterilized products.

Sterility testing is the standard used for product release and will likely remain so. Although new procedures and modifications of existing procedures are being developed, the basic tests will not change. Revisions of the USP take place as required, and current revisions should be reviewed before one attempts to comply with the intent of the USP.

Application of USP tests to a specific product may require modification of the tests to accommodate the product's unique characteristics. Sterilization process validation has become the standard of the medical products industry to provide an acceptable SAL. Selection of a validation process must be tailored to the specific product.

Numerous journal articles and professional publications have thoroughly discussed the various procedures for each sterilization process. Products that cannot be validated for any reason still require a strong knowledge of the acceptability of the process in order to obtain consistent SALs.

The use of biologic indicators for qualifying, validating, and monitoring sterilization processes is necessary to assure that the process produces biologic kill. The kill kinetics of BIs are specific to each process. Biologic indicators exposed to process parameters other than those that they are calibrated for may not perform in the expected manner or have the same resistance characteristics. Equipment and procedures for manufacturing and testing the resistance of BIs are being improved to provide less variability in their response. Standards such as those provided by the USP and AAMI are important in providing guidance for improvement in BI quality.

Chemical indicators are becoming more specific for the critical parameter of sterilization processes. Their use can aid in interpreting process acceptability. When used throughout the load, CIs can indicate the uniformity of process parameters.

Although pass-through type indicators indicate the presence of only one parameter, they provide assurance that the product has passed through the process. Improvements are being made in existing products, and new products are being developed that may make chemical indicators more important in the future.

The application of new sterilants and sporicides is becoming important to the medical products field as new materials and new applications of existing products are developed. They will find limited use for existing products, however, and are not likely to replace any of the major existing sterilization processes.

Testing of sporicides is likely to be improved, because much greater emphasis is being placed by the Food and Drug Administration on their effectiveness. The FDA has a draft protocol for the testing of sporicides/sterilants, which is being used by some manufacturers of products intended for use on items designed for single use that are now being reused. Additional evaluation is necessary to assure the reliability of the proposed tests.

REFERENCES

AAMI Recommended Practice (Draft). 1989. Guideline for Use of Industrial Ethylene Oxide and Steam Biological Indicators. AAMI, 1901 North Fort Meyer Drive, Suite 602, Arlington, VA, 22209, pp. 1–49.

AAMI Recommended Practice (Draft). 1989. Guideline for Electron Beam Radiation Sterilization of Medical Devices. AAMI, 1901 North Fort Meyer Drive, Suite 602, Arlington, VA, 22209, pp. 1–75.

AAMI Recommended Practice. 1984. Process Control Guidelines for Gamma

Radiation Sterilization of Medical Devices. AAMI, 1901 North Fort Meyer Drive, Suite 602, Arlington, VA, 22209, pp. 1–24.

AAMI Recommended Practice. 1988. Good Hospital Practice: Steam Sterilization and Sterility Assurance. AAMI, 1901 North Fort Meyer Drive, Suite 602, Arlington, VA, 22209, pp. 1–38.

AAMI Standard. 1982. BIER/EO Gas Vessels. AAMI, 1901 North Fort Meyer Drive, Suite 602, Arlington, VA, 22209, pp. 1–8.

AAMI Standard. 1982. BIER/Steam Vessels. AAMI, 1901 North Fort Meyer Drive, Suite 602, Arlington, VA, 22209, pp. 1–8.

AAMI Technical Information Report No. 3. 1988. Selection and Use of Chemical Indicators for Steam Sterilization. AAMI, 1901 North Ford Meyer Drive, Suite 602, Arlington, VA, 22209, pp. 1–49.

Akers, J.E., Charleton, F.J., Clements, W.C., and Woods, J.A. 1987. Survey on Sterility Testing Practices. J. Parenter. Sci. Technol., *41*(6), 197–209.

Anderson, R.A., and Rae, W.A. 1979. Stability of *Bacillus stearothermophilus* spore papers for use as biological indicators. Aust. J. Pharm. Sci., *8*(2), 55–56.

ANS, AAMI, 1987. Automatic, General-Purpose Ethylene Oxide Sterilizers and Ethylene Oxide Sterilant Sources Intended for Use in Health Care Facilities. AAMI, 1901 North Fort Meyer Drive, Suite 602, Arlington, VA, 22209, pp. 4–5.

ANS, AAMI. 1986. American National Standard for Biological Indicators for Ethylene Oxide Sterilization Processes in Health Care Facilities. AAMI, 1901 North Fort Meyer Drive, Suite 602, Arlington, VA, 22209, pp. 1–9.

ANS, AAMI. 1986. American National Standard for Biological Indicators for Saturated Steam Sterilization Processes in Health Care Facilities. AAMI, 1901 North Fort Meyer Drive, Suite 602, Arlington, VA, 22209, pp. 1–9.

ANS, AAMI. 1988. Guideline for Industrial Ethylene Oxide Sterilization of Medical Devices. AAMI, 1901 North Fort Meyer Drive, Suite 602, Arlington, VA, 22209, pp. 1–20.

ANS, AAMI. 1987. Guideline for Industrial Moist Heat Sterilization of Medical Products. AAMI, 1901 North Fort Meyer Drive, Suite 602, Arlington, VA, 22209, pp. 1–24.

Ascenzi, J.M., Ezzell, R.J., and Wendt, T.M. 1985. Evaluation of Carriers Used in the Test Methods of the Association of Official Analytical Chemists, Appl. Envir. Micro., Jan, 91–94.

Association of Official Analytical Chemists, Inc. 1980. Sporicidal Test. In *Official Methods of Analysis*. 13th Edition. Edited by W. Horowitz. Washington, D.C., AOAC, pp. 60–61.

Baird, R. 1988. Validation of dry heat tunnels and ovens. Pharm. Eng., *8*, 31–33.

Berube, R. 1981. Biological indicator resistometer equipment, the what, the why, and the how. Dev. Ind. Microbiol., *22*, 324–335.

Beyers, T. 1982. Validation, burden or benefit? D&CI, June, 43–44, 82, 86.

Blue Guide Review Panel. 1987. Guidance on Ethylene Oxide Sterilization. Supplies Technology Division DHSS. pp. 1–29.

Boris, C., and Graham, G.S. 1985. The effect of recovery medium and test methodology on biological indicators. MD&DI, *7*(2), 43–48.

Brewer, J.H. 1957. In *Antiseptics, Disinfectants, Fungicides, and Sterilization.* 2nd Edition. Edited by G.L. Reddish. Philadelphia, Lea & Febiger, pp. 160–161.

Broker, C.G. 1981. Validation in perspective. J. Parenter. Sci. Technol., *35*, 167–169.

Bunn, J.L., and Sykes, I.K. 1980. A chemical indicator for the rapid measurement of FO values. J. Appl. Bacteriol., *51*, 143–147.

Caputo, R.A., Odlaung, T.E., Wilkenson, R.L., and Mascoli, C.C. 1979. Biological validation of a sterilization process for a parenteral product—fractional exposure method. J. Parenter. Drug Assoc., *33*, 214–221.

Caputo, R.A., Rohn, K.J., and Mascoli, C.C. 1980. Recovery of biological indicator organisms after sublethal sterilization treatment. J. Parenter. Drug Assoc., *34*, 394–397.

Caputo, R.A., Rohn, K.J., and Mascoli, C.C. 1981. Biological validation of an ethylene oxide sterilization process. Dev. Ind. Microbiol., *22*, 357–362.

Christensan, E.A., and Kristensen, H. 1979. Biological indicators for the control of ethylene oxide sterilization. Acta Pathol. Microbiol. Scand., *3*, 147–154.

Code of Federal Regulations. 1980a. Chapter I of Title 21, Part 436, Test and Methods of assay of antibiotics and antibiotic containing drugs, Subpart B, Section 436.20; Sterility test methods and procedures. Office of Federal Registrar, National Archives and Records Adm.

Code of Federal Regulations. 1980b. Chapter I of Title 21, Subchapter F, Part 610, General Biological Products Standards, Subpart B General Provisions, Section 610.12; Sterility, Office of Federal Registrar, National Archives and Records Adm.

Code of Federal Regulations. 1980c. Chapter I of Title 21, Part 600, Biological Products: General Subpart B, Establishment, Standards, Section 600.11; Physical establishment, equipment, animals and care, Office of Federal Registrar, National Archives and Records Adm.

Code of Federal Regulations. 1980d. Chapter I of Title 9, Part 113, Animals and animal products; Animal and Plant Health Inspection Service, Sections 113.25 to 113.27, Office of Federal Registrar, National Archives and Records Adm.

Cole, E.C., Rutala, W.A., and Carson, J.L. 1987. Evaluation of penicylinders used in disinfectant testing: bacterial attachment and surface texture. J. Assoc. Off. Anal. Chem., *70*(5), 903–906.

Cooper, M.S. 1982. Evolving USP sterility test. J. Parenter. Sci. Technol., *36*, 256–259.

Cooper, M.S. 1986. Sterility Testing. The Microbiological Update. Microbiological Applications, Inc., 132 San Remo Drive, Islamorada, FL, 33036.

Dadd, A.H., Stewart, C.M., and Town, M.M. 1983. A standardized monitor for the control of ethylene oxide sterilization cycles. J. Hyg., *9*(1), 96–100.

Danielson, J., and Oxborrow, G.S. 1989. The Effects of Chemical Sterilants/Disinfectants on *Bacillus subtilis* Spores Under Various Conditions, Studies Conducted at the FDA Sterility Anlaysis Research Center.

Danielson, N.E. 1982. Sterilization process indicators: Biological vs. chemical. Med. Instr., Jan.–Feb., p. 52.

Department of Health and Social Security (DHSS) and United Kingdom Trade Associations. 1983. Guide to Good Manufacturing Practice for Medical Equipment. London, Her Majesty's Stationary Office, pp. 1–30.

Division of Small Manufacturers Assistance, Office of Training and Assistance. 1984. *Sterile Medical Devices: a GMP Workshop Manual*. 4th Edition. Washington, D.C., U.S. Department of Health and Human Services, Food and Drug Administration, National Center for Devices and Radiological Health, Rockville, MD, 20857, pp. 1–445.

Duberstein, R. 1979. Filter validation. II. Mechanisms of bacterial removal by filtration. J. Parenter. Drug Assoc., *33*, 250–256.

European Confederation of Medical Suppliers Association (EUCOMED). 1985. A General Guide to Good Manufacturing Practices for the Health Care Industry. EUCOMED, 551 Finchley Road, Hampstead, Lond, NW3 7BJ England, pp. 1–16.

EUCOMED. 1984. Recommendations for the Sterilization of Medical Devices and Surgical Products. EUCOMED, 551 Finchley Road, Hampstead, Lond, NW3 7BJ England, pp. 1–16.

EUCOMED. 1984. Guide to Good Manufacturing Practice for Sterile Medical Devices. EUCOMED, 551 Finchley Road, Hampstead, London, NW3 7BJ England, pp. 1–16.

EUCOMED. 1983. Guide to Good Manufacturing Practice for Sterile and Non Sterile Surgical Products. EUCOMED, 551 Finchley Road, Hampstead, Lond, NW3 7BJ England, pp. 1–16.

Everall, P.H. 1976. The quality control of sterilization. NatNews, Jan., 7–11.

Federal Standard 209D. 1988. Washington, D.C., General Services Admnistration.

Field, E.A., Field, J.K., and Martin, M.V. 1988. Time, steam, temperature (TST) control indicators to measure essential sterilization criteria for autoclaves in general dental practice and community dental service. Br. Dent. J., *164*, 183–186.

Fitzgerald, W.F. 1986. Validation of computerized sterilization measurement and control systems. MD&DI, *8*(2), 27–32.

Fogarty, M.G., Prince, D.L., and Morganstern, K.H. 1987. A study of sequential processing in sublethal sterilizing systems. MD&DI, 38–43.

Frieben, W.R., Kreiger, R.A., Juberg, D.L., and Enzinger, R.M. 1978. Validation of steam sterilization cycles used for sterile processing equipment. J. Parenter. Drug Assoc., *32*, 249–257.

Garfinkle, B., et al. 1985. Validation of a radiosterilization procedure for sterilization of a solidstate ophthalmic insert system. J. Parenter. Sci. Technol., *39*, 246–250.

Gee, L.W., Harvey, J.M.G.H., Olsen, W.P., and Lee, M.L. 1985. Sterility test systems for product recovery. J. Pharm. Sci., *74*, 29–32.

Genova, T.F., Hollis, R.A., Crowell, C.A., and Schady, K.M. 1987. A procedure for supplementing the AAMI BI method for validating radiation sterilized products. J. Parenter. Sci. Technol., *41*, 126–127.

Genova, T.F., Hollis, R.A., Crowell, C.A., and Schady, K.M. 1987. Procedure for validating the sterility of individual gamma radiation sterilized production batches. J. Parenter. Sci. Technol., *41*, 33–36.

Genova, T.F., Hollis, R.A., and Schady, K.M. 1985. Validation of products for cobalt sterilization: Microbiological considerations. J. Ind. Irrad. Tech., *3*, 3–4, 197–209.

Guilfoyle, D.E., and Yager, J.F. 1984. Procedures used for sterility testing of parenteral drugs by an FDA field laboratory. J. Parenter. Sci. Technol., *38*, 138–141.

Hennebert, P., Gillard, J., and Roland, M. 1986. New method of gaseous formaldehyde sterilization. S.T.P. Pharm., *2*, 536–542.

Hirsch, A., and Manne, S. 1984. Bioequivalent chemical steam sterilization indicators. Med. Instr., *18*(5), 272–275.

Hoborn, J. 1975. Steam sterilization: A comparison of steam-clox and some European biological indicators. Health Lab. Sci., *12*, 225–229.

Hoxey, E.V., Soper, C.J., and Davies, D.J.G. 1984. Biological indicators for low temperature steam formaldehyde sterilization: Effect of defined media and sporulation, germination index and moist heat resistance at 110°C of *Bacillus* strains. J. Appl. Bacteriol., *58*(2), 207–214.

Jones, A.T., and Pflug, I.J. 1981. *Bacillus coagulans*, FRR B666, as a potential biological indicator organism. J. Parenter. Sci. Technol., *35*, 82–87.

Jorkasky, J.F. 1987. Medical product sterilization: Changes and challenges. MD&DI, *9*, 33–37.

Joslyn, L. 1981. Sterilization process efficiency as measured by biological indicators vs. physical indicators. Dev. Ind. Microbiol., *22*, 341–348.

Juhlin, I., Lindquist, S.B., and Nystrand, R. 1986. Postcycle sporicidal effect of ethylene oxide—A new concept. J. Parenter. Sci. Technol., *39*(6), 223–230.

Kirk, B. 1987. Biological and chemical sterilization indicators—current concepts and future trends. J. Appl. Bacteriol., *63*(6), 167–171.

Korczynski, M.S. 1980. Concepts and issues–container/closure microbial validation. J. Parenter. Drug Assoc., *34*, 277–285.

Kotilainen, H.R., and Gantz, N.M. 1985. Biological sterilization monitors: A four-year in-use evaluation of two systems. Infect. Control, *6*, 451–455.

Kotilainen, H.R., and Gantz, N.M. 1987. An evaluation of three biological indicator systems in flash sterilization. Infect. Control, *8*, 311–316.

Leahy, T.J., and Sullivan, M.J. 1978. Validation of bacterial retention capabilities of membrane filters. Pharm. Tech., *2*, 65–75.

Lee, C.H., Montville, T.J., and Sinskey, A.J. 1979. Comparison of the efficacy of steam sterilization indicators. Appl. Environ. Microbiol., *113–117.*

Meyers, R.B. 1978. Practical system for validating heat sterilization processes. J. Parenter. Drug Assoc., *32*, 216–225.

Military Standard, Mil-Std-966. 1979. Monitoring Sterilization Systems for Medical Devices (Industrial). Defense Personnel Support Center Directorate of Medical Material, Code ATT, 2800 South 20 Street, Philadelphia, PA, 19101, pp. 1–14.

Military Standard, Mil-Std-969. 1980. Biological Indicators for Sterilization Processed. Defense Personnel Support Center Directorate of Medical Material, DPSC-Att, Philadelphia, PA, 19101.

Morris, B.G., Avis, K.E., and Bowles, G.C. 1980. Quality-control plant for intravenous admixture programs. II: Validation of operator technique. Am. J. Pharm., *37*, 688–692.

Odlaug, T.E., Caputo, R.A., and Graham, G.S. 1981. Heat resistance and population stability of lyophilized *Bacillus subtilis* spores. Appl. Environ. Microbiol., *41*, 1374–1377.

Odlaug, T.E. et al. 1984. Sterility assurance for terminally sterilized products without end-product sterility testing. P.D.A., *38*(4), July–Aug, 141–147.

Oxborrow, G.S., Kallander, K.D., and Mendelhall, G.R. 1983. Biological indicators for ethylene oxide sterilization performance evaluation. J. Parenter. Sci. Tech., *13–14.*

Oxborrow, G.S., Lanier, J.M., and Schawb, A.H. 1980. A survey of performance characteristics of biological indicators used for ethylene oxide sterilization. Dev. Ind. Microbiol., *2J*, 393–398.

Oxborrow, G.S., Placencia, A.M., and Danielson, J.W. 1983. Effects of temperature and relative humidity on biological indicators used for ethylene oxide sterilization. Appl. Environ. Microbiol., *45*, 546–549.

Oxborrow, G.S., Twohy, C.W., and Demetrius, C.A. 1989. BIER vessel performance for ETO and steam, in D&DI, *12*, 78–83.

Panezai, A.K. 1987. Validating environments for sterile maufacture. Manufact. Chem., July, 34–37.

Perkins, R.E., Bodman, H.A., Kundsin, R.B., and Walter, C.W. 1981. Monitoring steam sterilization of surgical instruments: A dilemma. Appl. Environ. Microbiol., *42*, 383–384.

Peterson, A.F., and Boris, C.A. 1981. The biological indicator restometer preliminary studies. Dev. Ind. Microbiol., *22*, 337–340.

Pflug, I.J., and Odlaug, T.E. 1986. Biological indicators in the pharmaceutical and medical device industry. J. Parenter. Sci. Technol., *40*(5), 242–248.

Placencia, A.M., Arin, M.L., Peeler, J.T., and Oxborrow, G.S. 1988. Physical tests are not enough. MD&DI, *10*, 72–78.

Placencia, A.M., and Oxborrow, G.S. 1984. Use of the Reuter Centrifugal Air Sample In Good Manufacturing Practices Investigations. Technical Report. U.S. Department of Health and Human Services, Public Health Service, Food and Drug Administration, Office of Regional Operations.

Placencia, A.M., Oxborrow, G.S., and Danielson, J.W. 1982. Batch-swirl method for detoxification of isopropyl myristate use for sterility testing of oils and ointments: Membrane selection. J. Pharm. Sci., *71*, 714–715.

Placencia, A.M., Oxborrow, G.S., and Danielson, J.W. 1982. Method of the sterility testing of 10% fat emulsions using membrane filtration and dimethyl sulfoxide. J. Pharm. Sci., *71*, 704–705.

Placencia, A.M., Oxborrow, G.S., and Peeler, J.T. 1986. Packaging integrity methodology for testing the biobarrier properties of porous packaging, part I: Exposure chamber method. MD&DI, *8*(4), 60–65.

Placencia, A.M., Oxborrow, G.S., and Peeler, J.T. 1986. Packaging integrity methodology for testing the biobarrier properties of porous packaging, part II: FDA exposure chamber method. MD&DI, *8*(5), 46–53.

Portner, D.M., and Hoffman, R.K. 1968. Sporicidal effect of peracetic acid vapor. Appl. Microbiol., *42*, 173–178.

Prince, H.N., and Rubino, J.R. 1984. Bioburden dynamics: The viability of microorganisms on devices before and after sterilization. MD&DI, *6*, 47–53.

Puleo, J.R., Bergstrom, S.L., Peeler, J.T., and Oxborrow, G.S. 1978. Thermal resistance of naturally occurring airborne bacterial spores. Appl. Environ. Microbiol., *33*, 374–479.

Reti, A.R., and Leahy, T.J. 1979. Filter validation, III, validation of bacterially retentive filters by bacterial passage testing. J. Parenter. Drug Assoc., *33*, 257–272.

Rhodes, P., Zelner, L., and Laufman, H. 1982. A new disposable Bowie-Dick-type test pack for prevacuum high-temperature sterilizers. Med. Instr., *16*(2), 117–120.

Robertson, T.H., et al. 1977. Validation of ethylene oxide sterilization cycles. Bull. Parenter. Drug Assoc., *31*, 265–273.

Shirtz, J.T. 1987. Sterility testing. Pharm. Eng., *7*(6), 35–41.

Skaug, N. 1983. Proper monitoring of sterilization procedures used in oral surgery. Int. J. Oral Surg., *12*(3), 153–158.

Skaug, N., and Berube, R. 1983. Comparative thermo resistance of 2 biological indicators for monitoring steam autoclave. 1. Comparison performed in a gravity BIER steam vessel. Acta Pathol. Microbiol. Immunol. Scand., *B91*(6), 435–441.

Simmons, P.L. 1979. Sterilizer validation. Pharm. Technol., April, *31*, 69–70.

Simmons, P.L. 1980. The secrets of successful sterilizer validation (Part I). Pharm. Eng., *9*(15), 43.

Simmons, P.L. 1981. The secrets of successful sterilizer validation (Part II). Pharm. Eng., *3*, 13–15.

Spicher, G. 1988. Biological indicators and monitoring systems for validation and cycle control of sterilization processes. Zentrabl. Sakt. Hyg., *A267*, 468–484.

Staines, L. 1984. Design control and validation of a facility for sterile clinical trial preparations. J. Parenter. Sci. Technol., *38*(3), 109–114.

Stellon, R.C. 1986. Sterile packaging process validation and good manufacturing practice requirements. MD&DI, *8*(10), 42–46.

The United States Pharmacopia (USP) XXI, the National Formulary (NF). 1985. 16th Edition. The United States Pharmacopeial Convention, Inc., 12601 Twinbrook Parkway, Rockville, MD, 20852, pp. 1156–1160 and 1347–1352.

The UPS-NF Supplement 5. 1987. Monographs, Biological Indicator for (Dry Heat), (Ethylene Oxide), (Steam) Sterilization, Paper Strip. The United States Pharmacopeial Convention, Inc., 12601 Twinbrook Parkway, Rockville, MD, 20852, pp. 2347–2353.

UK Panel on Gamma and Electron Irradiation. 1988. Validation and Routine Monitoring of Sterilization by Ionizing Radiation. British Standards Institute. UK Panel on Gamma and Electron Irradiation, pp. 1–12.

Van Asten, J., Dorpema, J.W., and Verweij, J.C. 1983. Analysis of factors influencing the Bowie-Dick-type test. Med. Instr., *17*(3), 206–210.

Ventura, D.A., and Shaffer, G.E. 1984. Unique aspects of steam sterilization validation of disposable syringe components. J. Parenter. Sci. Technol., *38*, 212–215.

Waldheim, B.J. 1988. Microbiological control of clean rooms. Pharm. Eng., *8*(1), 21–23.

Wallhauser, J.K. 1985. Sterility assurance based on valdiation and in-process control for microbial removal filtration and aseptic filling. Pharm. Ind., *47*(3), 314–319.

Wasynczuk, J. 1986. Validation of aseptic filling processes. Pharm. Technol., *10*(5), 36–38, 40, 42–43.

Watson, S.W., Levin, J., and Novitsky, T.J. 1987. Fixing and removing of bacterial endotoxin from glass surfaces for validation of dry heat sterilization. Prog. Clin. Biol. Res., *231*, 238–288.

Whitbourne, J.E., and Reich, R.R. 1979. Ethylene oxide biological indicators: Need for stricter qualification testing control. J. Parenter. Drug Assoc., *33*, 132–143.

Witonsky, R.J. 1977. New tool for the validation of the sterilization of parenterals. Bull. Parenter. Drug Assoc., *31*, 274–281.

CHAPTER 60

METHODS OF TESTING SANITIZERS
AND BACTERIOSTATIC SUBSTANCES

Robert Berube and Gordon S. Oxborrow

The terminology used to describe the control of microorganisms can be concise, confusing, and confounding. Dorland's (1988) and Steadman's (1988) medical dictionaries attempt to solidify terms that were private, descriptive, and sometimes contradictory—such as the definition that "sanitize" is "to clean and to sterilize" things such as eating and drinking utensils. The working definition of "sanitize" was, until recently, "to render sanitary, that is, to reduce the number of microbial contaminants to a safe or relatively safe level as may be judged by public health requirements or to a significant degree where public health standards have not been established or where the objective is not yet directly related to public health protection measures" (Asbury, 1983). A performance-related definition is now in place, viz., a sanitizer is an antimicrobial that kills 99.999% of specific test bacteria in 30 seconds under conditions of the official sanitizer test.

The following material may partially clarify the situation in which chemical agents are used to control microorganisms. First, two basic approaches are used to study the influence of chemical agents upon microorganisms: in one, the antimicrobial agent is added to the population of microbes and the effects on both metabolic functions and survival are observed; in the second, the antimicrobial agent is added to a developing culture and the effects on growth rate and crop yield are observed. The loss of viability, measured by the inability of the organisms to grow and to multiply when transferred into a fresh suitable growth environment, is referred to as a "bactericidal" or "germicidal" effect, depending on whether a bacteriologist or a salesperson is reporting the results. When the capability of a microorganism to reproduce is lost permanently, the effect is microbial death. If the loss of the ability to reproduce is temporary, or the rate of reproduction decreases, the effect is a "static" condition, and the agent is described as such: "bacteriostat," "fungistat," "microbiostat," etc. (Most of

these terms are described more fully in the Glossary of Terms and in the appropriate chapters of this book; this chapter will define the terms chemosterilant, disinfectant, and sanitizer.)

A *chemosterilant* is an antimicrobial agent that has as its function the killing of all microorganisms, including their spores (if any are produced); rapidity of action is implied but not specified. A *disinfectant* is an antimicrobial agent that is intended for application to inanimate objects or surfaces for the purpose of killing pathogenic organisms (excluding spore-forming bacteria); the official test organisms must be killed in 10 minutes under the defined conditions of the appropriate AOAC test. A *sanitizer* is an antimicrobial agent that is intended for application to inanimate objects or surfaces for the purpose of reducing the microbial count to safe levels; sanitizers must kill 99.999% of the test organisms in 30 seconds under the defined conditions of the appropriate AOAC test.

The distinction between disinfectant and sanitizer arose from the practical concerns of users. Users in the medical-care industry (e.g., doctors, nurses, hospitals, clinics) focused on applications that destroyed all pathogens. Therefore, tests on disinfectants and liquid sterilants centered on practical chemical contact times of 10, 30, or 60 minutes. Users in the public-health-related industries (e.g., food processing, dairy operations, restaurants, waste disposal activities) were not primarily concerned with pathogens, and complete kill was not economical. Therefore, the applications centered on decontamination procedures designed to reduce any real or potentially dangerous situation to a "safe" level, and a realistic chemical contact time of 30 to 60 seconds.

These considerations fostered the 10-minute use-dilution test method for evaluating hospital disinfectants and the 30-second count-reduction method for evaluating the sanitizers used by the public-health-related industries. The former is a go/no-go type of test (100% kill), and the latter seeks a 99.999% kill. Products with a sanitizer claim may not pass the disinfectant use-dilution test, and disinfectants may or may not pass the sanitizer test requirements.

Antimicrobial agents for medical devices are regulated under the authority of the Federal Food, Drug and Cosmetic Act by the Food and Drug Administration (FDA). Because these antimicrobial agents are for use on inanimate surfaces, they are also regulated by the Environmental Protection Agency (EPA) under the authority of the Federal Insecticide, Fungicide, and Rodenticide Act (FIFRA). Indeed, it was the enactment of FIFRA (1948–1972) that gave official recognition to the words sanitizer and sanitization. To satisfy the pertinent agency (EPA or FDA), any and all claims about sanitization, specific and implied, must be documented with appropriate data and completed details of the test protocol.

HISTORY

Sanitization

The following history on sanitization is a condensation of the reviews by Shaffer (1971, 1977) and Asbury (1983). Awareness of the variable resistance of microorganisms began in the 1880s, and these observations were reviewed in the early 1900s by Regenstein (1912). Conceptually, this study of resistance of microorganisms has been methodologically a study of the mode of action of a stimulus against the most sensitive site on a cell. The data that have accumulated show that microoganisms are complex systems adapted to continued survival in their available environment. When stresses are brought to bear upon the system, three responses are possible: (1) the system breaks down and the organism dies, (2) the system develops a means of resisting the stress, or (3) the system changes by accommodating itself to the presence of the stress.

Acceptance of chemicals as sanitizers occurred pragmatically. When those chemicals were successfully tested under "field-laboratory" conditions, the results were written up (by such as Speck et al., 1954). Some simulated-use programs were outlined by Stuart (1956) in order to generate data for regulatory evaluations of sanitizers and detergent-sanitizers. The fundamental premise was that a detergent-sanitizer must, in direct comparison, give an antimicrobial result significantly greater than that shown by controls (such as white floating soap or tetrasodium pyrophosphate) and that a sanitizing rinse should give an antimicrobial result significantly greater than that obtained by the use of cold water. Unfortunately, as observed by Weber (1949), the "significantly greater" stipulation was a bit vague.

In the absence of clear definitions of and roles for disinfectants and sanitizers, many public health officials expected a sanitizer to function as a disinfectant. In certain environments, when specific infectious pathogenic agents were (and are) suspected, a disinfectant was (and is) the appropriate antimicrobial. However, when large volumes of sanitizers are routinely used daily in various commercial operations–such as restaurants, dairies, and food plants—and where infectious organisms are not known or assumed to be present, and the need exists to prevent the adulteration of foods and beverages with residues from the various chemicals employed, there is the calculated risk noted by Dubois (1949): sanitizing operations result in marginal disinfection but give an acceptable level of sanitization. Further, in many industrial applications, the prime desire is for an economical reduction in the noninfectious microorganisms that might contaminate a product and lead to subsequent spoilage. Reductions in the numbers of these organisms may lead to a practical result either in terms of subsequent heat-processing times, as in canneries, in the shelf-life of fresh fish, dressed poultry, and shell eggs, or upon the market quality of beer, milk, butter, and even cosmetics. These different perspectives were largely responsible for the proliferation of terms that developed in the literature and on labels: sanitizer, germicide, bactericide, and disinfectant.

The method of Cade and Halvorson (1934) provided the basic screening test by which valuable comparative data were gathered on certain killing rates and on the influence of temperature, pH, and emulsifying agents. The phenol coefficient procedure was modified, by varying the inoculum and incorporating agar in the subculture medium so that plate counts could be made. Other advancements were the requirement for an arbitrary 99.9% reduction in the count over the control slides when exposed to 0.1% tetrasodium pyrophosphate as a control.

Attempts to develop a test procedure that would equate laboratory results with actual use-results were proposed by Johns (1947), using sterile microscope slides, and by Mallman and Hanes (1947), using sterile glass-rod carriers. Weber and Black (1948) outlined a dilution-tube procedure to determine the sanitizing efficiency of products recommended for use on food utensils, and could be correlated with actual use results (Weber, 1949). Chamber (1956) revised certain details and set the end-point at 99.999% reduction in the number of specified organisms within 30 seconds. This led to the AOAC Germicidal and Detergent-Sanitizer Test, a method that has been accepted for regulatory use in determining the effects of hard waters on sanitizers and detergent-sanitizers recommended for dairy, restaurant, and food plant applications. The test can be used to determine the minimum concentration of a chemical that can be permitted for use in sanitizing precleaned, nonporous, food-contact surfaces, and the maximum water hardness allowable for the various claimed concentrations of chemical.

Ortensio (1955) studied a procedure for determining the available chlorine concentrations of disinfecting solutions. A modification of the test, based on halide activity calculated as equivalent to available chlorine as hypochlorite (Ortensio, 1957; Ortensio and Stuart, 1959), culminated in the AOAC Available Chlorine Equivalent Concentration Test (1980). This test for determining chlorine germicidal equivalent concentrations, with *Salmonella typhi* as the test organism, is applicable to iodine, bromine, and organic chlorine products that are water-miscible disinfectants for use as sanitizing rinses for previously cleaned nonporous surfaces.

In sanitizing operations, where speed of action is a critical factor, the degree of hardness (principally by magnesium and calcium ions) in the available water supply can be a limiting factor in the use of certain sanitizers. Laws et al. (1964) reported that this effect was not restricted to inorganic ions and that quaternary ammonium compounds could form quaternary-protein complexes and exhibit less efficiency.

Bacteriostasis

Another aspect of microbial control is bacteriostasis, wherein the antimicrobial agent prevents the replications but not necessarily the metabolism of the affected microorganisms. The microbiostats control fungi and bacteria through the residual biostatic action of the agent. In certain prescribed applications, large quantities of these agents are sold to protect wood, fabrics, leather, paints, plastics, starch, and cutting oils from microbial invasion and deterioration. They have been successful in the protection of living plants and inanimate materials from fungi and bacteria.

When the residue of the sanitizer or microbiostat acts as a preservative (for such materials as hides, paper, wood, leather, plastics, and rubber), a wide variety of procedures may be employed to confirm the data of treatment efficacy. The residues are intended to be reactivated under moist conditions and affect the microorganisms that may be present or that may be deposited on the surface.

Because most hard surfaces are likely to remain dry or to be only briefly and intermittently moist under normal conditions of use, residual antimicrobial activity is difficult to document. Hence, as always, the type of test required for proper documentation will depend on the claims made and the recommended uses. For claims of residual bacteriostasis, the number of test microorganisms recovered from the treated surface must be fewer than the number recovered from untreated control surfaces. For claims of residual self-sanitization, there must be at least a 99.9% reduction in the number of test organisms on the treated surface compared to the untreated surface.

SCOPE OF SANITIZER USE

1. Mitigate the spread of nonpathogenic microorganisms of public health significance
2. Prevent the development of microbial malodors
3. Prevent the development of dangerous microbial end-products
4. Control of microorganisms in potential reservoirs of infection for living animals
5. Control of contaminants of economic significance (food, plants, and industrial establishments)
6. Prevent biologic decay and deterioration in materials (water-based paints, metal-working fluids)
7. Prevent microbial growth and spoilage in cane and beet sugar, other raw foodstocks
8. Control of airborne microorganisms.

TYPES OF SANITIZERS

The four most popular types of sanitizers are the chlorinated compounds, the iodophors or iodine compounds, the quaternary ammonium compounds, and the acid-anionic surfactant compounds. Soaps and phenol-based mixtures (such as pine oils) are also sanitizers.

Of these, the chlorine-based sanitizers are probably the most widely used because they are the most economical and have great killing power against a wide range of bacteria. In properly formulated products, they are relatively nontoxic, colorless, nonstaining, and easy to prepare and to apply. Characteristically, hypochlorites are active against all microorganisms, spores at high temperatures and long contact times, and bacteriophages; they do not form films; they have a short shelf-life; they have an odor; they are corrosive to many materials; and they affect the skin. The typical use-concentration is 200 to 500 ppm Cl_2 and must take the organic load into consideration.

The iodophors are basically a combination of iodine and a solubilizing agent that releases free iodine in aqueous solution, and they are highly bactericidal. Their effectiveness is not appreciably reduced by organic matter, provided that the product has been properly buffered to be on the acid side. Characteristically, iodophors are active against all microorganisms except bacterial spores and bacteriophage; they have a long shelf-life and good penetrative powers; they prevent and eliminate odors; they do not form films because of their acid nature; they are nonstaining, noncorrosive, relatively nontoxic, and non-irritating; they are stable in solution; and they require no potable water rinse when the use-concentration is less than 25 ppm available iodine. The storage temperature should be kept below the "gas-off" temperature of 120°F. The typical use-concentration is 25 ppm (or greater) I_2.

The quaternary ammonium sanitizers are equally effective againast many gram-positive bacteria but are slow to inactivate coliforms and pseudomonads. Characteristically, they are colorless, odorless, and nontoxic; they have a long shelf-life; and they are stable when heated and remain effective in the presence of hard water and organic soils. No potable water rinse is required if concentration is at or below 200 ppm active ingredients. They have good penetrative powers, form a bacteriostatic film, and are used with surfactants to form detergent-sanitizers. The typical minimum use-concentration is 200 ppm quat.

Acid-ionic surfactant germicides are combinations of organic or inorganic acids (usually phosphoric acid) with surface active agents (usually of the alkyl-aryl-sulfonate family). The antimicrobial effect is provided by the low pH. The activity of the surfactant, sodium dodecylbenzene sulfonate, when combined with phosphoric acid—a detergent-sanitizer—can provide a sanitizing-cleaning action that cleans and sanitizes in one step under certain conditions. Characteristically, they are active against a wide spectrum of microorganisms but only at acid pH (with pH 1.0 to 2.2 the optimum), leave a residual antibacterial film, and remain effective in the presence of organic and hard water, but are adversely affected by milk in combination with hard water. The typical use-concentration is generally not less than 100 ppm anion.

Selection of a Sanitizer

Efficient cleaning and sanitizing programs require the well-informed selection of the right detergent and sanitizer. The overall objectives are efficient cleaning, microbial kill, and safety. Proper cleaning of a surface is essential to remove all of the soils that protect microorganisms. Because effective cleaning of equipment is probably 90% of the overall sanitizing job and the application of sanitizers is the remaining 10%, the "cleaning" phase should receive some emphasis.

The selection of the detergent should take into consideration the equipment to be cleaned, the soils involved, and the method of application. For food-contact equipment, the effective detergent should contain surface-active agents for rapid wetting, penetration, and emulsification of fats and oils, plus a sequestering agent to permit effective performance in a variety of water conditions, and buffer capacity to keep the cleaning solution in the proper pH range for efficient cleaning.

When the use of soft water is not practical, an alkaline detergent compatible with the local water supply may be needed. (If very hard water is used, phosphoric acid-based cleaners or compounds utilizing acid sulfate may be necessary to prevent scale and to minimize pitting and corrosion of stainless steel and other sensitive materials.) With an alkaline detergent, the active alkalinity must deal with fat-containing residues (saponification into soap) and neutralize any acidic components. The active alkalinity should be balanced against the alkali demand to obtain soil removal and minimize surface corrosion.

Each type of surface-active agent has different properties: anionics are good detergents but poor bactericides, nonionics are good wetting agents, and cationics are good bactericides but have poorer detergency. Cationic and anionic detergents must not be used together. They are often more effective when used hot, but if the temperature exceeds 65°C, the ability to keep fat emulsified and rinsable is lost. Acid cleaners are usually used cold.

Desired Characteristics in a Sanitizer

1. Economical (price per use of "label-claim" concentrations of sanitizer)
2. Easy to apply; easy to use; easy to mix to use-concentrations. (Note: The ideal sanitizer is inadequate when improperly used. Proper training is essential, and this entails instruction, practice, and periodic inspection to review technique.)
3. Stable
4. Without harmful or offensive odor
5. Nontoxic
6. Good cleaning power
7. Good penetrative power
8. Demonstrates residual activity
9. Reduces vegetative organism count by 99.999% in 30 seconds
10. Active before and after dilution with hard water
11. Not influenced by presence of protein
12. Harmless (noncorrosive) to finish of contact surface
13. Destroys a wide variety of microorganisms: gram-positive and gram-negative bacteria, fungi, viruses
14. Acts rapidly
15. Compatible with other chemicals
16. Nondamaging to materials (rubber, plastic, cloth)

A PRECIS ON MICROBIOLOGIC EFFECTIVENESS

The biocidal effectiveness of a sanitizer is established by a test protocol. A scientific test is a test of a hypothesis, and the test results reject it or allow it to stand. At a minimum, test protocol must address the following factors:

1. The microbial strains must be identified, the inoculum and the culture conditions must be defined, and all materials used must be identified or described with precision. In addition, the inocula should meet validated performance criteria.
2. The inoculum for the test should be at a positive exponential growth phase. Two or three subcultures of the test strains in the same medium are recommended before the test, but this should be a part of the performance criteria for the inocula.
3. The size of the inoculum must allow for an assessment of survivors of significant statistical value.
4. The recovery culture medium should contain all the elements required for recovery of stressed organisms and for abundant growth, if these are not incompatible qualities.
5. Appropriate techniques should be employed to eliminate residual carry-over of the sanitizer in order not to inhibit the recovery and the growth of the surviving organisms for the quantitative determination of the survivors.
6. Tests should be performed on representative surfaces, with and without added organic soil, and with and without hard water.
7. Test methods must be validated, and must include positive and negative controls. A minimum of three replicate tests are required; replicating in triplicate a test on one product batch/lot is acceptable as one test.
8. The test method should be detailed and technically

sound, and could vary according to the type of product, its intended uses, the type of substrate to be treated, the label claims, the directions for use, and any other factors specific to the product. The technique developed should reasonably simulate the use conditions for the product, and must be precise, reproducible, and standardized.

9. The complete results for each individual replication should be reported, together with any pertinent observations and deductions. The composition and concentration of the sanitizer, the number of batches and the dates of preparation, the method of preparation and the manner of storage, and other pertinent observations should be a part of the evaluation of the product.

TEST ELEMENTS

Test Organisms

The test organisms should be representative of the principal groups found on the surfaces to be sanitized. Of the various organisms that have been used to study sanitizers, it appears that *Escherichia coli* (ATCC 11229) should be the principal test organism and that it should be complemented by a secondary test organism selected according to the specific use for which the sanitizer is recommended: for example, *E. coli* and *Staphylococcus aureus* (ATCC 6538) for a restaurant sanitizer; *E. coli* and *Micrococcus caseolyticus* for a dairy sanitizer; *E. coli* and *Pseudomonas aeruginosa* for a shell egg sanitizer; and *E. coli* and *Bacillus coagulans* for a cannery equipment sanitizer.

Testing should be performed using standard test organisms that have been cultivated in a standardized manner. This will allow comparisons of sanitizing systems and the development of standardized acceptance criteria. The use of product isolates may be informative but is not advocated for routine testing because of standardization problems. Regardless of the procedure used for culture maintenance, the difference in resistance or sensitivity to the antimicrobial agent by a product isolate, compared to a standard test organism, may be expected to disappear by in vitro maintenance through several subculture passages.

Resistance of bacteria to chemicals may vary considerably between different species, different strains of the same species, and different subcultures of the same strain. The age of a culture can influence resistance to a chemical, and there is an optimum age for each culture. The daily transfer of cultures probably should be restricted to seven passages because extended daily subculturing tends to lead to an altered resistance pattern. The mode of maintaining the test strains and the baseline resistance should be determined for the subculture(s) used.

The composition of the medium during culturing and variances in cultural conditions can be a major influence on the resistance of the organism. A practical way to control the vagaries of the culture medium is to first determine an acceptable lot of the dehydrated medium, and then to secure a large supply of that batch/lot and subsequently keep the bottles tightly sealed and cool. Similar considerations should be in effect for each component of a medium and for the quality of the water that is used in the preparation of a medium.

Inoculum

The harvest of microorganisms from a growth milieu and the preparation of the microbial suspension—the inoculum that will be used in sanitizer tests—should follow a written protocol that emphasizes reproducibility of technique and culture conditions. Microorganisms respond readily to many cultural stimuli: media composition, volume of medium, pH, ionic partial pressure of ambient gasses, harvesting procedures, and crop cleaning procedures. With microorganisms, "little things mean a lot."

Inoculum density should be adapted to the recovery technique for the survivors. Densities of 1.0×10^6 organisms per milliliter and greater are generally used with plate count techniques for assaying the degree of reduction of a population.

The use of mixtures of various test organisms is not advocated. First, microbial interaction and competition is a separate and complex field, and cannot be treated lightly; and second, it is seldom worth the aggravation of documenting the effectiveness of each batch/lot of each of the selective media, after the effectiveness of the procedure itself has been validated.

The choice of suspending medium and the manner in which the inoculum is prepared can influence the results of the test. Repeated washings of the organisms to eliminate traces of culture medium may be a waste. The addition of a small amount of peptone to a suspension medium (distilled or deionized water, physiologic or buffered sodium chloride) appears to allow bacteria to survive in the suspensions. Microbial suspensions give the most reproducible results when handled with tender, loving care; microorganisms respond to stimuli.

In general, the inoculum must be easy to prepare and give reproducible results. The procedure should require, in principle, the use of freshly prepared young cultures made from strains maintained on media or stock frozen in liquid nitrogen or lyophilized. The strains should be suspended and diluted in distilled water supplemented with a protective peptone to a suitable density based on count or photometric measurements. The viable population of the inoculum should be verified by a plate count made simultaneously with the test of the preparation. For greater accuracy in the deposition of inocula, the use of consistent technique with a calibrated precision syringe is recommended.

Application

Sanitizing agents may be applied by a variety of methods, as dictated by their nature, the surface to be treated, and the manufacturer's directions. The surface material(s), the surface type (porous or nonporous), the condition of the surface, the suspending medium, and the method of drying the organisms onto the test surface(s) can directly influence the test results. These factors should be standardized in laboratory testing, even though they will remain a wild card in field test, and particularly when organic material is present to absorb or decompose the agent.

To obtain the results claimed for the sanitizer by the manufacturer, it must be used as directed by the manufacturer. Sometimes, and perhaps only because of some small difference in the test techniques of manufacturer and user, the results of antimicrobial testing will not meet the label claims (Rutala and Cole, 1987). Test technique or antimicrobial controls are essential for clarity in interpretation of results.

Liquid sanitizing agents can be applied by:
1. *Spraying*, which is convenient for small surfaces.
2. *Wiping/Spreading*, which is also effective for small to medium-sized surfaces. Wiping combines the physical removal of organisms or debris by abrasion with the antibiologic activity of the agent. Wipes seem to have replaced the combination elbow grease with soap and water, but trained conscientious personnel remain a necessity.
3. *Mopping*, which is more appropriate for covering large environmental surfaces. Three mopping techniques are used: damp mopping, wet mopping, and flood and vacuum. Only the double-bucket wet mopping procedure and the flood and vacuum technique allow for adequate contact time with the at-use-dilution sanitizer.
4. *Submersion*, which is useful with small surfaces and equipment.

Once the efficacy of a sanitizer has been determined, applications can be considered and evaluated, and the efficacy can be documented.

Sanitizer

The relationship between a bactericidal concentration of a sanitizer and the rate of microbial destruction is an established principle with practical significance. The proper concentration must be great enough to sanitize within a period that is convenient for the user. This can only be determined by means of relevant tests, first in the laboratory and then in the field. Of practical note is the knowledge that it may take longer to sanitize a surface contaminated with a million bacteria than it does when only 100 are present. Optimism should always be tempered with the knowledge that microorganisms always "do their thing" when faced with adverse conditions.

Antimicrobial activity is profoundly influenced by pH. Some compounds may dissociate and become inactive, whereas others may become more active: at pH 8.2 only 100 ppm available chlorine is required to provide activity equivalent to 1000 ppm chlorine at pH 11.3. The antimicrobial activity of hypochlorites decreases with increasing pH, the active bactericidal factor being the un-

dissociated hypochlorous acid. Iodine is more effective at acid than at alkaline pH values but is less affected by acidity than chlorine.

The effect of pH can be three-fold: as an effect on the molecule of the antimicrobial agent, as an effect on the cell surface, and by influencing the partitioning of a component of a sanitizer between the product and the microbial cell. Organic materials—e.g., blood, serum, dirt, earth, food residues, and fecal materials—may reduce the effectiveness of sanitizers and disinfectants, either as a result of a chemical reaction between the sanitizer and the organic matter or through protection of the organisms from attack (Sykes, 1965). Phospholipids in serum, milk, and feces will reduce the antimicrobial activity of quaternary ammonium compounds. Organic matter decreases the effect of hypochlorites against bacteria, and there is a less marked effect with iodine and iodophors because of the lowered chemical activity.

Mathematical Modeling

The most commonly used model for inactivation of microorganisms by antimicrobials has been derived from the work of Chick and Martin (1908) and Walters (1917). The "Chick-Walters Law" is $(N/No) = -kCt$, where N/No is the ratio of surviving organisms to initial population at time t, C is the concentration of antimicrobial, and k and n are empirical constants; n is also called the coefficient of dilution and k is the slope of the response curve. The model implies that the concentration of antimicrobial and contact time are the two key variables governing the efficacy of disinfection/sanitization and sterilization. The equation is based on the observation that inactivation of microorganisms generally follows first-order kinetics. The report by Hoff (1986) describes the use of these mathematical concepts and the problems of extrapolating from the available laboratory data (chlorine-based model) to the application of data to field conditions.

The relation of antimicrobial concentration (C) and contact time (t) in microbial inactivation seems simple. However, the empirical C × t equation does not adequately predict the exponential rates of inactivation. Higher concentrations that can be less effective, differences in antimicrobial resistance between different isolates of the same species between different species within groups, aggregation, and prior growth conditions are some of the biological quirks that affect the model. Mixing intensity (complete and uniform), a constant sanitizer concentration, and the ionic status of the sanitizer are some of the technical quirks that confound the model. The real challenge has always been to make the laboratory data relevant to field operations (Hass and Karra, 1984; Noss and Olivieri, 1985).

The kinetics of the effects of concentrations of sanitizers/disinfectants on microbial activity have tended to use the dilution coefficient (concentration exponent), a measure of the effect of changes in concentration on cell death rate (Bean, 1972). The rate of inactivation of each challenge organism in the test sample is given by the decimal reduction time (D-value). The D-value is the time required to reduce the population by 90%, that is, a 1-log reduction when the population is subjected to a set of reproducible conditions; often, then, the D-value determination is more an art form than a science. Nonetheless, the rationale for the use of D-values is that every organism has a characteristic rate of inactivation when subjected to any lethal treatment, and the D-value provides a quantitative expression of the rate of inactivation of a specific organism in the test sample.

The D-value for a test organism in a given test sample is determined from the survivor curve plotted from the number of viable organisms recovered after various timed exposures to the sanitizer. The survivor curve is constructed by drawing a straight line through the points and onward to the X-axis, with the X-intercept representing the time for complete inactivation. The D-value is the positive expression of the slope of this curve. (Note: even though replicated D-value determinations can reveal reproducible D-values for a set of test conditions, indicating they are in "steady state" and that the suspension of test organisms is sufficiently clean and homogeneous to allow a "clean" regression line, the relativity of the inactivation rate to the effectiveness of the antimicrobial is not crystal clear.)

Of more immediate practicality is a calculator capable of least-squares linear regression analysis. A linear regression can be calculated directly from the data, as well as the Y-intercept (the theoretic population at the start of the inactivation), the slope of the survivor curve, and the correlation coefficient (r). As with all "massaged" data, certain nuances of the response of the microorganisms to the antimicrobial agent will be smoothed over (e.g., that an inactivation curve is seldom linear except for a portion of the curve, and that the "activation" and "tailing" effects can be of practical importance). Caution should be exercised to avoid great precision on inappropriately generated numbers or "much ado about nothing."

Use of linear regression method is suited to selecting the proper concentration of sanitizer to protect a product. First, samples of the test product containing different concentrations of the sanitizer are prepared. These samples are challenged with a test organism, and plate counts are determined at various times thereafter. Then the D-values are determined for the different sanitizer concentrations (formulations), resulting in a series of survivor curves. The curve that shows inactivation of the test organism at the desired rate provides the data to select the concentration of sanitizer that is efficacious against unattached bacteria.

The value of mathematical modeling has been shown in the studies on sanitization of unattached and biofilm (attached) bacteria. Unattached bacteria were quite susceptible, being reduced 99% by exposure to 0.08 mg of hypochlorous acid (pH 7.0) per liter (or to 94 mg/L monochloramine) for 1 minute. Biofilm bacteria, grown on the surfaces of granular activated carbon particles, metal cou-

pons, or glass microscope slides, were 150 to 3000 times more resistant to hypochlorous acid (free chlorine, pH 7.0) than were unattached cells. Resistance of biofilm bacteria to monochloramine ranged from 2 to 100 times more than that of unattached cells (Lechevalier et al., 1988).

Recovery System

The recovery system includes the diluent, the neutralizer (if necessary), the plating media, and the recovery procedure. Use of the proper recovery system is absolutely essential in sanitizer efficacy testing because the recovery system influences the accuracy and sensitivity of the plate count data. The commonly used diluents are distilled water, deionized water, physiologic saline, peptone water, Letheen broth, and Letheen Broth with Triton X-100. The commonly used plating media are Standard Methods Agar, Soybean Casein Digest Agar, and Soybean Casein Digest Medium with lecithin and Tween 80. The recovery procedures may be "stomaching," swabbing, shaking or sonication (or both), or a combination of these and other procedures (such as the kiss lift-off procedure techniques for fungi). The counting procedure may use spread plates, pour plates, or membrane filters, and each is placed into the appropriate recovery and growth environment.

Under use-conditions, the recovery of all organisms that may be on a product by the use of one recovery system is nearly impossible because different organisms have different growth requirements. All recovery procedures are selective to some degree. For example, one factor is the desirability of a low colony count (ideally 20 to 100 colonies per plate, according to the nature of the microorganisms, with variations in practice between 10 and 300 on 50-mm membranes and 90-mm agar plates). Another factor that enhances the threshold of detection of viable organisms is the elimination of residual antimicrobial effect. Thus, the sensitivity of the subculture techniques, including the important neutralization procedures (Favero et al., 1968; Engley and Day, 1970), should be validated. By differentiating between the "actual" and the "apparent" reduction in the numbers of organisms, the count reducing power of the sanitizing treatment could become more reproducible and, therefore, the data more usable.

The ideal recovery system possesses the following characteristics:

1. The diluent inactivates the active compounds of the sanitizer
2. The diluent is capable of dispersing materials
3. The diluent stabilizes injured (stressed) organisms and prevents them from drying out before they are introduced into the plating medium
4. The plating medium inactivates the active components of the sanitizer
5. The plating medium facilitates the repair and growth of the stressed cells
6. The plating medium encourages good growth so that colonies are readily observable after an incu-

bation period of 48 hours (for bacteria) and 7 days for fungi (yeasts and mold)

Note: The reliability of any test method should be established before it is used. Reliability depends on the precision, sensitivity, and accuracy of the method. In microbiologic testing, the precision generally depends on the skill and care used by the microbiologist, whereas the sensitivity and accuracy reflect the ability of the method to recover all viable organisms that are present. The reliability of the method used in sanitizer efficacy testing depends on the ability of the recovery system to neutralize any carry-over of active components of the sanitizer into the plating medium, and to facilitate repair and growth of the stressed organisms. Stressed organisms are injured cells. Microorganisms may be stressed by a number of agents, among which are antimicrobial compounds. Sublethal stress is characterized by a loss of selectivity of the semipermeable membrane of the cell and impaired ability to synthesize the macromolecules needed for repair and growth. The repair process typically requires several hours.

Microbiologists usually assume that each colony that is detected on a solid medium develops from a single cell in the inoculum. However, a cluster of cells on a solid medium will also produce a colony. Thus it can be important to know whether it was 10 one-cell colonies or 10 ten-cell colonies that were treated with the sanitizer or bacteriostat (or recovered after treatment). A 90% reduction of the former will leave one cell to proliferate, but a 90% reduction of the latter will leave 10 cells to multiply. (To assume is to be human, to test hypotheses is to be a competent scientist.)

Controls

Many different techniques have been used to study sanitizing agents, and the selection of one method over another is not critical. Regardless of the method employed, both the precision and the accuracy of the method must be known. Resistance of each culture to the known chemical or to boiling water should be determined concomitantly each time a test is run. Adequate control over the test requires standardization of equipment and materials, composition of media, pH, and stock culture and test culture handling; preparation of exact concentrations; accurate volume measurements; intense mixing of cells and agent; attention to manipulative detail; accurate timing; and appropriate neutralizers. (The required concentration of neutralizer varies with different test cultures and the active agent. Letheen broth is an appropriate subculture medium for cation surface-active agents such as quats and phenolics; thioglycolate medium works with oxidizing agents; sodium thiosulfate neutralizes residual chlorine; iodophors require lecithin and thiosulfate.)

CLAIMS FOR SANITIZER EFFICACY

Unless otherwise specified, antimicrobial pesticides must be performance-tested in the formulation(s) mar-

keted or to be marketed, for effectiveness, batch replicability, and shelf-life stability in expected "normal" conditions. Efficacy test data are required for all antimicrobial products with a claim of controlling microorganisms in the inanimate environment where the microorganisms may present a hazard to human health.

The test method should refer to and follow the appropriate AOAC test protocol. Basic test elements will vary according to the type of product, label claims, directions for use, and other factors peculiar to each product. Any modified method must reflect details of each modification that was used to meet specific requirements. Any product that claims effectiveness in hard water must be tested by the appropriate method in synthetic hard water (see AOAC citation for formulation and preparation) at the level claimed. Any product that bears claims for effectiveness as a "one-step" cleaner-sanitizer must be tested by the appropriate method in the presence of a representative organic soil, such as 5% blood serum or, if a specific type of soil is listed (such as soap film residue or hard water scum), in the presence of that specific soil. Before initiation of in-use or simulated-use studies, the proposed test protocols may be submitted to the appropriate agency for review and comment; sound reasoning and good, clear and detailed scientific protocols are always appreciated.

Verification of the Effectiveness of a Sanitizer

The methods used to evaluate sanitizing agents can be divided into two categories: standard laboratory tests and in-use tests. A combination of both of these methods can provide the most comprehensive documentation for a sanitizing procedure. The only requirement is that all elements of the test are under control.

Standard laboratory methods such as the AOAC Available Chlorine Germicidal Equivalent test, the AOAC Germicidal and Detergent Sanitizer test, and the AOAC Use-Dilution test are specifically designed for reproducibility in any laboratory by any operator. These standardized laboratory tests are useful for comparing the sanitizing activity of various products at various use-dilutions, exposure times, temperatures, etc; they can be made to work if appropriate modifications and controls are incorporated into the test procedure to document (and to clarify) any areas of difficulty. The sanitizer can be challenged in solution or on various test surfaces with microorganisms whose presence would be expected in the typical use-environment. By varying the exposure conditions, the kinetics of microbial death can be determined and the adequacy of the sanitizer can be judged.

The performance of a sanitizer under laboratory conditions can differ substantially from its performance in actual use. The strength of in-use testing is that the results reflect actual conditions, including personnel and procedures, soil, microbiologic load, contact time, water hardness, type of surface, type of applicator, temperature, and pH. The sanitizer is applied to a piece of equipment, a facility, or a surface, and the surviving microorganisms are recovered and enumerated by a validated method—swabbing, contact plates, elution, or whatever works and has been documented. Monitoring the sanitization process immediately after use-application gives some indication of the thoroughness of the process. Monitoring the effects of the sanitization process between times provides insight about the adequacy of the sanitizer (and any residual effect) and the frequency of sanitization.

When the method of testing the sanitizer or bacteriostatic agent gives reproducible data, and the data can be applied to sanitization procedures that will give predictable results and are reliable, then comes a potential reward—documented sanitization procedures. Once a sanitization procedure is properly and completely documented—with detailed written descriptions of the materials, methods, equipment, and critical sanitization parameters with appropriate controls—it needs to be monitored for effectiveness at periodic intervals. When a sanitization process is not documented, then the effectiveness of that process should be monitored each time it is used.

PRODUCTS FOR HARD SURFACES

Sanitizers (for Non–Food-Contact Hard Surfaces)

Products bearing label claims for effectiveness as sanitizers for inanimate hard surfaces, other than those which come in contact with food or beverage (e.g., floors, walls, furnishings), must show a reduction of at least 99.9% in the number of each test microorganism over the parallel control count.

Sanitizing Rinses (for Previously Cleaned Food-Contact Surfaces)

Any product with a label recommendation for treatment of previously cleaned food-contact surfaces (e.g., eating and drinking utensils and food-processing equipment) as a terminal sanitizing rinse, are defined as incidental food additives under the Federal Food, Drug, and Cosmetic Act, as amended (21 U.S.C. 201 et seq.), and are regulated as a food additive. Recommendation of a potable water rinse after treatment does not preclude this requirement.

Halide Chemical Products

Efficacy of sanitizing rinses formulated with iodophors, mixed halides, and chlorine-bearing chemicals must be demonstrated against *Salmonella typhi* (ATCC 6339) with data derived from the AOAC Chlorine Germicidal Equivalent Concentration Method, and the test results must show product concentrations equivalent in activity to 50, 100, and 200 ppm of available chlorine.

Other Chemical Products

The efficacy of sanitizing rinses formulated with quaternary ammonium compounds, chlorinated trisodium phosphate, and anionic detergent-acid formulations must be demonstrated against both *E. coli* (ATCC 11229) and *Staphylococcus aureus* (ATCC 6538) with data derived

from the AOAC Germicidal and Detergent Sanitizers Method. Test results must demonstrate a 99.999% reduction in the number of each test organism within 30 seconds. The results must be reported according to the actual count and percentage of reduction over the control.

Residual Self-Sanitizing Activity of Dried Chemical Residues on Hard Inanimate Surfaces

Products whose labels claim to provide residual self-sanitizing activity (e.g., significant reduction in numbers of infectious microorganisms that may be present or subsequently deposited) on treated surfaces that are likely to become and remain wet under normal conditions of use must demonstrate at least a 99.9% reduction in the number of test organisms on the treated surface(s) compared with parallel control surface(s).

Note: The test must be based upon an adequately controlled in-use study or simulated in-use study employing as test microorganisms those target pathogens likely to be encountered in the environment in which the product is to be used, and at a sufficient concentration to provide at least 1×10^4 survivors on the parallel control surface. The environmental conditions employed in the test, such as relative humidity and temperature, must be known. The residue on the treated surface(s) must be activated by the addition of moisture in a manner and over an exposure period identical to the use pattern for which the product is intended.

PRODUCTS REQUIRING CONFIRMATORY DATA

Sanitizers (for Previously Cleaned Food-Contact Surfaces)

The confirmatory test standard is as follows: one test on one sample, with or without hard water (depending on label claims), is required using either the AOAC Germicidal and Detergent Sanitizers Test against *E. coli* for quaternary ammonium compounds, chlorinated trisodium phosphate, and anionic detergent-acid formulations, or the AOAC Available Chlorine Germicidal Equivalent Concentration Test against *Salmonella typhi* for iodophors, mixed halides, and chlorine-bearing chemicals.

PRODUCTS FOR USE ON FABRICS AND TEXTILES (LAUNDRY ADDITIVES)

Antimicrobial products that bear label recommendations for use in the treatment of laundry (as a pre-soak treatment or in household and commercial laundry operations) to provide various levels of antimicrobial activity including disinfections, sanitization, or residual self-sanitization require specific documentation, as follows:

1. For disinfecting pre-soak treatment, the AOAC Use-Dilution Method modified to include organic

soil must be employed. The results must substantiate disinfection capability.

2. Sanitizing laundry additives (nonresidual), products that bear label claims as sanitizers for use in automatic or manual washing machine operations, must show at least a 99.9% reduction in bacteria over the control count for both laundry water and fabric against each test organism.

3. Self-sanitizing laundry additives (residual): products that bear label claims to provide residual self-sanitizing activity (e.g., significant reduction in numbers of infectious microorganisms that may contaminate the items) on treated fabrics when used in automatic or manual washing machine operations (usually in the final rinse), must demonstrate at least a 99.99% reduction of each test organism over the "0-time" control and parallel untreated inoculated control. (*Note:* Petrocci and Clarke (1969) have published an acceptable protocol.)

CARPET SANITIZERS

Products bearing label claims for effectiveness as carpet sanitizers must be tested against *S. aureus* and *Enterobacter aerogenes* (ATCC 13048) with two different types of representative synthetic carpeting, such as acrylic and polypropylene tufted-loop types. If the product is intended for use in hospitals or medical institutions, it must also be tested against *Pseudomonas aeruginosa* (ATCC 15442). If the product is also intended for use on wool carpeting, an additional representative sample of wool carpet must be tested; otherwise, the label must bear a disclaimer for use on wool. All of the types of carpet samples tested must be fully identified by the pile fiber, pile yarn weight of finished carpet, pile density, and tuft height. Test results must demonstrate a 99.9% reduction of test bacteria over the control.

AIR SANITIZERS

Products bearing label claims for treatment of air to temporarily reduce the numbers of airborne microorganisms should have data that show a viable count reduction of at least 99.9% over the parallel untreated control, after correcting for settling rates, in the air of the test enclosure with each of the test bacteria. (*Note:* There is considerable evidence that glycol vapors—triethylene, dipropylene, and propylene glycol—produce significant decreases in numbers of viable airborne bacteria under relatively wide conditions of relative humidity, temperature, and concentration (greater than 5%) when properly and continuously dispensed by a vaporizing device so as to maintain suitable concentrations in the air of enclosed spaces.

PRODUCTS FOR CONTROL OF MICROBIAL PESTS ASSOCIATED WITH HUMAN AND ANIMAL WASTES

Products bearing label claims as sanitizers for toilet bowl and urinal surfaces must show a reduction of at least 99.9% of each test microorganism over the parallel control count.

Products bearing label claims as sanitizers for toilet and urinal bowl water must show that the reduction of each test microorganism must be at least 99.9% over the 0-time control and the parallel untreated inoculated unit.

REFERENCES

Adair, F.W. 1982. Uses of water—nasal and oral liquid. In *Proceedings of the PMA Water Seminar Program*. Washington, D.C., PMA.

Anonymous. 1938. Modified technique of the Chick-Martin Test for Disinfectants. British Standard 808. London, British Standards Institution.

Anonymous. 1978. Foam sanitization. Am. Dairy Rev., *40*, 38–39.

Association of Official Analytical Chemists (AOAC). 1984. *Offical Methods of Analysis of the Association of Official Analytical Chemists*. 14th Edition. Washington, D.C., AOAC, pp. 65–77.

Asbury, E.D. 1983. Methods of testing sanitizers and bacteriostatic substances. In *Disinfection, Sterilization and Preservation*. 3rd Edition. Edited by S.S. Block. Philadelphia, Lea & Febiger, pp. 964–980.

American Type Culture Collection (ATCC). 1985. *Catalogue of Bacteria, Phages, rDNA Vectors*. 16th Edition. Edited by R. Gherna, W. Nierman, and P. Pienta. Rockville, MD, ATCC.

Ayliffe, G.A.J., Collins, B.J., and Deverill, C.E.A. 1974. Tests of disinfection by heat in a bed-pan washing machine. J. Clin. Pathol., *27*, 760–763.

Barkley, W.E., Wedum, A.G., and McKinney, R.W. 1983. The hazard of infectious agents in microbiologic laboratories. In *Disinfection, Sterilization and Preservation*. 3rd Edition. Edited by S.S. Block. Philadelphia, Lea & Febiger, pp. 566–576.

Bean, H.S., Heman-Ackah, S.M., and Thomas, J. 1965. The activity of antimicrobials in two-phase systems. J. Soc. Cosmet. Chem., *16*, 15–27.

Butterfield, C.T., Wattie, E., Megrogian, S., and Chambers, C.W. 1943. Influence of pH and temperature on the survival of coliforms and enteric pathogens when exposed to free chlorine. U.S. Public Health Rep., *58*, 1837–1866.

Cade, A.R., and Halvorson, H.O. 1934. Germicidal detergents, the synergistic action of soaps on the germicidal efficiency of alkalies. Part I, Soap, *10*(8), 17–19, 41–53; Part II, Soap, *10*(9), 25–26, 49.

Carr, R.H., Jr., Guest, G.A., and Cottone, J.A. 1987. Surface and equipment disinfection: an essential element in a comprehensive infection control program. Tex. Dent. J., *104*(4), 12–16, 70.

Chambers, C.W. 1956. A procedure for evaluating the efficiency of bactericidal agents. J. Milk Food Technol., *19*, 183–187.

Chick, H., and Martin, C.J. 1908. The principles involved in the standardization of disinfectants and the influence of organic matter upon germicidal value. J. Hyg., *8*, 654–697.

Costerton, J.W., and Lashen, E.S. 1984. Influence of biofilm on efficacy of biocides on corrosion-causing bacteria. Mater. Perform., *23*(2), 13–17.

Davis, J.G. 1973. Fundamentals of microbiology in relation to cleansing in the cosmetic industry. Soap Perfum. Cosmet., *46*, 37–46.

Dorland's Illustrated Medical Dictionary. 1988. 27th Edition. Philadelphia, W.B. Saunders.

Dubois, A.S. 1949. Meaning of "sanitization." Soap Sanit. Chem., *25*(5), 137, 147.

Engley, F.B., and Dey, B.P. 1970. A universal neutralizing medium for antimicrobial chemicals. Proc. Chem. Spec. Manuf. Assoc., 100–106.

Favero, M.S., et al. 1968. Microbiological sampling of surfaces. J. Appl. Bacteriol., *31*, 336–343.

Federal Pesticide Control Act of 1972. Amendments to the Federal Insecticide, Fungicide, and Rodenticide Act (7 USC 135 et seq.), (86 Stat. 973-999). Public Law 92-516, 92nd Congress, H.R. 10729. October 21, 1972.

The 1975 Amendment to the Federal Insecticide, Fungicide, and Rodenticide Act (7 USC 136 et seq.), (86 Stat. 973-999). Public Law 94-140, 94th Congress, H.R. 8841, November 28, 1975.

The 1978 Amendment to the Federal Insecticide, Fungicide, and Rodenticide Act (7 USC 136 et seq.), (86 Stat. 973-999). Public Law 95-396, 95th Congress, S. 1678, September 30, 1978.

Hass, C.N., and Karra, S.B. 1984. Kinetics of microbial inactivation by chlorine. I. Review of results in demand-free systems. Water Res., *18*, 1443–1449.

Hekmati, M., and Bradley, R.L., Jr. 1979. Effect of milk constituents on the persistence of sodium hypochlorite solution. J. Dairy Sci., 62, 47–48.

Hoff, J.C., and Geldreich, E.E. 1981. Comparison of the biocidal efficacy of alternative disinfectants. J. Am. Water Works Assoc., 73, 41–44.

Hoff, J.C. 1986. Inactivation of Microbial Agents by Chemical Disinfectants. EPA/600/2-86/067. PB86-232568, National Technical Information Service, Dept. Commerce, Springfield, VA.

Hoffman, P.N., Death, J.E., and Coates, D. 1981. The stability of sodium hypochlorite solutions. In *Disinfectants: Their Use and Evaluation of Effectiveness*. Edited by C.H. Collins, M.C. Allwood, S.F. Bloomfield, and A. Fox. New York, Academic Press, pp. 77–83.

Horsfal, J.G. 1956. *Principles of Fungicidal Action*. Waltham, Chronica Botanica.

Jeffrey, D.J., and Matthews, N.S. 1981. The effect of temperature and concentration on the antimicrobial effect of UK pine fluids. In *Disinfectants: Their Use and Evaluation of Effectiveness*. Edited by C.H. Collins, M.C. Allwood, S.F. Bloomfield, and A. Fox. New York, Academic Press, pp. 86–90.

Johns, C.K. 1947. Studies comparing the sanitizing efficiencies of hypochlorites and quaternary ammonium compounds. Can. J. Res., 26, 76–91.

Lange, K. 1975. AORN standards for OR sanitation. J. AORN, 21(7), 1223–1231.

Latlief, M.A., Goldsmith, M.T., Friedl, J.L., and Stuart, L.S. 1951. Germicidal and sanitizing action of quaternary ammonium compounds on textiles, prevention of ammonia formation from urea by Proteus mirabilis. J. Pediatr., 39, 730–737.

Law, A.B., and Claypotch, D.A. 1957. Turbidimetry as a technique for determination of Escherichia coli populations in Chambers test inoculum. J. Milk Food Technol., 20, 341–344.

Law, A.B., McNulty, P.J., and Rakus, L.M. 1964. Development of a procedure for chemical assay of the bactericidally active ingredient in quaternary ammonium sanitizing solutions. Proc. Chem. Spec. Manuf. Assoc., 154–160.

Lechevallier, M.W., Cawthorn, C.D., and Lee, R.G. 1988. Inactivation of Biofilm bacteria. Appl. Environ. Microbiol., 54(10), 2492–2499.

Lester, W., Jr., Kaye, S., Robertson, O.H., and Duklin, E.W. 1950. Factors of importance in the use of triethylene glycol vapor for aerial disinfection. Am. J. Public Health, 40, 813–820.

Mallison, G.F. 1980. Decontamination, disinfection, and sterilization. Nurs. Clin. North Am., 15(4), 757–767.

Mallman, W.L., and Hanes, M. 1945. The use-dilution method of testing disinfectants. J. Bacteriol., 49, 526.

Maurer, I. 1978. *Hospital Hygiene*. 2nd Edition. London, Edward Arnold.

McCoy, W.F. 1987. Fouling biofilm formation. In *Biological Fouling of Industrial Water Systems*. Edited by M.W. Mittelman and G.G. Geesey. San Diego, Water Micro Associates, pp. 24–55.

McCoy, W.F. 1987. Strategies for the treatment of biological fouling. In *Biological Fouling of Industrial Water Systems*. Edited by M.W. Mittelman and G.G. Geesey. San Diego, Water Micro Associates, pp. 247–268.

McCrea, A. 1931. Proposed standard method for the evaluation of fungicides. J. Lab. Clin. Med., 17, 72–74.

McGray, R.J. 1970. A test method for the evaluation of air sanitization. Proc. Chem. Spec. Manuf. Assoc., 106–111.

McRobbie, D.I., and Parker, M.S. 1974. Some aspects of the antifungal activity of esters of p-hydroxybenzoic acid. Int. Biodeter. Bull., 10, 109–112.

Miner, N.A., Whitmore, E., and McBee, M.L. 1975. A quantitative organic "soil" neutralization test for disinfectants. Dev. Indust. Microbiol., 16, 23–30.

Molinari, J.A. 1985. Chemical disinfection agents. J. Calif. Dent. Assoc., 13(10), 73–78.

Nishannon, A., and Pohja, M.S. 1977. Comparative studies of microbial contamination of surfaces by the contact plate and swab methods. J. Appl. Bacteriol., 42, 53–63.

Noss, C.I., and Olivieri, V.P. 1985. Disinfecting capabilities of oxychlorine compounds. Appl. Environ. Microbiol., 50, 1162–1164.

Ortensio, L.F. 1958. Report on fungicides and subculture media (Chambers modification of the Weber and Black test). J. AOAC, 41, 541–548.

Ortensio, L.F. 1957. Report on fungicide and subculture media (available chlorine germicidal equivalent concentration test). J. AOAC, 40, 755–758.

Ortensio, L.F. 1955. Report on fungicide and germicidal rinse testing methods. J. AOAC, 38, 274–280.

Ortensio, L.F., and Stuart, L.S. 1959. The behavior of chlorine-bearing organic compounds in the AOAC Available Chlorine Germicidal Equivalent Concentration. J. AOAC, 42, 630–633.

Orth, D.S. 1979. Linear regression method for rapid determination of cosmetic preservative efficacy. J. Soc. Cosmet. Chem., 30, 321–332.

Orth, D.S. 1980. Establishing cosmetic preservative efficacy by use of D-value. J. Soc. Cosmet. Chem., 31, 165–172.

Petrocci, A.N., and Clarke, P. 1969. Proposed test method for antimicrobial laundry additives. J. AOAC, 52, 836–842.

Prince, H.N. 1983. Disinfectant activity against bacteria and viruses. Partic. Microb. Control., 2, 55–62.

Prucha, J.J. 1929. Chemical sterilization of dairy utensils. Circular 332, Illinois Agric. Exp. Sta.

Prokop, A., and Humphrey, A.E. 1970. Kinetics of disinfection. In *Disinfection*. Edited by M.A. Bernarde. New York, Marcel Dekker, pp. 61–83.

Regenstein, H. 1912. Studien ueber die Anpassung von Bakterien an Disinfektionsmittel. Z. Bakt. Abtlg., 1, 63, 281–298. Cited by O. Wyss in "Bacterial resistance and dynamics of antibacterial activity." In *Antiseptics, Disinfectants, Fungicides, and Chemical and Physical Sterilization*. 2nd Edition. Edited by G.F. Reddish. Philadelphia, Lea & Febiger, pp. 205–222.

Scheusner, D.L. 1982. Methods to evaluate cleaners and sanitizers. J. Food Protect., 45, 1257–1260.

Shaffer, C.H., Jr. 1977. Methods of testing sanitizer and bacteriostatic substances. In *Disinfection, Sterilization and Preservation*. 2nd Edition. Edited by S.S. Block. Philadelphia, Lea & Febiger, pp. 78–99.

Shaffer, C.H., Jr. 1971. Methods of testing sanitizers and bacteriostatic substances. In *Disinfection, Sterilization and Preservation*. Edited by C.A. Lawrence and S.S. Block. Philadelphia, Lea & Febiger, pp. 159–178.

Sharpell, F.H. 1979. Development of test protocols for antimicrobial agents by the ASTM. Dev. Indust. Microbiol., 20, 73–80.

Speck, M.L., Murley, W.R., Lucas, H.L., and Aurand, L.W. 1954. Evaluation of a detergent-sanitizer for use on producer milking utensils. J. Milk Food Technol., 18, 71–76.

Stark, R.L., Ferguson, P., Garza, P., and Miner, N.A. 1975. An evaluation of the Association of Official Analytical Chemists Sporicidal Test Method. Dev. Indust. Microbiol., 16, 31–37.

Steadman's Medical Dictionary, Illustrated. 1988. 24th Edition. Baltimore, Williams & Wilkins.

Stuart, L.S. 1956. Labeling detergent-sanitizers. Soap Chem. Spec., 32(5), 49–51.

Stuart, L.S., Ortensio, L.F., and Friedl, J.L. 1955. The phenol coefficient number as an index to the practical use-dilution for disinfection. J. AOAC, 38, 465–478.

Stuart, L.S., Ortensio, L.F., and Friedl, J.L. 1957. Performance evaluation of quaternaries by the Chambers method. Proc. 44th Mid-Year Meeting Chem. Spec. Manuf. Assoc.

Sykes, G. 1965. Air disinfection and sterilization. In *Disinfection and Sterilization, Theory and Practice*. 2nd Edition. Edited by G. Sykes. London, E. and F.N. Spon, pp. 253–288.

Trimarchi, G. 1959. The bacterial control of food utensils in public service. Methods for the determination of the bacterial content. Igiene Moderna, 52, 95–111.

Tuley, L. 1988. Hygiene in the food plant. Food Manufact., 63(8), 27–28, 31, 33.

van Klingeren, B. 1978. Experiences with a quantitative carrier test for the evaluation of disinfectants. Zentralbl. Bakteriol. Mikrobiol. Hyg. [B], 167, 514–527.

Vesley, D., and Michaelson, G.S. 1964. Application of a surface sampling method technique to the evaluation of the bacteriological effectiveness of certain hospital housekeeping procedures. Health Lab. Sci., 1, 107.

Weber, G.R. 1949. Sanitization—another view. Soap Sanit. Chem., 25(6), 141.

Weber, G.R. 1948. Sterilization of dishes and utensils in eating establishments. J. Milk Food Technol., 11, 327.

Weber, G.R., and Black, L.A. 1948. Laboratory procedure for evaluating practical performance of quaternary ammonium and other germicides proposed for sanitizing food utensils. Am. J. Public Health, 38, 1405–1417.

CHAPTER 61

METHODS OF TESTING FUNGICIDES

C. George Hollis

The testing of fungicides may fall into three tiers. *Tier one* testing is an early series of tests designed to screen a large number of chemical compounds or products to determine their comparative efficacy as fungicides under strictly controlled laboratory conditions. *Tier two* testing is aimed at a particular type of application or end-use. In these tests the fungicide is applied to a substrate that needs protection, and the substrate is subjected to natural or simulated natural conditions of environment and inoculum. *Tier three* tests are actual in-use trials in which the treated material is placed into service on a small scale and exposed to end-use conditions to determine the level and length of time protection is afforded. As would be expected early screening in tier one and frequently in tier two testing there is a considerable amount of speculation as to the transference of data to actual field conditions. In addition, a major drawback of tier one testing is that it is often a test to exclude compounds from further testing, especially when performed and interpreted by personnel with little knowledge of end-use. The ideal situation for product development is to clearly define the end-use for a fungicide and then select or design a screening procedure to simulate that use. However, this is frequently labor intensive when a large number of potential fungicides are involved. Alsopp and Seal (1986) discussed these test categories as a preliminary screen, environmental simulation test, and field trial. They also suggested a fourth category of tests based on a national standard. However, standard tests are typically involved with tier two testing, and sometimes tier one.

Procedures used to test the efficacy of fungicides have to be involved with an inoculum, a contact substrate, the fungicide itself, the time of exposure, the environmental conditions for exposure, and frequently, a recovery medium. In general all of these factors come into play whether the procedure is one used for screening for general fungicidal activity of a chemical or whether the screen is designed to simulate actual end-use conditions.

In a chapter in the preceding edition of this book Czerkowicz (1983) reviewed the chemical and physical test methods for the prevention and reduction of the spread of pathogenic fungi via the environment. This chapter will retain much of the information provided by Czerkowicz but will also provide information on methods of testing fungicides for the preservation of wood, paper and paperboard, paint, leather, textiles, and plastics. As would be expected there is no one generalized test procedure to cover all possible applications of fungicides. The closest to it are such generalized tests as use-dilution evaluations, agar cup and seeded agar plate procedures, and some type of suspension test (Czerkowicz, 1983; Flynn and Taylor, 1986).

GENERAL FUNGICIDAL TESTING

Several general testing procedures are available that can be used as an initial screen (tier one) to test the effectiveness of candidate fungicides or fungistats. The tests may be carried out on solid media in dishes or bottles or they may be done in liquid. The former are typically called plate tests and the latter are suspension tests. In general, these tests are not aimed at a particular fungicidal application but are intended to compare fungicidal or fungistatic efficacy of different compounds and provide an early selection process for products to be further evaluated. These types of tests are used frequently to screen large numbers of chemicals at one time or to get some idea of the range of concentrations required for more elaborate testing of individual chemicals. Incidentally, these general tests are the ones most frequently used as instructional tools for college undergraduates in the applied microbiology laboratory. In other instances the agar plate test is used to determine the resistance of materials to attack by fungi. Hence these tests are applicable not only for disinfectant testing (Czerkowicz, 1983) but also for screening potentially useful antifungal agents against fungi of industrial importance.

Agar Plate Tests

One of the earliest types of screening procedures with fungi was used by Humphrey and Flemming (1915). They simply added the candidate control chemical to a melted nutrient agar medium in desired concentrations. The agar medium was poured into plates and allowed to solidify. The solid plates were surface inoculated with selected fungi. Treated plates were incubated at 28°C, and radial growth was measured on alternate days. If no growth occurred the inoculum on the plate was transferred to a slant of agar medium. If there was still no growth, the fungus was considered to be dead.

This method is still used for a quick screening procedure. However, because of the possibility of the inactivation of the chemical agent by the medium, results are generally unreliable. For example, most quaternary ammonium compounds, being cationic, are chemically bound by agar and are detoxified.

Seeded Agar Cup and Agar Plate Procedure

There are several variations of the seeded agar plate tests, all of which depend on the formation of a zone surrounding the test specimen. The agar cup procedure is used for the testing of liquids or emulsions that are free-flowing. Any fungus or mixture of fungi may be used for seeding the plates. The fungi should be grown on a suitable medium, usually slanted in tubes or bottles. The inoculum is prepared by the procedure or one similar to it that is described in the following section on disinfectant testing (AOAC, 1984). In this procedure the spores are washed or scraped from the surface of the agar in a 0.85% sodium chloride (physiologic saline) solution containing a drop or two of a wetting agent such as Triton X-100. The conidial suspension is shaken in a sterile flask with glass beads or dispersed by blending in a sterile stainless steel cup on an electric blender. After filtering and calibrating the number, the spores or conidia are added to 20 to 30 ml of cool (42 to 45°C) melted agar in a tube and mixed. The agar is poured into a standard 110-mm petri dish and allowed to solidify. In the agar cup procedure a small cup is formed in the agar. This can be accomplished by standing a sterile flat bottom cylinder, measuring 8 mm in diameter and 10 mm in height, in the center of the plate before the agar sets. After the medium is solidified the cylinder is removed, leaving a cup in the medium. An alternative procedure is to cut the cups out of the solidified medium with a sterile cork borer that is 15 mm in diameter. The cups so formed are filled (0.1 to 0.3 ml) with the various selections of the test chemical and incubated for 5 to 7 days at the desired temperature, usually room temperature or 30°C. The amount of fungistatic activity is indicated by the diameter of the clear zone around the cup.

Solid materials, creams, or semisolid products may be tested for their ability to withstand attack by the fungi in the plate. In such cases the material is placed on the surface of the seeded agar plates. Creams (and other semisolid materials) and powders are placed in the center of the dish and spread to cover an area of about 2 cm in diameter. Treated materials such as paper, plastics, textiles, leather, and painted surfaces are cut into standard sizes such as 1-inch squares and placed directly onto the surface of the seeded agar. A clear zone indicates that the substance has a soluble fungistatic agent in it capable of inhibiting the growth of the fungi in the test. In the case of treated materials, such as plastics, leather, paint and paper, it is preferable that the antifungal agent remain in the treated substrate. The formation of a zone of inhibition would indicate the loss of the protective chemical and the loss of some or all fungus resistance in the treated material itself. Therefore, a treated product that prevents the growth of the fungus on its edges or flat surfaces is ideally treated.

It is common to test antifungal agents by adding them to cellulose discs. The discs may be dried or partially dried and applied directly onto the surface of seeded agar. A clear zone, just as in the agar cup, indicates fungistatic activity. This procedure, although generally useful, requires that the chemical under test is not bound by the cellulose in the disc or bound by the medium as it attempts to diffuse, because as mentioned previously both monomeric and polymeric quats are discriminated against by these agar plate tests, which measure zone formation.

Suspension Tests

Suspension tests, as the name indicates, are procedures in which the test fungi are suspended in a medium or liquid that contains the fungicide/fungistat. The inoculum can be prepared by standard methods (AOAC, 1984). These can be simple. Tier one tests may use buffered water, 0.85% saline, mineral salts solution, or any other suspending liquid. The antifungal agents are dispersed in desired concentrations in the contact liquid, inoculated with a standard number of fungal propagules, and incubated. The temperature is a matter of choice, but usually incubation is at 28 to 30°C. If the contact liquid does not support growth the effectiveness of the chemical agent can be determined by placing an aliquot into a recovery medium and measuring survivors. This is a fungicidal test. By knowing the number of reproductive structures used in the inoculum and by counting the survivors, the percentage of kill can be determined. If the contact medium supports growth (e.g., mineral or basal salts) the fungistatic properties of the chemical agent can be approximated by visual evaluation. Numeric values can be assigned to the amount of growth if values between uninhibited and completely inhibited growth are important. Generally, the important value is the minimum inhibitory concentration of the chemical. This is the lowest concentration required to retard the growth of the fungus under the conditions of the test.

DISINFECTANT TESTING

Schamberg and Kolmer (1922) provided a method of testing disinfectants against dermatophytes, which are the primary target fungi for disinfectant testing even today. This procedure was designed to measure both the fungistatic and fungicidal activity of disinfectant. Three representative species of pathogens were used. To determine the fungistatic properties the disinfectant was added and mixed with Sabouraud's agar, which was subsequently tubed, slanted, and inoculated with the test fungi. The slants were inoculated and rated for growth or no growth. For the determination of fungicidal activity the fungi were grown on Sabouraud's slants. The disinfectants were dispersed at various concentrations, which were then inoculated with a physiologic saline dispersion of the slant culture. Transfers were made from this contact medium onto Sabouraud's agar slants at intervals of 15 minutes to 24 hours to determine viability of the fungi. This test is still used frequently as a tier one type test for screening a large number of compounds for application in industrial applications. However, the fungistatic portion of the test in which the fungicide is incorporated into the agar medium has drawbacks, chiefly the fact that many compounds are inactivated or neutralized by the agar or medium components. The principle of using a contact fluid in the fungicidal portion of the test is to be found in many tier one tests used in many applications. The test procedure of Emmons (1933), which has been adopted with minor modifications as the Fungicidal Test of the Association of Official Analytical Chemists (AOAC), uses an aqueous dilution of test compounds as the contact medium. The Association of Official Analytical Chemists (1984) procedure is reproduced here in its entirety, exactly as previously presented by Czerkowicz (1983) in the third edition of this book.

THE ASSOCIATION OF OFFICIAL ANALYTICAL CHEMISTS (AOAC) FUNGICIDAL TEST METHOD

(Applicable for Use with Water-Miscible–Type Fungicides Used to Disinfect Inanimate Objects)

Use as the test fungus a typical strain of *Trichophyton mentagrophytes* isolated from dermatophytosis of the foot. The strain must sporulate freely on artificial media, the presence of abundant conidia manifested by powdery appearance on the surface of 10-day cultures, particularly at the top of agar slants, and confirmed by microscopic examination. Conidia-bearing mycelium should peel easily from the surface of glucose agar. Conidia of required resistance survive 10-minute exposure at 20°C to phenol dilution of 1:70, but not to one of 1:60. (Strain No. 9533 (ATCC, replacing strain NIH 640, is suitable.)

Culture Medium

Carry the fungus on agar slants of the following composition: glucose 2%, Neopeptone (Difco) 1%, agar 2%, adjusted to pH 6.1 to 6.3. Use the same culture medium to prepare cultures for obtaining conidial suspensions, and use fluid medium of same nutrient composition

(without agar) to test the viability of the conidia after exposure to fungicide.

Care of Fungus Strain

Store stock culture of the fungus on glucose agar slants at 2 to 5°C. At intervals of not more than 3 months, transfer it to fresh agar slants, incubate 10 days at 25 to 30°C, and store at 2 to 5°C until the next transfer period. Do not use a culture that has been kept at or above room temperature for more than 10 days as a source of inoculum for the culture. (Cultures may be kept at room temperature to preserve the strain and to inoculate cultures if they are transferred at intervals of not more than 10 days.)

Preparation of the Conidial Suspension

Prepare petri-dish culture by planting the inoculum at the center of the agar plate and incubating the culture at 25 to 30°C for 10, but not more than 15, days. Remove the mycelial mats from the surface of five agar plate cultures, using a sterile spatula or a heavy flattened wire. Transfer to a heat-sterilized glass tissue grinder (Arthur H. Thomas Co., size B or equivalent) and macerate with 25 ml sterile physiologic NaCl solution (0.85% NaCl), or to a heat-sterilized Erlenmeyer flask containing 25 ml of sterile solution with glass beads, and shake thoroughly. Filter the suspension through sterile absorbent cotton to remove hyphal elements. Estimate the density of the conidial suspension by counting in a hemacytometer and store at 2 to 10°C as a stock spore suspension (125 to 155 million conidia/ml) for periods up to 4 weeks for use in preparing test suspension of conidia. Standardize the test conidial suspension with physiologic NaCl solution so that it contains 5 million conidia/ml.

Operating Technique

Prepare dilutions of the fungicide. Make 1% stock dilution of the substance to be tested (or make any other convenient dilution, depending on the anticipated concentration), in a glass-stoppered cylinder. Make the final dilutions from the 1% stock dilution directly into medication tubes and remove all excess over 5 ml (the range of dilutions should cover the killing limits of the disinfectant in 5 to 15 minutes and at the same time should be close enough for accuracy). From 5% stock phenol solution (1:20), dilute further to make 1:60 and 1:70 dilutions.

Place 5 ml of each fungicide solution and of the phenol control solution in 25 × 150 mm test-culture tubes, arrange the tubes in the order of ascending dilutions, place the tubes in a 20°C water bath, and let come to temperature. With a graduated pipette, place 0.5 ml of spore suspension in the first tube of fungicidal solution, shake, and immediately replace in the water bath; 30 seconds later add 0.5 ml of conidial suspension to the second tube. Repeat the procedure at 30-second intervals for each fungicidal dilution. If more convenient, run at 20-second intervals. After a 5-, 10-, and 15-minute exposure to the fungicide, remove the sample from each conidia-fungicide mixture with a 4-mm loop and place in 10 ml of glucose broth. To eliminate the risk of faulty results due to possible fungistatic action, make subtransfers from the initial glucose broth subculture tubes to fresh tubes of glucose broth, using the 4-mm loop before incubation, or make initial subcultures in glucose broth containing either 0.05% sodium thioglycolate, 1.5% iso-octylphenoxy-polyethoxyethanol, or a mixture of 0.07% lecithin (Azolectin) and 0.5% polysorbate 80 (Tween 80), whichever gives the lowest result. Incubate the inoculated tubes at 25 to 30°C. Read the final results after 10 days, although an indicative reading can be made in 4 days.

Note: The highest dilution that kills the spores within 10 minutes is commonly considered the highest dilution that could be expected to disinfect inanimate surfaces contaminated with pathogenic fungi.

Fungicidal formulations that are expected to disinfect in the presence of organic soils can be evaluated using the AOAC Fungicidal Test described previously. The procedure is modified by adding blood serum (5% v/v) in the fungicidal test solution before adding the conidial suspension (Schneider and Hitch, 1982).

* * * * *

OTHER TEST METHODS

The Use-Dilution and Germicidal Spray Products procedures of the AOAC (1984) are used to screen the activity of fungicides. The Germicidal Spray Products procedure recommends the use of *Trichophyton mentagrophytes* ATCC No. 9533 as the species for the test. This is the same organism used in the Fungicidal Test described previously. For nonstandardized screening, other organisms may be used in either of the Use-Dilution or Germicidal Spray procedures. It should be noted that among the most important facets of fungicidal testing is the preparation of the inoculum. It is for this reason the AOAC procedures stress the importance of the reduction of conidial masses to the unicellular level and the elimination, as much as possible, of hyphal elements of uncertain mass.

The Association Française de Normalisation (1981) has produced two procedures for the testing of fungicides that are useful in disinfectant testing. These tests (AFNOR NFT 72-200 and NFT 72-201) use four species, *Aspergillus versicolor* CNCM 1187-79, *Cladosporium cladosporoides* CNCM 1185-79, *Penicillium verrucosum* var. *cyclopium* CNCM 1186-79, and *Candida albicans* CNCM 1180-79 (ATCC 2091). These two procedures use the same kind of inoculum and contact times but differ in the amount of inoculum and in the method of recovery of the treated cells and neutralization of the disinfectant. In AFNOR NFT 72-200 the treated suspension of cells in passed through a neutralizing solution to detoxify the disinfectant followed by agar inclusion plating and counting of the resulting colonies. AFNOR NFT 72-201 recommends membrane filtration of the treated fungal elements, washing and placing the membranes on a plated agar medium which may or may not contain a neutralizer based on preliminary testing.

The Dutch Committee on Phytopharmacy (1974) includes yeast and fungi in their 5-5-5 Suspension Test Method for bactericidal, fungicidal, and sporicidal properties. This procedure is reviewed by Van Klingeren et al. (1977). In this test different species of microorganisms are used depending on whether the disinfectant is to be used in the food industry, in veterinary applications, or in hospitals. Among the fungi *Saccharomyces cerevisiae* is the representative strain for the food industry, *Aspergillus fumigatus* and *Candida albicans* for veterinary applications, and *Candida albicans* for hospital disinfectants. The lowest concentration that will reduce this population by a 5-log value in 5 minutes is interpreted as the effective level of the disinfectant.

INDUSTRIAL FUNGICIDES

The test procedures for evaluating the efficacy of fungal control agents against the variety of problems encountered in the industrial arena are varied. Fungi cause disfigurement, deterioration, spoilage, or a combination thereof in a tremendous variety of industrial products, including such common materials as paint, wood, paper, leather, metalworking fluids, fuels, textiles, adhesives, and aqueous dispersions and emulsions of all manner of liquid materials. For the most part the testing protocol for the protection of industrial products involves simulated end-use (tier two) tests or end-use (tier three) tests. In addition most test procedures provide for worst-case scenarios in that the tests are conducted under conditions to simulate the most severe situations likely to be encountered. As a result a large number of standardized tests have been suggested and many are in use across the world. Table 61–1 lists some of the testing procedures by the area of industrial application.

SURFACE PROTECTION

Disfigurement of surfaces caused by mold growth is a serious problem for many natural and synthetic products such as above-ground exposed wood, leather, paint films, textiles, and plastics. Disfigurement may be accompanied by deterioration, staining, or functional impairment. However, the mere presence of surface growth on many articles detracts from their esthetic value. Fungicides or fungistats are used for the prevention of this growth.

Tests designed to measure the amount of protection provided to surfaces usually are rather stringent and reflect the most severe conditions of exposure of the substrate. Two general types of tests that are commonly used to determine the resistance of materials to surface growth are the chamber exposure tests and the jar tests. The Environmental Chamber procedure is described in standards produced by the U.S. Department of Defense (1983) and by BSI (1985). In these two procedures the specimens are inoculated by spraying or dipping and

Table 61-1. *Standards Suggested for Testing Fungicides for Industrial Applications*

Pulp and Paper

ASTM. 1977. Efficacy of Slimicides for the Paper Industry. Philadelphia, American Society for Testing and Materials, E-599.

TAPPI. 1985. Fungal Resistance of Paper and Paperboard. Atlanta, Technical Association of the Pulp and Paper Industry, T 487-85.

BSI. 1967. Specification for Paper Jointing. Section 5.7. Resistance to Mold Growth. London, British Standard 4249.

Paint

ASTM. 1982. Standard Method of Evaluating Degree of Surface Disfigurement of Paint Films by Microbial (Fungal or Algal) Growth or Soil and Dirt Accumulation. Philadelphia, American Society for Testing and Materials DX-3274-82.

ASTM. 1986. Standard Test Method for Resistance to Growth of Mold on the Surface of Interior Coatings in an Environmental Chamber. Philadelphia, American Society for Testing and Materials, D3273-86.

Plastics

ASTM. 1985. Standard Practice for Determining Resistance of Synthetic Polymeric Material to Fungi, G21-70. Philadelphia, American Society for Testing and Materials, G21-70 (1985).

BSI. 1985. The Environmental Testing of Electronic Components and Electronic Equipment. London, British Standard 2011.

Textiles

SNV (Association Suisse Normalization). 1976. Examination of the Antimycotic Effect of Impregnated Textiles by the Agar Diffusion Test. St. Gallen, Switzerland, SNV 195.

BSI. 1981. Methods of Tests for the Determination of Textiles to Microbiological Deterioration. London, British Standard 6085.

AATCC. 1981. Fungicides, Evaluation of Textiles; Mildew and Rot Resistance of Textiles. Test Method 30. American Association of Textiles Chemists and Colorists Tech. Manual, 57, 304–306.

Wood

ASTM. 1986. Wood Preservatives by Laboratory Soilblock Cultures. Philadelphia, American Society for Testing and Materials, O1413-76.

NWMA. 1981. NWMA Soil Block Test. Park Ridge, IL, National Woodwork Manufacturers Association, NWMA-M-1-81.

ASTM. 1986. Standard Method of Evaluating Wood Preservatives by Field Tests with Stakes. Philadelphia, American Society for Testing and Materials D1758-86.

BSI. 1982. Wood Preservatives. Determination of the Toxic Values Against Wood Destroying Basidiomycetes Cultured on an Agar Medium. London, British Standard 6009 (EN 113).

BSI. 1968. Method of Test for Fungal Resistance of Manufactured Building Materials. London, British Standard 1982.

incubated in a chamber with elevated temperatures and humidity. Samples are exposed for 4 to 12 weeks. Resistance is determined by visual examination for the amount of mold growth. Where appropriate, tensile strength and other physical tests may be performed. The Tropical Chamber procedure is similar to that described for the Environmental Chamber Method with the exception that the inoculum is generally present in soil trays within the chamber and is circulated by induced air flow via a fan. For specifications for the two chambers and procedures, see ASTM (1986) and AFNOR (1962). These chambers operate at elevated temperatures and relative humidity and are used to measure the fungus resistance of wood, painted surfaces, leather, textiles, and plastics. Assessment of resistance is typically a visual companion to a standard. Ratings are on a scale of 1 through 10. The higher the numeric value, the less the growth.

The jar tests are so-called because a jar partially filled with water serves as the exposure chamber. Specimens of textiles, leather, wood, or other appropriate surfaces are sprayed with an inoculum of fungus. The samples are suspended in the jars above the water level and placed in an incubator. The degree of mold resistance is determined at appropriate intervals by visual inspection. This type of test was suggested by the U.S. Environmental Protection Agency as an acceptable method for demonstrating the efficacy of fungicidal treatments (Schneider and Hitch, 1982). The EPA no longer requires efficacy data for registration purposes. However, the methods are still in use as a means of determining resistance. One of these methods for measuring the resistance of leather is reproduced from the EPA Guidelines (Schneider and Hitch, 1982) to illustrate this form of testing.

Leather Mildew Fungistatic Test Method

1. Scope.
   1.1 Products intended for use to control, prevent or inhibit the growth of fungi which cause mildew on various articles or surfaces should be tested to demonstrate fungistatic effectiveness. This method is designed to determine effectiveness of products intended to control mildew and non-pathogenic fungal growth on indoor articles or surfaces of leather, such as book covers, luggage, shoes, and sporting goods. It also indicates duration of protection afforded, thereby providing a basis for recommending when to repeat applications.

2. Summary of Method.
   2.1 This method simulates use conditions by utilizing sections of vegetable tanned cowhide which, after treatment with the product, are artificially inoculated with a spore suspension of mildew-causing organisms and incubated at high humidity. Mildew growth on treated and untreated leather surfaces is rated during the 4-week test.

3. Apparatus.
   3.1 Glassware: Flasks with cotton plugs suitable for preparation of agar, diluent, and conidial suspensions. French square jars (500 ml) or equivalent screw cap containers. Screw caps adapted to allow suspension of leather sections 30 to 40 mm below the jar caps. Caps modified by center drilling cap and inserting appropriate size stainless steel or brass bolt to which a hook (formed from a 6- to 7-cm length of No. 22 nickel-chromium wire or other noncorrosive wire) is attached.
   3.2 Tissue grinder (homogenizer): No. 4288B, Arthur H. Thomas, Co.
   3.3 Atomizer: DeVilbiss No. 152 (or equivalent) operated at 69 kPa (10 psi).
   3.4 Counting chamber: Suitable for determining spore concentration.

4. Test Specimens.
   4.1 Leather: Squares (25 mm) of vegetable tanned cowhide (1.0 to 1.5 mm thick)[1] with a hole punched in the corner

of each square to permit it to be suspended from hook on modified French jar lid.

5. Test Fungi.

    5.1. *Aspergillus niger* (ATCC 6275)[2] and *Penicillium variabile* (NRRL-3765 or ATCC 32333).[3] Maintain stock cultures of each organism on neopeptone agar (10 g neopeptone, 20 g dextrose, 20 g agar, and 1 L distilled water) or Emmons agar. Incubate new stock cultures 7 to 10 days at 25°C, then store at 2 to 10°C.

6. Selection of Treatments:

    6.1 Test Fungistat: Dosages of the test fungistat evaluated should range from ineffective to effective levels so that the minimum effective dosage of test material can be determined. *Note:* Where both wipe-on and pump spray (i.e., nonpressurized containers) application methods are intended for the proposed formulation, only the wipe-on application method needs to be tested.

    6.2 Untreated Control: Ten untreated leather squares are required to establish the test validity and to ascertain the degree of control obtained with the test fungistat.

    6.3 Standard Fungistat: A fungistat registered for use on leather may be included in the test as a comparative treatment. The product selected must be used in accordance with label directions and should involve a method of application comparable to that of the test fungistat.

7. Procedures.

Note: Aseptic procedures must be followed throughout the course of the test.

    7.1 Preparation of conidial suspensions: Conidial suspensions of each fungal organism are prepared by washing spores from the surface of 7- to 10-day neopeptone agar cultures with sterile 0.85% saline solution containing a surfactant such as 0.05% isoctylphenoxypolethoxyethanol.[4] Spore chains should be broken up by transferring the suspension to the heat-sterilized tissue grinder and reciprocating the piston several times. Hyphal fragments should be removed by filtering the suspension through a thin layer of sterile cotton or other suitable material. Conidial suspension may be stored at 2 to 10°C for up to 4 weeks. Standardize test conidial suspensions to contain five million conidia per ml (determine spore concentration with a counting chamber[5]) by adding sterile saline solution.

    7.2 Treatment of Leather Squares: Treat both sides of ten leather test squares for each formulation, dosage, and method of application being evaluated. Wipe-on or spray application must simulate intended method of use. For spray applications, the type of sprayer and distance from nozzle to leather surface, as well as the degree of surface wetness, must be controlled and specified. Dip application of product to leather test squares is not an acceptable substitute for wipe-on or spray methods of application. If a standard fungistat is used, the leather squares should be treated in accordance with label directions for use. Immediately after treatment leather squares should be placed in a vertical or near-vertical position to permit excess liquid to drain. All treated leather should be allowed to dry before the mildew spore suspension is applied.

    7.3 Inoculation: Place equal volumes of well agitated *A. niger* and *P. variabile* conidial suspensions in a No. 152 DeVilbiss atomizer (or equivalent), maintain agitation,

and lightly spray both sides of each leather square with the mixture.

    7.4 Incubation: Suspend leather squares in individual modified 500-ml French square jars containing approximately 90 ml distilled water and incubate at approximately 28°C. Tighten the caps, then back off 1/8 turn to allow for some ventilation.

8. Determination of Results.

    8.1 Evaluation: Observations are recorded weekly for 4 weeks or until treatments fail and abundant growth occurs on all treated squares. The presence or absence of observable mold on leather squares is the criterion for determining the effectiveness of the test product. Where no visual growth is evident at the end of the test period, examination at approximately ×15 magnification is required to confirm the absence or establish the presence of subvisual fungal growth. The untreated control squares must have a minimum of 50% of their surface area covered with fungal growth after 7 days for the test to be valid.

    8.2 Interpretation: A product dosage is considered acceptable when all 10 treated replicates are free of fungal growth. The results of this test must be correlated to the intended label claims. The directions for use must specify retreatment every 7, 14, and 21 days, depending on the length of time all treated test squares remained free of mildew growth. Label directions for products which remain effective for the duration of the 4 weeks' test must specify a retreatment schedule, such as "repeat as necessary when new growth appears" and should indicate that treatments be effective for at least 28 days.

9. Data Reporting.

    9.1 Test reports must include all pertinent details of the test conditions and variables. Such information shall include at least the following types of information:

        9.1.1 Complete description of formulation(s) tested (type of formulation, name, and percentage of active ingredient(s), and EPA Registration Number of any standard fungistat used).

        9.1.2 Dosage rates (specify whether rate is in terms of product or active ingredient, and whether on a weight and/or volume basis).

        9.1.3 Complete description of all appropriate application procedures and materials including details such as the type of sprayer (pump versus pressurized spray), spray application distance and duration, applicator material used for wipe-on applications (damp cloth), degree of wetness to be obtained on surfaces (dampen, thoroughly wet, etc.), and time interval between application and rinsing.

        9.1.4 Test validity—the number of replicates with 50% or more of the surface area covered with fungal growth after 7 days.

        9.1.5 Effectiveness—The number of replicates with fungal growth at each observation date for each treatment being evaluated (including untreated controls). To demonstrate the differences among treatments it may be necessary to use additional criteria, such as the percentage of surface area covered with fungal growth or the density of fungal growth.

        9.1.6 Adverse effects data—describe the nature and

extent of any adverse effects noted on leather as a result of treatment.

9.1.7 Modification—describe the nature of any changes made in the test method and provide the rationale for each change.

Footnotes

[1]Vegetable tanned leather is available from Eberle Tanning Company, 360 Church Street, Westfield, Pennsylvania 16950.

[2]Cultures at *A. niger* (ATCC 6275) may be obtained from American Type Culture Collection, 12301 Parklawn Dr., Rockville, MD 20852.

[3]Cultures of *P. variabile* (NRRL 3765)(ATCC 32333) are available from ARS Culture Collection Investigations Fermentation Laboratory, USDA, 1815 North University Street, Peoria, IL 61604, or American Type Culture Collection, 12301 Parklawn Drive, Rockville, MD 20852.

[4]Triton-X-100, Rohm & Haas Company, Philadelphia, PA 19104, or other suitable wetting agent such as dioctyl sodium sulfosuccinate, as Aerosol OT solid A-349, Fisher Scientific Co.

[5]For detailed instructions see Tuite, John, *Plant Pathological Methods, Fungi and Bacteria,* 1969. Minneapolis, Burgess Publishing Company, pp. 183–184.

In addition to the Leather Mildew Fungistatic Test Method described in the foregoing, Schneider and Hitch (1982) described procedures for other tests. These include a Fabric Mildew Fungistatic Test Method, Hard Surface Mildew Fungistatic Test Method, Wood Block Mildew Fungistatic Test Method, Glass Slide Mildew Fungicidal Test Method, and Use-Dilution Mildew Fungicidal Test Method. In general, these procedures follow the same principles for the preparation and application of the inoculum and are applicable to many other forms of in-house tests where uniformity of inoculum is of paramount importance.

REFERENCES

AATCC. 1981. Fungicides, Evaluation of Textiles; Mildew and Rot Resistance of Textiles. Test Method 30. American Association of Textiles Chemists and Colorists Tech. Manual, *57*, 304–306.

AFNOR (Association Française de Normalisation). 1962. Methods of testing the resistance of plastic materials to attack. NFX 41-515. Paris, AFNOR.

AFNOR (Association Française de Normalisation). 1981. Recueil de Normes française des antiseptiques et desinfectants. In *Antiseptiques et Desinfectants.* 1st Edition (Bilingual). Paris, AFNOR.

Alsopp, O., and Seal, K.J. 1986. *Introduction to Biodeterioration.* London, Edward Arnold.

Association of Official Analytical Chemists. 1984. *Official Methods of Analysis of the Association of Official Analytical Chemists.* 14th Edition. Washington, D.C., AOAC.

ASTM. 1977. Efficacy of Slimicides for the Paper Industry. Philadelphia, American Society for Testing and Materials, E-599.

ASTM. 1982. Standard Method of Evaluating Degree of Surface Disfigurement of Paint Films by Microbial (Fungal or Algal) Growth or Soil and Dirt Accumulation. Philadelphia, American Society for Testing and Materials DX-3274-82.

ASTM. 1985. Standard Practice for Determining Resistance of Synthetic Polymeric Material to Fungi, G21-70. Philadelphia, American Society for Testing and Materials, G21-70.

ASTM. 1986. Standard Test Method for Resistance to Growth of Mold on the Surface of Interior Coatings in an Environmental Chamber. Philadelphia, American Society for Testing and Materials, D3273-86.

ASTM. 1986. Standard Method of Evaluating Wood Preservatives by Field Tests with Stakes. Philadelphia, American Society for Testing and Materials D1758-86.

ASTM. 1986. Wood Preservatives by Laboratory Soilblock Cultures. Philadelphia, American Society for Testing and Materials, O1413-76.

BSI. 1967. Specification for Paper Jointing. Section 5.7. Resistance to Mold Growth. London, British Standard 4249.

BSI. 1968. Method of Test for Fungal Resistance of Manufactured Building Materials. London, British Standard 1982.

BSI. 1981. Methods of Tests for the Determination of Textiles to Microbiological Deterioration. London, British Standard 6085.

BSI. 1982. Wood Preservatives. Determination of the Toxic Values Against Wood Destroying Basidimycetes Cultured on an Agar Medium. London, British Standard 6009 (EN 113).

BSI. 1985. The Environmental Testing of Electronic Components and Electronic Equipment. London, British Standard 2011.

BSI. 1985. Basic Environmental Testing Procedures. BS 2011, part 2.1. Test J. Mould Growth. London.

Czerkowicz, T.J. 1983. Methods of testing fungicides. In *Disinfection, Sterilization, and Preservation,* 3rd Ed. Edited by S.S. Block. Philadelphia, Lea & Febiger.

Dutch Committee for Phytopharmacy (Comissie voor Fytofarmacie.) 1974. Waardebepaling van disinfectie—middelen voor materiaal—ontsmitting in ziekenhmizen. Wageningen.

Emmons, C.W. 1933. Fungicidal action of some common disinfectants on two dermatophytes. Arch. Dermatol., *28*, 15–21.

Flynn, F.B., and Taylor, W.S. 1986. Biocides. In *Encylopedia of Polymer Science and Engineering.* Volume 2. New York, Wiley & Sons.

Humphrey, C.J., and Flemming, R.M. 1915. The toxicity to fungi of various oils and salts, particularly those used in wood preservation. Bull. 227. Washington, D.C., United States Dept. of Agriculture.

NWMA. 1981. NWMA Soil Block Test. Park Ridge, IL. National Woodwork Manufacturers Association, NWMA-M-1-81.

Schamberg, J.F., and Kolmer, J.A. 1922. Studies in the chemotherapy of fungus infections. Arch. Dermatol., *6*, 746–756.

Schneider, B.A., and Hitch, R.K. 1982. Pesticide assessment guidelines, Subdivision G, Office of Pesticides and Toxic Substances. Washington, D.C., EPA.

SNV (Association Suisse Normalization). 1976. Examination of the Antimycotic Effect of Impregnated Textiles by the Agar Diffusion Test. St. Gallen, Switzerland, SNV 195.

TAPPI. 1985. Fungal Resistance of Paper and Paperboard. Atlanta, Technical Association of the Pulp and Paper Industry, T 487-85.

U.S. Department of Defense. 1983. Military Standard 810 D. Method 508.3. Fungus. Washington, D.C., U.S. Department of Defense.

Van Klingeren, G., Leussink, A.B., and Wyngaarden, L.G. 1977. A collaborative study on the repeatability and the reproducibility of the Dutch Standard Suspension Test for the evaluation of disinfectants. Zentralbl. Bacteriol. Mikrobiol. Hyg. [B], *164*, 521–548.

CHAPTER 62

METHODS OF TESTING VIRUCIDES

John H.S. Chen

In recent years, with technical advances in cultivation of viruses in laboratory host systems and with the increased knowledge of the effects of disinfectants on viruses under various conditions, it has become possible to work out a number of procedures for assessing the virucidal efficacy of chemical disinfectants.

The virus inactivation of concern here is that which takes place outside the living host on inanimate objects. Although the viruses are obligate intracellular parasites, they are found in many environments—in dust and water and on inanimate objects—where they can survive but will not multiply. In environments of high viral contamination (hospital rooms, animal quarters, virus laboratories, and dairy plants that manufacture cultured products troubled by bacteriophages), some index as to the effectiveness of virucides is needed if they are to be used with confidence. Few viral therapeutic agents (except the host defense mechanism, which is beyond the scope of this chapter) have much effect on true viruses. The psittacosis-lymphogranuloma-trachoma group and the rickettsiae, however, which form two distinct biologic groups between bacteria and true viruses, are susceptible to therapeutic agents.

Because viruses vary in their resistance, chemical analysis of the virucidal agent alone is not sufficient to evaluate its effectiveness. Procedures employed by Klein and DeForest (1963) appear to give results that can be interpreted, in most instances, in terms of germicidal effectiveness in eliminating specific viruses in environmental disinfection programs. Their observations on the behavior of lipophilic and hydrophilic viruses in the presence of chemical disinfectants clearly point to the possibility of developing some standardized testing procedures with selected test viruses that will provide better estimates of the validity of virucidal claims.

FACTORS INVOLVED IN STANDARDIZING VIRUCIDAL TEST METHODS

Test methods must be selected or developed to provide useful results with sufficient precision for use in referee work. The selected methods must not be too complex or difficult, yet they must be adequately controlled so that by careful application they will be precise enough to be uniformly reproduced to yield consistent data for interpretation. Although the final criterion of effectiveness of virucides is the demonstration of effectiveness under conditions of practical application, the responsibility for primary evaluation and classification belongs to the laboratory. Only in the laboratory is it possible to establish control over the many factors encountered in actual performance that might help to eliminate fundamental uncertainties in the conclusions drawn. If controlled laboratory tests fail to yield a result that is a reliable index to practical value, then the tests are misleading. Therefore, interpretation of laboratory results in terms of practical virucidal values is a prime requirement for accuracy.

A number of factors must be controlled in the standardization of a virucide test method: apparatus, equipment, tissue culture media, indicator host systems, drying time and temperature for carriers, organic load in testing, time of contact between virus and virucide, exacting temperature controls, chemical standard as control to determine the resistance of each test virus at the time of testing, and description of mechanical manipulations in details.

Determining Levels of Inactivation

As related by Sykes (1965), in most cases the rate of inactivation of viruses appears to follow the death course of bacteria and, as with bacteria, there is often a fall in rate of inactivation near the end of the disinfection process. This general exponential form of the inactivation curve indicates that the number of surviving viruses at any given time is directly proportional to the initial concentration. The deviation from the regularity of inactivation occurs at the end of the disinfection process. This may be because the residual live viruses may consist of particles of varying resistance with varying degrees of aggregation.

It must be remembered that complete inactivation of a virus suspension cannot be determined, because the elimination of the last infective (active) virus particle cannot be detected. Different numbers of virus particles are needed to cause infection in vivo in different hosts, and previous exposure often influences the susceptibility of the host. The rate of decrease in activity, however, and the conditions under which a reasonable number of samples no longer causes infection can be determined with accuracy. Thus, the term *complete inactivation* is used to indicate a point below the level of infectivity. Negative findings (Vasington, 1965) or the failure to recover virus (for example, when a virus titered by dilution titering at 1×10^{-9} is employed and a dilution of 1×10^{-6} is necessary for subculture to avoid toxic effects of the medicant) would not indicate 100% kill even though it is the best measure for complete inactivation.

To accurately detect the extent of inactivation brought about by the virucidal agent, the focal lesion assay of plaque titration should be considered (Wolff, 1977). The plaque titration is able to reveal the action of a single virus but the Reed and Muench (1938) dilution end-point method was designed for use in toxicologic titrations where concentration effects are observed, not for viruses where a single particle can infect. The plaque titration can be shown to have greater accuracy or lowered standard deviation because this is equal to ± the square root of the number of plaques on a plate. The accuracy of 100 plaques is approximately 20%. To consider this to match that precision, it would be prohibitively expensive to use 100 tissue culture tubes for a $TCID_{50}$ (tissue culture infecting dose for 50% inoculated tubes) determination at each dilution level.

Toxicity of Germicides for Tissue Cultures

A major problem in determining inactivation is the problem of toxicity. This is usually resolved by dilution, removal, or neutralization of the germicide. With some classes of germicides, however, special procedures are required.

In instances of testing products containing formaldehyde, to which cell cultures are sensitive, Vasington (1965) suggests that dialysis would be effective in reducing the concentration of the formaldehyde in the mixture to a level that would not interfere with subsequent growth of cell cultures. If the virus was exposed for 1 or 10 minutes and the mixture dialyzed overnight, the formaldehyde could be removed and the virus tested for survival. The question of the significance of the exposure time should be considered, as there would be some exposure for the entire period that the mixture was being dialyzed, although the formaldehyde concentration would be reduced rather rapidly. Blackwell and Chen (1970) described a method employing Sephadex (Pharmacia Fine Chemicals, Inc., Piscataway, N.J.) that would remove the cytotoxic activity of some virus disinfectant mixtures. Their studies, using herpesvirus on Human Epidermoid Number 2 cell culture (H.Ep. 2), showed that Sephadex was an acceptable detoxicant for numerous low-molecular-weight compounds. The dry Sephadex beads, prepared as a slurry, swell and layer onto one another, forming a molecular sieve of such porosity that low-molecular-weight particles (e.g., water, disinfectant molecules, salts) are mechanically absorbed into the slurry, while high-molecular-weight particles (e.g., protein molecules, viruses) are excluded. The procedure is as follows.

Test Procedure

Add twice the germicidal chemical concentration to an equal volume of 2×10^6 plaque-forming units (pfu)/ml herpes simplex virus (HSV) in a 25×150-mm medication tube held at 20°C. After a 10-minute exposure, add the entire reaction mixture, using a pipette, to a Sephadex bed in filtration apparatus. Clarify the centrifugation apparatus for 3 to 5 minutes at $800 \times g$, then spin the sample 10 minutes at $1000 \times g$. Collect filtrate and make serial tenfold dilutions (five total) of filtrates using Dulbecco's phosphate-buffered solution (PBS, 2). Place 1 ml of each dilution on separate cell sheets of H.Ep. 2 culture prewashed with warmed PBS and held in plastic flask, and let adsorb 2 hours at 37°C. After 2 hours, remove the inoculum by pipette and add plaque medium No. 199 (e) (2) to cell sheets.

Incubate the flask cultures 48 hours at 37°C; then fix the cell sheet with absolute methanol and stain with Giemsa stain (1:20 dilution in Sorenson's buffer at pH 6.5). Air-dry the stained flask cultures and examine under 0.7 to $3 \times$ magnification of intactness of cell sheet, degree of lysis, general overall appearance for potential to support virus replication, and/or number of plaques of HSV present.

Unfortunately, cell cultures, which are the choice system for virus assay studies, are most affected by toxicity, because most germicidal chemicals are inherently toxic for them. Embryonated eggs, by contrast, support the growth of a smaller spectrum of viruses but are less affected by residual germicides.

Pancic et al. (1977) suggested that the excessive cytotoxicity for tissue culture also can be removed simply by tenfold dilution of the virus-virucide mixture in tissue culture medium and centrifugation of the mixture for an additional 2 hours at $159,000 \times g$. The supernatant is removed, and the virus pellets are resuspended for virus titration.

Selection of Standard Reference Viruses

According to a report of a general survey of virucide testing laboratories (independent 9; industry 7; university 3; and government 2) during the period of 1975–1976 summarized by Chen (1976), 39 types of viruses representing eight major virus groups (arbovirus; adenovirus; herpesvirus; myxovirus; papavovirus; picornavirus; poxvirus; reovirus) were practically employed as target viruses for virucide testing. It is, therefore, not surprising that no single laboratory could have available the necessary specific reagents, skills, and experience for the testing of such a great variety of viruses. Selection of a standard reference virus appears to be a reasonable approach.

In the selection of standard reference viruses for virucide testing, the work of Klein and DeForest (1963) is pertinent. They pointed out that there are at least 12 different classes of germicides with varying degrees of activity against the many viruses affecting man and animals. The testing of all classes of germicides against all viruses is a prohibitive task, and to generalize from a limited number of studies is precarious, since viruses are not homogeneous in their susceptibility to germicides.

Klein and DeForest (1963) found that antiviral powers of most germicides are determined by the chemical composition of the outer coats of the test viruses. They noted the work of Noll and Youngner (1959) on the interaction of viruses with lipids in which they observed that some viruses combine with lipids. These were called "lipophilic viruses," in contrast to "hydrophilic viruses" that do not combine with lipids. Klein and DeForest (1963) noted that the unusual resistance of enteroviruses to certain germicides is associated with the hydrophilic nature of the virus particle and the lipophilic nature of the germicide. Because bacteria are lipophilic and have been used in the past for evaluation of germicides, the limited activity of certain germicides against hydrophilic viruses escaped detection.

Klein (1965*b*) suggested "that the susceptibility of viruses to lipophilic germicides is related to a labile outer membrane and the presence of lipid that reacts with lipophilic germicides, thus allowing penetration into the virus particles. The susceptibility of the nonlipid-containing viruses may be related to the loose packing of the capsomeres and to an affinity for lipid and lipophilic compounds. Adenoviruses react more readily with cholesterol and hexadecylamine than do polioviruses. Assuming a lesser penetrability, the hypothesis is consistent with the additional and peculiar resistance of enteroviruses to isopropanol and their susceptibility to smaller non-lipophilic germicides, including methanol."

Klein and DeForest (1963) furthermore placed the viruses into three different categories based on the observation that the reaction of viral disease agents to chemical germicides can be predicted according to their solubility in lipids such as cholesterol. Representative test viruses could be selected from each of these categories. The first category contains the hydrophilic viruses composed of an inner core of nucleic acid and an outer protein shell. The picornaviruses belong to this group, as do the enteroviruses such as polio, Coxsackie, and ECHO viruses, which have been found to have a resistance to germicides somewhat greater than that of vegetative bacteria.

The second category is made up of the lipophilic viruses that have an outer envelope containing lipid or lipoprotein, and whether or not they are ether resistant, they are inactivated by germicides at levels similar to those inactivating vegetative bacteria. Examples of viruses in the lipophilic category would be herpes, vac-

cinia, and influenza viruses. The third category, called the "intermediate group," includes those viruses such as the adenoviruses that are medium in size, have no envelope and no lipid, and are considered to have a resistance similar to enteroviruses, but are found to have a pattern of resistance more similar to those containing a lipid envelope. The explanation of this is that these viruses are absorbed with lipids without having the structure or properties of the usual lipophilic viruses.

In evaluating germicides against representative viruses from each of the categories just described, Klein (1965*c*) found three of the oldest germicides, namely, phenol (5%), sodium hypochlorite (200 ppm), and ethyl alcohol (70 to 95%), to be effective in inactivating viruses from all three categories. His tests were made by combining suspensions of specific viruses and germicides in test tubes, allowing the combination to stand for 10 minutes and then injecting into mice, chick embryos, and various human cell cultures.

Vasington (1965), in commenting on the lipophilic and hydrophilic classification of Klein, indicated that he agrees with the hydrophilic part of the classification. He felt, however, that the lipophilic group of viruses was so variable that it would be necessary to reclassify this group into at least three or four subgroups for germicide testing.

A possible test virus to represent the hydrophilic group of viruses could be ECHO II, which can be grown in high titer, according to Vasington (1965). A possible representative of one of the subgroups of the lipophilic viruses for virucide testing could be Newcastle disease virus, which is quite hardy, can be obtained in high titer, and can be grown easily in embryonated eggs. A possible representative of the intermediate adenovirus group could be chick embryo lethal orphan (CELO) virus, which shares many properties with the adenovirus group and is a hardy virus that grows in the embryonated egg.

There is a need to study the relationship of the proposed test viruses to more pathogenic viruses within the lipophilic, hydrophilic, and intermediate groups of viruses, insofar as their susceptibility to germicides is concerned, before specific viruses can be recommended as standard test viruses. A selection of viruses for a complete virucidal program should also contain a bacteriophage, a representative of the psittacosis-lymphogranuloma-trachoma group, and a rickettsia to evaluate germicides against these organisms.

Bacteriophages, especially in dairy plants that manufacture cultured products, are an environmental sanitation problem. Bacteriophage inactivation in the dairy manufacturing industry is accomplished primary by spraying or fogging with germicidal solutions. Klein (1956) found the resistance of bacteriophages to germicides to be quite variable. Sing et al. (1964*a*) used *Streptococcus cremoris* 1445 and *Streptococcus diacetilactis* 18–16 phage in their comparisons of various germicidal aerosols.

Possibly, feline pneumonitis could be selected as a representative test organism of the psittacosis-lymphogranuloma-trachoma group, which forms a distinct biologic group between the true viruses and the rickettsiae. A member of this group should be included in testing programs as these antibiotic-susceptible, intracellular parasites are responsible for diverse, natural, clinical, and latent infections in birds, animals, and man.

The rickettsiae are structurally complex, closely resemble the gram-negative bacteria, and divide by binary fission. These microorganisms are so fastidious that their growth requirements are fulfilled only intracellularly. Their growth in vivo is inhibited by several drugs and antibiotics. The Gandt agent, which grows well in the yolk sac of embryonated eggs, is an organism that possibly can be used to represent the rickettsiae in germicide testing.

The following are some of the factors to consider in the selection of a series of prototype viruses for virucidal testing: (1) There should be a relatively low risk to personnel and animals in the surrounding environment. (2) The chosen prototype virus should be representative of a fairly well defined group of viruses. (3) The chosen agent should be stable, easy to handle, and one that can be grown in high titer. (4) The prototype virus should be one that can be obtained in a relatively pure form and grown on reasonably accessible growth media. (5) Although knowledge of the chemical composition of viruses is limited, prototype test viruses, whenever possible, should be those with known properties.

A major problem in testing virucides is that of obtaining satifactory virus preparations for test purposes. A part of this problem is obtaining virus preparations in high titer so that the exposed virus-medicant mixture may be diluted to a level where the carryover of the virucidal chemical will not interfere with growth of cell cultures or survival of chick embryos or animals. The combinations of a low-titer virus and a highly toxic compound that destroys the very tissue needed for virus growth is a problem frequently encountered in virucide testing.

If low-risk prototype viruses are unavailable to evaluate certain classes of viruses against germicides, and the use of pathogens is necessary, then adequate equipment, facilities, and safeguards must be employed to protect personnel and the surrounding environment.

Host System

Tissue culture, chick embryo, or murine models can be used as host assays in virucide testing. Tissue culture systems are the most commonly employed but are extremely susceptible to virucide cytotoxicity and produce variable results for the slowly replicating type of virus. Incubation time and refeeding (detoxifying schedule) have to be standardized. The chick embryo is the host of choice for the myxo- and para-myxoviruses and is less susceptible to toxicity than cell culture. It can also be used when pocks are produced on the chorioallantoic membrane (vaccinia and herpesviruses). Mice can be used in virucide assays when the host range does not include either cell culture or chick embryo, e.g., pseudorabies in suckling mice and encephalomyocarditis virus in adult mice.

As a general rule, the host system for which the test virus had the greatest infectivity should be the system of choice in virucide testing. Prince (1978) described the three host systems for testing as follows: The mice system (weanling mice weighing 9 to 12 g) was found to be susceptible to Coxsackie B1, influenza, ECHO 9, and herpes simplex type 2 viruses by intraperitoneal inoculation or intranasal instillation (two to three drops). The system was found to be particularly useful for screening against viral agents that propagate to low titers in toxicity-susceptible tissue cultures.

The tissue culture systems (rhesus monkey kidney or WI38) were susceptible to all of the viruses tested. With respect to depth of titration (sufficient virulence), cell cultures were used successfully to test phenolic compounds and iodophors against enterovirus and herpesvirus. The chick embryo system showed the most limited susceptibility spectrum. However, the system was the model of choice for myxoviruses.

Chang (1976) illustrated that evaluating the efficacy of virucide against influenza viruses was not possible in monkey kidney tissue culture because of low infectious titer for drying processes and high toxicity levels for disinfectants. The toxic level actually exceeded the viral infectious titer. These problems were not encountered when the tests were done in the developing chick embryos.

Drying Treatment Affecting the Survival of Viruses

The ability of viruses to survive in a potent state apart from their living host cells is a property that is quite variable for different groups of viruses. Some may remain virulent for weeks, whereas others seem to become innocuous almost at once under ordinary drying conditions. In testing a virucide, a dried viral culture prepared from an inanimate surface is usually required. Chen and Phebus (1977) found that the herpes simplex type 2 and influenza A_2/Hong Kong/8/68 viruses showed highly significant reduction ($p < 0.001$) in infectivity titer averaging from $10^{6.89}$ to $10^{4.47}$ of pfu and $10^{7.3}$ to $10^{5.4}$ of pfu respectively after drying on the bottom surface of a petri dish at 37°C for 60 minutes.

The stability of Coxsackievirus B3 (CB3) (McGeady et al., 1979) and human rhinovirus types 2 and 14 (HRV 2 and HRV 14) were studied under various laboratory conditions (Reagan et al., 1981). The effects on virus inactivation of temperature (6°, 23°, and 37°C), pH (7 and 9), protein content (0.25% bovine serum albumin—BSA), and ionic strength (buffered waster of saline) were compared under wet or drying conditions. In general, the addition of BSA in saline provided increased stability to the viruses, especially under conditions of drying. Although evaporation at 37°C reduced virus infectivity (CB3) over 24 hours by as much as 99.95% at pH 7, a residual amount of surviving infectious virus could pose a potential biohazard to nonimmune persons. The HRV immunotypes were more stable than the enterovirus (CBS) under all conditions tested. These studies provide evidence that selected picornaviruses survive conditions of evaporation on hard surfaces to permit their potential transmission to susceptible persons.

Influence of Organic Load

Organic contamination usually occurs in any form of disinfectant practice. The presence of extraneous organic substances frequently interferes with the reaction between a virus and virucidal agent. The concentration of virucide needed to inactivate a virus depends on the amount and kind of interfering organic matter. The viruses contaminated with organic materials sometimes cluster together to form aggregation clumpings of various sizes that may also interfere with antiviral activity of the virucidal agent. Chen and Phebus (1978) investigated the influence of organic load on virucide testing against influenza A₂/Hong Kong/8/68 viruses. In their study, 5% of heated inactivated calf serum, chick serum, filtered bovine albumin, and 2.5% mucin were added separately to the clarified virus suspension. The test protocol for evaluating the effectiveness of selected virucidal agents against the dried viruses from the bottom surface of a petri dish was based on the method recommended by Shannon (1976). The highest recovery of the virucide-treated viruses resulted when the viral culture contained 5% of bovine albumin (indicating high resistance to virucide). The second highest recovery was obtained for treated viruses containing 2.5% mucin, as previously expected. No protection advantages were observed when calf serum or chick serum was added to the viral culture before drying. The presence of 0.25% bovine albumin with salt (1 mM Tris-saline) also contributed significantly to the stabilization of dried Coxsackievirus B3 for virucide testing (McGeady et al., 1979).

Under environmental conditions, the viruses in nature obviously would vary. A poliovirus in a swimming pool would be in diluted suspension and reasonably vulnerable to disinfectants. The same viruses in undiluted feces would be surrounded by so much interfering organic matter that probably none of the commonly available disinfectants would inactivate them (Klein, 1976).

Slavin (1973) describes a test for evaluating disinfectants against both bacteria and viruses using yeast as the organic load, as follows.

Materials and Methods

Yeast is an accepted substance introduced into disinfectant tests to impede the action of the disinfectant in a way similar to one of the most important natural substances likely to interfere with disinfectant action, namely, feces. To form a coherent layer to contain the infective agent and the yeast, gelatin was selected because it is solid at the temperature of the test, 4°C, and at room temperature and soluble at the incubator temperature of 37°C.

In the first series of tests, the yeast and test organism were incorporated into a gelatin sausage, and slices 1 mm thick were cut from the sausage with a machine specially designed for the purpose. It was found difficult to prepare slices of consistent thickness, and there was

danger to the operator in preparing and handling them. The second method used a stainless steel disk with a circular cavity into which the gelatin containing the organisms and other ingredients was dropped in a liquid state and allowed to solidify. The disks were made of EN58J stainless steel, 0.376 mm thick. The diameter of the well was 7 mm, giving a thickness of layer of approximately 1.0 mm with 0.05 ml of the gelatin mixture. One edge of the steel disk was turned up to allow it to be easily picked up with forceps. A suitable punch was designed and made in the laboratory, and the disks could be produced in quantity. If the disks were carefully degreased before sterilizing, there was no difficulty in producing consistent layers. Degreasing was easily achieved by boiling in one of the commercial detergents used for laboratory glassware.

An aliquot, 0.05 ml, of a 15% gelatin solution containing 2.5% yeast suspension (BS No. 808: 1938), the organism or virus under test, plus Tween 80 at 0.05%, was dropped into the cavity of the degreased disks. It was sometimes necessary to concentrate the organisms by centrifugation to give 10⁸ per ml in the mixture of gelatin and yeast. The virus mixture had to be of a concentration high enough to allow a four-log drop to be demonstrated. The disks, contained in groups of three in a sterile 10-cm plastic petri dish, were chilled to 4°C to solidify the gelatin and held at this temperature throughout the test. The prepared disk was dropped into 20 ml of disinfectant contained in a small screw-capped jar for the desired time, picked out with forceps, drained, and transferred to 100 ml of distilled water in a crystallizing dish, which was rotated for 5 minutes on a mechanical rotator; the disk was then transferred to 5 ml of nutrient broth containing 5% horse serum in a screw-capped jaw. The nutrient broth was held at 37°C for 30 minutes prior to use. The disk of gelatin dissolved rapidly at this temperature, and further dilutions were made for plate counts by the Miles-Misra method (Slavin, 1973), or for titration of the virus in cell cultures. The exposure time was 30 minutes, except for *Mycobacterium fortuitum*, for which it was extended to 60 minutes. Normally, several dilutions of disinfectant were simultaneously tested.

The results of Slavin's (1973) tests against viruses are found in Table 62–1. This is a designed steel disk carrier test for evaluating disinfectants against viruses using yeast as the organic load. The disadvantage of the test procedure is that it is only workable within a certain range of various disinfectants, because it failed to carry the solidified viruses in the prepared disk for virus recovery after it had been dropped into disinfectant at high concentrations.

METHODS USED FOR TESTING VIRUCIDES

Methods of testing virucidal activity vary according to the possible combinations of virus and susceptible host system under a variety of simulated-use models. The principle employed is the same: the virus is exposed to

Table 62-1. *Results of Tests of Varying Concentration of Disinfectants Against Herpes Virus, Enterovirus, and Myxovirus Parainfluenzae*

| | Percentage Effective Disinfectant Concentration | | | |
Disinfectant	Bovine Herpes Virus IBR	Bovine Myxovirus Parainfluenza 3	Porcine Enterovirus	Percentage Concentration Not Effective†
4	1.5*	2.0*	—	5.0
5	1.0*	2.0*	—	5.0
6	2.0	2.0*	—	5.0
Hypochlorite (10.0% available chlorine)	4.0*	2.0*	2.0*	—
Sodium o-phenyl phenoxide	1.0	2.0*	—	4.0

*Lowest concentration tested

†Higher concentrations not tested

No. 4 Lysol, No. 5 and 6 selected phenols, No. 5 mainly C8 and No. 6 mainly C9 phenols

a chemical disinfectant under controlled conditions, and appropriate observations are made in order to determine the rate of virus inactivation with the chemical being investigated. The methods developed for evaluating virucides are generally of three types: (1) aqueous suspension test in which the test virus is suspended in a solution, (2) carrier test in which the test virus is dried on inanimate surfaces, and (3) aerosol test against airborne bacteriophages.

Aqueous Suspension Test Method

This method is used to evaluate the virucidal activity of disinfectant solutions against specific types of viruses. The virus suspension is diluted with disinfectant to give a final recommended-use concentration of this chemical in a sterilized tube for a specified exposure time and temperature.

Liquid Dilution Test (Hays and Elliker)

Hays and Elliker (1959) first described a suspension test method for evaluating the virucidal action of disinfectants against bacteriophage of *Streptococcus cremoris,* as follows:

Preparation of Bacteriophage. Bacteriophage culture was obtained by propagating the phage in skim milk culture of *Streptococcus cremoris.* The bacterial-free phage filtrate was standardized to a titer of 10^7 pfu/ml. The disinfectants were diluted with water so that the concentration was double that recommended for testing.

Test Procedure. At the beginning of the test, the bacteriophage suspension was diluted with equal volume of disinfectant solution and held at 25°C for 30 to 60 seconds (these exposure times are normally used for sanitizing food utensils). Following the designed exposure, 1 ml aliquot from an inactivated tube or appropriate dilution blank was transferred to a test tube containing 0.25 ml of a 5-hour-old broth culture of the sensitive host. After 1 minute, 3 ml of a soft agar (0.85%) cooled to 45°C were poured into the host-phage mixture. The contents were mixed by rotating the tube and then pouring into a petri

dish containing approximately 20 ml of hardened solid agar. After incubation of the plates at 30°C for 12 hours, the plaques were fully developed and countable. A complete inactivation of phage titer was required for determining the effectiveness of virucidal action.

Aqueous Suspension Test (Klein and DeForest)

Klein and DeForest (1963) described a procedure with the viruses in an aqueous suspension for determining inactivation of viruses using cell culture methods, as follows.

Determining Inactivation. Influenza virus was grown in the allantoic cavity of the chick embryo. Tests for infectivity were carried out by inoculating the virus into the allantoic cavity of the chick embryo and testing for viral hemagglutinins in the allantoic fluid. All other viruses were grown in cultures of HeLa cells, except herpes simplex, which was grown in freshly trypsinized rabbit kidney. The maintenance medium in which the viruses were harvested consisted of 2% chick serum, 20% trypticase soy broth, and 78% Eagle's medium (a mixture of amino acids and vitamins) in Earle's balanced salt solution. This medium, plus some tissue debris that remained after sedimenting the harvested virus preparations at 3000 rpm for 30 minutes, represents the interfering organic matter. All viral titers were in the range of 10^6 to 10^8 infectious doses per ml.

Viral inactivation was determined by mixing 0.9 ml of the test germicide with 0.1 ml of undiluted virus. In some studies, virus was diluted in saline at 1:100. After contact at room temperature for 1, 3, 5, and 10 minutes, viral inactivation was determined by titering the virus and comparing the titer with that of the untreated controls. Germicide carried over in the early dilutions was frequently toxic for tissue culture cells, and thus one could not determine complete viral inactivation.

The viruses used in Klein and DeForest's study are shown in Table 62-2.

In another study, Klein (1965a) described his procedure in more detail.

Table 62–2. *Viruses Included in Germicide Study*

Virus	Nucleic Acid	Size (mu)	Membrane	Lipid	Ether Susceptible	Adsorption by Cholesterol
Polio type 1	RNA	30				Hydrophilic
Coxsackie B-1	RNA	30				Hydrophilic
ECHO 6	RNA	25				Hydrophilic
Adeno type 2	DNA	72				Lipophilic
Herpes simplex	DNA	130	+	+	+	Lipophilic
Vaccinia	DNA	250	+	+		Lipophilic
Influenza (Asian)	RNA	100	+	+	+	Lipophilic

From Klein, M., and DeForest, A. 1963. The inactivation of viruses by germicides. Proc. Chem. Spec. Mfg. Assoc., 49th Mid-Year Meeting, pp. 116–118.

Armstrong and Froelich Germicidal Testing Method

Armstrong and Froelich (1964) tested a germicide against 13 different viruses as follows.

Materials and Methods. Viruses and strains used are shown in Table 62–3 together with details of their storage and assay. Tissue cultures used included the ATR and CATR lines of human amnion cells established in their laboratory. The 719 line of dog kidney cells, also established in their laboratory, as well as primary dog kidney cells, were used for the assay of canine hepatitis virus. The mice used were random-bred Swiss females. Embryonated hen's eggs were used for cultivation and assay of several viruses.

Virucidal Procedures. Benzalkonium chloride USP solutions were prepared at suitable concentrations in distilled water, phosphate-buffered saline, 0.5% bovine albumin, fraction V in distilled water, or 5 or 10% normal rabbit serum in buffered saline. Experiments were car-

ried out at room temperature or at 30°C in a water bath. In qualitative experiments, two or more virus dilutions were mixed with one or more dilutions of benzalkonium chloride, incubated for a suitable period (usually 10 minutes), rapidly diluted to avoid the inherent toxicity of benzalkonium chloride for cells, and injected into suitable hosts to determine the viability of the virus. In quantitative experiments, a single concentration of virus suspension was used. Treatment with benzalkonium chloride and dilution were followed by titration of residual virus in the treated sample.

Plaque-Formation Technique (Sykes)

Another method for testing virucidal agents is through the use of plaque-formation techniques as described by Sykes (1965), a description of which follows.

Methods employing direct plaque formation can also be employed. This is a result of the discovery by Dul-

Table 62–3. *Virus Strains and Culture Details*

Virus and Strain	Storage	Assay
Poliovirus type 2 (MEF₁)	Mouse brain and cord at 4°C Tissue culture fluid at −65°C	Mouse, intracerebral Tissue culture tube method; CATR cells
Encephalomyocarditis (MM)	Mouse brain at 4°C	Mouse, intraperitoneal
Influenza type A (PR₈ and Japan 305/57)	Allantoic fluid at −65°C	Egg, allantoic cavity, hemagglutination of allantoic fluids
Measles (Edmonston)	Tissue culture fluid at −65°C	Tissue culture tube method; CATR cells
Canine distemper (Onderstepoort)	Chorioallantoic membrane (50%) at −65°C	Egg, chorioallantoic membrane
Feline pneumonitis (No. 1)	Yolk sac (50%) at −65°C	Egg, yolk sac
Meningopneumonitis (Cal 10)	Mouse brain at −65°C	Mouse, intracerebral
Rabies (CVS and Flury LEP)	Mouse brain (20%) at −65°C	Mouse, intracerebral
Fowl laryngotracheitis (Lederle)	Chorioallantoic membrane (50%) at −65°C	Egg, chorioallantoic membrane
Semliki forest	Mouse brain at 4°C Tissue culture fluid at −65°C	Mouse, intraperitoneal Tissue culture tube method; ATR cells
Vaccinia (HD)	Yolk sac (50%) at −65°C Tissue culture fluid at −65°C	Egg, yolk sac Tissue culture tube method; CATR cells
Infectious canine hepatitis (Cornell)	Tissue culture fluid at −20°C	Tissue culture tube method; dog kidney cells
Herpes simplex (HF)	Tissue culture fluid at −65°C	Tissue culture tube method; ATR cells

becco (1952) that such formations are not confined to the bacteriophages but, because of their cytopathogenicity, can be induced with several of the animal viruses growing in tissue culture. The principle of the method is that an established film of the host cells on a suitable agar medium is infected with the virus, and then small disks of filter paper carrying the disinfectant are applied. After a suitable incubation period, the disks are removed and the agar stained with a suitable dye to observe plaque suppression, and also possible toxicity to the host. In the method of Hermann et al. (1960), trypsinized chick embryo cells are suspended in a calf serum-salts medium and incubated for 48 hours to obtain a confluent growth. The medium is then discarded and the cell film inoculated with virus and overlaid with a thin layer of serum agar. After this, small paper disks carrying the disinfectant are put on the surface and the plates incubated for 3 days to allow plaque formation, which is detected by staining with a tetrazolium agar and reading after 2 to 4 hours. Vaccinia, herpes, Newcastle disease, and Nile disease viruses can be used and, as with antibiotic assay, a straight line ratio between log disinfectant concentration and zone of response is found.

In a slight modification of this method. Siminoff (1961) grew the chick cells on a tris buffer-Earle's medium agar and stained with neutral red to observe plaque inhibition.

Virucidal Testing Methods Using Both Cell Culture and Chick Embryo Systems (Avampato et al.)

Avampato et al. (1965) described the following virucidal testing methods for representatives of four major virus groups (i.e., adenovirus, herpesvirus, myxovirus, and picornavirus) using both cell culture and chick embryo systems.

Virus Preparation. Echo, adeno, and parainfluenza viruses were grown in primary rhesus monkey kidney cell cultures, while herpes simplex was grown in primary rabbit-kidney cell cultures. The cell cultures were maintained in 0.5% lactalbumin hydrolysate in Earle's balanced salt solution. To minimize organic interference due to cellular debris, the fluid containing the virus was either filtered through 0.22 μm millipore membrane or centrifuged at 2000 rpm for 30 minutes. Influenza viruses were cultured in embryonated chicken eggs, harvested as allantoic fluid, and used without further treatment. All virus preparations were stored at −60°C.

Cell Cultures. The choice of the cell culture system used depends on the virus being used in the test, and the virus used must be one that will cause a cytopathic effect (CPE) in the infected cells or be detectable by some other means such as hemadsorption. The most common alterations are (1) rounding of cells that become refractory, and (2) syncytia formation with multinucleated giant cells. Some viruses exhibit only one or the other of these properties, whereas some exhibit both. Hemadsorption is a phenomenon whereby red blood cells are adsorbed to the surface of cultured cells that are infected with certain viruses. Many myxoviruses can be detected this way.

Test Procedure. The virus suspension is diluted 1:10 with the recommended use concentration of disinfectant. The mixture is allowed to stand for 10 minutes, at which time further tenfold dilutions are made and the surviving virus is assayed for potency. A virus control and a toxicity control are included in the test.

Virus Infectivity Assay. Virus assays are made mostly in cell cultures grown in 16 × 150 mm tubes. Two-tenths of a milliliter of each of the tenfold dilutions is inoculated into each of four tubes of cell cultures containing 1.8 ml of nutrient medium. The inoculated cultures with appropriate controls are incubated at 37°C for a period determined by the virus used in the test anywhere from 3 to 7 days. Fifty-percent end points are determined by the method of Reed and Muench (1938). The 50% end point is the calculated dilution at which half the inoculated tubes show evidence of virus and half do not. The potency is expressed as the log $TCID_{50}$, TCID being the abbreviation for tissue culture infective dose. Today, the use of 96 well microtiter plates would be more convenient for virus infectivity assays than test tube cultures.

Virucide Test Procedure in Suckling Mice (Fellowes)

Fellowes (1965) described a procedure for determining the virucidal action of some surface-active agents against foot-and-mouth-disease virus (FMDV) in suckling mice, as follows.

Virucide Procedure. The FMDV type O, strain M11, was prepared from cultures of primary calf kidney cells growing as monolayer in Povitsky bottles according to the method of Patty and May (1961). Unfiltered and uncentrifuged virus (viral titer: 7.3-log LD_{50}/ml) was used in this study.

The representative anionic and cationic surface-active agents were prepared as 0.5%, 1.0%, 2.0%, and 5.0% concentrations in undiluted virus suspension based on their declared active ingredient content. The pH adjustment of the mixture was made with 1 N NaOH or 1 N HCl. The virus-chemical mixture (20 ml) was agitated for 2 hours at 28°C with a magnetic stirring device. The potency of each compound was tested twice, and the mean value of activity was determined.

Determining Inactivation. The infectivity of the various chemical-virus mixtures after 2 hours at 28°C, as well as that of the controls, was assessed in suckling mice by the intraperitoneal inoculation of dilutions of the mixture. Each of 10 mice was inoculated with 0.05 ml of each dilution. A virus control was included to test the effect of the temperature of 28°C for 2 hours on the virus; controls were also used to determine the effect of pH on the virus infectivity over the range of pH 5, 6.5, and 9 under the conditions of the test. The number of mouse LD_{50} units of infectivity inactivated by a chemical was determined by substracting the mouse LD_{50} value of the heated (28°C) virus control from the mouse LD_{50} value of the virus-chemical mixture similarly heated. The mice were observed for a period of 7 days. In this study with

FMDV, the cationic or anionic effects of chemical, pH, and temperature must be considered important factors in inactivation of the virus. Perhaps this approach could be applied to testing virucides against the Coxsackieviruses, where an in vivo assay is desired to avoid virucide toxicity for tissue cultures.

Fluorescent Antibody Technique (Wright)

Wright (1970*b*, 1976) described a virucidal test method for the hog cholera virus using a fluorescent antibody technique. He states:

> Virucide evaluation depends on a reliable assay system. A direct test in cell culture would be most desirable, but hog cholera virus was not cytopathic. Therefore, an indirect means of detecting live virus in cell culture was required. Fluorescein isothiocyanate-labeled globulin from serum of immune swine was used to determine if cell culture contained live virus. The virucide test was completed by mixing a suspension of virus in a disinfectant for several time intervals and then diluting the mixture with cell culture medium. The disinfectant virus mixture was then placed on swine kidney cell culture. Several disinfectant types were tested using this method and were found to be virucidal. The system appears to be a useful model for other noncytopathic viruses.

Wright's (1970*b*) test method follows.

Virucide Test. A 20 × 125 mm screw-capped test tube with 9 ml of disinfectant at 1.11 times the concentration to be tested was placed in a water bath at 20°C. A 1-ml amount of virus suspension (1.0 × 10⁶ pfu/ml or greater) was added to the disinfectant. The contents of the test tube were mixed by gentle shaking. At 1, 5, and 10 minutes after introduction of the virus into the disinfectant, 0.5 ml was removed and placed in a test tube with 4.5 ml Earle's balanced salt solution containing lactalbumin hydrolysate and calf serum. When this procedure was completed, four Leighton tubes containing swine kidney cells were inoculated with 1 ml per tube of the diluted virus-disinfectant. The cell cultures were incubated at 37°C for virus adsorption. After 1 hour, the Earle's medium was decanted from the Leighton tube, and 1 ml of fresh Earle's medium with lactalbumin and calf serum was added. The cell culture was then incubated for an additional 15 to 19 hours.

Staining Cell Culture. The coverslip cultures were removed from the Leighton tubes and rinsed in phosphate-buffered saline (PBS—pH 7.2—.01 M), fixed in acetone for 5 minutes at room temperature, and air dried. The cell cultures were stained with fluorescent antibody conjugate for 20 minutes in a moist chamber at 37°C. After staining, the coverslip cultures were washed with PBS for 3 minutes, rinsed in distilled water, air dried, and mounted on slides in an equal volume of glycerine and double-strength PBS.

Microscopy. Coverslip cultures were examined by fluorescence using a cardioid condenser and illuminated by an Osram lamp HBO 200. The primary light filter was a BG-12, and the barrier filter was an OG-1. The coverslip cultures were examined at 100 or 250 × magnifications.

Antigen Capture ELISA Technique (McDougal et al.)

A description of a new disinfectant test method for the lymphadenopathy associated virus (LAV) using antigen capture ELISA procedures described by McDougal et al. (1985) follows. These assays should be performed in safety cabinets to avoid becoming accidently infected with this agent.

Virus Preparation. Lymphadenopathy associated virus, or the human immunodeficiency virus (HIV-1), is the etiologic agent of the acquired immunodeficiency syndrome (AIDS). The virus was propagated in phytohemagglutinin-stimulated lymphoblasts (PHA blasts) as follows (Barre-Sinoussi et al., 1983). Ficoll-Hypaque–separated mononuclear cells were cultured in "medium A" containing 10 μg/ml PHA for 3 days at 37°C in 6% CO_2 in a humidified incubator. "Medium A" is RPMI 1640 containing 100 U/ml penicillin, 50 μg/ml streptomycin, 2 mM L-glutamine, and 10% heat-inactivated (56°C for 30 minutes) fetal calf serum. The PHA blasts were harvested by centrifugation (300 × g for 7 minutes) and resuspended to 2 × 10⁶ viable cells/ml in "medium B." "Medium B" is "medium A," which also contains 10% v/v interleukin 2 (IL-2, Cellular Products, Buffalo, NY) and 0.04% v/v sheep anti-interferon. Cells were inoculated with LAV in the form of an LAV + culture supernate (10,000 reverse transcriptase cpm per 2 × 10⁶ cells determined by the method described by Poiesz et al., 1980) and incubated for 18 to 24 hours. The cells were then pelleted by centrifugation and resuspended at 1 × 10⁶/ml in medium B. Cultures were monitored by the ELISA capture assay and supernate reverse transcriptase activity (Poiesz et al., 1980). Supernates were harvested by sequential centrifugation (300 × g for 7 minutes followed by 1500 × g for 20 minutes) and stored at −70°C until assayed.

Preparation of Anti–HIV-1 Reagents. Serum with high titer antibody to HIV-1 was obtained from a homosexual man with chronic unexplained lymphadenopathy. The IgG fraction of serum was purified by ammonium sulfate precipitation and diethylaminoethyl cellulose chromatography in 0.01 M phosphate buffer, pH 8.0. A portion of IgG fraction was coupled to horseradish peroxidase (HPO, type VI, Sigma, St. Louis, MO) (Wilson and Nakane, 1978). The IgG was stored at −70°C in 0.01 M PO_4, 0.15 M NaCl, pH 8.0 (PBS). The HPO conjugate was stored in PBS containing 10 mg/ml bovine serum albumin, 50% v/v glycerol, and 0.2% NaN_3 at −70°C. The working ampule was stored at −20°C.

Test Procedure for HIV-Capture ELISA.
Step 1: Flat-bottom, 96-well microtiter tray wells were coated with 0.1 ml of anti-HIV IgG (25 μg/ml) for 4 hours at room temperature. The wells were rinsed four times with PBS containing 0.05 triton-X.
Step 2: One-tenth milliliter volumes of culture supernates to be tested were mixed with 0.1 ml PBS and 0.2%

v/v triton-X, and added to the wells. The plates were held overnight at 4°C.

Step 3: After the wells had been again washed four times with 0.5% triton-X PBS, 0.1 ml of HPO-conjugated anti-HIV IgG (4 µg/ml) 0.05% triton-X was added, and the plates were incubated at 4°C for 4 hours.

Step 4: A solution containing 0.1 mg/ml o-phenylenediamine (OPD) and 0.006% v/v H_2O_2 was prepared by dissolving the OPD in methanol (10 mg/ml), diluting in H_2O, and adding H_2O_2.

Step 5: After the wells had been washed four times, 0.2 ml of the OPD/H_2O_2 solution was added. Color reactions developed over 30 to 45 minutes and were stopped by adding 0.05 ml 8N H_2SO_4.

Step 6: The optical density (OD) at 490 nm was read in an automatic ELISA plate Reader (Dynatech, Alexandria, VA). Resultant optical densities are proportional to the relative amount of viral antigen (HIV) occurring in the test samples.

ID-50 Assay. Three-day PHA blasts (2×10^6) were suspended in 1 ml of medium B containing serial tenfold dilutions of HIV inoculum in 12×75 mm culture tubes. Initial incubation was for 18 hours. The tubes were centrifuged ($300 \times$ g for 7 minutes) and the cells were resuspended in 2 ml of medium B. One-tenth milliliter volumes were dispensed into 20 U-bottom microculture wells containing an additional 0.15 ml of medium B (1×10^5 cells in 0.25 ml). Every 3 days, 100 µl of culture supernate was removed and replaced with fresh medium. One-tenth of 1 ml of PBS containing 0.1% v/v Tween-20 was added to the culture supernates, which were stored at $-20°C$ until assayed in the HIV-capture ELISA. Twenty uninfected cell cultures were included in all assays.

Disinfectant Test Procedure. An undiluted HIV-1 + culture supernate with an ID-50 of $10^{5.24}$ was treated 10 to 20 seconds with various concentrations of sodium hypochlorite. NaOCl was formulated as household bleach (100% bleach equals 5.25% or 52,500 ppm NaOCl). Treated virus was then serially diluted and inoculated into indicator cells, and ID-50 was determined. Reduction in ID-50 was compared with that in bleach toxicity controls. For toxicity controls, separate tubes of virus and bleach were first serially diluted and then inoculated together into cell cultures. Each dilution of bleach used for virus inactivation had its own ID-50 control.

In this study with HIV-1, a dose of 0.1% v/v household bleach resulted in a greater than 4-log reduction in virus titer in 10 to 20 seconds.

Carrier Test Method

This method is used to evaluate the virucidal activity of disinfectant solutions or of pressurized disinfectant sprays against specific types of viruses dried on inanimate surfaces according to the directions for use on the product label.

Use-Dilution Method (Lorenz and Jann)

Lorenz and Jann (1964) described a method entitled "Use-Dilution Method and Newcastle Disease Virus" that was a modification of the AOAC Use-Dilution Test for bacteria. The Materials and Methods section of their paper is as follows:

Materials and Methods. The bacterial use-dilution test procedure is outlined here to orient the description of the modifications. In the bacterial use-dilution test, 20 sterile carrier rings were placed in a standard, liquid culture of bacteria. After 15 minutes, ten rings were removed and dried at 37°C for 20 to 60 minutes. Subsequently, one ring was placed in a tube of disinfectant. The disinfectant was diluted to that concentration at which the manufacturer specifies its practical application. After 10 minutes, a ring was transferred to a tube containing 10 ml of standard broth, and this tube was incubated in a standard manner. Ten carrier rings manipulated in this manner constituted a bacterial use-dilution test. If the ten tubes showed no evidence of bacterial growth, the disinfectant was judged to be effective at use-dilution, i.e., the dilution at which it is to be used as prescribed by the manufacturer.

This procedure was modified for testing the activity of disinfectants against viruses in the following way. Instead of using a standard bacterial culture, a standard allantoic fluid suspension of Newcastle disease virus (NDV) was used. The carrier rings were placed in the virus suspension. They were then dried and transferred to the disinfectant tubes in the exact manner described in the bacterial use-dilution test. But, instead of transferring a ring from the disinfectant to 10 ml of broth, it was transferred to 1 ml of broth. Subsequently, 0.1 ml of this broth was inoculated into the allantoic sac of each of six 10-day embryonated chicken eggs. If none of the inoculated embryos was killed by viral infection within 5 days after inculation, the disinfectant was judged effective at the dilution tested.

The details of these modifications are as follows:

Reagents and Apparatus. The reagents and equipment required for the viral use-dilution test are the same as those listed for the bacterial use-dilution test described by the Association of Official Analytical Chemists (1960). Additional material required includes: screw-capped Pyrex tubes (150 by 20 mm) for storing virus suspensions, 100 by 15 mm tubes, 1-ml syringes graduated in 0.1 ml, 25-gauge hypodermic needles (5/8 inches long), an egg shell punch or electric drill with carborundum burr, egg racks, flexible collodion, normal saline, tincture of iodine, and fertile chicken eggs.

Fertile eggs may be purchased from commercial hatcheries and arranged in the papier-mâché holders in which they are obtained from the hatcheries. The eggs were incubated at 37°C and were turned once a day during incubation.

Standard Suspension of Virus. An allantoic fluid suspension of NDV, California strain 11914, obtained from R.A. Bankowski, Davis, California, was used in these tests. Stock suspensions of the virus were prepared as follows: A stock allantoic fluid suspension of the virus was diluted 1:1000 in normal physiologic saline. One-tenth of a milliliter of this diluted suspension was inoculated into the allantoic sac of each of 50 or more 10-day embryonated eggs. One day after inculation, the eggs were candled, and all nonviable embryos were discarded. On the second day, eggs were then chilled by placing them in a refrigerator for several hours.

The allantoic fluid was harvested first by removing the shell above the air space of the egg. By use of a sterile blunt instrument, such as forceps, the membranes were depressed and held away from the pipette that was used to withdraw the clean allantoic fluid. If the yolk sac was broken or excessive bleeding occurred, the contents of such an egg were discarded. The amount of infectious allantoic fluid from individual eggs varied from 2 to 10 ml depending on the size of the egg and the success of avoiding the various membranes, which tend to clog the pipette. All allantoic fluid was pooled in a single sterile flask. Subsequently, 22-ml samples were transferred to screw-capped tubes and stored at $-20°C$. Before use in a viral use-dilution test, a tube of virus suspension was melted and centrifuged at $1500 × g$ for 10 minutes to remove insoluble precipitates that formed when the fluid was frozen. Only the clear supernatant fluid was used in the test.

The LD_{50} values of NDV suspensions were determined by the method described by the National Academy of Sciences (1959). The LD_{50} of an average pool of NDV was normally greater than 10^{-8}, and no change was encountered in storage for 6 months at $-20°C$.

The method of inoculating eggs was as follows: The site of inoculation was marked with a small pencil mark at the time of handling the eggs. The site was at the junction of the air space and the chorioallantoic membrane in an area of minimal vasculation. The site was swabbed with tincture of iodine and a small hole was made in the shell without damaging the shell membrane underneath. The material to be inoculated was drawn into a syringe and then, holding the syringe vertically, the needle was plunged blindly into the allantoic sac. After 0.1 ml of material had been inoculated and the needle removed, the hole in the shell was sealed with collodion and the eggs were returned to the incubator.

Test Proper. Twenty carrier rings were placed in 20 ml of clear allantoic fluid suspension of NDV, which was incubated at 20°C. After 15 minutes, the rings were transferred to a petri dish and dried for 20 to 60 minutes at 37°C. Then a ring was transferred to a tube containing 10 ml of diluted disinfectant, which was also incubated at 20°C. After 1 minute, the second ring was transferred to a second tube of disinfectant. This procedure was continued until ten rings had been transferred to disinfectant. At 10 minutes after the first ring had been transferred, it was removed and placed in 1 ml of nutrient broth contained in a tube (100 × 15 mm). This procedure was repeated until the ten rings were transferred to 1-

ml portions of broth. The tubes of broth were also incubated at 20°C. Immediately after the last ring had been transferred, 0.1 ml of each broth suspension was inoculated into each of six 10- to 12-day embryonated eggs as described previously. A different syringe was used for each broth suspension. The eggs were made ready for inoculation before the test was begun. With a minimum of experience, the 60 eggs could be inoculated in less than 15 minutes. All procedures, except those involving the inoculations of eggs, were conducted as prescribed by the Association of Official Analytical Chemists (1960).

On the day after inoculation, the eggs were candled, and all dead embryos were discarded from the test. Such deaths occurred from the trauma of inoculation. If more than one embryo in a set of six was killed nonspecifically, the test was considered invalid because only 40% or less of the 1-ml broth suspension was being sampled for active virus. The eggs were candled each day for an additional 4 days. If any embryos died during the period from the second to the fifth postinoculation day, the disinfectant was judged ineffective at the dilution tested. If all embryos survived except those killed nonspecifically, the disinfectant was judged effective at the dilution tested.

The obvious shortcoming in the method of Lorenz and Jann (1964), as pointed out by them, was that their method is restricted to viruses that cause death to the chick embryo. However, other viruses could be used that cause plaques on the chorioallantoic membrane, or dwarfing of the embryo. The approach of Lorenz and Jann was also adopted to test the disinfectant against herpes simplex and polio viruses in tissue culture system by Gaustad (1976) and Mahl (1976).

Modifications of Lorenz and Jann Method

Wright (1970*a*) repeated the test procedure of Lorenz and Jann using porcelain carriers and vesicular stomatitis virus. He found the LD_{50} titers of virus recovered from the carriers, when dried for 20 minutes, to be $10^{0.6}$, $10^{1.5}$, $10^{1.74}$ in three separate experiments. The LD_{50} titer of virus on a comparable carrier not dried was $10^{6.5}$. He concluded that the test method using porcelain penicylinders as a vehicle for carrying viruses was unsuccessful.

Chen and Phebus (1979) also found that the stainless steel penicylinders used in bactericide testing failed to carry a sufficient titer of herpes simplex virus for virucide test purposes. In the case of poliovirus type 1, the calculated input virus on the penicylinder carrier before drying had a titer of $10^{6.69}$ of pfu. The poliovirus that were actually recovered from the carrier after drying and soaking treatment had a titer of $10^{4.72}$ of pfu. The polioviruses recovered from the soaking water indicate the loss of viruses by rinsing action 5, and not by virucidal action of disinfectant.

Glass Surface Spray Method (Klein)

Other AOAC tests such as the Glass Slide Spray Test have been used in virucide testing. Klein (1971) described a modified spray test for evaluating the virucidal activity of influenza virus A, using an embryonated egg technique, which is as follows.

Preparation and Assay of Test Viruses. The influenza virus A_2 was grown in the allantoic sac of 10-day-old chick embryos. The virus was harvested after 40 hours' incubation at 37°C. The titer of the virus was 10^8 egg infectious doses per 0.1 ml as determined by hemagglutination of 0.5% suspension of chicken red blood cells by the infected allantoic fluid. The titer of the virus recovered from the test surface was close to that obtained by the tube assay. Six chick embryos were inoculated with each dilution.

Test Procedure for Evaluation of Disinfectant Spray. One tenth of a milliliter of virus was swabbed over the back surface of petri dishes 10 cm in diameter. The plates were allowed to dry. Control plates were left untreated. Treated plates were sprayed with test compound for 3 seconds holding the spray approximately 8 inches from the plate. After 10 minutes' contact, the degree of viral inactivation was determined. A single swab moistened in broth was thoroughly rubbed over each treated or control plate in a uniform fashion with a three-time interval rinsing in 0.9 ml of broth. This broth was called a 1-10 dilution of virus and tenfold dilutions in broth were made from this tube. The presence of virus was determined in each of the broth dilutions by inoculating 0.1 ml of each dilution into the allantoic cavity of six 10-day-old embryos. A similar approach to this method was also adopted to test the disinfectant against Newcastle disease virus by Brown (1976).

Glass Crushing Spray Method (Chen)

Chen (1975) introduced the cover glass crushing technique to be used in the spray test for viral recovery. The herpes simplex virus and the H.Ep. 2 cell line as an indicator host system were used. The cover glass crushing technique for viral recovery is as follows:

Spread three tenths (0.3 ml) of undiluted HSV suspension over the surface of a 24 × 60-mm cover glass and allow to dry 1.5 hours at 37°C. Crush cover glass completely in a glass homogenizer 30 × 120-mm (Guerra Technical Sales, Rockville, Maryland) containing 2.7 ml of PBS solution (Dulbecco's type). This Dulbecco's PBS is considered a 10^{-1} dilution of virus. Thoroughly mix the entire reaction preparation by an aspirating sterile pipette. Tenfold dilutions in Dulbecco's PBS are made from this tube. The quantitative assay of recovered HSV is based on the cytopathogenic effect of virus in H.Ep. 2 cell culture. Since the tissue cultures are more uniform in their response, five tissue culture flasks are inoculated with each virus dilution. The virus titer is calculated from the proportion of cell culture flasks observed to become infected when inoculated with an appropriate series of consecutive virus dilutions. The Reed and Muench method was used for the calculation of virus titer. Based on this study, the titer of the original HSV suspension was $10^{6.9}$ per ml. After drying 1.5 hours at 37°C, the titer in the recovered glass surface averaged $10^{5.57}$ per ml. Thus, the virus titer had been reduced by 1.33.

Carrier Disinfectant Test Method (Gaustad et al.)

A modified AOAC use-dilution test method for the evaluation of virucidal efficacy of liquid surface disinfectants against herpes simplex virus (MP strain), poliovirus type 1 (Brunhilde strain), vaccinia virus (WR strain), and adenovirus type 3 (G.B. strain) in H.Ep. 2 cell culture system was described by Gaustad et al. (1974), as follows.

Preparation of Cells and Viruses. H.Ep. 2 cells were cultured in TC medium 199 supplemented with 10% calf serum plus antibiotics. All four viruses were grown in monolayer cultures of H.Ep. 2 cells processed by freezing and thawing four times in a dry ice-cold bath. The virus cell suspensions were then centrifuged at 1000 × g for 20 minutes to remove cell debris, the supernatant fluid was drawn off, and the virus stock pool was concentrated by negative-pressure ultrafiltration according to Craig (1965) and Smith (1973) and stored at −90°C until use.

Virus Titer Assay. The titer of each test virus was determined by making serial tenfold dilutions and inoculating 48- to 72-hour-old H.Ep. 2 cell cultures. Virus concentration was expressed as the 50% tissue culture infective dose ($TCID_{50}$) and calculated by the technique of Reed and Muench (1938). The $TCID_{50}$ varied from $10^{5.9}$ for adenovirus, $10^{6.2}$ for vaccinia virus, $10^{7.9}$ for herpes simplex virus, to $10^{8.8}$ for poliovirus after negative-pressure ultrafiltration.

Test Proper. Five sterile cylinders (penicylinders of type 304 stainless steel) were placed in the concentrated stock pool of the virus, exposed 15 minutes to the virus, placed in a sterile petri dish containing matted filter paper, and put into a 37°C incubator until dry (approximately 20 to 25 minutes). Each carrier was placed separately into a sterile tube (20 × 150 mm) containing 10 ml of a use dilution of the test disinfectant, exposed for 10 minutes, and placed separately in a sterile tube containing 1.8 ml of letheen broth and shaken vigorously for 5 minutes. Serial tenfold dilutions (10^{-1} through 10^{-7}) were made by adding 0.2 ml of the previous dilution into 1.8 ml of maintenance medium 199 (5% calf serum only) in the next dilution. Each dilution (0.2 ml) was inoculated onto a monolayer of H.Ep. 2 cells in a tissue culture tube (16 × 125 mm). Each dilution was adsorbed on the cells for the equivalent time required for adequate adsorption of the virus. The equivalent adsorption times were 2 hours for herpes simplex, 30 minutes for poliovirus, 45 minutes for adenovirus, and 1 hour for vaccinia virus. The temperature of adsorption for all portions of the test method was 37°C. After the adsorption time was complete, 2.0 ml of maintenance medium 199 was added to each tissue culture tube. They were then incubated at 37° for 3 to 5 days, examined for end point of cytopathic effect, and calculated as the $TCID_{50}$ by the technique of Reed and Muench (1938). Virus control and cytotoxicity control of test disinfectant were run concurrently with each of the experiments. The average $\log_{10}$ of virus concentration retained on the cylinders varied from 4.7 for vaccinia virus, 4.8 for adenovirus, 5.3 for poliovirus, to

6.3 for herpes simplex virus after drying at least 20 minutes at 37°C.

Convenient In Vitro Method for Testing Rhinoviruses (Pancic et al.)

Pancic et al. (1977) described a convenient in vitro method for the testing of virucidal agents against rhinoviruses, as follows.

Test Procedure. Stock pool of rhinoviruses (type 2, 14, or 17) were grown in HeLa Cells and had a titer of 6 to 7 logs per 0.2 ml. To test the virucidal activity of chemical compounds against rhinoviruses dried on hard surfaces, 0.1 ml of undiluted virus was spread on the inner surface of a sterile, 10-cm diameter glass petri dish by means of a sterile microscope pipette. For convenience and rapidity, the virus was dried by passing a jet of filtered dry air over the surface of the dish for 1 minute, followed by 10 minutes of standing at room temperature. Nine-tenths of a milliliter of appropriate compound dilution was added and spread over the surface of the petri dish and allowed to dry at room temperature for 10 minutes. A 0.9-ml volume of Medium 199 was then added to the dish and was drawn and expelled from a pipette 10 times. The virus-test chemical mixture was diluted tenfold in M-199, and centrifuged for 2 hours at 159,000 × g centrifuge gravity force. The recovered virus pellets were resuspended in M-199 to be serially diluted, and added to the tissue cultures. Cultures were incubated at 33°C for 48 and 72 hours, examined microscopically, and scored on a scale of 0 to 4+ for virus-induced cytopathic effect (CPE). Appropriate cultures of virus alone recovered from the hard surface as well as chemical compound alone for cytotoxic purpose were also included in each test.

Determining Virucidal Activity. At the nontoxic levels of chemical compound, the absence of any virus-induced cytopathology was indicative of virucidal activity. Comparison was then made at this point between the titer of the "virus control" and titer of the virus-compound set. A reduction in virus titer of 3 logs (99.9%) or greater for test compound was generally required.

Virucide Floating Technique (Van der Groen et al.)

Van der Groen et al. (1980) described a new method for virucide testing against some arboviruses using the virucide floating technique, as follows.

Preparation of Viruses. Virus stock of vesicular stomatitis virus (VSV), chikungunya virus (CHIK), West Nile (WN) virus, Bangyi (BGN) virus, and a bunya-like virus were prepared in Vero cells. AnY 1444, an orbivirus, was prepared in BHK-21-cells. Vero and BHK-21 cells were cultured in TC-medium 199 supplemented with 7% and 10% inactivated calf serum, respectively, buffered with 13 mM sodium bicarbonate.

Virucide Floating Test Procedure.
Step 1: A block of 2% agarose of about 1 cm² was cut and mounted on the edge of a glass slide.
Step 2: A known quantity of virus suspension was put on the surface of the agarose and allowed to diffuse and

evaporate until the surface was completely dry; this usually took about 10 minutes.
Step 3: Two drops of 0.5% (w/v) formvar (BDH) dissolved in 1,2-dichloroethane (Merck) were then added and left for a few seconds. Excess formvar was then removed by placing the slide vertically against blotting paper.
Step 4: When the film was dry, the edges of the block were cut with a sharp knife.
Step 5: The block was dipped gently into the disinfectant solution; this moment of virus-disinfectant contact was noted.
Step 6: After a known time of contact the virus film was removed from the disinfectant solution by picking up the film with a sealed pipette. Any excess disinfectant still present was removed by gently touching the side wall of a tube.
Step 7: The film was transferred into 1 ml of tissue culture medium and disrupted with the sealed Pasteur pipette to release residual virus particles into suspension.
Step 8: This suspension was inoculated into tissue cultures in order to determine residual infectious virus. In control experiments the disinfectant was replaced by tissue culture medium.

Virus Assay. All viruses, except AnY 1444, were assayed in Vero cells by the 50% end-point method as previously described (Van der Groen et al., 1976). Serial tenfold dilutions of AnY 1444 virus in TC medium 199 with 2% inactivated calf serum were inoculated into four wells of microtissue culture plates, each well containing 5×10^3 BHK-21 cells.

The virus control titers ($TCID_{50}$/ml) recovered from the floating virus film varied from $10^{4.7}$ for WN virus, $10^{5.2}$ for BGN virus, $10^{5.7}$ for VSV and CHIK, to $10^{6.0}$ for AnY 1444 virus. Therefore, the virus to be tested in this method need not be a high-titered one. However, the method is limited by the chemical resistance of the formvar sheet to the disinfectant. Ethanol cannot be tested.

Aerosol Test Method

Sing, Elliker, and Sandine (1964b) described a procedure that simulated conditions applicable to circumstances where air-borne phages were being controlled by germicidal aerosols, whereby resistance of phages and effectiveness of germicidal aerosols could be measured. Their procedure is as follows.

Experimental. In order to evaluate various aerosols, a confined area was needed. This was provided by selecting a chamber lined with transite cement board. This chamber had a volume of 29.25 ft³, could be vented adequately, contained an observation window (2.5 × 5 ft), and was so constructed that all manipulations inside could be made through rubber glove ports.

A nebulizer (Fisher Catalog No. 5–719–5) was used to infect the chamber with a given amount of bacteriophage. This type of sprayer was chosen because it was constructed entirely of glass, could readily be cleaned and sterilized, and produced an ultrafine mist. The germicide sprayer was a simpler air-pressure type of sprayer that operates by means of an air flow directed horizontally across the orifice of a vertical feed tube dipping into the germicide solution. It was constructed using a 125-ml Erlenmeyer flask fitted with a No. 5 rubber stopper. The size of the droplets could be controlled by the size of the orifice of the supply tube. The orifice size was approximately 0.75 mm in diameter.

An air sampler developed by Andersen (1958) was incorporated in this study for collecting and enumerating viable air-borne phage particles. The instrument consists of a series of six sieve-type samplers through which the sample of air is drawn. The device is pressure sealed with gaskets and three adjustable spring fasteners. Each stage contains a plate perforated with 400 holes resting above an exposed petri dish of culture medium. Air is drawn through the device at the rate of 1 cubic foot per minute (cfm), and a jet of air from each of these holes plays on the surface of the medium. The size of the holes is constant for each stage but decreases in each succeeding lower stage. Consequently the air velocity increases in each succeeding stage so that the larger particles are impacted on the medium surface from the larger openings in the first stages and the smaller particles, depending on their size and inertia, are impacted on the last stages in the lower part of the sampler.

The collection medium used in the Andersen sampler was 5% gelatin containing an appropriate inactivator. For inactivation of iodine and chlorine compounds, 144 mg of sodium thiosulfate per 100 ml of 5% gelatin was used. Quaternary ammonium compound was inactivated by addition of 6.66 g of asolectin, 46.8 ml of Tween 80, and 80 ml of 4M phosphate buffer per liter of 5% gelatin adjusted to pH 7.2. A 5% gelatin in 50M phosphate-buffered solution at pH 7.2 was used to inactivate phosphoric acid wetting agent. All collection media were sterilized and stored in sterile bottles prior to use.

The organisms used in the host-phage system were *Streptococcus cremoris* strain 144F and *Streptococcus diacetilactic* strain 18–16. These organisms were activated from lyophilized stocks maintained in the Department of Microbiology at Oregon State University, and they were propagated by daily transfer in 10% sterile nonfat milk. Corresponding strains of bacteriophages were used. These were maintained as filtrates in whey having a titer of 10^{10} pfu/ml. The whey, prepared from infected milk cultures, was assayed for pfu/ml by the overlay method of Adams (1959) using semisolid lactic agar seeded with about 10^7 host cells. In preparing the phage for trials the filtrate was standardized to a concentration of 5×10^4 phage/ml with sterile milk whey.

In evaluating the effectiveness of any germicide either in aqueous solution or applied as an aerosol, certain fixed constants must prevail in order to measure accurately the gross effects. Many of these factors such as application of phage and germicide, type of collecting substances and appropriate collection times had to be established by trial and error. Once established, however, these factors had to remain constant throughout the trials made

on different germicides. The comparative results were then used as an index of their effectiveness.

The establishment of an optimum time and interval for taking the air sample was determined from a phage "fallout curve" within the test chamber. The percentage of the number of phage particles that had fallen out in the chamber was determined from the curve. From these data, a period of 5 minutes was selected as the air sample collection time. This period would commence immediately after the application of the experimental germicide or control solution. This was considered an appropriate period because at least 92 to 93% of the phage particles would be airborne during the first 5 minutes after application of experimental germicide or control solution and would facilitate the removal of a representative sample of air containing viable phages.

Procedure Adopted. The method employed for evaluating the effectiveness of germicidal aerosols on airborne phage was standardized after several modifications that involved variation of level of infection of test chamber method of spraying test agents and germicides, type of collection medium and periods of sampling. Following considerable experimentation discussed previously, the adopted method was as follows.

The collection plates from the Andersen sample: were poured with 10 ml of 5% gelatin containing an inactivator and placed at refrigeration temperature (2°C) to solidify the gelatin. The phage infection mixture was standardized in the sprayer with sterile whey to a volume of 50 ml with a titer of 5×10^4 pfu/ml. Just prior to the trial, respective germicide solutions at desired concentrations were weighed into 125-ml Erlenmeyer flasks (the germicide spray reservoir) to provide 80 g total net weight of germicide. Both the infection and germicide sprayers were weighed before and after each trial to ensure constant application into the test chamber.

The Andersen sampler was loaded with six petri plates, each containing previously cooled, solidified 5% gelatin, and placed in the test chamber. The chamber containing the Andersen sampler, the infection sprayer, and the germicide sprayer was sealed off. The chamber then was infected with the standardized whey suspension of phage for 4 minutes. Immediately following the infection, the experimental germicide was sprayed for 45 seconds. The chamber was now completely saturated with vapor. Following the application of the germicide, the vacuum hose was attached to the sampler and suction applied at the rate of 1 cfm for 5 minutes. The air flow was regulated by a flowmeter. The chamber then was opened and the plates removed from the sampler. Each plate was covered with a sterile lid. These gelatin collection plates were melted, aliquots removed, and appropriate dilutions made.

The plaque count method was used to assay for the remaining phages. Plates were incubated upright for 12 to 14 hours at 30°C, and plaques were counted on each collection stage of the sampler; these were summated and reported as total number of phages collected per trial. The magnitude of recovery using this procedure with phage strains 144F and 18–16 in the absence of any aerosol germicide was in excess of 10^6 pfu/ml.

PROTOCOL FOR TESTING DISINFECTANTS AGAINST FOWL PEST (NEWCASTLE DISEASE VIRUS AND FOWL PLAQUE VIRUS) APPROVED BY THE MINISTRY OF AGRICULTURE, FISHERIES AND FOOD (ENGLAND, 1970)

The Ministry of Agriculture, Fisheries and Food (1970) in Weybridge, Surrey, England, also has a method for testing disinfectants against Newcastle disease virus and fowl plaque virus using yeast as the organic load. The test (consisting of a single or a triple dilution test), to be carried out at the Central Veterinary Laboratory, Weybridge, will be similar to that laid down for general purpose disinfectants except that the test organisms will be Newcastle disease virus, strain Herts, 1933. The test mixtures will be held at 4°C ± 0.5° for 30 minutes, and at the end of this time a dilution will be made in 5% inactivated horse serum. Further dilutions will be made for titrations of the virus in embryonated eggs. The disinfectant under test must give a reduction of at least 10^4 in virus titer.

The test will consist of (a) a toxicity test and (b) a virus test, using 9-day-old embryonated eggs.

(a) Toxicity Test

(To determine if the disinfectant under test is toxic to embryonated eggs at the lowest dilution to be used in the test, i.e., at a 1 in 400 dilution of the manufacturer's lowest recommended dilution.)

Test Protocol

(i) The recommended dilutions (manufacturer's recommended dilution) of the disinfectant are prepared using WHO hard water.

(ii) 2.5 ml of each of these dilutions of disinfectant is added to an equal volume of a 5% dry-weight suspension of yeast prepared as directed in BS 808:1938.

(iii) After thorough mixing, the test mixture is held at 4°C ± 0.5° for 30 minutes, with shaking at intervals.

(iv) The test mixture is then further diluted 1 in 200 in 5% inactivated (56°C for 30 minutes) horse serum prepared using sterile distilled water.

(v) 0.2 ml of this dilution is then inoculated into the allantoic cavity of each of 10 embryonated eggs. Ten control eggs are similarly inoculated with the yeast suspension diluted with an equal volume of hard water.

(vi) All the eggs are examined daily for 7 days, and the disinfectant is regarded as nontoxic if the embryos remain alive at the end of this period.

(b) Virus Test

The test virus is the Herts, 1933 strain of Newcastle disease virus stored at −55°C. The infectivity titer of the virus used must be $10^{6.6} \pm 0.4$ EID$_{50}$/0.1 ml allantoic fluid.

Test Protocol

(i) Add 1.0 ml virus (allantoic fluid) to 24.0 ml 5% dry weight yeast suspension.

(ii) Add 2.5 ml yeast-virus mixture to 2.5 ml disinfectant dilution (manufacturer's recommended dilutions prepared in WHO hard water).

(iii) Mix thoroughly and transfer to a fresh container.

(iv) Hold at 4°C ± 0.5° for 30 minutes, shaking at intervals.

(v) Dilute 1 in 200 in 5% inactivated horse serum in sterile distilled water.

(vi) Prepare further dilutions for virus titration in log dilution steps, using 5% inactivated horse serum.

(vii) Titrate in embryonated eggs, using 7 eggs per dilution and inoculating 0.2 ml into the allantoic cavity of each egg and incubating at 37.5°C.

Titrate: undiluted.

10^{-1} dilution 10^{-3} dilution 10^{-5} dilution
10^{-2} dilution 10^{-4} dilution 10^{-6} dilution

(viii) All eggs are examined daily for 7 days.

(ix) All eggs that die or remain alive after 7 days are tested for the presence of viral hemagglutinin. The titration end point is determined by the method of Reed and Muench (1938).

To determine drop in infectivity titer, the titer of test material is subtracted from the titer of control material. If this is 10^4 or greater than 10^4, the disinfectant passes; if less than 10^4, the disinfectant fails.

EPA EFFICACY DATA REQUIREMENTS FOR VIRUCIDES

None of the present methods for testing virucides has been accepted as an official method. The Environmental Protection Agency (1981), however, will accept adequate data developed by any virologic technique that is recognized as technically sound, and that simulates to the extent possible in the laboratory the conditions under which the product is intended for use. For virucides whose use-directions identify the product as one intended for use upon dry, inanimate, environmental surfaces (such as floors, tables, and cleaned and dried medical instruments) carrier methods, which are modifications of either the AOAC Use-Dilution Method (for liquid surface disinfectants) or the AOAC Germicidal Spray Products Test (for surface spray disinfectants), must be used in the development of the virologic data. To simulate in-use conditions, the specific virus to be treated must be inoculated onto hard surfaces, allowed to dry, and then treated with the product according to the directions for use on the product label. One surface for each of two different batches of disinfectant must be tested against a recoverable virus titer of at least 10^4 from the test surface (e.g., petri dish, glass slide, steel cyl-

Table 62–4. *Test Results*

Dilution of Virus	Virus—Disfectant*	Virus—Control*	Cytotoxicity—Control
10^{-1}	T T T T	+ + + +	T T T T
10^{-2}	T T T T	+ + + +	T T T T
10^{-3}	T 0 0 0	+ + + +	T 0 0 0
10^{-4}	0 0 0 0	+ + + +	0 0 0 0
10^{-5}	0 0 0 0	+ + + +	0 0 0 0
10^{-6}	0 0 0 0	+ + + 0	0 0 0 0
10^{-7}	0 0 0 0	+ 0 0 0	0 0 0 0
10^{-8}	0 0 0 0	0 0 0 0	0 0 0 0

*Recovery of virus from surface demonstrated by cytopathogenic effect, fluorescent antibody, plaque count, animal response, or other recognized acceptable technique.

Note: T = toxic; + = virus recovered; 0 = no virus recovered.

inder) for a specific exposure period at room temperature. The virus is then assayed by an appropriate virologic technique. The protocol for the viral assay must provide the following information:

1. The virus recovery from a minimum of 4 determinations per each dilution in the assay system (tissue culture, embryonated egg, animal infection, or whatever assay system is employed).
2. Cytotoxicity controls: The effect of the germicide on the assay system from a minimum of 4 determinations per each dilution.
3. The activity of the germicide against the test virus from a minimum of 4 determinations per each dilution in the assay system.
4. Any special methods that were used to increase the virus titer and to detoxify the residual germicide.
5. The ID-50 values calculated for each assay.
6. The test results shall be reported as the reduction of the virus titer by the activity of the germicide (ID-50 of the virus control less the ID-50 of the test system), expressed as $\log_{10}$ and calculated by a statistical method (Reed and Muench, 1938; Litchfield and Wilcoxon, 1949).
7. For virucidal data to be acceptable, the product must demonstrate complete inactivation of the virus at all dilutions. When cytotoxicity is evident (as in Tables 62–4 through 62–6) at least a 3-log reduction in titer must be demonstrated beyond the

cytotoxic level. The calculated viral titers must be reported with the test results.

A typical laboratory report of a *single* test with *one* virus (recovered from a treated surface) involving a tissue culture, therefore, would include the details of the method employed and the information in Tables 62–4, 62–5, and 62–6.

Claims of virucidal activity for a product must be restricted to those viruses that have actually been tested. Separate studies on two batches of product are required for each virus.

ACKNOWLEDGMENTS

I am grateful to Dr. Richard L. Crowell, Professor and Chairman, Department of Microbiology and Immunology, Hahnemann University Medical School, for his valuable suggestions and critical comments in preparing the manuscript, and to Dr. J. Steven McDougal, Chief of Immunology Branch, Centers for Disease Control, U.S. Public Health Service, for his generous advice in disinfectant testing against AIDS virus. I would also like to thank Dr. Morton Klein, Professor of Temple University School of Medicine, for his continued support and encouragement.

Table 62–5. *Calculation of the Tissue Culture Infective Dose 50 (TCID₅₀)**

Virus Dilution Inoculated	No. Infected/ No. Inoculated	No. Infected	No. Not Infected	Accumulated Values			
				No. Infected	No. Not Infected	No. Infected/ No. Inoculated	Percent Infected
10^{-1}	4/4	4	0	24	0	24/24	100
10^{-2}	4/4	4	0	20	0	20/20	100
10^{-3}	4/4	4	0	16	0	16/16	100
10^{-4}	4/4	4	0	12	0	12/12	100
10^{-5}	4/4	4	0	8	0	8/8	100
10^{-6}	3/4	3	1	4	1	4/5	80
10^{-7}	1/4	1	3	1	4	1/5	20
10^{-8}	0/4	0	4	0	8	0/8	0

$TCID_{50} = 10^{6.5}$

*Based on method of Reed and Muench, 1938.

Table 62–6. *Calculation of the Tissue Culture Infective Dose 50 (TCID$_{50}$)**

Virus Dilution Inoculated	No. Toxic/ No. Inoculated	No. Toxic	No. Not Toxic	Accumulated Values			
				No. Toxic	No. Not Toxic	No. Infected/ No. Inoculated	Percent Toxic
10^{-1}	4/4	4	0	9	0	9/9	100
10^{-2}	4/4	4	0	5	0	5/5	100
10^{-3}	1/4	1	3	1	3	1/4	25
10^{-4}	0/4	0	4	0	7	0/7	0
10^{-5}	0/4	0	4	0	11	0/11	0
10^{-6}	0/4	0	4	0	15	0/15	0
10^{-7}	0/4	0	4	0	19	0/19	0
10^{-8}	0/4	0	4	0	23	0/23	0

TCID$_{50}$ = $10^{2.7}$

Therefore: Virus inactivation = TCID$_{50}$ − TCLD$_{50}$ = $10^{3.8}$ log$_{10}$. Claims for virucidal activity for a product must be restricted to those viruses that have actually been tested.

*Based on method of Reed and Muench, 1938.

REFERENCES

Adams, N.H. 1959. Bacteriophages. New York. Interscience Publishers, Inc.

Andersen, A.A. 1958. New sampler for the collection, sizing and enumeration of viable airborne particles. J. Bacteriol., *76*, 471–484.

Armstrong, J.A., and Froelich, E.J. 1964. Inactivation of virus by benzalkonium chloride. Appl. Microbiol., *12*, 132–137.

Association of Official Analytical Chemists. 1970. Official Methods of Analysis 59–72 (W. Horwitz, Ed.). Association of Official Analytical Chemists, Washington.

Association of Official Analytical Chemists. 1960. Official Methods of Analysis 63–66 (W. Horwitz, Ed.). Association of Official Analytical Chemists, Washington.

Avampato, J.E., Amundsen, S.M., and Vasington, P.J. 1969. Virucidal testing methods. Proc. 55th Meet. Chem. Specialties, Mfgs. Asso., New York, pp. 126–129.

Barre-Sinoussi, F., et al. 1983. Science, *220*, 868.

Blackwell, J.H., and Chen, J.H.S. 1970. Effects of various germicidal chemicals on H.Ep.2 cell culture and Harpes simplex virus. J. Assoc. Off. Anal. Chem., *53*, 1229–1236.

Brown, W.E. 1976. Virucide testing of disinfectants against Newcastle disease virus using chick embryo techniques. Paper presented at ASTM Antiviral Agents Group Memphis-Meeting (October 28).

Chang, T.W. 1976. Problems associated with testing virucide against influenza viruses by using tissue culture techniques. Paper presented at ASTM antiviral Agents Group Memphis-Meeting (October 28).

Chen, J.H.S., and Phebus, D.E. 1979. Study of viral recovery from the carrier used in disinfectant testing. Paper presented at ASTM Antiviral Agents Group Philadelphia-Meeting (April 4th).

Chen, J.H.S., and Phebus, D.E. 1978. The influence of organic load on the efficacy of virucide against influenza virus A2. Paper presented at ASTM Antiviral Agents Group Philadelphia-Meeting (March 16).

Chen, J.H.S., and Phebus, D.E. 1977. Effect of virus culture by drying treatment in testing virucide. Paper presented at ASTM Antiviral Agents Group Philadelphia-Meeting (March 31).

Chen, J.H.S. 1973. Comparison of virus recovery techniques for assessing the virucidal activity of disinfectant spray products. J. Assoc. Off. Anal. Chem., *5*, 130–132.

Chen, J.H.S. 1976. A survey of virucide testing laboratories. Paper presented at ASTM Antiviral Agents Group Memphis-Meeting (October 28).

Craig, L.C. 1965. Differential dialysis. In *Advances in Analytical Chemistry and Instrumentation*. Volume 4. Edited by C.N. Reilly. New York, Interscience Publishers.

Dahlgren, C.M., Decker, H.M., and Harstad, J.B. 1961. A slit sampler for collecting T-3 bacteriophage and Venezuelan equine encephalomyelitis virus. Appl. Microbiol., *9*, 103–107.

Devos, A., Viaene, N., and Deviriese, L. 1969. Tijdschr., Diergeneeskd., *38*, 266.

Dulbecco, R. 1952. Production of plaques in monolayer tissue cultures by single particles of an animal virus. Proc. Natl. Acad. Sci., *38*, 747–752.

Environmental Protection Agency. 1977. Methods for evaluating the virucidal activity of disinfectants.

El Mekki, A.A., Nieuwenhuysen, P., Van der Groen, G., and Pattyn, S.R. 1979. In Proc. Belgian Biophysical Society 10, Universitaire Instelling Antwerpen, to be published in Arch. Intern. Biochim. Physiol.

Fellowes, O.N. 1965. Some surface active agents and their virucidal effects on foot-and-mouth disease virus. Appl. Microbiol., *13*, 694–697.

Gaustad, J.W., McDuff, C.R., and Hatcher, H.J. 1974. Test method for the evaluation of virucidal efficiency of three common liquid surface disinfectants on a simulated environmental surface. Appl. Microbiol., 748–752.

Gaustad, J.W. 1976. Modified AOAC use-dilution techniques for determining the virucidal activity of liquid surface disinfectants. Paper presented at ASTM Antiviral Agents Group Memphis-Meeting (October 28).

Hays, H.A., and Elliker, P.R. 1959. Virucidal activity of new phosphoric acid wetting agent sanitizer against bacteriophage of Streptococcus cremoris. J. Milk Food Technol., *22*, 109–111.

Herrmann, E.C., Gabliks, J., Engle, C.G., and Perlman, P.L. 1960. Agar diffusion method for detection and bioassay of antiviral antibiotics. Proc. Soc. Exp. Biol. Med., *103*, 625–628.

Klein, M. 1976. Susceptibility of viruses to germicides. Paper presented at ASTM Antiviral Agents Group Memphis-Meeting (October 28).

Klein, M. 1971. Personal communication. Temple University, Philadelphia.

Klein, M. 1965a. Unpublished report. Temple University School of Medicine, Philadelphia.

Klein, M. 1965b. The chemical inactivation of viruses. Fed. Proc., *24*, abst. 1052.

Klein, M. 1965c. Viruses elude most germicides. World Med. News, *6*, 54.

Klein, M. 1956. The evaluation of the virucidal activity of germicides. Proc. Chem. Spec. Mfg. Assoc., 98–100.

Klein, M., and DeForest, A. 1963. The inactivation of viruses by germicides. Proc. Chem. Spec. Mfg. Assoc., 49th Mid-Year Meeting, pp. 116–118.

Litchfield, J.T., Jr., and Wilcoxon, F. 1949. A simplified method of evaluating dose-effect experiments. J. Pharm. Exp. Ther. *96*, 99–113.

Lorenz, D.E., and Jann, G.J. 1964. Use-dilution test and Newcastle disease virus. Appl. Microbiol., *12*, 24–26.

Mahl, M.C. 1976. Testing disinfectant products against viruses by a method similar to AOAC use dilution method. Paper presented at ASTM Antiviral Agents Group Memphis-Meeting (October 28).

McDougal, J.S., et al. 1985. Immunoassay for the detection and quantitation of infectious human retrovirus, lymphadenopathy-associated virus (LAV). J. Immunol. Methods, *76*, 171–183.

McGeady, M.L., Siak, J-S, and Crowell, R.L. 1979. Survival of coxsackievirus B3 under diverse environmental conditions. Appl. Environ. Microbiol., *37*, 972–977.

Ministry of Agriculture, Fisheries and Food. 1970. Protocol of test for approval of disinfectants for use against fowl pest (Newcastle disease virus, fowl plaque virus). Central Veterinary Laboratory, Weybridge, Surrey.

Ministry of Agriculture, Fisheries and Food. 1969. Explanatory note on the approval of disinfectants for the purposes of the Diseases of Animals Act 1950. Department of Agriculture and Fisheries for Scotland.

National Academy of Science. 1959. Methods for the examination of poultry biologicals. National Research Council, Washington, Publication *705*, 37–65.

Noll, H., and Youngner, J.S. 1959. Virus-lipid interactions. II. The mechanisms of adsorption of lipophilic viruses to water-insoluble polar lipids. Virology, *8*, 319–343.

Pancic, F., et al. 1977. Convenient in vitro methods for the testing of virucidal agents. Paper presented at ASTM Antiviral Agents Group Philadelphia Meeting (March 31).

Patty, R.E., and May, H.J. 1961. The production of high concentrations of foot-

and-mouth disease virus in cultures of cells on glass. Am. J. Vet. Res., *22*, 926–931.

Poiesz, B.J., et al. 1980. Proc. Natl. Acad. Sci. U. S. A., *77*, 7415.

Prince, H.N. 1976. Mouse as a host system for virucide activity. Paper presented at ASTM Antiviral Agents Group Memphis-Meeting (Octover 28).

Reagan, K.J., McGeady, M.L., and Crowell, R.L. 1981. Persistence of human rhinovirus infectivity under diverse environmental conditions. Appl. Environ. Microbiol., *41*, 618–620.

Reed, L.J., and Muench, H.A. 1938. A simple method of estimating fifty per cent endpoints. Am. J. Hyg., *27*, 493–497.

Shannon, W.A. 1976. The use of cell culture technique in virucide testing. Paper presented at ASTM Antiviral Agents Group Memphis-Meeting (October 28).

Siminoff, P. 1961. A plaque suppression method for the study of antiviral compounds. Appl. Microbiol., *9*, 66–72.

Sing, E.L., Elliker, P.R., and Sandine, W.E. 1964*a*. Comparative destruction of airborne lactic bacteriophage by various germicides applied as aerosols. J. Milk Food Technol., *27*, 129–134.

Sing, E.L., Elliker, P.R., and Sandine, W.E. 1964*b*. A method for evaluating the destruction of airborne bacteriophages. J. Milk Food Technol., *27*, 125–128.

Slavin, G. 1973. A reproducible surface contamination method for disinfectant tests. Br. Vet. J., *129*, 1–13–18.

Smith, J.D., and DeHarven, E. 1973. Concentration of herpesviruses. J. Virol., *2*, 325–328.

Sykes, G. 1965. Disinfection of viruses. In *Disinfection and Sterilization*. 2nd Edition. Philadelphia, J.B. Lippincott, pp. 291–306.

Van der Groen, G., Van den Berghe, D.A.R., and Pattyn, S.R. 1976. J. Gen. Virol., *34*, 353–361.

Van der Groen, G., El Mekki, A.A., and Pattyn, S.R. 1980. New method for virucide testing. J. Virol. Methods, *1*, 27–31.

Vasington, P.J. 1965. Personal communication. Lederle Laboratories, Pearl River.

Wilson, M.D., and Nakane, P.K. 1978. In *Immunofluorescence and Related Techniques*. Edited by W. Knapp, K. Holubar, and G. Wick. Amsterdam, Elsevier, p. 215.

Wolff, D.A. 1977. Quantitation of viruses for antiviral testing. Paper presented at ASTM Antiviral Agents Group Cleveland-Meeting (November 3rd).

Wright, H.S. 1976. A virucide test method by using tissue culture and immunofluorescence. Paper presented at ASTM Antiviral Agents Group Memphis-Meeting (October 28).

Wright, H.S. 1970*a*. Test method for determining the virucidal activity of disinfectant against vesicular stomatitis virus. Appl. Microbiol., *19*, 92–95.

Wright, H.S. 1970*b*. Hog cholera virucide testing method using a fluorescent antibody technique. ASTM Annual Meeting 1970. Boston.

CHAPTER 63

METHODS OF TESTING PROTOZOACIDES AND ANTIHELMINTICS

S.E. Leland, Jr.

Certain (but not all) protozoan and helminth parasites spend a portion of their life cycles outside of the host in nonparasitic situations. These nonparasitic stages provide the parasite with the opportunity for transmission to a new host or reinfection of the same host. Where such free-living or nonparasitic stages occur, the use of chemical agents to interrupt the life cycle at these stages or at least to reduce the level of contamination is particularly desirable, since prevention of infection is preferable to treatment of the host. However, nature has arranged things such that the nonparasitic stages in general are the most resistant and protected stages in the life cycle. Evaluating chemicals for activity against these stages requires complete knowledge of the life cycle of the particular species used in order to make valid interpretations.

Standardized testing methods in general are not available for each of the many widely varying organisms in these groups. Each investigator has detailed the procedure employed for the specific organism used, and these have required modification where the test organism is changed or in some cases with a change in the chemicals being tested.

Basically, test procedures consist of the following elements:

1. The particular nonparasitic stage is selected for challenge by the chemical agent, taking into account any innate vulnerability and considering ultimate practical application. It is then necessary to produce this selected stage in a sufficient quantity and in a viable state so that adequate numbers are available for experiments at regular intervals. This usually represents a major portion of the effort invested in the testing. Since, in most cases, in vitro culture techniques are not available, it may be necessary to maintain the organism in the host and preferably with a monospecific infection.

2. The organism is then subjected to the chemical agent in a manner simulating projected practical application. It should be noted at this point that these organisms may be vulnerable to a chemical agent in the naked or exposed state of the testing procedures, but in their natural environment in association with feces, soil, plant material, or large quantities of water, the agent may prove to be ineffective.

3. After exposure to the chemical agent, the organism is examined for obvious cytopathologic changes and cessation of normal development, and is tested for viability. Tests for viability will vary with the organisms being used and the availability of normal hosts. In some cases, survival and continued development following exposure are sufficient evidence that a chemical agent is ineffective. It may be necessary to wash the organism free of the chemical agent and introduce it into a suitable culture system to establish viability. In some cases, culture systems do not exist, and viability must be tested in a susceptible host that has been raised in a special manner to preclude natural infection.

4. A chemical agent showing activity is then tested under practical or field conditions. In the transition from laboratory experience to practical field application, problems may arise, many of which are unpredictable or difficult to control. Considerable effort may be necessary to solve these problems at the practical or applied level.

In specific experimental designs, isolation and concentration of the nonparasitic stage(s) may be required; such techniques as gradient-centrifugation for nematode eggs (Marquardt, 1961; Leland, 1967), the baermann procedure for nematode larvae (Baermann, 1917), cesium chloride gradient purification for *Cryptosporidium* (Upton et al., 1988), and sucrose flotation-percoll sedimentation for *Giardia* spp. (Marchin et al., 1983) have been used.

Of the pathogenic organisms where transmission by water has been established, the cysts of *Entamoeba histolytica* are apparently the most resistant to destruction by the chemical disinfectants. Chlorination, for example, has little effect on the cysts. The severe epidemic of amebic dysentery in Chicago in 1933 dramatically demonstrated the importance of transmission by cyst-containing chlorinated water. Thus, tests to detect a suitable chemical disinfectant have been set forth, and the method of Kessel and Moore (1946) is detailed here as an example of a test for a protozoacide:

1. Multiple geometric dilutions, in distilled water, of the test antiseptic are prepared in volumes of 9 ml in capped centrifuge tubes, brought to 20°C in a water bath and inoculated with 1 ml of a standard cyst suspension. It should be noted that cultures of *Entamoeba histolytica* must be induced by culture manipulation (Kessel et al., 1944) to form cysts, since the more vulnerable trophozoites afford no test significance at this point. The trophozoites are destroyed by distilled water. In addition, a good cyst-producing strain of *Entamoeba histolytica* should be obtained to ensure a large quantity of cysts for testing.

2. After 8 minutes, the solutions are removed and the cysts washed with distilled water by centrifugation.

3. The entire sediment is inoculated into Ringer's egg-serum medium containing starch and bacteria present in the original amebic culture.

4. Cultures are examined over a 5-day period for the appearance of viable trophozoites that would have developed from the cysts. If none is found, the authors conclude that the antiseptic killed the cysts.

5. The end points or dilutions (ED_{50}) that are cysticidal in half the trials are calculated according to the method of Reed and Muench (1938).

In recent years water-borne giardiasis has become a well established public health problem; the efficacy of chlorination for inactivation of *Giardia lamblia* cysts is a matter of concern to those responsible for water quality. Procedures used in determining inactivation of *Giardia* cysts following exposure to a disinfectant are recorded by Jarroll et al. (1981), Rice et al. (1982), and Marchin et al. (1983). The Environmental Protection Agency has adapted a protocol for testing all microbiologic water purifiers with *G. muris* as one of the test organisms (Marchin and Fina, 1989). The protocol provides for testing a proposed water purifier with the test organism under a variety of pHs, flow rates, and temperatures in waters containing added organic carbon and particulate matter. Successful halogen-containing water purifying units are required to effect a 3-log reduction in viability of *G. muris* cysts at 4°C with a chemical reductant being introduced as water exits the device. Marchin and Fina (1989) point out that all chemical disinfectants that in-

activate *Giardia* cysts require a discrete contact time; thus, this particular requirement precludes any device that depends solely on chemical disinfection for water purification.

Both the asexual and sexual stages of the pathogenic avian coccidial species *Eimeria tenella* have been cultivated successfully in cell culture (Strout and Ouellette, 1969; Doran, 1970). Thus it becomes possible to test in vitro the viability of free-living sporulated oocysts that have been subjected to various experimental disinfectants. Strout and Ouellette (1973) utilized the cell culture procedure to evaluate anticoccidial activity of compounds against the parasitic stages of *Eimeria tenella*.

Viability of *Giardia lamblia* (the human parasite) following exposure to a prospective disinfectant was determined by in vitro excystation (Rice and Schaefer, 1981). Viability of *G. muris* and *Cryptosporidium parvum* was determined by in vitro excystation and infectivity to mice (Marchin et al., 1985; Upton et al., 1988).

In the case of helminths, Leiper (1963) has reviewed the techniques used in evaluating chemical agents against nonparasitic species and the nonparasitic stages of parasitic species.

The eggs of cestodes or trematodes have not been used extensively to study the effects of chemical agents, whereas the nematodes have been used to evaluate interference with the development of the egg or the lethal effect on various nonparasitic larval stages. Egerton (1968) describes procedures for determining ovicidal or larvicidal effects of thiabendazole on nematodes of the genera *Ascaris*, *Haemonchus*, *Nematodirus*, *Necator*, *Ancylostoma*, *Oesophagostoma*, *Trichuris*, and *Strongyloides*. Other examples of nematodes used for testing include: horse strongyles (Parnell, 1936), infective larvae of horse strongyles (Leiper, 1937), various stages of sheep trichostrongyle larvae (Tiner, 1958), *Haemonchus contortus* larvae (Deschiens, 1954) and infective larvae of *Ancylostoma braziliense* (Blank et al., 1959). The chemical agent may be incorporated in a culture medium with the eggs and incubated at 24° to 27°C, or the test may be carried out on developed infective larvae. The effect of the chemical agent is judged by the concentration necessary to suppress development of the egg to the infective stage where cultures are used, but the larvicidal effect must be used in the case of infective larvae since, in the latter case, development normally is suspended unless the infective larvae reach a susceptible host. In order to determine whether infective larvae have retained infectivity, it may be necessary to introduce them into a susceptible host or into an in vitro cultivation system capable of supporting growth of the parasitic stages. Leland (1970) has reported the in vitro cultivation of a number of nematode species through their parasitic stages. Leland et al. (1971, 1975) also described procedures where parasitic stages of *Cooperia punctata*, an intestinal nematode of cattle, grown in vitro were used to detect direct anthelmintic activity of various classes of compounds. Compounds were tested over a range of concentrations in tenfold increments of drug per ml of medium to establish the concentration at which approximately 50% of the nematodes in a culture were dead 1 week after exposure. Two in vitro testing procedures evolved and were designated as presumptive and confirmatory. The former is relatively rapid and requires only seconds for evaluation, whereas the latter involves live-dead worm counts and is more informative. Thus, the nonparasitic stages of *C. punctata*, and particularly the infective larvae, could be exposed to a chemical agent and a quantitative or comparative measure of the agent's activity obtained by subsequent in vitro culturing. Mechanical or thermal stimulation or the use of the Baermann (1917) technique may be helpful in establishing motility of infective larvae after exposure to a chemical agent. However, the presence of active motile infective larvae does not necessarily indicate retained infectivity.

Leland (1964) utilized the following procedure to evaluate chemical agents for activity against the nonparasitic stages of *Strongyloides ransomi*, a pathogenic nematode of young swine.

1. Feces with a high concentration of worm eggs are collected from experimentally infected donor pigs with monospecific infections of *S. ransomi*.
2. Each batch of feces is homogenized by adding sufficient water so the eggs of the resulting semisolid mixture are evenly distributed.
3. Each batch is divided into 50-g (occasionally 100-g) portions. The chemical agent is added in decreasing amounts (tenfold) to 50-g portions and mixed. Two 50-g portions from each batch are not treated with the chemical agent and serve as controls.
4. Each 50-g portion is mixed with 14 g of sphagnum moss or vermiculite, packed in the lower one fourth of a jar and incubated 3 to 7 days at 24°C.
5. After incubation, the cultures are subjected to the Baermann (1917) technique to recover any nematodes.
6. The various stages of larvae are counted by a dilution technique and the control cultures compared with those exposed to the chemical agent.

By varying the age of the feces used, a chemical agent may be tested against the egg, larvae, and, in the case of *Strongyloides*, against the nonparasitic adults.

Thus, the very nature of these nonparasitic stages, with their naturally protected and resistant forms and their wide variation in habits and development, makes testing procedures highly specific and standardization of utmost importance.

REFERENCES

Baermann, G. 1917. Eine einfache methode zur auffindung von ankylostomum—(Nematoden)—larven in erdproben. Ned. Tijdschr. Geneeskd.—Indie, 57, 131–137.

Blank, H., Winter, M.W., and Beck, J.W. 1959. The effects of chemical and physical agents on filariform larvae of *Ancylostoma braziliense*. Am. J. Trop. Med. Hyg., 8, 401–404.

Deschiens, R. 1954. Sur un test d'activité anthelminthique des medicaments. Bull. Acad. Natl. Med., 3e Serie 138, 184–185.

Doran, D.T. 1970. *Eimeria tenella*: From sporozoites to oocysts in cell culture. Proc. Helm. Soc. Wash., 37, 84–92.

Egerton, J.R. 1968. The ovicidal and larvicidal effect of thiabendazole on various helminth species. Texas Rep. Biol. Med., 27, 561–580.

Jarroll, E.L., Bingham, A.K., and Meyers, E.A. 1981. Effect of chlorine on *Giardia lamblia* cyst viability. Appl. Environ. Microbiol., 41, 483–487.

Kessel, J.F., and Moore, F.J. 1946. Emergency sterilization of drinking water with heteropolar cation antiseptics. I. Effectiveness against cysts of *Endamoeba histolytica*. Am. J. Trop. Med., 26, 345–350.

Kessel, J.F. et al. 1944. The cysticidal effects of chlorine and ozone on cysts of *Endamoeba histolytica*, together with a comparative study of several encystment media. Am. J. Trop. Med., 24, 177–183.

Leiper, J.W.G. 1937. On the value of various chemical substances as a means of destroying infective larvae of horse sclerostomes in the field. J. Helminthol., 15, 153–166.

Leiper, J.W.G. 1963. The evaluation of potential anthelmintics by in vitro techniques. In *The Evaluation of Anthelmintics*. New York, Merck, Sharp, & Dohme International, pp. 14–17.

Leland, S.E., Jr. 1967. In vitro cultivation of *Cooperia punctate* from egg to egg. J. Parasitol., 53, 1057–1060.

Leland, S.E., Jr. 1970. *In vitro* cultivation of nematode parasites important to veterinary medicine. Adv. Vet. Sci. Comp. Med., 14, 29–59.

Leland, S.E., Jr., and Bogue, J.H. 1964. Laboratory tests on the anthelmintic activity of thiabendazole against the free-living states of *Strongyloides ransomi*. J. Parasitol., 50(Suppl.), 61.

Leland, S.E., Jr., Ridley, R.K., Slonka, G.F., and Zimmerman, G.L. 1975. Detection of activity for various anthelmintics against in vitro-produced *Cooperia punctata*. Am. J. Vet. Res., 36, 449–456.

Leland, S.E., Jr., et al. 1971. Anthelmintic activity of trichlorfon, coumaphos, and naphthalophos against the in vitro grown parasitic stages of *Cooperia punctata*. J. Parasitol., 57, 1190–1197.

Marchin, G.L., and Fina, L.R. 1989. Contact and demand release disinfectants. In *Critical Reviews in Environmental Control*. Edited by C.P. Straub. Boca Raton, FL, CRC Press. 19, 277–290.

Marchin, G.L., Fina, L.R., and Lambert, J.L. 1985. The biocidal properties of the pentacide/demand-type resin -I₅. Proc. Am. Water Works Assoc. Water Quality Technology Conf., Dec 8–11, pp. 461–472.

Marchin, G.L., Fina, L.R., Lambert, J.L., and Fina, G.T. 1983. Effect of resin disinfectants -I₃ and -I₅ on *Giardia muris* and *Giardia lamblia*. Appl. Environ. Microbiol., 46, 965–969.

Marquardt, W.C. 1961. Separation of nematode eggs from fecal debris by gradient centrifugation. J. Parasitol., 47, 248–250.

Parnell, I.W. 1936. Studies on the bionomics and control of the bursate nematodes of horses and sheep. II. Technique. Can. J. Res., 14, 71–81.

Reed, L.J., and Muench, H. 1938. A simple method of estimating fifty per cent endpoints. Am. J. Hyg., 27, 493–497.

Rice, E.W., Hoff, J.C., and Schaefer III, F.W. 1982. Inactivation of Giardia cysts by chlorine. Appl. Environ. Microbiol., 43, 250–251.

Rice, E.W., and Schaefer III, F.W. 1981. Improved in vitro excystation procedure for *Giardia lamblia* cysts. J. Clin. Microbiol., 14, 709–710.

Strout, R.G., and Ouellette, C.A. 1973. *Eimeria tenella*: Screening of chemotherapeutic compounds in cell culture. Exp. Parasitol., 33, 477–485.

Strout, R.G. and Ouellette, C.A. 1969. Gametogony of *Eimeria tenella* (coccidia) in cell cultures. Science, 163, 695–696.

Tiner, J.D. 1958. A preliminary in vitro test for anthelmintic activity. Exp. Parasitol., 7, 292–305.

Upton, S.J., Tilley, M.E., Marchin, G.L., and Fina, L.R. 1988. Efficacy of a pentaiodide resin disinfectant on *Cryptosporidium parvum* (Apicomplexa: Cryptosporidiidae) oocytes in vitro. J. Parasitol., 74, 719–721.

CHAPTER 64

Effective Use of Liquid Chemical Germicides on Medical Devices: Instrument Design Problems

W.W. Bond, B.J. Ott, K.A. Franke, and J.E. McCracken

The purpose of this chapter is twofold: (1) to augment a number of other chapters in this book, and (2) to outline several current problem areas that have significant effects on the choice and efficiency of liquid chemical germicidal procedures widely used to reprocess heat-sensitive instruments used in a variety of medical speciality areas such as endoscopy, dentistry, urology, and gynecology. Health-care workers in these and other specialty areas are confronted with an increasing array of technologically advanced reusable instruments, many of which are physically complex, fragile, and expensive. Unfortunately, both the design and manufacture of a number of these instruments have centered almost entirely on the intended function of the device with insufficient consideration given to pertinent questions such as easy physical access to all potentially contaminated components, physical and chemical stability, verifiable methods for cleaning, disinfecting, or sterilizing, and clear, adequate instruction materials to ensure safe and effective use of the instruments. Further, there is a paucity of epidemiologic and laboratory data to either firmly identify real or potential infection risks with a particular instrument or procedure or to verify the adequacy of a wide variety of methods and materials or products used to reprocess these instruments. For example, numerous types of infections (bacterial, viral, and fungal) have been associated with the use of flexible fiberoptic endoscopes, but the exact causes and extent of these infections are not known because of under-reporting of such incidents in the literature (Axon et al., 1991; Gorse and Messner, 1991). This under-reporting could be due to factors such as a lack of adequate disease surveillance or outbreak investigation, reluctance of health-care workers to write papers, or fear of medicolegal consequences. Also, the majority of endoscopic procedures are done on an outpatient basis, and patients infected in this setting are seldom followed up and documented as are patients in a conventional hospital setting. The current reality is that health-care workers responsible for maintaining and reprocessing a significant number of complex, expensive, heat-sensitive medical instruments must make many of their own choices and rely, at least in part, on individual "institutional policy" (as indicated in several instruction manuals for instruments in this category) rather than on specific, data-based recommendations from the instrument manufacturer.

SELECTION OF APPROPRIATE GERMICIDAL PROCEDURES: GENERAL CONSIDERATIONS

The most effective method of ensuring the success of a disinfection or sterilization procedure is consistent adherence to an established, written protocol for cleaning and disinfection or sterilization by specifically trained health-care workers. Before establishing such a protocol or "institutional policy," a number of basic variables must be considered. These include (1) the relative infection risks inherent to the instrument, the medical procedure, or the patient, (2) the relative resistance levels of a variety of microorganisms, (3) the comparative powers of a variety of germicidal chemicals, and (4) a number of procedural factors that can influence the effectiveness of germicidal procedures. Depending on the clinical situation, some of the variables might be more important than others. Nevertheless, all should be considered in the planning of a reprocessing strategy.

Various types of medical instruments, because of differences in degree of patient contact and the particular medical procedure being done, can have substantially different risks of disease transmission if they are contaminated with viable microorganisms at time of use. For instance, a flexible fiberoptic endoscope used for a visual examination of the gut might have only a low to moderate degree of infection risk if the instrument is contaminated with microorganisms from previous patients or from environmental sources such as contaminated water used in the reprocessing procedure. However, if the instrument is used for an invasive diagnostic or surgical procedure such as an examination of the bile duct or a biopsy, the risk of infection will be high. Gram-negative septicemia after endoscopic manipulation of the bile duct is perhaps the most frequently reported infectious hazard of flexible endoscopy, and many of these episodes have been traced to inadequately disinfected instruments (Axon et al., 1991). Certain microorganisms are more invasive than others; also, patient factors such as the status of immune function and general health will affect the degree of infection risk under a given set of circumstances.

Microorganisms vary widely in their resistance levels to a given liquid chemical germicide, and these resistance levels can vary even within the same general group or genus. Other factors, such as the number of microorganisms in a given population, can affect the extent of a germicidal process necessary to accomplish disinfection or sterilization. However, the most important factor influencing the effectiveness of any germicidal procedure is the amount of organic material on the surface being treated; increasing amounts of this material will result in larger and more diverse microbial populations. Also, there will be added negative effects of physical occlusion of microorganisms and direct inactivation of germicidal chemicals.

We are aware of few data indicating the effectiveness of a variety of manufacturer-suggested methods for the cleaning of delicate, physically complex medical instruments. Similarly, effectiveness data are lacking for many postmarket devices or products marketed for use in cleaning, disinfecting, or sterilizing heat-sensitive instruments. It has been recently suggested that certain "washer/disinfector" devices specifically designed to reprocess flexible fiberoptic endoscopes are not only ineffective as washers, but have contributed to microbial contamination of reprocessed instruments as well as patient infection (Allen et al., 1987; Alvarado et al., 1990; Axon et al., 1990; Moore et al., 1990; Struelens et al., 1990; Wheeler et al., 1989).

The generic type of chemical germicide, the appropriate concentration, and the appropriate exposure time during a germicidal regimen are all pertinent and interrelated considerations, but are currently among the most confusing choices to be made by the health-care worker. A wide variety of brand-name products promoted for use in reprocessing medical instruments is available. Some have the same basic active ingredient as others but with different additives, supposedly to increase the efficiency or stability of the product. Unclear label claims or instructions for use, as well as advertising for a variety of products, can add to the user's confusion (Gurevich et al., 1990).

The importance of establishing consistently appropriate and reproducible laboratory test methods to evaluate and compare the germicidal capabilities of liquid chemical agents cannot be overstated. If these test methods are not appropriate and verifiable, or if the resulting data are not reflective of various in-use conditions, then the overall effectiveness of many generic recommendations and guidelines for selection and use of liquid chemical germicides will be weakened.

Regulation of germicidal chemicals is discussed in detail in Chapters 35 and 54. Briefly, however, the Environmental Protection Agency (EPA) is responsible for the initial registering (licensing) of disinfectant germicides before they are marketed. Currently, the EPA requires manufacturers to submit laboratory test data to substantiate label claims on products, but the EPA does not conduct confirmatory tests to ensure the accuracy of this data. According to a recent government study, the EPA cannot be certain whether label claims on many currently marketed disinfectants are accurate (U.S. General Accounting Office, 1990). The study identified several serious problem areas in the registration and regulation of disinfectants and estimated that up to 20% of disinfectants on the market might be ineffective. In addition to the EPA, other federal agencies have direct or indirect regulatory authority over disinfectant chemicals. If a disinfectant is marketed for use on a medical device, the Food and Drug Administration (FDA) has regulatory authority over these products because it considers the disinfectant (or even devices to deliver the disinfectant) an accessory to the medical device being reprocessed. A second level of regulatory control, in addition to that of the EPA, might be required by the FDA for products in this category. The FDA has recently gained increased levels of authority over medical devices through the Safe Medical Devices Act of 1990, which includes a provision requiring users of the medical devices (or accessories to the devices) to report adverse device events.

There are few well defined policies regarding commercial advertising of chemical germicides or medical devices. The Federal Trade Commission (FTC) has specific regulatory authority over truth in advertising and frequently pursues instances of false or misleading advertising of food, drug, or medical device products, including disinfectant chemicals. Printed or verbal commercial advertising claims made without substantiating data are considered by the FTC to be false and misleading to the user or potential user.

DEVICE-RELATED RISKS OF DISEASE TRANSMISSION

Many current guidelines and recommendations for the selection and use of liquid chemical germicides for reprocessing medical instruments are based on concepts and terminology first developed over 20 years ago by Dr. Earle Spaulding (Spaulding, 1968). His clear and logical principles for selection of methods for disinfecting and sterilizing were incorporated into the basic infection control guidelines of the Centers for Disease Control soon after he developed them, and they have been retained in original form and intent to date (Centers for Disease Control, 1985). These concepts and terminology have been incorporated into many other guidelines worldwide and have literally become part of the language in the infection control community (American Society for Gastrointestinal Endoscopy, 1988; Axon et al., 1990, 1991; British Society for Gastrointestinal Endoscopy, 1988; Rutala, 1990; Society for Gastroenterology Nurses and Associates, 1990). Detailed discussions of applying the Spaulding concepts to the selection of appropriate germicidal procedures are presented in Chapter 35 and elsewhere (Centers for Disease Control, 1985; Favero and Bond, 1991; Rutala, 1990). Briefly, however, the concepts are initially based on the fact that medical instrument surfaces can differ in their degree of contact with the patient and therefore carry different levels of disease transmission risk. The levels of risk are reflected in the categories of medical instrument surfaces: critical, semicritical, and noncritical.

Critical instruments are those that routinely penetrate the skin or mucous membranes during use, e.g., needles, scalpels, or other surgical instruments. Because the infection risk is high if these items are contaminated with any microorganism at the time of use, they must be sterilized between uses (i.e., it is "critical" that they be free of all forms of viable microorganisms, that is, sterile). The methods most often used for sterilization of heat-stable items are steam autoclaving and, to a lesser extent, dry heat cycles in forced air ovens. These procedures are penetrating and reliable in killing even large numbers of highly resistant bacterial spores. Also, each cycle is capable of being monitored biologically for effectiveness, and the items being processed can be wrapped or otherwise contained to maintain sterility before use. Heat-sensitive reusable instruments can be reliably sterilized by low-temperature exposures to gaseous agents such as ethylene oxide. These procedures share many of the advantages of heat processes, for example, cycle efficiency monitoring with biologic indicators and the capability of wrapping items to maintain sterility. Alternatively, heat-sensitive instruments may be sterilized by prolonged exposures (up to 10 hours) to liquid chemical agents such as glutaraldehyde-, hydrogen peroxide-, peracetic acid-, or chlorine dioxide-based products. However, these procedures do not have the same levels of reliability ("overkill") as the procedures that are capable of being monitored biologically. Sterilization cycles using liquid chemicals have the added disadvantages of comparatively high expense, potential toxicity problems with both patients and personnel, potential problems of recontamination during rinsing and drying, and the inability to wrap items to maintain sterility. Consequently, products in this class of liquid chemical germicides are rarely used as sterilants, but are used most frequently as disinfectants.

Semicritical instruments such as flexible fiberoptic endoscopes, laryngoscopes, and vaginal specula normally come into contact with intact mucous membranes during use. The risk of transmitting infection during the use of this category of instrument is comparatively low if the items are free from all groups of microorganisms with the possible exception of low numbers of bacterial spores (i.e., it is "semicritical" that these instruments be sterile at time of use). If instruments in this category are heat-stable, the most reliable and least expensive procedure of choice would be steam autoclave sterilization. However, the minimum procedure generally recommended for reprocessing heat-sensitive semicritical instruments is high-level disinfection. By the Spaulding definition, high-level disinfection is done with a chemical germicide capable of killing resistant bacterial spores but with a contact time significantly less than is necessary for sterilization. Once a germicide has lost the capacity for sporocidal activity (by age of the solution, dilution prior to or during use or by organic contamination), then the chemical no longer qualifies as a "high-level" disinfectant. The process, if conducted properly, can be expected, with a high level of confidence, to eliminate all vegetative bacteria (including mycobacteria), all viruses, and all fungi. The degree of confidence that this level of germicidal activity has occurred even in the presence of a moderate microbial challenge is related directly to the relative power and demonstrated microbicidal spectrum of the germicide used. This inference is necessary, because liquid chemical germicidal procedures cannot be monitored biologically for effectiveness. Monitoring the concentration of a chemical agent during its term of use is a useful tool with which to infer its continued effectiveness.

Noncritical instruments are those that normally come into contact only with intact skin during use, such as blood pressure cuffs, physical measurement devices, stethoscopes, and electrocardiogram electrodes. The risk of disease transmission is very low with this category of instrument if they are contaminated, even with a variety of microorganisms at the time of use (i.e., it is "noncritical" that these instruments be sterilized between uses). Depending on the nature and amount of contamination, appropriate methods for reprocessing range from intermediate- to low-level disinfection to simple soap and water washing. The intermediate- or low-level germicides (phenolics, iodophors, chlorine compounds, alcohols, and quaternary ammonium compounds) might, depending on the formulation, have various levels of activity against fungi, viruses, vegetative bacteria, and, in some instances, mycobacteria. None of these formulations is classed as sterilants; in most instances, these types of germicides are appropriate for disinfecting environmental surfaces rather than medical instruments. Germicides designed for use on skin (antiseptics) are not appropriate in any instance for disinfecting inanimate surfaces.

LEVELS OF MICROBIAL RESISTANCE AND LEVELS OF GERMICIDE ACTIVITY

Figure 64–1 depicts a general descending order of microbial resistance levels, ranging from highly resistant bacterial spores unique to the genera *Bacillus* and *Clostridium* to relatively sensitive lipid-containing viruses

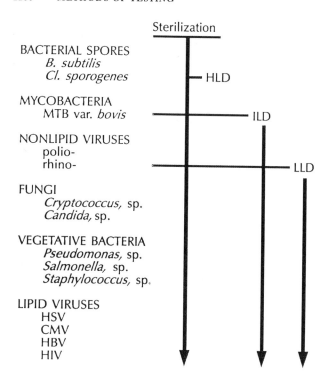

Fig. 64–1. Descending order of resistance to germicidal chemicals related to levels of germicidal activity. HLD, High-level disinfection; ILD, Intermediate-level disinfection; LLD, Low-level disinfection; MTB, *Mycobacterium tuberculosis;* HSV, Herpes simplex virus; CMV, Cytomegalovirus; HBV, Hepatitis B virus; HIV, Human immunodeficiency virus.

such as herpes viruses, cytomegalovirus, hepatitis B virus, and human immunodeficiency virus. As indicated, this general order is directly related to the levels of germicidal activity in the Spaulding classification system (sterilization and high-, intermediate-, and low-level disinfection). Also, the general activity spectrum of each level is reflected by the length of the descending arrows. Conveniently, the Spaulding terminology is consistent with and can be directly related to current label claim terminology used by the EPA for registration of liquid chemical disinfectants in the United States (Chapter 35; Favero and Bond, 1991; Society of Gastroenterology Nurses and Associates, 1990). The "sterilants" are obviously "sporocides," but they are also "tuberculocidal," "virucidal," "fungicidal," and "bactericidal," as indicated on the product labels.

The Spaulding category of **high-level disinfectant** ("HLD" in Fig. 64–1) is exactly the same type of chemical as in the sterilant category except that the use pattern is different. The sterilant is used as a high-level disinfectant by reducing the exposure time within its effective range of tuberculocidal, virucidal, fungicidal, and bactericidal activity (e.g., a 10-min. exposure for high-level disinfection instead of a 10-hr exposure for sterilization). As stated previously, when a liquid chemical sterilant is used as a disinfectant and reused multiple times for this purpose, the effective life of the product as a high-level disinfectant is limited by the remaining concentration of

its sporocidal component. Manufacturers of some sterilant products supply test kits to monitor effective concentrations of active components, which allows users to tailor replenishment intervals to their own unique use patterns.

The Spaulding category of **intermediate-level disinfectant** ("ILD" in Fig. 64–1) corresponds predominantly with the EPA label designations of "hospital disinfectant" (by virtue of demonstrated activity against *Pseudomonas aeruginosa, Staphylococcus aureus,* and *Salmonella choleraesuis*) and "tuberculocidal." The majority of the "tuberculocidal hospital disinfectants" are either phenolics, iodophors, or chlorine compounds, but products in this category do not have the demonstrated capacity for use as sterilants ("sporocides"). They are, therefore, not appropriate for use as high-level disinfectants.

The Spaulding category of **low-level disinfectant** ("LLD" in Fig. 64–1) includes products that are EPA-registered as "hospital disinfectants" but that are not effective tuberculocides. Products in this category are predominantly quaternary ammonium-based products, but certain phenolic or iodophor formulations might also lack the capacity for inactivating mycobacteria.

DEVICE-RELATED FACTORS AFFECTING THE EFFICIENCY OF GERMICIDAL PROCEDURES

Among such factors as numbers of microorganisms, the innate resistance of different types of microorganisms, the type and concentration of germicide, and the time and temperature of exposure, the amount of organic material present has perhaps the most decided effect on the efficiency of a liquid chemical disinfecting or sterilizing procedure. Increasing amounts of residual patient material remaining on or in a medical instrument prior to any germicidal procedure will require adjustment of other factors to ensure success of the procedure (e.g., use of a more powerful germicide, a higher concentration of germicide, a longer exposure time, an increase in the temperature of exposure, or a combination thereof). The general assumption of guidelines for selection and use of disinfecting or sterilizing procedures, as well as of the EPA-approved label instructions on germicidal products, is that a surface will be adequately precleaned before a germicidal product is applied. In this regard, the overall physical design as well as the stability of materials used in the production of medical instruments are the primary determinants of the exact methods necessary for the most efficient reprocessing between patients. Instruments designed to include (in any degree) lumens, crevices, loosely mated or occluded surfaces, knurled or textured surfaces, and fragile (heat-sensitive or easily corroded or abraded) materials present the greatest challenges to effective cleaning as well as to disinfecting or sterilizing. Flexible fiberoptic endoscopes and their accessories, as well as a variety of dental instruments, are among a number of medical instrument categories incorporating one or more of these physical or design characteristics. For illustrative purposes, the following discussion will

Table 64–1. *General Categories and Uses of Flexible Fiberoptic Gastrointestinal (GI) Endoscopes.*

Instrument Category*	Site(s) of Use†
Upper GE (EGD)‡	Esophagus, stomach, duodenum
Colonoscope	Colon, terminal ileum
Sigmoidoscope	Sigmoid colon
Duodenoscope (ERCP)§	Pancreatic and bile ducts

*Each category may have one or more models or configurations depending on the manufacturer (only three major companies worldwide) or the intended use, e.g., pediatric, therapeutic, or diagnostic.
‡Uses may include diagnostic and therapeutic procedures using a wide range of accessories such as biopsy forceps, snares, sclerotherapy needles, and cytology brushes.
‡EGD, Esophagogastroduodenoscopy.
§ERCP, Endoscopic retrograde cholangiopancreatography.

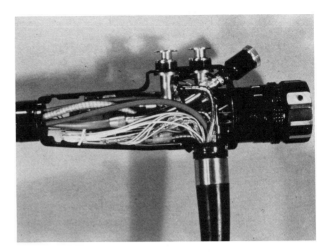

Fig. 64–2. Control head of a flexible fiberoptic endoscope with outer covering removed.

center on endoscopic equipment used in gastroenterology settings.

REPROCESSING OF FLEXIBLE FIBEROPTIC ENDOSCOPES AND ACCESSORIES

The clinical use of flexible fiberotic endoscopes is highly beneficial to patient health, because a wide variety of clinical and diagnostic procedures can be done without resort to conventional major surgical techniques. The two major groups of flexible endoscopic devices are bronchoscopes and upper or lower gastrointestinal (GI) endoscopes. Although the basic configurations and materials of the two groups are similar, the GI devices are more physically complex, having multiple and sometimes interconnected internal channels and valves. A brief listing of general categories and uses of flexible fiberoptic GI endoscopes is given in Table 64–1. Bronchoscopes usually have only a single internal channel (suction/biopsy) and are comparatively less difficult to clean and disinfect or sterilize. Physically complex accessories (e.g., biopsy forceps, snares, cytology brushes) are similar in both groups.

Flexible endoscopes are physically complex and fragile, very expensive, heat-sensitive (cannot be steam autoclaved), easily damaged by prolonged immersion in liquids (especially corrosive liquids), and accordingly, are difficult to clean and disinfect or sterilize. The humidity, temperature, and chemical effects of repeated ethylene oxide sterilization cycles will eventually damage the devices. According to a variety of generic guidelines, the minimum standard for reprocessing the optic portions of endoscopic sets is high-level disinfection (American Society for Gastrointestinal Endoscopy, 1988; Axon et al., 1990, 1991; British Society for Gastrointestinal Endoscopy, 1988; Centers for Disease Control, 1985; Rutala, 1990; Society of Gastroenterology Nurses and Associates, 1990). However, recent surveys have indicated a wide variation in practices used for reprocessing these devices,

many of which are inconsistent with current recommendations from either the manufacturers of the devices or medical specialty organizations (Axon et al., 1991; Gorse and Messner, 1991; Moore et al., 1990; Rutala et al., 1990a; Wheeler et al., 1989). Also, a survey of published literature, as well as a number of anecdotal observations, suggests that there is significant confusion among users regarding the structure, function, and inter-relationships among various components of flexible endoscopic equipment, in particular, the complex array of internal channels and valves (Ott and Nelson, 1987). Data confirming the efficacy of specific, manufacturer-recommended procedures for reprocessing (including recommendations for ethylene oxide sterilization) are lacking. Generally, precleaning of endoscope channels (before subsequent germicidal procedures) is done using initial air or water flushes (or both), flushing with detergent or soap solutions, scrubbing with brushes, or brief soaking in commercial enzyme-containing products designed to loosen or dissolve organic material. These precleaning methods may be used singly or in combination depending on the circumstance and the judgment of endoscopy personnel.

Figure 64–2 shows the control head of a flexible fiberoptic endoscope with the covering removed to show the complex internal configuration and array of valves, channels, fiberoptic bundles, and other components. The objective (eyepiece) lens (right), and insertion tube (left) are in the horizontal plane of the photograph; the air/water (top, right), suction (top, left), and biopsy (top, oblique) valves and universal cord (bottom; connection to light, air, and water sources) are in the vertical plane of the photograph. Figure 64–3 shows the external configuration of a typical flexible GI endoscope before connection to the light/air/water sources (insertion tube to the right of the control head and universal cord to the left). In Figure 64–4, the insertion tube of a similar endoscope is being sampled for residual hepatitis B surface antigen during an early study to determine the efficiency of commonly used methods for reprocessing endoscopic

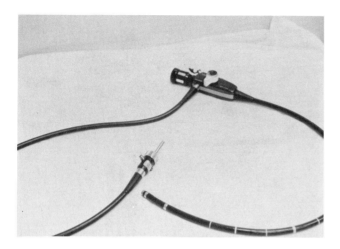

Fig. 64–3. External configuration of a flexible fiberoptic GI endoscope (not connected to the light/air/water source).

equipment (Bond and Moncada, 1978). Figure 64–5 is a simplified cutaway drawing showing the internal configuration of the insertion tube which, depending on the model of instrument, can vary in diameter (approximately 9 to 14 mm) and length (relatively short or up to a meter or more). Control wires for articulation of the distal section, fiberoptic bundles, channels, and other functional components are tightly confined and covered with metal braid and an outer plastic sheath. The air and water channels are approximately 1.0 to 1.2 mm in diameter and cannot be cleaned by physical means other than flushing with liquids or air between uses. These two channels are frequently connected slightly above a common exit port in the distal tip of the insertion tube; other points of access to either of these channels include the universal cord at the light source connection, the control head air/water valve, and the universal cord water bottle connection site. Access to the water channel is more difficult than to the air channel. In certain colonoscopes, yet another small-diameter channel/valve system is connected to the air/water system to supply carbon dioxide gas to the distal tip of the insertion tube. There is retrograde movement of patient material into all of the small-diameter channels during use, and frequent block-

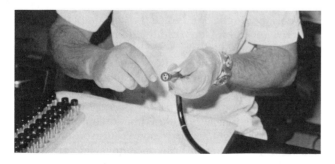

Fig. 64–4. Sampling of a flexible endoscope insertion tube for residual hepatitis B surface antigen. From Bond, W.W., and Moncada, R.E. 1978. Viral hepatitis B: infection risk in flexible fiberoptic endoscopy. *Gastrointest. Endosc., 24,* 225–230.

age of these channels is a common problem in many endoscopy units.

The biopsy/suction channel is a shared function system with a biopsy valve (entry port for biopsy forceps and a variety of accessories) and a suction valve connected to the same channel in the control head. The channel tubing in the insertion tube and universal cord is approximately 2.8 mm in diameter and is accessible from four locations: the universal cord at the suction source, the suction and biopsy valves in the control head, and at the distal tip of the insertion tube. This channel system is the only one in the instrument that will accept cleaning brushes during cleaning and reprocessing.

Figure 64–6 indicates the complex physical arrangement of the various channels and valve systems. The inter-relationships among the systems and methods for most optimal access and reprocessing are beyond the scope of this chapter but are discussed in detail elsewhere (Axon et al., 1990, 1991; Ott and Nelson, 1987; Society of Gastroenterology Nurses and Associates, 1990). Each instrument, however, should be considered separately, and manufacturers' instructions should be examined thoroughly but questioned where any doubt or uncertainty exists. Reliance on so-called "automatic" machines or other devices or products supplied by endoscope manufacturers or accessory product companies to solve difficulties in cleaning, disinfecting, or sterilizing these instruments should be approached with deliberate, informed caution. Producers or suppliers of these items should be able to provide convincing data to substantiate recommended procedures or advertising and product label claims. An increasing body of independent scientific literature suggests that a number of these devices and products marketed for instrument reprocessing fall short of their stated claims (Allen et al., 1987; Alvarado et al., 1990; Best et al., 1990; Cole et al., 1990; Leong et al., 1987; Moore et al., 1990; Pitzurra et al., 1990; Power and Russell, 1989, 1990; Rutala, 1990b; Struelens et al. 1990; Tyler et al., 1990; U.S. General Accounting Office, 1990; Wheeler et al., 1989).

VISUAL EXAMINATION OF A FIBEROPTIC ENDOSCOPE AND ACCESSORY

To illustrate potentially serious deficiencies in currently used methods for cleaning and reprocessing flexible fiberoptic endoscopes, a brief examination of internal channel and valve surfaces, as well as of the internal structure of a representative accessory to the endoscopic set (biopsy forceps), was conducted. The endoscopes and biopsy forceps had been cleaned and reprocessed using methods and materials either supplied or recommended by the endoscope manufacturer. The subsequent illustrations are typical representations of the patient-ready state in models of devices currently used in GI endoscopy.

A rigid arthroscopic endoscope (2 mm in diameter) was used to examine and photograph internal surfaces in the biopsy/suction channel systems of several flexible

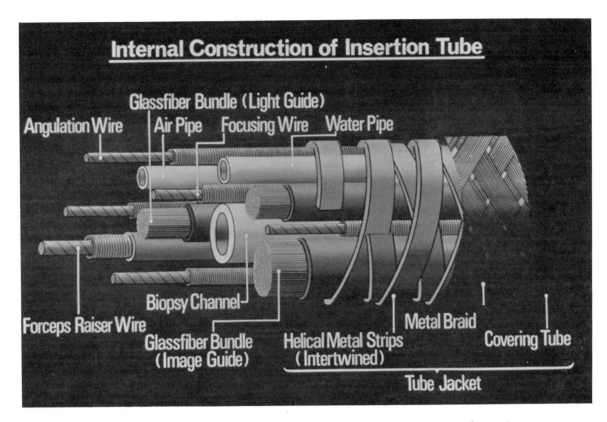

Fig. 64–5. Cutaway diagram of a flexible fiberoptic endoscope insertion tube (approximately 9 to 14 mm in diameter).

GI endoscopes (Figs. 64–7 through 64–9). Conventional photographic techniques were used to record the appearance of a biopsy/suction channel removed from an endoscope during repair (Fig. 64–10). A scanning electron microscope was used to examine the interior surfaces of a section taken from the spring-like shaft of a biopsy forceps (Fig. 64–11).

Figure 64–7 is a view inside the body of a suction valve housing of an unused instrument. Shown is the point of attachment between the valve housing and the suction channel tubing in the universal cord. The white coloration is the normal appearance of a "clean" channel. In this instance, however, the method of valve/channel attachment resulted in an irregular, kinked channel surface at the interface rather than a smooth, circular junction.

Figure 64–8 is an equivalent view of a suction valve housing in an endoscope that had been used and reprocessed (in the recommended manner) several times. Shown here is an accumulation of patient material at the irregular junction of the channel and the housing. Subsequent uses and reprocessing of similar endoscopes occasionally result in total blockage (not shown) of the channel by accumulated patient material, presumably due to the structural features of the channel shown here.

Figure 64–9 shows residual patient material on and around the valve seat in a suction valve housing (valve removed). The cleaning brush supplied by the endoscope manufacturer was too small and of inappropriate config-

uration to adequately clean the housing and valve seat during the cleaning process. The spring-loaded valves themselves (not shown) have been implicated in disease transmission in a bronchoscopy setting even after being repeatedly cleaned and disinfected using methods or materials recommended by the endoscope manufacturer. The disease outbreak ceased after valves were routinely steam autoclaved, an intervention specifically recommended against by the manufacturer, because the valves were supposedly heat-sensitive (Wheeler et al., 1989).

Figure 64–10 shows the interior surface of a segment from a suction channel removed during repair of a flexible endoscope after internal leakage was detected. The channel was sectioned longitudinally and pinned open to expose the interior channel surface. Holes in the channel are visible in the center and upper left portions of the segment, and apparently a raised area in the intact channel had caused the distal tips of cleaning brushes to be deflected away from a central course down the channel during cleaning operations. Over time, the deflected brushes not only resulted in holes being abraded in the channel wall but also left areas in the vicinity of the abrasions untouched during the cleaning process. Shown here are heavy encrustations (visible in upper right and lower left portions of the segment) of patient material (e.g., feces, blood, gastric mucin). It is noteworthy that the instrument from which this channel segment was taken had been routinely flushed and rinsed immediately

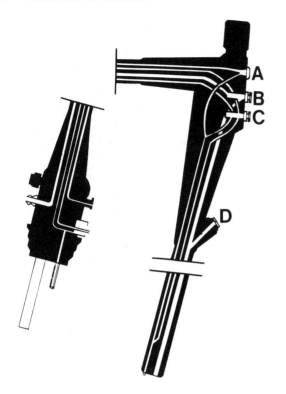

Fig. 64–6. Diagram showing the interrelationship of valves and channels in a flexible fiberoptic colonoscope. *A*, CO_2 valve. *B*, Suction valve. *C*, Air/water valve. *D*, Biopsy and accessory port. Valves activate use of the respective channels.

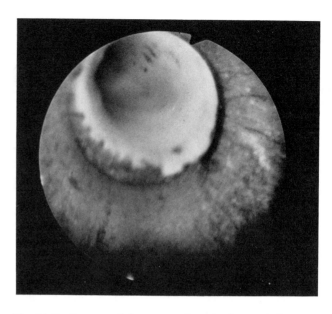

Fig. 64–8. Juncture of the suction channel tubing and the suction valve housing in a used but patient-ready (reprocessed) flexible fiberoptic endoscope (see text).

after each use and before brushing and subsequent disinfection. Also, the segment is from the only channel system in flexible GI endoscopes that is accessible with cleaning brushes (2.8 mm diameter suction/biopsy channel). Residual contamination such as that shown here and in the previous figures would present severe challenges to the effectiveness of any disinfecting or sterilizing procedure.

Figure 64–11 is a scanning electron micrograph showing interior components in the shaft of a biopsy forceps, an accessory to the flexible endoscopic set designed to

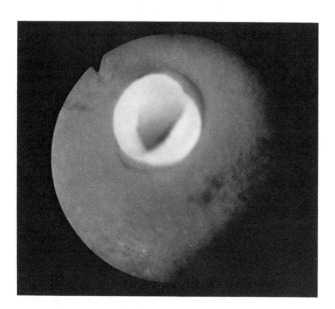

Fig. 64–7. Juncture of the suction channel tubing and the suction valve housing in an unused flexible fiberoptic endoscope.

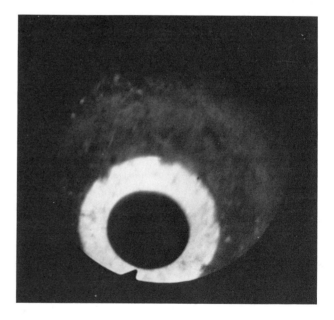

Fig. 64–9. Valve seat in the suction valve housing of a patient-ready (reprocessed) flexible fiberoptic endoscope (see text).

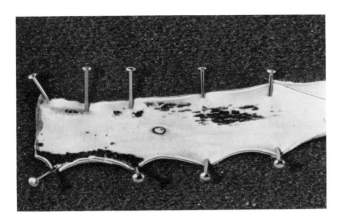

Fig. 64–10. Flexible fiberoptic endoscope suction channel (2.8 mm in diameter) removed during leak repair (see text).

break mucosal or skin barriers during use (i.e., a "critical" instrument). A segment of the spring-like forceps shaft (2.4 mm diameter) was taken near the distal tip (forceps jaw) of the instrument. The forceps had been sent for repair because of increasing difficulty in opening and closing of the jaws. Reprocessing between uses had been done according to manufacturer's instructions and consisted of cleaning the external surfaces with detergent and brushes and then immersing the instrument in a liquid chemical germicide (presumably the same germicide as used to disinfect the endoscope). The micrograph clearly accounts for the difficulty in operation of the instrument: the twisted wire shaft core (responsible for movement of forceps jaws) and the lumen of the spring-like shaft are impacted with residual patient material. The exterior surfaces of the spring coils appeared bright and clean by direct visual examination, but destructive sampling and microscopic examination showed residual material not only in the spring core but on the loosely mated areas between the spring coils. Transmission of disease by "cleaned and disinfected" biopsy forceps has been demonstrated (Dwyer et al., 1987); other

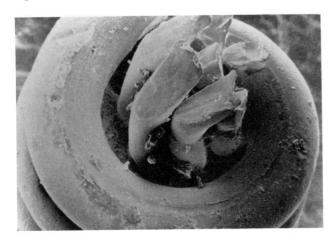

Fig. 64–11. Scanning electron photomicrograph of a segment taken from the spring-like shaft of a reprocessed but nonfunctioning flexible endoscope biopsy forceps, 2.4 mm in diameter (see text).

studies have shown that patient material (Bond and Moncada, 1978) and microorganisms (Karim et al., 1989) are not removed from biopsy forceps (and presumably from other accessories with similar design and physical structure) by routine cleaning methods alone. Recent guidelines suggest that biopsy forceps and similar accessories to the endoscopic set be cleaned using ultrasonic baths and then wrapped and sterilized by steam autoclaving (Axon et al., 1990, 1991; Society of Gastroenterology Nurses and Associates, 1990). A number of current instruction manuals from endoscope manufacturers suggest disinfection as an option for this category of instrument. This is clearly an inappropriate method of reprocessing an instrument that is, in effect, a scalpel.

Adequate rinsing of flexible endoscopes after cleaning and disinfecting procedures can also be difficult. A recent report has described toxic reactions in patients linked to inadequate rinsing of disinfectant chemicals (Jonas et al., 1988). In this report, it was not clear whether residual germicide was due to insufficient volumes of rinse fluid, failure to gain access to all channels of the instrument during rinsing, or physical occlusion of residual germicide in loosely mated or other irregular surfaces. Other workers have observed that materials used in the construction of flexible endoscopes can absorb and slowly release glutaraldehyde, the most often used disinfectant for these instruments (Power and Russell, 1989).

CONCLUSION

It is beyond the scope of this chapter to comprehensively address and propose solutions for many of the current problems related specifically to between-patient reprocessing of delicate, heat-sensitive medical instruments. Our purpose is to bring attention to some of these problems, and clearly, the solutions will be realized only through a multidisciplinary approach, including many areas of expertise ranging from epidemiology to biomedical engineering to education.

The appropriate choice of chemicals for sterilizing or disinfecting medical instruments depends highly on both the accuracy of microbiologic test data submitted to regulatory agencies during the premarket registration of these germicides and the clarity and accuracy of label instructions for the products. Also, one of the most important factors that can influence the in-use effectiveness of a given germicidal procedure is the amount of organic material remaining in or on an instrument before reprocessing. Certain medical instruments (e.g., flexible fiberoptic endoscopes and their accessories, dental instruments) have, for the most part, been designed functionally, and many are physically complex, expensive, delicate, difficult to clean, and not steam autoclavable. Methods of instrument reprocessing are not consistent within certain medical disciplines. This inconsistency could be due to not only the lack of data but to the lack of adequate instruction on verifiably effective procedures for cleaning, disinfecting, and post-process rinsing and storage. Future considerations of the in-use efficacies of germicidal chemicals for medical instruments should include both the accurate assessment of the germicidal activity spectrum of the chemicals and the availability of effective, implementable precleaning procedures appropriate for each type of instrument.

REFERENCES

Allen, J.I., et al. 1987. *Pseudomonas* infection of the biliary system resulting from the use of a contaminated endoscope. Gastroenterology, *92*, 759–763.

Alvarado, C.J., Stolz, S.M., and Maki, D.G. 1990. Nosocomial *P. aeruginosa* infections from contaminated endoscopes (abstract). *In* Abstr. Third International Conference on Nosocomial Infections, 31 July–3 Aug., 1990, Atlanta, GA, Abstract 74, p. 32.

American Society for Gastrointestinal Endoscopy. 1988. Infection control during gastrointestinal endoscopy: guidelines for clinical application. Gastrointest. Endosc., *34*(Suppl.), 37–40.

Axon, A.T.R., et al. 1990. Endoscopic disinfection. In *Working Party Reports of the World Congresses of Gastroenterology, Sydney, Australia, August, 1990.* Melbourne/Boston, Blackwell Scientific Publications, pp. 46–50.

Axon, A.T.R., et al. 1991. Disinfection and endoscopy: report and recommendations of an international working party. J. Gastroenterol. Hepatol., in press.

Best, M., Sattar, S.A., Springthorpe, V.S., and Kennedy, M.E. 1990. Efficacies of selected disinfectants against *Mycobacterium tuberculosis.* J. Clin. Microbiol., *28*, 2234–2239.

Bond, W.W., and Moncada, R.E. 1978. Viral hepatitis B: infection risk in flexible fiberoptic endoscopy. Gastrointest. Endosc., *24*, 225–230.

British Society for Gastrointestinal Endoscopy. 1988. Cleaning and disinfection of equipment for gastrointestinal flexible endoscopy: interim recommendations of a working party. Gut, *29*, 1134–1151.

Centers for Disease Control. 1985. Guidelines for handwashing and hospital environmental control. Atlanta, GA, Centers for Disease Control, HHS publication No. 99-1117.

Cole, E.C., et al. 1990. Effect of methodology, dilution, and exposure time on the tuberculocidal activity of glutaraldehyde-based disinfectants. Appl. Environ. Microbiol., *56*, 1813–1817.

Dwyer, D.M., et al. 1987. *Salmonella newport* infections transmitted by fiberoptic colonoscopy. Gastrointest. Endosc., *33*, 84–87.

Favero, M.S., and Bond, W.W. 1991. Sterilization and disinfection in the hospital. In *Manual of Clinical Microbiology.* 5th Ed. Edited by A. Balows, et al. Washington, D.C., American Society for Microbiology, pp. 183–200.

Gorse, G.J., and Messner, R.L. 1991. Infection control practices in the United States: a national survey. Infect. Control Hosp. Epidemiol., in press.

Gurevich, I., Yanelli, B., and Cunha, B.A. 1990. The disinfectant dilemma revisited. Infect. Control Hosp. Epidemiol., *11*, 96–100.

Jonas, G., Mahoney, A., Murray, J., and Gertler, S. 1988. Chemical colitis due to endoscope cleaning solutions: a mimic of pseudomembranous colitis. Gastroenterology, *95*, 1403–1498.

Karim, Q.N., Rao, G.G., Taylor, M., and Baron, J.H. 1989. Routine cleaning and the elimination of *Campylobacter pylori* from endoscopic biopsy forceps. J. Hosp. Infect., *13*, 87–90.

Leong, D., Dorsey, C., and Klapp, M. 1987. Dilution of glutaraldehyde by automatic endoscope washers: a need for a quality control program (abstract). Am. J. Infect. Control, *15*, 86.

Moore, R.M., Kaczmarek, R.G., and McCrohan, J. 1990. Multi-state investigation of the actual disinfection/sterilization of gastrointestinal endoscopes (abstract). *In* Abstr. Third International Conference on Nosocomial Infections. 31 July–3 Aug., 1990, Atlanta, GA, Abstract No. B/38, p. 55.

Ott, B.J., and Nelson, B. 1987. Understanding the structure and function of endoscope channels: the inside story. Soc. Gastrointest. Assist. J., *9*, 184–187.

Pitzurra, M., et al. 1990. What about the sporocidal activity of glutaraldehydes? (abstract). *In* Abstr. Second International Conference of the Hospital Infection Society, London, England, Sept. 4, 1990, p. 144.

Power, E.G.M., and Russell, A.D. 1989. Glutaraldehyde: its uptake by sporing and non-sporing bacteria, rubber, plastic, and an endoscope. J. Appl. Bacteriol., *67*, 329–342.

Power, E.G.M. and Russell, A.D. 1990. Sporocidal action of alkaline glutaraldehyde: factors influencing activity and a comparison with other aldehydes. J. Appl. Bacteriol., *26*, 261–268.

Rutala, W.A. 1990. APIC guideline for selection and use of disinfectants. Am. J. Infect. Control, *18*, 99–117.

Rutala, W.A., Clontz, E.P., Weber, D.J., and Hoffman, K.K. 1990a. Disinfection practices for endoscopes and other semicritical items (abstract). *In* Abstr. Third International Conference on Nosocomial Infections, 31 July–3 Aug., 1990, Atlanta, GA, Abstract No. B/36, p. 54.

Rutala, W.A., Cole, E.C., Wannamaker, N., and Weber, D.J. 1990b. Inactivation of *Mycobacterium tuberculosis* (Mtb) and *M. bovis* (Mb) by 13 hospital disinfectants (abstract). *In* Abstr. Third International Conference on Nosocomial Infections, 31 July–3 Aug., 1900, Atlanta, GA, Abstract No. 71, p. 31.

Society of Gastroenterology Nurses and Associates. 1990. *Recommended Guidelines for Infection Control in Gastrointestinal Endoscopy Settings.* 2nd Ed. Rochester, NY, Society of Gastroenterology Nurses and Associates.

Spaulding, E.H. 1968. Chemical disinfection of medical and surgical materials. In *Disinfection, Sterilization, and Preservation.* Edited by C.A. Lawrence and S.S. Block. Philadelphia, Lea & Febiger, pp. 517–531.

Struelens, M.J. 1990. Septicemia after ERCP: outbreak linked to an automatic endoscope disinfecting machine (abstract). *In* Abstr. Third International Conference on Nosocomial Infections, 31 July–3 Aug., 1990, Atlanta, GA, Abstract No. 73, p. 32.

Wheeler, P.W., Lancaster, D., and Kaiser, A.B. 1989. Bronchopulmonary cross colonization and infection related to mycobacterial contamination of suction valves of bronchoscopes. J. Infect. Dis., *159*, 954–958.

United States General Accounting Office. 1990. Disinfectants: EPA lacks assurance they work. Doc. No. GAO/RCED-90-139, August, 1990, Gaithersburg, MD, 68 pp.

Tyler, R., Ayliffe, G.A.J., and Bradley, C. 1990. Virucidal activity of disinfectants: studies with poliovirus. J. Hosp. Infect., *15*, 339–345.

CHAPTER 65

Microorganisms, Sick Buildings, and Building Related Illnesses

Seymour S. Block

Figure 65–1 presents a picture of a sick building. It may not look sick but it suffered a severe case of sick building syndrome (SBS). It seems to be well now, but its recovery took 5 years and cost 4.5 million dollars. The trouble started in February of 1985 when 4 people in the histopathology laboratory of the College of Veterinary Medicine at the University of Florida complained of eye irritation and skin rashes. An examination of the premises revealed fixing baths with volatile solvents stored in open containers in the lab. Furthermore, work using these chemicals was done in the open lab, not in the hood. These conditions were remedied but the people's symptoms did not disappear. In fact, people all over the building developed symptoms, which included headache, stuffy nose, dry throat, fatigue, cough, nausea, trouble in concentrating, and sensitivity to odors. In the next few months the situation got worse, until 160 of the 450 building occupants had been affected (Properzio, 1991). The situation was so bad that many people had to be moved to other buildings. Temporary buildings were set up. A series of consultants were called in to study the building. The building was thoroughly cleaned and renovated. The whole ventilating system was reconstructed, the animal quarters were separated and modified, chemicals that might be offending were removed, and many other changes were made. The cost for absenteeism, interrupted work, inefficient work, medical costs, legal matters, etc., was never calculated. No scientific study was reported and no cause of the problem was identified (Friedenberg, 1990). In the investigation of this case, occurrences of SBS at the University of South Florida, University of Georgia, and Virginia Polytechnic Institute also came to the writer's attention.

Consider another case of a sick building, reported by Hodgson et al. (1987). This outbreak occurred in 1981 in a seven-story office building occupied by the Tennessee Valley Authority (TVA) in Tennessee. There were 3 outbreaks in 2 months, after which the building was vacated and remained empty for at least 5 years, when the report was written. At the time of the first attack, 45.4% of the 335 people in the building became ill. The symptoms most frequently reported were muscle pain, fever, headache, chills, cough, fatigue, nausea, and tight chest. The problem was related to the air cooling system because the attacks occurred, in all 3 incidents, immediately following the time the system was turned on after it had been off for a period following a prior attack (see Table 65–1). The authors stated, "Because of difficulties with demonstrating safety for reoccupancy, the building was vacated and remains empty at this time." Despite a comprehensive investigation, no etiologic agent could be identified.

It should be noted that not all cases of SBS were so devastating. Whorton et al. (1987) tell of employee complaints following relocation of a business to a new office building in California. The new building was occupied in July of 1984 over a one week period during which time the symptoms developed. A questionnaire was sent to the 180 employees: their symptoms and frequency are reported in Table 65–2. It is interesting to note in this episode that the complaints decreased each week over a period of 5 weeks until the problem effectively disappeared. The health complaints experienced appeared to be neither persistent nor pervasive enough to constitute an ongoing health and safety hazard at the facility. As in the other cases, no causative agent was isolated.

Sick building syndrome, sometimes called tight building syndrome or building-related illness (BRI), is defined by the World Health Organization (WHO) as the excessive reporting by building occupants of headaches, fatigue, nasal congestion, eye irritation, etc. SBS is no rare phenomenon. WHO stated that 30% of new and refurbished public buildings worldwide have been affected by SBS. In a British study of 4373 office workers in 46 buildings, 29% reported 5 or more SBS symptoms. A study by Woods (1989) of 600 office workers in the United

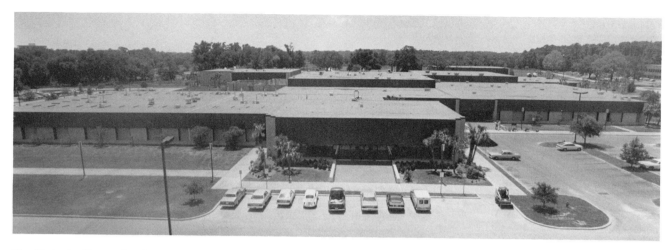

Fig. 65–1. Building with sick building syndrome (SBS).

Table 65–1. *Sequence of the Epidemic and Steps in the Investigation: Hypersensitivity Pneumonitis in Office Workers, Tennessee, 1981*

Date	Event
1940–1975	Tennessee Valley Authority (TVA) occupies the building.
1975–1981	Building is empty.
1981	
April	The TVA reoccupies the building.
September 18	Air cooling system turned off for the first time since April.
September 21	Air cooling system turned on again; the first outbreak occurs.
September 22	Knoxville County Health Department and TVA Industrial Hygiene Branch contacted.
September 23	First (TVA) questionnaire survey; air cooling system subsequently turned off.
October 12	Air cooling system turned on again.
October 13	Second outbreak; air handling system turned off.
October 14	Serum for precipitin titers drawn.
October 15	Air handling system turned on again; third outbreak occurs.
October 16	TVA removes employees from the building.
October 25–28	Industrial hygiene survey.
1982	
March 2–4	Second questionnaire survey.

From Hodgson, M.J., Morey, P.R., Simon, J.S., et al. 1987. Am. J. Epidem., *125*, 631–638.

Table 65–2. *Frequency Distribution of Symptoms for 154 Employees Who Worked in Building Within First 2 Weeks*

Symptom	Total	Frequency Rate (%)
Headache	98	63.6
Fatigue/drowsiness	84	54.5
Noticeable odors	78	50.6
Sore throat	74	48.1
Nasal/sinus congestion	68	44.2
Nausea	64	41.6
Dizziness	64	41.6
Sneezing	57	37.0
Eye irritation	54	35.1
Chest tightness	50	32.5
Back pain	44	28.6
Trouble sleeping	43	27.9
Unusual taste	41	26.6
Disorientation	41	26.6
Other	37	24.0
Chest congestion	30	19.5
Aching joints	28	18.2
Rapid heartbeat	27	17.5
Skin irritation/itching	25	16.2
Chest pains	25	16.2
Unusual vaginal discharge	21	13.6
Contact lens problems	19	12.3
Tongue/lip numbness	16	10.4
Bladder infections/dysuria	13	8.4
Nosebleed	8	5.2
Total symptoms	**1,109**	
No. of Employees in Area	154	

From Whorton, M.D., Lawson, S.R., Gordon, N.J. and Morgan, R.W. 1987. Investigation and work-up of tight building syndrome. J. Occup. Med., *29*, 142.

States showed that 20% of employees experienced symptoms of SBS and 7 to 11% reported that they were a serious problem. The problem has been extensively reported in the United States and Europe (European Community, 1989). Woods (1989) has estimated that 800,000 to 1,200,000 commercial buildings in the United States, with 30 to 70 million exposed occupants, have problems that manifest themselves as SBS.

The National Institute for Occupational Safety and Health (NIOSH) has responded to over 1000 requests for air quality health hazard investigations in buildings in the United States as a result of complaints from office workers (NIOSH, 1989). These are separate from asbestos-related investigations. Of the air quality investigations, 80% were of government and business office buildings, 13% were schools, and 7% were health care facilities. Statistics show that of 1200 health hazard investigations by NIOSH on all types of complaints made between 1971 and 1978, only 0.5% were for indoor air quality matters. Of the 1000 requests for air quality investigations, 99% were made after 1978, with 720 requests for assistance in 1988 alone. This demonstrates that SBS is a recent problem that occurs principally in buildings constructed within the past 20 years. It should be pointed out that 47.2% of United States office building space has been constructed since 1971 (Levin, 1991) and 25% of American workers are office workers. New construction following the Arab oil embargo of the early 1970s attempted to be energy efficient, with less use of outside air and more recirculation of inside air through internal heating, ventilating, and air conditioning systems (HVAC). Where buildings or parts of buildings were well supplied with fresh air the occupants did not suffer symptoms of SBS. These tight buildings generated savings by reducing HVAC costs because 40% of the energy used in the United States is used to air condition office buildings. It may have been a false economy because a study in Stockholm indicated that the cost of a 1% rate of absenteeism (and absenteeism due to SBS is estimated to be much greater than 1%) is 8 times greater than the potential savings through reduced energy consumption (Levin, 1989). The report fails to consider the further cost of reduced working efficiency caused by SBS.

POSSIBLE CAUSES

Peculiar to SBS and BRI, the symptoms of illness appear rapidly, 2 to 6 hours after people enter the building, and are usually temporary, disappearing in a few hours or overnight when people leave the building and get fresh air. They are respiratory-initiated ailments with unidentified cause or causes, although they appear to be related to the air supply system in air-tight buildings. The HVAC system apparently acts as a conduction vehicle to transport the offending material to the susceptible victim. It is possible that there are many causes for SBS and BRI, and that they could be different for different people and for different buildings. Chemical, biological, and physical causes have been proposed.

Actually SBS is only one and the least serious, in terms of the patient, of a number of building related respiratory-acquired illnesses. There are the hypersensitivity diseases: hypersensitivity pneumonitis (allergic alveolitis), humidity fever, allergic rhinitis, and office building-related asthma. Further, there are the infectious diseases, which are frequently disseminated in buildings. These include Legionnaire's disease, tuberculosis, chicken pox, and measles. Other infectious diseases have, on occasion, been spread through the ventilation system in a building. Microorganisms are the known causative agents for infectious diseases but they may be responsible, in whole or in part, for SBS and the hypersensitivity diseases.

THE HYPERSENSITIVITY DISEASES

Hypersensitivity diseases result from antigens that stimulate an antibody response. Hypersensitivity pneumonitis (HP) causes the body to produce antigen-specific immunoglobulin G (IgG) and symptoms are most likely in people with a specific immune defect. Allergic asthma and allergic rhinitis occur in people with a genetic makeup that allows the production of antigen-specific IgE. Since an immunological reaction is required for a hypersensitivity disease to occur, attack rates among exposed building occupants are usually low; only 5 to 10% of individuals regularly exposed to the etiologic agents of HP contract the disease. Attack rates for asthma and allergic rhinitis may reach 20%. Most building-related antigens are believed to be of fungal, bacterial, or protozoan origin, although the evidence to date is far from convincing.

Hypersensitivity Pneumonitis (HP)

HP is an occupational disease better known in agriculture as Farmer's lung, Mushroom worker's lung, and Bagassosis. It is also identified with ventilation systems. Clinically, it is characterized by intermittent episodes of chills, fever, cough, and shortness of breath occurring 4 to 8 hours after inhalation of a specific sensitizing agent. These symptoms sound very much like those of SBS. Hodgson et al. (1987), in reporting on the TVA office building condition in Tennessee, termed it an outbreak of acute and chronic HP. When the disease has progressed, chest x-rays may reveal diffuse modular infiltrates or interstitial fibrosis. HP from HVAC ventilation systems has been reported from inhaling thermophilic actinomycetes, *Micropolyspora faeni*, *Thermoactinomycetes vulgaris*, *T. candidus*, and *Saccharomonospora viridis*. Occasionally patients do not show antibodies to any of these organisms since HP sensitization allows reaction to concentrations of antigen too low to measure (Kurup et al., 1984). They may, however, develop precipitins against humidified water. The disease may be reproduced by challenging the patient with water from the humidifier, indicating that unidentified antigens may be present (Arnow et al., 1978). Hodgson et al. (1987) suggest that the disease may not be a reaction to one organism alone but a cumulative reaction to a number of organisms in the air. The antigens involved in HP are not only microbial but may be organic dusts (Farmer's lung) and may be even simple chemical molecules (Kurup et al., 1984), and the presence of some of these may play a part in producing the reaction.

Humidifier Fever (HF)

HF is characterized by fever, chills, and malaise but displays no prominent pulmonary symptoms. Flu-like symptoms usually arise within 4 to 8 hours of exposure and subside within 24 hours without long term effects (H.A. Burge et al., 1989). Additional symptoms may be cough, chest tightness, and shortness of breath. This disease was associated with cold aerosol humidifiers in enclosed environments. Edwards et al. (1977) reported at a symposium on HF that humidity control systems requiring the introduction of water into a moving current of air use baffle plates to eliminate large droplets. Organic dust that is drawn into the system, settles on the wet plates, and is utilized by microorganisms from the atmosphere, which build up a biomass. Microbial material is then voided into the working atmosphere by the ventilation system. The disease is more common in the winter since there is more recirculated air and less fresh air than in the summer, although in hot climates air-cooling systems produce a condensation of water which may give rise to the growth of microbes. The similarity of symptoms, relationship to recycled air and fresh air, humidifier or other source of water, and presence of microorganisms suggest a similarity and overlap between SBS, HP, and HF, if indeed there is a hard distinction in all cases. In a classic case of HP and HF there would be demonstrable immunologic response to the specific antigen and differences in chest x-rays. Unfortunately, there are few classic cases in these building attacks, for although most affected individuals responded when challenged by the suspected material, no microorganism or other agent could be identified with the disease (Hodgson et al., 1987, Arnow et al., 1978). Edwards et al. (1977), investigating cases of HP, noted, "The relationship between disease and precipitins did not hold for the factory workforce, where approximately 44% sera tested had precipitins in absence of the disease. When investigations of the source of the antigenic material were made, many bacteria and fungi were isolated from ceiling dust and humidifier material. Extracts of the organisms were antigenically negative. An exception was an amoeba, *Naegleria gruberi*, which produced consistently positive with sera from infected individuals. However, Hodgson and co-workers (1985) tested amoeba and many other microorganisms as antigens and found no significant differences between cases and noncases in rates of precipitin reactions to individual agents.

Allergic Rhinitis

This is the common allergy known as hay fever. The symptoms are nasal obstruction, nasal discharge, postnasal drip, sneezing, redness, itching, tearing eyes, and hawking cough. Pollen, mold spores, dust, and danders may be responsible for this condition in sensitive persons. Building-related rhinitis is common and may overlap with SBS complaints, but it has been poorly documented (Robertson and Burge, 1985).

Asthma

Bronchial asthma is found in individuals with an inherited allergic constitution. Attacks may be brought on by pollen, mites, fungi, and insect emanations. Building-related asthma is characterized by complaints of chest tightness, wheezing, coughing, and shortness of breath. Symptoms may occur within an hour of exposure or may be delayed 4 to 12 hours. A work-related pattern of reduced peak air flows may indicate that asthma is related to building exposure. Office building-related asthma has only recently been documented. Some case reports show asthma to be related to humidifier use (Burge et al., 1985). Asthma without complications is not identified with the flu symptoms of chills, fever, and muscle pain noted in HP, HF, and SBS.

INFECTIOUS DISEASES

Legionnaire's disease, or Legionellosis, a building-related disease was named after the causitive organism, *Legionella pneumophilia*, and the fact that 182 cases, with 29 fatal, of this disease occurred in Legionnaires attending a convention in a hotel in Philadelphia in 1976. Legionellosis is a bacterial pneumonia that may involve the gastrointestinal tract, kidneys, and central nervous system. The incubation period is 5 to 6 days, with only a small percentage of exposed persons contracting it. The bacteria were traced to aerosols from cooling towers, evaporative condensers, whirlpools, and shower heads.

Another form of Legionellosis is known as Pontiac fever after Pontiac, Michigan, where the organism infected 95 percent of the 144 member health department. About half became ill in 24 hours and the rest within 48 hours. Most recovered in 2 to 5 days. Their symptoms were chills, fever, headache, and muscle pain. A contaminated ventilation system was implicated in the dissemination of the bacteria through cracks in the ducts which allowed outlet air to mix with inlet air. Legionella occurs in the environment in bodies of water and builds up its numbers in water-handling systems for buildings such as cooling tower ponds. Guinea pigs breathing air from air ducts got the disease. In a London police station, six members in one wing of the building contracted Legionnaire's, the infection coming from aerosols from the air-conditioning system. Of further interest, the symptoms suggestive of SBS were also associated with working in the same wing (O'Mahoney et al., 1989).

Measles epidemics have occurred through building ventilation systems. Riley et al. (1978) reported on a sharp outbreak of measles in an elementary school in which 70% of the air was recirculated. Measles was introduced by a girl in second grade. After about 10 days incubation period 28 children in 14 classrooms developed the disease. None had been in the same classroom as the girl but all the rooms were served by the same recirculated air. Wells et al. (1942) gave an account of a measles epidemic in schools in Pennsylvania. Children in the same town in schools equipped with ultraviolet air disinfection did not contract measles. In an Asian influenza pandemic, a hospital with ultraviolet air disinfection had an incidence of 2%, whereas, in adjacent buildings without irradiation, the incidence was 19% (McLean, 1961). Airborne transmission of other viral infections are reported by Knight (1973). Experiments with guinea pigs showed that tubercle bacilli had been carried through the ventilating ducts of a tuberculosis ward in a hospital and infected the lungs of the animals (Riley et al., 1957). In specialized buildings such as research labs and hospitals, Burge et al. (1989) mentioned the dissemination of Q-fever from rickettsia, anthrax from bacteria, and histoplasmosis and cryptococcosis from fungi.

INITIATING AGENTS

Chemicals

As mentioned earlier, except in the case of known infectious diseases which may be positively diagnosed, the causative agent or agents of sick buildings has not been identified. That does not mean that there are not many ideas on the subject. An article in *Indoor Pollution* (1989) features two articles side by side in which the authors, Broughton and Thrasher, claim chemicals are the cause, and authors, White and Kemper, make a case for microbes. The chemical argument is that building furnishings, like new carpets, upholstery, etc., put small quantities of volatile organic chemicals in the ventilation system, which are below the OSHA permissible levels but which act synergistically to sensitize building occupants. They are said to act as irritants to the mucous membranes and can cause central nervous system symptoms. The authors cite antibodies to formaldehyde, toluene diisocyanate, and trimellitic anhydride in 14 subjects in a case of building-related illness, with several persons having antibodies to all 3 chemicals. One of the volatile chemicals in new carpet, 4-phenylcyclohexene, is said to be a neurotoxin in concentrations of 30 parts per billion. Multiple health complaints, Broughton and Thrasher (1989) said, are associated with the chemical outgassing from newly installed carpets. NIOSH (1989), in its investigations of air quality problems, attributed about 4 times as many problems to chemicals as to microorganisms. These include off-gases from building materials (foam insulation, particle board, glues, and silicone caulking) with acetic acid, formaldehyde, and organic solvents, and chemicals like methyl alcohol, butyl methacrylate, ammonia, diethylethanolamine, from operations equipment such as copying machines, blueprint machines, and boiler additive, as well as toxics from pesticides and cleaning agents. EPA (1989) found 350 volatile organics in a home for the elderly in Washington, D.C. In a paper on the sources of air contaminants in the office environment, Holt (1984) lists many chemicals, organic and inorganic, deriving from construction materials, building equipment, maintenance materials, and those chemicals brought in by the inhabitants of the building, in addition to those from outside air. Yet, in many careful studies no one has yet been able to relate any one or combination of chemicals to the symptoms of SBS, HP, or HF. Holt adds inconclusively that "all sources are important contaminants, but the lesser ones will drive you just as crazy."

While it is true that the known volatile toxic chemicals in these air contaminants are well below the OSHA permitted levels, and are only detected by sensitive analytic procedures, there are many whose toxicity has never been determined. Furthermore, it has been generally observed that building-related illnesses are associated with moisture somewhere in the system (Morey et al., 1984). This being the case, high humidity in the air would increase the volatility of many chemicals by the process of steam distillation. Since vapor pressure of immiscible liquids is additive, this allows steam to vaporize water-immiscible chemicals at temperatures below their boiling point. Many of the organic chemicals listed by Holt (1984) are immiscible with water and could be increased in their concentration in the air under non-equilibrium high humidity conditions. Apart from the many chemicals in the air in micro quantities, the major known ones, like carbon dioxide, carbon monoxide, tobacco smoke, radon, and asbestos which can have damaging health effects, do not produce the typical symptoms of SBS or other BRIs. The lack of fresh air in tight buildings is associated with SBS (NIOSH, 1989) but this factor cannot be tied to lack of oxygen for the amount of oxygen in the tight buildings is more than enough for comfort and well being and in other tight buildings the same conditions prevail without producing SBS.

Microorganisms

White and Kemper (1987) attribute SBS to antibodies produced by the body's immune system in response to the continuous exposure to excessive levels of airborne fungi or bacteria. These microorganisms are brought into the building with the building materials and furnishings, air, water, and the occupants. If the moisture and temperature are condusive to growth, they find homes on almost all surfaces including airborne dust. They require very small quantities of organic matter and minerals as nutrients, which are readily available in buildings. Moisture, which must be in the liquid form for bacteria or protozoa, or as high humidity in the air for fungi, can come from condensation on windows, sweaty pipes, a leaky roof, or the water spray humidifiers and pooled water from the dehumidifiers in the HVAC system. The microorganisms reproduce rapidly to great numbers under favorable conditions and are distributed around the building by the HVAC system. In their studies White and Kemper attributed 10 sick buildings to fungi growing in carpets, or to the HVAC system, since a biocide treatment appreciably lowered the fungal count and the complaints as well.

Morey of NIOSH and co-workers (1984) stated that microbial agents are involved in the etiology of most HP illnesses. They carried out health hazard evaluations on 5 large office buildings where HP and other respiratory diseases were alleged or reported in the literature (Table 65–3). They found that several buildings were characterized by a history of repeated flooding and that all contained mechanical systems with pools of stagnant water and microbial slimes. As seen in Table 65–3, the organisms identified as the etiologic agents in the cases presented included actinomycetes, a flavobacterium, penicillium, and an amoeba. Table 65–4 lists the organisms found in slimes in the HVAC system of another office building (the TVA building discussed earlier). Note

Table 65–3. *Sources of Microbial Contamination, Disease Agents, and Remedial Actions Associated with Past Outbreaks of HP or Allergenic Respiratory Disease*

Author	No. Persons Ill/Total Exposed	Source of Building Contamination	Etiologic Agent	Remedial Action
Weiss & Soleymani	Case report	Dust in HVAC system ductwork	Thermophilic actinomycetes	Tried unsuccessfully to clean occupied space; replaced HVAC system
Banaszak et al.	4/27	HVAC system water spray	Thermophilic actinomycetes	Unknown
Scully et al.	1/40	Dust in HVAC system ductwork	Thermophilic actinomycetes	Clean ductwork
Arnow et al.	48/4023	HVAC system water spray	Unknown	HVAC system replaced; all furnishings in occupied space replaced
Ganier et al.	26/50	Stagnant water in humidifier	Unknown	Tried unsuccessfully to decontaminate humidifier with fungicide; removed humidifier from HVAC system.
Rylander et al.	3/7	Aerosol from humidifier reservoir	*Flavobacterium spp.* or their endotoxins	Unknown
Edwards	20/50	Microbial slime in reservoir	Nonpathogenic amoebae	Filter air entering humidifier; water in humidifier run to waste; replaced furnishings in occupied spaces
Bernstein et al.	2/14	Contaminated fan coil units	*Penicillium*	Clean fan coil units; replace filters

From Morey, P.R., Hodgson, M.J. et al. 1984. Environmental studies in moldy office buildings: biologic agents, sources and preventative measures. Annals of Am. Conf., Govtl. Hygienists, 10, 21–35.

Table 65–4. *Microorganisms Found in Slimes in HVAC System of Building*

Bacteria:	*Bacillus* spp.* (including 55°C thermophiles)
	Flavobacterium spp.*
	Pseudomonas spp.
	55°C Actinomycetes*
Fungi:	*Penicillium* spp.*
	Cladosporium spp.
	Cephalosporium spp.*
	Aspergillus spp.*
	Trichoderma spp.
	Mucor spp.
	Ostracoderma spp.
	Rhodotorula spp.
	Cryptococcus spp.
	Fusarium spp.
	Harposporium spp.
Protozoa:	*Acanthamoeba* spp.*
	Vorticella spp.
Nematodes:	*Rhabditis* spp.

*Organisms which have been implicated as etiologic agents in previous outbreaks of HP or humidifier fever.

From Morey, P.R., Hodgson, M.J. et al. 1984. Environmental studies in moldy office buildings: biologic agents, sources and preventative measures. Annals of Am. Conf., Govtl. Hygienists, 10, 21–35.

the many types of organisms, and that many had been identified as etiologic agents in other outbreaks of HP or HF. In an attempt to quantify airborne microbial levels that might cause trouble, the authors suggest that levels greater than $10^3/m^3$ may indicate an indoor environment in need of improvement. This figure is based on evidence that has shown that, during an outbreak of HF, levels of *Flavobacterium spp.* of $3000/m^3$ were associated with the operation of a contaminated humidifier and were absent from the air when the unit was turned off (Rylander et al., 1978). Threshold levels for producing allergenic symptoms for *Cladosporium spp.* and for *Alternaria ssp.* spores were 3000 and 100 CFU/m³, respectively, (Graveson, 1979) and fungus levels of 5000 to 10,000 CFU/m³ were associated with an outbreak of HP (Bernstein et al., 1983). Morey et al. (1984) stated that their studies showed that two other parameters may be helpful in deciding if an indoor environment needs improvement. These are counts of microorganisms in stagnant water and in dusts in HVAC systems. In two buildings with BRI problems, the air handling units emitting a water spray and four cooling units had microbial loads of 10^5 to 10^7/ml. Well-maintained cooling tower reservoirs had only 10^3 to 10^4/ml. House dust contains about 2×10^5 fungi/g whereas dust from filters in a sick building contained 3×10^7 fungi/g. From these figures, the authors propose an upper level of 10^5/ml bacteria or fungi in stagnant water and a level 10^6/g fungi in dusts.

Edwards et al. (1977) suggest the steps in the generation of HF in buildings to be: (1) the introduction of water into a moving current of air; (2) organic dust is drawn into the system and settles on baffle plates (used to eliminate large droplets of water) and (3) in the mixing chamber, this dust is used by microorganisms from the air or water to build up a biomass, which is distributed throughout the building by the ventilation system.

Microbial Products

Microbial products include mold and bacterial spores, mycotoxins, endotoxins, enzymes (Edwards et al., 1977) and innumerable chemical products, most of which have never been identified. Mold spores are well known respiratory allergins (Al-Doory and Domson, 1984). They are light and are carried with the dust floating in the air. Prior to modern air conditioning, which produces dehumidification as well as cooling, considerable visible mildew growth was apparent in homes in Florida and other southern states during the warm, humid, summer months when allergy problems were common caused by inhalation of mold spores. Spores do not have to be viable to produce these symptoms. According to Miller (1990), fungi make up approximately one quarter of the biomass of the planet and molds are capable of producing very large quantities of spores in a short time. Miller also points out that 10 to 15% of the population is allergic to fungi. Since we breathe 10 liters of air per minute and over 15,000 liters per day, it is not surprising that 63% of all illnesses are respiratory (National Research Council, 1981) and that fungi and spores claim their share of that toll.

Fungi may cause health problems due to infection and allergy, but also as a result of the toxicity of the many products they produce. Over 500 volatile organic chemicals have been described from fungi of various kinds (Miller et al., 1988). Some of these compounds, namely the mycotoxins, are extremely poisonous. The spores and sclerotia of these toxigenic fungi contain large quantities of these toxins. *Asperigillus flavus* spores have been reported to contain 1100 ppm of aflatoxins (Wicklow and Shotwell, 1983). Aflatoxins are so toxic that their allowable concentration in food is only 30 ppb. They are known as food poisons but there are suggestions that they may also cause pulmonary mycotoxicosis (Sorenson, 1990). Individuals developed HP following massive exposure to fungal spores (Emanuel et al., 1975). *Stachybotrys atra*, which contains a number of trichothecenes (potent immunosuppressors and inhibitors of protein synthesis) has been associated with BRI on a number of occasions. Dust and lint in air conditioning ducts became extensively colonized by this fungus. People suffered from a variety of maladies including cold and flu symptoms, sore throat, headache, fatigue, dermatitis, and general malaise. Removal of the contamination relieved the distress (Croft et al., 1986). P.S. Burge (1990), in searching for the causes for BRI, feels that the problems relate to mycotoxins or endotoxins. H.A. Burge et al. (1989) suggest that HF may be caused by endotoxin exposure rather than being a hypersensitivity disease.

Endotoxins are produced by gram-negative bacteria in their cell membranes. Endotoxins are composed of lipopolysaccharides and, as found in the environment, include membrane protein. Endotoxins are highly toxic. They cause fever and malaise, respiratory distress, changes in white cell count, and even death. In experimental inhalation studies, the effects of endotoxins were fever, cough, aches, nausea, shortness of breath, and acute air flow obstruction (Pernis et al., 1961). Rylander et al. (1978) investigated three cases of HF in an office environment. They found acute symptoms of fever, shivering, and a general malaise. The three office employees had experienced repeated attacks of fever and slight respiratory symptoms which were connected with the operation of a humidifier. Bacteriological examination of the water in the humidifier showed that more than 90% of the colonies were gram-negative bacteria. When the humidifier was running, $3000/m^3$ Flavobacteria were found in the air, whereas none were found when the humidifier was not running. The authors indicated that endotoxins might be the causative agent. Rylander and Haglind (1984) investigated another case where 20 of 50 workers in a printing plant reported symptoms of HF, fever, chills, tight chest, breathing difficulty, headache, and weariness when the humidifier was operating. Most had the symptoms several times in previous years. The water in the humidifier was contaminated with Pseudomonas. The amount of airborne endotoxin when the humidifier was operating was 0.13 to 0.39 $\mu g/m^3$. The estimated inhaled dose of endotoxin of 0.25 $\mu g/70$ kg person/8 hr day was found to be sufficient to cause the observed symptoms.

People

People are responsible for murders, wars, and other undesirable events and perhaps they may take the blame for indoor pollution and BRIs as well. They bring into the building many volatile chemicals in the form of perfumes, tobacco smoke, toothpaste, cosmetics, aerosol sprays, insecticides, etc. (Holt, 1984). They are carriers of bacteria and viruses, pathogenic and nonpathogenic. They carry them on their clothes, on their bodies, and in their bodies. According to the National Research Council (1981), the primary source of bacteria in most indoor places is the human body. The major source is the respiratory tract. These organisms are distributed through sneezing, coughing, and speaking (Leedom and Loosli, 1979). Edmonds (1979) mentions an experiment in which a dental patient was seeded with a tracer microbe and viable bacteria were recovered from air in the adjoining waiting room 3 minutes after the start of dental operations. The skin is another productive source of microorganisms. According to Clark and Cox (1973), 7 million skin scales are shed per minute per person, with an average of 4 viable bacteria per scale. In an office building with 300 people, that would add up to some 4 trillion bacteria per day emitted from the skin alone; a figure that rivals the national debt. Flushing the toilet produces aerosols containing bacteria which becomes a source of potential deposition of particles in the respiratory tract.

The average flush was found to produce 10^5 airborne bacteria/m^3 and several investigators concluded that the flush toilet and urinal represent important public health problems (Edmonds, 1979). The human body is also a generator of volatile chemicals that produce unpleasant odors which are a source of annoyance and complaint if not disease, and in case of SBS can be a contributing factor in worker discontent. Ventilation requirements to provide minimum physiological needs for health, and an ambient CO_2 level below 0.5% by volume, are 4.5 m^3/h (10.5 cfm) or one-sixth of an air change per person per hour for sedentary work. Pleasant, comfortable conditions require the control of body odor, relative humidity, and cigarette smoke. Ventilation requirements to eliminate body odor are dependent upon the bathing habits of the room occupants: those who bathe weekly need approximately 50% more air than for those who bathe daily (Yaglou et al., 1936). Body size is also important for adults, although children are more odorous. For non-smoking conditions ASHRAE recommends 5 cfm of outside air per occupant and greater than 20 cfm for smoking (NIOSH, 1989).

Imagination

A not uncommon reaction to SBS is that some of the building occupants have colds, allergies, or other illnesses acquired at home, or somewhere other than the workplace, but believe that symptoms originated at the office. Others, helped along by psychological association and mass hysteria, imagine their symptoms. Still others are thought to have taken advantage of the situation to slow down on the job or take off from work. Black et al. (1990) (Letters, 1991) described a preponderance of psychiatric symptoms in 26 patients with environmental illness and proposed that commonly recognized psychiatric disorders explain some or all of the symptoms. Dr. Richard Lockey, Director of the Division of Allergy and Immunology at the University of South Florida at Tampa, states that symptoms attributed to SBS can be attributed to any illness and that many more allergens can be found at home than in the workplace, which is usually very clean (Friedenberg, 1990). He maintains further that true instances of BRI, such as the deaths due to Legionellosis that occurred at the Legionnaire's Convention at the Philadelphia hotel, are rare.

Can we assume then that BRI problems are essentially psychological in nature? Hodgson and fellow investigators (1987), who reported on the TVA building and other cases of HP, think not. To quote them: "This outbreak does not fit the pattern of mass hysteria, classical criteria for which include 'transmitting by sight or sound,' sex-specific attack rate differential, an index case with social power, and nonspecific symptoms. The median time of symptom onset was similar from floor to floor, and the problem was noted only the day after occurrence, making the first point—'transmission by sight or sound'—unlikely. Sex specific attack rates were no different for either acute or chronic disease, addressing the second point, sex-specific attack rate differential. There was no index

case as a source of transmission. Last, the symptoms were not dizziness, fainting, and weakness as have been described in mass hysteria."

Furthermore, as discussed previously regarding the TVA case, clear-cut evidence that the disease was associated with the air-handling system has been shown, as in other cases of BRI. In the TVA building, no one in the computer room, which had a separate supply of air, was ill. There is ample data in cases all over the country and Europe that demonstrate that tightly-closed buildings produce more respiratory problems than open buildings. A 47 month U.S. Army study in 4 Army training centers compared the occurrence of respiratory disease of recruits housed in new, tight, energy-conserving buildings versus those housed in old "leaky" barracks (Brundage et al., 1988). The men living in the tight buildings showed a 51% increase in febrile acute respiratory disease at the 4 training centers over the trainees in the old barracks. Higher increases to 250% were documented in the residents of the tight barracks during epidemic years when trainees were not immunized against adenovirus infection. Rates of respiratory disease increased as training progressed in the modern barracks in comparison to the old barracks, consistent with more efficient transmission of respiratory pathogens. The statistics in this study do not suggest that imagination played a part in these results. Reanalysis by Mendell and Smith (1990) of 6 European studies of SBS in tight air-conditioned office buildings might also be mentioned. Their work indicates that sealed buildings with air conditioning are associated with higher prevalence of work-related headache, lethargy, and eye, nose, and throat symptoms than unsealed buildings with no air conditioning, even in the absence of humidification. It also suggests that although air-conditioned buildings with steam humidification are associated with symptom prevalence no higher than air-conditioned buildings without humidification, air-conditioned buildings with water-based humidification may be associated with higher prevalence of eye, nose, and throat symptoms than those with steam humidification. Such findings tend to fortify the belief that microorganisms or their products are initiating these ailments.

PREVENTION AND CONTROL

Can we prevent or control an occurrence when we can't identify the cause? Edward Jenner in 1799 developed a vaccine for smallpox long before we knew the cause for that disease. Many similar cases give us reason to believe that empirical efforts and good hunches will allow us to succeed.

If volatile organic chemicals are causing the trouble one might filter the circulating air through activated charcoal filters to remove the offending agents, but Dr. B.C. Wolverton of NASA's Stennis Space Center in Mississippi had a more original idea; he used potted plants (Blomberg, 1990). In experiments originally designed for the enclosed environment of space stations, ordinary house plants like philodendron, spider plant, and aloe vera were able to remove organics like benzene, carbon monoxide, and formaldehyde from the air. One 10 to 12 inch potted plant such as a dieffenbachia was effective in removing dangerous levels of formaldehyde from a 10 × 10 room. Chrysanthemum and gerbera daisy were rated superior in removing benzene. They also removed 50% of the formaldehyde in the atmosphere of an airtight chamber in 6 to 24 hours.

If microorganisms are the offending agents, biocides would appear to be more suitable for prevention and control. Biocides have been used in humidification and dehumidification units of air-conditioning systems to prevent microbial growth and the slime that occurs in the drainage basins wherever water collects. The results are not always satisfactory, as reported by Nagorka et al. (1990). They employed methylisothiazolone (Kathon WT), made microbiological analyses, and analyzed the concentration during operation. They found that the concentration of the biocide varied widely and in some cases there was marked contamination with pathogens, including *Legionella pneumophilia*, free amoeba, and high aerobic colony counts. They measured 3.4 micrograms/m³ of the biocide in ambient indoor aerosols, which led them to conclude that both the unsatisfactory hygienic status of many circulatory spray humidifiers and the exposure to the biocides contained in the humidifier fluids may be responsible for some of the symptoms of SBS. The European Community in its report "Sick Building Syndrome" is quite emphatic when it states that biocides currently used in most cold water spray humidifiers to control microbial growth are highly irritating in concentrated form and may cause mucous membrane irritation when dispersed in indoor air at low concentrations, especially in susceptible individuals. And the American Conference of Governmental Industrial Hygienists (H. A. Burge et al., 1989) puts in heavy print, "The aerosolization of antimicrobial chemicals into the occupied space must be avoided." P.S. Burge (1989) quotes literature showing that numerous antimicrobial agents cause respiratory, nasal, and skin problems at low concentration.

Antimicrobial chemicals, however, may have a place in buildings to help prevent SBS. On the premise that microbial reservoirs exist in buildings, other than in the ventilation system, Kemper, White, and Gettings (1990) made a study of 10 office buildings and schools where the carpeting was treated with a non-volatile antimicrobial. The chemical, known as Sylgard, produced by Dow Corning Corp., was an immobilized silane quaternized amine, 3-trimethoxysilylpropyldimethyloctadecyl ammonium chloride, which was shown to be resistant to washing and to provide long-lasting, broad-spectrum antimicrobial surfaces on key building substrates. The authors mention a previous study in a Campbell County school in Kentucky where more than 200 students and staff complained of illness. Within 2 weeks of the treatment of the school's carpeting with the surface-bonded antimicrobial agent, they reported a substantial reduc-

tion in the microbioaerosol presence and the complaints ceased. These results led to more extensive tests with treated carpeting in 10 SBS/BRI buildings of different designs in different locations all over the country. The authors report a uniform reduction of microbial count of 71 to 98% and similar reduction in workers' symptoms following treatment of the carpeting.

Another antimicrobial, named Intersept, has been applied to interior surfaces as a treatment for SBS. This chemical biostat, produced by Interface Research Corporation, is a complex of polysubstituted imine salts and trialkyl phosphate esters with free alkylated phosphoric acid. It is incorporated in paints, carpet, carpet tiles, flooring, and cooling coil coating. Rhodes and Gilyard (1990) reported on its use in a case of SBS at Virginia Polytechnic Institute. Following a new roofing job on the Architecture building, numbers of people began complaining of throat irritation, burning eyes, rashes, and lethargy. The problem was thought to be caused by volatile roofing compounds getting into the ventilation system. Extensive chemical tests using gas chromatography-mass spectrophotometry could not relate any chemical to the problem. A microbial search was then made with samples taken from the air, the ductwork, and many interior surfaces, that led to the conclusion that the trouble resulted from a heavy infestation of fungi—the building being contaminated from years of use without a proper maintenance program. The most prevalent organisms were Cladosporium, Penicillium, Mucor, Rhizopus, and Aspergillus. These organisms are widely found in nature but were highly concentrated in the interior environment. The building was closed (Fig. 65–2) and thoroughly cleaned; ceiling tiles were removed and cleaned (Fig. 65–3), the ducts were vacuumed and wiped with detergent, and the inside surfaces of the ducts, mixing boxes, and air-handler plenum walls were coated with antimicrobial latex or polyvinylacetate paint containing 2% Intersept based on the weight of the dissolved solids. Books from the library were dusted and aired in the sunlight, filter medium was changed (Fig. 65–4), and the floors were scrubbed and waxed. Mold counts following the cleanup showed a dramatic reduction in numbers. The authors credit the antimicrobial latex, for they state that at the University of Texas the effectiveness of this agent over and above the effect of cleaning and housekeeping was more than three orders of magnitude, and it had not diminished after 2.5 years. The investigators blame the cause of this SBS on an accumulation of dirt and molds from lack of regular cleaning and maintenance; when the fungus habitat is disturbed, as in the roofing job, or when a filter is touched, the organisms "bloom," emitting a burst as many as 5 orders of magnitude above the background level from these reservoirs of fungus spores.

The American Conference of Governmental Industrial Hygienists (H.A. Burge et al., 1989) have listed some valuable do's and don't's for keeping buildings healthy and remedying sick ones:

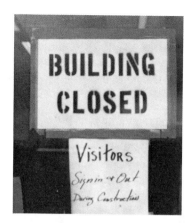

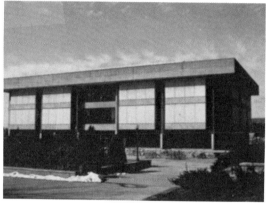

Fig. 65–2. Building being treated for SBS. From Rhodes, W.W. and Gilyard, Y.O. 1990. A sick building. Its diagnosis and treatment. Engineered Systems, July–Aug.

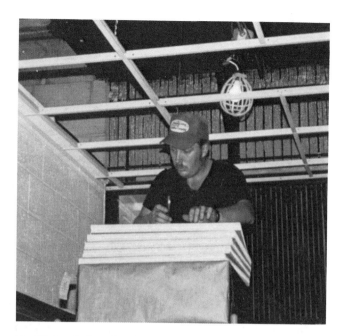

Fig. 65–3. Ceiling tiles of sick building being removed for cleaning and better access to the air handling system. From Rhodes. W.W. and Gilyard, Y.O. 1990. A sick building. Its diagnosis and treatment. Engineered Systems, July–Aug.

1. *Building Design.* Buildings should be designed to prevent entry of outdoor and proliferation of indoor aerosols. This should take into account:

A. Preventing entry of aerosols.
1) Air Intake. Outdoor air intakes should be put in the predominant upwind direction and at least 25 feet from external bioaerosol sources. The intakes should not be located in an architectural fence area which houses cooling towers or evaporative condensers. Neither should they be located at grade level where they can take in microorganisms from soil and vegetation.
2) Filtration. Filters with a moderate dust spot efficiency of 50 to 70% will adequately remove microorganisms larger than 2 μm from the air. Low efficiency prefilters should be used to remove coarse dust and prolong the life of the efficient microbial filters. Special absorbent filters are necessary for removing volatile organic compounds.

B. Preventing proliferation of indoor bioaerosols.
Building design should make provision for maintaining conditions within the building for providing comfort but discouraging microbial growth. The following factors should be considered in this endeavor.

1) Dilution. To insure sufficient fresh outdoor air to dilute aerosols from building occupants a rate of at least 15 cfm per occupant should be provided to the breathing zone.

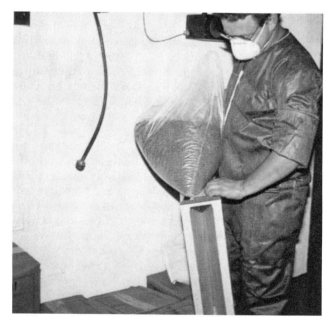

Fig. 65–4. Filter medium in heating-ventilating-air-conditioning system of sick building being changed. From Rhodes, W.W. and Gilyard, Y.O. 1990. A sick building. Its diagnosis and treatment. Engineered Systems, July–Aug.

2) Maintenance. Air handling units should be kept clean and free from stagnant water. To facilitate this aim, they should be equipped with access doors for cleaning purposes, and the drain pan below the cooling coils should be inclined toward a drain exiting at the bottom of the pan.

3) Substrates. It is important not to provide substances for microbial growth in areas where there is high moisture. Fiberglass insulation and carpeting are examples of such substrates. Fiberglass itself does not support microbial growth but the dust and moisture it collects makes it a substrate, therefore it should not be used where the ducts are subject to high humidity. Thermal and acoustical insulation on the inside surface of the housing of air-handling, fan-coil, and induction units should have a smooth surface to prevent microbial contamination. Carpeting should never be used on concrete floors or other places where persistent moisture is present. The adhesive backing and dust that accumulates in the pile of carpets provides nutrients for microorganisms and dust mites.

4) Humidification. Humidifiers as sources of water can be suspect as causes of HF and other BRIs. Those using recirculated water are not recommended since they can become sites for microbial proliferation. Instead, humidifiers in office buildings should use clean steam as a source of moisture. The steam should not contain amine-type corrosion inhibitors, such as morpholine, since amines are known allergens. If cold water is used for the humidifier it should be potable water and should be drained off after being used. Vaporizers and console humidifiers should not be used in the workplace. In residences, or wherever they are used, they should be emptied and thoroughly scrubbed and treated with a hypochlorite or peroxide disinfectant.

Since water spray humidifiers and air washers are almost always microbial amplifiers and have been associated with outbreaks of HF and HP, they are not recommended for use in office building HVAC systems. They were designed to be used with sterile water treated with disinfectants but the possible toxic hazard and odor of the latter makes the use of water spray humidifiers in office buildings undesirable.

5) Dehumidification. Both for comfort and to prevent mold growth, the relative humidity in the building should be maintained below 60%. Most office building HVAC systems remove moisture or latent heat from the air with an adequately-sized cooling coil section. The water removed from the air must be drained away and not allowed to accumulate. Another method for controlling humidity is to use reheat coils or dessicants downstream from the heat exchanger.

6) Filtration. The location of filters in the HVAC system is of critical importance in protecting building occupants from bioaerosols generated in the system. If filters are located upstream of the heat exchanger section, as with most air handling units, the people will not be protected from bioaerosols generated downstream in cooling deck coils, humidifiers, and water spray systems. In hospitals, and wherever protection is critical, it may be necessary to provide downstream filtration.

2. Maintenance

In existing buildings preventative maintenance is probably the most important factor in controlling bioaerosols. This involves maintaining a clean environment and maintaining equipment so that conditions favorable to microbial proliferation do not occur.

A. Cleaning

1) Routine cleaning. A regular schedule must exist for removal of dirt and debris from the internal components of air handling units, fan-coil units, and induction units. Carpeting should be maintained free of accumulated dirt with regular once a week vacuuming. Carpets must be kept dry, for cleaning alone will not prevent contamination with microbes and mites. If steam or water is used to clean the carpet, heat and fans should be used to quickly dry it. Duct cleaning is necessary when excessive dirt has accumulated but this should not be necessary in large buildings with adequate filtration, providing the filters are kept clean and are maintained.

2) Emergency cleaning. Emergency spills and floods should be cleaned up as soon as possible. Prompt repair and prevention of leaks is essential. Porous materials of construction, like ceiling tiles, thermal insulation, wall coverings, carpets and furnishings should be dried out quickly or discarded.

B. Equipment maintenance

1) Heat exchange systems. Stagnant water should not be allowed to accumulate in drain pans of air-handling and fan-coil units. Cooling coils should be operated during the summer so that spores and substrate impacted on the coils are washed away by condensed water.

2) Humidifiers. Cold water humidifiers should receive fastidious maintenance which would include removal of stagnant water and slime as well as regular inspection of the mechanical equipment.

3) Dehumidification. In offices the dew point temperature should be kept below 62°F (17°C)

and the relative humidity below 60%. (A lower limit for comfort would be 20%.) Moisture levels in the air must be low enough to prevent condensation on cold interior surfaces, such as cold water pipes. In buildings where large amounts of cool outdoor air are taken in, the ventilation air may have to be dehumidified even though the dry bulb temperature is satisfactory. Scheduled replacement of filters and protection against moisture damage is essential for proper maintenance. A static pressure gauge can be used to determine when filters need replacement.

3. Cleanup of Existing Contamination

An intensive onsite examination of the building should be made and potential bioaerosol sources that are revealed should be cleaned or removed. Contaminated cooling towers should be cleaned and oxidizing compounds (chlorine disinfectants and peroxides) used to prevent recolonization. Cooling towers and air intakes should be positioned so that human exposure is prevented. HVAC system mechanical components should be turned off during cleaning. Mechanical cleaning, steam cleaning, and use of detergents may be required prior to treatment with disinfectants. Chlorine compounds, hydrogen peroxide, or proprietary biocides may be used for disinfection but must be removed prior to reactivation of the HVAC system. Smooth-surface materials that have become contaminated can be cleaned with a biocide that is washed off after disinfection.

Vacuuming with a machine equipped with a high-efficiency particulate air filter (HEPA) may be used to physically remove microbial surface contamination. However, care must be used so that the surface of porous insulation is not damaged. Vacuuming may be used on valuable materials such as books to remove the loose, dry fungus once the organisms have been killed, but the HEPA filter must be used or the spores will be spread around to all locations by the process. Since contaminated ceiling plenums are almost impossible to clean they have to be bypassed using ductwork. Contaminated insulation, including duct lining, must be removed and discarded. Cleaning should be performed with adequate ventilation and masks may be desirable.

PERSPECTIVE

Building related illness is a result of indoor pollution and pollution has been with us for a long time. According to Greek mythology, Pandora, the first woman, was given a box by Zeus, the king of the gods, to be presented as a gift to her husband on the occasion of their marriage. When the groom opened the box, all the evils of the world flew out and were distributed by air currents all over the world. Thus air pollution and respiratory illnesses had their beginning.

Up to Colonial times, with the absence of large man-ufacturing plants, indoor pollution was more severe than outdoor pollution. Heating within a building was provided by the fireplace but most of the heat went up the chimney. By closing down the flue more heat was obtained inside but with it came smoke and indoor pollution. Benjamin Franklin's stove, invented in 1740, which acted as a house furnace as well as a stove for cooking, provided heat without smoke and helped alleviate indoor pollution. All was well until lately when air conditioning came on the scene and buildings were sealed up to conserve energy. The first paper on the subject of SBS was by Pestalozzi in 1959.

The seriousness of the problem is now recognized by all major health agencies such as the World Health Organization, the U.S. Department of Health and Human Services, The National Institute of Occupational Safety and Health, and The American Society for Microbiology, to mention a few. To emphasize the importance of indoor pollution and the resultant building-related illnesses, the National Academy of Sciences, the most prestigious U.S. organization and the one that advises the government, recently held a special meeting to decide what to do about "Populations affected by events involving a toxic exposure—for example, in airtight buildings, industrial workplaces, and contaminated communities" (Chemical Engineering News, 1991).

Why is this problem of indoor pollution so important? Because, according to the EPA's report to Congress (1989), the United States population spends 93% of its time indoors. Can the problem of sick buildings be solved? The answer is obviously in the affirmative. If we take the EPA figures in its 1989 report to the Congress, 65% of all buildings since 1970 have had SBS, and at least 10% of all people have had symptoms at one time or another, yet there is still a sizable number of buildings that remain free of it. Kreiss (1990) points out that we have inadequately studied the sick buildings and we have not studied well buildings at all, to be able to find differences that will give us clues to the causes of the problem. To take an extreme case of confinement in an indoor environment, consider the nuclear submarine where men spend as many as 70 days under water without access to natural outdoor air. As reported by Morris (1972) for the Polaris-type nuclear submarines the crews on these underwater patrols remained in better health and spent less time in sick bay than during land duty. This was confirmed to the writer by a naval officer who had spent 10 years in the submarine service. This indicates not only that the problem of SBS can be solved but that with its solution we may also expect to reduce the amount of colds, flu, and other infectious respiratory diseases that are contracted during the 93% of the time we spend indoors. Dr. Michael McCawley of NIOSH states (Broughton and Thrasher, 1989) "office air quality will be one of the big problems of the 1990s." Let us hope that with proper investigation this decade will also bring its solution.

REFERENCES

Al-Doory, Y., and Domson, J.F. 1984. Mould Allergy. Philadelphia, Lea & Febiger.

American Conference of Governmental Industrial Hygienists. 1984. Evaluating Office Environmental Problems. Ann. of the Am. Conf. Govtl. Ind. Hygienists, 5, 136.

Arnow, P.M. et al. 1978. Early detection of hypersensitivity pneumonitis in office workers. Am. J. Med., *64*, 236–242.

Banaszak, E.F., Thide, W.H., and Fink, J.N. 1970. Hypersensitivity pneumonitis due to contamination of an air conditioner. N. Engl. J. Med., *283*, 271–276.

Bernstein, R.S., Sorenson, W.G., and Garabrant, D., et al. 1983. Exposures to respirable, airborne *Penicillium* from a contaminated ventilation system. Clinical, environmental and epidemiological aspects. Am. Ind. Hyg. Assoc. J., *44*, 161–169.

Black, D.W., Rathe, A., Goldstein, R.B. 1990. Environmental illness: A controlled study of 26 subjects with 20th century disease. JAMA, *264*, 3166–3170.

Blomberg, M. 1990. A natural solution. Tests by NASA confirm plants purify the air. Gainesville (FL) Sun. p. 1F. July 29. (See also Wolverton, B.C. 1989. Interior landscape plants for pollution abatement. John C. Stennis Space Center, Miss. Final Rept., Sept.)

Broughton, A., and Thrasher, J. 1989. BRI. Which is the primary culprit: Microbes or Toxic Chemicals? Chemicals. Indoor Pollution, 2, March.

Brundage, J.F., Scott. R. McN., Lednar, W.M., et al. 1988. JAMA, *259*, 2108–2112.

Burge, H.A. 1989. Guidelines for the Assessment of Bioaerosols in the Indoor Environment. Am. Conf. Govtl. Ind. Hygienists, Cincinnati.

Burge, P.S. 1990. Building sickness—A medical approach to the causes. Indoor Air 90. Proc. 5th Intl. Conf. on Indoor Air Quality and Climate. Toronto. July 29. Vol. 5, 3–14.

Burge, P.S., Finnegan, M., Horsfied, N., et al. 1985. Occupational asthma in a factory with a contaminated humidifier. Thorax, *40*, 248–254.

Chemical & Engineering News. 1991. Chemical sensitivity. Experts agree on research protocol. Vol. 69, 4–5, April 1.

Clark, R.P., and Cox, R.N. 1973. The generation of aerosols from the human body. Edited by J.F.P. Hers, and K.C. Winkler. *In* Airborne Transmission and Airborne Infection. New York, John Wiley & Sons, p. 413–426.

Croft, W.A., Jarvis, B.B. and Yatawara, C.S. 1986. Airborne outbreak of trichothecene toxicosis. Atmosph. Environ., *20*, 549–552.

Edmonds, R.L. 1979. Aerobiology. The Ecological Systems Approach. Stroudsburg, PA. Dowden, Hutchinson & Ross.

Edwards, J.H. 1980. Microbial and immunological investigations and remedial action after an outbreak of humidifier fever. Brit. J. Ind. Med., *37*, 55–62.

Edwards, J.H. et al. 1977. Humidifier fever. Thorax, *32*, 653–663.

Emanuel, J.A., Wenzel, F.J. and Lawton, B.R. 1975. Pulmonary mycotoxicosis. Chest, *67*, 293–297.

EPA. 1989. EPA Report to Congress on Indoor Air Quality. U.S. Environmental Protection Agency. EPA/400/1-89/001B.

European Community. 1989. Sick Building Syndrome, A Practical Guide. European Community Concerted Action, Indoor Quality and Its Impact on Man. 36 pp.

Friedenberg, R. 1990. What makes a building sick? Gainesville (FL) Sun. p. 8–9 Business Monday Section. July 9.

Ganier, M, Lieberman, P., Fink, J. and Lockwood, D.G. 1980. Humidifier lung: An outbreak in office workers. Chest, *77*, 183–187.

Graveson, S. 1979. Fungi as a cause of allergic disease. Allergy, *34*, 135–154.

Hodgson, M.J. et al. 1985. Pulmonary disease associated with cafeteria flooding. Arch. Environ. Health, *40*, 96–101.

Hodgson, M.J., Morey, P.R., Simon, J.S., Waters, T.D. and Fink, J.N. 1987. Am. J Epidemiol, *125*, 631–638.

Holt, G.L. 1984. Sources of air contaminants in the office environment. Annals Am. Conf. Govtl. Hygienists, *10*, 15–19.

Kemper, R.A., White, W.C. and Gettings, R.L. 1990. Sustained aeromicrobiological reductions utilizing silane-modified quaternary amines applied to carpeting: preliminary data from an observational study of commercial buildings. Dev. Ind. Microbiol., *31*, 237–244.

Knight, V. 1973. Airborne transmission and pulmonary deposition of respiratory viruses. pp. 1–9. Edited by V. Knight. *In* Viral and Mycoplasmal Infections of the Respiratory Tract. Philadelphia, Lea & Febiger.

Kreiss, K. 1990. The sick building syndrome: Where is the epidemiologic basis? Am. J. Pub. Health, *80*, 1172–1173.

Kurup, V.P., John, K.V., Ting, E.Y., et al. 1984. Immunochemical studies of a purified antigen from *Micropolyspora faeni*. Mol. Immunol., *21*, 215–221.

Leedom, J.M. and Loosli, C.G. 1979. Airborne pathogens in the indoor environment with special reference to nosocomial (hospital) infections. Edited by R.L. Edmonds. *In* Aerobiology. The Ecological Systems Approach. Stroudsburg, PA. Dowden, Hutchinson, & Ross, Inc.

Letters. 1991. Environmental illness. JAMA, *265*, 2325–2327.

Levin, H. 1989. European Community Releases SBS Report. Indoor Air Quality Update, 2, No. 11. Nov.

Levin, H. 1991. An HVAC system perspective on IAQ. Indoor Air Quality Update, 4, No. 2. Feb.

McLean, R.L. 1961. The effect of ultraviolet radiation upon the transmission of epidemic influenza in long-term hospital patients. Am. Rev. Respir. Dis., (Suppl. 83), 36.

Mendell, M.J. and Smith, A.H. 1990. Consistent pattern of elevated symptoms in air-conditioned office buildings: A reanalysis of epidemiologic studies. 1990. Am. J. Pub. Health, 80, 1193–1199.

Miller, J.D. 1990. Fungi as contaminants of indoor air. Proc. 5th Intl. Conf. on Indoor Air Quality and Climate. Toronto. Aug. 3. Vol. 5, Plenary Lectures. 51–64.

Miller, J.D., Laflamme, A.M., Sobol, Y., La Fontaine, P. and Greenhalgh, R. 1988. Fungi and fungal products in some Canadian houses. Internat. Biodeterior., *24*, 103–120.

Morey, P.R., Hodgson, M.J., et al. 1984. Environmental studies in moldy office buildings: biologic agents, sources and preventative measures. Annals of Am. Conf. Govtl. Hygienists, *10*, 21–35.

Morris, J.E.W. 1972. Microbiology in the submarine environment. Proc. Roy. Soc. Med., *65*, 799–780.

National Research Council. 1981. Indoor Pollutants. National Academy Press. Washington, D.C. 537 pp.

NIOSH. 1989. Indoor Air Quality. Selected References. Nat. Inst. for Occupat. Safety and Health. Cincinnati. Sept.

O'Mahony, M., Lakhani, A., Stephens, A., Wallace, J.G., Youngs, E.R. and Harper, D. 1989. Legionnaires' disease and the sick building syndrome. Epidemio. Infect., *103*, 285–292.

Pernis, B., Vigliani, E.C., Cavagna, C. and Finulli, M. 1961. The role of bacterial endotoxins in occupational diseases caused by inhaling vegetable dusts. Br. J. Ind. Med., *18*, 120–129.

Pestalozzi, C. 1959. Fever illness in a model carpentry through inhalation of mildew contaminated moisture ("Moisture fever"). Schweiz Med. Wochenschr., *89*, 710–714.

Properzio, W.S. 1991. Personal Communication. Director, Division of Health and Safety. University of Florida.

Rhodes, W.W. and Gilyard, Y.O. 1990. A sick building. Its diagnosis and treatment. Engineered Systems. July–Aug.

Riley, R.L., Wells, W.F., Mills, C.C., Nyka, W. and McLean, R.L. 1957. Air hygiene in tuberculosis: Quantitative studies of infectivity and control in pilot ward. Am. Rev. Tuberc Pulm. Dis., *75*, 420–431.

Robertson, A.S. and Burge, P.S. 1985. Building sickness. Practitioner, *229*, 531–534.

Rylander, R. and Haglind, P. 1984. Airborne endotoxins and humidifier disease. Clin. Allergy, *14*, 109–112.

Rylander, R., Haglind, P., Lundholm, M., Mattsby, I. and Stenqvist, K. 1978. Humidifier fever and endotoxin exposure. Clin. Allergy, 8, 511–516.

Scully, R.E., Galdabini, J.J. and McNeely, B.U. 1979. Case records of the Massachusetts General Hospital, Case 47–1979. N. Engl. J. Med., *301*, 1168–1174.

Sorenson, W.G. 1990. Mycotoxins as potential occupational hazards. Dev. Ind. Microbiol., *31*, 205–211.

Weiss, N.S. and Soleymani, Y. 1971. Hypersensitivity lung disease caused by contamination of an air conditioning system. Ann. Allergy, *29*, 154–156.

Wells, W.F., Wells, M.W. and Wilder, T.S. 1942. The environmental control of epidemic contagion. I. An epidemiologic study of radiant disinfection of air in day schools. Am. J. Hyg., *35*, 97–121.

White, W.C. and Kemper, R.A. 1987. Building related illness: new insight into causes and effective control. Am. Specialists in Cleaning and Restoration, Ann. Meetg. Dow Corning Form No. 24-640-89.

White, W.C. and Kemper, R.A. 1989. BRI. Which is the primary culprit: Microbes or Toxic Chemicals? Microbes. Indoor Pollution, 2, March.

Whorton, M.D., Lawson, S.R., Gordon, N.J. and Morgan, R.W. 1987. Investigation and work-up of tight building syndrome. J. Occup. Med., *29*, 142.

Wicklow, D.T. and Shotwell, O. 1983. Intrafungal distribution of aflatoxins among condidia and sclerotia of *Aspergillus flavus* and *Aspergillus parasiticus*. Can. J. Microbiol., *29*, 1–5.

Woods, J.E. 1989. Cost avoidance and productivity in owning and operating buildings. Edited by J.E. Cone and M.J. Hodgson *In* Problem Buildings: Building Associated Illness and the Sick Building Syndrome. Occup. Med. State. of Art Rev., *4*, 753–770.

Yaglou, C.P., Riley, E.C. and Coggins, D.I. 1936. How much outside air is necessary for ventilation? Heating and Ventilating, *33*, 31–35. March.

Index

Page numbers in *italics* indicate illustrations; numbers followed by "t" indicate tables